Selected Typical Reference Intervals

SOME TYPICAL CLINICAL CHEMISTRY REFERENCE INTERVALS CONVENTIONAL AND SI UNITS

Component	System	Typical Reference Intervals		
		in Conventional Units	Factor*	in SI Units*†
Albumin	Serum	3.8–5.0 gm/dl	10	38–50 g/l
Bicarbonate	Plasma	21–28 mM	1	21–28 mmol/l
Bilirubin	Serum			
direct		<0.3 mg/dl	17.1	<5.1 μmol/l
indirect		0.1–1.0 mg/dl		1.7–17.1 μmol/l
total		0.1–1.2 mg/dl		1.7–20.5 μmol/l
Calcium	Serum	9.2–11.0 mg/dl	0.25	2.3–2.8 mmol/l
		4.6–5.5 mEq/l	0.5	
Chloride	Serum	95–103 mEq/l	1	95–103 mmol/l
Cholesterol	Serum	150–250 mg/dl	0.026	3.90–6.50 mmol/l
Creatinine	Serum	0.6–1.2 mg/dl	88.4	53–106 μmol/1
Globulins	Serum	2.3–3.5 gm/dl	10	23–35 g/l
Glucose	Serum	70–110 mg/dl	0.055	3.85–6.05 mmol/l
Iron	Serum	60–150 μg/dl	0.179	11–27 μmol/l
Lactate dehydrogenase	Serum	80–129 units at 25°C. (lactate→pyruvate)	0.48	38–62 U/l at 25°C.
		185–640 units at 30°C. (pyruvate→lactate)	0.48	90–310 U/l at 30°C.
Phosphatase, alkaline	Serum	20–90 IU/l at 30°C. (p-nitro phenylphosphate)	1	20–90 U/l at 30°C.
Phosphorus	Serum	2.3–4.7 mg/dl	0.323	0.78–1.52 mmol/l
Potassium	Plasma	3.8–5.0 mEq/l	1	3.8–5.0 mmol/l
Protein, total	Serum	6.0–7.8 gm/dl	10	60–78 g/l
Sodium	Plasma	136–142 mEq/l	1	136–142 mmol/l
Thyroxine	Serum	5.0–11.0 μg/dl	13.0	65–143 nmol/l
Transferases:	Serum			
aspartate amino-		16–60 U/ml (Karmen) at 30°C.	0.48	8–29 U/l at 30°C.
alanine amino-		8–50 U/ml (Karmen) at 30°C.	0.48	4–24 U/l at 30°C.
Triglyceride	Serum	10–190 mg/dl	0.011	0.11–2.09 mmol/l
Urea nitrogen	Serum	8–23 mg/dl	0.357	2.9–8.2 mmol/l
Uric acid	Serum			
male		4.0–8.5 mg/dl	0.059	0.24–0.5 mmol/l
female		2.7–7.3 mg/dl		0.16 mmol/l

*Factor = Number factor (the units are not presented).
†Value in SI units = Value in conventional units × factor.

SOME TYPICAL HEMATOLOGY REFERENCE INTERVALS IN CONVENTIONAL AND SI UNITS

Component	Typical Reference Intervals		
	in Conventional Units	Factor	in SI Units*
Complete Blood Count (CBC)			
Hematocrit			
male	40–54%	0.01	0.40–0.54
female	38–47%		0.38–0.47
Hemoglobin			
male	13.5–18.0 gm/dl	0.155	2.09–2.79 mmol/l
female	12.0–16.0 gm/dl		1.86–2.48 mmol/l
Erythrocyte count			
male	$4.6–6.2 \times 10^6/\mu l$	10^6	$4.6–6.2 \times 10^{12}/l$
female	$4.2–5.4 \times 16^6/\mu l$		$4.2–5.4 \times 10^{12}/l$
Leukocyte count	$4.5–11.0 \times 10^3/\mu l$	10^6	$4.5–11.0 \times 10^9/l$
Erythrocyte indices			
mean corpuscular volume	80–96 cu. microns	1	80–96 fl
mean corpuscular hemoglobin	27–31 pg.	1	27–31 pg
Platelet Count	$150–440 \times 10^3/\mu l$	10^6	$0.15–0.4 \times 10^{12}/l$
Reticulocytes	0.5–1.5% of erythrocytes	0.01	0.005–0.015
	25,000–75,000 cells/μl	10^6	$25–75 \times 10^9/l$

*Value in SI units = Value in conventional units × factor.

(Tables continue on back cover)

the magnitudes of such biases, and to test if statistically significant analytical biases are present. In linear regression analysis, two associated variables are analyzed. One variable, "x," which in this case would be the stated concentration value of the control specimen, is called the independent variable, and the other, "y," which in this case would be the concentration value measured by the method, is called the dependent variable. In this analysis a linear equation relating the two variables is determined such that the sum of the squares of the deviations of "y" from the line, $\hat{y} = bx + a$, is minimized; "b," the slope of the line, and "a" are constants which are estimated from the data. The correct interpretation of a classical regression analysis requires that the following assumptions be fulfilled:

1. The relationship between "x" and the expected value of "y" is linear throughout the range of "x."
2. The observed "y" follows a Gaussian distribution for any given value of "x."
3. The variances of these Gaussian distributions are the same (homoscedasticity) for all "x."
4. The value of "x" is known exactly. In practice one would require that the random analytical variance corresponding to

each x-value is negligible as compared to that of "y."

For the following discussion we will accept the premise that the aforementioned assumptions are fulfilled. Thus, we will assume that the quantity is known with negligible random analytical variation in a number of control specimens. This may be achieved, e.g., by performing a large number of determinations of the quantity in the control specimen using an independent and generally accepted method and then using the average of these measurements as "x." Since the random analytical variation decreases with increasing number of determinations, the random analytical variation of the average may be reduced sufficiently if the number of observations is large enough.

Provided that the biases of the specimens are linearly related to the stated values (and this may be tested statistically), we may distinguish three cases: (1) the biases are constant; (2) the biases are proportional to the stated values over the range examined; or (3) the biases comprise a constant component and a proportional component. To illustrate these concepts, we will show four constructed examples where 11 control specimens have been assayed for the quantity in question using four different methods. For the sake of

Table 1-8. COMPARISON OF RESULTS DETERMINED BY FOUR DIFFERENT METHODS

VALUE OF x*	VALUE OF y†			
	Method I	Method II	Method III	Method IV
0.0	0.0	2.0	0.00	1.00
1.0	1.0	3.0	0.75	1.75
2.0	2.0	4.0	1.50	2.50
3.0	3.0	5.0	2.25	3.25
4.0	4.0	6.0	3.00	4.00
5.0	5.0	7.0	3.75	4.75
6.0	6.0	8.0	4.50	5.50
7.0	7.0	9.0	5.25	6.25
8.0	8.0	10.0	6.00	7.00
9.0	9.0	11.0	6.75	7.75
10.0	10.0	12.0	7.50	8.50

RESULTS OF LINEAR REGRESSION ANALYSIS

Method	Equation	Constant Bias	Proportional Bias
I	$y = 1.0 \cdot x$	no	no
II	$y = 1.0 \cdot x + 2.0$	yes	no
III	$y = 0.75 \cdot x$	no	yes
IV	$y = 0.75 \cdot x + 1.0$	yes	yes

*x = Concentration of analyte actually present.
†y = Concentration of analyte determined by either Method I, Method II, Method III, or Method IV.

simplicity we will assume that the random analytical variations are zero so that we are determining the actual biases instead of estimating them.

Table 1–8 presents 11 different "x" values and the corresponding observed "y" values determined by each of four methods. If there were no analytical biases present (a constant bias of zero), the observed value "y" and the corresponding "x" value would be identical; this is the case for Method I. We can display the data graphically (Figure 1–5A), with the "x" values being the abscissa and the observed "y" values being the ordinate. We construct a line of identity (y = x) which makes a 45 degree angle with the "x" axis. The "slope of the line" is computed as the difference in "y" (Δy) divided by the corresponding difference in "x" (Δx); and for Method I, the slope is 1.0. The "y-intercept" is the expected value of "y" when the value of "x" is zero; and for Method I, the y-intercept is 0.0. The value of "a" is equal to the constant bias, while the deviation of "b" from 1.0 (i.e., b − 1) multiplied by "x" is equal to the proportional bias corresponding to the x-value. For Method I, there are no constant biases and no proportional biases.

Figure 1–5B displays the data points for Method II. Note that although the computed slope is 1.0, the observed "y" values are consistently 2 units greater than the corresponding "x" values. Linear regression anal-

ysis gives the equation: y = 1.0x + 2.0. Method II suffers from constant biases of 2.0, but it has no proportional biases. Method III consistently underestimates the quantity value in that the observed value of "y" is always equal to three fourths of the "x" value (Fig. 1–5C). Thus, Method III has proportional biases where each bias is equal to (0.75 − 1)x = −0.25x. Note that there is no constant bias. The linear equation for Method III is: y = 0.75x. Finally, Method IV (Fig. 1–5D) demonstrates both proportional and constant biases. The linear equation for Method IV is: y = 0.75x + 1.0. For example, when the "x" value is 6, the observed value is (0.75)(6) + 1.0 or 5.5.

Recovery experiments

In recovery experiments assays are made on each of two samples obtained from a specimen with a measured amount of substance having been added to one of the samples. The expected difference between the results can be calculated from the amount of substance added. This difference is then subtracted from the observed difference and is used as an estimate of the bias. Recovery experiments can be applied only to methods for the measurement of concentration, and they will detect only proportional biases and not constant biases. Recovery experiments should be made with as large a number of specimens as possible so as to include specimens with potentially interfering substances. In the statistical analysis of the data, regression analysis may be applied. The independent variable then is the increase in concentration computed from the volumes and the amount of substance added, and the dependent variable "y" is the difference between measurements before and after the substance has been added to the specimen (Barnett, 1967).

Vickelsöe (1974) proposed a method which may be considered a variant of the recovery principle. By this method, two specimens, one with a relatively high quantity value and one with a much lower quantity value, are mixed in various proportions, and the resulting mixtures are assayed several times each. Since the proportions may be determined without appreciable error, it is reasonable to assume that "x" is known without random analytical variation and one may utilize the technique of the classical regression analysis to test for the presence of significant proportional biases.

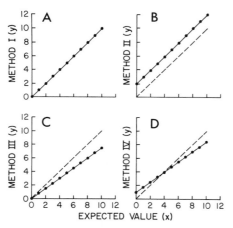

Figure 1–5. Relationship of observed values (y) to expected values (x). *A*, There is no bias evident. *B, C,* and *D,* The relationship seen in *A* is depicted by the broken line. In *B*, we note a constant bias of +2.0 units; in *C*, we observe a proportional bias of −0.25x; and in *D*, we compute a constant bias of +1.0 unit and a proportional bias of −0.25x. The actual data are presented in Table 1–8.

Comparison with a proven method

Selection of Specimens. By this technique a number of specimens are assayed using the new method and a comparison method. Preferably a large number (e.g., about 100) of patient specimens are assayed in replicate by each of the two methods. The specimens chosen should span the analytical ranges of both methods, and notes should be made of characteristics which may possibly give rise to interference or non-specificity.

Selection of Comparison Method. The IFCC expert panel on Quality Control defines accuracy (inaccuracy) as the agreement (lack of agreement) between the best estimate of a quantity and its true value. Using this definition, it proceeds to define four types of methods: (1) a *definitive method* is a method which, after exhaustive investigation, is found to have no known source of inaccuracy or ambiguity; (2) a *reference method* is a method which, after exhaustive investigation, has been shown to have negligible inaccuracy in comparison with its degree of random analytical variation; (3) a *method with known inaccuracy* is a method in which the amount of inaccuracy has been established; and (4) a *method with unknown inaccuracy.* Furthermore, the IFCC document recommends that a definitive method be used in the assessment of reference methods, and that reference methods rather than methods with known inaccuracy be used as comparison methods for new methods. If a reference method is not available, they recommend that the candidate method be compared with two or more methods of known inaccuracy (Büttner, 1976).

Statistical Analysis of Data. Prior to the statistical analysis, any result obtained on specimens contaminated with known interfering substances should be recorded and then removed before proceeding with the statistical analysis of the data. The statistical analysis presents a problem, since the results obtained by the comparison method are usually not without appreciable random analytical error. It may be shown that using the usual least square estimates, the true slope, i.e., the slope relating the expected values of "y" to those of "x," will be underestimated. This statistical bias may be corrected by computing a new slope $b' = b(1 + \lambda)$, where "b" is the least square slope obtained from the raw data and λ is the ratio between the random analytical variance of the comparison method as estimated from replicate measurements by the comparison method over the variance of the observed x values. Thus, it is critical to perform replicate measurements to estimate the random analytical variance of the comparison method for the range of concentration included in the experiment. It is also worth noting that the larger the range of "x" is, the larger will be the variance of the x-values and the smaller will be λ and thereby the bias of the slope (Bauer, 1975).

The reason why it is important to obtain replicate measurements of the "y" variable is two-fold. First, we want to estimate the random analytical variation of the candidate method, and second, we want to assess the validity of the assumption that the random analytical variance is independent of the quantity value. This is rarely the case, for typically the variance of "y" increases as the quantity value increases. If there is more than a five-fold increase in the variance of "y" over the range of "x," it may be necessary to transform the values or use a so-called weighted regression analysis. The interested reader is referred to standard statistical textbooks (Snedecor, 1967).

Specificity, sensitivity, dynamic range, and interference

In addition to estimating the magnitude of random analytical variations and of the analytical biases of a new method, one must also attest to its specificity, sensitivity, dynamic range, and freedom from interferences. A method is considered *specific* when it measures only the analyte it was designed to measure. Older methods of measuring glucose were not very specific, as they measured other reducing agents as well. The advent of glucose methods employing very specific glucose enzymes as reagents produced substantially greater specificity. The *sensitivity* of a method is established by determining the lowest concentration of the analyte which will be detected by the procedure. The *dynamic range* is the set of continuous values of the analyte which will give a linear signal response with the method without need for dilution of the sample or special treatment of the specimen. The effects of known common *interferences* on the performance of the method should be established. Here one should consider the effects of anticoagulant, preservatives, lipemia, icterus, and hemolysis on the result obtained using the new method.

MAINTAINING THE RELIABILITY OF AN ANALYTICAL METHOD PERFORMED UNDER ROUTINE OPERATING CONDITIONS

Until now we have examined the performance of the new analytical method when it is under careful control; i.e., the experienced developmental technologist is performing the assay, and the instrument is in good working condition. However, after the new method is introduced into routine operation, there may be a tendency for the quality of the performance to decline. In order to maintain the reliability of an analytical method's performance under routine day-to-day operating conditions, the following should be adhered to:

1. The method should be written so that all steps in the procedure can be followed without any confusion.

2. All technologists who may be called upon to use the method should be well trained in the method, understanding the critical steps and all possible precautions.

3. The laboratory director should provide a satisfactory working environment, i.e., adequate space, good lighting and ventilation, comfortable temperature, and freedom from interruptions.

4. There should be an established program of preventive maintenance of all instruments used in the laboratory.

5. The use of high-purity materials for standards, calibrators, and reagents should be encouraged. The National Bureau of Standards (NBS) has produced a number of primary and secondary standards of high purity. A primary standard is one in which the concentration is determined solely by dissolving a weighed amount of standard material in an appropriate solvent to make a stated volume or weight of the standard. The accuracy of a primary standard solution depends solely on the purity of the standard material and other components and the accuracy with which the solution is prepared. Since primary standards may not be available, one often relies on secondary standards. A secondary standard is one in which the concentration or other quantity is determined by an analytical method of stated reliability. The accuracy of a secondary standard therefore depends on the accuracy of the analysis, which in turn will involve a standard; ultimately there must be a primary standard. With this classification, both a potassium permanganate solution and serum can function as secondary standards (Büttner, 1976).

6. The laboratory should subscribe to both internal and external quality control programs. (See Chapter 63.)

CONCLUSION

The total variation in results obtained from healthy subjects over time can be partitioned into four components: (1) analytical variation, (2) preparation of the subject, (3) intra-individual physiologic variation, and (4) inter-individual biologic variation of mean values. The first two issues have been covered in this chapter, while the next chapter, "Reference Values," will deal with the intra-individual physiologic variations and the inter-individual variations. Appreciating these expected, non-pathologic sources of variations is critical in being able to discriminate a patient's value as signifying pathology vs. merely being evidence of some usual variation in the value of an analyte.

REFERENCES

Applegarth, D. A., and Poon, S.: Interpretation of elevated blood glycine levels in children. Clin. Chim. Acta, 63:49, 1975.

Barnett, R. N.: Medical significance of laboratory results. Am. J. Clin. Pathol., 50:671, 1968.

Barnett, R. N., and Youden, W. J.: A revised scheme for the comparison of quantitative methods. Am. J. Clin. Pathol., 54:454, 1970.

Barrett, P. V. D.: Hyperbilirubinemia of fasting. J.A.M.A., 217:1349, 1971.

Bauer, S., et al.: NCCLS Document: Protocol for Establishing the Precision and Accuracy of Automated Analytic Systems, 1975.

Belfrage, P., Berg, B., Hagerstrand, I., et al.: Alterations of lipid metabolism in healthy volunteers during long-term ethanol intake. Eur. J. Clin. Invest., 7:127, 1977.

Bellet, S., Kershbaum, A., and Aspe, J.: The effect of caffeine on free fatty acids. Arch. Intern. Med., 116:750, 1965.

Bishop, C., and Talbot, J. H.: Uric acid: its role in biological process and the influence upon it of physiological, pathological and pharmacological agents. Pharmacol. Rev., 5:231, 1953.

Bodansky, A., Jaffe, H. L., and Chandler, J. P.: Experimental factors influencing blood phosphatase values. J. Biol. Chem., 97:66, 1932.

Bokelund, H.: Analysis of variation in automated determination of sodium, potassium, and calcium ions in human serum. Clin. Chem., *22*:993, 1976.

Bokelund, H., Winkel, P., and Statland, B. E.: Factors contributing to intra-individual variation of serum constituents: 3. Use of randomized duplicate serum specimens to evaluate sources of analytical errors. Clin. Chem., *20*:1507, 1974.

Burtis, C. A., Begovich, J. M., and Watson, J. S.: Factors influencing evaporation from sample cups, and assessment of their effect on analytical error. Clin. Chem., *21*:1907, 1975.

Büttner, J., Borth, R., Boutwell, J. H., and Broughton, P. M. G.: Provisional recommendations on quality control in clinical chemistry. Part 1. General principles and terminology. Clin. Chim. Acta, *63*:F25, 1975.

Büttner, J., Borth, R., Boutwell, J. H., Broughton, P. M. G., and Bowyer, R. C.: Provisional recommendations on quality control in clinical chemistry. Part 2. Assessment of analytical methods for routine use. Clin. Chim. Acta, *69*:F1, 1976.

Calam, R. R.: Reviewing the importance of specimen collection. J. Am. Med. Technol., *39*:297, 1977.

Campbell, D. G., and Owen, J. A.: The analytical error. Clin. Biochem., *1*:3, 1967.

Caraway, W. T.: Accuracy in clinical chemistry. Clin. Chem., *17*:63, 1971.

Caraway, W. T., and Kammeyer, C. W.: Chemical interference by drugs and other substances with clinical laboratory test procedures. Clin. Chem. Acta, *41*:395, 1972.

Carlsten, A., et al.: Arterial concentration of free fatty acids and free amino acids in healthy individuals at rest and at different work loads. Scand. J. Clin. Lab. Invest., *14*:185, 1962.

Cotlove, E., Harris, E. K., and Williams, G. Z.: Biological and analytical components of variation in long-term studies of serum constituents in normal subjects: 3. Physiological and medical implications. Clin. Chem., *16*:1028, 1970.

Dybkaer, R. (chairman), Commission on Quantities and Units, Section on Clinical Chemistry, IUPAC, and Expert Panel on Quantities and Units, Committee on Standards, IFCC: Quantities and units in clinical chemistry. Recommendation 1973. Pure and Appl. Chem., *37*:517, 1974a.

Dybkaer, R. (chairman), Commission on Quantities and Units, Section on Clinical Chemistry, IUPAC, and Expert Panel on Quantities and Units, Committee on Standards, IFCC: List of quantities in clinical chemistry. Pure and Appl. Chem., *37*:547, 1974b.

Dybkaer, R., and Jørgensen, K.: Quantities and units in clinical chemistry, including recommendation 1966 of the Commission on Clinical Chemistry of the International Union of Pure and Applied Chemistry and of the International Federation of Clinical Chemistry. Copenhagen, Munksgaard, 1967.

Dybkaer, R., Jørgensen, K., and Nyboe, J.: Statistical terminology in clinical chemistry reference values. Scand. J. Clin. Lab. Invest., *35* (Suppl. 144):45, 1975.

Eisenberg, S.: Postural changes in plasma volume in hypoalbuminemia. Arch. Intern. Med., *112*:544, 1963.

Fawcett, J. K., and Wynn, V.: Effects of posture on plasma volume and some blood constituents. J. Clin. Pathol., *13*:304, 1960.

Freer, D. E., and Statland, B. E.: The effects of ethanol (0.75 g/kg body weight) on the activities of selected enzymes in sera of healthy young adults: 1. Intermediate-term effects. Clin. Chem., *23*:830, 1977.

Galteau, M. M., Siest, G., and Poortmans, J.: Continuous *in vivo* measurement of creatine kinase variation in man during an exercise. Clin. Chim. Acta, *66*:89, 1975.

Gambino, S. R., and Schreiber, H.: The measurement of CO_2 content with the Auto-Analyzer. Am. J. Clin. Pathol., *45*:406, 1966.

Glenn, G. C., and Hathaway, T. K.: Effects of specimen evaporation on quality control. Am. J. Clin. Pathol., *66*:645, 1976.

Hagebusch, O. I.: Automation in the private practice of laboratory medicine. Automat. Anal. Chem., Technicon Symposium, 1965. Technicon, 1966, p. 417.

Keys, A., and Parlin, R. W.: Serum cholesterol response to changes in dietary lipids. Am. J. Clin. Nutr., *19*:175, 1966.

King, S., Statland, B. E., and Savory, J.: The effects of a short burst of exercise on activity values of enzymes in sera of healthy subjects. Clin. Chim. Acta, *72*:211, 1976.

Laessig, R. H., Hassemer, D. J., Paskey, T. A., et al.: The effects of 0.1 and 1.0 per cent erythrocytes and hemolysis on serum chemistry values. Am. J. Clin. Pathol., *66*:639, 1976a.

Laessig, R. H., Hassemer, D. J., Westgard, J. O., et al.: Assessment of the serum separator tube as an intermediate storage device within the laboratory. Am. J. Clin. Pathol., *66*:653, 1976b.

Larsson-Cohn, U.: Differences between capillary and venous blood glucose during oral glucose tolerance tests. Scand. J. Clin. Lab. Invest., *36*:805, 1976.

Laurell, C. B., Killander, S., and Thorell, J.: Effect of administration of a combined estrogen-progestin contraceptive on the level of individual plasma proteins. Scand. J. Clin. Lab. Invest., *21* (Suppl.):337, 1967.

Levi, L.: The effect of coffee on the function of the sympathoadrenomedullary system in man. Acta Med. Scand., *181*:431, 1967.

Lubran, M.: The effects of drugs on laboratory values, Med. Clin. North Am., *53*:211, 1969.

Maclin, E.: Considerations of analytical goals for the clinical laboratory. An industrial perspective and a systems view. Presented at the Aspen Conference on Analytical Goals in Clinical Chemistry, August, 1977, College of American Pathologists.

Marley, E., and Blackwell, B.: Interactions of monoamine oxidase inhibitors, amines and foodstuffs. Advan. Pharmacol. Chemother., *8*:185, 1970.

Martin, H. F., Gudzinowicz, B. J., and Fanger, H.: Normal Values in Clinical Chemistry: A Guide to Statistical Analysis of Laboratory Data. New York, Merkel Dekker, Inc., 1975.

Martin, T. J.: The pharmacologic interactions with laboratory test values. August 1970, 596 Burnhamthorpe, Etobicoke, Ontario, Canada.

McGeachin, R. L., Daugherty, H. K., Haryan, L. A., and Potter, B. A.: The effect of blood anticoagulant on serum and plasma amylase activities. Clin. Chim. Acta, *2*:75, 1957.

Musiala, T. S., and Dubin, A.: Effects of chylomicrons and their removal on spectrophotometric analyses. Clin. Chem., *23*:1121, 1977.

Olusi, S. O., McFarlane, H., Osunkoya, B. O., and Adesina, H.: Specific protein assays in protein-calorie malnutrition. Clin. Chim. Acta, *62*:107, 1975.

Pragay, D. A., et al.: Evaluation of an improved pneumatic-tube system suitable for transportation of blood specimens. Clin. Chem., *20*:57, 1974.

Schiele, F., et al.: The effects of drugs on enzyme reference values. Clin. Chem., *23*:1120, 1977.

Schwartz, M. K.: Interferences in diagnostic biochemical procedures. Adv. Clin. Chem., *16*:1, 1973.

Snedecor, G. W., and Cochran, W. G.: Statistical Methods. Ames, The Iowa State University Press, 1967.

Statland, B. E., and Winkel, P.: Problems of precision and accuracy related to specimen collection and handling. Technical Improvement Service, *24*:60, 1976.

Statland, B. E., and Winkel, P.: Effects of non-analytical factors on the intra-individual variation of analytes in the blood of healthy subjects: Consideration of preparation of the subject and time of venipuncture. CRC Critical Reviews in Clinical Laboratory Science, *8*:105, 1977.

Statland, B. E., Winkel, P., and Bokelund, H.: Factors contributing to intra-individual variation of serum constituents: 2. Effects of exercise and diet on variation of serum constituents in healthy subjects. Clin. Chem., *19*:1380, 1973a.

Statland, B. E., Winkel, P., and Bokelund, H.: Serum alkaline phosphatase after fatty meals: The effect of substrate on the assay procedure. Clin. Chim. Acta, *49*:299, 1973b.

Statland, B. E., Winkel, P., and Bokelund, H.: Factors contributing to intra-individual variation of serum constituents: 4. Effects of posture and tourniquet application on variation of serum constituents in healthy subject. Clin. Chem., *20*:1513, 1974.

Statland, B. E., Young, D. S., and Nishi, H. N.: Serum alkaline phosphatase: Total activity and isoenzyme determinations made by use of centrifugal fast analyzer. Clin. Chem., *18*:12, 1972.

Steige, H., and Jones, J. D.: Evaluation of pneumatic tube system for delivery of blood specimens. Clin. Chem., *17*:160, 1971.

Sunderman, F. W., Jr.: Drug interference in clinical bio-chemistry. CRC Crit. Rev. Clin. Lab. Sci., *1*:427, 1970.

Swanson, J. R., and Wilkinson, J. H.: Measurement of creatine kinase activity in serum. Stand. Meth. Clin. Chem., *7*:33, 1972.

Tonks, D. B.: A study of the accuracy and precision of clinical chemistry determination in 170 Canadian laboratories. Clin. Chem., *9*:217, 1963.

Vikelsöe, J., Bechgaard, E., and Magid, E.: A procedure for the evaluation of precision and accuracy of analytical methods. Scand. J. Clin. Lab. Invest., *34*:149, 1974.

Wakkers, P. J. M., et al.: Applications of statistics in clinical chemistry: A critical evaluation of regression lines. Clin. Chim. Acta, *64*:173, 1975.

Weindling, H., and Henry, J. B.: Drug interaction and clinical laboratory data. Lab. Med., *6*:24, 1975.

Westgard, J. O., and Hunt, M. R.: Use and interpretation of common statistical tests in method-comparison studies. Clin. Chem., *19*:49, 1973.

Whitehead, T. P.: Quality Control in Clinical Chemistry. New York, John Wiley & Sons, Inc., 1977.

Wilkinson, E. J., Cherayil, G. D., and Borkowf, H. I.: L/S ratio and the "g-force" factor. N. Engl. J. Med., *296*:286, 1977.

Wilson, S. S., Guillan, R. A., and Hocker, E. V.: Studies of the stability of 18 chemical constituents of human serum. Clin. Chem., *18*:1498, 1972.

Winsten, S.: Collection and preservation of specimens. Stand. Meth. Clin. Chem., *5*:1, 1965.

Young, D. S.: Standardized reporting of laboratory data: The desirability of using SI units. N. Engl. J. Med., *290*:368, 1974.

Young, D. S., Pestaner, L. C., and Gibberman, V.: Effects of drugs on clinical laboratory tests. Clin. Chem., *21*:1D, 1975.

2

REFERENCE VALUES

Per Winkel, M.D., Doc. Med. Sci., and
Bernard E. Statland, M.D., Ph.D.

The product of the analytical procedure ultimately is a result referring to a patient specimen. The clinician interprets this result as indicating a change, a lack of change, or potential change in the health status of a patient. In order to make this interpretation meaningful, a clinician compares the given result with some interval of values. We shall refer to such an interval as a "reference interval." In the clinical setting, a reference interval is generally constructed so as to include the range of values found in 95 per cent of a reference population of healthy subjects. Unfortunately, the clinician usually interprets this interval to signify the lower and upper limits between which the patient's values should fall, assuming he is in a certain state of health.

CONCEPT OF REFERENCE VALUES

Prior to this present decade, the term "normal values" was most often used to characterize the values of healthy subjects. The word "normal" is confusing in that in the context of clinical chemistry, it has been assumed both to represent the normal (healthy) subject and to signify the normal (Gaussian) distribution. Martin (1975) has reviewed the mathematical basis for early applications of normal values. Galen (1977) reviews reference intervals among other alternatives to the normal range in a discussion of the normal range in transition.

Grasbeck (1969) introduced the concept of "reference values" and recommended that the term "normal values," which is ambiguous and impossible to define, be abolished. Reference values can be defined as a set of values of a measured quantity obtained from a group of individuals (or a single individual) in a defined state of "health."

We will consider two types of reference values in this chapter: group-based reference values and subject-based reference values.

How is either type of reference value used in the clinical setting? When evaluating a laboratory result, the physician often compares the present result with some interval. In this manner, he wants to estimate the probability that the subject (patient) from whom the given laboratory result was obtained belongs to a "group" of healthy subjects from whom the reference values were obtained (i.e., *grouped-based reference values*). If the reference values are those obtained from the "same subject" when he was in a defined state of health (i.e., *subject-based reference values*), the clinician compares the present value with past values to estimate whether the subject is still in the same state of health.

A common error occurring in the clinical setting is the practice of using the lower and upper limits of the interval as rigid boundaries within which the patient is considered "normal," and beyond which the patient is termed "abnormal" and thought to be suffering from some pathologic process. This approach may be very misleading for many reasons. For one thing, having a value outside the stated interval might be a sign of *good* health rather than a cause for concern, e.g., a patient having a serum cholesterol value *below* the lower reference limit. For another patient, having a value within the stated interval might *not* be a sign of good health, e.g., a diabetic with a "normal blood glucose."

Since the alternatives are not usually explicitly defined in the clinical setting, the isolated use of a reference interval may lead to erroneous conclusions. The only question that can be answered when using these intervals is the following: if the subject belongs to the reference group (or in the case when we use the subject as his own reference, if he is in the same state of health as when the reference values were obtained), what is the probability that we would observe the result which we have actually observed? For this reason we want to discourage the determination and utilization of group-based reference intervals independent of alternative reference intervals for relevant "disease groups."

We will first define the statistical terms that are commonly used to characterize reference values; second, we will explicitly list the steps that one must perform to obtain and to characterize the data base of reference values; third, we will compare group-based reference values with subject-based reference values.

SOME BASIC STATISTICAL CONCEPTS AND DEFINITIONS

SETS, SUBSETS, AND RANDOM SELECTION

It is often desirable for various purposes to know certain information about a very large number (set) of subjects. Usually it is not feasible to obtain observations from all the subjects; therefore, we must rely on information obtained from a smaller subset of the larger set of subjects. In the following we shall define and develop some of the more basic statistical terminology necessary to approach the above problem in a quantitative way. In the statistical sense of the word, a *set* (also called a population) is a collection of items, e.g., the set of all healthy females living in a certain location at a particular time. We may be interested in a particular quantity of the subjects, e.g., their weight as measured at a particular point in calendar time. When the total population of values (the set of values) is very large or infinite, we may obtain a smaller sample (or subset) of values upon which to generalize about the values in the original set. To characterize a finite set of values, we may examine a simple, randomly chosen *subset* of observed values obtained from the set. To obtain a simple, *randomly* chosen subset of a given size from a finite set, we must be assured that every possible subset of the given size has an equal chance of being selected. If the subset is a simple, randomly chosen one, it may be used for making inferences about (1) certain derived quantities (parameters) characterizing the set and (2) future random subsets obtained from the set. Table 2–1 presents the important distinctions between the "set" and a randomly chosen "subset" obtained from the set.

CHARACTERIZING A FINITE SET OF VALUES

In characterizing a finite set of values we want to obtain a measure of (1) what has been

Table 2–1. TERMS AND SYMBOLS USED TO CHARACTERIZE A FINITE SET OF VALUES AND A RANDOMLY CHOSEN SUBSET OF VALUES OBTAINED FROM THE SET

TERMS AND SYMBOLS[a]	SET[b]	SUBSET[c]
Number of observations	N	n
Sum of values	$\sum\limits_{i=1}^{N} x_i$	$\sum\limits_{i=1}^{n} x_i$
Mean of values	$\mu = \left(\dfrac{1}{N}\right) \sum\limits_{i=1}^{N} x_i$	$\bar{x} = \left(\dfrac{1}{n}\right) \sum\limits_{i=1}^{n} x_i$
Variance	$\sigma^2 = \left(\dfrac{1}{N}\right) \sum\limits_{i=1}^{N} (x_i - \mu)^2$	$s^2 = \left(\dfrac{1}{n-1}\right) \sum\limits_{i=1}^{n} (x_i - \bar{x})^2$
Standard deviation	$|\sqrt{\sigma^2}|$ or σ	$|\sqrt{s^2}|$ or s

[a] Examples of some symbols used:

$\sum\limits_{i=1}^{3} x_i =$ the sum of $x_1 + x_2 + x_3$

$\bar{x} =$ mean of all "x values"

$|\sqrt{y}| =$ the absolute value of the square root of y

[b] A set is defined here as a population of values.

[c] A subset is defined here as a *finite* sample of values obtained from the population of values.

called a typical value or alternatively the location of the values and (2) the extent to which the various observations differ from the typical value, i.e., the variation of the observations, also called the dispersion of the values.

Location of the Values. The mean (average value) or the median is often used as a typical or representative value of a set of N observations. The *mean* (μ) and the corresponding quantity, $\bar{x}$, are defined in Table 1–1. If we order the observations according to size, the *median* is defined as the middle observation. If there is no middle observation, that is, if the number of observations is even, the median is defined as the average value of the two middle observations. It follows from the definition of the median of an even numbered set that 50 per cent and no more of the observations are less than or equal to the median. A value fulfilling this condition we denote as the fiftieth percentile. A tenth percentile then is a value which fulfills the condition that 10 per cent and no more of all the observations are less than or equal to that value. In general, we define a *P-percentile* as a value which has the quality that P per cent and no more of the observations are *less than* or *equal to* the value. Obviously, percentiles are very helpful when

we want to characterize a set in greater detail than that obtained by computing the mean and median alone. The *mode* of a set of observations is that value which occurs most frequently.

Variation of the Values. The variation of the values comprising a set may be assessed by computing the range, the variance, or the standard deviation (Table 2–1). When the variance is a parameter characterizing a *set*, it is computed as $\sum\limits_{i=1}^{N} (x_i - \mu)^2/N$; i.e., the denominator is the total number of values (N) in the set, and the numerator is the sum of the squares of the deviations. However, if we wish to obtain an estimate of the variance based on a random *subset* obtained from the set, we use the quantity $s^2 = \sum\limits_{i=1}^{n} (x_i - \bar{x})^2/(n-1)$; i.e., we divide the sum of squares of deviations by the number of values (n) in the subset minus one (Table 2–1).

Distribution of the Values. A set can also be characterized by various distributions. A *distribution* is a summary of the relationship between one type of quantity (a univariate

Table 2–2. VALUES OF GLUCOSE CONCENTRATION IN PLASMA*

fP-GLUCOSE (mmol/l)	NUMBER OF SUBJECTS HAVING THE STATED VALUE	CUMULATIVE NUMBER OF VALUES	CUMULATIVE NUMBER FRACTION OF VALUES
3.7	1	1	0.005
3.8	0	1	0.005
3.9	2	3	0.015
4.0	1	4	0.020
4.1	2	6	0.030
4.2	2	8	0.040
4.3	6	14	0.070
4.4	9	23	0.115
4.5	15	38	0.190
4.6	20	58	0.290
4.7	19	77	0.385
4.8	21	98	0.490
4.9	19	117	0.585
5.0	20	137	0.685
5.1	22	159	0.795
5.2	18	177	0.885
5.3	10	187	0.935
5.4	5	192	0.960
5.5	2	194	0.970
5.6	1	195	0.975
5.7	1	196	0.980
5.8	0	196	0.980
5.9	1	197	0.985
6.0	0	197	0.985
6.1	1	198	0.990
6.2	0	198	0.990
6.3	1	199	0.995
6.4	1	200	1.000

computed mean: $\bar{x}$ = 4.865 mmol/l
computed standard deviation: s = 0.388 mmol/l

*One value was obtained from each of 200 fasting healthy subjects. The values are presented in ascending order.

distribution) and number of elements (or a derivative, e.g., the number fraction of elements or the cumulative number fraction of elements). A distribution may be given in the form of a table or a graph or in the form of an algebraic equation. Throughout the following discussion, the symbol "x" will represent the value of the clinical chemistry quantity under consideration and will be depicted on the abscissa (horizontal axis).

Table 2–2 presents a tabulation of 200 plasma glucose values, one value determined on each of 200 healthy fasting subjects. Note that the units correspond to the IUPAC/IFCC recommendations (p. 4) in that the "substance concentration" rather than the conventional "mass concentration" is used. (The conversion factor used to go from SI units to conventional units is $18 \, mg \cdot l \cdot mmol^{-1} \cdot dl^{-1}$; i.e., 5.0 mmol/l corresponds to [5.0 mmol $\cdot l^{-1}$ × $18 \, mg \cdot l \cdot mmol^{-1} \cdot dl^{-1}$] or 90 mg/dl.) Also note that the "fP" before the quantity name represents the system, i.e., plasma obtained from a fasting patient. The glu-

cose values (quantity/unit) are arranged in ascending numerical order. The second column presents the number of subjects having the stated value. For example, the number of subjects having the x-value 4.2 is 2 (Table 2–2). The number fraction is defined as the number divided by the total number of observations. The third column presents the cumulative number of values, i.e., the number of observations that are equal to or less than the particular value of "x." For the x-value of 4.2, the cumulative number is equal to the number of observations of the values: 3.7, 3.9, 4.0, 4.1, and 4.2; i.e., $1 + 2 + 1 + 2 + 2 = 8$. Finally, the fourth column presents the cumulative number fraction of values: i.e., the cumulative number divided by the total number of observations in the set. The total range of the number fraction and the cumulative number fraction must be 0.0 to 1.0 by definition. For the example of the x value of 4.2, the number fraction is 2/200 or 0.01, and the cumulative number fraction is 8/200 or 0.04. A term related to the cumulative number fraction is the cumulative probability distribution, which here is denoted as P(X ≤ a). In the example, P(X ≤ a) is the probability that we will obtain an observation from the set which is equal to or less than "a." When we pick a single observation from the set of 200 observations, X denotes a variate or a random variable (quantity). A variate is defined as a quantity which by chance may take any one of a specified set of values. P(X ≤ a) can be assessed only when the procedure by which we obtain a subset (comprising one observation) from the set is specified. In this example, we assume that the observation is picked by simple random sampling such that each of the 200 observations has the same chance of being picked. Therefore, the cumulative probability is identical with the cumulative number fraction. For example, the cumulative number fraction at 4.1 in the example shown in Table 2–2 is 6/200 or 0.03. In that all observations have the same probability of being picked, the probability for each observation of being picked is 1/200. Since there are six observations that are equal to or less than 4.1, the probability of picking one of these observations is equal to 6/200, which again is equal to the cumulative number fraction at 4.1. The computed mean and the computed standard deviation for the set of 200 plasma glucose values are presented in Table 2–2 as well.

CHARACTERIZING A SUBSET OF VALUES

A simple, randomly chosen subset may be characterized in the same way as the finite set from which it was obtained, namely by a mean, a median, various P-percentiles, a variance, a standard deviation (see Table 2–1), a number distribution, a number fraction distribution, a cumulative number distribution, and a cumulative number fraction distribution. A simple, randomly chosen subset may be used to make inferences about the various distributions and the parameters of the set (population of values) from which the subset was obtained. The mean, the median (or other percentiles), the variance, and standard deviation of the random *subset* (sample) are used as the best guesses or estimates of the corresponding quantities characterizing the *set* (population of values). Similarly, the various distributions are the best approximations to the corresponding distributions characterizing the set. While the values computed on a subset of ob-

servations are termed estimates, the analogous values computed on a set of values are called parameters. Thus, we distinguish between the parameters (μ and σ) of the set and the statistical terms (x̄ and s) determined on a random subset of values.

THE CUMULATIVE GAUSSIAN PROBABILITY DISTRIBUTION

The cumulative Gaussian probability distribution refers to a hypothetical probabilistic mechanism according to which the observed values are assumed to be generated.

It is defined as follows:

$$P(X \le a) = \int_{-\infty}^{a} f(x)\, dx = \int_{-\infty}^{a} \frac{1}{\sigma \sqrt{2\pi}} e^{-[(x-\mu)^2/2\sigma^2]}\, dx$$

where: $\pi = 3.1416$
  $e = 2.7183$ (base for the natural logarithm)
  σ = hypothetical standard deviation (see Table 2–1)
  μ = hypothetical mean (see Table 2–1)
  $f(x)$ = the Gaussian probability density function

Figure 2–1*A* represents the Gaussian probability density. Strictly speaking, the cumulative Gaussian (normal) probability distribution is only applicable for sets of infinite numbers of observations, for observations which are continuous, and for observations which theoretically can be infinitely large or infinitely small. In practice, the Gaussian model may be useful in most cases where the cumulative number fraction distribution of a large, finite set of discontinuous observations approximates the cumulative Gaussian probability distribution. As will be noted below, the blind application of the Gaussian model for all sets of chemical and hematologic quantities is subject to criticism; thus, each case must be examined individually to demonstrate reasonable adherence to the model. It may be shown that the integral (summation) of the probability density over all possible values (i.e., from −∞ to +∞) is equal to one. This is in accordance with the fact that the probability that a quantity will attain a value between −∞ and +∞ is equal to one. Thus, the total area under the curve in Figure 2–1*A* then is equal to 1.000, and the area bounded by the x-axis, the curve, and any two vertical lines is equal to the probability that the value of X would fall on the abscissa between the two vertical lines. The area bounded by the vertical lines per-

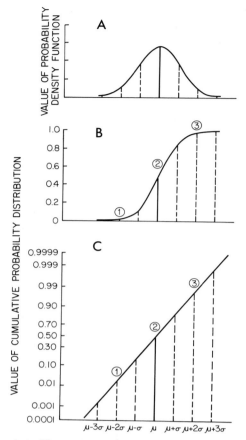

Figure 2-1. The uppermost frame (*A*) presents the Gaussian probability density function. The middle frame (*B*) depicts the Gaussian cumulative probability distribution on conventional graph paper. The lowermost frame (*C*) presents the Gaussian cumulative probability distribution on probability graph paper.

but that the values near 0.500 are much closer together than are the values at either end. Probability graph paper is used to depict the cumulative number fraction distribution (see Tables 2-2 and 2-3) of a subset of values obtained from the set (population) of values that one wants to characterize. The spacing of the values on the ordinate is such that the probability graph paper makes a cumulative Gaussian probability distribution linear and conversely will indicate to what extent the cumulative number fraction distribution of the observed X values deviates from a normal (Gaussian) distribution. Points labeled ①, ②, and ③ in Figures 2-1*B* and 2-1*C* are located at the x-values of $\mu - 2\sigma, \mu$, and $\mu + 2\sigma$.

In a clinical situation, one computes $\bar{x}$ and s from the subset of observations and on probability graph paper plots a straight line corresponding to a Gaussian distribution with mean $= \bar{x}$ and variance $= s^2$. This is achieved by setting the values $\bar{x} - 2s, \bar{x}, \bar{x} + 2s$ on the abscissa to correspond to the ordinate values

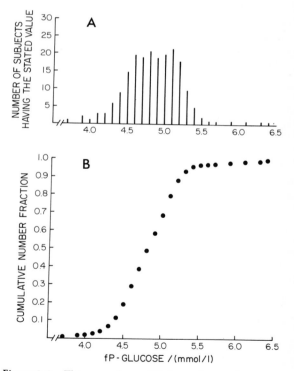

Figure 2-2. The upper frame (*A*) shows the number distribution (i.e., the number of subjects having the stated value) of 200 plasma glucose values with one value determined on each of 200 healthy fasting subjects (see Table 2-2). The lower frame (*B*) shows the corresponding cumulative number fraction distribution.

pendicular to the values $(\mu - \sigma, \mu + \sigma)$, i.e., the probability of a value being in the range of the mean ± one standard deviation, is 0.6826; for $(\mu - 2\sigma, \mu + 2\sigma)$, it is 0.9554; and for $(\mu - 3\sigma, \mu + 3\sigma)$, it is 0.9974.

Figure 2-1*B* is the cumulative Gaussian probability distribution corresponding to the probability density in Figure 2-1*A*. Note that at $X = \mu - 2\sigma$, the value of the cumulative Gaussian probability distribution is equal to 0.022; at $X = \mu$, it is 0.500; and at $X = \mu + 2\sigma$, it is equal to 0.978. These three points are labeled ①, ②, and ③ respectively in Figure 2-1*B*.

In Figure 2-1*C* the cumulative Gaussian probability distribution is depicted on "probability graph paper." Note that the values on the ordinate (y-axis) are not equally spaced,

0.022, 0.5, and 0.978 respectively. The cumulative number fraction distribution of the data base is then plotted on the probability paper. If the data have a Gaussian (normal) distribution, the cumulative number fraction distribution should show only small and unsystematic deviations from the above-mentioned idealized straight line. The hypothesis that the deviations are due only to chance effects may be evaluated for statistical purposes using a so-called chi-square test. The interested reader is referred to statistical textbooks for details (Snedecor, 1967). We will apply the graphic approach to the 200 observations of plasma glucose concentration (Table 2-1). Figure 2-2A depicts the number distribution of the values. The number distribution appears relatively symmetrical and resembles the familiar bell-shaped Gaussian probability density curve. Figure 2-2B depicts the cumulative number fraction distribution of the plasma glucose concentration values. The points in this figure correspond closely to the idealized cumulative Gaussian probability distribution curve seen in Figure 2-1B.

Figure 2-3 shows the cumulative number fraction distribution of the observations depicted on probability graph paper. Based on the mean and standard deviation of the observations, the straight line of the corresponding theoretical Gaussian distribution has also been plotted for comparison on the probability paper. The actual cumulative number fraction distribution between 0.1 and 0.9 on the y-axis does not differ substantially from the straight line drawn in the figure, thus suggesting that the values of plasma glucose concentration from fasting healthy subjects follow the Gaussian distribution rather closely.

The number fraction distribution of observations may be more peaked (positive kurtosis) than the theoretical Gaussian probability density function or more flat (negative kurtosis). When the peak is tall and narrow, the distribution is called *leptokurtic*, and when flat, *platykurtic*. It may be shown that where a data set is generated according to the Gaussian probability mechanism, the mean (aver-

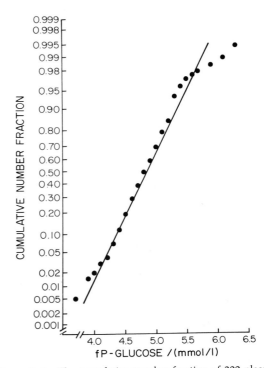

Figure 2-3. The cumulative number fraction of 200 plasma glucose values is depicted on probability graph paper. The straight line depicts the Gaussian cumulative probability distribution with a mean and a standard deviation as computed on the 200 plasma glucose values.

age value), the median (central value), and the mode (most frequent value) should be identical. When the mean, the mode, and the median of a data set are grossly different from each other, the number fraction distribution is said to be skewed. A distribution may be skewed to the right (positive skewness) with a mean being larger than the median, and the median being greater than the mode; or the distribution may be skewed to the left (negative skewness) with a mean being smaller than the median, and the median being smaller than the mode (Fig. 2-4). The magnitudes and signs of these deviations may be assessed, and the probability that observed deviations are

Figure 2-4. These two distributions represent negative skewness (left) and positive skewness (right). Modified from Martin, Gudzinowicz and Fanger (1975).

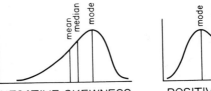

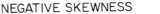

NEGATIVE SKEWNESS   POSITIVE SKEWNESS

Table 2-3. VALUES OF TRIGLYCERIDE CONCENTRATION IN SERUM

fS-TRIGLYCERIDES (mmol/l)	NUMBER OF SUBJECTS HAVING THE STATED VALUE	CUMULATIVE NUMBER OF VALUES	CUMULATIVE NUMBER FRACTION OF VALUES
0.3	1	1	0.005
0.4	4	5	0.025
0.5	10	15	0.075
0.6	29	44	0.220
0.7	26	70	0.350
0.8	27	97	0.485
0.9	23	120	0.600
1.0	16	136	0.680
1.1	14	150	0.750
1.2	12	162	0.810
1.3	9	171	0.855
1.4	8	179	0.895
1.5	6	185	0.925
1.6	4	189	0.945
1.8	2	191	0.955
1.9	1	192	0.960
2.1	1	193	0.965
2.6	1	194	0.970
2.7	1	195	0.975
3.0	2	197	0.985
3.4	1	198	0.990
3.8	1	199	0.995
4.2	1	200	1.000

computed mean: $\bar{x} = 0.996$ mmol/l
computed standard deviation: $s = 0.544$ mmol/l

*One value was obtained from each of 200 fasting healthy subjects. The values are presented in ascending order.

due to chance may be computed. For details on how skewness and kurtosis are calculated, textbooks on statistics should be consulted (Snedecor, 1967).

If a data set does not follow a Gaussian distribution, the data may be transformed, e.g., log x, log (x + c), $\sqrt{x}$, and the transformed data examined to determine whether they follow the Gaussian distribution. Wooton (1953) examined the distribution of values for 16 serum constituents in healthy subjects and found that 7 of the 16 were normally (Gaussian) distributed, namely: serum chloride, sodium ion, calcium ion, glucose, urate, total protein, and albumin; eight followed a Gaussian distribution after logarithmic transformation (serum potassium ion, creatinine, cholesterol, alkaline phosphatase, acid phosphatase, bilirubins, urea, and amylase), and one (globulin) was negatively skewed.

Table 2-3 presents the serum triglyceride values for the same 200 fasting subjects on whom we evaluated the plasma glucose concentrations. Figure 2-5A presents the number distribution of the 200 triglyceride values. It should be obvious that the distribution of the triglyceride values clearly deviates from that which one would expect if the data adhered to the Gaussian model in that the distribution of values is asymmetric with a tail to the right (positive skewness). Figure 2-5B presents the cumulative number fraction of the serum triglyceride concentration values. Figure 2-6 depicts the same distribution graphed on probability graph paper. It also presents the line corresponding to the idealized Gaussian distribution. It is clear that the actual observations do not follow the Gaussian distribution very closely. Next, serum triglyceride values are transformed using the logarithmic transformation. In Figure 2-7A and B the scale of the abscissa (x-axis) is logarithmic, thus enabling us to evaluate the number distribution and cumulative number fraction distribution of the logarithms of the serum triglyceride values. As seen in Figure 2-7A, the number distribution of log-transformed values more closely approximates the shape of the Gaussian probability density function than was the case for the untransformed values (Fig. 2-5A). Furthermore, the cumulative number fraction values of the log-transformed results more

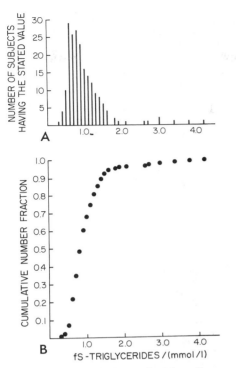

Figure 2–5. This figure represents selected results presented in Table 2–3. The upper frame (*A*) shows the number distribution (i.e., the number of subjects having the stated value) of 200 serum triglyceride values with one value determined on each of 200 fasting subjects. The lower frame (*B*) shows the corresponding cumulative number fraction distribution.

Gaussian or log-Gaussian distribution (i.e., a distribution such that the logarithms of the values follow a Gaussian distribution) when computing a reference interval is discussed by Reed (1971). He compares various methods for the computation of a so-called "normal range," i.e., the computation of reference intervals using parametric (Henry, 1964) or non-parametric methods (methods where no assumptions are made about the distribution of the set (Brunden, 1970)) and the computation of estimates of percentiles. He recommends the latter approach, which was originally proposed by Herrera (1958). To estimate a 95 per cent "normal range" according to this method, the 2.5 and 97.5 percentiles of the set are estimated. The estimated 95 per cent "normal range" then is the interval delimited by the estimated 2.5 and 97.5 percentiles. In our case of 200 values, we locate the 5th and the 195th values (in ascending order) to estimate the limits of the 95 per cent interval.

closely correspond to the calculated line (Fig. 2–7*B*) than was the case for the untransformed results as seen in Fig. 2–6. It should be noted, however, that even after log transformation the upper end of the cumulative number fraction distribution does deviate from the line (Fig. 2–7*B*).

THE COMPUTATION OF REFERENCE INTERVALS BASED ON NON-PARAMETRIC METHODS

It is often the case that none of the commonly used transformations will succeed in changing the data to correspond to a theoretical Gaussian model. An alternative approach for evaluating data is to make no assumptions about the distribution. This general approach is termed "non-parametric." The effect of the bias introduced by wrongly assuming a

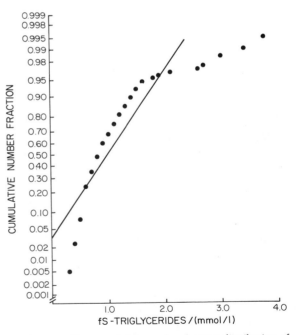

Figure 2–6. The cumulative number fraction distribution of 200 serum triglyceride values (one value determined on each of 200 healthy fasting subjects) is depicted on probability graph paper. The straight line depicts the Gaussian cumulative probability distribution with mean $\bar{x}$ and standard deviations, as computed on the 200 serum triglyceride values. Note how much the values of the cumulative number fraction deviate from the theoretical Gaussian distribution.

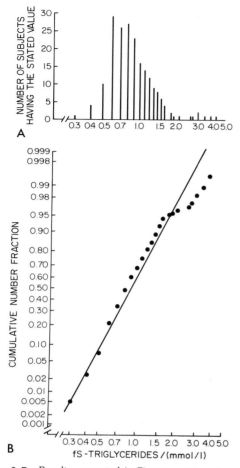

Figure 2-7. Results presented in Figures 2–5*A* and 2–6 for the values of 200 serum triglycerides are depicted here with the abscissa log-transformed. In *A* we are comparing the number of the subjects having the stated value, and in *B* the cumulative number fraction, with the logarithm of the triglyceride value. In *B*, note how much closer (as compared with Fig. 2–6) the values of the cumulative number fraction approximate the theoretical Gaussian distribution, although the values still deviate at the upper end of the distribution.

Table 2-4 compares the interval determined by the parametric approach, i.e., $\bar{x} - 2s$, $\bar{x} + 2s$, for the 200 plasma glucose values versus the 95 per cent interval on the same data using the non-parametric method. Note the very good agreement between both methods. Table 2-4 also presents the intervals on the 200 serum triglyceride values and on the logarithmically transformed serum triglyceride values, as determined by the parametric and non-parametric methods respectively. When we assume that the data follow a Gaussian distribution, we obtain a negative lower limit, i.e., -0.09 mmol/l, which is meaningless, of course. Note that the parametric approach

using the logarithmically transformed serum triglyceride values and the non-parametric method both yield similar results for the lower limit but differ markedly on the upper limit. These results are consistent with the information presented in Figure 2-7*B*.

CONFIDENCE INTERVALS, TOLERANCE INTERVALS, AND PREDICTION INTERVALS

Thus far, we have been concerned with so-called point estimates, e.g., the estimation of the mean of a set using the data of a randomly selected subset of the larger set. Based on statistical reasoning, we may also construct various intervals for a number of purposes. Here we shall define three types of intervals: (1) confidence intervals, (2) tolerance intervals, and (3) prediction intervals.

Hahn (1970) has categorized these intervals on the basis of the characteristic of interest, i.e., location (mean), dispersion (standard deviation), and enclosure region, as well as on the basis of whether the interval is used to enclose a proportion of the population or to predict the results of future observations. Table 2-5 summarizes these intervals (Hahn, 1973).

The first two intervals (*confidence interval* and *tolerance interval*) are useful when the main interest is in describing a set, whereas a *prediction interval*, as the name indicates, pertains to the prediction of the values of future observations obtained from the set.

Confidence Intervals. An interval that can be claimed to contain a set parameter or other set property (e.g., a mean, a standard deviation, or a specified percentile) with a stated degree of confidence is known as a *confidence interval*. In computing a *confidence interval of the mean*, we first must specify the wanted confidence. Often 95 per cent is chosen. What is meant by 95 per cent confidence may be expressed as follows: In the long run (i.e., many samplings) 95 per cent of all "95 per cent confidence intervals" will contain the unknown set parameter. The width of the interval depends on the standard deviation s, the number of observations n, and the specified degree of confidence; if the corresponding distribution is symmetrical, the interval is usually computed as: $\bar{x} \pm ks$, where k is a constant, the magnitude of which depends on n and on the degree of confidence. The larger n

Table 2–4. COMPARISON OF INTERVALS*

TECHNIQUE USED	fP-GLUCOSE/(mmol/l)	
	Lower Value	Upper Value
parametric (Gaussian distribution)	4.09	5.64
non-parametric	4.05	5.60
	fP-TRIGLYCERIDE/(mmol/l)	
	Lower Value	Upper Value
parametric (Gaussian distribution)	−0.09	2.08
parametric (log-Gaussian distribution)	0.39	2.09
non-parametric	0.40	2.70

* Intervals determined by parametric approaches ($\bar{x} - 2s, \bar{x} + 2s$) vs. intervals delimited by the 2.5 and 97.5 percentile values determined by a nonparametrical method for a set of 200 plasma glucose values and for a set of 200 serum triglyceride values.

is, the smaller k will be (k approaches zero as n approaches infinity); and the larger the wanted confidence is, the larger k will be.

Tolerance Intervals. A *tolerance interval* is defined as an interval which can be claimed to contain at least a specified proportion p of the set with a specified degree of confidence. Unless otherwise specified, we will assume in the following that the observations follow a Gaussian distribution. A tolerance interval is usually computed in a manner analogous to that for the confidence interval, that is, $\bar{x} \pm k_1s$. However, in this case another factor

k_1 is used, which depends on n, the specified proportion p of the population to be contained, and the specified confidence with which we want to be sure that at least the proportion p of the population is contained within the interval. In Table 2–6, we present the computed tolerance intervals for various values of n to contain the proportion, 0.95, of the population with a confidence of 95 per cent for an observed subset with a mean of 10 units and a standard deviation of 1.0 unit. Note that as n increases, the width of the tolerance interval decreases; but unlike a confidence interval, it

Table 2–5. CATEGORIZATION OF SOME STATISTICAL INTERVALS*

CHARACTERISTIC OF INTEREST	AREA OF INFERENCE	
	Description of Population	Prediction of Results of Future Samples
Location (measured by the mean)	*Confidence interval* to contain the population mean	*Prediction interval* to contain the mean of m future observations.
Dispersion (measured by the standard deviation)	*Confidence interval* to contain the population standard deviation	*Prediction interval* to contain the standard deviation of m future observations
Enclosure region	*Tolerance interval* to contain a population proportion	*Prediction interval* to contain all of m future observations

*Modified from Hahn, G. J. and Nelson, W.: J. Qual. Tech., *5*:178, 1973.

Table 2-6. COMPUTED TOLERANCE INTERVALS AND PREDICTION INTERVALS*

NUMBER OF OBSERVATIONS	TOLERANCE INTERVAL	PREDICTION INTERVAL
4	6.4–13.6	3.6–16.4
5	7.0–13.0	5.0–15.0
6	7.2–12.8	5.6–14.4
7	7.4–12.6	6.0–14.0
8	7.5–12.5	6.3–13.7
10	7.6–12.4	6.6–13.4
15	7.8–12.2	7.0–13.0
20	7.9–12.1	7.2–12.8
30	7.9–12.1	7.4–12.6
40	7.9–12.1	7.5–12.5
60	8.0–12.0	7.7–12.3
∞	8.04–11.96	8.04–11.96

*Tolerance intervals contain 0.95 of the population with 95 per cent probability, and prediction intervals contain the *next observation* with 95 per cent probability. For a subset of observations with $\bar{x} = 10$ and $s = 1.0$.

approaches a constant length, e.g., $\bar{x} \pm 1.96s$, rather than zero.

Prediction Intervals. The term "prediction interval" signifies the upper and lower limits between which some future value(s) should fall. One can compute prediction intervals to contain the mean of m future observations, the standard deviation of the m future observations, or all m future observations (see Table 2-5). However, here we will be concerned only with a *prediction interval* to contain a single future observation, i.e., $m = 1$, with a specified probability, since a prediction interval to contain a single future observation is of most interest in a clinical situation.

We can construct a prediction interval from a set of reference values, assuming that the cumulative number fraction distribution of values follows the Gaussian distribution (either directly or after transformation), based upon n (number of previous observations), $\bar{x}$ (mean of the n observations), and s (their standard deviation). In addition, we must decide on what the probability should be that a new observation will fall within the interval subject to the condition that the new observation belongs to the set from which the reference values were obtained. The reader is referred to Hahn (1970) for the exact formulas and constants to use. However, in Table 2-6 we present the prediction intervals for the situation where the mean of the previous values is 10.0 units, the computed standard deviation is 1.0 unit, and the desired probability of containing the future observation is 0.95. We compare in this table the prediction intervals for various numbers n of previous observations. Note that the width of the prediction

interval is inversely dependent upon the magnitude of n. By contrast, we include the tolerance intervals computed for a 95 per cent confidence level and 0.95 fraction of the population. As n approaches infinity the widths of the two kinds of intervals both approach $\bar{x} \pm 1.96s$ (or in this case 8.04 to 11.96 units).

Bauer (1976) has suggested that we use a *prediction interval* rather than a *tolerance interval* in the clinical setting, since in the clinical situation we are not especially interested in describing the whole population, but rather are concerned with deciding on how likely a particular patient's value is, subject to the condition that it originated from the set of values from which the original data base (reference values) was obtained (or as we have heard so often: Is the patient's value normal?). It should be apparent that the term *reference interval* is very ambiguous, as it has no statistical meaning. One should preferentially construct a prediction interval based upon the desired probability.

REFERENCE VALUES CHARACTERIZING A GROUP OF HEALTHY SUBJECTS

The process of obtaining and characterizing reference values includes (1) defining the population of subjects, (2) the selection of subjects, (3) the obtaining, processing, and assaying of the specimens, and (4) the statistical analysis of the data.

The level of health should be specified based on criteria for inclusion or exclusion of subjects from whom reference values are obtained. The population from which reference subjects are selected should be clearly defined, and one of the components of this definition should be the criteria for good health. The latter criteria may have to be established prospectively, as, for example, in a geriatric population based on survival time subsequent to the collection of the specimen (Grasbeck, 1969).

SELECTION OF SUBJECTS

A comparison between an observed value and some reference values obtained from a group of reference individuals is meaningful only if the observed individual sufficiently resembles the reference individuals in all respects other than those under investigation. This condition is usually impossible to fulfill completely in the clinical setting. Even though compatibility can be assured with regard to all easily recognized demographic factors such as sex, age, and race, other factors may be overlooked and or may be impractical to control. For instance, reference values are obtained only from those subjects who are willing to contribute biologic specimens. Such a subset would *not* be a simple, randomly chosen subset of the population of healthy subjects we wish to characterize.

Age. Winsten (1976) has divided the various age groups into the following categories: *newborns, the prepubertal group, the adult population* (post-pubertal and pre-menopausal), and *the older adult population* (post-menopausal female and the male after the sixth decade). Table 2-7 from Winsten (1976) lists eight analytes in which there is a significant

difference between reference values obtained from neonates and from adult subjects. A comparison between a group of subjects in prepuberty and a comparable group of adults showed that the prepubertal subjects exhibited higher values of serum alkaline phosphatase, inorganic phosphate, aspartate aminotransferase, and lactate dehydrogenase, but significantly lower serum urate, cholesterol, creatinine, and total protein values. The mean activity value of alkaline phosphatase in the sera of a group of healthy prepubertal subjects was found to be four times higher than that for a group of healthy young adults (Statland, 1972). The difference was attributed solely to the higher bone isoenzyme activities found in the younger group (Kattwinkel, 1973).

The effects of advanced age upon the mean values of biochemical constituents in serum of adults often depend on the sex of the subjects. After the onset of menopause, the changes observed in females as a function of age are especially pronounced for a number of constituents. Wilding (1972) noted that changes due to or associated with menopause in females include increases in the serum concentrations of cholesterol, urate, and inorganic phosphate, and the serum activity of alkaline phosphatase. For both males and females there are common changes noted with advancing age—a decrease in serum albumin and total protein and an increase in serum urea, creatinine, glucose, cholesterol, and alkaline phosphatase. In the case of alkaline phosphatase the increase is mainly due to an increase in the serum concentration of the liver isoenzyme (O'Carroll, 1975).

Sex. The mean values for serum urate, creatinine, and urea are higher in healthy males than in female counterparts. Before the sixth decade males have higher values for serum triglycerides, cholesterol, sodium, and calcium; however, after the fifth decade of life, females generally have higher serum values of cholesterol, calcium, inorganic phosphate, and alkaline phosphatase (Leonard, 1973; Werner, 1975).

Race. Blacks demonstrate a higher mean value than whites for serum immunoglobulin IgG (20 per cent higher), IgM (35 per cent higher), and IgA (20 per cent higher). Oriental adults are reputed to have lower serum cholesterol values and higher serum urate values as compared with both whites and blacks (Winsten, 1976).

Pregnancy. Pregnant women were found

Table 2-7. RATIO OF ANALYTES IN THE BLOOD OF NEONATES TO THOSE IN ADULTS*

ANALYTE	RATIO OF MEAN VALUES
Bilirubin	7.5
Alkaline phosphatase	2.5
Ammonia	2.0
Phosphorus	1.9
Potassium	1.5
Cholesterol	0.5
Immunoglobulin IgM	0.1
Amylase	0.1

*Blood specimens obtained from healthy neonates and healthy adults. Modified from Winsten, S.: CRC Crit. Rev. Clin. Lab. Sci., *6*:319, 1976.

to have significantly lower mean values of serum calcium, glucose, urea, total protein, and albumin as compared with age-matched non-pregnant women; however, the pregnant group's mean values for serum urate, cholesterol, lactate dehydrogenase, aspartate aminotransferase, and alkaline phosphatase were higher (O'Kell, 1970). The difference in alkaline phosphatase values is due to the presence of the placental alkaline phosphatase isoenzyme in the serum of the pregnant woman.

Other Factors. The degree of obesity has been correlated positively with urate, glucose, and triglyceride concentration values in serum (Lellouch, 1973) and with the activity value in serum of alanine aminotransferase (Siest, 1975). The mean value of intestinal alkaline phosphatase isoenzyme activity in serum is higher in subjects who are blood type O, Lewis positive secretors. It should be noted that, theoretically at least, many of the observed differences between demographically different groups of subjects may be caused by factors other than those under investigation. For instance, observed differences between races may be caused by socioeconomic factors correlated with the racial differences among the subjects.

OBTAINING AND ASSAYING SPECIMENS

Having selected an appropriate group of subjects, both the preparation of the subject

Table 2–8. CLASSICAL STATISTICAL APPROACH FOR CALCULATING THE ESTIMATED HYPOTHETICAL POPULATION PARAMETERS BASED ON A RANDOMLY CHOSEN SUBSET OF VALUES*

1. Arrangement and inspection of subset of random observed values.
2. Hypothesis about distribution type of set of possible values.
3. Testing of fit between observed and hypothetical distribution. Assuming the hypothesis (Step 2) is accepted, Steps 4, 5, and 6 are ignored.
4. Rejection of hypothesis.
5. Transformation of observed values (log x; log (x + c); $1/x$; $\sqrt{x}$).
6. New hypothesis and testing.
7. Acceptance of hypothesis.
8. Calculation of estimates of hypothetical parameters (e.g., arithmetic mean; standard deviation).

*Modified from Dybkaer, R.: Automatisation and Prospective Biology, 1973.

prior to specimen collection and the analytical process, including the pre-instrumental and instrumental components, should be specified with the reference values. Factors known to influence the quantity should be controlled when the reference values are obtained only if it is at all practical to control them also in the clinical situation. In addition, compatibility with the clinical situation should be assured. For instance, in the case of serum albumin, reference values obtained from blood specimens drawn from subjects in the sitting position should not be used when assessing the serum albumin of a blood specimen drawn from a patient in the supine position, since albumin concentration in serum is markedly influenced by the body position (see p. 12).

STATISTICAL ANALYSIS OF THE DATA OBTAINED FROM HEALTHY SUBJECTS—THE USE OF DIRECT METHODS TO COMPUTE GROUP-BASED REFERENCE INTERVALS

Table 2-8 presents the classical statistical approach used to analyze the data obtained from a group of healthy subjects. As presented earlier in this chapter, one first attempts to fit a parametric probability distribution to the data. If the cumulative number fraction distribution of the data does not fit a cumulative Gaussian probability distribution, one of a number of transformations may be successful in changing the data to correspond to a Gaussian distribution, and the mean and standard deviation of the subset of values are computed on the transformed data. Alternatively, one may elect to use a non-parametric technique in analyzing the data.

Harris (1972a) has discussed various reasons why the data often do not correspond to the classical Gaussian probabilistic model. In obtaining reference values from a group of healthy subjects, usually only a single determination of the analyte is performed for each subject. The distribution of such values (a single sample distribution) reflects both inter-individual and intra-individual variances. The intra-individual variance (i.e., the variation over time of the quantity value measured in the same subject) includes the analytical variance and the physiologic variance. The inter-individual variance reflects the differences among the subjects' particular individual distributions. In principle, these distributions may vary from subject to subject with regard to shape, location, and variance or dispersion. Based on the assumption that a given quantity follows the same type of distribution for all subjects in a group of reference subjects, Harris (1972b) derived general expressions for the mean, variance, kurtosis, and skewness of the single sample distribution. Each individual's distribution is characterized by a mean (μ_i) and a variance (σ_i^2) where i refers to subject No i. If the intra-individual variances σ_i^2 are positively correlated with the individual's mean values (μ_i), the resulting single sample distribution will be positively skewed (a tail of high values) even if the distribution of μ_i is perfectly symmetric; and if the correlation is negative, it will be negatively skewed. Most single sample distributions of chemical constituents tend toward positive skewness and peakedness. On this basis, Harris (1972b) suggested a general two-step procedure for transforming laboratory data to eliminate or at least to reduce non-Gaussian characteristics. Assuming a simple functional relationship between the mean μ_i and the variance (σ_i^2), a general type of transformation which removes this dependency may be derived. Since the amount of data necessary to estimate the best transformation is quite large, he recommended using the best of the following transformations: $\sqrt{x}$, log x, and log (x + C), where C is a constant to be estimated from the data. Inter-subject variation in the σ_i^2's results in peakedness of the single sample distribution (positive kurtosis). Therefore, if a symmetric distribution results from the first transformation with a positive kurtosis due to residual inter-subject variation in the σ_i^2 independent of the mean values, a second transformation may be indicated and justified on theoretical grounds (Harris, 1972b).

STATISTICAL ANALYSIS OF THE DATA OBTAINED FROM UNSELECTED PATIENTS—THE USE OF INDIRECT METHODS TO COMPUTE GROUP-BASED REFERENCE INTERVALS

Two major problems present themselves to the investigator interested in producing reliable reference values from a group of healthy subjects: (1) being able to obtain specimens from a sufficiently large number of healthy subjects—Martin (1975) recommends a minimum of 300 subjects, and (2) being certain that the factors involved in the preparation of the subject and in the analytical procedure noted during the production of the reference values are the same (i.e., no bias) as the factors present during the day-to-day routine of obtaining and assaying patient specimens. To overcome these problems, an alternative approach for producing reference values has been recommended, namely obtaining and assaying specimens from each of a number of unselected patients and analyzing the results using indirect methods to characterize a hypothetical subset of the data which is compatible with data obtained from healthy subjects. The unselected patient population may consist of all individuals entering the outpatient department over a stated time interval or all patients admitted to the inpatient ward. The reasoning behind this approach is based on the observation that the number fraction distribution of patient data often has a peak near one end with skewing toward the other end where pathologic values predominate. Based on the assumption that the majority of values stem from subjects whose values are compatible with those of healthy subjects (in the sense that their values have not been altered by disease), various attempts have been made to devise methods to characterize the data set corresponding to these subjects. A number of graphical methods are based on the assumption that the values obtained from the mentioned population, which are compatible with those of healthy subjects, follow a Gaussian distribution and are fairly well separated from the pathologic values (Hoffman, 1963; Neumann, 1968; and Curnow, 1963).

Cichinelli (1963) assumed that patient data comprise a mixture of two data sets, each of which can be fitted to a Gaussian distribution. He fitted a composite probability density function to the data, based on a method programmed for a digital computer. Amador (1969) compared the results obtained by the above-mentioned methods in a hospital setting with the results obtained using healthy volunteers of both sexes covering a wide age span (17 to 82 years). The serum specimens from the latter group were obtained and processed by the same personnel, with the same reagents and equipment, and in the same analytical batches as were the serum specimens from the patients. The estimated means based on patient values were shifted towards pathologic values, and the standard deviations were larger as compared with the estimates based on the results obtained from the healthy subjects. Thus, it is likely that the indirect methods failed for one reason or another. However, theoretically, the discrepancy may be due to differences with regard to preparation of the subjects and/or demographic factors.

Martin (1975) suggested using a computerized least square technique by which clinical data are fitted to two or more probability density functions. Each function is allowed to have only one peak (i.e., one maximum). But it should be noted that the probability density functions do not have to be Gaussian. The proposed technique allows for various degrees of skewness of the probability density functions assumed to generate the data, and is thus made more general than the previously mentioned methods. The data set to be analyzed then is considered to comprise a mixture of data subsets, each of which is generated by a hypothetical probabilistic mechanism characterized by a probability density function. It should be noted that in order for this program to work, the number of data subsets, their relative representation in the total data set, and the parameters of the corresponding probability density functions should first be guessed by the user of the program and these estimates should then be used as input to the program in addition to the patient data. Furthermore, the guesses, which are usually based on inspection of the number fraction distribution of the data, should not be too much off if the program is to function. This requirement may be difficult or impossible to fulfill as soon as more than two probability density functions are postulated to generate the data. Thus, in practice, the applicability of the method is probably limited to the case of two, or at most three, functions.

Table 2-9. RELATIONSHIP OF "EXPECTED ABNORMAL" RESULTS TO NUMBER OF MEASURED CONSTITUENTS*

NUMBER OF MEASURED CONSTITUENTS	EXPECTED PERCENTAGE OF ONE OR MORE "ABNORMAL" RESULTS
1	5
2	10
4	19
6	26
10	40
15	54
20	64

*Calculated by $1 - (0.95)^n$, where n is equal to the number of tests.

The validity of all indirect statistical attempts to characterize a subset of values unaffected by disease may be questioned on the following grounds: first, since many diseases are represented in a sample of patients, it is likely that a large number of different data subsets are represented in the data, and second, the fact that a subgroup of patient results may fit a Gaussian or other probability density function does not in itself guarantee that it represents a group of patients whose values are unaffected by their disease.

MULTIVARIATE PREDICTION REGIONS

If one quantity is measured in a healthy subject, there is a 5 per cent chance that the observed value will be "abnormal" in the sense that it will fall outside the 95 per cent prediction interval. The more assays we perform on a healthy subject, the more likely we are to find an "abnormal" result. Assuming independence of the measured constituents, it can be demonstrated that for "n" constituents, the probability that at least one of "n" constituents will fall outside its 95 per cent prediction interval is: $1 - (0.95)^n$. Table 2-9 indicates the probability of obtaining an "abnormal" result as we increase the number of assays performed. This is a theoretical presentation and assumes independence of laboratory measurements and in this case is based upon the 95 per cent prediction interval. The introduction of multi-assay analyzers into the clinical laboratory has brought this theoretical issue into practical considerations, e.g., how can one justify the apparent occurrence of one or more "abnormal" results in a battery of 20 chemical measurements in 64 per cent of the population of healthy subjects? (Table 2-9). A number of approaches have been offered to resolve this dilemma: first, decrease the number of abnormal results by using a wider interval, e.g., a 99 per cent prediction interval. In the case of a 99 per cent prediction interval for 10 independent quantities, the per cent of "abnormal" results would be: $1 - (0.99)^n$, or approximately 9 per cent as compared to 40 per cent when we use a 95 per cent prediction interval. Second, assume *a priori* that 5 per cent of the population of healthy subjects should be outside the 95 per cent prediction interval irrespective of the number of assays performed. Thus, for "n" assays, we solve the equation: $0.05 = 1 - (x)^n$, with "x" being the probability used for each of "n" prediction intervals. Thus for 40 separate assays (n = 40), the computed probability for each quantity would be 99.86 per cent, in that, $1 - (0.9986)^{40} = 0.05$.

The Multivariate Gaussian Model. Both of the approaches presented above ignore the relationships among the quantities, i.e., the correlations of the various pairs of quantities. We will consider the case of two variates: X and Y, and assume that their joint distribution is Gaussian. The two-dimensional Gaussian distribution is characterized by five parameters, namely, the mean values of the two quantities and their variances, which together characterize the expected location of the observations, as well as their scatter and the correlation coefficient, which characterizes the expected relationship between the values of the two quantities. The means and the variances are estimated from the data in the same way as were those of the univariate Gaussian distribution. The correlation coefficient is estimated from the data by the following equation:

$$r_{xy} = \frac{\sum\limits_{i=1}^{n} [(x_i - \bar{x})(y_i - \bar{y})]}{\sqrt{\sum\limits_{i=1}^{n} (x_i - \bar{x})^2 \cdot \sum\limits_{i=1}^{n} (y_i - \bar{y})^2}}$$

where r_{xy} is the estimated correlation coefficient, x_i symbolizes the i'th observation of the first quantity, $\bar{x}$ is the average x value, y_i symbolizes the i'th observation of the second quantity, and $\bar{y}$ is the average y value. It is noted that the expression within the summation sign in the numerator is positive when both quantities are either above their mean values or below their mean values. Otherwise, the expression is negative. Thus, when the quantities are positively correlated the sum is positive and when they are negatively correlated it is negative.

As in the univariate case, where we compute a tolerance interval, in an analogous manner we can compute a tolerance *region*, which is defined to include, at least, a stated proportion of the population of pairs of values with a specified degree of confidence. Although such models have been examined from a theoretical perspective (Grams, 1972; Winkel, 1972), their applicability in practice has yet to be demonstrated.

REFERENCE VALUES CHARACTERIZING A SINGLE SUBJECT

An alternative to the use of reference values characterizing a *group* of subjects is to use the subject's previous values as a reference for any future value. In this latter approach a number of specimens are obtained from a subject over a stated period of time during which the subject is in the same well-defined state of health. All specimens are assayed for the analyte in question, and the results are used to compute an interval which will contain the measured value as assayed in a future specimen with a specified probability, assuming that the individual is still in the same state of health. We shall refer to such an interval as a subject-based prediction interval.

BIOLOGIC TIME-SERIES MODELS

Before we can define and compute a subject-based prediction interval, we must adopt some notion as to the appropriate model of biologic time-series which the concentration of the analyte follows. Must we assume a constant mean value (set point) over a long time interval (homeostatic model)? Should we allow a changing set point over time in a healthy subject (non-stationary model)? If we assume that the former model (fixed set point) is the more correct biologic model, then we should place equal weight on all values observed in a subject over past time. If we assume a non-stationary set point, then we would rely most heavily on the more recent values.

Harris (1975, 1976) reviewed three major statistical time-series models which belong to the class of so-called "auto-regressive models." Two extreme models, the "homeostatic model" and the "random-walk model," as well as an "intermediate (more general) model" were introduced. For many analytes, we may assume that the values obtained from healthy subjects follow the homeostatic model. In the homeostatic model it is assumed that the observed values fluctuate at random around a fixed set point. It is also postulated that these fluctuations are independent of each other. Such models are called *deterministic*, since random components in the models do not create any dependency among the measurements. Random biologic fluctuations relative to a fixed set point take place. However, the organism responds to these fluctuations by changing the concentration back to the set point. The salient point is that this counter-regulation is so fast relative to the time interval between consecutive measurements that the fluctuation reflected in any given measurement is without influence on the value of the subsequent measurement. However, if we shorten the length of the time interval sufficiently (i.e., increase the frequency of timed measurements), we will eventually reach a point at which measurements are no longer independent.

THE CHOICE OF A MODEL AND THE PROBLEM OF SPECIFYING AN ALTER-NATIVE HYPOTHESIS TO THAT IMPLIED BY THE MODEL

Once a model has been chosen, the next step is to predict future measured values on the basis of values already observed in a given subject. The clinician may have introduced a factor, e.g., a new therapeutic maneuver, that may cause a change of the measured value in addition to that induced by random biologic and analytical factors, or alternatively he may suspect that a significant shift has occurred in a patient secondary to a change in the course of the disease. In either of the two situations, the observed value would be compared with that predicted by the model chosen and a decision be made whether or not one should act on the assumption that the observed change is due to the influence of random biologic and analytical factors alone. For the model-specific computations involved in this process, the reader is referred to Harris (1975, 1976) for a detailed derivation and application. The results of such computations should not be accepted without some reservations, in that too many absurd, albeit statistically significant, changes may be encountered. Before the results are accepted, at least two conditions should be fulfilled: (1) a well-defined hypothesis alternative to that implied by the model should be formulated by the clinician, and (2) the preparation of the patient and the specimen, as well as the analytical procedure, should be under good control. When assuming either the random-walk model or the interme-

diate model, it is necessary for the time intervals between consecutive measurements to be constant. Furthermore, in the case of the intermediate model a considerable number of observations must be obtained because one must estimate a parameter specifying the dependency among observations in addition to estimating the usual parameters. The three models discussed above apply to the clinical situation, assuming that the disturbances of the physiologic mechanisms which influence the quantity values in blood probably occur more or less at random. However, in many cases, we do have some knowledge about the physiologic response to various types of disturbances, and this knowledge *should* be built into the models in some way. Ideally a physiologic model should be formulated. An example is the model stated by Winkel (1976). He relates the changes in plasma progesterone values during pregnancy to changes in the growth rate of the placenta and suggests that this model be used for the prediction of spontaneous abortion.

INTRA-INDIVIDUAL VARIA-TION IN HEALTHY SUBJECTS

Over 60 years ago, Rietz pointed out that under apparently identical conditions the quantitative measurement of physiologic functions shows considerable variability within the same subject. An assessment of the magnitude of this intra-individual variation may be obtained from the results determined on multiple specimens obtained from the same individual over time. Using the homeostatic model one would compute the intra-individual variation from the standard deviation of the quantity values as measured in the specimens. The magnitude of the observed intra-individual variation depends, of course, on the particular subject selected but also on the magnitude of the analytical variation and on the control of preparation of the subject prior to specimen collection described in Chapter 1.

For a given quantity, a given individual, a given analytical procedure, and a defined preparation of the subject, the magnitude of the intra-individual variation may also depend on the times at which the specimens are obtained as well as the total time period over which the specimens are obtained. Thus, the term "intra-individual variation" should be further qualified to be meaningful. Accepting the homeostatic model, variation around the subject's set point may still be partially systematic in nature. However, as long as we do not have a meaningful physiologic theory as to what the nature of such a variation may be, the most practical and clinically relevant approach seems to be to relate the variation to time of day and to date of collection of specimen. Therefore, we partition the intra-individual variation into two major components: (1) a within-day variation relative to the daily mean value and (2) a day-to-day variation of the daily mean value relative to the set point.

Within-day Variation. The within-day variation may be systematic in the sense that the same pattern of variation is repeated from day to day for all the reference subjects (group-specific diurnal variation) and/or for each particular subject (subject-specific diurnal variation). In the latter case each person has a particular pattern of changes that is repeated from day to day. However, the patterns vary from individual to individual. The pattern is a function of the number of specimens obtained from each subject per day as well as the specific times of day at which the specimens are obtained. The remaining nonsystematic within-day biologic variations are referred to as random biologic fluctuations. Thus, the within-day variation is partitioned into three components: (1) group-specific diurnal variation, (2) subject-specific diurnal variation, and (3) random biologic fluctuations.

Winkel (1975) found that for the majority of the more commonly ordered serum constituents (hormones excluded) as measured in healthy subjects, the systematic diurnal components of variation are unimportant from a quantitative point of view as compared with the day-to-day variation or to the random biologic fluctuations. The case of serum potassium is the notable exception. Over 70 per cent of the total biologic variation for potassium is related to the subject's personal diurnal variation, which is consistent from day-to-day and also independent of any group diurnal variation. A clinically important within-day variation (mainly random biologic variation) has been seen for the serum concentration of iron, triglycerides, fatty acids, bilirubin, and amino acids as well as for a number of hormones in the sera of healthy subjects (Halberg, 1975; Statland, 1977b).

Day-to-day Variation. Fawcett (1956) assessed the day-to-day variation of the plasma concentrations of electrolytes and total proteins. Williams (1970), using the statistical technique of analysis of variance, examined the day-to-day variation of a number of quantities in healthy subjects. This latter study, as well as the majority of other studies of the intra-individual variation in healthy subjects, is based on assaying multiple specimens obtained from each of a number of subjects with one specimen obtained per subject per day and always at the same time of day (usually in the morning). Using such an experimental design, the observed intra-individual physiologic variation will reflect the variation of the subject's daily means relative to his set point plus any random biologic fluctuations, excluding systematic diurnal variations. Table 2-10 summarizes the results of a number of such studies. The results presented in the table are based on studies where the duration varied from two to four weeks and the time interval between the collection of consecutive specimens from the same subject varied from one to seven days. For each serum constituent and for each study the reported average intra-individual variation is expressed in terms of coefficient of variation (i.e., $(s/\bar{x})) \times 100$. It is noteworthy that for the majority of constituents, the intra-individual physiologic variation is remarkably consistent from study to study (Table 2-10).

The electrolyte concentrations in serum are controlled within narrow limits by healthy subjects. For electrolytes, the intra-individual physiologic day-to-day variation is relatively small, generally less than 5 per cent. Note how much tighter creatinine is maintained as compared to urea (Table 2-10). The pronounced day-to-day physiologic variations in urea and triglyceride probably reflect inconsistencies in dietary habits. Figure 2-8 illustrates the dramatic day-to-day variation in serum iron values in two healthy young adults. This variation is almost exclusively of a biologic nature (Statland, 1977). Apart from alkaline phosphatase and gammaglutamyl transferase, most enzymes in serum which we commonly measure in the laboratory vary greatly from day to day. This may be explained by inconsistent patterns of physical activity from day to day and possibly by variation in food intake and/or ethanol consumption. Furthermore, these enzymes, as well as bilirubin and urea, for example, should probably be regarded as waste products that have no function to carry out in the extracellular space. Therefore, from

Table 2–10.   INTRA-INDIVIDUAL PHYSIOLOGIC DAY-TO-DAY COEFFICIENT OF VARIATION × 100 OF COMMONLY ORDERED CLINICAL CHEMICAL ANALYTES*

ANALYTE	COEFFICIENT OF VARIATION × 100					REFERENCE†
Electrolytes						
Sodium	0.7,	1.4,	0.5			a, d, f
Potassium	4.3,	5.0,	4.6,	6.2		a, c, d, f
Calcium	1.7,	1.7,	1.6,	1.6		a, c, d, f
Magnesium	1.3,	2.3				c, d
Chloride	2.1,	1.4,	2.1			a, c, d
Phosphate	5.8,	7.5,	9.6,	6.8		a, c, d, f
Metabolites						
Urea	12.3,	13.3,	11.9,	13.6,	11.1	a, b, c, d, f
Creatinine	4.3,	7.5,	4.4			a, b, d
Urate	7.3,	8.3,	10.1,	8.5		a, b, c, d
Bilirubin	22.0,	26.0				a, f
Glucose	5.6,	6.5				c, d
Iron	26.6,	24.5,	29.3			a, g, h
Cholesterol	5.3,	6.4,	4.2,	4.8,	6.6	a, c, d, e,
Triglycerides	25.0,	18.0,	15.9			e, i, j
Enzymes						
Acid phosphatase	9.9					a
Alkaline phosphatase	4.8,	7.0,	5.7,	3.5,	6.4	a, b, d, e, f
γ-Glutamyl transferase	3.9					e
Lactate dehydrogenase	12.1,	4.7,	9.0,	7.3,	5.5	a, b, c, d, e
Aspartate aminotransferase	24.2,	8.3,	7.8,	10.9		a, b, d, e
Alanine aminotransferase	26.4,	13.2				a, e
Creatine kinase	25.7					e
Proteins						
Total protein	2.9,	2.8,	2.2,	3.0		a, c, d, f
Albumin	2.8,	3.9,	3.0,	3.2		a, c, d, f
Transferrin	2.5					e
α$_1$-antitrypsin	2.9					e
α$_2$-macroglobulin	3.1					e
IgG	2.7					e
IgA	3.5					e
IgM	3.1					e
Complement C3	3.8					e
Complement C4	5.9					e
Haptoglobin	8.8					e
Orosomucoid	11.1					e

*Analytes measured in the serum of healthy subjects.
†References:
(a) P. Winkel, H. Bokelund, and B. E. Statland: Clin. Chem., *20:*1520, 1974.
(b) P. Winkel, and B. E. Statland: Clin. Chem., *22:*1855, 1976.
(c) G. Z. Williams, D. S. Young, M. R. Stein, and E. Cotlove: Clin. Chem., *16:*1016, 1970.
(d) D. S. Young, E. K. Harris, and E. Cotlove: Clin. Chem., *17:*403, 1971.
(e) B. E. Statland, and P. Winkel: CRC Crit. Rev. Clin. Lab. Sci., *8:*105, 1977.
(f) J. F. Pickup, E. K. Harris, M. Kearns, and S. S. Brown: Clin. Chem., *23:*842, 1977.
(g) K. Hoyer: Acta Med. Scand., *119:*562, 1944.
(h) B. E. Statland, and P. Winkel: Am. J. Clin. Pathol., *67:*84, 1977.
(i) G. R. Warnick, and J. J. Albers: Lipids, *11:*203, 1975.
(j) L. E. Hollister, W. G. Beckman, and M. Baker: Am. J. Med. Sci., *248:*329, 1964.

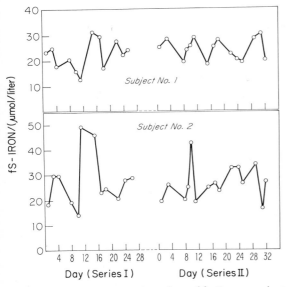

Serum Iron Values in Two Subjects
over Two Series

Figure 2–8. Mean concentration values of fasting serum iron in each of two healthy subjects on each of 12 days in Series I and on each of 15 days in Series II. (Modified from Statland, B.E., and Winkel, P.: Am. J. Clin. Pathol., *67*:84, 1977.)

a teleologic point of view at least, there is no reason for the body to regulate the concentration of these constituents very closely. Note the narrow limits within which the human organism controls specific protein concentrations in serum. This fact, coupled with the relatively large inter-individual variation for specific proteins in serum, demonstrates the insensitivity of group-specific reference intervals for detecting changes in these constituents due to pathologic processes.

ASSESSING THE NEED FOR USING THE SUBJECT AS HIS OWN REFERENT

The homeostatic model assumes that for a given healthy subject the mean of the observed values over time is constant. Using this model, one is able to determine the variation occurring within an individual over time over a series of values. The *ratio value* (Harris, 1974) is defined as the ratio of the physiologic intra-individual variation over the biologic inter-individual variation (for statistical details the reader is referred to Harris (1974)). The analytical variation should be separated

in the computations. The inter-individual variation reflects the variation among the subjects with regard to their mean values or set points, and the intra-individual variation is the average variation over time of the observed values relative to the set point.

Table 2–11 shows the ratio values compiled from two different studies (Winkel, 1975; Statland, 1977a). As noted, we have arranged the ratios in ascending order and have divided the analytes into four groups on the basis of ratio values: group I, 0.01–0.20; group II, 0.21–0.40; group III, 0.41–1.00; group IV, 1.01–10.00. The ratio values should be used only as rough guidelines, since the magnitude of the inter-individual variation depends on the demographic characteristics of the group examined, and, as mentioned previously, the magnitude of the intra-individual variation is dependent upon the times at which the specimens were obtained, the time period of the study during which the subjects were observed, and the degree of control of the preparation of the subjects prior to specimen collection. Figure 2–9, which presents the actual values of serum concentrations of immunoglobulin IgM for nine healthy subjects, illustrates the small magnitude of the intra-individual variation relative to the inter-individual variation for serum IgM.

Use of Subject-based Prediction Intervals. For those analytes demonstrating a very low ratio value (groups I and II in Table 2–11), there should be a considerable gain in sensitivity when relying on subject-based prediction intervals rather than on group-based prediction intervals. For the analytes in groups I and II, the group-based prediction interval would be too insensitive as compared with the subject-based prediction interval in identifying a subject in whom a "present value" is outside of his personal, subject-based interval. As noted in Table 2–11, the analytes found in groups I and II consist of the specific proteins, the enzymes—alkaline phosphatase and γ-glutamyl transferase—and the lipids—cholesterol and triglycerides. Among the analytes found in group IV are those quantities known to affect physiologic functions when they are only "slightly abnormal," e.g., calcium, potassium, sodium, and albumin. Although the values of the intra-individual variation are relatively consistent from study to study (Table 2–10), the ratio values (Table 2–11) may show a good deal of variation from study to study, probably owing to demo-

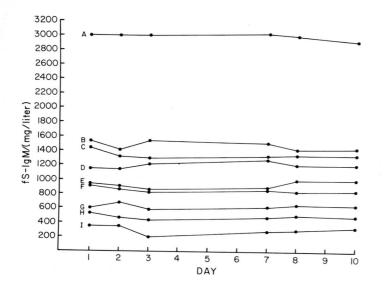

Figure 2–9. Mean concentration values of serum IgM from each of nine fasting healthy subjects (A–I) over a ten-day period. (Modified from Statland, B.E., Winkel, P., and Killingsworth, L.: Clin. Chem., *22:*1635, 1976.)

graphic differences among the groups of subjects studied (Winkel, 1977).

PRESENTATION OF CLINICAL LABORATORY RESULTS

As described previously in Chapter 1, the final product of the analytical procedure is the written (or printed) report. The report must include patient-identification data, the date and time of day when the specimen was obtained, the type of specimen obtained, the component assayed, the analytical result, and the units. Additional information which may be helpful in interpreting the results includes pertinent demographic data (e.g., age, sex) and relevant factors relating to the preparation of the patient (e.g., fasting, posture). Finally, the report may also contain the relationship of the given analytical result to the results obtained from a set of reference values. Three major approaches have been advocated for this last purpose: (1) merely printing

Table 2-11. RATIO VALUES* FOR SELECTED ANALYTES IN THE BLOOD OF HEALTHY SUBJECTS†

ANALYTE	RATIO VALUE	ANALYTE	RATIO VALUE
Group I		*Group III*	
IgM	0.06	Lactate dehydrogenase	0.44
IgA	0.09	Alanine aminotransferase	0.45
Haptoglobin	0.12	Creatinine	0.47
Alkaline phosphatase	0.14	Creatine kinase	0.56
IgG	0.15	Urea	0.73
γ-Glutamyl transferase	0.16	Aspartate aminotransferase	0.90
Complement C3	0.17	Urate	1.00
Complement C4	0.19		
α_1-antitrypsin	0.19	*Group IV*	
α_2-macroglobulin	0.19	Total protein	1.04
		Chloride	1.05
Group II		Iron	1.15
Cholesterol	0.25	Potassium	1.19
Transferrin	0.26	Sodium	1.75
Orosomucoid	0.26	Calcium	2.83
Hemoglobin	0.29	Albumin	5.60
Triglycerides	0.36		

*Physiologic intra-individual standard deviation over biologic inter-individual standard deviation.
†Modified from Winkel, P., and Statland, B. E.: Contemp. Topics Anal. Clin. Chem., *1:*287, 1977.

a suitable tolerance interval (should be *prediction interval*—see earlier discussion) computed from the reference values so that the clinician will be able to note if the present value is outside the stated limits; (2) computing the distance from the given result to the mean of the reference values using the standard deviation of the reference values as a unit, e.g., assuming a mean of 10, standard deviation of 2, and a given result of 16, the distance would be equal to $\frac{16 - 10}{2} = \frac{6}{2} = $ "+3" standard deviations; and (3) determining the smallest interval of percentile values (as determined from the reference values) which contains the observed value and then reporting the corresponding two percentiles.

CONCLUSION

Any of the methods used to determine group-based or subject-based reference intervals should be validated on the basis of additional clinical confirmation. This confirmation can be gained by looking at the patient's chart for variates relating to historical findings, physical examination, and/or other supporting data. In addition, prospective studies should be undertaken to validate the usefulness of producing subject-based prediction intervals. Such information would be invaluable to allow us to go from our statistical formulations to verified clinical utility.

REFERENCES

Amador, E., and Hsi, B. P.: Indirect methods for estimating the normal range. Am. J. Clin. Pathol., *52*:538, 1969.

Bauer, S.: Precognition in the laboratory: Prediction intervals and their applications. Clin. Chem., *22*:1183, 1976.

Brunden, M. N., Clark, J. J., and Sutter, M. L.: A general method of determining normal ranges applied to blood values of dogs. Am. J. Clin. Pathol., *53*:332, 1970.

Cichinelli, A. L.: The composite of two Gaussian distributions as a model for blood pressure distribution in man. Ph.D. Thesis, University of Michigan, 1963.

Curnow, D. H., and Sheard, K.: The use of probability paper in analyzing frequency distribution. Clin. Chem., *9*:462, 1963.

Dybkaer, R.: Production and presentation of reference values. Proc. 2nd Int. Colloquium "Automatisation and Prospective Biology," Pont-à-Mousson, 1972. Basel, Karger, 1973, p. 2.

Fawcett, J. K., and Wynn, V.: Variation of plasma electrolytes and total protein levels in the individual. Br. Med. J., *2*:582, 1956.

Galen, R. S.: The normal range. Arch. Pathol. Lab. Med., *101*:561, 1977.

Grams, R. R., Johnson, E. A., and Benson, E. S.: Laboratory data analysis system: Section III—Multivariate normality. Am. J. Clin. Pathol., *58*:133, 1972.

Grasbeck, R., and Saris, N. E.: Establishment and use of normal values. Scand. J. Clin. Lab. Invest., *24*(Suppl. 110):62, 1969.

Hahn, G. J.: Statistical intervals for a normal population, Part I. Tables, examples, and applications, J. Qual. Tech., *2*:115, 1970.

Hahn, G. J. and Nelson, W.: A survey of prediction intervals and their applications. J. Qual. Tech., *5*:178, 1973.

Halberg, F.: Biological rhythms, Adv. Exp. Med. Biol., *54*:1, 1975.

Harris, E. K.: Effects of intra- and inter-individual variation on the appropriate use of normal ranges. Clin. Chem., *20*:1531, 1974.

Harris, E. K.: Some theory of reference values. I. Stratified normal ranges and a method for following an individual's clinical laboratory values. Clin. Chem., *21*:1457, 1975.

Harris, E. K.: Some theory of reference values: II. Comparison of some statistical models of intra-individual variation in blood constituents. Clin. Chem., *22*:1343, 1976.

Harris, E. K., and DeMets, D. L.: Effects of intra- and inter-individual variation on distributions of single measurements. Clin. Chem., *18*:244, 1972a.

Harris, E. K., and DeMets, D. L.: Estimation of normal ranges and cumulative proportions by transforming observed distributions to Gaussian form. Clin. Chem., *18*:605, 1972b.

Henry, R. J.: Clinical Chemistry Principles and Technics. New York, Hoeber, 1964, p. 364.

Herrera, L.: The precision of percentiles in establishing normal limits in medicine. J. Lab. Clin. Med., *52*:34, 1958.

Hoffman, R. G.: Statistics in the practice of medicine. J.A.M.A., *185*:864, 1963.

Kattwinkel, J., Taussing, L. M., Statland, B. E., and Verter, J. I.: The effects of age on alkaline phosphatase and other serologic liver function tests in normal subjects and patients with cystic fibrosis. J. Pediatr., *82*:234, 1973.

Lellouch, J., and Claude, J. R.: A study of several biological parameters measured in a large population of a single profession. II. Factors which may affect the 'normal values.' Proc. 2nd Int. Colloquium "Automatisation and Prospective Biology," Pont-à-Mousson, 1972. Basel, Karger, 1973, p. 100.

Leonard, P. J.: The effect of age and sex on biochemical parameters in blood of healthy human subjects. Proc. 2nd Int. Colloquium "Automatisation and Prospective Biology," Pont-à-Mousson, 1972. Basel, Karger, 1973, p. 134.

Martin, H. F., Gudzinowicz, B. J., and Fanger, H.: Normal Values in Clinical Chemistry: A Guide to Statistical Analysis of Laboratory Data. New York, Marcel Dekker, Inc., 1975.

Neumann, G. J.: Determination of normal ranges from laboratory data. Clin. Chem., *14*:979, 1968.

O'Carroll, D., Statland, B. E., Steele, B. W., and Burke, M. D.: Chemical inhibition method for alkaline phosphatase isoenzymes in human serum. Am. J. Clin. Pathol., *63*:4, 564, 1975.

O'Kell, R. T., and Ellott, J. R.: Development of normal values for use in multitest biochemical screening of sera. Clin. Chem., *16*:161, 1970.

Reed, A. H., Henry, R. J., and Mason, W. B.: Influence of statistical methods used on the resulting estimate of normal range. Clin. Chem., *17*:275, 1971.

Rietz, H. L., and Mitchell, H. H.: On the metabolism experiment as a statistical problem. J. Biol. Chem., *8*:297, 1910.

Siest, G., Schiele, F., Galteau, M-M., et al.: Aspartate aminotransferase and alanine aminotransferase activities in plasma: Statistical distributions, individual variations, and reference values. Clin. Chem., *21*:1077, 1975.

Snedecor, G. W., and Cochran, W. G.: Statistical Methods. Ames, Iowa, The Iowa State University Press, 1967.

Statland, B. E., and Winkel, P.: Effects of non-analytical factors on the intra-individual variation of analytes in the blood of healthy subjects: Consideration of preparation of the subject and time of venipuncture. CRC Crit. Rev. Clin. Lab. Sci., *8*:105, 1977a.

Statland, B. E., and Winkel, P.: The relationship of the day-to-day variation of serum iron concentration values to the iron binding capacity values in a group of healthy young women. Am. J. Clin. Pathol., *67*:84, 1977b.

Statland, B. E., Young, D. S., and Nishi, H. N.: Serum alkaline phosphatase: Total activity and isoenzyme determinations made by use of centrifugal fast analyzer. Clin. Chem., *18*:12, 1972.

Werner, M., and Marsh, W. L.: Normal values: Theoretical and practical aspects. CRC Crit. Rev. Clin. Lab. Sci., *6*:81, 1975.

Wilding, P., and Rollason, J. G.: Detection of menopausal changes in biochemical constituents in well population screening. Scand. J. Clin. Lab. Invest., *29*(Suppl. 126):21, 1972.

Williams, G. Z., et al.: Biological and analytical components of variation in long-term studies of serum constituents in normal subjects. I. Objectives, subject selection, laboratory procedures, and estimation of analytical deviation; II. Estimating biological components of variation; III. Physiological and medical implications. Clin. Chem., *16*:1016, 1022, 1028, 1970.

Winkel, P., and Statland, B. E.: Using the subject as his own referent in assessing day-to-day changes of laboratory test results. Contemp. Topics Anal. Clin. Chem., *1*:287, 1977.

Winkel, P., Gaede, P., and Lyngbye, J.: Method for monitoring plasma progesterone concentrations in pregnancy. Clin. Chem., *22*:422, 1976.

Winkel, P., Lyngbye, J., and Jørgensen, K.: The normal region—a multivariate problem. Scand. J. Clin. Lab. Invest., *30*:339, 1972.

Winkel, P., Statland, B. E., and Bokelund, H.: The effects of venipuncture on variation of serum constituents: Consideration of within-day and day-to-day changes in a group of healthy young men, Am. J. Clin. Pathol., *64*:433, 1975.

Winsten, S.: The ecology of normal values in clinical chemistry. CRC Crit. Rev. Clin. Lab. Sci., *6*:319, 1976.

Wootton, I. D. P., and King, E. J.: Normal values for blood constituents. Lancet, *1*:470, 1953.

3

THEORY AND PRACTICE OF LABORATORY TECHNIQUE

E. George Linke, Ph.D.,
John Bernard Henry, M.D.,
and Bernard E. Statland, M.D., Ph.D.

The clinical laboratory worker undertakes a wide variety of maneuvers to obtain an end result. An adequate understanding of each process enables the investigator to achieve more nearly optimum experimental conditions and, consequently, to improve the accuracy and precision of each measurement. Collection, processing, and preparation of the specimen prior to analysis must receive prime consideration. Validity of data obtained on the specimen itself is highly dependent upon the excellence of laboratory technique, including proper manipulation of equipment, use of reagents of specified purity, and environmental control. The purpose of this chapter is to equip the laboratorian with fundamental knowledge prerequisite to skillful technique in each step of an analysis, keeping always in mind resultant improved patient care.

SPECIMEN COLLECTION

BLOOD

Chemical analysis of blood and other body fluids requires special attention to specimen collection and processing (Winsten, 1965). Since blood is the most frequent specimen analyzed in clinical chemistry and other body fluids are reviewed in appropriate chapters, this specimen merits special consideration. Various sources of bias presenting during the preparation of the subject for venipuncture are reviewed in Chapter 1.

Venipuncture with vacuum containing systems is ideal in terms of direct sampling, economy, and efficiency. These systems provide flexibility in terms of specimen volume (2, 3, 5, 7, or 10 ml per tube) and anticoagulant

Table 3–1. GUIDE FOR PROPER SPECIMEN TUBE SELECTION*

Blood Bank—7 ml Plain Tube (red top)
  Antibody detection (screen) (2 tubes)
  Antibody identification (2 tubes)
  Antiglobulin (direct & indirect) (DAG & IAG)
  Erythrocyte typing (ABO & Rh)
  Erythrocyte typing (extended)
  Open heart evaluation (ABO, Rh genotype, DAG,
    IAG) (3 tubes)
  Prenatal evaluation (ABO, Rh genotype, IAG) (2
    tubes)
      (ABO, Rh) and crossmatch (compatibility) (1 tube
        for 3 units)
      (ABO, Rh) and screen (antibody detection) (2
        tubes)

Blood Bank—Histocompatibility—7 ml Na Heparin
  (green top)
  HLA (A & B) lymphocyte typing
  HLA (cytotoxic) antibody detection
  MLC (HLA-D) mixed lymphocyte culture

Chemistry—7 ml Plain Tube (red top)*
  Acetaminophen† (Tylenol)
  Acetone
  Albumin
  Aldolase
  Alanine aminotransferase (ALT) or (GPT)
  Alcohol (do not use alcohol swab)
  Amylase (AMS)
  Aspartate aminotransferase (AST) or (GOT)
  Barbiturate screen
  Bilirubin
  Bromide
  BUN (blood urea nitrogen)
  Calcium (total)
  Carotene
  Cholesterol
  Cholinesterase (CMS)
  Copper
  Cortisol
  Creatine kinase (CK) and CK isoenzymes
  Creatinine
  Digoxin
  Digitoxin
  Electrolytes (Na, K, Cl, CO_2)
  Electrophoresis
  Ethosuximide (Zarontin)
  Folate

  FSH (follicle stimulating hormone)
  Free thyroxine (free T_4)
  Glucose
  Growth hormone
  Iron and iron binding capacity
  Lactate dehydrogenase (LD) & LD isoenzymes
  Leucine aminopeptidase (LAP)
  Lipase (LPS)
  Lipoprotein electrophoresis
  Lithium
  Long acting thyroid stimulator (LATS)
  Luteinizing hormone (LH)
  Magnesium
  Osmolality
  Parathyroid hormone (2 full tubes)
  Phenobarbital
  Phenytoin (Dilantin)
  Phosphorus
  Phosphatase, acid (ACP)
  Phosphatase, alkaline (ALP)
  Primidone (Mysoline)
  Procainamide
  Prolactin
  Propranolol
  Pseudocholinesterase
  Salicylate
  SMA 6-60 (Na, K, Cl, CO_2, BUN, Glu)
  T_3-RIA
  Testosterone
  Theophylline
  Thiocyanate
  Thyroid binding globulin (TBG)
  Thyroid stimulating hormone (TSH)
  Total protein
  Total thyroxine (T_4-RIA)
  Triglyceride
  Uric acid
  Vitamin B_{12}
  Vitamin B_{12} (unsaturated binding capacity)

Chemistry—5 ml Na Heparin (green top)
  Ammonia (on ice)
  Carboxyhemoglobin and oxygen saturation
  Cholinesterase (CHS)
  Erythrocyte potassium (K)
  Methemoglobin
  pH
  Plasma hemoglobin

Table 3-1. GUIDE FOR PROPER SPECIMEN TUBE SELECTION* (continued)

Chemistry—5 ml NaF Oxalate (gray top)
    Glucose
    Glucose tolerance
    Lactate (on ice)
    Lactose tolerance

Chemistry—7 ml Versene Tube EDTA (lavender top)
    Carcinoembryonic antigen (CEA) (2 tubes)
    Renin (2 tubes, on ice)

Chemistry—10 ml Chemically Clean (red top)
    Lead

Hematology—4.5 ml Na Citrate Tube (blue top)—must
        be full
    Factor assays (coagulation)
    Fibrinogen level
    G-6-PD assay (also 1 lavender top)
    Partial thromboplastin time (PTT)
    Prothrombin time (PT)
    Thrombin time (TT)

Hematology—7 ml Versene Tube (lavender top)
    CBC (WBC, RBC, Hgb, Hct, MCV, MCH, MCHC)
    Differential count
    Erythrocyte sedimentation rate (ESR)—tube must be
        full (Westergren)
    Glucose-6-phosphate dehydrogenase screen (G-6-PD)
    Hgb electrophoresis
    Platelet count
    Reticulocyte count
    Sickle cell preparation
    Total eosinophil count
    Zeta sedimentation rate (ZSR)—tube must be full

Hematology—7 ml (red top)*
    Haptoglobin
    LE preparation
    Serum viscosity (3 full tubes)

Immunology-Serology—7 ml (red top)
    Alpha-1-antitrypsin
    Alpha-1-fetoprotein
    Anti-DNA
    Anti-DNAse B
    Antihyaluronidase (AHA)
    Antinuclear antibody (ANA)
    Antistreptolysin O (ASO)
    Antithyroid antibody

Immunology-Serology—7 ml (red top) (continued)
    Aspergillus antibody
    Brucella antibody
    Candida antibody
    Ceruloplasmin
    C_1 esterase inhibitor
    CH_{50} (total hemolytic complement)
    Cold agglutinins
    Complement
        C_3
        C_4
        C_3A (Factor B)
    Cryoglobulin
    Extractable nuclear antibodies
        Anti-Sm
        Anti-DNP
    Farmer's lung antibodies
    Fluorescent treponemal antibody absorption (FTA-
        ABS)
    Franciscella agglutinins
    Hepatitis associated antigen (HAA, HB_sAg)
    Heterophile antibody
    IgE
    Immunoelectrophoresis
    "Lung" antibodies
    Lysozyme
    Monospot
    Muramidase
    Proteus agglutinins
    Rheumatoid factor
    Rubella antibodies
    Salmonella agglutinins
    Thyroid antibody
    Toxoplasma IFA
    VDRL

Immunology-Serology—7 ml Na Heparin (green top)
    (*Note:* These tests must be scheduled with the Im-
        munology Laboratory)
    Nitroblue tetrazolium (NBT)
    Phagocytosis—2 tubes (1 plain tube must accompany)
    T and B cells—3 tubes (1 versene tube must accom-
        pany)

Immunology-Serology—Special tubes from Immunology
    Lymphocyte proliferation
    Phytohemagglutinin (PHA)

---

*No additive, silicone coated.
†2 to 3 tests can be done per tube, unless otherwise specified.

(heparin, oxalate, citrate, or ethylenediamine-tetraacetic acid salts), as well as chemically clean or sterile glassware. Disposable needles eliminate the hazard of serum hepatitis transmission, and an adapter with holder may be used for selection of appropriate gauge needle when necessary. While rubber stoppers are color-coded to distinguish whether the test tube contains a specific anticoagulant, is a plain tube, or is a special tube made chemically clean (e.g., for lead, iron, and iodine determinations), a color-coded label may also be applied to insure appropriate tube selection and proper identification of specimen in terms of patient's name, hospital number, date, and time of collection. Serum is used for many analyses because of potential interference by the various anticoagulants (see Chap. 1). Whole blood with anticoagulant yields the frequently analyzed blood component known as plasma. Heparin in the form of a lithium salt is an effective anticoagulant in small quantities without significant effect on many determinations and is the ideal universal anticoagulant for blood from which plasma may be harvested (Table 3-1). For glucose measurements fluoride may be added to heparin. Fluoride inhibits glycolysis of the blood cells that may otherwise destroy glucose at the rate of about 5 per cent per hour. In the presence of bacterial contamination of blood specimens, fluoride inhibition of glycolysis is neither adequate nor effective in preserving glucose concentration. Furthermore, prompt separation of plasma or serum from cells is important to yield a proper specimen for most chemical determinations.

While a pediatric vacuum system is practical for single or occasional blood specimen collections from infants after three months of age with small (2 or 3.5 ml) volume tubes, a micro-sampling technique is required for newborn infants and children as well as for adults who require frequent blood specimen collections to evaluate repetitive sequential measurements and examinations (Fig. 3-1). With aseptic technique, a deliberate skin puncture sufficient in depth to assure free blood flow from finger, big toe, or heel is made with either a long point microlance or regular microlance (Becton-Dickinson, Rutherford, N.J. 07070), depending on the amount of blood to be collected (Fig. 3-2). When 70 per cent alcohol-soaked sponges are used to prepare puncture site, a sterile 2 by 2-inch gauze pad should be applied to the site subsequently for final removal of all alcohol (when area is not dry) in order to prevent hemolysis of specimen and ensure that reasonable spherical bubbles of blood exude from the puncture site. Anhydrous ether or Wescodyne (West Chemical Products, Inc., Long Island City, N.Y.) may be substituted for alcohol in preparation of skin; the latter is preferred when oxygen is being used in the area. From the puncture site, free-flowing blood may be collected in capillary tubes or a B-D Microtainer (Fig. 3-1) capillary blood serum separator by capillary attraction and gravity.

We have found the Caraway micro blood-collecting tube No. A-2934 satisfactory (Clay Adams, Inc., 141 E. 25th Street, N.Y. 10010)—length, 75 mm; inside diameter, 2 mm; outside diameter, 4 mm. However, microsampling techniques are best evolved to meet specific or predominant patient care requirements. This is especially true in regard to the selection of capillary tubes or other microcontainers. For the infant who requires a single total bilirubin measurement, a single capillary collection tube may suffice, but if several measurements are to be performed with a microsimultaneous

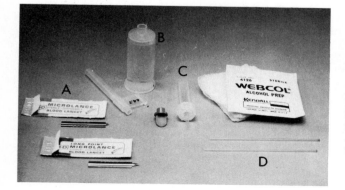

Figure 3-1. Equipment for Fingerstick Blood Drawing, observing from left to right: *A,* Regular lancet over long lancet (Becton-Dickinson and Company, Rutherford, New Jersey 07070); *B,* Unopette, No. 5840—for Hematology CBC (complete blood count) (Becton-Dickinson and Company); *C,* Microtainer Capillary Blood Serum Separator (Becton-Dickinson and Company) with cap; and *D,* Micro-Hematocrit Tubes (Clay Adams/Becton-Dickinson, Parsippany, New Jersey 07054).

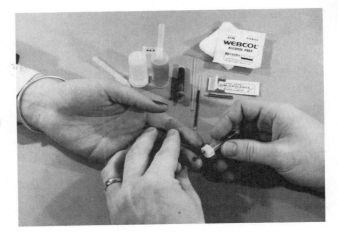

Figure 3–2. Collecting blood specimen in micro blood collecting tube with related micro sampling items (Courtesy of Ray Wassel).

automated system, a different type of micro-container may be preferred. The skill or frequency of use by personnel is another factor that may prompt selection of other than capillary tubes, which are difficult to fill completely without entrance of air bubbles and are fragile in processing. The specimen collection technique is a greater challenge than analysis of microliter measurements for many of the clinically useful determinations requiring 0.1 ml (100 μl) or less of specimen in the form of plasma, serum, or whole blood. Indeed, such a policy should prevail that all analyses be performed on minimal specimen volumes such as 20 to 100 μl or less where possible and with maximal accuracy, precision, and efficiency, as well as compatibility with semiautomated or automated single or simultaneous measurements (Mabry, 1966). This approach has obvious advantages to patients and personnel.

Integrated serum separator tubes are available for isolating serum from whole blood (Corning Glass Works, Corning, N.Y. 14830; Becton-Dickinson, Div. Becton-Dickinson & Company, Rutherford, N.J. 07070). An evacuated glass tube serves as a closed system for both collection and processing of the blood specimen. During centrifugation blood is forced into a silicone gel material located at the base of the tube, causing a temporary change in viscosity. The specific gravity of the gel is intermediate to that of the red cells and serum, so that the gel rises and lodges between the packed cells and the top serum layer (Spencer, 1976). The gel hardens and forms an inert barrier. Pediatric-sized tubes are also available with the same concept (Fig. 3–1). Advantages of serum separator tubes are

(1) ease of use, (2) shorter processing time through clot activation, (3) a higher serum yield, (4) only one centrifugation step, (5) use of the same tube as that into which the patient specimen is drawn, and (6) ease of labeling. A unique advantage for the reference laboratory is that the centrifuged specimen can be transported without disturbing the separation. These tubes must not be spun down in an angle-head centrifuge, as the barrier will not be horizontal, allowing red blood cells to escape back into the serum in a relatively short time.

Arterial punctures are reviewed in Chapter 5, p. 111.

URINE

Collection and preservation of urine for analytical testing must follow a carefully prescribed procedure to insure valid results. Laboratory testing of urine generally falls under three categories, i.e., chemical, bacteriologic, and microscropic examination. In this section, obtaining the specimen for chemical testing is stressed.

There are three kinds of collection for urine specimens: (1) random, (2) timed, and (3) 24-hour total volume. Random specimens are collected any time. Test results for a random collection are expressed per unit volume if the result is a quantitative analysis. Much reporting of testing on a random collection is expressed as "positive" or "negative," indicating the presence or absence of a particular constituent, such as glucose. Random urine specimens should be collected in a chemically clean receptacle, either glass or plastic. The vessel is tightly sealed, labeled with the patient's name and date of collection, and submitted for analysis. Timed specimens are obtained at designated intervals, starting from "time zero." For example, in the glucose tolerance test, collections are made at 0, 30, 60, 120, and 180 minutes. It is important to note the time of collection on each specimen container. Urine specimens for a 24-hour total volume collection are most difficult to obtain and require the utmost cooperation from the patient. Incomplete collection is the major problem. In some instances, overcollection occurs. As in-hospital collection is usually under the supervision of the nursing staff, it is more reliable than outpatient collections. Collection of urine specimens from pediatric patients requires special attention to avoid contamination from the stool. One can avoid problems by giving patients complete instructions with a warning that the test can be invalidated by incorrect sampling. One should give the patient a one-gallon (approximately 4 liters), chemically clean bottle with the correct preservative already added. An unbreakable plastic container is preferred. Some compounds to be tested are light-sensitive; thus, for these tests one should use an amber glass bottle or a plastic bottle wrapped with aluminum foil. One should remind the patient to *discard* the first morning specimen, record time, and collect every voiding for the next 24 hours, with the last to be 24 hours after timing commenced. Overcollection occurs if the first morning specimen is included in this routine. Measure the total volume collected, record on the request form, thoroughly mix the entire 24-hour collection, and submit for analysis. A 40-ml aliquot is adequate for this purpose. Completeness of collection is difficult to determine. If results appear clinically invalid, this is cause for suspicion. Since creatinine excretion is based on muscle mass, and since a patient's muscle mass is relatively constant, creatinine excretion is also reasonably constant. Therefore, one should measure creatinine on several 24-hour collections and should keep this as part of the patient's record. Another approach is to express results relative to the concentration of creatinine when collecting a specimen other than a 24-hour one.

Preservation of a urine specimen is essential in order to maintain its integrity. Unpreserved urine specimens are subject both to microbiologic decomposition and to inherent chemical changes. To prevent growth of microbes, the specimen should be refrigerated during and after collection, and when necessary should contain the indicated chemical preservative. For some determinations, where a chemical additive will affect the assay, use only refrigeration if necessary. The preservative is added to the empty bottle and a warning label is placed on the bottle as well. Warnings are necessary, e.g., acid burns to patient's genitals is not an unknown occurrence with the use of concentrated acids as preservatives. Light-sensitive compounds are protected in either amber glass bottles or plastic bottles wrapped in aluminum foil. Precipitation of calcium and phosphorus occurs unless the urine is acidified adequately before analysis.

A useful guide for the collection and preservation of urine specimens according to the chemical analyte measured is presented in Table 3-2.

SPECIMEN PROCESSING

Processing of specimens embraces that phase between collection of specimen and actual analysis. Ideally all measurements should be performed within one hour after collection. Whenever this is not practical, the specimen should be processed to a point at which it can be properly stored in order to preclude alterations of constituents to be measured. However, some whole blood specimens are initially processed by preparation of a protein-free filtrate with tungstic acid, trichloroacetic acid, or barium sulfate; such filtrates may be stored in a refrigerator at 4 to 6°C. if the interval prior to analysis exceeds 30 minutes. Plasma or serum is preferred to whole blood for most determinations because many constituents are distributed differently in erythrocytes versus serum or plasma; also, the results in the whole blood are different from those obtained in plasma because of a difference in water content between erythrocytes and plasma. Plasma or serum contains about 93 per cent water, whereas whole blood contains about 81 per cent water. The most efficient processing system generates a single or as few as possible blood fractions for analyses.

In clinical chemistry, serum and plasma are interchangeable except for very few measurements, e.g., ACTH by radioimmunoassay requires plasma with heparin as anticoagulant. In fact, if serum can be used, it is preferred over plasma because of simplicity of specimen collection and handling. A further advantage

Table 3–2. URINE DETERMINATION WITH RECOMMENDED COLLECTION AND PRESERVATION*

DETERMINATION	COLLECTION†	NO PRESERVATIVE	BORIC ACID (10–15 g)	GLACIAL ACETIC ACID (15 ml)	HYDROCHLORIC ACID (15 ml)	REFRIGERATION—NO PRESERVATIVE
ALA (delta-aminolevulinic acid)	24				X	
Albumin	24		X			
Alpha-amino nitrogen	24		X			
Aldosterone	24			X		
Amino acids	24		X			
Amylase	2					X
Arsenic	24	X				
Barbiturates	R					X
Bence-Jones protein	24		X (mail)			X
Calcium	24				X	
Catecholamines	24			X		
Chloride	24		X			
Chorionic gonadotropin	24					X
Copper	24	X				
Coproporphyrin (see under porphyrins)						
Cortisol	24		X			
Creatine	24		X			
Creatinine	24		X			
Drug abuse screen	R					X
Electrolytes (Cl, K, Na)	24					X
Estriol, pregnancy	24	X	X (Kober)			
Estrogens, total	24		X			
Follicle stimulating hormone	24					X
Glucose	24		X			
Heavy metals	24	X				
5-Hydroxyindoleacetic acid (5-HIAA)	24		X			
17-Hydroxycorticosteroids	24			X		
Hydroxyproline	24		X			
17-Ketogenic steroids (17-KGS)	24			X		
17-Ketosteroids (17-KS)	24			X		
Lead	24	X				
Lithium	24			X		
Metanephrines	24			X		
Mercury	24	X				
Osmolality	24				(mail or store frozen) X	
Phosphorus	24				X	
Porphobilinogen (see under Porphyrins)						
Porphyrins, Total	24					
Coproporphyrin	24		5 g Na$_2$CO$_3$			
Porphobilinogen	24		(protect from light;			
Protoporphyrin	24		ship frozen)			
Uroporphyrin	24					X
Potassium	24					X
Pregnanediol	24			X		
Pregnanetriol	24			X		
Protein	24		X (mail)			X
Protoporphyrin (see under Porphyrins)						
Sodium	24					X
Tetrahydro compound "S" (THS)	24			X		
Uric acid	24		X			
Uroporphyrin (see under Porphyrins)						
Vanillylmandelic acid (VMA)	24			X		

*Courtesy of International Clinical Laboratories, Inc., Nashville, Tennessee.
†Time of collection: 24 = 24 hour; 2 = 2 hour; R = Random.

is that serum poses no possible interference from anticoagulant. One should not refrigerate blood which is to be used for preparation of serum or plasma, as refrigeration inhibits the sodium-potassium pump, leading to increased potassium in the separated serum or plasma.

The actual steps in processing that must be followed for separation of whole blood into its fractions, components, or derivatives are as follows:

1. Blood should be kept in the stoppered original container until ready for analysis, which should begin within one hour after drawing blood specimen.

2. For plasma preparations, centrifuge blood within one hour after collection, preferably in the original container, for 10 minutes at a relative centrifugal force (RCF) of 850 to 1000 g, keeping the container stoppered to prevent evaporation. Label plasma container and store in refrigerator at 4 to 6°C. until plasma is analyzed, or freeze at −20°C. if analysis is to be delayed more than four hours. The Caraway microcapillary tubes with a maximum volume of 350 μl are occluded with microcaps or vinyl plaster putty at the tapered end prior to centrifugation for one minute at 5000 g; this will yield about 150 μl of plasma.[*]

3. For serum preparations, allow blood to clot in the original closed container at room temperature (usually 20 to 30 minutes). When clot has formed, gently loosen it at the top ("rim") with a fine glass rod or applicator stick, if necessary. Centrifuge blood 10 minutes at an RCF of 850 to 1000 g in the stoppered container. Label and store the serum in a refrigerator at 4 to 6°C. until analyzed or freeze at −20°C. if analysis is to be delayed more than four hours.

CENTRIFUGATION

A centrifuge is a machine which uses centrifugal force to separate phases of different densities. The centrifuge has multiple specific uses in the clinical laboratory. One of the most frequent uses of primary importance is in blood processing to derive plasma or serum fractions. Conditions for centrifugation should

specify both the time and centrifugal force. In selecting a centrifuge, one should look for the highest possible centrifugal force and not be misled by the high rotational speed. When the radius (r) is known, calculation of the relative centrifugal force (g) may be made from a nomogram (Fig. 3–3) or by the use of the following formula:

$$RCF = 1.118 \times 10^{-5} \times r \times (rpm)^2$$

in which RCF is the relative centrifugal force in units of g, i.e., multiples of the gravitational force; 1.118×10^{-5} is a constant; r is the radius, expressed in centimeters, between the axis of rotation and the center of the centrifuge tube; and rpm is the speed in revolutions per minute. Several principles must be observed to avoid damage to the centrifuge or the specimen and danger to personnel.

The principle of "balance" must be observed. Tubes and carriers or shields of equal weight, shape, and size should be placed in opposing positions in the centrifuge head, with regard for a geometrically symmetrical arrangement, using water-filled tubes when necessary.

Equipment. A wide variety of centrifuges and accessories are available to meet specific needs in the clinical laboratory. Table-top general laboratory centrifuges develop forces up to about 3000 g, depending on the type of centrifuge head. Angle centrifuge heads are high-speed heads with drilled holes which hold the tubes at a fixed angle. Horizontal centrifuge heads allow the tubes to swing from a vertical to horizontal position during centrifugation. Portable floor-type models, nonrefrigerated, are capable of accepting both angle and horizontal heads, with up to 36 places for the angle heads. Horizontal heads may have 4 to 16 places. By number of places is meant the number of cups or tubes which the head can accept. Generally, the lower the number of places, the larger the volume or capacity of each cup. These portable floor models operate at a RCF (g forces) of 800 to 3500, depending on the type of head. A microhematocrit centrifuge is a special version of a table-top centrifuge which very rapidly generates g forces in the range of 12,000 and also can be stopped in seconds. Tiny capillary tubes fit into a fixed head which may be specially cooled. Refrigerated centrifuges are heavy-duty, non-portable, floor-type centrifuges capable of generating g forces up to 50,000, if angle heads are used. These centrifuges are

---

[*]International Micro-Hematocrit, Centrifuge Model MB with 16-place head. Sample slots are milled down to base. An embroidery hoop may be used as a gasket; tapered ends of Caraway tubes may cut standard rubber gasket (Mabry, 1967).

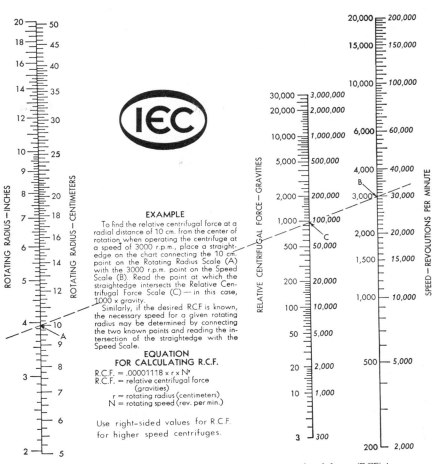

Figure 3-3. Nomogram for calculation of relative centrifugal force (RCF) in g.

utilized in the blood bank, and to very good advantage in the radioimmunoassay laboratory, i.e., for spinning down protein precipitates and for handling large numbers of tubes in temperature-sensitive charcoal separations. Ultracentrifuges, generating g forces in the hundreds of thousands, are finding routine clinical use in tissue receptor assays and clarifying lactescent serum for electrolyte and other measurements (Chap. 6).

Calibration of Centrifuge. For every procedure requiring a centrifuge operation there should be a written specification in the procedure manual. It is important to define which particular centrifuge to use, at what temperature, the g forces required, and the length of time for spinning. In order to calculate the g forces, the rpm and radius must be known (Fig. 3-3). Therefore, a centrifuge has to be calibrated. Hamlin (1974) provides an excellent review of function, verification, and ad-

justment for a centrifuge. To do this, the centrifuge must have a built-in tachometer or a dial on its rheostat. Otherwise, it can be calibrated only at maximum speed. It is very important to calibrate the instrument each time under as nearly identical conditions as possible. Use the same head loaded with the same number of empty cups. Any significant change will indicate deterioration effects, such as wearing of brushes, incipient bearing problems, or a defective tachometer (Hamlin, 1974).

REFRIGERATION AND FREEZING

A myriad of changes occurs in clinical specimens once removed from the patient. Bacterial growth and enzymatic activity can alter drastically the value of blood components. Many biologic compounds are of themselves unstable. Refrigeration or freezing of the biologic specimen is an effective means of retarding many of these degradative reactions. In fact, preservation of specimens is a prime consideration, and increases in importance with increasing time of delay before the analysis is performed.

Effect on Specimen. Generally, the Q_{10} of a reaction, or the increase in reaction rate with an increase in temperature of 10°C., is about two. If we consider that the difference in temperature between room and refrigerated storage is about 20°C., it is immediately apparent that a reaction will occur about four times as fast at room temperature.

The effect of bacterial degradation may be much more dramatic. With long-term storage in the refrigerator, bacterial populations reach significant levels with severe degradative effects on biologic components. These effects are extremely variable, since entirely different bacterial populations may predominate in serum specimens.

Even under frozen storage (-20°C.) a biologic system is unstable. For example, enzymatic reactions occur to alter the concentration of substrate. The enzyme molecule itself may be unstable, so that enzyme activity will change with long standing. Some fairly simple molecules, like folic acid, are unstable at -20°C. The most practical consequence is that control specimens stored at -20°C. can and sometimes do change in concentration with long-term storage. This effect will be seen by a gradually decreasing mean on control charts (Chap. 63). The question of the effect of freeze/thaw cycles on stability comes up often. In specimens such as plasma and serum the ice crystals which form cause shear effects which are disruptive to molecular structure, especially large molecules like proteins. Slow freezing allows larger crystals to form, with more serious degradative effects. Therefore, for optimum stability quick freezing is preferred. As for the extent of degradation in freeze/thaw cycles, actual experimentation is necessary to demonstrate the quantitative effect.

PERFORMING THE ASSAY

The validity of clinical laboratory data is dependent not only upon proper manipulation of equipment, but also upon use of specific reagents and materials and upon environmental control. An understanding of these fundamental issues embracing materials and essential measurements is a prelude to an appreciation of analytical procedures.

WATER

Purification. The two methods in general use for preparation of laboratory reagent grade water are distillation and deionization. To meet standards for reagent water specified by the College of American Pathologists, it will generally be necessary to further purify distilled water. This is most often done by deionization. Many laboratories use deionization without prior distillation for preparation of reagent grade water. Deionizers work on the principle of ion exchange. Insoluble resin polymers are prepared with acid or amine functional groups on the molecule. A cation exchange resin, for example, a phenolformaldehyde polymer with $-SO_3H$, $-CH_2COOH$, $-COOH$, or $-OH$ radicals, will react in the following manner, with R— representing the insoluble backbone of the polymer, and Na^+ as an example:

$$R-\underset{\underset{O}{\|}}{\overset{\overset{O}{\|}}{S}}-OH + Na^+ \rightleftharpoons R-\underset{\underset{O}{\|}}{\overset{\overset{O}{\|}}{S}}-O-Na + H^+ \quad (1)$$

In this reaction, sodium ions are removed from solution and hydrogen ions are ejected into solution. Thus, there is an exchange between sodium and hydrogen ions. In a similar manner, an anion exchange resin such as formed by the condensation of formaldehyde with various amines, for example, m-phenylenediamine and urea, will exchange hydroxyl ions for negatively charged ions in solution. One such reaction will be:

$$R_4NOH + Cl^- \rightleftharpoons R_4NCl + OH^- \quad (2)$$

A commercially installed system usually will have a cationic exchange resin followed by an anionic exchange resin, a charcoal filter to remove organic compounds, and a final filter to remove particulate matter. This type can be monitored, for example, at 1 megohm-cm specific resistance with a light to indicate that the system is producing water at least equal to the indicated quality. At peak operation this system will generate water at 10 megohm per cm specific resistance or better.

Table 3–3. CONDUCTANCE AND RESISTANCE SPECIFICATIONS

SPECIFICATION	WATER GRADE		
	Type I	Type II	Type III
Specific conductance, microhms, maximum	0.1	2	5
Specific resistance, megohms, minimum	10	0.5	0.2

Specifications. The College of American Pathologists has drawn up specifications and methods of quality control for reagent water (Stier, 1974). Three grades of water are defined, Types I, II, and III, with conductance and resistance specifications shown in Table 3–3.

Each test established in the laboratory must be judged for the type of water necessary to avoid interference with specificity, accuracy, and precision. It is known, for example, that metal contaminants can have profound effects on enzyme values (Winstead, 1967). The following are recommendations of the Commission on Inspection and Accreditation of the College of American Pathologists (Stier, 1974) for reagent water requirements:

Type I Reagent Water
  For methods intended to give maximum accuracy and precision:
    Atomic absorption spectrometry.
    Flame photometry.
    Enzymology.
    Blood gas and pH determinations.
    Electrolytes and inorganic ions.
    Reference buffer solutions.
Type II Reagent Water
  For general laboratory testing.
  Chemical methods not specifically stated or proven to require Type I water; may include most of the procedures listed under Type I water depending upon the methodology, the reagents used, and the sensitivity. The only group of procedures determined to require Type I water specifically are those performed by atomic absorption. Most hematologic, serologic, and microbiologic procedures are also included.
Type III Reagent Water
  For general laboratory testing.
  Satisfactory for most qualitative analysis procedures:

Most urinalyses, parasitology, and histologic procedures.
Rinsing glassware.

Carbon dioxide (CO_2) free water (reagent water, free of CO_2) is used where such gases as CO_2, ammonia, and oxygen may affect analysis. Boiled type II water is adequate for such use.

REAGENTS

Grades. Chemicals exist in varying degrees of purity. Even sodium chloride may contain a small amount of potassium sulfate or iodide. Meticulous attention to the label on a bottle as well as to the supplier's catalogue will frequently reveal the maximum limits of impurities in chemicals. Several companies show on the label the actual analysis so that one may identify the exact amount of an impurity present in a particular batch or bottle. For quantitative measurements and preparation of accurate standard solutions, it is important to use pure chemicals and to identify exact amounts of compound or elements desired, as well as amounts of contaminants. The use of "reagent-grade" chemicals, although more expensive than less pure grades of chemicals, is essential for accuracy. Because several grades of chemicals are available, an awareness of the terms used widely is necessary. For the most highly purified chemicals, "reagent grade," "analytical grade," or "ACS" for having met the established standards of purity by the American Chemical Society are terms that should be identified on a label or in the catalogue. Less pure grades are referred to as "purified" and "technical."

U.S.P. and N.F. represent other grades of purity and mean that these chemicals meet the stipulations listed in the United States Pharmacopeia or the National Formulary; while they are adequate for human consumption, they may not be pure enough for specific chemical applications. Radin (1967) has reviewed the use and availability of standards with the limitations of so-called standards.

N.B.S., or National Bureau of Standards, and the College of American Pathologists (C.A.P.), along with several suppliers who list the exact composition or maximum limits of impurities in their chemicals, are preferred sources for preparation of many standards used in medical chemistry (Meinke, 1971).

Proprietary reagents (such as drugs) of undisclosed composition should be avoided, even though they may give satisfactory results under the usual conditions. With abnormal specimens or under abnormal conditions, confusing results as well as invalid data may be produced by use of such proprietary reagents. It is important to know what compounds are being used in a specific determination to understand what reaction is taking place and to identify as well as anticipate and evaluate abnormal reactions or interferences.

Techniques of Use and Storage. A reagent or chemical will arrive in the laboratory with a certain guarantee of purity. Once the seal is broken, the guaranteed analysis is strictly in the hands of the receiving laboratory. Definite steps must be taken to insure that the chemical or reagent is handled under optimum conditions: (1) It is extremely important to read the label for proper storage. While most chemical compounds are stable at room temperature without desiccation, some must be refrigerated, frozen, or even stored at $-70°C$. Light-sensitive chemicals and reagents must be stored in brown bottles. (2) Absolutely never sample directly from the reagent bottle. An entire bottle of reagent grade chemical can become contaminated by an unclean spatula or a dirty pipette. Pour slightly more than the required amount of reagent into another vessel, such as a beaker, and sample from that vessel. Discard the excess. It is a common practice to sample directly from standard solutions, largely as a matter of convenience. This can lead to contamination of the standard and a change in its value.

MEASUREMENT OF MASS

In the modern clinical laboratory, measurements of mass are seldom performed. Reagents, standards, and controls come ready for use, or simply need reconstituting. However, since the measurement of mass is fundamental to every analysis, the technologist will eventually use some sort of balance. It is usual for the toxicologist to prepare his/her own drug standards from pure authentic material. Fecal fats may be measured by gravimetric analysis. It is prudent to prepare in-house many laboratory reagents which are much less expensive than if purchased. Of course, volumetric equipment is calibrated by measurement of mass.

Theory and Technique (Natelson, 1971; Fritz, 1974; Hackler, 1970). The basic principle in the measurement of mass is to balance an unknown mass with a known mass. Modern balances, though extremely sophisticated, use the basic concept of a simple lever which pivots on a knife-edge fulcrum placed at the center of gravity of the lever. From this concept, balances are designed in a variety of ways. *Two pans* of equal mass may be suspended from the ends of the lever, or beam. In this case, *calibrated* weights are placed on one pan to counterbalance an object of unknown mass on the other pan. A rider and/or a chain weight device is generally utilized to avoid fractional weights. Motion of the beam is indicated by a pointer traversing a scale much like a ruler. Macrobalances of this sort generally have a capacity of 200 g and a sensitivity of 0.1 mg. It is necessary to determine the rest point by a method of swings with the balance both empty and loaded. From the sensitivity the mass of an object is calculated to the nearest 0.1 mg.

Single-pan balances offer the speed and accuracy necessary in the clinical laboratory. These balances encompass a range from 1 μg to 1000 g in both analytical and top-loading balances. Although single-pan balances work on the principle of weighing by substitution, they still utilize the basic concept of a lever and fulcrum. The balance is first set at the zero point. In this configuration one end of the beam has a built-in mass just equal to the mass on the other end of the beam, which includes the single pan and a set of built-in calibrated weights. These weights are nonmagnetic chrome-nickel steel rings or cylinders standardized against prototype weights at the National Bureau of Standards. The sample is placed on the pan. As selector knobs are adjusted, weights on the beam corresponding to the sample weight are removed until the zero point is again reached. Therefore, the mass of the sample is exactly substituted for an equivalent mass of weights originally on the sample side of the beam. Single-pan analytical balances suitable for the clinical laboratory are available as semimicro or macro balances with a scale from 0 to 160 g and a precision (standard deviation) of 0.01 mg or 0.1 mg. An air-release system provides damping for rapid attainment of equilibrium. Optical range taring or full range taring permits container weights to be dialed off so that weight read-out begins at zero.

The guiding principle in weighing technique is to regard a balance as a delicate, precision instrument which will function properly only if it is not abused. The knife edge located at the fulcrum of the beam is a synthetic sapphire and can be injured by lowering the beam too hard or through excessive vibration. Make gross weight changes with the balance in the beam arrest position. Release the beam gently. Avoid chemical spills; if these occur, immediately clean up the area. Never weigh a sample directly on the pan. One must not overload the balance.

The sequence in weighing a sample using a single-pan balance is as follows:

1. Check that the balance is level by observing the level indicator. Make appropriate adjustments to the feet.
2. Observe that the balance is not in direct sunlight and is in a draft-free location.
3. Set the balance to its zero point. If taring is used, set the read-out at zero. For the analytical balance, this setting is made with the sliding windows closed and the beam resting on the knife edge.
4. Lock the beam of the analytical balance. Open the window of the balance case and place the object to be weighed on the pan. Close the window.
5. Set the beam arrest knob in the intermediate position.
6. Make gross weight changes until the weight of the object is in the range of the optical scale.
7. Fully release the beam and allow the pan to come to its final point of rest.
8. Record the mass of the object.
9. Fully arrest the beam and remove the object from the pan.

Hygroscropic materials and volatile liquids are difficult to weigh accurately. Solids which have been dried *in vacuo* and placed in a desiccator are often hygroscopic and should be weighed in weighing bottles with ground-glass stoppers.

Calibration. The weights in a typical single-pan analytical balance meet individual and group tolerances for Class S weights established by the National Bureau of Standards. These tolerances are defined in the NBS Circular 547 (Lashof, 1954). In order to calibrate a balance, weights conforming to Class S tolerances are available commercially. One such set consists of 12 fractional weights: 1-2-3-5-10-20-30-50-100-200-300-500 mg; and 9 rhodium-plated bronze gram weights: 1-2-3-5-10-20-30-50-100 g. These weights must be handled with forceps supplied with the set. A balance out of calibration will usually require a specialist for adjustment and realignment.

Top-Loading Balances. Single-pan top-loading balances operate on the same principle as single-pan analytical balances, i.e., weighing by substitution. Damping is magnetic rather than air-release. There is an entire line of these balances available covering a dynamic weighing range up to 10,000 g. These balances are especially suitable for rapidly weighing larger masses which do not require as much analytical precision, such as large volume reagent preparation.

Balance Maintenance. The two most important factors in balance maintenance are to keep the balance scrupulously clean and to avoid excessive vibrations. The more rugged general utility balances can be taken apart to clean the knife edges, which can become clogged with dust accumulation. Intricate, internal maintenance of analytical and top-loading balances is best left to qualified factory-trained service personnel.

MEASUREMENT OF VOLUME

Types of Glassware. By far the most common type of glassware encountered in measurement of volume is borosilicate glass. It is essentially a sodium-aluminum borosilicate with an excess of silica. This glass is characterized by a high degree of thermal resistance. Commercial brands are known as Pyrex (Corning) and Kimax (Kimble). The glass has a low alkali content and is free from the magnesia-lime-zinc group of elements, heavy metals, arsenic, and antimony. It is very poor technique to store concentrated alkaline solutions in borosilicate glass. The caustic conditions will etch, or dissolve, the glass and destroy the calibration. Also, glass stoppers become frozen and are extremely difficult to remove without breaking the neck of the flask. Borosilicate glassware with heavy walls, such as bottles, jars, and even larger beakers, should not be heated with a direct flame or hot plate. Be careful not to heat any glass above its strain point, which for Pyrex is 515°C. If this occurs, and the glass is cooled too quickly, strains will develop and the glass cracks easily when again heated. Also, in the case of volumetric glassware, heating can destroy the calibration.

Corex brand glassware is a special alumina-silicate glass strengthened chemically rather than thermally. Corex is at least six times stronger than borosilicate glass, e.g., Corex pipettes have a typical strength of

30,000 psi, compared to 2,000 to 5,000 psi for borosilicate pipettes. Corex brand cylinders will outlast conventional cylinders by at least 10 times. Corex is also better able to resist clouding and scratching.

Alkali-resistant glassware should be used to handle strongly alkaline solutions. However, it has only about half the thermal shock resistance of Pyrex glassware and therefore must be heated and cooled more carefully.

Low actinic glassware is a glass of high thermal resistance with a red color added as an integral part of the glass. The density of the red color is adjusted to permit adequate visibility of the contents, yet give maximum protection to light-sensitive materials, such as bilirubin standards.

Specifications.   Volumetric glassware is classed A, B, and Student Grade. The tolerances for accuracy of Class A glassware meet or exceed the strict requirements specified by the National Bureau of Standards in Circular C-602. All Class A volumetric ware is the only type acceptable by the College of American Pathologists for use in an approved clinical laboratory.

Pipettes.   There are many kinds of pipettes available for use in a clinical laboratory, each intended to serve a specific function. In general, pipettes fall into two classes, volumetric or transfer pipettes and graduated or measuring pipettes. The volumetric pipette is calibrated for one specified volume measurement, either "to deliver" (T.D.) or "to contain" (T.C.). For class A pipettes this distinction is clearly indicated on the pipette. A "to deliver" pipette calibrated for blow-out has an opaque ring near the top. In this case the small amount of liquid remaining in the tip after free delivery has ceased is blown out and added to the initial volume. "To deliver" pipettes are calibrated for the volume delivered, with no attempt to wash out the film which adheres to the inside glass surface. "To contain" pipettes are calibrated for the total volume of liquid held in the pipette, and must be washed out completely for delivery of the correct volume. Most micropipettes, in the range up to 0.5 ml, are calibrated "to contain." Graduated pipettes are long, cylindrical tubes drawn out to a tip and are calibrated in uniform fractional volume measurements. The Mohr type is calibrated between two marks on the stem, while the serologic type is calibrated to the tip. All serologic pipettes are therefore calibrated for blow-out, and accordingly have an opaque ring at the top for identification.

Before using a pipette, be sure it is the correct size, is clean, and is free of chips. Without careful inspection, a broken tip may go unnoticed. Absolutely never pipette by mouth. This is especially critical in the clinical laboratory. There is no guarantee that the stem of the pipette is sterile, so that pathologic organisms can be taken in by this route. Also, in pipetting sera it is very easy to suck serum into the mouth. The same applies for strong acids and alkalis.

The steps in good pipetting procedure include the following:

1. Place a safety pipette filler on the stem of the pipette.
2. Lower the pipette into the solution. Allow sufficient depth to fill the pipette above the calibration mark.
3. Apply suction and load the pipette to a point above the calibration mark. In cases of a critically low volume of solution, fill the pipette slowly and watch carefully to avoid aspiration of air.
4. Remove the pipette from the solution. Wipe the tip with a tissue or gauze.
5. Hold the pipette in a vertical position. Empty the pipette slowly until the lower meniscus just touches the calibration mark. Pay attention to parallax errors.
6. Touch the tip to a clean, dry receptable to remove any pendant drop.
7. Drain the pipette freely in a *vertical* position. The pipette has been calibrated to deliver its specified volume in a vertical position with a constant rate of delivery. Changing the angle of the pipette changes the rate of delivery and hence the volume of liquid left behind in the pipette. For the same reason, do not attempt to force the liquid from the pipette at a faster rate than free drainage permits.
8. When the liquid enters the stem just below the bulb, touch the tip to the side of the receiving vessel, but not into the liquid. Allow several seconds for the pipette to drain. For blow-out pipettes, manipulate the small bulb of the safety pipette filler to force a gentle blast of air through the pipette. This removes the last bit of liquid from the tip.

Semiautomatic and Automatic Pipettes.
Automatic pipetting devices permit rapid, repetitive measurement and delivery of equal volumes. Automatic pipetting and diluting devices have evolved for insuring the more efficient delivery of equal volumes of specimens followed by diluent at a constant ratio to specimen. Commercial automatic pipettes are either of the sampling type, usually manually operated (Table 3-4), or of the sampling-diluting type, usually electrically operated (Table 3-5). Manually operated automatic pipettes are generally of the air-displacement variety.

Table 3-4. AUTOMATIC MANUAL PIPETTES

	TRADEMARK	RANGE*
Brinkman Instruments, Inc. Cantiague Road Westbury, N.Y. 11590	Eppendorf	1-1000 μl
Centaur Chemical Co. 4 West Kenosia Avenue Danbury, Conn. 06810	Centaur	5-1000 μl
Clay-Adams 141 E. 25th Street New York, N.Y. 10010	Aupette	10 μl-10 ml
Medical Laboratory Automation, Inc. 500 Nuber Ave. Mount Vernon, N.Y. 10550	MLA Precision Pipettes	5-1000 μl
Labindustries 1802 Second Street Berkeley, Calif. 94710	Repipet	0.1 μl-50 ml
Monostat 20 No. Moore Street New York, N.Y. 10013	Vari-pet	10 μl-30 ml
Oxford Laboratories 1149 Chess Drive Foster City, Cal. 94404	Sampler	1-5000 μl
Pfizer Diagnostics Division 300 W. 43rd Street New York, N.Y. 10036	Micro Pipet	20-1000 μl
Rainin Instrument Company 1030 Commonwealth Avenue Boston, Mass. 02215	Pipetman	0-1000 μl
Schwarz/Mann Orangeburg, N.Y. 10962	Biopette	0.025-1.0 ml
Scientific Manufacturing Industries 1399 Sixty-Fourth Street Emeryville, CA 94608	Micro/pettor	1-3000 μl

*More than one model may be required to accomplish range indicated.

Since proper care and calibration are essential to precise, accurate sampling, it is important to read and follow the manufacturer's instructions. Two common errors include allowing a sample to aspirate into the barrel of the pipette and ignoring lubrication of the piston. The sampling-dispensing automatic pipettes fall into three general classes: (1) the peristaltic type, (2) the piston type, and (3) the Seligson type, which uses a vacuum to aspirate, gravity to dispense, and a manually operated stopcock to separate the two phases of the cycle. Again, it is very important to follow the manufacturer's instructions in the operation and maintenance of these machines.

Automatic pipettes remove much of the tedium associated with repetitive sampling and dilution. Even for a limited number of samples, the speed of an automatic pipette is an advantage. Because operator fatigue is minimized, precision of multiple sampling and dilution is often improved with the automatic pipette. The micro-automatic pipettes, which can sample as little as 2 to 5 μl, offer a unique advantage, especially for the expanding field of radioimmunoassay.

Manufacturers generally claim a pipetting and dilution accuracy in the range of 0.1 to 1.0 per cent. However, it is essential that automatic pipettes be calibrated when new and at regular intervals thereafter. Never assume that factory calibrations are accurate! The random analytical variation of an automatic manual pipette can be established by repetitive pipetting of a radioactive solution in counting the activity of each sample. Calculations are made to determine the mean and standard deviation of the counts. The total variance includes both the variance of the counter and the variance of the pipette. The variances are additive (see Chap. 1). Therefore, the variance of pipetting is calculated as:

$$\sigma^2 \text{ Total} = \sigma^2 \text{ Counter} + \sigma^2 \text{ Pipetting}$$

In using an automatic pipette, the tip wiping technique is important in obtaining repro-

Table 3–5. AUTOMATIC SAMPLER-DILUTERS

		VOLUME RANGE*	
	PRINCIPLE OF SYSTEM	Sampling	Diluting
Brinkman Instruments, Inc. Cantiague Road Westbury, N.Y. 11590	Piston	0.1-5000 μl	1-5000 μl
Cordis Laboratories P.O. Box 684 Miami, Fl. 33137	Piston	20-100 μl	5-15 ml
DADE Miami, Fl. 33152	Piston	20-50 μl	5-10 ml
Fisher Scientific Co. 52 Fadem Road Springfield, N.J. 07081	Piston	10-1000 μl	1-10 ml
General Diagnostic Division Warner-Lambert Co. Morris Plains, N.J. 07950	Peristaltic	5 μl-10 ml	5 μl-10 ml
Hobbs Scientific, Inc. P.O. Box 600 S. Miami, Fl. 33143	Piston	20-200 μl	5-15 ml
Micromedic Systems, Inc. Rohm and Haas Building 6th and Market Streets Philadelphia, Pa. 19105	Piston	2-1000 μl	2-5000 μl
Oxford Laboratories 1149 Chess Drive Foster City, Cal. 94404	Piston	10-100 μl	0.5-20 ml
Arthur H. Thomas Co. Vine Street at Third Philadelphia, Pa. 19105	Thomas-Seligson Pipette Vacuum Sampling- Gravity Dilution	0.02-1.0 ml	Unspecified
York Instrument Corp. 150 Fifth Avenue New York, N.Y. 10011	Piston	0-1 ml (microliter ranges available)	0-25 ml

*More than one model may be required to accomplish range indicated.

ducibility. Aspirate the sample into the tip. Then wipe the tip with absorbent cloth or tissue with two downward strokes at 90 degrees with respect to one another. Each stroke should start above the level that the tip was immersed into the fluid sample and proceed downward past the tip. Do not actually touch the fluid in the tip, as this will draw the fluid out of the tip.

With an automatic sampling-diluting pipette, the operator must always beware of possible carry-over. When a sample is introduced into the tip, diffusion of sample occurs. The washout by diluent may be insufficient to remove all the sample, and this then becomes mixed with the succeeding sample. The result is that any analyses performed on the first sample dilution are too low, and those done on the second are too high. In general, the ratio of diluent to sample must be at least 5:1 for quantitative washout. This must be increased if the sample is viscous or oily and the diluent is of an aqueous base. Also, certain components are adsorbed by the tip construction, and the washout must be increased. In general, a Teflon tip adsorbs less than a glass tip. Some hormones, for example, have a high affinity for glass.

Volumetric Flasks. Inspect the flask to be sure that it is clean, dry, and not cracked. For glass-stoppered flasks, be sure the stopper fits properly so as not to leak. It is usually possible to tell by how well the stopper seats in the joint. The steps in using a volumetric flask are as follows:

1. Add to the flask the solution to be diluted or the solid to be dissolved and diluted to volume. A solid is best added to the flask by having first weighed the material in a beaker. Then add enough solvent to the beaker to dissolve the solid. Hold a glass rod across the beaker with one end over the lip. Tip the beaker and allow the solution to pour down the glass rod into the opening of the flask. Keep adding small volumes of solvent to wash the beaker. This will result in a quantitative transfer to the flask.

2. Bring nearly to volume with solvent.

3. Use a Pasteur pipette to wet the neck of the flask. Add solvent drop by drop to bring the meniscus to the final calibration mark.

4. Stopper the flask and mix thoroughly. For adequate mixing turn the flask upside down and shake. Then turn the flask upright. Repeat this four more times. In the case of solutions which foam, mixing must be done more slowly with many more revolutions of the flask. In extreme cases of foaming, the flask can only be rotated, not tipped upside down. Magnetic stirrers may be used.

Calibration. According to the strictest of standards, every piece of volumetric glassware in the clinical laboratory should be coded and a record kept of its calibration. Any piece of glassware which does not meet Class A tolerances should be rejected. To prepare a piece of glassware for calibration, rinse with tap water followed by a thorough rinsing with reagent grade water.

Cleaning of Glassware. Glassware from general laboratory use should be rinsed and immediately placed into a weak detergent solution. Never leave corrosive chemicals in glassware which is later to be picked up by washroom personnel. Serious chemical burns may occur in handling. The glassware will usually be rinsed and placed in a completely automatic glassware washer, which will prewash, wash, rinse, and finally rinse with reagent grade water from a separate plumbing system. The glassware will then be placed in a glassware dryer before distribution to laboratory glassware storage.

The surface of a thoroughly clean glass apparatus will become uniformly wet, with no adhering water droplets. Special treatment is required in cases of stubborn grease and other organic residues. Let the glassware stand overnight in a sulfuric acid–dichromate mixture, prepared by pouring 1000 ml of concentrated sulfuric acid into 35 ml of saturated sodium dichromate. Avoid contact with the flesh or clothing. Rinse the glassware *thoroughly* after removal from the mixture.

Bacteriologic glassware should be soaked in 2 to 4 per cent cresol, or a weak Lysol solution. Follow by autoclaving, then pass the glassware through the normal washing procedure.

Glassware used for iron determinations must be soaked in hydrochloric acid solution (concentrated HCl diluted 1:2) or nitric acid solution (concentrated HNO_3 diluted 1:3) and then rinsed with reagent grade water.

CONTROL OF TEMPERATURE

Precise temperature control in many clinical measurements is an absolute prerequisite. The dependence of enzyme activity on temperature and the requirement for precise temperature control is a classic example. Indeed, any measurement which includes a time/temperature-dependent reaction must be rigorously controlled with respect to these two variables.

Constant Temperature Baths. For general clinical laboratory use, constant temperature water baths must offer variable temperature control from $+5°C$. above ambient temperature to $100°C$., with a precision of $\pm0.2°C$. No refrigeration capabilities are required in this type of unit. For precise temperature control at room temperatures or below, a refrigerated bath is necessary. These are available with a temperature range from $0°$ to $100°C$., at a constancy of $\pm0.2°C$. A compressor and heater work in tandem to offer temperature control over this range. An important consideration in the selection of a constant temperature bath is that the model be large enough to accomodate the desired working volume. Models which have independent controlled agitation to maintain a uniform bath temperature are desirable. Heating blocks are more useful for high temperature use.

Maintenance. Maintenance of a constant temperature water bath is improved by filling it with distilled or deionized water. This prevents the accumulation of mineral deposits from regular tap water which can affect the temperature sensing elements and generally lead to poor heat transfer. However, if an accumulation of these minerals does occur, a weak hydrochloric acid solution will dissolve the deposits. Overheating can occur if the bath goes dry, so this should be avoided. At higher temperatures the bath should be covered, both to maintain proper temperature control and to prevent rapid evaporation to dryness.

Quality Control. A thermometer calibrated against another certified by the National Bureau of Standards must be a component of any constant temperature bath. The temperature should be noted and recorded for each assay. This function by the operator insures that indeed the temperature of the bath is the same as the reading of the thermometer.

EVAPORATION AND SPECIMEN CONCENTRATION

Evaporation as a batch or unit process is an essential step in many analytical procedures. Solvent extraction is almost always followed by evaporation of solvent to recover the extracted material for further processing. Cerebrospinal fluid, urine, and even serum specimens must be concentrated to bring certain compounds within the range of analytical sensitivity.

Large-volume solvent evaporation is best accomplished with a thin-film rotary vacuum evaporator. Evaporation of test-tube quantities of solvent, in the range of 10 to 15 ml or less, is handled conveniently in an evaporator which concentrates by blowing a stream of an inert gas, usually nitrogen, across the surface of the solvent. Using the same principle, evaporators to handle large numbers of tubes such as required in high volume radioimmunoassay or toxicology laboratories can be designed and constructed from plastic.

Polymer films, or membranes, constructed with an effective pore size to retain solutes above a selected molecular weight, can be utilized to concentrate proteins, including enzymes, isoenzymes, and hormones. Typical molecular weight cut-off values for these ultrafiltration membranes are 15,000, 25,000, 75,000, and 125,000. Amicon Corporation (21 Hartwell Avenue, Lexington, Mass. 02173) utilizes these films in the construction of clinical sample concentrators.

Ultrafiltration membranes constructed in the form of a cone can be supported in a tube and placed in a centrifuge. The force of centrifugation will drive liquid and solute past the membrane, below a critical molecular weight cut-off value. Protein-free filtrates can be prepared by this technique. Therefore, it becomes possible to determine the free, or non-protein-bound, fraction of blood components. For instance, using this technique it is possible to measure the concentration of free phenytoin in serum (Booker, 1973).

FILTRATION

Filtration may be used in place of centrifugation to separate solids from liquids. This is usually performed with filter paper, folded properly, and a funnel. A funnel containing glass wool may be substituted for paper when acids or bases too strong for filter paper require filtering. Many types of filter paper with different degrees of porosity are available for selection according to requirements of separation by filtration.

DIALYSIS

Dialysis is a technique for the separation of substances in molecular or ionic solution from colloidally dispersed molecules. A dialyzing membrane is a porous diaphragm which acts like a sieve. When an aqueous system to be dialyzed is placed on one side of the membrane, and pure water is placed on the other side, the substances in molecular or ionic solution diffuse through the pores of the membrane. Colloidally dispersed molecules are too large to pass through the pores and therefore are held back. Diffusion of the smaller molecules or ions in solution continues until at equilibrium their respective concentrations on each side of the membrane are equal. Therefore, if the side originally containing the pure water is continuously replaced with pure water, a condition will be reached where the colloidally dispersed molecules are practically free of all diffusable molecules. The material which passes through the membrane during the process of dialysis is referred to as diffusate. The term dialysate applies to the substance which does not pass through the membrane.

Membranes used in dialysis are most commonly made of regenerated cellulose, using cotton linters for the source of cellulose. The membrane may be constructed as a tube or sheet. Cellulose membranes are available with a molecular weight cut-off specification ranging from 2,000 MWCO (molecular weight cut-off) to 12,000 to 14,000 MWCO. The 12,000 MWCO film will have an average pore diameter of 4.8 nanometers. The 12,000 to 14,000 MWCO membrane has a dialysis rate about three times that of the 6000 to 8000 MWCO membrane. After processing, cellulose membranes have glycerol added as a humectant to keep the film supple. Small amounts (0.1 per cent) of polysulfides are also generally present as a contaminant. Both the glycerol and polysulfide may be removed by proper washing.

Dialysis is a unit process for determinations employing continuous flow analyzers. One such dialyzer component consists of two flat, spirally grooved plates; one is a mirror image of the other. The two plates, separated by a cellulose membrane, are clamped together with the grooves matched. The standard or specimen stream enters the dialyzer and flows parallel to a stream of reagent; the two streams (specimen and reagent) are separated by the cellulose membrane. The constituent for analysis dialyzes through the membrane and enters the reagent stream. A specific color reaction occurs under precisely timed conditions, controlled by the rate of flow.

Dialysis is a key step in the analysis for CEA (carcinoembryonic antigen) by radioimmunoassay (Roche Diagnostics, Nutley, N.J. 07110). It is critical that the dialysis be conducted under controlled conditions with uniform adequate agitation during the dialysis. Dialysis is used to remove interfering substances in the radioimmunoassay of FSH and LH in urine. A simplified, reproducible procedure for the determination of serum-free thyroxine by equilibrium dialysis is available (Wilson, 1974).

Dialysis bags must be prewetted before use. Do this by cutting a desired length of dialysis tubing from the roll and lowering the tubing into a beaker of distilled water. Change the water at intervals to wash away impurities. An hour is adequate time for prewetting. The bag must then be tied off at one end, *using a double knot*. Fill the bag with the solution to be dialyzed. Care must be taken at this point because the solution can be easily spilled. Rub the untied end of the prewetted tube between the thumb and forefinger. The end of the tube will open

up. By rubbing the tube further and further down from this initial opening a large air space can be made. Bring the beaker, test tube, or pipette to the opening of the bag. The liquid will now easily enter the bag and run to the bottom. It is important to remove all air from the dialysis bag, since the presence of air will retard the rate of dialysis and cause the bag to float. Tie off the bag with a double knot, leaving room for expansion of the liquid volume. Immerse the sac in the dialyzing medium.

EXTRACTION

Theory. Extraction is a separation technique in which a solute is transferred from one solvent to a second immiscible solvent by allowing the solute to form an equilibrium distribution between the two solvent phases. For increased separation efficiency the solute is transferred a fraction at a time by a series of single extractions. The distribution of solute between the two immiscible solvents is quantitatively expressed by the distribution, or partition, coefficient, K, according to equation (3):

$$K = \frac{\text{concentration of A in solvent 1}}{\text{concentration of A in solvent 2}} \quad (3)$$

Let us consider that X_0 g of compound A is being extracted from V ml of solution by repeated extraction with v ml of an immiscible solvent. The number of grams, X_n, of compound A remaining in solution after n extractions can be shown to be

$$X_n = X_0 \left(\frac{KV}{KV + v} \right)^n \quad (4)$$

where K is the partition coefficient. The important principle which this illustrates is that extraction with several smaller volumes of an extracting solvent is more efficient than using the same total volume of solvent in one extraction.

Technique. A separatory funnel is commonly used in the laboratory for extraction, especially for larger volumes. Screw-capped or glass-stoppered centrifuge tubes are convenient for extractions involving large numbers of samples. An entire rack of tubes can be placed in a shaker to rapidly equilibrate the solute being extracted.

The main problem in using screw-capped or glass-stoppered centrifuge tubes for extraction is leakage during the shaking operation. Caps of screw-capped tubes must be lined with Teflon, and

Table 3–6. CHEMISTRY AND ACTIVITY OF DESICCANTS*

DRYING AGENT	ACTIVITY†	CAPACITY	DELIQUE-SCENCE	EASY REGENERATION	CHEMICAL REACTION
Phosphorus pentoxide	0.02	very low	yes	no	acidic
Barium oxide	0.6–0.8	moderate	no	no	alkaline
Alumina	0.8–1.2	low	no	yes	neutral
Magnesium perchlorate (anhydrous)	1.6–2.4	high	yes	no	neutral
Calcium sulfate (Drierite)	4–6	moderate	no	yes	neutral
Silica gel	2–10	low	no	yes	neutral
Potassium hydroxide (stick)	10–17	moderate	yes	no	alkaline
Calcium chloride (anhydrous)	330–380	high	yes	no	neutral

*From Bermes, E. W., Jr., and Forman, D. T.: Basic laboratory principles and procedures. *In* Tietz, N. W. (ed.) Fundamentals of Clinical Chemistry, 2nd ed. Philadelphia, W. B. Saunders Company, 1976.

†Micrograms residual water per liter of air at 30°C.

the rim of the glass tube must not be chipped. These rims must be examined before each use, as breakage in washing happens frequently. Similarly, the stoppers for glass-stoppered centrifuge tubes must fit properly and must be held firmly in place during shaking. If both layers must be saved, use a Pasteur pipette to draw off the top layer; otherwise, aspirate.

DRYING

Desiccants or drying agents have a variety of applications in the laboratory (Bermes, 1976). It is apparent from Table 3-6 that several are alkaline and one is strongly acidic. Selection of an appropriate desiccant or drying agent for absorption of moisture depends on the composition of materials or gases to be dried, convenience, efficiency, and cost. Some desiccants can be regenerated easily, e.g., silica gel by heating in a drying oven at 120°C.

MIXING

Mixing as an operation is intended to form a homogeneous mass, or to create a uniform heterogeneous system. Mixing is used to bring solids into solution; to bring phases into intimate contact, for instance, in extraction procedures; to wash suspended solids; to homoge-nize liquid phases; and to perform many other operations too numerous to mention. Mixing and centrifuging accomplish opposite objectives. A serious consequence of inadequate mixing can be failure to completely resuspend protein which settles out under long-term frozen storage of serum controls. The result might be a run invalidated because the control is "off." In some instances, mixing must be carefully controlled to avoid protein denaturation. The importance of mixing serum and plasma specimens before sampling for analysis cannot be overly stressed. A phase separation occurs when these specimens stand for a period of time, as can be noted by careful visual observation. The concentration of even small molecules in such a system will be heterogeneous. The reason is that as protein settles and becomes more concentrated at the bottom of the specimen, the effective water concentration decreases in this layer. This produces a water concentration gradient throughout the system and, consequently, a concentration gradient of all components.

Single-tube Mixers. A vortex mixer is capable of a variable speed oscillation which results in a swirling motion to liquid contents of a test tube or other container. The angle of contact and degree of pressure can be regulated for optimum mixing action. A very effective mixing action is created by a multiple touch sequence, i.e., touching and withdrawing the tube from the neoprene oscillating cup of the mixer. The operator must be careful not to fill the container too full or to mix the liquid contents too fast, since spillage can occur.

Multiple-tube Mixers. A whole line of mixers is available to handle a variable number of tubes, with several different types of motion. A Thermolyne Maxi-Mix^R (Sybron Corporation, Dubuque, Iowa) can conveniently be used for vortex mixing one tube or several tubes at one time. Mixing action is varied by changing the pressure of the container against the foam rubber top, which is replaceable. Circular motion on a tilted disc provides continuous inversion of contents in tubes which are clipmounted at the circumference of the rotating disc. Rotational speed can be varied to provide gentle or more vigorous mixing. Control sera are conveniently reconstituted on this type of mixer. Tube shakers which tilt back and forth at variable speeds provide thorough mixing of, for example, whole blood samples.

MATHEMATICS AND CHEMICAL CALCULATIONS

Errors in patient or specimen identification as well as transcription errors may well constitute major problems, but errors in arithmetic warrant equal attention. A brief review of the mathematics most frequently utilized by laboratory personnel should clarify and identify principles so essential for accurate work (Rice, 1960).

Significant Figures. In addition, subtraction, multiplication, and division, calculation of data should retain as many significant figures as are contained in the quantity having the least number of significant figures.

Example: Sum of   65.12
                      2.115
                      1.2222
                     68.4572

Answer: 68.46

Exponents. The use of exponential forms permits simple calculation involving large or small numbers.

$$5^2 = 5 \times 5 = 25$$
$$5^{-2} = \frac{1}{5^2}$$

$$5^0 = 1$$
$$5^2 \times 5^3 = 5^5$$
$$5^{1/2} = \sqrt{5^1} = \sqrt{5} = 2.23$$
$$5^{2/3} = \sqrt[3]{5^2} = \sqrt[3]{25} = 2.92$$

Logarithms. The common logarithm of a number is the exponent which must be applied to the base 10 in order to produce the number.

Example: $10^3 = 1000$. The exponent 3 is the common logarithm of 1000, since 3 applied as an exponent to $10 = 1000$.

In terms of logarithms, this is written as follows:

$\log_{10} 1000 = 3$ (logarithm of 1000 to the base 10 equals 3)

Exponents and Logarithms

$\log_{10} 1 = 0$	$1 = 10^0$
$\log_{10} 10 = 1$	$10 = 10^1$
$\log_{10} 100 = 2$	$100 = 10^2$
$\log_{10} 1000 = 3$	$1000 = 10^3$
$\log_{10} 0.1 = -1$	$0.1 = 10^{-1}$
$\log_{10} 0.01 = -2$	$0.01 = 10^{-2}$
$\log_{10} 0.001 = -3$	$0.001 = 10^{-3}$

A logarithm is composed of two parts: (1) the mantissa (found in logarithm tables), which is placed to the right of the decimal point, and (2) the characteristic, which is placed to the left of the decimal point. The mantissa gives the antilogarithm, or the number of which it is the logarithm. The characteristic identifies the decimal point in the antilogarithm. Logs simplify arithmetical calculations. For example:

1. To multiply two or more numbers, add their logs, then look up the antilog (antilog is the number which corresponds to a log).

2. To divide, subtract logs, then look up the antilog.

3. For roots and fractional exponents, multiply the log by the fractional exponent, then look up the antilog.

Examples:

$$\log(5 \times 2) = \log 5 + \log 2$$
$$\log 47/2 = \log 47 - \log 2$$
$$\log 76^{3/8} = \tfrac{3}{8} \log 76$$

To find the characteristics:

Digits to the left of decimal point:		1 2 3 4 5 6
Characteristic is:		0 1 2 3 4 5

Zeros to right of decimal point and preceding first significant figure:	0 1 2 3 4
Characteristic is:	-1 -2 -3 -4 -5

Aqueous Solution. The concentration of a solution may be expressed in a variety of ways, e.g., molarity, normality, and weight/volume (w/v). These are concentrations based on volume. Solutions based on weight and expressed as molality and weight/weight (w/w) are used less frequently in the laboratory.

Molarity (M) is equal to the number of moles of solute per liter of solution. One gram molecular weight of a substance (GMW) is also called 1 mole of the substance. One mole of water (H_2O) = 18.015 g.

$$\text{Moles} = \frac{g}{\text{GMW}}$$

A 1-molar (M) solution contains 1 mole of solute per liter of finished solution.

$$\text{Molarity} = \text{moles/liter} = \frac{\text{grams/liter}}{\text{GMW}}$$

A millimole (m mole) is 1/1000 of a mole.

$$\text{Millimoles per liter} = \frac{\text{milligrams/liter}}{\text{GMW}}$$

Avogadro's
number = number of molecules per g-mole
= number of atoms per g-atom
= number of ions per g-ion
= 6.023×10^{23}

In practice though, one Avogadro's number of particles (i.e., 1 g-mole, 1 g-atom, or 1 g-ion) is called a "mole" regardless of whether the substance is ionic, monoatomic, or molecular in nature. Thus, 39.0 g of K^+ ion may be called a "mole," instead of a "gram-ion." To make 1 liter of a 1M NaCl solution (mol. wt. = 58.5), 58.5 g of NaCl is dissolved in enough water to make 1 liter.

When small concentrations are used, they are frequently expressed in millimoles/liter (1000 millimoles = 1 mole). For example, to prepare 10 ml of a 10 mM (0.01M) NaOH solution, 4 mg NaOH are diluted to 10 ml.

Normality (N) is equal to the number of equivalents of solute per liter of solution. One gram equivalent weight of an element or compound equals the gram molecular weight divided by valence.

$$\text{Gram equivalent weight} = \frac{\text{GMW}}{\text{valence}}$$

One gram equivalent weight of a substance is also called one equivalent of the substance.

$$\text{Number of equivalents} = \frac{\text{grams}}{\text{gram equiv. wt.}}$$

Example: $Ca(OH)_2$ (GMW = 74)
Equivalent wt. = 74/2 = 37
1 mole = 2 equivalents

H_2SO_4 (GMW = 98)
Equivalent wt. = 98/2 = 49
1 mole = 2 equivalents

Therefore, one equivalent (i.e., the equivalent weight) of an acid or base is the weight that contains 1 g-atom (1 mole) of replaceable hydrogen, or 1 g-ion (1 mole) of replaceable hydroxyl.

To prepare 1 liter of 1N H_2SO_4 from pure (96.2 per cent) concentrated sulfuric acid having a specific gravity* of 1.84, dilute 27.7 ml H_2SO_4 to 1 liter.

Appendix 2 contains useful information about various acids and bases commonly used in the laboratory.

Weight/volume per cent (% w/v) is equal to the number of grams of a solid dissolved in enough solvent to bring the final volume to 100 ml.

A 10 per cent NaOH solution is prepared by dissolving 10 g NaOH in enough water to make a final volume of 100 ml.

Molality (M) is equal to the number of moles of solute per 1000 g of solvent. A molal solution is used in certain physical chemical calculations, e.g., calculations of boiling-point and freezing-point depression.

Weight/weight per cent (% w/w) is equal to the weight in g of a solute per 100 g of solution. The concentrations of many commercial acids are given in terms of % w/w.

Acids, Alkalis, and pH. An acid molecule yields hydrogen ions (protons) in aqueous solutions; an alkali accepts these. At room temperature in pure water:

$$[H^+] = [OH^-] = 1 \times 10^{-7} \text{ molar}$$

In all aqueous solutions, both acid and alkaline:

$$K_w = [H^+] \times [OH^-] = 10^{-14}$$

In an acid solution $[H^+]$ is greater than 10^{-7} M. In an alkaline solution, $[H^+]$ is less than 10^{-7} M.

---

*specific gravity (sp. gr.) = $\dfrac{\text{weight in g}}{\text{volume in ml}}$

pH is the exponent which must be applied to 10 in order to give the value of $1/H^+$. That is,

$$pH = \log_{10} 1/H^+$$

When pH is 1, H^+ is 10^{-1} and OH^- is 10^{-13}
   2   10^{-2} 10^{-12}
   4   10^{-4} 10^{-10}
   6   10^{-6} 10^{-8}
  10   10^{-10} 10^{-4}
  13   10^{-13} 10^{-1}

A change of one pH unit indicates a tenfold change in H^+ concentration.

Buffer Solutions. The theory of buffers and their preparation can be found in Appendix 2. A more extensive description of various buffer solutions is reviewed by Gomori (1955).

LABORATORY SAFETY

The Psychology of Safety. Injuries affect the morale and threaten the emotional health of the party involved. Injuries are expensive in terms of lost wages and medical treatment. An injured person cannot work at peak efficiency. Persons in the professions of health care are vital to the needs of others. Injuries impair this ability to serve (see Chap. 58).

In an excellent study, Stout (1972) investigated the cause of accidents. These findings have important implications for the medical professional. It was discovered that accidents were not caused by inexperience. Rather, accidents occurred when experienced operators consciously accepted *risks* that inexperienced operators would avoid. Contributory causes to accidents were found to be (1) the conscious acceptance of an obvious and familiar risk; (2) hurrying to meet deadlines, some imaginary; (3) carelessness and fatigue; (4) mental preoccupation—planning, worrying, day dreaming.

Accident prevention can therefore be broken down into two components, namely, knowledge factors and emotional factors. It is important to *know* the rules of safety. However, Stout (1972) found in his study that the injured parties knew the rules of safety. Therefore, this is not enough. The knowledge factor must be accompanied by emotional or psychological factors. The worker must maintain a constant, cautious, attentive *alertness*. *Concentration* on the job is imperative. This attitude of safety which encourages an awareness of hazards can help insure the continued health and productivity of all personnel.

REFERENCES

Bermes, E. W., Jr., and Forman, D. J.: Basic laboratory principles and procedures. *In* Tietz, N. W. (ed.): Fundamentals of Clinical Chemistry, 2nd ed. Philadelphia, W. B. Saunders Company, 1976.

Booker, H. E., and Darcey, B.: Serum concentrations of free diphenylhydantoin and their relationship to clinical intoxication. Epilepsia, *14*:177, 1973.

Corning/Pyrex Labware (catalog), Laboratory Products Department, Corning Glassworks, Corning, New York 14830. 1967.

Fritz, J. S., and Schenk, G. H.: Quantitative Analytical Chemistry, 3rd ed. Boston, Allyn and Bacon, Inc., 1974.

Gomori, G.: Preparations of buffers for use in enzyme studies. Meth. Enzymol., *1*:138, 1955.

Hackler, M.: How to choose a laboratory balance. Am. Lab., March, 1970.

Hamlin, W. B., Duckworth, J. K., Gilmer, P. R., and Stevens, M. V.: Laboratory Instrument Maintenance and Function Verification. College of American Pathologists, 230 North Michigan Avenue, Chicago, Illinois, 60601. 1974.

Lashof, T. W., and Macurdy, L. B.: Precision laboratory standards of mass and laboratory weights. National Bureau of Standards Circular 547. Washington, D.C., United States Department of Commerce, 1954.

Mabry, C. C., Gevedon, R. E., Roeckel, I. E., and Gochman, N.: Automated submicrochemistries. A system of rapid sodium, potassium, chloride, carbon dioxide, sugar, urea nitrogen, total and direct-reacting bilirubin, and total protein. Am. J. Clin. Pathol., *46*:265, 1966.

Mabry, C. C., Roeckel, I. E., Gevedon, R. E., and Koepke, J. A.: Recent Advances in Pediatric Clinical Pathology. Lexington, Kentucky, The University of Kentucky Medical Center, 1967.

Meinke, W. W.: Standard reference materials for clinical measurements. Anal. Chem., *43*:28A, 1971.

Natelson, S.: Weighing the sample. *In* Techniques of Clinical Chemistry, 3rd ed. Springfield, Ill., Charles C Thomas, Publisher, 1971.

Radin, N.: What is a standard? Clin. Chem., *13*:55, 1967.

Rice, E. W.: Principles and Methods of Clinical Chemistry for Medical Technologists. Springfield, Ill., Charles C Thomas, Publisher, 1960.

Segel, I. H.: Biochemical Calculations, 2nd ed. New York, John Wiley & Sons, Inc., 1976.

Spencer, W. W., Nelson, G. H., and Konicki, K. A.: Evaluation of a new system ("Corvac") for separating serum from blood for routine laboratory procedures. Clin. Chem., *22*:1012, 1976.

Stier, A. R., Miller, L. K., and Smith, R. J.: Water Specifications. Commission on Laboratory Inspection and Accreditation. College of American Pathologists, 230 North Michigan Avenue, Chicago, Illinois, 60601. 3rd printing, 1974.

Stout, T. T., and Darby, B. I.: Disabling form accidents. Ohio Rep. Res. Devel., 57:35, 1972.

Weast, R. C. (ed.): Handbook of Chemistry and Physics. Cleveland, The Chemical Rubber Co., 1976, pp. D147–D152.

Wilson, F., Rankel, S., Linke, E. G., and Henry, J. B.: Free-thyroxine—an abbreviated assay. Am. J. Clin. Pathol., 62:383, 1974.

Winstead, M.: Reagent grade water: How, when and why? Austin, Texas, The Steck Company, 1967.

Winsten, S.: Collection and preservation of specimens. In Meites, S. (ed.): Standard Methods of Clinical Chemistry, Vol. 5. New York, Academic Press, Inc., 1965.

4

PRINCIPLES OF INSTRUMENTATION

Merle A. Evenson, Ph.D.

Prior to the 1930's most measurements in clinical chemistry were gravimetric, volumetric, or manometric. Most information was only semiquantitative, and instrumentation was centered on the analytical balance and was very limited. The introduction of the visible photoelectric colorimeter to replace the color comparator was the first major advance in clinical chemistry instrumentation. The introduction of the flame photometer for the measurement of sodium and potassium instead of the slow, inaccurate, troublesome gravimetric methods in serum was a significant advance. In the early 1940's a spectrophotometer that could operate in the ultraviolet range opened new vistas to clinical laboratories. In the late 1950's the AutoAnalyzer by the Technicon Company (Tarrytown, New York) produced the largest impact up to that time upon the field of clinical chemistry in the United States. In the early 1960's multichannel analyzers became available and that technologic development had another enormous impact upon the field. The volume of work in the clinical laboratory increased exponentially as a result of newly available laboratory measurements. Discrete sample analyzers were also introduced in the 1960's, a development that improved emergency analysis availability and afforded more accurate and precise answers. Also in the 1960's atomic absorption spectrophotometers and gas chromatographs designed for chemical measurements began to appear in clinical laboratories. In the 1970's radioimmunoassays, high-performance liquid chromatography, ion-selective electrodes, and micro-processor-controlled instrumentation are being used frequently in clinical chemistry laboratories.

The major purpose of this chapter is to provide a brief nonmathematical explanation of the general physical and chemical principles involved in the measurements commonly made in clinical laboratories, and particularly in clinical chemistry. The discussion will use only simple mathematical equations to describe some of the physical laws upon which the analytical measurements are based. It will be only moderately involved with a description of specific analytical methods for individual analytes. Since the analytical procedures range widely in a modern clinical laboratory and most of the different types of available instrumentation are used daily, it is important for the personnel in the clinical laboratory to be well acquainted with the principles of the different measurements. Electronics, physics, inorganic chemistry, organic chemistry, physical chemistry, analytical chemistry, biochemistry, and immunology are all important disciplines that are blended together in a functioning clinical laboratory; hence, personnel in the laboratory should be knowledgeable in all these areas to understand more fully the analytical methodology and instrumentation used in the laboratory.

Because analytical methodologies and instrumentation change so rapidly, specific examples will not be included in this chapter, nor will performance criteria on specific analytical procedures be considered. The major purpose of this chapter is to introduce the generalized principles of the various fields that will serve as a basis for the analytical methodology used in clinical laboratories. Textbooks on instrumentation that should be helpful to the interested reader include those by Ewing (1969), Skoog (1971), and Strobel (1973).

SPECTROPHOTOMETRIC AND PHOTOMETRIC MEASUREMENTS

The term *photometric measurement* was originally defined as measurement of light intensity of multiple wavelengths, while *spectrophotometric measurements* formerly meant measurement of light intensity in a much narrower wavelength range. It has recently become common usage to refer to instruments that use filters for isolation of part of the spectrum as photometers or colorimeters, whereas instruments that use gratings and/or prisms are called spectrophotometers. The range of light measured is no longer a valid distinction between colorimeters and spectrophotometers.

Electromagnetic radiation (EMR) includes radiant energy from short wavelength gamma rays to long wavelength radio waves. Frequently, a white light source for the visible region or a deuterium source for ultraviolet (UV) light will provide the wavelengths used. The wavelength of light is defined as the distance between peaks as the light is envisioned to travel in a wavelike manner. The distance between peaks in the ultraviolet and visible ranges is measured either in Angstroms (Å), nanometers (nm), or millimicrons (mμ). There are 10^{10} Å, 10^9 nm, or 10^9 mμ in one meter. A recent trend is to use nanometer (nm) for expressing the wavelength of light. There are 10 Å per nm and a nm numerically equals a mμ. The nm is the preferred SI unit. In addition to possessing wavelength characteristics, light also has properties that indicate its composition to be discrete energy packets called photons. The relationship between the energy of photons and their frequency is given by the equation:

$$E = h\nu$$

E refers to the energy in ergs when the frequency ν is given in hertz (cycles per sec.) and h, Planck's constant, is given as 6.62×10^{-27} erg-second. The frequency of light is related to the wavelength by an equation:

$$\nu = \frac{c}{\lambda}$$

where ν is the frequency in cycles per second, c is the speed of light in a vacuum (3×10^{10} cm/sec.), and λ the wavelength in cm. By looking at the above equations we can readily see that as the frequency of light increases, so does the energy. If we substitute the value of ν from the second equation into the first equation we obtain:

$$E = \frac{hc}{(\lambda)}$$

This equation shows that the energy of light is inversely proportional to the wavelength. For example, UV radiation at 200 nm possesses greater energy than infrared radiation at 750 nm.

Table 4-1 shows the relationship of the wavelength to the name assigned to certain areas in the electromagnetic radiation spectrum and also shows relationships between the various units that are used in the measurement of wavelength. Table 4-2 shows similar relationships except that it is limited to the UV and visible range of the spectrum. The areas are classified as to the name of the region, its wavelength, its color, and its complementary color.

If a solution absorbs light between 400 and 480 nm (blue), it will appear yellow to the eye. Therefore, yellow is the complementary color of blue. Likewise, if the green color is absorbed, the solution will appear purple. The human eye responds to radiation only between

Table 4-1. ELECTROMAGNETIC RADIATION CHARACTERISTICS

	Gamma Rays	X-Rays	Ultraviolet	Visible	Infrared	Micro Waves	Radio Waves
	WAVELENGTH INTERVAL WHERE THE TYPE OF EMR BEGINS						
Wavelength							
Angstrom (Å)	1	10	1800	3400	7000		
Nanometer (nm) (millimicron) (mμ)			180	340	700		
Micrometer (micron) (μ)					0.7	400	
Centimeter (cm)						0.04	25

350 and 800 nm, but laboratory instrumentation permits measurements at both shorter wavelength—ultraviolet (UV)—and longer wavelength—infrared (IR)—portions of the spectrum.

PRISMS FOR WAVELENGTH ISOLATION

In spectrophotometry, generally the wavelength under consideration is isolated by means of gratings or prisms. Prisms are wedge-shaped pieces of glass, quartz, sodium chloride, or some other material that allows transmission of light. Because of the variation of the refractive index with wavelength, the light that enters the prism is dispersed to varying degrees, depending upon the wavelength of the light. The red end of the spectrum is refracted least by the prism, while the blue or violet end of the spectrum is refracted the most as it passes through the prism.

GRATINGS FOR WAVELENGTH ISOLATION

A grating is a device that has small grooves cut into it at such an angle that each groove

Table 4-2. COLORS AND COMPLEMENTARY COLORS OF THE ULTRAVIOLET AND VISIBLE SPECTRUM

WAVELENGTH (nm)	REGION NAME	COLOR ABSORBED	COMPLEMENTARY OR SOLUTION COLOR
180–220	short UV	not visible	–
220–340	UV	not visible	–
340–430	visible	violet	yellow green
430–475	visible	blue	yellow
475–495	visible	green blue	orange
495–505	visible	blue green	red
505–555	visible	green	purple
555–575	visible	yellow green	violet
575–600	visible	yellow	blue
600–620	visible	orange	green blue
620–700	visible	red	blue green

behaves like a very small prism. Light is reflected or transmitted from or through the grating in such a manner that white light is again separated into its various color components throughout the spectrum. A grating may have 3000 or more small grooves per mm cut into the grating surface. Each little groove functions like a prism in resolving white light into its components except that usually the light is reflected off the grating rather than transmitted through the prism, thereby reducing loss of energy.

SELECTION OF WAVELENGTH FOR MEASUREMENT

When a measurement is made in a spectrophotometer, the color of light that shows maximum or near maximum absorption should be passed through the solution to obtain maximum sensitivity. A blue solution absorbs red strongly; therefore a wavelength in the red portion of the spectrum would be chosen for measurements of blue solutions. Occasionally an absorption measurement will intentionally be made at a wavelength off the absorption maximum to minimize absorption of interfering substances. Although less than ideal, a reduction in sensitivity is often less critical than the interference. This reduction in sensitivity will frequently linearize or extend the linear portion of a working curve. Many chemical methodologies in clinical chemistry use the above approach to reduce non-linearity in non-specific color reactions.

Most analyses performed in the clinical chemistry laboratory depend upon making measurements of the amount of light absorbed for each of the particular substances being measured. Most of the measurements are made in the visible range of the spectrum, some in the ultraviolet range, and even fewer in the infrared region. However, new instruments and improved methodology are making more and more applications practical in the field of infrared spectrophotometry. In clinical laboratories, infrared instruments are used to determine the composition of renal stones and gallstones and to analyze for purified toxicologic substances.

BEER'S LAW

Beer's law states that the concentration of a substance is directly proportional to the amount of light absorbed or inversely proportional to the logarithm of the transmitted light.

The mathematical relationship between absorption of radiant energy and the concentration of a solution is shown by Beer's law:

$$A = abc = \log \frac{100}{\%T} = 2 - \log \%T$$

where A = absorbance
    a = absorptivity
    b = light path of the solution in cm
    c = concentration of the substance of
        interest
  %T = per cent transmittance

Transmittance (T) is defined as the ratio of transmitted light (I) to incident light (I_o).

The above relationship is the basis for all spectrophotometric absorption measurements and results from contributions from several individuals. Lambert, Bouguer, and others independently contributed to the above formula, commonly called "Beer's law."

Beer's law is an ideal mathematical relationship that contains several limitations in practice. There are three areas where deviations from Beer's law can occur—simultaneous absorption at multiple wavelengths, absorption of light by other species, and transmission of light by other mechanisms. Strictly speaking, the absorptivity (a) is different for each wavelength of light. Unless the absorptivity is constant over the range of wavelengths being used, Beer's law will not be followed.

If two or more chemical species are absorbing the wavelength of light being used, each with a different absorptivity, Beer's law will not be followed.

Finally, if the absorption of a fluorescent solution is being measured, Beer's law may not be followed.

Deviations from Beer's law also occur when

a very wide range of concentrations is measured. The range of concentrations that are linear with absorbance varies with each substance.

Figure 4-1 shows a plot of per cent transmittance (%T) vs. concentration, illustrating that %T is inversely and logarithmically related to concentration. Also shown is a plot of absorbance vs. concentration, where the absorbance is directly and linearly related to the concentration of interest. From the figure, notice that the absorbance decreases by 50 per cent when the concentration (or light path) decreases by 50 per cent, while %T shows a non-linear relationship to the same condition. Since %T has a reciprocal log relationship to concentration, a decrease in concentration produces a logarithmic increase in %T. Most laboratory instruments produce an electrical signal that is proportional to %T. If one wants to take advantage of the linear relationship between absorbance and concentration, the %T values have to be converted to absorbance either electronically or with the aid of logarithmic scales or tables. Usually the conversion is electronic, and a digital read-out or printer gives the values in absorbance.

In summary, Beer's law will only be followed if the incident radiation on the substance of interest is monochromatic, if the solvent absorption is insignificant compared to the solute absorbance, if the solute concentration is within "linear limits," and if a chemical reaction does not occur between the molecule of interest and another solute or solvent molecule.

Spectrophotometric measurements have gained significantly in popularity in recent years. The principal advantages of spectrophotometric measurements are relatively high sensitivity, ease with which rapid measurements can be made, and a relatively high degree of specificity. Specificity is obtained by reacting the substance of interest with the proper reagents, thus producing different colors, or by analytical separations prior to color forming reactions. Spectral isolation of interferences by the monochromators in spectrophotometers is also used but may alone be inadequate for high accuracy measurements. Spectrophotometric methods are widely applicable for both qualitative and quantitative analyses. Nearly all substances of interest will either absorb energy of a specific wavelength themselves or can be chemically converted to compounds which will then absorb energy of a

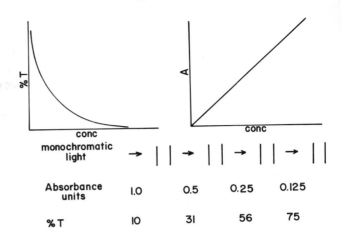

Figure 4–1. The relationship of absorbance (A) and percent transmittance (%T) to concentration (conc).

specific wavelength. The specificity of many spectrophotometric procedures used in measurements is not always adequate, and continuous efforts to improve methods are being made. At the same time, other physical measurements are being developed so that dependence of clinical laboratories on spectrophotometric measurements will probably decrease in the future.

COMPONENTS OF SPECTROPHOTOMETERS

Figure 4–2 shows the basic components of a spectrophotometer. All spectrophotometers need a light source and an entrance slit so that the light that enters the monochromator will come from a common, well-defined point. The monochromator consists of a system of prisms or gratings by which white light is resolved into the various wavelengths. The exit slit is used to control the size of the beam (incident light) that passes to the analytical cell or cuvette. The analytical cell or cuvette is a glass, quartz, or plastic container that holds the solution whose absorption is to be meas-

ured. The detector is the module that measures the intensity of light that passes through the cuvette (emergent light). The output of the detector is related to the concentration of the substance of interest.

THE LIGHT SOURCE

The function of the light source is to provide radiant energy in the form of visible or non-visible light that may be passed through the monochromator to be separated into discrete wavelengths. The light of the proper wavelength is then made to be incident on the analytical cell holding the solution whose absorption is to be measured.

In the conventional spectrophotometer commercially available 15 to 20 years ago, a tungsten light bulb was usually the only source of visible light. Today other sources are commonly used and these will be mentioned later in this section. The tungsten bulb was and is acceptable for making measurements in moderately dilute solutions where the difference in color intensity varies significantly with small changes in concentration. A common disadvantage with some early photome-

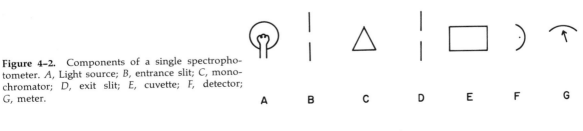

Figure 4–2. Components of a single spectrophotometer. *A,* Light source; *B,* entrance slit; *C,* monochromator; *D,* exit slit; *E,* cuvette; *F,* detector; *G,* meter.

A   B   C   D   E   F   G

single beam

ters is that a considerable amount of electrical energy was necessary to maintain a constant high energy output from such a source. As a result, significant heat may be generated by the source, which may cause measurement problems. The generated heat may change the geometry of the optical system as well as the sensitivity of the detectors. The thermal change can shift the optics (lenses) so that a different wavelength of light is incident on the cuvette between the standardization and analysis steps. This wavelength change and/or the sensitivity change of the detectors may produce significant errors.

A tungsten light source does not supply sufficient radiant energy for measurements in the ultraviolet region below 320 nm. For this purpose a mercury-arc, hydrogen, or deuterium lamp is suitable, since adequate energy is supplied over the usually used ultraviolet range. Recently the deuterium light source has come into more frequent use and although it does not possess as much intensity as the mercury arc, it has approximately three times as much intensity as a hydrogen lamp.

Tungsten iodide sources are frequently used for visible and UV measurements and are mounted in a quartz envelope so that they may also be used in the ultraviolet region of the spectrum. These sources are high intensity and long lasting. They will frequently operate two to three thousand hours before replacement is necessary.

THE ENTRANCE SLIT

The function of the entrance slit is to minimize stray light and prevent scattered light from entering the monochromator system. Stray light must be excluded from passing through the cuvette; otherwise Beer's law will not be followed and significant errors may be introduced depending upon how compensations for such design deficiencies are handled.

MONOCHROMATORS

The function of the monochromator in spectrophotometers is to isolate specific wavelengths of light emitted by the source. This is achieved by the use of prisms or gratings or both in spectrophotometry. The prism or grating may be tilted or rotated in the light beam so as to permit the proper wavelength to be incident upon the cuvette and the detector. Still other spectrophotometers obtain the proper wavelength of light incident on the cuvette by moving the light source. In visible spectrophotometry, glass prisms are frequently used, but quartz is required for ultraviolet region measurements. Prisms made of sodium chloride or potassium bromide were frequently used in infrared spectrophotometers before gratings became popular. Some spectrophotometers designed years ago contained only prisms, while certain high-quality, high-performance ultraviolet-visible recording spectrophotometers contained both prisms and gratings. In many of the medium-price-range, medium-quality spectrophotometers, prisms have been replaced with gratings. Detailed descriptions of how gratings are made are available elsewhere in the literature, so only a brief discussion will be included here.

Generally, a master grating is made by carefully controlled etching of grooves into a metal surface. A thin layer of aluminum is then deposited on the master grating and an optically flat surface is glued to the aluminized grooves deposited in the master grating. When hardened, the replica grating is removed from the master grating and performs nearly as well as an original. Such a grating frequently costs only one per cent or less of the cost of the master grating and performs adequately. Gratings are inexpensive and can increase the amount of energy available by using reflection instead of transmittance techniques. Light must always pass through a prism, but a grating may be used in either reflectance or transmittance modes of operation.

INTERFERENCE FILTERS

Filter photometers use devices called *interference filters* to obtain spectral purity instead of using prisms or gratings. Interference filters are made by depositing thin semitransparent silver films on each side of a dielectric such as magnesium fluoride. A dielectric is an insulating material that does not allow electric current to flow. When light perpendicular to the silvered surface enters the interference filter, it will pass through the dielectric and be reflected from the second silver surface back through the dielectric to the first silver layer to be reflected again. Finally, the light is transmitted through the semitransparent silver film and into the photometer. Constructive and destructive interference will occur as the light is reflected between the transparent silver films. Constructive interference will occur only when the wavelength of the light is equal to the thickness of the magnesium fluoride layer or a multiple of that thickness. Interference filters will allow transmission of a range of wavelengths between 10 and 20 nm wide and will allow 40 to 60 per cent of incident light to be transmitted. The band of wavelengths allowed to pass is called the "band path." The thickness of the magnesium fluoride can be carefully controlled, and filters of different wavelengths are made by varying this thickness. Multilayer interference filters can be prepared by depositing several layers of dielectrics on each other, each of which is a fraction of a wavelength thick. Multilayer interference filters such as this will have a band path of 5 to 10 nm and will allow 60 to 95 per cent of the incident light to be transmitted. Interference filters are inexpensive individually, but several sets are required to work at different wavelengths. The Technicon Auto-Analyzer colorimeter contains interference filters of this type with individual specifications on the filters. For example, the identification number 530 on a filter means that the peak transmittance occurs at 530 nm. A second number, e.g., 18, that appears below the first number refers to the band path transmitted by that filter at one half the height of maximum transmission, i.e., 18 nm.

Gelatin Filters

Less expensive photometers may use gelatin or colored glass filters in order to obtain some spectral resolution. The colored gelatin is layered between two plates of glass. The gelatin filter can be used to absorb light of wavelengths other than that of the color of the gelatin. Likewise, colored glass can be prepared which functions in the same way as the gelatin filters. Glass and gelatin filters permit only a small percentage of incident light to be transmitted and have relatively wide band paths of up to 50 nm.

Analytical Cell or Cuvette

The function of the cuvette is to hold the solution in the instrument where the absorption is to be measured. Cells are made of soft or borosilicate glass, quartz, or plastic. The soft glass cells are used for solutions that are acidic and do not etch glass. Strongly alkaline solutions should be measured in borosilicate cells because of their higher resistance to alkali. As soon as measurements are completed, alkaline solutions must be rinsed from the cells. Glass cells are unsuitable for measurements in the short ultraviolet region of the spectrum. Some glass cells (Corex) can be used to make measurements at 340 nm. Only quartz or plastics that do not absorb ultraviolet radiation can be used for measurements at wavelengths below 320 nm. Recently, some plastic materials have been developed that show little or no absorption of radiant energy from 200 to 700 nm. Generally, these cells are inexpensive and in some cases disposable and will most certainly find increased usage in the near future.

Common errors in handling cuvettes are failure to position the cell properly in the photometer and failure to match absorbance readings of the cells. When round cuvettes are used, they should be marked near the top and always positioned in a predetermined manner. If inexpensive unmatched cells are used, blank readings should be taken to measure the tolerance of each cuvette at each wavelength used.

Detectors

The two most commonly used devices for measuring light intensity in the UV and visible regions of the spectrum are barrier layer cells and photomultiplier tubes. The barrier layer cells are rugged and are used in inexpensive instruments, while photomultipliers are almost always used in the higher quality, more expensive spectrophotometers.

Barrier layer cells

Barrier layer cells operate on the principle that when light falls on certain metals or semiconductors, electrons will flow in proportion to the intensity of the light. The barrier layer cell consists of a thin layer of silver on a layer of the semiconductor selenium. The silver and selenium metals are then mounted on an iron backing or support. The iron backing is deficient in electrons and is therefore the positive electrode. The silver mounted on top of the selenium where the light will be incident is the negatively charged electrode. When light falls on the thin semitranslucent silver metal, electron flow from the semiconductor selenium into the iron backing occurs. Electrons cannot flow in the reverse direction in a barrier layer cell.

The sensitivity to wavelength of the barrier layer cell is similar to that of the human eye. The maximum sensitivity of both occurs at 550 nm. Barrier layer cells are usually used at high levels of illumination and the output from these photo cells is generally not amplified. Barrier layer cells are very stable, but are slow in responding to changes of light intensity. Because of their slow response time, barrier layer cells are not suitable as detectors in instruments that employ interrupted (chopped) light beams falling on the detectors. Another disadvantage of this photo cell is that it tends to show fatigue. Fatigue occurs in a barrier layer cell when at a constant extremely high level of intensity, the electrical output of the photo cell decreases with time. Therefore, barrier layer cells should not be used at extremely high illumination.

The Coleman spectrophotometer (Coleman Instrument Division, Perkin-Elmer Corporation, Oak Brook, N.J.) and older Technicon Auto-Analyzer interference filter colorimeters contain photo cells of this type. The cells are very rugged, last for years, and perform well as inexpensive detectors. A potential problem with barrier layer cells is that their electrical output is very temperature dependent. If a heat-producing high intensity lamp or flame is used for the light source, instrument design must be such that thermal stability and rapid temperature equilibrium of the photo cell is achieved. This is accomplished in the Auto-Analyzer colorimeter by having the light source far removed from the photo cell. Use of heat shields or plastic materials which do not conduct heat readily are other ways of improving thermal stability of instruments.

Photomultiplier tubes

A photomultiplier is an electron tube that is capable of significantly amplifying a current. It is constructed by using a light-sensitive material that emits electrons in proportion to the radiant energy which strikes the surface of the light-sensitive material. The electrons produced by this first stage go to a secondary stage (surface) where each electron produces between four and six additional electrons. Each of these electrons from the second stage go on to another stage, again producing four to six electrons. Each electron produced cascades through the photomultiplier stages; thus, the final current produced by such a tube may be one million or more times as much as the initial current. As many as 10 to 15 stages or dynodes are present in common photomultipliers.

To operate such a tube, voltage is applied between the photocathode and each successive stage. The normal increment of voltage increase of each photomultiplier stage is from 50 to 100 volts larger than that of the previous stage. A common photomultiplier tube will have approximately 1500 volts applied to it.

Photomultiplier tubes have extremely rapid response times, are very sensitive, and do not show as much fatigue as other detectors. Because of their excellent sensitivity and rapid response, all stray light and daylight must be carefully shielded from the photomultiplier. A photomultiplier with the voltage applied should never be exposed to room light because it will burn out. Because of the fast response time of the photomultiplier, this detector is applicable to interrupted light beams such as those produced by choppers and thus provides significant advantages when used as a UV-visible detector in spectrophotometers. The rapid response times are also needed when a spectrophotometer is being used to determine an absorption spectrum of a compound. The photomultiplier also has adequate sensitivity over a wider wavelength range than do photo cell detectors.

When voltage is applied to photomultipliers and all light has been blocked from them, some current will usually be produced. This current is called *dark current*. It is desirable to have the dark current of photomultipliers at their lowest level, as it would also be amplified and would appear as background noise.

DOUBLE-BEAM SPECTROPHOTOMETERS

There are several optical and electrical configurations used in commercially available spectrophotometers. Each configuration has advantages for certain applications.

Double-beam instruments have been classified as double beam in space (Fig. 4-3) or double beam in time (Fig. 4-10). Notice in the double beam in space instrument that all components are duplicated except the light source. The two beams pass at the same time through different components separated in space. This arrangement would compensate for changes in intensity of the light source and also compensate for changes in absorbance of the reagent blank as the wavelength is changed in a scanning operation.

A double-beam instrument in time usually uses the same components as a single-beam instrument. The two beams pass through the

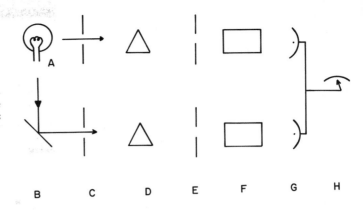

Figure 4-3. Double beam in space spectrophotometer. *A*, Light source; *B*, mirror; *C*, entrance slits; *D*, monochromators; *E*, exit slits; *F*, cuvettes; *G*, photomultipliers; *H*, meter.

same components but not at the same time. Duplication of cuvette compartments is sometimes used. A light beam chopper (a rotating wheel with alternate silvered sections and cut-out sections) is inserted after the exit slit. A system of mirrors would pass the reflected portion of the light off the chopper through a reference cuvette and then onto the common detector. Just as a single-beam instrument is adjusted to zero absorbance with the blank before and between sample readings, the double-beam system makes these adjustments automatically. The detector, as in Figure 4-10, is made to look alternately at the sample and then the reference beam of light. The difference or ratio of the timed signals is then amplified and is proportional to the substance of interest in the sample cuvette. The double-beam-in-time approach using one detector compensates for light source variation as well as for sensitivity changes of the detector.

Various other combinations of components and parts of the two approaches presented above have been used in double-beam spectrophotometers. Usually the design is conceived to solve a specific problem.

Although more expensive, double-beam instruments provide increased quality measurements. Some double-beam instruments use a recorder for the output. The recorder traces a plot of the absorbance or per cent transmittance (%T) versus wavelength as the operator desires. The recording double-beam spectrophotometer has its greatest advantage when scanning the spectrum. It automatically compensates when the absorbance of the blank and the intensity of the light source vary with wavelength.

SELECTION OF AN INSTRUMENT FOR PHOTOMETRY

The most important consideration in the selection of an instrument for spectrophotometric or photometric analysis is the intended use of the instrument. If a high-precision scanning instrument is required, a high quality recording double-beam spectrophotometer is needed. If, on the other hand, it is necessary to measure changes in concentration at a limited number of wavelengths where it is not critical to have spectral purity and wavelength isolation, an inexpensive instrument would work well.

If a UV spectrophotometer is to be used for measuring a barbiturate, it is desirable to have a double-beam recording scanning instrument for such a determination. The advantage of a double-beam instrument is that a continuous correction for optical errors or deficiencies can be made automatically as the wavelength changes. In the case of the barbiturate determinations, if a known negative serum sample is inserted in the reference beam and the sample to be analyzed is placed in the sample beam, the instrument automatically makes the correction for unwanted extracted substances and presents to the operator a corrected peak which is directly related to concentration without further calculations. This technique of using a serum sample in the reference beam of double-beam UV-visible recording spectrophotometers also has the advantage of increasing the sensitivity for all measurements. A spectrum scan will usually detect interferences owing to other drugs.

The method of *ultimate precision* may be

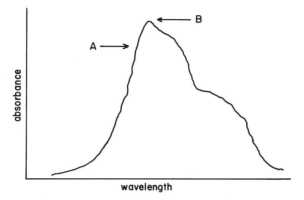

Figure 4-4. Example of an absorption spectrum (see text).

applied in absorption spectroscopy. This is accomplished by closely bracketing the unknown solution with two solutions of known concentration, then adjusting the darker colored solution to read zero transmittance and the lighter colored solution to read 100 per cent transmittance. The per cent transmittance of the unknown is read and the result obtained by interpolation. The maximum sensitivity and smallest error in measurement are achieved by using this method of *ultimate precision*.

Figure 4-4 is an example of an absorption spectrum showing the plot of absorbance vs. wavelength. If a single well-defined absorption spectrum is obtained, the amount of absorption that occurs at the "peak" wavelength (B) (Fig. 4-4) is to be preferred over an absorption measurement on the "shoulder" (A) of the peak. An increase in sensitivity and specificity results from a measurement at peak absorption. However, if interferences are present, it may be necessary, although less desirable, to make measurements of absorption off the peak wavelength and relate this measurement to concentration. If the absorption peak is sharp or if a shoulder wavelength is selected for absorbance readings, great care must be used in adjusting the proper wavelength each time the instrument is used. Shoulder operation can easily introduce large measurement errors and should be avoided.

Occasionally, by not measuring at the peak absorption, the linear working range of a method can be expanded. This occurs because of the reduction in sensitivity and is frequently used in cholesterol and glucose methods.

A method to correct for background inter-

ferences is to measure absorbance at the peak wavelength and at two other wavelengths, usually equidistant from the peak. Values for the latter are averaged to obtain a baseline under the peak, which is then subtracted from the peak reading. The value so obtained is known as a "corrected" absorbance and can be related to the concentration, provided that the background absorbance is linear with wavelength over the region in which readings are made. This technique of making corrections for interfering substances is called the *Allen correction* and is illustrated in Figure 4-5.

Salicylate extracted from acidified serum, for example, shows a peak absorbance at 300 nm (see curve A of Figure 4-5). An extract of salicylate-free serum also exhibits appreciable absorbance at this wavelength, but the absorbance is linear between 280 and 320 nm (line B of Figure 4-5). The corrected absorbance at 300 nm is obtained from the Allen equation:

$$A_{Corr} = A_{300} - \frac{(A_{280} + A_{320})}{2}$$

Similar corrections are applied in procedures for spectrophotometric determinations of porphyrins, steroids, and other compounds.

Before using the Allen correction, knowledge of the shape of the absorption curve for the substance of interest and of the interferences must be obtained. The linearity of the baseline shift should be verified by measuring the absorption spectrum of commonly encountered interferences. Care should be exercised in use of the Allen correction. If not properly used, it may introduce larger errors than

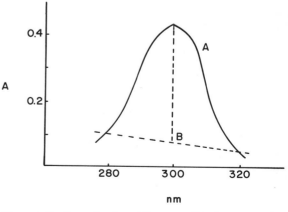

Figure 4-5. Example of an Allen correction for a measurement of salicylate in serum (see text).

would be observed without correction. For example, such a situation may occur if the background reading is not linear over the region measured.

FLAME PHOTOMETRY

The flame emission spectrophotometer is one of the most important instruments used in clinical laboratories. It offers one of the most convenient, accurate, and precise measurements made in laboratories today. The basis of the measurement was illustrated in preliminary chemistry courses where qualitative analysis was performed using the flame spot test, in which the color of a burning flame is different for certain cations.

The principle behind flame photometry involves the excitation of electrons in an atom by the heat energy of a flame. The electrons, being unstable in this excited stage, then give up their excess energy to the environment as they change from the higher energy state (excited) to a lower energy state. If the energy is dissipated as light, the light may consist of one or more than one energy level and therefore may possess different wavelengths. These different wavelengths or lines of the spectrum are individually characteristic for each element. The wavelength to be used for the measurement of an element—as in spectrophotometry—depends upon the selection of a spectral line of strong enough intensity to provide adequate sensitivity. It also depends upon freedom from other interfering lines at or near the selected wavelength.

Alkali metals are comparatively easy to excite in the flame of an ordinary laboratory burner. Lithium produces a red, sodium a yellow, potassium a violet, rubidium a red, and magnesium a blue color in a flame. These colors are characteristic of the metal atoms that are present as cations in solution.

Under constant and controlled conditions, the light intensity of the characteristic wavelength produced by each of the atoms is directly proportional to the number of atoms emitting energy, which in turn is directly proportional to the concentration of the substance of interest in the sample. Thus, flame photometry lends itself well to direct concentration measurements of some metals.

Other cations, like calcium, are less easily excited in the ordinary flame. In these cases, the amount of light given off may not always provide adequate sensitivity for analysis by flame emission methods. The sensitivity can be improved slightly by using higher temperature flames. Of the more easily excited alkali metals like sodium, only 1 to 5 per cent of the atoms present in solution become excited in a flame. Even with this small percentage of excited atoms, the method has adequate sensitivity for measurement of alkali metals for most bioanalytical measurements. Most metal ions are not as easily excited in a flame, and flame emission methods are not as applicable for their measurement.

ESSENTIAL PARTS OF THE FLAME PHOTOMETER

Figure 4-6 shows a schematic diagram of the basic parts of a flame photometer. A supply of gases, two-stage pressure regulators, and high-pressure tubing must be used to lead the gases to the flame. An atomizer is needed to spray the sample as fine uniform droplets into the flame. The monochromator entrance and exit slits and detectors are similar to those previously discussed in the spectrophotometer section.

GASES FOR FLAME PHOTOMETRY

Various combinations of gases and oxidants have been proposed and are being used in flame photometers. A mixture of hydrogen and oxygen gas produces a hot temperature commonly used on conventional flame pho-

Figure 4–6. Essentials of a flame photometer. *A*, Flame; *B*, atomizer; *C*, aspirator; *D*, entrance slit; *E*, monochrometer; *F*, exit slit; *G*, detector.

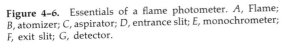
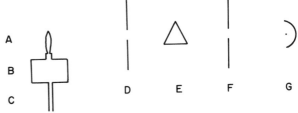

tometers. In addition, natural gas, acetylene, and propane using either air or oxygen are other combinations of gases frequently used. All of these fuel gases and their various oxidants work well, the difference being in the flame temperature and therefore the sensitivity that each combination provides. It is essential that the flame temperature be held constant; otherwise sensitivity changes will result. High quality gas regulation to maintain constant flame temperature is also essential for proper operation.

The Atomizer

The atomizer and the flame are the two most critical components in a flame photometer. The function of the atomizer is to break up the solution into fine droplets so that the atoms will absorb heat energy from the flame and become excited. There are basically two types of atomizers commonly used in flame photometers. In one type of burner, the gases are passed at high velocity over the end of a capillary suspended in the solution, causing liquid to be drawn up through the capillary into the flame. This type of burner is called the total consumption burner and details of it can be found in the section on atomic absorption (p. 90). A second kind of burner involves the gravitational feeding of solution through a restricting capillary into an area of high-velocity gas flow where small droplets are produced and passed into the flame. The large droplets in this type of burner are usually taken to waste and not all the sample is forced to go into the flame as in the capillary type burner.

The Flame

The purpose of the flame is to transfer energy to the unexcited atoms, as explained above. The single most important variable of the flame is the temperature. Frequent standardization of flame photometers is essential because thermal changes do occur and affect the response of the flame photometer.

Monochromator

The monochromator, including the entrance and exit slits, are similar to those previously described for spectrophotometers. Their function is to isolate the wavelength of interest from interfering light before it passes on to the detector. Ideally, monochromators in flame photometers should be of higher quality than those found in absorption spectrophotometers. When non-ionic materials are burned, light of various wavelengths is given off. This is known as *continuous emission* and will be added to the *line emission* of the element being measured. For this reason, the narrowest band path that is achievable should be used to eliminate as much of the extraneous, continuous emission as possible but still permit a maximum amount of the line emission to pass through to the detector.

Detectors

Detectors used in flame photometers operate by the same principle and in the same way as those previously described in the spectrophotometry section. In designing a flame photometer, compensation or design features must be incorporated so that thermal equilibrium is achieved rapidly. Flame photometers that use photomultipliers for detectors have improved sensitivity and, because of improved design, seldom require long times to come to thermal equilibrium. However, even this type of flame photometer usually requires aspirating water and standards to establish flame thermal equilibrium before measurements are taken.

OPERATION OF FLAME PHOTOMETERS

The major problem associated with flame photometers involves inadequate control over the flame and the aspirator. Slight variations in gas pressure will change both the rate of aspiration of the sample and the temperature of the flame. A significant amount of design effort has been exerted to assure constant flame and aspirator conditions. A flame photometer is available that uses an internal standard of lithium. A single flame and multiple detectors are used to monitor the same flame. The ratio of the sample and reference (lithium) detectors is proportional to the sample concentration. Therefore, any change in flame characteristics and aspirator conditions would simultaneously affect the signal to both the lithium reference detector and the sample detector. By using the ratio of the two signals, errors due to flame fluctuations or changes in the aspiration rate are minimized.

The ratio between the lithium and sodium and the lithium and potassium channels is taken, amplified, and fed to a direct digital read-out displayed on the front of the instrument. In addition, the lithium acts as a *radiation buffer*. If potassium is measured, for example, the potassium signal is critically dependent upon the amount of sodium present unless a high concentration of another easily excited cation such as lithium is present. In the absence of a high concentration of lithium, energy will be transferred from an excited sodium atom to a potassium atom. This would produce different percentages of potassium atoms excited, depending upon sodium concentration. The amount of potassium excited would vary and analytical errors would result. A means of compensating for this error is to dilute the samples with an excessively high concentration of lithium, so that the same percentage of potassium becomes excited regardless of the sodium concentration in the sample. The use of an internal standard and radiation buffer, the direct read-out for sodium and potassium concentrations, and the simple dilution of serum make the modern flame photometer highly suitable for use in the clinical laboratory.

ATOMIC ABSORPTION SPECTROPHOTOMETRY

The principle of atomic absorption had been known for a century before a useful analytical application evolved. Allan Walsh, an Australian physicist, suggested the idea as an analytical procedure for measuring metals in 1955. Soon after 1955, the production of commercial equipment resulted in a rapid expansion of applications.

Later, in the middle 1960's, the graphite furnace attachments increased the sensitivities of atomic absorption two or three orders of magnitude for some metals. Recently, some investigators have observed that matrix effects and other interferences can cause inaccurate analyses in biologic materials.

The reason for this rapid growth in atomic absorption spectrophotometry is that, instrumentally, the most advanced atomic absorption spectrophotometer is very simple compared to other analytical tools such as mass spectrometry, neutron activation analysis, x-ray fluorescence, and arc or laser emission spectroscopy.

Atomic absorption spectrophotometry is basically the inverse of emission methods. In all emission methods—arc, spark, laser, flame, x-ray fluorescence, or neutron activation analysis—the sample is excited in order to measure the radiation energy of interest given off as the sample returns to its lower energy level. Extraneous radiation must be isolated from the energy of interest if interference by these signals is to be avoided.

In atomic absorption spectrophotometry, the process opposite of emission takes place. The element is not excited in the flame, but merely dissociated from its chemical bonds and placed in an unexcited, un-ionized, neutral atom ground state. This statement means that the atom is at a low energy state in which it is capable of absorbing radiation at the very narrow band path width between 0.001 and 0.01 nm. The source emitting such radiation is the hollow cathode lamp. The energy of the absorbed radiation is equal to that which would be emitted if the element in question were excited. While only a small percentage of atoms in the flame are excited (1 to 5 per cent), nearly all are converted to the dissociated form in which they are capable of absorbing light emitted by the hollow cathode lamp.

Figure 4-7 shows the basic components of an atomic absorption spectrophotometer. The hollow cathode lamp is the light source; the nebulizer (atomizer) sprays the sample into the flame; and the monochromator, the slits, and the detectors have their usual function, as described previously in the spectrophotometer sections.

THE HOLLOW CATHODE LAMP

Figure 4-7 also shows schematically the components of a hollow cathode lamp. The

Figure 4-7. Essentials of an atomic absorption instrument. *A,* Hollow cathode; *B,* chopper; *C,* flame; *D,* entrance slit; *E,* monochromator; *F,* exit slit; *G,* detector.

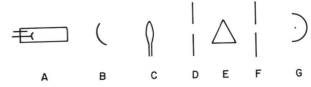

A   B   C   D   E   F   G

hollow cathode lamp produces a wavelength of light specific for the kind of metal in the cathode. In some cases, an alloy is used to make a multielement cathode.

Neon or argon gas at a few millimeters of mercury pressure is usually used as a filler gas. A neon-filled lamp produces a reddish orange glow during operation, while the argon produces a blue to purple glow inside the hollow cathode lamp. Quartz or special glass that allows transmission of the proper wavelength is used as a window.

A current is applied between the two electrodes inside the hollow cathode lamp, and metal is sputtered from the cathode into the bases inside the glass envelope. When the metal atoms collide with the gases, neon or argon, they lose energy and emit their characteristic radiation. Calcium has a sharp, intense, analytical emission line at 422.7 nm. This line is the most frequently used for calcium analysis. In an interference-free system, only calcium atoms will absorb the calcium light from the hollow cathode as it passes through the flame.

THE BURNER

Until now, only two types of burners have been used in most clinical applications. One is a *total consumption burner*, as illustrated by the Beckman burner and shown in Figure 4–8. With this burner, the gases—hydrogen and air—and the sample are not mixed before entering the flame. One disadvantage of this type of burner is that relatively large droplets are produced in the flame, which cause signal noise by light scattering. Another disadvantage of this type of burner is that the amount of acoustical noise produced is very high and may become uncomfortable after a few hours of operation. An advantage of this type of burner is that the flame is more concentrated and can be made hotter, causing molecular

dissociations which may be desirable to minimize some chemical interferences.

A modification of this type of burner is to split the liquid stream aspirated into 10 to 20 smaller streams prior to injection into the flame. This usually results in a flame that may be about 2.0 cm in diameter at the base. This modification produces much less noise than the single-jet total-consumption burner.

Figure 4–9 shows a *pre-mix burner* and illustrates how the sample is aspirated, volatilized, and burned. Notice that the gases are mixed and the sample atomized *before* being burned. An advantage of this system is that the large droplets go to waste and not into the flame, thus producing a less noisy signal. Another advantage of this type of burner is that the path length of the burner is longer than that of the total consumption burner. This produces greater absorption and increases the sensitivity of the measurement. A disadvantage of the pre-mix type of burner is that its flame is usually not as hot as that of the total-consumption burner and cannot sufficiently dissociate certain metal complexes in the flame (e.g., calcium phosphate complexes). Another disadvantage of this type of burner is that as much as 90 per cent of the sample may be discarded; hence, the sensitivity may be less than desirable. Recently, nitrous oxide pre-mix burners have been developed. These burners produce higher temperatures and will dissociate some calcium complexes. This makes unnecessary the addition of competing cations, e.g., lanthanum or strontium, to the solutions. However, an error can be introduced into the calcium determination by the use of the high-temperature nitrous oxide burner. Calcium becomes excited to a significant extent and thus emits ions in the flame. The use of this burner produces a new problem, and further studies must be conducted.

THE MONOCHROMATOR AND DETECTOR

All atomic absorption systems use monochromators and photomultipliers for isolating a spectrally pure light signal and measuring the intensity of that signal, respectively. The monochromator filters out extraneous light from the flame, while the photomultiplier converts that part of the light from the hollow cathode which was not absorbed in the flame to an electrical current and amplifies this cur-

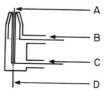

Figure 4–8. Total consumption burner. *A,* Capillary tip; *B,* fuel inlet; *C,* oxidant inlet; *D,* capillary.

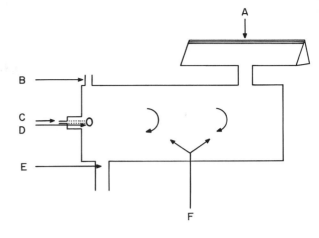

Figure 4–9. Laminar flow burner. *A*, Bolin head; *B*, fuel inlet; *C*, sample capillary; *D*, oxidant inlet; *E*, drain; *F*, spoilers.

rent to drive a read-out device or recorder. The monochromators and the photomultipliers have been discussed previously in the spectrophotometric section of this chapter (p. 82 and p. 84).

INTERFERENCES IN ATOMIC ABSORPTION SPECTROPHOTOMETRY

There are three general types of interferences in atomic absorption spectrophotometry—chemical, ionization, and matrix effects.

Chemical interference refers to the situation when the flame cannot dissociate the sample into neutral atoms so that absorption can occur. An example of a chemical interference is the phosphate interference in the serum determination of calcium caused by the formation of calcium phosphate complexes. These calcium phosphate complexes do not dissociate in the flame unless a special high-temperature burner is used. The phosphate interference is overcome by adding a cation which will displace the calcium from phosphate. Usually in atomic absorption determinations of calcium in serum, lanthanum or strontium is added to the serum, releasing the calcium from the phosphate in solution and replacing it. The free neutral calcium atoms are then capable of absorbing the calcium light from the hollow cathode. The freeing of calcium occurs because lanthanum and strontium form more stable complexes with phosphate than does calcium.

Ionization interference results when atoms in the flame become excited instead of only dissociated and then emit energy of the same wavelength as that being measured. Compensation for this condition can be achieved by adding an excess of a more easily ionized substance that will absorb most of the flame energy so that the substance of interest will not become excited. Another way to correct for ionization interference is to operate the flame at a lower temperature.

A third type of interference is the *matrix interference*. One example of a matrix effect is the enhancement of light absorption by organic solvents. An atom may absorb between two and five times more energy when dissolved in an organic solvent instead of an aqueous solvent. A second kind of matrix effect is the light absorption caused by formation of solids from sample droplets as the solvent is evaporated in the flame. This will usually occur only in concentrated solutions of greater than 0.1 mol/l. Refractory oxides of metals formed in the flame can also be classified as matrix interferences.

COMMERCIAL ATOMIC ABSORPTION SPECTROPHOTOMETERS

Figure 4–10 is a schematic diagram of a type of atomic absorption spectrophotometer manufactured by a number of instrument companies. If one traces the light path in Figure 4–10 from the hollow cathode lamp, we see that the chopper either reflects the light beam or allows the light beam to pass through the flame as the reference beam in the rear (top of Figure 4–10). The beams then pass alternately through the same monochromator to the one detector. When the beams arrive at the detector, they are out of phase with each other.

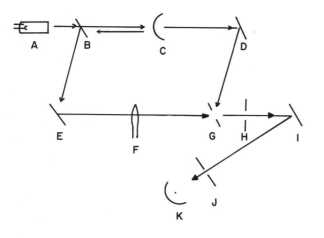

Figure 4-10. Schematic diagram of a double beam in time atomic absorption spectrophotometer. *A*, Hollow cathode lamp; *B*, half silvered mirror that reflects and transmits light; *C*, chopper; *D* and *E*, mirrors; *F*, flame; *G*, half silvered mirror; *H*, slit; *I*, grating; *J*, slit; *K*, detector.

In other words, the photomultiplier looks first at the reference beam and then uses this value to compare the reference and the sample beams. When more atoms are present in the flame, more light will be absorbed, and the greater the difference will be in light intensity between the sample and reference beams. This difference is then amplified and fed into a read-out device. Note that in the double-beam system, differences between the sample and reference beams are continuously being measured. This double-beam arrangement compensates for changes in the output of the hollow cathode lamp and for changes in the detector system. However, it does not correct for variations in the sample beam that may occur between the sample beam and the reference beam.

Atomic absorption spectrophotometry provides the analyst with a technique that is accurate and precise. To achieve comparable selectivity, sensitivity, and versatility with other instrumentation, the cost would be several times that of atomic absorption spectrophotometers.

Atomic absorption spectrophotometry is sensitive, accurate, precise, and high in specificity. One of the reasons for these advantages is that the method does not require excitation of the sought-for substance, and thus it is less affected by temperature variations in the flame and the transfer of energy from one atom to another. The high specificity results from the fact that the light used has an extremely narrow band path (0.01 nm) which is selectively absorbed by atoms being measured.

The disadvantages of atomic absorption spectrophotometry are few. The most significant difficulty is the elimination of interferences. Although some suggestions have been presented to compensate partially for some of these factors, more work is needed to study and to explain some of the interference problems that remain in atomic absorption spectrophotometry.

OTHER APPROACHES

FLUOROMETRY

Fluorescence is a physical energy process that occurs when certain compounds absorb electromagnetic radiation, become excited, and then return to an energy level slightly higher than or equal to their original energy level. Since the energy given off is less than or equal to that absorbed, the wavelength of the light being given off will be longer or equal to that absorbed for excitation. A delay time of between 10^{-8} and 10^{-4} second occurs between the absorption of the energy and the releasing of part of the energy in the form of light.

If the length of time is longer than 10^{-4} second from the time the chemical species absorbs the energy until the light is emitted, this process is called phosphorescence. The remainder of this discussion will be centered on fluorescence, since it is the more common process used in the laboratory.

Fluorometric Instrumentation

Figure 4-11 shows a schematic diagram of the components of a fluorometer. The energy source of a fluorometer is generally a mercury arc lamp or xenon lamp that will produce enough energy that when absorption occurs,

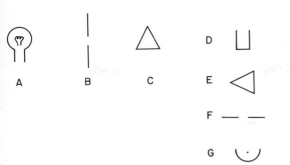

Figure 4–11. Essentials of a fluorometer. *A*, Light source; *B*, slit; *C*, primary monochromator or filter; *D*, cuvette; *E*, secondary monochromator or filter; *F*, slit; *G*, detector.

electron transitions to higher energy within the molecule will occur. In a fluorometer, the entrance and exit slits are similar to those described in spectrophotometers, except that the exit slit is usually perpendicular to the entrance slit. Fluorometers that use a continuous source like a xenon lamp have a monochromator so that isolation of wavelengths can occur before excitation of the substance in the cell occurs. All fluorometers have another monochromator system that will selectively remove unwanted wavelengths before they fall upon the detector. Fluorometers are designed so that the secondary monochromator and the detector are at right angles to the incident light beam into the cuvette. This arrangement prevents the light from the high-energy source of the mercury or xenon lamp from reaching the detector.

The single most important advantage of fluorometry is its extreme sensitivity. Sometimes the sensitivity may be one thousand times that of colorimetric methods. Some molecules fluoresce directly, but a larger percentage must be complexed or chemically reacted to transform them into fluorescent compounds. The fluorescence of the new compound is then measured. By selection of different complexers, fluorescence of different wavelengths may be produced, making it possible to work at a wavelength significantly removed from interferences.

Fluorescent spectra are not as valuable for qualitative identification as are absorption spectra. Other disadvantages of fluorometry are quenching interferences, extreme sensitivity to pH change, temperature change, and interferences owing to the presence of other foreign undefined fluorescent materials in reagents. Frequently, energy is transferred from one molecule to another in solution and is dissipated in this manner rather than being given off directly as fluorescence energy. Quenching sometimes occurs when foreign materials form unwanted non-fluorescent complexes with the substance of interest.

TURBIDIMETRY

The principle of the turbidity measurement is to determine the amount of light blocked by particulate matter as light passes through the cuvette. Several problems are inherent in making turbidimetric measurements, problems associated mostly with sample and reagent preparation rather than with the operation of the instrument. Turbidimetric measurements can be made with either a regular colorimeter or a spectrophotometer.

The amount of light that is blocked by a suspension of particles in a cuvette depends not only upon the number of particles present, but also upon the cross-sectional area of each particle. If the particle size of the standards is not the same as the particle size in the samples being measured, errors in turbidimetric measurements result. Another problem with the turbidimetric measurement is the need to keep the length of time between sample preparation and measurements as constant as possible. Particles may settle out of solution while the measurements are being made, thus producing an error. Control of the rate of settling is usually accomplished by using gum arabic or gelatin. These materials provide a viscous medium which retards particle settling while measurements are being made.

Turbidimetric measurements are acceptable provided that the number of particles and their size are in a reasonably narrow range. A high-intensity light or a very low-intensity light should not fall on the photo detector because errors in instrumentation would then augment other errors in the measurement.

NEPHELOMETRY

Nephelometric measurements are similar to turbidimetric measurements. In nephelometry, the light that is scattered by the small particles is measured at right angles to the beam incident to the cuvette. The amount of scatter that occurs is related to the number and to the size of particles in the light beam.

The particle size and shape and the wavelength of the incident light are important variables to control. The shorter the wavelength of the incident light, the greater the degree of dispersion. Nephelometry has an advantage over turbidimetric measurements in that nephelometric measurements are usually capable of somewhat greater precision. Specific antigen-antibody complexes and a laser source have been combined to provide high specificity with high precision. As a result turbidimetric and especially nephelometric measurements will be used more in clinical laboratories in future years.

ELECTROCHEMISTRY

Analytical electrochemistry for the clinical laboratory includes potentiometry, amperometry, and coulometry. Generally amperometry and potentiometry are the most commonly used techniques, and these center on blood gas measurements. Potentiometry is the measurement of the potential of a solution, while amperometry refers to the measurement of the amount of current that flows when a constant voltage is applied to the measuring electrode. Ion-selective electrodes for sodium, potassium, calcium, and many other substances of medical importance have increased the amount of interest in electrochemistry for the clinical laboratory (Pelleg, 1975).

POTENTIOMETRY

The measurement of the potential (voltage) between two electrodes in solution forms the basis for a variety of measurements that can be used to quantitate concentrations of the substance of interest.

Both an indicator and a reference electrode are necessary to measure the potential (E) of a solution. The potential of the indicator electrode can be made to respond proportionally to the concentration of the substance of interest, while the reference electrode must maintain a constant voltage under controlled conditions for a significant length of time. The most frequently used reference electrode in electro-analytical measurements is the saturated calomel electrode (SCE). Figure 4-12 shows the schematic diagram of the components of an SCE reference electrode. A porous plug shown at the bottom of the figure stoppers the outside glass jacket yet allows solution contact with the inner part of the calomel electrode. A

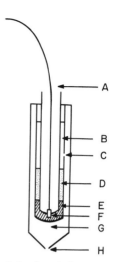

Figure 4–12. Saturated calomel electrode. *A*, Wire; *B*, inner jacket; *C*, port for saturated KCl; *D*, Hg, Hg_2Cl_2, KCl paste; *E*, Hg; *F*, platinum tip; *G*, saturated KCl; *H*, a porous plug.

small platinum tip is sealed on the end of the inner glass jacket, which is submerged in a saturated solution of potassium chloride. A paste is made of mercury and saturated mercurous chloride. Potassium chloride is next inserted into the inner jacket. Finally, electrical contact is made to the mercury-mercurous chloride interface and the platinum tip electrode by a wire to the measuring device. The standard reduction potential (E_o) of the calomel electrode versus a normal hydrogen electrode is −0.242 volts.

A silver-silver chloride electrode is another common reference electrode and may be easily constructed using a low-voltage (less than 6 volts) battery, a platinum wire, and a silver wire. The silver wire is usually coiled, connected to the positive pole of the battery, and submerged in a dilute chloride solution. The platinum wire is connected to the negative pole of the battery, then submerged in the same solution containing the coil of silver wire. Hydrogen will be liberated at the platinum cathode and silver chloride will be deposited on the silver anode when connected to the battery.

The silver wire will develop a rose to purple color in a few minutes. The silver-silver chloride wire is then placed in a standard chloride solution that has been saturated with silver ions to decrease the solubility of silver chloride and maintain a stable reference potential. A silver-silver chloride electrode has the advantage over the calomel electrode of being less sensitive to temperature changes.

The normal hydrogen electrode (NHE) consists of a platinized platinum electrode in a 1.228 N HCl solution with hydrogen at atmospheric pressure bubbled over the platinum surface. This reference electrode has an assigned E_o of 0.000 volts. Owing to difficult maintenance problems, the NHE is not frequently used in routine measurements.

There are several types of indicator electrodes that can be used with reference electrodes like those described above. Indicator electrodes can be a platinum wire, a planar surface of almost any other metal, a carbon rod, or a thin stream of mercury flowing into the solution where a measurement will be made.

In potentiometry the potential is measured and the relationship between the measured voltage and the sought-for concentration is shown by the Nernst equation:

$$E = E_o + \frac{0.059}{n} \log \frac{[C_{ox}]}{[C_{red}]} \qquad (1)$$

where E = the potential measured at 25°C.
  E_o = the standard reduction potential
  n = the number of electrons involved in the reaction
  C_{ox} = the molar concentration of the oxidized reaction form
  C_{red} = the molar concentration of the reduced reaction form

Measurement of pH

The pH of a solution is defined by the equation:

$$pH = -\log [H_3O^+] \qquad (2)$$

where $[H_3O^+]$ = hydrogen ion concentration in moles/liter.

In buffer solutions, the pH is related to the concentrations of the undissociated acid and its corresponding anion according to the following equation:

$$pH = pK_a + \log \frac{[A^-]}{[HA]} \qquad (3)$$

where $[A^-]$ = the molar concentration of anion
  $[HA]$ = the molar concentration of acid
  K_a = the acid dissociation constant
  pK_a = $-\log K_a$

Notice the similarities and relationships between (1) the Nernst equation, (2) the definition of pH, and (3) the buffer equation. A

single potential measurement under proper conditions can be directly related to the H_3O^+ concentration in solution.

A pH measurement is usually made with the aid of a glass indicator electrode. One type consists of a bulb of special glass filled with 0.1 mole/liter HCl in contact with a suitable metallic electrode. When immersed in solution, a potential difference develops between the solution inside the glass electrode and the solution being measured for H_3O^+. The magnitude depends upon the hydrogen-ion concentration of the solution. This potential difference is measured by combining the glass electrode with some standard reference electrode, such as the saturated calomel electrode, and measuring the voltage of the system.

Calibration is achieved by using a known buffer solution that has a pH value assigned by the National Bureau of Standards. The pH of an unknown solution is compared to the known buffer solution by potential measurements using a pH meter. A pH meter simply measures the potential produced in a solution using electrodes described above.

The electrode arrangement for a pH measurement may be considered as a special type of concentration cell. A modification of equation (1) that can be used for a concentration cell is:

$$\Delta E = \frac{RT}{nF} \ln \frac{C_1}{C_2} \qquad (4)$$

where ΔE = measured change in potential
  R = gas constant
  T = temperature in degrees Kelvin
  n = number of electrons in electrochemical reaction
  F = value of the Faraday constant
  C_1 = concentration of unknown (outside of glass electrode)
  C_2 = concentration of known (inside glass electrode)

At 25°C. for a one-electron reaction and with C_2 equal to one mole/liter, equation (4) becomes $\Delta E = 0.059$ pH. In other words, a 59 millivolt (mv) change will occur when the pH changes 1 unit.

A schematic diagram for a pH meter is shown in Figure 4-13. While making the pH measurement, it is important that the amount of current drawn from the measuring electrodes be very small. Generally 10^{-10} to 10^{-12} ampere or less is drawn. The principle behind the pH measurement involves the adjustment of the high-impedance potentiometer poten-

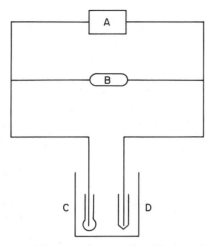

Figure 4–13. Schematic diagram of a pH meter. In making pH measurements one adjusts the potentiometer (*A*) until the voltage across the glass electrode (*C*) and the reference electrode (*D*) is zero, which is indicated by the null meter (*B*).

tial to be equal to and in the opposite direction from the potential of the measuring electrodes (Noonan, 1976).

Coulometric Measurements

Coulometry involves the measurement of the quantity of electricity (in coulombs) at a fixed potential where:

$$Q = I \times T \qquad (5)$$

Q = coulombs of electricity
I = the current in amperes
T = the time in seconds that the current is flowing

Two approaches can be used in coulometric measurements. When the current is kept constant, the elapsed time is proportional to the total coulombs consumed. Alternatively, the current may be changed in a known manner for a fixed time and the area beneath the current curve integrated with respect to time to obtain the number of coulombs. A coulomb is equal to a current flow of one ampere per second. A Faraday is defined as 96,500 coulombs and corresponds to the electrical charge carried by one gram equivalent of substance. One equivalent is equal to one mole if only one electron is involved in the electrochemical reaction. Thus, the number of coulombs consumed can be related directly to the concentration of the unknown.

In the chloride determination using the

Cotlove titrator (Buchler Instruments, Inc., Fort Lee, N.J.), a constant current is applied across silver electrodes, which liberates silver ions into the solution at a constant rate. When all of the chloride ions in solution have been complexed by the liberated silver ions, a pair of indicator electrodes senses the excess silver ions and activates a relay which shuts the timer off and stops the titration. The length of time that the titrator generates silver ions is directly proportional to the chloride ion concentration, since the current has been kept constant.

Polarography

Another amperometric technique frequently used in electroanalytical chemistry is polarography. The technique involves making a current measurement as the potential is varied. A polarographic measurement in its simplest form involves a two-electrode system consisting of a reference electrode and an indicator electrode. Many kinds and combinations of indicator and reference electrodes may be used for polarographic measurements. The indicator electrode frequently consists of a thin ribbon of mercury metal flowing slowly through a small glass capillary and dropping into the solution to be measured. Generally, a linearly increasing cathodic voltage is applied to the dropping mercury electrode (DME); the current that flows between the two electrodes is measured and is proportional to the concentration of the substance of interest.

The current measured is called the diffusion current (i_d) because it is at the applied potential where the maximum amount of current can flow in the system. The i_d is limited by the rate of diffusion of the electroactive species to the surface of the DME and can be related to the concentration. The quantitative relationship between the i_d and the concentration is given by the Ilkovic equation:

$$i_d = 607 \, nD^{1/2} \, M^{2/3} \, t^{1/6} \, C \qquad (6)$$

where n = number of Faradays per mole of substance reduced
D = diffusion coefficient in cm^2sec^{-1}
M = rate of flow of mercury in mg/sec
t = drop time in seconds
C = millimolar concentration of substance reduced

For a given substance, n and D will be constant, and under experimental conditions, M and t are kept constant. Hence, from the above equation, it is apparent that the concentration of the electroactive species is directly proportional to the diffusion current (i_d).

As with other electroanalytical methods, polarography is not widely used at present in clinical laboratories. The reason is probably the complicated uncontrolled interferences in biologic samples. Increased usage of these techniques will almost certainly occur in the near future when separations are used to purify the matrix containing the substance of interest (Ryan, 1975; Brooks, 1975).

ION-SELECTIVE ELECTRODES

For many years ion-selective electrodes have been used in clinical laboratories with varying degrees of success. Early glass electrodes used to measure pH produced erroneously high results in the presence of high concentrations of sodium when the pH was above 9 or 10. Today, newer glasses used to make the pH electrode have reduced the sodium error significantly so that at pH 12 errors less than 10 per cent are common.

In addition to glass ion-selective electrodes, two other types of electrodes are common. There are the liquid ion-exchange electrodes that have membranes isolating the organic exchangers from the solution being measured. Metal ions outside the membrane and the same metal ions bound to the ion-exchange material inside the electrode will produce a potential that can be related to the solution activity using the Nernst equation. The third type of electrode is the solid-state electrode by which enzymes or substrates can be trapped in gels or bound to membranes but still remain active. Products of the enzyme reaction can then be measured electrochemically and can be used to measure substrate or enzyme activity.

These last types of electrodes, which have been developed and tested for 10 years, continue to hold high promise for the future but have not contributed significantly to service clinical laboratories (Schwartz, 1976).

ELECTROPHORESIS

Electrophoresis for protein fractionation has been a valuable separation and quantitation technique in the clinical laboratory. The moving-boundary technique developed by Tiselius led to the use of solid supports for protein electrophoresis in the late 1940's. Papers, cellulose acetate, gels, starch, dextrans, and other materials were used as supports for the separation of the electrically charged molecule-like proteins.

The usual technique for protein electrophoresis is to pass current through a buffer in the pH 8 range. At this pH most proteins will be negatively charged and will move toward the positively charged end (anode) of the cell. The rate of movement (mobility) of the individual proteins will be determined by their overall charge and size (charge density). The greater the charge density the faster the protein will move. Usually a few microliters of serum are applied to the solid support saturated with buffer. A voltage is applied so as to produce a few milliamperes for nearly an hour or longer. The power is then turned off and the support removed from the buffer solutions. Next the solid support is placed into a dye solution to stain the protein bands; then the excess stain is rinsed away. Quantitation of the fractions is usually achieved by using a densitometer to measure either the intensity of the light reflected from the dyed fractions or the amount of light transmitted through the solid support. The peak areas of the densitometer read-out are considered proportional to the concentration of the protein in that band.

Paper electrophoresis for amino acid analysis is no longer commonly used in service laboratories. The usual procedure was to use organic solvents to run paper chromatography in one direction, then dry the paper and run electrophoresis perpendicular to the direction of chromatography. This technique was very important for isolation of peptides and amino acids before column chromatography was fully developed. With paper chromatography, up to 2500 volts is applied and about 200 ma of current flows for about one hour.

Usually agarose gel electrophoresis is conducted in a flat slab of the gel that was poured into a mold and formed.

Disc gel electrophoresis usually is combined with polyacrylamide mixtures that range from 7.5 to 13 per cent acrylamide. These gels are usually poured into glass tubes and allowed to harden prior to use. The electrophoresis is run with the gel still in the glass tube. The gel is carefully removed from the glass tube for staining, destaining, and further handling when the electrophoresis is complete.

Cellulose acetate is perhaps the most widely used support for routine protein electrophoresis in clinical laboratories. The separation of lactate dehydrogenase (LDH) isoenzymes as well as creatine kinase (CK) isoenzymes is a widely used application of electrophoresis techniques.

INSTRUMENTATION CHARACTERISTICS

The instrumentation for electrophoresis consists basically of a power supply, an electrophoresis cell, electrodes submerged in a buffer compartment isolated physically but not electrically from the gel or cellulose acetate strip, and the densitometer for measuring the amount of each of the fractions after the separation. Staining and destaining are optional. The power supply commonly requires an output of about 200 volts with about 4.5 milliamperes of current being drawn. The buffer is usually a carefully controlled ionic strength buffer causes heat to be generated within the cell while a high ionic strength does not permit good separation of fractions. The electrodes that are immersed in the buffer are usually placed in separate compartments connected to the cell by salt bridges so that pH changes that occur in the electrode chambers do not alter the pH of the buffer saturating the matrix. Significant care must be taken by the operator to prevent contamination of the cell, the electrodes, or the matrix with fingerprints or any foreign substance that will disturb the even current flow throughout the matrix. Most commercial apparatuses have built-in safety features to protect the operators from the potentially dangerous voltages present in such devices. however, the laboratorian must frequently check to see that these safety features are working properly.

OSMOMETRY

The *osmolality* of a solution is dependent only on the *number* of particles in solution. The size or charge of the ion or molecule does not affect the measurement. One *osmol* of a substance is equal to the gram-molecular weight divided by the number of particles or ions into which the substance dissociates in solution. Thus, since glucose molecules do not dissociate in aqueous solution, 1 osmol of glucose = 1 mole = 180 gm. For NaCl, which dissociates into 2 ions in aqueous solution, 1 osmol = 0.5 mole or $\frac{58.5}{2}$ = 29 grams = 1 osmol. For Na_2SO_4, 1 osmol = 0.33 mole, etc.,

assuming 100 per cent dissociation for ions in solution.

A solution containing 1 osmol of solute per kilogram of solvent has a concentration of 1 osmolal. This concentration is independent of temperature, since it is based on weight only. A solution containing 1 osmol of solute per liter of solution has a concentration of 1 osmolar. Osmolar concentrations vary with temperature, since the volume varies with temperature. For aqueous solutions of low concentrations, such as body fluids, the difference between osmolality and osmolarity becomes negligible and it is customary to use milliosmols per liter (1 osmol = 1000 milliosmols).

The freezing point of water is depressed 1.86° C. when solute is added to make a 1 osmolal solution; hence, 1 osmol of any solute is that amount which will depress the freezing point of 1 kg of water by 1.86° C. An osmolality measurement in clinical chemistry provides an estimate of the effective number of particles in solution even though we do not know either the nature or the concentration of the individual substances dissolved in the solution.

Osmolality is determined by measuring the freezing point depression. The apparatus consists of a cooling bath to freeze the specimen and a thermistor. A thermistor is a device whose electrical resistance decreases as the temperature decreases. With a constant current source and a balancing circuit, the resistance of a potentiometric balance bridge is adjusted to equal the resistance of the thermistor. This resistance of the thermistor is directly related to the temperature being measured. Thus, a thermistor is an electrical thermometer.

The measurement is very accurate and precise and is easily calibrated. The precision of an osmometer is usually of the order of 0.3 per cent or less.

The amount that the freezing point is depressed is related to the concentration by the following equation:

$$\Delta T = \frac{RT_o{}^2M_1W_2}{H_fW_1M_2} \qquad (7)$$

where ΔT = the change in the freezing point
 R = the gas constant, 1.987 cal/mol
 T_o = the freezing point of the solvent in °K.
 M_1 = the molecular weight of the solvent
 W_2 = the grams of the solute

H_f = the heat of fusion of the solvent in cal/mol
W_1 = the grams of the solvent
M_2 = the molecular weight of the solute

The weight of solute (W_2) divided by the molecular weight of the solute (M_2) is equal to the number of moles of solute present; hence, from the equation above, the depression in freezing point is directly proportional to the number of moles of solute and is independent of the molecular weight.

The heat of fusion of water is 1436 calories per mole and the freezing point of water is 273.1 °K. A 1 molal solution of urea, for example, contains 60 g of urea dissolved in 1000 g of water. The change in freezing point, calculated from the above equation, is:

$$\Delta T = \frac{(1.987)(273.1)^2(18.02)(60)}{(1436)(1000)(60)} = 1.86°$$

Based on equation (7), the number of moles (m) of solute dissolved in 1000 gm of water is:

$$m = \frac{\Delta T}{1.86}$$

Freezing point depression is a colligative property of a solution; that is, its magnitude depends on the number of solute particles per kg of H_2O. Other colligative properties include boiling point elevation and vapor pressure depression. This latter property is exploited by instruments that use dew point (vapor pressure) change to measure osmolality.

CHROMATOGRAPHY

Chromatography began when a Russian botanist named Tswett ground up some green leaves, extracted them, and placed the extract on a sorbent in a column. He observed that the green color was separated into various color bands that were adsorbed onto the solid support in the column. It was because of this experiment and the separation of colors that the word "chromatography" was coined. Today most applications of this technique do not involve separation of substances of different colors, but the term chromatography remains.

The purpose of chromatography in all cases involves separation of a mixture on the basis of specific differences of the physical-chemical characteristics of the components. The types of chromatography that will be discussed include ion-exchange chromatography, paper chromatography, gas-liquid chromatography, liquid-liquid chromatography, gel-permeation chromatography, and thin-layer chromatography.

In paper chromatography the physical characteristics that determine separations are the rate of diffusion, the solubility of the solute, and the nature of the solvent. In liquid-liquid chromatography, separation is based on differences in solubility between two liquid phases. One of the liquids is often aqueous, while the other is an organic solvent. Solubility can be modified by changes in ionic strength or pH of each of the liquid phases. In gel-permeation chromatography, the molecular weight, the size and charge of the ions, and the hydrophobicity of the molecules are the characteristics that are responsible for separation. In ion-exchange chromatography, the separation of substances depends principally upon the sign and ionic charge density. Ions with greatest charge density will be held most strongly on an ion-exchange material. In an electrophoresis separation, the physical characteristic that differentiates between components is the mobility of the substance of interest in an electric field. In gas-liquid chromatography, the sample volatility, its rate of diffusion into the liquid layer of the column packing, and the solubility of the sample gas in the liquid layer (partition coefficient) determine the separation capabilities of this technique. Thin-layer chromatography, like paper chromatography, depends upon the rate of diffusion and solubility of the substance of interest in solvents as the components migrate through media such as silica gel.

ION-EXCHANGE
CHROMATOGRAPHY

Ion-exchange chromatography is a very well-established procedure that has been studied intensively. The natural purification of water as it percolates through soil is an example of this process. Ion-exchange chromatography potentially has many uses in clinical chemistry.

Figure 4-14 shows the functional groups that are attached to the styrene structure cross-linked with divinyl benzene, used in constructing a synthetic strong *anion*-exchange resin. Nitrogen is bonded to the styrene, and three methyl groups are bonded to the nitrogen. The chloride anion is electrostatically attracted to the positive charge that remains on the nitrogen atom. Any anion passing through

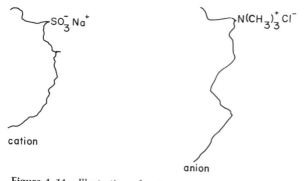

cation

anion

Figure 4–14. Illustration of a strong anion and cation resin with functional groups.

the solution that has greater affinity for the nitrogen than the chloride ion causes a displacement of the chloride from the resin. The amount and the rate of exchange depend upon the relative affinities of the nitrogen atom for the chloride ion or the other anion in solution. This is a technique to remove an unwanted anion from solution by exchanging it for other more desirable anions.

Figure 4–14 also shows a typical strong *cation*-exchange resin, again with the styrene structure, but with SO_3^- groups bound to the styrene. In this example, any cation that would be more strongly held to the SO_3^- than sodium would be preferentially adsorbed from solution and the sodium ion would be discharged into the solution. As with the anion-exchange material, a cation-exchange process serves to separate unwanted substances from solution. In certain cases, very large volumes of dilute solutions may be passed through ion-exchange materials to effectively concentrate the solute of interest. Ion-exchange chromatography will find increasing uses in the clinical chemistry laboratory, since it materially improves the specificity and accuracy of the method by removal of interfering substances.

GEL-PERMEATION (SIZE-EXCLUSION) CHROMATOGRAPHY

Gel-permeation chromatography became widely used in the early 1960's. The trade name of a material that appeared on the market is Sephadex (Pharmacia, Inc., Piscataway, N.J.). Polyacrylamide gels are also often used in size-exclusion chromatography. Sephadex is a dextran material that has been modified so

that it contains pores of accurately controlled size. Various pore size materials are currently commercially available. When a mixture of small and large molecules is allowed to pass over small particles in a column, the smaller molecules and ions diffuse into the gel. Larger molecules such as proteins are too large to diffuse into the interstitial cavities of the material and pass rapidly through the column. The smaller molecules and ions are then temporarily retained until they have time to diffuse back out of the gel. Thus, the large molecular weight materials will appear in the effluent first and the smaller molecular weight materials will be delayed in the dextran packing of the column.

The use of gels makes it possible to separate compounds by their molecular weight, provided the pore size of the material is properly selected for the separation.

Gel-permeation chromatography was further improved by introducing ion-exchange groups on the dextran. The ion-exchange characteristics of the dextran, in addition to the size-exclusion chromatography, greatly expanded the separation capability of this material. With the additional ion-exchange characteristics, not only the size of the molecule, but the ionic charge of the molecule, became important for the separation. Recently, Sephadex has been further modified to allow it to be used with organic solvents. Hydroxy-propylation of G-25 produces a dextran material capable of performing separations of compounds dissolved in highly non-polar organic systems.

Agarose gels (Sepharose) are commonly used for the separation of larger molecular proteins, polysaccharides, and nucleic acids. These agarose gels are often the starting material that is modified to produce affinity columns. The use of agarose and six molar guanidine hydrochloride will allow an estimate of the molecular weight of proteins and is a widely used technique.

In addition to Sephadex, other materials have been used in gel-permeation chromatography. Polyacrylamide gels have been manufactured that, like dextran, have a closely controlled pore size. These materials are more suitable for use in a wider pH range. The rate of hydrolysis of Sephadex becomes significant at high pH values, while polyacrylamide gels are more suitable for this type of application. Polyacrylamide has the additional advantage that it will not support bacterial growth, which is frequently a problem when working with biologic fluids.

Gel-permeation chromatography has been used principally for the separation of proteins from lower molecular weight molecules and ions. In addition, gel-permeation chromatography has been used quite extensively in the study of isoenzymes and enzyme chemistry.

HIGH-PERFORMANCE LIQUID CHROMATOGRAPHY (HPLC)

Since the early 1970's the development of pumps, columns, flow monitors, and other instrumentation has allowed aqueous or organic solutions to be pumped through columns with pressures between 500 and 5000 pounds per square inch. Additional technologic advances allowed the preparation of controlled pore size porous glasses for size-exclusion chromatography. The glass beads are spherical and are very small (5 to 8 microns). For size exclusion chromatography glass beads with pore sizes of 60, 100, 500, or 1000 Angstroms (10^{-10} meter) are commercially available.

Very carefully controlled spherical silica gel beads of the same size as mentioned above are also available for adsorption chromatography. Because different molecules adsorb differently often a separation can be completed in a few minutes using the types of solvents used for silica gel thin-layer chromatography plates. The thin-layer method may take up to an hour to allow separation to occur, while a few minutes is often enough with HPLC. A disadvantage of HPLC adsorption chromatography is that the extent of hydration of the silica gel is critically important. The degree of hydration can easily change as various amounts of solvent are pumped through the column. Hence, exactly reproducing separation conditions is often difficult and equilibration time may be long.

A still more recent development in HPLC is the "reverse phase" column packings that are now commercially available. A very common, widely useful, and universal packing involves the covalent bonding of octadecyl silane (ODS) to small porous spherical glass beads. This ODS material is non-polar, and non-polar molecules will dissolve in the non-polar liquid phase bound to the glass support beads packed in a column. The sample containing a mixture of non-polar molecules (benzene, naphthalene, anthracene, etc.) is dissolved in a solvent like methanol. Using a mobile phase mixture of about 75 per cent methanol and 25 per cent water, the sample is injected on the top of the column. Because of the different solubilities (partition coefficients) between the mobile phase and the liquid phase on the solid support of the different components, the individual components will separate on a pass through the reverse phase column. This same column can be used for many drug analyses as well as for phenylthiohydantoin derivatives of amino acids.

Anion- and cation-exchange coated glass beads are also available in the small bead sizes that are suitable for use in the HPLC instruments. Other types of cyano derivative functional groups and C_8 phases are also becoming commercially available, but their use in clinical laboratories remains to be developed (Molnar, 1976).

GAS-LIQUID CHROMATOGRAPHY

Gas-liquid chromatography (GLC) was developed by a crash program instituted by one of the large industrial chemical companies during World War II. The first published work on GLC appeared in the early 1950's. Today GLC is one of the most versatile, powerful analytical tools available. This technique is capable of separating and measuring nanogram and picogram amounts of volatile substances. It is used for the measurement and fractionation of steroids, lipids, barbiturates, drugs, blood alcohol, and measurements of other toxicologic substances. Gas-liquid chromatographic methods are rapid, sensitive, and accurate when compared with other separation techniques.

The basic components of a gas-liquid chromatograph are schematically shown in Figure 4–15. Although the basic principles are not

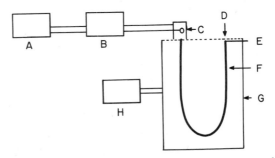

Figure 4–15. Essentials of a gas-liquid chromatograph. A, Strip chart recorder; B, electrometer to measure and amplify detector current; C, hydrogen flame detector; D, sample input; E, carrier gas input; F, column; G, temperature-controlled oven; H, programmer to control oven temperature.

difficult to understand, the technologic requirements for columns, electronics, and temperature control were difficult to achieve until a few years ago.

The carrier gas is introduced near the top of the column near the point where the sample is to be injected. The carrier gas is an inert gas such as helium, nitrogen, or argon that flows at a constant rate through the column. The column is usually glass or an inert metal and is packed with an inert solid support such as diatomaceous earth that has been coated with a thin layer of a liquid phase. The liquid phase is usually some silicon oil that is non-volatile and does not chemically react with the substance of interest.

The detectors of gas-liquid chromatographs generally are of three basic types: the hydrogen flame, nitrogen-phosphorous, and the electron capture detectors. Since the hydrogen flame detector is most commonly used in the clinical laboratory, it will be discussed in some detail. It consists of a small platinum loop mounted approximately 1 cm above the hydrogen flame. A metal gas jet is mounted directly over the exit port of the column, and a flammable gas such as hydrogen is passed through the gas jet. A small flame is ignited and burns at the tip of the jet where the column effluent and the hydrogen mix. A voltage is applied between the gas jet and the platinum ring mounted above it. The platinum ring is maintained at a voltage of 50 to 125 volts or more. When the hydrogen flame is burning, ions that are formed by burning the effluent in the flame will be collected by the platinum ring and produce a small current between the gas jet and the platinum loop. This current is detected by the electrometer, amplified, and the signal fed to the recorder.

The electrometer

Basically, the electrometer is an electronic device that is capable of measuring very small currents and amplifying them linearly. The amplified signal is then fed to the read-out device which is a strip chart recorder, an integrator, or a printer.

The programmer

The programmer is a combination of electronic controls whose basic function is to provide temperature control of the column oven. The oven is usually controlled to within a tenth of a degree and is usually capable of being changed at a linear and constant rate ranging from 1°C. to 50°C. per minute. This change in temperature during a determination is useful in producing separations of materials that have penetrated the liquid phase. The respective components of the sample are then selectively eluted from the column in accordance with their differences in volatility as the temperature changes.

The recorder

The recorder is simply an electrical mechanical device that measures the voltage output of the electrometer and presents it on a strip chart for interpretation by the operator. The size of the voltage signal introduced to the recorder is usually 1 to 10 millivolts.

Principles of operation

In a gas-liquid chromatography determination, either the substance of interest must be volatile or a new compound (derivative) must be formed that is volatile. The derivative, in addition to being more volatile, may protect the compound of interest from thermally decomposing by binding with heat-labile groups. A small quantity of the liquid material to be measured is injected onto the column and is immediately volatilized in the entrance port to the column. The carrier gas then transports the volatilized sample to the liquid phase on the solid support within the column. Separation occurs owing to the different solubility and the different diffusion rates of the various components of the sample gas into and out of the liquid phase. Thus, the various fractions of the gaseous sample tend to move through the column at different rates and appear at different times at the detector. This process of going into the liquid phase by solubility, diffusing back out, and going back into the liquid phase is usually repeated 6000 to 8000 times during the one pass through the column. The column is said to have 6000 to 8000 theoretical plates.

As these bands are eluted from the column by the carrier gas, the burning flame produces a large number of ions. The surge of ions causes an increase in detector current, which is amplified by the electrometer and sent to the recorder. Peaks will then appear on the strip chart recording. As each of the bands is eluted from the column, successive peaks will be presented on the strip chart recorder. The length of time for each of the peaks to appear on the strip chart recorder from the injection time is the *retention time* and is usually characteristic for the substance of interest. Two substances in a mixture generally do not have identical retention times. The retention time, therefore, *qualitates* the substance in the sample while the peak area *quantitates* the amount of each of the fractions present. If good resolution in the gas chromatograph is achieved and if the peaks formed on the strip chart recorder are very sharp, then the peak height may be found to be proportional to the concentration. Temperature changes, type or concentration of the liquid phase, volatility of different derivatives, or some other parameter can be introduced to effect an adequate fractionation of the sample.

In summary, because the gas chromatograph separates, detects, qualitates, and quantitates several fractions of a volatilized sample in a single step, its use has great potential in clinical chemistry, especially in drug analyses (Huffman, 1976).

LIQUID-LIQUID CHROMATOGRAPHY

When two liquid phases are mixed, as is commonly done in a separatory funnel, substances will distribute themselves between the two phases. The solubility principally determines the distribution of the species into the aqueous or the organic layer in a two-phase system. Generally, the solubility will be determined largely by the relative polarity of the substance of interest and the polarity of the two liquid phases. A highly polar substance tends to be more soluble in a highly polar solvent such as water, while the less polar substances tend to be more soluble in the less polar solvents such as organic solvents ("like dissolves like").

The solubility of a species and therefore the control of what phase the species will be found in is most easily managed by changing the pH of the aqueous solution. For example, if an anion is found in the aqueous phase and if that anion is to be extracted into the organic phase, addition of hydrogen ion will usually produce the transfer. When H^+ is added to the aqueous layer and the anion becomes protonated, the polarity of that molecule is much less (less ionic) than it was as an anion. Its solubility

will be much greater in the organic phase because of its reduced polarity and the lower polarity of the organic phase compared with the water phase.

An example of how liquid-liquid chromatography is applied to clinical chemistry is the UV barbiturate method. The acid form (non-ionized, non-polar) of the barbiturate is first extracted from the aqueous phase (blood, urine) into an organic phase like chloroform. Next, the chloroform layer is contacted with a NaOH solution and the anion of the barbiturate goes into the alkaline aqueous phase, which then can be analyzed for barbiturates.

The distribution ratio ($D_{o/w}$) defines the amount of material found in each phase at equilibrium.

$$D_{o/w} = \frac{[C_{org}]}{[C_{water}]}$$

where $[C_{org}]$ = concentration in the organic phase
$[C_{water}]$ = concentration in the aqueous phase

A column liquid-liquid chromatography system can be established by impregnating a solid support with one liquid phase, then allowing another liquid to percolate through the column. A solid phase frequently is silica gel, the liquid phase is water, and an organic solvent is allowed to percolate through the column. Separations will occur with such an arrangement in a manner similar to other column chromatographic separations.

PAPER CHROMATOGRAPHY

In ascending paper chromatography, a strip of filter paper is usually hung vertically into a solvent. The solvent moves up through the paper by capillary action, with the paper serving as a wick. A spot of the substance to be fractionated is placed on the paper just above the solvent level and permitted to dry before the paper is inserted in the jar containing the solvent. As the solvent moves up through the paper, various fractions in the sample move at different rates. The relative solubilities of the components of the sample in the solvent mixture, the polarity of the solvent, and the polarities of the solutes of interest all affect the rate at which different components move. After the separation has taken place, the paper is removed, dried, and sprayed with a chemical for color development. The spots may then be quantitated by measuring their area or intensity or both. In certain cases, the spots may be visible in the ultraviolet region of the spectrum, in which case the paper is examined under such light. In descending chromatography the papers are inserted into a tray and clamped into position to allow the solvent to rise over the edge of the tray by capillary action, then pass down through the paper and drop to the bottom of the tank.

Paper chromatography has been used in clinical laboratories in the past for fractionation of sugars and amino acids and for barbiturates. Today amino acid analyzers involving ion-exchange chromatography are more frequently used for amino acid separations, while barbiturates are usually identified by UV spectrophotometry, HPLC, or thin-layer or gas chromatography. Sugars are usually separated by column chromatography.

THIN-LAYER CHROMATOGRAPHY

The principles of thin-layer chromatography (TLC) are similar to those described above for ascending paper chromatography. The main difference between the two techniques is that glass or plastic plates to which is attached a thin layer of silica gel, alumina, polyacrylamide gel, or starch gel are used for the matrix instead of filter paper. The edges of the plates are then placed on edge into a solvent solution and the solvent passes up through the thinly layered material on the glass plate in the same manner as it passes up the paper—by capillary action. Again, separation occurs because of differences in solubility, polarity of the solvent, polarity of the substance of interest, and rate of diffusion.

One advantage of thin-layer chromatography is that the spot may be scraped from the plate, easily redissolved in a solvent, and then analyzed on an instrument such as a gas chromatograph or a fluorometer. Another advantage of TLC is that separation can often be completed in 30 to 90 minutes, as compared with 12 to 24 hours for paper chromatography. The main functions of thin-layer chromatography are the identification and separation of unknown substances in one step or preliminary purification of mixtures prior to performing the final analysis by another technique. Several samples can be spotted on the same plate and a standard can be placed on

each plate to test whether the whole system is working properly.

RADIOCHEMICAL TECHNIQUES

Perhaps 50 different compounds important in clinical medicine have been measured using radioimmunoassay (RIA) methods. The largest number of analyses has been in the area of hormones for endocrinology. Peptide hormones and steroids are ideal candidates because of their size and concentration for RIA analysis and account for the focus in endocrinology. Several drug analyses are becoming commercially available that use immunochemical techniques. Several companies are using radioactive labels for these types of methods; hence, radioactivity counting is an important instrumental technique for clinical laboratories (see also Chap. 14).

We will discuss only liquid scintillation counting for beta radiation and sodium iodide activated with thallium for gamma radiation counting. There are higher resolution gamma counters that consist of lithium-drifted germanium solid state detectors. These detectors have lithium metal deposited on one side of a germanium block. The whole detector must be operated at liquid nitrogen temperatures, so clinical laboratories usually do not use these solid state detectors.

When a gamma ray penetrates the NaI (Tl) crystal, a flash of light is generated as the energy is absorbed. These flashes of light can then be measured by a typical photomultiplier (PM) tube. The PM amplification plus additional electronic amplification makes the counting a highly sensitive technique. The NaI (Tl) crystal must be sealed from the air because it is hygroscopic. Another disadvantage is that large amounts of lead shielding are usually necessary, so the counter is heavy and occupies substantial space.

Beta counting, on the other hand, involves mixing the radioactivity directly with a solvent and an organic compound that will absorb the much weaker beta radiation and then give off a flash of light. Two common scintillators are 2,5-diphenyloxazole (PPO) and 2,2-p-phenylene bis-5-phenyl-oxazole (POPOP). Today most service laboratories purchase the scintillation "cocktails" already prepared. When the flash of light is given off by the liquid scintillation fluid again, as with the gamma counter, a photomultiplier detects the signal, amplifies it 10^6 to 10^8 times, and feeds that signal to the electronics.

By adjusting the amplification it is possible to minimize the background count, select a narrow energy range of only the isotope to be counted, or conduct pulse height analysis of the radiation measured by the counter. Quenching is a problem in liquid scintillation counting but usually is not troublesome for gamma counting. Quenching may be the absorption of the light within the sample cocktail prior to PM detection. Most often cleaner glassware, a cleaner sample, or additional separations prior to counting will correct some of the quenching problems.

Several companies now provide excellent counters, have training courses for operators, and offer various types of service contracts. Hence, today radiation counting is not a difficult measurement to make in most service clinical laboratories.

SUMMARY

Since the introduction of the AutoAnalyzer into the clinical chemistry laboratory by the Technicon Corporation in the late 1950's, quantum jumps in instrumental capabilities have occurred. The single-channel instruments, the 12-channel instruments, and the 20-channel instruments, all from Technicon (Technicon Instrument Corporation, Tarrytown, New York) have allowed enormous improvements in analytical consistency without being slowed by accuracy problems.

The large analyzers from Hycel (Hycel, Inc., Houston, Texas), DuPont (E.I. DuPont de Nemours & Company, Inc., Wilmington, Delaware), Union Carbide (Union Carbide Corporation, Rye, New York), Aminco (Aminco, Silver Spring, Maryland), AGA (AGA, Sweden), Instrumentation Laboratory, Inc. (Instrumentation Laboratory, Inc., Lexington, Mass.), Abbott (Abbott Laboratories, No. Chicago, Ill.), Coulter (Coulter Electronics, Inc., Hialeah, Florida), Damon (Damon/IEC, Needham Heights, Mass.), Perkin-Elmer (Perkin-Elmer Corporation, Wellesley, Mass.), Electro-Nucleonics (Electro-Nucleonics, Inc., Fairfield, N.J.), Greiners (Greiners Electronics, Switzerland), and others have made enormous contributions to the improvement of analytical capabilities in clinical laboratories. Principles of operation, some performance data, and testimonials on the above instruments and others is a monthly feature in the magazine *Laboratory World* (Laboratory World, North American Publishing Company, Philadelphia, Pa.). The series is written by Dr. Nelson L. Alpert, and interested readers are urged to examine these articles dealing with instruments. General instruments such as scanning ultraviolet and visible spectrophotometers, gas chromatography, liquid chromatographs, fluorometers, atomic absorption spectrophotometers, and computers have been adapted successfully into clinical laboratories. Recently these general purpose instruments have begun to come equipped with their own micro-processors. These micro-computers can correct for baseline drift and non-linearity in standard working curves and can help with other operating tasks (Pesce, 1975). The near future will find more micro-processors in more instruments in clinical laboratories.

A significant contribution to instrumentation was made with the introduction of the fast centrifugal analyzer into the clinical laboratory (Anderson, 1969). In principle, the instrument relies on centrifugal force to transfer sample and reagent into one of a number of rotating cuvettes. The optical absorption of each cuvette is monitored on-line. A small computer is interfaced with the analyzer so that the rate of the reactions can be evaluated depending on the program entered into the computer. Numerous applications, e.g., enzyme activity rates, kinetic analyses of substrates, and antigen-antibody reaction monitoring have been developed for use with commercial fast centrifugal analyzers (Tiffany, 1974).

In future years clinical chemistry laboratories may see optical instruments with echelle gratings and with Vidicon detectors under computer control (Pardue, 1975). Laser nephelometry for specific protein analyses using antibodies has already become available (Laser Nephelometer PDQ, Hyland Division, Travenol Laboratories, Inc., P.O. Box 2214, 3300 Hyland Avenue, Costa Mesa, California 92626).

Microcalorimetry, the measurement of very small amounts of heat during chemical reactions, also may make some contribution to clinical chemistry, provided enough specificity and separations can be supplied prior to the analysis steps (Goldberg, 1976).

More HPLC instruments, specific small mass spectrometers, and electrochemical measurements can be expected in the near future. Emission methods for trace metals using very hot excitation devices can also make significant contributions in clinical laboratories because of their potential for multi-element analyses. Finally, circular dichroism and optical rotatory dispersion are techniques that can provide significant and new information on biologic molecules. Exciting new instrumental developments will continue to improve the accuracy, precision, and speed of analyses in the future in clinical laboratories.

Other instrumentation is reviewed elsewhere, i.e., Chapters 9, 13, and 15.

Portions of this chapter previously published in Tietz, N. W.: Fundamentals of Clinical Chemistry. Philadelphia, W. B. Saunders Company, 1976.

REFERENCES

Anderson, N. G.: Analytical techniques for cell fractions. XII: A multiple-cuvet rotor for a new microanalytical system. Anal. Biochem., *28*:545, 1969.

Brooks, M. A., and Hackman, M. R.: Trace level determination of 1,4-benzodiazepines in blood by differential pulse polarography. Anal. Chem., *47*:2059, 1975.

Ewing, G. W.: Instrumental Methods of Chemical Analysis, 3rd ed. New York, McGraw-Hill Book Company, 1969.

Goldberg, R. N.: Microcalorimetric determination of glucose in reference samples of serum. Clin. Chem., *22*:1685, 1976.

Huffman, D. H., and Hignite, C. E.: Serum quinidine concentrations: Comparison of fluorescence, gas-chromatographic, and gas-chromatographic/mass-spectrometric methods. Clin. Chem., *22*:810, 1976.

Molnar, I., and Horvath, C.: Reverse-phase chromatography of polar biological substances: Separation of catechol compounds by high-performance liquid chromatography. Clin. Chem., *22*:1497, 1976.

Noonan, D. C., and Komjathy, Z. L.: Long-term reproducibility of a new pH/blood-gas quality-control system compared to two other procedures. Clin. Chem., *22*:1817, 1976.

Pardue, H. L., McDowell, A. E., Fast, D. M., and Milano, M. J.: Applications of a vidicon spectrometer to analytical problems in clinical chemistry. Clin. Chem., *21*:1192, 1975.

Pelleg, A., and Levy, G. B.: Determination of Na^+ and K^+ in urine with ion-selective electrodes in an automated analyzer. Clin. Chem., *21*:1572, 1975.

Pesce, M. A., Bodourian, S. H., and Nicholson, J. F.: Rapid kinetic measurement of lactate in plasma with a centrifugal analyzer. Clin. Chem., *21*:1932, 1975.

Ryan, M. D.: Comments on the polarographic determination of metal-bilirubin formation constants. Anal. Chem., *47*:1717, 1975.

Schwartz, H. D.: New techniques for ion-selective measurements of ionized calcium in serum after pH adjustment of aerobically handled sera. Clin. Chem., *22*:461, 1976.

Skoog, D. A., and West, D. M.: Principles of Instrumental Analysis. New York, Holt, Rinehart and Winston, Inc., 1971.

Strobel, H. A.: Chemical Instrumentation: A Systematic Approach, 2nd ed. Reading, Mass., Addison-Wesley Publishing Company, 1973.

Tiffany, T. O.: Centrifugal fast analyzers in clinical laboratory analysis. CRC Crit. Rev. Clin. Lab. Sci., *5*:129, 1974.

5

SPIROMETRY AND BLOOD GASES

Robert Gilbert, M.D.

WITH A SECTION ON COLLECTION, PROCESSING,
AND MEASUREMENT OF BLOOD GASES BY
Michael Lapinski, M.D.

Although a number of pulmonary function tests are available, only two are needed for most problems in clinical medicine. These are spirometry and arterial blood gas analysis; discussion will be limited to these.

The primary function of the lung is that of gas exchange; arterial blood gases are the best guide to this function. In order for gas exchange to be a continuous process, alveolar air must constantly be exchanged with environmental air. This is the ventilatory function, the act of breathing. Spirometry is the best guide to mechanical impairment that may impede this function.

SPIROMETRY

EQUIPMENT

The spirogram is a graph with volume of air on the ordinate and time on the abscissa. In its simplest form a spirometer consists of a hollow cylinder open at the bottom, floating in a water jacket (Fig. 5-1).

The subject breathes in and out of the cylinder, causing it to move up and down. The vertical motion of the cylinder is transcribed

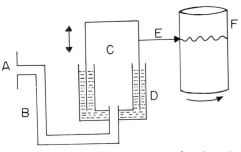

Figure 5-1. Schematic diagram of a simple spirometer. *A*, Mouthpiece; *B*, conducting tubing; *C*, hollow cylinder floating in waterjacket, *D*; *E*, pen; *F*, rotating drum containing calibrated paper.

onto calibrated paper fixed to a rotating drum, providing a record of volume of air versus time.

A large number of electronic spirometers are available which work on a variety of principles. Some of these provide only a digital read-out without a graphic display. Since they are more expensive, less accurate, and provide less information than the simple mechanical model described, they cannot be recommended. The Collins Survey Spirometer (Warren E. Collins, Inc., Braintree, Mass. 02184) works exactly as shown in Figure 5-1; it costs only a few hundred dollars and is very satisfactory for routine purposes. For more sophisticated testing, including flow-volume loops, a Wedge Spirometer (Med-Science Electronics, Inc., St. Louis, Mo. 63132) recording on a Tektronix oscilloscope (Tektronix, Inc., Beaverton, Ore., 97005) with a dual time base may be used, (Peppi, 1975). Simultaneous volume-time and flow-volume spirograms are provided by this method. Many commercially packaged systems are available, usually at a higher cost.

PERFORMANCE

Proper instruction of the patient is vital. Spirometry is a performance test; the patient must understand the test and must be willing to perform at a maximum level. If the patient has not been tested before, both a forced inspiratory and forced expiratory effort should be recorded.

What is required is a maximum inspiratory effort from a full expiratory position, and a maximum expiratory effort from a full inspiratory position. This can be done in one or two stages. For a one-stage test, the nose is oc-cluded with a nosepiece and the mouthpiece is placed in the patient's mouth. One or two normal breaths are recorded and the patient then expires easily to his residual volume. At this point, he breathes in as forcibly as he can to full inspiration, holds his breath briefly, then breathes out as forcibly as possible to full expiration (Fig. 5-2). If the test is performed in two stages, the patient inhales to full inspiration before placing the mouthpiece in his mouth, then inserts the mouthpiece and performs a forced expiration. After a few seconds rest, again with the mouthpiece out, he expires fully, inserts the mouthpiece, and makes a maximum inspiratory effort. (In a two-stage test, the order of inspiration and expiration can of course, be reversed). It is usually necessary to encourage the patient very strongly to produce maximum efforts, and the test should be repeated several times to assure that maximum values have been obtained.

INTERPRETATION

The spirogram contains two basic types of information—the total amount of air which can be moved in or out of the lung (the vital capacity, VC) and the rate of air flow. The three most useful measurements of rate of air flow are the volume of air expired during the first second of the forced expiration (FEV_1), the volume of air inspired during the first second of the forced inspiration (FIV_1), and the average flow rate over the middle half of the forced expiratory curve, the maximum mid-expiratory flow rate (MMF). Figure 5-2 demonstrates these measurements in a normal spirogram; the volume of air expired is shown equal to the volume inspired. In cases of severe airway obstruction there may be air

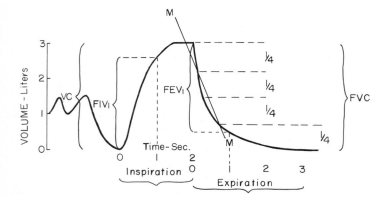

Figure 5-2. Normal shaped spirogram. Slope of line MM is the maximum mid-expiratory flow rate. VC = vital capacity; FVC = forced vital capacity; FEV_1 = one second forced expiratory volume; FIV_1 = one second forced inspiratory volume.

trapping with forced expiration, so that the total volume expired during this forced expiration, forced vital capacity (FVC), may be smaller than the vital capacity recorded during inspiration. This is especially likely to be true if the inspiratory effort was started from a residual volume reached from a slow, nonforceful expiration. If both the inspiratory and expiratory vital capacities are measured, the larger should be reported as the vital capacity.

Reference values for vital capacity and MMF are based on age, height, and sex; the prediction formulas of Cherniack (1972) are satisfactory, and many others are available in textbooks of pulmonary disease. The predicted value must always be considered in relation to the statistical confidence limits of the prediction, and these limits must accompany the prediction formulas. Prediction formulas for FEV_1 are available, but the FEV_1 is usually related to the FVC as the ratio FEV_1/FVC, often abbreviated $FEV_1\%$. The lower reference limit for $FEV_1\%$ is 75 per cent. It tends to decline slightly with age, but this can be ignored for most purposes. Reference values for FIV_1 are not available, but FIV_1 is normally equal or nearly equal to the vital capacity.

It is customary to classify abnormal spirograms as "obstructive" or "restrictive." The *restrictive* pattern or defect refers to a reduced vital capacity with normal or relatively normal flow rates. "Relatively normal" is a vague term, but certainly the $FEV_1\%$ should be above 75 per cent. The absolute value of FEV_1, FIV_1, MMF, or any other measurements may be low, especially if the vital capacity is severely reduced. In such cases the FEV_1 may equal the vital capacity. *The spirogram of a restrictive defect looks like a normal spirogram with all volumes reduced proportionally.*

The term "restrictive *disease*" should not be used, since a wide variety of diseases produce a restrictive pattern. These include heart failure with or without acute pulmonary edema, pneumonia, pulmonary fibrosis and other types of interstitial lung disease, pulmonary embolism, atelectasis, pneumothorax, pleural effusion, crushed chest injuries, and neurologic diseases such as poliomyelitis, myasthenia gravis, and Guillain-Barré syndrome. (Rarely, during a severe attack of asthma, clearly a disease involving airway obstruction, a restrictive pattern is seen.) The spirogram therefore indicates that a restrictive ventilatory defect is present, provides information as to the severity of the defect but not its etiology, and will usually but not always rule out significant airway obstruction.

The *obstructive* pattern or defect refers to airway obstruction, and its most common cause is the asthma-bronchitis-emphysema group of diseases. FEV_1 and MMF will be reduced and the $FEV_1\%$ will be below 75 per cent. VC and especially FVC are usually reduced, but this is primarily the result of an increase in residual volume plus air trapping, rather than loss of lung tissue, increased stiffness of the lung, or chest wall or neuromuscular disease, as in the case of a restrictive defect. A spirogram showing severe airway obstruction with a low vital capacity, therefore, should not be referred to as a combined restrictive and obstructive defect. The interpretation of a combined restrictive and obstructive defect should be limited to spirograms showing a reduction in vital capacity with only mild airway obstruction. Figure 5–3 shows a spirogram of a moderately severe obstructive defect.

The obstructive defects we have been describing are those of so-called lower airway obstruction, that is, obstruction of airways within the lung parenchyma. In these cases

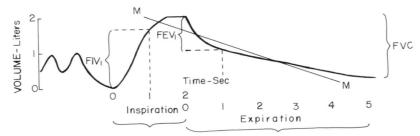

Figure 5–3. Spirogram demonstrating moderately severe airway obstruction. Note that the FVC is less than the vital capacity recorded during inspiration. Note also the difference in slope of line MM compared to that in Figure 5–2.

expiratory flow rates are always more severely affected than inspiratory flow rates; FIV_1 should always be greater than FEV_1. If both FIV_1 and FEV_1 are reduced, and FIV_1 is smaller than FEV_1, so-called upper airway obstruction must be strongly considered. The most common causes of this are tracheal stenosis and diseases of the larynx and epiglottis. Tracheal tumor, thyroid compression of the trachea, and obstruction in the posterior pharynx are rarer causes of upper airway obstruction.

A special warning is necessary in the interpretation of the inspiratory spirogram. Although the entire spirogram is effort-dependent, this is especially true for inspiration. In advanced airway obstruction, in fact, the FEV_1 may be relatively independent of the force applied by the patient. This is never true for FIV_1, and the inspiratory part of the spirogram must always be interpreted with caution if there is any reason to suspect less than a maximum effort.

With very severe ventilatory impairment of either type, for example, with a vital capacity of only a few hundred milliliters in a normal-sized adult, it may be difficult to distinguish between a restrictive and an obstructive defect. In these cases it is preferable simply to note that a severe ventilatory defect is present; its exact nature will usually be evident from clinical considerations.

The earliest manifestations of chronic bronchitis and emphysema are probably in the small airways, arbitrarily defined as those with an internal diameter of less than 2 mm. In the interval between attacks, the asthmatic patient may have obstruction limited to these small airways. Because they are so numerous, their total cross-sectional area is large, and considerable disease can be present in these small airways without contributing significantly to overall airway obstruction. In this case, the volume-time spirogram may be normal. There has been considerable effort in recent years to develop more sensitive tests for "early" or small airway obstruction. Many have been reported, but over the course of time they have been found to be too complex, too expensive, too uncomfortable, too unreliable, too time consuming, or any combination of these for routine use. At this writing, the MMF in the volume-time spirogram is probably as good as any measurement for routine clinical purposes for detecting early airway disease. If the $FEV_1\%$ is low, the MMF will always be reduced. If the MMF is low in the presence of a normal $FEV_1\%$ and normal vital capacity, small or early airway disease can be suspected.

There has also been a great deal of recent interest in the flow-volume spirogram. It provides an excellent visual display; at a glance one can tell if a defect is present and the nature of the defect. For quantitative measurements for clinical purposes, however, its value in place of or in addition to the volume-time spirogram described here has yet to be proven. Flow-volume loops, as they are usually called, seem most useful for the detection of upper airway obstruction and small airway disease. A detailed description is beyond the scope of this discussion, but a good review has recently been provided by Kryger (1976).

COLLECTION, PROCESSING, AND MEASUREMENT OF BLOOD GASES

Michael Lapinski

SPECIMEN COLLECTION RECEPTACLES

Many types of blood specimen collection receptacles have been evaluated and recommended for blood gas determinations. One of the first and still preferred is the glass syringe, which should probably be considered a "reference" receptacle. All others, such as regular plastic syringes, "specialized plastic syringes," vacuum tubes, and capillary tubes should be compared with glass syringes. The glass syringe and plunger should be matched for best fit. Approximately 1 ml of heparin (1000 or 5000 U/ml) is drawn into the syringe and the barrel lubricated. The plunger is tested to insure easy mobility, and the heparin should be expelled, leaving the dead space filled with residual heparin (Winkler, 1974). Advantages of the glass syringe include the most accurate results obtainable, a glass plunger that moves upward because of arterial pressure (if 23 gauge or larger needle is used), and reusability. Disadvantages of the glass syringe include relatively high initial cost, need for proper sterilization between patients, and easy breakage. Alternative devices include standard plastic (polypropylene) syringes, special plastic syringes designed especially for blood gases, and vacuum tubes. Plastic syringes eliminate the need for resterilization, are low in cost, readily available in any hospital setting, and relatively unbreakable. Unfortunately, standard plastic syringes have their own disadvantages. A valid question concerns accuracy because of gas leakage through the plastic. A major technical disadvantage is that the plunger will not rise owing to arterial pressure, and a minor problem is that air bubbles are harder to remove.

Leakage of gases through plastic can pose a major problem or a relatively minor problem depending on the type of plastic and the oxygen and carbon dioxide tensions of the blood specimen collected. The greater the difference between the partial pressures of oxygen and carbon dioxide in the blood and the partial pressures in room air, the larger is the leakage. Scott (1971a and b) does not recommend the use of plastic syringes. Polypropylene plastic syringes are superior to polystyrene plastic syringes (Scott, 1971b). Other authors (Evers, 1972; Winkler, 1974) conclude that plastic syringes are acceptable for patient management, and most clinical problems are not affected by relatively small differences that may exist between glass and plastic syringes.

Recently a new type of plastic syringe has been developed featuring a plunger which will rise owing to arterial pressure. An example is the Terumo syringe (Terumo Corporation, Tokyo, Japan), which we have been evaluating. Our initial data suggest that these syringes do not show significant leakage for up to three hours. However, before this type of syringe can replace the glass syringe, more experience with it is necessary.

Controversy has surrounded the use of vacuum tubes such as the Vacutainer. Fleisher (1971) reported the successful use of a special Vacutainer tube (Becton-Dickinson and Company, Rutherford, N.J.) filled with nitrogen gas at a pressure of 152 mm Hg and containing 143 units of sodium heparin. A special adapter was used to obtain arterial blood gases. Although these specialized vacuum tubes were shown to produce accurate results, the large air space at the top of standard heparin vacuum tubes can produce erroneous results by equilibrating with the blood.

The last type of acceptable container for blood collection and transport is special capillary tubes. However, their accuracy and deficiencies cannot easily be separated from the arterialized capillary blood which they contain.

BLOOD SPECIMEN COLLECTION AND PATIENT PREPARATION

The brachial and radial arteries are the preferred vessels for arterial puncture. The femoral artery is relatively large and easy to puncture, but care must be taken in older individuals, in whom the femoral artery tends to bleed more than the radial or brachial. Since the bleeding site is hidden by bedcovers, it may not be noticed until bleeding is massive. The radial artery is more difficult to puncture but exhibits a lower incidence of complications (Mortensen, 1967). When using the radial artery it is possible to test the collateral circulation of the hand using the Allen test (Bedford, 1974; Greenhow, 1972). The Allen test consists of elevating the hand to empty it of blood, occlusion of the radial artery, and observation of the return of blood flow through the ulnar artery as the hand is lowered. This test insures collateral circulation should the radial artery become occluded as a consequence of manipulation. The major complications of arterial puncture include thrombosis and hemorrhage (Siggaard-Anderson, 1968). Petty (1966) reported no complications except for minimal hematomas with 475 arterial punctures. Using trained registered nurses to perform radial arterial punctures, Sackner (1971) reported 1541 punctures with no morbidity.

The artery to be punctured is identified by its pulsations. The skin is properly cleansed to prepare an aseptic site for puncture. Although a local anesthetic wheal may be made, an anesthetic is not required. The use of butterfly infusion sets is not recommended (Bageant, 1975). Using 19 vs. 25 gauge needles does not vary the Pco_2 or Po_2 more than 1 mm Hg (Bageant, 1975).

The needle (18 or 20 gauge for brachial artery) should pierce the skin at an angle of approximately 45 to 60 degrees and should approach the artery slowly. Some degree of dorsiflexion of the wrist is necessary with the radial artery for which a 23 to 25 gauge needle is used. The pulsations of blood into the syringe confirm that arterial blood has been obtained. Usually, if a 23 gauge or larger needle has been used, the syringe will fill by arterial pressure alone. If the plunger is pulled back there is a possibility of aspirating air into the syringe. Any air that is accidently aspirated should be immediately expelled (Ishikawa, 1974). After the blood specimen is obtained, the needle should be removed and an airtight cap placed over the tip of the syringe. Although it is common practice to force the point of the needle into a cork or rubber stopper, this practice should be avoided owing to the danger of the needle's puncturing hospital personnel handling the specimen. After the arterial puncture, compression on the puncture site should be applied for a minimum of two minutes and preferably for five minutes (timed).

The recommended volume of arterial blood obtained varies with different authors, but certainly the greater the specimen volume, the less dilution effect from the heparin. With a 10 ml syringe, the dead space is 1.2 to 2.4 per cent of the maximal volume (Siggaard-Anderson, 1961). The heparin dilution primarily affects the P_{CO_2}. Siggaard-Anderson (1961) reports a 16 per cent fall in P_{CO_2} with a dilution of 12 to 13 per cent, while Bradley (1972) reports an error of 28 per cent on the same dilutional factor.

At times, it is either impractical or impossible to obtain arterial blood from a patient. Under these circumstances, another source of blood can be obtained, but it should be remembered always that the most accurate results are achieved with arterial blood.

The most readily obtainable blood is venous blood. However, venous blood usually reflects the acid-base status of an extremity, not the body as a whole. Venous blood properly collected will yield adequate pH values, but venous blood yields incorrect values for arterial oxygen saturation and alveolar P_{CO_2}. (Gambino, 1959; 1961).

Arterialized capillary blood from the finger has been recommended as a suitable substitute for arterial blood for pH and P_{CO_2} but is not acceptable for P_{O_2} (Jung, 1966). In order for it to be a satisfactory substitute for arterial blood, some estimation of the P_{O_2} must be available. The recommended site for obtaining arterialized capillary blood is the earlobe (Langlands, 1964; 1965) because of its vascularity, low metabolic requirements, and the ease with which it can be "arterialized." The earlobe can be arterialized by heat, by flicking with the index finger until definite flushing is observed, or by chemical means of Trafuril paste (Ciba A-G, Basle, Switzerland).

To obtain a blood specimen, the earlobe is cleansed with alcohol and punctured. The puncture area should be adequate to obtain a free flow of blood and the lobe wiped dry. Two heparinized capillary tubes (100 μl) are placed in the center of the drop and filled to capacity without air bubbles. Both ends are sealed in clay after the insertion of a rustproof metal stirrer. Blood in the tubes is stirred by the use of a magnet, thus mixing specimen with heparin (Sadove, 1973). Whenever the cardiac output is severely restricted (Laughlin, 1964), there is a systolic pressure below 95 mm Hg (Koch, 1968), or there is vasoconstriction (Sadove, 1973), capillary blood yields unreliable data.

The greatest value of capillary blood is in the pediatric age group. In the older pediatric population, earlobe blood is available, but in neonates and infants in whom it is impractical to sample the earlobe it is often used. A deep heel prick is made at the distal edge of the calcanean protuberance following a 5 to 10 minute period in 45 to 47°C. water (Koch, 1967). The specimen is then handled as described for the earlobe specimen. Capillary blood obtained in this manner is unacceptable for P_{CO_2} and P_{O_2} determination in the first day of life, probably owing to vasoconstriction and poor perfusion of the extremities (Koch, 1967). In infants with respiratory distress syndrome, heel blood deviates significantly from arterial blood in all parameters except base excess and standard bicarbonate (Gandy, 1964; Bigen, 1975). The best method for blood gas collection in the newborn still remains the indwelling umbilical artery catheter.

New methods for determining pH, P_{CO_2}, and P_{O_2} are being investigated. Attempts to measure P_{CO_2} and P_{O_2} through the use of transcutaneous electrodes have been reported (Huch, 1977). Also, *in vivo* pH and P_{CO_2} sensors have been used in experimental animals (Coon, 1976).

The patient's temperature may be taken into account in the determination of blood gas values. For P_{O_2}, there is about a 6 per cent change per degree centigrade (Nunn, 1962).

Although correction factors are available for fever (Kelman, 1966), they are rarely used in clinical medicine but should be; with automatic blood gas analyzers, a patient's temperature can be included in the analysis.

BLOOD SPECIMEN HANDLING AND TRANSPORT

All blood specimens in sealed receptacles should be placed in ice water immediately after they are obtained from the patient. Blood will consume oxygen and liberate carbon dioxide at a rate which is temperature-dependent. When the Po_2 of the original blood is above 150 mm Hg the decay at $37°C$. is 2.7 mm Hg/min (Newball, 1973). Although room temperature does not produce as large an error, it is not an acceptable mode of transport. One can appreciate the importance of blood cooling when one considers that in most large hospitals, blood gas determinations require between 10 and 15 minutes after blood collection for completion; this means an error of 27 to 40 mm Hg lower for Po_2 at $37°C$.

When a specimen is received in the laboratory, it should be placed in ice water, properly identified, and scrutinized for clots and air bubbles. If all these conditions are not met, the specimen should not be analyzed. A clotted specimen aspirated or injected into a modern gas analyzer may necessitate a major cleaning of the instrument. If a specimen arrives only in water, without visible ice, one should be very suspicious of the elapsed time for transport, and possible errors from room temperature storage.

BLOOD GAS INSTRUMENTATION

Blood gas instrumentation has advanced tremendously since the development of specific electrodes within the last 20 years. Every modern blood gas instrument contains pH, Pco_2, and Po_2 electrodes (see Chapter 4, p. 95).

A glass electrode system is used for pH measurement. This system consists of two halves, the calomel or reference electrode and the glass electrode. The calomel electrode maintains a constant potential, while the glass electrode membrane develops a potential proportional to the hydrogen ion concentration in the solution. This electrode is calibrated by using two phosphate buffers of known pH (Dowd, 1973).

The Severinghaus electrode is used commonly for Pco_2. This is a pH electrode surrounded by an electrolyte solution separated from the blood by a membrane permeable to carbon dioxide. The pH of the solution is dependent on the Pco_2 that comes to an equilibrium with the blood. The membrane can be of silicone rubber or Teflon (Severinghaus, 1962; 1968).

For O_2 determination, the polarographic Clark oxygen electrode is used. A constant polarizing voltage is applied to the silver-silver chloride anode and the platinum wire cathode. The anode and cathode are in a KCl electrolyte solution. The blood is separated by an oxygen-permeable membrane of polypropylene or polyethylene. Oxygen is reduced at the electrode, and the potential change is proportional to the rate of oxygen reduction. This rate varies directly with the oxygen tension of the blood.

To calibrate Po_2 and Pco_2 electrodes, either a gas or a liquid of known oxygen partial pressure must be used. If a gas is used, problems arise because of calibration of the O_2 electrode. Most Po_2 electrodes yield a lower Po_2 for blood than for the gas with which the electrode was equilibrated. This discrepancy is in the range of 1.8 to 5.6 per cent (Bird, 1974). It is known as the "blood gas factor" and holds the greatest significance at a Po_2 over 150 mm Hg (Bird, 1974). Protein contamination of the membranes must periodically be removed; membranes have only limited life before they develop leaks.

The differences among various available blood gas analyzers or instruments center on the degree of automation. A manual instrument properly used will yield results as accurate and reliable as the most automated instrument. In a very busy laboratory where instruments tend to be abused and the number of specimens is great, the more automated analyzer tends to reduce error owing to technical personnel carelessness and abuse; however, they may suffer more from disturbances of electronic circuitry and mechanical parts, which require maintenance and repair. The manual instrument is usually simpler to repair, and repairs can often be accomplished by a well-trained technologist in the laboratory. Usually, most repairs on the automatic instruments necessitate a factory authorized repair person. All automatic analyzers have automatic calibration. Some of the more advanced instruments have incorporated barometers (strain gauge type) and a photometer to measure hemoglobin. Often the operator can make corrections for patient's temperature by proper programming. The more manual analyzer generally reports only measured values; thus, the operator uses nomograms for the other parameters such as bicarbonate, base excess, oxygen saturation, total carbon dioxide, standard bases excess, and standard bicarbonate. Usually the top-of-the-line instruments will calculate these parameters.

A very important consideration in the choice of an instrument is the service of the company. In Table 5-1 a comparison of selected manual and top-of-the-line automatic models reveals several types of blood gas analyzers available. Because of space limitation, we have not included many fine, dependable instruments, nor do we recommend any one instrument.

QUALITY CONTROL

Quality control is difficult to perform adequately. The most accurate instrument is worthless if the specimen is incorrectly obtained or transported. It is imperative that the laboratory receive a proper specimen in every case that is reported. Quality control and preventive maintenance must be performed on a regular schedule. In one large community involving several laboratories, instruments initially showed inaccuracies ranging from -30.8 per cent to $+17.3$ per cent for Po_2 and from -14.0 per cent to $+42.9$ per cent for Pco_2; by the conclusion of the quality control study, these inaccuracies were greatly reduced (Delaney, 1976).

One method of quality control for a laboratory consists of duplicate determinations of each blood specimen. In our laboratory, all abnormal blood gas results are confirmed on a different instrument and results recorded. If these results agree, we report the results of the first instrument; if they do not agree within 5 per cent, the specimen is analyzed on a third instrument. We then report the results of the two instruments which coincide within 5 per cent. The necessary investigative steps are then taken to correct the instrument yielding an unacceptable value. All results are maintained as a permanent written record.

This method, because of its frequent use, discloses problems which may take hours to identify by other quality control measures. Although duplicate analyses of a single specimen for quality control are useful, they should only supplement another accepted method of quality control.

Other methods of quality control include measuring room air injected into the machine, measuring water equilibrated at 37°C. with room air, and checking the CO_2 channel by another method.

Three major methods of quality control that should be used employ commercial ampules containing aqueous buffered bicarbonate solutions, equilibrated tonometer blood, or bicarbonate solutions. Aqueous buffered bicarbonate solutions equilibrated with known high, normal, and low gas tensions are sealed in glass ampules. An example is GAS controls (General Diagnostics—Division of Warner Lambert Company, Morris Plains, N.J.). The coefficient of variation of these aqueous controls is as follows: Po_2 3.2 to 5.4 per cent; Pco_2 2.6 to 4.4 per cent; and pH 0.18 to 0.24 per cent (Noonan, 1976). A major problem with these controls is their relatively quick equilibration with room air once the ampule is opened. Within four minutes, GAS control level III equilibrated with room air from an initial Po_2 of 58.3 mm Hg to 62.1 mm Hg, while level I change was from 163.5 to 163.2 mm Hg in four minutes (Komjathy, 1976).

Recently, Instrumentation Laboratories (Lexington, Mass.) has released ampules of aqueous buffered bicarbonate solutions similar to those offered by General Diagnostics. Also a new type of ampule control based on whole human blood is being introduced by Dade (Dade Division, American Hospital Supply Corporation, Miami, Fl.).

In our opinion, the best method of quality control is through use of a tonometer. A tonometer equilibrates blood with a known analyzed mixture of gas at a constant temperature of 37°C. (Chalmers, 1974). An example of this type of instrument is the Instrumentation Laboratory Tonometer 237 (Laboratory Instrumentation, Lexington, Mass.), which equilibrates blood with a gas phase using thin-film methodology. Major advantages of equilibrated blood from a tonometer include: blood is a biologic specimen, which is usually measured in a blood gas instrument; the blood can be equilibrated to specific Po_2 and Pco_2 values which the laboratory desires, and the blood is

Table 5–1. COMPARISON OF SELECTED BLOOD GAS INSTRUMENTATION

BLOOD GAS ANALYZER	INSTRUMENTATION LABORATORY MICRO 13*	RADIOMETER MICROSYSTEM BGA2, 3M53, MK2/PHM 73§	CORNING 165-2‡	INSTRUMENTATION LABORATORY 813*	TECHNICON BG 11†	RADIOMETER ABL II§	CORNING 175‡
APPROXIMATE PRICE	$6,200	$6,375	$7,950	$13,500	$15,450	$15,900	$17,900
MEASURES Po_2, Pco_2, pH	yes	yes	yes	yes	yes	yes, plus barometric pressure and hemoglobin	yes, plus barometric pressure
CALCULATES BICARBONATE, BASE EXCESS, AND TOTAL CARBON DIOXIDE	no	no	yes	yes	yes, plus standard bicarbonate, standard base excess, oxygen saturation, and oxygen content	yes, plus oxygen saturation, standard base excess, and standard bicarbonate	yes, plus oxygen saturation and content
CORRECTIONS	none	none	hemoglobin[1]	temperature	temperature, hemoglobin; liquid-gas	temperature	temperature
CALIBRATION	manual	manual	manual	automatic	automatic	automatic	automatic
SAMPLE SIZE	100 or 300 μl	130 μl	150 or 500 μl	175 or 450 μl	130 or 500 μl	200 μl	125[2] or 500 μl
AUTOMATIC POINT DETECTION	no	no	no	no	true end point with peak monitoring	timed end point	continuous delta check
SELF DIAGNOSIS	partial	partial	partial	yes	yes	yes	yes
TIME TO PERFORM ANALYSIS	120 sec	120 sec	90 sec	72 sec	150 sec	150 sec	60 sec[2] or 180 sec
COMMENTS	1 of 3 manual systems	1 of 6 manual systems: separate units; printer optional	[1]patient hemoglobin necessary, incorporated by operator printer to become available		printer is standard	liquid calibration, gasmixer, printer, and computer interface are standard	printer standard computer interface, and/or teletype optional [2]without calculated parameters

* Instrumentation Laboratory Inc., Lexington, Massachusetts 02173
† Technicon Instruments Corp., Tarrytown, New York 10591
‡ Corning Medical, Medfield, Massachusetts 02052
§ Radiometer, DK2400, Copenhagen NV, Denmark

relatively stable. The disadvantages are that a bulk buffer must be used for pH quality control and technical time must still be allocated to prepare a blood sample in a tonometer.

The coefficient of variation with tonometer blood for Pco_2 varies from 2.9 to 6.2 per cent and for Po_2 from 1.2 to 3.6 per cent (Leary, 1977). Blood obtained from a tonometer is very stable in a plastic syringe for up to 1.5 hours, and for all except the very high Po_2 range most samples remain stable for up to 6 hours (Leary, 1977). Our data essentially agree with that of Leary (1977). For example, we use equilibrated blood from a tonometer with a Pco_2 and Po_2 at 49.2 to 49.8 mm Hg depending on barometric pressure, and have set up 95 per cent confidence limits for our Radiometer ABL II blood gas analyzer (Copenhagen, Denmark) at 46 to 53 mm Hg. We can usually anticipate major mechanical failure two to three days in advance through quality control efforts, i.e., 95 per cent confidence limits not obtained during that interval.

ARTERIAL BLOOD GASES

OXYGEN

TRANSPORT OF OXYGEN IN THE BLOOD

Partial pressure

Oxygen and carbon dioxide are generally reported in units of partial pressure. *The partial pressure of a gas in a liquid is the partial pressure of that gas with which the liquid is in equilibrium.* Consider a glass of water in a room. Assuming a barometric pressure of 760 mm Hg, the partial pressure of oxygen (Po_2) in room air is approximately 21 per cent of 760, or 160 mm Hg. Since the water is in equilibrium with the room air, the Po_2 in the water is also 160 mm Hg.

A glass of blood stands next to the glass of water. Since both the water and the blood are in equilibrium with the same gas, in this case room air, the Po_2 of the blood must also be 160 mm Hg. The actual quantity of oxygen in the blood is far greater than in the water. The *amount* of a gas in a liquid depends on the solubility of the gas in the liquid, as well as on the partial pressure, but the partial pressure of the gas in the liquid depends only on the partial pressure of the gas with which the liquid is in equilibrium.

Oxygen saturation

Although the *quantity* of oxygen in the blood can be expressed in absolute terms such as volumes per cent, it is usually reported as oxygen saturation (So_2). Today blood oxygen saturation is measured by spectrophotometry, but the concept of saturation is best understood by considering the original method of measurement. A sample of blood is drawn anaerobically and divided into two parts. One part is introduced into a Van Slyke apparatus and all the gases liberated from the blood. The oxygen is then absorbed and its volume calculated from the gas laws by noting the pressure change resulting from the absorption. This is the oxygen content. The second part of the sample is equilibrated with room air (which will allow full saturation), and the amount of oxygen in this blood is measured in a similar manner (oxygen capacity). The oxygen saturation is calculated as: So_2 = oxygen content $\times$ 100/oxygen capacity. The oxygen saturation is a measure of the amount of oxygen in the blood that is combined with hemoglobin compared with the total amount of oxygen that can combine with hemoglobin. Oxygen saturation and oxygen content are linearly related through the oxygen capacity, which in turn depends on the amount and type of hemoglobin in the blood.

Oxygen dissolved in physical solution

The oxygen saturation refers to the oxygen carried by the hemoglobin. A very small amount of oxygen will dissolve in the plasma in physical solution, 0.003 ml of oxygen in each 100 ml of plasma for each mm Hg of the Po_2. This amount is ordinarily of no significance; it may assume importance during the breathing of 100 per cent oxygen (approximately 1.95 volumes per cent) and is the key factor in hyperbaric oxygenation.

The oxyhemoglobin dissociation curve

The amount of oxygen combined with hemoglobin is related to the Po_2 by the oxyhe-

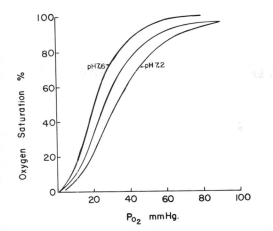

Figure 5–4. Oxyhemoglobin dissociation curve for normal adult hemoglobin. The center curve is a so-called standard curve for a pH of 7.4.

moglobin dissociation curve (Fig. 5–4). Oxygen saturation rather than oxygen content is used for the ordinate so that the curves will apply to any hemoglobin concentration. The reasons for the shape of the curve are complex and will not be discussed here. The implications of the shape are of great importance in the interpretation of blood gas data and will be discussed in the appropriate sections.

The center curve in Figure 5–4 is the so-called standard curve, representing a pH of 7.40 and Pco_2 of 40 mm Hg. Alkalemia shifts the curve to the left, acidemia to the right. A left shift increases the affinity of the hemoglobin for oxygen; for a given Po_2 the content and saturation are greater. A right shift decreases the affinity. Increase in CO_2 will shift the curve slightly to the right; a decrease shifts the curve to the left. This effect is independent of the effect of CO_2 on the pH.

These shifts have physiologic value. Acidity increases when blood reaches the tissue level, thereby facilitating release of oxygen from the blood to the tissues. As carbon dioxide is eliminated in the lungs, the blood becomes more alkaline, increasing the affinity for oxygen, and thereby facilitating oxygen uptake by the blood.

Recent work has shown that the red cell concentration of 2,3-diphosphoglycerate (DPG), and other organic phosphates as well, will also alter the position of the curve; an increase in DPG shifts the curve to the right, for example. These shifts occur in a wide variety of diseases, and therefore there is no standard dissociation curve in clinical medicine. Most of these shifts are minor, however, at least as regards the interpretation of blood gas data; hence it is still useful to think in terms of the standard curve.

The position of the curve can be indicated by a single number, the P50. This is the Po_2 at which the hemoglobin is 50 per cent saturated with oxygen. The value of P50 for the so-called standard curve is approximately 26 mm Hg.

If the laboratory reports both Po_2 and So_2, these should represent independent determinations and not merely determination of one and recourse to the standard curve to determine the other. There are several reasons for this in addition to the lack of a true standard curve. First, because of the flat shape of the curve at saturations above 95 per cent, the Po_2 cannot be estimated accurately from the saturation above this level. Second, on the steep portion, So_2 cannot be estimated accurately from the Po_2 for similar reasons. Finally, independent determinations of So_2 and Po_2 with instruments utilizing entirely different principles serve as useful checks against gross errors in measurement.

THE ALVEOLAR-ARTERIAL OXYGEN DIFFERENCE

The partial pressure of a gas in a liquid is the partial pressure of the gas with which the liquid is in equilibrium. For the arterial blood, what is this gas? The obvious answer is the alveolar air; if this were true, the partial pressures of the arterial blood gases would be the same as those of the alveolar air. This is not the case, however. An understanding of the difference between the partial pressure of oxygen in the alveolar air (P_AO_2) and in the arterial blood (P_aO_2), the alveolar-arterial (A-a) oxygen difference ($P_{A-aD}O_2$), is vital for the interpretation of arterial blood gas data. This difference is always positive; that is, P_AO_2 is always higher than P_aO_2.

Mixing of blood

The Po_2 resulting from the mixture of blood samples with different values of Po_2 cannot be calculated directly from the Po_2 values of the original blood. Only oxygen content or saturation, representing actual quantities or concentrations of gas, can be directly manipulated mathematically. The calculation of resulting Po_2 values requires working through the dissociation curve. For example, if equal quantities of two blood samples are mixed, one with a P_{O_2} of 300 mm Hg and one with a P_{O_2} of 40 mm Hg, the P_{O_2} of the resulting mixture is *not* (300 + 40)/2. Instead, the oxygen content or saturation of the two blood samples must be obtained from the dissociation curve, averaged, and the P_{O_2} then obtained from the resulting content or saturation by referring again to the dissociation curve. When this is done, the P_{O_2} resulting from equal mixtures of blood at 300 mm Hg and 40 mm Hg is found to be 61 mm Hg.

When *gases* mix, the P_{O_2} values can be calculated directly, since the concentration or quantity of gas is directly proportional to the partial pressure. Thus, if equal volumes of two gases are mixed with partial pressures of 300 mm Hg and 40 mm Hg, the resulting P_{O_2} would be 170 mm Hg.

We can now proceed to a discussion of those factors which produce $P_{A\text{-}aD}O_2$.

Diffusion gradient

To reach the interior of the red cell from the alveolus, oxygen must pass through the alveolar membrane, an interstitial fluid-filled space, the capillary membrane, the plasma, and the red cell membrane. If these structures are normal, little pressure gradient is required to move the oxygen across this barrier. The normal oxygen pressure gradient between the alveolar air and the *mean* pulmonary capillary blood is about 10 mm Hg, and the gradient between the alveolar air and the *end* pulmonary capillary blood (pulmonary vein) is less than 1 mm Hg. Several factors may increase these gradients: (1) the barrier may be thickened by fibrous or granulation tissue (alveolar capillary block syndrome); (2) the total surface area available for diffusion may become reduced; (3) exercise or other high cardiac output states may reduce the time that the blood spends in the pulmonary capillary bed.

There is a wide margin of safety. A severe reduction in diffusing capacity will lead to an increase in the alveolar-to-*mean* pulmonary capillary gradient, but will produce only a minor increase in the alveolar-to-*end* pulmonary capillary gradient. At or near sea level, under resting conditions and breathing room air, the diffusion gradient makes only a minor contribution to the total $P_{A\text{-}aD}O_2$. Furthermore, if the concentration of oxygen in the inspired gas is raised above that of room air, any hypoxemia owing to a diffusion defect will be abolished.

Ventilation/perfusion (V/Q) inequalities

The normal alveolar ventilation ($\dot{V}A$) is approximately 4 l/min and the normal cardiac output ($\dot{Q}$) is approximately 5 l/min. The overall V/Q ratio of the lung is therefore approximately 0.8. This ratio, however, does not necessarily apply to every discrete area of the lung. Even in normal lungs, both ventilation and perfusion are unevenly distributed. Part of this is a gravitational effect. In the upright position, there is a gradient of both ventilation and perfusion from the top to the bottom of the lung, so that the lung bases receive more ventilation and more perfusion than the apices. The gradient is much more pronounced for perfusion than for ventilation (West, 1962). At the apex the V/Q ratio is approximately 3.3, in the midportion 0.90, and at the base 0.63. In the supine position a similar condition applies, with the ventilation and perfusion gradients running from ventral to dorsal regions. The magnitude of these gradients would obviously not be as large.

These regional inequalities in V/Q ratios are responsible in part for the normal $P_{A\text{-}aD}O_2$ of about 10 mm Hg. In many diseases, but most prominently in chronic obstructive airway disease, there are marked regional differences in ventilation and perfusion in addition to the gravitational gradients. This non-uniform distribution of ventilation, perfusion, or both leads to a wide spectrum of V/Q ratios throughout the lung. The areas where the ratio is low are under-ventilated in relation to the blood flow; the P_AO_2 will be low and the blood leaving these areas will have a relatively low P_{O_2} and oxygen content compared with that of normal arterial blood. The areas with a high V/Q ratio are over-ventilated in relation to the blood flow; the P_AO_2 will be high as will be the P_{O_2} of the blood leaving these areas. However, the under-ventilated, over-perfused areas contribute a larger proportion of blood to the final mixed arterial blood than do the over-ventilated, under-perfused areas. Furthermore, the blood leaving the over-ventilated areas is on the high, flat portion of the dissociation curve; although the P_{O_2} is high, the oxygen content is increased very little above the normal value for arterial blood. Thus, when the blood from areas of low and high V/Q ratios mix, the resulting blood will have a lower P_{O_2} than if the V/Q ratios were normal. The result will be an increase in $P_{A\text{-}aD}O_2$.

Shunting

Normally, 2 to 5 per cent of the cardiac output is shunted from the right to the left side of the heart without traversing ventilated alveoli. This includes contributions from the thebesian veins which drain directly into the left ventricle, the more distal branchings of the bronchial arteries which drain into the pulmonary rather than the bronchial veins, and blood traversing alveoli that are not ventilated. This venous blood, when mixed with oxygenated blood, will lower the oxygen content and P_{O_2} of the resulting arterial blood.

In pneumonia, atelectasis, pulmonary edema, and shock, for example, many lung units may lose their ventilation while retaining their blood supply. In addition, new vascular channels may open which bypass ventilated alveoli. The blood traversing these areas is effectively shunted from the venous to the arterial side of the circulation. This type of right-to-left shunting is an important factor in the extreme widening of $P_{A-aD}O_2$ in critically ill patients. Since these lung units receive no ventilation, breathing even 100 per cent oxygen does little to improve the hypoxemia resulting from shunting.

Relative contribution of diffusion, V/Q inequalities, and shunting to $P_{A-aD}O_2$

Although the diffusion gradient may assume importance during exercise and at high altitudes, even in severe cases of so-called alveolar-capillary block (with the possible exception of the adult respiratory distress syndrome), this gradient makes only a minor contribution to $P_{A-aD}O_2$ at or near sea level if the patient is at rest breathing at least 21 per cent oxygen. In normal subjects breathing room air, V/Q inequalities and shunting contribute about equally to the normal $P_{A-aD}O_2$. In chronic obstructive airway disease the abnormally wide $P_{A-aD}O_2$ is due primarily to the wide spectrum of V/Q ratios. The widened $P_{A-aD}O_2$ in most critically ill patients is due to varying combinations of V/Q inequalities and shunting.

Effect of cardiac output on $P_{A-aD}O_2$

Cardiac output, oxygen consumption ($\dot{V}O_2$), and arterial-venous oxygen content difference ($C_aO_2 - C_{\bar{v}}O_2$) are interrelated through the Fick equation: $C_aO_2 - C_{\bar{v}}O_2 = \dot{V}O_2/\dot{Q}$. If $\dot{Q}$ decreases without a fall in $\dot{V}O_2$, the arterial-venous oxygen content difference widens as the tissues, receiving less blood, extract more oxygen from the blood that is delivered. This results in a fall in the mixed venous oxygen content. Obviously, the lower the oxygen content of the shunted blood, the greater will be its effect on lowering the P_aO_2 and widening the $P_{A-aD}O_2$.

The alveolar air equation

$P_{A-aD}O_2$ is the difference between the partial pressure of oxygen in the alveolar air (P_AO_2) and the partial pressure of oxygen in the arterial blood (P_aO_2). P_aO_2 is measured directly. To calculate $P_{A-aD}O_2$ it is necessary to calculate a value of P_AO_2, since this is cumbersome to measure directly.

There is no single value for P_AO_2, since even in normal lungs the uneven distribution of ventilation and perfusion will cause regional variations in P_AO_2. An average or "ideal" value can be calculated using the ideal alveolar air equation; the derivation for this equation can be found in most textbooks of pulmonary physiology. In clinical medicine the equation is used in a simplified form: $P_AO_2 = P_IO_2 - (1.25 \times P_aCO_2)$, where P_IO_2 is the partial pressure of oxygen in the inspired air. The 1.25 is the reciprocal of an assumed respiratory quotient (R) of 0.8.

Example: A subject breathing 40 per cent oxygen at a barometric pressure of 750 mm Hg has the following arterial blood gas values: $P_aO_2 = 110$ mm Hg, $P_aCO_2 = 56$ mm Hg; Calculate $P_{A-aD}O_2$. $P_AO_2 = ((750 - 47) \times 0.40) - (1.25 \times 56) = 211$ mm Hg. (47 mm Hg is the vapor pressure of water in the alveolar air. In respiratory medicine it is customary to calculate in terms of dry gas.) $P_{A-aD}O_2$ therefore will equal $211 - 110$, or 101 mm Hg. A final simplification: for practical purposes at or near sea level, barometric pressure $- 47$ can be assumed to equal 700 mm Hg.

To calculate the P_AO_2, the inspired oxygen concentration must be known. It should be noted on the request form submitted with the blood specimen for gas analysis. In patients breathing room air, this value is 0.21. The various types of high-flow Venturi masks provide reasonably precise oxygen concentrations. For patients on ventilators, the more sophisticated models allow the inspired concentration to be set by the operator, and this is usually accurate. For ventilators without precise mixing controls, the inspired oxygen concentration can be measured from the inspiration line with one of the inexpensive paramagnetic oxygen analyzers. Unfortunately, with nasal cannulas and catheters, the precise inspired oxygen concentration cannot be determined and $P_{A\text{-}aD}O_2$ cannot be estimated.

The a/A ratio

$P_{A\text{-}aD}O_2$ as an estimate of gas exchange is conceptually appropriate and widely used. A major drawback, however, is that $P_{A\text{-}aD}O_2$ increases with increasing inspired oxygen concentration ($F_{I}O_2$), even with all other factors remaining stable. Unfortunately, the precise normal limits for $P_{A\text{-}aD}O_2$ at different values of $F_{I}O_2$ have not been reported.

Gilbert (1974) has described the use of the ratio of P_aO_2 to P_AO_2 (a/A) as a substitute for $P_{A\text{-}aD}O_2$. In normal subjects this ratio remains relatively constant for values of $F_{I}O_2$ from 21 to 100 per cent, with the lower limit of normal approximately 0.75. In subjects with pulmonary disease, the ratio is more variable with changing levels of $F_{I}O_2$, but more stable than $P_{A\text{-}aD}O_2$. a/A therefore can be used (1) to compare gas exchange among patients recieving different inspired oxygen concentrations, (2) to compare gas exchange in the same patient as $F_{I}O_2$ is changed, and (3) to estimate the P_aO_2 expected at a given value of $F_{I}O_2$ if blood gas data are available at another level of $F_{I}O_2$. For example, if P_aO_2 and P_aCO_2 are known for a patient receiving 40 per cent oxygen, the P_aO_2 expected if he were breathing 30 per cent oxygen can be estimated by assuming that P_aCO_2 and a/A will not change as $F_{I}O_2$ is lowered. Although this is a rough estimate and these assumptions are not necessarily valid, the calculation is useful for clinical purposes.

Even for a patient breathing room air, calculation of the a/A ratio or $P_{A\text{-}aD}O_2$ may uncover an unsuspected defect in gas exchange. For example, consider the following blood gas data for a patient breathing 21 per cent oxygen: $P_aO_2 = 80$ mm Hg, $P_aCO_2 = 24$ mm Hg. The P_aO_2 appears to be normal. However, $P_AO_2 = 147 - 1.25 \times 24 = 117$ mm Hg. a/A = 80/117 = 0.68, and $P_{A\text{-}aD}O_2 = 117 - 80 = 37$ mm Hg. These are both abnormal values indicating defective gas exchange despite the apparently normal P_aO_2.

DANGEROUS LEVELS OF HYPOXEMIA

Unlike all other substances that must be obtained from the environment, body stores of oxygen are virtually non-existent and death occurs within a few minutes following complete oxygen deprivation. Any level of hypoxemia, therefore, should be cause for some concern. So long as a continuous supply of oxygen is available, however, the defense mechanism can compensate for surprising degrees of hypoxemia.

The shape of the dissociation curve provides one important line of defense. A fall in P_aO_2 from a normal value of 90 mm Hg to 55 mm Hg produces less than a 10 per cent fall in the oxygen content. Fifty-five mm Hg is the shoulder of the dissociation curve; below this level there is a precipitous fall in oxygen content with further decreases in P_aO_2 (Fig. 5-4). For this reason, 50 to 55 mm Hg for P_aO_2 is usually considered the minimum value to aim for in the treatment of respiratory failure; values higher than this are preferable since they provide a wider margin of safety.

The arterial oxygen content is only one factor in oxygen delivery to the cells. The cardiac output, regional blood flow, regional oxygen uptake, oxygen extraction, position of the dissociation curve, and hemoglobin concentration all play a role in this vital process. Survival has been reported following values of P_aO_2 as low as 7.5 mm Hg. It is difficult to predict, therefore, in the individual case, at what level hypoxemia becomes life threatening. Additional factors may be decisive. Hypoxemia increases the susceptibility to cardiac glycoside intoxication and may precipitate intractable arrhythmias in patients with severe pre-existing cardiac or pulmonary disease. Since oxygen delivery is the product of cardiac output and arterial oxygen content, the combination of hypoxemia and low cardiac output is particularly dangerous.

REFERENCE VALUES

For young healthy subjects breathing 21 per cent oxygen (room air), 80 mm Hg can be considered the lower limit for P_aO_2; for older subjects 70 mm Hg is an appropriate lower limit. For $P_{A\text{-}aD}O_2$, 5 to 20 mm Hg can be considered a reasonable value during room air breathing. On 100 per cent oxygen, values as high as 200 mm Hg have been reported in young healthy subjects, although 35 to 50 mm Hg is generally considered the upper limit. Reference values for $P_{A\text{-}aD}O_2$ while breathing intermediate levels of $F_{I}O_2$ are not available. The lower limit for the a/A ratio can be considered to be 0.75 for all values of $F_{I}O_2$.

CONCLUSION: GAS EXCHANGE AND VENTILATION

Ventilation is the process by which air moves in and out of the lungs; gas exchange is the process by which oxygen and carbon dioxide are exchanged between alveolar air and pulmonary capillary blood. The defects we have been discussing—V/Q inequalities, shunting, and diffusion defects—produce abnormalities in gas exchange. They result in a wide $P_{A-aD}O_2$ and a low a/A ratio, which may produce hypoxemia, depending on the F_IO_2 and the severity of the defect. They will also produce an elevated P_aCO_2 (hypercapnia), but only if ventilation is also defective. This will be reviewed next.

VENTILATION AND CARBON DIOXIDE

THE ALVEOLAR VENTILATION

The partial pressure of a gas in a liquid is the partial pressure of gas with which the liquid is in equilibrium. For oxygen in arterial blood, the alveolar air is not quite this gas; in fact, there is no single equilibrating gas. Venous to arterial shunting, V/Q inequalities, and to a lesser extent, the diffusion gradient, all lower P_aO_2 and produce a positive $P_{A-aD}O_2$. This occurs even in normal lungs; in disease the difference is accentuated. The classic approach to blood gas interpretation is that these three factors do not alter P_aCO_2 and that $P_ACO_2 = P_aCO_2$. Since P_ACO_2 (partial pressure of alveolar CO_2) is under control of the alveolar ventilation, P_aCO_2 (partial pressure of arterial CO_2) is considered to give direct information about the state of the ventilation.

The following relationship, the alveolar ventilation equation, exists between carbon dioxide production ($\dot{V}CO_2$), P_ACO_2, and the alveolar ventilation ($\dot{V}_A$): $\dot{V}CO_2 = \dot{V}_A \times P_ACO_2/0.863$. For simplicity, the constant 0.863 will be omitted subsequently). Rewriting the equation as $P_ACO_2 = \dot{V}CO_2/\dot{V}_A$, P_ACO_2 emerges as the outcome of the relationship between CO_2 production and alveolar ventilation. A rise in $\dot{V}CO_2$ or a fall in $\dot{V}_A$ without a commensurate change in the other will raise P_ACO_2, and changes in the opposite direction will lower P_ACO_2. Since the classic approach assumes $P_ACO_2 = P_aCO_2$, these statements also apply to P_aCO_2. Thus, P_aCO_2 becomes the indicator of the adequacy of the alveolar ventilation in rela-

tionship to the metabolic load; a high P_aCO_2 indicates relative alveolar hypoventilation and a low P_aCO_2 indicates alveolar hyperventilation.

But what is the alveolar ventilation? It cannot be measured directly; it can be calculated as the total ventilation minus the dead space ventilation, but dead space cannot be measured directly either. Furthermore, there are several different dead spaces, depending on how the calculation is made.

The alveolar ventilation equation can also be written as $\dot{V}_A = \dot{V}CO_2/P_ACO_2$. In this form $\dot{V}_A$ becomes a clearance ratio similar to those used in renal physiology; the alveolar ventilation (V_A) is the (theoretical) ventilation necessary to excrete the metabolically produced CO_2 at a concentration equal to $P_aCO_2/$(barometric pressure −47).

We have been arguing in a circle. P_aCO_2 is high because the alveolar ventilation is low in relationship to the CO_2 production. Since we cannot measure the alveolar ventilation, how do we know that it is low? Answer—because P_aCO_2 is high. Alveolar ventilation, therefore, should not be looked on as the cause of hypercapnia. Hypercapnia, rather, should be considered to be synonymous with alveolar hypoventilation.

HYPERCAPNIA AND HYPOCAPNIA

Despite the circuitous reasoning, P_aCO_2 remains the best clinical guide to the effectiveness of ventilation *and the functioning of the ventilatory control system*. P_aCO_2 is normally kept within narrow limits (32 to 45 mm Hg) by this rigid control system. The presence of hypo- or hypercapnia indicates a serious defect in ventilatory control.

Any one of three general disturbances may lead to hypercapnia:

1. *The respiratory control centers which set the level of P_aCO_2 may be defective.*

2. *The neuromuscular apparatus of breathing may be defective.*

3. *The work of breathing may be markedly increased.* Under this last circumstance, normal respiratory control centers may not be able to force a normal neuromuscular breathing apparatus to maintain the ventilation necessary to excrete, at a normal CO_2 concentration, the CO_2 produced by tissues; the P_aCO_2 will rise until a new equilibrium is established at the elevated P_aCO_2. Such an increase in the work of breathing is usually the result of se-

vere airway obstruction such as is seen in the asthma, chronic bronchitis, and emphysema group of diseases. It is also common in severe kyphoscoliosis, but is only rarely seen in restrictive defects such as occur in pulmonary fibrosis.

A comparison can be drawn between the control system for P_aCO_2 regulation and a thermostatically controlled home heating system. Both systems are designed to maintain a parameter within narrow limits. Hypercapnia can be compared to the condition in which the house is too cold. For the house, there are three possibilities: (1) The thermostat may be defective—comparable to a defect in the respiratory control centers such as might occur with depressant drugs, cerebral disease, or occasionally idiopathically. (2) The furnace may be defective—comparable to a defect in the neuromuscular apparatus of breathing such as might occur with Guillain-Barré syndrome, myasthenia gravis, crushed chest, etc. (3) Both the thermostat and the furnace may be intact, but the system may be forced to work under conditions more extreme than those for which it was designed. If a house built for temperate climates were transported to Antarctica, it is doubtful whether the normally functioning furnace and thermostat could maintain the inside temperature at 72° F. The system was not designed to operate under such an excessive workload. This is comparable to the hypercapnia seen in advanced obstructive pulmonary disease with a marked increase in the work of breathing.

With severe hypercapnia a combination of these factors is often present. Carbon dioxide narcosis in patients with chronic obstructive airway disease is associated with a high work of breathing owing to the airway obstruction, plus respiratory control centers acutely depressed by oxygen and perhaps chronically depressed by a high P_aCO_2.

We have reviewed the relationship of P_aCO_2 to the alveolar ventilation and pointed out the rather elusive nature of the concept of alveolar ventilation. The total minute ventilation, which is the product of the ventilatory frequency and the tidal volume, however, is a clearly definable quantity that can be measured directly. Hypocapnia is always associated with an increase in the total minute ventilation above the normal resting level. With hypercapnia, the total minute ventilation may be low, normal, or high. If the metabolic rate is increased with fever or restlessness, for ex-

ample, more CO_2 is presented to the lungs fo excretion, and a normal ventilation will no keep P_aCO_2 normal. With rapid shallow breath ing, the dead space ventilation constitutes greater proportion of the tidal volume an P_aCO_2 may rise despite a rise in the total min ute ventilation. Finally, in many diseas states the dead space may be increased. Unde all these circumstances only an increased tota minute ventilation will keep P_aCO_2 at a norma level. If the ventilatory control system is in tact and the work of breathing not prohib tively high, this increased ventilatory require ment will be met and P_aCO_2 will remai normal. If the work of breathing is excessiv or the ventilatory control system defective only a partial attempt at compensation ma occur. In this case, both P_aCO_2 and the tota minute ventilation may be high.

The hypocapnic patient always has a tota minute ventilation above the normal restin value, whereas the hypercapnic patient ma have a ventilation which is low, normal, o high. The importance of hypercapnia is no that it indicates hypoventilation, but that indicates a serious derangement in the respi ratory control centers, a defective breathin apparatus, an overwhelming increase in th work of breathing, or any combination of these

Hyperventilation with resulting hypocapni is seen in a wide variety of clinical disorders Hyperventilation may be secondary to hypox emia, compensatory to metabolic acidosis, o psychological. In many critical illnesses hyper ventilation occurs without acidosis or hypoxe mia; if hypoxemia is present, the hyperventi ation may persist despite correction of th hypoxemia by oxygen administration. Thes illnesses include head injuries, liver failure shock from various causes, and septicemi The exact stimulus for the hyperventilation i unknown.

EFFECTS OF V/Q INEQUALITIES AND SHUNTING ON P_aCO_2

For several decades, it has been axiomati that V/Q (ventilation/perfusion) inequalitie do not raise P_aCO_2 because the CO_2 dissociatio curve is relatively linear in the physiologi range. Furthermore, since the CO_2 dissocia tion curve is relatively steep (Fig. 5–5) com pared with the oxygen dissociation curve, th difference between P_aCO_2 and mixed venou CO_2 ($P_{\bar{v}}O_2$) is only a few mm Hg, compare with approximately 50 mm Hg for oxyge

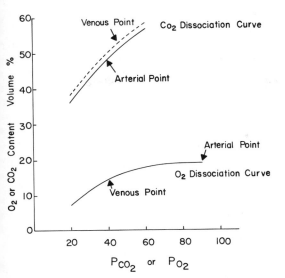

Figure 5–5. Oxygen and carbon dioxide dissociation curves drawn to same scale. The A-V difference for both is approximately the same, but the resulting change in partial pressure is much greater for oxygen than for carbon dioxide.

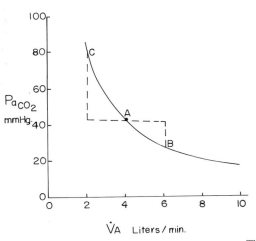

Figure 5–6. Plot of the alveolar ventilation equation. The absolute magnitude of the change in ventilation from A to B and A to C is the same, but the resulting change in P_{CO_2} is much greater on the lower ventilation side.

Shunting, therefore, has been considered to play an insignificant role in elevating P_aCO_2.

Although superficially this reasoning seems logical, it does not hold up under close scrutiny. West (1971) has explored these concepts using computer models of the lung. His results show that V/Q inequalities interfere with CO_2 excretion to approximately the same extent as with oxygen uptake and will produce hypercapnia unless compensatory mechanisms intervene. The argument that shunting will not raise P_aCO_2 is also deceptive. If shunting produces a small rise in P_aCO_2, $P_{\bar{v}}CO_2$ will also rise, producing another increment in P_aCO_2, and so on until a new steady state is achieved.

Why then is hypercapnia so much less common than hypoxemia and so intimately bound by tradition to the ventilation? There are several reasons: (1) Because of the steep slope of the CO_2 dissociation curve, an increase in ventilation toward normal of poorly ventilated lung units will lower the CO_2 content of the blood leaving these units to a much greater degree than it will raise the oxygen content. (2) Because the CO_2 dissociation curve does not flatten out at low values of P_aCO_2, overall hyperventilation will lower P_aCO_2 of blood leaving well-ventilated lung units to compensate for the elevated CO_2 of shunted blood. The hyperbolic nature of the P_aCO_2-$\dot{V}_A$ curve (Fig.

5-6 and see below) will make this an inefficient process, but it will occur. The flat shape of the oxygen dissociation curve at high levels of P_{O_2} will preclude the well-ventilated units from adding appreciable oxygen to the blood (see Fig. 5-5). (3) Hypercapnia is a much more powerful stimulus to ventilation than is hypoxemia. If the respiratory control centers are intact, there will be a strong drive to increase the ventilation so long as hypercapnia persists. Once hypercapnia has been corrected, the remaining hypoxemia will offer less inducement to further increase in ventilation, especially if work of breathing is high.

V/Q inequalities and shunting will lower P_aO_2 and raise P_aCO_2. The important distinction between hypercapnia and hypoxemia in this regard is that an increase in ventilation will correct the hypercapnia but not the hypoxemia.

VENTILATION AND
CARBON DIOXIDE

Granting that alveolar ventilation is more a conceptual than an actual quantity, it remains a useful tool for defining the relationship between ventilation and carbon dioxide. Figure 5-6 is a plot of the alveolar ventilation equation substituting P_aCO_2 for P_ACO_2. Hyperventilation is seen as a relatively inefficient process and hypoventilation as a rather critical one. To lower P_aCO_2 from 40 mm Hg to 20 mm

Hg requires an increase of 4.1 l/min in alveolar ventilation; to raise P_aCO_2 from 40 mm Hg to 60 mm Hg requires a fall in alveolar ventilation of only 1.4 l/min. From a level of 60 mm Hg, a fall in alveolar ventilation of only 0.7 l/min will raise the P_aCO_2 to 80 mm Hg. Thus, the more hypercapnic the patient becomes, the more sensitive the P_aCO_2 is to further decreases in ventilation.

VENTILATION AND OXYGEN

Hypoxemia, not hypercapnia, is the main threat in respiratory failure. P_AO_2 and P_ACO_2 are related through the alveolar air equation reviewed previously (p. 119) for oxygen. The simplified form of this equation can be rearranged: $P_ACO_2 = R(P_IO_2 - P_AO_2)$ when R is respiratory quotient. If constant values are assigned to R and P_IO_2, the equation will be a straight line with the slope equal to $-R$, an X intercept equal to P_IO_2, and a Y intercept equal to $R \times P_IO_2$. In Figure 5–7 the solid line is a plot of this equation for an R of 0.8 and a P_IO_2 of 147 mm Hg (room air). If a $P_{A-aD}O_2$ of 20 mm Hg is assumed, the arterial blood line will be 20 mm Hg to the left, as indicated by the dotted line. With a value of R below 1, the usual case, a rise in P_aCO_2 will produce a fall in P_aO_2 greater than the rise in P_aCO_2. The graph shows why severe hypercapnia rarely occurs in patients breathing room air. With a $P_{A-aD}O_2$ of even 20 mm Hg, as P_aCO_2 reaches 90 mm Hg, P_aO_2 has fallen to 20 mm Hg, a level often (but not invariably) incompatible with life. The patient may thus die of hypoxia before severe hypercapnia can occur. Furthermore, at very low values of P_aO_2, hypoxemia

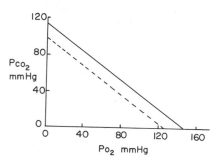

Figure 5–7. The simplified form of the alveolar air equation plotted on an O_2-CO_2 diagram for an F_IO_2 of 21 per cent. The solid line represents alveolar air, and the dotted line represents arterial blood with a $P_{A-aD}O_2$ of 20 mm Hg. Note that for arterial blood, when the Pco_2 reaches 90 mm Hg, the P_aO_2 has fallen to 20 mm Hg.

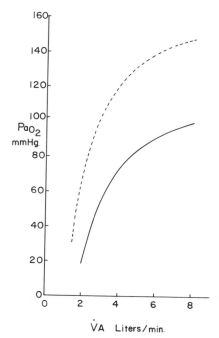

$\dot{V}A$ Liters/min.

Figure 5–8. A combination of the alveolar air equation and alveolar ventilation equation. The solid line represents an F_IO_2 of 21 per cent with a $P_{A-aD}O_2$ of 20 mm Hg. The dotted line is for an F_IO_2 of 30 per cent with a $P_{A-aD}O_2$ of 35 mm Hg. Note the precipitous drop in P_aO_2 as alveolar ventilation falls below 4 l/min. Note also that although breathing 30 per cent oxygen does not prevent this precipitous fall in P_aO_2, the absolute level of P_aO_2 is maintained in an acceptable range down to values of $\dot{V}A$ as low as 2 l/min.

will become a significant ventilatory stimulus tending to prevent severe hypoventilation. If the patient breathes an enriched oxygen mixture, two things happen. First, the hypoxic stimulus to ventilation will be lessened or abolished, and second, high levels of P_aCO_2 can occur without accompanying severe hypoxemia (the line is shifted to the right).

If $(\dot{V}CO_2 \times 0.863/\dot{V}_A)$ is substituted for P_aCO_2 in the alveolar air equation, this equation becomes: $P_AO_2 = (P_IO_2 - \dot{V}CO_2 \times 0.863)/R \times \dot{V}_A$. With a value of 200 ml/min for $\dot{V}CO_2$, 147 mm Hg for P_IO_2, and a $P_{A-aD}O_2$ of 20 mm Hg, the curve of P_aO_2 vs $\dot{V}_A$ is shown by the solid line in Figure 5–8. As with hypercapnia, hypoventilation produces an ever-increasing tempo of hypoxemia.

A moderate increase in F_IO_2 provides good protection against the hypoxemia produced by hypoventilation. The broken line in Figure 5–8 shows the same data for an F_IO_2 of 30 per cent an a $P_{A-aD}O_2$ of 35 mm Hg.

PATIENTS ON VENTILATORS

Although it might at first be thought that the P_aCO_2 of a patient on a ventilator depends only on the ventilator settings, this is not necessarily the case. If the respirator is used in the patient-triggering mode, and the automatic cycling is not set so high that it overrides the patient's own ventilatory frequency, the patient's ventilatory control system usually maintains control of P_aCO_2. If the tidal volume setting of a patient-triggered volume-limited ventilator is doubled, the patient will drop his ventilatory frequency in half and P_aCO_2 will not change (Levine, 1972). If the ventilator is of the fixed-cycle, constant-volume type delivering controlled rather than assisted ventilation, or if the patient has received medication to suppress his respiratory control centers or paralyze the muscles of breathing, these remarks, of course, do not apply.

Surprisingly high values of tidal volume (above 1 l) and high values of total minute ventilation (above 12 l/min) may be delivered to patients on assisted ventilation without producing hypocapnia (Pontoppidan, 1965). This high ventilatory requirement is due at least in part to an increase in metabolic activity plus a marked increase in dead space. Some of it may also be related to an inefficiency in distribution of ventilation by positive pressure breathing. After removal from a ventilator a patient can often maintan the same P_aCO_2 which was present while on the ventilator but with a much lower total minute ventilation (Gilbert, 1974).

DANGEROUS LEVELS OF HYPOCAPNIA AND HYPERCAPNIA

With the rigid control system for P_aCO_2 which is normally in effect, any abnormal value of P_aCO_2 should cause some concern. In contrast to hypoxemia, hypercapnia is important to recognize more for what it indicates about underlying pathophysiology than for its harmful effects per se.

For hypercapnia, there are two aspects to consider. First, what levels indicate a rapidly deteriorating disease process requiring immediate action? This depends on the nature of the disease. When pulmonary function was previously normal, any level of hypercapnia is cause for alarm. In Guillain-Barré syndrome or myasthenia gravis, for example, even mild hypercapnia indicates need for immediate action. During an acute attack of bronchial asthma in a patient known to have normal pulmonary function between attacks, mild hypercapnia (P_aCO_2 of 45 to 55 mm Hg) is cause for concern; moderate to severe hypercapnia often is an indication for intubation and assisted ventilation. In contrast, patients with chronic obstructive airway disease in an acute exacerbation of respiratory failure can usually be managed without intubation or assisted ventilation despite severe elevations of P_aCO_2.

With regard to the harmful effects of hypercapnia per se, it is difficult to be dogmatic for at least two reasons. First, the effects are difficult to separate from hypoxemia and acidosis, which often accompany hypercapnia, and, second, the effects correlate poorly with the level of P_aCO_2. Seiker (1956) found no significant abnormalities in mental state if P_aCO_2 was below 90 mm Hg and pH above 7.25. Coma or a semicomatose state always accompanied P_aCO_2 values above 130 mm Hg and pH below 7.14. Within these limits, however, there was great variability.

A rapid lowering of P_aCO_2 from hypercapnia levels by assisted ventilation has been associated with seizure, coma, and death; the accompanying alkalosis undoubtedly plays an important role. Values of P_aCO_2 above 65 mm Hg have been shown to reduce renal function (Kilburn, 1966) and may account in part for the fluid retention seen in respiratory failure.

Hypocapnia and respiratory alkalosis imposed on the patient by controlled ventilation can cause cardiac arrhythmias refractory to the usual antiarrhythmic measures until the respiratory alkalosis is corrected (Ayres, 1969). In the reported cases, P_aCO_2 varied from 13 to 23 mm Hg and pH from 7.51 to 7.74. Many critically ill patients have spontaneous hyperventilation with resulting hypocapnia. The leftward shift in the oxygen dissociation curve would be expected to interfere with oxygen utilization at the tissue level. Since these patients are critically ill, it is difficult to assign a specific harmful effect to the alkalosis or hypocapnia alone. It is difficult to find convincing evidence that *spontaneously* occurring, as opposed to iatrogenically induced, hypocapnia has significant harmful effects. It is usually unwise to try to treat hyperventilation per se; the attention should be directed to the underlying cause.

CONCLUSION: P_aO_2 AND P_aCO_2

Hypoventilation will lower P_aO_2 and raise P_aCO_2. V/Q inequalities, shunting, and, to a lesser extent, diffusion defects will also lower P_aO_2. V/Q inequalities and shunting have the *potential* to raise P_aCO_2, but will do so only if there is a failure of a compensatory increase in ventilation. P_aO_2 is, therefore, a more sensitive but less specific indicator of abnormal pulmonary function compared to P_aCO_2; hypoxemia is much more common than hypercapnia. When P_aO_2 is low, there is unquestionably an abnormality in gas exchange, ventilation, or both; the P_aO_2 alone indicates neither the nature of the abnormality nor the underlying disease. A high P_aCO_2 is much more specific: it indicates a defect in the respiratory control centers, a defective breathing apparatus, an overwhelming increase in the work of breathing, or any combination of these.

ACID-BASE BALANCE

This presentation will not follow traditional lines. The Henderson-Hasselbalch equation, base excess, the Singer-Hastings nomogram, the Siggaard-Anderson diagrams, the Bronsted theory, and most of the other familiar concepts will not be considered. Instead, this approach is based on the use of whole body titration curves. This method has been chosen because from personal experience the author has found it to be the best method for identification of abnormalities, and it appears to be the way of the future. Only the recognition (or diagnosis) of the abnormalities will be reviewed. The various states of acidosis and alkalosis will not be presented in detail, nor will treatment be considered. This section emphasizes interpretation of arterial blood gas data, and the recognition of the acid-base state as reflected by the blood gases alone. Acid-base balance is discussed further in Chapter 6, and many other standard texts are available to the interested reader.

pH AND H+

There appears to be a gradual replacement of the use of pH by the use of hydrogen ion concentration. Logarithmic notation is convenient when large changes in H^+ occur, but for the narrow range encountered in blood its usefulness is questionable. Furthermore, the carbonic acid dissociation equation is more simply manipulated without the logarithmic notation of the Henderson-Hasselbalch equation. The equation is: $H^+ = 24 \times P_{CO_2}/$

Table 5–2. pH vs H+ (nmol/1)

pH	H+	pH	H
7.00	100	7.40	40
7.05	89	7.45	35
7.10	79	7.50	32
7.15	71	7.55	28
7.20	63	7.60	25
7.25	56	7.65	22
7.30	50	7.70	20
7.35	45	7.75	18

HCO_3^-. In this equation P_{CO_2} is in millimeters of mercury, HCO_3^- in mmol/l, and H^+ in 10^{-9} mol/l, or nanomoles/liter (nmol/l). The reference value for H^+ is 40 nmol/l, corresponding to a pH of 7.40. The scales along the abscissa in Figures 5–9 to 5–12 will give the reader a general idea of the relationship between H^+ and pH in the physiologic range. Table 5–2 presents a more detailed comparison.

NOMOGRAMS

A nomogram is a graphic display of an equation; it contains no information that is not present in the equation itself. Many nomograms have been proposed for the carbonic acid dissociation equation; none are used in this chapter. The acid-base diagram to be presented is not a nomogram, and the whole body titration curves are not expressions of the Henderson-Hasselbalch equation. They are empirical observations that could not have been calculated from any equation; as such they bring additional information to bear on each blood gas determination with which they are compared.

TERMINOLOGY

We will follow the terminology of Winters (1967). The suffix *-emia* will refer to the state of the blood, e.g., acidemia is a condition of excess blood acidity as indicated by the $H+$ or pH. The suffix *-osis* will refer to a pathologic process in which acid or base is gained or lost from the body. These processes may or may not be accompanied by acidemia or alkalemia depending upon the degree of compensation. *Compensation* is the physiologic process in response to the primary disturbance which tends to restore the blood acidity toward normal. The normal or expected physiologic response to a primary disturbance will not be nsidered a second primary process. Thus, the etention of bicarbonate as a compensation or a respiratory acidosis will not be considred a metabolic alkalosis. The acute changes n the blood buffers owing to mass action will ot be considered part of the compensation rocess. Two primary processes occurring toether will be considered a *mixed* disturbance.

WHOLE BODY TITRATION CURVES

A whole body titration curve is a graphic epresentation of the *in vivo* changes in H^+ Pco_2, and HCO_3^- which occur in the arterial lood in response to a primary acid-base disurbance. The data are obtained by one of two nethods. The first involves subjecting normal ndividuals to an imposed artificial disturbnce, for example, breathing a high CO_2 mixure. Blood specimens are drawn at the new steady state. In the second method, arterial lood specimens are obtained from patients with naturally occurring disturbances. It is important that these subjects not have diseases of the organ system responsible for compensation and that they have only a single primary disturbance. With both methods, data are obtained from a group of subjects and the results expressed as 95 per cent confidence bands. These represent the mean ±2 standard deviations of the group data at several points, or ±2 standard errors of estimate of the regression line representing the data. *The 95 per cent confidence band thus represents the primary disturbance plus the expected or normal physiologic response to this disturbance.*

The confidence bands will be displayed on a Pco_2-H^+ diagram. These axes have been chosen because they are the two components actually measured by electrodes in blood gas analyzers (p. 112). Both Pco_2 and H^+ will be displayed as linear scales; pH will also be shown on the same axis as H^+, but will be logarithmic. The normal range will be shown as a square in the center. With one exception, bicarbonate isopleths will not be shown; the value for bicarbonate can be derived easily from the carbonic acid dissociation equation presented earlier.

ACUTE RESPIRATORY ACIDOSIS

Brackett (1965) studied seven normal young subjects exposed to 7 and 10 per cent CO_2 in 21 per cent oxygen in an environmental

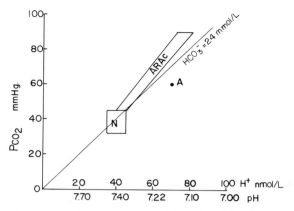

Figure 5-9. A 95 per cent confidence band for the acute respiratory acidosis (ARAc) whole body titration curve. The box labeled N is the normal range. Point A is a mixed disturbance, respiratory and metabolic acidosis. The line is the HCO_3^- isopleth for 24 mmol/l.

chamber for periods up to 90 minutes. The 95 per cent confidence band for this disturbance is labeled ARAc in Figure 5-9. Blood gas values falling within this area are compatible with an acute respiratory acidosis.

Values such as point A in Figure 5-9 which lie to the acid side of area ARAc represent a respiratory acidosis (because the P_aco_2 is high), but are too acidotic to be explained by the respiratory acidosis alone. Some other primary disturbance must be adding to the acidity, and this can only be a metabolic acidosis. This area, then, represents a mixed disturbance—that is, two primary disturbances, respiratory acidosis and metabolic acidosis.

If a normal value of 24 mmol/l for bicarbonate is entered into the equation $H^+ = 24\, Pco_2/HCO_3^-$, the equation becomes $H^+ = Pco_2$. Thus the $HCO_3^- = 24$ isopleth shown in Figure 5-9 is an identity line with a slope of 45 degrees. This line approximates the right margin of the ARAc confidence band, and therefore almost all blood gas determinations in the mixed respiratory and metabolic acidosis area will have a bicarbonate equal to or below 24 mmol/l.

CHRONIC RESPIRATORY ACIDOSIS

Brackett (1969) studied 20 patients with chronic hypercapnia in a relatively stable condition. The H^+-P_aco_2 values for these subjects plus 7 normal subjects were used to establish the 95 per cent confidence band labeled CRAc

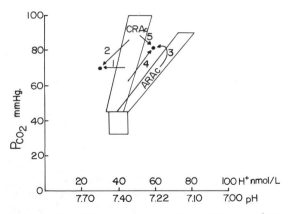

Figure 5–10. CRAc is the chronic respiratory acidosis confidence band. For explanation of points and arrows, see text.

in Figure 5-10. Blood gas values within this area are compatible with a *maximally compensated respiratory acidosis*, also referred to as chronic respiratory acidosis. The bicarbonate will always be above 24 mmol/l.

Blood gas values within the chronic respiratory acidosis confidence band will have a high bicarbonate and a high base excess, features common to a metabolic alkalosis. For this reason such values are often considered to represent a mixed disturbance, respiratory acidosis plus metabolic alkalosis. In this case, however, the metabolic alkalosis is not a primary disturbance, but an expected physiologic response to the primary respiratory acidosis, produced by renal retention of bicarbonate. It would seem preferable to reserve the term "mixed disturbance" for two primary disturbances.

Many patients develop acute CO_2 retention superimposed on a background of chronic hypercapnia. This condition has been duplicated in dogs in an environmental chamber (Goldstein, 1971): the blood gases start from within the CRAc confidence band and change along lines approximately parallel to the ARAc band.

Points to the left (alkalotic side) of the chronic respiratory acidosis confidence band represent a respiratory acidosis but are too alkalotic to be explained even by maximal compensation. A separate primary disturbance must be present, in this case metabolic alkalosis. This will be a true mixed disturbance, metabolic alkalosis and respiratory acidosis. Patients with chronic obstructive airway disease often have blood gas values in this

area, the result of CO_2 retention plus a metabolic alkalosis secondary to potassium loss brought on by chronic diuretic therapy. Arrow (1) in Figure 5-10 demonstrates this course.

Rapid correction of hypercapnia may also result in an acid-base disturbance of this type. Patients with severe chronic CO_2 retention with a compensatory elevation of bicarbonate may, when placed on a ventilator, change as shown by arrow (2) in Figure 5-10. This occurs because the kidney cannot excrete bicarbonate fast enough to compensate for the rapid fall in P_aCO_2 resulting from effective assisted ventilation. The chloride depletion which invariably accompanies the bicarbonate expansion accentuates this abnormality, and administration of chloride will help speed the normalization of the acid-base disturbance (Schwartz, 1968).

Values between the acute and chronic respiratory acidosis bands demonstrate the inability to make a specific diagnosis from a single set of blood gas values. Arrow (3) in Figure 5-10 represents a partially compensated respiratory acidosis starting from normal values. Arrow (4) is an acute respiratory acidosis arising from a chronic respiratory acidosis. Arrow (5) shows a metabolic acidosis superimposed on chronic respiratory acidosis. All three clinical disturbances will have the same blood gas analysis at the point shown. It is important to realize that clinical data must be added to the blood gas data to make an accurate diagnosis.

CHRONIC METABOLIC ACIDOSIS

Albert (1967) studied 60 patients with metabolic acidosis; most were infants or children with diarrhea, diabetes, or renal disease. The duration of the acidosis exceeded one day in every case, a time sufficient for respiratory compensation by hyperventilation. They had received no medication and had no pulmonary disease. The 95 per cent confidence band for this group is labeled CMAc in Figure 5-11. This is considered to be chronic metabolic acidosis, and the slope of the band compared to the slope of the CRAc band indicates that compensation is much less complete in metabolic acidosis compared with respiratory acidosis.

About 24 hours is required for the maximum ventilatory response to metabolic acidosis. Therefore points *above* the metabolic acidosis confidence band may represent an acute met-

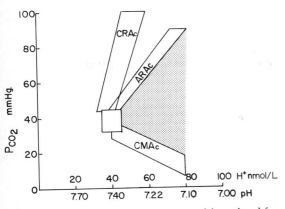

Figure 5–11. CMAc is the 95 per cent confidence band for chronic metabolic acidosis. The shaded area represents a mixed disturbance, respiratory acidosis and metabolic acidosis.

abolic acidosis with insufficient time for the full ventilatory response. Statistical confidence limits for a very acute metabolic acidosis are not available.

If the clinical data suggest that enough time has elapsed for maximum ventilatory compensation, the area above the metabolic acidosis confidence band will then represent an inadequate or defective ventilatory response, and such patients should be suspected of having pulmonary disease. Does this represent a mixed disturbance, metabolic and respiratory acidosis, even when the P_aCO_2 is below 32 mm Hg? If a respiratory acidosis is defined simply as a P_aCO_2 above normal, then the normal P_aCO_2 for a metabolic acidosis is set by the confidence band and any P_aCO_2 above this band represents a respiratory acidosis. The entire area, then, between the metabolic acidosis band and the acute respiratory acidosis band can be considered an area of mixed respiratory and metabolic acidosis (shaded area in Figure 5–11). The most critically ill patients will usually be found to have arterial blood gas data within this area.

ACUTE RESPIRATORY ALKALOSIS

Arbus (1969) studied 12 patients who were hyperventilated during general anesthesia; metabolic, endocrine, cardiovascular, pulmonary, and renal diseases were excluded. The 95 per cent confidence band is labelled ARAlk in Figure 5–12; it is essentially a continuation of the band for acute respiratory acidosis. Points to the left (alkalotic side) of this band repre-

sent a mixed disturbance, respiratory and metabolic alkalosis. Figure 5–12, incidentally, represents the completed diagram suitable for clinical use.

Metabolic compensation would move the blood gas values to the right (acid side) of the acute respiratory alkalosis band toward normal H^+. Residents at high altitudes and pregnant women have low values of P_aCO_2 with a normal H^+; obviously, complete metabolic compensation for respiratory alkalosis is possible. No confidence limits have been reported for this compensation, however, and complete compensation is unusual in clinical medicine. Patients with blood gas values between the acute respiratory alkalosis confidence band and the $H^+ = 40$ line should be considered to have a mixed disturbance, respiratory alkalosis and metabolic acidosis, rather than a compensated respiratory alkalosis. By taking this approach, one is less likely to miss an important clinical disturbance such as unsuspected uremia or diabetes. If no cause for metabolic acidosis is found and it appears that compensated respiratory alkalosis is the correct diagnosis, no harm has been done.

METABOLIC ALKALOSIS

An acute, uncompensated metabolic alkalosis would move the blood gas values to the left (alkalotic side) along the $P_aCO_2 = 40$ line. Respiratory compensation would involve a rise in P_aCO_2; does this occur? Kildeberg (1963) has shown that it does occur in infants with persistent vomiting due to pyloric stenosis; com-

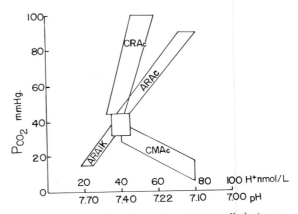

Figure 5–12. ARAlk is the acute respiratory alkalosis confidence band. This is the completed diagram which can be used for blood gas interpretation. Data for its construction are given in Table 5–2.

Table 5-3. COORDINATES FOR CONSTRUCTING ACID-BASE CONFIDENCE BANDS

DISTURBANCE	LEFT BOUNDARY LINE			RIGHT BOUNDARY LINE		
	P_{CO_2}	H^+	pH	P_{CO_2}	H^+	pH
Acute respiratory acidosis	50	43.5	7.36	50	49.5	7.31
	90	73.6	7.15	90	81.2	7.09
Chronic respiratory acidosis	50	34	7.47	50	45	7.35
	100	45	7.35	100	58	7.24
Metabolic acidosis	30	40	7.40	30	58	7.24
	10	72	7.14	20	75	7.13
Respiratory alkalosis	30	29.4	7.53	30	35.7	7.45
	15	18.3	7.74	15	24.6	7.61

parable data for adults are not available. Data collected up until a few years ago suggested that P_aCO_2 did not rise in adults purely on the basis of metabolic alkalosis. Several recent reports, however, suggest that hypercapnia secondary to severe metabolic alkalosis may be more common than would appear from previous studies. Regardless of the exact incidence, there seems little doubt that respiratory compensation for metabolic alkalosis (which would require hypoventilation) is much less common than respiratory compensation for metabolic acidosis (requiring hyperventilation).

CONSTRUCTING THE DIAGRAM

The diagram is best constructed on graph paper. The normal area can be a box running from P_{CO_2} 32 to 45 and H^+ 35 to 45 (pH 7.35 to 7.45). The confidence bands are bound by straight lines; Figure 5-12 can be used as a guide. Table 5-3 gives the coordinates for these lines.

Several other acid-base diagrams have been published using whole body titration curves. Some have bicarbonate as one of the axes; others have P_aCO_2 on the abscissa and pH on the ordinate. Once the reader has learned the principles behind the use of whole body titration curves, he will have no trouble adapting to any of the published diagrams.

PRECISION

The precision of blood gas analysis on a day-to-day basis in a clinical laboratory is difficult, if not impossible, to judge; as soon as an assessment begins, techniques tighten up. Reports of reproducibility from research labo-

ratories reflect a minimal workload with special care exerted. Two standard deviations about the mean of replicated samples have been reported as 0.026 for pH, 4.6 mm Hg for P_{CO_2}, and 2.2 mm Hg for P_{O_2} (Lumley, 1971). Considering that 95 per cent of the values lie within ± 2 standard deviations, these results are disappointing. For example, by these standards, blood with a true P_{CO_2} of 45 mm Hg could, on a single analysis, have a measured P_{CO_2} anywhere between 40.5 and 49.5. As noted previously (p. 114), however, rigorous quality control coupled with preventive maintenance of instruments and meticulous technical attention can yield improved precision and accuracy in blood gas analyses (Leary, 1977).

WHAT ARTERIAL BLOOD GASES WILL NOT TELL YOU

Although the blood gases will demonstrate certain abnormalities, they will not indicate how much the patient is suffering from the abnormality. A low P_aO_2 does not necessarily imply tissue hypoxia, nor does a normal P_aO_2 assure adequate tissue oxygenation. The cardiac output, regional blood flow, affinity of hemoglobin for oxygen, capillary perfusion, and tissue oxygen consumption are all important in oxygen utilization. The vital signs and level of mental function are good clinical guides to the adequacy of tissue oxygenation. Mixed venous P_{O_2} reflects tissue oxygenation much better than does arterial P_{O_2}.

Arterial blood gas values should not be expected to correlate with dyspnea. Dyspnea is a mechanical problem, not a chemical one, usually related to an increase in work of breathing. Unless this work becomes extreme, or the respiratory control system is defective, dyspnea will occur but not hypercapnia. Hypoxemia is more related to the distribution of ventilation and blood flow than to abnormalities in the mechanical properties. During an attack of asthma, patients as dyspneic as any which a physician is likely to see may have normal or only mildly abnormal arterial blood gas values.

Arterial blood gas values cannot give a specific etiologic diagnosis. For example, patients with chronic obstructive airway disease and respiratory failure may have the same blood gas values as cardiac patients with acute pulmonary edema; patients with asthma may have values similar to those of patients with pneumonia.

Resting arterial blood gases are poor screening tests for the exclusion of pulmonary disease. The primary function of the lung is to make arterial blood out of venous blood, and the arterial blood gases therefore are an excellent indication of overall pulmonary function. But like all organ systems, considerable disease can be present before the system fails. A careful history and physical examination, spirometry, and the chest x-ray are the proper screening procedures for pulmonary disease.

UNCERTAINTY AS TO REFERENCE VALUES

In a survey of 73 laboratories (Leiner, 1969), the accepted lower reference limit for pH varied from 7.35 to 7.39; the upper limit varied from 7.42 to 7.46. The accepted lower reference limit for P_aCO_2 varied from 32 to 38 mm Hg; the accepted upper limit varied from 36 to 46 mm Hg. For P_aO_2 the accepted lower reference limit varied from 68 to 95 mm Hg.

PATTERNS OF ARTERIAL BLOOD GAS ABNORMALITIES IN SPECIFIC DISEASES

CHRONIC OBSTRUCTIVE PULMONARY DISEASE

A wide variety of patterns of blood gas values is seen in this group of diseases, ranging from normal to severe hypoxemia and hypercapnia. In the type A (pink puffer or emphysematous) variety, the most common pattern is mild to moderate hypoxemia with a normal P_aCO_2. In the type B (blue bloater or bronchitic) variety, more severe hypoxemia with hypercapnia is the rule. In both groups V/Q (ventilation/perfusion) inequalities are the primary cause for the hypoxemia.

The hypercapnia is usually ascribed to hypoventilation but, as noted previously (p. 112), this is an oversimplification. It is more likely that the V/Q inequalities produce hypercapnia and the marked increase in the work of breathing precludes the ventilatory response required to keep the P_aCO_2 normal.

BRONCHIAL ASTHMA

In the symptom-free intervals the blood gases are normal. During a moderately severe attack, hypoxemia with a normal or low P_aCO_2 is the usual finding. Hypercapnia may be seen during a severe attack and indicates a rapidly deteriorating clinical state, often with exhaustion. Intubation and assisted ventilation are often required at this stage.

DIFFUSE INTERSTITIAL PULMONARY DISEASES

This group of diseases has a wide variety of names (pulmonary fibrosis, fibrosing alveolitis, chronic interstitial pneumonitis, Hamman-Rich disease). Although the diffusion defect (alveolar capillary block) has received a great deal of attention, at rest the P_aO_2 is usually normal or only mildly reduced. A marked fall in P_aO_2 may occur with exercise. The P_aCO_2 is usually normal or low.

SHOCK

Hypoxemia with normal or slightly low P_aCO_2 is the usual finding in septic and hemorrhagic shock (Bredenberg, 1969); the hypoxemia is primarily the result of shunting. Hypercapnia may occur terminally despite high minute ventilation delivered by a ventilator. Metabolic acidosis is a frequent finding.

MYOCARDIAL INFARCTION

There has been a great deal of recent interest in the arterial blood gases in this disease. One of the unexpected findings has been mild hypoxemia even in patients without complications. This mild hypoxemia results from V/Q imbalance, with poor aeration of the lung bases a major factor. When shock, pulmonary edema, or pulmonary embolism occur in the course of myocardial infarction, these complications will dominate the blood gas picture.

PULMONARY EDEMA

Moderate to severe hypoxemia with normal or low P_aCO_2 are frequent findings. However, Anthonisen (1965) reported four cases of severe respiratory acidosis in pulmonary edema. This type of disturbance has subsequently been shown to be a mixed respiratory and metabolic acidosis, and to be much more common than previously thought.

PULMONARY EMBOLISM

Szucs (1971) reported the results of 50 patients with pulmonary embolism. P_aO_2 ranged from 38 to 80 mm Hg. Values of $P_{a}O_{2}$ above 80 mm Hg are seen occasionally, but there is no doubt that hypoxemia is the rule. Respiratory alkalosis is the usual acid-base disturbance. Only six of Szucs' patients had a $P_{a}CO_{2}$ above 40 mm Hg; three of these had chronic obstructive airway disease.

EXERCISE

In normal subjects and cardiac patients the $P_{a}O_{2}$ is normal even at the breaking point of severe exercise, and higher than the resting $P_{a}O_{2}$ (Gilbert, 1970). By contrast, patients with type A emphysema show a fall in $P_{a}O_{2}$ with severe exercise; patients with type B disease usually show a slight rise, presumably the result of more uniform distribution of blood flow and ventilation during exercise. Normal subjects invariably show a metabolic acidosis, often uncompensated, at the breaking point of severe exercise; cardiac and pulmonary patients have less severe degrees of metabolic acidosis than do normal subjects, presumably because they are unwilling or unable to push themselves to extreme limits of endurance. A respiratory alkalosis at the exercise breaking point usually indicates a hyperventilation syndrome or neurocirculatory asthenia.

ADULT RESPIRATORY DISTRESS SYNDROME

This syndrome has also been called post-traumatic pulmonary insufficiency and shock lung. The best description is that of Moore and associates (1969). The syndrome follows a variety of severe body insults with the common denominator often but not invariably a period of low cardiac output. If the patient survives the initial episode, circulatory stabilization occurs, and there may be a period of a few hours or a few days when no pulmonary problem is apparent. There then follows progressive respiratory failure, often fatal. Early in the disease the arterial blood gases show mild hypoxemia, hypocapnia, and a mixed respiratory and metabolic alkalosis. Later more severe hypoxemia develops, the result of shunting plus an extreme reduction in diffusing capacity. Metabolic and respiratory acidosis are seen in the terminal stages.

ASPIRIN INTOXICATION

Within the first few hours there is a respiratory alkalosis due presumably to a direct effect of salicylate on the central nervous system. This is followed (especially in infants and young children) by a metabolic acidosis. This does not appear to be compensation in response to the respiratory alkalosis, but rather a defect in intermediary metabolism, and therefore represents a true mixed disturbance, respiratory alkalosis and metabolic acidosis. A low $P_{a}CO_{2}$ with a normal pH, especially in a young child, should immediately bring to mind the possibility of aspirin intoxication.

RESPIRATORY FAILURE

This commonly used term has no generally accepted meaning. It is often defined in terms of the blood gases; that is, respiratory failure is present when the arterial blood gases are abnormal. Since the major function of the respiratory system is that of gas exchange, there is certainly justification for this usage. But does it require both an abnormal $P_{a}O_{2}$ and $P_{a}CO_{2}$? Many critically ill patients with severe pulmonary disease have a low $P_{a}O_{2}$ and a low or normal $P_{a}CO_{2}$. This implies defective gas exchange but a ventilatory control system sufficiently intact to prevent hypercapnia. Certainly hypercapnia implies ventilatory failure, that is, a ventilation either abnormally low or one that has not or is unable to respond sufficiently to the hypercapnia produced by defective gas exchange, increased metabolic activity, or both. The reader should be aware of the various facets of so-called respiratory failure and of the imprecise nature of the term.

SUMMARY

The arterial blood gas interpretation should answer three questions:

(1) Is gas exchange defective? This is determined by the $P_{a}O_{2}$ in conjunction with the a/A ratio or $P_{A-aD}O_{2}$.

(2) What is the state of the ventilatory control system? This is determined by the $P_{a}CO_{2}$ with consideration of the acid-base state.

(3) What is the state of acid-base balance? This is determined by reference to appropriate whole body titration curves plus all other available clinical and laboratory findings.

REFERENCES

Albert, M. S., Dell, R. B., and Winters, R. W.: Quantitative displacement of acid-base equilibrium in metabolic acidosis. Ann. Intern. Med., 66:312, 1967.

Anthonisen, N. R., and Smith, H. J.: Respiratory acidosis as a consequence of pulmonary edema. Ann. Intern. Med., 62:991, 1965.

Arbus, G. S., Hebert, L. A., Levesque, P. R., Etsten, B. E., and Schwartz, W. B.: Characterization and clinical application of the "significance band" for acute respiratory alkalosis. N. Engl. J. Med., 280:117, 1969.

Ayres, S. M., and Grace, W. J.: Inappropriate ventilation and hypoxemia as causes of cardiac arrhythmias. Am. J. Med., 46:495, 1969.

Baegeant, R. A.: Variations in arterial blood gas measurements due to sampling techniques. Resp. Care, 20:565, 1975.

Bedford, R. H., and Wollman, H.: Arterial puncture for blood gas studies: Sites, complications, personnel. J.A.M.A., 228:763, 1974.

Bigen, R., Racine, T., and Roy, J. C.: Value of capillary blood gas analysis in the management of acute respiratory distress. Am. Res. Respir. Dis., 112:879, 1975.

Bird, B. D., Williams, J., and Whitwam, J. G.: The blood gas factor: A comparison of three different oxygen electrodes. Br. J. Anaesth., 46:249, 1974.

Brackett, N. C., Jr., Cohen, J. J., and Schwartz, W. B.: Carbon dioxide titration curve of normal man. N. Engl. J. Med., 272:6, 1965.

Brackett, N. C., Jr., Wingo, C. F., Muren, O., and Solano, J. T.: Acid-base response to chronic hypercapnia in man. N. Engl. J. Med., 280:124, 1969.

Bradley, J. G.: Errors in the management of blood Pco_2 due to dilution of the sample with heparin solution. Br. J. Anaesth., 44:231, 1972.

Bredenberg, C. E., James, P. M., Collins, J., Anderson, R. W., Martin, A. M., Jr., and Hardaway, R. M.: Respiratory failure in shock. Ann. Surg., 169: 392, 1969.

Chalmers, C., Bird, B. D., and Whitwam, J. G.: Evaluation of a new thin film tonometer. Br. J. Anaesth., 46:253, 1974.

Cherniack, R. M., and Raber, M. E.: Normal standards for ventilation function using an automated wedge spirometer. Am. Rev. Resp. Dis., 106:38, 1972.

Coon, R. L., Lai, N. C. J., and Kampine, J. P.: Evaluation of a dual-function pH and Pco_2 in vivo sensor. J. Appl. Physiol., 40:625, 1976.

Delaney, C. J., Leary, E. R., Raisys, V. A., and Kenny, M. A.: Proficiency testing for blood gas quality control. Clin. Chem., 22:1675, 1976.

Dowd, F., and Jenkins, L. C.: Some problems associated with measurement of physiological blood gases. Can. Anaesth. Soc. J., 20:129, 1973.

Evers, W., Racz, G. B., and Levy, O. A.: A comparative study of plastic (polypropylene) and glass syringes in blood gas analysis. Anesth. Analg., (Cleve.), 51:92, 1972.

Fleisher, M., and Schwartz, M. K.: Use of evacuated collection tubes for routine determination of arterial blood gases and pH. Clin. Chem., 17:610, 1971.

Gambino, S. R.: Comparisons of pH in human arterial, venous and capillary blood. Am. J. Clin. Pathol., 32:298, 1959.

Gambino, S. R.: Collection of capillary blood for simultaneous determinations of arterial pH, CO_2 content, Pco_2 and oxygen saturation. Am. J. Clin. Pathol., 35:175, 1961.

Gandy, G., Grann, L., Cunningham, H., Adamson, K., and James, L. S.: The validity of pH and Pco_2 measurements in sick and healthy newborn infants. Pediatrics, 34:192, 1964.

Gilbert, R., and Auchincloss, J. H.: Arterial blood gases and acid-base balance at the exercise breaking point. Arch. Intern. Med., 125:820, 1970.

Gilbert, R., Auchincloss, J. H., Jr., Peppi, D., and Ashutosh, K.: The first few hours off a respirator. Chest, 65:152, 1974.

Gilbert, R., and Keighley, J. F.: The arterial/alveolar oxygen tension ratio. Am. Rev. Resp. Dis., 109:142, 1974.

Goldstein, M. B., Gennari, F. J., and Schwartz, W. B.: The influence of graded degrees of chronic hypercapnia on the acute carbon dioxide titration curve. J. Clin. Invest., 50:208, 1971.

Greenhow, D. E.: Incorrect performance of Allen's test ulnar-artery flow, erroneously presumed inadequate. Anesthesiology, 37:356, 1972.

Huch, A., Secter, D., Meinzer, K., Huch, R., Galster, H., and Fubbers, D. W.: Transcutaneous Pco_2 measurement with a miniaturized electrode. Lancet, 1:982, 1977.

Ishikawa, S., Fornier, A., Borst, E., and Segal, M.: The effects of air bubbles and time delay on blood gas analysis. Ann. Allergy, 331:72, 1974.

Jung, R. C., Balchum, O. J., and Massey, F. J.: The accuracy of venous and capillary blood for the prediction of arterial pH, Pco_2 and PO_2 measurements. Am. J. Clin. Pathol., 45:129–138, 1966.

Kelman, G. R., and Nunn, J. F.: Nomograms for correction of blood PO_2, PCO_2, pH, and base excess for time and temperature. J. Appl. Physiol., 21:1484, 1966.

Kilburn, K. H., and Dowell, A. R.: Renal function in respiratory failure. Arch. Intern. Med., 127:754, 1971.

Kildeberg, P.: Respiratory compensation in metabolic alkalosis. Acta Med. Scand., 174:515, 1963.

Koch, G., and Wendel, H.: Comparison of pH, carbon dioxide tension, standard bicarbonate and oxygen tension in capillary blood and in arterial blood during the neonatal period. Acta Paediatr. Scand., 56:10, 1967.

Koch, G.: The validity of PO_2 measurements in capillary blood as a substitute for arterial blood. Scand. J. Clin. Invest., 21:10, 1968.

Komjathy, Z. L., Mathies, J. C., Parker, J. A., and Schreiber, H. A.: Stability and precision of a new ampuled quality control system for pH and blood gas measurements. Clin. Chem., 22:1399, 1976.

Kryger, M., Bode, F., Antic, R., and Anthonisen, N.: Diagnosis of obstruction of the upper and central airways. Am. J. Med., 61:85, 1976.

Langlands, J. H. M., and Wallace, W. F. M.: Small bloodsamples from earlobe puncture. Lancet, 2:315, 1965.

Laughlin, D. E., McDonald, J. S., and Bedell, G. N.: A microtechnique for measurement of Po_2 in "arterialized" earlobe blood. J. Lab. Clin. Med., 64:330, 1964.

Leary, T. E., Delaney, C. J., and Kenny, M. A.: Use of equilibrated blood for internal blood-gas quality control. Clin. Chem., 23:493, 1977.

Leiner, G. C., Abramowitz, S., and Small, M. J.: Pulmonary function testing in laboratories associated with residency training programs in pulmonary diseases. Am. Rev. Resp. Dis., 100:240, 1969.

Levine, M., Gilbert, R., and Auchincloss, J. H., Jr.: A comparison of the effects of sighs, large tidal volumes, and positive end expiratory pressure in assisted ventilation. Scand. J. Res. Dis., 53:101, 1972.

Lumley, J., Potter, M., Newman, W., Talbot, J. M., Wakefield, E., and Wood, C.: The unreliability of a single estimation of fetal scalp blood pH. J. Lab. Clin. Med., *77*:535, 1971.

Moore, F. D., Lyons, J. H., Jr., Pierce, E. C., Morgan, A. P., Drinker, P. A., MacArthur, J. D., and Dammin, G. J.: Post-traumatic Pulmonary Insufficiency. Philadelphia, W. B. Saunders Company, 1969.

Mortensen, J. D.: Clinical sequelae from arterial puncture, cannulation and incision. Circulation, *35*:1118, 1967.

Newball, H.: Arterial blood samples should be stored in ice for gas analysis. J.A.M.A., *223*:696, 1973.

Noonan, D. C., and Komjathy, Z. L.: Long term reproducibility of a new pH/blood-gas quality control system compared to two other procedures. Clin. Chem., *22*:1817, 1976.

Nunn, J. F.: Measurement of blood oxygen tension: Handling of samples. Br. J. Anaesth., *34*:621, 1962.

Peppi, D., Gilbert, R., and Auchincloss, J. H., Jr.: Simultaneous recording and display of the volume-time spirogram and flow-volume loop. Analyzer, *5*:13, 1975.

Petty, T. L., Bigelow, D. B., and Levine, B. E.: The simplicity and safety of arterial puncture. J.A.M.A., *195*:181-183, 1966.

Pontoppidan, H., Hedley-Whyte, J., Bendixen, H. H., Laver, M. B., and Radford, E. P., Jr.: Ventilation and oxygen requirements during prolonged artificial ventilation in patients with respiratory failure. N. Engl. J. Med., *273*:401, 1965.

Sackner, M. A., Avery, W. G., and Sokolowski, J.: Arterial punctures by nurses. Chest, *59*:97, 1971.

Sadove, M. S., Thompson, R. D., and Jobsen, E.: Capillary versus arterial blood gases. Anesth. Analg. (Cleve.), *52*:724, 1973.

Schwartz, W. B., van Ypersele de Strihou, C., and Kassirer, J. P.: Role of anions in metabolic alkalosis and potassium deficiency. N. Engl. J. Med., *279*:630, 1968.

Scott, P. V., Horton, J. N., and Mapleson, W. W.: Mechanism and magnitude of leakage from blood and water samples stored in plastic syringes. Br. J. Anaesth., *43*:717, 1971a.

Scott, P. V., Horton, J. N., and Mapleson, W. W.: Leakage of oxygen from blood and water samples stored in plastic and glass syringes. Br. Med. J., *3*:512, 1971b.

Severinghaus, J. W.: Electrodes for blood and gas P_{CO_2}, P_{O_2} and blood pH. Acta Anaesth. Scand. (Suppl. XI):207, 1962.

Severinghaus, J. W.: Measurement of blood gases, P_{O_2} and P_{CO_2}. Ann. N.Y. Acad. Sci., *148*:115, 1968.

Sieker, H. O., and Hickan, J. B.: Carbon dioxide intoxication: The clinical syndrome, its etiology and management with particular reference to the use of mechanical respirators. Medicine, *35*:389, 1956.

Siggaard-Anderson, O.: Acid-base and blood gas parameters—arterial or capillary blood. Scand. J. Clin. Lab. Invest., *21*:289, 1968.

Siggaard-Anderson, O.: Sampling and storing of blood for determination of acid-base status. Scand. J. Clin. Lab. Invest., *13*:196, 1961.

Szucs, M. M., Brooks, H. L., Grossman, W., Banas, J. S., Meister, S. G., Dexter, L., and Dalen, J. E.: Diagnostic sensitivity of laboratory findings in acute pulmonary embolism. Ann. Intern. Med., *74*:161, 1971.

West, J.: Regional differences in gas exchange in the lung of erect man. J. Appl. Physiol., *17*:893, 1962.

West, J. B.: Causes of carbon dioxide retention in lung disease. N. Engl. J. Med., *284*:1232, 1971.

Winkler, J. B., Huntington, C. B., Wells, D. E., and Befeler, B.: Influence of syringe material on blood gas determinations. Chest, *66*:518, 1974.

Winters, R. W., Engel, K., and Dell, R. B.: Acid Base Physiology in Medicine. Cleveland, The London Company, 1967.

6

EVALUATION OF RENAL FUNCTION, AND WATER, ELECTROLYTE, AND ACID-BASE BALANCE

John E. Murphy, M.D., and
John Bernard Henry, M.D.

In order for intracellular metabolism to occur optimally, the internal environment of the cells must be constant in composition. The intracellular environment is a direct reflection of the composition of the extracellular fluid (ECF), which is regulated by the lungs and kidneys. The lungs control the concentration of the blood gases and the respiratory component of the acid-base system. These parameters and their corresponding measurements are discussed in Chapter 5. The kidneys, in addition to eliminating metabolic wastes, control the tonicity, volume, and chemical composition of the ECF, including the metabolic component of the acid-base system, by the formation of urine (see Chap. 17).

THE KIDNEYS

The kidneys are paired structures that are on either side of the vertebral column in the retro-peritoneal space between the levels of the twelfth thoracic and third lumbar vertebrae. In the adult, each kidney weighs approximately 150 g and measures 12 cm in length (Fig. 6-1). Medial aspects of the kidneys are indented to form hili which receive renal arteries and veins. The ureters, which transport urine from each kidney to the bladder, exit from the hilar regions. Kidney parenchyma is composed of two distinct zones: the outer cortex and the inner medulla, which form the renal pyramids.

The microscopic functional unit is the nephron. It consists of a capillary plexus called the glomerulus and a complex tubule divided into Bowman's capsule and the proximal and distal convoluted tubules that are connected by the loop of Henle (Fig. 6-2). The glomerulus is enclosed in a blind, invaginated, and dilated end of the tubule which is called Bowman's capsule. Between the endothelial cells and visceral epithelial cells of the tubule is a distinct basement membrane. Bowman's capsule tapers to form the proximal convoluted tubule, which has a prominent luminal brush border. This part of the tubule repeatedly turns upon itself and then narrows and straightens out to form the thin descend-

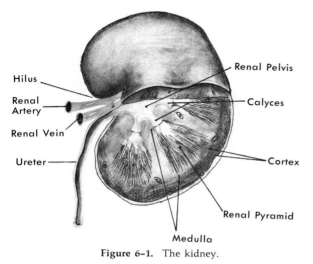

Hilus

Renal
Artery

Renal Vein

Ureter

Renal Pelvis

Calyces

Cortex

Renal Pyramid

Medulla

Figure 6-1. The kidney.

ducts which terminate at the tips of the renal pyramids. The glomerulus and convoluted tubules are present in the cortices; the loops of Henle and collecting ducts are present in the medullae. There are approximately one million nephrons in each kidney.

Afferent arterioles connect the glomeruli to the arterial system. The glomeruli are also connected to efferent arterioles that have thicker walls and smaller lumens than do afferent arterioles. This part of the vascular system is lined by specialized granulated cells called juxtaglomerular cells, which together with the adjacent macula densa form the juxtaglomerular apparatus. The efferent arterioles join the glomeruli to capillaries which surround the tubules as a branched network. Those capillaries that originate in the juxtamedullary portion of the cortex form distinct loops called vasa recta which parallel several adjacent loops of Henle.

The ureters and their dilated proximal portions called calyces (which surround the pyramids) and the collecting tubules are derived from the Wolffian ducts. The nephrons are derived from primitive mesoderm called the metanephros.

As a result of the complicated embryogenesis, congenital malformations of the kidney are frequent. More common are duplications of the larger blood vessels and of the ureters. Agenesis, hypoplasia, ectopic development, and fusion (horseshoe kidney) also occur. Dilations of the tubular systems

ing loop of Henle. This makes a 180 degree turn to form the straight ascending loop of Henle, which is at first thin but then abruptly thickens. The thick portion of the ascending loop, in the region of the glomerulus, bends upon itself to form the distal convoluted tubule. The junction between the ascending loop of Henle and the distal convoluted tubule is called the macula densa. Several adjacent convoluted tubules join together to form collecting

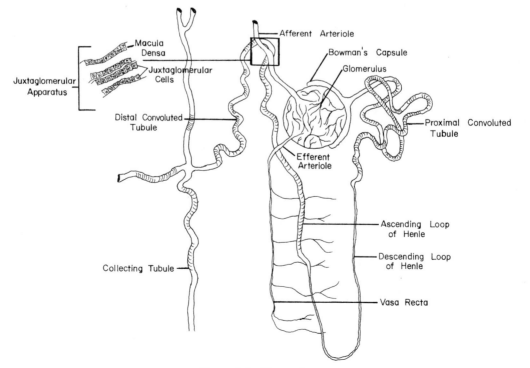

Macula
Densa

Afferent Arteriole

Bowman's Capsule

Glomerulus

Juxtaglomerular
Apparatus

Juxtaglomerular
Cells

Distal Convoluted
Tubule

Proximal Convoluted
Tubule

Efferent
Arteriole

Ascending Loop
of Henle

Descending Loop
of Henle

Collecting Tubule

Vasa Recta

Figure 6-2. The nephron.

may be present which can progressively enlarge to form large cysts (polycystic kidney disease). Many of these abnormalities can result, over varying periods of time, in extensive obstruction and consequently destruction of parenchyma with loss of renal function.

FORMATION OF URINE

Urine is a modified ultrafiltrate of plasma. As a result of the extensive vasculature of the kidneys, these organs receive 20 to 25 per cent of the entire cardiac output under basal conditions. The amount of plasma that passes from the glomeruli into Bowman's capsules—the glomerular filtrate—is regulated by differences between the net hydrostatic pressures and net oncotic pressures (Wallin, 1977). The glomerular hydrostatic pressure is 45 mm Hg (i.e., approximately 40 per cent of the systemic arterial pressure) and the tubular hydrostatic pressure is 10 mm Hg. The hydrostatic pressure gradient is therefore 35 mm Hg, and this difference does not change throughout the entire glomerulus. The tubular oncotic pressure is zero, and the capillary oncotic pressure increases from 20 mm Hg at the end of the afferent arteriole to 35 mm Hg at the beginning of the efferent arteriole. This is a result of the progressive increase in the concentration of plasma proteins secondary to the filtration process. Therefore, the filtration pressure at the beginning of the glomerulus is 15 mm Hg and decreases to 0 mm Hg at the end of the glomerulus.

An imbalance in the hydrostatic pressures secondary to vascular collapse, renal arterial occlusive diseases, inflammatory disease with increased interstitial pressure, or obstruction of the urinary outflow system can result in a marked decrease in glomerular filtration with scanty urine formation (oliguria) or no urine formation (anuria). Similarly, imbalances in the oncotic pressures secondary to hypoproteinemia or glomerular basement membrane damage with proteinuria can result in increased glomerular filtration (see Chap. 17).

By measuring the concentration of a small molecular weight substance like inulin (see discussion of clearance below) in the plasma and proximal convoluted tubule, it is found that this substance, which infiltrates freely but is neither absorbed nor secreted by the tubules, increases in concentration four times in the lumen of the proximal convoluted tubule (Ganong, 1975a). This is a result of 75 per cent

of the filtered water and its contained solute being absorbed in this part of the nephron. Sodium (Na^+), chloride (Cl^-), and water diffuse passively into the tubular cells. Sodium, then, is actively pumped out of the cells into the intercellular spaces. Cl^- and water follow to maintain electrical and osmotic equilibriums (Wallin, 1977). The intercellular contents are reabsorbed into adjacent capillaries. The ultrafiltrate remaining in the tubules at this point is isosmotic with plasma.

Other electrolytes and organic substances are actively transported from the urine into the proximal convoluted tubular cells and then into the microcirculation (Ganong, 1975a). These substances (glucose, amino acids, creatine, sulfate, uric acid, ascorbic acid, ketone bodies, potassium, and phosphate) are conserved, in order that efficient body metabolism may occur. Conversely, conjugated steriods and 5-hydroxyindoleacetic acid are actively secreted into the urine by the same tubular cells. Drugs, such as penicillin, are also secreted.

Inherited or acquired proximal tubular enzymatic defects can result in the loss of nonabsorbed substances into the urine. This is referred to as Fanconi syndrome (Kramer, 1974). There is failure to reabsorb glucose, phosphate, and amino acids. Cystinuria with failure to reabsorb the basic amino acids—lysine, cystine, ornithine, and arginine—and consequent formation of cystine urinary stones may occur with Fanconi syndrome in children.

In the descending loop of Henle, which is permeable to water only and not to solute, an additional 5 per cent of the filtered water is reabsorbed. As a consequence of this selective reabsorption, urine becomes progressively hyperosmotic. However, the thin ascending limb of Henle is permeable to both sodium and urea, and chloride is actively pumped out of the filtrate by the thick portion of ascending loop, with sodium passively following to maintain electrical neutrality (Kokko, 1977). Both parts of the ascending loop are impermeable to water and, as a result, urine as it reaches the macula densa becomes hyposmotic compared with plasma. The process of selective removal of solute by the ascending loops, creating an interstitium with a high osmolality that is responsible for the absorption of water from both the descending loops of Henle and from the collecting ducts, is called countercurrent multiplication. This mechanism would not exist if it were not for the fact that the vasa recta allow only solute and not water to remain in the interstitium. Solute diffuses from the interstitium into the descending limb of the vasa recta and then out of the ascending limb into the interstitium. Water diffuses in the reverse direction: out of the descending limb and into the ascending limb. This process is called countercurrent exchange.

In the distal convoluted tubule, sodium (Na^+) (with H_2O) in the urine is exchanged for either potassium (K^+) or hydrogen ion (H^+). The reabsorption of Na^+ and water in this part of the tubule is regulated by the levels of circulating mineralocorticoids (i.e., aldosterone and deoxycorticosterone). In response to decreased renal arterial pressure, to decreased urinary sodium in this part of the nephron, or to hypokalemia, the juxtaglomerular cells synthesize and release into the circulation increased amounts of a proteolytic enzyme called renin. This, in turn, acts upon an α_2 globulin synthesized in the liver, called angiotensinogen, to convert it to a decapeptide called angiotensin I (Chap. 14). Angiotensin I is converted into angiotensin II by the action of another proteolytic enzyme called converting enzyme, which is manufactured in the endothelial cells of lung capillaries. Angiotensin II is a potent vasoconstrictor and causes the release of aldosterone from the adrenal cortex (Chap. 14). Angiotensinases are made in the kidney and other tissues and are released into the plasma; these enzymes prevent excessive or prolonged effects of this regulatory sequence. Approximately 8 per cent of the filtered water is reabsorbed by the distal convoluted tubules.

Another hormone, vasopressin or antidiuretic hormone (ADH), is responsible for further reabsorption of water by collecting ducts. This substance is made in the hypothalamus and stored in the posterior pituitary. The amount of circulating hormone (ADH) is determined by osmoreceptors present in the hypothalamus; these are stimulated by high plasma osmolality and/or low plasma volume (hypovolemia). Vasopressin causes pores in the collecting ducts to increase in diameter, permitting an increasing amount of water to be osmotically reabsorbed into the renal medulla. An additional 11 to 12 per cent of the filtrate can be reabsorbed, with the resulting urine having an osmolality almost five times that of plasma. Conversely, in the absence of vaso-

pressin (e.g., diabetes insipidus) or a nonresponse of the collecting tubules to vasopressin (e.g., nephrogenic diabetes insipidus) large volumes of dilute urine result (polyuria).

LABORATORY ASSESSMENT OF RENAL FUNCTION

Initial laboratory evaluation of renal function begins with the basic examination of the urine or complete urinalysis with particular attention to protein and specific gravity (Chap. 17). This should be followed with a measurement of serum creatinine and/or urea nitrogen (Chap. 10). In the event that an abnormality is identified in the urinalysis, this should be studied further, including measurement of 24-hour urine protein and perhaps concentration-dilution evaluations. Massive proteinuria warrants examination of serum proteins (electrophoresis) (Chap. 9) and blood lipid determinations (Chap. 8). An elevated serum creatinine should be followed by additional measurements to delineate an alteration in glomerular filtration, i.e., creatinine clearance. In the event that there is a significant decrease in glomerular filtration rate, i.e., azotemia and/or uremia, appropriate measurements of electrolytes and acid-base are in order. Special emphasis should be placed on blood pH as well as on potassium, sodium, and carbon dioxide. Serum potassium is most significant because of the potentially fatal consequences of hyperkalemia. Radiographic studies provide estimates of renal size via pyelogram studies, intravenous and/or retrograde. Renal scans may also be helpful in this regard. When urine sediment examination is abnormal, more careful urine sediment examinations, including special stains, may be indicated (Chap. 17). Finally, renal biopsy to delineate the specific pathologic lesion of renal failure is important. This may require immunopathologic examinations (Chap. 36).

Long-term evaluation and management of patients with chronic disorders of renal function, including renal failure, are achieved through periodic urinalysis, serum creatinine, creatinine clearance, and electrolyte measurements, as well as estimates of rate of urine formation. All of these parameters are used together to determine appropriate fluid and electrolyte replacement therapy.

CLEARANCE

Overall renal function as well as individual aspects of kidney physiology can be determined by simultaneously measuring concentrations of substances in both the blood and the urine that are selectively filtered and/or secreted. By measuring the volume of urine formed during a set time interval, the volume of plasma which contained the measured substance excreted in the urine during this time can be determined. This volume, expressed in ml/min, is called clearance. The formula for determining clearance is:

$$\text{Clearance} = \frac{V \times U}{P}$$

where U = concentration of measured substance in urine

P = concentration of same substance in plasma

V = urine volume converted to ml/min

It is necessary that the concentration units for U and P be identical so that they cancel. Clearance is proportional to renal parenchymal mass, and in order for values to be comparable, it is necessary to correct for differing kidney masses by multiplying the clearance by the factor 1.73/A. 1.73 is the external surface area in square meters of the average person; A is the body surface area of the patient. This correction is used because kidney mass is roughly proportional to body surface area. This correction is definitely necessary if the body surface area of the patient (e.g., child) differs greatly from the average. The corrected formula for clearance is:

$$\text{Clearance (std. surface area)} = \frac{U \times V}{P} \times \frac{1.73}{A}$$

A is determined from nomograms or from formulae relating surface area to weight and height (see Appendix C).

Substances that are freely filtered but are neither reabsorbed nor secreted by the tubules are used to determine glomerular filtration rate (GFR) which is equal to the clearance values of these substances. Inulin, a polysaccharide with a molecular weight of 5100 daltons, is such a substance. Although used for very accurate investigation work, it is not routinely employed in a clinical setting because of the necessity of using a continuous intravenous infusion (Faulkner, 1976). The average value for inulin clearance is 125 ml/min in men and 115 ml/min in women. GFR is lower in children (corrected for surface area) until the age of two years and also decreases progressively as individuals pass middle age (Renkin, 1974).

It is easier to perform a creatinine clearance. Creatinine, the degradation product of creatine, is formed at a constant rate in the body and is freely filtered but is not transported by the tubules (endogenous test). However, if plasma creatinine levels increase markedly above normal, creatinine is also secreted by the tubules into the urine (Chap. 10). Therefore, clearance tests employing exogenously administered creatinine will overestimate the GFR. This will also occur in renal pathologic states with impaired renal circulation (Smith, 1964). However, even though this will falsely elevate the GFR, it does not invalidate the usefulness of creatinine clearance for monitoring a patient with renal impairment (Tobias, 1962). Precisely timed urine collections are required. Varying periods of collection (i.e., 1 hr., 2 hr., 4 hr., 6 hr., and 24 hr.) have been found to be adequate (Tobias, 1962). However, if the shorter time intervals are used, it is necessary that the patient be well hydrated and urine flow be unimpaired.

Creatinine clearance reference intervals or normal values are 85 to 125 ml/min for males and 75 to 115 ml/min for females. The difference is due to the difference between GFR's. If a more specific method is used to measure creatinine concentrations (i.e., use of aluminum silicate or Lloyd's reagent) (Chap. 10) reference intervals are 97 to 137 ml/min for males and 88 to 128 ml/min for females. The greater values are due to the elimination of non-specific chromogens that are present in much lower concentrations in urine than in plasma but are measured by the non-specific Jaffe reaction (see Chap. 10, p. 000). Falsely low values will be obtained if the collected urine is not refrigerated and/or a bacterial inhibitor (e.g., thymol) is not added to the urine container. The urine creatinine concentration should be determined no later than 24 hours after collection. Acidity or alkalinity of the urine (a result of bacterial metabolism) promotes the conversion of creatinine to creatine, which is not measured directly by the Jaffe reaction. Bacteria, in addition to causing a change in pH of the urine, also produce creatininases which destroy creatinine.

To evaluate secretory function of the tubules, exogenous substances, which are secreted predominantly by the tubules, can be injected into the circulation and clearance values determined. Ninety per cent of p-aminohippurate (PAH), if injected so that the resultant plasma concentration does not exceed its threshold limit, is cleared from the plasma in a single passage through the kidneys (Berliner, 1973). In order for the test accurately to reflect changes in renal function, the renal circulation has to be unimpaired. If tubular function is normal, the clearance value is a measurement of the plasma flow that is in direct contact with renal tubules, the effective renal plasma flow (ERPF). The reference interval is 600 to 700 ml/min. The actual renal plasma flow (RPF) is approximately 10 per cent greater owing to the fact that 10 per cent of the blood does not directly bathe the tubules. The GFR/RPF ratio is called the filtration fraction and is normally 0.16 to 0.20. PAH clearance tests are used only for very accurate investigational purposes because of the need to prime the patient and to maintain a constant blood level using a continuous intravenous infusion. A simpler measurement of secretory function that is employed clinically is the phenolsulfonphthalein (PSP) test (Cannon, 1974). PSP, a pH indicator, is injected in a single bolus intravenously. Sixty to seventy per cent of this dye is removed during a single passage through the kidneys, with active tubular secretion accounting for almost 95 per cent of that which is cleared. If secreting function is optimal, 25 to 50 per cent of the amount injected is secreted in the first 15 minutes and an additional 15 to 25 per cent is secreted in the next 15 minutes. The dye concentration is measured colorimetrically (540 nm) after alkalizing the urine.

An infrequently used clinical measurement of total renal function (i.e., glomerular and tubular function) is the urea clearance test. Urea is a very small molecule with a molecular weight of 60. It is freely filtered by the glomerulus but then is variably reabsorbed by the tubules, depending upon the transit time of the filtrate in the tubules. The greater the rate of urine flow through the kidneys, the less urea is reabsorbed and vice versa. Therefore, in order to interpret the urea clearance value, the rate of urine flow also has to be determined. If the flow rate is 2 ml/min or greater, the normal urea clearance is 64 to 99 ml/min. This is called the maximal clearance (C_m). If the flow rate is less than 2 ml/min, the normal

urea clearance is 41 to 68 ml/min. This is called the standard clearance (C_s). The standard clearance is calculated by substituting $\sqrt{V}$ for V in the formula for clearance (p. 139). Mathematically, these two clearance values can be compared by dividing each by the average value for each respective clearance (i.e., mean $C_m = 75$ ml/min; mean $C_s = 54$ ml/min) and converting to per cent by multiplying by 100. The reference intervals for both clearances expressed as per cent of normal are 75 to 125 per cent. Accuracy decreases with decreasing urine flow, and if the urinary flow rate is less than 1 ml/min, the urea clearance test should not be done (Tietz, 1976). Because of the wide range of reference values owing to the variable effect of urine flow, this test has been largely replaced by the creatinine clearance test.

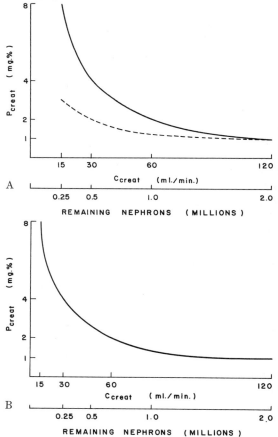

Figure 6–3. A, Plasma creatinine concentration (P_{creat}) as a function of creatine clearance (C_{creat}) and number of residual nephrons. The graph does not allow for nephron hypertrophy. B, Plasma creatinine concentration (P_{creat}) as a function of creatinine clearance (C_{creat}) and number of residual nephrons. Graph assumes progressive nephron hypertrophy with advancing disease.

Although clearance tests are technically demanding, requiring accurately timed and complete urine collections and measurements simultaneously of both serum and urine solute concentrations, they are useful as very sensitive parameters of kidney function. Measurements of metabolic waste substances in the serum are very insensitive guidelines of renal function. Sixty-five to seventy-five per cent of the kidney parenchyma has to be destroyed or become non-functional before the various non-protein nitrogen substances (creatinine, urea, uric acid) that are excreted into the urine become elevated in the blood (Fig. 6–3).

MEASUREMENTS OF URINARY SOLUTE CONCENTRATION

The ability of the kidney to maintain both the tonicity and water balance of the ECF requires that energy be expended by the tubules. These functions can be evaluated by measuring the solute concentration of the urine either routinely or under artificial conditions (i.e., concentration or dilution tests). Solute concentrations of fluids are most conveniently quantitated by measuring either specific gravity or osmolality.

Specific gravity

Specific gravity is the ratio of the mass of a solution compared with the mass of an equal volume of water. It is a comparison of weights and therefore is a directly related but *not* an exact measurement of the number of solute particles, since different atoms and molecules have different weights. The specific gravity of plasma is very constant and ranges from 1.010 to 1.012. Urine specific gravity can vary from 1.003 to 1.035, reflecting either a dilution or a concentration of the glomerular ultrafiltrate. Concentrating ability is one of the first functions to be lost as a result of renal tubular damage.

Specific gravity can be measured by a calibrated urine hydrometer called a urinometer. It is necessary to correct the specific gravity reading for temperature effects, adding 0.001 to the observed specific gravity reading for each 3°C. above the calibration temperature and subtracting 0.001 for each 3°C. below the calibration temperature. It is also necessary to correct for proteinuria and glycosuria, subtracting 0.003 for each 1 g of protein/dl of

urine and 0.004 for each 1 g of glucose/dl of urine from the temperature-compensated value.

Specific gravity can also be measured by using a refractometer. This is discussed in Chapter 17 (p. 579).

Osmolality

Osmolality is a measure of the number of dissolved solute particles in solution. Dissolved solutes change four physical properties of solutions, called colligative properties. They are osmotic pressure, vapor pressure, boiling point, and freezing point. The extent of these changes at a constant temperature is determined only by the number and *not* by the nature of the particles in solution. Osmotic pressure is the pressure that must be exerted on a solution on one side of a semipermeable membrane to oppose the net movement of solvent into the solution owing to the presence of a non-permeable solute in the solution. Osmotic pressure is increased by the presence of solute, as is the boiling point, the temperature at which the vapor pressure of the solution is equal to the atmospheric pressure owing to lowering of the vapor pressure of the solution. The freezing point, the temperature at which the vapor pressure of the solution equals the vapor pressure of its solid phase, is for the same reason lowered. One gram molecular weight (mole) of a non-electrolyte like glucose which contains 6.023×10^{23} particles (Avogadro's number), if dissolved in 1 kg of H_2O, will increase the boiling point of water 0.52°C. and the osmotic pressure 17,000 mm Hg and lower the vapor pressure 0.3 mm Hg and the freezing point 1.858°C. This solution is defined as having an osmolality of 1 (or 1 osmol/kg H_2O). A related expression is osmolarity, defined as 1 osmol of non-electrolyte dissolved in 1 liter of water. Osmolality is the preferred unit of measurement, since it is a constant weight/weight relationship. In contrast, osmolarity varies owing to the volume-expanding effect of dissolved solute and the direct proportional effect of temperature on fluid volume.

The osmolality of a one-molal solution of an electrolyte (e.g., NaCl) is greater than one owing to dissociation of electrolyte into component atoms when in solution. The osmolality of an electrolyte solution is determined by the following formula:

$$\text{osmolality} = \Phi nC$$

where n is the number of atoms that dissociate

in solution (e.g., n for NaCl is 2); C is the concentration of the electrolyte in mol/kg H_2O; and Φ is the osmotic coefficient. This factor, which is different for each electrolyte, is necessary because the dissociation of electrolyte into individual atoms may not be complete and the individual particles may form secondary chemical bonds with solvent molecules. Φ is derived by dividing the measured osmolality by the theoretical osmolality of the electrolytic solution. Φ for NaCl is 0.93.

The electrolytes Na^+, Cl^-, and HCO_3^-, because they are present in high concentrations in the ECF and are monoionic, contribute to over 92 per cent of the serum osmolality. The other ECF electrolytes, serum proteins, glucose, and urea are responsible for the remaining 8 per cent. The normal osmolality of the serum is between 285 and 310 mosmol/kg H_2O. Many simple formulae can be used to estimate serum osmolality (Weisberg, 1971). The one that is used most often is:

osmolality (mosmol/kg H_2O)

$$= 1.86\,[Na^+] + \frac{[glucose]}{18} + \frac{[BUN]}{2.8}$$

The number 1.86 is derived from 0.93×2 (Φn), since each Na^+ in solution is balanced by a corresponding anion (Cl^- or HCO_3^-) in order to conserve electrical neutrality. The number 18 is used because the molecular mass of glucose is 180 daltons and the expression $\dfrac{[glucose]}{18}$ converts the units from mg/dl to mmole/l. Similarly, 2.8 is used because the molecular mass of the 2 nitrogen atoms in urea is 28 daltons and the expression $\dfrac{[BUN]}{2.8}$ converts the units from mg/dl to mmole/l. The above formula can be further simplified to:

osmolality (mosmol/kg H_2O)

$$= 2\,[Na^+]\frac{[glucose]}{20} + \frac{[BUN]}{3}$$

The ratio of serum sodium concentration to serum osmolality is normally between 0.43 and 0.50 (Ganong, 1975a). This ratio remains unchanged in uncomplicated dilutional or dehydration states. A decreased ratio can be seen in pathologic states in which there is an increase in osmotically active substances (e.g., diabetes, uremia, salicylate poisoning).

Urine osmolality is much more variable, with a reference interval extending normally from 300 to 900 mosmol/kg H_2O. If the renal tubules are able to maximally dilute and concentrate the urine, osmolalities between 50 and 1400 mosmol/kg H_2O may be encountered. Urine osmolality corresponds fairly well with urinary specific gravity in non-disease states. However, urinary specific gravity does not correlate well with urine osmolality in renal disease states owing to the greater contribution of high molecular weight substances like glucose and protein to specific gravity than to osmolality (Holmes, 1962).

More information concerning the state of renal function and type of renal pathology can be obtained if urine osmolality is compared to serum osmolality and if urine electrolyte studies are performed. Normally the ratio of urine osmolality to serum osmolality is between 1.0 and 3.0. In acute tubular dysfunction (including necrosis) and in chronic renal insufficiency the U/P osmol ratio is equal to or less than 1.2 and the urinary Na^+ is greater than 20 mEq/l (mmol/l) (Levinsky, 1976). In diseases in which the GFR is primarily impaired (e.g., congestive heart failure, acute glomerulonephritis, acute obstructive uropathy), the U/P ratio is greater than 1.2 and the urinary Na^+ is less than 20 mEq/l (mmol/l) (Levinsky, 1976).

The U/P osmol ratio can also be useful in differentiating among etiologies of polyuria. The U/P osmol ratio is always greater than 1 in osmotic diuresis and less than 1 in water diuresis. In idiopathic or nephrogenic diabetes insipidus, the ratio is less than 1 and remains unchanged even with water deprivation. In contrast, in psychogenic diabetes insipidus, the ratio increases with fluid restriction (Utiger, 1969).

Free water clearance

The U/P osmol ratio can be expressed as a clearance value by multiplying by the urinary volume (V). This clearance value is the osmol clearance (C_{osmol}).

$$C_{osmol} = \frac{U_{osmol} \times V}{P_{osmol}}$$

The osmol clearance is a measure of the amount of water that is cleared from the plasma, resulting in urine that has the same osmolality as plasma. A different measure of the dilution or concentrating ability of the renal tubules can be obtained by comparing this value to the total amount of urine formed.

The difference between the total urine volume and osmol clearance is called the free water clearance (C_{H_2O}).

$$C_{H_2O} = V - C_{osmol}$$

If the value is positive, this indicates that the urine is dilute compared with serum (i.e., hyposthenuria), and conversely, if the value is negative, this indicates that the urine is more concentrated than serum (i.e., hypersthenuria). If there is no net difference, then a urine isosmotic with plasma is being produced (i.e., isosthenuria) and no work is being done by the tubules either to concentrate or to dilute the ultrafiltrate.

Urinary specific gravity, osmolalities, and free water clearance values can all be measured after restricting fluids (concentration tests) or after fluid overloading (dilution tests). These provocative tests, performed under controlled conditions, can yield more sensitive information in the presence of minimal or early renal disease.

Cryoscopy

The most convenient method to measure osmolality in the clinical laboratory is to measure the freezing point depression of a solution using a cryoscope (see Chap. 4, p. 98). Serum or heparinized plasma may be used, but plasma anticoagulated with chelating or precipitating agents is unsuitable. Urine is centrifuged to remove all large particulate matter. The solution is supercooled (i.e., cooled below its freezing point) in an insulated freezing bath and then crystallized, using a vibrator which agitates the solution. As crystallization occurs, heat of fusion is produced and the temperature of the solution increases, reaching a plateau which is slightly below the freezing point. This temperature is compared with plateau temperatures obtained with known standards; therefore, no correction is necessary. A thermistor, Wheatstone bridge, and galvanometer convert the temperature changes into osmolality values in mosmol/kg H_2O. An alternative method for measuring osmolality is to measure vapor pressure depression. Instrumentation for this purpose is now available in the routine chemistry laboratory (Wescor, Inc., Logan, Utah 84321).

WATER BALANCE

Water constitutes approximately 70 per cent (50 liters) of the total body weight in an average adult male (70 kg). This percentage decreases to 60 per cent in the average adult female owing to the fact that women have more subcutaneous fat which contains less water than does non-fatty tissue. Similarly, overweight individuals have a decreased proportion of their weight composed of water. Two thirds of the body water is intracellular (ICF), with the remaining one third being extracellular (ECF). Three fourths of ECF is within the tissues proper and is called interstitial fluid. The rest of the ECF is contained within the vascular spaces and constitutes the aqueous portion of the plasma.

In non-disease states, the body loses in excess of 2400 ml of H_2O per day (Koushanpour, 1976), with 1500 ml being lost as urine because of the necessity of eliminating metabolic waste solute molecules in solution. An additional 800 ml is lost as insensible or non-visible evaporation from the lungs, owing to the formation of water vapor in the lungs and tracheobronchial tree and from the skin surfaces. A further 100 ml is lost in the stool. Fluid losses are replaced by eating and drinking. Oxidation of solid food supplies approximately 300 ml of H_2O per day and the remainder of the fluid losses are replaced, and generally exceeded, by the ingestion of liquid.

Water balance is controlled by the same mechanisms that are responsible for the constancy of the tonicity of the ECF. These are (1) the effect of ADH on the collecting tubules, (2) the renin-angiotensin-aldosterone system, and (3) the thirst center. The first two mechanisms have been discussed previously in this chapter. The thirst center is located in the hypothalamus and is stimulated by either an increased osmotic pressure in the interstitial fluid or a decreased ECF volume via adjacent osmoreceptors and possibly centers that are stimulated by angiotensin (Ganong, 1975c).

If losses exceed replacement, dehydration or hypovolemia develops. Sodium (Na^+) is usually lost with water, but the relative amount may vary depending on the Na^+ content of the fluid lost. The most common causes of volume depletion are vomiting, diarrhea, surgical drainage, internal pooling of the fluids (e.g., peritonitis, ileus), renal disease, diuretic administration, and hypoadrenocorticism (i.e., Addison's disease).

There are *no* laboratory measurements that can quantitate the amount of fluid loss. It must be remembered that concentration measurements are relative measurements (i.e., comparison of amounts of substances in specific volumes of fluid). The hematocrit and serum protein concentrations rise, and these changes may be helpful in estimating a change in plasma volume. Blood urea nitrogen (BUN) is usually increased to a greater extent than the serum creatinine, the U/P osmol ratio is greater than 1, and the urine Na^+ concentrations less than 20 mEq/l (mmol/l) except in Addison's disease and renal diseases in which there is Na^+ loss. Treatment consists of administration of appropriate fluids to correct both fluid and electrolyte losses.

The opposite situation, an increase in total body H_2O or volume overload, is associated with an increase in total body water. This occurs in cardiac failure and in conditions associated with hypoalbuminemia such as cirrhosis or the nephrotic syndrome. The common denominators in all of these conditions are decreased renal blood flow and renal congestion. The net result is an increase in aldosterone production and Na^+ and H_2O retention. As a result of impaired hemodynamics, this fluid is retained in the interstitial spaces, resulting in edema, ascites, and pleural effusions.

For the reason discussed above, there is *no* practical laboratory measurement to quantitate the amount of overhydration. Treatment is directed at correcting the underlying pathology and is aided in some cases by the use of diuretics.

ELECTROLYTES AND ELECTROLYTIC BALANCE

Electrolytes are free ions that exist in body fluids. In the ECF, the major cations are Na^+ and K^+ and the major anions are Cl^- and HCO_3^-. All metabolic events are affected to some degree by the relative and absolute concentrations of these electrolytes, which are important determinants of osmolality, state of hydration, and pH of both ICF and ECF. In addition, membrane potentials and normal functioning of nervous tissue and muscle are regulated by the concentration differences between ICF and ECF electrolytes. Electrolyte concentrations, formerly expressed as milliequivalents/liter (mEq/l) are now expressed in S.I. units. In the S.I. units of measurement, the units are millimoles/liter or mmol/l (Lehmann, 1976). Since 1 mEq is equal to 1 mmol for monovalent ions, the numerical values for the four major electrolytes are the same using either system of units.

SODIUM

Na^+ is the major cation present in the ECF. Serum sodium concentration varies between 135 and 148 mmol/l in healthy individuals. The normal daily intake of Na^+ is 100 to 250 mmol. If serum sodium concentration levels exceed 110 to 130 mmol/l, which is the normal situation, Na^+ is excreted into the urine. The normal Na^+ level in urine varies from 30 to 280 mmol/day. If the sodium intake is less than 30 mmol/day and/or the sodium concentration decreases to less than 110 mmol/l, all of the Na^+ in the urinary ultrafiltrate is reabsorbed by the tubules, as discussed previously.

Hyponatremia, or low serum Na^+, can be found in a variety of unrelated conditions. It can occur with sodium (solute) loss or water (solvent) excess. Excess Na^+ loss relative to water loss can occur in the following disease states: (1) diarrhea, (2) nephrosis, (3) Addison's disease, (4) metabolic acidosis with excretion of cations with increased anions, (5) diuretic therapy, and (6) polyuric states. If the water and salt losses are replaced with water alone, a dilutional hyponatremia develops. If excess water is administered to a patient who is not able to excrete a water load (e.g., renal disease), water intoxication may develop as a result of the decreased osmotic pressure of the ECF. The central nervous system symptomatology in this syndrome is a result of the increase of ICF in the neurons. Hyponatremia also occurs in conditions in which there is an increase in total body water, or hypervolemia. Although the amount of total body Na^+ is increased in these diseases, the ratio (Na/H_2O) is not as great as the amount of water retained in the body.

Hyponatremia is also a component of the syndrome of inappropriate ADH secretion, or the Schwartz-Bartter syndrome. The hyponatremia is due to H_2O retention secondary to a continuous secretion of ADH which is not related to serum osmolality. Other laboratory parameters of this syndrome are (1) decreased serum osmolality, (2) U/P osmol ratio greater than 1, and (3) urinary Na^+ more than 25 mmol/l. Clinically, there is absence of peripheral edema or of volume depletion. This syndrome is encountered in malignancies, inflammatory lung disease. CNS diseases, and following various drug therapies, including anticancer agents and thiazide diuretics (Streeten, 1974) (see Chap. 14).

Artifactual hyponatremia is encountered in the laboratory in two situations. Hyperglycemia may result in an increase in serum osmolality, with a subsequent shift of ICF to the ECF, decreasing ECF solute concentration. A blood glucose of 180 mg/dl may cause an artifactual decrease of the serum sodium concentration of 5 mmol/l (Costrini, 1977). Hyponatremia is also found in lactescent specimens containing high levels of triglycerides. This is a result of the restriction of Na^+ to the aqueous phase only and therefore the serum (aqueous plus lipid phases) Na^+ concentration is correspondingly less. Actual or true Na^+ values can be found by redrawing the serum after fasting, by using non-polar solvents to extract the lipids, or by using an ultracentrifuge to separate the aqueous from lipid phases (Steffes, 1976).

Hypernatremia, or elevated serum Na^+, is seen in those conditions in which water is lost in excess of salt (e.g., profuse sweating, prolonged hyperpnea, diarrhea, renal disease, and polyuric states). Hypernatremia may also result from lack of sufficient water intake owing to lack of an adequate thirst mechanism (e.g., coma, hypothalmic disease). High Na^+ levels are also encountered in Cushing's disease and in hyperaldosteronism.

Treatment of these conditions is directed at correction of the electrolyte imbalance (and tonicity), taking into consideration the state of hydration and the cause(s) for the deviated Na^+ values.

POTASSIUM

K^+ is the major intracellular cation, with only 2 per cent of the total body potassium being extracellular. The diet normally contains 50 to 150 mmol K^+/day. Kidneys usually excrete 80 to 90 per cent of the ingested K^+, regulating the ECF concentration. Expected serum potassium concentration is 3.8 to 5.5 mmol/l. Unlike Na^+, however, there is no renal threshold for K^+, and it continues to be excreted into the urine even in K^+ depleted states. In normal subjects, daily urinary excretion is 25 to 120 mmol.

Hypokalemia, or depressed serum K^+, occurs with gastrointestinal fluid losses (e.g., vomiting, diarrhea), in renal diseases, with diuretic administration, in mineralocorticoid excess (e.g., Cushing's disease, hyperaldosteronism), and in alkalemia. The hypokalemia associated with alkalemia is due to the exchange of ECF K^+ for intracellular H^+ and the increased exchange of K^+ (attributed to the lack of renal tubular cell H^+) for Na^+ in the distal convoluted tubules.

Hyperkalemia, or elevated serum K^+ concentration, is seen in acute and sometimes in chronic renal diseases, in renal tubular acidosis in which the exchange of Na^+ for K^+ and/or H^+ is impaired, and in extensive tissue injury with release of intracellular K^+ into the ECF, and in acidotic states.

Artifactual hyperkalemia may be encountered in disease states in which the platelet count is elevated (Weissman, 1974). As clotting occurs in the test tube, intraplatelet K^+ is released and measured in the serum. In these cases heparinized plasma can be used for K^+ determination. False high potassium values are also seen if a tourniquet is left on too long with juxtavenular cellular injury and leakage of K^+ into the plasma (Skinner, 1961). This effect is markedly enhanced if the fist is repeatedly clenched prior to and during drawing. A hemolyzed specimen will yield an elevated value owing to the high concentration of K^+ within erythrocytes (105 mmol/l).

Elevated and depressed serum potassium concentrations may have profound adverse effects on the neuromuscular system (apathy, weakness, paralysis) and especially on the myocardium. Serious arrhythmias can develop and death ensue. Hypokalemia is treated by parenteral and/or non-parenteral administration of K^+. Depending on the acuteness or seriousness of the situation, hyperkalemia is treated by Ca^{++} infusion, which antagonizes the effect of K^+ on cardiac tissue; by $NaHCO_3$ infusion, which causes the movement of K^+ into cells; by glucose infusion, which stimulates insulin production with resultant intracellular sequestration of glucose and K^+; by renal dialysis; by oral or rectal administration of resins which bind K^+ (removing it from the ECF); and by use of diuretics.

Measurement of Na^+ and K^+

The most frequently used means to measure Na^+ and K^+ in the clinical laboratory is *emission photometry* (Chap. 4). Na^+ and K^+, both being alkali metals, are easily excited in a low-temperature flame. As their electrons return to their normal stable shells, characteristic photons are given off which can be isolated by separate monochrometers and the intensities of the radiation quantitated by photomultiplier tubes connected to Wheatstone bridge circuitries (Chap. 4). In order for the intensity of the emitted photons to be proportional to the number of atoms in the flame, the flame temperature has to be held constant. This is accomplished directly by the use of pressure regulators on the gas lines and indirectly by the use of the internal standard, lithium (Li^+), which is added to the specimen in a diluent. Li^+ is also an alkali metal and the ratio of Na^+/Li^+ and K^+/Li^+ emission intensities are determined electronically. If a small fluctuation in flame temperature exists, the ratios will remain virtually constant and thus be accurate indicators of Na^+ and K^+ concentrations in the sample. Li^+ also acts as a "radiation buffer": being present in high concentrations, it prevents the proportional mutual excitation of K^+ by different concentrations of Na^+ in the samples and in the standards.

Na^+ and K^+ can also be measured by atomic absorption, but it is not necessary to use this more complex instrumentation owing to the fact that such a large proportion of these alkali atoms is excited and emits light in a flame (Sunderman, 1976).

Ion-specific electrodes have been developed for Na^+ and K^+ activity measurements in the clinical laboratory, and some have been adapted to automated systems. The most practical Na^+ electrode is made of a specialized glass which is highly selective for Na^+. A liquid ion-exchange membrane electrode using the antibiotic valinomycin as the K^+ binder is the most selective for K^+. As technology continues to develop in this area, these electrodes will likely become more commonplace in the laboratory.

CHLORIDE

Cl^- is the major extracellular anion. Most of the ingested chloride is absorbed and the excess excreted along with cations into the urine. The normal serum concentration is 98 to 106 mmol/l. Slightly lower values are encountered if the serum sample is drawn soon after eating; this is a result of the increased synthesis of hydrochloric acid (HCl) by the parietal cells of the stomach. The daily urinary output of chloride is 110 to 250 mmol.

Low serum Cl^- values are observed in prolonged vomiting with loss of HCl, in metabolic acidotic states in which there is an increased accumulation of organic anions (see below under Anion Gap), in Addisonian crises, and in salt-losing renal diseases.

Elevated serum Cl^- values are seen in metabolic acidosis associated with prolonged diarrhea with loss of $NaHCO_3$ and in renal tubular diseases in which there is a decreased excretion of H^+ and therefore a decreased reabsorption of HCO_3^-. Elevated serum chloride values have been reported in some cases of hyperparathyroidism (Wells, 1971). This may be due to the effect of parathormone on renal tubular reabsorption of HCO_3^-.

Measurement of Cl^- concentration in sweat is useful in the diagnosis of the exocrine glandular disorder, cystic fibrosis. In these patients, the secretion of Cl^- in sweat is increased to two to five times reference values. The Cl^- concentration in non-diseased individuals is 5 to 35 mmol/l, while in affected infants after the age of 1 month, the concentration is 60 to 160 mmol/l (di Sant' Agnese, 1967). The patient is induced to sweat, usually by iontophoresis (the introduction of pilocarpine into the skin by electrical stimulation). Sweat is collected and weighed, and the Cl^- concentration measured. Sweat Cl^- concentrations in the cystic fibrosis range have been reported also in patients with Addison's disease (di Sant' Agnese, 1967). False normal values may be observed if affected patients are deficient in electrolytes, which can occur after prolonged or profuse sweating (see Chap. 23).

Measurement of chloride

Cl^- is measured by mercurimetric titration, by coulometric-amperometric titration, by colorimetry using $Hg(SCN)_2$, and by the use of ion-specific electrodes.

In the mercurimetric method, Cl^- combines with added Hg^{++} to form the soluble complex $HgCl_2$. Excess added Hg^{++} combines with the indicator, diphenylcarbazone, to form a blue color which is the endpoint of the titration.

In the coulometric-amperometric titration, two separate electrical circuits are involved: a coulometric circuit that generates Ag^+ and an amperometric indicator circuit (Chap. 4). As silver ions (Ag^+) are generated, they combine with Cl^- in the sample to form AgCl; when the Cl^- is exhausted, free Ag^+ creates an increased current between the indicator electrodes, which is able by a relay circuit to stop the generation of Ag^+ and also a stop clock. The time registered is proportional to the

crease in pH instead of a large one. The blood buffers in descending order of importance are (1) bicarbonate/carbonic acid, (2) hemoglobin, (3) plasma proteins, and (4) erythrocyte and plasma phosphate. The bicarbonate/carbonic acid equilibrium ($H_2O + CO_2 \rightleftarrows H_2CO_3 \rightleftarrows H^+ + HCO_3^-$) can be conveniently expressed as the derived Henderson-Hasselbalch equation:

$$pH = pK_a + \log \frac{[HCO_3^-]}{[H_2CO_3]}$$

pH is the negative logarithm of the hydrogen ion concentration and pK_a is the negative dissociation constant, K_a, of H_2CO_3. The pK' of normal plasma at 37°C. is 6.1.* The pK' varies inversely with both pH and ionic strength and directly with temperature (Severinghaus, 1956). This equation can also be expressed as

$$pH = pK_a' + \log \frac{[total\ CO_2] - 0.03\ Pco_2}{0.03\ Pco_2}$$

In normal plasma, 0.03 is the solubility coefficient (α) of CO_2 gas at 37°C. This value (0.03) times the Pco_2 is equivalent to the small amount of H_2CO_3 found in plasma. The solubility coefficient varies inversely with temperature and/or concentration of salt or protein and varies directly with lipid concentration (Tietz, 1976). The product, $0.03 \times Pco_2$, subtracted from the total CO_2 value is a close approximation of the HCO_3^-. Although the pK_a' of this buffer system is low (6.1) compared with the pH of plasma (7.4), it is an extremely effective buffer because the ratio of base to acid is finely regulated by respiration.

Hemoglobin is the second most important blood buffer owing to the fact that each hemoglobin molecule contains 38 histidine residues that are able to bind with H^+ and owing to the high concentration of hemoglobin (15 g/dl) (Ganong, 1975b).

Plasma proteins act as buffers because both their free carboxyl and amino groups are able to bind H^+.

Least important is the buffering capacity of the inorganic and organic phosphates present in blood. At a pH of 7.4, the $HPO_4^=/H_2PO_4^-$ ratio is 80/20 or 4/1.

The sum of all blood buffers is called the buffer base. The reference values are between 46 and 52 mmol/l, with an average value of 49 mmol/l. If this average value is subtracted from the actual buffer base, base excess is derived. The reference interval for base excess is ±3.0 mmol/l. A negative base excess, or

decrease in blood buffering capacity, is sometimes referred to as base deficit.

Although the blood buffers act instantaneously to minimize the change in pH, their capacity to do so is limited. Ultimate regulation of acid-base balance, together with the regeneration of free buffers, is a function of the renal tubular cells (de Wardener, 1973). Normally, 85 to 99 per cent of the filtered HCO_3^- is reabsorbed by the proximal tubular cells. CO_2 present in the cells as a result of cellular metabolism and diffusion from the blood and urine binds with H_2O in a reaction catalyzed by carbonic anhydrase to make H_2CO_3. This dissociates to form HCO_3^-, which is absorbed into the microcirculation along with Na^+, and H^+, which is excreted into the lumen. The H^+ combines with the filtered HCO_3^- to produce H_2CO_3, which is broken down to CO_2 and H_2O in the presence of carbonic anhydrase, present on the surface of the epithelial brush border. CO_2 diffuses into the tubular cell and the cycle continues. The net effect is the indirect reabsorption of urinary HCO_3^-, with the generated tubular HCO_3^- actually being absorbed into the circulation. At plasma concentrations below 25 mmol/l, the process is virtually complete; if the levels are greater than this, HCO_3^- is excreted into the urine.

In the distal convoluted tubules, the H^+ that is generated by the cells is actively exchanged for Na^+. However, if the luminal hydrogen ion concentration increases with a decrease of pH to 4.5, the gradient is such that no further secretion of H^+ can take place. This extreme pH, however, is not usually seen, owing to the buffering capacity of the filtered $HPO_4^=$ and the secreted NH_3. Dibasic phosphate ($HPO_4^=$) combines with H^+ to form monobasic phosphate ($H_2PO_4^-$). At the pH extreme of 4.5, the ratio of $HPO_4^=/H_2PO_4^-$ is 1/100 with up to 10 to 30 mmol of H^+ excreted per day (Pitts, 1945). This is referred to as titratable acidity. NH_3 is produced in the distal tubular cells from deamination of glutamine by glutaminase. The NH_3 combines with H^+ in the urine to form NH_4^+, with the elimination of 30 to 50 mmol of H^+ per day (Pitts, 1945). The mechanisms of respiration which control the Pco_2 and therefore the H_2CO_3 concentration are discussed in Chapter 5.

Acidemia. Acidemia is defined as a blood pH of less than 7.35. It can result from the accumulation of CO_2 in the body. This is called respiratory acidosis because it is due to a failure of pulmonary ventilation. The term *acido-*

---

*pK' refers to the pK_a for given conditions (i.e., pH, ionic strength, temperature, etc.).

sis is used to signify the altered physiologic state resulting in acidemia. The kidney, by reabsorbing base and secreting fixed acids, is able to compensate for the lowering of pH, the degree of compensation depending on the chronicity of the ventilatory insufficiency and the function of the renal tubules. This is reflected by an increase in total CO_2 and in buffer base, and a positive base excess. Etiologies are discussed in Chapter 5.

Acidemia can also occur from an accumulation of fixed acids or a decrease in base (e.g., HCO_3^-). This results in a primary decrease in total CO_2 and buffer base and a negative base excess (base deficit). This is referred to as metabolic acidosis. Clinically, metabolic acidosis can be divided into two types: acidemia with an increased anion gap (>17 mEq/l) and acidemia with a normal anion gap (≤ 17 mEq/l) or hyperchloremic metabolic acidosis. Causes of an increased anion gap have been noted previously (p. 148). Hyperchloremic acidemia can result from the ingestion of ammonium chloride but is most commonly seen in severe diarrhea (or enteric fistulae) with loss of HCO_3^- or in inherited or acquired (e.g., hypokalemia, drug-induced carbonic anhydrase inhibition) renal tubular defect in which HCO_3^- is not able to be reabsorbed from the urine. This is called renal tubular acidosis. The rate and depth of respiration is increased, with the degree of compensation dependent on the adequacy of respiratory function. Treatment is directed at correction of the underlying disease process(es), with administration of HCO_3^- to acutely ill and symptomatic patients and simultaneous correction of existing electrolyte and fluid imbalance.

Alkalemia. Alkalemia is defined as a blood pH greater than 7.45. Alkalemia can occur as a result of a decreased PCO_2 concentration in the blood. This is called respiratory alkalosis because it is secondary to hyperventilation. The term *alkalosis* is used to signify the altered physiologic state resulting in alkalemia. The kidney is able to compensate to varying degrees depending on the chronicity of the alkalemia by decreasing the secretion of fixed acids and the reabsorption of HCO_3^-. Correspondingly, the total CO_2, buffer base, and base excess are decreased. Etiologies are discussed in Chapter 5.

Alkalemia also occurs when there is a loss of fixed acids or an increase in blood alkali (e.g., HCO_3^-). There is therefore a primary increase in total CO_2, buffer base, and base excess. This is called metabolic alkalosis. Loss of fixed acid is most often due to prolonged vomiting or to nasogastric suctioning. Alkali excess can occur in excessive ingestion of basic substances such as antacids. Metabolic alkalosis can also occur in disease states in which there is excessive intracellular accumulation of H^+ and/or excess excretion of H^+ into the urine. This occurs in the mineralocorticoid excess syndromes (e.g., hyperaldosteronism, Cushing's syndrome, prolonged administration of corticosteroids) and in hypokalemia. Respiratory rate decreases in metabolic alkalosis with a compensatory increase in PCO_2. Treatment, as in all acid-base imbalances, is directed toward the correction of the underlying disease process(es) with the replacement of K^+ deficits with KCl and correction of fluid imbalances.

Laboratory Measurement of Acid-base Parameters. In order to evaluate the acid-base status of the patient and to both identify and quantitate any causes (i.e., metabolic, respiratory, or both) responsible for the imbalances that may exist, it is necessary to determine, besides pH, one or more of the following parameters: (1) total CO_2, (2) PCO_2, (3) base excess, or (4) buffer base.

The arteriovenous pH difference is extremely small (0.01 to 0.03), except in patients in congestive heart failure and in shock (Gambino, 1959). This small change is due to the fact that the increased CO_2 concentration of venous blood is balanced by the increased buffering capacity of deoxygenated or reduced hemoglobin. Total CO_2 values average 5 to 7 mm Hg higher in venous blood than in arterial blood. Both arterial and venous blood can be used to determine these acid-base parameters even in severe respiratory disease (Fleischer, 1972). It is necessary, though, that the skin of the arm and hand be warm, that the tourniquet not be applied too tightly or for too long, and that the fist not be repeatedly clenched prior to and during the drawing of the blood sample (Gambino, 1959). Arterial blood, however, has to be used to accurately measure PO_2 and oxygen saturation (SO_2) (Fleischer, 1972). Capillary blood can be "arterialized" by warming a fingertip, earlobe, heel, or toe, with measurement of the blood gases unaffected by local metabolism.

Only heparinized blood is used for PCO_2 and PO_2 measurements. Heparinized blood and plasma and serum can be used for pH determination. Heparin is the anticoagulant of choice, since it does not cause a shift of electrolytes and water between plasma and blood cells and does not cause a change in pH as do the other anticoagulants (i.e., oxalate, citrate, or EDTA) (Gambino, 1959).

If serum is used, it is necessary that the separation from the clot or from the cells be done at body temperature. If the separation occurs at a lower temperature, an alkaline error will result owing to the fact that the change in pH/°C. is greater for whole blood (0.0147 to 0.0150 pH/°C.) than for plasma or serum (0.0110 to 0.0120 pH/°C.) (Hamilton, 1970). In other words, the pH of blood will increase when blood is cooled below 37°C.; and if serum or plasma is obtained and then warmed to 37°C., there will be a drop in the pH. However, it will not decrease to what it was in the whole blood sample. In actuality, the measured pH of whole blood is approximately 0.01 unit lower than the pH of plasma (or serum) separated at body temperature owing to the effects of the red cells on the liquid junction potential of the glass electrode (Severinghaus, 1956).

The pH is determined directly in the laboratory by a glass electrode (Chap. 5).

Pco_2 can be determined indirectly from the Henderson-Hasselbalch equation if the pH and total CO_2 are known, from various nomograms, or by interpolation (Astrup method) using a Siggaard-Anderson Curve Nomogram. In this latter method, gases with known Pco_2 are equilibrated with the sample and the corresponding pH's determined. The actual pH of the unequilibrated sample is also determined and the Pco_2 is interpolated from the line connecting the two derived points.

The direct measurement of CO_2, however, is preferable in that it is much simpler and less time-consuming. The Pco_2 electrode, a modified pH electrode, is described in Chapter 5.

Base excess and buffer base can be derived from nomograms (e.g., Siggaard-Anderson) or can be read directly from some gas instruments having computer capabilities (Astrup, 1960; Siggaard-Andersen, 1976).

REFERENCES

Astrup, P., Siggaard-Andersen, O., Jørgensen, K., and Engel, K.: The acid-base metabolism—a new approach. Lancet, *1*:1035, 1960.

Berliner, R. W. (ed.): Renal excretion. *In* Best and Taylor's Physiological Basis of Medical Practice, 9th ed. Baltimore, The Williams and Wilkins, Co., 1973, vol. 5, p. 14.

Cannon, D. C.: Kidney function tests. *In* Henry, R., Jr. (ed.): Clinical Chemistry—Principles and Technics, 2nd ed. Hagerstown, Md, Harper and Row, Publishers, Inc., 1974, pp. 1548–1551.

Costrini, W. V., and Thompson, W. M.: Fluid and Electrolyte Disturbances. *In* Manual of Medical Therapeutics, 22nd ed. Boston, Little, Brown and Co., 1977, p. 34.

De Wardener, H. E.: Tubular Function and Tests of Tubular Functional Integrity. *In* The Kidney, An Outline of Normal and Abnormal Structure and Function, 4th ed. Edinburgh, Churchill Livingstone, 1973, pp. 68–81.

di Sant' Angnese, P. A., and Lalamo, R.C.: Pathogenesis and pathophysiology of cystic fibrosis of the pancreas. N. Engl. J. Med., *277*:1287. 1967.

Driscoll, J. L., and Martin, H. F.: Detection of brominism by automated chloride method. Clin. Chem., *12*:314, 1966.

Faulkner, W. R., and King, J. W.: Renal function. *In* Tietz, N. W.: Fundamentals of Clinical Chemistry, 2nd ed. Philadelphia, W. B. Saunders Company, 1976, p. 985.

Faulkner, W. R., and Martin, H. F.: Detection of brominism by automated chloride method. Clin. Chem., *12*:989, 1966.

Fleischer, W., and Gambino, S. R.: Blood, pH, PO_2, and oxygen saturation. ASCP Commission on Continuing Education, Council on Clinical Chemistry, 1972, pp. 11–50.

Gambino, S. R.: Heparinized vacuum tubes for determination of plasma pH, plasma CO_2 content, and blood oxygen saturation. Am. J. Clin. Pathol., *32*:285, 1959a.

Gambino, S. R.: Normal values for adult human venous plasma pH and pCO_2 content Am. J. Clin. Pathol., *32*:294, 1959b.

Gambino, S. R., and Schreiber, H.: The measurement of CO_2 content with the AutoAnalyzer. Am. J. Clin. Pathol., *45*:406, 1966.

Ganong, W. F.: Formation and excretion of urine. *In* Review of Medical Physiology, 7th ed. Los Gatos, Cal., Lange Medical Publications,1975a, pp. 514–536.

Ganong, W. F.: Gas transport between lungs and tissues. *In* Review of Medical Physiology, 7th ed. Los Gatos, Cal., Lange Medical Publications, 1975b, pp. 489–490.

Ganong, W. F.: Neural centers regulating visceral function. *In* Review of Medical Physiology, 7th ed. Los Gatos, Cal., Lange Medical Publications, 1975c, p. 163.

Hamilton, L. H.: Respiratory and blood gas analysis. *In* Progress in Clinical Pathology, vol. II. New York, Grune & Stratton, Inc., 1970, pp. 284–319.

Holmes, J. H.: Measurement of osmolality in serum, urine, and other biological fluids by the freezing point determination. *In* Workshop Manual on Urinalysis and Renal Function Studies. ASCP—Commission on Continuing Education, 1962.

Kokko, J.: The role of the renal concentrating mechanisms in the regulation of serum sodium concentration. Am. J. Med., *62*:165, 1977.

Koushanpour, E.: Renal Physiology: Principles and Functions. Philadelphia, W. B. Saunders, Company, 1976, pp. 35–39.

Kramer, H. J., and Burgard, U. G.: Further studies on epithelial transport defect in experimental and human Fanconi syndrome. Clin. Chim. Acta, *55*:57, 1974.

Lam, C. W. K., and Tan, I. K.: Evaluation of the Harleco micro CO_2 system for measurement of total CO_2 in serum or plasma. Clin. Chem., *24*:143, 1978.

Lehmann, H. P.: Metrication of clinical laboratory data in SI units. Am. J. Clin. Pathol., *65*:2, 1976.

Levinsky, N. G., and Alexander, E. A.: Acute renal failure *In* Brenner, B. M., and Rector, F. C. (eds.): The Kidney. Philadelphia, W. B. Saunders Company, 1976, p. 809.

Pitts, R. F.: The renal regulation of acid-base balance with special reference to the mechanism for acidifying the urine. Science, *102*:81, 1945.

Renkin, E., and Robinson, R.: Glomerular filtration in physiology in medicine. N. Engl. J. Med., *290*:785, 1974.

Schwartz, A. B.: Differential diagnosis of metabolic acidosis using anion gap. *In* Schwartz, A. B., and Lyons, H. (eds.): Acid-Base and Electrolyte Balance. New York, Grune & Stratton, Inc., 1977, pp. 23-38.

Severinghaus, J. W.: Variations of serum carbonic acid pK with pH and temperature. J. Appl. Physiol., *9*:197, 1956.

Severinghaus, J. W., and Bradley, A. F.: Accuracy of blood pH and pCO$_2$ determinations. J. Appl. Physiol. *9*:189, 1956.

Siggard-Anderson, O.: The Acid-Base Status of the Blood, 3rd ed., Baltimore, William & Wilkins Co., 1976.

Skinner, S. L.: Cause of erroneous potassium levels. Lancet, *1*:478, 1961.

Smith, H. W.: Clearances involving tubular excretion. *In* The Kidney—Structure and Function in Health and Disease. New York, Oxford University Press, 1951, pp. 182-194.

Smithline, N., and Gardner, K. D.: Gaps—Anionic and Osmolal. J.A.M.A., *236*:1594, 1976.

Steffes, M. W., and Frier, E. F.: A simple and precise method of determining true sodium, potassium and chloride concentrations in hyperlipemia. J. Lab. Clin. Med., *88*:683, 1976.

Streeten, D. H. P., et al.: Disorders of the neurohypophysis *In* Harrison's Principles of Internal Medicine, 8th ed. New York, McGraw-Hill Book Company, 1974, pp. 498-500.

Sunderman, F. W., Sr., and Sunderman, F. W. Jr.: Survey of methods for analysis of sodium and potassium. Proficiency Test Service—Institute for Clinical Science, September, 1976. p. 4.

Tietz, N. W.: Blood gases and electrolytes. *In* Tietz, N. W.: Fundamentals of Clinical Chemistry, 2nd ed. Philadelphia, W. B. Saunders Company, 1976.

Tobias, G. J., et al.: Endogenous creatinine clearance. N. Engl. J. Med., *266*:317, 1962.

Utiger, R.: Diabetes insipidus. J.A.M.A., *207*:1699, 1969.

Valtin, H.: Renal Function: Mechanisms Preserving Fluid and Solute Balance in Health. Boston, Little, Brown and Co., 1973, p. 149.

Wallin, J. D.: The Kidney and the Urine. *In* Review of Physiological Chemistry, 16th ed. Los Gatos, Cal., Lange Medical Publications, 1977. pp. 609-632.

Weisberg, H. F.: Osmolality, Clinical Chemistry Check Sample No. CC71 (Critique). ASCP—Commission on Continuing Education, 1971, pp. 25-28.

Weissman, N., and Pileggi, V. J.: Inorganic ions. *In* Henry, R. J., et al. (eds.): Clinical Chemistry, Principles and Technics, 2nd ed. Hagerstown, Md., Harper and Row, Publishers, Inc., 1974, p. 645.

Wells, M. R.: Value of plasma chloride concentration and acid-base status in the differential diagnosis of hyperparathyroidism from other causes of hypercalcemia. J. Clin. Pathol. *24*:219, 1971.

7

CARBOHYDRATES

Peter J. Howanitz, M.D., and Joan H. Howanitz, M.D.

Starches, which are widespread in nature and serve as reserve food for plants, are the major carbohydrate source for humans. About 50 to 90 per cent of the carbohydrates consumed come from grain, vegetables, and legumes such as rice, wheat, corn, and potatoes, where they are in the form of starch. Other important sources of carbohydrates include fruits, which are high in glucose, fructose, and pentoses; milk and milk products, which contain lactose; and cane and sugar beets, which are the chief source of sucrose. Animal sources of carbohydrates are negligible, since they contain less than 1 per cent glycogen. These various carbohydrates, when ingested, are all interconverted to glucose, which is the predominant carbohydrate fuel.

CLASSIFICATION OF CARBOHYDRATES

Carbohydrates are all compounds of carbon, hydrogen, and oxygen, generally with the hydrogen and oxygen present in a proportion of two hydrogen atoms to one oxygen atom, as in water. These "carbohydrates" (carbon hydrates) have the general molecular formula $C_n(H_2O)_n$. Those carbohydrates that cannot be hydrolyzed into "simpler compounds" are called simple sugars or "monosaccharides." The presence of an aldehyde or ketone group and the number of carbon atoms are the basis of the nomenclature. Some of the important monosaccharides are as follows:

NUMBER OF CARBONS	GENERIC NAME	FORMULA	ALDEHYDE	KETONE
3	(Triose)	$C_3H_6O_3$	Glyceraldehyde	Dihydroxyacetone
4	(Tetrose)	$C_4H_8O_4$	Erythrose	Erythrulose
5	(Pentose)	$C_5H_{10}O_5$	Ribose	Ribulose
6	(Hexose)	$C_6H_{12}O_6$	Glucose	Fructose
7	(Heptose)	$C_7H_{14}O_7$		Sedoheptulose

Many carbohydrates contain the same number of atoms and the same kind of groups, yet they are distinctly different. For example, the formula $C_6H_{12}O_6$ may be represented in 16 different ways, since there are four different asymmetric carbon atoms. These spatial arrangements of groups on the carbon atoms result in *stereoisomers*; the arrangement of the end carbon atom is not significant.

Of all other monosaccharides, the hexoses are the most important physiologically. The structures of the three most important aldoses and the ketose fructose are shown in *A* at the bottom of the page.

If the OH group on the carbon next to the last (in the case of hexose, carbon 5) is on the right, by convention this is called a D sugar, while those with the OH on the left are L sugars. The majority of sugars in the body are of the D configuration.

Since carbohydrates contain both aldehyde and alcohol groups, they can react to form hemiacetals. In the case of glucose, the aldehyde group reacts with the hydroxyl carbon in position 5, as pictured below, to form a six-membered ring form (pyra-

nose). If the hydroxyl on carbon 1 is written to the right, it is then called α, while if it is on the left, it is in the β configuration. This is noted by the amount of optical rotation of the two different forms. In solution, about two-thirds of glucose exists in the α form, one-third is in the β form, and the chain form is present only in trace amounts (see *B* at bottom of page).

With fructose, two rings are formed, a six-membered ring (pyranose) and a five-membered ring (furanose) (see *C* at bottom of page).

Haworth proposed that the ring structures more accurately represent the actual configuration of sugars than do other configurations. When using these structures, it is customary to leave out the carbon atoms. In the D series, a terminal primary alcohol group CH_2OH projects above the plane of the ring, while in the L series it lies below the ring. The hydroxyl group on C1 in the α-D and β-L forms lies below the plane of the ring, while in the β-D and α-L forms, the hydroxyl group lies above the plane of the ring (see *A* on page 155).

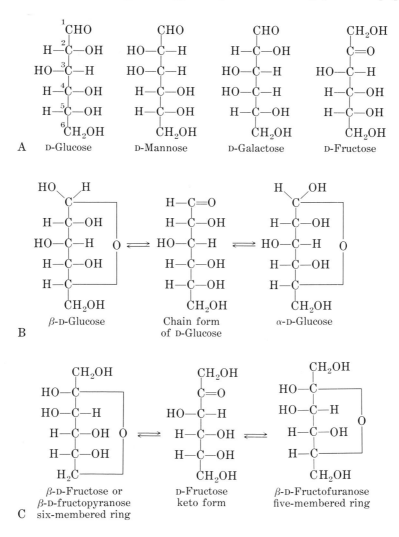

A   D-Glucose   D-Mannose   D-Galactose   D-Fructose

B   β-D-Glucose   Chain form of D-Glucose   α-D-Glucose

C   β-D-Fructose or β-D-fructopyranose six-membered ring   D-Fructose keto form   β-D-Fructofuranose five-membered ring

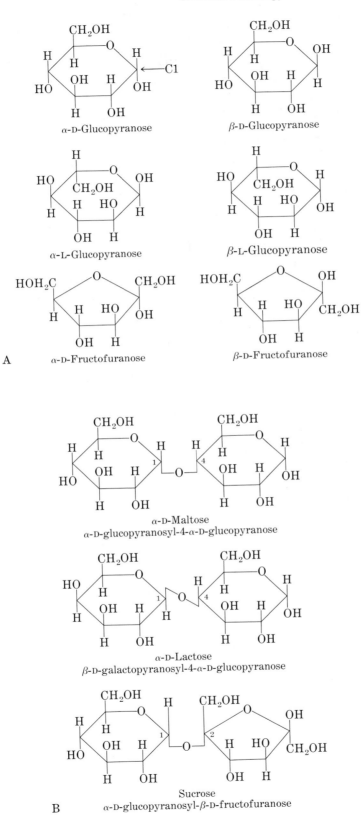

α-D-Glucopyranose

β-D-Glucopyranose

α-L-Glucopyranose

β-L-Glucopyranose

α-D-Fructofuranose

β-D-Fructofuranose

A

α-D-Maltose
α-D-glucopyranosyl-4-α-D-glucopyranose

α-D-Lactose
β-D-galactopyranosyl-4-α-D-glucopyranose

Sucrose
α-D-glucopyranosyl-β-D-fructofuranose

B

Disaccharides are sugars that can be hydrolyzed into two monosaccharides. The structures of three important disaccharides (maltose, lactose, and sucrose) are depicted in *B* on the previous page.

Raffinose, the most important of the trisaccharides, is found in sugar beets and molasses. When completely hydrolyzed it yields one molecule each of glucose, galactose, and fructose.

The polysaccharides are composed of many molecules of monosaccharides. The most important ones occurring in nature are the starches, which characteristically yield glucose when hydrolyzed. The starches, with molecular weights approaching 50,000, contain 80 to 90 per cent amylopectin and 10 to 20 per cent amylose. Both are composed of many glucose units joined through an α-glucoside linkage, as found in maltose. The glucose units of amylose are linked in an unbranched chain, with the amylose structure considered as an expanded maltose structure with a free sugar group at one end. It can be represented as:

α1,4 linkage

0000000000000000000000000000000000000000000000

Amylopectin, while containing chains of glucose units like those of amylose, also has branches of these glucose chains linked through the OH group of carbon 6 to give an α1,6 linkage and a branched point in the chain. It can be represented as:

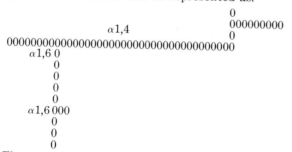

The substances that are formed in the course of the hydrolytic breakdown of starches are called dextrins.

Glycogen is a polysaccharide of glucose occurring widely in animal tissue such as liver. It is more highly branched and therefore more compact than the amylopectin molecule, but it contains the same α1,4 and α1,6 linkages. The arrangement of glucose molecules in glycogen has been represented as a tree-like shape.

Cellulose is the chief constituent of the framework of plants. Although made up of D-glucose molecules, the linear arrangement of these β1,4 linkages into the polymer makes this compound virtually resistant to digestive enzymes of man.

Polysaccharides, which are associated with the structure of animal tissue, are analogous to the cellulose of plant cells. Examples are hyaluronic acid (in which the predominant recurring disaccharide units consist of glucuronic acid linked to

the N-acetyl glucosamine) and chondroitin sulfate. Heparin, which is used as an anticoagulant, is also a carbohydrate.

GLUCOSE METABOLISM

The diet of the average adult in the Western Hemisphere is about 45 per cent carbohydrate, 45 per cent fat, and the remainder protein. Of the carbohydrate ingested, 60 per cent is starch, 30 per cent sucrose, and the remainder lactose. Salivary and gastrointestinal enzymes break down starch and other polysaccharides to monosaccharides, of which about 80 per cent are glucose, 15 per cent fructose, and 5 per cent galactose. These are absorbed in the small intestine by active transport and simple diffusion. Most of the saccharides in the peripheral blood are glucose and are taken up through simple diffusion by hepatic cells. Cells of the liver and the kidney metabolize glucose, as shown in Figure 7-1. Glucose enters the cells under the influence of insulin to form glucose 6-phosphate intracellulary. Glucose 6-phosphate then occupies a strategic position and is metabolized further to glycogen. It is also metabolized through the hexose monophosphate shunt or through the glycolytic scheme for energy production.

Glucose 6-phosphate can be converted by a complex enzymatic pathway to glycogen. Phosphoglucomutase acts on glucose 6-phosphate to form glucose 1-phosphate. After a series of reactions involving uridine triphosphate (UTP), UDP glucose is formed, which is then condensed with a glycogen molecule by a 1,4 linkage. Further modification of glycogen involves the construction of a branched point by a "branching enzyme." This enzyme modifies the glycogen molecule by detaching a glucose molecule from the 1,4 linkage and adding it on in a 1,6 linkage. In liver and muscle, this pathway is induced by insulin.

Glycogen is broken down to glucose by the phosphorylase system. This complex enzyme group is induced by various hormones in different tissues: epinephrine and glucagon in liver, epinephrine in muscle, and norepinephrine and epinephrine in adipose tissue. Cyclic AMP (cyclic 3',5'-adenosine monophosphate) is the activator of this enzyme. This enzyme system is depicted in detail in Figure 7-2.

Intermediary metabolism of glucose involves the formation of glucose 6-phosphate by phosphoglucoisomerase. Phosphofructokinase then adds another phosphate to form fructose 1,6-diphosphate. This reaction can be reversed by fructose 1,6-diphosphatase, an enzyme which forms fructose 6-phosphate. The diphosphatase is found in the highest concentration in the liver and is induced during starvation.

After the formation of fructose 1,6-diphosphate, the hexose unit is split into two interconvertible

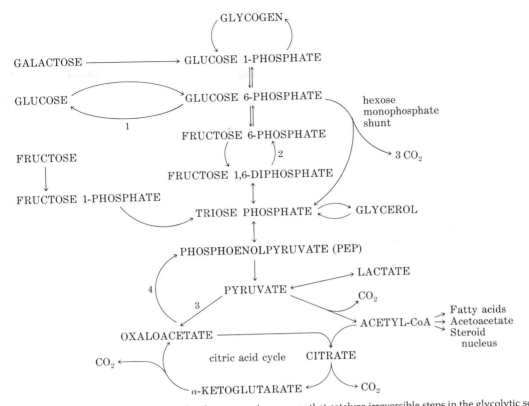

Figure 7-1. Metabolism of carbohydrates. The gluconeogenic enzymes that catalyze irreversible steps in the glycolytic scheme are:
1. glucose 6-phosphatase
2. fructose 1,6-diphosphatase
3. pyruvate carboxylase
4. PEP carboxykinase

three-carbon phosphorylated sugars, glyceraldehyde 3-phosphate and dihydroxyacetone phosphate. These can be further metabolized by a complex series of reactions that finally yield pyruvate. The final step in the formation of pyruvate is irreversible. If conditions are anaerobic, then lactate is formed from pyruvate by the enzyme lactate dehydrogenase. However, when aerobic conditions predominate, pyruvate is formed.

When pyruvate is metabolized, it must be decarboxylated into acetyl-CoA. There are four main pathways involved in the further metabolism of acetyl-CoA: (1) acetyl-CoA can be converted to a long chain fatty acid (fat synthesis from carbohydrates); (2) two acetyl-CoA units can condense to form acetoacetate; (3) acetyl-CoA can be incorporated by a series of steps into a steroid nucleus; and (4) acetyl-CoA can be condensed in the tricarboxylic acid (TCA) cycle with oxaloacetate to form citrate. Citrate then can be metabolized by a series

of enzymes in the TCA cycle to yield energy in the form of ATP with the regeneration of oxaloacetate.

During the fasting state, plasma glucose concentrations are maintained by two compensatory mechanisms. The first mechanism, glycogenolysis, occurs in minutes; it breaks down existing glycogen in liver ultimately to glucose. The other mechanism for the maintenance of blood glucose is gluconeogenesis, which involves the transformation of non-sugar precursors to glucose (e.g., protein via amino acids and the TCA cycle). A specific group of gluconeogenic enzymes, among them fructose 1,6-diphosphatase and glucose 6-phosphatase are induced; these are involved in the metabolism of glucose precursors back through the glycolytic scheme to glucose (see Fig. 7-1).

A number of hormones also play important roles in the regulation of blood glucose concentration. Insulin, glucagon, and somatostatin are involved intimately in a minute-to-minute maintenance of

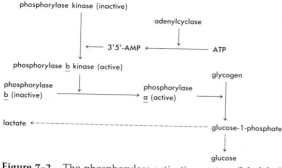

Figure 7–2. The phosphorylase activating system (Modified from Fernandes, 1974).

plasma glucose; these are described on page 162. Other hormones, such as growth hormone, have antagonistic actions on insulin and tend to raise plasma glucose concentrations. An elevated growth hormone concentration is responsible for the hyperglycemia in acromegaly. Hydrocortisone and other glucocorticoids also stimulate gluconeogenesis. Frequently in syndromes of glucocorticoid excess, such as Cushing's syndrome, an elevated plasma glucose concentration is found. Epinephrine, secreted by the adrenal medulla, stimulates glycogenolysis, resulting in increased plasma glucose levels. Physical or emotional stress increases production of epinephrine, subsequently increasing plasma glucose concentrations. Tumors of the adrenal medulla, e.g., pheochromocytomas, secrete excessive epinephrine and norepinephrine and produce moderate hyperglycemia. Thyroid hormones appear to stimulate glycogenolysis and also increase the rate of absorption of glucose from the intestine. For these reasons, hyperthyroid patients may be hyperglycemic. All these hormones acting on a minute-to-minute basis are responsible for maintaining the plasma glucose concentration.

GLUCOSE METHODOLOGY

The diagnosis of disorders of carbohydrate metabolism rests in part on the measurement of plasma glucose either in the fasting state or following stimulative or suppressive testing. Although early manual determinations of glucose were performed on whole blood, this is no longer practical for a number of reasons. Because some of the criteria for the laboratory diagnosis of diabetes mellitus were developed utilizing whole blood glucose, it is important to have at least some knowledge of these determinations. Whole blood values vary with the hematocrit; as the hematocrit decreases, the aqueous content of the blood increases (erythrocytes contain 73 mg/dl of water, while plasma contains 93 mg/dl). For example, if whole blood glucose is 100 mg/dl (5.5 mmol/l) when the hematocrit is 45 per cent, then decreasing the hematocrit to 20 per cent or increasing it to 60 per cent would result in a whole blood glucose of 104 and 91 mg/dl (5.77 and

5.05 mmol/l), respectively. Other reasons for abandoning the measurement of whole blood glucose include lack of an easy automated approach and the interference by non-glucose reducing substances from erythrocytes (called saccharides). Another important consideration is that if an inhibitor of glycolysis is not included in a specimen, erythrocytes and leukocytes continue to metabolize glucose at a rate of about 7 mg/dl/hr (0.4 mmol/l/hr) (Weissmann, 1958).

CHEMICAL METHODS OF GLUCOSE ESTIMATION

Glucose methodology can be divided into two groups, chemical and enzymatic. Most chemical measurements of glucose depend upon its reducing properties. Glucose exists in several forms, one of which is the enediol; this gives glucose its strong reducing property. The enediol form is favored in alkaline conditions and appears as follows:

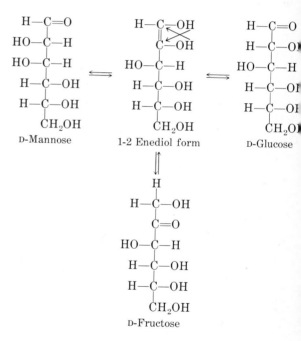

It will be noted that glucose, mannose, and fructose form the same enediol. Thus mannose and fructose will react in methods that depend on the reducing property of glucose. Several methods have been developed. Most are non-specific and depend on the reduction of selective heavy metals (Cu^{++} or Fe^{+++}) or the nitroaromatic acids by the aldehyde group of glucose. Some modifications are discussed subsequently.

The earliest method, called Folin-Wu, utilized an alkaline copper solution that was reacted with whole blood after it was subjected to the protein precipitating agent, tungstic acid. The cuprous ion (cupric ion is reduced to cuprous ion by glucose) produced was measured by the addition of an excess of phosphomolybdic acid, which forms phosphomolybdenum blue. Red cell constituents such as glutathione, glucuronic acid, ergothioneine, and ascorbic acid, which are commonly referred to as the "saccharoids," and other reducing sugars also reduced the cupric ion, leading to an overestimation of glucose. Reference interval of 80 to 120 mg/dl (4.4 to 6.6 mmol/l) has been obtained.

Modification by Nelson (Nelson-Somogyi) included the precipitation of proteins by barium hydroxide and zinc sulfate. The cuprous ion that formed from the reaction of glucose with alkaline copper solutions was coupled to arsenomolybdic acid and the color quantitated. Since saccharides were not measured, this method was referred to as measuring "true glucose." The reference interval is 60 to 100 mg/dl (3.3 to 5.6 mmol/l). Folin-Wu and Nelson-Somogyi methodologies are now considered to be obsolete.

Neocuproine (2,9,dimethyl 1,10-phenanthroline hydrochloride) specifically complexes to cuprous ions to form a yellow color. The cuprous ions were formed by the reduction of cupric ions with glucose. This methodology is used with some of the continuous-flow analyzers. When results are compared with those of an enzymatic method such as glucose oxidase, neocuproine is 4 to 5 mg/dl (0.2 to 0.3 mmol/l) higher.

Ferricyanide methodology depends on the reduction of a yellow ferricyanide ion to a colorless ferrocyanide by glucose. Since ferricyanide oxidizes substances other than sugars, glucose values are higher than in the copper reduction methodology and about 5 to 10 mg/dl (0.3 to 0.6 mmol/l) higher than in the enzymatic methods. Of chief concern are the elevated values found in uremia from uric acid and creatinine: values up to 40 mg/dl (2.2 mmol/l) higher than in glucose oxidase methods may occur.

Ortho-toluidine methods are based on the condensation of aldosaccharides such as glucose with various aromatic amines and glacial acetic acid (Dubowski, 1962). The stable green color that developed was then measured spectrophotometrically. This method can be used on plasma, urine, or cerebrospinal fluid without protein precipitation (Ceriotti, 1971). Galactose and mannose were found to react as well as glucose, while lactose, maltose, sucrose, and fructose, among others, react to a much lesser extent. The values for this methodology are higher than for the enzymatic method, but about 9 per cent lower than for ferricyanide methods. A major disadvantage of ortho-toluidine is the corrosiveness of the reagent to laboratory equipment as well as its toxicity (Indriksons, 1975). Reference values for the ortho-toluidine method are essentially the same as those for other enzyme methods: 65 to 115 mg/dl (3.6 to 6.8 mmol/l); however, with uremia, they may be slightly higher.

ENZYMATIC METHODS OF GLUCOSE ESTIMATION

Enzymatic methods yield maximum specificity for glucose estimations. Glucose can be measured by the reaction with glucose oxidase, in which gluconic acid and hydrogen peroxide (H_2O_2) are formed. Hydrogen peroxide then reacts with an oxygen receptor such as ortho-tolidine or ortho-dianisadine in a reaction catalyzed by peroxidase to form a blue color. This reaction is shown at the bottom of the page.

Glucose oxidase is highly specific for beta D-glucose, and any glucose present in the alpha form must be converted before reacting. Some preparations of glucose oxidase contain the enzyme mutarotase, which accelerates this process. The second step involving peroxidase is less specific than the first, and numerous reducing substances inhibit the chromogens used in the peroxidase reaction. Ortho-tolidine is no longer utilized, since it is a known carcinogen. New peroxide receptors have been described, such as 3-methyl-2-benzothiazolinone-hydrozone with N-N-dimethylaniline (Gochman, 1972) or phenylamine-phenazone, Trinder's reagent (Lott, 1975). Although uric acid and creatinine cause little interference in either of these methods, ascorbic acid leads to falsely decreased values. Reference interval of venous plasma is 65 to 115 mg/dl (3.6 to 6.4 mmol/l). Glucose oxidase (Trinder), when applied to a centrifugal analyzer, was found to be precise and accurate and to correlate well with hexokinase (Sonowane, 1976). One of the chief advantages of a glucose oxidase method is its inexpensiveness.

A useful approach to glucose methodology has been the glucose oxidase-oxygen automated method (Kadish, 1968). In this method glucose is measured by the use of an oxygen-sensing electrode that determines the rate of oxygen consumption, resulting in the series of reactions at the top of the next page. The electrode measures the rate

$$\beta\text{-D-Glucose} \xrightarrow[\text{Oxidase}]{\text{Glucose}} \text{Gluconolactone} \xrightarrow[\text{O}_2]{\text{H}_2\text{O}} \text{Gluconic Acid} + \text{H}_2\text{O}_2$$

$$\text{H}_2\text{O}_2 + \begin{array}{c} \text{Ortho-tolidine} \\ \text{or} \\ \text{Ortho-dianisidine} \\ \text{(chromogenic O}_2 \text{ receptors)} \end{array} \xrightarrow{\text{Peroxidase}} \text{blue color (chromogen)} + \text{H}_2\text{O}$$

$$\beta\text{-}\text{D-Glucose} + O_2 \xrightarrow{\text{Glucose Oxidase}} \text{D-glucono-}\delta\text{-lactone} + H_2O_2$$

$$H_2O_2 + \text{ethanol} \xrightarrow{\text{catalase}} \text{acetaldehyde} + H_2O$$

$$H_2O_2 + 2H^+ + 2I^- \xrightarrow{\text{molybdate}} I_2 + 2H_2O$$

of oxygen consumption in the first reaction, while H_2O_2 is captured in the last two reactions (above).

This method was found to be precise, linear, and free from interferences. Results approximate those of the Proposed Product Class Standard hexokinase glucose method (Passey, 1977).

A hexokinase method has been introduced which provides the ultimate degree of specificity in estimating true blood glucose (Neeley, 1972). This reaction is:

$$\text{Glucose} + \text{ATP} \xrightarrow[\text{Mg}^{++}]{\text{Hexokinase}}$$
$$\text{Glucose 6-phosphate} + \text{ADP}$$

$$\text{Glucose 6-phosphate} + \text{NADP} \xrightarrow{\text{G6PD}}$$
$$\text{6-phosphogluconate} + \text{NADPH} + H^+$$

For every mole of glucose reduced, one mole of NADPH is formed; it is measured spectrophotometrically. Hexokinase has been proposed as the reference method for glucose by the Department of Health, Education and Welfare (1974). The main disadvantage is its cost; in an extended comparison, it produced the best between-run and within-run precision. It also demonstrated no major interferences from a long list of substances that interfere with other methods (Passey, 1977).

Niejadlik (1973) addressed the problem of the discrepancy among glucose values determined by various methods. He found that plasma glucose by the copper reduction method was approximately 17 per cent higher than whole blood glucose by the Somogyi-Nelson method. Plasma glucose measured by the copper reduction method was consistently 5 mg/dl (0.3 mmol/l) higher than that measured by the hexokinase method, and in azotemic patients this discrepancy sometimes was as great as 25 mg/dl (6.3 mmol/l). He points out that the discrepancies in glucose values may be enough to alter the interpretation of the glucose tolerance test. For further information on glucose methodology, see Cooper (1973).

The current state of the art for glucose methodology prompts our selection of an enzymatic method for plasma glucose measurements. The glucose oxidase methods employing Trinder's reagent are relatively specific and less costly than hexokinase. However, hexokinase is favored because of its specificity and its application to cen-

trifugal analyzers, continuous flow equipment, and other large instruments such as the DuPont aca.

GLUCOSE SPECIMEN COLLECTION

Although in infants and others presenting difficulties with venipuncture, capillary blood can be utilized, venous blood is the specimen of choice for glucose analysis. After an overnight fast, capillary values are only 2 to 3 mg/dl (0.1 to 0.2 mmol/l) higher than venous concentrations, but after carbohydrate loading, the capillary values may be up to 20 to 30 mg/dl (1.1 to 1.7 mmol/l) higher. The glucose concentrations in arterial and capillary blood are quite similar.

At room temperature, glucose in a blood specimen is metabolized at approximately 7 mg/dl/hr (0.4 mmol/l/hr); at 4°C., the loss is approximately 2 mg/dl (0.1 mmol/l). Although erythrocytes and platelets utilize glucose, leukocytosis and bacterial contamination are the usual causes of glycolysis. A serum specimen is appropriate for glucose analysis if separated from the cells within one half hour, but if blood is in contact with cells for longer than one half hour, a preservative such as fluoride must be added. If blood is refrigerated, 2 mg of sodium fluoride per ml of blood prevents glycolysis for up to 48 hours. If refrigerated, glucose is stable in a cell-free environment for a period of 48 hours.

HYPERGLYCEMIA

Over 200 years ago it was found that the sweetness in blood and urine in patients with diabetes mellitus was due to glucose. Diabetes mellitus affects about 10 million Americans (5 per cent of the population) and is the third leading cause of death in the United States. One in 600 children has diabetes mellitus. People with diabetes have an increased risk of blindness, kidney disease, peripheral vascular disease, and heart disease. Diabetes mellitus is a chronic disease characterized by abnormally

Table 7–1. CLASSIFICATION OF
HYPERGLYCEMIA

Primary
  Maturity-onset (Adult) diabetes mellitus
  Growth-onset (Juvenile) diabetes mellitus
Secondary
  Hyperglycemia resulting from disease of the pancreas
    Inflammation
      Acute pancreatitis (rare)
      Chronic pancreatitis
      Pancreatitis due to mumps
      ? Cell damage due to Coxsackie-B_4 infection
      ? Autoimmune disease
    Pancreatectomy
    Infiltration (hemochromatosis)
    Tumors
    Trauma to pancreas (rare)
  Hyperglycemia related to other major endocrine diseases
    Acromegaly
    Cushing's syndrome
    Thyrotoxicosis
    Pheochromocytoma
    Hyperaldosteronism
    Glucagonoma
    Somatostatinoma
  Hyperglycemia caused by drugs
    Steroids
    Thiazide diuretics and diazoxide
    Oral contraceptives
    Alloxan and streptozotocin
  Hyperglycemia related to other major disease states
    Chronic renal failure
    Chronic disease of the liver
  Hyperglycemia related to insulin receptor antibodies
    Acanthosis nigricans

high concentrations of plasma glucose, resulting in its excretion in the urine and a specific form of microangiopathy. This angiopathy involves a thickening of the basement membranes of almost every capillary in the body.

Hyperglycemia may result from a total absence of insulin secretion, such as a surgical pancreatectomy; it may occur from the delayed development of the pancreas as in transient neonatal diabetes, or occur intermittently during periods of stress, such as severe infection, dehydration, and pregnancy. Hyperglycemia may be secondary to other endocrine diseases, or even be due to an antibody to the insulin receptor (Kahn, 1977). Some drugs, such as propranolol, thiazide diuretics, and phenytoin, block insulin release and cause hyperglycemia. A classification of hyperglycemia appears in Table 7–1.

Diabetes mellitus is clinically divided into two groups, non-insulin-dependent or maturity onset, and insulin-dependent or juvenile onset. In juvenile onset patients, who are usually thin, diabetes mellitus appears at an early age (usually before 30), with a rapid onset; it has occasional remissions and ketosis is prominent. In contrast, maturity onset diabetics are usually obese: diabetes appears at an age over 40, with an insidious onset, and ketosis is rare. In juvenile onset diabetics there is an increased incidence of histocompatibility antigen HLA-B8 and W15, while HLA-B7 is significantly less common (Nerup, 1974). There is some evidence that the D locus, which is involved in cellular immunity, has a close association with juvenile diabetes (Pyke, 1977). There appears to be no association with the HLA antigens and adult onset diabetes (see Chap. 41). Although it may have a number of causes, maturity onset diabetes apparently is predominantly inherited and appears to be genetically different from juvenile onset diabetes.

FASTING PLASMA GLUCOSE

The diagnosis of diabetes mellitus can be made by the measurement of plasma glucose in the fasting state. Plasma that is collected after a 12- to 14-hour fast shows less variation among individuals than specimens collected at any other time during the day. Plasma glucose results can be classified as either hyperglycemic or hypoglycemic, but both these definitions are rather arbitrary, with no clear-cut distinction between what is normal and abnormal. An overnight fasting glucose level between 50 and 110 mg/dl (2.8 to 6.2 mmol/l) is accepted by most as being normal, but the upper limit of what is considered normal rises with increasing age. Currently, a plasma glucose of 140 mg/dl (7.7 mmol/l) is considered abnormal; if it is abnormal on two or more occasions, the diagnosis of diabetes mellitus can be made (Siperstein, 1975). Because the diagnosis of diabetes mellitus may damage a patient's life, perhaps causing him to lose his job or have his insurance policy changed, this upper limit is not strictly adhered to in all circumstances. Since there still is no conclusive evidence that an early diagnosis of diabetes mellitus is of any benefit in preventing the subsequent difficulties to which a diabetic is subject, there appears to be no urgency in its diagnosis by relatively sensitive but nonspecific procedures.

This point of view is in marked contrast to that taken by the American Diabetes Association. Because of the insensitivity of the fasting glucose measurements, it does not recommend their use (American Diabetes Association, 1975).

RANDOM PLASMA GLUCOSE

Plasma glucose concentration varies only slightly throughout the day and generally is in the range of 45 to 130 mg/dl (2.5 to 7.3 mmol/l). The only rise that occurs is found after a meal, but even then there is rarely a rise of more than 10 to 15 mg/dl (0.6 to 0.8 mmol/l) (Alberti, 1975a). This degree of elevation is quite different from that obtained during a glucose tolerance test. When healthy middle-aged and older subjects are given a load of glucose, plasma glucose concentrations may range from 20 to 50 mg/dl (1.1 to 2.8 mmol/l) higher than when the same subjects are given a breakfast with 75 grams of carbohydrate (Alberti, 1975b).

Values below 45 mg/dl (2.2 mmol/l) are unusual and warrant further investigation, especially if the individual is symptomatic. Low values may reflect normal physiologic response in plasma glucose concentrations following the ingestion of a meal, or they could be the first and only clue to a disorder in glucose homeostasis. (For details regarding the diagnosis of hypoglycemia, see p. 171.) It is unlikely that symptoms of hypoglycemia occur when plasma glucose concentrations are greater than 45 mg/dl (2.5 mmol/l).

In insulin-treated diabetics, the plasma glucose concentration may be grossly abnormal during the day, with swings in plasma glucose as great as 150 mg/dl (8.3 mmol/l). Although 130 mg/dl (7.3 mmol/l) is considered the upper normal for plasma glucose, individuals who are 65 years old or older commonly have values of up to 180 mg/dl (10.0 mmol/l).

PANCREATIC HORMONES

The cells of the endocrine pancreas secrete three hormones involved in glucose homeostasis: insulin, glucagon, and somatostatin. Each hormone is made by an individual cell type physically contiguous with the other types of endocrine cells. It is thought that secretion of a hormone by one cell type can somehow influence the secretion of the other cells.

Under physiologic circumstances the availability of energy sources necessitates release of glucagon, or insulin, such that a reciprocal relationship occurs between them. Insulin acts to store energy and inhibits mobilization of energy stores from endogenous sources, such as liver, fat, and muscle. In contrast, during the postprandial and fasting periods, glucagon enhances catabolic functions such as hepatic glycogenolysis and stimulates the formation of glucose in conjunction with other catabolic hormones. Usually glucose is controlled within narrow limits by insulin and glucagon. This bihormonal control of glucose regulation requires the appropriate secretion of varying amounts of these two hormones, which act in concert on such distant sites as adipose tissue, liver, and muscle, to maintain a steady concentration of plasma glucose.

Fluctuations in circulating energy sources are the primary determinates of both synthesis and release of insulin and glucagon (Unger, 1977c). For example, glucose stimulates insulin and suppresses glucagon secretion, while protein ingestion stimulates both glucagon and insulin. In diabetic ketoacidosis, in which insulin is absent, glucagon is markedly elevated. Additional control of pancreatic secretion which is provided by other hormones and the central nervous system, is mediated through the adrenergic, cholinergic, and possibly peptinonergic mechanisms. Somatostatin may act locally to regulate the release of insulin and glucagon in the pancreas as well as in the gastrointestinal tract.

Somatostatin

Somatostatin, a tetradecapeptide with a disulfide bridge, was isolated first from the hypothalamus (Fig. 7–3). It was originally thought that somatostatin was strictly a hypothalamic hormone that inhibited growth hormone secretion, but the discovery of somatostatin in the islets of Langerhans provided new impetus for investigation of its function in the endocrine pancreas. Subsequently, somatostatin also was found in the gastric mucosa and intestine. It has been found to inhibit pituitary hormones (GH, TSH, ACTH), gastrointestinal hormones (gastrin and secretin), and pancreatic hormones (glucagon and insulin) as well as to possess non-endocrinologic activities. Listed in Table 7–2 are some of the functions attributed to somatostatin.

D cells of the pancreas, which make up 10 per cent of the total islet mass, are thought to be the site of somatostatin synthesis (Gerich, 1977b). The D cells generally are distributed asymetrically such that they are in close prox-

SOMATOSTATIN

H-ALA-GLY-CYS-LYS-ASN-PHE-PHE-TRP-LYS-THR-PHE-THR-SER-CYS-OH

Primary sequence of somatostatin

Figure 7–3. Primary sequence of the tetradecapeptide somatostatin.

imity to the glucagon-producing or A cells. The infusion of somatostatin into insulin-requiring diabetics has been shown to cause a reduction of elevated glucagon levels, with a decrease in plasma glucose concentrations. When insulin is withdrawn in these patients, somatostatin infusion can prevent the appearance of ketosis (Gerich, 1977a). From these data and other studies, it has been concluded that somatostatin predominantly affects glucagon by diminishing its release. In diabetics with essentially no beta (insulin-producing) cells, D cells account for perhaps one-third of all pancreatic islet cells (Gerich, 1977b). It has been proposed that this may reflect a compensatory, albeit inadequate, mechanism to correct the hyperglycemia. That is, through increased somatostatin secretion, glucagon-related glucose formation is reduced (Unger, 1977b). In normal patients infused with somatostatin, the levels of glucose, insulin, and glucagon fall. This is taken as evidence that the D cells, by means of direct within-islet action, influence insulin and glucagon, which in turn influence glucose formation.

In addition to the actions on pancreatic islets, there is evidence that somatostatin, perhaps originating from the somatostatin-containing cells in the gut and acting on gastric, duodenal, and pancreatic secretion, also may involve nutrient entry in the portal vein. Since somatostatin secretion is stimulated by most of the same stimuli as insulin (Unger, 1977a), it appears likely that its effects are mediated through cyclic AMP.

A short half-life of one minute, its diverse

actions, and the failure to detect it in the peripheral circulation argue against the function of somatostatin as a circulating hormone and point to its action as a local modulator. Somatostatin may be measured by radioimmunoassay, but this assay is not widely available (Patel, 1977).

Tumors of the somatostatin-producing D cells of the pancreas have been described (Larsson, 1977; Ganda, 1977); in both of these cases, patients presented with hyperglycemia and hypoglucagonemia.

Glucagon

Glucagon is formed by the alpha-2 (or A cells) of the pancreas, which are derived embryologically from the neuroectoderm. At one time it was thought that glucagon was synthesized by both the pancreas and the gastrointestinal tract and that it was a polypeptide consisting of 29 amino acids. Subsequent work has indicated that pancreatic glucagon differs from gut glucagon. Gut glucagon is a material found in the stomach of man (Munoz-Barragan, 1977) that reacts with certain glucagon antisera but has few of the biologic actions of pancreatic glucagon.

There appears to be heterogeneity of circulating plasma pancreatic glucagon: four fractions include a component with a mass greater than 40,000 daltons, others with a mass of 9,000 and 3,500, and one component with a mass less than 2,000 daltons. The latter has been found in the plasma of normals and is thought to be a degradation product of glucagon (Jaspan, 1977). The various components show marked differences in the response to agents that are known to stimulate or suppress pancreatic glucagon secretion. Normal plasma immunoreactive glucagon concentration is about 115 pg/ml, with 54 per cent comprising the 40,000 dalton component and the remainder the 3,500 dalton fraction (Kuku, 1976). In patients with renal failure, glucagon levels are increased fivefold, with the 9,000 dalton component predominating. Further studies have confirmed that the kidneys are a major site of glucagon metabolism and probably responsible for removal of the 9,000 dalton

Table 7–2. ACTIVITIES OF SOMATOSTATIN

ENDOCRINE	NON-ENDOCRINE
Inhibition of secretion or diminution of	
Growth hormone	Gastric acid secretion
Thyrotropin	Gastric emptying time
Gastrin	Gallbladder contraction
Secretin	Pancreatic bicarbonate release
Vasointestinal peptide	
Glucagon	Pancreatic enzyme release
Insulin	Acetylcholine release from peripheral nerve endings

fraction. Although not characterized chemically, the 3,500 dalton glucagon is thought to be the physiologically important fraction. It increases more with stimulation than do any other fractions and is suppressed by hyperglycemia and somatostatin.

Glucagon concentrations are important in the diagnosis of the alpha cell tumor of the pancreas (glucagonoma). This tumor is associated with mild diabetes mellitus, and plasma glucagon concentrations ranging from 900 to 7800 pg/ml. The presence of a very high glucagon level in a diabetic suggests this diagnosis. Clinically these patients present with a characteristic necrolytic migratory rash, weight loss, anemia, stomatitis, and glossitis (Mallinson, 1974). About two thirds of patients present with metastatic disease (Jaspan, 1977). An autosomal dominant disorder, familial hyperglucagonemia, also has been described in which glucagon is elevated, mainly owing to increase of the 9000 dalton component. A member of one of these families has developed a glucagonoma (Boden, 1977).

In juvenile diabetics, immunoreactive glucagon levels are normal but inappropriate to plasma glucose concentration, and they show an exaggerated response to such stimuli as protein loading.

An interesting cause of the aberrant glucagon results has been reported by Jaspan (1976). In juvenile onset diabetics, an impurity in some insulin preparations may result in the formation of anti-glucagon antibodies in a small percentage of the patients treated. These antibodies then compete with certain glucagon antibodies employed to measure glucagon by radioimmunoassay. Depending on the separation step used in the assay, falsely high or low glucagon levels will be obtained because of this competing antibody.

Since glucagon is relatively unstable, it should be collected in cold tubes containing a protease inhibitor such as Trasylol, centrifuged immediately in the cold, and frozen until assayed (Eisentraut, 1968).

Insulin

Insulin is a small peptide with a mass of about 6000 daltons consisting of a so-called alpha chain of 21 amino acids connected by two S-S bonds to a chain of 30 amino acids, designated beta. The classic work of Steiner (1967) reported that the polypeptide precursor of insulin, termed proinsulin, is synthesized in the microsomal fraction of the pancreatic beta cell as a long single chain with a mass of 9000 daltons. It then is transported to the Golgi apparatus, where it is stored. The 9000 dalton peptide chain folds back on itself, aligning sulfhydryl groups so that a disulfide bond is formed within the alpha chain. In addition, two disulfide bonds are formed between the alpha and beta chains. Proinsulin is subjected to continuous conversion to insulin in secretory granules of the beta cell. It is shortened to a double-chain molecule by a proteolytic process that removes the central protein or "C" chain, thus forming insulin (Fig. 7-4). It is believed that the connecting peptide or "C" chain, along with native insulin, is secreted into the blood in equimolar amounts. *In vivo* studies on the activity of proinsulin have shown that it has about 10 per cent of the biologic activity of insulin; however, it has a half-life that is three times as long. A molecule even larger than proinsulin has been identified and is called pre-proinsulin; this may be a precursor for proinsulin (Steiner, 1977a).

In the fasting state, insulin secretion is minimal and proinsulin secretion is only about 15 per cent that of insulin. This ratio stays about the same when there is an acute stimulus to insulin secretion. However, in older patients, pregnant diabetics, obese diabetics, patients with insulinomas, some cases of functional hypoglycemia, and a rare syndrome called hyperproinsulinemia, an increased percentage of circulating proinsulin is found (Kitabchi, 1977).

The reference value of fasting serum insulin by radioimmunoassay is from 4 to 10 μ units/ml. It has been shown that antibodies produced in laboratory animals for use in the radioimmunoassay of insulin cross-react with proinsulin (Wright, 1970; Rubenstein, 1970). This is not surprising, since insulin and proinsulin share a common sequence. The extent of cross-reactivity depends on individual antiserum but usually is in the range of 30 per cent. Proinsulin and "C" peptide also may be measured by radioimmunoassay. Since proinsulin antiserum is directed against the antigenic determinants of the connecting peptide sequence, the proinsulin radioimmunoassay will cross-react with "C" peptide assays.

Measurements of insulin appear to have little clinical value except in the diagnosis of spontaneous hypoglycemia (Marks, 1976). The utility of this assay is discussed in the sections on insulinomas and hypoglycemia (p. 171 and 173). In general, the sensitivity of the insulin

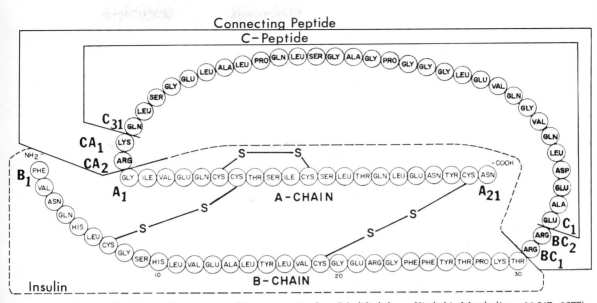

Figure 7-4. Proposed amino acid sequence of human proinsulin. (Modified from Kitabchi, Metabolism, 26:547, 1977). Connecting peptide is the amino acid residue connecting the carboxy end of the B chain to the amino end of the A chain of insulin. "C" peptide is formed when two basic residues BC_1-BC_2 and CA_1-CA_2 have been removed from connecting peptide. Insulin (broken line) consists of the A and B chain.

radioimmunoassay is such that it is impossible to differentiate normal insulin levels from low levels. Thus, at glucose levels less than 30 mg/dl (1.7 mmol/l), insulin cannot be detected. Assays for proinsulin are not readily available.

Insulin Antibodies. The measurement of insulin antibodies in the serum has been utilized in the diagnosis of "factitious hypoglycemia." When insulin is injected into patients with a normal beta cell function, glucose levels are depressed and hypoglycemia may occur. Insulin-related peptides, which are invariably present in most "crystalline" insulin preparations, are the major immunogenic components in insulins that are used therapeutically (Chance, 1976). Since these peptides result in formation of antibodies, their presence in patients who are not treated with insulin is strong evidence for exogenous insulin injection. The introduction of a more purified insulin, monocomponent insulin, should reduce the incidence of insulin antibodies and thus decrease the value of this test. "C" peptide measurements are currently replacing insulin antibody measurements in "factitious" hypoglycemia (Scarlett, 1977).

"C" Peptide. Human "C" peptide is the 31 amino acid chain that is part of the connection of the alpha and beta chains of insulin within the proinsulin molecule (see Fig. 7-4). Insulin is rapidly removed by its initial passage through the liver; however, the hepatic extraction of "C" peptide is negligible. Therefore, it is not surprising that the half-life of "C" peptide in the circulation is more than twice that of insulin. Although the secretory ratio of "C" peptide to insulin is 1:1, in plasma the ratio is about 5 to 15:1. The function of "C" peptide in the peripheral circulation is unknown.

The measurement of "C" peptide has been used in a few clinical settings, which are listed in Table 7-3. In selected hypoglycemic states, such as insulinoma, "C" peptide is elevated. A diagnostic test for insulinoma has been developed in which insulin is injected and "C" peptide quantitated (Horwitz, 1976). This is dis-

Table 7-3. CLINICAL INDICATIONS FOR "C" PEPTIDE MEASUREMENT

Hypoglycemic States
  Diagnosis of insulinoma
  Diagnosis of surreptitious injection of insulin
Euglycemic States
  Demonstration of remission phase or "recovery" from diabetes
Hyperglycemic State
  Follow-up evaluation after pancreatectomy
  Evaluation of the "brittle" diabetic patient

cussed in the section on insulinoma (p. 173). The most important use of "C" peptide measurement is in the diagnosis of surreptitious injection of insulin, resulting in "factitious" hypoglycemia (Couropmitree, 1975). Since the "C" peptide has been removed during the purification of commercial insulin preparations, those patients who have injected insulin will have demonstrable insulin by radioimmunoassay, but no "C" peptide. The absence of "C" peptide, high insulin, and hypoglycemia point to the injection of exogenous insulin. Other uses of the "C" peptide assay include follow-up evaluation of total pancreatectomy for carcinoma, and demonstration of the remission phase of "recovery" from diabetes (Block, 1973). Patients with complete loss of beta cell capacity have no "C" peptide and are frequently "brittle" diabetics, while diabetics with residual beta cell function and thus "C" peptide tend to have stable diabetes mellitus. The assay of "C" peptide is useful in distinguishing these groups.

Fasting serum "C" peptide concentrations in healthy subjects range between 0.9 and 3.9 ng/ml. After administration of a glucose load, the levels rise five- to sixfold. In diabetics, the "C" peptide may be decreased or absent; in diabetic acidosis, "C" peptide is not present. The cross-reactivity of proinsulin with the "C" peptide antiserum may be up to one fifth that of "C" peptide. However, since the concentration of proinsulin is about one tenth that of "C" peptide in a reference population, less than 5 per cent of the "C" peptide immunoreacting material is proinsulin. In insulin-requiring diabetics, antibodies are produced to insulin which also react with proinsulin. Some beta cell function in the presence of these antibodies results in accumulation of proinsulin in the circulation. It has been found that in some diabetics, up to 80 per cent of the "C" peptide immunoreactivity may be proinsulin. Thus, "C" peptide immunoreactivity indicates only that beta cell secretion is taking place, and the values which are obtained cannot be compared with those in a normal population to quantitate insulin secretion (Horwitz, 1976).

GLUCOSE TOLERANCE TESTING

Diabetes mellitus is a disease characterized by hyperglycemia occurring from a relative or absolute decrease in insulin secretion and associated with a specific form of microangiopathy. The morbidity and mortality of this disease result from vascular, renal, and neurologic complications. In order to define diabetes chemically, clinicians have commonly used the response of a patient to a glucose load or challenge. This challenge has been standardized: after either an oral or an intravenous load of glucose, plasma glucose values are determined and, in addition, insulin levels sometimes are obtained. Although the glucose tolerance test is very sensitive, it suffers from lack of specificity. It is abnormal in a wide variety of diseases and influenced by diet as well as other variables. The most widely used of these procedures is the oral glucose tolerance test, yet there is no consensus as to what constitutes an abnormal response. In an effort to standardize glucose tolerance testing, the Committee on Statistics of the American Diabetes Association (ADA) has recommended standardized conditions under which the test should be performed (Klimt, 1969). Unfortunately, many glucose tolerance tests are carried out without regard to these requirements.

Preparatory phase

If meaningful data are to be obtained, the conditions of performing the test must be controlled rigidly. It is important that the patient consume a diet adequate in carbohydrates. For three days prior to the glucose tolerance test, a diet of at least 150 grams per day of carbohydrate is required. Two more days of this diet are essential if the patient has not been on a diet sufficient in carbohydrates. The presence of anorexia or any other condition precluding adequate food intake automatically invalidates the test. Inactivity, such as bed rest, has been reported to reduce glucose tolerance. A glucose tolerance test thus should not be performed in non-ambulatory patients. During the 12 hours prior to a test, the patient must fast and avoid even black coffee. In addition, smoking and even mild exercise are not permitted. The test should not be performed in those patients who have had an illness during the prior two weeks. Many endocrine disorders resulting from excessive or inadequate hormonal secretion may be associated with abnormal glucose tolerance. Thus, any dysfunction of the endocrine system should be evaluated, and only after it has been corrected should a glucose tolerance test be performed. Many drugs such as salicylates, diuretics, and anticonvulsants have been reported to decrease insulin secretion. They should be avoided for at least three days prior to the performance of the test. Oral contraceptives should be omitted for one complete cycle prior to the test.

Procedures

The size of the glucose load employed is variable. Some workers utilize a 50-gram load, others 75 grams, while still others use 100 grams. Since pure glucose is extremely unpalatable, a synthetic product called Glucola, which consists of a hydrolyzable saccharide of corn syrup and carbonated water with cola or cherry flavoring, commonly is used. Although not recommended because of possible differences in intestinal absorption, it is better tolerated in patients who experience gastrointestinal upset with glucose. Seven ounces of Glucola are equivalent to 75 grams of glucose. Some workers recommend a glucose load of 1.75 g/kg body weight; this has been advocated in pediatric patients. The American Diabetes Association, however, recommends a dose of 40 grams of glucose per square meter of body surface, using a nomogram to relate weight to square meters of body surface.

Between 7 and 9 A.M. and after 30 minutes of rest, a blood sample for baseline glucose is obtained and the patient ingests the glucose load. The glucose is taken over 5 minutes, and the first blood specimen drawn at a specified time after baseline depending on the criteria used for interpretation (see Table 7-4). If nausea, fainting, sweating, or other autonomic nervous system overactivity occurs, a specimen for glucose should be drawn immediately and the procedure discontinued and repeated at a later date if indicated. If a glucose tolerance test is performed in the morning and repeated 12 hours later, some of those patients who are judged normal in the morning would be called "mild" diabetics, based on the evening test (Carroll, 1973). Other patients tested on alternate days may be found to be diabetic on one day and normal on the second test.

Evaluation of results

Most of the data utilized to establish the criteria for glucose tolerance testing are based on measurements of whole blood glucose. However, it is current practice to perform glucose determinations only on serum or plasma samples. Many different glucose methodologies have been utilized in determining reference values for the glucose tolerance test.

These different methodologies result in small changes in comparative glucose values and add further confusion to the interpretation of the glucose tolerance test. The most widely used recommendations are those criteria provided by the Wilkerson point system or the Fajans-Conn criteria, which are listed in Table 7-4. Also listed there are the other criteria provided by Danowski and those by Siperstein. Many other criteria have been proposed, but for the sake of brevity they have been omitted. The Fajans-Conn criteria were developed utilizing whole blood as the specimen source, but they have been modified so that plasma values of more than 185 mg/dl (10.3 mmol/l) at one hour, 160 mg/dl (8.9 mmol/l) at one and a half hours, and 140 mg/dl (7.8 mmol/l) at two hours are required to diagnose diabetes during the glucose tolerance test. More liberal criteria are those of Danowski (1973), in which the plasma glucose concentrations of fasting, one hour, two hours, and three hours are summed. A summed value of 501 to 800 mg/dl (27.8 to 44.1 mmol/l) represents an equivocal range, and values above 800 mg/dl (44.1 mmol/l) are in a diabetic range. Six of the commonly used criteria for the diagnosis of diabetes were compared in a study by Valleron (1975). He found that only 48 per cent of the subjects were classified in the same way by any of the commonly used diagnostic criteria. This study emphasizes the importance of the criteria used in the identification of glucose intolerance and the fact that all the commonly used ones are susceptible to errors in interpretation.

Criticism of the glucose tolerance test has been made by Siperstein (1975). He has pointed out that the reference population used for the Fajans-Conn criteria were young subjects and that glucose intolerance increases with age. Other studies of tolerance testing have utilized similar types of controls. If these commonly used criteria are accepted, from 35 to 60 per cent of the general population over the age of 40 would be labeled diabetic. Siperstein recommends that a glucose of greater than 260 mg/dl (14.4 mmol/l) at one hour and 220 mg/dl (12.2 mmol/l) at two hours should be the criteria used for the diagnosis of diabetes mellitus. He recommends that a fasting plasma glucose of 140 mg/dl (7.7 mmol/l) on two and preferably three separate occasions also can be used to establish the diagnosis of diabetes mellitus.

Other non-specific factors such as inactivity,

obesity, and race have been reported to affect the glucose tolerance test. In a study of over 100,000 people it was found by Dales (1974) that there are racial differences in glucose levels following glucose tolerance testing. Blacks seem to have lower glucose values than whites, and Orientals have values significantly higher than either of the other groups.

In many laboratories urine is collected at frequent intervals during the test for the measurement of urine glucose. While this practice may be of some value in detection of renal glycosuria, it is of no significance in the diagnosis of diabetes and may actually be an additional stress on the patient, thereby adversely affecting the performance of the test. For these reasons, it should not be utilized (Sherwin, 1977).

In its statement on glucose tolerance testing, the American Diabetes Association recommends that the Fajans-Conn or the Wilkerson point system or "other methods at the author's discretion" should be used to interpret the glucose tolerance test (Meinert, 1972). Some of the more common ones are listed in Table 7-4.

At present, it is difficult to recommend which criteria, if any, are most acceptable. The recent trend has been away from the criteria established by Fajans and Conn and toward more liberal criteria, similar to those proposed by Siperstein. However, Siperstein (1975) recommends that the glucose tolerance test be abandoned. Although the diagnosis will be missed in some early diabetics, there does not appear to be any evidence that this delay in diagnosis will affect morbidity from the disease.

Perinatal infant mortality in mild or gestational diabetic pregnancies exceeds that observed in non-diabetic pregnancies, and treatment significantly decreases this loss. To find those pregnant patients, glucose determinations have been performed. Throughout pregnancy, normally a lower fasting glucose is found, but during the second and third trimester glucose intolerance is increased. Diabetic patients have been identified by the presence of an abnormal glucose tolerance, using a 100-gram glucose load. Reference values during pregnancy were determined by O'Sullivan (1964), who established a fasting glucose at 105 mg/dl (5.8 mmol/l), and one-, two-, and three-hour specimens at 190, 165, and 145 mg/dl (10.6, 9.2, and 8.1 mmol/l), respectively. If two of these values are exceeded,

then the diagnosis of diabetes is made (Table 7-4). A one-hour glucose value greater than 150 mg/dl (8.3 mmol/l) following an oral glucose load has been utilized as screening evidence for performing the glucose tolerance test in pregnant women (O'Sullivan, 1973). It has been recommended that in pregnancy the intravenous glucose tolerance test not be performed (see below) (Lavine, 1977).

The glucose tolerance test is of questionable value because of potential pitfalls in making the diagnosis of diabetes mellitus and the variability of the response in non-obese fasting patients. The diagnosis may even lead to unnecessary anxiety in some patients who have been told that they are diabetic. Sherwin (1977) recommends that the glucose tolerance test be reserved for the management of obese and pregnant patients. An abnormal glucose tolerance test may provide the stimulus for weight reduction, while in pregnancy the proper management of gestational diabetes may lead to improved rate of fetal survival.

Glucose tolerance testing with insulin levels

Insulin determinations have been used in conjunction with glucose measurements in order to improve the diagnostic accuracy of the glucose tolerance test (GTT). The values have been expressed in a number of ways, such as the ratio of insulin to glucose or increments of glucose and insulin expressed as a ratio.

The upper reference limit for the ratio of insulin (μ units/ml) to glucose (mg/dl) was established to be about 0.30 in a group of fasting healthy subjects (Fajans, 1975). During a glucose tolerance test the mean fasting ratio was found to be 0.10 and to increase about eightfold, peaking at one hour (Chiles, 1970). Most diabetic patients have a nearly normal ratio in the fasting state. During a GTT, severe diabetics show little increase in the insulin-to-glucose ratio, while in early diabetes, the ratio is increased and the peak is delayed.

Other criteria for the use of insulin levels during glucose tolerance testing have been established by Danowski (1973). Data obtained during the GTT are expressed in terms of increases in glucose levels over baseline, compared with increments in serum insulin. Two abnormal patterns were found: those in which the ratio was normal at one-half hour but thereafter was elevated, and those in which

Table 7-4. DIAGNOSTIC CRITERIA FOR DIABETES MELLITUS

MEASUREMENT SYSTEM	PLASMA GLUCOSE LEVELS (mg/dl)*						Criteria
	Fasting	½ hour	1 hour	1½ hours	2 hours	3 hours	
Fajans-Conn	-	-	185 (10.3)	160 (8.9)	140 (7.8)	-	All values equal to or greater than shown.
Wilkerson Point System (USPHS)	125 (6.9) 1 point	-	195 (10.8) ½ point	145 (7.8) 0 points	– ½ point	125 (6.9) 1 point	A total of two or more points.
Siperstein	140 (7.8)	-	260 (14.4)	-	220 (12.2)	-	1. Fasting 140 on two occasions. 2. One-hour 260 and two-hour 220.
O'Sullivan (Gestational diabetes mellitus)	105 (5.8)	-	190 (10.6)	-	165 (9.5)	145 (8.1)	Two or more values equal to or greater than shown.
Danowski (Sum of plasma glucose at 0, 1, and 2 hours)	501 (27.8) Non-diabetic		501-800 (27.8-44.4) Equivocal		800 (44.4) Diabetes mellitus		

*Values in parentheses are in mmol/l.

the ratio was low at one-half hour and normal at one hour but persistantly elevated thereafter. Although extremely high ratios were found in diabetics, some healthy subjects and obese individuals also showed an elevated ratio.

Other methods of data expression and interpretation have been proposed by Kraft (1975). A normal fasting level of insulin was considered between 0 and 30 μ units/ml. During the GTT, it peaks at one half to one hour, and the second hour value is less than 50 μ units/ml. Insulin levels during the third hour are lower than in the second. Kraft's criteria for diabetes are as follows: if the sum is greater than 60 μ units/ml, a probable diagnosis of diabetes can be made; if it is greater than 100 μ units/ml, patients are considered to be diabetic. Additional criteria considered to be diagnostic of diabetes include delayed insulin peak occurring between two and three hours, a fasting insulin level of greater than 50 μ units/ml, or the persistence of insulin levels in the fasting range.

The glucose tolerance test for determining insulin levels has not been widely used. Expense of performing multiple insulin measurements and difficulties in data interpretation probably have been responsible for lack of its widespread use. The extreme variability of the insulin response to identical glucose loads also has cast doubt on the appropriateness of insulin measurements during a glucose tolerance test (Olefsky, 1974). However, use of insulin-glucose ratios remains indispensable for evaluating patients with hypoglycemia.

Other glucose tolerance tests

The intravenous glucose tolerance test (IVGTT) has been used to diagnose diabetes mellitus in patients who are unable to ingest an oral glucose load. It also circumvents the variability of glucose absorption. No recommendations for the standardization of the test have been made by the American Diabetes Association. Commonly, this test is performed using 0.5 g/kg body weight glucose given as a rapid intravenous infusion within a three-minute period. Blood is drawn for glucose before infusion and at 1, 3, 5, 10, 20, 30, 40, 60, and 120 minutes following the end of the infusion. Glucose disappearance constants (k values) are calculated from a plot of the log of the glucose concentration in relationship to time. A k value of less than 1.2 is considered to be diagnostic of diabetes mellitus. In a comparison of the oral glucose tolerance test and the intravenous test, Olefsky (1973) found that these two tests gave different diagnostic information 40 per cent of the time. These workers, using a very elegant experimental procedure, found that there was no correlation between their reference procedure and the IVGTT. They concluded that the intravenous glucose tolerance test is a poor method for estimating glucose disposal. For this reason, as well as lack of standardization, the results are even more difficult to interpret than are those of an oral glucose tolerance test.

Another test of glucose tolerance involves the use of cortisone and glucose (cortisone glucose tolerance test). Since cortisone promotes gluconeogenesis, it may accentuate carbohydrate intolerance in latent or mild diabetics. After two doses of cortisone, an oral glucose tolerance test is performed. A two-hour specimen yielding a plasma glucose value of greater than 140 mg/dl (7.8 mmol/l) is used to discriminate between diabetics and nondiabetics. Use of a single two-hour value for the upper limit of normal has proved to be unreliable, since it results in the diagnosis of diabetes mellitus in a large number of people (Pozefsky, 1965). The prognostic implication of this test is uncertain not only in the elderly but in other age groups as well.

Two-hour postprandial plasma glucose

Two-hour postprandial glucose levels have been used to screen for diabetes mellitus, to diagnose diabetes, and to monitor glucose control. Data from such studies as those of Valleron (1975) have shown that the two-hour plasma glucose is the most sensitive of the values of the glucose tolerance test in establishing a diagnosis of diabetes. Normally the maximal increase in plasma glucose after a meal occurs at about 60 to 90 minutes and by two hours the levels are similar to the fasting values. In older individuals, however, the two-hour level may be slightly higher than the fasting glucose level. Because of a delay or absence of insulin release, the maximal difference between the glucose concentration in a diabetic and a normal should occur at two hours. Thus, a single plasma glucose determination obtained two hours postprandially should be the most helpful in defining the insulin response.

A committee of the American Diabetes Association (1975) has recommended a 50 to 100 mg challenge of glucose, 75 g carbohydrate, or a meal containing 100 g carbohydrate be given before the two-hour postprandial specimen is obtained. If the plasma glucose is above 140 mg/dl (7.8 mmol/l), a "further evaluation" is required. To make the diagnosis of diabetes mellitus, a plasma glucose level above 200 mg/dl (11.1 mmol/l) on two occasions is necessary. Mirsky (1974) suggests that a formal glucose tolerance test should be performed if a two-hour postprandial glucose level greater than 140 mg/dl (7.8 mmol/l) is obtained. A study by Kopf (1973) found that the two-hour postprandial value was dependent not on sex or weight, but only on age. In his study, a value of 160 mg/dl (8.9 mmol/l) was the upper limit of normal for patients who were in their sixth decade. In addition, he proposed that for each decade away from the sixth, 6 mg/dl (0.3 mmol/l) should either be added or subtracted from the reference value.

The significance of the two-hour postprandial value is limited by the lack of rigidly controlled conditions such as the amount of carbohydrate, the age of the patient, and intercurrent infection. These factors are responsible for the differences in the interpretation of the results. As with the glucose tolerance test, the diagnostic value of the two-hour postprandial glucose is debatable.

The Joslin Clinic group recommends that when the two-hour postprandial glucose level is used for monitoring control in diabetic subjects, a value greater than 150 mg/dl (8.3 mmol/l) two hours after a meal should be considered poor control, while values less than 130 mg/dl (7.2 mmol/l) are considered good control (Ingelfinger, 1977). However, the criteria for control vary widely and, as emphasized by Valleron (1975), the common denominator observed in most evaluations has been the inconsistency of criteria.

HYPOGLYCEMIA

Hypoglycemia is a syndrome characterized by low plasma glucose and an associated group of symptoms. Two different groups of symptoms occur, depending on whether the hypoglycemia is acute or chronic. If low plasma glucose occurs rapidly, homeostatic mechanisms release epinephrine and symptoms of sweating, shakiness, trembling, weakness, and anxiety are produced. If the reduction of plasma glucose occurs slowly, headache, irritability, lethargy, and other central nervous system symptoms predominate. Widespread publicity in the news media has led the public to believe that there is an exceedingly common and unrecognized occurrence of hypoglycemia in this country. In a statement on hypoglycemia, the American Diabetes Association (1973) and other medical societies conclude that these claims are not substantiated. However, many patients continue to appear with the self-diagnosis of hypoglycemia. It is important that, if the diagnosis is not confirmed after a proper laboratory workup, these patients be assured that their initial notions of hypoglycemia were wrong. If, however, hypoglycemia has been documented, it is essential that a full investigation of its cause be undertaken.

Merimee (1974) has attempted to define the criteria for laboratory diagnosis of hypoglycemia during fasting. In a group of normal subjects who had fasted for 24 hours, lower reference limits of plasma glucose were found to be 55 mg/dl (3.1 mmol/l) in men and 35 mg/dl (1.9 mmol/l) in women. In men, fasting plasma glucose was 50 mg/dl (2.8 mmol/l) if the fast was continued for 72 hours. It became virtually impossible to define a reference plasma glucose that was meaningful in the discrimination of hypoglycemia in premenopausal women who had fasted for more than 36 hours. In these studies, after a 72 hour fast, a normal plasma glucose in this reference population was considered to be as low as 15 mg/dl (0.8 mmol/l). These and other studies have raised a question of the definition of hypoglycemia. Merimee (1977) concludes that what has been called "functional" hypoglycemia is in fact normal, and in this instance false standards have created a false disease. In a review of the treatment of hypoglycemia, Newmark (1975) defined a glucose level below 50 mg/dl (2.8 mmol/l) as hypoglycemic. Prior to this, hypoglycemia was considered to exist at a glucose level of less than 60 mg/dl (3.2 mmol/l).

During a fast, serum insulin values decline steadily to reach low levels as the glucose concentration falls. The ratio of immunoreactive insulin (μ units/ml) to glucose (mg/dl) after an overnight fast, or during a 72 hour fast, normally is less than 0.30 (Fajans, 1976). The use of insulin-to-glucose ratios has become important in the definition of inappropriate insulin secretion and the definition of hypoglycemia. These are discussed in the section on insulinomas (p. 173).

The temporal occurrence of hypoglycemia

Table 7–5. CLASSIFICATION OF SOME OF THE MORE COMMON CAUSES OF HYPOGLYCEMIA

NO ANATOMIC LESION PRESENT
  Fasting plasma glucose normal
    Reactive hypoglycemia
      "Functional" hypoglycemia
      Prediabetic or diabetic hypoglycemia
      Alimentary hypoglycemia
  Fasting serum glucose low
    Ethanol-induced hypoglycemia
    Drug-induced hypoglycemia
      Sulfonylurea
      Ethanol
      Salicylates
      Phenformin
      Insulin
      Combinations of the above
  Factitious—fasting glucose normal or low
ANATOMIC LESION PRESENT
  Insulinoma
  Adrenal cortical insufficiency
  Hypopituitarism
  Extrapancreatic neoplasms
  Massive liver disease

---

can give a clue to its diagnosis. For example, if hypoglycemia occurs after a meal, it is called reactive hypoglycemia and a definite anatomic lesion usually is not found. If hypoglycemia occurs distant to a meal, such as in the night, it is called fasting hypoglycemia and carries a much more severe prognosis.

Classification of the causes of syndromes presenting with hypoglycemia is seen in Table 7–5. In the first group there is no anatomic lesion, hypoglycemia usually occurs in relationship to a meal, and fasting plasma glucose is normal. Whereas a glucose tolerance test of three hours' duration has been utilized for the diagnosis of hyperglycemia, if it is continued for five hours, important information may be obtained regarding hypoglycemia. Since the symptoms of hypoglycemia are so transient, specimens should be obtained every 30 minutes and when the patient becomes symptomatic. Three classic patterns of hypoglycemia have been described from the five-hour glucose tolerance test (Fig. 7–5). Hypoglycemia that occurs following a meal is called "reactive" and is classified as (a) functional, (b) prediabetic or diabetic, and (c) alimentary. Reactive hypoglycemia during a five-hour glucose tolerance test is considered to occur when the plasma glucose falls below 40 to 45 mg/dl (2.2 to 2.4 mmol/l) (Fajans, 1973). Marks (1976), however, defines hypoglycemia as (1) a venous plasma glucose concentration below 40 mg/dl (2.2 mmol/l); (2) symptoms of neuroglycopenia; (3) a postnadir rise in cortisol of at least 10 μg/dl (275 nmol/l); and (4) a postnadir growth hormone concentration of 10 ng/ml or more. Functional hypoglycemia is quite common in adults and is characterized by hypoglycemia occurring two to four hours after a meal, with predominant epinephrine-induced symptoms occurring shortly thereafter. This syndrome is commonly seen in those who have emotional

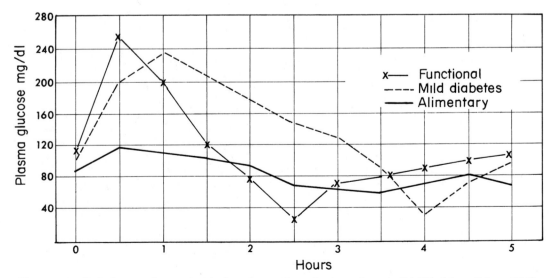

Figure 7–5. Oral glucose tolerance test in three types of reactive hypoglycemia (Modified from Fajans, 1973).

problems. The five-hour glucose tolerance test gives a characteristic pattern of low glucose levels at about three hours, with serum insulin levels throughout the test appropriate for glucose levels. These patients do not develop diabetes mellitus at a rate any greater than does the general population. Hypoglycemia in relationship to a meal is sometimes seen in prediabetics or diabetics. Here hypoglycemia occurs later than in the "functional" group, and insulin response is delayed and exaggerated. These patients may develop diabetes mellitus. The third type of reactive hypoglycemia, called "alimentary," occurs in those patients who have had gastrointestinal surgery, which leads to an accelerated absorption of glucose. Marked postprandial hyperglycemia with a corresponding insulin release results; the ensuing hypoglycemia occurs one-half hour to three hours after eating. The rapid rise in plasma glucose initiates an exaggerated insulin response, which then results in hypoglycemia. This pattern of the glucose intolerance and a history of gastrointestinal surgery are suggestive of this diagnosis. Some patients with the typical pattern of rapid glucose absorption and insulin release have been described who have not had gastrointestinal surgery (Permutt, 1973). It is exceedingly important to obtain plasma for a glucose determination if and when symptoms occur during a glucose tolerance test. During the glucose tolerance test a significant number of patients will experience the symptoms which resulted in their referral, but these symptoms may not occur in relationship to low plasma glucose values. These patients should be evaluated for anxiety states and should receive supportive psychotherapy with de-emphasis of hypoglycemia. True functional hypoglycemia should be documented with serum cortisol during the hypoglycemic episode and 90 minutes later. A positive physiologic response, which is a doubling of the cortisol, is evidence of functional hypoglycemia (Vinicor, 1975). These patients improve when their food intake is divided so that they eat many small meals rather than several large ones.

During the five-hour glucose tolerance test, Park (1972) demonstrated that about one fourth of normal patients had glucose values below 50 mg/dl (2.8 mmol/l), while prediabetics and early diabetics had about the same incidence. An occasional patient in all three groups had values below 35 mg/dl (1.9 mmol/l). It was concluded that there was very little justification for or diagnostic discrimination in a five-hour glucose tolerance test. This study has cast serious doubt on the diagnosis of hypoglycemia during the five-hour glucose tolerance test. The interpretation of the first three hours of this test is discussed at length in the hyperglycemia section (p. 160). The five-hour glucose tolerance test undoubtedly is one of the most poorly understood and misinterpreted tests currently used for investigating patients with suspected "hypoglycemia," and it is responsible for the epidemic of "non-hypoglycemia" prevalent in some parts of the world (Yager, 1974).

Other causes of hypoglycemia are ethanol and other drugs. Ethanol-induced hypoglycemia occurs only after prolonged ingestion of alcohol and when the liver supply of glycogen is depleted concurrently. The most common causes of drug-induced hypoglycemia are hypoglycemic agents (sulfonylureas, insulin, etc.), which account for more than half of the drug-induced causes; salicylates; sulfonamides; propranolol; or a combination of these (Seitzer, 1972). Factitious hypoglycemia is another phenomenon that may not occur in the relationship to meals.

Insulinomas or other tumors such as mesotheliomas, hepatic carcinomas, adrenal cortical tumors, and gastrointestinal carcinomas may cause hypoglycemia. The hypoglycemia caused by lesions such as tumors generally is profound and unremitting. About 30 to 50 per cent of tumors such as large mesenchymal tumors, hepatomas, and adrenocortical carcinomas produce insulin-like substances that cause hypoglycemia (Megyesi, 1974). The activity of these substances is not suppressed by insulin antibodies *in vitro;* therefore, this material has been appropriately called non-suppressible insulin-like activity (NSILA). This material can be quantitated by bioassay or radioreceptor assay, both of which are available on a research basis (Kahn, 1977). Other diseases that have commonly been found to present with hypoglycemia include adrenal cortical insufficiency, hypopituitarism, and diffuse liver disease.

INSULINOMA

The most important cause of spontaneous hypoglycemia is excessive and inappropriate secretion of insulin by pancreatic beta (islet cell) tumors. These tumors, called insulinomas, have been reported to occur at every age, but are most common in the fourth to sixth decades. The many clinical features associated with these tumors are caused by the hypoglycemia that they induce. The symptoms, which usually have an insidious onset, can mimic a wide variety of psychiatric and neurologic disorders. The diagnosis of hypoglycemia should be made using the criteria known as Whipple's triad: (1) hypoglycemic attacks precipitated by fasting, (2) plasma glucose less than 40 mg/dl (2.2 mmol/l) during the attack, (3) symptoms relieved promptly by the administration of glucose. Approximately 80 per cent of insulinomas are benign, 10 per cent are multiple, and another 10 per cent are malignant. Malignant insulinomas also have been reported to produce other hormones, including ACTH, glucagon, and gastrin.

Since the cause of hypoglycemia is the excessive and inappropriate production of insulin, the use of the insulin radioimmunoassay is essential in confirming the diagnosis. Normally fasting is associated with progressive fall in serum insulin concentrations; however, patients with insulinoma fail to show a fall of insulin with hypoglycemia. Since an overnight fast may not be sufficient to separate completely those patients with tumor from the non-tumor patients, fasting for up to 72 hours may be necessary. Although the absolute insulin concentration in the patient with an insulinoma may actually be within the normal range, the values are inappropriately high for the degree of hypoglycemia. Apart from factitious hypoglycemia, the only disorder in which inappropriate insulin secretion has been documented by RIA during fasting is idiopathic hypoglycemia of childhood.

A ratio of insulin to glucose has been developed that corrects for the technical problems involved in the insulin assay and has led to an "amended" insulin-to-glucose ratio. Since insulin secretion from the normal beta cell is reduced to basal levels with hypoglycemia, insulin will be non-detectable by radioimmunoassay at glucose concentrations of about 30 mg/dl. Therefore, a value of 30 mg/dl is subtracted from the glucose value. This amended ratio is seen below (in μ units/ml):

$$\frac{100 \times \text{Insulin } (\mu \text{ units/ml})}{\text{glucose (mg/dl)} - 30 \text{ mg/dl}}$$

A ratio for a reference population extends up to $100\,\mu$ units/mg, while in insulinoma patients a mean ratio of 180 was found (Frerichs, 1976). A similar study by Fajans (1976) has suggested that an amended ratio up to $50\,\mu$

units/mg is normal. In both these studies some of the patients with insulinomas have been found to have normal ratios. Manifestations of inappropriate insulin release are exaggerated by responses to insulin secretagogues such as tolbutamide. Tolbutamide, an oral hypoglycemic agent, when given as a rapid intravenous infusion, normally causes an immediate release of insulin, resulting in hypoglycemia. The depth and length of the hypoglycemia have been used to indicate the presence of an insulinoma. The criteria that are used are (1) a decrease in plasma glucose of more than 65 per cent or below 30 mg/dl (1.7 mmol/l), (2) plasma glucose of less than 40 mg/dl (2.2 mmol/l) persisting up to 180 minutes or longer, and (3) significant increase of serum insulin concentrations above the upper limit of normal (Frerichs, 1976). A false positive tolbutamide test may occur in obese subjects, while false negative tests occur in up to 50 per cent of patients with insulinomas (Schein, 1973). A stimulatory test utilizing leucine is capable of causing insulin secretion in about 50 per cent of insulinoma patients. Although other secretagogues such as glucagon and calcium infusions have been used, experience with them is still limited.

The glucose tolerance test is of little use in the diagnosis of an insulinoma, since a normal, diabetic, functional pattern may be found. However, the five-hour glucose tolerance test may be of some help in the differentiation of patients with reactive hypoglycemia from those with insulinomas. Patients with reactive disorders will have a rebound elevation of plasma glucose from the hypoglycemic range, while in those with an insulinoma this may not occur.

Diazoxide, an inhibitor of insulin secretion, has been used in the diagnosis of insulinomas. A rise in the plasma glucose level in response to oral administration of diazoxide is strong supportive evidence that the glucose-insulin axis is intact. A failure of the glucose to rise is circumstantial evidence that an insulinoma is present (Schein, 1973).

The use of the "C" peptide assay also has been helpful in the diagnosis of insulinomas: the suppressibility of beta cell secretion with insulin-induced hypoglycemia is monitored by "C" peptide measurements. Since commercial insulin preparations have "C" peptide removed during purification, the presence of "C" peptide in the circulation is good evidence of autonomous insulin secretion. Normal patients will suppress their insulin and "C" peptide secretion, but some of those with insulinomas also will show decreased or absent "C" peptide secretion (Horwitz, 1974).

In conclusion, fasting hypoglycemia may be diagnosed when glucose levels are less than 55 mg/dl (3.1 mmol/l) in men and less than 40 mg/dl (2.2 mmol/l) in women during the first 12 hours of fasting and are associated with an inappropriately high insulin-to-glucose ratio. If the insulin-to-glucose ratio is normal, the workup should be terminated; but if the index of suspicion is still high, the overnight fast with glucose and insulin levels can be repeated. Tumors producing NSILA are exceedingly rare but yield a normal ratio when insulin levels are determined by immunoassay. If an inappropriately high insulin-to-glucose ratio is found, diagnostic investigation should be pursued to locate an anatomic lesion or a metabolic cause for the hypoglycemia, and only then should a stimulatory or suppressive test of pancreatic function be performed.

If symptoms of hypoglycemia occur in relation to a meal, it is less important to pursue the cause. However, a five-hour glucose tolerance test with appropriate cortisol determinations can be used to document functional hypoglycemia.

The individual glucose values of the five-hour glucose tolerance test should not be utilized for the diagnosis of hypoglycemia, but rather the pattern of the test should receive attention. It should be remembered that patients with an "alimentary pattern" need not have had gastrointestinal surgery, nor need those patients with a "prediabetic" or "diabetic" pattern be differentiated from normals on the basis of hypoglycemia alone. What usually has been called hypoglycemia during this test should not be so classified unless the patient is symptomatic when the plasma glucose is at least below 45 mg/dl (2.5 mmol/l) and this is accompanied by an adequate rise in cortisol. If used with these limitations, the five-hour glucose tolerance test still remains of value for the diagnosis of reactive hypoglycemia. If a "low" glucose is not followed by a rebound elevation, or if a cortisol response is not detected, then these patients should have further investigative studies.

DIABETIC KETOACIDOSIS

Diabetic ketoacidosis is a syndrome whose main features are hyperglycemia, hyperosmo-

lality, dehydration, and ketoacidosis, which occurs because of an absolute or relative insulin deficiency. In the normal state, there is a balance between effects of insulin and those of the catabolic hormones—glucagon, cortisol, catecholamines, thyroid hormones, and growth hormone. An imbalance may arise because of an absolute insulin deficiency, as in a juvenile diabetic. If insufficient insulin is present, plasma glucose concentrations rise as a result of both enhanced gluconeogenesis and decreased extrahepatic utilization. The increased production is due both to the removal of the restraint on gluconeogenesis by insulin and to the activation of the enzymes glucose 6-phosphatase, fructose 1,6-diphosphatase, pyruvate carboxylase, and phosphoenolpyruvate (PEP) carboxykinase (see Fig. 7-1). At the same time, the relative or absolute excess of glucagon and epinephrine promotes glycogenolysis, while glucagon and cortisol also enhance the uptake of the gluconeogenic substances such as alanine. The hyperglycemia leads to hyperosmolality, and to osmotic diuresis with renal loss of glucose, electrolytes, and water.

The non-esterified fatty acids that are released from the adipose tissue are assimilated by the liver at a rate dependent on their plasma concentration. These long chain fatty acids are converted to their CoA derivatives and transported to the mitochondrial system and oxidized to acetyl-CoA. The disposition of acetyl-CoA depends on the availability of oxaloacetate. In diabetic ketoacidosis, acetyl-CoA is diverted almost entirely to ketone body formation with the formation of acetoacetyl-CoA; acetoacetyl-CoA is then converted to acetoacetate and hydroxybutyrate, while the third ketone, acetone, arises from the spontaneous decarboxylation of acetoacetate, as shown at the top of the next page. These ketone bodies cannot be utilized by the liver, and they enter the circulation to be utilized by other tissues.

The mortality of diabetic ketoacidosis is in the range of 5 to 15 per cent (Alberti, 1977b). Most signs and symptoms of ketoacidosis are easily recognized. Thirst, polyuria, weight loss, anorexia, fatigue, hyperventilation, dehydration, and drowsiness are the usual presenting signs and symptoms. Persistent hyperglycemia will cause the loss of intracellular water and an osmotic diuresis with fluid loss leading to hypovolemia, hypotension, and tachycardia. The rate and depth of respirations increase, causing further loss of fluid. About 10 per cent

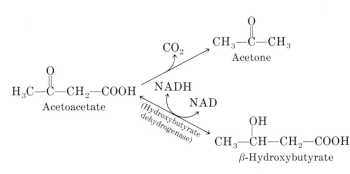

of cases present in true coma, and 20 per cent have no clouding of consciousness.

Treatment of diabetic ketoacidosis can be divided into fluid replacement, insulin replacement, potassium replacement, and treatment of the predisposing factors.

Fluid replacement is probably the single most important factor in the treatment: an average deficit of about 5 liters has been found. Fluids should be replaced with isotonic saline to prevent too rapid a fall in extracellular osmolality.

The major change in the therapy of ketoacidosis has occurred since about 1974 and has concerned the use of insulin. Many groups have suggested the use of much smaller doses of insulin given as a constant intravenous infusion, but the advantages of this still remain controversial. The advantages and disadvantages of low dose insulin have been reviewed by Alberti (1977a). However, it has been concluded that the incidence of hypokalemia and hypoglycemia is certainly less than with high dose infusion.

Total body potassium deficits range from 400 to 1000 mEq/l (400 to 1000 mmol/l) in patients with severe diabetic ketoacidosis. When insulin is replaced, potassium enters cells, resulting in a lowering of the plasma concentration. As this potassium deficit is replaced, potassium levels must be monitored closely. The replacement of alkali remains controversial and because of possible paradoxial fall in cerebrospinal fluid pH, extreme caution is advised. However, in cases in which blood pH is below 7.0 or in which distressing hyperventilation occurs, administration of alkali is advisable. Underlying causes of diabetic ketoacidosis include infection, trauma, or failure to take insulin.

The frequency of laboratory determinations in diabetic ketoacidosis is dependent on many factors, among them the clinical setting and the severity of the ketoacidosis. In addition to the routine diagnostic determinations, those specific for the treatment of severe ketosis should include plasma glucose, acetone, and electrolytes. As a minimum, they should be followed every two to three hours until recovery is well established. Early in the course of treatment plasma glucose should be measured more frequently until a therapeutic response is seen, while late in the treatment potassium measurements should be monitored more frequently for the development of hypokalemia. Venous pH measurements should be performed to document the degree of acidemia and its improvement. A less severe presentation will require less frequent laboratory determinations.

Occasionally an alcoholic patient will present with hyperketonemia and a metabolic acidosis in the absence of hyperglycemia (Levy, 1973). About 25 per cent of these patients are hypoglycemic. This syndrome is differentiated from diabetic ketoacidosis by plasma glucose levels of less than 200 mg/dl (11.1 mmol/l) and the absence of glucosuria. Contrary to treatment for diabetic ketoacidosis, these patients should not be treated with insulin.

HYPEROSMOLAR NON-KETOTIC COMA

Decreased or absent insulin secretion may manifest itself in a spectrum of presentations from pure ketoacidosis to one without ketosis. If ketosis is absent, the osmotic diuresis from the hyperglycemia is prolonged, and severe dehydration with coma finally occurs. But if ketosis is severe, marked dehydration and coma rapidly supervene and medical help must be sought quickly (Foster, 1974). Many of the causes of coma, including intracranial disease and toxic metabolic encephalopathy, such as hepatic insufficiency, anoxia, uremia, or disturbances in body temperature, can be substantiated by their associated signs noted on physical and neurologic examination. If the odor of acetone is not present in the breath of the subject, the diagnosis of diabetic coma is usually discarded and hyperosmolar non-ketotic coma may be overlooked. This perhaps is the reason for the extremely high mortality.

Altered consciousness with very high serum osmolality does not always imply severe dehydration and hyperosmolar coma. Since ethyl alcohol is osmotically active, a high plasma osmolality may accompany coma due to ordinary drunkenness. However, in a middle-aged or elderly mild diabetic who presents in coma without Kussmaul respirations and without the odor of alcohol or ketones on the breath, the physician should be alerted to the likelihood of hyperosmolar non-ketotic coma.

Laboratory diagnosis of hyperosmolar non-ketotic coma rests on the presence of 3+ to 4+ glycosuria and extreme hyperglycemia, usually greater than 1000 mg/dl (55.5 mmol/l) in the absence of ketoacidosis (McCurdy, 1970). Occasionally some patients are found with mild acetonemia (2+), but these can be regarded as either non-ketotic, ketotic, or a "mixture" of both (Arieff, 1972). Patients with the hyperosmolar syndrome have modestly elevated levels of lactate even in the absence of frank lactic acidosis; however, the amount of lactate that accumulates does not explain the mild acidosis. Although a number of precipitating causes, such as peritoneal dialysis, acute burns, ketoacidosis, and a variety of drugs, which include propranolol, phenytoin, steroids, immunosuppressive drugs, thiazide diuretics, and diazoxide, have been identified, usually the etiology cannot be determined.

HEMOGLOBIN A_{Ic}

Current methods of assessing diabetic control include the measurement of plasma and urine glucose. These measurements reflect acute changes and may not be adequate indicators of the long-term aspects of diabetic control. A more useful technique for assessing diabetic control may prove to be the identification of hemoglobin A_{Ic}, a hemoglobin A with a glucose moiety on the amino terminal valine of the beta chain (Peterson, 1977b).

When hemolysates of human red cells are chromatographed using cation-exchange resins, three or more minor peaks elute before the main hemoglobin A peak. This hemoglobin is made by a postsynthetic modification of hemoglobin A at a slow, constant rate during the 120-day life span of the red cell. Levels of hemoglobin A_{Ic}, which composes 3 to 6 per cent of the total hemoglobin in normals, are increased up to 12 per cent in diabetics. The other hemoglobin variants, Hb_{Ia} and Hb_{Ib}, which are the other minor hemoglobins eluting before the main peak, normally account for about 1.6 and 0.8 per cent of the total hemoglobin, respectively. These hemoglobins also are increased in diabetics (Gabbay, 1977).

The synthesis of the increased amounts of hemoglobin A_{Ic} has been shown to correlate with glucose intolerance in diabetics (Koenig, 1976a); with good diabetic control, the amount of hemoglobin A_{Ic} returns to the normal range (Koenig, 1976b). Peterson (1977a) has postulated that hemoglobin A_{Ic} is proportional to the time-averaged concentration of glucose within the cell; thus, A_{Ic} assays may provide a useful means of evaluating the extent to which satisfactory diabetic control has been achieved.

A column chromatography method for the measurement of hemoglobin A_{Ic} is available in the kit form. Since the hemoglobin variants A_{Ia} and A_{Ib} elute with the A_{Ic} fraction in this method, they are measured as well (Trivelli, 1971). A high performance liquid chromatographic method has been developed which allows for the quantitation of each hemoglobin A variant (Davis, 1978).

LACTIC ACIDOSIS

Lactic acid, which is a strong acid with a pK of 3.9, is dissociated at physiologic pH. Therefore, practically all of plasma lactic acid will be in the form of lactate and hydrogen ion. Lactate is the end product of anaerobic metabolism and its level is related to oxygen availability (see Fig. 7-1). When the supply of oxygen is limited, the cytochrome system is unable to function as an intermediate in the transfer of hydrogen to molecular oxygen. In this situation, reduced nicotinamide adenine dinucleotide (NADH) accumulates and is oxidized by the lactate dehydrogenase system with the production of lactate. Lactate dehydrogenase catalyzes the following reaction:

$$\text{pyruvate} + \text{NADH} + \text{H}^+ \rightleftharpoons \text{lactate} + \text{NAD}$$

Lactate is a dead-end branch of the energy metabolism chain, and following its accumulation, it can be easily metabolized back to pyruvate when oxygen again becomes abundant. As the lactate increases in such tissues as skeletal muscle, liver, and erythrocytes, diffusion out of these tissues occurs and concentrations of blood lactate begin to rise. In non-exercising man, the liver and to a certain extent the kidneys are the chief organs responsible for the lactate metabolism to glucose, or its oxidation to CO_2 and H_2O. In the presence of elevated concentrations, cardiac and skeletal muscle also may oxidize lactate.

Shock is perhaps the most widely recognized cause of lactic acidosis; however, in some cases, excess lactate production may precede shock. Such conditions as myocardial infarction, severe congestive heart failure, pulmonary edema, and blood loss are the common causes of shock which may produce lactic acidosis. Phenformin, a drug that is used in the treatment of diabetes mellitus, is by far the most commonly reported direct cause of lactic acidosis. In his personal experience and review of the literature, Cohen (1976) has estimated that phenformin accounts for 50 per cent of the reported cases of lactic acidosis. The majority of these cases occur shortly after the initiation of phenformin therapy or after the dose has been increased. Other causes of lactic acidosis include intravenous infusions of substances such as fructose, sorbitol, or epinephrine, and large doses of drugs such as ethanol or acetaminophen (Table 7-6). Hepatic necrosis, neoplasms, lymphomas, and various forms of leukemia have been reported to cause lactic acidosis. In diabetic coma, lactic acidosis is common. In some cases, the lactic acidosis is secondary to some common cause such as shock, phenformin ingestion, or epinephrine

Table 7-6. COMMON CAUSES
OF LACTIC ACIDOSIS

Shock
Drugs
  Phenformin
  Sorbitol
  Fructose
  Ethanol
  Epinephrine
  Acetaminophen
Hepatic disease
Neoplasms
Diabetic ketoacidosis
Idiopathic
Congenital
  Glucose 6-phosphatase deficiency
    (Type I glycogen storage disease)
  Fructose 1,6-diphosphatase deficiency

release, but in other instances it has been reported secondary to the ketoacidosis (Marliss, 1970). Although it has been reported that up to 30 per cent of all cases of lactic acidosis may be classified as idiopathic, in a recent study and review of the literature, Fulop (1977) concluded that lactic acidosis rarely, if ever, lacks an identifiable cause.

An anion gap in a patient with metabolic acidosis suggests the diagnosis of lactic acidosis. Hence, the diagnosis can be suspected when the sum of anions minus the sum of cations $((Na^+ + K^+) - (Cl^- + HCO_3^-))$ exceeds 18 mmol/l in the absence of other causes of an anion gap, such as renal failure, salicylate ingestion, methanol poisoning, or significant ketonemia.

Lactate values are determined by enzymatic methods employing lactate dehydrogenase (Westgard, 1972). Several precautions are necessary in the collection of a satisfactory specimen for lactate analysis. Although a venous blood specimen may yield higher results than an arterial sample, venous samples often are used for convenience. If prior to obtaining the specimen the patient remains at complete rest, venous and arterial levels are virtually alike. The venostasis formed from applying a tourniquet has little effect, but such minor movements as hand clenching can raise blood lactate significantly (Braybrooke, 1975). Blood should be collected in a syringe and deproteinized immediately, for example, by adding the blood to a tube containing perchloric acid (Marks, 1976). Plasma kept at 25°C. is also a satisfactory specimen if tubes containing sodium fluoride and potassium oxalate are used for the blood collection and separation of the plasma is completed within 15 minutes (Westgard, 1972). If blood is not collected by these or comparable methods, lactate will increase rapidly from glycolysis by the red cell enzymes. When blood is not collected in the correct tube and is kept at 25°C., increases may be as great as 20 per cent in 3 minutes or 70 per cent within 30 minutes.

A normal venous blood lactate concentration is usually 0.6 to 1.7 mEq/l (0.6 to 1.7 mmol/l), but even mild exercise will increase lactate levels substantially. In lactic acidosis, values exceeding 7 to 8 mEq/l (7 to 8 mmol/l) usually are associated with a fatal outcome (Oliva, 1970).

The absence of a rise in lactate levels after mild exercise is an important criterion in the diagnosis of patients with McArdle's disease

(Type V glycogen storage disease), as discussed elsewhere (p. 182).

Although the measurement of pyruvate in conjunction with the measurement of lactate clearly indicates the state of tissue oxidation, methods of pyruvate measurement are laborious. For this reason they are not widely used.

DISORDERS OF FRUCTOSE METABOLISM

Disorders of fructose metabolism are divided into three groups: essential fructosuria, hereditary fructose intolerance, and fructose 1,6-diphosphatase deficiency. All are transmitted as autosomal recessives. Only in essential fructosuria are there no outward signs or symptoms and the patient leads an essentially normal life.

Normally fructose is found in small quantities in the serum, usually in the range of 1 to 6 mg/dl (0.1 to 0.3 mmol/l). A major source of fructose is the disaccharide sucrose, which contains 1 molecule of glucose and 1 molecule of fructose and is present in fruits and vegetables. The average daily ingestion of about 50 to 100 grams is one fifth to one third of the daily carbohydrate load. The relationship of the enzymes involved in fructose metabolism is shown in Figure 7-6. After fructose loading, values as high as 100 mg/dl (5.5 mmol/l) may be seen in patients with disorders of fructose metabolism.

ESSENTIAL FRUCTOSURIA

Essential fructosuria, usually occurring in Jewish families, is a benign condition which has an incidence of 1 in 130,000 (Froesch, 1972). The enzymatic defect is a relative lack of hepatic fructokinase, the enzyme which is responsible for phosphorylation in the 1 position. This results in high levels of fructose after meals containing either sucrose or fructose. About 10 times more fructose than the normal 1 to 2 per cent is found in the urine of patients with this disorder. The presence of the reducing sugar fructose in the urine has been detected by non-specific glucose methods (Chap. 17). With the replacement of reducing methods by more specific glucose methods, these patients are not being detected. Neither serum glucose nor serum phosphorus falls in these patients following a glucose load.

HEREDITARY FRUCTOSE INTOLERANCE

Hereditary fructose intolerance is characterized by the development of nausea, abdominal pain, hypoglycemia, amino aciduria, hyperuricemia, uricosuria, and fructosuria following ingestion of fructose or sorbitol. Babies with hereditary fructose intolerance exhibit vomiting and hypoglycemia when fed formulas high in fructose or fruit juices. If they are continued on this diet, many may die; if fructose is stopped the babies cease vomiting and start to gain weight, and the enlarged liver

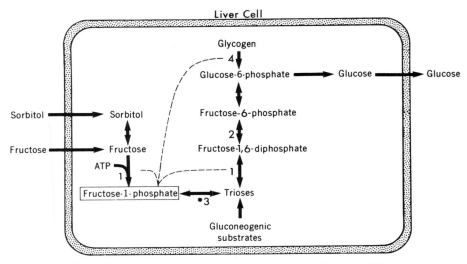

* Primary defect in Hereditary Fructose Intolerance, deficiency of fructose-1-phosphate aldolase.

Figure 7-6.   Hereditary defects in fructose metabolism (Modified from Steiner, 1977b).
   1—Primary defect in fructosuria (fructokinase).
   2—Primary defect in fructose 1,6-diphosphatase.
   3—Primary defect in hereditary fructose intolerance (fructose diphosphate aldolase).
Defects secondary to accumulation of fructose 1-phosphate
   1—Fructokinase.
   4—Phosphorylase and phosphoglucomutase.
   3—Fructose diphosphate aldolase.

becomes normal in size. In older children and adults, strong aversion to sweets and fruits is characteristic. Diagnosis of hereditary fructose intolerance is made by the intravenous (IV) fructose tolerance test (Marks, 1976). After the IV infusion of 0.25 g/kg body weight of fructose, blood is obtained at frequent intervals, such as 0, 10, 20, 30, 45, 60, 75, and 90 minutes thereafter, and glucose as well as phosphorus is measured. A normal response is a small but definite rise in plasma glucose and a small, short-lived fall in phosphorus concentrations. Patients with hereditary fructose intolerance show a persistent decrease in the plasma concentrations of glucose and phosphate and usually become hypoglycemic. This diagnostic procedure is of extreme value in older children and adults and may indicate that hereditary fructose intolerance is present. A definitive diagnosis can be made by liver biopsy and the measurement of fructose 1-phosphate aldolase, the enzyme that is markedly decreased in this disease. In newborns, the fructose tolerance test may not be as helpful as in the adult.

Other enzymatic defects have been associated with hereditary fructose intolerance and account for hypoglycemia (Fig. 7-6). They are fructose diphosphate aldolase deficiency, the inhibition of aldolase, the inhibition of phosphorolysis of glycogen to glucose 1-phosphate, and the inhibition of fructokinase, all of which occur because of the accumulation of glucose 1-phosphate (Perheentupa, 1972). During the hypoglycemic period, insulin secretion is appropriately low. Renal tubular acidosis (Type I or the distal type) has been described in some patients, while in others a proximal defect (Type II) occurs during periods of hyperfructosemia (Steiner, 1977b). An interesting facet of this disease is that adults with hereditary fructose intolerance tend not to have dental caries.

FRUCTOSE 1,6-DIPHOSPHATASE DEFICIENCY

These patients tend to present with symptoms indistinguishable from those of type I glycogen storage disease. Lactic acidosis, ketoacidosis, hyperlipidemia, hyperuricemia, and hepatomegaly occur, but skeletal and mental growth are normal. This disease results from a total lack of functioning fructose 1,6-diphosphatase (Baker, 1970). Since fructose 1,6-diphosphatase is absent, fructose 6-phosphate cannot be formed, and glyconeogenesis cannot occur. The liver can produce glucose as long as glycogen is present, but once glycogen is depleted, the child becomes hypoglycemic. Symptoms usually occur in response to an infection or a prolonged fast. In contrast to hereditary fructose intolerance, hypoglycemia without vomiting may occur in response to a large fructose load. Lactic acidosis is found because fructose enters the glycolytic scheme below the enzyme deficiency (Fig. 7-6). Once this disease is recognized, the patient is treated with frequent meals. The hepatomegaly is

secondary to lipid storage and not excessive glycogen deposition (Pagliara, 1973).

GLYCOGEN STORAGE DISEASES

Glycogen storage diseases result from a specific deficiency of enzymes involved in the metabolism of glycogen. As a consequence of this deficiency, glycogen accumulates in the liver, but with some of the defects this deposition is generalized. The incidence of all forms of glycogen storage diseases combined is about 1 in 40,000 (Mahler, 1976). There are ten distinct types of glycogen storage disease; however, several are extremely rare. Most are inherited as an autosomal recessive, with only a few also exhibiting other forms of inheritance. In some of these, bacterial or fungal enzymes have been used as replacement for the deficient enzyme, but very little clinical success has resulted. In all glycogen storage diseases, definitive diagnosis can be made by the assay of the enzyme from the appropriate tissue and by a characteristic microscopic appearance of the affected tissues. A prenatal diagnosis can be made in those in which the defect is present in all tissues. Generally, in those in whom the defect is present in one or two tissues, a prenatal diagnosis is not possible. The classification presented in Table 7-7, with a Roman numeral for each type, is that used by Mahler (1976). In the many descriptions of these diseases, eponyms are used; they also are listed. Glycogen storage diseases have been extensively reviewed; for further details see Huijing (1975) or McAdams (1974).

Type I. Von Gierke's disease is caused by a deficiency of glucose 6-phosphatase, an enzyme found only in the liver, kidney, and small intestine. In this disease, plasma glucose cannot be maintained and severe fasting hypoglycemia, with glucose approaching 20 mg/dl (1.1 mmol/l) occurs after an overnight fast. Since glucose 6-phosphate produced by glycogen breakdown cannot be transported out of the liver as glucose, it is metabolized to lactic acid, then released, resulting in lactic acidosis. The clinical picture is one of massive liver enlargement, retardation of growth and development, osteoporosis, and in about 50 per cent of the cases, death in early childhood. Gout, which results from the decreased renal clearance of uric acid, is also present.

There is genetic heterogeneity found in glucose 6-phosphatase deficiency. Most patients have no detectable enzyme, while in others immunoreactive material is found by an antibody to this enzyme (Collipp, 1974). Patients with the immunoreactive material appear to be less clinically affected than those without the enzyme. Diagnosis can be made by the intramuscular injection of 0.5 mg of glucagon. A normal response is a glucose rise of 60 to 80 mg/dl (3.3 to 4.4 mmol/l) in 10 to 20 minutes with no change in lactate, while in von Gierke's disease, lactate increases by 3 to 6 mEq/l (3 to 6 mmol/l)

Table 7-7. CLINICAL GUIDE TO GLYCOGEN STORAGE DISEASES

TYPE	MAJOR CLINICAL FEATURES	ENZYME DEFICIENCY	FASTING HYPOGLYCEMIA	PLASMA GLUCOSE RESPONSE TO I.M. GLUCAGON (0.5 mg)
I von Gierke's	Hepatomegaly, lactic acidosis, hyperlipidemia	Glucose 6-phosphatase Liver (kidney)	Severe	No response
II Pompe's	a. Cardiomegaly, muscle weakness. Death in infancy b. Adult	Alpha 1,4-glucosidase All tissues Muscle	None None	Normal Normal
III Cori-Forbes	Variable degrees of hepatomegaly and muscle weakness	Debrancher All tissues	Moderate to severe	Normal after food; poor after fasting
IV Anderson	Portal cirrhosis. Usually death in infancy	Brancher All tissues	None	Normal
V McArdle's	Pain and stiffness after exertion. Myoglobinuria in 50% of cases	Phosphorylase Muscle	None	Normal
VI Hers	Hepatomegaly	Phosphorylase Liver	Absent to mild	No response fasting or after food
VII Tarui	Pain and stiffness on exertion	Phosphofructokinase Muscle (? liver)	None	Normal
VIII	Spasticity, decerebration, high urinary catecholamines, death in infancy	Adenyl kinase Liver, brain	None	Normal
IX	Hepatomegaly	Phosphorylase kinase Liver	None, moderate	Normal, poor
X	Hepatomegaly only	Cyclic AMP-dependent kinase Liver, muscle	None	Normal

but a glucose increment is absent. By frequent feedings, the immediate risks of hypoglycemia can be avoided. The use of portacaval shunting has resulted in remarkable improvement in some of these patients (Starzl, 1973).

Type II. Pompe's disease reflects a deficiency of lysosomal alpha 1,4-glucosidase, resulting in the increase of glycogen in all organs. Glycogen is taken up by the lysosomal enzymes and cannot be degraded, resulting in abnormally large lysosomes. Several variants of the deficiency are becoming apparent. In the infantile form of the deficiency, the enzyme is missing from all tissues analyzed, and a rapid progression to death occurs by age one. There is massive accumulation of glycogen in the heart, skeletal muscle, and brain. The clinical symptoms are characterized by profound weakness, cardiomegaly, and heart failure, which differentiate it from Type I glycogen storage disease. The term *Pompe's disease* is restricted to the infantile form, since a more benign form called acid maltase deficiency has been recognized in adult life (Di-Mauro, 1977). In these adult patients, the decreased enzyme activity is usually restricted to skeletal muscle, resulting in a syndrome simulating muscular dystrophy or polymyositis with no cardiac or neuronal disorders. Weakness, generally of the trunk and proximal limb muscles, is slowly progressive, eventually involving respiratory muscles in about half the cases. Serum creatine kinase (CK) is consistently elevated, and histopathologic features are those of vacuolar myopathy on skeletal muscle biopsy. Glucose, lipids, and uric acid are normal, and there is a normal response to glucagon. Homozygotic and heterozygotic adults can be detected by measuring acid maltase in the urine (Mehler, 1976). Since there have been no families with both the infantile and the late onset forms, it appears that there are two different genetic disorders affecting the same enzyme.

Type III. Type III, one of the most common forms of the disease, results from the absence of a debrancher enzyme. It presents in the full range of the clinical spectrum, from those who are severely affected to those who are asymptomatic. The clinical syndrome is dominated by hepatomegaly, hypoglycemia, seizures, and growth retardation. Plasma glucose levels do not drop as low as in Type I (von Gierke's disease), since the outer branches of glycogen can be degraded. Since fasting blood lactate concentrations are not elevated as in the phosphatase deficiency, the brain does not have an available source of energy in the form of lactate. As a result, when compared with von Gierke's disease, seizures are seen at a much higher glucose concentration than in the phosphatase deficiency, where the brain is able to use the elevated concentrations of lactate or pyruvate as the energy source. Diagnosis is made by injection of glucagon (Table 7–7). With fasting, glucagon results in no rise in glucose, but with refeeding and testing two hours later, there is a normal elevation in glucose. There is no change in lactate with either one of these tests. Prognosis for Type III is fairly good if the child lives through the first four years and mental retardation has not occurred. The muscular weakness and wasting regress considerably. Some patients have a defective enzyme, others the absence of the enzyme, while a third group has small amounts of enzyme. This latter group has been treated with the enzyme-inducing drug phenytoin with considerable success (Jubiz, 1974). Since this disorder is systemic, leukocytes, erythrocytes, and cultured skin fibroblasts can be used for diagnostic enzyme assays (Huijing, 1976).

Type IV. Brancher deficiency is extremely rare and one of the least understood of the glycogen storage diseases. The glycogen that has accumulated has a structure superficially similar to amylopectin (predominantly 1,6 linkages), giving the disease the name of amylopectinosis. However, it is not understood why unbranched amylopectin (1,6 linkages) rather than amylose (1,4 linkages of glucose) accumulates in this disease. There is no storage glycogen found, and cirrhosis or progressive liver enlargement and muscle weakness occur by the age of two months. Death usually occurs before the age of three. Skin fibroblasts or leukocytes can be used for the diagnosis.

Type V. McArdle's disease, inherited as a deficiency of skeletal muscle phosphorylase, is approximately four times as prevalent in males as in females. The clinical picture is characterized by exercise intolerance. Soon after beginning exercise, muscle stiffness and aching occur, and if the exercise is continued, pain and stiffness disappear. The exercise then may be continued symptom-free for some time before the symptoms reoccur. This "second wind" phenomenon, characteristic of this disorder, may be due to the increased blood flow through the muscle, and the increase of fatty acids provides an alternate source of energy to glycogen (Lubran, 1975). Prolonged exercise, however, results in muscle necrosis and myoglobinuria. Some cases have been described in which acute tubular necrosis has resulted (Grünfeld, 1972). McArdle's disease is transmitted as an autosomal recessive, but at least in some families an autosomal dominant transmission has been documented. Laboratory diagnosis is made by applying a blood pressure cuff inflated above the systolic pressure on the exercising forearm and sampling blood lactate one minute after the exercise has begun. In this disease, there is no rise in blood lactate with exercise. The definitive diagnosis can be made by the measurement of phosphorylase in a muscle biopsy specimen.

Type VI. Liver phosphorylase deficiency, due to the absence of phosphorylase A and B, presents primarily with hepatomegaly and mild hypoglycemia. Following glucagon injection, there is no rise in plasma glucose in these patients. The phosphorylase deficiencies can be further divided into a number of enzyme deficiencies, which represent deficiencies of the enzyme activators of the phosphorylase complex. The remainder are classified as Types VIII, IX, and X. Liver phosphorylase deficiency seen in this disease is mild, with patients showing asymptomatic liver enlargement and occasional growth retardation. Since leukocytes possess the hepatic type of phosphorylase, they can be used in the diagnosis of this disorder. In Figure 7-2, the relationship of the various enzymes involved in the phosphorylase activation is seen.

Type VII. Muscle phosphofructokinase is absent, and the exercising forearm muscle test is used for the diagnosis. As in Type V, there is no increase in lactate. A mild hemolytic anemia may be present, but the other symptoms are similar to those of Type V: exercise intolerance, myoglobinuria on strenuous exercise, and the "second wind" phenomenon with ischemic exercise. Because the metabolic block affects glycolysis rather than gluconeogenesis, there is no rationale for the administration of glucose or other hyperglycemic agents in this condition. This condition is extremely rare.

Type VIII. This is an extremely rare form in which central nervous system symptoms dominate the clinical picture. Phosphorylase activity is extremely low, but the defect is probably the result of incomplete activation of adenyl kinase.

Type IX. This is also a deficiency of liver phosphorylase, originating from the genetic deficiency of liver phosphorylase kinase. There are two forms, one an autosomal recessive and the other a sex-linked recessive. Whereas patients with the autosomal recessive syndrome have a normal response of plasma glucose to glucagon, poor response is seen in those with the sex-linked recessive trait.

Type X. Only one case of Type X has been found, with increased glycogen demonstrated in the liver and muscle. All phosphorylase was in the inactive form in this disorder, and cyclic AMP-dependent kinase was absent.

GALACTOSEMIA

Galactosemia is a rare genetic disorder transmitted as an autosomal recessive. The prevalence of the homozygotic state is between 1 in 18,000 and 1 in 180,000 (Shih, 1971). It is characterized by low plasma glucose and the inability to metabolize galactose, a monosaccharide that is contained in milk as a constituent of the disaccharide lactose. The classic syndrome develops in infants who appear normal at birth but, after ingestion of milk, develop vomiting, cirrhosis, cataracts, and mental retardation. The metabolism of galactose involves three enzymatic steps; defects at any one of these steps cause a syndrome of galactosemia. Galactose is metabolized as follows:

The three enzymes involved in the metabolism of galactose are galactokinase (I), galactose 1-phosphate uridyl transferase (II), and UDP glucose 4-epimerase (III), with almost all defects involving the transferase. The symptoms of classic transferase (II) deficiency include mental retardation, failure to thrive, jaundice, and juvenile cataracts, while in the galactokinase (I) deficiency, juvenile cataracts are the only manifestation (Beutler, 1973). Epimerase (III) deficiency is rare and relatively asymptomatic (Gitzelman, 1972). There is some evidence that the liver and lens changes that occur in the transferase deficiency are reversible but that mental retardation resulting from the low glucose is not. Since dietary restriction of galactose intake is very effective treatment if it is started before irreversible damage has occurred, it is imperative that a diagnosis be documented early in the course of the disease and treatment begun.

The diagnosis of the homozygotic state is suggested by low plasma and urine glucose values detected by specific enzymatic glucose methods. Since galactose is a reducing sugar, its presence will yield elevated glucose levels in both blood and urine if the analysis is carried out by methods that depend on the reducing properties of glucose. A specific galactose urine dipstick impregnated with galactose oxidase, the enzyme peroxidase, and the oxygen acceptor ortho-toluidine now is available (Galactostix, Ames Company, Elkhart, Ind. 46514).

Widespread screening programs for galactosemia are based on measuring transferase (II) activity in red blood cells utilizing the method of Beutler (1966). The enzyme is monitored by the generation of the fluorescent, reduced pyridine nucleotide NADPH with a coupled enzymatic reaction. The glucose 1-phosphate formed by the transferase is converted to glucose 6-phosphate and then to 6-phosphoglutamate by glucose 6-phosphate dehydrogenase with the formation of NADPH. The absence of the transferase results in the failure to produce glucose 1-phosphate and subsequently fluorescent NADPH. With this methodology, false positives (absence of fluorescent NADPH) occur with a frequency of 1 in 100 to 1 in 5000 (Shih, 1971). The presence of other enzyme deficiencies such as glucose 6-phosphate dehydrogenase or phosphoglucomutase is a known cause of false positive results. These two enzymes are required in the coupled enzymatic assay that forms NADPH. Since the specimens are usually sent to a specialized laboratory for analysis, false positives may be caused by heat inactivation of the transferase occurring during the shipping process (Schön, 1977). A positive by this method thus requires a quantitative measurement of either substrate, UDP glucose or galactose 1-phosphate, for confirmation of the diagnosis (Kirkman, 1976). Most recently it has been reported that prenatal diagnosis of galactosemia is possible by measuring transferase activity in cultured amniotic cells (Ng, 1977).

If a patient is found to have galactosemia and transferase activity is present, the Guthrie test can be utilized to diagnose galactokinase deficiency.

$$\text{Galactose} \xrightarrow{\text{I}} \begin{array}{c} \text{Galactose 1-PO}_4 \\ + \\ \text{UDP Glucose} \end{array} \xrightarrow{\text{II}} \begin{array}{c} \text{Glucose 1-PO}_4 \\ + \\ \text{UDP Galactose} \\ \text{III} \diagdown \\ \text{UDP Glucose} \end{array}$$

The Guthrie test is a simple screening test for galactosemia which involves growth inhibition of *Escherichia coli* by elevated galactose concentrations. The measurement of the enzyme galactokinase is a more specific technique available for making this diagnosis (Beutler, 1971).

In an infant who is suspected of having galactosemia, the use of the galactose tolerance test is absolutely contraindicated, since a violent intestinal reaction to galactose will occur.

PENTOSURIA

In essential pentosuria, an innocuous condition transmitted as autosomal recessive, from 1.0 to 4.0 grams of the pentose L-xylulose is excreted into the urine daily. The incidence of pentosuria in the general population is about 1 in 50,000; however, almost all cases have been reported in Jews, and in this population the incidence may be as high as 1 in 2,000 (Hiatt, 1972).

Essential pentosuria results from a defect in metabolism of glucuronic acid. Glucuronic acid is metabolized by a series of reactions to the pentose L-xylulose, and then to L-xylitol by the enzyme xylitol dehydrogenase. L-Xylitol is subsequently metabolized to a hexose. The absence of a xylitol dehydrogenase in essential pentosuria results in the excessive excretion of L-xylulose (Hiatt, 1972).

The diagnosis of essential pentosuria can be suspected by the presence of reducing substances in the urine. Specific chromatography procedures are necessary for the identification of the individual

sugar. Since xylulose is present in serum in quantities of less than 2 mg/dl (0.1 mmol/l), plasma glucose measurements employing the reducing methods show no interference by xylulose. Although L-xylulose excretion is increased in patients with cirrhosis, the amount is much less than that in patients with essential pentosuria (Oka, 1976).

OXALOSIS

Oxalosis, which can be divided into primary and secondary types, is characterized by the soft tissue deposition of oxalate salts, resulting in chronic inflammation and fibrosis. The most obvious deposition of oxalate salts occurs in the kidney and bladder, where the occurrence of these stones may result in renal failure. Since two thirds of all kidney stones are at least in part calcium oxalate, the association of oxalosis and kidney disease is of considerable importance.

Primary oxalosis is a rare metabolic disorder transmitted as an autosomal recessive and characterized by continued excessive synthesis as well as excretion of oxalic acid (COOH—COOH). Oxalic acid is a metabolic end product that normally is excreted almost entirely in the urine. In primary oxalosis serum oxalic acid is normal, but an excessive amount is found in the urine. The metabolism is seen in Figure 7-7. The main intermediate precursors of oxalic acid are ascorbic acid and glyoxylic acid (COOH—CHO), each accounting for about 40 per cent of its total endogenous production. The remainder is derived from glycolic acid (COOH—

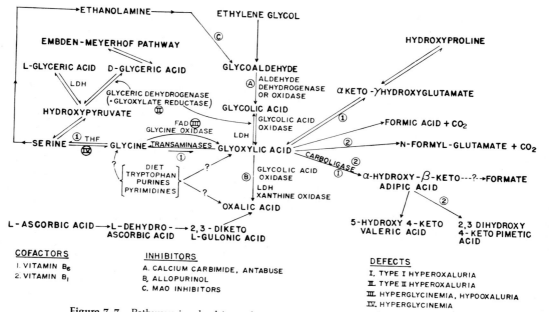

Figure 7-7. Pathways involved in oxalate metabolism (Modified from Hagler, 1973a).

CH$_2$OH), other glyoxate-forming reactions, and dietary ingestion. In type I, or glycolic aciduria, the enzyme carboligase, which catalyzes the breakdown of glyoxylic acid, has been found to be decreased, resulting in the increased synthesis and excretion of glycolate and glyoxalate in addition to oxalate. Recently a second type (glyceric aciduria or type II) has been described, in which oxalate and glycerate are increased in the urine. Primary hyperoxaluria of both types is manifested by nephrolithiasis, nephrocalcinosis, and widespread deposition of oxalate crystals throughout the organs of the body. The onset of symptoms usually occurs before the age of 5; 80 per cent of the patients die before reaching the age of 20. A few cases have been described presenting in adulthood. For additional information, the extensive review by Hagler (1973a, b, c, and d) should be consulted.

Secondary hyperoxaluria has been reported in a variety of diseases, including diabetes mellitus, cirrhosis, pyridoxine deficiency, and sarcoidosis; and with ethylene glycol (antifreeze) ingestion and methoxyfluothane anesthesia. Recently, excessive urine excretion of oxalate has been found to be a frequent complication of diseases presenting with steatorrhea, such as pancreatic insufficiency, celiac disease, and bacterial overgrowth. Patients with Crohn's disease have an increased prevalence of calcium oxalate nephrolithiasis, probably from increased absorption of dietary oxalate (Chadwick,

1973). Oxalosis also has been documented following ileal resection and after jejunoileal shunt procedures (Gelbart, 1977). Since these groups of diseases require an intact colon and occur in the presence of steatorrhea, Dobbins (1977) recommends that these syndromes be called "colonic hyperoxaluria."

Diagnosis of oxalosis is made by the determination of oxalic acid in the urine. Because oxalate crystals may be present in normal urine, they are of no diagnostic significance. Patients with primary hyperoxaluria excrete at least 100 mg and occasionally even up to 600 mg of oxalate per 24 hours. In renal failure, however, as total urine volume drops, the excretion of oxalates also has been found to decrease. Since serum oxalates are normal, the diagnosis of primary oxalosis in the presence of renal failure can be made only by specific enzyme analysis (Hagler, 1973d). Measurements of these enzymes, however, are not widely available.

Methods for measuring oxalate have been reviewed by Hodgkinson (1970). Most of these involve the precipitation of oxalate prior to its chemical determination, and at best, these methods remain laborious. Recently an enzymatic approach has been developed in which the CO$_2$ generated from oxalate by the enzyme oxalate decarboxylase is measured (Hatch, 1977).

REFERENCES

Alberti, K. G. M. M.: Low-dose insulin in the treatment of ketoacidosis. Arch. Intern. Med., *137*:1367, 1977a.

Alberti, K. G. M. M., Dornhorst, A., and Rowe, A. S.: Metabolic rhythms in normal and diabetic man: Studies in insulin-treated diabetes. Isr. J. Med. Sci., *11*:571, 1975a.

Alberti, K. G. M. M., Dornhorst, A., and Rowe, A. S.: Metabolic rhythms in old age. Biochem. Soc. Transaction, *3*:132, 1975b.

Alberti, K. G. M. M., and Hockraday, T. D. R.: Diabetic coma: A reappraisal after five years. Clin. Endocrinol. Metabol., *6*:421, 1977b.

American Diabetes Association: Detection and diagnosis of diabetes: Plasma glucose procedures. 1975.

American Diabetes Association, Endocrine Society and American Medical Association: Statement on hypoglycemia. Diabetes, *22*:137, 1973.

Arieff, A. I., and Carroll, H. J.: Nonketotic hyperosmolar coma with hyperglycemia: Clinical features, pathophysiology, renal function, acid-base balance, plasma-cerebrospinal fluid equilibria and the effects of therapy in 37 cases. Medicine, *51*:73, 1972.

Baker, L., and Wingrad, A. I.: Fasting hypoglycemia and metabolic acidosis associated with deficiency of hepatic fructose-1,6-diphosphatase activity. Lancet, *2*:13, 1970.

Beutler, E., and Baluda, M.: A simple spot screening test for galactosemia. J. Lab. Clin. Med., *68*:137, 1966.

Beutler, E., Matsumoto, F., Kuhl, W., Krill, A., Levy, N.,

Sparkes, R., and Degnan, M.: Galactokinase deficiency in cataracts. N. Engl. J. Med., *288*:1203, 1973.

Beutler, E., Pariker, N. U., and Trinidad, F.: The assay of red cell galactokinase. Biochem. Med., *5*:325, 1971.

Block, M. B., Rosenfield, R. L., Mako, M. E., Steiner, D. F., and Rubenstein, A. H.: Sequential changes in beta-cell function in insulin-treated diabetic patients assessed by C-peptide immunoreactivity. N. Engl. J. Med., *288*:1144, 1973.

Boden, G., and Owen, O. E.: Familial hyperglucagonemia—an autosomal dominant disorder. N. Engl. J. Med., *296*:534, 1977.

Braybrooke, J., Lloyd, B., Nattrass, M., and Alberti, K. G. M. M.: Blood sampling techniques for lactate and pyruvate estimation: A reappraisal. Ann. Clin. Biochem., *12*:252, 1975.

Carroll, K. F., and Nestel, P. J.: Diurnal variation in glucose tolerance and in insulin secretion in man. Diabetes, *22*:333, 1973.

Ceriotti, G.: Blood glucose determination without deproteinization, with use of *o*-toluidine in dilute acetic acid. Clin. Chem., *17*:201, 1971.

Chadwick, V. S., Modha, K., and Dowling, R. H.: Mechanism for hyperoxaluria in patients with ileal dysfunction. N. Engl. J. Med., *289*:172, 1973.

Chance, R. E., Root, M. A., and Galloway, J. A.: The immunogenicity of insulin preparations. Acta Endocrinol., (Suppl. 205), *83*:185, 1976.

Chiles, R., and Tzagournis, M.: Excessive serum insulin response to oral glucose in obesity and mild diabetes: Study of 501 patients. Diabetes, *19*:458, 1970.

Cohen, R. H.: Disorders of lactic acid metabolism. Clin. Endocrinol. Metabol., *5*:613, 1976.

Collipp, P. J., Chen, S. Y., Maddaiah, V. T., Thomas, J., and Huijing, F. J.: Diagnosis of glycogen storage disease type I by serum immunodiffusion. Pediatrics, *53*:71, 1974.

Cooper, G. R.: Methods for determining the amount of glucose in blood. *In* CRC Critical Reviews of Clinical Laboratory Science, vol. 4. Cleveland, The Chemical Rubber Co., 1973.

Couropmitree, C., Freinkel, N., Nagel, T. C., Horwitz, D. L., Metzger, B., Rubenstein, A. H., and Hahnel, R.: Plasma C-peptide and diagnosis of factitious hyperinsulinism: Study of an insulin-dependent diabetic patient with "spontaneous" hypoglycemia. Ann. Intern. Med., *82*:201, 1975.

Dales, L. G., Sieglaub, A. B., Feldman, R., Friedman, G. D., Seltzer, C. C., and Collen, M. F.: Racial differences in serum and urine glucose after glucose challenge. Diabetes, *23*:327, 1974.

Danowski, T. S., Khurana, R. C., Nolan, S., Stephan, T., Gegick, C. G., Chae, S., and Vidalon, C.: Insulin patterns in equivocal glucose tolerance test (chemical diabetes). Diabetes, *22*:808, 1973.

Davis, J. E., McDonald, J. M., and Jarett, L.: A high performance liquid chromatography by method for hemoglobin A_{Ic}. Diabetes, *27*:102, 1978.

Department of Health, Education and Welfare, Food and Drug Administration: In vitro diagnostic products for human use, proposed establishment of Product Class Standard for detection or measurement of glucose. Fed. Reg., *126*:24136-24147, 1974.

DiMauro, S., and Eastwood, A. B.: Disorders of glycogen and lipid metabolism. Adv. Neurol., *17*:123, 1977.

Dobbins, J. W., and Binder, H. J.: Importance of the colon in enteric hyperoxaluria. N. Engl. J. Med., *296*:298, 1977.

Dubowski, K. M.: An *o*-toluidine method for body-fluid glucose determination. Clin. Chem., *8*:215, 1962.

Eisentraut, A. M., Whissen, N., and Unger, R. H.: Incubation damage in the radioimmunoassay for human plasma glucagon and its prevention with Trasylol^R. Am. J. Med. Sci., *255*:137, 1968.

Fajans, S. S., and Floyd, J. C.: Fasting hypoglycemia in adults. N. Engl. J. Med., *294*:766, 1976.

Fajans, S. S., and Floyd, J. C.: Hypoglycemia: How to manage a complex disease. Mod. Med., *41*:24, 1973.

Fajans, S. S., Floyd, J. C., and Vij, S. K.: Differential diagnosis of spontaneous hypoglycemia. *In* Krystem, L. J., and Shaw, R. A. (eds.): Endocrinology and Diabetes: The Thirtieth Hahnemann Symposium. New York, Grune and Stratton, Inc., 1975, p. 453.

Fernandes, J., Koster, J. F., Grose, W. F. A., and Sorgedrager, N.: Hepatic phosphorylase deficiency: Its differentiation from other hepatic glycogenoses. Arch. Dis. Child., *49*:186, 1974.

Foster, D. W.: Insulin deficiency in hyperosmolar coma. Adv. Intern. Med., *19*:159, 1974.

Frerichs, H., and Creutzfeld, W.: Hypoglycemia. I. Insulin secreting tumors. Clin. Endocrinol. Metabol., *5*:747, 1976.

Froesch, E. R.: Disorders of fructose metabolism. Clin. Endocrinol. Metabol., *5*:599, 1976.

Froesch, E. R.: Essential fructosuria and hereditary fructose intolerance. *In* Stanbury, J. B., Wyngaarden, J. B., and Fredrickson, D. S. (eds.): The Metabolic Basis of Inherited Disease, 3rd ed. New York, McGraw-Hill Book Company, 1972.

Fulop, M., and Hoberman, H. D.: Is lactic acidosis "spontaneous"? N.Y. State J. Med., *77*:24, 1977.

Gabbay, K. H., Hasty, K., Breslow, J. L., Ellison, R. C., Bunn, H. F., and Gallop, P. M.: Glycosylated hemoglobins and long term blood glucose control in diabetes mellitus. J. Clin. Endocrinol. Metabol., *44*:859, 1977.

Ganda, O. P., Weir, G. C., Soeldner, J. S., Legg, M. A., Chick, W. L., Patel, Y. C., Ebeid, A. M., Gabbay, K. H., and Reichlin, S.: "Somatostatinoma": A somatostatin-containing tumor of the endocrine pancreas. N. Engl. J. Med., *296*:963, 1977.

Gelbart, D. R., Brewer, L. L., Fajardo, L. F., and Weinstein, A. B.: Oxalosis and chronic renal failure after intestinal bypass. Arch. Intern. Med., *137*:239, 1977.

Gerich, J. E.: Somatostatin. Am. Fam. Physician, *15*:149, 1977a.

Gerich, J. E.: Somatostatin—its possible role in carbohydrate homeostasis and the treatment of diabetes mellitus. Arch. Intern. Med., *137*:659, 1977b.

Gitzelman, R.: Deficiency of uridine diphosphate galactose 4-epimerase in blood cells of an apparently healthy infant. Helv. Pediatr. Acta, *27*:125, 1972.

Gochman, N., and Schmitz, J. M.: Application of a new peroxide indicator reaction to the specific automated determination of glucose with glucose oxidase. Clin. Chem., *18*:943, 1972.

Grünfeld, J. P., Ganeval, D., Chanard, J., Fardeau, M., and Dreyfus, J. C.: Acute renal failure in McArdle's disease; report of two cases. N. Engl. J. Med., *286*:1237, 1972.

Hagler, L., and Herman, R. H.: Oxalate metabolism I. Am. J. Clin. Nutr., *26*:758, 1973a.

Hagler, L., and Herman, R. H.: Oxalate metabolism II. Am. J. Clin. Nutr., *26*:882, 1973b.

Hagler, L., and Herman, R. H.: Oxalate metabolism III. Am. J. Clin. Nutr., *26*:1006, 1973c.

Hagler, L., and Herman, R. H.: Oxalate metabolism IV. Am. J. Clin. Nutr., *26*:1073, 1973d.

Hatch, M., Bourke, E., and Costello, J.: New enzymic method for serum oxalate determination. Clin. Chem., *23*:76, 1977.

Hiatt, H.: Pentosuria. *In* Stanbury, J. B., Wyngaarden, J. B., and Fredrickson, D. S. (eds.): The Metabolic Basis of Inherited Disease, 3rd ed. New York, McGraw-Hill Book Company, 1972.

Hodgkinson, A.: Determination of oxalic acid in biological material. Clin. Chem., *16*:547, 1970.

Horwitz, D. L., and Rubenstein, A. H.: Insulin suppression. Lancet, *2*:1021, 1974.

Horwitz, D. L., Kuzuya, H., and Rubenstein, A. H.: Circulating serum C-peptide: A brief reveiw of diagnostic implications. N. Engl. J. Med., *295*:207, 1976.

Huijing, F.: Glycogen metabolism and glycogen-storage diseases. Physiol. Rev., *55*:609, 1975.

Indriksons, A.: Hazards of *o*-toluidine. Clin. Chem., *21*:1345, 1975.

Ingelfinger, F. J.: Debates on diabetes. N. Engl. J. Med., *96*:1228, 1977.

Jaspan, J. B., and Rubenstein, A. H.: Circulating glucagon-plasma profiles and metabolism in health and disease. Diabetes, *26*:887, 1977.

Jaspan, J. B., Kuku, S. F., Locker, J. D., Huen, A. H.-J., Emmanouel, D. S., Katz, A. I., and Rubenstein, A. H.: Heterogeneity of plasma glucagon in man. Metabolism, *25*:1397, 1976.

Jubiz, W., and Rallison, M. L.: Diphenylhydantoin treatment of glycogen storage diseases. Arch. Intern. Med., *134*:418, 1974.

Kadish, A. H., Litle, R. L., and Sternberg, T. C.: A new and rapid method for determination of glucose by measurement of rate of oxygen consumption. Clin. Chem., *14*:116, 1968.

Kahn, C. R., Megyesi, K., Bar, R. S., Eastman, R. C., and Flier, J. S.: Receptors for peptide hormones. Ann. Intern. Med., *86*:205, 1977.

Kirkman, H. N., Lanier, D. C., Clemons, E. H., and Sanderford, J. L.: Estimation of galactose-1-phosphate in blood spotted on filter paper. J. Lab. Clin. Med., *83*:515, 1976.

Kitabchi, A. E.: Proinsulin and C-peptide: A review. Metabolism, *26*:547, 1977.

Klimt, C. R., Prout, T. E., Bradley, R. F., Dolger, H., Fisher, G., Gastineau, C. F., Marks, H., Meinert, C. L., and Schumacher, O. P.: Standardization of the oral glucose tolerance test. Report of the Committee on Statistics of the American Diabetes Association, June 14, 1968. Diabetes, *18*:299, 1969.

Koenig, R. J., Peterson, C. M., Kilo, C., Cerami, A., and Williamson, J. R.: Hemoglobin A_{Ic} as an indicator of the degree of glucose intolerance in diabetes. Diabetes, *25*:230, 1976a.

Koenig, R. J., Peterson, C. M., Jones, R. L., Saudek, C., Lehrman, M., and Cerami, A.: Correlation of glucose regulation and hemoglobin A_{Ic} in diabetes mellitus. N. Engl. J. Med., *295*:417, 1976b.

Kopf, A., Tchobroutsky, G., and Eschwege, E.: Serial postprandial blood glucose levels in 309 subjects with and without diabetes. Diabetes, *22*:834, 1973.

Kraft, J. R.: Detection of diabetes mellitus in situ (Occult diabetes). Lab. Med., *6*:10, 1975.

Kuku, S. F., Jaspan, J. B., Emmanouel, D. S., Zeidler, A., Katz, A. I., and Rubenstein, A. H.: Heterogeneity of plasma glucagon; circulating components in normal subjects and patients with chronic renal failure. J. Clin. Invest., *58*:742, 1976.

Larsson, L. I., Holst, J. J., Kühl, C., Lundqvist, G., Hirsh, M. A., Ingemansson, S., Lindkaer-Jensen, S., Rehfeld, J. F., and Schwartz, T. W.: Pancreatic somatostatinoma—clinical features and physiologic implications. Lancet, *1*:666, 1977.

Lavine, R. L.: Diabetes and pregnancy. *In* Rose, L. I., and Lavine, R. L. (eds.): New Concepts in Endocrinology and Metabolism: Hahnemann Endocrinology Metabolism Symposium, 1976. New York, Grune and Stratton, Inc., 1977.

Levy, L. J., Duga, J., Girgis, M., and Gordon, E.: Ketoacidosis associated with alcoholism in non-diabetic subjects. Ann. Intern. Med., *78*:213, 1973.

Lott, J. A., and Turner, K.: Evaluation of Trinder's glucose oxidase method for measuring glucose in serum and urine. Clin. Chem., *21*:1754, 1975.

Lubran, M. M.: McArdle's disease: A review. Ann. Clin. Lab. Sci., *5*:115, 1975.

Mahler, R. F.: Disorder of glycogen metabolism. Clin. Endocrinol. Metabol., *5*:579, 1976.

Mallinson, C. N., Bloom, S. R., Warin, A. P., Salmon, P. R., and Cox, B.: A glucagonoma syndrome. Lancet, *2*:1, 1974.

Marks, V., and Alberti, K. G. M. M.: Selected test of carbohydrate metabolism. Clin. Endocrinol. Metabol., *5*:805, 1976.

Marliss, E., Ohman, J. L., Aoki, T. E., and Kozak, G. P.: Altered redox state obscuring ketoacidosis in diabetic patients with lactic acidosis. N. Engl. J. Med., *283*:978, 1970.

McAdams, A. J., Hug, G., and Bove, K. C.: Glycogen storage disease, Types I to X. Hum. Pathol., *5*:463, 1974.

McCurdy, D. K.: Hyperosmolar hyperglycemic nonketotic diabetic coma. Med. Clin. North Am., *54*:683, 1970.

Megyesi, K., Kahn, C. R., Roth, J., and Gorden, P.: Hypoglycemia in association with extrapancreatic tumors: Demonstration of elevated plasma NSILA-s by a new radioreceptor assay. J. Clin. Endocrinol. Metabol., *38*:931, 1974.

Mehler, M., and DiMauro, S.: Late onset acid maltase deficiency: Detection of patients and heterozygotes by urinary enzyme assay. Arch. Neurol., *33*:692, 1976.

Meinert, C. L.: Standardization of the oral glucose tolerance test, criticism and suggestions invited. Diabetes, *21*:1197, 1972.

Merimee, T. J.: Spontaneous hypoglycemia in man. Adv. Intern. Med., *22*:301, 1977.

Merimee, T. J., and Tyson, J. E.: Stabilization of plasma glucose during fasting: Normal variations in two separate studies. N. Engl. J. Med., *291*:1275, 1974.

Mirsky, S.: Adult-onset diabetes. Primary Care, *1*:53, 1974.

Munoz-Barragan, L., Rufener, C., Srikant, C. B., Shannon, A., Beatens, D., and Unger, R. H.: Immunohistologic identification of glucagon-containing cells in the human fundus. Horm. Metabol. Res., *9*:37, 1977.

Neeley, W. E.: Simple automated determination of serum or plasma glucose by a hexokinase/glucose-6-phosphate dehydrogenase method. Clin. Chem., *18*:509, 1972.

Nerup, J., Platz, P., Ortved-Anderson, O., Christy, M., Lyngsoe, J., Poulsen, J. E., Ryder, L. P., Staub-Nielsen, L., Thomsen, M., and Svejgaard, A.: HL-A antigens and diabetes mellitus. Lancet, *2*:864, 1974.

Newmark, S. R.: Hyperglycemia and hypoglycemia crisis. J.A.M.A., *231*:185, 1975.

Ng, W. G., Donnell, G. N., and Alfi, O.: Prenatal diagnosis of galactosemia. Lancet, *1*:43, 1977.

Niejadlik, D. C., Dube, A. H., and Adamko, S. M.: Glucose measurements and clinical correlations. J.A.M.A., *224*:1734, 1973.

Oka, H., Suzuki, S., Suzuki, H., and Oda, T.: Increased urinary excretion of L-xylulose in patients with liver cirrhosis. Clin. Chim. Acta, *67*:131, 1976.

Oliva, P. B.: Lactic acidosis. Am. J. Med., *48*:209, 1970.

Olefsky, J. M., Farquhar, J. W., and Reaven, G. M.: Do the oral and intravenous glucose tolerance tests provide similar diagnostic information in patients with chemical diabetes mellitus? Diabetes, *22*:202, 1973.

Olefsky, J. M., and Reaven, G. M.: Insulin and glucose response to identical oral glucose tolerance test performed forty-eight hours apart. Diabetes, *23*:449, 1974.

O'Sullivan, J. B., and Mahan, C. M.: Criteria for the oral glucose tolerance test in pregnancy. Diabetes, *13*:278, 1964.

O'Sullivan, J. B., Mahan, C. M., Charles, D., and Dandrow, R. V.: Screening criteria for high-risk gestational diabetic patients. Am. J. Obstet. Gynecol., *116*:895, 1973.

Pagliara, A. S., Karl, I. E., Haymond, M., and Kipnes, D. M.: Hypoglycemia in infancy and childhood, Part II. J. Pediatr., *82*:558, 1973.

Park, B. N., Kahn, C. B., Gleason, R. E., and Soeldner, J. S.: Insulin-glucose dynamics in non-diabetic reactive hypoglycemia and chemical diabetics. Diabetes, *21*:373, 1972.

Passey, R. B., Gillum, R. L., Fuller, J. B., Urry, F. M., and Giles, M. L.: Evaluation and comparison of 10 glucose methods and the reference method recommended in the Proposed Product Class Standard (1974). Clin. Chem., *23*:131, 1977.

Patel, Y. C., Rao, K., and Reichlin, S.: Somatostatin in human cerebrospinal fluid. N. Engl. J. Med., *296*:529, 1977.

Perheentupa, J., Raivio, K. O., and Nikkitä, E. A.: Hereditary fructose intolerance. Acta Med. Scand. (Suppl.), *542*:65, 1972.

Permutt, M. A., Kelly, J., Bernstein, R., Alpers, D. H., Siegel, B. A., and Kipnis, D. M.: Alimentary hypoglycemia in the absence of gastrointestinal surgery. N. Engl. J. Med., *288*:1206, 1973.

Peterson, C. M., and Jones, R. L.: Minor hemoglobins, diabetic "control", and diseases of post synthetic protein modification. Ann. Intern. Med., *87*:489, 1977a.

Peterson, C. M., Jones, R. L., Koenig, R. J., Melvin, E. T., and Lehrman, M. R.: Reversible hematologic sequelae of diabetes mellitus. Ann. Intern. Med., *86*:425, 1977b.

Pozefsky, T., Colker, J. L., Langs, H. M., and Andres, R.: The cortisone-glucose tolerance test: The influence of age on performance. Ann. Intern. Med., *63*:988, 1965.

Pyke, D. A.: Genetics of diabetes. Clin. Endocrinol. Metabol., *6*:285, 1977.

Rubenstein, A. H., Welbourne, W. P., Mako, M., Melani, F., and Steiner, D. F.: Comparative immunology of bovine, porcine and human proinsulins and C-peptides. Diabetes, *19*:546, 1970.

Scarlett, J. A., Mako, M. E., Rubenstein, A. H., Blix, P. M., Goldman, J., Horwitz, D. L., Tager, H., Jaspan, J. B., Stjernholm, M. R., and Olefsky, J. M.: Factitious hypoglycemia: Diagnosis by measurement of serum C-peptide immunoreactivity and insulin-binding antibodies. N. Engl. J. Med., *297*:1029, 1977.

Schein, P. S., DeLellis, R. A., Kahn, C. R., Gorden, P., and Kraft, A. R.: Islet cell tumors: Current concepts and management. Ann. Intern. Med., *79*:239, 1973.

Schön, R., and Thalhammer, O.: False-positive galactosemia screening. Lancet, *1*:43, 1977.

Seltzer, H. S.: Drug-induced hypoglycemia: A review based on 473 cases. Diabetes, *21*:955, 1972.

Sherwin, R. S.: Limitations of the oral glucose tolerance test in diagnosis of early diabetes. Primary Care, *4*:255, 1977.

Shih, V. E., Levy, H. L., Karolkewicz, V., Houghton, S., Efron, M. L., Isselbacher, K. J., Beutler, E., and MacCready, R. A.: Galactosemia screening of newborns in Massachusetts. N. Engl. J. Med., *284*:753, 1971.

Siperstein, M. D.: The glucose tolerance test: A pitfall in the diagnosis of diabetes mellitus. Adv. Intern. Med., *20*:297, 1975.

Sonowane, M., Savory, J., Cross, R. E., Heintges, M. G., and Chester, B.: Kinetic measurement of glucose with a centrifugal analyzer: Hexokinase and glucose oxidase procedures compared. Clin. Chem., *22*:1100, 1976.

Starzl, T. E., Putnam, C. W., Porter, K. A., Halgrimson, C. G., Corman, J., Brown, B. I., Gotlin, R. W., Rodgerson, D. O., and Greene, H. L.: Portal diversion for the treatment of glycogen storage disease in humans. Ann. Surg., *178*:525, 1973.

Steiner, D. F.: Insulin today. Diabetes, *26*:322, 1977a.

Steiner, D. F., and Oyer, P. E.: The biosynthesis of insulin and a probable precursor of insulin by a human islet cell adenoma. Proc. Natl. Acad. Sci. U.S.A., *57*:473, 1967.

Steiner, G., Wilson, D., and Vranic, M.: Studies of glucose turnover and renal function in an unusual case of hereditary fructose intolerance. Am. J. Med., *62*:150, 1977b.

Trivelli, L. A., Ranney, H. M., and Lai, H. T.: Hemoglobin components in patients with diabetes mellitus. N. Engl. J. Med., *284*:353, 1971.

Unger, R. H.: Somatostatinoma. N. Engl. J. Med., *296*:998, 1977a.

Unger, R. H., and Orci, L.: Role of glucagon in diabetes. Arch. Intern. Med., *137*:482, 1977c.

Unger R. H., Ipp. E., Schuszdziarra, V., and Orci, L.: Hypothesis: Physiologic role of pancreatic somatostatin and the contribution of D-cell disorders to diabetes mellitus. Life Sci., *20*:2081, 1977b.

Valleron, A. J., Eschwege, E., Papoz, L., and Rosselin, G. E.: Agreement and discrepancy in the evaluation of normal and diabetic oral glucose tolerance test. Diabetes, *24*:585, 1975.

Vinicor, F., Faulkner, S., and Clark, C. M.: Reactive hypoglycemia. Hosp. Med., *11*:65, 1975.

Weissman, M., and Klein, B.: Evaluation of glucose determinations in untreated serum samples. Clin. Chem., *4*:420, 1958.

Westgard, J. V., Lahmeyer, B. L., and Birnbaum, M. L.: Use of the DuPont "automatic clinical analyzer" in direct determination of lactic acid in plasma stablized with sodium fluoride. Clin. Chem., *18*:1334, 1972.

Wright, P. H., and Makulu, D. R.: Reactions of proinsulin and its derivatives with antibodies to insulin. Proc. Soc. Exp. Biol. Med., *134*:1165, 1970.

Yager, J., and Young, R. T.: Non-hypoglycemia as an epidemic condition. N. Engl. J. Med., *291*:907, 1974.

8

MEASUREMENT OF LIPIDS AND EVALUATION OF LIPID DISORDERS

Israel Tamir, M.D.
Basil M. Rifkind, M.D.
and Robert I. Levy, M.D.

With a Section on Lipid Storage Diseases
by Robert Calhoun, M.D.

GENERAL CHARACTERISTICS

LIPIDS—STRUCTURE, COMPOSITION, AND FUNCTION

Lipids are organic substances composed primarily of carbon and hydrogen as well as some oxygen. Several of the compound lipids also contain nitrogen and phosphorus. They are by definition insoluble in water, but are soluble in such organic solvents as hydrocarbons (petroleum ether and benzene), halogenated hydrocarbons (chloroform, carbon tetrachloride, and dichloroethane), and ether. Table 8–1 details a simplified classification of the lipids.

Table 8–1. CLASSIFICATION OF LIPIDS

Simple lipids—esters of fatty acids and an alcohol
    Fats (true or neutral fats)—alcohol is glycerol
        Triglycerides
    Waxes—alcohol other than glycerol
        Sterol esters (cholesterol)
Compound or conjugated lipids—esters of fatty acids that contain groups in addition to an alcohol and fatty acid such as phosphoric acid, nitrogenous moiety, or carbohydrate
    Phospholipids
        Lecithins—one fatty acid esterified to glycerol is replaced by phosphoric acid and choline (nitrogenous moiety)
        Cephalins—nitrogenous moiety is serine or ethanolamine in place of choline
        Sphingomyelins—no glycerol present
    Glycolipids (cerebrosides)—fatty acids and carbohydrates (galactose or glucose) with nitrogen but no glycerol
    Others (aminolipids and sulfolipids)
    Lipoproteins
Derived lipids—hydrolytic derivatives of the above substances
    Fatty acids
        Saturated
        Unsaturated
    Glycerol alcohol
    Other alcohols
        Sterols
        Steroids

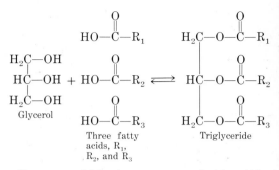

Figure 8–1. Molecular components of triglyceride.

The main lipids present in human plasma are triglycerides, cholesterol (free and esterified), phospholipids, and non-esterified fatty acids (NEFA).

The aqueous insolubility of lipids necessitated the evolution of transport systems that would permit their passage through different body compartments. Thus, hydrophobic lipids, in association with hydrophilic phospholipids, combine with unique plasma proteins (apoproteins) to form macromolecular complexes known as lipoproteins, which are the transport form of the lipids in the blood.

Triglycerides (Triacylglycerol)

Triglycerides are formed by esterification (Fig. 8-1) of glycerol and three fatty acids. They are the main storage lipids in man and constitute about 95 per cent of adipose tissue lipids. They are also found in plasma as part of the lipoproteins. Most triglycerides in humans are mixed; that is, three different fatty acids are esterified to glycerol or only two of the three are the same. The fatty acids of plasma triglycerides almost always have straight chains and an even number of carbon atoms.

Triglycerides are found in various concentrations in all plasma lipoproteins (Table 8-2); in general, the higher the concentration of triglyceride, the lower the density of the lipoprotein. The main triglyceride-carrying

Table 8–2. HUMAN PLASMA LIPOPROTEINS

	MOBILITY (PAPER)	DENSITY (g/ml)	S_f†	Mol. wt.	LIPID COMPOSITION (mg/100 mg lipoprotein lipid)			MOLAR RATIO	
					TG‡	CH‡	PL‡	ESTERIFIED: FREE CHOLESTEROL	LECITHIN: SPHINGOMYELIN
Chylomicrons	Origin	0.95	400	100×10^6	87.7	3.0	8.8	0.88	5.85
VLDL*	Pre-beta	0.95–1.006	20–40	6×10^6	55.7	16.8	19.3	1.30	4.02
LDL*	Beta	1.019–1.063	0–12	1.8×10^6	7.3	19.3	27.8	2.33	2.46
HDL$_2$*		1.063–1.125		0.4×10^6	6.1	42.5	42.8	2.81	5.08
HDL$_3$*	Alpha-1	1.125–1.210		0.2×10^6	6.7	38.4	40.9	4.38	8.38

*VLDL = very low density lipoprotein; LDL = low density lipoprotein; HDL = high density lipoprotein
†Flotation rate, S_f, is expressed in Svedberg flotation units (negative sedimentation Svedberg units, 10^{-13} cm/sec-dyne-g).
‡TG = triglyceride; CH = cholesterol; PL = phospholipids

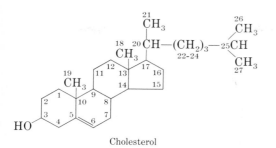

Figure 8-2. Molecular structure of cholesterol.

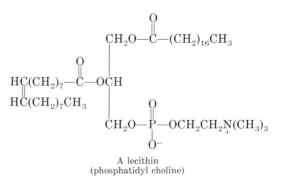

A lecithin
(phosphatidyl choline)

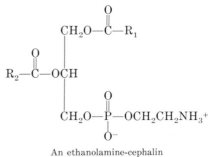

An ethanolamine-cephalin
(phosphatidyl ethanolamine)

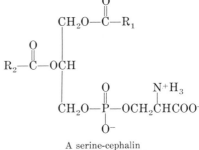

A serine-cephalin
(phosphatidyl serine)

Figure 8-3. Molecular structures of selected phospholipids.

lipoproteins are the chylomicrons and the very-low-density lipoproteins (VLDL) (see Lipoproteins—Structure, Composition, and Function) (p. 192).

Cholesterol

Cholesterol is an unsaturated steroid alcohol whose structure is based on the cyclopentanoperhydrophenanthrene nucleus (Fig. 8-2). In humans it is a key intermediate in the biosynthesis of related sterols such as bile acids, adrenocortical hormones, androgens, and estrogens. Cholesterol exists both in free (non-esterified) and ester forms. Normally about two thirds of total plasma cholesterol is esterified. Sixty to seventy-five per cent of the plasma cholesterol is transported by low-density lipoprotein (LDL); a small but significant amount (15 to 25 per cent) is bound to high-density lipoprotein (HDL).

Phospholipids

This class of complex lipids is derived from phosphatidic acid (Fig. 8-3). In human plasma the main phospholipids are sphingomyelin, phosphatidyl choline or lecithin, phosphatidyl ethanolamine, and phosphatidyl serine (the last two are sometimes termed cephalins). Like cholesterol and triglyceride, phospholipids are found in several different lipoproteins. About 20 to 25 per cent of the LDL (low-density lipoprotein) mass is composed of phospholipids with a lecithin:sphingomyelin ratio of 2:1. HDL (high-density lipoprotein) contains about 30 per cent phospholipids by weight, with a lecithin:sphingomyelin ratio of 5:1.

Non-esterified fatty acids (NEFA)

Also known as free fatty acids or FFA, NEFA represent that small proportion of the plasma fatty acids not esterified with glycerol

Table 8-3. SELECTED FATTY ACIDS WITH VARIABLE NUMBERS OF CARBONS AND DOUBLE BONDS (REFLECTING UNSATURATION)

NAME	NO. OF CARBONS	NO. OF UNSATURATED DOUBLE BONDS
Myristic acid	14	0
Palmitic acid	16	0
Palmitoleic acid	16	1
Stearic acid	18	0
Oleic acid	18	1
Linolenic acid	18	2
Linolenic acid	18	3
Arachidonic acid	20	4

or cholesterol. Naturally occurring NEFA usually have an even number of carbon atoms and are straight-chained (Table 8-3). NEFA are transported in the plasma complexed with albumin. In the fasting state they are derived mainly from hydrolysis of triglyceride in adipose tissue, and to a smaller degree from circulating triglyceride-rich lipoproteins. Postprandially, chylomicrons and VLDL are the main sources of circulating NEFA. Since the rate of removal of NEFA from circulation is very rapid and their concentration in plasma is low (0.405 to 0.780 mmol/l), they contribute relatively little to the total circulating plasma lipid level at any particular time.

LIPOPROTEINS—STRUCTURE, COMPOSITION, AND FUNCTION

Lipoproteins are macromolecular complexes that serve in the plasma as the transport vehicle of insoluble lipids. For descriptive purposes they have been classified into five classes (Table 8-2) on the basis of their density (g/ml), flotation characteristics, and mobility on paper or agar gel electrophoresis. Apoprotein content is still another characteristic that varies among the lipoproteins (Table 8-4).

Despite the descriptive and diagnostic utility of these classifications, it is important to remember that all lipoproteins are *metabolically* closely related.

Chylomicrons

In these lipoproteins the arrangement of lipids and proteins takes place in two phases: the "core" or center of the particle is occupied by neutral lipids (triglyceride, cholesterol) and the "surface" or water-lipid interface is occupied by apoproteins, phospholipids, and unesterified cholesterol. Triglycerides constitute 85 to 95 per cent of total chylomicron lipid mass, and phospholipids and cholesterol 5 to 10 per cent and 3 to 5 per cent, respectively. Their apoprotein content is 1 to 2 per cent of particle mass and consists predominantly of apo B and some apo A and the various C apoproteins (Tables 8-2 and 8-4).

However, the lipid and apoprotein composition depends on the source of the chylomicrons. Those isolated from lymph contain less protein and more phospholipid than do those obtained from plasma. Similarly, larger chylomicrons contain relatively less protein and more triglyceride than do smaller particles.

Very-low-density lipoprotein (VLDL)

The internal structure of the VLDL particle is similar to that of the chylomicron and follows the general core model of lipoproteins VLDL particles contain 60 to 70 per cent triglyceride (of endogenous origin), 10 to 15 per cent cholesterol (with an esterified:free cholesterol molar ratio of about 1.0), 10 to 15 per cent phospholipids (lecithin:sphingomyelin ratio of about 4.0), and about 10 per cent protein. The apoprotein composition varies with the particle size. It averages about 40 per cent apo B, 50 per cent apo C, and 10 to 15 per cent other apoproteins, primarily the arginine-rich apoprotein (apo E). As with chylomicrons, the bigger VLDL particles contain relatively less apoprotein, phospholipids, and cholesterol (surface material) and more triglyceride (core constituent) than the smaller particles. The "increased" apoprotein content of smaller particles is largely *relative* owing to the loss of triglyceride.

Recent studies have shown that with decreasing particle size the relative content of the different apoproteins also changes. Al

Table 8-4. APOPROTEIN CONCENTRATIONS IN HUMAN PLASMA LIPOPROTEINS*

LIPOPROTEIN	APOPROTEIN (mg/100 mg LIPOPROTEIN)	PER CENT OF TOTAL PROTEIN					
		Apo B	Apo A-I	Apo A-II	Apo C-I	Apo C-II	Apo C-II
Chylomicrons	1-2	5-20	11.6%†		15	15	40
VLDL	10	40	Trace	Trace	10	10	30
LDL	25	95	Trace	Trace	Trace	Trace	Trace
HDL	50	Trace	65	25	2	2	6

*Adapted From Eisenberg, S.: Atheroscl. Rev., *1*:23, 1976.
†Apo A-I and Apo A-II account for 11.6 per cent of apoprotein content of chylomicrons isolated from human thoracic duct lymph.

though apo B content remains constant, apo C content decreases, resulting in an increased apo B:apo C ratio in the smaller particles.

Intermediate-density lipoprotein (IDL)

This fraction is not usually considered a separate species of lipoprotein but rather occurs during the transition of VLDL to LDL (see Metabolism, p. 199). IDL is not normally identified in plasma because of its rapid turnover of 2 to 6 hours.

Each particle of IDL contains approximately 40 per cent triglyceride, 30 per cent cholesterol, and 20 per cent phospholipids. The ratio of esterified to free cholesterol is lower than in VLDL. The sphingomyelin:lecithin ratio is about three times that found in the VLDL particle.

IDL has been best characterized in the rat, where it was found to be almost devoid of apo C (only about 7 per cent of the original apo C content of VLDL was recovered in IDL), but contained all the apo B that was initially present in VLDL.

Low-density lipoprotein (LDL)

LDL constitutes about 50 per cent of the total lipoprotein mass in human plasma. The approximate lipid composition is 45 per cent cholesterol (esterified:non-esterified molar ratio, 2.3), 20 to 30 per cent phospholipids (lecithin:sphingomyelin ratio, 2.5), and 5 to 10 per cent triglyceride.

More than 95 per cent of the protein of LDL is accounted for by apo B, whereas only very small amounts of apo C are found in the LDL density range.

It is likely that the proteins and phospholipids of the LDL particle are located mainly at the surface. This may explain why all the apo B of LDL can be identified immunochemically and why most of the phospholipids are hydrolyzable by phospholipase. Because delipidated apo B is insoluble in water, guanidine, or urea, and becomes soluble only after chemical modification (e.g., succinylation), the basic structure of the LDL particle is not yet fully understood.

High-density lipoprotein (HDL)

Of the total HDL mass, 50 per cent is accounted for by protein; of that, the A apoproteins (A-I, A-II, and A-III) constitute 90 to 95 per cent and apo C, about 5 to 10 per cent. Cholesterol constitutes about 20 per cent of

HDL mass (esterified:free cholesterol molar ratio, about 3.0) and phospholipids 30 per cent (lecithin:sphingomyelin ratio, 5.0). Normally, only traces of triglyceride are present.

HDL is often separated into two subclasses: HDL_2 (density, 1.063 to 1.125 g/ml) and HDL_3 (density, 1.125 to 1.210 g/ml), which differ in composition and particle size. The physiologic importance of these differences has not yet been determined.

Several models for the structure of HDL have been proposed (Eisenberg and Levy, 1976). All assume that apoproteins and phospholipids are present at the surface of the HDL particle. They differ, however, in the structural arrangements of lipid and apoprotein in the particle. Whether all HDL particles contain all the A apoproteins is not known. HDL particles containing only apo A-II were recently isolated from the plasma of patients with Tangier disease (Assmann, 1974).

LP(a) lipoprotein (HDL₁—"sinking pre-beta-lipoprotein")

This lipoprotein is found in the density interval of 1.055 to 1.085 g/ml. It is composed of 27 per cent protein, 65 per cent lipid, and 8 per cent carbohydrate (Albers, 1974). It is characterized by a disproportionately high molecular weight as compared to its sedimentation properties. The apoprotein content of LP(a) consists of 65 per cent apo B, about 20 per cent LP(a) protein, and the rest albumin (Ehnholm, 1972). On electrophoresis, the LP(a) protein migrates between LDL and albumin; however, variability in its electrophoretic mobility has been demonstrated in preparations from different individuals. This protein is rich in carbohydrate which is probably linked to serine and threonine.

The LP(a) lipoprotein cross-reacts with LDL immunochemically but residual antigenicity is identified after absorption of the antiserum with LDL (Eisenberg and Levy, 1976). LP(a) lipoproteins differ from LDL in chemical composition and physical properties.

LP(a) lipoprotein is found in varying concentrations (20 to 760 mg/l) in most individuals (Albers, 1977). Increased levels are sometimes found in several members of the same family, often following a pattern of autosomal dominant inheritance. When present in increased concentrations in the plasma, LP(a) appears as a lipid-staining pre-beta lipoprotein band and may be confused with VLDL.

Lipoprotein-x (L_p-x—lipoprotein of obstructive jaundice)

L_p-x is an abnormal lipoprotein found in patients with obstructive jaundice. It contains about 65 per cent lecithin, 25 to 30 per cent unesterified cholesterol, 2 per cent cholesterol ester, and 6 per cent protein.

The structural arrangement of L_p-x, determined by its unusual lipid composition, is that of disc-shaped particles made of bilayered sheets 5 to 6 nm thick. Electron microscopy shows that these particles have a major axis of about 50 nm.

About 80 per cent of the protein in L_p-x is apo C, and the rest is albumin. Apo C is believed to be located on the surface of the L_p-x particle, since it can be identified immunochemically on the intact particle. The albumin, on the other hand, is presumably located in the interior of the particle; it can be identified in L_p-x only after delipidation or attack by phospholipases.

APOPROTEINS—STRUCTURE, COMPOSITION, AND FUNCTION

The apoproteins constitute the protein portion of the lipoproteins. Although no general agreement has been reached on their nomenclature, the A, B, C nomenclature suggested by Alaupovic (1971) is useful and will be employed here. Table 8-5 shows the differential characteristics of the apoprotein groups.

Apoprotein A (Apo A)

Three apoproteins, designated apo A-I, apo A-II, and apo A-III, can be isolated from human HDL. They are easily separated by various chromatographic techniques. They differ in aminoterminals, amino acid composition, and immunologic properties, but they are all soluble in water and urea solutions and contain glutamine at their carboxyterminals.

Apo A-I and Apo-II. Almost 90 per cent of these apoproteins are found in HDL; only trace amounts appear in the other lipoproteins. Apo A-I has a molecular weight of 28,300 and its protein content consists of 245 amino acids. Reported mean normal levels of apo A-I range from 1000 to 1540 mg/l. These differences in mean normal values may be due to differences in methods and antisera used. Apo A-I is thought to be an activator of the lecithin:cholesterol acyltransferase (LCAT) enzyme system (see below).

Apo A-II has a molecular weight of 17,000. Each molecule consists of two identical peptides linked by a single disulfide bond. Each peptide has a molecular weight of 8500 and consists of 77 amino acid residues. Reported mean normal plasma levels of apo A-II range from 340 to 830 mg/l.

The site of apo A synthesis in man is not yet determined. Intestinal perfusion studies in the rat indicate that this organ may be the major source of apo A, although liver perfusion studies have shown that the liver secretes particles in the HDL density range. These particles differ, however, from plasma HDL in that they are richer in apo E and poorer in apo A-I content.

Table 8-5. APPROXIMATE METABOLIC PARAMETERS OF SELECTED APOPROTEINS IN HUMANS

APOPROTEIN	MEAN PLASMA LEVEL (mg/dl)	MASS SYNTHESIS (mg/day)	PLASMA HALF-LIFE (days)	SITE OF SYNTHESIS	POSSIBLE SITE OF CATABOLISM	FUNCTION
A-I	120	450–600	5.0	Intestine, liver	Liver, kidney lysosomes	Activate LCAT*
A-II	40	150–200	5.0	Intestine, liver	Liver, kidney lysosomes	?
B	90	850	3.0	Liver, intestine	Peripheral tissue, liver	Transport triglyceride
C-I C-II C-III	25	850	0.6	Liver	Liver	Affect lipase activity

*LCAT = Lecithin: cholesterol acyltransferase

Apo A catabolism is closely related to HDL catabolism. Labeled apo A-I, when associated with unlabeled HDL, has been reported to have a plasma half-life of 4.5 days in normal subjects. In contrast to apo C and apo B in VLDL, apo A-I and A-II in HDL appear to decay together. Animal studies suggest that the liver and kidney lysosomes play an important role in HDL catabolism.

Apo A-III (Apo D, thin-line peptide).

This apoprotein is isolated as a minor constituent from human HDL, especially HDL_3. It has different antigenic properties, amino acid composition, and migration on polyacrylamide gel than apo A-I and apo A-II. The molecular weight of apo A-III is about 22,100. It may participate in the activation of the LCAT system and may be a specific carrier of the lysolecithin formed after LCAT has acted on HDL.

Apoprotein B (Apo B)

Apo B constitutes more than 95 per cent of LDL and about 40 per cent of VLDL protein. Its concentration in human plasma ranges between 700 and 1000 mg/l. Carbohydrates (mannose, fucose, glucosamine, glucose, galactose, and sialic acid) constitute about 5 per cent of the mass of apo B. Neither the nature of the basic protein subunit nor the molecular weight of the apo B monomer is known (estimates range between 24,000 and 250,000). Insoluble in water, apo B is maintained in solution only in the presence of detergents (sodium dodecyl sulfate or sodium decyl sulfate) and is rendered soluble following maleation or succinylation.

In the rat, apo B is synthesized both in the liver and in the intestine and enters the circulation in either chylomicrons or VLDL. This also appears to be true for man. Normally about 850 mg apo B/day is synthesized. The apo B of VLDL is converted to LDL through a chain of delipidation steps (see Metabolism). The clearance of apo B from the circulation in normals occurs *only* in LDL particles, whereas in dyslipoproteinemic individuals variable amounts of apo B may be cleared from the plasma while particles are still in the VLDL or IDL density range. The specific sites of apo B removal in man are not clear. The biologic half-life of apo B in normal humans varies between 2.25 and 3.58 days.

Apoprotein C (Apo C)

At least three different apoproteins belong to this group: C-I, C-II, and C-III. Their masses range between 8 and 10×10^3 dal-tons. These apoproteins are best separated by ion-exchange chromatography by use of DEAE cellulose.

Apo C-I.
Apo C-I contains 57 amino acids, has an aminoterminal threonine and carboxyterminal serine. It contains no carbohydrates and lacks histidine, tyrosine, and cysteine. Apo C-I makes up about 3.5 per cent of VLDL and about 2 per cent of HDL protein.

Apo C-II (apo-LP-glu).
Apo C-II has a carboxyterminal glutamine and aminoterminal threonine. This apoprotein contains no carbohydrate and lacks histidine and cysteine. It constitutes about 7 per cent of VLDL protein and less than 2 per cent of HDL protein.

Apo C-III.
This protein is isolated in several polymorphic forms, depending on the molar content of sialic acid. Each apo C-III molecule contains a carbohydrate sidechain attached to threonine, has aminoterminal serine and carboxyterminal alanine, but contains no cysteine or isoleucine. Apoprotein C-III makes up about 30 per cent of the protein mass of VLDL and about 5 per cent of HDL protein mass.

In fasting human plasma, the C apoproteins are found mainly in VLDL and HDL (predominantly HDL_2). They play an important role in the metabolism of triglyceride-rich lipoproteins. Apo C-II is a specific co-factor essential for triglyceride hydrolysis by extrahepatic lipoprotein-lipase. Apo C-III may serve as a specific inhibitor of the lipoprotein-lipase system (it should, however, be noted that all C apoproteins, when present in excess, may inhibit triglyceride hydrolysis).

The concentrations of apo C-II and apo C-III in normal plasma are about 50 mg/l and 140 mg/l, respectively. The concentration of apo C-I has not been reported but is probably similar to that of apo C-II.

Very little is known about apo C metabolism in man. In animal (rat) experiments it was shown that apo C is synthesized and secreted by the liver, but not the intestine. Whether apo C is secreted from the liver with VLDL or HDL or both is not clear. The half-life of apo C in the normal human circulatory system is less than 24 hours. HDL seems to serve as a major vehicle for the clearance of apo C.

Apoprotein D (Apo D)

See Apo A-III.

Apoprotein E (Apo E)

Also found in human plasma is an argine-rich apoprotein (apo E), with a molecular weight of 33,000. It has an aminoterminal of lysine and a carboxyterminal sequence of leucine-serine-alanine. Arginine-rich apoprotein is isolated by DEAE ion-exchange chromatography from VLDL. It constitutes about 5 to 10 per cent of normal VLDL and is found in excess amounts in patients with Type III hyperlipoproteinemia. It is also present, in minor quantities, in LDL and HDL. Analytical isoelectric focusing in 8M urea shows this apoprotein to be composed of three major polypeptides with pI values of 5.5, 5.6, and 5.75. It is not currently known whether these three different polypeptides are "isoproteins" or unrelated polypeptides. However, it has been suggested that one of these polypeptides (apo E-III) is missing in patients with Type III hyperlipoproteinemia and that this may be the underlying defect of this disorder. Apo E has been shown in rats to be secreted from the liver with newly synthesized HDL. However, it rapidly transfers to VLDL once in the plasma.

LIPOPROTEIN-LIPASES

In fasting human plasma, lipolytic activity is barely detectable. A few minutes following the intravenous injection of heparin, several lipolytic activities are discerned. At least two triglyceride hydrolases are detected in this so-called post-heparin plasma. They differ in their pH optimum, inhibition by protamine or concentrated saline solution, and activation by specific apoprotein co-factors.

Extrahepatic lipoprotein-lipase

This enzyme, derived mainly from adipose tissue, is operative in the hydrolysis of chylomicron and VLDL triglyceride. It is normally located on the surface of endothelial cells of adipose tissue and of skeletal and heart muscles. Hydrolysis of chylomicron triglyceride occurs following the attachment of these particles to the capillary endothelial cells. Phospholipids and apo C-II are essential co-factors for triglyceride hydrolysis by this enzyme. In familial Type I hyperlipoproteinemia there is a complete absence of extrahepatic lipoprotein-lipase activity.

Hepatic lipoprotein-lipase

This enzyme is predominantly associated with the hepatocyte outer membrane. It has only a limited capacity to hydrolyze significant amounts of triglyceride from intact glyceride-laden lipoproteins. It has been postulated (Eisenberg and Levy, 1976) that this enzyme is operative in the conversion of IDL into LDL particles. Since the activity of hepatic lipoprotein-lipase is independent of the presence of apo C, it can proceed in the apo C-poor IDL.

Post-heparin phospholipase

Another lipolytic activity present in post-heparin plasma is a phospholipase which hydrolyzes fatty acids in the 2-position of phosphatidylcholine and phosphatidylethanolamine. The enzymatic activity results in formation of lysophosphatide compounds, mainly lysolecithin. In the rat most of the phospholipase activity originates in the liver. Recent studies have indicated that hydrolysis of lecithin to lysolecithin may account for the disappearance of some phospholipids from VLDL after interaction of this lipoprotein with post-heparin plasma (Eisenberg and Levy, 1976).

LECITHIN:CHOLESTEROL ACYLTRANSFERASE (LCAT)

Normally present in human plasma, this enzyme system catalyzes the esterification of cholesterol by promoting transfer of fatty acids from lecithin to cholesterol, which results in the formation of lysolecithin and cholesterol ester. The enzyme is synthesized in the liver and circulates in plasma with HDL, which seems to be the preferred substrate. It is activated by apo A-I. Recently, it was suggested that this enzyme system also plays a role in removing surface material of chylomicrons and VLDL. LCAT may also be involved in removal of excess free cholesterol and lecithin from the circulation.

METABOLISM

SYNTHESIS AND DEGRADATION OF CHOLESTEROL

Total body cholesterol is derived from two sources: (a) dietary cholesterol (exogenous), and (b) synthesis (endogenous) (Fig. 8–4). The average daily diet of North American adults currently contains approximately 450 mg of cholesterol. In contrast, about 1 g cholesterol

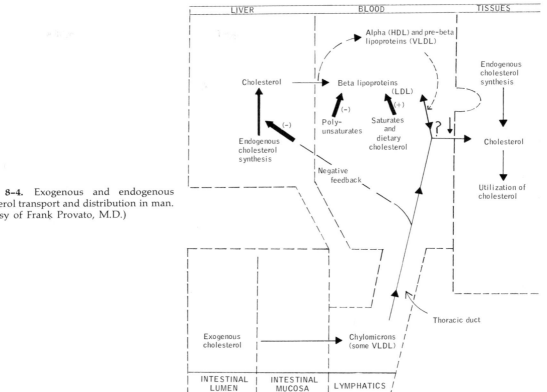

Figure 8-4. Exogenous and endogenous cholesterol transport and distribution in man. (Courtesy of Frank Provato, M.D.)

per day is synthesized by the body. All of the endogenously synthesized cholesterol is derived from acetate, with mevalonic acid and squalene the key intermediates in the biosynthesis.

In terms of plasma output, the liver and intestine are the major sites of cholesterol synthesis, although active cholesterol synthesis probably takes place in all tissues. Cholesterol is transported in the plasma only in the lipoproteins (mainly LDL), and only the liver and intestine synthesize lipoproteins capable of transporting cholesterol out of the cells.

The liver is the major excretory pathway of cholesterol from the body. Most of the cholesterol is converted in the liver to bile acids. Some of the cholesterol is excreted untransformed in the bile and is partially reabsorbed (together with bile acids and dietary cholesterol) from the intestine (enterohepatic cycle).

ABSORPTION AND SYNTHESIS OF TRIGLYCERIDE

About 1 to 2 g of glyceride per kg body weight is ingested daily. In the intestinal lumen the glycerides are partially hydrolyzed to monoglycerides and NEFA, absorbed in the form of micelles, and in the intestinal mucosa, reformed into triglycerides. The triglycerides are then incorporated mainly into chylomicrons, although small amounts of VLDL are also formed. The triglyceride-rich chylomicrons are released into the mesenteric lymphatics and carried via the thoracic duct to the bloodstream for distribution to most tissues. Triglycerides containing shorter-chain fatty acids (medium-chain triglycerides—MCT) do not result in chylomicron formation but are absorbed directly into the portal circulation.

Endogenous triglycerides derived from the

liver constitute the major source of plasma triglycerides in the fasting state. Triglycerides are synthesized from NEFA taken up by the liver or from acetyl coenzyme A derived from carbohydrate metabolism. These triglycerides are released from the liver in the form of VLDL. A very small amount of the endogenously synthesized triglyceride is transported in HDL and LDL.

SYNTHESIS, INTRAVASCULAR METABOLISM, AND CATABOLISM OF LIPOPROTEINS

Structurally, the lipoproteins can be differentiated into two discrete classes: (1) the apo B-containing chylomicrons, VLDL, IDL, and LDL, and (2) HDL with apo A as its basic structural unit.

Functionally, however, the lipoproteins are dynamically interrelated, mainly because of exchange and interaction among their constituent apoproteins. (For descriptive purposes, the metabolism of each lipoprotein "class" will be described separately.)

Chylomicrons

Chylomicrons, synthesized in the intestinal epithelium during fat absorption, contain newly synthesized cellular lipids assembled from free fatty acids, monoglycerides, and cholesterol ester derived from intraluminal hydrolysis of dietary fats and bile acids. These lipids are formed in the endoplasmic reticulum and intestinal microsomal fractions. The endoplasmic reticulum, a site for active protein synthesis, is the first place where newly synthesized lipoproteins can be identified. The lipoproteins are then transferred via the Golgi cisternae to the basal border of the cell and secreted by reverse pinocytosis. The subsequent mode whereby these particles are channeled into the lymphatic vessels is not known. It is important to remember that intestinal mucosal cells do not synthesize apo C, and therefore this apoprotein derived from HDL and partially degraded lipoproteins is attached to the surface of chylomicrons in the circulation.

Inside the Golgi apparatus, carbohydrates are attached to the lipoprotein and possibly play an important role in the mechanism of their release from the intestinal cells.

The catabolism of chylomicrons begins with their interaction with extrahepatic lipoprotein-lipase at the capillary endothelial surface of adipose tissue and muscle. Though it is not proven, apoproteins, primarily apo C-II, may enhance the binding of the chylomicrons to the enzyme. This interaction of chylomicrons with extrahepatic lipoprotein-lipase initiates a process of delipidation. Triglyceride and phospholipids are hydrolyzed, and apo C is transferred to HDL. The subsequent steps in the degradation of chylomicrons are not known; it may proceed along similar lines of degradation as VLDL particles (see VLDL below), but there is no direct proof of this, at least in humans. In the rat, sheep, and dog, it has been shown that after injected labeled chylomicrons have been delipidated by extrahepatic lipase, a triglyceride-poor, cholesterol-rich "remnant" remains in circulation and is probably subsequently metabolized by the liver.

The rate of disappearance of the chylomicron triglyceride is very rapid. The half-life of radioactively labeled chylomicrons injected into humans is less than one hour and is directly related to particle size.

VLDL and IDL

VLDL is secreted from the liver and intestine. Data in humans are limited almost exclusively to the intestine. Lipoproteins are first identified in smooth endoplasmic reticulum vesicles at the luminal portion of the cell, a site of active acylation of monoglyceride with acyl-CoA derivatives of fatty acids. The lipoprotein particles are then transferred to Golgi organelles and leave the cells by reverse pinocytosis. VLDL synthesis in the liver was studied extensively in the rat and was found to be essentially similar to VLDL synthesis by the human small intestine.

Nascent VLDL contains very little apo C, indicating that it is not a necessary constituent for VLDL synthesis. On the other hand, apo B is essential for the synthesis of VLDL. VLDL is one of the lipoproteins not identified in the plasma of patients with abetalipoproteinemia.

The triglycerides of VLDL are newly synthesized, in the intestine and liver, from endogenous NEFA. Carbohydrate feeding and insulin may increase hepatic VLDL synthesis by increasing the synthesis of NEFA.

VLDL triglyceride has a half-life in normal humans of 2 to 4 hours. It is hydrolyzed by the extrahepatic lipoprotein-lipase system and, as in the catabolism of chylomicrons, the larger VLDL particles are more susceptible than the

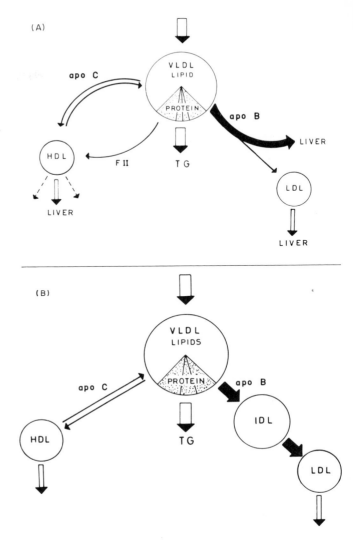

Figure 8–5. Schematic representation of probable pathways for VLDL apoprotein metabolism in rats (A) as compared with that in humans (B). In humans, as in the rat, the liver is the probable site of HDL and LDL clearance from the bloodstream. (From Eisenberg, S., and Levy, R. I.: Lipoprotein metabolism. Adv. Lipid Res., *13*:1, 1976.)

smaller particles to the action of this enzyme system. Following the hydrolytic action of lipoprotein-lipase, the large VLDL loses about 80 per cent of its triglyceride and about 60 per cent of its free cholesterol and phospholipids. At the same time, marked changes also occur in the apoprotein constituents of VLDL. Apo C is transferred to other lipoproteins, predominantly HDL. This transfer to HDL occurs in direct relation to the relative concentration of these two lipoproteins in the plasma (Fig. 8–5).

The first stage of VLDL degradation terminates with the formation of IDL. The particles formed during this stage of VLDL degradation contain the original amount of apo B,

with a much higher ratio of apo B:apo C and a lower concentration of all lipids. These particles probably represent the end of the first stage of VLDL metabolism.

The metabolic pathways leading to the further degradation of IDL in humans are not known. In the rat, IDL is cleared from the circulation primarily by the liver, probably after specific interaction with hepatic cell surfaces. The binding of IDL particles to hepatocytes may be a function of the apoprotein composition on the particle surface. Following delipidation and further loss of protein, the IDL particles in the rat are interiorized into the hepatocyte and degraded.

Although the exact metabolic pathways for

the degradation of IDL in man are not known, it is clear that IDL is the main precursor of LDL.

LDL

Although LDL is derived mainly from VLDL, other possible sources for LDL (or IDL?) are chylomicrons and direct synthesis of this lipoprotein in the liver and/or intestine.

Because the liver is the major pathway for excretion of cholesterol, it has been assumed that this organ also plays a major role in the degradation of LDL. Recent studies, however, have cast some doubt on this assumption. In hepatectomized dogs and swine, the fractional catabolic rate of LDL were actually increased.

Goldstein and Brown (1974) have shown that cultured fibroblasts are capable of catabolizing the protein moiety of LDL and that this process is dependent on the binding of LDL to specific receptors on the cell surface. By use of electron microscopy, the binding sites of LDL have been localized to short indented segments of the cell membrane. Following binding to the receptors, the LDL enters the cell by endocytosis and undergoes hydrolysis by lysosomal enzymes. The resulting free intracellular cholesterol then regulates several activities: (1) it suppresses the activity of 3-hydroxy-3-methyl-glutaryl coenzyme A reductase (HMG-CoA reductase), probably by reducing enzyme synthesis; (2) it further activates acyl-CoA:cholesteryl acyltransferase, which in turn re-esterifies the free cholesterol; and (3) it reduces the synthesis of the LDL receptors. Therefore, degradation of LDL in humans may proceed mainly at extrahepatic sites, involving factors as yet undiscovered (Eisenberg, 1976).

HDL

This lipoprotein is synthesized in both the liver and the intestine, but the relative importance of these two sites is not known. Similarly, the factors that influence HDL synthesis are not known. The level of HDL varies considerably among individuals but is much more constant in any individual than are levels of LDL, VLDL, or chylomicrons. HDL is altered by several physiologic and pathologic conditions. HDL levels are decreased by diets very rich in carbohydrate (80 per cent of calories). Higher levels are found in adult females than in males of comparable age. In males a decline

in HDL concentration occurs during adolescence, and the concentration of HDL remains lower in adult males than in pre-adolescent boys. No such change occurs in females during adolescence (LRC Data Book, 1978).

The HDL particle undergoes continuous exchange in the circulation. A constant exchange of protein (mainly apo C) occurs between HDL and newly formed VLDL. Moreover, an exchange of free cholesterol and phospholipids apparently occurs between HDL particles and the tissues, and cholesterol ester is generated within the lipoprotein through the action of LCAT.

Although the metabolism of each lipoprotein has been described separately, it must be re-emphasized that metabolically all major lipoproteins are closely related and participate in the physiologic process of triglyceride transport. For additional information, the reader is referred to the recent review of Eisenberg and Levy (1976).

METHODS FOR CLINICAL PRACTICE

SAMPLING CONDITIONS

Concern with precision and accuracy in laboratory methodology is essential for the proper diagnosis and long-term management of patients with abnormalities in lipoprotein metabolism. Since some inaccuracies are inherent in the various methods, the clinician and pathologist should be informed regarding different methods and select the most appropriate ones. Erroneous results may also be obtained owing to improper sampling conditions; hence, it is essential to be familiar with the effects that differences in sampling procedures may have on plasma lipids and lipoproteins, and to standardize as much as possible the conditions under which a blood specimen is drawn.

Total cholesterol and triglyceride can be measured in either plasma or serum, although the concentrations of these lipids in EDTA plasma are about 3 per cent lower than in serum (Bachorik, 1977). When plasma is used, EDTA is the preferred anticoagulant because of its stabilizing effect on the lipoproteins. If electrophoresis of lipoproteins is to be included and the cholesterol content of the various lipoproteins is to be measured, EDTA plasma is preferred over heparin plasma because lipoprotein mobility can be altered by heparin. If whole blood is allowed to stand at room temperature, spontaneous redistribution of cholesterol may occur among the lipoproteins. Furthermore, at room temperature changes may also occur in the relative concentration of cholesterol, cholesterol ester, and phospholipids through the action of the LCAT system. To avoid changes after the collection of the samples, blood should be cooled to 4°C. and the cells separated as soon as possible. If only cholesterol and/or triglyceride will be analyzed, plasma or serum can be frozen. This should not be done if lipoprotein analysis is also to be performed on the specimen.

Posture affects the concentrations of the various plasma constituents by changing circulating plasma volume. As much as a 10 per cent drop in plasma lipid concentration can be observed in subjects who, after standing for 30 minutes, assume a recumbent position. It is therefore necessary to standardize the specimen-obtaining posture as much as possible.

Precaution must be taken to avoid *in vitro* hemolysis. This is particularly important when "direct" methods are used for cholesterol analysis, because in these methods plasma or serum is analyzed without elimination of hemoglobin and other possible interfering substances. On the other hand, enzymatic or other methods that incorporate extraction and absorption stages are less susceptible to interference from hemoglobin.

Feeding has only a slight effect on plasma cholesterol levels. However, depending on the type and amount of food ingested, it may have a considerable effect on the plasma triglyceride concentration. It must be remembered that chylomicrons will usually be present in postprandial plasma, but their presence in fasting plasma is considered abnormal. Hence, it is necessary to obtain blood specimens not earlier than 12 to 14 hours after the last meal.

Lipoprotein concentrations are readily influenced by factors such as weight change, drugs, and intercurrent illness, especially if accompanied by fever. Dramatic changes occur following a myocardial infarction, with an immediate drop of 10 to 60 per cent in LDL and a more gradual (within 10 to 30 days) increase in the concentration of VLDL.

ESTIMATION OF CHOLESTEROL

Several methods are available for the determination of total plasma cholesterol, each of which has certain advantages, and, unfortunately, disadvantages. Hence, the laboratorian must be familiar with the principles of each group of methods and select the most appropriate method for the specific task. Generally, it may be said that the more accurate a method is, the more laborious it will be. The most accurate methods usually require several isolation and purification steps or special equipment, whereas the rapid and simple ("direct" i.e., without saponification) methods are easy to perform but usually lack specificity.

If the sample load is relatively small and great accuracy and specificity are required, methods should be used that involve preliminary saponification of cholesteryl ester and removal of interfering substances. For greater sample loads, such as for population screening, or in the routine clinical laboratory, methods that reduce sample handling may be used.

Colorimetric methods

These are the classic methods used for the estimation of cholesterol. They depend on the reaction of cholesterol with one of three mixtures: acetic anhydride-sulfuric acid (Liebermann-Burchard); ferric chloride-sulfuric acid; or *p*-toluene sulfonic acid. A major source of error in these methods is the different production of color by cholesterol and cholesteryl ester with these reagents. Unesterified cholesterol produces less color with the acetic anhydride-sulfuric acid reagent than does free cholesterol, but produces slightly more color with the ferric chloride-sulfuric acid reagent. No difference exists in color production between free and esterified cholesterol when *p*-toluene sulfonic acids are used. Different color production by other plasma steroids (e.g., 7-dehydrocholesterol) with different reagents can also add to the error in analysis.

Another source of error in cholesterol determinations is the presence of interfering substances such as bilirubin, hemoglobin, salicylate, iodide, or vitamins A and D; of these, the most important are bilirubin and hemoglobin. It is imperative, therefore, to avoid hemolysis in blood sampling and to use a method that involves prior removal of interfering substances in all samples in which the presence of one of these substances is suspected.

A relatively simple reference method and probably the most widely used for estimation of total cholesterol is the Abell-Kendall procedure. This method involves saponification of cholesteryl ester by alcohol potassium hydroxide, extraction of the cholesterol by petroleum ether, and color development with acetic anhydride-sulfuric acid. This method avoids interference by bilirubin, protein, and hemoglobin.

The Schoenheimer-Sperry method was the accepted reference method until it was replaced largely by the Abell-Kendall. It is an accurate but laborious method and is not suitable for large numbers of samples. In the Schoenheimer-Sperry procedure esterified cholesterol is saponified and proteins and other interfering substances are extracted by organic solvents. An additional step, which eliminates bilirubin, is the precipitation of cholesterol by digitonin and quantitation of the cholesterol by means of the Liebermann-Burchard reaction.

Chromatographic methods

The use of gas-liquid chromatography (GLC), with the addition of internal standards, has recently been introduced for measuring total plasma cholesterol. This method begins with saponification of esterified cholesterol by alkaline hydrolysis and the extraction of unesterified cholesterol into an organic medium. The advantage of using an internal standard, instead of direct calibration of the instrument with a standard cholesterol solution, is that evaporation of the extraction solution during handling will not affect the samples with the internal standard. Very specific and highly sensitive, this method can be applied to determine total cholesterol concentrations in as little as 5 μl of plasma. It must be noted, however, that results obtained by the GLC method are lower (by about 3 per cent) than by the reference Abell-Kendall method.

Automated "direct" methods

Several methods for the estimation of total cholesterol in plasma omit saponification. These methods, which are easily automated, are frequently employed for screening procedures and for use in the clinical laboratory, where large numbers of samples have to be analyzed. They are, however, subject to several sources of error such as the presence of bilirubin and other interfering substances, freezing, etc.

The most widely used of the automated methods without prior saponification is the ferric chloride-sulfuric acid method (Lipid Research Clinics Program, 1974). This method uses an isopropanol extract of plasma (extraction of proteins) while bilirubin, hemoglobin pigments, and other materials are removed by a "zeolite mixture" (zeolite, copper sulfate, calcium hydroxide, and Lloyd's reagent). Following centrifugation the supernatant isopropanol extract is analyzed on the AutoAnalyzer by use of a pure cholesterol standard. One possible error of this method is the sensitivity of the reaction to water, which is present in about 5 per cent of the isopropanol extract; thus, an equal amount of water must be added to the standard. Furthermore, since the zeolite mixture removes water from the samples, the cholesterol standard must be treated identically.

The less intense color developed by cholesteryl ester present in the plasma will produce slightly lower results when this method is compared with the Abell-Kendall procedure. Moreover, long-term frozen samples give somewhat higher results than do fresh plasma samples (Bachorik, 1977).

An automated procedure that uses the ferric perchlorite-ethylacetate sulfuric acid reagent has recently been introduced. In addition to eliminating saponification, this method also omits extraction. Therefore, hemoglobin and bilirubin interfere with this method, as do high concentrations of gamma globulin.

In many clinical laboratories total serum cholesterol is estimated as a part of a battery of 12 chemical tests analyzed by the Technicon SMA 12/60 or the Technicon SMA automated system (Technicon methods SF4-0026FC4 and SG4-0026PM4 1974). These are direct methods that require unextracted serum samples in which cholesterol is determined by use of the acetic anhydride-sulfuric acid mixture. They are subject to various sources of error such as the presence of bilirubin, hemoglobin, etc., and may result in overestimating plasma cholesterol by 0.75 to 1.0 mmol/l or 30 to 40 mg/dl. Another potential source of error is the use of commercially available serum with a stated cholesterol concentration as a standard, because differences may exist between stated values and reference values. Thus, if absolute quantification is needed, these methods should be calibrated with one of the accepted reference methods.

Enzymatic methods

Probably the simplest yet most specific and accurate methods for the estimation of cholesterol are the enzymatic methods, whereby cholesteryl esters are hydrolyzed with cholesteryl-ester hydrolase and cholesterol is oxidized with cholesterol oxidase obtained from *Nocardia* species. Hydrogen peroxide is formed and quantitated colorimetrically (Fig. 8-6). It should be noted, however, that not even these methods are absolutely specific, because cholesterol oxidase will react with other plasma sterols. Interference by substances other than sterols

$$\text{CHOLESTEROL ESTER} + H_2O \xrightarrow{\text{cholesterol ester hydrolase}} \text{CHOLESTEROL} + \text{FATTY ACID}$$

$$\text{CHOLESTEROL} + O_2 \xrightarrow{\text{cholesterol oxidase}} \text{CHOLEST-4-EN-3-ONE} + H_2O_2$$

$$2H_2O_2 + \text{4-AMINOANTIPYRINE} + \text{PHENOL} \xrightarrow{\text{HPOD}} \text{QUINONEIMINE DYE} + 2H_2O$$

Figure 8-6. Schematic representation of reactions involved in enzymatic estimation of cholesterol.

(such as bilirubin and hemoglobin) is negligible (Allain, 1974).

Kit methods

Several commercially available kits are in use for estimating cholesterol. Although some may furnish clinically useful information, their accuracy and reproducibility vary. The performance of a particular kit should always be evaluated by comparison with reference methodology. The long-term precision of analyses should be monitored by inclusion of samples of known cholesterol content.

ESTIMATION OF TRIGLYCERIDE

The wide variety of methods still in use for the estimation of plasma triglyceride suggests that no one method is completely satisfactory. It is beyond the scope of this chapter to describe in detail the technical procedure for each of the many methods available (for this the reader is referred to the excellent review by Witter, 1972). Here, only the basic principles of the most commonly used methods will be discussed in terms of their relative merits and disadvantages.

Although most methods currently employed measure plasma glyceride glycerol by chemical or enzymatic methods, another group of methods can determine intact plasma triglyceride without prior hydrolysis.

The estimated triglyceride is expressed as the concentration of glycerol liberated from glyceride, i.e., in terms of mmol/liter. Anyone using methods that give the actual mass of triglyceride must remember that this number is influenced by the type of fatty acids attached to the glycerol; triglyceride mass is usually related to triolein, which is the most commonly used standard. The presence of fatty acids other than oleic acid in the plasma triglyceride molecule will result in some error in the expression of the triglyceride mass.

Triglycerides are carried in the bloodstream as a part of the lipoproteins (primarily in chylomicrons and VLDL). Less polar solvents, such as diethyl ether or petroleum ether, which usually dissolve free triglyceride easily, are not suitable for dissolving triglyceride from lipoproteins, and more polar solvents must be used.

Colorimetric methods

The most widely used method for extracting and washing triglyceride from plasma is that of Folch (1957), followed by silicic acid column chromatog-

raphy to separate the glyceride from other lipids. Other methods use isopropanol as the extracting solution, and any unwanted components are then removed by adsorbents such as alumina or a "zeolite mixture." However, when such adsorbents are used, the standard must be subjected to identical treatment in order to compensate for any removal of water by these materials. Substances that may interfere with the estimation of triglycerides are those having adjacent hydroxyl, or hydroxyl and amino, groups such as glucose and phospholipids; they interfere because oxidation of glycerol to formaldehyde is not specific for glycerol but occurs in all of these substances.

Release of glycerol is achieved by saponification with isopropanolic or ethanolic potassium hydroxide or by transesterification with sodium methoxide in isopropanol. The reaction mixture obtained contains cholesterol and either methyl esters or potassium soaps of fatty acids. As these substances may interfere in the subsequent steps of the analysis, they may have to be removed, depending on the methods employed (Bachorik, 1977). The presence in the plasma of free glycerol and/or partial glyceride may also be a source of error in the estimation of triglycerides. Under ordinary circumstances the contribution of both of these is very small, but free glycerol in high concentrations is sometimes encountered in patients with uncontrolled diabetes and in samples that have been allowed to stand for a prolonged time at room temperature. Therefore, when the presence of these substances in high concentrations is suspected, methods should be used that will remove them (at least partially) from the reaction. In one method, plasma is extracted into isopropanol and nonane or heptane, and following separation the nonane or heptane layer contains essentially glycerol-free triglycerides.

The presence of free glycerol and/or partial glycerides will most often interfere with the oxidation of glycerol to formaldehyde. None of the methods is specific for triglyceride glycerol; thus, any substance that has adjacent hydroxyl groups or adjacent amino and hydroxyl groups should be removed prior to the oxidation step. Usually dilute solutions of sodium periodate are used to oxidize the glycerol molecule to two molecules of formaldehyde and one molecule of formic acid.

As mentioned above, under normal conditions none of these substances will contribute appreciably to the results obtained. However, anyone dealing with unusual physiologic conditions must keep in mind the possibility of falsely elevated triglycerides. A triglyceride "blank" should be run with materials present in plasma extracts that react similarly to, but are not, triglyceride. These should be estimated and subtracted from the total triglyceride obtained (Mather, 1975). The most common way to run a triglyceride "blank" is to eliminate the step of saponification and thus measure the fluorescence obtained from substances present in plasma other than triglyceride.

The formaldehyde obtained from the oxidation

$$\text{GLYCEROL} + \text{ATP} \xrightarrow{\text{glycerokinase}} \alpha\text{-GLYCEROPHOSPHATE} + \text{ADP}$$

$$\text{ADP} + \text{PHOSPHOENOLPYRUVATE} \xrightarrow{\text{pyruvate kinase}} \text{ATP} + \text{PYRUVATE}$$

$$\text{PYRUVATE} + \text{NADH} + \text{H} \xrightarrow{\text{lactate dehydrogenase}} \text{LACTATE} + \text{NAD}$$

Figure 8–7.   Schematic representation of reactions involved in enzymatic estimation of triglycerides.

of glycerol is estimated colorimetrically following reaction with chromotropic acid in strong sulfuric acid, or with ammonium ions and acetyl acetone at pH 5.5 to 6.5. Several manual and semiautomated methods that use these procedures are available. The various methods for estimation of triglyceride were recently reviewed by Bachorik (1977).

Enzymatic methods

In recent years, enzymatic methods have also been used to determine plasma triglycerides. Most are based on the enzymatic hydrolysis of triglycerides by bacterial lipase (Fig. 8-7). These methods, which have the advantage of high specificity for plasma triglycerides, have been automated (Bucolo, 1975) and adapted to the Technicon SMAC (SG4-0037PM4, 1974).

ESTIMATION OF PHOSPHOLIPIDS

Clinicians are less likely to request determination of total plasma phospholipids than measurement of other lipid substances, because measurement of this class of lipids adds little information in most cases. However, the estimation of total phospholipids or their major constituents may be required in cases such as obstructive jaundice or the hypolipoproteinemias (see Disorders with Deficient Lipoprotein Levels (p. 218).

Methods for their estimation involve extracting the lipids and washing them by means of the Folch (1957) procedure; after evaporation, the total phosphorus in the lipid extract is determined. This quantity, when multiplied by 25, expresses plasma total phospholipids.

The major individual phospholipids constituting the "total phospholipids" are phosphatidylcholine, sphingomyelin, phosphatidylethanolamine, and lysophosphatidylcholine. Since measurement of these individual phospholipids is rarely required in clinical medicine, a detailed discussion here of the various methods is unwarranted (see review by Nelson, 1972).

ESTIMATION OF NON-ESTERIFIED FATTY ACIDS (NEFA)

In most cases measurement of NEFA adds little information to the assessment and management of the patient with disorders in lipid and lipoprotein metabolism. However, on occasion, it is of diagnostic interest to measure their concentration. A reliable titrimetric method has been developed by Trout (1960) and a colorimetric method by Duncombe (1963).

ESTIMATION OF LIPOPROTEINS

For most clinical and epidemiologic studies, measurement of plasma total cholesterol and triglyceride is all that is needed. However, in many patients additional information is required and the quantitative and qualitative measurement of at least some of the lipoproteins, combined with estimation of plasma lipids, is necessary. Though many methods for measuring lipoproteins are available, most require special skills and elaborate equipment not readily accessible to the majority of clinical laboratories. Fortunately for the day-to-day work of the clinical laboratory, these measurements are not required but lie more in the province of the research and specialized laboratories. In this chapter we will mention only briefly the more sophisticated methods such as ultracentrifugation and isoelectric focusing; instead, we will concentrate on description of the more basic methods available to and needed by every clinical laboratory dealing with disorders in lipids and lipoproteins.

Selection of the method(s) best suited to the specific laboratory depends on several factors such as expense, technical difficulty, and accuracy required. If large numbers of specimens are expected, a moderately accurate method that is suited to analyze this heavy load must be selected. If, on the other hand, effects of drug or diet in individual patients are to be followed, accuracy is of prime importance to indicate even modest changes over time.

The methods used for separation and analysis of the lipoproteins are based on some of their physicochemical properties, such as density, particle size, electrical charge, and antigenicity.

"Standing plasma" test

To determine the presence or absence of chylomicrons, the "standing plasma" test (Lipid Research Clinics Program, 1974) provides a very simple qualitative method. Although plasma containing chylomicrons will be turbid, this may also be due to the presence of high concentrations of VLDL. However, if the plasma is stored at 4°C. for 16 hours, any chylomicrons present will float to the surface, leaving a clear infranatant. Turbidity remaining in the infranatant is due to VLDL.

Electrophoretic separation

Electrophoretic separation of lipoproteins by use of various media such as paper, agarose gel, and cellulose acetate is widely employed, although its contribution to the diagnosis of hyperlipoproteinemia is limited (see Rational Approach to the Detection and Diagnosis of Abnormalities in Lipoprotein Metabolism). The separation of the various lipoprotein classes is a function of their negative net surface, their electrical charge, their interaction with the media employed in electrophoresis, and the size of the lipoprotein particle. The electrophoretically separated fractions of lipoproteins are named according to the plasma protein band with equal mobility. Thus, LDL are found in the beta-protein region (beta-lipoprotein), VLDL in the $alpha_2$ position, and HDL in the alpha region. This order of migration may, however, vary according to the medium employed.

Following separation, the lipoproteins are visualized by dyes taken up by the lipid component of lipoproteins. As different lipids have differential dye uptakes, the intensity of staining of the various lipoprotein classes may be according to their specific lipid content and not just according to their actual quantity. Therefore, most attempts to quantitate lipoproteins after electrophoretic separation have failed.

Paper Electrophoresis. The most widely used media for electrophoretic separation of lipoproteins are paper and agarose gel. Electrophoresis on paper is a simple method, yet it requires 16 hours for complete separation of lipoproteins. Moreover, the resolution between beta and pre-beta bands is not always complete. A third disadvantage of paper is the high background uptake of dye.

Agarose Gel Electrophoresis. The advantages of agarose gel over paper as the separation medium are the speedy separation (60 to 90 min), sharp separation between bands (especially important for separation between beta and pre-beta bands), and colorless background. Semimicro methods that use commercial kits and agarose gel as the separating medium are available. By use of "internal standardization" techniques, agarose gel electrophoresis has been converted into a quantitative method, but this method has not yet gained universal acceptance.

Cellulose Acetate Electrophoresis. Since chylomicrons may show pre-beta mobility on cellulose acetate, this medium is not advocated for lipoprotein separation.

Precipitation methods

A useful method for the quantitative determination of LDL is the "indirect beta-quantification" (Lipid Research Clinics Program, 1974; Friedewald, 1972), which eliminates the need for an ultracentrifuge. VLDL and LDL are precipitated from whole plasma by a sulfated polysaccharide such as heparin in the presence of metal ions (e.g., dextran sulfate-calcium chloride), and the amount of HDL (expressed as HDL cholesterol or HDL_c) is estimated. In the absence of chylomicrons or increased concentrations of IDL, almost all plasma triglycerides are carried in VLDL. The molar ratio of triglyceride:cholesterol in VLDL is 5 (for plasma triglyceride < 4.4 mmol/l). Therefore, it is possible to calculate the concentration of VLDL cholesterol by dividing plasma triglyceride (TG) by 5.

It follows that:

$$LDL_c = \text{Total cholesterol} - \left(HDL_c + \frac{TG}{5}\right).$$

This method should not be used when plasma triglyceride exceeds 4.4 mmol/l or when triglyceride-carrying lipoproteins other than VLDL (e.g., IDL, chylomicrons) are present.

Ultracentrifugation methods

Preparative Ultracentrifugation. These methods constitute the reference procedure for plasma lipoprotein separations. Because of the expensive equipment and special skills needed, they are not usually within the reach of most clinical laboratories. With the introduction of simpler and less expensive methods, the need for ultracentrifugal separation has remained largely with the specialized or research laboratory. Ultracentrifugation is based on two unusual properties of lipoproteins: (1) they have densities lower than any other naturally occurring macromolecules, and (2) each class of the lipoproteins has a different density. Thus, VLDL will float at the density (d) of plasma (1.006 g/ml), whereas VLDL and LDL float at d 1.063 g/ml. All lipoproteins float at d 1.210 g/ml.

The preparative ultracentrifuge is used for the quantitative separation of the lipoproteins.

Two basic methods are used. In the first, a sample is centrifuged at d 1.006 when VLDL floats. The density of the infranatant is then adjusted to d 1.063 for the separation of LDL. If it is necessary to separate HDL from other lipoproteins, a third adjustment of d 1.210 is made.

The second method employs simultaneous ultracentrifugation of plasma aliquots that have previously been adjusted in solution to the various fractions. They are brought to a known volume with saline, and the total cholesterol is estimated in each fraction.

Beta-quantification. The most widely used method for quantitating the plasma lipoproteins for clinical purposes is this combined ultracentrifugal-precipitation method. Plasma is ultracentrifuged at d 1.006. The cholesterol content of the bottom fraction ($d > 1.006$; LDL + HDL) is determined, as well as HDL cholesterol (obtained following precipitation of whole plasma with heparin sodium and manganese chloride).

The cholesterol content of the various fractions can then be calculated as follows:

(a) HDL cholesterol: directly estimated
(b) LDL cholesterol: $d > 1.006$ cholesterol minus HDL cholesterol
(c) VLDL cholesterol: total cholesterol minus $d > 1.006$ cholesterol

VLDL cholesterol can also be measured directly in the $d < 1.006$ fraction, but it tends to be inaccurate when triglyceride concentrations are greater than 300 mg/dl or less than 100 mg/dl.

Analytical Ultracentrifugation. Although this is the most accurate procedure for determination of lipoprotein classes in plasma, it is used only in a few research centers. It is also used in suspected type III patients to obtain VLDL to identify floating beta on electrophoresis. For additional reading see Lindgren, 1972.

Density Gradient Ultracentrifugation. In this procedure a continuous density gradient is established by overlaying plasma with sodium chloride solutions of decreasing density (Lindgren, 1972). This method seems particularly useful when fractionation of larger VLDL particles is undertaken, and for the isolation of particles that have a $S_f > 400$.

Immunoelectrophoresis and immunodiffusion methods

The ability of proteins to stimulate the production of specific antibodies is useful for quantification and identification of lipoproteins. The sensitivity of these methods permits the detection of very low concentrations of lipoproteins, which makes these methods particularly useful for the diagnosis of such disorders as abetalipoproteinemia and Tangier disease. It should, however, be remembered that the immunologic cross-reactivity of various lipoproteins (owing to the presence of the same apoproteins in various lipoproteins) complicates the quantitative immunologic analysis of specific lipoproteins in whole plasma. Thus, anti-B lipoproteins will react with both VLDL and LDL.

Specific antilipoprotein antisera may be purchased commercially, although if continuous use of these methods is contemplated, the preparation of one's own antisera has certain advantages, particularly for obtaining large quantities of a uniform antiserum at a relatively low cost.

A detailed description of the various immunologic methods appears in the review by Verbruggen (1975).

INDIVIDUAL VARIATION OF PLASMA LIPID AND LIPOPROTEIN CONCENTRATIONS

Plasma lipid and lipoprotein concentrations vary within and among populations, and under different conditions, within a given individual.

Limited space precludes a detailed description of all demographic, environmental, genetic, and physiologic determinants of blood lipids and lipoproteins. Nonetheless, it should be noted that this variability in the concentrations of lipids and lipoproteins makes the use of universally accepted "upper reference limits" difficult (see Chap. 2).

The relative contribution of genetic and environmental factors to the distribution curve for cholesterol concentration cannot be assessed with certainty in any population. However, family and twin studies have shown that genetic components (including polygenic effects as well as the mutant allele responsible for familial hypercholesterolemia) may account for as much as 40 per cent of the total variability. On the other hand, environmental factors, although not clearly understood, also markedly influence the variability in the distribution of cholesterol between populations. For example, immigrants who come to the United States from countries where the mean cholesterol level is low usually acquire the high levels characteristic of North America. Nutritional factors have important effects upon lipid metabolism in man and probably play the dominant role in the pathogenesis of hyperlipidemia so commonly found in western populations.

In healthy subjects cholesterol of dietary origin contributes to elevation of LDL cholesterol. The total amount of dietary fat and the type of fat (saturated or polyunsaturated) also have a well-documented effect upon plasma lipid and lipoprotein concentrations. In general, it may be stated that saturated fat elevates and polyunsaturated fat decreases the plasma cholesterol levels. The mechanisms by which such fats influence plasma lipid levels are unclear.

The amount and type of carbohydrate consumed have little long-term effect upon plasma lipid levels (Connor, 1977). In short-term (a few days to a few weeks) experimental studies, an increase of carbohydrate intake (to about 75 per cent of total calories) has usually resulted in a sharp increase in plasma triglyceride. Long-term studies, however, have indicated, that in spite of continuation of the high carbohydrate diet, triglyceride concentrations will return to baseline levels.

Excessive caloric consumption of any source of food with an associated weight gain may lead to hypertriglyceridemia through VLDL increase; this is particularly true in individuals with already elevated triglycerides. Even moderate reduction in caloric intake in hypertriglyceridemic overweight patients usually leads to lower VLDL levels.

Various medications are known to influence plasma lipid distribution. Of these, sex hormones (oral contraceptives and estrogen replacement therapy) are epidemiologically the most important. For example, the Lipid Research Clinics Program of the National Heart, Lung, and Blood Institute recently reported that in an aggregate of 11 U.S. populations, 50 per cent of the women in the 20-to-24-year-old age group used sex hormones and that sex hormone use was associated with increases in plasma cholesterol and triglyceride levels. Mean plasma triglyceride concentration was 48 per cent higher in hormone users under age 40 than in non-users in the same age group. Use of sex hormones is undoubtedly the most common cause of hypertriglyceridemia in women 20 to 50 years old. On the other hand, in postmenopausal women the use of estrogen replacement therapy is accompanied by a decrease in plasma cholesterol.

REFERENCE VALUES FOR PLASMA LIPIDS AND LIPOPROTEINS

The variability in plasma lipids and lipoproteins precludes the establishment of universally acceptable limits of "reference intervals." What may be considered normal for one population group may not necessarily be applicable to another. Even within a country, these reference intervals may vary from one region to another and are markedly age- and sex-dependent.

Table 8–6. PLASMA TOTAL CHOLESTEROL (mg/dl)* IN 11 FREE-LIVING NORTH AMERICAN POPULATIONS OF WHITE PARTICIPANTS

| | MALES (n = 3580) | | | FEMALES (n = 3413) | | |
| | | Percentiles | | | Percentiles | |
AGE	Mean ± SEM†	10th	90th	Mean ± SEM†	10th	90th
5–9	155.3 ± 1.8	131	183	164.0 ± 1.8	135	189
10–14	160.9 ± 1.5	132	191	160.1 ± 1.5	131	191
15–19	153.1 ± 1.4	123	183	159.5 ± 1.6	126	198
20–24	162.2 ± 2.5	126	197	170.3 ± 2.5	132	220
25–29	178.7 ± 2.1	137	223	179.5 ± 1.7	142	217
30–34	193.1 ± 1.8	152	237	179.2 ± 1.7	141	215
35–39	200.6 ± 1.9	157	248	189.6 ± 2.1	149	233
40–44	205.2 ± 1.9	161	251	197.5 ± 1.9	156	241
45–49	213.4 ± 1.9	171	258	206.2 ± 2.0	162	256
50–54	213.2 ± 1.9	168	263	217.3 ± 2.4	171	267
55–59	215.0 ± 2.2	172	260	228.7 ± 2.4	182	278
60–64	216.6 ± 3.3	170	262	232.3 ± 3.7	186	282
65–69	221.0 ± 3.8	174	275	234.1 ± 4.0	179	282
70+	210.3 ± 3.4	160	253	224.5 ± 2.8	181	268

Source: LRC Data Book (1978). By permission.

*Multiply by 0.026 $\frac{mmol \cdot dl}{liter \cdot mg}$ to transform to SI Units.

†SEM = Standard error of the mean.

Table 8–7. PLASMA TRIGLYCERIDES (mg/dl)* IN 11 FREE-LIVING NORTH AMERICAN POPULATIONS OF WHITE PARTICIPANTS

| | MALES (n = 3580) | | | FEMALES (n = 3413) | | |
| | | Percentiles | | | Percentiles | |
AGE	Mean ± SEM†	10th	90th	Mean ± SEM†	10th	90th
5–9	51.9 ± 1.7	34	70	63.8 ± 2.5	37	103
10–14	63.4 ± 1.6	37	94	72.0 ± 1.7	44	104
15–19	78.2 ± 2.4	43	125	72.8 ± 1.9	40	112
20–24	89.3 ± 3.7	50	146	87.3 ± 2.9	42	135
25–29	104.2 ± 4.2	51	171	87.4 ± 2.8	45	137
30–34	122.1 ± 3.7	57	214	86.0 ± 2.8	45	140
35–39	140.8 ± 5.5	58	250	98.3 ± 3.2	47	170
40–44	152.4 ± 6.9	69	252	98.1 ± 2.6	51	161
45–49	143.4 ± 5.9	65	218	112.5 ± 3.4	55	180
50–54	153.4 ± 5.5	75	244	116.0 ± 3.4	58	190
55–59	134.3 ± 4.2	70	210	133.1 ± 4.8	65	229
60–64	130.6 ± 8.7	65	193	132.1 ± 9.1	66	210
65–69	138.6 ± 11.1	61	227	136.5 ± 6.8	64	221
70+	132.8 ± 7.2	71	202	128.3 ± 6.5	68	189

Source: LRC Data Book (1978). By permission.

*Multiply by 0.026 $\frac{mmol \cdot dl}{liter \cdot mg}$ to transform to SI Units.

†SEM = Standard error of the mean.

It should also be mentioned here that a "normal" lipid level, i.e., less than the upper 5 per cent of the distribution, is not synonymous with "healthy" and does not necessarily imply absence of risk. Therefore, different cut-off points may be used for different purposes. Traditionally the 90th or 95th percentile is used. However, this is arbitrary, since no clear cut-off point for coronary heart disease exists, and in fact the relationship between plasma cholesterol and coronary heart disease risk is that of a continuous variable. Tables 8–6 through 8–10 give the means and selected percentiles of the mean concentration values of plasma cholesterol and triglycerides, demonstrating the effects of age and sex.

Table 8–8. PLASMA VLDL-CHOLESTEROL (mg/dl)* IN 11 FREE-LIVING NORTH AMERICAN POPULATIONS OF WHITE PARTICIPANTS

| | MALES (n = 3539) | | | FEMALES (n = 3374) | | |
| | | Percentiles | | | Percentiles | |
AGE	Mean ± SEM†	10th	90th	Mean ± SEM†	10th	90th
5–9	8.2 ± 0.5	2.0	15.0	9.7 ± 0.7	1.0	19.0
10–14	9.9 ± 0.4	2.0	18.0	10.9 ± 0.4	3.0	20.0
15–19	12.8 ± 0.5	3.0	23.0	11.8 ± 0.5	3.5	21.5
20–24	13.7 ± 0.8	4.8	24.0	13.5 ± 0.6	4.0	24.0
25–29	17.4 ± 0.9	6.0	30.7	13.4 ± 0.5	3.4	24.0
30–34	21.3 ± 0.9	8.0	36.0	12.2 ± 0.5	3.0	21.0
35–39	24.1 ± 1.0	7.0	45.8	15.4 ± 0.7	3.0	29.0
40–44	25.5 ± 1.2	8.0	42.5	14.7 ± 0.5	4.9	28.0
45–49	24.4 ± 1.1	7.6	40.0	17.4 ± 0.7	4.0	32.6
50–54	26.8 ± 1.1	10.0	49.0	17.2 ± 0.7	5.0	32.0
55–59	21.6 ± 1.1	6.0	39.0	20.7 ± 1.0	4.0	37.0
60–64	18.9 ± 1.3	4.0	34.8	16.7 ± 1.8	3.0	29.0
65–69	19.7 ± 2.0	2.5	39.5	17.0 ± 1.3	3.0	36.0
70+	17.0 ± 1.2	2.9	31.1	15.6 ± 1.2	0.6	31.7

Source: LRC Data Book (1978). By permission.

*Multiply by 0.026 $\frac{mmol \cdot dl}{liter \cdot mg}$ to transform to SI Units.

†SEM = Standard error of the mean.

Table 8-9. PLASMA LDL-CHOLESTEROL (mg/dl)* IN 11 FREE-LIVING NORTH AMERICAN POPULATIONS OF WHITE PARTICIPANTS

| | MALES (n = 3540) | | | FEMALES (n = 3374) | | |
| | | Percentiles | | | Percentiles | |
AGE	Mean ± SEM†	10th	90th	Mean ± SEM†	10th	90th
5–9	92.5 ± 1.8	69	117	100.4 ± 2.1	73	125
10–14	96.8 ± 1.4	73	123	97.4 ± 1.3	73	126
15–19	94.4 ± 1.3	68	123	95.7 ± 1.5	66	129
20–24	103.3 ± 2.4	73	138	103.7 ± 2.2	65	141
25–29	116.7 ± 1.9	75	157	110.2 ± 1.6	75	148
30–34	126.4 ± 1.6	88	166	111.3 ± 1.5	77	146
35–39	133.2 ± 1.7	92	176	119.7 ± 2.0	81	161
40–44	135.6 ± 1.6	98	173	125.1 ± 1.8	84	165
45–49	143.7 ± 1.8	106	185	129.4 ± 1.9	89	173
50–54	142.3 ± 1.7	102	185	138.1 ± 2.3	94	186
55–59	145.8 ± 2.1	103	191	146.1 ± 2.4	97	199
60–64	146.3 ± 3.1	106	188	152.0 ± 3.6	105	191
65–69	150.4 ± 3.5	104	199	153.8 ± 4.1	99	205
70+	142.9 ± 2.9	100	182	148.6 ± 2.7	108	189

Source: LRC Data Book (1978). By permission.

*Multiply by 0.026 $\frac{mmol \cdot dl}{liter \cdot mg}$ to transform to SI Units.

†SEM = Standard error of the mean.

CLINICOPATHOLOGIC CORRELATION

Coronary heart disease (CHD) is one of the major health problems in modern society. In 1967, the United States ranked second highest in mortality rates for young adult and middle-aged men (Task Force on Arteriosclerosis, 1971). Although a decline in mortality has been observed over recent years, it still maintains epidemic proportions. For every fatal event at least one, and probably more, nonfatal events occur.

During recent years, strong evidence has accumulated to indicate that both constitutional and environmental factors exert an im-

Table 8-10. PLASMA HDL-CHOLESTEROL (mg/dl)* IN 11 FREE-LIVING NORTH AMERICAN POPULATIONS OF WHITE PARTICIPANTS

| | MALES (n = 3573) | | | FEMALES (n = 3407) | | |
| | | Percentiles | | | Percentiles | |
AGE	Mean ± SEM†	10th	90th	Mean ± SEM†	10th	90th
5–9	55.8 ± 1.0	43	70	53.2 ± 1.0	38	67
10–14	54.9 ± 0.7	40	71	52.2 ± 0.7	40	64
15–19	46.1 ± 0.6	34	59	52.3 ± 0.7	38	68
20–24	45.4 ± 1.0	32	57	53.3 ± 1.0	37	72
25–29	44.7 ± 0.7	32	58	56.0 ± 0.8	39	74
30–34	45.5 ± 0.6	32	59	56.0 ± 0.7	40	73
35–39	43.5 ± 0.6	31	58	55.0 ± 0.8	38	75
40–44	44.2 ± 0.6	31	60	57.8 ± 0.9	39	79
45–49	45.5 ± 0.6	33	60	59.4 ± 1.0	41	82
50–54	44.1 ± 0.6	31	58	62.0 ± 1.0	41	84
55–59	47.6 ± 0.9	31	64	62.2 ± 1.1	41	85
60–64	51.5 ± 1.3	34	69	63.8 ± 1.4	44	87
65–69	51.1 ± 1.5	33	74	63.3 ± 1.8	38	85
70+	50.5 ± 1.7	33	70	60.7 ± 1.4	38	82

Source: LRC Data Book (1978). By permission.

*Multiply by 0.026 $\frac{mmol \cdot dl}{liter \cdot mg}$ to transform to SI Units.

†SEM = Standard error of the mean.

portant influence on the incidence of CHD. Genetic factors, manifested as inborn errors of lipoprotein metabolism, are responsible for premature atherosclerosis in some families. But these account for only a small percentage of all affected individuals.

Several risk factors, defined as those habits, traits, and abnormalities associated with a sizable increase in susceptibility to CHD, have been recognized. These factors may be classified into those involving social environment and life style (e.g., diet, smoking); those involving endogenous biochemical-physiologic regulatory mechanisms (e.g., pharmacologic agents, diet, etc.); and those involving fundamental biology, such as age and sex.

Among the major risk factors identified so far are elevated plasma cholesterol and LDL cholesterol, cigarette smoking, and elevated blood pressure. Recently, low levels of HDL have been found to make a significant contribution to risk. Weaker associations with coronary heart disease have been demonstrated for obesity, hyperglycemia, elevated triglyceride, hyperuricemia, etc.

The evidence of the association between serum cholesterol level and arteriosclerosis is extensive and unequivocal. It is derived from a variety of sources, including (a) production of atherosclerotic lesions in animals by hypercholesterolemia-inducing diets, (b) the nature and dynamics of the human atherosclerotic plaque, (c) the occurrence of hyperlipidemia in groups of subjects with clinically manifested atherosclerotic disease, (d) the study of genetic hyperlipidemias associated with premature atherosclerosis, and (e) epidemiologic studies of populations with differing serum lipid levels.

In prospective studies (Kannel, 1972), it was clearly demonstrated that in a healthy population, the risk of coronary heart disease is directly related to the plasma cholesterol concentration (Fig. 8-8). One of the most important results that emerged from these studies was the demonstration that although a greater risk for developing coronary heart disease is experienced by subjects with the highest cholesterol levels, no level encountered in these studies seems to be immune. The accuracy of predicting the risk of coronary heart disease (CHD) from cholesterol concentrations is higher in the young than in the old.

This continuous relationship between cholesterol and the incidence of CHD is of the utmost importance. There is little justification to use the Gaussian distribution to define reference intervals (see Chap. 2). The practicing physician should remember that the higher the cholesterol, the greater the probability for CHD and hence, the greater the need is for prophylaxis; but no single level of plasma cholesterol separates those who need prophylaxis from those who do not.

Plasma LDL concentrations correlate closely with plasma cholesterol concentrations, as would be expected, since 60 to 70 per cent of the total cholesterol is normally transported in this lipoprotein. They thus carry more or less the same predictive power.

LDL and HDL are both potent risk factors for CHD, but whereas LDL cholesterol is directly related to risk, HDL cholesterol apparently shows an even stronger but inverse relationship.

In spite of numerous studies in the past that demonstrated this inverse relationship between HDL and atherosclerosis, HDL is only now becoming part of a standard coronary risk

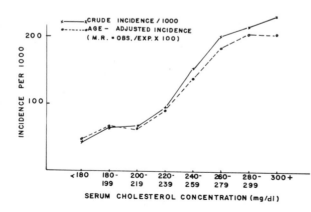

Figure 8-8. Risk of CHD (coronary heart disease) according to serum cholesterol concentration in men 30 to 49 years of age. (From Kannel, W. B., and Dawber, T. R.: Contributors to coronary risk implications for prevention and public health. The Framingham Study. Heart Lung, 1:797, 1972.)

considered diagnostic of Type III, with ratios of 0.25 to 0.29* representing a zone of uncertainty.

Recently an immunochemical test has been described for detecting increased apo E in frozen as well as fresh plasma (Kushwaha, 1977). However, the specificity of this apo E assay for the diagnosis of Type III is still to be fully tested. Perhaps promising in this regard is the report by Utermann (1975) of a lack of isoapolipoprotein E_3 in subjects with Type III hyperlipoproteinemia.

The genetic transmission of Type III is not clear. It seems that the disorder is transmitted as an autosomal recessive trait and that patients with the phenotypic expression are homozygous. An extremely high prevalence of heterozygosity explains reports of vertical transmission. In recent years, it has been shown that multiple lipoprotein patterns may co-exist in kindred of Type III patients. For a detailed discussion the reader is referred to the recent paper by Levy (1977).

Disorders with increased VLDL (Type IV Hyperlipoproteinemia)

Type IV hyperlipoproteinemia is defined in chemical terms as an abnormal increase in plasma triglycerides produced by the liver and transported in the VLDL (Beaumont, 1970). It is fairly common and usually fairly easy to diagnose, although at times this is complicated by wide fluctuations in triglyceride concentrations caused by changes in diet, body weight, or alcohol consumption. It should also be remembered that a patient with the Type IV pattern who consumes a high-fat diet can quickly, though temporarily, convert to the Type V pattern.

The diagnosis of Type IV hyperlipoproteinemia is based on the finding of increased concentrations of triglycerides in the absence of chylomicrons (turbid infranatant in the "standing plasma" test without a cream layer at the top) and normal or only slightly elevated plasma cholesterol (Table 8–12). Paper or agarose gel electrophoresis, although not essential for diagnosis, will confirm it by demonstrating an increase in pre-beta lipoproteins. It should be remembered, however, that an increased pre-beta band in the absence of hypertriglyceridemia denotes "sinking pre-beta" or LP(a).

Type IV hyperlipoproteinemia may be secondary to many disorders (Table 8–11). It is most prevalent in women between 20 and 50 years of age who are taking oral contraceptives (Levy, 1976). It may also be secondary to diabetes mellitus, glycogen storage disease, the nephrotic syndrome, and alcoholism.

The primary Type IV patient may represent a sporadic or familial case. In most of the families studied the disorder was transmitted as an autosomal dominant trait with late penetrance, the clinical form being infrequently encountered in childhood. Hypertriglyceridemia can be detected in no more than 20 per cent of the children born to a parent with familial Type IV hyperlipoproteinemia, but it is detected in higher numbers of adult first-degree relatives.

Glucose intolerance, found in about 50 per cent of the Type IV cases, is often associated with hyperuricemia. When the VLDL are greatly elevated, eruptive xanthomas may appear. The lipoproteins of patients with Type IV are very susceptible to body weight changes; obesity, which aggravates the disorder, is often present, whereas reduction to ideal weight will result in lowering of plasma VLDL. The exact mechanism responsible for the increase in VLDL in Type IV patients is not known. Delay in the removal rate of triglycerides has been shown in some patients with endogenous hypertriglyceridemia.

Premature vascular disease of the coronary vessels is the most important of the clinical manifestations of Type IV hyperlipoproteinemia. Of the Type IV patients over the age of 25 studied by Fredrickson and Levy (1972), 38 per cent gave a history of angina or myocardial infarction. As early as 1954, Gofman showed that both S_f 0-12 and S_f 12-400 lipoprotein classes were significantly elevated in patients with documented myocardial infarction, as compared with age- and sex-matched controls. A high frequency of prominent pre-beta band was described in patients with myocardial infarction.

While several case-control studies have substantiated that hypertriglyceridemia with the Type IV electrophoretic pattern is common in patients with coronary heart disease, prospective studies have generally not identified either triglycerides or VLDL as an independent risk factor. Thus, evidence on the role of hypertriglyceridemia as an independent risk factor is as yet inconclusive.

Type IV hyperlipoproteinemia is distributed

---

*0.63 − 0.74 = ratio of values in mmol/l.

in many kindred along autosomal dominant inheritance lines, with the expression in late childhood or early adult life.

TREATMENT OF HYPERLIPOPROTEINEMIA

Any discussion on the treatment of hyperlipidemia must stress that substantial evidence relates hyperlipidemia to coronary heart disease (CHD) risk and that appropriate therapy can partially or totally correct most forms of hyperlipidemia. However, the evidence to date has not proved that lowering elevated blood lipid levels in man is of specific benefit for the prevention of coronary heart disease or the regression of atherosclerosis.

In the secondary forms of hyperlipidemia, treatment is mainly aimed at the underlying disease, since correction of the primary disorder will usually be followed by a lowering of lipid levels. The treatment of hyperlipoproteinemia falls into one or more of three categories (Table 8–14): correction of dietary intake, medication, and surgical intervention. The first always takes precedence. (For detailed reviews of the treatment of hyperlipi-

demia, see Rifkind and Levy, 1976, and Fredrickson, 1974.)

DISORDERS WITH DEFICIENT LIPOPROTEIN LEVELS

Disorders with deficient LDL

Abetalipoproteinemia. This is a rare disorder characterized by the absence of all three lipoproteins that contain apo B (LDL, VLDL, and chylomicrons). Clinically it is manifested by steatorrhea, retinitis pigmentosa, and ataxic neuropathic disease (Table 8–15). An additional characteristic feature is the presence of acanthocytes in wet preparations of fresh blood.

Plasma cholesterol is very low in all patients, rarely exceeding 1.2 mmol/l (50 mg/dl); plasma triglycerides are usually less than 0.2 mmol/l (20 mg/dl), and phospholipids less than 1000 mg/l (Table 8–16). The fatty acid composition of plasma lipids is abnormal, with a marked decrease in linoleic acid concentration.

Profound changes are also seen in plasma lipoproteins. With electrophoresis, only alpha lipoproteins are seen. In the preparative ul-

Table 8–14.   TREATMENT OF FAMILIAL HYPERLIPOPROTEINEMIA

TYPE/PATTERN OF HYPERLIPOPROTEINEMIA	DIET*	PREFERRED DRUGS	SURGERY†
I	Low fat (25–35 g/day) MCT‡ supplement No alcohol	–	–
IIa	Low cholesterol (300 mg/day) Low saturated fat (P:S§ = 2.0)	Biliary sequestrant Nicotinic acid	Ileal bypass Portacaval shunt
IIb	Low cholesterol (<300 mg/day) Low saturated fat (P:S = 2.0), ≤40% of calories; Caloric control Alcohol restriction	Biliary sequestrant Nicotinic acid	Ileal bypass Portacaval shunt
III	Low cholesterol (<300 mg/day) Low saturated fat (P:S = 2.0), ≤40% of calories; Alcohol restriction	Clofibrate Nicotinic acid	–
IV	Moderate cholesterol (300–500 mg/day) Low saturated fat (P:S = 1.0); Alcohol restriction	Clofibrate Nicotinic acid	–
V	Moderate cholesterol (300–500 mg/day) Low carbohydrate (50% of calories) Low fat (30% of calories) No alcohol	Nicotinic acid Progestogens	–

*For detailed dietary treatment, see Fredrickson, 1974.
†May be undertaken under certain circumstances in homozygotes and severe heterozygotes.
‡MCT = medium-chain triglyceride.
§P:S = polyunsaturated fat:saturated fat.

Table 8–15. MAJOR FEATURES OF FAMILIAL LIPOPROTEIN DEFICIENCY STATES*

FEATURES	LDL† DEFICIENCY		HDL† DEFICIENCY (Tangier disease)	LCAT† DEFICIENCY
	Abetalipopro-teinemia	Hypobetalipopro-teinemia		
Malabsorption	+	Rarely	−	−
Rectal infiltration	−	−	+	−
Hepatic involvement	−	−	+	−
Tonsillar infiltration	−	−	+	−
Lymphadenopathy	−	−	+	−
Splenomegaly	−	−	+	−
Retinopathy	+	Rarely	−	−
Corneal opacity	−	−	+	+
Neurologic involvement	+	Rarely	+	−
Renal involvement	−	−	−	+
Hematologic changes	+	Rarely	−	+
	(Acanthocytes)			(Anemia + target cells)

*Adapted from Lloyd, J. K.: Lipoprotein deficiency disorders. Clin. Endocrinol. Metabol., 2:127, 1973.
†LDL = low density lipoprotein; HDL = high density lipoprotein; LCAT = lecithin:cholesterol acyltransferase.

tracentrifuge only HDL is detected, although in some cases, small quantities of $d < 1.063$ lipoprotein are found. Immunochemically, this lipoprotein is identical to normal HDL, as is the small amount of lipid that is sometimes precipitated by heparin manganese or other precipitation methods.

The most likely genetic defect in abetalipoproteinemia is complete absence of synthesis of apo B. Of all the plasma apoproteins present in normal plasma, only this apoprotein is missing, which results in the absence of all the apo B-containing lipoproteins.

The mode of transmission is that of an autosomal recessive; the presumed heterozygotes are not detectable by any marker. A gene frequency of 1 in 20,000 has been calculated. The clinical picture varies with the age of the

Table 8–16. COMPOSITION OF PLASMA LIPIDS AND LIPOPROTEINS IN LIPOPROTEIN DEFICIENCY STATES

TYPE OF DEFICIENCY	PLASMA LIPIDS*						PLASMA LIPOPROTEINS		
	Total cholesterol (mg/dl)	Trigly-cerides (mg/dl)	Phospho-lipids (mg/dl)	Choles-terol ester	Phospha-tidyl choline (% distribution)	Sphingo-myelin	VLDL	LDL	HDL
LDL									
Abetalipo-proteinemia	19–72	1–12	33–96	61	48–51	37–39	Absent	Absent	Decreased
Hypobetalipo-proteinemia	55–146	20–140	110–170	Normal	71–73	13–18	Decreased	Markedly decreased	Normal
HDL									
Tangier disease	30–117	118–332	68–148	Normal	58–72	5–22	Increased	Increased	Normal HDL absent; small quantities of HDL_T present†
LCAT	140–600	120–1800	160–800	5–27	82–86	7–12	Increased	Increased	Decreased; abnormal lipoproteins present in HDL & LDL ranges

*Data on lipids taken from Lloyd, 1973.
†Detectable by preparative ultracentrifugation or immunochemical methods.

patients; in infancy the dominant picture is that of malabsorption of fat and fat-soluble vitamins, and failure to thrive.

Steatorrhea (unrelated to gluten) is present from early infancy with loose, pale, bulky stools and abdominal distention. By the fourth to fifth year, the steatorrhea becomes less marked. Small intestinal biopsy reveals a pathognomonic mucosal abnormality. In abetalipoproteinemia, unlike gluten-induced enteropathy, the structure of the villi is normal, with many triglyceride droplets scattered throughout the cytoplasm of the mucosal cell. This intracellular accumulation of fat is due to a defective process of removal of the fat from the cells into the lymphatics. The processes of intraluminal digestion and assimilation of fat into the cells are normal.

Neuromuscular abnormalities usually appear in the second and third years of life, the first manifestation often being unsteadiness in walking; progressively, other neuromuscular symptoms and signs appear: areflexia, cerebellar signs, muscle weakness, and proprioceptive defects. Visual and retinal changes, which appear in late childhood and adolescence, include visual field defects, night blindness, and pigmentary degeneration of the retina. A characteristic finding in all patients is the presence of high numbers of acanthocytes in the blood. These cells are best seen in wet preparations of fresh blood suspended in Dacie's solution (Fredrickson, 1972).

The diagnosis of abetalipoproteinemia should be suspected in all patients who have acanthocytes in the peripheral blood, atypical retinitis pigmentosa, or ataxic neuropathy. The demonstration of acanthocytes in fresh blood films, together with a plasma cholesterol of less than 1.2 mmol/l (50 mg/dl) and clear serum, is virtually diagnostic. However, the diagnosis should be confirmed by electrophoretic, ultracentrifugal, or immunochemical methods.

Familial Hypobetalipoproteinemia. The beta lipoprotein deficiency was first described by Van Buchem (1966). This is a genetically determined disorder transmitted as an autosomal dominant and is probably due to a primary reduction in the synthetic rate of beta lipoprotein. This disorder was initially considered to be a variant of abetalipoproteinemia, but it now appears to be quite distinct from that disorder (Fredrickson, 1972). LDL is considerably reduced but of normal composition; plasma phospholipid concentration is reduced, but triglyceride values are generally within the normal range (Table 8–16).

Although the lipoprotein disorder is not usually associated with any clinically detectable abnormality, occasionally some of the features of abetalipoproteinemia have been noted.

Disorders with deficient HDL

Familial HDL Deficiency (Tangier Disease). This rare genetic disorder was first described in a five-year-old boy and his sister from Tangier Island, Virginia (Fredrickson, 1961). It is inherited as an autosomal recessive; affected individuals are homozygous for the gene defect.

It is characterized by reduced concentrations of plasma cholesterol and phospholipids (Table 8–16), with normal or raised triglycerides. Clinically, the main features of this disorder are orange or yellowish gray coloration of the tonsils or residual tonsillar tissue, hepatosplenomegaly, and enlargement of lymph nodes (Table 8–15). In one patient severe neurologic abnormalities were the presenting symptoms.

The basic defect concerns the synthesis of normal HDL. Electrophoretic separation does not permit visualization of HDL, but immunochemical and ultracentrifugal studies show that small amounts (<10 per cent) of HDL are present. It was shown that this lipoprotein (referred to as HDL_T) is immunochemically related to, but otherwise different from, normal HDL. In HDL_T the proportion of triglyceride to protein is increased and the proportion of cholesterol to protein is decreased. It was further shown that both of the major A apoproteins are present, albeit in greatly reduced concentrations and that apo A-I is disproportionately decreased with respect to apo A-II.

The pathogenesis of most lesions can be explained by the deposition of cholesterol esters. However, the mechanism of this selective storage of cholesterol ester and its relationship to the lipoprotein abnormality are not clearly understood.

Lecithin:cholesterol acyltransferase (LCAT) deficiency

Deficiency of this enzyme was described in several patients who were clinically characterized by corneal opacities, anemia, and proteinuria. The corneal opacities are the most easily

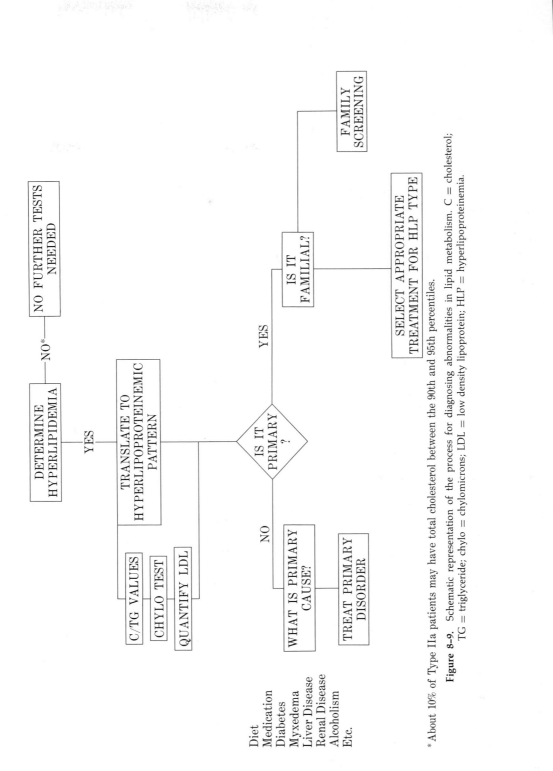

Figure 8–9. Schematic representation of the process for diagnosing abnormalities in lipid metabolism. C = cholesterol; TG = triglyceride; chylo = chylomicrons; LDL = low density lipoprotein; HLP = hyperlipoproteinemia.

*About 10% of Type IIa patients may have total cholesterol between the 90th and 95th percentiles.

detectable clinical signs. They are in the form of grayish infiltrates in all layers of the stroma but are most marked near the limbus. The clinical signs and biochemical findings in these patients are shown in Tables 8–15 and 8–16. In the plasma, abnormal lipoproteins similar to the lipoprotein of obstructive jaundice are found. These very large lipoproteins are in the density range of LDL and HDL and contain mainly cholesterol (unesterified) and lecithin.

The presence of the enzyme can be demonstrated by measuring the changes in plasma lecithin or cholesterol following incubation of plasma at 37°C., or by measurement of radioactive cholesterol ester following incubation of plasma with radioactive cholesterol (Glomset, 1964).

Although this disorder seems to be the expression of a homozygous autosomal recessive trait, only the study of more cases will establish the exact mode of inheritance.

RATIONAL APPROACH TO THE DETECTION AND DIAGNOSIS OF ABNORMALITIES IN LIPOPROTEIN METABOLISM

The diagnosis of hyperlipidemia is based on the measurement of plasma cholesterol and triglyceride concentrations. Two important questions must be resolved when concentrations of cholesterol and/or triglyceride outside the accepted "reference" values are detected: (1) What is the precise lipoprotein pattern underlying the hyperlipoproteinemia? (2) Is this pattern a secondary or a primary (possibly genetically determined) disorder? Some simple procedures will usually enable the laboratory and the physician to define the lipopro-

tein pattern. The combination of cholesterol and triglyceride values will usually indicate the lipoprotein pattern underlying the hyperlipidemia. Thus, a high cholesterol concentration in the presence of normal triglyceride almost invariably indicates the Type II pattern. On the other hand, high cholesterol accompanied by moderately elevated triglyceride (4.4 mmol/l or 400 mg/dl) may indicate Type IIb, III, or IV patterns. To distinguish between Types IIb and IV, LDL must be quantified. If the presence of Type III is suspected because of the presence of a slight chylomicron layer in the "standing plasma" test and/or the presence of unusual palmar deposits or tuberoeruptive xanthoma, further diagnostic tests should be done in a specialized laboratory to confirm the diagnosis.

The presence of a Type IV or V pattern should be suspected when a high plasma cholesterol is accompanied by very high plasma triglyceride (4.4 to 11 mmol/l or 400 to 1000 mg/dl). To distinguish between these two patterns, a "standing plasma" test is performed. The presence of a creamy supernatant indicates the Type V pattern. If slight to markedly elevated plasma triglyceride is the only abnormality, then Type IV is nearly always present, although infrequently it may be Type III.

Once the pattern of the lipoprotein abnormality has been defined, the clinician should request appropriate laboratory measurements that are designed to define the diseases most commonly associated with the abnormal lipoprotein pattern. The results should provide the answer to the second question: Is the lipoprotein abnormality primary or secondary?

Figure 8–9 summarizes the various steps to be taken in the diagnosis of patients with hyperlipidemia.

LIPID STORAGE DISEASES

Robert Calhoun, M.D.

In general, the abnormal metabolism and accumulation of lipids in the central nervous system involves the sphingolipids. As a group these substances are characterized by the presence of sphingosine. Within the last 20 years much exciting work has delineated these disorders, variously called sphingolipidoses, lipid storage diseases, cerebral lipidoses, lysosomal storage diseases, or gangliosidoses. Sev-

eral excellent reviews are available (Rapin, 1976; Brady, 1975; Malone, 1976).

For the most part these diseases have been shown to result from inherited defects in the catabolism of sphingolipids, resulting in the accumulation of various lipids in the central nervous system and other organs (Fig. 8–10; Table 8–17). Recently a single case of a deficiency in ganglioside synthesis leading to ab-

Table 8–17. THE SPHINGOLIPIDOSES*

DISEASE	ENZYME DEFICIENCY	COURSE	SYSTEMIC FEATURES	NEUROLOGIC FEATURES	MATERIAL STORED
GM₁† gangliosidosis	β-galactosidase	Rapid, severe (infantile: death by 2 years; later infantile: death by 10 years)	Infantile only: hepatosplenomegaly, downy hirsutism, hernias, coarse loose skin, bony changes	Profound dementia, seizures, myoclonus, optic atrophy (cherry red spot in 50% of infantile type)	GM₁ ganglioside in CNS, keratan sulfate-like material in viscera
GM₂ gangliosidosis Tay-Sachs disease	Hexosaminidase A	Rapid, severe, onset in infancy, death by 5 years	Head enlarged after 2 years	Profound dementia, seizures, myoclonus, cherry red spot	GM₂ ganglioside in CNS and viscera
Other infantile variants (non-Jewish)	(a) Hexosaminidase A and B	Same as Tay-Sachs	Same as Tay-Sachs	Same as Tay-Sachs	GM₂ ganglioside in CNS, globoside in viscera
	(b) No deficiency of hexosaminidase A and B on artificial substrates	Same as Tay-Sachs	Same as Tay-Sachs	Same as Tay-Sachs	GM₂ ganglioside in CNS
Non-infantile variants	Partial deficiency of hexosaminidase A	Severe, childhood going into adolescence	None	Dementia, seizures, cerebellar tremor, dystonic posture	GM₂ ganglioside in CNS
Adult (chronic) variant	Partial deficiency of hexosaminidase A	Onset childhood, life expectancy indefinite	Pes cavus	Spinocerebellar picture, distal muscle atrophy, no dementia, no seizures	GM₂ ganglioside in CNS
GM₃ gangliosidosis	Enzyme synthesizing GM₂ ganglioside from GM₃ ganglioside	Infancy, acute	Like infantile GM₁	Like infantile GM₁	GM₃ ganglioside in CNS
Fabry's disease (sex-linked recessive)	Trihexosyl ceramide, α-galactosidase	Chronic, late adolescence, young adults	Kidney failure, angiokeratoma	Lightning pains, strokes	Trihexosyl ceramide
Metachromatic leukodystrophy	Sulfatide sulfatase (arylsulfatase A)	Late infantile variant: rapid death by 10 years	None	Severe dementia, cerebellar signs, neuropathy, optic atrophy	Sulfatide
		Juvenile variant: slower, death in second decade	None	Same	Sulfatide
		Adult variant, chronic	None	Schizophreniform dementia	Sulfatide
	Multiple sulfatases (arylsulfatase ABC, steroid sulfatase)	Late infantile, death in first decade	Mild visceromegaly, mild bony changes	Dementia, cherry red spot	Sulfatide, ganglioside, mucopolysaccharide
Globoid cell leukodystrophy (Krabbe's disease)	Cerebroside β-galactosidase	Acute onset in infancy, death preschool	None	Severe dementia, spasticity, seizures	Galactosyl ceramide (galactose-cerebroside), psychosine

Table continued on the following page

†GM = Ganglioside metabolism.

Table 8-17.   THE SPHINGOLIPIDOSES* (Continued)

DISEASE	ENZYME DEFICIENCY	COURSE	SYSTEMIC FEATURES	NEUROLOGIC FEATURES	MATERIAL STORED
Gaucher's disease	Cerebroside β-glucosidase	Infantile: acute, severe, death by 2 years	Hypersplenism, splenomegaly (all types), ± hepatomegaly, bony deformity and fractures (juvenile type)	Only in infantile type: brainstem signs, dysphagia, cranial nerve anomalies, spasticity	Glucosyl ceramide (glucocerebroside)
		Juvenile: chronic, death in adulthood (Ashkenazic Jews)	Failure to thrive (infantile type), Gaucher cells in bone marrow		Glucocerebroside
Niemann-Pick disease	Sphingomyelinase	Infantile (A): rapid, severe; juvenile and atypical types (B, C, D): variable	Hepatosplenomegaly (all types), jaundice, failure to thrive, lymphadenopathy (infantile type), bony infiltration, vacuolated lymphocytes and histiocytes, Niemann-Pick cells in bone marrow	Hypotonia, moderate dementia (infantile type and Nova Scotia variant), paralysis of upward gaze (juvenile variant)	Sphingomyelin (ceramide phosphorylcholine)
Farber's disease (ceramide lipidosis, lipogranulomatosis)	Ceramidase	Infantile, death in childhood	Periarticular joint swelling, stiff joints, hoarseness, fevers	Hypotonia, dysphagia, cherry red spot	Ceramide

*Reproduced with permission from Rapin, I.: Progressive genetic-metabolic diseases of the central nervous system in children. Pediatr. Ann., 5:313, 1976.

normal storage of lipid was reported. Apparently this is the first reported example of abnormal synthesis of sphingolipids (Fishman, 1975). Defective catabolism may take the form of a lack of a specific enzyme. Alternatively the enzyme may be present, as measured immunologically, but in a non-functional form. This seems to occur in metachromatic leukodystrophy (Brady, 1975).

The accumulated material may include more than sphingolipids. When a defective enzyme is also involved with the catabolism of other substances, they also may accumulate. Increased amounts of both sphingomyelins and mucopolysaccharides are found when arylsulfatase is defective (Kolodny, 1976). This obscures the boundary between the lipidoses and the mucopolysaccharidoses. These patients show signs and symptoms of both types of disorders.

Sphingolipids are associated with cell membranes throughout the body. Recently, evidence has accumulated supporting the theory that sphingolipids may play a role as cell surface membrane receptors. Specifically, the effects of glycoprotein hormones may be partially mediated by cell membrane sphingolipids (Fishman, 1976).

Other lipid storage diseases have been described which include mucolipidoses, Refsum's disease, and ceroid lipofuchsinoses (Rapin, 1976). Specific enzyme defects have been described for several of the mucolipidoses, but this area is not as clearly delineated as are the sphingolipidoses. Specific assays are available in research laboratories for intrauterine diagnosis of those disorders which have been well-defined enzymatically. The ceroid lipofuchsinoses as a group are poorly defined chemically. They are described in terms of

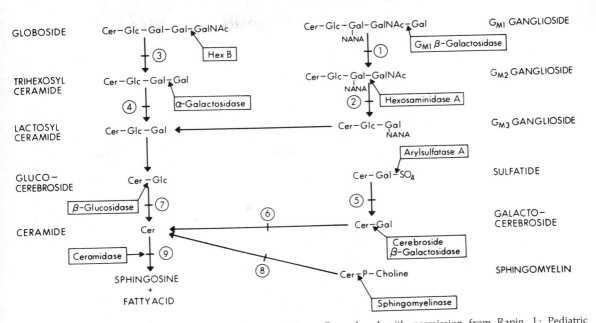

Figure 8–10. Schematic pathways for sphingolipid catabolism. Reproduced with permission from Rapin, I.: Pediatric Neurology II. Pediatr. Ann., 5:313, 1976.

their gross and microscopic pathology, and by clinical findings. Laboratory diagnosis is not available (Rapin, 1976). In Refsum's disease there is an accumulation of the fatty acid, phytanic acid, owing to decreased amounts of phytanic acid oxidase. Prenatal and heterozygous detection is possible with assays of amniotic fluid cells and cultured skin fibroblasts (Burton, 1974).

The clinical manifestations of the lipidoses vary considerably, with mental retardation usually presenting as the most outstanding and serious problem (Table 8–17). The earlier the disease manifests itself, generally the more severe will be the outcome. Therapeutic attempts have focused on enzyme replacement and organ transplantation. These have been virtually unsuccessful; however there have been some promising results so that further studies are in progress (Rapin, 1976; Brady, 1975). Therefore, the most important maneuver available to the physician is to detect the heterozygous state, aiding in genetic counseling, and to diagnose the disease in utero early enough to perform a therapeutic abortion if needed.

The laboratory determinations now available to perform these tasks developed as a direct result of the original biochemical research on these diseases (Brady, 1975). Moreover, the final diagnosis essentially rests upon these diagnostic laboratory procedures, although the clinical picture is often fairly specific. Generally these tests are constructed to reveal the activity of the specific enzyme which is thought to be deficient. The substrate for the enzyme analysis may be either the naturally occurring sphingolipid, labeled with a radioisotope, or a synthetic compound which may be either radioactively labeled or a chromogenic compound. This allows use of well-established radioassays or spectrophotometric measurements (Brady, 1975; Volk, 1976). The use of simpler synthetic compounds as substrate depends upon the fact that these enzymes are fairly specific for certain types of linkages and the terminal oligosaccharide components of these large molecules. The remainder of the molecule is less important for enzyme activity (Kolodny, 1976). This simplifies and reduces the cost of the determination. However, this is not always possible but depends on the specificity of the particular enzyme.

The specimen for analysis may be leukocytes, cultured skin fibroblasts, or amniotic fluid cells. Some of the lysosomal enzymes occur in plasma, tears, and urine, and may be measured directly (Brady, 1971; Carmody, 1973). An abnormal accumulation of various sphingolipids may be detected both intracellularly and in such fluids as plasma, urine, and amniotic fluid for certain diseases. In view of this, automated techniques may evolve for determining enzyme activity or abnormal amounts of lipids, thus providing a reasonable method for large screening programs. However, to date these determinations are still being evaluated, and, in general, the assay of particular enzymes in cell cultures is the most specific determination available (Burton, 1974; Volk, 1976).

These procedures are performed, as a rule, in research laboratories actively involved in this area, or in certain reference laboratories, (e.g., New York State Department of Health, Birth Defects Institute, Albany, New York). There are procedures available for essentially all of the biochemically well-characterized lipidoses for determining heterozygosity, for prenatal detection, and for primary diagnosis

(Brady, 1975; Rapin, 1976). Experience in laboratories doing this work has shown that technical competence must be well-developed in order to obtain reliable results (Lowden, 1975). This is especially important because cell culturing technique is often needed for accurate results. Amniotic fluid cells should be obtained by 16 weeks gestation. A safe therapeutic abortion, if indicated, would have to be performed before 20 weeks. Therefore, failure of the cell culture results in the loss of valuable time, and less accurate determinations may have to be relied upon. Expertise from experience is necessary to avoid such difficulties.

Future developments may include, among others, isolating fetal cells from the maternal circulation for enzyme analysis and the use of high-performance liquid chromatography to improve methods for detecting sphingolipids and phospholipids (Volk, 1976).

REFERENCES

Alaupovic, P.: Apolipoproteins and lipoproteins. Atherosclerosis, 13:141, 1971.

Albers, J. J., Adolphson, J. L., and Hazzard, W. R.: Radioimmunoassay of human plasma Lp(a) lipoprotein. J. Lipid Res., 18:331, 1977.

Albers, J. J., and Hazzard, W. R.: Immunochemical quantification of human plasma Lp(a) lipoprotein. Lipids, 9:15, 1974.

Allain, C. C., Poon, L. S., Chan, C. S. G., Richmond, W., and Fu, P. C.: Enzymatic determination of total serum cholesterol. Clin. Chem., 20:470, 1974.

Assmann, G., Fredrickson, D. S., Herbert, P., Forte, T., et al.: An A-II lipoprotein particle in Tangier disease. Circulation, 50 (Suppl. III):259, 1974.

Bachorik, P. S., and Wood, P. D. S.: Laboratory considerations in the diagnosis and management of hyperlipoproteinemia. In Rifkind, B. M., and Levy, R. I. (eds.): Hyperlipidemia: Diagnosis and Therapy. New York, Grune & Stratton, 1977.

Beaumont, J. L., Carlson, L. A., Cooper, G. R., et al.: Classification of hyperlipidaemias and hyperlipoproteinaemias. Bull. WHO, 43:891, 1970.

Brown, M. S., and Goldstein, J. L.: Familial hypercholesterolemia: A genetic defect in the low-density lipoprotein receptor. N. Engl. J. Med., 294:1386, 1976.

Bucolo, G., Yabut, J., and Chang, T. Y.: Mechanized enzymatic determination of triglycerides in serum. Clin. Chem., 21:420, 1975.

Connor, W. E., and Connor, S. L.: Dietary treatment of hyperlipidemia. In Rifkind, B. M., and Levy, R. I. (eds.): Hyperlipidemia: Diagnosis and Therapy. New York, Grune & Stratton, 1977.

Duncombe, W. Y.: The colorimetric microdetermination of long chain fatty acids. Biochem. J. (Lond.), 88:7, 1963.

Ehnholm, C., Garoff, H., Renkonen, O., et al.: Protein and carbohydrate composition of Lp(a) lipoprotein from human plasma. Biochemistry, 11:3229, 1972.

Eisenberg, S.: Lipoprotein metabolism and hyperlipemia. Atheroscl. Rev., 1:23, 1976.

Eisenberg, S., and Levy, R. I.: Lipoprotein metabolism. Adv. Lipid. Res., 13:1, 1976.

Fredrickson, D. S., Altrocchi, P. H., Avioli, L. V., Goodman, D. S., et al.: Tangier disease. Ann. Intern. Med., 55:1016, 1961.

Fredrickson, D. S., Gotto, A. M., and Levy, R. I.: Familial lipoprotein deficiency. In Stanbury, J. B., Wyngaarden, J. B., and Fredrickson, D. S. (eds.): The Metabolic Basis of Inherited Diseases, 3rd ed. New York, McGraw-Hill Book Company, 1972.

Fredrickson, D. S., and Levy, R. I.: Familial hyperlipoproteinemia. In Stanbury, J. B., Wyngaarden, J. B., and Fredrickson, D. S. (eds.): The Metabolic Basis of Inherited Diseases, 3rd ed. New York, McGraw-Hill Book Company, 1972.

Fredrickson, D. S., Levy, R. I., Bonnell, M. B., and Ernst, N.: Dietary management of hyperlipoproteinemia. A Handbook for Physicians and Dietitians. DHEW Publication No. (NIH) 76-110, 1974.

Friedewald, W. T., Levy, R. I., and Fredrickson, D. S.: Estimation of the concentration of low-density lipoprotein cholesterol in plasma, without use of the preparative ultracentrifuge. Clin. Chem., 18:499, 1972.

Glomset, J. A., and Wright, J. L.: Some properties of a cholesterol esterifying enzyme in human plasma. Biochim. Biophys. Acta, 89:266, 1964.

Goldstein, J. L., and Brown, M. S.: Binding and degradation of low density lipoproteins by cultured human fibroblasts. Comparison of cells from a normal subject and from a patient with homozygous familial hypercholesterolemia. J. Biol. Chem., 249:5153, 1974.

Gordon, T., Castelli, W. P., Hjortland, M. C., et al.: High density lipoprotein as a protective factor against coronary heart disease. The Framingham Study. Am. J. Med., 62:707, 1977.

Greenberg, B. H., Blackwelder, W. C., and Levy, R. I.: Primary Type V hyperlipoproteinemia. A descriptive study in 32 families. Ann. Intern. Med., 87:526, 1977.

Hazzard, W. R.: Primary Type III hyperlipoproteinemia.

In Rifkind, B. M., and Levy, R. I. (eds.): Hyperlipidemia: Diagnosis and Therapy. New York, Grune & Stratton, 1977.

Kannel, W. B., and Dawber, T. R.: Contributors to coronary risk implications for prevention and public health: The Framingham study. Heart Lung, *1*:797, 1972.

Kushwaha, R. S., Hazzard, W. R., Wahl, P. W., et al.: Hyperlipoproteinemia: Diagnosis in whole plasma by lipoprotein-E immunoassay. Ann. Intern. Med., *87*:509, 1977.

Levy, R. I.: Hyperlipoproteinemia. Concepts of diagnosis and management. Curr. Probl. Cardiol., *1*:1, 1976.

Levy, R. I., and Morganroth, J.: Familial type III hyperlipoproteinemia. Ann. Intern. Med., *87*:625, 1977.

Lindgren, F. T., Jensen, L. C., and Hatch, F. T.: The isolation and quantitative analysis of serum lipoproteins. *In* Nelson, G. J. (ed.): Blood Lipids and Lipoproteins: Quantitation, Composition and Metabolism. New York, Wiley-Interscience, 1972.

Lipid Research Clinics Program: Manual of Laboratory Operations, Volume 1—Lipid and Lipoprotein Analysis. DHEW Publication (NIH) 75-628, 1974.

Lipid Research Clinics (LRC) Program: LRC Data Book (in preparation), 1978.

Lipid Research Clinics (LRC) Program: Plasma lipid distributions in 11 North American populations: The Lipid Research Clinics Program Prevalence Study (in preparation), 1978.

Lippel, K., Ahmed, S., Albers, J., et al.: Analytical performance and comparability of the determination of cholesterol by 12 lipid research clinics. Clin. Chem., *23*:1744, 1977.

Mather, A.: Center for Disease Control. Proficiency Testing. Clin. Chem. Survey, *1*:66, 1975.

Nelson, G. J.: Quantitative analysis of blood lipids. *In* Nelson, G. J. (ed.): Blood Lipids and Lipoproteins: Quantitation, Composition and Metabolism. New York, Wiley-Interscience, 1972.

Rifkind, B. M., and Levy, R. I.: Present status of treatment in hyperlipidemia. *In* Varco, R. L., and Delaney, J. P. (eds.): Controversy in Surgery. Philadelphia, W. B. Saunders Company, 1976.

Starzl, T. E., Chase, H. P., Putnam, C. W., and Porter, K. A.: Preliminary communication: Portacaval shunt in hyperlipoproteinemia. Lancet, *2*:940, 1973.

Task Force On Arteriosclerosis of the National Heart and Lung Institute: Arteriosclerosis. Vol. 1, U.S. Dept. of Health, Education and Welfare, P.H.S. DHEW Publication No. (NIH) 72-137, 1971.

Technicon Method No. SG4-0037PM4. Tarrytown, N.Y., Technicon Instrument Corporation, 1974a.

Technicon Method No. SG4-0026PM4. Tarrytown, N.Y., Technicon Instrument Corporation, 1974b.

Technicon Method No. SF4-0026FC4. Tarrytown, N.Y., Technicon Instrument Corporation, 1974c.

Trout, D. L., Estes, H. E., Jr., and Friedberg, S. J.: Titration of free fatty acids of plasma: A study of current techniques, and a new modification. J. Lipid Res., *1*:199, 1960.

Utermann, G., Jaeschke, M., and Menzel, J.: Familial hyperlipoproteinemia Type III: Deficiency of a specific apolipoprotein (apo E-III) in the very-low-density lipoproteins. FEBS Lett., *56*:352, 1975.

Van Buchem, F. S. P., Pol, G., deGier, J., Böttcher, C. J. F., et al.: Congenital betalipoprotein deficiency. Am. J. Med., *40*:794, 1966.

Verbruggen, R.: Quantitative immunoelectrophoretic methods: A literature survey. Clin. Chem., *21*:5, 1975.

Witter, R. F., and Whitner, V. S.: Determination of serum triglycerides. *In* Nelson, G. J. (ed.): Blood Lipids and Lipoproteins: Quantitation, Composition and Metabolism. New York, Wiley-Interscience, 1972.

Lipid storage disease

Brady, R. O., Johnson, W. G., and Uhlendorf, W. F.: Identification of heterozygous carriers of lipid storage disease. Am. J. Med., *51*:423, 1971.

Brady, R. O.: The abnormal biochemistry of inherited disorders of lipid metabolism. Fed. Proc., *32*:1660, 1973.

Brady, R. O.: Inherited metabolic diseases of the nervous system. Science, *193*:733, 1976.

Brady, R. O.: Lipidoses. *In* Tower, D. B. (ed.): The Nervous System, vol. II. New York, Raven Press, 1975.

Burton, B. K., Gerbie, A. B., and Nadler, H. L.: Present status of intrauterine diagnosis of genetic defects. Am. J. Obstet. Gynecol., *118*:718, 1974.

Carmody, P. J., Rattazzi, M. D., and Davidson, R. G.: Tay-Sachs disease—the use of tears for the detection of heterozygotes. N. Engl. J. Med., *289*:1072, 1973.

Fishman, P. H., and Brady, R. O.: Biosynthesis and function of gangliosides. Science, *194*:906, 1976.

Fishman, P. M., Max, S. R., Tallman, J. F., Brady, R. O., MaClaren, N. K., and Cornblath, M.: Deficient ganglioside biosynthesis: A novel human sphingolipidosis. Science, *187*:68, 1975.

Kolodny, E. H.: Lysosomal storage diseases. N. Engl. J. Med., *294*:1217, 1976.

Lowden, J. A., Rudd, N., Cutz, E., and Doran, T. A.: Antenatal diagnosis of sphingolipid and mucopolysaccharide storage diseases. Can. Med. Assoc. J., *113*:507, 1975.

Malone, M. J.: The cerebral lipidoses. Pediatr. Clin. North Am., *23*:303, 1976.

Rapin, I.: Progressive genetic-metabolic diseases of the central nervous system in children. Pediatr. Ann., *5*:56, 1976.

Volk, B. W., and Schneck, L. (eds.): Current trends in sphingolipidoses and allied disorders. *In* Advances In Experimental Medicine and Biology. New York, Plenum Press, 1976.

9

SPECIFIC PROTEINS

Robert F. Ritchie, M.D.

TOTAL PROTEIN
METHODS
    Non-destructive Analysis
    Destructive Analysis
    Immunochemical Analysis
    Immunoelectrophoresis

SPECIFIC PROTEINS
    Carrier Proteins
    Acute Phase Reactants
    Complement Proteins

Clinical application of specific protein studies has resulted largely from a burgeoning interest in and awareness of protein chemistry. This chapter will describe a few specific proteins in some detail, attempting to relate them to one another and to give clinically relevant information about each. Other chapters also review specific proteins, e.g., immunoglobulins (36), complement (37), acute phase reactants (54), coagulation factors, including fibrinogen (33), and enzymes (11, 12, 23, and 24). Several chapters embrace protein measurements in other body fluids, including serum hormones (14), urine (17), cerebrospinal fluid (18), and amniotic fluid (20). Lipoproteins are reviewed in Chapter 8.

Literally speaking, the body's framework and substance is protein. All tissues are proteinaceous, and the *metabolism* of endogenous organic and inorganic substances (e.g., lipids, carbohydrates, nucleic acids, steroids), as well as a wide variety of exogenous substances, is mediated by individual proteins performing specific tasks. Specific functions, often reflecting an individual's genetic make-up, can now be measured through a variety of clinically applicable protein analyses involving such disciplines as hematology, immunology, and microbiology. This has fostered investigation at the molecular and submolecular levels (Boyer, 1964; Putnam, 1975a), culminating in the ability to study specific tissue proteins either in solution or in fixed tissue sections labeled by immunologic reagents. Many of these studies are now used routinely where the presence or distribution of a specific protein is important.

Several hundred proteins, including coagulation factors, enzymes, immunoglobulins, and hormones, exist in human plasma (Ritzmann, 1975). The study of specific proteins may utilize either of two philosophies. The first examines individually the species that are of special importance (e.g., alkaline phosphatase, IgE, alpha-fetoprotein) without correlating the resulting values with other analytes in the same sample. The second selects a group of proteins, examines each, and interprets the findings within the context of the group. Although the former approach is described in other chapters as noted, this chapter will discuss the latter, understanding that any attempt to synthesize a single picture even from among the 22 best understood and most highly concentrated body fluid proteins presents serious problems.

TOTAL PROTEIN

Expanding knowledge about individual proteins as measured immunochemically has documented the ambiguity of definition as well as the inaccuracy of measuring total protein. In spite of this, colorimetric measurement of total protein clearly will continue to be performed for some time to come.

A major problem with measuring total protein arises because individual proteins carry as part of the molecule a wide variety of other substances. Albumin, a material containing very low levels of carbohydrate and lipid, has been extensively employed as a reference material. Unfortunately, when albumin is used as a reference material for other purified proteins whose carbohydrate and lipid ratios are different, a high degree of accuracy is difficult. Several of the methods described below are used satisfactorily to measure total protein in spite of these inherent problems.

METHODS

Protein analysis, whether for a specific species or for total protein, is performed by procedures which fall into three major categories: *non-destructive* (of particular interest to the investigator), *destructive*, and *immunochemical* (theoretically non-destructive, but practically destructive).

NON-DESTRUCTIVE ANALYSIS

Mass

Efforts to establish an international reference material for several individual plasma proteins have been frustrated by the uncertainty in assigning mass values to purified preparations because the analytical approaches vary considerably from method to method (Reimer, 1978). The most direct analytical method is by weighing, but a considerable amount of dry, salt-free protein is required. Hence, this form of analysis has been used almost exclusively to assign values to whole serum reference materials. As expertise in purification has developed, it is now reasonable to consider preparing 10 to 100 mg batches of ultrapure protein to be given a primary mass value by direct weight. Re-analysis of the weighed material after dissolution becomes yet another serious problem, but at least an absolute mass measurement can act as a beginning reference point.

Refractive index (Kabat, 1974; Schultze, 1966; Haschemeyer, 1973)

Proteins in concentrations greater than 25 g/l (2.5 g/dl) may be measured most simply by refractive index as total dissolved solute. Unaffected by turbidity and non-protein pigments, the method provides an excellent and simple non-destructive measurement of total protein in serum or plasma because the great majority of dissolved substances in these fluids are proteins. However, high concentrations of glucose and cholesterol can cause significant biases.

Spectrophotometry (Kabat, 1974; Schultze, 1966; Haschemeyer, 1973)

This method is used extensively by immunologists, since with pure solutions of IgG the absorbance (OD_{280}) of a 1-cm light path is equivalent, for practical purposes, to the approximate concentration expressed as mg/ml. The method is reasonably sensitive and is acceptably precise in the concentration range of 50 to 1500 $\mu g/ml$. Most proteins include three aromatic amino acids that absorb ultraviolet light at 280 nm: tryptophan, tyrosine, and phenylalanine. Because amounts of these constituents vary considerably from protein to protein, the molar absorptivities for each protein in pure solution must be known in order to calculate concentration accurately when measured individually. Furthermore, molar absorptivities range over an order of magnitude, so that analysis of mixed solutions can be considered only as a crude estimate of protein concentration.

Salting-out

The precipitation of various fractions of plasma by the addition of neutral salts or organic liquids no longer has wide application in the clinical laboratory as an assay method. It remains valuable to the researcher who is interested in recovering fractions from large volumes of starting material. Ammonium sulfate, sodium sulfate, ethyl alcohol, and chloroform were used in crude protein fractionation prior to the advent of electrophoresis. More recently, precipitins such as polyethylene glycol and ethodin (Rivanol) have come into use. In general, the lowest salt concentration precipitates proteins with high isoelectric points, i.e., the immunoglobulins. As salt concentration increases, beta globulins, alpha globulins, and eventually albumin come out of solution.

DESTRUCTIVE ANALYSIS

Colorimetry

Analysis of the *nitrogen* content of protein is a major tool for the analyst. As in other methods, the extreme variability in the makeup of proteins presents serious standardization problems. The accepted value of nitrogen as 16 per cent of total protein mass is based upon the careful analysis of bovine serum albumin containing only traces of carbohydrate and lipid. Most other proteins contain between 12 and 18 per cent nitrogen, rarely as much as twice that concentration. The incorporation of nonprotein constituents into the protein molecule reduces the proportional amount of nitrogen. In the lipoproteins, the nitrogen-containing fraction is extremely low. Nitrogen analysis can be seriously distorted by the presence of free amino acids and nucleic acids.

The two most commonly used methods (Jacobs, 1965) are the Kjeldahl, in which nitrogenous compounds are converted to the ammonium ion by digestion with sulfuric acid, and the Nessler colorimetric reaction. Both techniques are exquisitely sensitive and require considerable care and practice to ensure precision. The Kjeldahl method is more complex but has application in the analysis of nitrogenous substances when other compounds which produce turbidity or insoluble char during digestion make the Nessler reaction unsuitable.

Perhaps the most widely used method for protein analysis in the intermediate range (20 to 400 μg) is the *biuret* reaction. Unlike nitrogen analysis, in which the analyte can be contributed from other sources within the sample, the biuret reaction requires the presence of at least three adjacent peptide bonds, thus restricting the color reaction to proteins. Amino acids do not interfere with the color reaction, but small peptides that may not be detectable by electrophoresis or immunoanalysis can give spurious results. The intense red-violet color of the biuret compound in the presence of alkaline copper sulfate is measured spectrophotometrically at 557 nm. This method can be used for the measurement of soluble proteins, but values must be corrected for the presence of non-protein carbohydrate or lipid. Some reference works give "biuret numbers" for individual purified proteins, with albumin being assigned the value 100 (Schultze, 1966). Since albumin is the predominant protein in serum, its analytical values roughly equal those of total protein. However, in states of severe hypoalbuminemia with a marked elevation of globulins, the analysis is in error.

A modification of the *Folin-Ciocalteau* phenol color reaction (Lowry, 1951) increases the sensitivity approximately 10 times (10 to 100 μg) over the original method by the addition of small amounts of copper ion (Herriott, 1941). The method depends upon the presence of tyrosine and tryptophan, two amino acids intrinsic to proteins characterized by their ability to absorb ultraviolet light. The considerable variation in concentration of these aromatic amino acids will affect the test values when different proteins are being analyzed. The color reaction, read at 720 nm or 660 nm, is not well suited to the measurement of insoluble proteins.

For greater sensitivity (1 to 20 μg N), the *Ninhydrin* reaction is recommended. In a modification described by Troll (1953), color variation produced by different proteins was minimized by allowing the color reaction to develop in organic solvents. The violet color generated with primary amino acids and the Ninhydrin reagent is measured at 440 nm, with various proteins producing results which range between 70 and 110 per cent of expected values.

Chemical precipitation

Introduction of certain chemicals to a protein solution renders them insoluble. The rapid development of light-scattering particles allows optical analysis in a variety of instruments. Trichloracetic acid and sulfosalicylic acid have been used to measure cerebrospinal fluid and urinary protein concentrations. Certain proteins vary in their resistance to these precipitating agents, and the method has not been examined to ascertain the degree of variability to be expected when purified proteins are tested. The traditional 3 per cent sulfosalicylic acid solution used to measure cerebrospinal fluid total protein fails to precipitate spinal fluid glycoproteins that make up a significant fraction of the total.

Dye binding

Largely applied to the determination of albumin, the dye binding techniques depend on the ability of albumin to bind low molecular weight substances. Many compounds, including bile pigments, salicylates, penicillin, and a variety of other drugs, interfere with test results by reducing albumin's capacity to bind the analytical dye. Nevertheless, the dye binding methods, largely in automated systems, are the predominant means by which serum albumin is determined. The BCG (Bromcresolgreen) method is the most commonly employed today.

Electrophoresis

Discussion of specific protein analysis must acknowledge the primacy of serum protein electrophoresis. It was introduced to clinical medicine in the 1950's as boundary electrophoresis and then in a supporting matrix—paper, cellulose acetate membrane, and eventually in gels, both acrylamide and agarose. The method fostered recognition of plasma proteins as an extremely complex family of substances systematically modulated by individual genetic differences and a variety of pathologic processes. The marriage of immunochemistry and electrophoresis produced immunoelectrophoresis, a technique making specific protein analysis practical for the first time.

Laboratories interested in implementing electrophoresis are faced with deciding among many systems. At present, the forms of agarose, cellulose acetate, paper, and polyacrylamide gel (PAGE) are the preferred methods. Moreover, paper and agar supports are no longer used to any degree in the clinical laboratory for routine serum protein electrophoresis (SPE). Only agarose and cellulose acetate are considered (Fig. 9-1). They are both technically simple, rapid, inexpensive, and relatively standardized. PAGE has less value in routine specimen screening. However, this elegant method with its capacity for high resolution is valuable for the research investigator. Recently, isoelectric focusing in PAGE has been utilized as a powerful tool for genetic polymorphism studies. In the United States, SPE is often subjected to densitometric scanning rather than critical visual inspection with interpretation. The former has serious limitations for comparison of many immunologically distinct species. Even the albumin peak includes several other proteins of varying concentration (Fig. 9-2). The alpha and beta glob-

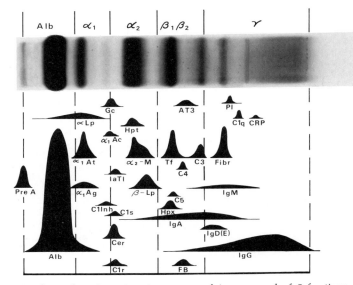

Figure 9-1. Plasma protein electrophoresis pattern in agarose gel is composed of 5 fractions, each composed of many individual species (see Figure 9-2). Some of the major proteins are shown here in an artist's rendition for clarity. (Adapted from Laurell, C. B., Clin. Chem., *19*:99, 1973.)

α_1Ac = Alpha$_1$-Antichymotrypsin
α_1Ag = Alpha$_1$-Acid Glycoprotein
α_1At = Alpha$_1$-Antitrypsin
α_2 − M = Alpha$_2$-Macroglobulin
αLp = Alpha Lipoprotein
Alb = Albumin
AT3 = Antithrombin III
β − Lp = Beta lipoprotein
Complement Components:
C1q, C1r, C1s, C3, C4, C5 = As designated
C1Inh = C1 Inhibitor

Cer = Ceruloplasmin
CRP = C-Reactive Protein
FB = Factor B
Fibr = Fibrinogen
Hpt = Haptoglobin
Hpx = Hemopexin
Immunoglobulins:
IgA, IgD, IgE, IgG, IgM = As designated
Pl = Plasminogen
Pre A = Prealbumin

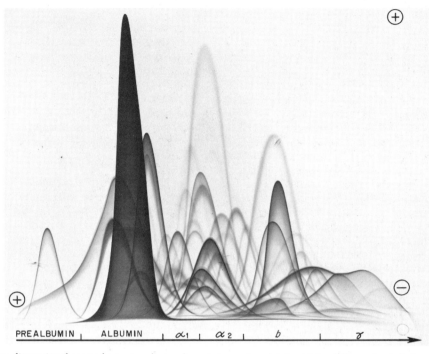

PREALBUMIN | ALBUMIN | α_1 | α_2 | b | γ

Figure 9–2. Two-dimensional crossed immunoelectrophoresis in a gel containing high quality anti-whole human serum shows a complex population of proteins spread from prealbumin to gamma globulin. Each electrophoretic fraction can be seen to contain all or part of many individual species each identified as separate "rocket". The dense peak at the left is albumin and the broadest peak at the right is IgG. Without specific studies it is impossible to unequivocally identify any of the others. (Plate courtesy of DAKOPATTES, A-F, DK-2000, Copenhagen, Denmark)

ulin peaks are composed of a dozen species which respond to disease processes, with disparate values at times, but yielding no other changes in densitometric values.

Serum protein electrophoresis, however, is not a method for the determination of specific proteins. In the previous edition of this text, considerable attention was given to the methodology. Since that time, interest in electrophoresis as such has reached a plateau and will probably decline as methods of specific protein analysis become widespread. However, serum protein electrophoresis (SPE) is the single most sensitive procedure for detection of monoclonal gammopathies (Fig. 9–3). SPE is also considered a valuable determination in organ panels or profiles, e.g., hepatic, renal. Furthermore, the method (SPE) is still commonly used to determine certain proteins such as albumin and even immunoglobulin G, since both these materials are largely responsible for the electrophoretic fractions that bear their names. Proteins other than albumin cannot be measured with certainty, because the individual electrophoretic fractions represent a composite of many species (Figs. 9–1 and 9–2). Furthermore, their mobilities vary depending upon the buffer system and the type of support matrix used. However, electrophoresis is capable of making the identification even when resolution is poor, since these proteins migrate as homogeneous bands. With well-resolved systems, even small monoclonal or oligoclonal bands can be easily identified visually, giving evidence of intense immunologic stimulation such as may accompany serious viral infections or tissue necrosis (Fig. 9–4).

IMMUNOCHEMICAL ANALYSIS

Strictly speaking, immunochemical analysis is non-destructive in that the antigen remains intact after the test is completed. For practical purposes, however, the material introduced into the assay vessel is lost. Quantitative precipitation with immunochemical reagents is the only method that can be broadly applied for specific protein analysis. Since individual proteins are indistinguishable from one another in chemical quantitative methods for protein, the technique must be capable of selecting only the species of interest from what

Clinical Impression: _____   Acc. No. _____

SERUM PROTEIN ELECTROPHORESIS

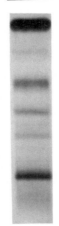

Guide for

Identification of

Electrophoretic Bands

prealbumin
albumin
alpha lipoprotein
alpha-1 antitrypsin

trypsin inhibitor and
    antichymotrypsin
alpha-2 macroglobulin
haptoglobin

transferrin

beta lipoprotein
C3 complement

application slit

immunoglobulins

Photograph of

Patient's Serum

Electrophoresis

COMMENTS:

    **Slightly increased total proteins,
with prominent monoclonal band in the
immunoglobulin region. Pattern suggests
a monoclonal gammopathy.**

Qualitative Evaluation

of Electrophoretic Zones

prealbumin	normal
albumin	normal
alpha lipoprotein	normal
alpha-1 antitrypsin	normal
alpha-2 macroglobulin	normal
haptoglobin	normal
transferrin	normal
beta lipoprotein	normal
C3 complement	normal
immunoglobulins	see comment

Total Protein __8.9__ gms/dl

Albumin __4.3__ gms/dl

Figure 9-3. Report form displaying serum protein electrophoresis (agarose) and interpretation.

may be an extremely complex population. The exquisite sensitivity and specificity of properly prepared antisera make possible quantification of a single protein species at a concentration at least as low as $1 \mu g/ml$ from a mass containing dozens of others with concentrations as much as 5×10^4 or higher. By the addition of labels such as ^{125}I, enzymes, or fluorochromes, the differential can be extended to 5×10^7.

Immunochemical analyses rely on the binding of specific antibody to the appropriate antigenic sequence or epitope on the antigen. Antibody recognition may require, in addition to the amino acid sequence, carbohydrates, steroids, drugs, or, not infrequently, a specific conformation. The various methods for detecting the reaction are the subject of an extensive literature. The antigen-antibody reaction can occur free in a liquid, in the liquid

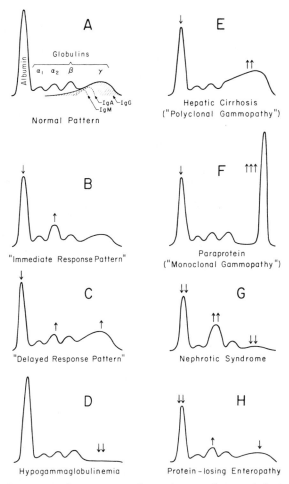

Figure 9-4. Serum protein electrophoresis: clinicopathologic correlations. (Courtesy of Dr. A. F. Krieg.)

phase of the gel-sol matrix, at the surface of a liquid-solid, or at a liquid-liquid interface. Quantification is by the observation of visible precipitates that may be either stained or observed directly by the naked eye or by an electro-optical device. For those methods that employ a secondary system such as a highly active label, quantification is by colorimetry, fluorimetry, or radiometry (see Chapters 35, 36, and 38, as well as Chapters 4 and 13).

Radial immunodiffusion (RID)
(Crowle, 1973)

There are several gel diffusion techniques of historical interest, but in the clinical laboratory the method first used to quantify specific proteins was radial immunodiffusion (RID)

(Feinberg, 1957; Mancini, 1964; Fahey, 1965). This extremely simple technique requires neither high titer nor strictly monospecific antiserum. A gel film of 1 to 2 mm thickness composed of 1.5 per cent agar or 0.8 to 1.5 per cent agarose in any of a variety of neutral buffers or salt solutions is cast in some form of supporting plate. Commercial kits for specific protein analysis are manufactured in plastic-covered containers that maintain a humid atmosphere during incubation. RID is reviewed in detail in Chapter 35, p. 1194.

Electroimmunoassay (EIA)
(Axelsen, 1973, 1975)

As a direct extension of RID, the application of an electric current through an antibody-containing gel film into which small wells have been punched and filled with serum obviates some of the problems inherent in the passive RID technique. This method, first described by Laurell in 1966, is called quantitative immunoelectrophoresis. Protein analytes in the beta-globulin to albumin electrophoretic zones can be analyzed by this technique. A variety of modifications have been described to make it possible to perform the assays for the immunoglobulins as well (Bjerrum, 1973; Renn, 1976). In contrast to RID, in which the wells punched in the gel need to be in no particular order, EIA requires that a row of holes no closer than 1 cm apart be punched across one side of the gel plate. Once these are filled, and filling should be done rapidly to minimize diffusion, the electric current is normally applied across the plate so that the positive electrode is on the opposite side of the plate from the sample wells. Proteins with high electrophoretic mobility such as the alpha$_1$-globulins and albumin move rapidly into the antibody-containing gel. Because of the dissolution of the initially formed precipitate as antigen moves from behind, a clear and gradually tapering central area bounded by precipitate is formed, culminating in a pointed rocket as the supply of antigen is exhausted. The amount of antibody in the gel must be tailored to the antigen concentration. Relatively large amounts of an antiserum will be required for whole serum, and much smaller amounts will be needed for spinal fluid analysis. Depending upon the dimensions of the plate, 10 to 30 samples can be run simultaneously, including calibrators and control samples. Because the protein movement in the gel toward the positive electrode is not passive, variations in molecular weight and configuration, viscosity, and gel temperature have less effect upon results.

Several commercial kits are available for EIA, some recommending staining of the films, others suggesting only that they be viewed by indirect lighting with an enhancing agent (Crowle, 1973; Renn, 1975).

The sensitivity of the EIA system, using equivalent reagents, is about three- to fivefold greater than for RID. With the analysis of amniotic fluid alpha-fetoprotein, the lower limit of acceptable precision is 400 to 700 ng/ml. This assay is unique, however, being two to three times more sensitive than other "rocket" assays.

Two maneuvers that can enhance sensitivity are (1) overlaying the washed plate with a second antibody before subsequent staining, and (2) incorporating a labeled antibody into the gel film and developing it rather than staining it.

As in RID, strictly monospecific antiserum is of only relative concern, since the operator is usually able to disassociate the precipitate produced by the contaminant antibody. For example, many workers performing coagulation Factor VIII related protein analyses by EIA have used antiserum which is of fairly high titer against the protein but contains a variety of additional antibodies that appear only as shadows. The precipitate that represents Factor VIII related protein is easily identified and measured. EIA is also reviewed elsewhere (p. 1192).

IMMUNOELECTROPHORESIS (CROWLE, 1973)

Immunoelectrophoresis (IMEL) has played an extraordinarily important role in exposing the complexity of the plasma protein system by demonstrating that, with appropriately heterospecific antiserum, human plasma can be shown to contain dozens of immunologically unique species (Grabar, 1953). The simple technique electrophoretically moves proteins from wells punched in a gel slab. After migration is complete, diffusion is allowed to occur in all directions (Fig. 9-5). Protein that moves laterally toward a trough containing antiserum produces a precipitin band in the same fashion as any of the diffusion-in-gel techniques. As the amounts of reactants increase per unit area, the intensity of the band increases. Visual observation with indirect

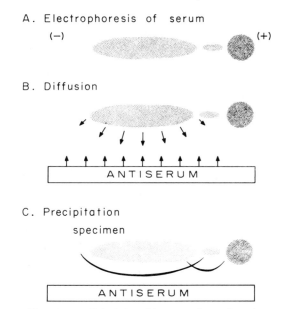

Figure 9-5. Principles of immunoelectrophoresis.

lighting is satisfactory only for the proteins at high concentration; staining with any of a number of dyes is superior. Interpretation of the results of IMEL requires considerable experience, and even an experienced observer is frequently unable to identify an abnormality seen by standard protein electrophoresis when using immunoelectrophoresis. The method has its chief application in detecting monogammopathies in which the antisera are directed against the various classes and subclasses of the immunoglobulins. Antisera against whole serum and against many of the alpha- and beta-globulins are chiefly applicable to research (see Chap. 35).

Immunofixation

Small bands representing monoclonal immunoglobulins visible on standard protein electrophoresis may become lost during diffusion, making interpretation of immunoelectrophoresis inconclusive. A method termed *immunofixation* by Alper (1969) and modified by Ritchie (1976) prevents diffusion of electrophoresed proteins during incubation by overlaying the electrophoretic strip with appropriate antisera. The unambiguous results are the product of the specific protein being trapped, in the same distribution as seen by electrophoresis, by precipitation immediately after termination of electrophoresis. Careful washing and staining after a relatively short incubation of $\frac{1}{2}$ to 1 hour results in only the precipitated protein being visualized. Agarose is the best medium for this procedure, since the resolution is considerably superior to that of cellulose acetate or paper. Immunofixation can be applied to other support media that are of coarse porosity, but application to acrylamide has been difficult because of the small gel pore size. Several attempts have been made to surface immunofix in acrylamide (Zeineh, 1973); however, the results have not been used to any degree. Recent work, however, suggests that a different approach to immunofixation in small pore gels may be very effective (Johnson, 1976; Viau, 1978).

Turbidimetry

Of the methods to measure the concentration of soluble antigen in a free aqueous medium, turbidimetry is the simplest. The reaction of the antigen with its specific antibody produces particulate complexes, initially in suspension, which precipitate as aggregation proceeds. While this method was considered to be inexact when first described in the early 1900's, several workers found that in fact the method was superior to other available methods (Boyden, 1947). In its simplest form, an amount of antiserum greater than that necessary to precipitate a given quantity of antigen completely is added to a measured volume of sample (Schultze, 1959). At a specified time, the reaction products are read in a simple colorimeter at 420 nm. The method is exactly analogous to the measurement of urinary and cerebrospinal fluid protein by chemical precipitation. In the optical instrument, the analytical light beam entering the cuvette is partially absorbed by the suspended material, either being scattered and lost on the absorbing surfaces of the cuvette holder, reflected toward the light source, or converted to heat. The suspended material absorbs the light energy directed into the solution and reduces the intensity of the beam. The amount of antigen-containing solution can be quite large, and therefore, concentrations of $1\,\mu g/ml$ are not difficult to analyze (Ritchie, 1967). Production of the immune precipitate in a free liquid medium allows it to be easily applied to automated techniques, as was successfully done in 1969 by Kahan. Turbidimetry is affected by even low concentrations of pigment that absorbs at the wavelength used and, like all immunologic tests performed in liquid, is extremely susceptible to the quality of the precipitating antiserum, particularly relating to monospecificity. While this method is usable, it requires relatively large amounts of antisera.

Nephelometry (Ritchie, 1975, 1978; Kusnetz, 1978)

Two modifications of turbidimetric analysis of immune precipitates improve the method considerably. By measuring the light reflected from the suspended particles, sensitivity can be extended greatly, the amounts of reactants reduced markedly, and the method applied to continuous-flow devices, performing the analysis in minutes rather than hours.

There are two basic approaches to optical analysis of light scatter from immune precipitates. At present, the most commonly employed method is endpoint analysis, in which the amount of light scattered from a suspension is measured at a specific time and angle. A newer technique involves the measurement of change in light scatter per unit time and employs the rate of immune complex development as the mode of analysis.

Endpoint nephelometry, originally described as a manual method (Alper, 1968) and later applied to continuous-flow analysis (Ritchie, 1969), has subsequently returned to the manual mode. Several current commercial instruments employ high-energy light sources and light scatter at angles other than the 90 degrees used by the initial workers. Sensitivity of end-point nephelometry is sharply restricted by the intrinsic light scatter of the specimen being analyzed. Human serum and plasma contain light-scattering materials, mainly lipoproteins, which in non-fasting specimens may make the measurement of soluble proteins virtually impossible at concentrations of less than $1\,g/l$. In normal fasting samples the sensitivity can be advanced so that a precise assay at $100\,mg/l$ is possible. In clear solutions such as cerebrospinal fluid and urine, antigen concentrations into the low microgram and high nanogram ranges can be analyzed effectively, especially in the manual mode, in which very large sample volumes of antigen in clear solution can be applied. Since most specific protein analyses are carried out on serum, endpoint nephelometry is primarily constrained by the normally occurring light-scattering materials and pigment.

Several commercially available manual instruments employ endpoint nephelometry. These flexible systems can measure almost as many plasma proteins as RID or rocket electrophoresis with reasonable accuracy. The shortened reaction time of one to two hours is partially offset by the increased complexity of the procedures. Nonetheless, the instruments can be considered as replacements for RID.

Certain antigen/antibody pairs combine rapidly and avidly to produce a heavy flocculent precipitate within minutes. Others, most notably IgM-anti-IgM, are slow to react. This phenomenon can be a significant problem in automated systems. Agents that enhance immune precipitation when applied to continuous-flow analysis by Hellsing (1978) have shortened the usual incubation time of 20 minutes to less than 3 minutes and markedly accelerated the reaction of IgM-anti-IgM. The addition of polyethylene glycol with an average molecular weight of 6000 has also extended the range of analysis and increased the expected signal in the lower portion of the concentration curve.

Because the specimen's intrinsic light scattering is a major factor in limiting endpoint nephelometry sensitivity, there is considerable advantage in analyzing the antigen-antibody reaction kinetically (Savory, 1974). Examination of the first derivative of the light-scattering signal significantly advances sensitivity and reduces analysis time (Anderson, 1978), producing sensitivity to less than 1 μg/ml with high-affinity antiserum. A wide range of antigens has thus been analyzed successfully, the only variable being sample and antigen dilution.

Since this technique measures the *change* in light scatter per unit time, the effect of intrinsic light-scattering material or pigments in the sample is markedly diminished. Depending upon the concentration of antigen, light scatter begins to increase within seconds, continuing until a maximum rate is reached, generally at between 15 and 70 seconds—the shortest times indicating optimum concentrations.

SPECIFIC PROTEINS

A discussion of specific proteins requires that the individual constituents that make up the plasma protein mass be addressed separately. Ideally, this chapter would include information on all the individual plasma proteins, placing each species in a major group and relating each to the total synthesis of the plasma proteins. Obviously, this is impossible, for there are hundreds already identified (Fig. 9-1). The section to follow selects certain proteins that, for reasons of concentration or location in a functional sequence, require discussion (Table 9-1). The proteins have been clustered into four groups according to their principal role as perceived at present: the carrier proteins, the acute phase reactants, the complement proteins, and the immunoglobulins. Immunoglobulins are reviewed in Chapter 36 and complement is considered in Chapter 37. In the many instances when an individual species is a member of more than one group, its discussion will appear under the group in which it appears to play the most important clinical role. In several instances, the author fully agrees that assigning a protein to a single group appears arbitrary and could be challenged. However, short of discussing each protein individually, some form of organization seems warranted.

CARRIER PROTEINS

The use of the word *transport* in the context of plasma proteins conveys a distorted image. The term implies that a moiety is carried from one location to another in an organized, uninterrupted, and controlled traffic pattern. An argument could be made that certain species are indeed transport proteins. Haptoglobin, for example, once loaded with a hemoglobin molecule, disappears from the circulation very rapidly. Protease inhibitors likewise, when complexed with an enzyme, remain in the circulation only a short time. A better term for most, however, is *carrier protein*, since they pick up a moiety, move it into a pool which may be the entire body, and allow it to be removed as required at one or more locations. Some carrier proteins provide a storage function, since their primary role is to receive a moiety from, for example, the vascular bed close to the intestinal wall, and to hold that material in circulation until it is released. One carrier protein may load and unload its respective compound repeatedly during its lifespan, while others bind moieties more permanently and still others home in on a substance, link with it, and are removed. This classification of carrier proteins includes some species which are primarily members of other groups,

Table 9-1. CHARACTERISTICS OF SPECIFIC PROTEINS

PROTEIN	PRIMARY SITE OF PRODUCTION	RANGE OF USUAL PLASMA VALUES	NO. OF VARIANTS/ SUBCLASSES	DEFICIENCY STATE	ELECTROPHORESIS AND LOCATION	MOLECULAR WEIGHT
Prealbumin	Liver	0.1–0.4 g/l	?	Not recognized	Prealbumin	62,000
Albumin	Hepatocyte	3.2–5.5 g/l	20+	Yes	Albumin	66,248
Alpha$_1$-lipoprotein (HDL)	? Liver	3–7 g/l lipid + protein	?	Yes	Albumin-alpha$_1$	360,000
Gc-globulin	Liver	?	2 (3)	Not recognized	Alpha$_1$	51,000
Beta-lipoprotein (LDL)	Liver	0.40–1.5 g/l	?	Yes	Beta	380,000 (apoprotein)
Transferrin	Liver; RE system	2.0–3.4 g/l	21+	Yes	Beta$_1$	76,500
Hemopexin	Hepatocyte	0.50–1.0 g/l	?	Not recognized	Beta$_1$	60,000
Alpha$_1$-acid glycoprotein (Orosomucoid)	Liver	0.35–1.40 g/l	2	Not recognized	Alpha$_1$	40,000
Alpha$_1$-antitrypsin	Liver	1.5–3.2 g/l	25+	Yes	Alpha$_1$	54,000
Alpha$_1$-antichymotrypsin	?	0.4–0.6 g/l	?	Not recognized	Alpha$_1$	70,000
Inter-alpha trypsin inhibitor	? Liver	0.2–0.7 g/l	?	Not recognized	Alpha$_1$-alpha$_2$	170,000
Ceruloplasmin	Liver	0.15–0.45 g/l	5+	Yes	Alpha$_2$	160,000
Antithrombin III	Liver	0.2–0.4 g/l	2	Yes	Alpha$_2$	62,300
Haptoglobin	Liver	0.4–1.8 g/l	Many	Yes	Alpha$_2$	100,000 (1-1) >100K (2-1, 2-2)
Alpha$_2$-macroglobulin	Liver	1.5–3.5 g/l age and sex dependent	?	?	Alpha$_2$	820,000
Fibrinogen	Liver	1.8–4.2 g/l	Many	Yes	Beta$_2$	340,000
Plasminogen	? Liver	0.1–0.25 g/l	?	Not recognized	Beta$_2$	92,000
C-reactive protein		0.07–8.2 mg/l	Several	Not recognized	Gamma	135,000
C1	Intestinal epithelium	C1q 1.8 g/l C1s 1.1 g/l C1r trace	?	Yes	q-Alpha$_2$ s-Alpha$_2$ r-Beta	400,000 90,000 170,000
C1 inhibitor	Liver and RE system	>0.11 g/l	? 2	Yes	Alpha$_2$	90,000
C4	Liver/ macrophage	0.10–>0.40 g/l	?	Not recognized	Beta	200,000
C2	Macrophage	10–30 mg/l	?	Yes	Beta$_1$	417,000
C3	Liver	0.90–2.30 mg/l	>20	Yes	Beta$_1$	185,000
Factor B	Liver	0.15–>0.60 g/l	4+	Yes	Beta$_2$	94,000
Immunoglobulin A	Lymphoid cells	0.4–3.5 g/l	2	Yes	Beta-gamma	160,000 SIgA- 400,000
Immunoglobulin D	Lymphoid cells	10–400 mg/l	2	Yes	Beta-gamma	180,000
Immunoglobulin E	Lymphoid cells	50–600 μg/l	2	Yes	Beta-gamma	180,000
Immunoglobulin G	Lymphoid cells	7–15 g/l	4	Yes	Alpha$_2$-gamma	150,000
Immunoglobulin M	Lymphoid cells	0.25–2.0 g/l	? (2)	Yes	Beta-gamma	850,000

e.g., acute phase reactants and immuno-globulins.

Circulating carrier proteins respond individually to the burden of the moiety to be complexed. Transferrin levels, for example, climb as available iron supplies decrease. Restoration of iron stores results in a lowering of the transferrin level. Beta-lipoproteins react in an opposite fashion to varying amounts of circulating lipids. In other cases, changes in protein levels represent a primary response to a disease process, with the material to be carried being affected secondarily. In circumstances in which the protein acts as a carrier for low molecular weight materials, the bound fraction remains in the body while the unbound may be rapidly excreted. In such cases the serum level of the carrier protein has a great effect upon the use and availability of the chemical.

Prealbumin

Synonyms. Thyroxine binding prealbumin (TBPA), vitamin A-transporting protein, tryptophan-rich prealbumin.

In most human sera, this protein is found to migrate faster than albumin in electrophoresis. One of the intermediate level plasma constituents, it plays a role in thyroxin metabolism and in the physiology of vitamin A or retinol (Peterson, 1971). This tetrameric protein is unusual in that it is specifically responsible for the transport of two plasma constituents (Nilsson, 1975).

Few studies examining prealbumin levels in serum have been published; however, it is known that levels moderately low at birth rise rapidly to adult levels during the first few weeks of life. Malnutrition and inflammatory processes adversely affect serum prealbumin levels. It is of relatively high concentration in cerebrospinal fluid.

Prealbumin is filtered through the glomerular membrane at low levels; however, the smaller associated retinol-binding protein (RBP) is readily filtered at the glomerulus and only partially reabsorbed through the renal tubule.

Prealbumin has two apparent roles: the first, a minor role as a carrier of thyroxin, is distinctly less important for this function than thyroxin-binding alpha-globulin (Oppenheimer, 1968). Secondly, prealbumin binds to RBP, transporting the complex through the vascular space to cell surfaces where the vitamin A-RBP complex is released to unload vitamin A onto the cell membrane. Virtually all RBP is associated with prealbumin. Even though prealbumin has four RBP binding sites, it complexes stoichiometrically in a ratio of 1:1. The binding sites for RBP-retinol are separate and distinct from the site for thyroxin, giving this protein its unique dual transport function (Rask, 1973). Each of the four prealbumin subunits simultaneously can bind one thyroxine molecule.

Negative nitrogen balance, whether due to malnutrition, the cachexia of malignancy, chronic infection, or hepatic disease, results in decreased levels of prealbumin and RBP. A fall in the levels of prealbumin is often an early indicator of hepatitis even before other protein constituents are affected, probably because of the protein's short half-life. Correction of the pathologic process is often accompanied by rapid production and release of prealbumin, RBP, and retinol. Administration of corticoids also results in an increase in serum prealbumin levels.

The most satisfactory means of analyzing prealbumin is by direct immunoassay. Serum levels are sufficiently high to make gel diffusion or nephelometry fully satisfactory. The presence of RBP bound to prealbumin theoretically should affect analysis of prealbumin in gel diffusion methods, but as yet this has not been observed.

Albumin

In man, the major serum protein is albumin (Peters, 1970, 1975), which normally makes up over 60 per cent of the total. Significantly decreased albumin levels in individuals not congenitally deficient accompany and are accompanied by many disturbances in homeostasis.

Concentration. Albumin synthesis occurs very early in fetal development (Gitlin, 1975). By the fourth to sixth week of gestation, yolk sac and liver cells produce proteins immunologically identifiable as albumin. Adult values are reached by the twentieth to twenty-sixth week of gestation, and cord serum, therefore, has a full complement of the protein. Serum values remain remarkably stable in the normal individual until late in life when a small but significant downward trend in serum values begins. Women in general have serum values slightly lower than those of men of the same age.

Albumin values drift downward with the progress of a pregnancy, and some women experience variations in plasma albumin during the menstrual cycle. Contraceptive medication does not affect albumin levels significantly (Horne, 1970; Laurell, 1970).

Hypoalbuminemia is a hallmark of protein malnutrition, whether it be due to kwashiorkor, alcoholism, malabsorption, parasitism, malignancy, or the "tea and toast" syndrome of an elderly person living alone. Low serum albumin levels most commonly are associated with chronic inflammation and severe acute disease. However, whether the process basically differs from the above, i.e., insufficient supply of amino acids, remains a topic for discussion. A variety of cytotoxic medications have a depressive effect upon the synthesis of plasma proteins, including albumin. In children, hypoalbuminemia and peripheral edema are closely associated; in the adult, edema is less predictable.

The time at which a specimen is drawn may also play an important role in establishing an adequate interpretation for serum albumin level (Winkel, 1975a, 1975b). Overnight fasting in preparation for phlebotomy not infrequently results in a significant increase in serum protein values for young males but not for young females. Dehydration caused by exercise can increase serum albumin levels in young men to 60 g/l. Serum specimens which are collected in the recumbent position will have a lower total protein and serum albumin than those taken after hours in the upright position.

Genetics. Many genetic variants of albumin, the alloalbumins, have been described with unusual physical properties such as stability, electrophoretic mobility, and the ability to transport low molecular weight substances (Gitlin, 1975). The common form of albumin is called albumin A, with many of the variants a result of minor alterations in the amino acid content. Some electrophoretic variants are common in populations with restricted ethnic backgrounds, such as in North American Indian tribes. In some instances, the variants are so limited as to have been identified only in a single kindred.

Congenital analbuminemia (Waldmann, 1964) is a very rare syndrome in which some patients are capable of synthesizing only very small amounts of albumin (<0.5 per cent of normal) measured by sensitive methods. Clinical interest in these patients centers on the fact that they have little difficulty attributable to the protein deficiency despite albumin's central role in maintenance of osmotic pressure and transport and storage of low molecular weight substances. Total serum protein in these individuals ranges from 45–57 g/l with plasma colloid osmotic pressure about one half of that expected; yet peripheral edema, when present, is mild. The unusual and unexpected benignity of the deficiency of such an important blood component has suggested to some that albumin may, in fact, not be as important as generally perceived.

Physiology. Synthesized almost totally by the liver, albumin has a half-life of 15 to 19 days. Synthesis of this protein is clearly tied to the delivery of amino acid building blocks to the liver, hence its sensitivity to protein malnutrition. Albumin synthesis rises within 30 minutes after protein-depleted individuals receive adequate levels of amino acids, suggesting that albumin synthesis may not be constant but occurs in relation to dietary supply and absorption of protein subunits (Rothschild, 1972).

Catabolism of the protein occurs primarily in organs with high metabolic rates, e.g., liver, spleen, kidney, muscle, etc. Cells incorporate plasma droplets by pinocytosis and digest the protein contents to amino acids, which are again available for protein synthesis.

For an average-size individual, 350 g of albumin are included in the body mass, with 140 g in the intravascular and 210 g in the extravascular space. Albumin is distributed throughout the body, including bone and skin, with only about 2 g within the liver, mostly in lymphatic channels. This large mass of protein plays a prominent role in fat metabolism in addition to being a nitrogen source. The action of lipoprotein lipase upon lipids releases unstable fatty acids which are then briefly bound to albumin in rapid transit from liver to peripheral tissues. The sole major biochemical defect in analbuminemic patients is a markedly disturbed lipid metabolism (Waldmann, 1964).

Transport and storage of a wide variety of low molecular weight substances such as cortisol, sex hormones, calcium, and a host of drugs is a major function of normal albumin. The qualification "normal" must be given, since there is information that some albumin variants may be altered in their ability to bind drugs such as warfarin. Binding and resulting detoxification represent other major functions of albumin in the newborn. Bilirubin bound to albumin is less likely to pass to the hydrophobic tissues of the brain than is free bilirubin. Certain heavy metals also are bound to albumin in a non-toxic form. During extensive hemolysis, a complex with heme, called methemalbumin, is formed.

Very low levels of albumin portend serious disease (Slater, 1975) either from increased loss and/or catabolism or decreased synthesis. Pathologic states such as alcoholic cirrhosis, accompanied by hypoalbuminemia, often result from protein malnutrition and a decrease in functional liver tissue. In patients whose disease is compounded by portal hypertension, malabsorption augments the problem. Given the necessary building blocks, the liver can maintain an adequate serum albumin level in spite of moderately large losses by the kidney; however, even well-nourished nephrotics may have low serum albumin levels if active inflammation persists.

Analysis. Because it is a stable protein with minimal problems of heterogeneity, albumin is easily analyzed by a variety of chemical or immunologic methods (Slater, 1978). Albumin's capacity to bind and transport small molecules is exploited in the dye-binding methods in widespread use today. Since patients may have their albumin already partially saturated by common drugs such as aspirin or metabolites such as bilirubin, the dye-binding methods may give falsely low values. Immunochemical methods for albumin appear unaffected by transported moieties and are receiving increasing attention in the clinical laboratory. Virtually every immunochemical method for assaying soluble proteins has been applied to albumin analysis.

Group-specific components (Gc)

Synonyms. Vitamin D-binding globulin, Gc globulin.

In the past, Gc globulin was of interest only because it had a pronounced and easily studied genetic polymorphism found in all human populations, with resulting forensic applications. It was recognized as being the vitamin D-binding globulin only in 1975 (Daiger).

Concentration. Gc is present in cord blood, but quantitative studies during maturation, health, and disease are not available.

Genetics. The common polymorphism, as demonstrated by electrophoresis, is determined by two autosomal codominant alleles, Gc^1 and Gc^2. As a result, there are three major permutations visible on well-resolved electro-phoresis: homozygous types 1-1, 2-2, and the heterozygous type, 2-1 (Johnson, 1975). Gc^1 is more common in the general population than is Gc^2 (see Chap. 44).

Physiology. Gc globulin, perhaps now more correctly called the vitamin D-binding globulin, clearly binds vitamin D_3, 25-hydroxy-vitamin D_3, and 1,25-dihydroxy vitamin D_3 *in vitro* and probably *in vivo*. Apparently the vitamin D-binding capacity is many times greater than that needed to bind physiologic levels of vitamin D, but no clinical data are available to indicate whether Gc globulin levels are related to disease.

Analysis. This protein can be readily measured by standard immunochemical procedures, manual or automated. Analytical problems have not been encountered. Immunofixation leads to a clear separation of the genetic variants, far superior to that experienced with immunoelectrophoresis.

Transferrin (Tf) (see also Chapter 9)

Synonyms. Siderophilin, beta$_1$-metalbinding globulin.

Without iron, the majority of living organisms cannot survive. In general, iron exists in three states: in transit, in use, or in storage. In man and most animals a single protein, transferrin, is responsible for transport of iron from absorptive surfaces to the bone marrow where it is incorporated into the heme portion of the hemoglobin molecule. Although apotransferrin is colorless, incorporation of iron into the protein produces a strong pink-red color that, because of its high concentration, contributes to the color of serum.

Concentration. The concentration of plasma transferrin is most affected by dietary intake of iron and, therefore, indirectly by socioeconomic factors. Nutritionally deficient but calorie-rich diets are generally lacking in iron. As a result, serum iron levels are low and transferrin levels are high, particularly among teenagers, in whom requirements are increased by rapid growth. In infancy, iron-supplemented formula (many formulae are not iron-supplemented), milk, or breast milk contain adequate levels of iron; therefore, high transferrin levels are not seen until weaning of the normal child. If protein malnutrition is severe, the synthesis of transferrin is significantly reduced in spite of iron deficiency (McFarlane, 1970). Parasitism, also common in underdeveloped nations where dietary iron is low, intensifies the deficiency through either blood loss or malabsorption (Saraya, 1970).

Contraceptive medications as well as pregnancy have been shown to produce an increase in plasma transferrin. Withdrawal of the medication or termination of a pregnancy results in a return to normal levels (Horne, 1970; Laurell, 1970). Administration of either oral or parenteral iron will lower the level of plasma transferrin in an individual suffering from iron deficiency. Once saturation of plasma transferrin exceeds 60 to 70 per cent, iron is deposited in the liver where it is available for future mobilization and use (Wheby, 1964). Any medication or condition which produces hemolysis exceeding the serum hemoglobin-binding capacity can lead to increased iron loss via the biliary tree and increased transferrin levels. Excessive acute oral doses of iron will result in toxicity if the plasma transferrin iron-binding capacity is exceeded.

Genetics.   With available electrophoretic techniques, the transferrin band (beta$_1$-globulin) sometimes appears reduplicated. The extra bands, usually of the same concentration as the fraction in the normal location, may appear either anodal or cathodal to the usual position and are evidence for genetic polymorphism of transferrin. At least 21 variants have been described (Giblett, 1969). Various racial groups have specific transferrin variants, e.g., American blacks, certain Indian tribes, Japanese, and Chinese. The incidence in North American blacks for one variant (D$_1$) approaches 10 per cent; other variants are less frequent except in certain isolated gene pools, e.g., Australian aborigines. The variants are unassociated with known clinical conditions and are fully capable of binding the full complement of iron. A rare genetic state of atransferrinemia has been described, accompanied by severe clinical problems leading to death as a result of the failure of proper iron transport (Riegel, 1956). These individuals, as a result of their inability to bind iron, suffer the complications of iron deposition disorders and anemia (Walbaum, 1971).

Physiology.   The total iron-binding capacity (TIBC) of the plasma can be equated with the transferrin concentration (Daigneault, 1978). A correction factor of 0.025 times the transferrin concentration in mg/l yields the total iron-binding capacity in μmol/l. Plasma transferrin serves as a reusable transport protein for trivalent iron *in vivo* and divalent iron *in vitro*. The 30 mg of iron required each day

for hemoglobin synthesis can be received by transferrin either near the absorptive surfaces of the GI tract or in proximity to the sites of hemoglobin degradation. Transferrin then makes iron available wherever hemoglobin synthesis is carried out and also delivers iron to the site of the synthesis of certain iron-containing enzymes. A large amount of plasma transferrin is ordinarily not saturated. Therefore, the total transferrin pool acts as a cushion to buffer large amounts of absorbed or released iron that would otherwise be toxic in the free trivalent form. Transferrin may also play an important role in trace element transport.

Transferrin is believed to play an important role in bacteriostasis (Putnam, 1975c). Trivalent iron is necessary for bacterial survival and replication. Individuals whose serum iron levels are low, but whose transferrin, i.e., TIBC, is high, may deal effectively with the infection in spite of anemia. Therapeutic administration of iron could result in prompt worsening of the infection. Individuals with low plasma transferrin levels have been noted to fare poorly with bacterial infections, and the few patients with congenital atransferrinemia have died of sepsis, which supports this hypothesis.

The interface of transferrin with the storage protein ferritin and the intracellular protein lactoferrin completes the normal iron cycle. Exchange of ferric iron from transferrin to intracellular lactoferrin found in secretions such as milk affects the delivery of iron to the breast-fed infant.

Hypotransferrinemia of variable degree can occur in a variety of disorders. Protein-losing states, most notably the nephrotic syndrome, can result in levels as low as 15 per cent of normal (0.4 g/l). In general, the transferrin level parallels that of albumin in protein-losing states. Severe liver disease (e.g., cirrhosis) also can result in marked depression of plasma transferrin levels, with values as low as 0.6 g/l. In chronic liver disease, low levels of low molecular weight proteins contrast with the normal or elevated levels of the immunoglobulins.

Elevated levels, occasionally as high as 7 g/l, occur as the result of severe iron deficiency and depletion of total body iron stores. Few references to hypertransferrinemia are found in the literature. The finding of a significant elevation of the protein, therefore, indicates a deficiency of available iron.

Analysis.   Although the electrophoretic

quantitation of transferrin is possible, its imprecision makes other techniques more desirable. The stability of the transferrin molecule and the lack of variations in molecular weight in genetic variants make quantitation by any of the gel diffusion or light-scattering methods precise and accurate. The degree of iron saturation does not appear to have any effect on the precision of the assays.

Hemopexin

Synonyms. Beta$_{1b}$-globulin, heme-binding globulin.

Another pigmented plasma protein, this red-brown beta-globulin found in normal plasma binds heme (Muller-Eberhard, 1970). It represents one of the three proteins involved with the binding, transport, storage, and conservation of hemoglobin/heme proteins after release into the circulation.

Concentration. Hemopexin is produced in the early fetus at very low levels. Cord blood contains a significant per cent of adult serum levels, which are eventually reached by the end of the first year (Gitlin, 1969).

Physiology. Produced in the liver by hepatocytes, hemopexin serum levels can be increased by the intravenous injection of heme. Certain drugs, including some carcinogens, have also been shown to increase hemopexin levels in animals. This may be related to the effect of these agents upon hepatic enzymes directed at the metabolism of porphyrins and porphyrogenic drugs (Wochner, 1974). Unlike the hemoglobin-binding protein haptoglobin, hemopexin is not an acute phase protein, a fact that may make the measurement of hemopexin valuable in interpreting certain acute phase reactants in the presence of hemolysis.

As its name implies, hemopexin's primary function is to bind heme. When the hemoglobin-binding capacity of circulating haptoglobin has been exceeded, hemoglobin dissociates either into two molecules, each containing two heme moieties, or into four heme molecules and globin. Oxidized heme (metheme) then complexes firmly with hemopexin. A less avid and probably transient complex is formed with albumin to form methemalbumin. Heme-hemopexin is believed to be degraded in the hepatocyte while the albumin complex circulates until it gives up its heme to unsaturated hemopexin. The heme-hemopexin complexes are found in the hepatocytes in contrast to the hemoglobin-haptoglobin complexes,

which are cleared by the reticuloendothelial system. The goal of hemopexin is iron conservation through the binding of free or loosely bound circulating heme.

Analysis. Measurement of hemopexin in serum or plasma is readily accomplished by gel diffusion or nephelometric methods, provided satisfactory antisera are available.

ACUTE PHASE REACTANTS (APR)

Clinicians have been resistant, even refractory, to the suggestion that the laboratory can predict future overt illness. Most existing laboratory studies, particularly those oriented toward acute illness, have been justifiably considered as of little value as an "early warning system" of evolving illness. The majority of APR studies of individual components of the APR group have been oriented toward changes occurring *after* a clinical diagnosis has been established rather than as an effective means of alerting the physician to subclinical problems (see Chap. 54).

Traditionally, clinical medicine views the inflammatory process as a response following an insult. Perhaps this highly variable constellation of events, including leukocytosis, fever, anorexia, and malaise, is the means by which an individual becomes aware of illness, but it is misleading to assume that biochemical abnormalities cannot precede clinical signs. For example, it is well known that biochemical indicators of inflammation, such as elevated sedimentation rate, may be present years before clinical illness becomes apparent. Furthermore, an abnormal sedimentation rate can be associated with disturbed levels of certain plasma proteins, notably fibrinogen, which, in addition to its role as a coagulation factor, also responds as an acute phase reactant. It is important to document these premonitory changes further, relating specific protein abnormalities known to be associated with clinical signs and symptoms to preclinical disease.

By definition, acute phase reactants are proteins whose concentrations increase or decrease in association with an inflammatory stimulus. These numerous non-specific reactors are found in the alpha and beta electrophoretic fractions. Those in highest concentration are: haptoglobin, alpha$_1$-antitrypsin, orosomucoid, C3, inter-alpha-trypsin inhibitor, ceruloplasmin, fibrinogen, and C-reactive protein. Most perform a specific function, which becomes increasingly important during inflammation. Teleologically speaking, elevated levels reflect the body's biochemical preparation to end and repair the process. There must be some final common pathway that allows such apparently diverse processes as neoplasia, rheumatoid arthritis, and sepsis to be expressed in a similar manner. Many substances, such as complement, kinins, and clotting and fibrinolytic factors, have been proposed as mediators of the inflammatory response. The immune system can also be involved as the initiator of the complement cascade with its resultant production of mediators. In addition, in animals at least, immunosuppression blunts the inflammatory process. Suppression of the inflammatory response can also follow the administration of corticosteroids, again suggesting that the cellular component—particularly the immunocyte—plays a decisive role. What is directly responsible for the increased synthesis of this family of glycoproteins by the liver? Individual substances associated with tissue damage, such as prostaglandins and lysosomal enzymes, have been shown to stimulate production of APRs, but the mechanism that elevates plasma levels of APRs is unknown (Weissmann, 1974).

While an inflammatory process results in increased synthesis of certain proteins by the liver, others often referred to as negative acute phase reactants manifest a decrease. Of the proteins discussed in this chapter, albumin, transferrin, and the thyroxin-binding prealbumin are examples of negative acute phase reactants. Decreasing serum levels during inflammation without a coexistent protein-losing state are generally brought about by a decrease in hepatic synthesis. Malnutrition and deficiency of amino acids have been directly implicated in hypoproteinemia; however, the mechanism whereby the liver selectively decreases production of some proteins —namely the negative acute phase reactants —while increasing production of others remains unclear. A humoral factor, associated with neoplasia and exerting its effect upon albumin synthesis, has been described (Toporek, 1973). It is likely that the final common pathway of protein synthesis reflects the sum of many factors. Furthermore, the effect upon individual plasma protein production ranges from marked depression through no change to marked increase, often with disparate results upon individual protein species.

The liver responds to a stimulus by *increasing* acute phase reactant synthesis and, therefore, serum levels. The time lag from the insult or the beginning of a process to a detectable change in concentration is different for each protein. C-reactive protein increases after only a few hours, while C3 and ceruloplasmin do not increase until several days later, if at all (Daniels, 1974; Fisher, 1976). All plasma proteins are presumably under genetic control. Therefore, it is not surprising that synthetic rates in some individuals would be different from those in others. For this reason, analyses for a single APR are to be discouraged (Milford-Ward, 1977).

Several of the acute-phase reactants have been shown to have plasma levels that reflect genetic control. The most notable is alpha$_1$-antitrypsin, whose polymorphism in man is related to the rate of synthesis and release of the protein into the circulation. Those gene combinations that result in markedly depressed (less than 30 per cent) protein concentration in the otherwise healthy individual are more detectable than those that result in moderate reduction (30 to 70 per cent). Very low levels will remain low even in the face of an extensive inflammatory drive. Those individuals with intermediate levels carry moderately depressed levels of alpha$_1$-antitrypsin in the steady state, but respond proportionally to their baseline levels, only reaching plasma levels within the normal range. Short of determining the phenotype (Pi) of each individual, the only means of detecting an inflammatory process in an individual of alpha$_1$-antitrypsin Pi type MZ is to analyze one or preferably several other APRs simultaneously.

The variable involvement of individual APR serum levels is a common and serious interpretive problem. Haptoglobin presents an excellent example. Its primary function is to bind irreversibly with free hemoglobin and to be removed by the reticuloendothelial system. A sudden release of hemoglobin results in a prompt reduction in plasma levels, often to zero. Since ordinary plasma levels are approximately 1 g/l and the monomeric protein (Hp phenotype 1-1) binds stoichiometrically with hemoglobin A, approximately 0.6 mg of hemoglobin will be bound per ml of normal plasma or about 0.4 mg of hemoglobin per ml of whole blood. Therefore, the release of 1.9 g of hemoglobin will effect the complete removal of plasma haptoglobin in an average adult male. This amounts to the destruction of 7 ml of red blood cells in a normal individual. It is common for normal, young adults to have steady-state haptoglobin values of approximately 0.3 to 0.5 g/l, giving a hemoglobin binding capacity of only 2 to 3.5 ml of red blood cells. If the individual is of the more common type 2-1 or 2-2 phenotype, where haptoglobin exists in polymeric form, substantially less hemoglobin would presumably be required to reduce the value to zero. It is presumed, therefore, that the haptoglobin deficiency seen in athletes and in musicians who use their hands vigorously is the result of low-level mechanical breakdown of circulating red cells. This is a common finding in a pediatric population, in whom physical restraint is necessary to obtain blood specimens, or in a population of patients with seizure disorders, whose violent muscular contractions result in hemolysis.

Selective loss of protein across membranes in the kidney or gut can result in canceling the effect of an inflammatory process on APR serum levels. Of the major APRs, haptoglobin (2-1, 2-2), fibrinogen, and CRP are of the highest molecular weight; others are considerably lower. Therefore, plasma exposed to a damaged and highly permeable membrane would be subjected to an ultrafiltration process favoring the passage of low molecular weight proteins (Weeke, 1973). Even though the synthesis of alpha$_1$-antitrypsin, for example, may be high, its loss across a membrane is also high, with the result that plasma levels may be normal or even depressed. At the same time, the high molecular weight APRs may be extraordinarily elevated. Values for fibrinogen of over 20 g/l and for haptoglobin of over 10 g/l have been seen in protein-losing states, while alpha$_1$-antitrypsin and orosomucoid levels have been less than 50 per cent of normal.

Dramatic changes in some of the APRs can occur in the absence of an inflammatory process. Pregnancy or the pseudopregnancy of contraceptive medication may produce marked elevations of certain APRs—notably ceruloplasmin—and lesser elevations of orosomucoid, plasminogen, and alpha$_1$-antitrypsin (Doe, 1967; Song, 1970). Haptoglobin levels are diminished by administration of estrogen. Unlike the inflammatory syndrome, albumin and transferrin levels are largely unchanged late in gestation in spite of the hydremia that occurs.

Special circumstances, in which the presence of an inflammatory process is of particular interest, may present a difficult interpretive situation. In the newborn and particularly the premature infant, certain globulin levels are normally low or absent, e.g., haptoglobin. Under these circumstances, evidence of inflammation can be retrieved only by careful definition of normal or reference values for the several acute phase proteins.

Alpha$_1$-acid glycoprotein (α_1 Gp) (Schmid, 1975)

Synonyms. Orosomucoid, alpha$_1$-seromucoid, uromucoid.

This acute phase alpha-globulin of plasma carries approximately 10 per cent of the serum protein-bound carbohydrate in spite of its modest concentration and low molecular weight.

Concentration. In general, mean values for children are considerably below those for adults. Similar observations have been made for other acute phase reactants. Limited clinical experience in late pregnancy indicates that α_1 Gp levels are increased (Good, 1975).

Genetics. Electrophoretic polymorphism of desialated α_1 Gp has been demonstrated at acid pH. Although no genetic pattern has been connected with low levels, a small percentage of normal individuals have α_1 Gp levels about one third to one half of the usual values.

Physiology. Any inflammatory condition increases α_1 Gp levels along with the other acute phase reactants. Significant elevations of serum levels can be detected within a day of a circumscribed insult, such as a simple surgical procedure (van Oss, 1975). Unlike several other acute phase reactants, the serum level falls rather abruptly after four to five days and in that regard resembles CRP* and the erythrocyte sedimentation rate. It has been suggested that conditions with cell proliferation stimulate α_1 Gp production. Therefore, it has been used to monitor patients with malignancies as though it were a tumor marker (Twining, 1977). The role of α_1 Gp remains uncertain. It has been shown to bind certain steroids such as progesterone, to interact with DNA, to influence prothrombin levels, and to modify platelet adhesive capacity. Alpha$_1$-acid glycoprotein may also exert control over the spacing of collagen fibers as they are assembled from collagen.

Analysis. The protein is an excellent antigen and can be assayed by a variety of immunologic techniques without difficulty. The staining of electrophoresis strips seriously misjudges α_1 Gp levels. Its high carbohydrate

---

*CRP = C reactive protein.

content results in resistance to fixation and poor binding with standard protein dyes used in electrophoresis, leading to serious underestimation of α_1 Gp levels. It lies beneath alpha$_1$-antitrypsin in both cellulose and agarose electrophoresis and under the leading edge of albumin in acrylamide gel electrophoresis.

Alpha$_1$-antitrypsin (α_1 AT) (Eriksson, 1965; Mittman, 1972; Laurell, 1975; Talamo, 1978)

Synonyms.   Alpha$_1$-trypsin inhibitor, alpha$_1$-protease inhibitor.

The release of proteolytic enzymes from plasma onto organ surfaces and into tissue spaces must inevitably result in the destruction of the host unless a control mechanism exists. In man, the highest concentration inhibitor of enzymatic proteolysis is alpha$_1$-antitrypsin.

Concentration.   At birth, and for a few days after, serum α_1AT concentrations may be significantly below adult normal levels, but rise rapidly (Sveger, 1975). There appears to be no significant change in concentration through life unless inflammatory conditions supervene. Pregnancy and contraceptive medication elevate the serum levels as determined by diffusion in gel methods (Laurell, 1970; Mendenhall, 1970; Lieberman, 1971). Cessation of medication produces a prompt fall of α_1AT to pretreatment levels. Since α_1AT is an acute phase protein, its serum levels can be expected to rise with an inflammatory process, provided the individual's genetically controlled synthetic mechanism can respond.

Several workers have indicated that the accepted reference values for α_1AT are as much as two times too high. Current mean values are said to be approximately 2.4 g/l, with a range from 1.5 to 3.2 g/l. Recent information suggests a range of 1.0 to 1.6 g/l for a healthy population.

Genetics.   Extensive studies on the polymorphism of α_1AT were stimulated by the discovery that a severe form of lung and/or liver disease afflicting children and young adults was associated with low circulating levels of α_1AT. The most common allele (Pi^M) is found as the homozygous phenotype (MM) in about 90 per cent of the white population. Therefore, approximately 10 per cent of the individuals are heterozygous for the M allele, or homozygous for the less common Pi^S, Pi^Z, or Pi^F alleles. This represents a major health problem, considering the incidence of the MZ state (approximately 2.5 per cent) and the fact that a child born of an MZ couple (MZ $\times$ MZ) yields a 25 per cent incidence of the homozygous state (ZZ) with attendant severe pulmonary and/or hepatic problems. The incidence of the ZZ state is estimated at between 1 in 500 and 1 in 700 individuals in Sweden. In American Caucasians the incidence is considerably less, and in blacks and Orientals still less common.

Alpha$_1$-antitrypsin serum levels in heterozygous MZ or MS individuals react proportionally to baseline serum levels with an inflammatory drive. Thus, interpretation of a single value or even a trend during disease may be impossible without the knowledge of the phenotype and of simultaneously measured levels of other acute phase reactants (Johnson, 1976).

Only the very low serum levels seen in the ZZ, Z-, and perhaps the SZ states have been linked with pulmonary and/or hepatic disease, but the expression is variable. Only a small percentage of infants with the genetic defect experience neonatal hepatitis, and some adults survive into the seventh decade with only moderate pulmonary disease. The ZZ protein appears fully capable of exerting its inhibition of proteolysis in proportion to its concentration. A level 10 per cent of normal, however, is insufficient to maintain control over the proteases constantly being elaborated, for example, by phagocytic cells in the alveolar spaces.

The hepatocyte's inability to secrete the ZZ protein plays an important role in hepatic manifestations of the disorder (Chap. 11). Transient neonatal hepatitis, progressive cirrhosis in infancy, or, occasionally, cirrhosis along with obstructive pulmonary disease may appear in adult life.

Physiology.   Serum levels appear to be at least related to the genetic form expressed in the phenotype, M > S > Z. Explaining the serum level of protein in the ZZ state is complicated by the fact that at least some of the protein produced does not escape from the hepatocyte. The periodic acid–Schiff (PAS) positive granules that are the hallmark of α_1AT-related liver disease are composed of unsialylated Z protein. The rare null state described in 1973 (Talamo, 1973; Sveger, 1974) results from an allele having no expression. Hence, values for serum α_1AT are one half of those expected in heterozygotes according to phenotype. An M- or M null genotype will exhibit a phenotype indistinguishable from an MM, but the absolute serum value will be significantly reduced in the absence of acute phase response, pregnancy, or estrogen therapy.

The primary function of α_1AT is to inhibit various proteolytic enzymes by forming firm but partially reversible complexes. Specificity of α_1AT is such that it can inhibit a broad spectrum of enzymes, including chymotrypsin, plasmin, thrombin, collagenase, and elastase. Alpha$_1$-antitrypsin is not the only protease inhibitor. It is, however, in highest concentration and has a broad inhibitory spectrum. It has limited ability to function at the pHs prevalent in the stomach and gut and exerts the greatest effect in areas near physiologic pH, e.g., the respiratory tract and the closed spaces of the body, including third-space compartments containing serious effusions of pH above 5 to 5.5.

Alpha$_1$-antitrypsin levels may rise to extraordinary heights during inflammatory conditions. Serum values over 400 per cent of normal have been observed. Following inflammatory insult such as an uncomplicated surgical wound, serum levels increase detectably within two to three days and remain elevated for a week or more. Apparently, any condition that produces the ill-defined constellation known as inflammation results in an increase in α_1AT, provided the individual possesses the proper genotype. Conditions such as rheumatoid arthritis, bacterial infection, vasculitis, and carcinomatosis—particularly if necrosis exists—are such examples.

Analysis. The first case of α_1AT deficiency was identified by visual inspection of paper electrophoresis. Many cases are still identified by this technique, but confirmation by quantitative and qualitative means is now imperative. It should be emphasized that the visual appearance of the electrophoresis strip should clearly show the abnormality regardless of the numerical information obtained by densitometry. In all cases of the ZZ state, the alpha$_1$ zone is visually "empty," although a substantial amount of protein can be identified by scanning. This inconsistency results from the presence of low concentration proteins in the same electrophoretic area. Other α_1AT phenotypes may be aberrant in agarose gel. Specimens which are improperly stored show a marked change in the electrophoretic mobility as a result of the loss of sialic acid. Radial-

immunodiffusion, electroimmunodiffusion, and nephelometry are the major quantitative techniques used for measuring α_1AT. The molecular configurations of the various phenotypes have no effect on the immunoassays, and there have been no convincing data to indicate that an immunologic distinction exists between the M and Z forms. Phenotyping of α_1AT is an important integral part of the laboratory examination of the protein. This is particularly important in reporting an abnormally low value, since an explanation is warranted. Acid starch gel electrophoresis followed by crossed antigen-antibody electrophoresis plays a major role in phenotyping, but because of its costs and complexity, few laboratories have developed the expertise. More recently, a simple technique employing immunofixation has made it possible to study phenotypes wherever electrophoresis is available (Ritchie, 1976). Commercial availability of special ampholytes for electrofocusing of α_1AT in polyacrylamide gels is now making it possible for laboratories having appropriate equipment to perform phenotyping by this elegant technique (Allen, 1974).

Functional assays for total trypsin inhibitory capacity of serum have been used in the past. Since 80 to 90 per cent of the trypsin inhibitory capacity (TIC) of serum is contributed by α_1AT, correlation of TIC and α_1AT are excellent. In conditions in which the levels of inhibitory proteins are severely distorted, TIC may be misleading.

Alpha$_1$-antichymotrypsin (α_1Ac)

Synonyms. Alpha$_1$-X-glycoprotein.

One of the first acute-phase proteins to respond is the carbohydrate-rich alpha-globulin, alpha$_1$-antichymotrypsin. Within hours, plasma levels double. As its name implies, it is an inhibitor of the proteolytic enzyme, chymotrypsin.

Concentration. Mean adult serum levels for both sexes are about 0.5 g/l (Kosaka, 1976).

Physiology. Despite its name, α_1Ac is a weak inhibitor of proteases including chymotrypsin, which is more effectively inhibited by alpha$_1$-antitrypsin and alpha$_2$-macroglobulin. As an acute phase reactant, α_1Ac is as sensitive as CRP to inflammation (Kosaka, 1976).

Analysis. Serum levels are sufficiently high to allow analysis by a variety of immunologic techniques. No special problems have been encountered in analysis.

Inter-alpha-trypsin inhibitor (IATI) (Steinbuch, 1975)

In addition to the major protease inhibitors, serum contains several low-concentration proteins that are weak inhibitors. Presumably, their role is similar to that of the major inhibitors. One of these, IATI, is in high enough concentration to allow easy analysis by gel diffusion or nephelometry, but clinical information is sparse. A single clinical study suggests that it may be a sluggish acute phase reactant. In vitro, it is a weak inhibitor of the pancreatic enzymes trypsin and chymotrypsin, but the inhibitory effect in vivo is unknown. It appears to be antigenically related to a low molecular weight acid stable proteinase inhibitor found in serum and urine (Hochstrasser, 1976; Bretzel, 1976).

Ceruloplasmin

Synonym. Copper oxidase.

Various metal ions play a critical role in enzyme performance. One whose enzyme activity has been well studied is the intensely blue, copper-containing protein, ceruloplasmin.

Concentration. Population studies of sufficient size to establish trends in ceruloplasmin levels during life are limited (Gitlin, 1969; Schultze, 1966). Copper and ceruloplasmin levels are low at birth. Pregnancy and the administration of contraceptive drugs (Burrows, 1971) result in an increase in serum copper (Schenker, 1971) and ceruloplasmin levels. A study of a patient with very low serum ceruloplasmin and copper levels demonstrated that administration of oral copper sulfate increased ceruloplasmin levels, the reverse of the situation seen in iron deficiency. The data of Al-Rashid (1971) indicate that in some fashion the synthesis of the protein requires adequate serum copper levels.

Genetics. Because of the effect of specimen aging on the protein and because of the infrequency of some of the variants, the genetics of ceruloplasmin expression are controversial, although its polymorphism has been well documented (Giblett, 1969). Wilson's disease (hepatolenticular degeneration) is inherited as an autosomal recessive trait whose manifestations rarely occur before six years of age and may be delayed into middle life (Sternlieb, 1968). Associated with the disorder is deficiency of ceruloplasmin and, therefore, the appearance of excessive levels of free or loosely bound serum copper (Klein, 1968).

Physiology. Both ceruloplasmin production and binding of eight atoms of Cu^{++} to apoceruloplasmin occur in the liver. The principal role of ceruloplasmin in man is still not established. Involvement in copper homeostasis and Wilson's disease is circumstantial, since hypoceruloplasminemia leads to elevated urinary copper levels and the deposition of copper in the cornea, brain, liver, and kidney, organs deranged in the pathologic process. That a dysfunctional ceruloplasmin is to blame has not been verified. Moderately depressed levels of ceruloplasmin secondary to decreased synthesis or increased loss lead to an anemia related to the second function of ceruloplasmin, that of acting as ferro-oxidase that converts ferrous iron to the usable ferric form (Roeser, 1970).

Ceruloplasmin (Cp) levels rise as the result of many disorders broadly categorized as inflammatory processes, including infection and malignancy, particularly those that contain foci of necrosis. Elevated estrogen levels as the result of either contraceptive medication or pregnancy will also produce elevated ceruloplasmin levels. Although estrogen levels are high in chronic liver disease, ceruloplasmin levels are often discordant as the result of organ failure to synthesize the protein.

Analysis. RID has been widely used to measure Cp levels and, to a lesser extent, electroimmunodiffusion and nephelometry. The specificity of the antiserum may produce confusing results when several precipitin rings are produced as the result of multiple antibody specificities. Analysis by immunologic techniques in gels should be performed on fresh specimens of sera. Ceruloplasmin levels can also be measured by the protein's enzymatic action upon paraphenylene-diamine and other substrates.

Antithrombin III (AT3)

Synonym. Heparin co-factor.

The delicate balance between fluid and clotted blood is normally maintained by regulators of the coagulation system exemplified by the plasma protein antithrombin III (Rosenburg, 1975; Musumeci, 1976).

Concentration. Because of the interest in thrombotic disorders associated with pregnancy and the side effects of contraceptive medications, the mechanisms of thrombosis under these conditions have been extensively studied and found to be associated with reduction in plasma concentration of AT3, sometimes to a marked degree (Peterson, 1970; Innerfield, 1976).

Genetics. Familial predilection to life-threatening thrombosis has been reported in association with AT3 deficiency. The production of the protein is under genetic control with autosomal codominant inheritance (Carvalho, 1976). As a rule, functional AT3 levels correlate with the immunochemically measured protein. There is a single report of an acquired functionally defective AT3 in spite of normal concentrations by immunochemical methods. Individuals heterozygous for the deficiency possess circulating AT3 levels 25 to 50 per cent of normal for immunochemical AT3 and 60 to 70 per cent of normal for functional AT3 and are at risk for deep vein thrombosis and pulmonary emboli. Homozygous AT3 deficiency has not been identified, suggesting that the defect is "lethal."

Expression of the defect has not been observed at less than 10 years of age, and individuals with low AT3 levels may never experience thromboses (von Kaulla, 1967). The incidence of the deficiency in Scandinavian and Boston populations is 1:2000. The prevalence in thrombotic disorders is estimated to be as high as 2 per cent.

Physiology. Individuals suffering from severe hepatic disorders such as cirrhosis or acute hepatitis have significantly depressed AT3 levels, while diseases accompanied by inflammation may show elevations. Serum levels are markedly depressed as the result of protein-losing syndromes, particularly in the protein-losing nephropathies (Kauffmann, 1976). The molecular weight of AT3 is approximately that of albumin.

The protein's primary function is to inactivate the proteolytic enzyme thrombin, preventing uncontrolled polymerization of fibrinogen and clot formation. Plasma levels of 50 per cent or less of reference values predispose to thrombosis. AT3 also functions to inhibit activated proteases such as coagulation factors IX, X, XI, and XII. The gradual inhibition of thrombin by AT3 is enhanced to almost instant neutralization by the presence of heparin. Heparin binds to AT3 at specialized lysine groups activating antithrombin activity.

Disorders such as the diffuse intravascular coagulation syndrome, in which proteases such as plasmin and thrombin are rapidly gener-ated, may markedly deplete AT3 levels (Chap. 33). Platelet lysis releases the AT3 inhibiting substance platelet Factor IV. In both conditions, heparin is incapable of controlling thrombus formation. Management requires attention to underlying disease, as well as the availability of AT3 from fresh plasma coupled with heparin to restore a new balance (Chap. 33).

Analysis. Antithrombin III levels can readily be analyzed immunochemically. RID, EID, and nephelometric methods have been described (Sas, 1975) in both serum or plasma. However, specimens that have been defibrinated with thrombin should not be used.

Many assays for AT3 function have been described. Some, based upon the progressive neutralization of thrombin by test plasma, are commercially available.

Haptoglobin (Hpt) (Putnam, 1975b)

Hemoglobin in the circulation can cause a variety of difficulties, particularly when release is coincident with other pathologic processes. The glycoprotein haptoglobin binds firmly and, under physiologic conditions, irreversibly with hemoglobin and results in its prompt removal by the reticuloendothelial system instead of its being lost via the kidney.

Concentration. At birth, and for up to several weeks after, little or no haptoglobin can be found by the usual immunochemical assays. When the protein is found in cord blood, it is often the result of maternal blood contaminating the sample, although values up to 1 g/l can be found in neonates suffering from infection acquired *in utero*. Within a few days of birth, haptoglobin appears in the circulation of the normal full-term infant. Values in infants and children are generally lower than those found in the adult.

Genetics (Giblett, 1969). Both qualitative and quantitative variants of haptoglobin have been well studied. Haptoglobins are separated into two major types, Hp 1 and Hp 2, and three major phenotypic variants, 1-1, 2-1, and 2-2. Rare genetic variants include anhaptoglobinemia, designated Hp 0. Anhaptoglobinemia is found in 3 to 5 per cent of American children and black adults. Sickle trait or other hemoglobinopathies could be responsible for the deficiency in blacks, but data have not supported this. Extensive population studies have shown that in western countries, the incidence of Hp 1:Hp 2 is approximately 1:2.

The ratio shifts to 1:4 for peoples from Southeast Asia and to 1:1 in Central and South American natives (Chap. 44).

Physiology. Haptoglobin is produced mainly by hepatocytes, with small amounts also produced in tissue cultures of reticuloendothelial (RE) tissues of the spleen, thymus, and lymph nodes. The rate of synthesis is transiently stimulated by inflammatory stimuli, resulting in increased circulating haptoglobin levels. The substances responsible for such stimulation are not known but are frequently and most dramatically associated with tissue necrosis. Values five to eight times normal are seen in malignancy, particularly when there are areas of necrosis, e.g., hypernephroma (McPhedran, 1972). Patients with extensive tissue damage from burns, abscess, and certain infections such as tuberculosis also may have enormous elevations of the protein.

Any process which damages blood cells, allowing hemoglobin to be released, can lower the level of haptoglobin. During sports, particularly contact sports, any part of the body can be subjected to blows, exaggerating the normal process of hemolysis. For this reason, caution must be exercised in interpreting low haptoglobin values in children.

Hypohaptoglobinemia frequently accompanies diseases complicated by severe liver involvement. Implantation of artificial heart valves always produces hypohaptoglobinemia through mechanical damage. Endothelial verrucae also mechanically damage red blood cells through turbulence, but subacute bacterial endocarditis can nevertheless produce extraordinary increases in haptoglobin levels, presumably when mechanical red cell damage is minimal.

Haptoglobin's primary function is to bind with hemoglobin, thus initiating removal from the circulation by the reticuloendothelial (RE) system. This being the case, individuals deficient for the protein should be subject to disorders associated with circulating hemoglobin. This apparently is not the case. Furthermore, calculations based upon the hemoglobin-binding capacity of the total haptoglobin mass indicate that only a portion of hemoglobin processed by the reticuloendothelial system can arrive complexed with haptoglobin. Free hemoglobin is rapidly picked up by the RE cell, but a small fraction may also be excreted in the urine. The haptoglobin-hemoglobin complex prevents significant loss of iron by preventing urinary hemoglobin excretion. How anhaptoglobinemic individuals conserve iron well remains unanswered.

Analysis. The variability of molecular weight found in haptoglobins from normal individuals seriously compromises passive gel diffusion forms of analysis. All passive diffusion methods require that the type of haptoglobin phenotype be known and a conversion factor be included in the calculation. Electroimmunoassay and light-scattering techniques are not significantly affected by this variable and, therefore, yield appropriate values.

Alpha₂-macroglobulin (α_2M)

Synonyms. Alpha₂-antiplasmin, alpha₂-trypsin binding globulin.

This large protein has been implicated in hormonal transport, but at present its only well-defined biologic function is inhibition of proteolytic enzymes.

Concentration. The range seen in the general population is very wide. For an individual, however, the excursion seen during adult life is rather narrow, complicating clinical interpretation of the serum values. This may be in part responsible for the paucity of clinical information available. Values are high in newborns and rise during childhood to become one of the principal plasma protein constituents. At puberty, values fall in an unpredictable fashion. Some teenagers develop adult values by 15 years of age; others at 22 may still retain childhood levels.

Alpha₂-macroglobulin is one of the few plasma proteins whose levels are affected by gender; levels are considerably higher in adult females than in adult males. Children have values far above those of adults of both sexes, but independent of sex, suggesting that high levels are suppressed by the development of either class of sex hormones—testosterone being more effective than progesterone.

Paradoxically, contraceptive medications or a developing pregnancy increase serum levels approximately 20 per cent. However, because of the extremely wide distribution of values in the population, explanation of a given value for an individual woman is often not possible.

Genetics. Based upon studies in lower animals, polymorphism of human α_2M is believed to exist. In human studies, the complexing of α_2M with substrate alters the electrophoretic mobility slightly, making predictable phenotypic patterns difficult to obtain.

Physiology. Hepatocytes synthesize the protein even in the early fetus. Because of the protein's large size, it is found primarily in the intravascular spaces, but lower levels can also be found in various body fluids such as the cerebrospinal and synovial fluids. Its presence at concentrations above 30 to 50 per cent of serum levels in these spaces suggests major leakage as a result of disturbed membranes (Chap. 18). The protein is known to be labile, reducing to subunits that conceivably could be responsible for the immunoreactive α_2M found in normal cerebrospinal and synovial fluids and urine.

As a protease inhibitor, α_2M is second only to alpha$_1$-antitrypsin. However, unlike α_1AT, its complex is rapidly removed by the reticuloendothelial system. The binding appears to be irreversible, initiated by the protease enzymatic attack on α_2M itself. Conformational changes then occur to entangle the protease. Trypsin, alpha-chymotrypsin, thrombin, plasmin, and kallikrein are effectively inhibited.

As noted above, hormonal shifts during normal maturation, pregnancy, and contraceptive management affect serum α_2M concentration. Serum levels are generally unaffected by most diseases; however, during processes that affect the glomerular filtration membrane, dramatic changes may occur. During, and for sometime after, resolution of the nephrotic syndrome, α_2M levels may reach remarkably high values. Levels of three to eight times normal have been observed during classic nephrotic syndrome in children and in an isolated instance, a level of 15 g/l was seen in a case of membranoproliferative glomerulonephritis in which the total serum protein was 32 g/l (3.2 g/dl), the balance having been made up of IgM and other very large molecules.

Analysis. Few problems have been encountered in the analysis of this protein. Concern has been voiced relating to its lability and possible disassociation in body fluids other than serum. The analyses being performed today are infrequent enough that perhaps problems are, as yet, not recognized. To my knowledge, in serum and plasma at least, gel diffusion and nephelometric methods of analysis are satisfactory.

Fibrinogen (Doolittle, 1975)

Synonyms. Clotting Factor I.
One of the major plasma proteins, fibrinogen is not present in any form in normal serum. This unusual, elongated protein, visible by electron microscopy, is the precursor of the fibrin clot and is also a sensitive indicator of inflammation. It plays a key role in the erythrocyte sedimentation rate.

Concentration. Present at all times of life, its values change little in healthy individuals. Although several workers suspected that fetal fibrinogen was a different molecule from that found in the adult, careful analysis of fibrinogen from the two sources has indicated that they are apparently identical. Fibrinogen levels are elevated during pregnancy and the pseudopregnancy of contraceptive medications.

Genetics. Although instances are rare, many different, inheritable variations of fibrinogen have been identified (Mammen, 1976; Menache, 1973). Most of the dysfibrinogenemic patients studied have little in the way of coagulation disorders and often have been detected only by chance to have a prolonged thrombin time in the face of a normal fibrinogen level (Chap. 33). This in itself presents a problem in clinical studies, making the population incidence indefinable. It is believed that the defects involve primarily abnormalities in the fibrinogen molecule, interfering with polymerization of fibrin monomer after interaction with thrombin. Immunochemical studies have not identified molecular differences, but electrophoretic differences have been seen.

Complete deficiency of fibrinogen or true afibrinogenemia can be detected immunochemically or functionally. In either case, familial instances of the disorders have been described.

Physiology. The liver produces fibrinogen in its final form. Production can be accelerated by hormones and by the development of an inflammatory process. Hence, fibrinogen has been considered a prominent acute phase reactant. The stimulus to release fibrinogen from within the hepatocyte has not been identified. Values may reach extreme levels in disorders such as membranoproliferative glomerulonephritis, in which prolonged massive proteinuria of small molecular species occurs. Levels as high as 15 g/l have been observed.

The polymerization of soluble "dimeric" fibrinogen to the insoluble fibrillar protein fibrin is the basis for hemostasis. Without adequate amounts of functional fibrinogen, clotting fails. Fibrinogen, described by many workers as a metastable protein on the brink of instability, converts to the thoroughly stable protein fibrin through a series of minor changes. The enzymatic attack of thrombin upon fibrinogen results in the release of two small peptides, A and B. Dissociation of peptide A and less so of peptide B leads to the interconnection of molecules to form a long intermediate polymer, several of which associate in parallel to form a fibril. Branching of fibrils in the presence of Factor XIII and calcium forms the tough, resilient network of clot. Further stabilization occurs through cross-linkages between chains, resulting in clot retraction or syneresis. The impermanence of the clot *in vivo* indicates that a mechanism for its dissolution is present (Pechet, 1965). Plasmin, a potent proteolytic enzyme, efficiently cleaves and dissociates the fibrin polymer, releasing "split products" of varying molecular sizes. Under ordinary circumstances, the formation and lysis of fibrin produces low levels of "split products." As fibrinolysis accelerates in certain disease states, these fragments become detectable in serum and urine by relatively insensitive methods.

Analysis. Normal fibrinogen has for years been assayed by its functional ability to form a clot or to alter the physical or optical characteristics of a fluid medium. These assays fail to detect unclottable fibrinogen or fibrin split products. Fibrinogen antisera will detect clottable and unclottable fibrinogen as well as fibrin split products, giving no indication of functional ability. Antisera have also been prepared that are believed to recognize only fibrinogen degradation products. Peptides A and B, while antigenic, require radioimmunoassay for detection, since their molecular weights are too low to permit precipitation by gel methods. Fibrinogen and its degradation products can be readily analyzed by gel diffusion and light-scattering methods. Care must be taken in the preparation of the specimen to account for the possibility of cold precipitable fibrinogen. Electrophoresis also is useful in detecting fibrinogen in plasma, since the protein migrates as a distinct band. Unfortunately, plasma cannot be recommended for routine electrophoresis, since the well-resolved beta band of fibrinogen occurs in the electrophoretic region where monoclonal proteins will be found.

Plasminogen

Synonym. Profibrinolysin.

Once formed within the body, fibrin must be removed, either to re-establish blood flow or to allow regrowth of new tissues. Plasmin, the active proteolytic enzyme derived from circulating plasminogen, is responsible.

Concentration. Produced by the fetus in the first trimester of pregnancy, plasminogen levels are close to adult levels at birth (Gitlin, 1969). Serum plasminogen levels rise during pregnancy (Lackner, 1973). Contraceptive medications also increase serum levels, although there had been some disagreement about this in earlier studies.

Genetics. While there has been no clear evidence of the mode of genetic inheritance for plasminogen, several workers have shown that there is electrophoretic polymorphism and multiple banding of purified preparations; several different molecular forms have been described.

Physiology. Plasminogen is the circulating proenzyme from which the fibrinolytic molecule, plasmin, is derived. The inactive protein can be converted to the enzymatically effective form by several endogenous activators found in many tissues, particularly within the vascular walls, and in the urinary tract, where the activator is specifically referred to as urokinase. Kallikrein also appears to induce plasminogen activation. Exogenous substances such as streptokinase are also potent activators of plasminogen. Selective cleavage of plasminogen results in the production of the active proteolytic enzyme. Endogenous and exogenous inhibitors of plasmin are known and act to control plasmin-induced fibrinolysis (Beattie, 1976). In blood, plasmin is largely inhibited by the protease inhibitors $alpha_1$-antitrypsin and $alpha_2$-macroglobulin, and to a lesser degree by antithrombin III, Cl-inhibitor, and $alpha_2$-antiplasmin, a protein distinct from $alpha_2$-macroglobulin. Plasmin cleaves fibrin into low molecular weight fragments no longer capable of repolymerizing and, if uninhibited, may produce bleeding disorders such as occur in prostate and thoracic surgery, obstetrical complications, and leukemia. Plasminogen recently has been successfully used therapeutically to ameliorate the course of respiratory distress syndrome (Ambrus, 1977).

Analysis. A variety of methods for the analysis of plasmin have been described, including those which capitalize on its functional ability to degrade substances such as casein. The conversion from plasminogen to plasmin has negligible effects upon the immunochemical properties of the protein so that precautions to prevent the activation of plasminogen before analysis do not appear to be important. Plasminogen is an excellent antigen, and high quality antisera can therefore be produced for the assay.

C-reactive protein (CRP)

Initially believed to be a specific indicator of infection by the pneumococcus, this interesting protein has proved to be a non-specific responder to inflammation. It probably is the most sensitive acute phase protein (Chap. 54).

Concentration. CRP is normally present at very low levels (10 to 370 ng/ml) in the fetus and in all normal individuals (Claus, 1976). An elevated CRP level in cord blood has been considered evidence of intrauterine infection. CRP is not transported across the placenta, and maternal infection or inflammation, provided it does not also affect the fetus, does not increase CRP synthesis in the infant (Saxstad, 1970). The sex of the fetus apparently does not affect concentration.

CRP levels increase early in pregnancy, but are not sustained throughout gestation. Most contraceptive medications induce elevated CRP levels (Connell, 1971). Intrauterine devices increase CRP levels, with the change being more pronounced in instances of long use.

Genetics. Polymorphism of CRP has been observed in gel electrophoresis, but no definite inheritance pattern has been described.

Physiology. CRP synthesis can increase by three orders of magnitude during illness. Serum levels range from a low of 10 ng/ml in some cord bloods to 256,000 ng/ml in inflammatory states.

One of the actions identified with CRP has been its ability to bind to pneumococcal C-polysaccharide in the presence of calcium. In addition, the involvement of CRP in the immune mechanism has recently begun to emerge. It is now known to activate the classic complement pathway, to bind to and interfere with certain T-lymphocyte functions, and to inhibit clot retraction and platelet aggregation. In addition to sharing several functional characteristics with immunoglobulins, sequence studies of the CRP molecule show significant homology with IgG and with the amyloid P-component. It is, however, antigenically distinct when studied with immunologic techniques.

Analysis. Measurement of CRP has increasingly employed immunologic means, replacing tests utilizing the protein's reactivity with C-polysaccharide. The insensitive gel diffusion techniques have been the predominant method used. Consequently, most normal individuals have been considered to have no CRP in their circulation. With improved methods, CRP is found to be a normal constituent of plasma (Claus, 1976). A deficient individual has not yet been identified.

In well-resolved agarose electrophoresis, the gamma migrating CRP band is frequently visible in the serum of individuals with inflammatory processes. Under such circumstances, levels may be so high as to produce a distinct band easily misinterpreted as a monoclonal immunoglobulin.

COMPLEMENT PROTEINS (RUDDY, 1972; ALPER, 1974A AND B; POLLY, 1975; TUCKER, 1975)

Unlike other groups of proteins, the complement proteins are an orchestrated family with each member tied either functionally or antigenically to the others. In simplest terms, the complement proteins link the antigen-antibody reaction to the inflammatory response.

Several aspects of complement action require integrity of the entire sequence; others, once the system is activated, act independently. The lysis of bacteria or red blood cells requires the entire chain of C1-C9 (see Chap. 37). However, preparation of a bacterium for immune adherence and phagocytosis requires only the enzymatic cleavage of C3 to produce fixed C3b, a protein that can apparently act alone to stimulate phagocyte activity.

Complement activation occurs via two pathways: the classic and the alternative. Both have the same C3-C9 sequence but are initiated differently in the early phase, one being triggered by antibody, the other by a variety of intrinsic and extrinsic substances not involving antibody. In either case the key action of complement is amplification at each step with recruitment of other proteins and cellular elements.

The complement proteins also participate in the acute phase response, albeit to a modest degree in comparison with the more familiar acute phase proteins. Difficulty in interpreting complement protein assays quantitatively is compounded by their susceptibility to simultaneous stimulation of production and consumption. Furthermore, a normal immunochemical concentration does not rule out pathology, since the protein may be converted. For this reason, some workers perform the assay for total hemolytic complement along with immunochemical quantification. Complement components, their interactions, and methods of analysis are described in further detail in Chapter 37.

C1

Concentration. C1 and its subcomponents are produced early in gestation, with adult levels being reached at about the time of birth. No information is yet available about the effect of pregnancy or contraceptive medications on C1 synthesis.

Genetics. Each of the subcomponents has occasionally been found deficient in individual patients. C1r deficiency in siblings has been reported, but there is little other evidence to indicate a possible mode of inheritance (Marden, 1976; Moncada, 1972).

C1 inhibitor (C1INH) (Frank, 1976)

Synonyms. C1s-inhibitor, C1-inactivator, C1-esterase inhibitor, alpha$_2$-neuroaminoglycoprotein.

Perhaps the most dramatic disorder related to the proteins involved in the complement system is the life-threatening disorder called hereditary angioneurotic edema (HANE or HAE). Localized swelling, often following minimal trauma or emotional stress, can affect the skin, GI, or GU tract as well as the upper airway. The latter gives rise to obstruction, requiring prompt surgical intervention.

Concentration. The clinical syndrome of HANE is transmitted as an autosomal dominant trait, heterozygotes being affected. The homozygous deficiency state may represent a lethal condition. Variable genetic defects are suggested by the fact that 15 to 25 per cent of HANE patients have a functional deficiency of C1INH but normal or even supranormal serum concentrations.

Physiology. C1INH, normally produced in hepatocytes, cannot be demonstrated in liver tissue from genetically deficient individuals in spite of serum levels of 10 per cent of normal. Small amounts of the protein may be synthesized also in cells of the reticuloendothelium system and in fibroblasts.

The activation of C1 and the release of C1s can be accomplished by reaction with surface-bound antibody and by proteolytic factors such as plasmin or products of the clotting system such as Hageman factor. The action of C1s on its natural substrates C2 and C4 is normally held in check by the inhibitory effect of C1INH. Therefore, in patients deficient in functional C1INH, there will be activation of C2 and C4 with a local release of vasoactive peptides, believed to be responsible for the painless, usually non-pruritic, edema of HANE.

Analysis. C1INH can be analyzed functionally or immunochemically. The functional test is based upon the protein's ability to block the hydrolysis of N-acetyl-tyrosine ethyl ester by C1s. It is clear from the preceding discussion that the functional assay is important. Immunochemical analysis can be performed by gel diffusion, electroimmunoassay, immunoelectrophoresis, and nephelometry.

C4

Synonyms. C'4, beta$_{1e}$ globulin.

Numbered out of sequence in complement activation, C4 is actually the second step in the process. It has the second highest serum concentration of the nine complement proteins.

Physiology. In various pathologic states C4 levels may be extremely low, indicating activation of the classic complement pathway. Normal C4 levels in the presence of significantly depressed C3 levels suggest that the alternative pathway is active. In many instances, both classic and alternative pathways may be activated simultaneously. Because C4 may bind to particles in analytical samples such as chylomicrons, care should be taken to document, by more than one technique, low serum C4 levels. Markedly elevated values of C4 are occasionally observed in apparently healthy individuals. C4 levels increase in response to an acute inflammatory process, further complicating the interpretation of C4 values in the presence of immunologic diseases that may be accompanied by inflammation. It is, strictly speaking, an acute phase reactant in addition to being a complement protein.

C2

Concentration. Homozygous deficiency of C2 in several kindreds has been reported (Osterland, 1975; Kim, 1977). Heterozygotes have one half normal serum C2 levels. The prevalence of the recessive gene is of the order of 1 per cent in the population, predicting the incidence of the homozygous state as approximately 0.01 per cent. The HLA system and C2 have been reported to be genetically associated (Wolski, 1975).

Physiology. C2 is synthesized by monocytes in man and released into tissue spaces and into the circulation (Colten, 1972). Enzymatic cleavage of C2 by activated C1 in the presence of magnesium ion produces two products, C2a and C2b. This action can occur on cell surfaces, in proximity to bound antiody, and also in the fluid phase. C2a, combined with the previous complex of antibody and portions of C1 and C4, produces the complex C142a (or EAC142), also known as C3 convertase, that is rapidly inactivated unless C3 is available. The residue, C2b, has not been isolated and may be rapidly degraded by the further action of C1s.

C3

Synonyms. B_{1A}, $B_{1C'}$, C'3.
Of the large number of plasma proteins integral to the complement cascade, C3 is in highest concentration. Its relationship to disease and its biochemistry have been the most extensively studied. Although it is primarily a complement protein, it also is an acute phase reactant, a feature which demands care for adequate interpretation.

Concentration. Production in the fetus begins in the first trimester, and none is transported across the placenta. At birth, mean values in cord blood are about 50 per cent of those of the normal adult, attaining full concentration within a few weeks. Very little is known about the effect of pregnancy or contraceptive medications on C3 levels. One study suggests that a small increment occurs with withdrawal of contraceptive medications (Laurell, 1970).

Genetics (*Alper, 1974b*). Like many other plasma proteins, C3 exhibits genetic polymorphism, best demonstrated on prolonged electrophoresis in agarose gel. The two most common alleles are the S and F (slow and fast), inherited as an autosomal codominant trait. However, there are over 20 different alleles. These common variations appear to have no effect on health. The discovery of a kindred with almost complete deficiency of C3 indicates that absolute levels of C3 may be under genetic control and inherited as an autosomal recessive with expression also in the heterozygote.

Analysis. In agarose gel electrophoresis with Ca^{++} or Mg^{++} containing buffers, the band of native C3 can be clearly seen in the slow beta region, and if degradation occurs, a faster moving fraction becomes prominent near transferrin in the fast beta zone (see also Chap. 37).

Factor B (Alper, 1974a)

Synonyms. C3PA, C3 proactivator, GBG, beta$_2$-glycoprotein II.

The properdin system, of which Factor B is a prominent member, was identified years before its true role in alternative pathway complement activation was proved. For a long time its very existence was seriously questioned. Now that the alternative complement pathway has been defined, only Factor B has been found in sufficient concentration to warrant consideration in this chapter. Factor B, a glycine-rich beta-globulin (GBG), allows entry into the common sequence of complement activation from the alternative pathway.

Concentration. Levels in cord serum average 120 mg/l, rising to adult concentrations by three months of age. At the end of the third trimester, maternal serum levels peak at 420 mg/l.

Genetics. Factor B demonstrates genetically controlled polymorphism. The major types consist of F (fast) and S (slow), with several infrequent subtypes. F_1 occurs primarily in blacks and S_1 in Caucasians. The gene frequencies in blacks and whites are 0.437 and 0.709 for F and 0.512 and 0.278 for S, respectively. There appears to be no functional or clinical significance for the different phenotypes. Control of Factor B, C2, and C4 is closely linked to the major histocompatibility locus on the sixth chromosome in man.

Physiology. The major role of Factor B is the enzymatic cleavage of C3 to form C3a and C3b, analogous to the action of C42 in the classic pathway. Factor B itself is activated enzymatically by Factor D (GBGase, C3Pase) in the presence of magnesium ions and C3b to produce two fragments: Bb (glycine-rich gamma-glycoprotein, GGG), and Ba (glycine-rich alpha-glycoprotein, GAG).

Analysis. Factor B degrades to subunits about half as large as the native molecule, having major implications in gel-diffusion immunoanalysis. The alpha (GAG) and gamma (GGG) fractions can confuse the gel pattern when aged serum or plasma is examined. Assays performed in liquid, e.g., nephelometry, provide the most reliable quantitative measurement. After prolonged electrophoresis and immunofixation with antiserum to Factor B (GBG), breakdown products as well as molecular variants can be visualized. In immunoelectrophoresis, Factor B and its two major breakdown products will produce three distinct arcs.

The immunoglobulins are discussed in Chapters 36 and 42.

REFERENCES

Allen, R. C., Russell, A. H., and Talamo, R. C.: A new method for determination of alpha-1-antitrypsin phenotypes using isoelectric focusing on polyacrylamide gel slabs. Am. J. Clin. Pathol., *62*:732, 1974.

Alper, C. A.: Complement. *In* Allison, A. C. (ed.): Structure and Function of Plasma Proteins, I. New York, Plenum Publishing Corporation, 1974a.

Alper, C. A., and Johnson, A. M.: Immunofixation electrophoresis: Technique for the study of protein polymorphism. Vox. Sang., *17*:445, 1969.

Alper, C. A., and Propp, R. P.: Genetic polymorphism of the third component of human complement (C'3). J. Clin. Invest., *47*:2181, 1968.

Alper, C. A., and Rosen, F. S.: Genetics of the complement system. *In* Harris, H., and Hirshhorn, K. (eds.): Advances in Human Genetics. New York, Plenum Publishing Corporation, 1974b.

Al-Rashid, R. A., and Spangler, J.: Neonatal copper deficiency. N. Engl. J. Med., *285*:841, 1971.

Ambrus, C. M., Choi, T. S., Cunnanan, E., Eisenberg, B., Staub, H. P., Winetraub, D. H., Courey, N. G., Patterson, R. J., Jockin, H., Pickrin, J. W., Bross, I. D., Okhee, S. J., and Ambrus, J. L.: Prevention of hyaline membrane disease with plasminogen: A cooperative study. J.A.M.A., *237*:1837, 1977.

Anderson, R. J., and Sternberg, J. C.: A rate nephelometer for immunoprecipitin measurement of specific proteins. *In* Ritchie, R. F. (ed): Automated Immunoanalysis. New York, Marcel Dekker, Inc., 1978.

Axelsen, N. H. (ed.): Quantitative immunoelectrophoresis. New developments and applications. Scand. J. Immunol., *4*:Suppl. 2, 1975.

Axelsen, N. H., Kroll, J., and Weeke, B. (eds.): A manual of quantitative immunoelectrophoresis. Methods and applications. Scand. J. Immunol., *2*:Suppl. 1, 1973.

Beattie, A. G., Ogston, D., Bennett, B., and Douglas, A. S.: Inhibitors of plasminogen activation in human blood. Br. J. Haematol., *32*:135, 1976.

Bjerrum, O. J., Ingild, A., Lowenstein, H., and Weeke, B.: carbamylated antibodies used for quantitation of human IgG. A routine method. Scand. J. Immunol., *2* (Suppl. 1): 145, 1973.

Boyden, A., Bolton, E., and Gemeroy, D.: Precipitin testing with special reference to the photoelectric measurement of turbidity. J. Immunol., *57*:211, 1947.

Boyer, IV, S. H.: Proteins, evolution and disease. Am. J. Med., *36*:337, 1964.

Bretzel, G., and Hochstrasser, K.: Liberation of an acid stable proteinase inhibitor from the human inter-alpha-trypsin inhibitor by the action of kallikrein. Hoppe-Seyler's Z. Physiol. Chem., *357*:487, 1976.

Burrows, S., and Pekala, B.: Serum copper and ceruloplasmin in pregnancy. Am. J. Obstet. Gynecol., *109*:907, 1971.

Carvalho, A., and Ellman, L.: Hereditary antithrombin III deficiency. Effect of antithrombin deficiency on platelet function. Am. J. Med., *61*:179, 1976.

Claus, D. R., Osmand, A. P., and Gewurz, H.: Radioimmunoassay of human C-reactive protein and levels in normal sera. J. Lab. Clin. Med., *87*:120, 1976.

Colten, H. R., and Frank, M. M.: Biosynthesis of the second (C2) and fourth (C4) components of complement in vitro by tissues isolated from guinea-pigs with genetically determined C4 deficiency. Immunology, *22*:991, 1972.

Connell, E. B., and Connell, J. T.: C-reactive protein in pregnancy and contraception. Am. J. Obstet. Gynecol., *110*:633, 1971.

Crowle, A. J. (ed.): Immunodiffusion, 2nd ed. New York,

Academic Press, Inc., 1973.

Daiger, S. P., Schanfield, M. S., and Cavalli-Sforza, L. L.: Group-specific component (Gc) proteins bind vitamin D and 25-hydroxy-vitamin D. Proc. Natl. Acad. Sc. U.S.A., *72*:2076, 1975.

Daigneault, R., and Vernet-Nyssen, M.: Transferrin. *In* Ritchie, R. F. (ed.): Automated Immunoanalysis, New York, Marcel Dekker, Inc., 1978, p. 253.

Daniels, J. C., Larson, D. L., Abston, S., and Ritzmann, S. E.: Serum protein profiles in thermal burns. II. Protease inhibitors, complement factors and C-reactive proteins. J. Trauma, *14*:153, 1974.

Doe, R. P., Mellinger, G. T., Swaim, W. R., and Seal, U. S.: Estrogen dosage effects on serum proteins. J. Clin. Endocrinol., *27*:1081, 1967.

Doolittle, R. F.: Fibrinogen and fibrin. *In* Putnam, F. W. (ed.): The Plasma Proteins, vol. II, 2nd ed. New York, Academic Press, Inc., 1975, p. 110.

Eriksson, S.: Studies in alpha₁-antitrypsin deficiency. Acta Med. Scand., *177*:Suppl. 432, 1965.

Fahey, J. L., and McKelvey, E. M.: Quantitative determination of serum immunoglobulins in antibody-agar plates. J. Immunol., *94*:84, 1965.

Feinberg, J. G.: Identification, discrimination and quantification in Ouchlterlony gel plates. Intern. Arch. Allerg. *11*:129, 1957.

Fisher, C. L., Gill, C., Forrester, M. G., and Nakamura, R.: Quantitation of "acute phase proteins" postoperatively. Value in detection and monitoring of complications. Am. J. Clin. Pathol., *66*:840, 1976.

Frank, M. M., Gelfand, J. A., and Atkinson, J. P.: Hereditary angioedema: The clinical syndrome and its management. Ann. Intern. Med., *84*:580, 1976.

Giblett, E. R. (ed.): Genetic Markers in Human Blood. Oxford, Blackwell Scientific, 1969.

Gitlin, D., and Biacacci, A.: Development of -G, -A, -M Bic/Bia, C'1 esterase inhibitor, ceruloplasmin, transferrin, hemopexin, haptoglobin, fibrinogen, plasminogen α₁-antitrypsin, orosomucoid, b-lipoprotein, α₂-macroglobulin, and prealbumin in the human conceptus. J. Clin. Invest., *48*:1433, 1969.

Gitlin, D., and Gitlin, J. D.: Genetic alterations in the plasma proteins of man. *In* Putnam, F. W. (ed.): The Plasma Proteins, vol. II, 2nd ed. New York, Academic Press, Inc., 1975, p. 321.

Good, W.: Maternal serum sialomucins during pregnancy and post-partum in patients with pre-eclampsia. Br. J. Obstet. Gynaecol., *82*:907, 1975.

Grabar, P., and Williams, Jr., C. A.: Méthode permettant l'étude conjuguée des propriétés électrophoretiques et immunochemiques d'un mélange de proteines. Application au sérum sanguin. Biochim. Biophys. Acta, *10*:19, 1953.

Haschemeyer, R. H., and Haschemeyer, E. V. (eds.): Proteins. A Guide to Study by Physical and Chemical Methods. New York, John Wiley & Sons, Inc., 1973.

Hellsing, K.: Enhancing effects of nonionic polymers on immunochemical reactions. *In* Ritchie, R. F. (ed): Automated Immunoanalysis. New York, Marcel Dekker, 1978, p. 67.

Herriott, R. M.: Reaction of Folin's reagent with proteins and biuret compounds in the presence of cupric ions. Proc. Soc. Exper. Biol. Med., *46*:642, 1941.

Hochstrasser, K., Bretzel, G., Feuth, H., Hilla, W., and Lempart, K.: The inter-alpha-trypsin inhibitor as precursor of the acid-stable proteinase inhibitors in human serum and urine. Hoppe-Seyler's Z. Physiol. Chem. *357*:153, 1976.

Horne, C. H. W., Weir, R. J., Howie, P. W., and Goudie,

R. B.: Effect of combined oestrogen-progestogen oral contraceptives on serum levels of α_2-macroglobulin, transferrin, albumin and IgG. Lancet, *1*:49, 1970.

Innerfield, I., Stone, M. L., Mersheimer, W., Clauss, R. D., and Greenberg, J.: Antithrombin and heparin antithrombin patterns in pre-thrombosis and thrombosis. Am. J. Clin. Pathol., *65*:384, 1976.

Jacobs, S.: The determination of nitrogen in biological materials. Meth. Biochem. Anal., *13*:241, 1965.

Johnson, A. M.: Genetic typing of alpha$_1$-antitrypsin by immunofixation electrophoresis. Identification of subtype Pi M. J. Lab. Clin. Med., *87*:152, 1976.

Johnson, A. M., Cleve, H., and Alper, C.: Variants of the group-specific component system as demonstrated by immunofixation electrophoresis. Report of a new variant, Gc Boston (GcB). Am. J. Hum. Genet., *27*:728, 1975.

Kabat, E. A., and Mayer, M. M.: Experimental Immunochemistry. Springfield, Ill., Charles C Thomas, Publisher, 1974.

Kahan, J., and Sundblad, L.: Immunochemical determination of beta-lipoproteins. Scand. J. Clin. Lab. Invest., *24*:61, 1969.

Kauffmann, R. H., De Graff, J., De La Riviere, G. B., and Van Es, L. A.: Unilateral renal vein thrombosis and nephrotic syndrome. Report of a case with protein selectivity and antithrombin III clearance studies. Am. J. Med., *60*:1048, 1976.

Kim, Y., Friend, P. S., Dresner, I. G., Yunis, E. J., and Michael, A. F.: Inherited deficiency of the second component of complement (C2) with membranoproliferative glomerulonephritis. Am. J. Med., *62*:765, 1977.

Klein, R., and Haddow, J. E.: Trace elements in health and disease. Practitioner, *201*:314, 1968.

Kosaka, S., and Tazawa, M.: α_1-antichymotrypsin in rheumatoid arthritis. Tohoku J. Exp. Med., *119*:369, 1976.

Kusnetz, J., and Mansberg, H. P.: Optical considerations: Nephelometry. *In* Ritchie, R. F. (ed): Automated Immunoanalysis. New York, Marcel Dekker, Inc., 1978.

Lackner, H., and Javid, J. P.: The clinical significance of the plasminogen level. Am. J. Clin. Pathol., *59*:175, 1973.

Laurell, C.-B.: Electrophoresis, specific protein assays, or both in measurement of plasma proteins? Clin. Chem., *19*:99, 1973.

Laurell, C.-B.: Quantitative estimation of proteins by electrophoresis in agarose gel containing antibodies. Anal. Biochem., *15*:45, 1966.

Laurell, C.-B., and Jeppsson, J.-O.: Protease inhibitors in plasma. *In* Putnam, F. W., (ed.): The Plasma Proteins, vol. I, 2nd ed. New York, Academic Press, Inc., 1975, p. 229.

Laurell, C.-B., Kullander, S., and Thorell, J.: Rate of plasma protein normalization after parturition and withdrawal of oral contraceptives. Scand. J. Clin. Lab. Invest., *26*:345, 1970.

Lieberman, J., Mittman, C., and Kent, J. R.: Screening for heterozygous α_1-antitrypsin deficiency. III. A provocative test with diethylstilbesterol and effect of oral contraceptives. J.A.M.A., *217*:1198, 1971.

Lowry, O. H., Rosebrough, N. J., Farr, L., and Randall, R. J.: Protein measurement with Folin phenol reagent. J. Biol. Chem., *193*:265, 1951.

Mammen, E. F.: Congenital dysfibrinogenemias: Molecular abnormalities of fibrinogen. Blut, *33*:229, 1976.

Mancini, G., Vaerman, J.-P., Carbonara, A. O., and Heremans, J. F.: A single-radial-diffusion method for the immunological quantitation of proteins. Protides. Biol. Fluids, Proc. Colloq., *11*:370, 1964.

Marden, R. J., Rent, R., Choi, E. Y. C., and Gewurz, H.: C1$_q$ deficiency associated with urticarial-like lesions and cutaneous vasculitis. Am. J. Med., *61*:560, 1976.

McFarlane, H., Reddy, S., Adcock, K. J., Adeshina, H., Cooke, A. R., and Akene, J.: Immunity, transferrin, and survival in kwashiorkor. Br. Med. J., *4*:268, 1970.

McPhedran, P., Finch, S. C., Nemerson, Y. R., and Barnes, M. G.: Alpha-2 globulin "spike" in renal carcinoma. Ann. Intern. Med., *76*:439, 1972.

Menache, D.: Abnormal fibrinogens: A review. Thromb. Diath. Haemorrh., *29*:525, 1973.

Mendenhall, H. W.: Serum protein concentrations in pregnancy. I. Concentrations in maternal serum. Am. J. Obstet. Gynecol., *106*:388, 1970.

Milford-Ward, A., Cooper, E. H., Turner, R., Anderson, J. A., and Neville, A. M.: Acute-phase reactant protein profiles: An aid to monitoring large bowel cancer by CEA and serum enzymes. Br. J. Cancer, *35*:170, 1977.

Mittman, C. (ed.): Pulmonary Emphysema and Proteolysis. New York, Academic Press, Inc., 1972.

Moncada, B., Day, N. K. B., Good, R. A., and Windhorst, D. B.: Lupus-erythematosus-like syndrome with a familial defect of complement. N. Engl. J. Med., *286*:689, 1972.

Muller-Eberhard, U.: Hemopexin. N. Engl. J. Med., *283*:1090, 1970.

Musumeci, V., Vincenti, A., and Bizzi, B.: A method for the differential determination of plasma antithrombins. J. Clin. Pathol., *29*:63, 1976.

Nilsson, S. F., Rask, L., and Peterson, P. A.: Studies on thyroid hormone-binding proteins. II. Binding of thyroid hormones, retinol-binding protein, and fluorescent probes to prealbumin and effects of thyroxin on prealbumin subunit self-association. J. Biol. Chem., *250*:8554, 1975.

Oppenheimer, J. H.: Role of plasma proteins in the binding, distribution and metabolism of the thyroid hormones. N. Engl. J. Med., *278*:1153, 1968.

Osterland, C. K., Espinoza, L., Parker, L. P., and Schur, P. H.: Inherited C2 deficiency and systemic lupus erythematosus: Studies on a family. Ann. Intern. Med., *82*:323, 1975.

Pechet, L.: Fibrinolysis. N. Engl. J. Med., *273*:966, 1965.

Peters, T., Jr.: Serum albumin. Adv. Clin. Chem., *13*:37, 1970.

Peters, T., Jr.: Serum albumin. *In* Putnam, F. W. (ed): The Plasma Proteins, vol. I, 2nd ed. New York, Academic Press, Inc., 1975, p. 133.

Peterson, P. A.: Studies on interaction between prealbumin, retinol-binding protein and vitamin A. J. Biol. Chem., *246*:44, 1971.

Peterson, R. A., Krull, P. E., Finley, P., and Ettinger, M. G.: Changes in antithrombin III and plasminogen induced by oral contraceptives. Am. J. Clin. Pathol., *53*:468, 1970.

Polley, M. J., and Bearn, A. G.: Genetics of diseases of complement: An explosion. Am. J. Med., *58*:105, 1975.

Putnam, F. W.: Perspectives—Past, present and future. *In* Putnam, F. W. (ed): The Plasma Proteins, vol. I, 2nd ed. New York, Academic Press, Inc., 1975a.

Putnam, F. W.: Haptoglobin. *In* Putnam, F. W. (ed.): The Plasma Proteins, vol. II, 2nd ed. New York, Academic Press, Inc. 1975b.

Putnam, F. W.: Transferrin. *In* Putnam, F. W. (ed.): The Plasma Proteins, vol. I, 2nd ed. New York, Academic Press, Inc., 1975c.

Rask, L., and Peterson, P. A.: Structure and function of the retinol binding protein: A protein characteristic of tubular proteinuria. Protides Biol. Fluids, *21*:485, 1973.

Reimer, C. B., Smith, S. J., Hannon, W. H., Ritchie, R. F., Van Es, L., Becker, W., Markowitz, H., Gauldie, J., and Anderson, S. G.: Progress toward international reference standards for human proteins. J. Biol. Stand., 1978, in press.

Renn, D. W., and Evans, E.: A rapid electroimmunoassay system. Anal. Biochem., *71*:588, 1976.

Renn, D. W., and Evans, E.: Use of heteropolyacids as immunological precipitin brighteners. Anal. Biochem., *64*:620, 1975.

Riegal, C., and Thomas, D.: Absence of beta-globulin

fraction in serum protein of patient with unexplained anemia. N. Engl. J. Med., *255*:434, 1956.

Ritchie, R. F.: A simple, direct, and sensitive technique for measurement of specific protein in dilute solution. J. Lab. Clin. Med., *70*:512, 1967.

Ritchie, R. F.: Automated immunoprecipitation analysis of serum proteins. *In* Putnam, F. W. (ed): The Plasma Proteins, vol. II, 2nd ed. New York, Academic Press, Inc., 1975, p. 376.

Ritchie, R. F.: Nephelometric analysis. *In* Rose, N., and Bigazzi, P. E. (eds.): Methods in Immunodiagnosis, 2nd ed. New York, John Wiley & Sons, Inc. 1978, in press.

Ritchie, R. F., and Smith, R.: Immunofixation. I. General principles and application to agarose gel electrophoresis. Clin. Chem., *22*:497, 1976.

Ritchie, R. F., Alper, C. A., and Graves, J. A.: Experience with a fully automated system for immunoassay of specific proteins. Arthritis Rheum., *12*:693, 1969.

Ritzmann, S. E., and Daniels, J. C. (eds.): Serum Protein Abnormalities. Diagnostic and Clinical Aspects. Boston, Little, Brown, and Co., 1975.

Roeser, H. P., Lee, G. R., Nacht, S., and Cartwright, G. E.: The role of ceruloplasmin in iron metabolism. J. Clin. Invest., *49*:2408, 1970.

Rosenburg, R. D.: Actions and interactions of antithrombin and heparin. N. Engl. J. Med., *292*:146, 1975.

Rothschild, M. A., Oratz, M., and Schreiber, S. S.: Albumin synthesis. N. Engl. J. Med., *286*:748, 816, 1972.

Ruddy, S., Gigli, I., and Austen, K. F.: The complement system of man. N. Engl. J. Med., *287*:489, 1972.

Saraya, A. K., Tandon, B. N., and Ramachandran, K.: A study of iron and protein deficiency in hookworm infestation. Indian J. Med. Res., *58*:1234, 1970.

Sas, G., Pepper, D. S., and Cash, J. D.: Investigations on antithrombin III in normal plasma and serum. Br. J. Haematol., *30*:265, 1975.

Savory, J., Buffone, G. J., and Reich, R.: Kinetics of the IgG–anti-IgG reaction, as evaluated by conventional and stopped-flow nephelometry. Clin. Chem., *20*:1071, 1974.

Saxstad, J., Nilsson, L.-A., and Hanson, L. A.: C-Reactive protein in serum from infants as determined with immunodiffusion techniques. Acta Paediatr. Scand., *59*:676, 1970.

Schenker, J. G., Jungreis, E., and Polishuk, W. Z.: Oral contraceptives and serum copper concentration. Obstet. Gynecol., *37*:233, 1971.

Schmid, K.: a_1-acid glycoprotein. *In* Putnam, F. W. (ed.): The Plasma Proteins, vol. I, 2nd ed. New York, Academic Press, Inc., 1975.

Schultze, H. E., and Heremans, J. F. (eds.): Molecular Biology of Human Proteins. Amsterdam, Elsevier, 1966, p. 568.

Schultze, H. E., and Schwick, G.: Quantitative Immunologische von Plasmaproteinen. Clin. Chim. Acta, *4*:15, 1959.

Slater, L., Carter, P. M., and Hobbs, J. R.: Measurement of albumin in the sera of patients. Ann. Clin. Biochem., *12*:33, 1975.

Slater, L.: Albumin. *In* Ritchie, R. F. (ed): Automated Immunoanalysis. New York, Marcel Dekker, Inc., 1978.

Song, C. S., Merkatz, I. R., Rifkind, A. B., Gillette, P. N., and Kappas, A.: The influence of pregnancy and oral contraceptive steroids on the concentration of plasma proteins. Studies with a quantitative immunodiffusion method. Am. J. Obstet. Gynecol., *108*:227, 1970.

Steinbuch, M., Audran, R., Lambin, P., and Fine, J. M.: New data concerning inter-alpha-trypsin inhibitor. Protides Biol. Fluids, *23*:115, 1975.

Sternlieb, I., and Scheinberg, H. I.: Presentation of Wil-

son's disease in asymptomatic patients. N. Engl. J. Med., *278*:352, 1968.

Sveger, T., Laurell, C.-B., and Ljunggren, C.-G.: a_1-antitrypsin deficiency: Pi genotype ZO, SO and MO. Protides Biol. Fluids, *22*:501, 1974.

Sveger, T., and Ekelund, H.: Variations of protease inhibitors in foetuses, newborn infants and in some neonatal disorders. Acta Paediatr. Scand., *64*:763, 1975.

Talamo, R. C., Bruce, R. M., Langley, C. E., Berninger, R. W., Brant, L. J., Duncan, D. B., and Pierce, J. A.: Alpha$_1$-antitrypsin Laboratory Manual, National Heart and Lung Institute, in press.

Talamo, R. C., Langley, C. E., and Reed, C. E.: a_1-Antitrypsin deficiency: A variant with no detectable a_1-antitrypsin. Science, *181*:70, 1973.

Toporek, M.: Effects of whole blood or albumin fraction from tumor bearing rats on liver protein synthesis. Cancer Res., *33*:2579, 1973.

Troll, W., and Cannan, R. K.: Modified photometric Ninhydrin method for analysis of amino and imino acids. J. Biol. Chem., *200*:803, 1953.

Tucker, E. S., and Nakamura, R. M.: Abnormalities of the complement system. *In* Ritzmann, S. E., and Daniels, J. C., (eds.): Serum Protein Abnormalities. Diagnostic and Clinical Aspects. Boston, Little, Brown and Co., 1975, p. 265.

Twining, S. S., and Brecher, A. S.: Identification of a_1-acid glycoprotein, a_2-macroglobulin and antithrombin III as components of normal and malignant human tissues. Clin. Chim. Acta, *75*:143, 1977.

Viau, M., Gouaillard, C., Bouissou, C., and Constans, J.: A practical method for immunofixation in acrylamide gel. Anal. Biochem., 1978, in press.

von Kaulla, E., and von Kaulla, K. N.: Antithrombin III and diseases. Am. J. Clin. Pathol., *48*:69, 1967.

van Oss, C. J., Bronson, P. M., and Border, J. R.: Changes in the serum alpha glycoprotein distribution in trauma patients. J. Trauma, *15*:451, 1975.

Walbaum, R.: Déficit congénital en transférrine. Lille Med., *16*:1122, 1971.

Waldmann, T. A., Gordon, R. S., and Rosse, W.: Studies on the metabolism of the serum proteins and lipids in patients with analbuminemia. Am. J. Med., *37*:960, 1964.

Weeke, E. O. B.: Urinary serum proteins. Protides Biol. Fluids, *21*:363, 1973.

Weissmann, G. (ed.): Mediators of Inflammation. New York, Plenum Publishing Corporation, 1974.

Wheby, M. S., and Umpierre, G.: Effect of transferrin saturation on iron absorption in man. N. Engl. J. Med., *271*:1391, 1964.

Winkel, P., Statland, B. E., Bokelund, H., and Johnson, E. A.: Correlation of selected serum constituents: 1. Inter-individual variation and analytical error. Clin. Chem., *21*:1592, 1975a.

Winkel, P., Statland, B. E., and Bokelund, H.: The effects of time of venipuncture on variation of serum constituents. Consideration of within-day and day-to-day changes in a group of healthy young men. Am. J. Clin. Pathol., *64*:433, 1975b.

Wochner, R. D., Spilberg, I., Atsushi, I., Liem, H. H., and Muller-Eberhard, U.: Hemopexin metabolism in sickle cell disease, porphyrias and control subjects—effect of heme injection. N. Engl. J. Med., *290*:822, 1974.

Wolski, K. P., Schmid, F. R., and Mittal, K. K.: Genetic linkage between HL-A system and a deficit of the second component (C2) of complement. Science, *188*:1020, 1975.

Zeineh, R. A., Mbawa, E., Pillay, V. K. G., Fiorella, B. J., and Dunea, G.: Immunocore electrophoresis of urinary albumins. J. Lab. Clin. Med., *82*:326, 1973.

10
METABOLIC INTERMEDIATES
AND INORGANIC IONS

Jannie Woo, Ph.D.,
John J. Treuting, Ph.D.,
and Donald C. Cannon, M.D., Ph.D.

NON-PROTEIN NITROGENOUS COMPOUNDS

There are more than 15 different non-protein nitrogenous (NPN) compounds in plasma with a total nitrogen concentration of 250 to 400 mg/l. The NPN of whole blood is approximately 75 per cent greater than that of plasma, largely because of the high glutathione content of erythrocytes. Urea is the major NPN constituent in plasma and composes about 45 per cent of the total. Other major constituents in decreasing order of nitrogen contribution are amino acids, uric acid, creatinine, creatine, and ammonia. Until about 15 years ago, the NPN determination was widely used as an index of renal function. Increased concentrations of several of the major components, i.e., urea, uric acid, and creatinine, do occur as a consequence of diminished renal function. The NPN, however, is a relatively non-specific index of renal disease because other diseases can cause significant alterations in the plasma concentrations of the various constituents. For example, gout or excessive catabolism of purines will increase the uric acid concentration in plasma. Liver disease can cause diminished amino acid metabolism and a corresponding rise in plasma amino acid nitrogen. In contrast, urea synthesis is diminished in severe liver disease. Consequently, most clinical laboratories no longer perform NPN determinations on a routine basis but instead offer determinations of serum urea nitrogen and creatinine, which are more sensitive and specific indices of renal function, uric acid, creatine, ammonia, and alpha amino nitrogen, which reflects the concentration of amino acids.

UREA

Physiologic Chemistry. Urea is the major end product of protein and amino acid catabolism and is generated in the liver through the urea cycle. A simplified diagram of this complex cycle is outlined as follows (Cantarow, 1967):

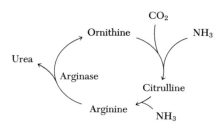

From the liver, urea enters the blood to be distributed to all intracellular and extracellular fluids, since urea is freely diffusible across most cell membranes. Most of the urea is ultimately excreted by the kidneys, but minimal amounts are also excreted in sweat and degraded by bacteria in the intestines.

Urea is freely filtered by the glomeruli. Depending upon the state of hydration and therefore the rate of urine flow, 40 to 80 per cent of the filtered urea is passively reabsorbed with water, mostly in the proximal tubules. There does not appear to be active tubular reabsorption or secretion of urea by mammalian kidneys. Urea ordinarily constitutes about half (25 g) of the total urinary solids and 80 to 90 per cent of the total urinary nitrogen. It is an interesting fact that the renal nephrons can concentrate urea with a gradient of up to 50-fold greater than plasma in view of the fact that urea freely crosses most cell membranes and capillary walls in the body.

In the United States, the urea concentration of blood is often expressed in terms of the blood urea nitrogen content (BUN). In Europe, however, urea is expressed as such. The molecular weight of urea is 60, including two nitrogen atoms with a weight of 28. Consequently, urea nitrogen can be converted to urea by multiplying by 60/28 or 2.14. Thus a BUN 20 mg/dl is equal to a urea of 20×2.14 or 42.80 mg/dl. The concentration of urea nitrogen in whole blood is somewhat less than that in plasma or serum, chiefly because of the lower water content of erythrocytes as compared with plasma. Plasma or serum is the specimen of choice for technical reasons. Nevertheless, the analytical measurement is still termed by convention the BUN. The normal BUN in adults is about 8 to 26 mg/dl (2.9 to 9.3 mmol/l) using either serum or plasma (Reed, 1972).

Clinicopathologic Correlation. The serum concentration of urea varies rather widely in health and is influenced by such diverse factors as dietary intake of protein and the state of hydration. Glucocorticoids have an anti-anabolic effect and the thyroid hormones have a catabolic effect on protein and thus tend to raise the BUN. Androgens and growth hormone have an anabolic effect and thus decrease the formation of urea.

Azotemia is a biochemical designation referring to any significant increase in the plasma concentration of non-protein nitrogenous compounds, principally urea and creatinine. Azotemia is frequently categorized as prerenal, renal, and postrenal. *Prerenal azotemia* is the result of inadequate perfusion of the kidneys and, therefore, diminished glomerular filtration in the presence of otherwise normal renal function. Important etiologies include dehydration, shock, diminished blood volume, and congestive heart failure. Although the increased serum urea or BUN accompanying many cases of massive gastrointestinal hemorrhage is sometimes explained on the basis of greatly increased absorption of amino acids following the digestion of blood proteins, it is probable that hypovolemia resulting from the hemorrhage is the single most important factor. An additional cause of increased serum urea (BUN) is increased protein catabolism, e.g. with fever, stress, and burns.

The pathogenesis of *renal azotemia* is primarily diminished glomerular filtration and, therefore, urea retention as a consequence of acute or chronic renal disease. Other complicating factors frequently present are dehydration or edema, which cause diminished renal perfusion, increased catabolism of proteins, and the general anti-anabolic effect of glucocorticoids. Uremia is a clinical syndrome that can occur with protracted severe azotemia and includes acidosis, water and electrolyte imbalance, nausea, vomiting, anemia, neuropsychiatric changes, and a variety of other clinical manifestations, including coma. The elevated BUN varies in magnitude but usually is in excess of 100 mg/dl, or approaching 200 mg/dl with deep coma or stupor. The progressively rising but at times fluctuating BUN is in contrast to the more slowly rising creatinine, which rarely exceeds 20 mg/dl, and uric acid which, in the absence of gout, does not usually rise above 12 mg/dl in chronic renal failure.

Post-renal azotemia is usually the result of urinary tract obstruction so that urea is reabsorbed into the circulation. An uncommon cause is perforation of the lower urinary tract with extravasation of urine into soft tissues.

From the foregoing discussion, it is evident that the BUN can at best be a rough guide to renal function. Even in the presence of normal dietary intake, hydration, renal perfusion, and integrity of the lower urinary tract, the BUN will ordinarily not be significantly increased until the glomerular filtration is decreased by at least 50 per cent (p. 140). This is a reflection of the fact that the glomerular filtration rate is related to the BUN in a hyperbolic instead of a linear fashion.

A significantly decreased BUN or serum urea occurs in only a few conditions. In addition to poor nutrition, high fluid intake or excessive administration of intravenous fluids in the presence of normal renal function will result in a decreased BUN because relatively little urea will be reabsorbed by the renal tubules. A tendency to a decreased BUN in pregnancy is probably the result of an augmented glomerular filtration rate. Severe liver disease can cause a decrease in urea synthesis because of diminished activity of the urea cycle.

There is some advantage in terms of clinical interpretation to determine both the serum urea and creatinine concentrations and calculate their ratio (Baum, 1975). Creatinine is affected very little by diet and minimally if at all by the state of hydration. Although there is slight tubular secretion of creatinine, tubular reabsorption is minimal if it occurs at all under normal circumstances. Ordinarily the BUN/serum creatinine ratio is about 10:1. Pre-renal azotemia typically results in a ratio greater than 15 because of augmented tubular reabsorption of urea in the presence of diminished glomerular filtration. Similarly, post-renal azotemia also results in a ratio greater than 15 because urea is reabsorbed to a much greater extent than creatinine, whether from the urinary tract in the case of acute obstructive uropathy or from the tissues in the case of extravasation of urine. In patients with reduced muscle mass, creatinine production is subnormal and the BUN/creatinine ratio will be high. A high BUN/creatinine ratio can occur in patients with compromised renal function who have a high protein diet, tissue destruction, thyrotoxicosis, or Cushing's syndrome.

A decreased BUN/creatinine can occur in any of the previously mentioned conditions in which urea production is decreased. Because of their greater creatinine formation, muscular individuals who develop renal failure can also have a low ratio. Renal dialysis causes a decreased ratio because urea is more readily dialyzed than creatinine.

Analytical Techniques. There are two general procedures used to determine urea nitrogen in biologic fluids. A direct method involves the condensation of diacetyl with urea to form a colored chromogen, which can be quantitated by photometry. An indirect procedure measures the ammonia released when urea is hydrolyzed by the enzyme urease.

The diacetyl-urea reaction is shown in Figure 10-1. The liberated hydroxylamine accompanying diacetyl formation inferferes with quantitation and is usually eliminated with appropriate oxidizing agents such as ferric ammonium sulfate, potassium persulfate, or arsenic acid. The diacetyl reaction, although simple to perform, is less specific than the enzymatic assay using urease, particularly at elevated urea concentrations (e.g., 100 mg/dl). Other limitations to this method include instability of the reaction color, deviation from Beer's law, and the irritating odor of the reagents, which may necessitate working in a fume hood.

The alternative procedure utilizes the action of enzyme urease on urea to produce ultimately ammonia and carbonic acid:

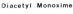

$$O{=}C\begin{smallmatrix}NH_2\\\\NH_2\end{smallmatrix} + 2\,H_2O \xrightarrow{\text{Urease}} O{=}C\begin{smallmatrix}OH\\\\OH\end{smallmatrix} + 2\,NH_3$$

Urea   Carbonic acid

Various methodologies have been developed for the measurement of the liberated ammonia, including acidimetric titration, coulometric titration with hypobromide, Nesslerization, and the indophenol reaction of Berthelot. In

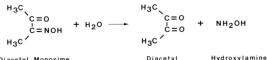

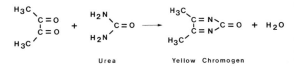

Figure 10-1. Diacetyl-urea reaction for the determination of urea nitrogen in biologic fluids.

the Berthelot procedure, catalysts such as nitroprusside are added to facilitate the conversion of ammonia to indophenol.

For ease of adaptation to automation, the ammonia released from the urease reaction is reacted with α-ketoglutaric acid in the presence of glutamic dehydrogenase. The decrease of absorbance at 340 nm, corresponding to the oxidation of NADH to NAD, is proportional to the ammonium concentration (Talke, 1965). This procedure is currently used on both the duPont Automatic Clinical Analyzer (ACA) and the Union Carbide Centrifugal Analyzer.

A semi-automated Beckman Analyzer for the measurement of urea nitrogen based on conductivity rate method has been developed (Horak, 1972). The NH_4^+ and HCO_3^- generated from the action of urease on urea cause an increased conductivity in the reaction mixture, which is monitored by a conductivity electrode. The ease of operation and its adequate precision make this analyzer amenable to stat analyses.

Another semi-automated analyzer, equipped with immobilized urease on an inert support column, measures the eluted ammonia with an ammonia-sensing electrode (Hanson, 1977).

The results have been favorable in terms of both precision and specificity.

Since hemoglobin causes colorimetric interference, measurement of urea nitrogen using serum or plasma is preferred over blood. The urease reaction has also been shown to be inhibited by a high concentration of sodium fluoride (Norkus, 1976). Although urea is stable in plasma, serum, or urine for several days under refrigeration, samples, especially urine, should be assayed within a few hours to avoid bacterial contamination, which can result in rapid loss of urea.

CREATINE AND CREATININE

Physiologic Chemistry. Creatine is important in muscle metabolism in that it provides storage of high-energy phosphate through synthesis of phosphocreatine. Creatine is synthesized in a two-step process involving the initial synthesis of guanidoacetate (glycocyamine), which takes place in the kidneys, small intestinal mucosa, pancreas, and probably the liver (Fig. 10-2). This reaction between glycine and arginine is catalyzed by a

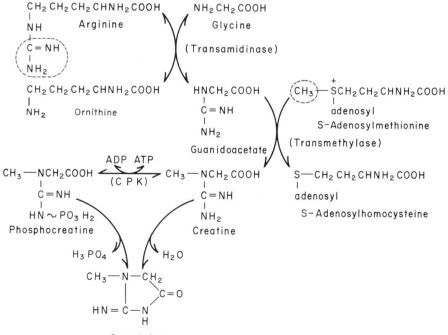

Figure 10-2. Synthesis of creatine and phosphocreatine and formation of creatinine. CPK = creatine phosphokinase. (Modified from Cantarow and Schepartz: Biochemistry, 4th ed., 1967.)

transaminidase, which is subject to feedback inhibition by increased creatine. Guanidoacetate is transported to the liver where it is methylated to creatine. Creatine then enters the blood to be widely distributed, chiefly to muscle cells. The body content of creatine is proportional to the muscle mass.

Creatinine is an anhydride of creatine and is formed by a spontaneous and irreversible reaction. Free creatinine is not reutilized in the body's metabolism and thus functions solely as a waste product of creatine. Formation of creatinine is reasonably constant, and about 2 per cent of the creatine is so transformed every 24 hours. Consequently, creatinine formation also has a direct relationship to muscle mass.

Creatine is filtered by the glomeruli but is largely or completely reabsorbed by the proximal tubules. Consequently, there is only a very small net excretion, i.e., from 0 to 40 mg/24 hours (0 to 0.30 mmol/24 h) for adult males and 0 to 100 mg/24 hours (0 to 0.76 mmol/24 h) for adult females. Creatinine is also freely filtered by the glomeruli but is not reabsorbed to any appreciable extent if at all under normal circumstances. A small but significant amount of creatinine is also excreted by active tubular secretion, which increases with increasing plasma creatinine concentration. Although ranges are frequently quoted for total creatinine excretion, e.g., 1.0 to 2.0 g/24 hours (8.8 to 17.6 mmol/24 h) for adult males and 0.6 to 1.5 g/24 hours (5.3 to 13.2 mmol/24 h) for adult females, a better index would relate creatinine excretion to muscle mass or lean body weight. A reasonable compromise is to relate creatinine excretion to total body weight, i.e., 21 to 26 mg/kg body weight/24 hours (0.18 to 0.23 mmol/kg/24 h) for adult males and 16 to 22 mg/kg body weight/24 hours (0.14 to 0.19 mmol/kg/24 h) for adult females. Although creatinine excretion is usually considered to be reasonably constant in a given individual, one study indicated an intraindividual coefficient of variation of 10 per cent (Scott, 1968). Severe exercise and a high meat diet will cause significantly increased creatinine excretion. Total creatinine measurement is commonly used as an index of the completeness of 24-hour urine collections. Some investigators have concluded, however, that this is an unreliable practice (Tocci, 1972).

The serum concentration of creatinine is relatively constant and somewhat greater in males than in females, i.e., 0.6 to 1.2 mg/dl (53–106 μmol/l) for males and 0.5 to 1.0 mg/dl (44 to 88 μmol/l) for females when specific analytical methods are used (true creatinine). Less specific, i.e., total chromogen, methods for creatinine result in ranges that are about 0.3 mg/dl higher. The plasma creatine concentration is more variable than creatinine and is higher in females than in males, i.e., 0.2 to 0.6 mg/dl (15 to 45 μmol/l) for males and 0.6 to 1.0 mg/dl (45 to 76 μmol/l) for females. Increased levels occur in children and pregnant women. Ingestion of creatine will cause a rapid rise in plasma concentration.

Clinicopathologic Correlation. Serum or plasma creatine concentration and urinary creatine excretion are increased significantly by skeletal muscle necrosis or atrophy (Pennington, 1971), e.g., trauma, the rapidly progressing muscular dystrophies, poliomyelitis, amyotrophic lateral sclerosis, amyotonia congenita, dermatomyositis, myasthenia gravis, and starvation. Methyltestosterone stimulates increased creatine synthesis by the liver. Increased creatine is also associated with hyperthyroidism, diabetic acidosis, and the puerperium.

The constancy of creatinine formation and excretion makes creatinine a useful index of renal function, primarily of glomerular filtration. By virtue of its relative independence from such factors as diet (protein intake), degree of hydration, and protein metabolism, the plasma creatinine is a significantly more reliable screening test or index of renal function than is the BUN. The plasma creatinine tends to increase somewhat more slowly than the BUN in renal disease but also decreases more slowly with hemodialysis. The usefulness of plasma creatinine and the creatinine clearance test are discussed in detail in Chapter 6.

Analytical Techniques. Most of the commonly used methods for the determination of creatinine and creatine are based on the Jaffe reaction, in which creatinine is treated with an alkaline picrate solution to yield a bright orange-red complex. This procedure, although extremely simple, is subject to interferences from a variety of substances, e.g., glucose, proteins, and other non-creatinine chromogens. The reaction is also sensitive to temperature and pH changes. Lloyd's reagent, an aluminum silicate, has been used to separate creatinine from other chromogens prior to the Jaffe reaction. This has rendered high specificity to this procedure (Owens, 1954), and this modification is commonly regarded as the reference method for measuring "true" creatinine. There are numerous modifications of the picrate reaction that are designed to improve assay specificity. One modification, based on the fact that the color resulting from true creatinine is less resistant to acid than the color from non-creatinine chromogens, involves measurement of the impact of acidification on color following total color development. In another approach, the change in color intensity of the picrate reaction is measured before and after bacterial-enzyme destruction of creatinine. In still another version, the proteins are removed by heat prior to treatment with Lloyd's reagent, purportedly to avoid loss of creatinine caused by protein precipitation with tungstic acid. Lloyd's reagent has also been replaced by other adsorbing agents such as Sephadex (Pharmacia Laboratories, Inc., Piscataway, N.J.) or cation-exchange resin. The eluted creatinine fraction is quantitated directly by ultraviolet absorption, usually at 234 nm.

More specific methods based on principles other than Jaffe's reaction have been developed in the last decade. They include colorimetric determinations of complexes formed with 3,5-dinitrobenzoic acid and with o-nitrobenzaldehyde. The use of 3,5-dinitrobenzoic acid as a complexing agent has recently been evaluated (Sims, 1977). These investigators found that methyl-3,5-dinitrobenzoate in an organic medium such as methyl sulfoxide optimizes complex formation and is superior to the picrate reaction in terms of linearity, precision, and susceptibility to interferences. Creatinine determinations based on enzymatic reactions have also been developed in recent years. One method involves the hydrolysis of creatinine to creatine using creatinine amidohydrolase, followed by a series of coupled-enzyme reactions in which creatine reacts with creatinine kinase, pyruvate kinase, and lactate dehydrogenase, culminating in the oxidation of NADH (Moss, 1975). The high cost and limited availability of specific enzymes may prevent widespread use of this procedure. An enzyme-selective electrode coupled to tripolyphosphate-activated creatininase has been described for measuring creatinine in both urine and serum (Meyerhoff, 1976). The activation mechanism is believed to improve electrode sensitivity.

A recently developed kinetic-rate modification of Jaffe's reaction is applicable to routine automation and is relatively free of interfering chromogens (Ward, 1976). It has been adapted for use on centrifugal analyzers. True creatinine determination by high-performance liquid chromatography has recently been described (Brown, 1977). Its validity is still to be tested against established criteria for true creatinine determination.

Creatine is usually measured by the difference in creatinine before and after conversion of creatine to creatinine, generally by heat.

Since considerable amounts of non-creatinine chromogens are present in the erythrocytes, plasma and serum are preferred over whole blood for measuring creatinine. While hemolysis does not affect the determination of creatinine, it increases the creatine value by 100 to 200 per cent. Because of the lability of creatine and creatinine, fresh specimens are recommended. Also, specimens should be maintained at pH 7 during storage to minimize interconversion. Substances which may interfere with creatinine determination by Jaffe's reaction include acetoacetate acetone, barbiturates, phenolsulfonephthalein, bromosulfonephthalein, and protein.

URIC ACID

Physiologic Chemistry.   Uric acid is the major product of purine catabolism in man and the anthropoid apes and is formed from xanthine by the action of xanthine oxidase (Fig. 10-3). In lower mammals uric acid is further oxidized by the action of uricase to allantoin, which is their main excretory product of purine catabolism. Interestingly, birds and reptiles synthesize uric acid as an end product of both purine and protein catabolism, with the distinct advantage that these animals can excrete the sparingly soluble uric acid as crystals and thereby conserve water. The metabolism of uric acid has been recently reviewed (Balis, 1976; Cartier, 1974).

The average adult has a total body content of about 1.2 g of uric acid, which may be considered to be a miscible pool with high turnover. Uric acid in this pool is derived from three sources: (1) catabolism of ingested nucleoproteins, (2) catabolism of endogenous nucleoproteins, and (3) direct transformation of endogenous purine nucleotides (Ryckewaert, 1974). Approximately 60 per cent of this pool is replaced daily by concomitant formation and excretion. Most uric acid formation occurs in the liver, which has a high activity of xanthine

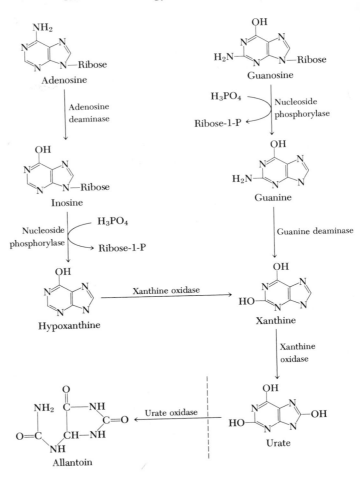

Figure 10–3. Catabolism of purine nucleosides. (From Cantarow and Schepartz: Biochemistry, 4th ed., 1967.)

oxidase, as does the intestinal mucosa. Only traces of xanthine oxidase are present in other tissues. On a low purine diet, about 275 to 600 mg of uric acid will be excreted by the average adult in a 24-hour period. This is somewhat less than the amount formed by endogenous metabolism. It is probable that most, if not all, of the remaining uric acid excretion occurs through biliary, pancreatic, and gastrointestinal secretions followed by degradation by the intestinal flora. Human tissues have very limited uricolytic capability.

Uric acid is a weak acid with a pKa_1 of 5.75 and a pKa_2 of 10.3. Consequently, at the pH of body fluids uric acid exists almost entirely as the urate anion. Although there is some difference of opinion, it appears that urate binding to plasma proteins is minimal. The stated normal range for serum or plasma urate varies considerably as a consequence of differences in analytical methods and in age, racial, sex, social, and geographic factors (Fessel, 1972). One

recent study of 1419 clinically healthy Americans revealed a 95 per cent non-parametric normal range of 4.0 to 8.5 mg/dl (0.24 to 0.50 mmol/l) for males and 2.7 to 7.3 mg/dl (0.16 to 0.43 mmol/l) for females when uric acid was analyzed by a phosphotungstate method (Reed, 1972). This study included adult subjects from age 20 to old age, but there was no statistically significant effect of age except for an increased upper limit of normal of about 0.5 mg/dl for females at the time of menopause. Urate concentration in male children is approximately 1 mg/dl less than that in adult males, but this difference disappears between ages 15 and 20 (Ryckewaert, 1974).

The average adult excretes approximately 0.4 to 0.8 g of uric acid in the urine every 24 hours. On a low purine diet, about 275 to 600 mg of uric acid will still be excreted as a result of catabolism of endogenous purines (Ryckewaert, 1974). Uric acid excretion can exceed 1.0 g/24 hours as a consequence of high purine diet or any of the various causes for increased synthesis or catabolism of endogenous purines. Urate is freely filtered by the glomeruli. The renal clearance of urate is, however, less than 10 per cent of inulin clearance, thus indicating considerable tubular reabsorption. The renal handling of urate is, however, extremely complex and involves not only glomerular filtration and active reabsorption by the proximal tubules but also active tubular secretion and a second tubular reabsorption. It has been estimated that 98 to 100 per cent of the filtered urate is actively reabsorbed in the tubules, as is 90 to 94 per cent of that subsequently secreted by the tubules (Rieselbach, 1977).

At least twice as much uric acid will dissolve in urine as in water at the same pH and temperature. Uromucoid is probably one of the most important solubilizers (Sperling, 1965).

Clinicopathologic Correlation. Numerous diseases, physiologic conditions, biochemical changes, and even social and behavioral factors are associated with alterations in the urate concentration of plasma. Increased serum urate concentration is much more frequent and clinically more significant than decreased concentration. Among the most common etiologies of hyperuricemia are renal failure, ketoacidosis, lactate excess, and the use of diuretics (Bendersky, 1975). Hyperuricemia also has a poorly understood but positive relationship to hyperlipidemia, obesity, atherosclerosis, diabetes mellitus, hypertension, social class, exercise, and achievement-oriented behavior (Fessel, 1972). Dietary intake of purine-rich foods, e.g., meat, viscera, leguminous vegetables, and yeast, causes mild hyperuricemia as well as significantly increased urinary excretion of urate.

Gout is a disorder of purine metabolism or renal excretion of uric acid characterized by (1) hyperuricemia, (2) precipitation of monosodium urate as deposits (tophi) throughout the body except for the central nervous system, but with a special predilection for joints and the periarticular cartilage, bone, bursae, and subcutaneous tissue, (3) recurrent clinical attacks of arthritis, which typically respond to colchicine, and (4) nephropathy and frequently nephrolithiasis. Although genetic in origin, fewer than one third of all patients have a family history of clinical gout. Hyperuricemia is frequently found in asymptomatic close relatives. Although some investigators have considered gout to be an autosomal dominant trait with incomplete penetrance, the mode of inheritance is not known with certainty. Gout may well be of polygenic origin. Males constitute more than 90 per cent of all cases. Gout is uncommon in females prior to menopause. The peak age of onset is in the fifth decade, and the disease is very rare prior to age 20.

Gout is frequently categorized as primary or secondary on the basis of whether the disease is presumed to be an inborn error of metabolism directly involving uric acid synthesis or excretion or whether it is associated with hyperuricemia from any of numerous other etiologies. Considering the frequency of hyperuricemia, secondary gout is a very uncommon complication. The miscible pool of uric acid is greatly increased in gout and can exceed 30 g. The concentration of urate in plasma is roughly correlated with clinical severity, but it is not known why one individual will have clinical gout while another in the same kinship with an equally elevated concentration of urate in the plasma can be asymptomatic. The increased body burden of uric acid is a result of significantly increased synthesis of uric acid from endogenous purines, diminished renal excretion of urate, or a combination of both defects. Most investigators have in the past emphasized the importance of overproduction of uric acid in the pathogenesis of gout, but more recently it has been suggested that cases of gout are about equally distributed in the three categories of overproduction, underexcretion, or a combination of the two defects (Klinenberg, 1977). The pathogenesis of the acute inflammation accompanying uric acid deposits in gout is unclear. It is possible that the monosodium urate crystals enhance bradykinin synthesis through activation of the Hageman factor.

A rare but interesting etiology for primary gout is a deficiency in the enzyme hypoxanthine-guanine-phosphoribosyl-transferase (HGPRT), which results in overproduction of purines and marked accumulation of uric acid. HGPRT is normally present in all tissues and converts hypoxanthine and guanine to their respective nucleotides, inosinic acid and guanylic acid. This disease, commonly termed the Lesch-Nyhan syndrome, is characterized by mental retardation, choreoathetosis, spastic cerebral palsy, aggressive behavior, and compulsive self-mutilation in addition to the pathologic manifestation of hyperuricemia, gouty arthritis, tophi, nephrolithiasis, and nephropathy (Nyhan, 1974).

Urate retention and hyperuricemia are early consequences of azotemic renal disease. Although previously considered to be a reflection of decreased glomerular filtration, the urate retention is more likely the result of decreased tubular secretion of urate or altered postsecretory reabsorption or both factors (Steele, 1975). The plasma urate seldom increases much above 10 mg/dl in renal failure, probably because of increased gastrointestinal secretion and uricolysis (Bendersky, 1975). Clinical gout is an uncommon complication of the hyperuricemia of renal disease and occurs in fewer than 5 per cent of all cases. There are two interesting exceptions, however. Chronic lead nephropathy is associated with gout (saturnine gout) in about half of all cases (Bendersky, 1975). Polycystic kidney disease predisposes to both hyperuricemia and secondary gout even before renal function deteriorates enough to cause azotemia.

Various drugs and chemical substances interfere with renal excretion of urate. Ethacrynic acid, furosemide, and the benzothiadiazide diuretics have a definite anti-uricosuric effect. p-Aminohippurate, lactate, acetoacetate, and β-hydroxybutyrate competitively inhibit tubular secretion of urate. Some drugs such as salicylate, probenecid, sulfinpyrazone, and phenylbutazone are of particular interest in that they inhibit uric acid excretion in low doses but have a marked uricosuric effect in high doses. This is explained by the fact that these drugs inhibit tubular secretion of urate in low doses but are able to inhibit tubular reabsorption only at significantly higher levels.

Increased nucleoprotein production and catabolism are important in the hyperuricemia occurring with leukemia, lymphoma, macroglobulinemia, polycythemia, multiple myeloma, neuroblastoma, and various other widely disseminated neoplasms. Chemotherapeutic agents and ionizing radiation therapy of malignant neoplasms can greatly increase the formation of uric acid. Psoriasis is also associated with hyperuricemia, which is the result of increased proliferation of epidermal cells. Hyperuricemia occurs frequently in sickle cell anemia.

Ethanol intake will frequently increase the plasma concentration of urate and can cause attacks of gout in susceptible patients. The pathogenesis is related to lactate excess, which is produced by the alcohol dehydrogenase catalyzed oxidation of ethanol to acetaldehyde

and which competitively inhibits renal excretion of urate. Lactate excess is also associated with hyperuricemia in severe exercise, toxemia of pregnancy, and ethylene glycol intoxication. Increased acetoacetate and β-hydroxybutyrate similarly contribute to hyperuricemia in diabetic ketoacidosis and starvation. Glycogen storage disease type 1 is regularly accompanied by hyperuricemia as a consequence of both lacticacidemia and increased formation of purines.

Hyperuricemia occurs in many other conditions in which the pathogenetic relationship is less well defined. Included are Down's syndrome, barbiturate overdose, chloroform, carbon monoxide, ammonia and beryllium poisoning, hypoparathyroidism, acromegaly, nephrogenic diabetes insipidus, sarcoidosis, and liver disease.

Causes for hypouricemia are relatively few. Renal tubular reabsorption defects, either congenital as in the Fanconi syndrome and Wilson's disease, or acquired, particularly through toxic damage, can cause increased urinary loss of urate and low plasma levels. Hypouricemia has also been described in association with malignant disorders, e.g., Hodgkin's disease, multiple myeloma, and bronchogenic carcinoma (Kay, 1973). Xanthinuria, a rare condition, is caused by a congenital deficiency of xanthine oxidase so that xanthine and hypoxanthine are excreted instead of uric acid (Watts, 1976). Vigorous treatment of gout with the xanthine oxidase inhibitor, allopurinol, can have a similar effect. Another rare congenital condition, phosphoribosylpyrophosphatase deficiency, also causes extremely low plasma urate concentrations. Severe liver disease can seriously impair the conversion of xanthine to uric acid.

Uric acid is an important constituent of renal calculi, but only a small minority of patients with either primary or secondary gout form renal calculi. The risk in primary gout is estimated to be 10 to 30 per cent (Fessel, 1972). In one series of 207 patients with renal calculi, 22 had uric acid calculi, but only four of these patients had primary gout (Melick, 1958). The most important factors in the formation of uric acid calculi are probably increasing concentration of uric acid in urine and increasing acidity of the urine (de Vries, 1974).

Analytical Techniques. Most methods are based on the oxidation of uric acid to allantoin by either chemical or enzymatic means. The older methods are mainly photometric procedures involving the reduction of tungstate to a blue complex. The most commonly used oxidizing agent is alkaline phosphotungstate, the reduction product of which, tungsten blue, can be measured photometrically at 700 nm. However, there are several inherent difficulties with this method, including the coprecipitation of uric acid with plasma proteins, the formation of turbidity during color development, and the presence of endogenous, potentially interfering substances such as ascorbic acid, free thiols, methylated purines, homogentisic acid, and glucose in very high concentrations. The use of protein-free filtrate for color formation has eliminated most of the interferences. The sodium carbonate reagent initially used to provide the alkaline medium has been replaced by sodium cyanide in order to increase assay sensitivity. Furthermore, the inclusion of urea has been shown to reduce turbidity in the final color solution. One modification of this method involves pretreatment of the sample with trisodium phosphate, precipitation of plasma proteins with phosphotungstic acid, and the use of a carbonate-urea-triethanolamine reagent in color development (Jung, 1970). The trisodium phosphate is intended to destroy the serum chromogens.

In spite of numerous modifications of the basic colorimetric method aimed at improving specificity, the oxidation of uric acid using the enzyme uricase remains the most specific method available. The enzymatic procedure is based on the fact that uric acid has a characteristic ultraviolet absorption spectrum at 293 nm, while the oxidation product, allantoin, does not absorb at this wavelength. Consequently, the difference in absorbance before and after treatment of the sample with uricase is proportional to the uric acid concentration. The advantages of this method are that it avoids protein precipitation and has superior sensitivity and specificity. The method has been adapted to both the AutoAnalyzer and centrifugal analyzers.

Several modifications are available whereby the H_2O_2 formed during the enzymatic reaction is coupled through another oxidation reaction to produce a colored compound. For example, the uricase reaction, when coupled to catalase, results in the formation of the chromophore, 3,5-diacetyl-1,4-dihydrolutidine (Kageyama, 1971). The self-coupling of p-hydroxyphenylacetic acid to form a fluorescent compound in the presence of the H_2O_2 system results in excellent sensitivity and specificity compared with spectrophotometric methods (Kamoun, 1976). The oxidation of homovanillic acid by H_2O_2 to yield a fluorescent compound has also been described (Kuan, 1975). Other methods have been extensively reviewed by Watts (1974). These include the measurement of oxygen uptake during the formation of H_2O_2, coulometric titration, and chromatographic determinations.

Uric acid is stable in both serum and urine for about three days at room temperature. Stability may be increased with the addition of fluoride or thymol. All anticoagulants may be used except potassium oxalate, which forms insoluble potassium phosphotungstate, resulting in turbidity.

AMMONIA

Physiologic Chemistry. Ammonia is a product of amino acid metabolism and therefore of protein catabolism. Considerable ammonia is also absorbed from the intestinal tract, where it is formed by bacterial degradation of dietary proteins and the urea present in gastrointestinal secretions. Ammonia is formed principally in the liver by the oxidative deamination of amino acids, chiefly by the glutamic dehydrogenase catalyzed deamination of L-glutamate to form α-ketoglutarate. Net synthesis of L-glutamate occurs as a result of transamination involving other amino acids, which are transformed in the reaction to their corresponding alpha-keto acids. Smaller amounts of ammonia are formed by non-oxidative deamination of amino acids and aerobic oxidation of various physiologic amines, such as epinephrine and dopamine.

Most ammonia is ultimately disposed of as urea, which is formed in the urea cycle subsequent to the synthesis of carbamyl phosphate. Considerable ammonia is temporarily stored as glutamine, which is formed from glutamic acid principally in the liver but also to some extent in the brain and in skeletal muscle. The kidneys take up glutamine from plasma and form ammonia by the action of glutaminase. The ammonia thus formed is excreted in the urine as one of the two most important urine buffers of hydrogen ions, the other being phosphate. The human kidneys excrete about 30 to 50 mmol (mEq) of ammonia each day, accounting for about 5 to 10 per cent of all nitrogen excreted and buffering most of the 40 to 80 mmol of metabolic acid produced and excreted by the body (Goldstein, 1976).

Ammonia concentration in plasma is ordinarily less than 120 $\mu g/dl$ (67 $\mu mol/l$).

Clinicopathologic Correlation. The most frequent etiology of altered ammonia metabolism is severe liver disease. It is also elevated in Reye's syndrome. When liver function is no longer adequate to metabolize ammonia, the plasma concentration increases, with various toxic manifestations, particularly in the brain. This is discussed in more detail in Chapter 11.

Deficiencies in any of the principal enzymes in the urea cycle, i.e., carbamyl phosphate synthetase, ornithine transcarbamylase, argininosuccinic acid synthetase, argininosuccinase, and arginase, are an important but rare cause for increased plasma ammonia and toxic manifestations (Levin, 1971; Shih, 1972).

In metabolic acidosis the renal excretion of ammonia rises precipitously, provided that normal renal function is maintained (Herns, 1975). In chronic renal disease the ability of the kidneys to secrete ammonia and, therefore, to excrete metabolic acid is compromised. This is discussed further in Chapter 6.

Analytical Techniques. The measurement of ammonia in blood involves the conversion of NH_4^+ to gaseous NH_3. This initial reaction may be conducted directly in blood or in a protein-free filtrate. The liberated NH_3 can be separated from the plasma or serum by reabsorption on a cation exchange resin followed by quantitation with either Nessler's reagent or by the indophenol reaction, in which NH_4^+ reacts with sodium phenoxide in the presence of hypochlorite and nitroprusside to yield a stable blue color. An alternate and more widely used procedure in separating ammonia from blood or plasma is isothermal diffusion. The isolated NH_3 can be measured by acidimetric titration, Nesslerization, photometric determination of the color produced with ninhydrin or with the indophenol reaction, coulometric titration with electrolytically produced hydrobromite, or a variety of other means. A recently introduced approach for determining blood ammonia is the enzymatic reaction of ammonia with α-ketoglutaric acid in the presence of glutamic dehydrogenase (Ishihara, 1972). The decrease of absorbance at 340 nm from the corresponding conversion of NADH to NAD is proportional to the ammonia concentration.

The *in vitro* formation of ammonia in blood, which results from the enzymatic determination of labile amides such as glutamine is an important problem in ammonia determinations. The ammonia content in freshly drawn blood has been reported to increase at the rate of 0.003 $\mu g/ml$ blood/min at room temperature (Seligson, 1957). The ammonia concentration will remain constant for at least 24 hours if the sample is frozen at $-20^\circ C$. If there is more than a few minutes delay in the analysis, quick freezing of arterial rather than venous blood samples in Dry Ice and acetone is recommended.

AMINO ACIDS

Physiologic Chemistry. An examination of Figure 10-4 reveals that the α-amino acid molecule contains an amino group (—NH_2), a carboxyl group (—COOH), and an R group or side chain, which is responsible for specific characteristics of the particular amino acid. Although more than 150 different amino acids are known biologically, only 21 are present in the body as significant constituents of proteins. Some of these amino acids must be supplied by dietary intake, while others can be synthesized by various metabolic pathways. Those amino acids which have to be supplied by dietary intake because endogenous synthesis is inadequate to meet normal requirements are termed essential amino acids. This distinction implies only a necessity for supply from an external source and does not imply that these amino acids are more important for metabolism and growth than the remaining non-essential amino acids. The essential and non-essential amino acids are shown structurally in Figure 10-5.

Amino acids that possess an asymmetric carbon atom, i.e., those with four different

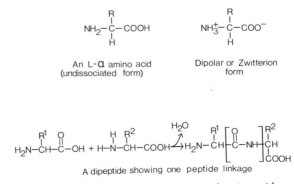

An L-α amino acid
(undissociated form)

Dipolar or Zwitterion form

A dipeptide showing one peptide linkage

Figure 10-4. Chemical characteristics of amino acids.

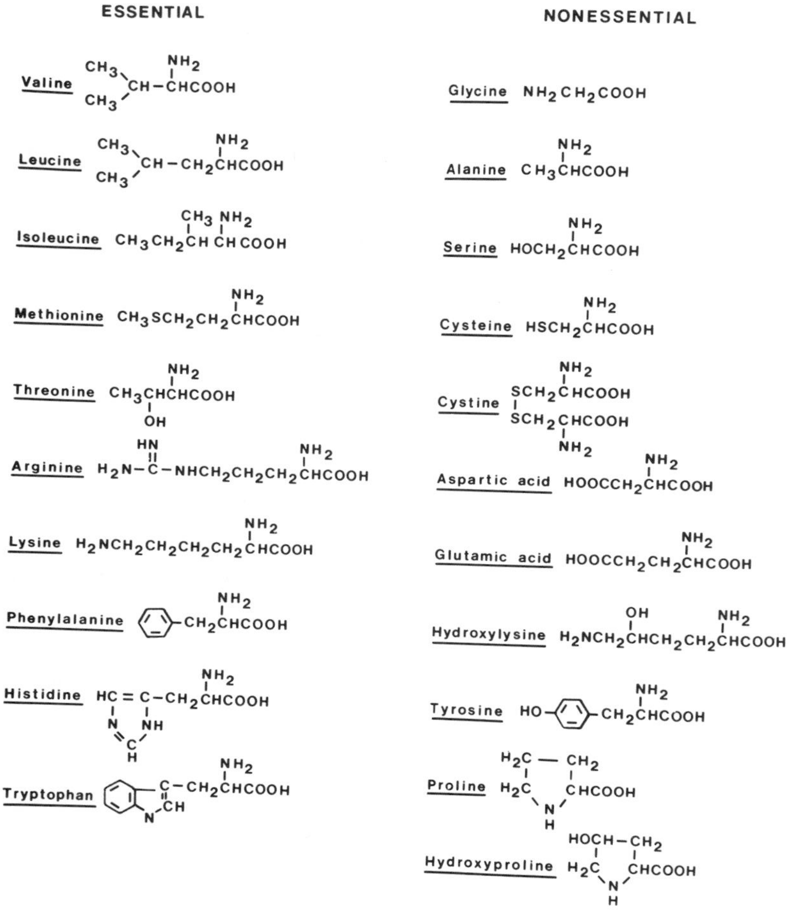

ESSENTIAL

Valine
$$CH_3\!\!-\!\!CH\!\!-\!\!\underset{NH_2}{CHCOOH}$$
$$CH_3$$

Leucine
$$CH_3\!\!-\!\!CH\!\!-\!\!CH_2\underset{NH_2}{CHCOOH}$$
$$CH_3$$

Isoleucine
$$CH_3CH_2\underset{CH_3}{CH}\ \underset{NH_2}{CH}\ COOH$$

Methionine
$$CH_3SCH_2CH_2\underset{NH_2}{CHCOOH}$$

Threonine
$$CH_3\underset{OH}{CHCHCOOH}\ \overset{NH_2}{}$$

Arginine
$$H_2N\!\!-\!\!\underset{HN}{C}\!\!-\!\!NHCH_2CH_2CH_2\underset{NH_2}{CHCOOH}$$

Lysine
$$H_2NCH_2CH_2CH_2CH_2\underset{NH_2}{CHCOOH}$$

Phenylalanine
$$\bigcirc\!\!-\!\!CH_2\underset{NH_2}{CHCOOH}$$

Histidine
$$HC = C\!\!-\!\!CH_2\underset{NH_2}{CHCOOH}$$
$$N\quad NH$$
$$C$$
$$H$$

Tryptophan
$$C\!\!-\!\!CH_2\underset{NH_2}{CHCOOH}$$
$$CH$$
$$N$$

NONESSENTIAL

Glycine NH_2CH_2COOH

Alanine $CH_3\underset{NH_2}{CHCOOH}$

Serine $HOCH_2\underset{NH_2}{CHCOOH}$

Cysteine $HSCH_2\underset{NH_2}{CHCOOH}$

Cystine
$$\underset{|}{SCH_2}\underset{NH_2}{CHCOOH}$$
$$\underset{|}{SCH_2}\underset{NH_2}{CHCOOH}$$

Aspartic acid $HOOCCH_2\underset{NH_2}{CHCOOH}$

Glutamic acid $HOOCCH_2CH_2\underset{NH_2}{CHCOOH}$

Hydroxylysine $H_2NCH_2\underset{OH}{CHCH}CH_2\underset{NH_2}{CHCOOH}$

Tyrosine $HO\!\!-\!\!\bigcirc\!\!-\!\!CH_2\underset{NH_2}{CHCOOH}$

Proline
$$H_2C\!\!-\!\!CH_2$$
$$H_2C\quad CHCOOH$$
$$N$$
$$H$$

Hydroxyproline
$$HOCH\!\!-\!\!CH_2$$
$$H_2C\quad CHCOOH$$
$$N$$
$$H$$

Figure 10–5. Essential and non-essential amino acids.

substituent groups, have dextrorotatory (D) and levorotatory (L) optical specificity. All amino acids in human proteins are of the L configuration, which is diagrammatically shown in Figure 10–4.

Amino acids in their crystalline state have melting points above 190°C. and are more soluble in water than in other less polar solvents. At a pH that is specific for each amino acid, the molecule is doubly charged, i.e., the carboxyl group is negatively charged and the amino group is positively charged, thus resulting in a net charge of zero. Dipolar ions of this type are referred to as zwitterions (Fig. 10–4). Amino acids thus behave as both weak acids and weak bases, i.e., they are amphoteric.

Proteins are composed of long chains of amino acids joined by peptide linkage. The peptide or amide linkage is formed by the condensation of the α-amino group of one amino acid with the carboxyl group of another. A molecule of water is removed in the forma-

tion of the amide bond (Fig. 10–4). After the peptide linkage has been formed, a carboxyl group of one amino acid and the amino group of the other are still available to form additional peptide linkages.

Proteins in ingested foods are not absorbed intact to any significant degree. In the process of digestion, enzymatic cleavage of peptide linkages occurs. In the stomach and proximal small intestine, endopeptidases hydrolyze the inner portions of the polypeptide chains while exopeptidases attack the terminal linkages.

The action of the endopeptidases, pepsin, trypsin, chymotrypsin, and elastase, and the exopeptidases, carboxypeptidases A and B, results in a mixture of amino acids and small peptides, which can be absorbed by the intestine. After absorption into the microvilli, further enzymatic hydrolysis converts oligopeptides into the constituent amino acids. The molecules of essentially all the amino acids are much too large to diffuse passively through the membrane pores of the intestinal mucosal cells. The amino acids are absorbed by at least three stereospecific active transport systems: (1) neutral amino acids are absorbed competitively by a single transport system, (2) basic amino acids are absorbed but at a slower rate by a second active transport system, and (3) proline and hydroxyproline are absorbed by a third transport system (Adibi, 1967; Schultz, 1970). After absorption, amino acids enter the portal venous blood to be transported to the liver, where some are utilized for protein synthesis while others enter the systemic circulatory amino acid pool. Protein synthesis throughout the body utilizes amino acids from the systemic pool, while protein catabolism contributes additional amino acids. The usual process of catabolism involves initial removal of the amino group (Fig. 10-6). The resultant keto acids enter the Krebs aerobic cycle to be oxidized to CO_2 and water with the production of energy, which can be stored as ATP (adenosine triphosphate). Amino acids exist in the systemic circulatory pool but cannot be stored as such. The adult normal range of plasma amino acids will vary according to the method of analysis. Goodwin (1968), using a method involving the formation of colored complexes, established an adult normal range of 3.6 to 7.0 mg amino acid nitrogen/dl (2.6 to 5.0 mmol/l).

Amino acids are filtered by renal glomeruli and are very efficiently reabsorbed by active transport processes in the proximal tubules. Ordinarily less than 5 per cent of the filtered amino acids is not reabsorbed and is thus ex-creted in the urine. In the normal adult, urinary excretion of amino acids is fairly constant and averages 200 mg of alpha-amino nitrogen per 24 hours. Disturbances in amino acid metabolic pathways can result in accumulation of amino acids in the blood and excessive excretion into the urine. These "overflow" aminoacidurias can be caused by either acquired or hereditary disturbances in amino acid metabolism. Transport defects in the renal tubules can cause excessive excretion of amino acids when plasma concentrations are normal. Aminoacidurias are discussed further in Chapter 17.

Clinicopathologic Correlations. This discussion will be concerned with abnormal amino acid metabolism that is reflected in increased plasma concentrations of one or more amino acids (p. 581). Excessive concentrations of a number of amino acids in plasma (as seen in severe liver disease) can be evaluated by measurement of total alpha amino nitrogen. As mentioned earlier, all biologically significant amino acids contain an amino group. Although some amino acids contain other amino groups as well, these do not react to any appreciable extent in the assay.

Analytical Techniques. A wide variety of methods has been used for the determination of total α-amino acids in plasma. Early methods include formol titration, formation with copper sulfate and analysis of copper in the soluble complex, and gasometry. These methods have not met with widespread acceptance because of their non-specificity and/or specialized equipment requirements. More

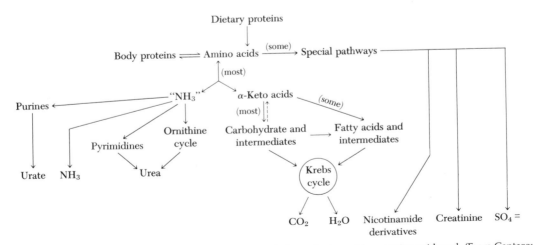

Figure 10–6. General pathways of protein and amino acid metabolism. Amino acids = amino acid pool. (From Cantarow and Schepartz: Biochemistry, 4th ed., 1967.)

recent approaches to the detection and quantitation of α-amino acids have employed color reactions. A reliable and rapid method, developed by Goodwin (1968) utilizes 1-fluoro-2,4-dinitrobenzene (FDNB), which forms a yellow dinitrophenyl derivative (see below) of the amino acids which can be quantitated spectrophotometrically at 420 nm.

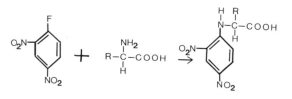

Alternative methods utilize 2,4,6-trinitrobenzene sulfonate (Palmer, 1969) and sodium β-naphthoquinone-4-sulfonate (Sobel, 1957).

In many metabolic disturbances, it is not the total concentration of amino acids that is of clinical importance, but rather the altered concentration of one amino acid or a group of related amino acids. In many such instances, the abnormalities can be readily detected by simple screening tests of urine using chromatography (paper or thin layer) or high voltage electrophoresis (HVE). These techniques, along with their interpretation, are fully discussed in Chapter 17. For more accurate quantitative studies, the amino acids in plasma or urine can be separated on an automated high-pressure column chromatography system (amino acid analyzer) using an ion-exchange resin followed by gradient elution. In the original amino acid analyzer, developed by Spackman (1958), quantitation was achieved by spectrophotometric analysis following ninhydrin derivatization. Refinements in the original procedure, particularly improved column technology and the development of new fluorescent detection systems (fluorescamine and phthaldealdehyde), have resulted in increased sensitivity and reduced analysis time (Hammond, 1976).

A combined gas chromatography (GC) mass spectrometry (MS) approach to amino acid analysis appears to be a potentially useful technique in the clinical laboratory (Hammond, 1976). In this approach, the amino acids are initially converted to their N-trifluoroacetyl-O-n-butyl ester (TFA-n-butyl) derivative before quantitation (Jellum, 1973).

Specific determinations of three amino acids are of particular clinical importance and will be considered briefly. The amino acid most often determined in blood is phenylalanine. A bacterial inhibition test, using dried blood, was developed by Guthrie and Susi (1963). For more accurate diagnosis and therapeutic monitoring, the concentration of phenylalanine can be accurately quantitated using the fluorometric method of McCaman and Robins (1962). The procedure is based upon the reaction between phenylalanine, copper, and ninhydrin with enhancement of the resultant fluorescent complex by any one of several dipeptides. Other chemical methods include gas-liquid chromatography (Steed, 1972), and ultraviolet spectrophotometry (La Du, 1960). The upper limit of normal for newborns may be considered to be 4.0 mg/dl (0.24 mmol/l). Infants with values greater than 4.0 mg/dl require further investigation. Phenylketonuria (PKU) is discussed further in chapter 17 (p. 599).

Determination of tyrosine (p-hydroxyphenylalanine) in blood is useful in the diagnosis of tyrosinosis. In this disease a deficiency of tyrosine transaminase (p-hydroxyphenylpyruvic acid oxidase) causes elevated plasma levels of tyrosine and hyperexcretion of p-hydroxyphenylacetic acid, p-hydroxyphenylpyruvic acid, and p-hydroxyphenylacetic acid. The quantitative method of choice for the specific determination of tyrosine is the fluorometric assay of Wong, (1964). Deproteinized serum reacts with 1-nitroso-2-naphthol to produce a fluorescent product that is measured at 545 nm after excitation at 470 nm. The normal range in fasting adults is 0.6 to 1.5 mg/dl (0.03 to 0.08 mmol/l).

Glutamine is the most abundant free amino acid in plasma and has the important role of acting as a storage and transport form of ammonia. Most of the ammonia secreted by the kidney is derived from glutamine. The most important application of glutamine assays, however, relates to cerebrospinal fluid and not to plasma. Glutamine concentration is significantly increased in the cerebrospinal fluid in association with hepatic encephalopathy (p. 329). The earliest method for the determination of glutamine in cerebrospinal fluid involves acid hydrolysis of the sample and the measurement of ammonia by Nesslerization (Whitehead, 1955). Hourani (1971) used Berthelot's phenolhypochlorite reaction to measure the ammonia in order to avoid the imprecision with Nessler's reagent. In normal individuals the cerebrospinal fluid glutamine is less than 20 mg/dl (1.4 mmol/l).

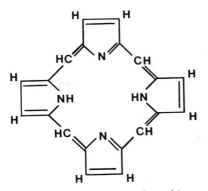

Figure 10-7.   Structure of porphin.

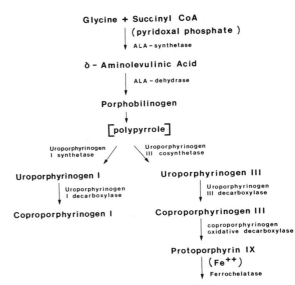

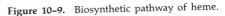

Figure 10-9.   Biosynthetic pathway of heme.

PORPHYRINS

PHYSIOLOGIC CHEMISTRY

The porphyrins are metabolic intermediates in the biosynthetic pathway that has heme as its principal product. Hence, porphyrins are in hemoglobin, myoglobin, cytochromes, etc. The basic structure common to all porphyrins is the porphin nucleus, which consists of one pyrrolenine, one maleimide, and two pyrrole type rings. These rings are joined together by four methene bridges, as shown in Figure 10-7. The porphyrins are differentiated by the substituents found in the eight peripheral positions. There are many kinds of porphyrins known, but very few are found in nature and only three are of clinical significance: uroporphyrins, coproporphyrins, and protoporphyrins (Fig. 10-8). Four isomeric forms can exist for each porphyrin (I, II, III, IV). All naturally occurring porphyrins are of either the I or III isomer type. Only the type III

isomers have been shown to play a functional role in the biosynthesis of heme.

The biochemistry of porphyrins and heme synthesis has been the subject of numerous reviews (Elder, 1972; Sinnott, 1976). A brief sequence of the heme biosynthetic pathway is shown in Figure 10-9. The formation of δ-aminolevulinic acid (ALA) requires the presence of pyridoxal phosphate and involves the enzyme, ALA synthethase. It is the rate-limiting step in hepatic porphyrin synthesis. The condensation of ALA to porphobilinogen (PBG) involves ALA dehydrase, which is present in relatively high levels in both hepatic and bone marrow cells. PBG undergoes self condensation to form a polypyrrole which spontaneously becomes either uroporphyrino-

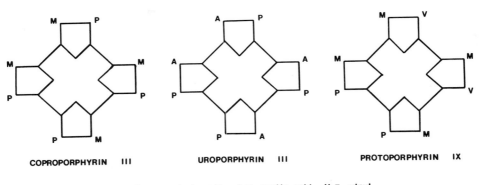

Where   M = methyl , P = propionic acid , A = acetic acid , V = vinyl

Figure 10-8.   Some examples of naturally occurring porphyrins.

gen I or uroporphyrinogen III. Both isomers undergo decarboxylation to yield the respective coproporphyrinogens. The type III isomer undergoes oxidative decarboxylation to form protoporphyrin, which reacts with ferrous ion to produce heme.

It is worth noting that the biosynthetic intermediates between PBG and protoporphyrin are not porphyrins but rather their reduced forms, the porphyrinogens. They are colorless non-fluorescent compounds readily converted to porphyrins by weak oxidizing agents, such as light in the presence of air. Thus uroporphyrin and coproporphyrin are merely the oxidation products of their respective porphyrinogens, which are the true substrates in the biosynthetic pathway.

CLINICOPATHOLOGIC CORRELATIONS

Porphyrin disorders, which may be either genetically determined or acquired, result from metabolic defects in heme biosynthesis. The separation of porphyrin disorders into erythropoietic and hepatic types according to the sites of biochemical and pathologic lesion was suggested by Schmid (1954). The classification that will be used (Table 10-1) is based on that of Elder (1972). This scheme categorizes the porphyrias as erythropoietic, hepatic, or erthyrohepatic, based on the sites of excessive or abnormal porphyrin production. Lead intoxication was not included in the original scheme of Elder (1972), but it can probably

Table 10-1. CLASSIFICATION OF DISORDERS OF PORPHYRIN METABOLISM

Erythropoietic Involvement
   Congenital erythropoietic porphyria
   Erythropoietic coproporphyria

Erythropoietic and Hepatic Involvement
   Erythrohepatic protoporphyria
   Lead intoxication

Hepatic Involvement
   Inherited hepatic prophyrias
     Acute intermittent porphyria
     Variegate porphyria
     Hereditary coproporphyria
   Symptomatic cutaneous hepatic porphyrias
     Familial
     Acquired, associated with:
       Alcoholism, liver disease, iron
        overload, estrogen therapy
       Hexachlorobenzene poisoning
       Hepatic neoplasms

best be categorized under erythrohepatic involvement. Erythrohepatic protoporphyria is a redesignation of the disease, originally named erythropoietic protoporphyria, because it is now known that this disease can involve both the liver and the bone marrow (Scholnick, 1971). A different classification has been suggested by some investigators whereby the porphyrin disorders are distinguished as porphyrias and porphyrinurias. The porphyrias include classic metabolic disorders, which are inherited and have clinical symptoms directly related to the elevated heme precursors in the body. The porphyrinurias, on the other hand, include disorders that are usually acquired or induced as a result of interference in the normal pathway of heme synthesis, the notable examples being lead intoxication and chronic alcoholism.

Congenital Erythropoietic Porphyria. This extremely rare autosomal recessive disorder is manifested shortly after birth. It is associated with red pigmented urine, erythrodontia, hemolytic anemia, and severe cutaneous photosensitivity. Splenomegaly and hemolytic anemia typically develop and early death usually occurs. The red urine is the result of excessive excretion of coproporphyrin and uroporphyrin, mainly of Type I. Although the exact nature of the defect is not known, overactivity of the ALA synthetase and/or uroporphyrinogen III cosynthetase has been suggested (Goldberg, 1971).

Erythropoietic Coproporphyria. This extremely rare disorder apparently can be totally asymptomatic. Clinical manifestations usually include mild skin photosensitivity associated with abnormal levels of coproporphyrin III in the erythrocytes (Goldberg, 1971).

Erythrohepatic Protoporphyria. This is thus far the only known inherited disorder in which the biochemical lesions are localized in both hepatic and erythropoietic cells. Transmitted as an autosomal dominant trait, it is associated with mild skin photosensitivity. The onset of disease occurs during the first few years of life or adulthood. Laboratory findings are those of abnormally high protoporphyrin in circulating erythrocytes and elevated fecal coproporphyrin and protoporphyrin, causing the feces to be fluorescent. Overactivity of ALA synthetase appears to be important in the pathogenesis of this disease. It has been proposed that deficient synthesis of heme from protoporphyrin results in deficient production of a specific heme protein that is important in a feedback suppression of ALA synthetase (Elder, 1972). Recent evidence revealed by Piomelli (1975) appears to indicate that all protoporphyrin excreted in the feces can be accounted for by the bone marrow cells. They have suggested that there is no need to postulate synthesis of protoporphyrin by the liver as a causative factor in this type of porphyric disorder.

Acute Intermittent Porphyria. This is the most common of the inherited porphyrias. It is transmitted as an autosomal dominant trait but affects three females to every two males. This disease typically presents with colicky abdominal pain often associated with vomiting, constipation, fever, and leukocytosis. Hypertension, peripheral neuritis, behavioral changes, and frank psychosis may occur.

Sassa (1974) proposed that three enzyme defects might account for this disorder—increased levels of ALA synthetase, decreased levels of uroporphyrinogen I synthetase, and a reduced activity of the enzyme, Δ^4-5α-reductase. Laboratory findings include elevated urinary ALA and PBG, inappropriate secretion of ADH, and overt liver function abnormalities, e.g., transient elevation of bilirubin and alkaline phosphatase.

Variegate Porphyria. This autosomal dominant porphyria affects females and males equally and is particularly prevalent in the white population of South Africa. The disease onset is usually in the third or fourth decade of life and is somewhat variable in its clinical manifestations. Cutaneous lesions are the most common manifestation, but some patients present with acute attacks that are indistinguishable from acute intermittent porphyria. Elevated urinary ALA, PBG, and porphyrins, and highly elevated fecal porphyrins may be found during acute attacks. Increases of ALA synthetase have also been demonstrated.

Hereditary Coproporphyria. This hepatic porphyria is transmitted in an autosomal dominant fashion. Patients afflicted with this condition either are asymptomatic or present with mild neurologic, abdominal, or psychiatric symptoms. Acute attacks have also been reported. Coproporphyrin III is excreted virtually constantly in the feces, while coproporphyrin, aminolevulinic acid, and porphobilinogen appear intermittently in the urine. A block in the conversion of coproporphyrinogen III to protoporphyrin and/or an induction of ALA synthetase have been implicated in the mechanism of this condition.

Symptomatic Cutaneous Hepatic Porphyrias. Except for rare familial cases this group of porphyrias is acquired. Skin lesions are the most obvious clinical feature. The condition has been reported in association with liver disease, particularly with alcohol as the inciting agent, with estrogen therapy, and with ingestion of hexachlorobenzene. Elevated urinary uroporphyrin is the characteristic biochemical finding, while excretion of PBG and ALA is usually normal.

Lead Intoxication. The clinical manifestations of lead intoxication are highly varied and may include acute colicky abdominal pains, constipation or diarrhea, nausea, vomiting, anorexia, neuromuscular weakness, behavioral changes, coma, or convulsions. Basophilic stippling of erythrocytes and anemia are common. Significant cutaneous manifestations do not occur. The clinical manifestations and laboratory tests of lead intoxication are discussed further in Chapter 15 (p. 513).

ANALYTICAL TECHNIQUES

A complete laboratory investigation of any disorder of porphyrin generally begins with screening tests for porphyrins or their precursors, ALA and PBG, in urine, feces, and blood. This is usually followed by the appropriate quantitative determinations should the preliminary investigation suggest further study. The typical biochemical findings associated with disorders of porphyrin metabolism are shown in Table 10-2.

All porphyrins have in common a characteristic type of absorption spectrum in the near ultraviolet and visible region, resulting primarily from the conjugated bond system of the tetrapyrrole ring. Hence, all porphyrins have an intense absorption band near 400 nm, known as the Soret band. When irradiated with light of this wavelength, all free porphyrins exhibit an intense red fluorescence. This property enables porphyrins to be detected and quantitated in the laboratory at concentrations of 2×10^{-4} μmol/l. Reference values for porphyrins and their precursors are listed in Table 10-3.

The solubility of both the porphyrins and their precursors decreases with decreasing number of hydroxyl and carboxylic groups. Consequently PBG and uroporphyrin are excreted mainly in the urine, while protoporphyrin is excreted exclusively in the bile and thus appears in the feces. Coproporphyrin is ex-

Table 10-2. TYPICAL BIOCHEMICAL FINDINGS ASSOCIATED
WITH DISORDERS OF PORPHYRIN METABOLISM

	ERYTHROCYTE			URINE				FECES		
DISORDER	UP	CP	PP	ALA	PBG	UP	CP	UP	CP	PP
Congenital erythropoietic porphyria	↑↑	↑↑	↑	N	N	↑↑	↑	N	↑	N
Erythropoietic copro- porphyria	N	↑↑	N	N	N	N	N	N	↑	N
Erythropoietic proto- porphyria	N	N	↑↑	N	N	N	N	N	↑	↑
Acute intermittent prophyria (AIP)	N	N	N	↑↑	↑↑	↑	↑ or N	N	N	N
Variegate porphyria (acute attacks)	N	N	N	↑	↑	↑ or N	↑ or N	N	↑	↑↑
Symptomatic porphyria	N	N	N	N	N	↑↑	↑	N	↑ or N	↑ or N
Lead poisoning	N	↑ or N	↑	↑	↑ or N	N	↑	N	N	N

UP = uroporphyrin; CP = coproporphyrin; PP = protoporphyrin; ↑ = increased; ↑↑ = large increase; N = normal.

creted mainly in the bile, but also in urine as coproporphyrinogen. The solubility difference plays an important role in the choice of specimen to be analyzed and in the method of measurement.

ALA and PBG. The most widely used screening procedure for excess ALA and PBG was first introduced by Watson (1941). PBG condenses with *p*-dimethylaminobenzaldehyde in hydrochloric acid (HCl) (Ehrlich's reagent) to form a magenta color complex. A description of the analytical techniques and possible interferences is presented in Chapter 17 (p. 601).

Porphyrins. The characteristic red fluorescence exhibited by all porphyrins serves as the basis for the screening tests of porphyrins in urine, feces, and blood. The general procedure involves the extraction of porphyrins into an organic solvent system, e.g., acetic acid/ethyl acetate, followed by re-extraction into

Table 10-3. REFERENCE VALUES OF PORPHYRINS AND THEIR PRECURSORS

ANALYTE	REFERENCE INTERVAL
Erythrocyte	
Coproporphyrin	0.5-2.0 µg/dl (0.75-3.00 nmol/l)
Protoporphyrin	4-52 µg/dl (7.2-93.6 nmol/l)
Urine	
ALA	1.5-7.5 ml/24 h (11.2-57.2 µmol/24 h)
PBG	<1.0 mg/24 h (<4.4 µmol/24 h)
Coproporphyrin	50-160 µg/24 h (0.075-0.24 µmol/24 h)
Uroporphyrin	10-30 µg/24 h (0.012-0.037 µmol/24 h)
Feces	
Coproporphyrin	0-500 µg/24 h (0-0.75 µmol/24 h)
Protoporphyrin	0-600 µg/24 h (0-1.08 µmol/24 h)

HCl. The fluorescence is read with an ultraviolet light source. Comprehensive and rapid porphyrin screening procedures applicable to urine, feces, and blood have been described by both Haining (1969) and Rimington (1971).

Most quantitative measurements of porphyrins are based on preliminary extraction and differentiation by solvent partition followed by spectrophotometric or fluorometric measurement. In recent years, improved resolution of porphyrin fractionation has been achieved by electrophoresis (Magnus, 1971) or by thin layer chromatography after extraction and esterification (Doss, 1971). These methods, though accurate and precise, are nevertheless time-consuming. With the advent of high-pressure liquid chromatography, rapid identification and quantitation of porphyrins have been possible in both urine (Carlson, 1976) and feces (Lim, 1976).

Although the determination of ALA dehydrase has been emphasized as a diagnostic test for lead intoxication, it has met with limited acceptance. Recent interest has focused on the use of erythrocyte protoporphyrin determination as a screening test for lead poisoning (Lamola, 1975). This was motivated in part by the discovery that erythrocyte protoporphyrin exists in "free" form in erythropoietic protoporphyria but is found as zinc protoporphyrin (ZPP) in lead intoxication and in iron deficiency anemias. Lamola (1975) has identified the prominent fluorescent porphyrin in erythrocytes in chronic lead intoxication as zinc protoporphyrin. He has also shown that it can be assayed fluorometrically in diluted whole blood and proposed this as a screening procedure for lead intoxication. Similar methodologies employing small sample volumes (10 to 40 μl whole blood) have been proposed by other investigators as screening procedures for lead exposure in children (Orfanos, 1977).

ALA Dehydrase. Clinical tests that have been used for the diagnosis of lead intoxication include blood lead, coproporphyrin, and ALA. Because of inadequate specificity these tests have in recent years been replaced by the determination of ALA dehydrase, particularly since the inhibitory action by lead on this enzyme has been shown to occur long before other biologic effects are measurable. The procedure of choice for measurement of ALA dehydrase appears to be that of Bonsignore or its modifications (Morgan, 1972). This method measures the amount of PBG formed in the crude enzyme assay. However, partial conversion of PBG to porphyrin during the crude enzyme assay has been shown to result in underestimation of its activity and an alternate procedure of measuring the ALA consumed has been proposed (Tomokuni, 1974).

CALCIUM AND PHOSPHORUS

PHYSIOLOGIC CHEMISTRY

Calcium Homeostasis. Calcium is the most abundant mineral element in the human body and the fifth most abundant of all elements. Approximately 98 per cent of the 1000 to 1200 g of calcium in the adult is present in the skeleton, primarily as hydroxyapatite, which is a crystal lattice composed of calcium, phosphorus, and hydroxide. Of the remaining calcium, about half is present in extracellular fluid and the remainder in a variety of tissues, particularly skeletal muscle. Of critical importance to calcium homeostasis is the fact that less than 1 per cent of the total skeletal reservoir of calcium is readily exchangeable with extracellular fluid (Russell, 1976). In addition to its obvious importance in skeletal mineralization, calcium plays a vital role in such basic physiologic processes as blood coagulation, neuromuscular conduction, maintenance of normal tone and excitability of skeletal and cardiac muscle, stimulus-secretion coupling in various exocrine glands, and preservation of cell membrane integrity and permeability, particularly in terms of sodium and potassium exchange.

The calcium level in serum is maintained within a relatively narrow range of about 9.2 to 11.0 mg/dl (4.6 to 5.5 mEq/l or 2.3–2.8 mmol/l) (Reed, 1972). Quoted normal ranges or reference values vary among laboratories, partly as a result of different analytical methods. Three distinct fractions compose the total calcium in serum: (1) free or ionized calcium accounts for about 50 per cent of total calcium; (2) about 5 per cent of total calcium is complexed with a variety of anions, particularly phosphate and citrate; (3) the remaining 45 per cent of calcium is bound to plasma proteins, especially to albumin but also to globulin to a limited extent. Both ionized calcium and the calcium complexes are freely dialyzable. Ionized calcium concentration in extracellular fluids is of far greater importance to homeostasis than total calcium. It is only ionized calcium that is important in such physiologic functions as neuromuscular conduction and blood coagulation. The relative distributions of the three calcium species are altered as a result of change in pH of either the extracellular fluids or the protein concentration. Acidosis promotes an increase in ionized calcium, while alkalosis causes a corresponding decrease. If ionized calcium is to remain within its normal physiologic range, an increased concentration of plasma proteins will result in a corresponding increase in total calcium, which reflects an increase in bound calcium. Similarly, decreased plasma protein concentration will ordinarily result in decreased total calcium.

The binding of calcium to plasma proteins is a freely reversible process, which is governed by a dissociation constant. The process is thus analogous to the dissociation of a weak acid or base. This was long ago recognized by McLean (1935), who represented the relationship as follows:

$$\frac{[Ca^{++}][Pr^{=}]}{[CaPr]} = K$$

where $[Ca^{++}]$ is the concentration of ionized calcium, $[CaPr]$ is the concentration of protein-bound calcium, $[Pr^{=}]$ is the concentration of free protein capable of binding calcium, and K is a constant that is specific for each protein species and varies with pH and temperature. Simple transposition of this equation serves to emphasize that the concentration of ionized calcium will remain constant and is thus independent of bound calcium as long as the ratio of the concentrations of protein-bound calcium to free protein remains constant:

$$[Ca^{++}] = K \frac{[CaPr]}{[Pr^=]}$$

Use has been made of this relationship to construct various equations and nomograms for estimating ionized calcium from measurements of total calcium and protein concentrations. Direct measurement of ionized calcium is now technically reliable and has many clinical applications (Robertson, 1976).

Maintenance of calcium homeostasis involves the participation of three major organs—the small intestine, the kidneys, and the skeleton. The mammary gland is also important during lactation, as are the placenta and fetus during gestation. Although usually ignored in balance studies, the sweat glands are responsible for a small but significant excretion of calcium. In the adult there is no persistent net gain or loss of calcium in health. During growth and pregnancy, a positive calcium balance must be maintained. Calcium homeostasis is regulated by various hormones that act principally upon the major organs involved in calcium metabolism (Lutwak, 1975). The most important hormones are parathyroid hormone and the hormones derived from renal metabolism of vitamin D_3, notably 1,25-dihydroxycholecalciferol. Quite possibly calcitonin plays a role in the regulating process, although its significance in man is still controversial. Other hormones that affect calcium metabolism but whose secretion is determined primarily by factors other than changes in plasma calcium and phosphate include thyroid hormones, growth hormone, adrenal glucocorticoids, and gonadal steroids.

Dietary calcium varies widely for adults from about 200 to 1500 mg/day, most of which in the American diet is derived from milk or other dairy products. The minimum daily dietary requirement for calcium is commonly stated to be 800 mg, but it has been sufficiently demonstrated that calcium balance can be maintained in adults who ingest as little as 200 to 400 mg of calcium daily. It is commonly recommended that the daily dietary intake of calcium should be about 1200 mg during pregnancy and lactation and 800 to 1200 mg during childhood.

Calcium is absorbed by an active transport process that occurs mostly in the duodenum and upper jejunum. The major stimulus to calcium absorption is vitamin D. Absorption is also enhanced by growth hormone, an acid medium in the intestines, and increased dietary protein. The ratio of calcium to phosphorus in the intestinal contents is also important in that a ratio greater than two tends to inhibit calcium absorption because of the formation of insoluble calcium phosphates. Phytic acid derived from various cereal grains can also form insoluble calcium compounds as can dietary oxalate and fatty acids. Cortisol and excessive alkalinity of the intestinal contents are both inhibitory to calcium absorption. The net absorption of calcium from the intestinal tract is only about 10 to 20 per cent of dietary intake. This approximation is grossly misleading, however, because considerable calcium is actively secreted into the intestines.

Estimates of the daily calcium excretion in sweat vary widely from 15 to more than 100 mg. The loss can greatly exceed this range during extreme environmental conditions. The major net loss of calcium is urinary excretion, which accounts for 50 to 200 mg or more each day, depending on dietary intake. Urinary calcium excretion is enhanced by hypercalcemia, phosphate deprivation, acidosis, and glucocorticoids. Urinary calcium excretion is diminished by parathyroid hormone, certain diuretics, and probably vitamin D.

Phosphorus Homeostasis. Phosphorus is also an abundant element in the body and is omnipresent in its distribution. About 85 per cent of the 500 to 600 g of phosphorus (measured as inorganic phosphorus) in the adult is present in bone as hydroxyapatite. The remaining phosphorus is mostly combined with lipids, proteins, carbohydrates, and other organic substances to fill vital roles as phospholipids, nucleic acids, nucleotides, constituents of cell membranes and cell cytoplasm, and compounds that are important in biochemical energy storage and exchange.

Most of the phosphorus in extracellular fluid is inorganic, predominantly as two species, $HPO_4^=$ and $H_2PO_4^-$. Negligible amounts of $PO_4^\equiv$ exist in the physiologic pH range. The relative amounts of the two phosphate ions are obviously pH-dependent (Table 10-4). At pH 7.4, the ratio of $HPO_4^=$ to $H_2PO_4^-$ is about 4:1. Because of the effect of pH on the relative concentrations of the two phosphate species, serum phosphorus should be expressed as milligrams per deciliter. In health, serum phos-

Table 10–4. pH CONVERSION FACTORS FOR INORGANIC PHOSPHORUS*

pH	FACTOR
7.10	0.537
7.15	0.546
7.20	0.555
7.25	0.563
7.30	0.570
7.35	0.577
7.40	0.583
7.45	0.589
7.50	0.594
7.55	0.599
7.60	0.603
7.70	0.611

*Milligrams per deciliter × factor = mEq. per liter. (With permission of Sunderman, F. W.: Inorganic Phosphorus, Proficiency Test Service, April, 1973, p. 3.)

phorus varies over a rather wide range of 2.4 to 4.7 mg/dl (0.78 to 1.51 mmol/l) (Reed, 1972). Higher phosphorus levels occur in growing children (4 to 7 mg/dl or 1.30 to 2.25 mmol/l). Serum phosphorus also has a distinct circadian rhythm (Goldsmith, 1972). Ingestion of food can significantly alter serum phosphorus concentration. Ingestion of phosphate-rich food can increase serum phosphorus, while a high carbohydrate meal can cause a significant decrease.

Three major organs are involved in phosphorus homeostasis, the small intestine, the kidneys, and the skeleton, which functions as a storage reservoir. Phosphorus is present in virtually all foods. Consequently, dietary deficiencies do not occur. The average dietary intake for adults is about 800 to 1000 mg, most of which is derived from milk and dairy products. About two thirds of ingested phosphate is absorbed, mostly in the jejunum. The remaining dietary phosphate is excreted in the feces, mostly as insoluble calcium compounds. Intestinal absorption of phosphate is an active, energy-dependent process. Absorption is increased in association with decreased dietary calcium and increased acidity of the intestinal contents. Absorption is also augmented by the action of vitamin D and growth hormone. The action of parathyroid hormone on the intestinal absorption of phosphate is probably purely indirect through its effect on the metabolism of vitamin D.

Most of the phosphorus absorbed from the intestines of adults who are in phosphorus balance is excreted in the urine. This is equivalent to about 0.35 to 1.0 g of inorganic phos-

phorus daily. About 90 per cent of plasma phosphorus is filterable by the glomeruli. Ordinarily about 85 to 95 per cent of the filtered phosphate is reabsorbed, almost all in the proximal tubules. Parathyroid hormone inhibits renal tubular reabsorption of phosphate. Whether phosphate is secreted at all by the renal tubules is open to conjecture.

Parathyroid Hormone. Parathyroid hormone (PTH) from various species is structurally similar but not identical. Bovine, porcine, and human PTH consists of 84 amino acid residues in a single peptide chain. The complete sequence of both bovine and porcine hormones is known, but that of the human hormone has been only partially elucidated. Synthesis of different segments of the chain has shown that the amino-terminal fragment of the molecule, which consists of the first 32 to 34 amino acid residues, contains the structural requirements for full biologic activity. Proparathyroid hormone, a biosynthetic precursor of PTH, has been found in the parathyroid glands of swine, cattle, rats, and humans. It differs from PTH in part by having an additional hexapeptide linked to the amino-terminal end of the PTH molecule (Cohn, 1974). This prohormone is believed to have been formed from a still larger molecule, prepro-PTH, consisting of a total of 115 amino acid residues (Habener, 1975). It is generally agreed that PTH is formed from these precursors. It is then secreted from the parathyroid glands into the blood stream, primarily as a biologically active peptide with a molecular weight of 9,500 and a relatively short half-life measured in minutes. In tissues and perhaps in blood PTH undergoes cleavage to yield a carboxy-terminal fragment with a molecular weight of approximately 7,000. This fragment has no biologic activity but is believed to have a long half-life measured in days and thus accumulates to greater concentrations in blood than does intact PTH. The corresponding amino-terminal fragment which retains biologic activity has a very brief half-life in blood (Arnaud, 1974). The carboxy-terminal fragment is usually the circulating PTH determined in radioimmunoassays. The existence of various precursors and cleavage products of PTH has complicated the development and application of radioimmunoassays for measuring PTH in plasma.

The primary physiologic function of PTH is to regulate the concentration of ionic calcium in extracellular fluids. PTH secretion ordinarily causes a rise in plasma ionic calcium concentration and a fall in phosphorus concentration. By way of an effective feedback mechanism, hypercalcemia leads to PTH suppression. The interaction between calcium and phosphorus is complex and involves magnesium in an incompletely understood manner. In severe hypomagnesemia, for example, the action of PTH is impaired. Patients with low plasma magnesium concentration require magnesium to increase the plasma PTH before the plasma calcium level can be restored to normal.

The most important effects of PTH on the kidney are to increase reabsorption of calcium, principally in the distal tubules, and to depress reabsorption of phosphorus both in the proximal and distal tubules. This results in a rise in plasma calcium concentration and a fall in plasma phosphorus concentration. Although the biochemical mechanisms involved in the renal handling of calcium and phosphorus reabsorption are still not completely understood, evidence accumulated thus far is consistent with the hypothesis that the action of PTH in kidney and in bone is mediated via the stimulation of adenyl cyclase activity, leading to enhanced cyclic AMP production. These effects precede and presumably mediate changes in phosphorus and calcium transport in kidney and in bone (Chase, 1968). PTH also diminishes the secretion of hydrogen ion, thus leading to an increased excretion of bicarbonate and to a hyperchloremic acidosis, which is often present in patients with primary hyperparathyroidism (Wills, 1971).

The major action of PTH on bone is the mobilization of both calcium and phosphorus to restore extracellular fluid calcium concentration to normal. The site of action of PTH on bone appears to be directed primarily to the stable or established component of bone rather than to the labile component. Bone resorption induced by PTH is mediated by increased activity of both osteocytes and osteoclasts. Increased conversion of osteoprogenitor cells to osteoclasts occurs as a consequence of more prolonged PTH stimulation. Additional effects of PTH on bone are increased formation of collagenase, which degrades the matrix of bone, and increased breakdown of the ground substance of bone. The end result of PTH action on bone is thus true bone resorption and not simply demineralization.

PTH promotes the intestinal absorption of calcium. With the discovery that PTH stimulates the renal synthesis of 1,25-dihydroxycholecalciferol, however, it appears more likely that the effect of PTH upon intestinal calcium transport is mediated indirectly via its effects upon calciferol metabolism.

Vitamin D Compounds. Vitamin D is a generic designation for a group of fat-soluble, structurally similar sterols, several of which are vitally important in calcium and phosphorus metabolism. Some of these sterols are appropriately termed provitamins because they can be transformed into physiologically active compounds by irradiation with ultraviolet light. The two most important vitamins are vitamin D_2 or ergocalciferol and vitamin D_3 or cholecalciferol. Ergosterol is present in yeast and a variety of plant substances and can be transformed into the antirachitic ergocalciferol by irradiation. Ergocalciferol is the active vitamin D in various commercial vitamin preparations and in irradiated bread. Cholecalciferol, in contrast, is found in certain animal tissues and products, particularly fish livers and viscera, the livers of fish-eating mammals, and irradiated milk.

Approximately 94 per cent of the vitamins D_2 and D_3 in plasma are bound to a specific inter-alpha globulin with a molecular weight of 60,000. Excess vitamin D may be stored in tissues, metabolized to inactive products, or excreted in the bile. One reduction product, dihydrotachysterol, is formed from either ergocalciferol or cholecalciferol and has therapeutic uses.

Vitamin D_3 is the major biosynthetic and degradative pathway in humans. In addition to dietary sources, cholecalciferol is synthesized in the skin by ultraviolet irradiation of 7-dehydrocholesterol (Fig. 10-10). Cholecalciferol is transported to the liver where it undergoes hydroxylation to produce 25-hydroxycholecalciferol (25-OH-D_3). Although 25-OH-D_3

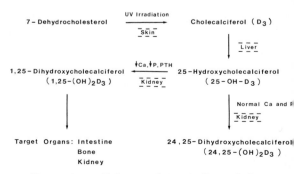

Figure 10-10. Pathways of vitamin D metabolism.

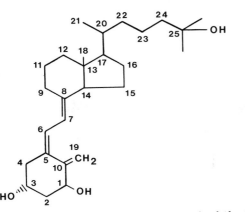

Figure 10–11. Structure of 1,25-dihydroxycholecalciferol.

Calcitonin. Calcitonin is a peptide hormone consisting of 32 amino acid residues with a molecular weight of 3,000. Structural differences in the hormone among various animal species are reflected in differences in relative potency. The complete structure of porcine, bovine, salmon, and human calcitonin has been elucidated. The intact molecule appears to be essential for biologic activity.

Calcitonin is produced and secreted by specialized C-cells, which are part of the APUD cell system derived embryologically from the neural crest (See p. 467). In man, the C-cells are represented predominantly as parafollicular cells in the lateral lobes of the thyroid gland. Small numbers of C-cells are also located in the thymus. Secretion of calcitonin is stimulated by an increase in the concentration of ionic calcium (Deftos, 1974). The fact that pentagastrin and glucagon are also potent stimuli to calcitonin secretion suggests a physiologic role for calcitonin in modulating postprandial hypercalcemia.

In experimental animals, the metabolic effect of calcitonin administration is most noticeable in young animals and in those older animals that are undergoing active bone remodeling. Following an initial transient release of calcium from bone, calcitonin causes a significant inhibition of calcium release. Consequently, the plasma concentrations of both calcium and phosphorus eventually decrease. Calcitonin decreases the activity of osteoclasts and osteocytes as well as the transformation of osteoprogenitor cells into these cell species. Long-term calcitonin administration thus results in a decrease of both bone resorption and bone remodeling.

The physiologic effects of calcitonin on the kidney are less well understood. Calcitonin causes increased renal excretion of phosphorus, sodium, and chloride in the promixal tubules. Calcitonin also inhibits the conversion of 25-OH-D$_3$ to 1,25-(OH)$_2$D$_3$ by PTH.

The exact physiologic role of calcitonin in man is still not established. Unfortunately, currently available data from radioimmunoassays have not yielded many definitive answers.

has limited biologic activity, it is the major circulating metabolite of vitamin D$_3$. In the kidney, 25-OH-D$_3$ undergoes a second hydroxylation to form either 1,25-dihydroxycholecalciferol (1,25-(OH)$_2$D$_3$) (Fig. 10–11) or 24,25-dihydroxycholecalciferol (24,25-(OH)$_2$D$_3$). These alternate pathways are reciprocally related. Formation of 1,25-(OH)$_2$D$_3$ is enhanced by decreased plasma phosphate, by PTH, and consequently by any factors that cause augmented secretion of PTH, e.g., hypocalcemia (DeLuca, 1974). Currently, the fate of 24,25-(OH)$_2$D$_3$ is unknown. Of known compounds, 1,25-(OH)$_2$D$_3$ is the most metabolically active form of vitamin D in terms of both calcium and phosphorus metabolism. Since it is endogenously produced and has specific target tissues, i.e., bone and intestine, 1,25-(OH)$_2$D$_3$ is appropriately considered a hormone rather than a vitamin (Norman, 1974).

There are two major metabolic effects of 1,25-(OH)$_2$D$_3$ on intestine and bone, and a relatively minor effect on the kidneys. Intestinal absorption of calcium and calcium-dependent phosphate transport are both enhanced by 1,25-(OH)$_2$D$_3$. The precise mode of action of 1,25-(OH)$_2$D$_3$ is not known, but existing evidence indicates that it stimulates the synthesis of proteins that are active in transcellular calcium transport (DeLuca, 1977). It has been clearly established that 1,25-(OH)$_2$D$_3$ facilitates the effect of PTH on bone, but it probably has no independent effect. The relatively minor effects of 1,25-(OH)$_2$D$_3$ on the kidneys are to promote calcium and probably also phosphorus reabsorption. The biochemistry of vitamin D has been extensively reviewed by DeLuca (1977).

CLINICOPATHOLOGIC CORRELATION

Although considerable progress has been made in recent years in elucidating the physi-

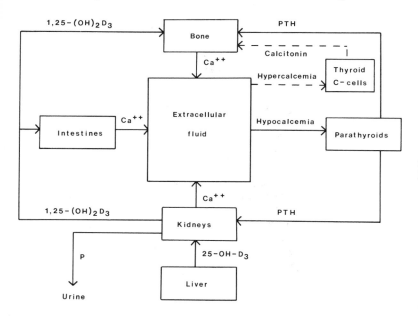

Figure 10–12. Major hormonal regulators of calcium metabolism.

ologic chemistry of calcium and phosphorus metabolism, relatively little is yet known about the biochemical and molecular biologic processes at the cellular level. It is a virtual certainty that some of the current concepts of diseases that affect calcium and phosphorus metabolism will be altered as cellular processes in both health and disease are better understood. Present concepts of the major hormonal regulations of calcium metabolism are summarized in Figure 10-12. A fall in serum calcium concentration stimulates the parathyroid glands to secrete PTH, which manifests its effects on the kidneys and bone. In the kidneys PTH promotes tubular reabsorption of calcium and phosphate diuresis. It also stimulates the biosynthesis of 1,25-$(OH)_2D_3$, which acts on the intestines to increase calcium absorption. Along with 1,25-$(OH)_2D_3$, PTH effects mobilization of both calcium and phosphorus from bone. This process continues until additional calcium from intestinal absorption, bone mobilization, and renal conservation is sufficient to restore the plasma concentration to normal. Hypercalcemia, on the other hand, probably stimulates the C-cells in the thyroid glands to secrete calcitonin, which acts on bone to inhibit resorption.

Scientific and technical advancements in clinical laboratory science have been such that precise and accurate determinations of calcium, inorganic phosphate, and alkaline phosphatase in serum are now commonly included in routine health screening or hospital admis-

sion profiles. This has resulted in an increasing challenge to the practicing physician, who is more frequently confronted with the interpretation of relatively minor abnormal variations of these analytes. Additional laboratory data are ordinarily required. Determinations of the timed urinary excretions of calcium and inorganic phosphate have long been available but are of limited diagnostic value unless the dietary intake is carefully controlled. Within the past few years, radioimmunoassay of parathyroid hormone has become readily available from reference laboratories. Improved instrumentation should facilitate the routine availability of ionized calcium determinations, at least in larger hospitals, in the very near future. Determination of various other analytes can provide valuable information in selected cases, e.g., growth hormone, cortisol, vitamin D metabolites, and hydroxyproline. Nevertheless, the entire constellation of laboratory data related to aberrations in calcium and phosphorus metabolism is seldom both pathognomonic of the disease etiology and indicative of its extent of involvement. Meaningful interpretation of the relevant laboratory data may require various special studies in addition to a complete history and physical examination. In particular, roentgenographic examinations can provide valuable information regarding both the etiology and extent of disease. Renal function tests and studies of acid-base balance may be indicated. Histopathologic examination of bone biopsies from

Table 10-5. TYPICAL CHEMICAL PATHOLOGY FINDINGS IN METABOLIC BONE DISEASES

DISEASE	SERUM			URINE	
	Ca^{++}	$HPO_4^=$	Alkaline phosphatase	Ca^{++}	$H_2PO_4^-$
Primary hyperparathyroidism	↑	↓	N, ↑	↑	↑
Renal osteodystrophy	↓, N	↑	↑	↓	↓
Vitamin D deficiency (rickets or osteomalacia)	N, ↓	↓	↑	↓	↑
Hypoparathyroidism	↓	↑	N	↓	↓
Pseudohypoparathyroidism	↓	↑	N	↓	↓
Vitamin D resistant rickets	N, ↓	↓	↑	↑	↑
Renal tubular acidosis	N, ↓	↓	↑	↑	↑
Fanconi syndrome	N, ↓	↓	↑	N, ↑	N
Idiopathic osteoporosis	N	N	↑	N, ↑	N
Paget's disease	N, ↑	N	↑	N	N
Hypophosphatasia	N, ↑	N	↓↓	N	N
Vitamin D intoxication	↑	N, ↕	N	↑	↑
Fibrous dysplasia	N	N	↑	N	N
Osteogenesis imperfecta	N	N	N	N	N
Osteopetrosis	N	N	N	↓	N

↑ = increase; N = normal; ↕ = increase or decrease; ↓ = decrease; ↓↓ = great decrease.

appropriate sites such as the iliac crest in generalized bone disease or directly from localized lesions can be of unique value in selected cases.

The effects of various diseases on calcium and phosphorus metabolism are shown in Table 10-5. It is to be emphasized that dietary inadequacies of calcium and phosphorus are seldom the cause of significant metabolic derangements. The high phosphate content of cow's milk can result in deficient calcium absorption and tetany in the newborn. Other factors incriminated in neonatal hypocalcemia include prematurity, vitamin D deficiency, transient physiologic hypoparathyroidism, and decreased ability of the kidneys to excrete inorganic phosphate.

A rare dietary problem affecting calcium and phosphorus metabolism is vitamin D intoxication, which is usually the result of excessive intake of vitamin supplements over a prolonged period of time. Large amounts of vitamin D can be stored in the body, since it is fat-soluble. Clinically the disease is manifested by weakness, irritability, nausea, vomiting, and diarrhea. Plasma calcium is typically elevated, while inorganic phosphorus is variable. The hypercalcemia is the result of both increased intestinal absorption of calcium and increased mobilization from bone. Metastatic calcification of soft tissues and viscera, compromised renal function with frank azotemia, and osteoporosis may occur.

Bone Disease. Most of the body content of calcium and phosphorus is present in bone as a highly structured crystal lattice similar to hydroxyapatite, the general formula of which is $Ca_{10}(PO_4)_6(OH)_2$. Bone minerals also include 70 per cent of the body content of magnesium, 30 per cent of the sodium, and smaller amounts of potassium, carbonate, citrate, and fluoride. The dry weight of compact bone consists of approximately 75 per cent inorganic mineral salts and 25 per cent organic matrix as shown in Table 10-6. Mineralization of bone matrix is not a simple precipitation of salts but rather is a complex, incompletely understood physiochemical process (Parfitt, 1976a). In previous times, the importance to bone mineralization of the solubility product of calcium phosphate, $Ca^{++} \times HPO_4^=$, was emphasized. Although the initial salt that is formed may well be $CaHPO_4$, the solubility product explanation is overly simplistic, particularly since extracellular fluid is supersaturated with these ions.

Even in adult life, bone is in a dynamic state, as evidenced by the fact that perhaps 3 to 5 per cent of the bone mass is undergoing active remodeling at any one time. The processes of bone formation and resorption are controlled by various hormonal and metabolic influences (Lutwak, 1975; Deftos, 1975). Bone is formed by the action of osteocytes and osteoblasts, the activity of which is reflected in the alkaline phosphatase level in serum. Bone resorption occurs predominantly as a result of the action of osteoclasts and ordinarily involves dissolution of both minerals and or-

Table 10-6. COMPOSITION OF BONE

Mineral inorganic crystalline salts (75 per cent of dry weight)	Phosphate and carbonate salts of calcium (compressional strength). Small amounts of magnesium, sodium, potassium, hydroxide, fluoride, and sulfate.
Organic matrix (25 per cent of dry weight)	94 per cent collagen fibers (tensile strength) (hydroxyproline and proline constitute a third of total amino acid composition of collagen fibrils). 5 per cent ground substance: Extracellular fluid Mucoprotein Chondroitin sulfate Hyaluronic acid 1 per cent citrate

ganic matrix. The urinary excretion of hydroxyproline is elevated in association with increased bone resorption, as it is in other etiologies of increased collagen turnover (Table 10-7). This is a result of the fact that collagen is the only mammalian protein that contains significant amounts of hydroxyproline.

Osteoporosis is the most common metabolic disease of bone. It is not a single etiologic entity but rather is associated with a variety of epidemiologic, clinical, and biochemical factors that result in decreased bone mass. The term bone atrophy is sometimes applied to this pathologic process, but this term is imprecise because osteoporosis can occur as a consequence of increased bone resorption, decreased bone formation, or a combination of both factors. Normal mineralization of existing osteoid is a critical feature that distinguishes osteoporosis from osteomalacia. The roentgenographic appearance of diffusely diminished bone density is reflected in the histopathologic appearance of thinned bone cortices and delicate trabeculae. Skeletal deformities, fractures, especially compression fractures of the vertebral bodies, and bone pain are common sequelae.

The various etiologies of osteoporosis are shown in Table 10-8. The most common type by far is postmenopausal or senile osteoporosis, which is far more common with aging and is three to four times more frequent in females than in males. There are various theories as to the etiologic factors in senile osteoporosis, including diminished physical activity, deficiency of gonadal hormones, and dietary inadequacies. Urinary calcium and hydroxyproline excretions are frequently increased. Other parameters of calcium and phosphorus metabolism are usually normal. In contrast, both calcium and inorganic phosphate in plasma can be elevated in rapidly developing osteoporosis of disuse such as occurs following

Table 10-7. ELEVATION OF URINARY HYDROXYPROLINE IN DISEASE*

Marked
  Paget's disease
  Fibrous dysplasia
  Osteomalacia
  Neoplastic bone disease
  Rickets
  Hyperthyroidism
  Hyperparathyroidism (primary and secondary)
  Severe burns
  Acute osteomyelitis
  Congenital hypophosphatasia

Moderate
  Acromegaly
  Marfan's syndrome
  Active rheumatoid arthritis
  Active scleroderma

Normal to slight
  Inflammatory skin diseases
  Osteoporosis
  Pregnancy
  Aseptic bone necrosis
  Diabetes mellitus
  Renal disease

*Niejadlik, D. C.: Postgrad. Med. *51* (No. 5):214, 1972.

Table 10-8. ETIOLOGIC CLASSIFICATION OF OSTEOPOROSIS

Primary (idiopathic, postmenopausal, senile)
Secondary
  Hyperparathyroidism
  Cushing's syndrome
  Hyperthyroidism
  Acromegaly
  Heparin therapy (prolonged high dosage)
  Vitamin D excess
  Immobilization
  Pregnancy (rare cause)
  Miscellaneous (diabetes, liver disease, sickle cell anemia, various lipid or carbohydrate storage diseases)

mmobilization or paralysis in a previously active individual.

Osteomalacia refers to deficient mineralization of bone resulting from various disturbances in calcium and phosphorus metabolism. Osteoid formation continues, but the bones become softened. Weakness, skeletal pain and deformities, and fractures can occur as the disease progresses. Roentgenographic examination reveals generalized rarefaction of the skeleton with an accentuated trabecular pattern. Rickets is the designation for osteomalacia that occurs prior to cessation of growth, i.e., closure of the epiphyses of bones. The skeletal deformities in rickets are accentuated as a consequence of compensatory overgrowth of epiphyseal cartilage, wide bands of which remain unmineralized and unresorbed. In severe cases of rickets, decreased growth may be associated with such evident deformities as swellings of the costochondral junctions of the ribs (rachitic rosary), a protuberant sternum, frontal bossing, and delayed closure of the anterior fontanelle.

There are various etiologies of osteomalacia. Vitamin D deficiency is particularly important in childhood and can be caused by inadequate dietary intake, intestinal malabsorption, or diminished synthesis of active metabolites as a consequence of inadequate exposure to sunlight. Dietary deficiency is very uncommon in America because of the widespread use of fortified milk and bread and vitamin supplements. When vitamin D deficiency occurs in adults it is usually a consequence of malabsorption. Since vitamin D is a fat-soluble vitamin, its absorption is impaired in sprue, biliary or pancreatic disease, or steatorrhea from other causes. A systemic resistance to vitamin D may be of major importance in the osteomalacia that accompanies chronic renal disease. Dietary inadequacy of calcium is a rare cause of osteomalacia, while dietary deficiencies of phosphorus do not occur. Increased loss of inorganic phosphorus in the urine occurs in various renal tubular disorders and can result in osteomalacia. These diseases include vitamin D-resistant rickets (phosphate diabetes), renal tubular acidosis, and the Fanconi syndrome.

A rare cause of osteomalacia is hypophosphatasia, an inherited autosomal recessive disease characterized by a significant depression of alkaline phosphatase in both plasma and tissues. Concentrations of calcium and phosphorus in plasma are normal or increased.

Urinary excretion of hydroxyproline is decreased. A curious finding is the presence of significant amounts of phosphoethanolamine in urine.

It is not currently possible to designate a common denominator in the pathogenesis of osteomalacia. Formerly, the criticality of the solubility product of calcium phosphate, $Ca^{++} \times HPO_4^{=}$, was emphasized. In chronic renal disease, however, osteomalacia can progress in the presence of a normal or even elevated solubility product. Other etiologies, including vitamin D deficiency, can cause severe osteomalacia in the presence of normal or only slightly decreased serum calcium concentration. Phosphate depletion is probably of greater importance than decreased calcium.

Osteitis deformans or Paget's disease of bone is an uncommon but not rare disorder characterized by irregular skeletal distribution and varying severity. The disease may involve only one bone or may be more or less generalized. Osteoclastic resorption of bone, extensive production of abnormal, poorly mineralized osteoid, and fibrous tissue proliferation result in bone that is structurally weak and prone to deformities and fractures. Osteogenic sarcoma is a late complication in a small percentage of cases. Serum calcium and inorganic phosphorus concentrations are usually normal but occasionally are elevated. Of particular significance is the greatly elevated alkaline phosphatase activity in plasma, which reflects the active but pathologic osteoblastic proliferation. Urinary excretion of calcium and phosphorus is normal or increased, while excretion of hydroxyproline is usually significantly increased.

Osteitis deformans frequently responds both clinically and pathologically to therapeutic administration of calcitonin.

Parathyroid Diseases. Primary hyperparathyroidism is characterized by excessive secretion of parathyroid hormone (PTH) in the absence of an appropriate physiologic stimulus, i.e., hypersecretion co-existent with normal or elevated serum ionized calcium. The etiologic frequency of primary hyperparathyroidism has been reported to be single parathyroid adenomas in 92 per cent, multiple adenomas in 4 per cent, hyperplasia in 3 per cent, and carcinoma in less than 1 per cent of cases (Goldman, 1971). Uncomplicated primary hyperparathyroidism is characteristically associated with elevated serum calcium and decreased serum inorganic phosphorus (Table

10–5) and frequently accompanied by a mild systemic acidosis. PTH acts directly on bone to cause increased resorption and consequent increase in serum calcium (Parfitt, 1976b). Two other factors also contribute to the elevated serum calcium. PTH stimulates increased renal biosynthesis of 1,25-$(OH)_2D_3$, which increases intestinal absorption of calcium. PTH also augments renal tubular reabsorption of calcium. The decreased concentration of inorganic phosphate is primarily the result of PTH-induced phosphate diuresis caused by decreased renal tubular reabsorption.

The bone lesions of hyperparathyroidism, often termed osteitis fibrosa cystica or von Recklinghausen's disease of bone, are of particular clinical and pathologic importance (Parfitt, 1976c). Increased osteoclastic activity leads to extensive bone resorption with thinning of both cortical and cancellous bone. In addition to severe osteoporosis, extensive fibroblastic proliferation occurs in the marrow spaces and can cause cystic lesions. Bone pain, skeletal deformities, and fractures can result.

In the past, the general assumption was that patients with primary hyperparathyroidism have autonomous PTH secretion. Data from PTH radioimmunoassays, however, clearly reveal that most if not all patients with primary hyperparathyroidism exhibit a suppression of PTH secretion with calcium infusion (Murray, 1972). It can thus be concluded that the set point in the feedback mechanism operates at a higher than normal level. Plasma PTH values obtained by radioimmunoassay cannot always differentiate between hyperparathyroidism and normals because considerable overlap occurs between the two groups. This discrepancy is resolved in most cases, however, when plasma PTH values are compared with plasma ionized calcium concentrations. The discrimination is made on the basis that in a normal individual, plasma calcium concentration bears an inverse relationship to the PTH concentration. Thus, while the plasma PTH concentration may be within the normal range for patients with primary hyperparathyroidism, this level is inappropriately high when coexistent with hypercalcemia (Arnaud, 1971). Hence, the demonstration of normal amounts of circulating PTH in the presence of elevated calcium is strongly indicative of primary hyperparathyroidism.

Detection of excessive phosphate diuresis can be helpful in distinguishing hyperparathyroidism from other etiologies of hypercalcemia (Gordan, 1968). This can be achieved by determining the tubular reabsorption of phosphate (TRP) or the renal phosphate clearance (C_p) according to the following equations:

$$\text{TRP}(\%) = 100 \left[1 - \frac{P_u \times Cr_s}{P_s \times Cr_u} \right]$$

$$C_p(\text{ml/min}) = \frac{V/t \times P_u}{P_s}$$

where P_u and P_s are the inorganic phosphate concentrations (mg/dl) in urine and serum.

Cr_u and Cr_s are the creatinine concentrations (mg/dl) in urine and serum

V is the urine volume collected in an established time interval (t).

The TRP is not applicable even in mild azotemia. The TRP is normally 80 to 90 per cent while the C_p is normally 5 to 15 ml/min. In hyperparathyroidism the TRP is usually less than 78 per cent, while the C_p is greater than 18 ml/min.

Secondary hyperparathyroidism is characterized by an appropriately excessive secretion of PTH in response to chronic hypocalcemia. In the United States and Europe most cases of chronic hypocalcemia are the result of either vitamin D deficiency or renal disease; hypocalcemia is rarely caused by an inadequate dietary intake of calcium. Vitamin D deficiency leads to decreased absorption of both calcium and phosphate so that both the serum calcium and inorganic phosphorus are low. Increased PTH secretion tends to increase calcium toward normal but to suppress inorganic phosphorus even further because of the increased renal loss of phosphate under the influence of PTH (Table 10–5).

Chronic renal failure can result in compensatory hyperparathyroidism, which in turn causes diffuse bone disease, including osteoporosis, osteomalacia, osteosclerosis (areas of increased bone density), osteitis fibrosa cystica and metastatic calcification. The disease complex is sometimes termed renal osteodystrophy or, when it occurs in children, renal rickets. The bone manifestations of chronic renal disease are seen more often now that life is prolonged with maintenance hemodialysis. The interrelationships in hyperparathyroidism secondary to chronic renal disease are very complex, as shown in Figure 10–13. The pathogenesis varies somewhat, depending upon the nature and severity of the renal disease. Decreased renal excretion of phosphate as a consequence of impaired glomerular filtration

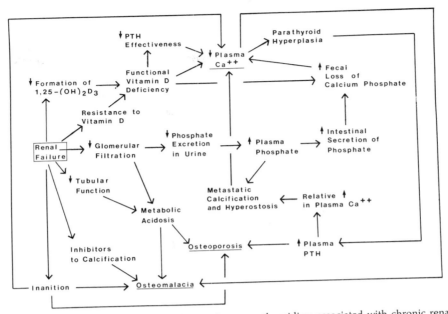

Figure 10–13. Pathophysiologic interrelationships in hyperparathyroidism associated with chronic renal disease.

is of paramount importance. Diminished responsiveness to vitamin D and probably decreased renal biosynthesis of 1,25-$(OH)_2D_3$ are also important. The effectiveness of PTH is compromised by the functional deficiency of vitamin D and the inability of the renal tubules to respond with a phosphate diuresis. Increased fecal loss of calcium also occurs. There is evidence that normal calcification is impeded by circulating inhibitors.

Hypoparathyroidism is usually the result of parathyroidectomy, frequently as an unintentional consequence of thyroidectomy. Uncommonly it can result from an idiopathic lack of parathyroid function. Lack of parathyroid hormone from whatever cause leads to a fall in plasma calcium and a corresponding rise in plasma inorganic phosphorus concentration. There is increasing evidence that the biosynthesis of 1,25-$(OH)_2D_3$ can be impaired as a result of PTH deficiency and perhaps also hyperphosphatemia. The most important clinical manifestations are directly attributable to decreased ionized calcium concentrations in plasma, which can cause increased neuromuscular excitability and tetany.

Pseudohypoparathyroidism is a rare genetic disorder characterized by signs and symptoms of hypoparathyroidism. It is, however, distinguishable from true hypoparathyroidism in that plasma calcium concentration is low and

plasma phosphorus high in spite of an increased concentration of PTH in plasma. Moreover, while infusion of PTH into patients with hypoparathyroidism generally results in a marked increase in both urinary cyclic AMP and inorganic phosphate excretion, PTH infusion into patients with pseudohypoparathyroidism causes a distinctly subnormal response in both urinary phosphate excretion and cyclic AMP production. This has been interpreted as a genetically determined inability of the renal tubules to respond to PTH. The term pseudo-pseudohypoparathyroidism has been used to describe patients with skeletal manifestation of the disease whose plasma calcium and phosphorus metabolism are normal. These are only variations in the same basic genetic defect, as evidenced by the fact that both manifestations can occur in a single kindred.

Hypercalcemia commonly accompanies the metastases of malignant neoplasms to bone, usually as a consequence of rapid bone resorption as the metastases enlarge. Occasional malignant neoplasms, particularly those of the lung, kidney, and ovary, may secrete parathyroid hormone to such an extent that true hyperparathyroidism develops. This condition has been termed the ectopic PTH syndrome. Hypercalcemia may also be caused by vitamin D-like compounds produced by tumor (e.g., breast). One feature that is sometimes useful in distinguishing the two neoplastic etiologies of hypercalcemia is the inorganic phosphorus level in plasma, which tends to be low in association with ectopic PTH production and normal or elevated in association with simple bone resorption secondary to metastases.

Hypercalcemia of malignancy versus hyperparathyroidism is an important differential diagnosis and often a difficult diagnosis to make.

Renal Diseases. Chronic renal failure, discussed previously as an important etiology of secondary hyperparathyroidism, is by far the most important renal disease affecting calcium and phosphorus metabolism. In addition, however, several uncommon or rare renal tubular defects can significantly affect calcium and phosphorus metabolism.

Vitamin D-resistant rickets, also termed familial hypophosphatemia and phosphate diabetes, is inherited, usually as a sex-linked dominant character. The exact cause of the disease is not known with certainty but is believed to be a primary defect in the ability of the renal tubules to reabsorb inorganic phosphorus. Renal phosphate clearance is definitely increased and accounts for the associated hypophosphatemia. Plasma calcium is usually normal, while alkaline phosphatase is moderately elevated. The disease may be asymptomatic or manifested by severe osteomalacia or rickets and growth retardation. The disease can be treated with some success using dietary phosphorus supplementation and high doses of vitamin D.

Renal tubular acidosis consists of both inherited and acquired conditions having in common a metabolic acidosis resulting from decreased ability of the renal tubules to secrete hydrogen ions. The defect can involve primarily either the proximal or distal tubules. The disease inherited as an autosomal dominant and involving the distal tubules is of particular importance to calcium and phosphorus metabolism. Increased calcium excretion occurs, but plasma calcium is usually normal, probably as a consequence of compensatory stimulation of the parathyroids to secrete PTH. Increased phosphate excretion typically leads to low plasma inorganic phosphorus. These factors lead to osteomalacia, which is aggravated by the systemic acidosis. Renal calculi are common sequelae.

The Fanconi syndrome consists of inherited renal diseases characterized by increased urinary excretion of phosphate, glucose, and amino acids, low plasma inorganic phosphorus and systemic acidosis. Acquired diseases can have identical manifestations. The pathogenesis of the osteomalacia that develops is not well understood.

Calcitonin and Other Hormones. No essential physiologic role has yet been established for calcitonin. The only known cause for excessive secretion of calcitonin is medullary carcinoma of the thyroid, which originates from the parafollicular C-cells. This neoplasm is frequently familial, and kindred of affected patients frequently have elevated levels of calcitonin in their plasma (Melvin, 1971). The elevated levels of calcitonin are associated with decreased skeletal remodeling, but there is no appreciable effect on plasma calcium and phosphorus.

Hyperthyroidism is associated with hypercalciuria, hyperphosphatemia, elevated alkaline phosphatase activity, and occasionally hypercalcemia. There is marked increase in bone turnover and in skeletal remodeling. It is believed that thyroxine acts directly on bone to cause greater bone resorption than formation. This results in a decreased PTH secretion, which accounts for the diminished renal reabsorption of calcium and enhanced reabsorption of phosphorus (Russell, 1976).

The effect of growth hormone upon skeletal growth has recently been revealed to be mediated indirectly via somatomedin (Van Wyk, 1974). In adults growth hormone is not necessary for the maintenance of mineral homeostasis. Growth hormone induces an increase in both intestinal absorption and renal reabsorption of calcium and phosphorus. Because of this positive balance with regard to skeletal mass, growth hormone has been proposed as a therapeutic agent for the treatment of osteoporosis.

Administration of glucocorticoids results in decreased intestinal absorption and renal tubular reabsorption of calcium. Consequently PTH secretion is stimulated and increased bone resorption occurs. Osteoporosis is indeed a prominent sign of Cushing's disease. However, the mode of action of cortisol, either in bone or in the intestine, is still unclear.

The effects of estrogens upon bone metabolism are still not clearly defined. While short-term estrogen administration seems to favor bone formation, long-term administration can apparently result in hypocalcemia and secondary hyperparathyroidism.

ANALYTICAL TECHNIQUES

Total Calcium. The oldest but still widely used procedure for the determination of total serum calcium concentration is that of Clark and Collip (1925). Calcium in serum is precipitated as calcium oxalate, which is subsequently redissolved with acidification. The resulting oxalic acid is titrated against potassium permanganate in a redox reaction, in which the purple $Mn_2O_7^=$ is reduced to the colorless Mn^{++}. This method, although highly reliable and regarded for many years as the reference procedure, requires meticulous attention in order to achieve good accuracy and is time consuming. The Clark-Collip procedure has in recent years been replaced by the more convenient and accurate methods involving photometry, fluorometry, and atomic absorption spectrophotometry.

Precipitation of calcium by chloranilic acid has been used as a method for plasma calcium determination. The precipitated calcium chloranilate is treated with ethylenediaminotetraacetic acid (EDTA), which complexes the calcium and thereby releases chloranilic acid. The latter is reddish purple and can be quantitated by spectrophotometry. This method, though accurate, is also time consuming and requires a large sample volume. It has now largely been replaced by atomic absorption and various automated procedures.

Direct determination of plasma calcium by chelation with EDTA, which is much less tedious, originated from the work of Schwarzenbach (1952). In one of the modified techniques, calcium in serum is titrated against EDTA using a fluorescent indicator, e.g., calcein, which complexes with calcium. The disappearance of the yellowish green fluorescence indicates the end point at which all the calcium is complexed to EDTA. The sensitivity and speed of this technique render it suitable as a micromethod. However, the change from fluorescence to non-fluorescence is so gradual that end point detection is difficult, particularly in the presence of elevated bilirubin, hemoglobin, jaundice, and lipemia. Other fluorescent indicators in use include murexide (ammonium purpurate), Cal-Red, and Eriochrome Black T. The presence of magnesium interferes in most of these reactions. The interference can be eliminated in some instances by titration at high pH at which magnesium precipitates as $Mg(OH)_2$.

Attempts at determining serum calcium concentration by flame photometry have not met with much success because of positive interference by sodium and potassium, inhibitory interference by phosphates and sulfates, and the fact that excitation of the calcium atom itself is difficult. Isolation of calcium as the oxalate to eliminate interfering substances has not been successful because oxalate itself lowers the emission, probably as a result of the introduction of degradation products with low excitation potential.

With the advent of the AutoAnalyzer (Technicon Instruments Corporation, Tarrytown, N.Y.), simple chemical methods for the determination of calcium based on color complex formation have found wide application. For example, color complex formation between calcium and o-cresolphthalein complex and its subsequent spectrophotometric quantitation is now the adapted procedure on the Technicon SMA 12/60. In this procedure, 8-hydroxyquinoline is added to bind magnesium, which otherwise would cause interference. Color complex formation of calcium with alizarin and subsequent quantitation by spectrophotometry has been adapted for use on the Union Carbide Centrifugal Analyzer (Union Carbide Corporation, New York, N.Y.). Other automated procedures include complex formation of calcium with calcein plasmo-corinth B and glyoxal-dis-(2-hydroxyanil)-GBHA. The precision obtained with automated instruments is in the magnitude of ± 3 per cent.

In terms of accuracy, precision, and speed, the determination of serum calcium concentration by atomic absorption spectrophotometry is undoubtedly the method of choice both for routine analysis and as a reference procedure. Calcium in serum and urine is diluted sufficiently with lanthanum chloride solution, which binds interfering substances such as protein and phosphates. When introduced into a flame, the dissociated free calcium atom absorbs light from the characteristic wavelengths (e.g., 422.7 nm) produced by a hollow cathode lamp with a calcium filament. A small fraction of calcium atoms (about 1/1,000) is raised to high energy level, and on returning to the ground state emits radiation, the intensity of which is proportional to the calcium concentration in the sample. Precision achievable on standard instruments is about ± 3.5 per cent.

In general, specimens for total calcium determination should be serum or heparinized plasma collected in the fasting state. Oxalate and EDTA interfere with most determinations, since the former causes precipitation and the latter results in chelation of calcium, thus rendering it unavailable for analysis. Total calcium concentrations are known to be affected also by prolonged venous occlusion and by posture. The former leads to hemoconcentration, thereby causing an increase in the calcium values while patients in a recumbent posture have lower calcium concentrations. Both factors, however, appear to affect mainly the protein-bound fraction of the calcium concentration.

Ionized Calcium. The physiologic importance of ionized calcium in extracellular fluid was first established by McLean (1935), who observed that the amplitude of contraction of the isolated frog heart was proportional to the ionized calcium concentration. Since then, numerous methods have been devised to measure the ionized fraction of calcium in serum. Prior to the advent of calcium-selective electrodes, the techniques for these measurements were mainly colorimetric determinations based on the color change produced in the metal ion indicator, murexide, when it complexes with calcium ions. This technique unfortunately has severe limitations because murexide itself binds to serum albumin, thus causing overestimation of the ionized calcium concentration. Furthermore, the sensitivity to pH changes and the temperature dependency necessitate stringent experimental conditions. Most of the difficulties, however, appear to be overcome by using the tetramethyl derivative of murexide, which does not bind to serum protein. Furthermore, its color formation is independent of pH within the physiologic range, and the precision has been reported to be greater than that with murexide.

The development of various calcium ion-selective electrodes in the late 1960's has helped make the determination of ionized calcium a procedure amenable to routine operation. Recently an automated system based on a flow-through sensor (Orion Model SS-20) has been developed. This instrument consists of a liquid ion-exchange flow-through electrode, the membrane of which is impregnated with a liquid ion-exchanger. The membrane selectively binds calcium and is normally saturated with that ion. During operation, serum is pumped through the electrode to make contact with the ion-exchange membrane, thus causing a potential difference between the ionized calcium of the serum and that of the liquid ion-exchanger.

Since the calcium concentration of the saturated ion-exchanger is constant, the resultant potential difference is proportional to the ionized calcium concentration of the serum. Potentiometric methods have the advantages that they are technically simple and require relatively small sample volumes (0.5 ml). The between-run precision is in the range of 2 to 3 per cent. The normal range is 2.0 to 2.4 mEq/l (1.0 to 1.2 mmol/l), which is in reasonable agreement with previously reported values.

Since the ionized calcium fraction is pH-dependent, the most important factor throughout the analysis is the maintenance of a constant pH. It is recommended that the blood collection and handling procedure be conducted anaerobically insofar as possible and that the red cells be separated as soon as clotting is complete to obviate pH changes, because a decrease in pH will result in dissociation of bound calcium. Conversely, increased pH resulting from loss of CO_2 will cause a fall in the ionized calcium concentration. It is possible to correct ionized calcium values for the effect of pH changes, provided that the pH values both at the time of collection of the blood sample and at the time of analysis are known (Wybenga, 1976). The requisite equation is applicable to wide fluctuations in pH and is independent of protein concentration. Hyperventilation sufficient to cause an increase of 0.1 to 0.2 pH units of blood pH is known to produce up to a 10 per cent reduction in ionized calcium concentration. It is therefore imperative that the state of ventilation be normal during sampling. Prolonged venous occlusion will influence the total serum calcium concentration if pH changes occur as a result. While short-term change in posture does not seem to affect the ionized calcium concentration, long-term bed rest has been shown to cause elevation in both the total and the ionized calcium concentration as a result of increased mobilization from bone.

Ionized calcium in serum is also temperature-dependent, and measurement at 37°C. is recommended. Heparinized blood should not be used for the analysis because heparin has been shown to complex calcium ions.

Phosphorus. Most methods for phosphorus determination are based on the principle that under suitable conditions molybdates react with phosphate to form various heteropoly compounds, such as ammonium phosphomolybdate, which is believed to have the formula $(NH_4)_3[PO_4(MoO_3)_{12}]$. Different techniques have been employed in the quantitation of this complex. An ultramicro-method has been described in which the phosphomolybdate is determined by acidimetric titration. Direct measurement of this complex at 340 nm is now adapted for use on the Union Carbide Centrifugal Analyzer. To improve assay sensitivity, the phosphomolybdate has also been extracted into xylene-isobutanol prior to spectrophotometric determination at 310 nm. However, most of the techniques for the determination of phosphorus involve photometric measurement of the molybdenum blue formed by reduction of phosphomolybdate under conditions that do not reduce the excess molybdate present. A variety of reducing agents have been introduced, including stannous chloride, p-aminonaphtholsulfonic acid, ascorbic acid, p-methylaminophenolsulfate (Elon), N-phenyl-p-phenylenediamine, and ferrous sulfate. Most procedures involve deproteinization with trichloroacetic acid. The protein-free filtrate is mixed with molybdic acid to form phosphomolybdate that is reduced with the appropriate reducing agent to produce molybdenum blue. Quantitation is usually carried out at 660 nm. A modification using iron (Fe^{++}) and thiourea is the method of choice because of its color stability, improved sensitivity, and conformity to Beer's law over a wide range of concentrations (Goldenberg, 1966). The precision of this method is reported to be in the range of ± 5 per cent.

Complex formation between phosphomolybdate and the triphenylmethane dye malachite green appears to be the most sensitive procedure known for phosphorus determination. Unfortunately, the high acidity at which complex is formed also causes hydrolysis of organic phosphates. An enzymatic method for phosphorus determination is also described whereby phosphorus undergoes successive enzymatic reactions catalyzed by glycogen phosphorylase, phosphoglucomutase, and glucose-6-phosphate dehydrogenase (Schultz, 1967). The NADPH produced can be quantitated by fluorescence or light absorption. The reaction takes place at neutral pH, thus permitting the measurement of inorganic phosphorus in the presence of unstable organic phosphates. Since organic phosphates exist principally in the erythrocytes, it is important to separate serum from the red cells as soon as clotting is complete.

Hydroxyproline. Since more than 90 per cent of the hydroxyproline in urine is present as a component of oligopeptides, almost all laboratory procedures begin with acid hydrolysis of the sample. The liberated hydroxyproline is then oxidized by chloramine T to pyrrole, which reacts with Ehrlich's reagent to form a red chromogen that is determined colorimetrically. However, most hydrolysates of urine also contain ammonium chloride, glucose, and mannitol, which interfere with color formation. Various modifications to this procedure have been developed in an effort to improve assay specificity. For example, the use of a cation-exchange resin is recommended for the separation of hydroxyproline from interfering contaminants prior to hydrolysis, oxidation, and color development (Goverde, 1972). Alternately, the isolation of the oxidized product by distillation or extraction with toluene has successfully eliminated interferences caused by non-volatile color compounds produced by tyrosine and tryptophan. This procedure is found to yield accurate results, provided care is taken to avoid loss of the volatile oxidation products (DuPont, 1967).

Another method using charcoal-butanol extraction of an acid hydrolysate of urine followed by colorimetric determination with p-dimethylaminobenzaldehyde has recently been described (Ritchie, 1977). Results obtained by this procedure compare favorably with those obtained from a more specific method requiring ion-exchange chromatography.

For the determination of free hydroxyproline, the initial acid hydrolysis step is omitted.

Parathyroid Hormone. Although the measurement of PTH by radioimmunoassay was first described by Berson in 1963, only in the last few years has this assay found widespread clinical application. The theoretical and technical problems contributing to this delay are many. An important consideration is that PTH exists in multiple forms in the circulation, thus complicating not only the development of a radioimmunoassay but also the interpretation of results. At present there are no supplies of highly purified human PTH for general use; hence assays of this peptide must rely on antisera to either bovine or porcine hormone. The fact that these antisera lack high affinity for the human hormone causes reduced sensitivity of the assay. Furthermore, the lack of any reference preparation of human PTH has made it impossible for direct comparison of assay results among laboratories.

It became obvious by 1972 that the conflicting results generated from different laboratories were not just a quantitative expression of interlaboratory precision but mainly a qualitative discrepancy engendered by the fact that various antisera had specificities for different fragments of PTH. It is generally agreed that antisera that recognize the carboxy-terminal fragment of the molecule are more suitable for routine clinical use because they provide a more clear-cut separation of normal and abnormal PTH concentrations. On the other hand, the slow turnover rate of the carboxy-terminal fragments may interfere with the study of the acute secretory dynamics of the parathyroid gland, such as in the stimulation and suppression tests of parathyroid function using induced hypo- and hypercalcemia (Arnaud, 1974). In this respect, an antiserum specific for the amino-terminal fragment would be more useful in detecting the rapid changes in PTH secretion.

With the improved immunologic techniques, it has become possible to produce antisera with the desired specificity for use in the assay. In conjunction with the measurement of ionized calcium in plasma, PTH determination by radioimmunoassay provides good differentiation of hyperparathyroidism from hypercalcemia of other etiologies as well as from normal individuals (Arnaud, 1971; Robertson, 1976).

Vitamin D Compounds. The classic bioassay of vitamin D was the rat-line test, which measures the concentrations of all vitamin D precursors and metabolites, including both active and potentially active forms. This time-consuming method has in recent years been replaced by specific assays for the individual metabolites because the parent vitamins have now been shown to function primarily as precursors of the more active 25-hydroxy derivative (25-$(OH)D_3$), which are the predominant circulating species. The measurement of 25-$(OH)D_3$ thus provides a more precise index both of nutritional status and of actual, rather than potential, vitamin D activity.

Measurements of 25-$(OH)D_3$ in plasma usually involve solvent extraction, chromatographic separation to remove other sterols, and subsequent competitive protein-binding assay using a binding protein derived from rat kidney (Haddad, 1973). The binding protein

in human plasma may find application in the competitive protein-binding assay in the future.

A radioreceptor assay for 1,25-$(OH)_2D_3$, the most active hormonal form of vitamin D_3, has been reported using as binder the intestinal chromatin of chicks (Brumbaugh, 1974). While the assay itself is simple to perform, the preparation of the receptor protein requires three separate chromatographic steps. It would appear that this assay has good potential application in the diagnosis of disorders of calcium homeostasis involving vitamin D metabolism.

Calcitonin. Calcitonin was previously measured by a bioassay based on the ability of calcitonin to lower serum calcium concentration in rats. This method has in recent years been replaced by a far more sensitive radioimmunoassay, which utilizes antisera prepared against calcitonin from extracts of thyroid medullary carcinoma.

Synthetic human calcitonin is used both as labeled antigen and as a standard. The synthetic preparation is immunologically indistinguishable from endogenous calcitonin. There is no immunologic cross-reactivity between the human hormone and either the bovine, ovine, porcine, or salmon calcitonin (Deftos, 1971).

Considerable controversy exists regarding measurement of circulating calcitonin in normal subjects, since the basal plasma concentrations of most are below the limits of assay sensitivity (< 100 pg/ml). Calcium infusion in normal individuals does not result in any detectable increase in circulating calcitonin.

Cyclic AMP. Two very sensitive assays are available for the determination of urinary cyclic AMP (Gilman, 1970). A competitive protein-binding procedure utilizes a binding protein from either the muscle or the adrenal cortex which is presumably cyclic AMP-activated protein kinase. The assay is based on the competition between cyclic AMP and the radioiodinated nucleotide for binding sites on the binder. Assay sensitivity is about 0.05 to 0.1 pmole. The binder, however, cross-reacts with cyclic GMP, which may be removed by separation on a Dowex 1 ion-exchange column. The chromatographic separation step can be eliminated if the measurement is performed using radioimmunoassay, since antisera prepared for this purpose have shown adequate specificity for cyclic AMP (Steiner, 1969). Assay sensitivity has been reported to be 0.01 pmole. Both assays are now available commercially in kit packages. However, cyclic AMP measurements have not proved to be as useful as projected for hyperparathyroidism.

OTHER INORGANIC IONS

MAGNESIUM

Physiologic Chemistry. Magnesium is one of the most abundant cations in the body and is essential to many physiochemical processes. The body of an adult contains 20 to 30 g of magnesium, about 50 per cent of which is present in bone, 45 per cent in intracellular fluid, and 5 per cent in extracellular fluid. As an intracellular cation, magnesium is second in abundance only to potassium, and its concentration in intracellular fluid is about 10 times that in the extracellular fluid. Magnesium is an activator of various enzymes including phosphatases, transphosphorylases, pyrophosphatases, carboxylases, and hexokinase. Magnesium is also essential for the preservation of the macromolecular structure of DNA, RNA, and ribosomes (Wacker, 1968a).

The dynamics of magnesium exchange and homeostasis are rather poorly understood. About one third of the average adult daily dietary intake of 20 to 40 mEq* is absorbed, predominantly in the small intestine, and excreted in the urine. The absorption process appears to be poorly controlled, and homeostasis is maintained largely by renal excretion, which is regulated by tubular reabsorption. The plasma concentration is not significantly affected by dietary intake over a rather wide range (Agarwal, 1976). The pharmacology of magnesium has been recently reviewed (Massry, 1977).

Reference serum levels vary somewhat depending on the analytical method employed. Using atomic absorption, the normal range is about 1.3 to 2.1 mEq/l (0.7 to 1.1 mmol/l). There appears to be no sex difference, but levels are somewhat higher in females during menstruation. The concentration in newborns is essentially the same as in adults. The concentration in erythrocytes is about three times that in serum. About 70 per cent of the magnesium in serum is freely diffusible and the remainder is bound to plasma proteins, largely albumin. The magnesium content of cerebrospinal fluid is about 2.0 to 2.7 mEq/l (1.0 to 1.4 mmol/l).

Clinicopathologic Correlation. Magne-

sium depletion is clinically more significant and frequent than an excess but is nevertheless relatively uncommon. Signs and symptoms of magnesium depletion do not usually appear until extracellular levels have fallen to 1 mEq/l* or less. Manifestations of significant magnesium depletion include weakness, irritability, tetany, delirium, and convulsions. Causes for symptomatic hypomagnesemia include malabsorption, severe diarrhea, nasogastric suction with administration of magnesium-free parenteral fluids, alcoholism, acute pancreatitis, early chronic renal disease, malnutrition, excessive lactation, chronic dialysis, digitalis intoxication, hyper- and hypoparathyroidism, hyperaldosteronism, diabetes mellitus, diuretic therapy (mercurial, thiazides, and ammonium chloride), and porphyria with inappropriate secretion of antidiuretic hormone (Wacker, 1968b, 1968c). Serious cardiac arrhythmias can also occur (Iseri, 1975).

Elevated serum concentrations of magnesium are rarely encountered, largely as a consequence of the ability of the kidneys to excrete systemic excesses. Signs of magnesium toxicity include anesthesia, flaccidity, paralysis of voluntary muscles, and hypotension. Symptomatic hypermagnesemia can be caused by advanced renal failure, acute diabetic acidosis, Addison's disease, severe dehydration, overly aggressive administration of magnesium sulfate enemas, or ingestion of excessive amounts of magnesium-containing antacids.

Analytical Techniques. Various analytical techniques have been introduced for the determination of magnesium in biologic fluids. The oldest method, but one which is occasionally still used, involves precipitation of magnesium as the ammonium phosphate salt after removal of calcium as calcium oxalate. Phosphorus in the precipitate is then quantitated by a variety of means, chiefly by photometry as molybdenum blue or as the molybdivanadate complex.

Precipitation of magnesium with 8-hydroxyquinoline is the basis for many procedures. The precipitate is quantitated by titrimetry, colorimetry, flame photometry, or fluorometry. Calcium, which will interfere, is eliminated by complexing with ethylene bis(oxyethylenenitrilo)tetraacetic acid (EGTA). In the fluorometric determination, the use of 8-hydroxyquinoline sulfonate is preferred because of its greater stability and enhanced sensitivity (Klein, 1967).

Photometric measurement of the red col-

---

* or 40–80 mmol/l

* or 2 mmol/l

ored complex formed with titan yellow in an alkaline medium was the first method for the direct determination of magnesium. Unfortunately this fast and simple method suffers from a series of limitations, including color instability, limited adherence to Beer's law, lack of sensitivity, and interference by calcium gluconate. Polyvinyl alcohol and gum ghatti have been used to potentiate and to stabilize color formation. This method also has serious inaccuracy with discrepancies of up to 10 to 15 per cent when compared with other methods.

In terms of accuracy, speed, and convenience, the determination of magnesium by atomic absorption spectrophotometry is the method of choice. After deproteinization and removal of phosphate ions with a lanthanum salt, the diluted filtrate is analyzed using the 285.2 nm line of a magnesium hollow cathode lamp (Hansen, 1967). The determination of magnesium in serum is sometimes performed directly without deproteinization.

Other methods for magnesium determination include complex formation with Magon, 1-azo-2-hydroxy-3-(2,4-dimethyl-carboxanilido)naphthalene-1-(2-hydroxybenzene) and a modification of Schwarzenbach's EDTA titration (1952). Flame photometry has not gained widespread application because of interferences from other anions.

IRON

Physiologic Chemistry. Iron is essential to most living organisms and participates in a variety of vital processes varying from cellular oxidative mechanisms to the transport of oxygen to the tissues. It is a constituent of the oxygen-carrying chromoproteins, hemoglobin and myoglobin, as well as various enzymes, e.g., cytochrome oxidase, xanthine oxidase, peroxidase, and catalase. The remaining body iron is present in the flavo-proteins (NADH dehydrogenase and succinic dehydrogenase), the iron-sulfur proteins, as well as the storage (ferritin) and transport (transferrin) forms of iron. The approximate distribution of iron in the normal adult male is presented in Table 10-9.

Unlike other trace elements, iron homeostasis is unique in that it is regulated primarily by absorption and not by excretion. Since the capacity of the body to excrete iron is very limited, its absorption from the intestine must

Table 10-9. APPROXIMATE DISTRIBUTION OF IRON IN THE NORMAL ADULT MALE

COMPOUND	IRON CONTENT (mg)	PER CENT
Hemoglobin	2800	68.3
Myoglobin	135	3.3
Ferritin	520	12.7
Hemosiderin	480	11.7
Transferrin	7	0.17
Enzyme iron	8	0.19
Remaining organic iron (by difference)	150	3.65
Total	4100	100

be controlled so that tissue accumulations do not reach toxic levels. For a review of iron metabolism, the reader is referred to Chapter 29. Salient features of iron homeostasis are presented in Figure 10-14.

In adult males, iron is lost by way of the gastrointestinal tract (0.6 mg), skin by sweat and exfoliation of squamous cells (0.2 mg), and the urinary tract (0.1 mg) for a total of 0.9 mg daily. In the female, losses through normal menstruation add an additional average daily increment of 0.4 mg, giving a total daily loss of 1.3 mg (Cook, 1973). During pregnancy and lactation additional demands of up to 4 mg/day are placed on maternal iron stores.

The recommended allowance of 10 mg/day for adult males is readily obtainable from a well-balanced diet. It is difficult for women to obtain the recommended allowances (18 mg/day) from dietary sources unless fortified foods or supplements are included. The richest dietary source of iron is animal viscera, e.g., liver, kidney, heart, and spleen. Other good sources include egg yolk, fish, oysters, clams, and dried legumes (Anderson, 1977).

Since the body conserves iron extremely well, only 6 to 12 per cent of dietary intake need be absorbed in order to maintain iron equilibrium. However, in iron deficiency states and during growth and pregnancy, the normal gastrointestinal absorption will be increased from 1.3 mg daily to perhaps 4 mg/day. For a comprehensive review of iron absorption and nutrition, several excellent articles may be consulted (Munro, 1977; Linder, 1977; Jacobs, 1977; Cook, 1977).

Aside from a small amount of iron that is absorbed from the stomach, most iron absorption takes place in the duodenum and jejunum. In order to be absorbed, iron must be in its reduced or ferrous form. The acid pH of the stomach, along with reducing substances and

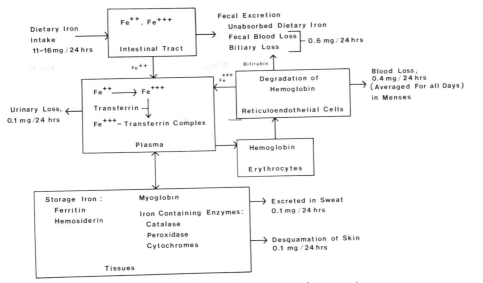

Figure 10-14. Interrelationships in iron homeostasis.

ascorbic acid, enhances iron absorption by maintaining iron in a reduced, more soluble form and by forming a chelate with ferric iron, which remains soluble as the pH rises in the small intestine (Cook, 1977). The regulation of iron absorption is largely carried out by the intestinal epithelial cells. Linder (1977) has proposed a mucosal control mechanism in which solubilized ionic iron in the intestinal lumen adsorbs to specific receptors in the brush border of the mucosal cells. The iron then passes from these receptors into the cytosol of the mucosal cell by an energy-dependent process. Controversy still exists concerning the mechanism of transport across the mucosal cell to the serosal surface. Several possible explanations of the process have been proposed. In addition to the classic apoferritin theory described by Hahn (1943), Saltman (1976) recently suggested that iron is solubilized by chelation to low molecular weight endogenous substances. Linder (1977) suggests that transport of iron across the cell is effected by chelation to amino acids. Most absorbed iron becomes attached to the plasma protein, transferrin, for transport in the plasma. Any remaining iron is retained within the cell, where it combines with the protein apoferritin (M.W. 460,000) to form ferritin. Ferritin also occurs in hepatic parenchymal cells and reticuloendothelial cells of the bone marrow, liver, and spleen. If the amount of apoferritin is insufficient to bind the remain-

ing iron, it is deposited in tissues as small iron oxide granules known as hemosiderin. Approximately 25 per cent of the iron in the body is in the storage forms of ferritin and hemosiderin. These storage forms represent a ready reserve of iron which can be mobilized to meet homeostatic needs.

The plasma iron transport protein, transferrin (formerly known as siderophilin), has the electrophoretic mobility of a β_1 globulin and is formed in the liver. It has a molecular weight of approximately 90,000. Each molecule is able to bind two atoms of ferric iron. The half-life of this protein is about 10 days. By contrast, the iron in the plasma pool has a half-life of 60 to 120 minutes.

Iron is carried to storage sites and to the bone marrow. Transferrin is not itself assimilated by the target tissues. Indeed, transferrin may bind briefly to normoblast membranes where the iron is passed directly into the developing erythrocyte for incorporation into heme (Fairbanks, 1971). Subsequently, transferrin returns to plasma to take up unbound iron. From effete erythrocytes, iron is split from hemoglobin by reticuloendothelial system cells and returns to plasma, where it is again bound to transferrin. A small portion of the emergent iron may enter the plasma in the form of ferritin (Siimes, 1974). Free iron is extremely toxic and little, if any, is present in the body.

Clinicopathologic Correlations. Trans-

Table 10-10. SERUM IRON, TIBC*, AND PERCENT SATURATION IN VARIOUS CONDITIONS

	SERUM Fe	TIBC	SATURATION (%)
NORMAL	60-150 (µg/dl)	300-360 (µg/dl)	20-50
Iron deficiency	↓	↑	↓
Chronic infections	↓	↓	↓
Malignancy	↓	↓	↓
Menstruation	↓	N	↓
Iron poisoning	↑	↓	↑
Hemolytic anemia	↑	N, ↓	↑
Hemochromatosis	↑	N, ↓	↑
Pyridoxine deficiency	↑	N	↑
Late pregnancy	↓	↑	↓
Oral contraceptives	N, ↑	↑	N
Viral hepatitis	↑	↑	N, ↑
Nephrosis	↓	↓	↑
Kwashiorkor	↓	↓	↑
Thalassemia	↑	↓	↑

↓ = decrease; ↑ = increase; N = normal.
*TIBC = Total iron binding capacity.

ferrin is usually measured indirectly by the amount of iron that it can bind; this is referred to as the total iron-binding capacity (TIBC). The total circulating apo-transferrin (protein capable of binding additional iron) is generally about a third saturated with iron; this iron is measured in the serum iron determination. The unsaturated iron-binding capacity (UIBC) is that amount of additional iron which transferrin can bind above that which is already complexed. This relationship can be expressed as TIBC = UIBC + serum Fe.

Another useful expression of this relationship is percentage saturation, which relates the amount of iron present in the serum to the amount of transferrin present (TIBC). The formula for this relationship is:

$$\% \text{ saturation} = \frac{\text{serum Fe}}{\text{TIBC}} \times 100$$

Percentage saturation is a better index of iron stores than serum iron alone. It is a useful clinical concept but must always be reported along with both the iron and TIBC for optimal clinical interpretation. The relationship between serum iron, transferrin (TIBC), and per cent saturation as it occurs in various conditions and diseases is presented in Table 10-10. Additional clinicopathologic correlations are reviewed in Chapter 29.

Normal values for the TIBC in healthy adults average between 300 and 360 µg/dl (54 to 64 µmol/l). There is no diurnal variation in the level of the TIBC as there is for serum iron. TIBC values tend to decrease with age (250 µg/dl in individuals above 70 years of age). At birth the average newborn levels are about 275 µg/dl and reach a peak by the eighth month.

Common causes for an increase in TIBC include iron deficiency anemia, infancy, ingestion of oral contraceptives, and possibly hepatitis (Table 10-10). Decreased transferrin and, therefore, TIBC can be found in association with a generalized decrease in plasma proteins from various causes, e.g., reduced protein synthesis, nephrosis or other direct loss, and increased catabolism (malignancy or starvation). In common with albumin, but unlike many of the glycoproteins of plasma, transferrin tends to be decreased by chronic inflammatory conditions. Patients with iron overload from repeated blood transfusions also have a depression of transferrin. The average serum iron level is about 125 µg/dl in adult males and 100 µg/dl in adult females. The range varies between 60 and 150 µg/dl (11 to 27 µmol/l). There is no seasonal variation in iron levels, although a diurnal variation has been observed. Serum iron levels may be one third higher in the morning than at night. The average plasma and serum iron levels at birth approach 200 µg/dl. There is a drop to about 45 µg/dl during the first few hours of life and then an increase to 125 µg/dl after the first three weeks of life. In the elderly, the serum iron level decreases to 40 to 80 µg/dl (7 to 14 µmol/l). In pathologic states, elevations of serum iron may be seen in (1) conditions of increased erythrocyte destruction (hemolytic anemia), (2) decreased blood formation (lead poisoning or pyridoxine deficiency), (3) increased release of iron from the body stores (release of ferritin in acute hepatic cell necrosis), (4) defective iron storage (pernicious anemia), and (5) increased rate of absorption (hemochromatosis and transfusion siderosis).

Decreased serum iron occurs in association with (1) generalized iron deficiency (lack of sufficient dietary iron), inadequate absorption, or chronic loss as a result of bleeding or nephrosis, and (2) impaired release of iron from the reticuloendothelial system (infection). Moderate depression of serum iron may occur in association with conditions such as malignancies and rheumatoid arthritis.

The ratio of serum iron level to plasma

transferrin level (percentage saturation) is altered in various diseases (Table 10-10). An increase in the saturation can occur in conditions of decreased circulating protein (chronic liver disease, nephrosis, kwashiorkor), in conditions associated with ineffective erythropoiesis or blocks in hemoglobin synthesis (thalassemia, lead poisoning, pyridoxine deficiency anemia), in disease associated with iron overload (idiopathic hemochromatosis and hemosiderosis), and in acute blood loss. A decrease in the percentage of saturation (less than 15 per cent) is present in iron deficiency anemia and in late pregnancy. In conditions such as infection and malignancies, both serum and total iron-binding capacity are decreased, but the serum iron depression is proportionately greater, so the percentage of saturation is lower.

In evaluating patients for iron deficiency or iron overload, the work-up should include a complete hematologic profile, including an examination of peripheral blood smear, as well as measurements of serum ferritin, serum iron, and iron-binding capacity (TIBC), with calculation of percentage saturation. A single measurement of serum iron, except in iron poisoning, is inadequate for confirmation of iron overload or iron deficiency.

Analytical Techniques. Measurement of iron may evolve as an important indicator of total body iron. A simplified deferoxamine test has been reported by Rosen (1966) that may prove helpful in the detection of iron overload (hemochromatosis). Deferoxamine is a chelating agent with a high affinity for iron. It has been used therapeutically in the treatment of iron poisoning and in a variety of diagnostic tests for excessive iron stores (Rosen, 1966). Two six-hour urine specimens are collected for iron analysis, one before and one after intramuscular injection of a 500-mg dose of deferoxamine mesylate. With iron overload, patients have increased iron excretion in both specimens, but a more striking increase in the post-deferoxamine urine sample.

The serum ferritin concentration may be used to monitor changes in iron stores. The mean concentration is higher in males than in females, and the range is 12 to 300 μg/l, although on occasion a higher level may be found in subjects who are otherwise normal. In iron deficiency anemia, serum ferritin is ordinarily less than 12 μg/l. In iron overload, serum ferritin may reach 10,000 μg/l. Serum ferritin

concentrations appear to provide a better reflection of body iron stores than does the traditional method of visual assessment of stainable iron in bone marrow (Jacobs, 1977). Although some investigators have recently suggested that serum ferritin concentrations may be useful in the detection or follow-up of malignancy or as an index of liver damage, this estimation is not yet in general use, and its overall value is still being assessed. Accurate measurements of serum ferritin are attainable using radioimmunoassay (Marcus, 1975).

In the various colorimetric methods for the analysis of serum iron, the initial step involves splitting iron from its protein combination (transferrin) by exposure to strong acids. In manual methods this is accomplished either by removal of proteins by precipitation with hot trichloroacetic acid (Trinder, 1956) or by providing conditions that allow the protein to remain in solution without interfering with subsequent analytical manipulations (White, 1973). In automated methods iron is dialyzed from the transferrin (Zak, 1965). The next step in most procedures is the reaction of the reduced iron with a chromogen to produce an iron-chromogen complex. Reagents with superior sensitivity for complexing with iron include sulfonated bathophenanthroline (Zak, 1965) 2,4,6-tripyridyl-S-triazine (TPTZ), ferrozine (Carter, 1971), and terosite (Zak, 1971). Addition of the color reagent results in the formation of a deeply colored Fe-chromogen complex with an absorbance maximum in the visible region of the electromagnetic spectrum.

Measurements of serum iron and iron binding capacity may also be determined by atomic absorption spectrophotometry. Although one would assume that atomic absorption would be a popular method for serum iron determination, this has not been the case. Several methods have been published claiming good results. Sunderman (1973) recommends the flame atomization method of Olsen (1969), or the flameless atomization method of Olsen (1973), for routine use. However, limitations of sensitivity, matrix interferences, and the inability of atomic absorption to distinguish hemoglobin iron from transport iron make the rapid and sensitive colorimetric methods more desirable and practical.

While serum iron determination reflects iron bound to transferrin, the TIBC is usually only 30 per cent saturated with iron. The latent or unsaturated iron-binding capacity

(LIBC or UIBC) is estimated also in measurements of total iron-binding capacity. Most commonly the UIBC is determined indirectly by subtracting the serum iron from the TIBC. TIBC is determined by saturating the transferrin with iron, removing the excess, unbound iron with an iron absorbent, and measuring the iron in the filtrate. Absorbents serve to remove any unbound iron excess and ideally should not remove iron which has become bound to the transferrin molecule (Cook, 1970). Effective absorbents include activated charcoal, magnesium carbonate, and Amberlite resin.

COPPER

Physiologic Chemistry. Copper is an essential trace element that is a constituent of certain metalloenzymes and proteins. Copper is required for hemoglobin synthesis and is a constituent of cytochrome oxidase, tyrosinase, monoamine oxidase, ascorbic acid oxidase, uricase, galactose oxidase, and amino-levulinate dehydratase.

The major portion of copper in the erythrocyte (at least 80 per cent) occurs as a constituent of the enzyme superoxide dismutase (erythrocuprein). This enzyme, also found in liver (hepatocuprein) and brain (cerebrocuprein), has the unique role of protecting cells by catalytically scavenging the toxic-free radical superoxide ion (O_2^-) generated during aerobic metabolism (Fridovich, 1975). The remainder of erythrocyte copper is dialyzable and is believed to consist of complexes with amino acids, which function to maintain dismutase activity (Evans, 1973). The total copper content of erythrocytes tends to remain constant, on the average 98 μg/dl (15 μmol/l), despite deficiencies of dietary copper or increases in plasma or hepatic copper (Burch, 1975).

The concentration of copper in the plasma is somewhat higher than in the erythrocyte. In a study of 28 patients, Rosenthal (1974) found mean plasma levels of 119 μg/dl, which is significantly different from the mean serum levels of 127 μg/dl. The normal range for serum copper in adults is 70 to 140 μg/dl (11 to 22 μmol/l) for males and 80 to 155 μg/dl (13 to 24 μmol/l) for females. Copper in plasma occurs in two main forms, one loosely bound and the other firmly bound to plasma proteins. Only trace amounts of copper remain free or dialyzable in plasma. Loosely bound copper is a minor fraction and includes copper bound predominantly to serum albumin.

The albumin-bound copper probably represents copper in transit and increases promptly after copper is ingested, then falls exponentially as a result of hepatic uptake. Firmly bound copper, composing 80 to 95 per cent of the total plasma copper, is incorporated into an α_2-globulin, which is called ceruloplasmin because of its blue color (Harper, 1977). Serum ceruloplasmin concentration increases as albumin-bound copper decreases. Ceruloplasmin, a multifunctional enzyme, aids in the mobilization of iron from storage sites. It functions as a ferroxidase enzyme during the conversion of iron from its ferrous state to the ferric form (Frieden, 1973). Reference values for ceruloplasmin range from 25 to 43 mg/dl (250 to 430 mg/l).

Clinicopathologic Correlation. The most important abnormality in copper metabolism is Wilson's disease or hepatolenticular degeneration. This disease is of autosomal recessive inheritance with onset usually in the second or third decade but occasionally as early as four or five years of age. As suggested by the name, the disease is characterized by degenerative changes, particularly in the liver and the basal ganglia of the brain as a result of excessive deposition of copper. The most common presenting signs and symptoms are those of central nervous involvement—rigidity, dysarthria, dysphagia, tremor, incoordination, choreoathetotic movements, and ataxia. Some patients, especially those in the younger age ranges, may present with liver insufficiency ranging from weakness and anorexia to jaundice and progressing to ascites and other features of portal hypertension as a consequence of cirrhosis (Sass-Kortsak, 1975). Other patients present with a combination of central nervous system and hepatic disease. A pathognomonic finding is a brown ring near the limbus of the cornea, termed the Kayser-Fleischer ring, which results from deposition of copper in Descemet's membrane.

The biochemical defect in Wilson's disease has not been elucidated. Plasma ceruloplasmin is ordinarily greatly decreased, usually to less than 20 mg per dl. It is unlikely, however, that the depression of ceruloplasmin is a causative factor in the disease because a few patients with Wilson's disease have normal levels of ceruloplasmin. Furthermore, 10 to 20 per cent of heterozygote carriers and other patients with the nephrotic syndrome or sprue have significantly decreased ceruloplasmin but are free of the manifestations of Wilson's disease. Plasma copper is correspondingly decreased. Patients with Wilson's disease have a persistently positive copper balance in spite of increased renal excretion. The fact that biliary and, therefore, fecal excretion of copper is abnormally low may be of pathogenetic importance. Copper is also increased in the cerebrospinal fluid.

Prompt diagnosis of Wilson's disease is important so that therapy can be instituted. Progression of the disease can be abated and manifestations at least partially reversed by a diet low in copper and therapy with D-penicillamine, which promotes copper excretion, probably by chelation (Goldstein, 1974).

Hypercupremia is usually observed during pregnancy, with ceruloplasmin concentrations in serum reaching values at parturition that are twice those found in non-pregnant women. Extremely high concentrations of ceruloplasmin, and therefore of copper, have been found in various lymphomas, particularly Hodgkin's disease. Increased ceruloplasmin also occurs in acute and chronic infections, rheumatoid arthritis, biliary cirrhosis, and thyrotoxicosis. The concentration of copper in serum, urine, and hair is also increased in patients with pellagra (Krishnamachari, 1974). The high content of leucine in pellagra-associated cereal grains may be responsible for the increase, because administration of leucine produces similar increases in copper levels.

There are several other conditions in which subnormal concentrations of copper are found in the serum. Hypocupremia has been observed in conditions associated with hypoproteinemia, e.g., protein malnutrition (kwashiorkor), protein malabsorption syndrome (sprue), and nephrosis (Burch, 1975).

Hypocupremia is also a characteristic feature of Menkes' kinky hair syndrome or trichopoliodystrophy, a sex-linked recessive disorder characterized by progressive mental deterioration, retardation of growth, defective keratinization and pigmentation of hair ("kinky hair or pili torti"), hypothermia, degenerative changes in aortic elastic, scorbutic bone changes, and cerebral gliosis with cystic degeneration (Menkes, 1972). Danks (1973) showed that in addition to hypocupremia this syndrome is associated with profound hypoceruloplasminemia and diminished concentrations of copper in the hair. The copper deficiency may be responsible for the alterations

in the elastic fibers of arterial walls and the scorbutic bone deformities, as well as the changes in hair. Although orally administered copper was ineffective, parenteral administration of copper was therapeutically beneficial as a result of stimulation of ceruloplasmin formation.

Analytical Techniques. While spectrophotometry, neutron activation, and radioisotopic dilution techniques have been used to determine copper in biologic fluids, atomic absorption spectrometry remains the method of choice for the determination of copper in serum, plasma, or urine (Sunderman, 1973). Atomic absorption spectrometry provides the sensitivity, specificity, speed, and ease of analysis required for routine clinical use. Methods of sample preparation for measurements of copper in serum, plasma, and/or whole blood by flame atomic absorption include: (1) simple dilution and aspiration in the flame (Sinha, 1970); (2) dissociation of copper from the proteins (albumin and ceruloplasmin) by treatment with acid followed by protein precipitation and aspiration of the supernatant (Sunderman, 1967); or (3) liberation of plasma and erythrocyte copper by acid digestion followed by chelation with ammonium pyrrolidine dithiocarbamate (APDC) and extraction into an organic solvent (methyliobutylketone, MIBK) for flame atomic absorption measurement (Berman, 1965). Evenson (1975) introduced a method using flameless atomic absorption in a graphite tube. This analytical approach is especially useful when only small amounts of material are available, since it requires less than 5 ml of body fluid.

ZINC

Until recent years zinc metabolism received relatively little attention in clinical medicine although it is known to be an essential component of many important enzymes, including alcohol dehydrogenase, carbonic anhydrase, alkaline phosphatase, procarboxypeptides, and superoxide dismutase. The importance of zinc in several diseases has now been clearly established.

Low plasma levels of zinc occur as a nonspecific finding in association with a variety of diseases, including alcoholic cirrhosis, sickle-cell anemia, carcinoma of the lung, acute myocardial infarction, corticosteroid therapy, and oral contraceptive therapy. A pathogenetic relationship between zinc deficiency and disease is suggested by the observation that patients who develop decreased tastes and olfactory acuity without any apparent cause have shown improvement following zinc supplementation (Burch, 1975). Improvement in healing of extensive burns or wounds has been observed following administration of zinc sulfate to patients with zinc depletion or dietary inadequacy. A therapeutic response to zinc has also been noted in some patients with bedsores (Cohen, 1968). Zinc deficiency in children is associated with anorexia, impaired taste perception, pica, lethargy, failure to thrive as infants, growth retardation of older children, and delayed sexual maturation (Hambridge, 1977).

Acrodermatitis enteropathica is a disease with onset in early childhood characterized by various gastrointestinal and cutaneous manifestations including alopecia, diarrhea, and vesiculopustulous dermatitis, particularly of the extremities and around mucous membranes. This disease, which is inherited as an autosomal recessive trait, has been attributed to a defect related to zinc metabolism (Hambridge, 1977).

Although deficiencies of zinc have received greater attention than overdoses, acute zinc intoxications from industrial exposure, consumption of acidic foods or beverages from galvanized containers, illicit spirits, or children's toys have been reported. Symptoms from accidental ingestion include gastrointestinal irritation with fever, nausea, vomiting, diarrhea, abdominal pain, and a metallic taste in the mouth. With industrial exposure via inhalation, metal fume fever is the predominant symptom. Other toxic effects include dry throat, cough and chest discomfort, tachycardia, hypertension, and pulmonary edema. Considerable discrepancies exist in the literature concerning normal zinc levels. Improper specimen collection and/or non-specific colorimetric methods may partially explain the disparity. The normal plasma concentration of zinc by atomic absorption is approximately 100 μg/dl, with a range of 55 to 150 μg/dl (8.42 to 22.95 μmol/l). Platelet disintegration is thought to account for the higher level in serum.

CHROMIUM

Only recently has chromium been recognized as an essential trace element. Chromium is a component of several enzyme systems and may be important in nucleic acid metabolism. Its major physiologic role, however, is related to its action in insulin. Chromium is required as a cofactor for the initiation of the action of insulin on peripheral tissues (Hambridge, 1974). The biologically active form of chromium has been termed "glucose tolerance factor" or GTF, which is thought to be a low molecular weight, naturally occurring nicotinic acid-chromium complex. Reduced chromium intake in humans can be an aggravating factor in the disturbed glucose tolerance of marasmic infants, of maturity-onset diabetics, and of elderly people (Fox, 1975).

Chromium toxicity is seen primarily in occupational exposure to chromium compounds. Toxic exposure to the skin results in dermatitis and persistent ulceration. Accidental ingestion has resulted in vertigo, abdominal pain, vomiting, anuria, convulsions, shock, and coma. Chromium levels in blood are extremely low. Using atomic absorption spectrophotometry, Pekarek (1974) observed a serum level of 1.58 $\pm$ 0.08 μg/l in a group of 15 healthy adults. Levels of chromium in hair are substantially higher than in serum and may be used as an index of chromium nutrition (Hambridge, 1974).

REFERENCES

Adibi, S., and Gray, S. J.: Intestinal absorption of essential amino acids in man. Gastroenterology, *52*:837, 1967.

Agarwal, B. N., and Agarwal, P.: Magnesium deficiency in clinical medicine—a review. J. Am. Med. Wom. Assoc., *31*:72, 1976.

Anderson, C. E.: Minerals. *In* Schneider, H. A., Anderson, C. E., and Coursin, D. B. (eds.): Nutritional Support of Medical Practice. Hagerstown, Md., Harper and Row Publishers, 1977.

Arnaud, C. D., Goldsmith, R. S., Bordier, P. J., and Sizemore, G. W.: Influence of immunoheterogeneity of circulating parathyroid hormone on results of radioimmunoassays of serum in man. Am. J. Med., *56*:785, 1974.

Arnaud, C. D., Tsao, H. S., and Littledike, T.: Radioimmunoassay of human parathyroid hormone in serum. J. Clin. Invest., *50*:21, 1971.

Balis, M. E.: Uric acid metabolism in man. Adv. Clin. Chem., *18*:213, 1976.

Baum, N., Dichoso, C. C., and Carlton, C. E., Jr.: Blood urea nitrogen and serum creatinine: Physiology and interpretations. Urology, *5*:583, 1975.

Bendersky, G.: Etiology of hyperuricemia. Ann. Clin. Lab. Sci., *5*:456, 1975.

Berman, E.: Application of atomic absorption spectrometry to the determination of copper in serum, urine, and tissue. At. Absorp. News, *4*:296, 1965.

Berson, S. A., Yalow, R. S., Aurbach, G. D., and Potts, J. T., Jr.: Immunoassay of bovine and human parathyroid hormone. Proc. Natl. Acad. Sci. USA, *49*:613, 1963.

Brown, N. D., Sing, H. C., Neeley, W. E., and Koetitz, S. E.: Determination of "true" serum creatinine by high-performance liquid chromatography combined with a continuous-flow microanalyzer. Clin. Chem., *23*:1281, 1977.

Brumbaugh, P. F., Haussler, D. H., Bressler, R., and Haussler, M. R.: Radioreceptor assay for 1,α,25-dihydroxyvitamin D₃. Science, *183*:1089, 1974.

Burch, R. E., Hahn, H. K. J., and Sullivan, J. F.: Newer aspects of the roles of zinc, manganese, and copper in human nutrition. Clin. Chem., *21*:501, 1975.

Cantarow, A., and Schepartz, B.: Biochemistry, 4th ed. Philadelphia, W. B. Saunders Company, 1967.

Carlson, R. E., and Dolphin, D.: High pressure liquid chromatographic techniques for the separation of complex mixtures of naturally occurring porphyrins. *In* Doss, M. (ed.): Porphyrins in Human Diseases. Basel, S. Karger, 1976.

Carter, P.: Spectrophotometric determination of serum iron at the submicrogram level with a new reagent (ferrozine). Anal. Biochem., *40*:450, 1971.

Cartier, P., and Hamet, M.: The normal metabolism of uric acid. Adv. Nephrol., *3*:3, 1974.

Chase, L. R., and Aurbach, G. D.: Cyclic AMP and the mechanism of action of parathyroid hormone. *In* Talmage, R. V., and Belanger, L. F. (eds.): Parathyroid Hormone and Thyrocalcitonin (Calcitonin). Amsterdam, Excerpta Medica, 1968.

Clark, E. P., and Collip, J. B.: A study of the Tisdall method for determination of blood serum calcium with a suggested modification. J. Biol. Chem., *63*:461, 1925.

Cohen, C.: Zinc sulphate and bedsores. Br. Med. J., *2*:561, 1968.

Cohn, D. V., MacGregor, R. R., Chu, L. L. H., Huang, D. W. Y., Anast, C. S., and Hamilton, J. W.: Biosynthesis of proparathyroid hormone and parathyroid hormone. Chemistry, physiology and role of calcium in regulation. Am. J. Med., *56*:767, 1974.

Cook, J. D.: An evaluation of adsorption methods for measurement of plasma iron-binding capacity. J. Lab. Clin. Med., *76*:497, 1970.

Cook, J. D.: Absorption of food iron. Fed. Proc., *36*:2028, 1977.

Cook, J. D., Barry, W. E., Hershko, C., Fillet, G., and Finch, C. A.: Iron kinetics with emphasis on iron overload. Am. J. Pathol., *72*:337, 1973.

Danks, D. M., Cartwright, E., Stevens, B. J., and Townley, R. R. W.: Menkes' kinky hair disease: Further definition of the defect in copper transport. Science, *179*:1140, 1973.

Deftos, L. J.: Immunoassay for human calcitonin. I. Method. Metabolism, *20*:1122, 1971.

Deftos, L. J.: Radioimmunoassay for calcitonin in medullary thyroid carcinoma. J.A.M.A., *227*:403, 1974.

Deftos, L. J., Roos, B. A., and Parthemore, J. G.: Calcium and skeletal metabolism. West. J. Med., *123*:447, 1975.

DeLuca, H. F.: Vitamin D: The vitamin and the hormone. Fed. Proc., *33*:2211, 1974.

DeLuca, H. F.: Vitamin D endocrine system. Adv. Clin. Chem., *19*:125, 1977.

DeVries, A., and Sperling, O.: Recent data on uric acid lithiasis. Adv. Nephrol., *3*:89, 1974.

Doss, M., Ulshofer, B., and Philipp-Dormston, W. K.: Quantitative thin-layer chromatography of porphyrins by in situ fluorescence measurements. J. Chromatogr., *63*:113, 1971.

DuPont, A.: On the determination of hydroxyproline in urine. Clin. Chim. Acta, *18*:59, 1967.

Elder, G. H., Gray, C. H., and Nicholson, D. C.: The porphyrias: A review. J. Clin. Pathol., *25*:1013, 1972.

Evans, G. W.: Copper homeostasis in the mammalian system. Physiol. Rev., *53*:535, 1973.

Evenson, M. E., and Warren, B. L.: Determination of serum copper by atomic absorption, with use of the graphite cuvette. Clin. Chem., *21*:619, 1975.

Fairbanks, V. F., Fahey, J. L., and Beutler, E.: Clinical Disorders of Iron Metabolism. New York, Grune & Stratton, Inc., 1971.

Fessel, W. J.: Hyperuricemia in health and disease. Semin. Arthritis Rheum., *1*:275, 1972.

Fox, F. W.: The trace elements—a new chapter in nutrition. S. Afr. Med. J., *49*:1629, 1975.

Fridovich, I.: Superoxide dismutases. Ann. Rev. Biochem., *44*:147, 1975.

Frieden, E.: The ferrous to ferric cycles in iron metabolism. Nutr. Rev., *31*:41, 1973.

Gilman, A. G.: A protein binding assay for adenosine 3':5'- cyclic monophosphate. Proc. Natl. Acad. Sci. USA, *67*:305, 1970.

Goldberg, A.: Porphyrins and porphyrias. *In* Goldberg, A., and Brain, M. C. (eds.): Recent Advances in Haematology. Edinburgh, Churchill Livingston, 1971.

Goldenberg, H., and Fernandez, A.: Simplified method for the estimation of inorganic phosphorus in body fluids. Clin. Chem., *12*:871, 1966.

Goldman, L., Gordan, G. S., and Roof, B. S.: The parathyroids: Progress, problems and practice. Current Problems in Surgery, 1, August, 1971.

Goldsmith, R. S.: Laboratory aids in the diagnosis of metabolic bone disease. Orthop. Clin. North Am., *3*:545, 1972.

Goldstein, L.: Ammonia production and excretion in the mammalian kidney. *In* Thurau, K. (ed.): Kidney and Urinary Tract Physiology II. Baltimore, University Park Press, 1976.

Goldstein, N. P., and Owen, C. A.: Symposium on copper metabolism and Wilson's disease. Mayo. Clin. Proc., *49*:363, 1974.

Goodwin, J. F.: The colorimetric estimation of plasma amino nitrogen with DNFB. Clin. Chem., *14*:1080, 1968.

Gordan, G. S., and Roof, B. S.: Laboratory tests for hyperparathyroidism. J.A.M.A., *206*:2729, 1968.

Goverde, B. C., and Veenkamp, F. J. N.: Routine assay of total urinary hydroxyproline based on resin catalysed hydrolysis. Clin. Chim. Acta, *41*:29, 1972.

Guthrie, R., and Susi, A.: A simple phenylalanine method for detecting phenylketonuria in large populations of newborn infants. Pediatrics, *32*:338, 1963.

Habener, J. F., Kemper, B., Ernst, M., Rich, A., and Potts, J. T.: Preproparathyroid hormone. Partial sequence determination of a 115-amino acid polypeptide precursor of parathyroid hormone. Clin. Res., *23*:321A, 1975.

Haddad, J. G., Jr., Chyu, K. J., Hahn, T. J., and Stamp, T. C. B.: Serum concentrations of 25-hydroxyvitamin D in sex-linked hypophosphatemic vitamin D-resistant rickets. J. Lab. Clin. Med., *81*:22, 1973.

Hahn, P. F., Bale, W. F., Ross, J. F., Balfour, W. M., and Whipple, G. H.: Radioactive iron absorption by gastrointestinal tract: Influence of anemia, anoxia, and antecedent feeding distribution in growing dogs. J. Exp. Med., *78*:169, 1943.

Haining, R. G., Hulse, T. E., and Labbe, R. F.: Rapid porphyrin screening of urine, stool, and blood. Clin. Chem., *15*:460, 1969.

Hambridge, K. M.: Nutrition in man. Am. J. Clin. Nutr., *27*:505, 1974.

Hambridge, K. M.: The role of zinc and other trace metals in pediatric nutrition and health. Pediatr. Clin. North Am., 24:95, 1977.

Hammond, J. E., and Savory, J.: Advances in the detection of amino acids in biological fluids. Ann. Clin. Lab. Sci., 6:158, 1976.

Hansen, J. L., and Freier, E. F.: The measurement of serum magnesium by atomic absorption spectrophotometry. Am. J. Med. Technol., 33:158, 1967.

Hanson, D. J., and Bretz, N. S.: Evaluation of a semi-automated blood urea nitrogen analyzer. Clin. Chem., 23:477, 1977.

Harper, H. A.: Review of Physiologic Chemistry. Los Altos, Cal., Lange Medical Publications, 1977.

Herns, D. A.: Biochemical aspects of renal ammonia formation in metabolic acidosis. Enzyme, 20:359, 1975.

Horak, E., and Sunderman, F. W., Jr.: Measurement of serum urea nitrogen by conductivimetric urease assay. Ann. Clin. Lab. Sci., 2:425, 1972.

Hourani, B. T., Hamlin, E. M., and Reynolds, T. B.: Cerebrospinal fluid glutamine as a measure of hepatic encephalopathy. Arch. Intern. Med., 127:1033, 1971.

Iseri, L. T., Freed, J., and Bures, A. R.: Magnesium deficiency and cardiac disorders. Am. J. Med., 58:837, 1975.

Ishihara, A., Kurahasi, K., and Uehara, H.: Enzymatic determination of ammonia in blood plasma. Clin. Chim. Acta, 41:255, 1972.

Jacobs, A.: Serum ferritin and iron stores. Fed. Proc., 36:2024, 1977.

Jellum, E., Stokke, O., and Eldjarn, L.: Application of gas chromatography, mass spectrometry and computer methods in clinical biochemistry. Anal. Chem., 45:1099, 1973.

Jung, D. H., and Parekh, A. C.: An improved reagent system for the measurement of serum uric acid. Clin. Chem., 16:247, 1970.

Kageyama, N. A.: A direct colorimetric determination of uric acid in serum and urine with uricase-catalase system. Clin. Chim. Acta, 31:421, 1971.

Kamoun, P., Lafourcade, G., and Jerome, H.: Ultramicromethod for determination of plasma uric acid. Clin. Chem., 22:964, 1976.

Kay, N. E., and Gottlieb, A. J.: Hypouricemia in Hodgkin's disease. Report of an additional case. Cancer, 32:1508, 1973.

Klein, B., and Oklander, M.: The automated fluorometric determination of serum magnesium. Clin. Chem., 13:26, 1967.

Klinenberg, J. R.: Hyperuricemia and gout. Med. Clin. North Am., 61:299, 1977.

Krishnamachari, K. A. V. R.: Some aspects of copper metabolism in pellagra. Am. J. Clin. Nutr., 27:108, 1974.

Kuan, J. C., Kuan, S. S., and Guilbault, G. G.: An alternative method for the determination of uric acid in serum. Clin. Chim. Acta, 64:19, 1975.

La Du, B. N., and Michael, P. J.: An enzymatic spectrophotometric method for the determination of phenylalanine in blood. J. Lab. Clin. Med., 55:491, 1960.

Lamola, A. A., Joselow, M., and Yamane, T.: Zinc protoporphyrin (ZPP): A simple, sensitive, fluorometric screening test for lead poisoning. Clin. Chem., 21:93, 1975.

Levin, B.: Hereditary metabolic disorders of the urea cycle. Adv. Clin. Chem., 14:65, 1971.

Lim, C. K., Gray, C. H., and Stoll, M. S.: Separation of porphyrins from biological materials by high pressure liquid chromatography. In Doss, M. (ed.): Porphyrins in Human Diseases. Basel, S. Karger, 1976.

Linder, M. C., and Munro, H. N.: The mechanism of iron absorption and its regulation. Fed. Proc., 36:2017, 1977.

Lutwak, L.: Metabolic and biochemical considerations of bone. Ann. Clin. Lab. Sci., 5:185, 1975.

Magnus, I. A., and Wood, M.: X-porphyrins and the porphyrias. Trans. St. John's Hosp. Derm. Soc., 57:105, 1971.

Marcus, D. M., and Zinberg, N.: Measurement of serum ferritin by radioimmunoassay: Results in normal individuals and patients with breast cancer. J. Natl. Cancer Inst., 55:791, 1975.

Massry, S. G.: Pharmacology of magnesium. Ann. Rev. Pharmacol. Toxicol., 17:67, 1977.

McCaman, M. W., and Robins, E.: Fluorimetric method for the determination of phenylalanine in serum. J. Lab. Clin. Med., 59:885, 1962.

McLean, F. C., and Hastings, A. B.: The state of calcium in the fluids of the body. 1. The conditions affecting the ionization of calcium. J. Biol. Chem., 108:285, 1935.

Melick, R. A., and Henneman, P. H.: Clinical and laboratory studies of 207 consecutive patients in a kidney-stone clinic. N. Engl. J. Med., 259:307, 1958.

Melvin, K. E. W., Miller, H. H., and Tashjian, A. H., Jr.: Early diagnosis of medullary carcinoma of the thyroid gland by means of calcitonin assay. N. Engl. J. Med., 285:1115, 1971.

Menkes, J. H.: Kinky hair disease. Pediatrics, 50:181, 1972.

Meyerhoff, M., and Rechnitz, G. A.: An activated enzyme electrode for creatinine. Anal. Chim. Acta, 85:277, 1976.

Morgan, J. M., and Burch, H. B.: Comparative tests for diagnosis of lead poisoning. Arch. Intern. Med., 130:335, 1972.

Moss, G. A., Bondar, R. J. L., and Buzzelli, D. M.: Kinetic enzymatic method for determining serum creatinine. Clin. Chem., 21:1422, 1975.

Munro, H. N.: Iron absorption and nutrition—introduction. Fed. Proc., 36:2015, 1977.

Murray, T. M., Peacock, M., Powell, D., Monchik, J. M., and Potts, J. T., Jr.: Non-autonomy of hormone secretion in primary hyperparathyroidism. Clin. Endocrinol., 1:235, 1972.

Norkus, N. S., Kubasik, N. P., and Sine, H. E., Jr.: Four commercial urease reagents and a laboratory-prepared reagent compared for analysis of blood urea nitrogen with the Beckman analyzer. Clin. Chem., 22:683, 1976.

Norman, A. W., and Henry, H.: 1,25-dihydroxycholecalciferol—a hormonally active form of vitamin D₃. Rec. Prog. Horm. Res., 30:431, 1974.

Nyhan, W. L.: The Lesch-Nyhan syndrome. Adv. Nephrol., 3:59, 1974.

Olsen, E. D., Jatlow, P. I., Fernandez, F. J., and Kahn, H. L.: Ultramicro method for determination of iron in serum with the graphite furnace. Clin. Chem., 19:326, 1973.

Olson, A. D., and Hamlin, W. B.: A new method for serum iron and total iron-binding capacity by atomic absorption spectrophotometry. Clin. Chem., 15:438, 1969.

Orfanos, A. P., Murphey, W. H., and Guthrie, R.: A simple fluorometric assay of protoporphyrin in erythrocytes (EPP) as a screening test for lead poisoning. J. Lab. Clin. Med., 89:659, 1977.

Owens, J. A., Iggo, B., Scandrett, F. J., and Stewart, C. P.: The determination of creatinine in plasma or serum, and in urine; a critical examination. Biochem. J., 58:426, 1954.

Palmer, D. W., and Peters, T.: Automated determination of free amino groups in serum and plasma using 2,4,6, trinitrobenzene sulfonate. Clin. Chem., 15:891, 1969.

Parfitt, A. M.: The actions of parathyroid hormone on

bone: Relation to bone remodeling and turnover, calcium homeostasis, and metabolic bone disease. Part I. Mechanisms of calcium transfer between blood and bone and their cellular basis: Morphological and kinetic approaches to bone turnover. Metabolism, 25:809, 1976a.

Parfitt, A. M.: The actions of parathyroid hormone on bone: Relation to bone remodeling and turnover, calcium homeostasis, and metabolic bone diseases. Part II. PTH and bone cells: Bone turnover and plasma calcium regulation. Metabolism, 25:909, 1976b.

Parfitt, A. M.: The actions of parathyroid hormone on bone: Relation to bone remodeling and turnover, calcium homeostasis, and metabolic bone disease. Part III. PTH and osteoblasts: The relationship between bone turnover and bone loss, and the state of the bones in primary hyperparathyroidism. Metabolism, 25:1033, 1976c.

Pekarek, R. S., Hauer, E. C., Wannemacher, R. W., and Bersel, W. R.: The direct determination of serum chromium by an atomic absorption spectrophotometer with a heated graphite atomizer. Anal. Biochem., 59:283, 1974.

Pennington, R. J.: Biochemical aspects of muscle disease. Adv. Clin. Chem., 14:409, 1971.

Piomelli, S., Lamola, A. A., Poh-Fitzpatrick, M. B., Seaman, C., and Harber, L. C.: Erythropoietic protoporphyria and lead intoxication: The molecular doses for difference in cutaneous photosensitivity. I. Different rates of disappearance of protoporphyrin from the erythrocytes both *in vivo* and *in vitro*. J. Clin. Invest., 56:1519, 1975.

Reed, A. H., Cannon, D. C., Winkelman, J. W., Bhasin, Y. P., Henry, R. J., and Pileggi, V. J.: Estimation of normal ranges from a controlled sample survey. 1. Sex- and age-related influence on the SMA 12/60 screening group of tests. Clin. Chem., 18:57, 1972.

Rieselbach, R. E.: Renal handling of uric acid. Adv. Exp. Med. Biol., 76B:1-22, 1977.

Rimington, C.: Quantitative determination of porphobilinogen and porphyrins in urine and porphyrins in faeces and erythrocytes. Broadsheet No. 70 (revised Broadsheet 36), Assoc. Clin. Pathol., 1971.

Ritchie, J. C., Smith, S. F., and Castor, C. W.: Measurement of urinary and serous-fluid glycosaminoglycans and urinary hydroxyproline. Am. J. Clin. Pathol., 67:585, 1977.

Robertson, W. G.: Measurement of ionised calcium in body fluids: A review. Ann. Clin. Biochem., 13:540, 1976.

Rosen, B. J., and Tullis, J. L.: Simplified deferoxamine test in normal, diabetic, and iron-overload patients. J.A.M.A., 195:261, 1966.

Rosenthal, R. W., and Blackburn, A.: Higher copper concentration in serum than in plasma. Clin. Chem., 20:1233, 1974.

Russell, R. G. G.: Regulation of calcium metabolism. Ann. Clin. Biochem., 13:518, 1976.

Ryckewaert, A., and Kuntz, D.: Etiologic varieties of hyperuricemia and gout. Adv. Nephrol., 3:29, 1974.

Saltman, P., Hegenauer, J., and Christopher, J.: Tired blood and rusty livers. Ann. Clin. Lab. Sci., 6:167, 1976.

Sass-Kortsak, A.: Wilson's disease—a treatable liver disease in children. Pediatr. Clin. North Am., 22:963, 1975.

Sassa, S., Granick, S., Bickers, D. R., Bradlow, H. L., and Kappas, A.: A microassay for uroporphyrinogen I synthase, one of the three abnormal enzyme activities in acute intermittent porphyria, and its application to the

study of the genetics of this disease. Proc. Natl. Acad. Sci. USA, 71:732, 1974.

Schmid, R., Schwartz, S., and Watson, C. J.: Porphyrin content of bone marrow and liver in the various forms of prophyria. Arch. Intern. Med., 93:167, 1954.

Scholnick, P., Marver, H. S., and Schmid, R.: Erythropoietic protoporphyria: Evidence for multiple sites of excess protoporphyrin formation. J. Clin. Invest., 50:203, 1971.

Schultz, D. W., Passonneau, J. V., and Lowry, O. H.: An enzymic method for the measurement of inorganic phosphate. Anal. Biochem., 19:300, 1967.

Schultz, S. G., and Curran, P. F.: Coupled transport of sodium and organic solutes. Physiol. Rev., 50:637, 1970.

Schwarzenbach, G.: Chelate couplex formation as a basic for titration processes. Anal. Chim. Acta, 7:141, 1952.

Scott, P. J., and Hurley, P. J.: Demonstration of individual variation in constancy of 24-hour urinary creatinine excretion. Clin. Chim. Acta, 21:411, 1968.

Seligson, D., and Hirahara, K.: The measurement of ammonia in whole blood, erythrocytes, and plasma. J. Lab. Clin. Med., 49:962, 1957.

Shih, V. E., and Efron, M. L.: Urea cycle disorders. In Stanbury, J. B., Wyngaarden, J. B., and Fredrickson, D. S. (eds.): The Metabolic Basis of Inherited Disease, 3rd ed. New York, McGraw-Hill Book Co., Inc., 1972.

Siimes, M. A., and Dallman, P. R.: New kinetic role for serum ferritin in iron metabolism. Br. J. Haematol., 28:7, 1974.

Sims, C., and Parekh, A. C.: Determination of serum creatinine by reaction with methyl-3,5-dinitrobenzoate in methyl sulfoxide. Ann. Clin. Biochem., 14:227, 1977.

Sinha, S. N., and Gabrieli, E. R.: Serum copper and zinc levels in various pathologic conditions. Am. J. Clin. Pathol., 54:570, 1970.

Sinnott, J. L.: The laboratory investigation of the porphyrin disorders: A review. Med. Lab. Sci., 33:133, 1976.

Sobel, C., Henry, R. J., Chiamori, N., and Segalove, M.: Determination of α-amino acid nitrogen in urine. Proc. Soc. Exp. Biol. Med., 95:808, 1957.

Spackman, D. H., Stein, W. H., and Moore, S.: Automatic recording apparatus for use in the chromatography of amino acids. Anal. Chem., 30:1190, 1958.

Sperling, O., De Vries, A., and Kedem, O.: Studies on the etiology of uric acid lithiasis. IV. Urinary non-dialyzable substances in idiopathic uric acid lithiasis. J. Urol., 94:286, 1965.

Steed, E., Pereira, W. E., Halpern, B., Solomon, M. D., and Duffield, A. M.: An automated gas chromatographic analysis of phenylalanine in serum. Clin. Biochem., 5:166, 1972.

Steele, T. H.: Renal excretion of uric acid. Arthritis Rheum., 18:793, 1975.

Steiner, A. L., Kipnis, D. M., Utiger, R., and Parker, C.: Radioimmunoassay for the measurement of adenosine 3',5'-cyclic phosphate. Proc. Natl. Acad. Sci. USA, 64:367, 1969.

Sunderman, F. W.: Atomic absorption spectrometry of trace metals in clinical pathology. Hum. Pathol., 4:549, 1973.

Sunderman, F. W., and Roszel, N. O.: Measurements of copper in biologic materials by atomic absorption spectrometry. Am. J. Clin. Pathol., 48:286, 1967.

Talke, H., and Schubert, G. E.: Enzymatische Harnstoffbestimmung in Blut und Serum in optischen test nach Warburg. Klin. Woch., 43:174, 1965.

Tocci, P. M., Phillips, J., and Sager, R.: The effect of diet upon the excretion of parahydroxyphenylacetic acid and creatinine in man. Clin. Chim. Acta, *40*:449, 1972.

Tomokuni, K.: New method for determination of aminolaevulinate dehydratase activity of human erythrocytes as an index of lead exposure. Clin. Chem., *20*:1287, 1974.

Trinder, P.: The improved determination of iron in serum. J. Clin. Pathol., *9*:170, 1956.

Van Wyk, J. T., Underwood, L. E., Hintz, R. L., Clemmons, D. R., Voina, S. J., and Weaver, R. P.: The somatomedins: A family of insulinlike hormones under growth hormone control. Rec. Prog. Horm. Res., *30*:259, 1974.

Wacker, W. E. C., and Parisi, A. F.: Magnesium metabolism. N. Engl. J. Med., *278*:658, 1968a.

Wacker, W. E. C., and Parisi, A. F.: Magnesium metabolism. N. Engl. J. Med., *278*:712, 1968b.

Wacker, W. E. C., and Parisi, A. F.: Magnesium metabolism. N. Engl. J. Med., *278*:772, 1968c.

Ward, P., Ewen, M., Pomeroy, J. A., and Leung, F. Y.: Kinetic urine creatinine determination with the Gemsaec analyzer. Clin. Biochem., *9*:225, 1976.

Watson, C. J., and Schwartz, S.: A simple test for urinary porphobilinogen. Proc. Soc. Exp. Biol. Med., *47*:393, 1941.

Watts. R. W. E.: Determination of uric acid in blood and in urine. Ann. Clin. Biochem., *11*:103, 1974.

Watts, R. W. E.: Uric acid biosynthesis and its disorders. J. R. Coll. Physicians Lond., *11*:91, 1976.

White, J. M., and Flashka, H. A.: An automated procedure, with use of Ferrozine, for assay of serum iron and total iron binding capacity. Clin. Chem., *19*:526, 1973.

Whitehead, T. P., and Whittaker, S. R. F.: A method for the determination of glutamine in cerebrospinal fluid and its results in hepatic coma. J. Clin. Pathol., *8*:81, 1955.

Wills, M. R.: Value of plasma chloride concentration and acid-base status in the differential diagnosis of hyperparathyroidism from other causes of hypercalcemia. J. Clin. Pathol., *24*:219, 1971.

Wong, P. W. K., O'Flynn, M. E., and Inouye, T.: Micromethods for measuring phenylalanine and tyrosine in serum. Clin. Chem., *10*:1098, 1964.

Wybenga, D. R., Ibbott, F. A., and Cannon, D. C.: Determination of ionized calcium in serum that has been exposed to air. Clin. Chem., *22*:1009, 1976.

Zak, B., and Epstein, E.: Automated determination of serum iron. Clin. Chem., *11*:641, 1965.

Zak, B., Baginski, E. S., Epstein, E., and Weiner, L. M.: Determination of serum iron with a new color reagent. Clin. Toxicol., *4*:621, 1971.

EVALUATION OF THE FUNCTION AND INTEGRITY OF THE LIVER

Hyman J. Zimmerman, M.D.

The liver is a complex organ which performs many metabolic functions. More than 100 measurements of hepatic functions have been based on the hundreds of reactions that have been shown to occur in the liver. Many of these have been abandoned after early study. A few tests have been found to be clinically useful. Table 11-1 contains a classification of the hepatic tests arranged according to their physiologic basis.

Classic experiments in hepatic physiology have shown that removal of large portions of the liver of normal animals may leave some types of hepatic function unimpaired. This has led many authors to emphasize the great reserve power of the liver and to suggest that mild hepatic disease will not be exposed by examination of hepatic function. The relevance of such experiments to clinical problems, however, is questionable. Diffuse though mild disease, such as viral hepatitis or early cirrhosis of the liver, produces impairment of several measurements of hepatic function, with the severity of disease reflected in the degree of hepatic dysfunction. Indeed, disturbed hepatic function does not necessarily mean hepatic disease, since physiologic effects of some non-hepatic diseases also may produce apparent impairment of liver function. Nevertheless, the occurrence of abnormal hepatic function can usually be found to have a rational basis when considered in the light of the clinical problem.

Clinicians tend to refer to all biochemical determinations that reflect hepatic disease as "liver function tests." Only some, however,

Table 11-1. PHYSIOLOGIC CLASSIFICATION OF HEPATIC FUNCTION AND RELATED DETERMINATIONS

PHYSIOLOGIC BASIS	MEASUREMENTS	COMMENTS
Excretion and detoxification		
Bilirubin determinations	Serum bilirubin (direct & indirect)	Very useful
	Urine bilirubin	Very useful
	Urine urobilinogen	Useful
	Fecal urobilinogen	Useful, but neglected
Clearance of exogenous load		
Dye excretion	Sulfobromophthalein (BSP)	Very sensitive test of hepatic function; largely abandoned because of reactions.
	Indocyanine green (ICG)	Has been used extensively in research to measure hepatic function and blood flow. Recommended as replacement for BSP.
	Rose bengal (RB)	Obsolete test; recently revived as radioactive RB and used for differential diagnosis of infantile jaundice.
Other	^{14}C-bilirubin	
	^{14}C-cholic acid	Experimental
	Galactose tolerance	See carbohydrate tests.
Clearance of endogenous load	Bile acid levels (fasting & postprandial)	Very promising, but limited by technology
	Bilirubin levels	Depends on other factors; see bilirubin metabolism.
	NH$_3$ levels	See protein metabolism.
Xenobiotic metabolism		
Conjugating ability	Hippuric acid excretion	Formerly widely used; now obsolete
Drug metabolism (mixed-function oxidase activity)	Drug metabolism measured by $^{14}CO_2$	Promising; experimental
Metabolic and synthetic		
Carbohydrate metabolism	Glucose tolerance test	Not useful
	Fructose tolerance test	Not useful } in measuring
	Lactate tolerance test	Not useful } hepatic function
	Galactose tolerance test	Used little in U.S.A. Still used in other countries.
	Epinephrine tolerance tests	Of some use for diagnosis of glycogenoses but used little for diagnosis of other liver disease
	Glucagon tolerance tests	
Lipid metabolism	Plasma or serum cholesterol level	Limited usefulness
	Plasma or serum cholesterol ester level	Little clinical value
	Cinnamic acid tolerance	Of physiologic interest, but no clinical use
Protein metabolism		
Protein levels of blood	Serum protein levels	Very useful in analysis of hepatic and non-hepatic diseases
	Albumin, globulin, electrophoretic fractions; gamma globulin levels, immunoglobulins	
	Mucoproteins and haptoglobin	Have seen little use
	Flocculation and turbidimetric tests	Largely obsolete
	Lipoprotein-x	Marker of cholestasis; of research interest
	Alpha-1-antitrypsin	Specific value for diagnosis of metabolic error
	Alpha-fetoprotein	Specific value for hepatic carcinoma
	Amino acid levels of blood & urine	Of research interest
	Blood ammonia levels	Useful in understanding, diagnosis and management of hepatic encephalopathy
	CSF (cerebrospinal fluid) glutamine	

Table 11-1. PHYSIOLOGIC CLASSIFICATION OF HEPATIC FUNCTION AND RELATED DETERMINATIONS (continued)

PHYSIOLOGIC BASIS	MEASUREMENTS	COMMENTS
Biosynthetic activity	Albumin level	See protein metabolism.
	Blood urea levels	Of clinical value, but not useful to measure liver function
	Rate of urea synthesis	Research interest thus far
	Prothrombin time & response to Vitamin K	Very useful
	Plasma level of other coagulation factors	Reflected in prothrombin time. Individual factor measurement of research interest
Serum enzyme levels		
Large number of enzymes normally present in the liver because of multiple metabolic reactions that occur there; enzymes released to blood as a result of hepatocyte injury, biliary tree impatency, or both	Alkaline phosphatase (and related tests)	Very useful
	Aspartate aminotransferase (AST) or GOT	Very useful
	Alanine aminotransferase (ALT) or GPT	Very useful See Chapter 12 for other serum enzymes.
Other substances released from damaged liver	Iron	Limited use
	Vitamin B_{12}	Limited use
Determinations that reflect special hepatic diseases		
Serum levels of	Alpha-fetoprotein	Hepatocellular carcinoma*
	Alpha-1-antitrypsin	Alpha-1-antitrypsin-liver disease*
	Iron, transferrin, and ferritin	Hemochromatosis*
	Ceruloplasmin	Wilson's disease*
	Serologic tests for	
	Viral hepatitis	See Table 11-13.
	"Autoimmune" liver disease	See Chapter 38.

*Condition for which determination is particularly helpful.

actually measure hepatic function. For example, the imposition of an exogenous load for clearance by the liver (e.g., foreign dyes, galactose, or infused bile acid) or the estimation of the ability of the liver to excrete an endogenous load (e.g., bilirubin, bile acids, ammonia) are indeed tests of liver function. Measurement of the ability of the liver to metabolize a drug, to conjugate a foreign compound with glycine, and to synthesize prothrombin, albumin, or urea also comprise measurements of hepatic function, although factors other than liver function can affect the results. Distortions of intermediary metabolism wrought by hepatic disease are of physiologic interest, and some hepatic function determinations have been based on the distortions.

Another group of biochemical determinations are of great help in the recognition of hepatic disease but do not measure liver function. These include measurement of blood constituents that, when elevated, reflect hepatocyte injury or biliary tree impatency. Serum activity of several enzymes (aminotransfer-

ases or transaminases, ornithine carbamoyl transferase, etc.), iron, ferritin, and vitamin B_{12} are elevated in patients with hepatic necrosis, to a degree that may assist in diagnosis. Conversely, the levels of other enzymes (alkaline phosphatase, 5'-nucleotidase, etc.), cholesterol, trihydroxy bile acids, and lipoprotein-X are elevated to a diagnostically helpful degree in patients with biliary tree obstruction.

A third group of biochemical and serologic measurements are useful for the diagnosis of specific hepatic diseases. In this group, for example, are serum alpha-fetoglobulin, alpha-1-antitrypsin, ceruloplasmin, iron and transferrin, serologic markers of viral hepatitis, antimitochondrial antibodies, anti-smooth muscle antibodies, and immunoglobulins (IgM, IgG, and IgA).

No one measurement or test of liver function is sufficient for clinical analysis of most problems. From the available measurements and examinations, a group of procedures that are most applicable to a particular clinical problem should be selected. These determinations and the various radiographic, radioisotopic, ultrasonic, and endoscopic procedures, as well as liver biopsy, constitute a panel of measurements and examinations that should permit diagnosis of almost all patients with hepatic disease.

In the following pages, the physiologic basis for examination of hepatic functions is discussed, a number of individual tests are analyzed, and the batteries of tests that are considered useful are presented. The results obtained in various diseases also are described.

HEPATIC TESTS BASED ON EXCRETORY FUNCTION

An important physiologic role of the liver is the removal from the blood of potentially noxious endogenous and exogenous substances, and, thereafter, excretion into the bile or conversion to products suitable for excretion by the kidney or lung. Measurement of the concentrations of some of the endogenous substances in the blood, urine, or feces, or of the rate of uptake and excretion of exogenous substances, has provided useful tests of hepatic function (Table 11-1). Some of these are discussed in this section (related to bilirubin metabolism, dye excretion, bile acid metabolism). Others are discussed in the section devoted to intermediary metabolism (tests based on uptake by the liver of galactose, ammonia, and amino acids).

BILIRUBIN METABOLISM

Knowledge of bilirubin metabolism (Fig. 11-1) is essential for the proper understanding of hepatic disease. Bilirubin is a product of the catabolism of hemoglobin, from which it is formed in the cells of the reticuloendothelial system. Here the protoporphyrin is separated from the iron and globin portions of the molecule, and the ring is opened oxidatively, leading to the quantitative release of the α-carbon bridge as carbon monoxide* and to the formation of biliverdin. The biliverdin is rapidly

_____
* Measurement of CO production can serve as a measure of heme catabolism.

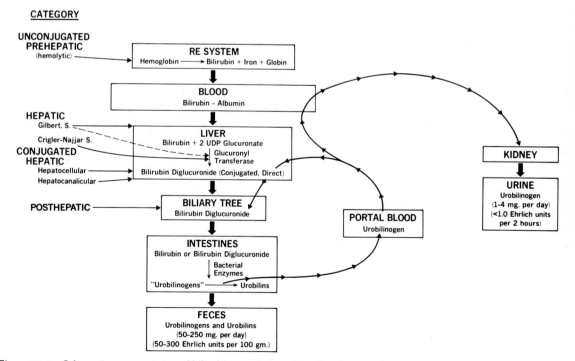

Figure 11-1. Schematic representation of bilirubin metabolism. The classification of jaundice (see Table 11-3) is shown on the left, the arrows pointing to the site of the physiologic defect responsible for the respective category of jaundice.

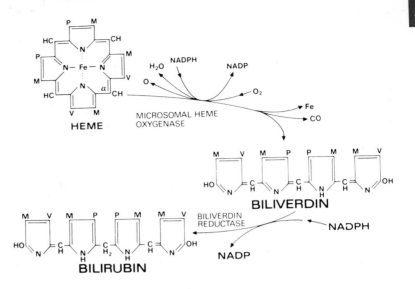

Figure 11-2. Biochemical pathway for conversion of heme to bilirubin via the intermediate biliverdin. From Tenhunen (1976) with permission.

reduced to bilirubin (Fig. 11-2). Approximately 85 per cent of the bilirubin is derived from senescent erythrocytes. Most of the remainder is produced by intracorpuscular degradation of the hemoglobin of immature erythrocytes in the bone marrow (ineffective erythropoiesis). Very small amounts are derived from the degradation of heme-containing enzyme proteins derived from the liver and, perhaps, from other organs.

Bilirubin is transported through the blood (bound to albumin) to the liver. Transport of bilirubin from sinusoidal blood into the hepatocyte depends on mechanisms which are currently under intensive study. It involves dissociation of bilirubin from albumin and is facilitated by or depends on specific transport proteins described by Arias (1969) and by Fleischner (1976). The process is saturable and shows mutually competitive inhibition by other organic ions, such as sulfobromophthalein (BSP), indocyanine green, and iodipamide, suggesting that bilirubin uptake is a carrier-mediated transport process.

In the liver, bilirubin is conjugated with glucuronic acid* to form the diglucuronide (Fig. 11-3). In addition, some of the monoglucuronide is also formed (Billing, 1975).

In the intestines bacterial enzyme action converts bilirubin through a group of intermediate compounds to several related com-

pounds collectively referred to as "urobilinogen" (Fig. 11-1). A portion (estimated to be 10 per cent or more) of the urobilinogen is reabsorbed into the blood and re-excreted by the liver. Normally, small amounts (1 to 4 mg/24 hr) are excreted in the urine. Fecal urobilinogen levels in normals range from 50 to 250 mg/day. Some of the urobilinogen is oxidized to urobilin in the intestines or later in the feces. Measurement of fecal urobilinogen

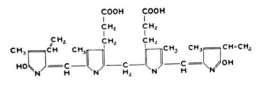

Indirect

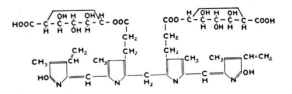

Direct

Figure 11-3. The structure of indirect and direct bilirubin. Note that direct bilirubin is bilirubin diglucuronide and that indirect is unconjugated bilirubin. Conversion of bilirubin to the diglucuronide is catalyzed by glucuronyl transferase. (This schematic representation of bilirubin as a linear tetrapyrrole is the conventional model, although a ring-shaped structure is more accurate.)

---

*A fraction of the bilirubin excreted by the liver is conjugated with other groups. The conjugates of bilirubin that are formed differ in different species.

usually includes the sum of urobilinogens and urobilins. The metabolism of bilirubin is summarized in Figure 11-1.

Bilirubin was first demonstrated in serum by van den Bergh and Muller. They found that bilirubin in normal serum reacted with the Ehrlich diazo reagent (diazotized sulfanilic acid) only when alcohol was added. Their observation that bile pigment in human bile reacted with the diazo reagent without the addition of alcohol led to the recognition that some change in bilirubin had been effected by the liver. Van den Bergh called the form of bilirubin that reacted with the diazo reagent without the addition of alcohol "direct" and the variety that reacted only in the presence of alcohol "indirect." Serum from patients with jaundice caused by hemolysis gave the indirect reaction, while in the serum of patients with jaundice due to obstruction of the biliary tree the increased serum bilirubin levels gave the direct reaction. The response of the serum to the van den Bergh test has been the basis for several classifications of jaundice.

The properties of indirect and of direct bilirubin are summarized in Table 11-2. It is clear that the indirect bilirubin is "free" or unconjugated bilirubin bound to albumin en route to the liver from the reticuloendothelial system, where it has been formed. The unconjugated bilirubin is non-polar and therefore not soluble in water. Consequently it will react with the diazo reagent only in the presence of an agent (alcohol) in which it and the diazo reagent are soluble.* The non-polar nature of unconju-

---

*The alcohol also enhances the intensity of the color formed by the bilirubin reaction with the van den Bergh reagent.

gated bilirubin bound to albumin is also the basis for the failure of indirect bilirubin to appear in the urine in more than trace amounts. Unconjugated bilirubin is so tightly bound that it cannot be filtered at the glomerulus, and there appears to be no known tubular secretion of bilirubin. Accordingly, unconjugated bilirubin is not excreted in the urine. Direct (conjugated) bilirubin is a polar compound. It is therefore soluble in water solution, reacting directly with the diazo reagent and able to appear in the urine when the blood levels are increased. Conjugated bilirubin is, in large part, not protein-bound; hence, it can be filtered at the glomerulus and excreted in the urine.

Qualitative analysis of serum bilirubin as indirect or direct according to the type of van den Bergh reaction has long been replaced by quantitative determination of the amount of direct and of total bilirubin, the difference being presumed to represent indirect bilirubin. Commonly used procedures for measuring bilirubin and its fractions are modifications of the method of Malloy (1937). These methods depend on the speed of the reaction with the diazo reagent and on the solvent in which it occurs. The pigment that reacts promptly without the addition of ethanol or methanol is "direct," and that which reacts later and with the addition of the alcohol is the "total" bilirubin (indirect plus direct). Many laboratories supplement their diazotization method with one of the direct spectrophotometric techniques. An excellent review of bilirubin methodology which is complete and extensive is available (Sunderman, 1978).

The level of bilirubin in the serum is less than 1.0 mg/dl in 99 per cent of normals. This is almost entirely unconjugated. Up to 20 per cent of the unconjugated bilirubin, however, can react with the van den Bergh reagent, simulating the presence of up to 0.2 mg/dl of conjugated bilirubin in normal plasma. Accordingly, values for direct bilirubin above 0.2 mg/dl by the method of Ducci (1945) are suspect. The upper reference limit for direct bilirubin may, however, vary from 0.2 to 0.4 mg in different laboratories, and each laboratory should determine the reference interval for its method and conditions. Levels of total serum bilirubin above 2.5 mg/dl usually produce jaundice.

Jaundice has been classified by various authors according to pathophysiology, etiology, or both. The classification of McNee (1923),

Table 11-2. COMPARISON OF PROPERTIES OF DIRECT AND INDIRECT BILIRUBIN

	DIRECT (CONJUGATED)	INDIRECT (UNCONJUGATED)
Structure	Bilirubin diglucuronide	Bilirubin
Type of compound	Polar	Nonpolar
Solubility		
Water	+	−
Alcohol	+	+
Van den Bergh reaction	Direct	Indirect
Affinity for brain tissue	Low	High*
Presence in urine of patients with jaundice	+	−

* Kernicterus (deposition of bilirubin in brain tissue) occurs only in association with very high levels of unconjugated bilirubin.

Table 11-3. CLASSIFICATION OF JAUNDICE

CLASSIFICATION OF HYPERBILIRUBINEMIA	PHYSIOLOGIC DEFECT	EXAMPLES OF ETIOLOGY	TESTS OF BILIRUBIN METABOLISM*			
			Serum Bilirubin Direct: Total in %	Urine Bilirubin	Urobilinogen†	Fecal Urobilinogen‡
Unconjugated Prehepatic	Excessive production of bilirubin	Hemolytic states Extensive hematoma	<20	–	(↑)	↑
Hepatic	Defective transport of bilirubin from sinusoidal blood into hepatocyte	Gilbert syndrome§	<20	–	N	N
	Inability to conjugate	Some toxins (e.g., flavaspidic acid) Crigler-Najjar syndrome Neonatal jaundice Some drugs (e.g., Novobiocin)	<20	–	N	N
Conjugated Hepatic Hepatocellular	Hepatocyte injury	Viral or toxic hepatitis, cirrhosis, alcoholic hepatitis, other causes of hepatocyte injury	>40	+	N, ↑, or ↓	↓
Hepatocanalicular	Intrahepatic cholestasis owing to defective transport of bilirubin into canaliculus	Some drugs (e.g., chlorpromazine, anabolic steroids), viral hepatitis, primary biliary cirrhosis, some forms of familial jaundice	>50	+	N, ↑, or ↓	↓
Posthepatic	Mechanical obstruction of biliary tree	Carcinoma of pancreas or common bile duct Choledocholithiasis Other anatomic obstruction	>50	+	↓	↓

*Arrow indicates direction of change. Parentheses indicate that change may or may not occur. N = normal; ↑ = elevated; ↓ = depressed; + = positive reaction or present.

†Normal urine contains very small amounts of urobilinogen.

‡Normals show a very wide range of fecal urobilinogen content. Levels above 250 mg/day are considered increased and those below 5 mg/day are decreased to a diagnostically useful degree.

§May also include impaired conjugation.

which was based on etiology, that of Rich (1930), which was based on mechanisms, and that of Ducci (1947), which was based on both, are now mainly of historic interest.

The currently employed classification of jaundice (Table 11-3; Fig. 11-1) is rational and simple. It divides hyperbilirubinemia into the two categories of *unconjugated* and *conjugated*. The *unconjugated* category includes the forms of jaundice in which at least 80 per cent of the serum bilirubin is indirect. This may be *prehepatic*, in which excess bilirubin production (hemolysis) is responsible, or *hepatic*, in which either removal of bilirubin from the blood or conjugation of bilirubin by the liver is defective. The *conjugated* category also includes two groups: *hepatic*, which includes a number of genetic and acquired defects of the

liver, and *posthepatic*, which refers to anatomic obstruction of the extrahepatic biliary tree.

The *prehepatic* type of unconjugated hyperbilirubinemia commonly referred to as hemolytic jaundice occurs because excessively rapid destruction of erythrocytes results in the production of bilirubin at a rate exceeding the ability of the liver to conjugate and excrete it. It may result from any of the genetic or acquired types of hemolytic disease. The hyperbilirubinemia, accordingly, is largely the indirect (unconjugated) type. The increased production of bilirubin usually results in an increase in the amount of fecal urobilinogen, a characteristic of hemolytic jaundice. Often there is also an increase in the urine content of urobilinogen. Presumably this results from the reabsorption from the intestines of greater amounts of urobilinogen than can be re-excreted by the liver. Bilirubin does not appear in the urine in hemolytic jaundice, since the elevated level of blood bilirubin consists largely of the unconjugated (bound to albumin) type.

The *hepatic* type of unconjugated hyperbilirubinemia includes the Gilbert syndrome (constitutional hepatic dysfunction) and the Crigler-Najjar syndrome (constitutional hyperbilirubinemia with kernicterus). The Gilbert syndrome is a mild condition that appears to result from a genetic defect in the transport of bilirubin from sinusoidal blood into the hepatocyte. (The Gilbert syndrome probably includes several different conditions, all of which present a similar benign syndrome of mild unconjugated hyperbilirubinemia.) The Crigler-Najjar syndrome is a severe disease with marked hyperbilirubinemia that results from a genetic deficiency of the hepatic microsomal enzyme, glucuronyl transferase, which is needed for the conjugation of bilirubin. Another form of glucuronyl transferase deficiency, which is a clinically much more benign syndrome, has been described. Hepatic unconjugated hyperbilirubinemia resembles that of hemolytic (prehepatic) hyperbilirubinemia in that it is largely unconjugated. The fecal and urine urobilinogen content in the hepatic type of *unconjugated* hyperbilirubinemia, in contrast to that of the prehepatic type, is normal or reduced, since the rate of bilirubin entry into the duodenum is depressed rather than increased (Fig. 11-4*B* and *C*).

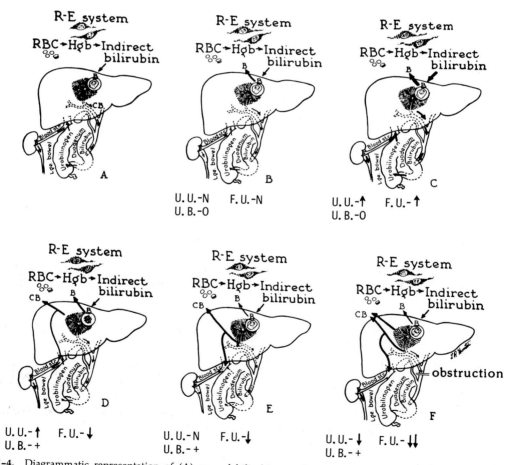

Figure 11-4. Diagrammatic representation of (A) normal bilirubin metabolism and the type of defect in (B) Gilbert or Crigler-Najjar syndrome, (C) hemolytic jaundice, (D) hepatocellular jaundice, (E) hepatocanalicular jaundice (intrahepatic cholestasis), and (F) posthepatic jaundice. In the diagrams, B represents unconjugated and CB conjugated bilirubin; U.U. represents urine urobilinogen, U.B. urine bilirubin, and F.U. fecal urobilinogen. N represents normal; + indicates present; 0 indicates absent; number of upward or downward-directed arrows indicates increase or decrease, respectively.

Posthepatic jaundice, commonly called obstructive jaundice, usually is the result of obstruction of the common bile or hepatic duct by carcinoma of the head of the pancreas, papilla of Vater, or common duct, by choledocholithiasis, or by pancreatitis. Rarely, diseased lymph nodes surrounding the duct or neoplastic invasion of the *porta hepatis* may produce posthepatic jaundice. Obstruction of the biliary tree produces jaundice by preventing the entry into the duodenum of bilirubin that has been conjugated. The bilirubin is "regurgitated" into the blood, raising the serum level of direct-reacting bilirubin, which then appears in the urine. The exclusion of bilirubin from the duodenum results in clay-colored feces and very low levels of urobilinogen in the feces and urine (Fig. 11-4F).

Hepatic (conjugated) jaundice or hyperbilirubinemia can be divided into two subcategories: the hepatocellular and hepatocanalicular types. *Hepatocanalicular jaundice* closely resembles posthepatic jaundice in its clinical and biochemical features. This is also commonly referred to as *intrahepatic cholestasis.*

The hepatocellular types of hepatic jaundice result from injury to the parenchyma (viral hepatitis, toxic hepatitis, cirrhosis). Hepatic damage theoretically might be expected to produce an unconjugated hyperbilirubinemia because of (theoretically) impaired conjugating ability. Indeed, late in convalescent hepatitis, the jaundice may be of the unconjugated type. During the more deeply jaundiced phase of hepatitis, however, there are features similar to those of posthepatic jaundice. Thus, in viral hepatitis there is a distinct increase in the direct-reacting bilirubin fraction of the blood and there is bilirubin in the urine. The degree of exclusion of bilirubin from the duodenum, however, is much less marked than in posthepatic jaundice. Stools usually are only somewhat lighter than normal but may be clay-colored. The urobilinogen content of the stool is usually decreased, but rarely to the levels characteristic of posthepatic jaundice. Even though amounts of bilirubin entering the duodenum are less than normal, liver damage prevents adequate hepatic clearing from the blood of the urobilinogen reabsorbed from the duodenum. Urine urobilinogen, therefore, is often increased in some stages of hepatocellular jaundice (Figs. 11-4D and 11-5).

It has been presumed, therefore, that in hepatitis (as in posthepatic jaundice) much of the bilirubin presented to the liver cell is conjugated, excreted into the canaliculi, and then regurgitated into the blood. In this concept, the regurgitation has been assumed to be via necrotic cells or increased canalicular permeability. There is little to support this view, however, and some other mechanism may well be responsible, perhaps impaired synthesis of bile acids necessary to permit adequate transport of conjugated bilirubin into the canaliculus.

The hepatocanalicular type of hepatic jaundice simulates posthepatic jaundice very closely (Fig. 11-4E). It has also been called "cholangiolitic," a term based on the theory that jaundice occurs because bilirubin regurgitates into the blood through inflammatory defects in the cholangioles. It is better called *intrahepatic cholestasis,* a term that describes the fact that bile flow into the duodenum is inhibited by intrahepatic disease. This type of jaundice is seen most commonly with certain drug reactions (chlorpromazine, organic arsenicals, methyltestosterone); it is thought to occur occasionally as a result of viral hepatitis or it may be "idiopathic."

DETERMINATIONS

Total serum bilirubin level is useful in evaluating the depth and progress of jaundice. Direct and indirect bilirubin measurements have been of some value in the differential diagnosis of jaundice. When the direct fraction is less than 20 per cent of the total bilirubin value, the jaundice is considered to be a manifestation of unconjugated hyperbilirubinemia—due either to hemolysis or to one of the types of constitutional hyperbilirubinemia (Table 11-3). Little specific aid in the distinction of hepatic from posthepatic causes of conjugated hyperbilirubinemic jaundice can be obtained from the relative levels of direct and indirect bilirubin. The direct fraction may constitute 40 to 60 per cent of the total bilirubin in either hepatic or posthepatic jaundice. Levels of the direct fraction that constitute between 20 and 40 per cent of the total bilirubin, however, are more characteristic of hepatic than of posthepatic jaundice. Levels in excess of 50 per cent of the total are somewhat more characteristic of posthepatic than of hepatic jaundice.

Most commonly used methods are the Malloy and Evelyn (1937) or modifications of it

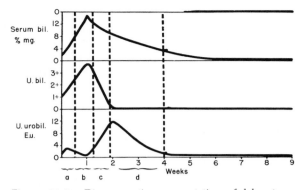

Figure 11–5. Diagrammatic representation of laboratory abnormalities during the course of viral hepatitis. Note that early in the course (phase *a*) there is presence of bilirubin and increased amounts of urobilinogen in the urine with elevated serum bilirubin levels. This is followed by the phase (*b*) of deepening jaundice with decreased urine urobilinogen and increased urine bilirubin, after which there is an increase in urine urobilinogen (phase *c*) as the serum and urine bilirubin begin to decrease. In phase *d* bilirubin often disappears from the urine, but serum bilirubin levels are still distinctly elevated. Most patients show or are observed only in phases *c* and *d*, but some show this complete pattern. (Modified from Watson: Ann. Intern. Med., 25:195, 1947.)

such as Ducci and Watson (1945) or Michaelson (1961). In these methods the bilirubin reacts with diazotized sulfanilic acid to form azobilirubin, the intensity of the purple color being proportional to the quantity of bilirubin. In the Ducci and Watson method, the amount of bilirubin that reacts with the diazo reagent (in aqueous solution) at the end of one minute is determined. This "one-minute" bilirubin is equivalent to the "prompt," direct-reacting bilirubin of van den Bergh. The total bilirubin is measured 15 minutes after the addition of methanol. The difference between the total and the direct is the indirect. Other methods employ the same principle.

Urine bilirubin (urine "bile") measurements are useful in the differential diagnosis of jaundice. The presence of bilirubin in the urine of a patient with jaundice shows that the hyperbilirubinemia is of the conjugated type, i.e., hepatic or posthepatic. Bilirubin may also be present in the urine of patients without jaundice, as in early or anicteric hepatitis, in metastatic carcinoma, or in early obstruction of the biliary tree.

A number of methods have been devised for the measurement of bilirubin in the urine. The most sensitive depend on concentration of bilirubin by absorption, followed by oxidation or diazotization to yield a characteristic color

reaction. In this country, simplified methods involving tablets or "dip-sticks" impregnated with diazo reagent have superseded other procedures. The impregnated tablets can detect bilirubin concentrations of 0.05 to 0.1 mg/dl. Dip-sticks are somewhat less sensitive. There should be no bilirubin demonstrable by any of these methods in normal urine (see Chap. 17).

Decreased *fecal urobilinogen* is characteristic of obstructive (posthepatic) jaundice but may also be found in patients with hepatocellular jaundice. An extremely low level (below 5 mg or 5 Ehrlich units per day) of fecal urobilinogen is evidence that the jaundice is posthepatic. An increased level (above 250 mg or 300 Ehrlich units per day) is evidence of hemolysis. When fecal urobilinogen levels are being determined as measures of hemolysis, they should be correlated with the degree of anemia (see Chap. 29).

Measurement of urobilinogen content of feces and urine can be useful but has lost popularity in recent years. The several compounds which are collectively referred to as urobilinogens give the same cherry-red color with Ehrlich's aldehyde reagent. The intensity of the color permits ready quantitation of total urobilinogen content. Urine urobilinogen can be measured by the simple two-hour test of Watson (1944) and even more simply with Ehrlich's aldehyde reagent. By the method of Watson, normal urine should contain less than 1 Ehrlich unit (1 mg urobilinogen) per two-hour specimen. Measurement of fecal urobilinogen involves the same color reaction but is somewhat more arduous and less aesthetic.

Urine urobilinogen levels are decreased in posthepatic jaundice and in some phases of hepatic jaundice. Increased levels are observed usually in hemolytic jaundice and with subsiding hepatitis. Increased levels may also be a sensitive measure of hepatic damage even in the absence of jaundice, as in some patients with cirrhosis of the liver, metastatic carcinoma, or congestive heart failure.

Studies of urine and stool pigments are extremely useful to the clinician, but there are several pitfalls in the application of bile pigment study to the analysis of jaundice. Very low levels of urobilinogen in the stool are characteristic of posthepatic jaundice but may also occur in patients who have received "broad-spectrum" antibiotics. These agents suppress the intestinal bacteria which convert bilirubin to urobilinogen. On the other hand, normal levels of urine urobilinogen may be found in patients with incomplete obstructive jaundice. During the course of acute viral hepatitis (Fig. 11-5), urobilinogen and bilirubin content of the urine may be characteristic of hepatocellular jaundice (phases a and c) and of obstructive jaundice (phase b) and may even simulate prehepatic icterus (phase d). Mixed forms of jaundice may yield potentially confusing patterns. For example, hemolytic icterus may be complicated by hepatic necrosis (as in sickle cell anemia) and thus by hepatocellular jaundice or by pigment stones obstructing the common duct and producing posthepatic jaundice.

Other tests based on bilirubin metabolism have been devised but have found little clinical application. The *bilirubin tolerance test* consists of administering a known amount of bilirubin and observing the rate of disappearance from the blood. This test is a sensitive measure of hepatic function but has not been adopted widely because it is laborious and expensive. Use of ^{14}C-bilirubin makes the test far easier to perform, but it is used only in research.

Excretion of foreign dyes

It has been recognized for many years that extraction of foreign dyes from the blood by the liver can be applied to the testing of hepatic function. The three dyes which have been employed for this purpose are rose bengal, sulfobromophthalein (BSP), and indocyanine green (ICG). BSP and ICG also have been used to measure hepatic blood flow. The technique, which is used primarily as a research tool, involves hepatic vein catheterization, measurement of the fraction of dye extracted by the liver per unit volume of blood perfusing it, and application of the Fick principle.

Rose Bengal Excretion. Rose bengal excretion was the first test of liver function, based on the elimination of dyes by the liver, that received significant clinical application. In this test the dye is administered parenterally, and either excretion of the dye into the duodenum or retention in the blood is measured. For technical reasons, this procedure was considered inferior to the BSP test and abandoned. Rose bengal excretion has been revived recently with the introduction of rose bengal "tagged" with ^{131}I. The rate of accumulation of the radioactivity over the liver and its rate of disappearance from the liver have been used to help detect hepatic disease. A test based on the fecal and urinary excretion of injected radioactive rose bengal and its products has been helpful in distinguishing hepatocellular from obstructive jaundice, particularly in infants. It is of little assistance in distinguishing intrahepatic cholestasis from extrahepatic obstruction, particularly in adults. I-131-rose bengal clearance has found little use as a test of liver function. The use of this and other radioactive substances for scanning of the liver surface is discussed elsewhere in this chapter (p. 339).

Sulfobromophthalein (BSP) Excretion. The BSP excretion test has been one of the most widely used and most sensitive tests of liver function. Normal results with this procedure virtually rule out a significant degree of parenchymal hepatic disease.

Recent years have seen decreased use of the procedure, in part because of adverse reactions and in part because the information sought is provided by other tests. Nevertheless, it has been so widely used that an adequate description of its physiologic basis is in order.

The dye is administered intravenously and its disappearance from the blood is determined. The BSP is almost completely cleared from the blood by the normal liver. (In hepatectomized animals, up to 20 per cent of the dye may be removed by extrahepatic tissue.) The two factors involved in BSP excretion by the liver are normal hepatic function and an adequate hepatic circulation.

Excretion of BSP by the liver involves four steps: (1) The dye is transferred from the blood to the hepatic parenchymal cell. (2) It is stored there briefly bound to ligandin and the z protein. (3) It is *conjugated* with glutathione. (4) The conjugate* is excreted by active transport into the bile. Refined techniques are available for the measurement of clearance from the blood and excretion into the bile and for the estimation of storage capacity. Excretion into the bile is the rate-limiting step for which a transport maximum (Tm) has been defined. These measurements and the determination of blood levels of conjugated and unconjugated BSP are research tools useful for unraveling the relative roles of hepatic uptake, conjugation (and storage), and biliary excretion in the clearance of BSP. They are, however, too elaborate for ordinary clinical use. Simplified techniques have been used to demonstrate defective transport of conjugated BSP into the bile in the Dubin-Johnson syndrome and in individuals with impaired hepatic function induced by methyltestosterone and other C-17 alkylated steroids.

Several standardized tests have been based on the ability of the liver to remove BSP from the blood. In the most widely used procedure a dose of 5 mg/kg of body weight is administered intravenously, and a blood specimen is obtained 45 minutes later. The level of dye at 45 minutes is expressed as the per cent of dye "retained," i.e., not

---

* A small fraction (<30 per cent) of the dye is excreted in the unconjugated form.

Table 11–4. DISEASES CHARACTERIZED
BY ABNORMAL BSP EXCRETION

I. Parenchymal hepatic disease
   A. Cirrhosis
   B. Fatty metamorphosis
   C. Viral hepatitis
   D. Toxic hepatic injury
   E. Infectious mononucleosis
II. Biliary tract disease
   A. Common bile duct obstruction (with or without
      jaundice)
   B. Cholelithiasis and cholecystitis
III. Extrahepatic disease
   A. Circulatory
      1. Congestive heart failure
      2. Hepatic vein occlusion (Chiari's syndrome)
      3. ? Shock
      4. Spinal cord injuries
   B. Systemic disease producing infiltrative lesions of
      liver
      1. Metastatic carcinoma
      2. Lymphomas and leukemias
      3. Granulomatous disease (tuberculosis, histo-
        plasmosis, sarcoidosis)
      4. Amyloidosis
   C. Nonspecific (fever, chronic and debilitating dis-
      eases)

excreted. A level of 10 mg/dl is considered to represent 100 per cent retention.

The determination of the rate of disappearance (percentage disappearance rate (PDR)) by obtaining multiple serum samples after administration of the dye provides a greater degree of accuracy than does the single-specimen method. It is too elaborate for routine clinical application, however.

Healthy individuals can remove from the blood over 95 per cent of the injected dose by 45 minutes. "Retention" in the blood of over 5 per cent of the dose, accordingly, is evidence of abnormal hepatic function or impaired blood flow.

Abnormal retention occurs in a number of hepatobiliary and systemic conditions. In hepatic and posthepatic jaundice, values are abnormal. In unconjugated hyperbilirubinemia, however, whether of the prehepatic (hemolytic) or hepatic (Crigler-Najjar and Gilbert's syndromes) type, BSP excretion is usually normal. (One form of Gilbert's syndrome is associated with impaired BSP excretion.)

Excretion of BSP also is abnormal in non-jaundiced patients with hepatic, biliary tract, or extrahepatic disease (Table 11–4). In patients with cirrhosis, excretion is rarely normal. Those with ascites or portal hypertension usually show a high degree of BSP retention. Nevertheless, in rare instances of inactive cirrhosis,* even when accompanied by severe portal hypertension, hepatic function, as measured by BSP excretion, may be normal or only slightly abnormal.

_____
* Absence of necrosis and little or no inflammation.

In most (75 per cent) patients with fatty metamorphosis of the liver, the ability to excrete BSP is impaired, and, in general, the degree of impairment parallels the intensity of the steatosis. Indeed, impaired BSP excretion may be the only abnormal hepatic function in patients with hepatic steatosis.

In patients with viral or toxic hepatitis, BSP excretion is, of course, abnormal during the icteric phase. It may remain abnormal, however, for a period after jaundice has subsided and usually becomes abnormal before jaundice has appeared. Most patients with infectious mononucleosis have impaired BSP excretion.

Patients with non-hepatic disease may also have impaired BSP excretion. In patients with heart failure, the degree of BSP retention is proportional to the severity of right-sided failure, as reflected in the degree of venous pressure elevation. In hepatic vein occlusion (Budd-Chiari syndrome) the mechanisms for impaired excretion, presumably, are similar to those of heart failure. Impaired hepatic blood flow and hepatocyte anoxia appear to contribute to the dysfunction. Shock also may lead to a moderate degree of impairment of BSP excretion. The impairment of BSP excretion observed in paraplegic patients has been ascribed to alterations in hepatic blood flow.

Certain extrahepatic diseases impair liver function by producing infiltrative lesions in the liver. These include metastatic carcinoma, the lymphomas, leukemia, the systemic granulomatous diseases (disseminated tuberculosis, sarcoidosis), and amyloidosis. Almost all patients with metastatic carcinoma of sufficient involvement to produce hepatomegaly have impaired BSP excretion, ranging in degree from 5 to 50 per cent retention. In the other diseases cited, the degree of retention is less.

Other non-hepatic diseases lead to impaired BSP excretion by different mechanisms. Febrile illnesses with fever of more than 103° F. usually produce some abnormality of this function. Certain chronic and "debilitating" diseases, such as rheumatoid arthritis, may also lead to moderate impairment of BSP excretion.

It is apparent that the BSP excretion test is of greatest value in the patient with little or no jaundice. A normal result is helpful in excluding the presence of hepatic parenchymal disease. The test has been useful in the identification of the cause of gastrointestinal hemorrhage, since patients with esophageal varices owing to cirrhosis usually have moderate to marked degrees of BSP retention (15 to 50 per cent.† Patients with gastrointestinal hemorrhage owing to a peptic ulcer, however, usually have normal or only slightly abnormal BSP

_____
† Advances in endoscopy have permitted precise identification of the site of gastrointestinal bleeding and have made the approximating role of the dye excretion test obsolete.

excretion. This test is also useful in measuring the severity of liver disease and in assessing the completeness of recovery (e.g., in hepatitis). It is of aid in detecting early hepatic damage in patients who have been exposed to hepatotoxins. It is of help in recognizing the presence of metastatic hepatic carcinoma.

The BSP excretion test is particularly helpful in diagnosing the Dubin-Johnson syndrome and in distinguishing it from the Rotor syndrome, which it resembles. In the Dubin-Johnson syndrome a genetic defect leads to impaired transport of BSP, after conjugation, into the canaliculus and, consequently, regurgitation of conjugated BSP into the blood. Removal from blood and hepatic storage, however, are normal. Accordingly, in the Dubin-Johnson syndrome the BSP values at 45 minutes may be normal or only slightly increased, while the value subsequently (90, 120, or 150 minutes after administration) may be much higher. In the Rotor syndrome, also due to a genetic defect in bilirubin metabolism, storage and excretion of BSP are abnormal and the BSP value in the blood is abnormal at 45 minutes and less abnormal thereafter.

Pitfalls in the application of this test lie in its great sensitivity and, accordingly, in the large number of extrahepatic causes of abnormal values, although clinical correlations are of help in this regard, of course. Conversely, some forms of intrinsic hepatic disease may be associated, though infrequently, with normal BSP excretion. These include occasional instances of hemochromatosis, polycystic disease of the liver, amyloidosis, and inactive macronodular cirrhosis. An additional source of error in interpreting results of the BSP test is the interference with excretion of the dye induced by some gallbladder dyes. Accordingly, an unexpectedly abnormal value within 24 hours of a cholecystogram should not be accepted until confirmed by repetition at another time. Some drugs (e.g., rifampin) also compete with hepatic uptake of BSP.

The irritative effect of BSP on extravascular tissue is great. Extravasation of the dye in the course of intravenous administration can lead to a severe cellulitis and slough. This can be prevented by meticulous technique in administration.

The most important disadvantage is the extremely rare but serious complication of anaphylactic (or anaphylactoid) shock caused by BSP administration. Although this test will probably disappear, it is implicit from foregoing comments that this author considers the BSP test valuable.

Indocyanine Green Excretion. Excretion of indocyanine green (ICG) has been utilized as a test of hepatic function during the past few years. Excretion of this dye by the liver does not involve conjugation. Furthermore, there is virtually no extrahepatic removal from the blood of ICG, which is removed almost exclusively by the liver. Accordingly, this dye has been studied as a possible substitute for BSP. Results of the ICG excretion test in the dose ordinarily used (0.5 mg/kg) are comparable to those of the BSP test in patients with severe hepatic disease, but the BSP test appears to be a more sensitive indicator of mild hepatic abnormality than does the ICG in this small dose. The larger dose of ICG (5 mg/kg) appears to be as sensitive as BSP, but is far more expensive. It is probable that the ICG test will prove to be useful in the settings which have employed the BSP. Nevertheless, a large amount of clinical experience and testing will be required to validate the assumption that results with the ICG test can be considered equivalent to those formerly obtained with the BSP test.

Serum bile acids

Bile acids are generally referred to as *primary* and *secondary* (Fig. 11-6). The principal *primary* bile acids, cholic and chenodeoxycholic acid, are synthesized in the liver from cholesterol (Chap. 8). Cholic acid is a trihydroxy (3-α, 7-α, 12-α) and chenodeoxycholic acid is a dihydroxy (3-α, 7-α) bile acid. The primary bile acids are conjugated with glycine and taurine prior to their active transport into the bile. The conjugated primary bile acids, after secretion into the bile, are stored in the gallbladder during the fasting state. During digestion the bile acids are excreted into the lumen of the intestinal tract.

The bile acids undergo an efficient enterohepatic circulation involving the following three pathways: (1) passive jejunal reabsorption of the conjugate of chenodeoxycholic acid; (2) active ileal reabsorption of conjugated bile salts; (3) passive colonic reabsorption of "secondary" bile acids formed by bacterial deconjugation and chemical alteration of the conjugated bile salts. Of the many secondary bile acids formed in the colon, deoxycholic and lithocholic (LCA) acids are the most important. The pathophysiologic ramifications of bile acid metabolism are great and beyond the scope of this chapter. The promise that bile acid measurement offers for evaluation of liver function, however, warrants further discussion.

Small amounts of primary bile acids are present in the portal blood at any time. Bile acids are almost completely removed from the portal blood by hepatocyte extraction and are then rapidly re-excreted into the bile. Accordingly, the quantity of bile acids present in the peripheral or portal blood or within the liver normally represents a very small fraction of the total bile acid pool. Almost all of the bile acid pool is within the gallbladder in the fast-

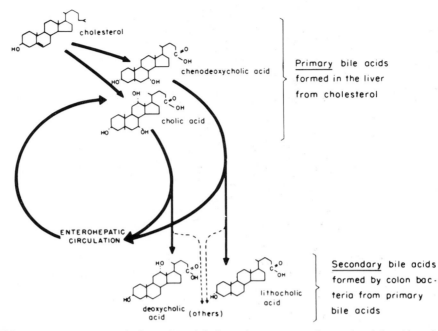

Figure 11-6. Schematic representation of relationship of cholesterol to primary and secondary bile acids and of enterohepatic circulation of bile acids. From Javett (1975) with permission.

ing state and within the intestinal lumen during digestion (Hofman, 1976).

Removal of bile acids from sinusoidal blood is a concentrative, saturable, and carrier-mediated process (Erlanger, 1976). It resembles in some ways the uptake and excretion of bilirubin, BSP, and ICG but differs in that the uptake of bile acids appears not to depend on the y and z carrier proteins. The highly efficient uptake of bile salts by the normal hepatocyte permits this phenomenon to be utilized as a test of liver function. Indeed, hepatic bile salt uptake and peripheral bile salt concentration have turned out to be highly sensitive indicators of hepatocellular dysfunction. It is clear that decreased or altered hepatic blood flow, such as can occur in cirrhosis, also would lead to abnormalities of this function.

It has long been recognized that levels of bile acids are increased in the blood and urine of patients with obstructive (posthepatic) jaundice, as shown in the past by simple qualitative methods (Hay's and Pettenkofer's tests). The lack of satisfactory quantitation in the past and the demonstration that bile acids may also be found in the urine of patients with hepatocellular jaundice had prevented the clinical application of these procedures. Quantitative methods which have been applied

recently, however, have yielded characteristic patterns in patients with hepatobiliary disease. Unfortunately, the methods for the measurement of total serum bile acid and of the individual bile acids thus far available are too difficult and time-consuming for regular clinical application. Nevertheless, rapid advances in the theory and technology of bile acid measurement indicate that assay of bile acid levels will become a routine clinical determination.

There have been four approaches to the utilization of bile acid levels for the diagnosis of hepatobiliary disease. Two of these have involved measurement of total bile acid levels, another has consisted of measuring removal from the blood of an infused bile acid, and the fourth has involved fractionation into the di- and trihydroxy acids.

Total Bile Acid Level. Measurements of total bile acid levels of the serum have been done in the fasting and postprandial states. Fasting levels are elevated in patients with acute and chronic hepatitis, alcoholic hepatitis, cirrhosis, posthepatic jaundice, and intrahepatic cholestasis. Indeed, as a measurement of acute and chronic hepatic disease, the total bile acid level has appeared to be almost as sensitive as the 45-minute BSP excretion test.

Thus far three types of methods have been employed. One has involved the enzymatic measurement employing 3-hydroxysteroid dehydrogenase. Another method has utilized gas liquid chromatography. The third has employed radioimmunoassay (RIA). Of the three, the one which will probably prove to be most suitable for routine application is RIA, once it has been properly refined.

Postprandial Serum Bile Acid Levels. Measurement of serum bile acid concentrations two hours after a meal may be considered an endogenous loading test. The presence during the fasting state of the major portion of the bile acid pool in the gallbladder, the postprandial contraction of the gallbladder, and the efficient enterohepatic recirculation of bile acids provide a setting in which the postprandial bile acid level appears to be an extremely sensitive measure of hepatobiliary disease. Clinical testing suggests that the postprandial value is more sensitive than the fasting concentration. Sufficient clinical application to evaluate the usefulness of the procedure, however, remains to be conducted.

Bile Acid Tolerance Test. Exogenous bile acid load tests have utilized infusion of unlabeled cholylglycine or of radiolabeled bile acids. The cholylglycine or other bile acid tolerance tests have involved measuring a fractional disappearance rate or a 10-minute "retention" value utilizing RIA for measurement of the cholylglycine levels. This has been reported to be a sensitive indicator of impaired hepatic function. Indeed, it has been alleged to be more sensitive than serum levels of bilirubin, aspartate aminotransferase (AST or GOT) or alkaline phosphatase, and more sensitive than the levels of cholylglycine. These clearance tests, however, have not been subjected to any significant clinical evaluation, and it remains to be seen whether clinical use will endorse their value.

Ratio of Serum Trihydroxy to Dihydroxy Bile Acids. Theoretically this ratio has much to recommend it. Synthesis of the trihydroxy bile acids requires adequate hepatic function. Patients with posthepatic jaundice or intrahepatic cholestasis are likely to have elevated serum total bile acid concentrations because of excretory blockade, and, because hepatic function is preserved, to have a high ratio of serum trihydroxy to dihydroxy bile acids. The patient with hepatocellular jaundice, however, who may be expected to have impaired hepatocellular function, will have a lesser proportion of bile acids in the trihydroxy form. Accordingly, the ratio may be of help in the differential diagnosis of jaundice. The technical difficulties involved in measuring bile acid levels, however, have precluded extensive efforts to apply this determination.

Accordingly, despite the promise of clinical value of measuring bile acid levels of endogenous and exogenous "tolerance" tests and of fractionating them, clinical application has been delayed. Problems of technology and the lack of a sufficient body of clinical data supporting the applicability preclude their being a part of routine batteries of liver function tests.

DETOXIFICATION AND DRUG METABOLISM

The liver has long been recognized to effect metabolic changes in foreign compounds. Viewed broadly, these changes consist of conversion of non-polar to polar compounds to permit their excretion. While enzymatic machinery for metabolic changes in xenobiotics can be found in extrahepatic tissues, the liver accounts for almost all of the biotransformation of foreign compounds.

The biotransformation consists of two phases. *Phase I* involves oxidation or other reactions that introduce a polar group into the molecule. *Phase II* consists of conjugation of the product of Phase I or the original compound, if it already has a polar group, with glucuronate, glycine, or other moieties. *Phase II* reactions have long been recognized and termed the *conjugating* or *detoxifying* function of the liver. It is the basis of an obsolete measure of hepatic function, the *hippuric acid excretion* test. Conjugation of bilirubin with glucuronide to form "direct" bilirubin and formation of conjugates of steroids and other endogenous substances are other examples of Phase II xenobiotic metabolism. During the past several years, hepatic function tests based on Phase I metabolism also have been introduced.

Hippuric acid excretion test

Over 40 years ago, a test based on the hepatic synthesis of hippuric acid by the conjugation of benzoic acid with glycine was introduced. With several modifications, it remained in use for a number of years. The test consisted of administering a standard amount of benzoic acid orally or of sodium benzoate intravenously and determining the amount of hippuric acid excreted during a specific period of time. Excretion of hippuric acid after a standard dose of benzoic acid had been found to be decreased in patients with intrinsic hepatic disease, such as cirrhosis or severe hepatitis. In early obstructive jaundice, however, excretion of hippuric acid was generally normal. Accordingly, it was advocated for use in the differential diagnosis of jaundice. The ability to synthesize hippuric acid, however, depends not only on the conjugating enzyme systems of the liver but also on the hepatic stores of glycine. Furthermore, the hippuric acid formed is measured by its concentration in the urine. Accordingly, renal function must be intact in order for hippuric acid excretion to reflect hepatic function. For these reasons, and because the test is cumbersome, it has fallen into disuse. It is now mainly of historic interest.

Tests based on drug metabolism

Experimental hepatic disease in animals impairs drug-metabolizing ability, and the degree of impairment reflects the severity of hepatic injury and parallels other measures of hepatic failure (Plaa, 1968). Studies in humans utilizing a variety of indirect measures, including rate of clearance of drugs from the blood and appearance of metabolic products in the blood and urine, also have demonstrated adverse effects of hepatic disease on drug metabolism. These measurements, however, are too cumbersome for regular clinical use and pose problems of interpretation.

The recently introduced "breath analysis" test permits quantitative measurement of

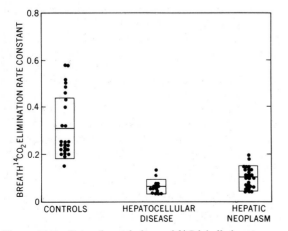

Figure 11-7. Rate of metabolism of ^{14}C-labelled aminopyrine in patients with hepatocellular disease and hepatic neoplasm compared with that of normals as reflected in elimination of $^{14}CO_2$. From Hepner and Vesell (1976) with permission.

drug metabolism and appears to provide a useful type of hepatic function test. It consists of administration by mouth of a drug labeled with a trace dose of ^{14}C. Expired $^{14}CO_2$ is a measure of the metabolic conversion of the drug. Most extensively studied thus far has been aminopyrine labeled at the 2 N-methyl positions. In the studies of Hepner (1976) it has appeared to be a useful and simple measure of hepatic function (Fig. 11-7). Further experience with this test using this and other drugs and correlating the results with other tests of hepatic function are required to appraise fully the clinical usefulness of this promising approach to hepatic function testing.

TESTS OF HEPATIC SYNTHETIC ABILITY

The liver is responsible for a variety of synthetic activities. Some (e.g., conjugations) have been discussed in the preceding section. Others, e.g., synthesis of serum proteins and urea, are discussed in Chapters 9 and 10. A synthetic activity useful for the testing of hepatic function and of clinical importance is the role of the liver in the manufacture of plasma coagulation factors. For testing of hepatic function, the *prothrombin time* and related assays described in Chapter 33 (p. 1156) are used.

PROTHROMBIN TIME AND VITAMIN K RESPONSE

It has been known for a long time that patients with severe hepatic disease, as well as those with obstructive jaundice, may have coagulation defects. The pathogenesis of the clotting defect is complex and may include deficient or defective platelets, circulating anticoagulants, intravascular coagulation, and deficiency in plasma clotting factors. Demonstration of deficiency of plasma clotting factors, as reflected in the one-stage prothrombin time, has been a valuable tool for the diagnosis of liver disease.

Identification of vitamin K in 1940 and the demonstration that vitamin K deficiency leads to coagulation defects and to hypoprothrombinemia were promptly followed by the recognition that bleeding tendencies in obstructive jaundice could be repaired by the parenteral administration of vitamin K. Vitamin K is fat-soluble and requires bile salts for absorption. The hypoprothrombinemia of obstructive (posthepatic) jaundice, accordingly, was clearly attributable to the deficiency of vitamin K resulting from lack of its absorption. Hypoprothrombinemia, found in patients with parenchymal hepatic disease, however, was not restored to normal by parenteral administration of vitamin K and was recognized to reflect defective hepatic synthesis.

These observations led to the formulation of a test which has been used for the differential diagnosis of jaundice for several decades. The test employs the one-stage prothrombin time (PT). If it is abnormally prolonged, the effect of vitamin K administration can distinguish between deficiency of vitamin K or deficient hepatocyte synthetic ability as the cause of the abnormal PT. Administration of a standard dose of vitamin K to a patient with posthepatic jaundice usually restores a prolonged PT to normal, whereas it fails to do so in patients whose abnormal values are due to intrinsic hepatic diseases. The test is usually performed by measuring the PT, and, if it is prolonged, by administering 10 mg of vitamin K intramuscularly daily for one to three days. In a patient with deep jaundice, the restoration of an abnormal PT to normal by this regimen provides helpful evidence that the abnormality is due to malabsorption of vitamin K and that the jaundice is obstructive. Lack of normalization of a markedly prolonged PT strongly suggests that jaundice is hepatocellular in origin.

There are several pitfalls in the application of this procedure. Patients with obstructive jaundice may have only a mildly prolonged PT; the difference after administration of vitamin K, therefore, may be insufficient to provide a conclusive answer. Furthermore, in intrinsic hepatic disease which mimics posthepatic jaundice (intrahepatic cholestasis), parenchymal dysfunction may be relatively slight, and the response of the "hypoprothrombinemia" may be similar to that of posthepatic jaundice. Also, a patient with a cause for malabsorption other than posthepatic jaundice or one who had been taking an oral antibiotic that inhibits bacterial flora may have an abnormal PT response to vitamin K.

The degree of prolongation of the PT in a patient with parenchymal hepatic disease is a useful measure of the severity of the hepatic injury. In patients with acute hepatitis, marked prolongation of the value is an ominous sign and may herald a fatal outcome. In cirrhosis it is also a reflection of severely impaired parenchymal function.

Originally the one-stage PT was considered to be a specific measurement of prothrombin (factor II). We now know that it depends on factors I (fibrinogen), II (prothrombin), V (proaccelerin), VII (proconvertin), and X (Stuart factor). All of these factors are synthesized in the liver and all but factors I and V require adequate amounts of vitamin K in the liver for their synthesis. Indeed, we now speak of the "prothrombin complex," referring to factors that affect the one-stage PT (Table 11-5).

Coagulation defects in patients with hepatic disease or with obstructive jaundice usually include deficiency of other factors as well as prothrombin (Table 11-5), and the prolonged one-stage PT reflects depression of multiple factors of the prothrombin complex (Chap. 33). Measurable deficiency of factor V, however, is found only in association with severe liver disease. Deficiency of fibrinogen synthesis is a preterminal event and of little clinical significance. Indeed, measurement of individual plasma coagulation factors (Chap. 33), while useful in the management of hemorrhagic phenomena, has not been applied to the diagnosis of hepatic disease.

Excess fibrinolysis, either as a direct reflection of liver disease or more probably as the result of the disseminated intravascular coagulation syndrome (DIC), may be responsible for a hemorrhagic tendency in patients with terminal cirrhosis (Chap. 33). Thrombocytopenia secondary to hypersplenism and decreased platelet adhesiveness also contributes to hypocoagulability of the blood. In spite of these difficulties, response of the PT to parenteral vitamin K may be a useful ancillary measure in the differential diagnosis of jaundice.

Table 11-5. CLOTTING ABNORMALITIES IN PATIENTS WITH LIVER DISEASE

Deficiency of plasma factors
  Prothrombin
  Factors VII, X, V — Measured by one-stage prothrombin time
  Fibrinogen
  (XIIIa)

Thrombocytopenia (as result of hypersplenism)
Decreased platelet adhesiveness
Disseminated intravascular coagulation (DIC)
Fibrinolysins

METABOLIC TESTS

A number of hepatic function tests have been based on the role of the liver in intermediary metabolism. Those tests related to carbohydrate metabolism have been least useful and those related to protein metabolism most useful. Only one commonly used test relates to lipid metabolism.

CARBOHYDRATE METABOLISM

Patients with hepatic disease may have hypoglycemia. They also may show diminished tolerance for administered glucose, galactose, fructose, or lactate. Their hepatic glycogen stores may be decreased as measured by plasma glucose response to administered epinephrine or glucagon.

Hypoglycemia occurs regularly in hepatectomized animals. It occurs in about 10 per cent of patients with acute hepatic necrosis. The incidence of hypoglycemia in other forms of hepatic disease, however, is low. It has been described in rare instances of biliary cirrhosis, in primary or metastatic carcinoma of the liver, and in the hepatic congestion of heart failure. Hypoglycemia is particularly characteristic of two peculiar forms of fatty livers, one associated with a febrile state in children referred to as *Reye's syndrome*, and the other, the rare *fatty liver of pregnancy*. The hypoglycemia that occurs in alcoholic patients results from acute direct and indirect metabolic effects of alcohol, not from the liver disease of alcoholism.

Glucose tolerance is characteristically abnormal in patients with cirrhosis of the liver. There is a rapid rise of plasma glucose to values above the upper reference limit and then a slow return to normal. This pattern in patients with liver disease can be distinguished from that of diabetes mellitus by the normal or low fasting plasma glucose in liver disease and the occurrence of subnormal values by the fifth hour after the glucose has been given. The oral or intravenous glucose tolerance test is of little value in diagnosis of hepatic disease.

The *galactose tolerance test* has been applied to the study of liver for many years. The normal liver is able to convert galactose to glucose, which is stored as glycogen. In patients with hepatic disease, this ability is defective. Administration of galactose results in persistence of abnormal blood levels for several hours and in urinary excretion of abnormal amounts of galactose. This test yields abnormal results in patients with hepatocellular jaundice but normal results in patients with obstructive jaundice of brief duration (less than three weeks). Although formerly recommended by some authors for the differential diagnosis of jaundice, this test was never widely employed and today is used in few centers in this country. It continues to be employed in some European centers.

The *fructose tolerance test*, based on a principle similar to that of galactose tolerance, has found no clinical application. Elevated blood levels of lactic acid have been described in patients with severe liver disease. This observation and a *lactic acid tolerance test* have been described as tests of hepatic function but also have found no regular clinical application.

The *epinephrine tolerance test* has been used to estimate hepatic glycogen stores by observing the plasma glucose response to a standard dose of epinephrine. Normal individuals show a blood glucose rise of 40 to 60 mg/dl within one hour after the epinephrine has been given. Patients with hepatic disease (cirrhosis, hepatitis) and patients with genetic deficiency in glycogenolytic enzymes (glycogen storage disease) show a subnormal response. The test has found little use in the diagnosis of liver disease but has been useful in clinical research and for the diagnosis of glycogen storage disease. The *glucagon tolerance test*, a modification of this test, has involved the use of glucagon instead of or combined with epinephrine to produce glycogenolysis. In either epinephrine or glucagon tolerance tests the subject should receive a high-carbohydrate diet for at least three days before the test.

LIPID METABOLISM

The liver is importantly involved in many phases of lipid metabolism, including the synthesis, esterification, and excretion of cholesterol. Only the determination of serum-free and esterified *cholesterol* has been applied intensively to the study of hepatic disease. In normal individuals (in the United States) the serum cholesterol level ranges between 150 and 250 mg/dl,* approximately 70 per cent of which is esterified. Esterification of cholesterol is largely catalyzed by lecithin-cholesterol acyltransferase (LCAT), an enzyme found in the blood and liver.

In general, serum cholesterol is normal or depressed in hepatocellular jaundice and elevated in obstructive jaundice. In patients with hepatitis, the serum cholesterol may be mildly depressed or normal, but the level of esterified cholesterol is usually moderately decreased. In severe hepatitis or cirrhosis the serum cholesterol (total and esterified) levels may be markedly depressed. In patients with posthepatic jaundice or intrahepatic cholestasis, the serum

---

*4.9–6.5 mmol/l

cholesterol value is usually elevated as high as 500 mg/dl.* Greater elevations occur occasionally but are more characteristic of hepatocanalicular jaundice (intrahepatic cholestasis) than of posthepatic jaundice. In "primary biliary cirrhosis," levels up to 1800 mg/dl† may be observed. It is generally stated that patients with obstructive jaundice usually have a normal (2/3) serum cholesterol-ester/total cholesterol ratio. Strictly speaking, this is not true. Although the degree of depression of the ratio is characteristically less than that seen in hepatic disease, moderate degrees are regularly seen. Determination of total serum cholesterol is widely used in the diagnosis of hepatic disease, but determination of the ester fraction is of little diagnostic value.

Abnormal values of other plasma lipids occur in patients with hepatic and biliary tract disease. Increased plasma levels of triglycerides are observed in patients with obstructive jaundice, in alcoholic patients with hemolytic anemia, hyperlipemia, and fatty liver (the Zieve syndrome), and in those with pancreatitis. Values of plasma non-esterified or free fatty acids are increased in patients with all forms of parenchymatous hepatic disease. Plasma concentrations of phospholipids are increased in obstructive jaundice and in biliary cirrhosis. While measurement of the several lipid fractions has been of investigative interest, it is too time-consuming and complex for routine clinical application.

The *cinnamic acid* tolerance test is an interesting test of hepatic function that couples two reactions known to occur in the liver. One is a measure of lipid metabolism (fatty acid oxidation) and the other involves conjugation. The normal liver oxidizes (beta oxidation) cinnamic acid to benzoic acid, which in turn is conjugated with glycine to form hippuric acid. Abnormal hepatic function is reflected in the decreased excretion of hippuric acid. Although this test has found no clinical application, it is cited here as an interesting approach to the measurement of hepatic function.

PROTEIN METABOLISM

Amino acid metabolism, urea synthesis, and protein metabolism occur in the liver. Evidence of defects in each of these areas may be observed in patients with hepatic disease. These include abnormal plasma levels of

* 13 mmol/l
† 47 mmol/l

amino acids, proteins, urea, and ammonia as well as abnormal urine (and cerebrospinal fluid) levels of amino acids. Several measurements of hepatic function and disease have been based on these phenomena.

Plasma Protein Values. A number of plasma proteins are formed in the liver. These include albumin, fibrinogen, and some of the alpha and beta globulins. Accordingly, changes in the plasma (or serum) proteins form the basis for important laboratory aids to the diagnosis of hepatic disease. Changes in the plasma concentration of an individual protein, however, may be due to altered rate of synthesis or catabolism, to dilution by an expanded plasma volume, or to abnormal losses into the gut. Indeed, the expanded plasma volume associated with cirrhosis exaggerates the hypoalbuminemia owing to impaired synthesis. Nevertheless, the depressed serum albumin level which is characteristic of chronic hepatic disease is a valuable clinical tool. The *serum globulin* level is often elevated in patients with chronic hepatic disease (cirrhosis) and chronic hepatitis, representing mainly the immunoglobulins or gamma globulin fractions and reflecting largely immune responses.

The procedures which have been used to evaluate serum protein changes in patients with liver disease include determination of serum albumin and globulin levels, serum electrophoresis, and several turbidometric ("flocculation") tests. The turbidometric tests reflect largely changes of the gamma globulin and albumin levels. Immunochemical methods have been used to measure the various immunoglobulins.

The *serum albumin* level is an index of severity and prognosis in patients with chronic hepatic disease. In patients with cirrhosis there is a positive correlation between the degree of hypoalbuminemia and the severity of the ascites. Patients who show a rise of serum albumin have a more favorable prognosis than those whose levels remain low. In patients with acute hepatic disease (viral or toxic hepatitis), serum albumin levels are usually normal or only mildly depressed. Those who develop subacute hepatic necrosis ("subacute yellow atrophy") frequently have moderate to marked hypoalbuminemia.

The total serum globulin level is often elevated in patients with cirrhosis. The degree of elevation is usually moderate in alcoholic and in biliary cirrhosis, with levels of 3 to 4 g/100 ml. In active postnecrotic cirrhosis and

Table 11-6. ABNORMALITIES OF SERUM PROTEINS IN LIVER DISEASE*

	ACUTE HEPATITIS	CIRRHOSIS (LAENNEC'S)	CAH† WITH OR WITHOUT CIRRHOSIS	CIRRHOSIS (BILIARY)	OBSTRUCTIVE JAUNDICE	PRIMARY OR METASTATIC CARCINOMA
Albumin	N or ↓	↓↓	↓↓	↓	N or ↓	↓
Globulin	N or ↑	↑	↑	↑	N	N
Alpha-1‡						↑
Alpha-2		N	N	↑	↑	↑↑
Beta	↑	↑	↑	↑↑↑	↑↑	N
Gamma§	↑	↑↑	↑↑↑	↑	N	N
	(IgG or IgM)¶	(IgA or IgM)	(IgG)	(IgM)		

*Direction and magnitude of change indicated by number of arrows.
†Chronic active hepatitis (CAH).
‡Alpha-1-antitrypsin low in one type of familial liver disease (see text). A majority of patients with primary hepatic carcinoma have the abnormal protein, alpha-fetoglobulin, in their serum (see text).
§Main type of immunoglobin (Ig) shown in parentheses.
¶Mainly IgG in virus B hepatitis; mainly IgM in virus A hepatitis.

in chronic active hepatitis (CAH), elevations also may be moderate but at times are marked, with values in the range of 6 to 9 g/dl occasionally observed. Such very high levels of serum globulin are particularly likely to be seen in patients with the hepatitis B antigen (HbsAG)-negative, "autoimmune" type of chronic active hepatitis. Levels in patients with acute hepatitis are usually normal or only mildly elevated, but in occasional patients may exceed levels of 4 g/100 ml. In patients with posthepatic jaundice the globulin level is usually normal, although it may be elevated.

The *total serum protein* level in patients with cirrhosis is occasionally low, often normal, and at times even elevated. Reversal of the albumin·globulin (A/G) ratio has been emphasized in this and in other hyperglobulinemic diseases. Reference to the A/G ratio, however, is needlessly awkward and imprecise. A low A/G ratio may occur because there is hyperglobulinemia or hypoalbuminemia or both. The term should be abandoned and the depression or elevation of the respective protein values described.

Serum protein electrophoresis (Chap. 9) is useful to demonstrate the globulin fraction which is elevated. In postnecrotic cirrhosis and in chronic active hepatitis, hyperglobulinemia represents largely increases in the immunoglobulins of the gamma globulin fraction. In biliary cirrhosis the alpha-2 and beta fractions are prominently increased, and often the gamma fraction also shows an increase. In posthepatic jaundice, the gamma globulin level is usually normal but may be increased; the alpha-2 and beta fractions are increased.

The patterns of abnormality of serum proteins in patients with hepatic disease are outlined in Table 11-6.

Application of quantitative immunochemical techniques (Chap. 38) has demonstrated characteristic changes in the gamma globulin fractions among the several forms of chronic liver disease. The increased gamma globulin level of chronic active hepatitis (CAH), cryptogenic cirrhosis, and "subacute" viral hepatitis consists mainly of the immunoglobulin gamma (IgG) proteins and includes only minor elevations of other immunoglobulins (Ig). In alcoholic cirrhosis, IgA and to a lesser extent IgM and IgG proteins are increased. In primary biliary cirrhosis (PBC), the elevated gamma globulin value consists mainly of IgM accompanied by minor elevations of IgG and IgA proteins. While the patterns of abnormality are suggestive rather than diagnostic, they can be clinically useful. Thus, an elevated gamma globulin level which consists mainly of IgM protein would favor the diagnosis of primary biliary cirrhosis (PBC) in a difficult-to-distinguish clinical setting.

SPECIAL PROTEIN TESTS

Flocculation Tests. A large number of tests which reflect abnormality of plasma proteins have been developed. These reactions, which have been called the "flocculation tests," "globulin reactions," or tests of the "serum colloidal stability," have been useful to the clinician. In Table 11-7 are listed a few of these procedures with an indication of the presumed related protein abnormalities.

These tests have in common the tendency to be abnormal in patients with intrinsic hepatic disease

Table 11–7. SOME FLOCCULATION TESTS INCLUDING SERUM PROTEIN ABNORMALITIES THAT THEY REFLECT*

TEST	PRECIPITATING REAGENT	PROTEIN FRACTIONS PRODUCING ABNORMALITY	ALBUMIN† INHIBITION
Cephalin flocculation	Cephalin-cholesterol emulsion	γ	+
Thymol turbidity	Supersaturated solution thymol	$\gamma\ (\beta)$	(+)‡
Colloidal gold	Colloidal gold	γ	+
Zinc sulfate turbidity	$ZnSO_4$	γ	(+)
Takata-Ara	$HgCl_2$	$\gamma\ (\beta)$	+
Cadmium sulfate	$CdSO_4$	$\gamma\ (\alpha\beta)$	+

*Modified from Maclagan, N. F., J. Clin. Pathol., 5:1, 1952. γ = gamma globulins; β = beta globulins; α = alpha globulins.

†Indicates that addition of albumin *in vitro* can convert a positive to a negative result.

‡(+) Indicates that addition of albumin is less effective in decreasing the degree of abnormal results.

(hepatitis, cirrhosis) and to be normal in patients with obstructive jaundice. Indeed, serum from patients with obstructive jaundice has the property of inhibiting the flocculation or turbidity tests when mixed with serum that gives a positive reaction. The responsible factor for this inhibition may be a phospholipid. In patients with various systemic diseases characterized by hyperglobulinemia (Table 11–8), the flocculation tests also may yield abnormal results. The various tests differ in the relative incidence of abnormality in various diseases.

The *cephalin-cholesterol flocculation* test is positive in approximately 90 per cent of patients with hepatitis and in approximately 60 per cent of patients with cirrhosis (Fig. 11–8). It depends on hypergammaglobulinemia and the degree of inhibition produced by the serum albumin. Decreased albumin contributes to a "positive" cephalin-cholesterol flocculation. It has been stated that a qualitative change in the albumin molecule also contributes to a positive cephalin flocculation result.

Table 11–8. CLASSIFICATION OF DISEASES ASSOCIATED WITH HYPERGLOBULINEMIA

I. Infections (especially chronic)
   A. Bacterial (subacute bacterial endocarditis, chronic suppurative infections, granulomatous infections)
   B. Spirochetal (syphilis)
   C. Viral (lymphogranuloma venereum, psittacosis)
   D. Fungal (histoplasmosis, coccidioidomycosis)
   E. Protozoal (leishmaniasis, malaria)
   F. Helminthic
II. Liver disease (cirrhosis, chronic hepatitis)
III. Collagen disease (rheumatoid arthritis, lupus erythematosis, polyarteritis nodosa, scleroderma)
IV. Neoplastic (multiple myeloma, macroglobulinemia, lymphomas, and leukemia, but rarely in carcinoma except for bronchogenic carcinoma)
V. Miscellaneous (sarcoidosis)

The *thymol turbidity* test also depends on the degree of elevation of gamma globulin. The beta globulin fraction has also been considered to play a role, since the precipitate is a thymol-globulin lipid complex. The degree of turbidity has been expressed in arbitrary units (Maclagan units), which may be determined by visual comparison with a turbidity standard or by use of a spectrophotometer.

Levels are elevated 80 to 90 per cent in patients with acute viral hepatitis and in 20 to 70 per cent of patients with cirrhosis, depending on the stage and type (Fig. 11–9). During the course of the viral hepatitis the thymol turbidity becomes abnormal a few days after the cephalin flocculation test but may remain abnormal after the latter has reverted to normal.

Abnormal values for the thymol turbidity and cephalin flocculation tests occur in a number of other hyperglobulinemic diseases (Figs. 11–8 and 11–9). Technical "false-positive" results may be obtained with sera that have a high lipid content. In fact, the thymol turbidity test has been applied to the estimation of fat absorption by observing changes after ingestion of a fat-containing meal.

Today the flocculation tests are generally regarded as too non-specific for clinical application, and they have been abandoned in most centers. Nevertheless, they are interesting reflections of changes in serum protein fractions which are not completely exposed by electrophoretic techniques. Their physiologic interest and their continued use in some clinics warrant this brief description.

Turbidimetric Estimation of Gamma Globulin Levels. There are several turbidimetric procedures in which the turbidity produced correlates quantitatively with the gamma globulin concentration of the serum. Some of these tests depend on the tendency for gamma globulin to be precipitated by low concentrations of metallic or other ions in solutions of low total ionic strength or by high

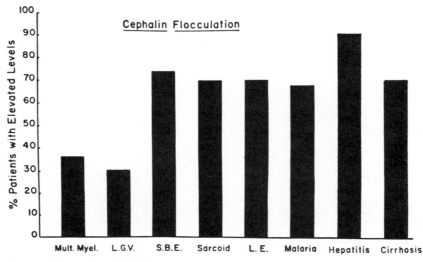

Figure 11–8. Incidence of abnormal cephalin flocculation results in various hyperglobulinemic diseases and in hepatitis and cirrhosis. S.B.E. = Subacute bacterial endocarditis; L.G.V. = lymphogranuloma venereum; L.E. = lupus erythematosus.

concentrations of salts. One of these, the zinc sulfate turbidity test (Kunkel test), has been applied to the distinction of hepatocellular from obstructive jaundice and in following the levels of gamma globulin in cirrhosis and other hyperglobulinemic diseases. Most laboratories today, however, choose to measure gamma globulin electrophoretically.

Serum Haptoglobin. This protein migrates with the alpha-2 globulins. Serum haptoglobin is elevated in patients with posthepatic jaundice and depressed in those with hepatocellular disease. Accordingly, measurement of serum haptoglobin level has been suggested as an aid to the differential diagnosis of jaundice, but it has seen little clinical testing.

Lipoprotein-x (L_P-x). This abnormal lipoprotein is found in the serum of patients with cholestatic jaundice, whether owing to hepatic disease or to obstruction of the biliary tree. It is also found in patients with deficiency of the enzyme lecithin-cholesterol acyltransferase (LCAT). While presence of L_P-x in the serum is a sensitive measure of cholestasis (in the absence of LCAT deficiency), it is of no aid in distinguishing intrahepatic cholestasis from posthepatic jaundice (see Chap. 8).

Alpha-fetoprotein (AFP). This alpha-globulin is present in appreciable amounts in the serum of the fetus, infant, and normal pregnant female. The serum of normal adults

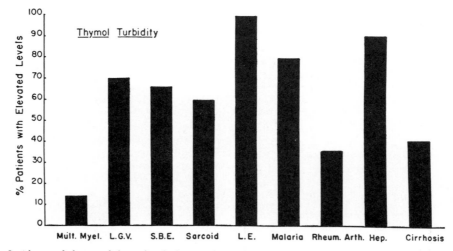

Figure 11–9. Incidence of abnormal thymol turbidity results in various hyperglobulinemic diseases and in hepatitis ("Hep.") and cirrhosis. S.B.E. = Subacute bacterial endocarditis; L.G.V. = lymphogranuloma venereum; L.E. = lupus erythematosus.

and children beyond the age of one year contains less than 30 ng/ml, an amount that is detectable only by radioimmunoassay. High values in amounts detectable by the relatively insensitive technique of Ouchterlony gel diffusion (>1000 ng/ml) are almost diagnostic of hepatocellular carcinoma in adults. In children, such high values may reflect teratoblastomas of the testes and ovary. A small proportion of patients with carcinoma of the pancreas, stomach, colon, and lung have also been reported to show elevated serum AFP, but usually below 1000 ng/ml.

Hepatocellular carcinoma is the entity which, among adults, is most characteristically associated with increased levels of AFP. Studies using radioimmunoassay have demonstrated increased levels in over 70 per cent of patients with this tumor, and values in excess of 3000 ng/ml in two thirds of those with elevated levels. Even higher values are found in patients from parts of Asia, Africa, and the Mediterranean littoral who have hepatocellular carcinoma.

Measurement of alpha-fetoprotein (AFP), of course, is not a test of hepatic function or even of hepatic injury *per se*. It is a useful clue in adults to the presence of hepatocellular carcinoma. If the relatively insensitive method of gel diffusion yields a positive result, indicating a probable value above 1000 ng/ml, the likelihood of hepatocellular carcinoma is increased, and a value above 3000 ng/ml as demonstrated by radioimmunoassay is virtually diagnostic. A very low value or absence of AFP from the serum does not exclude the diagnosis of hepatocellular carcinoma, since 30 to 50 per cent of patients may lack the abnormal protein.

Levels of AFP may also serve to monitor the course of hepatic carcinoma in response to treatment. Surgical removal can lead to a dramatic fall from a high value, as may effective chemotherapy.

Non-neoplastic hepatocellular disease can lead to modestly elevated serum AFP levels, almost always below 500 ng/ml (e.g., chronic active hepatitis; alcoholic cirrhosis, especially after a period of abstention; and the early convalescent phase of severe acute hepatitis). Indeed, some of the data from patients with non-neoplastic hepatic disease are consistent with the concept that elevated serum AFP levels reflect regenerative activity of hepatocytes. The impression that presence of elevated levels in patients with fulminant hepatic failure augurs a favorable prognosis, however, has not been confirmed.

Alpha-1-antitrypsin. A recently discovered genetic disease is characterized by a markedly depressed plasma level of alpha-1-antitrypsin, apparently the result of defective assembly of the molecule. The abnormal protein formed, which lacks the sialo groups present in the normal alpha-1-antitrypsin, is not released to the blood from its site of synthesis, the hepatocyte. The accumulated protein can be seen in periportal hepatocytes as diastase-resistant, periodic acid-Schiff-positive inclusion bodies. Indeed, their presence provides the histologic hallmark of alpha-1-antitrypsin deficiency.

The manifestations of the condition include liver disease of infancy, childhood, or even maturity, and in some of the involved adults precocious pulmonary emphysema. Deficiency of alpha-1-antitrypsin is reflected in a low or absent alpha-1-globulin peak on a serum protein electrophoretogram (Chap. 9, p. 231).

Measurement of the serum concentration of alpha-1-antitrypsin cannot be considered a test for liver disease, in the ordinary sense. It is a test useful in identifying liver disease in an infant with unexplained cholestasis or in a patient of any age with chronic liver disease of unknown cause. Even more useful for diagnosis is demonstration of the "antitrypsin bodies" in the periportal hepatocytes.

If a low serum concentration of alpha-1-antitrypsin is found, it is desirable to determine the patient's phenotype with respect to the molecular form of the alpha-1-antitrypsin, protease inhibitor (Pi) phenotype (Sharp, 1976). The molecular forms of alpha-1-antitrypsin revealed by special electrophoretic techniques have been designated F (fast), M (medium), S (slow), and Z (ultra-slow) according to their relative electrophoretic mobilities. The patterns specific for particular Pi phenotypes are designated by two of these letters. Most normal people are of the Pi phenotype MM. Patients with hepatic lesions owing to alpha-1-antitrypsin deficiency usually have the rare Pi phenotype ZZ, although subjects with other rare Pi phenotypes (MZ, FZ, and SZ) may have hepatic lesions which are similar to those associated with the Pi ZZ phenotype.

Serum alpha-1-antitrypsin is usually normal or somewhat increased in other forms of liver disease. Indeed, a well-maintained or increased value in fulminant liver failure has been interpreted as a clue to hepatic regenerative activity and, hence, possibly a favorable prognosis.

Ceruloplasmin. Ceruloplasmin is the copper-containing protein in plasma. It also has enzymatic (oxidase) activity. The latter property is utilized in one of the standard methods of measuring the concentration of this protein. Its main function is presumed to be transport of copper (Chap. 9). A low serum concentration of ceruloplasmin (less than 0.2 g/l) occurs in about 95 per cent of patients who are homozygous and in about 10 per cent of subjects who are heterozygous for Wilson's disease (Scheinberg, 1973). Low serum concentrations of ceruloplasmin in these individuals presumably reflect a selective defect in the synthesis of this protein in the liver cell.

Other forms of liver disease (viral hepatitis, cirrhosis) can lead to increased serum levels of ceruloplasmin. As a similar phenomenon, the level may become normal in Wilson's disease once liver damage is advanced. Accordingly, a normal value for this protein in the presence of overt liver disease does not exclude the diagnosis of Wilson's disease. A low value, of course, offers strong support for the diagnosis.

TESTS RELATED TO DISORDERED NITROGEN METABOLISM

Aminoaciduria. It has been known for a long time that patients with acute hepatic necrosis ("acute yellow atrophy") have leucine and tyrosine crystals in the urine. These amino acids represent, at least in part, products of autolyzed hepatic tissue. Other amino acids are found in the urine of patients with severe cirrhosis or hepatitis (toxic or viral). This aminoaciduria reflects the elevated levels of blood amino acids that result from impaired amino acid metabolism by the liver as well as from the release from necrotic tissue.

These observations may be applied to the study of hepatic disease. Demonstration of aminoaciduria by paper chromatography is preferable to and more reliable than the laborious search for characteristic tyrosine and leucine crystals. Amino acid content of the blood and urine, however, has found less routine than research application. Tests of hepatic function that have been based on the impaired ability of the damaged liver to metabolize amino acids include the *tyrosine tolerance*, the *methionine tolerance*, the *glycine tolerance*, and the *protein hydrolysate tolerance* tests. Each of these procedures may reveal a defect in the disappearance of administered amino acids from the blood of patients with hepatic disease, but they have not been applied to the study of clinical problems.

Blood Ammonia Determination. A relationship between elevated levels of blood ammonia and liver disease has been recognized for the past 30 years and suspected for over 60 years. It is uncertain whether ammonia, as measured in the blood, represents this substance as such or is ammonia released from some bound state by chemical manipulation.[*] At any rate, the amount of ammonia released from blood or plasma by treatment with alkali has been shown to be related to the severity of the liver disease.

A variety of methods are available for ammonia determination. A simple and widely used method is that of Seligson (1951), which uses whole blood. By that method, as modified by Bessman (1959), the normal levels are under $100 \mu g/dl$[†] of whole blood. An adaptation of the glutamate dehydrogenase enzymatic method of van Anken (1974) employing ACA (Dupont Automatic Clinical Analyzer, Dupont Instruments, Wilmington, Del.) has been satisfactory and efficient.

Studies have shown conclusively that the major source of blood ammonia is the gastrointestinal tract, although a minor contribution is made by the kidney. Bacteria, particularly those in the area of the cecum, release ammonia from nitrogen-containing foods. This ammonia, as well as ammonia ingested as ammonium salts or released from urea by bacterial or other urease, is absorbed into the portal vein. The liver normally removes most of the ammonia from the portal vein blood, converting it to urea. Little ammonia normally escapes from the liver into the hepatic vein to be carried to the systemic circulation.

Elevated blood ammonia levels in patients with hepatic disease appear to depend on two mechanisms, "shunting" of portal blood past the liver and impaired parenchymal function (Fig. 11-10). In patients with cirrhosis and extensive collateral portal circulation, elevation of the ammonia levels has been ascribed largely to the shunting of portal blood past the liver. Hepatic vein catheterization studies have shown that patients with severe hepatitis or cirrhosis remove less than normal amounts

---

[*] Almost all the blood "ammonia" is present as NH_4^+ ion rather than NH_3 at the pH of normal blood. Alkalosis increases the levels of free NH_3 by its effect on the equilibrium

$$NH_4^+ \rightleftarrows NH_3 + H^+$$

This has a bearing on the effect of alkalosis on the neurotoxicity of hyperammonemia, since free NH_3 crosses cell membranes more readily than does NH_4^+ ion.

[†] $55 \mu mol/l$

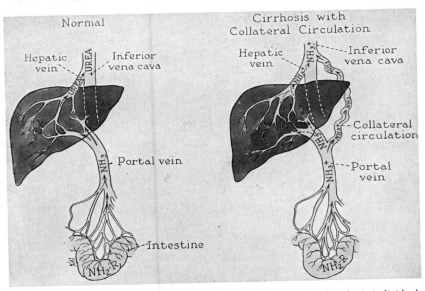

Figure 11–10. Pictorial representation of intestinal formation of ammonia in normal and cirrhotic individuals and of the role of the normal liver in removing ammonia brought to it by the portal blood. Figure also shows the production of elevated plasma ammonia levels by "shunting" of blood through the collateral circulation or by impaired hepatic parenchymal function.

of ammonia from the portal blood, perhaps as a manifestation of defective urea synthesis.

Elevated ammonia levels are seen in impending or fully developed hepatic coma, owing to cirrhosis or severe hepatitis, and occasionally in severe heart failure, azotemia, cor pulmonale, and erythroblastosis fetalis. They have also been described in animals and humans with Eck fistulae and in animals in shock.

The use of the blood ammonia determination has been of assistance in the recognition of impending or established hepatic coma (Chap. 10). As much or more, however, can be learned by proper clinical appraisal of the patient or by use of electroencephalography. Blood ammonia determination may be useful for monitoring the efficacy of treatment of hepatic coma. In Reye's syndrome the level of ammonia appears to relate directly to level of consciousness and survival (Glasgow, 1972). An additional application has been suggested. In patients with cirrhosis and hemorrhage from esophageal varices or from any other source in the esophagus, stomach, or small intestine, blood ammonia levels are elevated, whereas in non-cirrhotic patients with gastrointestinal bleeding the ammonia levels are usually normal. Combining the ammonia level with the determination of sulfobromophthalein excretion is of assistance in recognizing gastrointestinal bleeding in cirrhotic patients. Measur-

ing the plasma ammonia level after a standard dose of an ammonium salt has been recommended as an aid in estimating the patency of a portacaval shunt.

Cerebrospinal Fluid Glutamine. A number of authors have shown that the level of cerebrospinal fluid (CSF) glutamine correlates well with the degree of hepatic encephalopathy (Chap. 18). Glutamine is synthesized in brain tissue from ammonia and glutamic acid. As more and more glutamic acid is diverted toward the synthesis of glutamine, intermediates of oxidative metabolism such as α-ketoglutaric acid are depleted. Depletion of these intermediary metabolites of cerebral metabolism is thought to be one of the etiologic factors in hepatic encephalopathy. The upper reference limit for CSF glutamine is 20 mg/dl (1.5 mmol/l). Glutamine levels can be measured by a simple method involving hot acid hydrolysis which releases ammonia, in turn measured by a colorimetric reaction (Hourani, 1971).

SERUM ENZYME VALUES*

A large number of enzymes are found in normal serum or plasma, to which they gain access from the tissues. The characteristically

---

* References relevant to this section will be found at the end of Chapter 12.

Table 11–9. CATEGORIES OF SERUM ENZYMES* ACCORDING TO THEIR
BEHAVIOR IN HEPATITIS AND OBSTRUCTIVE JAUNDICE

	CHARACTERISTICS	PROTOTYPE	OTHER ENZYMES IN GROUP
I	Higher in obstructive jaundice than in hepatitis	ALP	LAP, 5'-N, GGT
II	Higher in hepatitis than in obstructive jaundice	AST (GOT), ALT (GPT)	OCT, ICD, IdD, Ald
III	Normal or only slightly elevated in hepatitis and obstructive jaundice	LD, CPK	Lipase Lecithinase Amylase
IV	Depressed in hepatitis and normal in obstructive jaundice	Cholinesterase	LCAT

*See Table 12–1, p. 349, for meaning of abbreviations.

abnormal serum enzyme levels produced by various diseases and the general aspects of serum enzymology are considered in Chapter 12. The following discussion describes the type of change in serum enzyme levels caused by hepatic disease and deals with the clinical usefulness of a few enzyme assays for the diagnosis of disease of the liver and biliary tree.

Serum enzymes can be arranged into four categories according to the changes in their levels produced by posthepatic jaundice and acute hepatitis (Table 11–9). *Group I* includes enzymes whose levels are higher in obstructive jaundice than they are in acute hepatitis. The prototype of this group is alkaline phosphatase (ALP). This category also includes leucine aminopeptidase (LAP), 5'-nucleotidase (5'-N), and gamma glutamyl transpeptidase (GGT). *Group II* includes enzymes whose levels are much higher in acute hepatitis than in obstructive jaundice. The best known members of this group are the glutamate oxaloacetic (GOT)* and the glutamate pyruvate (GPT)† transaminases. Ornithine carbamoyl transferase (OCT), isocitric dehydrogenase (ICD), aldolase (Ald), iditol (sorbitol), dehydrogenase (IdD), and a number of other enzymes are also in this category. In *Group III* are enzymes whose levels are elevated only slightly or not at all in hepatitis and in posthepatic jaundice. This group includes lactate dehydrogenase (LD), creatine phosphokinase (CPK), lipase, lecithinase, and a number of other enzymes. A fourth main type of serum enzyme response to hepatic disease (*Group IV*) is seen with cholinesterase, the levels of which are *decreased*

in acute hepatitis and normal or only slightly decreased in obstructive jaundice.

The selection of serum enzyme assays for the diagnosis of hepatic and biliary disease has been based on sufficient experience in correlating the serum values with other measures of hepatic function and disease to assure adequate sensitivity and specificity, and on the technical ease of performing the procedure. These considerations have led to the widespread adoption of alkaline phosphatase, aspartate aminotransferase (AST or GOT), and alanine aminotransferase (ALT or GPT) for the diagnosis of hepatic and related disease. These virtually routine hepatic tests and a few related enzyme tests are discussed in the following pages. The levels of other serum enzymes in hepatic and other types of diseases are considered in Chapter 12.

ALKALINE PHOSPHATASE (ALP)

Alkaline phosphatase (ALP) (EC 3.1.3.1), formally designated orthophosphoric monoester phosphohydrolase, was the first serum enzyme to be studied in hepatic disease. It has been extensively applied to the differential diagnosis of jaundice. Early interest in this enzyme focused on the elevated levels seen in patients with osteoblastic bone disease, presumably as a reflection of increased activity of the osteoblasts, which are rich in phosphatase. This was soon followed, however, by the observation that values were also increased in patients with obstructive (posthepatic) jaundice. When the obstruction is complete, the serum enzyme activity is almost always increased to levels that are three to eight times the upper reference limit. Lower values, however, may be observed in obstructive jaundice,

---

*Also referred to as aspartate aminotransferase (AST).

†Also referred to as alanine aminotransferase (ALT).

especially when the obstruction is incomplete. Biliary obstruction resulting from carcinoma produces higher values than those observed in patients with gallstones producing obstruction. One variety of posthepatic jaundice with normal ALP levels in the serum is that seen in infants with congenital atresia of the extrahepatic biliary tree. In these patients the serum alkaline phosphatase (ALP) activity may not be elevated unless bony lesions of hepatic rickets develop. In contrast, infants with intrahepatic biliary atresia show striking elevations of serum ALP activity (Table 11-10).

Elevated levels of serum ALP also occur in hepatocellular jaundice. Approximately 90 per cent of patients with viral hepatitis or with toxic hepatocellular jaundice have elevated values. Almost all these have values that are elevated less than three-fold and often less than two-fold. Approximately 5 per cent of patients with hepatocellular jaundice, how-

ever, have values that are increased more than three-fold. Nevertheless, values in this range should lead to the suspicion that the jaundice may be posthepatic. In jaundiced patients with higher levels, posthepatic jaundice should be considered.

Some forms of hepatic disease may present a laboratory and clinical picture simulating that of posthepatic jaundice. This has been called "intrahepatic cholestasis" or *hepatocanicular jaundice* (Table 11-3). Although it has been considered to be a form of viral hepatitis ("cholangiolitic hepatitis"), more often it is a manifestation of drug-induced hepatic injury or is cryptogenic. Patients with intrahepatic cholestasis have values of ALP at least as high as those observed in patients with posthepatic jaundice.

The serum alkaline phosphatase (ALP) activity is of value in the differentiation of hepatocellular from posthepatic jaundice, but there are several caveats. As stated previously, ALP activity in the "obstructive" jaundice range may occur in intrinsic hepatic disease, and levels in the "hepatocellular" range may be seen in patients with incomplete biliary obstruction. When taken with other measurements of liver disease and clinical features, however, the ALP level is a useful diagnostic aid.

Serum alkaline phosphatase (ALP) elevation may also occur in non-jaundiced patients with hepatobiliary disease. In patients with "space-occupying" lesions of the liver, such as granulomatous disease, metastatic or primary carcinoma of the liver, liver abscess, and amyloidosis, the degree of alkaline phosphatase elevation may at times be striking (up to 20-fold), with little or no rise in the serum bilirubin values. This pattern of hepatic dysfunction is useful in the recognition of these "space-occupying" lesions, particularly in the recognition of metastases to the liver in patients with carcinomatosis (Table 11-10).

There is another type of disease associated with normal or only slightly elevated serum bilirubin levels but with distinctly increased alkaline phosphatase levels. This is occlusion of one hepatic duct or incomplete occlusion of the common bile or hepatic duct. This condition should be kept in mind, particularly in dealing with patients with cholelithiasis who develop this "dissociated" pattern of hepatic dysfunction.

Levels of ALP in micronodular cirrhosis are usually normal or only mildly elevated. In

Table 11-10. ALKALINE PHOSPHATASE VALUES (ALP) IN HEPATOBILIARY DISEASE

DISEASE	INCIDENCE ALP ELEVATION	USUAL RANGE OF VALUES*
Jaundiced states		
Hepatic jaundice		
Hepatocellular	80-100%	1-3 ×
Hepatocanalicular	100%	3-8 ×
Posthepatic		
Obstruction due to neoplasm	95-100%	3-8 ×
Obstruction due to gallstone	95-100%	1-8 ×
Congenital atresia of bile ducts		
Intrahepatic	100%	10-15 ×
Extrahepatic	20-30%	1-4 ×
Jaundice absent or present		
Infectious mononucleosis	60-70%	1-8 ×
Cirrhosis, Laennec's	40%	1-3 ×
Cirrhosis, postnecrotic	50%	1-5 ×
Cirrhosis, biliary, primary	100%	3-20 ×
No jaundice		
Space-occupying lesions		
Carcinoma	80%	1-10 ×
Tuberculosis	50%	1-10 ×
Sarcoidosis	40%	1-10 ×
Amyloidosis	Frequent	1-10 ×
Stone in common duct or in one hepatic duct	Frequent	1-10 ×

*Degree of increase over normal (upper reference limit).

macronodular cirrhosis the levels are generally somewhat higher. In primary biliary cirrhosis elevated levels of alkaline phosphatase are regularly seen. They range from 3- to 20-fold the normal or upper reference limit. In obstructive biliary cirrhosis, the elevations are modest, usually elevated less than three- or four-fold, except during bouts of ascending cholangitis.

Most patients with hepatic steatosis have only slightly elevated levels. The occasional instances of deep jaundice in alcoholics with fatty liver accompanied by high ALP levels are probably due to common bile duct obstruction by alcoholic intrahepatic cholestasis caused by severe steatosis. In alcoholic hepatitis, usual values for ALP are also less than three-fold elevated (Zimmerman, 1970).

The basis for elevated serum levels of ALP in patients with hepatobiliary disease is obscure. Impaired hepatic excretion of enzyme formed in bone or liver or both was considered formerly to be the mechanism. *Increased formation* of the enzyme by hepatic parenchymal or ductal cells, perhaps supplemented by impaired disposition, is the apparent mechanism.

Alkaline phosphatase is found in many tissues. In a number of these tissues the molecular form of the enzyme is distinctive. Recognition that hepatobiliary rather than osseous disease is responsible for an elevated ALP level is relatively simple in the patient with jaundice or other overt clinical or laboratory evidence of hepatic or biliary tree disease. In patients whose clinical and biochemical data provide inconclusive evidence for liver disease as the cause of the hyperphosphatasemia, or who show evidence of both hepatic and osseous disease, elucidation of the cause of the elevated ALP level may be difficult. Distinction of ALP isoenzymes by electrophoresis or by the effects of chemical or physical factors on the ALP activity has found selected, if not limited, clinical application. Indeed, of the four isoenzymes of ALP that appear in the serum, the hepatic and osseous are the most difficult to distinguish from each other (see Chap. 12, Table 12-8). Several other serum enzymes, however, are helpful in identifying the source of an elevated ALP level to be hepatic or biliary tree disease. Serum values of leucine aminopeptidase (LAP), 5'-nucleotidase (5'-N), and gamma glutamyl transferase (GGT)* appear to parallel those of ALP in

_____
*Gamma glutamyl transpeptidase.

hepatobiliary disease and have been considered to approximate the degree of elevation of the hepatic isoenzyme of ALP.

AMINOTRANSFERASES (TRANSAMINASES)*

Enzymes that catalyze the reversible transfer of an alpha amino group from an amino acid to an alpha keto acid (Fig. 11-11) were first demonstrated in animal tissue by Braunshtein in 1937. He called the enzymes *aminopherases.* Although a large number of substrate-specific transaminases have been demonstrated in various animal tissues, only two have been described in the serum, *aspartate aminotransferase* (AST) or *glutamate oxaloacetic transaminase* (GOT), and *alanine aminotransferase* (ALT) or *glutamate pyruvate transminase* (GPT). Abnormal levels of AST (GOT) are seen in patients with hepatic disease, myocardial and skeletal muscle necrosis, and other diseases to be described. ALT (GPT) elevations are absent or slight in disease that does not involve the liver primarily or secondarily.

Aspartate aminotransferase (AST) or *glutamate oxaloacetic transaminase* (GOT) (2.6.1.1) catalyzes the reversible transfer of the amino group from aspartate to α-ketoglutarate (Fig. 11-12). It has been demonstrated in the serum and tissues of all animals studied. In man it is found in cardiac, hepatic, skeletal muscle, renal, and cerebral tissue in decreasing concentrations. The recognition of the high myocardial content of this enzyme led to the observation, in 1953, that patients with acute myocardial infarction had elevated levels in the serum for a few days after the infarction. Shortly thereafter, studies in several laboratories showed high serum levels of this enzyme in patients and animals with acute hepatic necrosis.

The activity of this serum enzyme was first demonstrated by a chromatographic technique, which was too laborious for routine use.

_____
*See Chapter 12 for further discussion of transaminases and other enzymes.

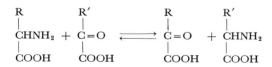

Figure 11-11. Prototype of aminotransferase (transamination) reactions.

ALANINE AMINOTRANSFERASE (ALT) OR GLUTAMATE
PYRUVATE TRANSAMINASE (GPT)

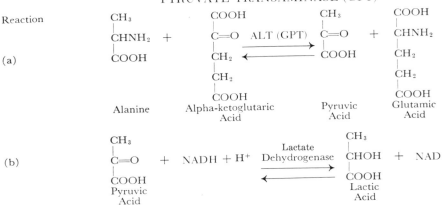

Figure 11–14. Reaction catalyzed by ALT (GPT) principles of assay methods, and conditions in which increased serum levels are observed.

Method of assay is based on measurement of rate of formation of product (pyruvic acid) of reaction. This may be done (1) indirectly by the coupled reaction (b) in which the rate of NADH oxidation, in the presence of added lactate dehydrogenase, is a measure of pyruvic acid formed (method of Karmen), or (2) directly, by one of several colorimetric methods that depend on formation of the dinitrophenylhydrazone of pyruvate.

Conditions in which abnormal serum levels of enzyme are observed, arranged in the order of decreasing levels:

A. *Hepatic Disease Abnormalities*
    Hepatic necrosis; e.g., hepatitis (infectious, toxic), infectious mononucleosis, cirrhosis
    Obstructive jaundice
    Metastatic carcinoma
    Hepatic congestion (centrilobular liver cell necrosis) secondary to heart failure or hepatic vein thrombosis

B. *Other Abnormalities* (*Slight*)
    Myocardial infarction
    Acute pancreatitis

ployed. The reference interval for this enzyme is almost the same as that for the serum AST (GOT) (4 to 24 U/l at 30°C.).

Patients with viral hepatitis and other forms of hepatic necrosis usually show striking elevations of the serum ALT (GPT) level (200 to 4000 U/l). Values of ALT (GPT) are modestly elevated (<200 U/l) in most patients with posthepatic jaundice and intrahepatic cholestasis. They are even lower (<50 U/l) in most patients with metastatic carcinoma, cirrhosis, or alcoholic steatonecrosis (alcoholic hepatitis). Values for ALT (GPT) are as high as or higher than those of AST (GOT) in most patients with viral hepatitis, posthepatic jaundice, or intrahepatic cholestasis, while they are much lower than the respective values for AST (GOT) in patients with cirrhosis, alcoholic hepatitis, or metastatic carcinoma. Levels of ALT (GPT) are normal or only minimally elevated in patients with myocardial infarction (Fig. 11–15).

Clinical Value of Serum Aminotransferase (Transaminase) Measurements. The determination of serum aminotransferases is of distinct clinical aid. Differentiation of hepatic

(hepatocellular) from posthepatic jaundice is facilitated by determining serum AST (GOT) and ALT (GPT) values, since values above 200 U/l are rare in patients with posthepatic jaundice. In the hepatocanalicular type of hepatic jaundice (intrahepatic cholestasis), the serum AST (GOT) or ALT values are like those of posthepatic jaundice. Likewise, in cirrhosis of the liver, even with deep jaundice, the moderate AST (GOT) level and the lower ALT (GPT) level are in contrast to the high levels of both transaminases* observed in acute viral hepatitis. Determination of AST, ALT, or both is useful in the early recognition of viral or toxic hepatitis and is, therefore, helpful in studying patients exposed to hepatotoxic drugs. Elevations of the ALT (GPT) activity appear to reflect acute hepatic disease somewhat more specifically than is true of the AST (GOT) values. The level of either enzyme, particularly the AST, may be elevated in patients with extrahepatic disease (see Chap. 12).

The levels of alkaline phosphatase (ALP), AST, and ALT are individually helpful in the differential diagnosis of hepatic disease. Their diagnostic usefulness may be enhanced by

_____
*Aminotransferases.

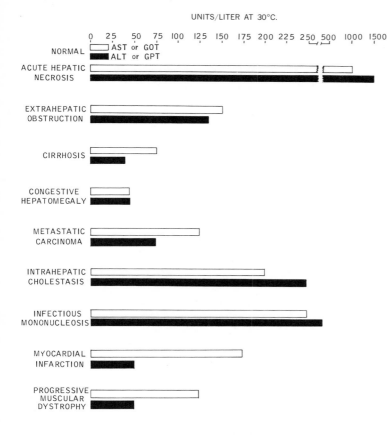

UNITS/LITER AT 30°C.

Figure 11–15. Relative levels of aspartate aminotransferase (AST) or glutamate oxaloacetate transaminase (GOT) and alanine aminotransferase (ALT) or glutamate pyruvate transaminase (GPT) in patients with hepatic, biliary, and other diseases.

Figure 11–16. Patterns of abnormality in various types of hepatic and biliary disease provided by levels of alkaline phosphatase (AP), aspartate aminotransferase (AST), alanine aminotransferase (ALT), and lactate dehydrogenase (LD).   HEPATOCELL = Hepatocellular; INFECT MONO = Infectious mononucleosis; JAUND = Jaundice; CA 1° or 2° = Primary or metastatic carcinoma; P.B.C. = Primary biliary cirrhosis; ALC = Alcoholic; CHR. HEP ± CIRRHOSIS = Chronic active hepatitis with or without cirrhosis.

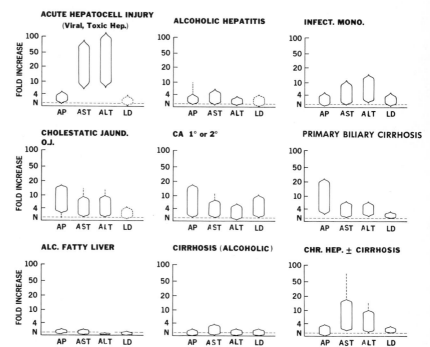

observing the patterns of abnormality obtained by measuring all three, especially when combined with lactate dehydrogenase (LD) levels (see Chap. 12). In Figure 11-16 are shown diagrammatically the patterns obtained with a variety of hepatic lesions. The very high values for AST (GOT) and ALT (GPT) and relatively slightly elevated ones for alkaline phosphatase (ALP) observed in acute hepatitis and other necroinflammatory diseases of the liver differ sharply from the lower transaminase* and higher alkaline phosphatase values of posthepatic jaundice. The pattern of the "incomplete" posthepatic jaundice of choledocholithiasis overlaps with that of hepatitis, while the pattern of acute hepatocanalicular jaundice or of biliary cirrhosis simulates that of posthepatic jaundice.

The patterns of cirrhosis are characteristically different. In alcoholic cirrhosis, AST elevations are slight, ALT values even lower, and lactate dehydrogenase (LD) and alkaline phosphatase (ALP) values very slightly elevated or normal. In inactive postnecrotic cirrhosis, the values resemble those of alcoholic cirrhosis; but in active postnecrotic cirrhosis and chronic active hepatitis, the AST (GOT) values may be as low as those of alcoholic cirrhosis or as high as those of acute hepatitis, and the values of the two transaminases* may be approximately equally elevated. The pattern of metastatic or primary carcinoma of the liver is distinctive in that the transaminase levels resemble those of alcoholic cirrhosis, while the LD and alkaline phosphatase levels are much higher. (See Chapter 12 for LD values in carcinomatosis.)

The various patterns are not necessarily pathognomonic of the respective entity, since overlapping of values and patterns may be observed. Nevertheless, when taken with other diagnostic measures they may be of great diagnostic assistance.

SERUM "METALS"

Abnormal serum values of certain metallic substances are found in patients with some hepatic diseases. Elevated serum *iron* levels and reduced iron-binding capacity are observed in patients with hemochromatosis and transfusion hemosiderosis and may be of aid in diagnosis. Acute elevations of serum iron levels are observed in patients with viral hepatitis and in others with acute hepatic necrosis. It has been observed that patients with

---

* Aminotransferase.

posthepatic jaundice usually have normal serum iron levels. This has led to the application by European and South American workers of the serum iron level determination to the differential diagnosis of jaundice. This application, however, has not been adopted widely in the United States.

Elevated blood levels of "free" *copper* and increased amounts of tissue copper have been observed in patients with Wilson's disease (hepatolenticular degeneration). The levels of free copper are increased in most patients with this disease, accompanied by decreased levels of ceruloplasmin, a copper-carrying protein that is also an enzyme (copper oxidase). Diagnosis of Wilson's disease is aided by the demonstration of depressed levels of ceruloplasmin in the plasma. Increased levels of serum and tissue copper are also observed in primary biliary cirrhosis.

Abnormal levels of other metallic ions of the blood have been described in patients with chronic hepatic disease. Depressed serum levels of *zinc* have been reported in patients with alcoholic cirrhosis. The significance of this observation remains to be determined. Lower than normal serum *magnesium* levels have been reported in alcoholic patients with delirium tremens and with cirrhosis. Among the factors considered responsible is malnutrition. In cirrhotics with ascites the *hyponatremia* commonly observed is considered to be a manifestation of water retention, not sodium loss. *Hypokalemia* is frequent in patients with severe hepatic disease (Zimmerman, 1973).

TESTS BASED ON THE ROLE OF LIVER IN VITAMIN ECONOMY

Deficiency in a number of vitamins is prone to occur in the malnourished alcoholic patient. Accordingly, in alcoholic cirrhosis evidence of beriberi, pellagra, and scurvy may be observed. In addition, abnormal levels of vitamins A and B_{12} have been described in patients with hepatic disease.

Depressed plasma levels of vitamin A are characteristic of patients with parenchymal hepatic disease. The observation that patients with early obstructive jaundice usually have normal levels has led to the application of vitamin A determination to the differential diagnosis of jaundice. The dependence of the absorption of this fat-soluble vitamin on an adequate concentration of bile salts in the duodenum, however, also leads to depressed levels in posthepatic jaundice; accordingly, this determination is of little value in the differential diagnosis of jaundice.

Vitamin B_{12} is stored in the liver. In patients with acute viral hepatitis very high plasma levels of this vitamin are observed, presumably resulting from release by necrotic hepatic cells. Somewhat elevated values are observed in cirrhosis also. A test of hepatic function based on the estimation of the hepatic "uptake" of an oral dose of vitamin B_{12} labeled with radioactive cobalt has been described. None of these tests has been used extensively in the clinical setting.

SPECIAL PROCEDURES

The diagnostic armamentarium of hepatology consists of some of the biochemical tests described in the foregoing pages and a few special procedures (Table 11–11). These include percutaneous biopsy of the liver, scintiscan-

Table 11–11. USUAL PANEL OF MEASUREMENTS AND EXAMINATIONS AVAILABLE FOR DIAGNOSIS OF HEPATIC DISEASE*

Bilirubin	Serum levels, direct and total
	Urine bilirubin (and urobilinogen)
Dye excretion tests	BSP or ICG (role in clinical medicine needs re-evaluation).
Serum protein levels and electrophoresis	Immunoglobulins (Alpha-1-antitrypsin) (Alpha-fetoglobulin) (Ceruloplasmin)
Serum enzyme activity	ALP (5'-N, LAP, GGT) AST (GOT) ALT (GPT)
Prothrombin time (+vitamin K) Serum cholesterol	
Special procedures	Serology for viral hepatitis (see Table 11–13). Serology for "autoimmune" factors (see Chap. 38). Liver biopsy Scintiscanning Cholangiography Ultrasound Arteriography

*List includes only those available at most hospitals in U.S.A. Tests in parentheses used only for special procedures.

ning employing radionuclides, and serologic tests. Not discussed in this chapter, but of great usefulness in the study of special hepatologic problems, are cholangiography (intravenous, percutaneous, or endoscopic), ultrasonography, peroral endoscopy, laparoscopy, and celiac axis arteriography.

LIVER BIOPSY

Needle biopsy of the liver, a procedure which has been widely used for three decades, is very helpful in the diagnosis of hepatic and non-hepatic disease (Table 11–12). It is useful in defining the cause of hepatocellular jaundice and of hepatomegaly and in demonstrating the presence of cirrhosis, steatosis, alcoholic hepatitis, chronic hepatitis, biliary cirrhosis, and carcinoma. Indeed, it serves to define the hepatic disease, attention to which has been drawn by clinical or biochemical clues. It is an important part of the evaluation of poorly resolving hepatitis. Biopsy may also be of help in distinguishing between intrahepatic cholestasis and posthepatic jaundice, although the distinction is at times difficult and the safety of needle biopsy in the face of posthepatic jaundice somewhat controversial. Liver biopsy is particularly useful in establishing the diagnosis of systemic disease, e.g.,

Table 11–12. INDICATIONS AND CONTRAINDICATIONS FOR LIVER BIOPSY

I. Possible applications
   A. Finding the cause of hepatomegaly, jaundice, ascites, gastrointestinal bleeding, or abnormal liver function or serum enzyme values
   B. Establishment of precise diagnosis in patients with probable hepatic disease, e.g., chronic hepatitis, cirrhosis, fatty liver, or carcinoma (metastatic or primary)
   C. Recognition of systemic disease, e.g., hematogenous tuberculosis, sarcoidosis, amyloidosis, and lymphoma (may be helpful in "staging" in known Hodgkin's disease)
   D. Evaluation of response to therapy of acute or chronic liver disease
II. Relative contraindications
   A. Clotting defects (abnormal bleeding time, coagulation time, or partial thromboplastin time), prothrombin time (>5 seconds greater than control), or history of recent hemorrhagic tendency
   B. Firm clinical diagnosis of posthepatic jaundice
   C. Severe anemia
   D. Uncooperative or unduly apprehensive patient
   E. Bacterial infection in area to be traversed by biopsy needle, e.g., right lower lobe pneumonia

tuberculosis, sarcoidosis, amyloidosis. The indications and contraindications for liver biopsy, as we view them, are shown in Table 11–12.

RADIOISOTOPES IN DIAGNOSIS OF LIVER DISEASE

The availability of radioisotopes has contributed much to the study of hepatic physiology and disease. They have been used to measure liver function and blood flow, to define the configuration and size of the liver and spleen, to demonstrate "space-occupying" lesions in the liver (tumor, cysts, and abscesses), and to provide indirect evidence of the presence of portal hypertension.

Four types of radiopharmaceuticals are available. One group consists of tagged molecules that are taken up by normal hepatocytes. A second group consists of substances phagocytized by reticuloendothelial (RE) cells. A third group remains in the blood, and a fourth group is selectively taken up by malignant hepatocytes and by the leukocytes of an abscess.

Tagged molecules taken up by hepatocytes include such substances as ^{14}C-bilirubin, ^{14}C-cholylglycine, ^{58}Co- or ^{60}C-labeled cyanocobalamine, ^{131}I-rose bengal (RB), and ^{131}I-BSP. These have been used to measure hepatic function by the rate of disappearance of the radioactive molecule from the blood or by the rate of its accumulation in the liver. These tests of hepatic function, however, have been largely of research interest. None has found regular clinical use. To a limited degree, ^{131}I-RB has been applied to the differential diagnosis of jaundice, especially in infants. The demonstration that the radioactivity is taken up by the liver but fails to enter the duodenum and instead appears in the urine is taken as evidence of biliary obstruction. Even for this limited purpose, the value of ^{131}I-RB is controversial. For visualization of the diseased liver, agents that are selectively accumulated by normal hepatocytes, are, of course, satisfactory. Rose bengal, which was used in the early years of scintiscanning, was discarded after it was found not to be adequately accumulated by diseased hepatocytes.

Radioactive colloids taken up by RE cells are most suitable for nuclear imaging, since parenchymal hepatic disease would not preclude concentration of the agent by the liver. Those which have been used include radioactive gold (^{198}Au or ^{199}Au), indium (^{113m}In), and technetium sulfur colloid (^{99m}Tc). Today ^{99m}Tc is the most widely used in hepatology; and gamma camera imaging is, by far, the most useful application of radiopharmacology to the study of liver disease.

Nuclear imaging with a scintillation camera provides a pattern of the radioactivity concentrated in the liver. Areas within boundaries of the organ that fail to accumulate radioactivity ("cold" areas) represent pathologic processes. They may be produced by primary or metastatic tumors of the liver, cysts, abscesses or the broad scars of macronodular cirrhosis. "Cold" areas also may be caused by a normal gallbladder fossa or some prominent portal veins in the hepatic hilus rather than by an intrahepatic mass. Multiple small cold areas usually represent diffuse disease (cirrhosis), although they may be caused by diffuse carcinomatous involvement. This pattern of diffusely decreased hepatic uptake, accompanied by splenomegaly and increased uptake by the spleen and bone marrow, is common in moderate to advanced cirrhosis.

Gallium (^{67}Ga) citrate is taken up selectively by neoplastic and inflammatory tissues. Areas that appear "cold" with ^{99m}Tc sulphur colloid may concentrate ^{67}Ga if due to primary or metastatic carcinoma or abscess.

Radioactive agents that remain in the blood are useful to measure hepatic perfusion. ^{131}I-labeled albumin, ^{99m}Tc albumin, and ^{133}Xe have been used, largely for research purposes.

Nuclear imaging is an important diagnostic procedure for the study of hepatic disease. Like ultrasonography, it is useful for the detection of masses in the liver, such as metastatic carcinoma, hepatoma, cysts, or abscesses. In a patient suspected of having one of these lesions or with unexplained hepatomegaly, imaging may confirm the diagnosis or indicate the site for biopsy if a carcinoma is suspected. Recognition of a single mass in the liver is possible if it is 2 cm in diameter or greater. Smaller masses cannot be recognized unless they are coalescent. Even larger masses, if multiple, may escape identification, since multiple infiltrative masses and cirrhosis may give a similar pattern. Conversely, the scan of a coarse nodular (postnecrotic) cirrhosis may be mistaken for that of multiple infiltrative masses.

Scanning of the liver is also useful in defining hepatic size, contours, and extent. This is especially important in patients who are extremely obese, in those with marked ascites, and in those with an abnormal contour of the right leaflet of the diaphragm observed on chest roentgenography.

SEROLOGIC TESTS

A number of serologic tests for the diagnosis and prevention of hepatic disease are available. The most important ones are those used to detect current or past infection with hepatitis B virus (HBV). The serologic aspects of HBV infection are being uncovered at so rapid a rate, however, as to make any generalizations regarding their status hazardous. However, a summary is shown in Table 11-13, with further consideration in Chapter 52 (p. 1866).

The increasingly complex series of antigens of HBV include the surface antigen (HBsAg), the "core" antigen (HBcAg), and the "e" antigen (HBeAg), to each of which demonstrable antibodies are formed. The antigens and antibodies demonstrated in the serum can be correlated with the type of hepatic disease produced by the infection (Table 11-13).

Acute HBV hepatitis is characterized by presence of HBsAg and anti-HBc in the blood and often by HBeAg. Recovery is attended by disappearance of HBsAg and HBeAg, persistence of anti-HBc, and appearance of anti-HBs and often of anti-HBe. Persistence of HBsAg beyond three months of onset of acute illness is a hallmark of chronic hepatitis or of the carrier state. Presence of HBeAg in a presumed carrier of HBsAg enhances the likelihood that the "carrier" is actively infective. The observation that many patients with hepatocellular carcinoma have HBsAg in their blood

(and liver) has led to renewed attention to the probable hepatocarcinogenic role of HBV.

Testing for HBsAg is available in almost all medical centers for the diagnosis of acute and chronic virus B hepatitis and in blood banks for the detection of carriers of HBV. It has also served to demonstrate a probable role of HBV infection in the etiology of hepatocellular carcinoma. Presence of anti-HBs, anti-HBc, and anti-HBe is evidence of former infection with HBV and probably immunity. Of these, anti-HBc is the first to appear during acute infection.

Tests for hepatitis A virus (HAV) infection have also become available. Early in the disease, HAV can be identified in the feces by immunoelectron microscopy or immunofluorescent techniques. More widely applied to diagnosis, thus far, has been the demonstration of rising titers of anti-HA antibodies. The procedure, however, is available in only a few laboratories.

Circulating antibodies to various tissue components have been found in patients with chronic hepatic disease. These "autoantibodies" in patients with chronic active hepatitis (antinuclear antibodies, LE factor, anti-smooth muscle antibody) and in patients with primary biliary cirrhosis (antimitochondrial antibody) provide indirect evidence of autoimmune pathogenesis of these syndromes, and are clinically useful. They are discussed in Chapter 38, p. 1265.

CLINICAL APPLICATION OF LIVER FUNCTION TESTS

Some of the clinical settings in which hepatic tests are applied are listed in Table 11-14. They are useful for the diagnosis of hepatic disease and specifically for the differential di-

Table 11-13. SEROLOGIC FACTORS RELATED TO HEPATITIS B VIRUS*

	HBsAg†	Anti-HBs	Anti-HBc†	HBeAg†	Anti-HBe
Acute hepatitis					
Early acute phase	+	−	+	±	−
Early convalescence	−	−	+	−	−
Recovery	−	+	+	−	−
Chronic HBV hepatitis	+	−	+	±	−
Carrier state	+	−	+	±	±
Hepatocellular carcinoma	+	−	+	±	±

*Dr. Jay Hoffnagle provided advice in preparation of this table.
†HBsAG = hepatitis B antigen; HBc = "core" antigen; HBeAg = "E" antigen. HBV = hepatitis B virus.

Table 11–14. APPLICATION OF LIVER FUNCTION TESTING

I. Diagnosis
  A. Recognition of presence or absence of hepatic disease
  B. Differential diagnosis
    1. Hepatomegaly
    2. Jaundice
    3. Ascites
    4. Gastrointestinal hemorrhage
  C. Testing for hepatotoxicity of drugs or industrial hepatotoxins
  D. Recognition of non-hepatic disease, e.g., hematogenous tuberculosis, sarcoidosis, amyloidosis, and infectious mononucleosis
II. Estimating severity in known hepatic disease
  A. Monitoring convalescence (hepatitis, cirrhosis)
  B. Preoperative evaluation
    1. In patients with recent hepatic disease
    2. In patients with extrahepatic disease that may affect liver status and function, e.g., hyperthyroidism, cholelithiasis, ulcerative colitis

agnosis of jaundice, hepatomegaly, ascites, and gastrointestinal hemorrhage. Systematic monitoring of selected tests of hepatic function is necessary in testing for the hepatotoxicity of new drugs or of industrial exposure to chemicals. Characteristic patterns of abnormality are observed in extrahepatic diseases and assist in their recognition. Estimation of the severity of known hepatic disease and response to treatment is facilitated by testing of liver function.

A large number of tests have been described or mentioned in the preceding material. Only some of these are readily applicable to clinical problems. A "battery" or panel of tests, which we use regularly in the diagnosis of hepatic disease, is shown in Table 11–11. With this group, patterns of hepatic dysfunction are observed that are useful in the differential diagnosis of jaundice (Table 11–15), hepato-

Table 11–15. LABORATORY APPROACH TO DIFFERENTIAL DIAGNOSIS OF JAUNDICE[a,b]

| TYPE OF HYPERBILIRUBINEMIA | BILIRUBIN TESTS | | | SERUM CHOLEST. | SERUM ENZYMES | | | PROTHROMBIN TIME | |
	Serum (Dir/Tot) ×100	Urine B U	Feces U		ALP	AST (GOT)	ALT (GPT)	1°	+K
Unconjugated									
Prehepatic	20	0 ↑	↑↑	N	N	N	N	N	NA
Hepatic		N	N						
Conjugated[c]									
Hepatic—Hepatocellular									
Viral or toxic hepatitis	40	+ ↑	N	N	↑	↑↑↑	↑↑↑↑	(↑)	
Alcoholic hepatitis						↑↑	(↑)		
—Hepatocanalicular									
Acute—drug or viral[d]		(↑)	(↓)	↑↑	↑↑	↑↑	↑↑	↑	+
Chronic (primary biliary cirrhosis[e])	50	+ (↑)	N	↑↑↑↑	↑↑↑	↑	↑	↑	+
Familial cholestatic jaundice		N	N	N	N	N	N	N	NA
Posthepatic—Complete (carcinoma)	50	+ N	↓↓↓	↑↑	↑↑↑	↑↑	↑↑	↑↑	+
—Incomplete (stones)		(↑)	↓	(↑)	↑–↑↑↑	↑↑↑	↑↑↑	↑↑↑	

[a] Dir/Tot. = direct/total bilirubin; B = bilirubin; U = urobilinogen; cholest. = cholesterol; ALP = alkaline phosphatase; GOT = glutamate oxaloacetate transaminase; GPT = glutamate pyruvate transaminase; 1° = prior to administration of vitamin K; +K = after administration of vitamin K.

[b] Arrows indicate direction, degree, and incidence of abnormal results. Arrow in parentheses indicates that abnormality may or may not occur. N indicates normal. NA = not applicable.

[c] Distinction between hepatic and posthepatic jaundice may at times require special procedures, e.g., biopsy, ultrasound, cholangiography.

[d] Serologic studies helpful in diagnosis.

[e] The Dubin-Johnson syndrome is a genetic disorder characterized by a black pigment in the hepatocytes and a special form of "dissociated" intrahepatic cholestasis in which there is defective excretion of bilirubin into the canaliculus but other components of bile apparently are normally excreted, thus differing from other forms of hepatic canalicular jaundice. The Rotor syndrome resembles the Dubin-Johnson syndrome in some but not all features. Other familial forms of hepatocanalicular jaundice include "benign intermittent juvenile cholestatic jaundice" and cholestatic jaundice of pregnancy.

Table 11-16. LABORATORY AIDS IN THE DIFFERENTIAL DIAGNOSIS OF HEPATOMEGALY OR OTHER PRESENTATIONS SUGGESTING HEPATIC DISEASE IN THE ANICTERIC PATIENT*

				GLOBULIN							
	BSP	BILIRUBIN	ALB	Tot.	Fract.	Ig.†	ALP	AST (GOT)	ALT (GPT)	LD	SPECIAL‡ PROCEDURES
Acute hepatitis	↑↑↑	↑	N	(↑)	β,γ	IgG	↑	↑↑-↑↑↑↑	↑↑-↑↑↑↑	↑	Serol (V) B
Chronic active hepatitis ± cirrhosis	↑↑↑	(↑)	↓	↑-↑↑↑	γ	IgM	↑-↑↑	↑-↑↑	↑-↑↑	(↑)	Serol (V)
Primary biliary cirrhosis	↑↑↑	(↑)	(↓)	(↑)	α₂,β,γ	IgG	↑↑↑	↑	↑	(↑)	Serol (A-I) B / AMA, B
Alcoholic cirrhosis	↑↑↑	(↑)	↓	↑,N,↓	γ	IgM IgA N	↑	↑↑	(↑)	(↑)	B
Steatosis	(↑)	(↑)	N	N				↑	N	N	B
Alcoholic hepatitis	↑↑↑	↑	↓	↑,N,↓	γ	IgM IgA	↑-↑↑	↑↑	↑	(↑)	B
Carcinoma, primary	↑↑	(↑)	(↓)	↑,N,↓	α₂	N	↑-↑↑↑	↑↑	↑	↑↑	Scan, US
Carcinoma, metastic or lymphoma	↑↑↑	(↑)	(↓)	(↓)	α₂	N	↑-↑↑↑	↑↑	↑	↑-↑↑↑	Art, B; AFP / Scan, B
Infectious mononucleosis	↑↑	(↑)	N	N	β,γ	IgG	↑-↑↑	↑↑	↑-↑↑	↑-↑↑	Serol
Amyloidosis	↑↑	(↑)	↓	↑,N,↓	α₂,γ	IgG	↑-↑↑↑	↑		N,(↑)	B
Congestive heart failure	↑↑↑	(↑)	(↓)	(↓)	-	N	↑	↑↑	↑-↑↑	↑↑	Clinical
Granulomatous disease	(↑)	(↑)	N	↑↑	γ	IgG	↑-↑↑↑	↑	↑	(↑)	B

*Arrows indicate direction, degree, and incidence of abnormal results. N indicates normal. ( ) = may or may not be elevated.

†IgG in virus B hepatitis. IgM in virus A hepatitis.

‡Special procedures: serol = serology; V = viral; A-I = autoimmune; B = biopsy; AMA = Antimitochondrial antibody; Scan = scintiscanning; Art = arteriography; AFP = alpha-fetoprotein. ALB = albumin; Tot. = total.

Table 11-17. LABORATORY AIDS IN THE DIAGNOSIS OF ASCITES*

	BSP	Bil.	Alb.	Glob.	ALP	AST (GOT)†	ALT (GPT)†	LD
Cirrhosis	↑↑	↑	↓	↑	↑	↑↑	(↑)	(↑)
Carcinomatosis‡	(↑)	N	(↓)	N	↑↑↑	↑↑	(↑)	(↑)
Tuberculosis	(↑)	N	(↓)	↑	↑↑↑	↑↑	(↑)	↑↑↑
Heart failure	↑↑	↑	(↓)	N	↑↑ / ↑	↑ / ↑-↑↑	↑ / ↑-↑↑	↑ / ↑-↑↑

*Decisive procedures include biopsy and laparoscopy.

†Transaminases (AST/GOT, ALT/GPT) add little to this differential diagnosis.

‡Degree of abnormality depends on presence of lesions in liver; results will be normal if only peritoneum is involved.

Table 11-18. LABORATORY AIDS TO THE DIFFERENTIAL DIAGNOSIS OF GASTROINTESTINAL HEMORRHAGE*

	BSP	Bilirubin	Albumin	Globulin	NH₃	AST (GOT)	ALT (GPT)
Peptic ulcer	N	N	N	N	N	N	N
Alcoholic gastritis	(↑)	(↑)	(↓)	N	(↑)	N	N
Esophageal varices							
Intrahepatic portal obstruction							
Alcoholic cirrhosis	↑	(↑)	↓	(↑)	↑	↑↑	(↑)
Alcoholic hepatitis	↑	↑	↓	(↑)	↑	↑↑	(↑)
Cryptogenic cirrhosis (= CAH)	↑	(↑)	(↓)	↑	↑	↑↑↑	↑↑
Extrahepatic portal obstruction	N	N	N	N	(↑)	N	N

*Radiography, endoscopy, and at times arteriography are the diagnostically decisive procedures.

Table 11-19.   PATTERNS OF HEPATIC DYSFUNCTION AND RELATED
BIOCHEMICAL ABNORMALITIES IN NON-HEPATIC DISEASE

PATTERN	EXAMPLES
I. Resembling hepatic disease	
A. Generalized abnormalities involving BSP, bilirubin, flocculation tests, serum proteins, enzymes with or without jaundice	Pneumococcal pneumonia Infectious mononucleosis
B. Jaundice	
Hepatocellular	Hemoglobin-S disease
Hepatocanalicular	Gram-negative systemic infection in infants
II. Dissociated abnormalities	
A. Mainly impaired BSP excretion; elevated ALP levels; minor AST (GOT)-ALT (GPT) increases	Right ventricular failure Hypernephroma (without hepatic metastases) Granulomatous disease
B. Mainly abnormal serum proteins with gamma globulin increase and abnormal flocculation tests	Subacute bacterial endocarditis (SBE) Disseminated tuberculosis Sarcoidosis Lymphopathia venereum Systemic lupus erythematosus
III. Combinations of dissociated patterns (IIA & IIB)	
A. Hyperglobulinemic disease with granulomas in liver	Sarcoidosis Brucellosis Disseminated tuberculosis
B. Hyperglobulinemic disease and heart failure	Subacute bacterial endocarditis

megaly (Table 11-16), ascites (Table 11-17), and gastrointestinal hemorrhage (Table 11-18) and that can even be helpful in the recognition of extrahepatic disease (Table 11-19). The patterns shown represent those most frequently observed in each instance. Exceptions occur, and the patterns should be regarded only as guides.

HEPATIC FUNCTION IN NON-HEPATIC DISEASE

Abnormal results with one or more tests of hepatic function may be obtained in patients with a variety of extrahepatic diseases. These have been considered at times to reflect on the value and specificity of liver function testing. Even in non-hepatic disease, however, fairly consistent patterns of hepatic function may be observed. In Table 11-19 is shown a classification of non-hepatic diseases in terms of the type of hepatic dysfunction observed and the presumed basis for it.

CONCLUSIONS

The foregoing dicussion has attempted to review the basis for liver function testing and has listed a large number of laboratory proce-

dures for this purpose. A small number of useful determinations have been selected from this group and their applications in a clinical setting have been considered.

It should be recalled that there are a number of pitfalls in the application of the tests to the diagnosis and management of hepatic disease (Table 11-20). Correlation of laboratory re-

Table 11-20.   SOME COMMON PITFALLS
IN APPLICATION OF LIVER TESTS

1. Dependence on results of one test rather than patterns of abnormality.
2. Assumption that normal results signify no parenchymal disease (e.g., values for AST (GOT) normal in 25 per cent and for ALT (GPT) normal in 50 per cent of patients with alcoholic cirrhosis).
3. Assumption that abnormal values for "liver function" tests mean only liver disease.
4. Failure to recognize acute jaundice as:
   a. *Hepatocellular* because AST (GOT) and ALT (GPT) values are unexpectedly low (below 200 U/l in 20 per cent of patients with acute viral hepatitis) or because ALP values are unexpectedly high (more than three times the ULN* in 5 per cent of patients with acute hepatitis).
   b. *Posthepatic* because values for AST (GOT) and ALT (GPT) are unexpectedly high (above 200 U/l in 15 per cent of patients with choledocholithiasis) or because values for ALP are unexpectedly low.
5. Failure to reconcile results of tests with clinical features.

*ULN = upper limit of normal or upper reference limit.

sults with clinical features should obviate most of these potential difficulties. In Chapter 16, an algorithm is presented to aid in classifying patients suspected of having hepatic disease, given the knowledge of several chemical pathology variates.

REFERENCES

Liver function (General)

Burke, M. D.: Liver function. Human Pathol., *6*:273, 1975.

Combes, B., and Schenker, S.: Laboratory tests. *In* Schiff, L. (ed.): Diseases of the Liver, 4th ed. Philadelphia, J. B. Lippincott Co., 1975, pp. 204-246.

Gabrieli, E. R., Kawasaki, H., Orfanas, A., and Sinka, S. O.: Computer-oriented laboratory testing of hepatic status. *In* Popper, H., and Schaffner, F. (eds.): Progress in Liver Diseases, vol. III New York, Grune & Stratton, 1970, pp. 147-163.

Grand, R. J., and Ulshen, M. H.: Clinical and physiological abnormalities in hepatic function. Pediatr. Clin. North Am., *22*:897, 1975.

Hargreaves, T.: The Liver and Bile Metabolism. New York, Appleton-Century Crofts, 1968.

Kew, M. C., Dos Santos, H. A., and Sherlock, S.: Diagnosis of primary cancer of the liver. Br. Med. J., *4*:408, 1971.

Plaa, G. L.: Evaluation of liver function methodology. *In* Burger, A. (ed.): Medical Research Series, vol. III. New York, Marcel-Dekker, 1968, pp. 255-258.

Reinhold, J. G.: Chemical evaluation of the functions of the liver. Clin. Chem., *1*:351, 1955.

Rosoff, L., Jr., and Rosoff, L., Sr.: Biochemical tests for hepatobiliary disease. Surg. Clin. North Am., *57*:257, 1977.

Sherlock, S.: Diseases of the Liver, 5th ed. Oxford, Blackwell Scientific Publications, 1975.

Tygstrup, N.: The prognostic value of laboratory tests in liver disease. Scand. J. Gastroenterol., *8* (Suppl. 19):47, 1973.

Zimmerman, H. J.: The differential diagnosis of jaundice. Med. Clin. North Am., *52*:1417, 1968.

Zimmerman, H. J.: Hepatic failure. *In* Gall, E. A., and Mostofi, F. K. (eds.): The Liver. Baltimore, Williams and Wilkins, 1973, pp. 384-405.

Bilirubin metabolism and jaundice

Arias, I. M., Gartner, L. M., Cohen, M., et al.: Chronic non-hemolytic unconjugated hyperbilirubinemia with glucuronyl transferase deficiency. Clinical, biochemical, pharmacologic and genetic evidence for heterogeneity. Am. J. Med., *47*:395, 1969.

Berk, P. D., and Berlin, N. I. (eds.): Chemistry and Physiology of Bile Pigments. Fogarty International Proceedings No. 35, DHEW Publication No. (NIH) 77-1100, 1977.

Bernstein, R. B.: Comparison of serum clearance and urinary excretion of mesobilirubinogen-H^3 in control subjects with liver disease. Gastroenterology, *61*:733, 1971.

Billing, B. H.: Bilirubin metabolism. *In* Schiff, L. (ed.): Diseases of the Liver, 4th ed. Philadelphia, J. B. Lippincott, 1975, pp. 287-313.

Bradley, B. W. D.: A physiological approach to jaundice. Clin. Biochem., *9*:144, 1976.

Ducci, H.: Contribution of the laboratory to the differential diagnosis of jaundice. J.A.M.A., *135*:694, 1947.

Fleischner, G. M., and Arias, J. M.: Structure and function of ligandin (Y protein, GSH transferase B) and Z protein in the liver: A progress report. *In* Popper, H., and Schaffner, F. (eds.): Progress in Liver Diseases, vol. V. New York, Grune & Stratton, 1976, pp. 172-182.

Israels, L. G.: The bilirubin shunt and shunt hyperbilirubinemia. *In* Popper, H., and Schaffner, F. (eds.): Progress in Liver Diseases, vol. III. New York, Grune & Stratton, 1970, pp. 1-12.

Jendrassik, L., and Grof, P.: Vereinfachte photometrische Methoden zur Bestimmung des Blutbilirubins. Biochim. Z., *297*:81, 1938.

Malloy, H. T., and Evelyn, K. A.: The determination of bilirubin with the photoelectric colorimeter. J. Biol. Chem., *119*:481, 1937.

McNee, J. W.: Jaundice: A review of recent works. Q. J. Med., *16*:390, 1923.

Michaelsson, M.: Bilirubin determination in serum and urine. Scand. J. Clin. Lab. Invest., *13* (Suppl. 56):5, 1961.

Poland, R. L., and Odell, G. B.: Physiologic jaundice: The enterohepatic circulation of bilirubin. N. Engl. J. Med., *284*:1, 1971.

Rich, A. R.: Pathogenesis of forms of jaundice. Bull. Johns Hopkins Hosp. *47*:338, 1930.

Schmid, R.: Hyperbilirubinemia. *In* Stanbury, J. B., Wyngaarden, J. B., and Frederickson, D. S. (eds.): The Metabolic Basis of Inherited Disease, 3rd ed. New York, McGraw-Hill Book Company, 1972, pp. 1141-1178.

Sunderman, F. W.: Proficiency test service. Bilirubin, January, 1978.

Tenhunen, R.: Microsomal heme oxygenase. *In* Berk, P. D., and Berlin, N. I. (eds.): Chemistry and Physiology of Bile Pigments. Fogarty International Proceedings No. 35, DHEW Publication No. (NIH) 77-1100, 1977.

Thompson, R. P. H.: Recent advances in jaundice: Physiology. Br. Med. J., *1*:223, 1970.

Watson, C. J.: The importance of the fractional serum bilirubin determination in clinical medicine. Ann. Intern. Med., *45*:351, 1956.

Watson, C. J., Schwartz, S., Sborov, V., and Bertie, E.: Studies of urobilinogen V. A simple method for the quantitative recording of the Ehrlich reaction as carried out with urine and feces. Am. J. Clin. Pathol., *14*:605, 1944.

Serum proteins and related abnormalities

Alpert, E.: Human alpha-1-feto protein (AFP). *In* Popper, H., and Schaffner, F. (eds.): Progress in Liver Diseases, vol. V. New York, Grune & Stratton, 1976, pp. 337-349.

Eliakim, M., Zlotnik, A., and Slavin, S.: Gammopathy in liver disease. *In* Popper, H., and Schaffner, F. (eds.): Progress in Liver Diseases, vol. IV. New York, Grune & Stratton, 1972, pp. 403-418.

Glynn, L. E.: Immunopathology of liver disease. *In* Popper, H., and Schaffner, F. (eds.): Progress in Liver Diseases, vol. V. New York, Grune & Stratton, 1976, pp. 311-325.

Hobbs, J. R.: Serum proteins in liver disease. Proc. R. Soc. Med., *60*:1250, 1967.

Maclagan, N. F., Martin, N. H., and Lunnon, J. B.: The mechanism and interrelationships of the flocculation tests. J. Clin. Pathol., 5:1, 1952.

Osserman, E. F., and Takatsuki, K.: The plasma protein in liver disease. Med. Clin. North Am., 47:679, 1963.

Owen, J. A., Padangi, R., and Smith, H.: Serum hepatoglobins and other tests in the diagnosis of hepatobiliary disease. Clin. Sci., 21:189, 1961.

Purves, L. R., Bersohn, I., and Geddes, E. W.: Serum alpha-feto-protein and primary cancer of the liver in man. Cancer, 25:1261, 1970.

Scheinberg, I. H.: Adult Wilson's disease. Arch. Neurol., 29:449, 1973.

Seidel, D., Gretz, H., and Ruppert, C.: Significance of the LP-X test in differential diagnosis of jaundice. Clin. Chem., 19:86, 1973.

Sharp, H. L.: Current status of α-1-antitrypsin, a protease inhibitor, in gastrointestinal diseases. Gastroenterology, 70:611, 1976.

Smith, J. B.: Alpha-feto-protein, occurrence in certain malignant diseases and review of clinical applications. Med. Clin. North Am., 54:797, 1970.

Blood ammonia levels and related abnormalities

Bessman, S. P.: Blood ammonia. In Sabotka, H., and Stewart, C. P. (eds.): Advances in Clinical Chemistry, vol. 2. New York, Academic Press, Inc., 1959, pp. 135–166.

Breen, K. J., and Schenker, S.: Hepatic coma: Present concepts of pathogenesis and therapy. In Popper, H., and Schaffner, F. (eds.): Progress in Liver Diseases, vol. IV. New York, Grune & Stratton, 1972, pp. 301–332.

Fischer, J. E., and Baldesserani, R. J.: Pathogenesis and therapy of hepatic coma. In Popper, H., and Schaffner, F. (eds.): Progress in Liver Diseases, vol. V. New York, Grune & Stratton, 1976, pp. 363–397.

Gabuzda, G. J.: Ammonium metabolism and hepatic coma. Gastroenterology, 53:806, 1959.

Galambos, J. T., Warren, W. D., and Rudman, D.: Portal surgery and liver function. A new look at an old problem. Mt. Sinai J. Med., 43:219, 1976.

Glasgow, A. M., Cotton, R. B., and Dhiensiri, K.: Reye's syndrome. Blood ammonia and consideration of the nonhistologic diagnosis. Am. J. Dis. Child., 124:827, 1972.

Hourani, B. T., Hamlin, E. M., and Reynolds, T. B.: Cerebrospinal fluid glutamine as a measure of hepatic encephalopathy. Arch. Intern. Med., 127:1033, 1971.

Seligson, D., and Seligson, H.: A microdiffusion method for the determination of nitrogen liberated as ammonia. J. Lab. Clin. Med., 38:324, 1951.

Steigmann, F., Kazemi, F., Dubin, A., and Kissane, J.: Cerebrospinal fluid glutamine in the diagnosis of hepatic coma. Am. J. Gastroenterol., 40:378, 1963.

Summerskill, W. H. L., and Wolpert, E.: Ammonia metabolism in the gut. Am. J. Clin. Nutr., 23:633, 1970.

Van Anken, H. C., and Schiphorst, M. E.: A kinetic determination of ammonia in plasma. Clin. Chim. Acta, 56:151, 1974.

Galactose tolerance and other tests related to carbohydrate metabolism

Blaauwen, D. H., and Thijs, L. G.: The bromosulfalein and galactose tolerance tests in patients with various liver diseases. Acta Gastro-Enterologica Belgica, 36:345, 1973.

Felig, P., and Sherwin, R.: Carbohydrate homeostasis,

liver and diabetes. In Popper, H., and Schaffner, F. (eds.): Progress in Liver Diseases, vol. V. New York, Grune & Stratton, 1976, pp. 149–171.

Menesholme, E. A.: Role of the liver in integration of fat and carbohydrate metabolism and clinical implications in patients with liver disease. In Popper, H., and Schaffner, F. (eds.): Progress in Liver Diseases, vol. V. New York, Grune & Stratton, 1976, pp. 125–135.

Tengstrom, B.: An intravenous galactose tolerance test and its use in hepatobiliary diseases. Acta Med. Scand., 183:31, 1968.

Van Itallie, T. B., and Bentley, W. B.: Glucagon-induced hyperglycemia as an index of liver function. J. Clin. Invest., 34:1730, 1955.

Verhaegen, H., Verhaegen-Declercq, M. L., DeBeukelar, A., and Krug, F.: The double glucagon test, a new liver function test. Postgrad. Med. J., 47:108, 1971.

Drug metabolism as a measure of hepatic function

Bircher, J., Küpfer, A., Gikalov, I., and Preisig, R.: Aminopyrine demethylation measured by breath analysis in cirrhosis. Clin. Pharmacol. Ther., 20:484, 1976.

Hepner, G. W., and Vesell, E. S.: Aminopyrine disposition: Studies on breath, saliva, and urine of normal subjects and patients with liver disease. Clin. Pharmacol. Ther., 20:654, 1976.

Schenker, S., Hoyumpa, A. M., and Wilkinson, G. R.: The effect of parenchymal liver disease on the disposition and elimination of sedatives and analgesics. Med. Clin. North Am., 59:887, 1975.

Dye excretion tests

Bircher, J., and Häcki, W.: A practical approach to quantitate hepatic excretory function. Yale J. Biol. Med., 3:196, 1974.

Jablonski, P., and Owen, J. A.: The clinical chemistry of bromosulfophthalein and other cholephilic dyes. In Bodansky, O., and Stewart, C. P. (eds.): Advances in Clinical Chemistry, vol. 12. New York, Academic Press, Inc., 1969, pp. 309–386.

Javitt, N.: Clinical and experimental aspects of sulfabromophthalein and related compounds. In Popper, H., and Schaffner, F. (eds.): Progress in Liver Diseases, vol. III. New York, Grune & Stratton, 1970, pp. 110–117.

Leevy, C. M., Smith, F., Longueville, J., et al.: Indocyanine green clearance as a test for hepatic function: Evaluation by dichromatic or densitometry. J.A.M.A., 200:236, 1967.

Paumgartner, G.: The handling of indocyanine green by the liver. Schweiz. Med. Wochenschr., [Suppl.] 105, 1975.

Serum bile acid levels

Barnes, S., Gallo, G. A., Trash, D. B., and Morris, J. S.: Diagnostic value of serum bile acid estimations in liver disease. J. Clin. Pathol., 28:506, 1975.

Carey, J. B., Jr.: The serum trihydroxy-dihydroxy bile acid ratio in liver and biliary tract disease. J. Clin. Invest., 37:1494, 1958.

Demers, L. M., and Hepner, G.: Radioimmunoassay of bile acids in serum. Clin. Chem., 22:602, 1976.

Erlanger, S.: Hepatocellular uptake of taurocholate in the dog. J. Clin. Invest., 55:419, 1975.

Fausa, D.: Serum bile acid concentrations after a test meal. Scand. J. Gastroenterol., 11:229, 1976.

Hofman, A. F.: Enterohepatic circulation of bile acids in man. Adv. Intern. Med., *21*:501, 1976.

Javitt, N. B.: Bile acid and hepatobiliary disease. *In* Schiff, L. (ed.): Diseases of the Liver, 5th ed. Philadelphia, J. B. Lippincott, 1975, pp. 111–145.

Korman, M. G., Hofman, A. F., and Summerskill, W. H. J.: Assessment of activity in chronic active liver disease: Serum bile acids compared with conventional tests and histology. N. Engl. J. Med., *290*:1399, 1974.

Williams, C. N.: Bile acid metabolism and the liver. Clin. Biochem., *9*:149, 1976.

Blood clotting in liver disease

Aledort, L. M.: Blood clotting abnormalities in liver disease. *In* Popper, H., and Schaffner, F. (eds.): Progress in Liver Diseases, vol. V. New York, Grune & Stratton, 1976, pp. 350–362.

Dymock, I. W., Tucker, J. S., Woolf, I. L., Poller, L., and Thomson, J. M.: Coagulation studies as a prognostic index in acute liver failure. Br. J. Hematol., *29*:385, 1975.

Green, G., Poller, L., Thomson, J. M., and Dymock, I. W.: Factor VII as a marker of hepatocellular function in liver disease. J. Clin. Pathol., *29*:971, 1976.

Ratnoff, O. D.: Disordered homeostasis in liver disease. *In* Schiff, L. (ed.): Diseases of the Liver, 4th ed. Philadelphia, J. B. Lippincott, 1975, pp. 184–203.

Radioisotopic and other special procedures employed in diagnosis of hepatobiliary disease

Bekerman, C., and Gottschalk, A.: Diagnostic significance of the relative uptake of liver compared with spleen in ^{99}Tc-sulphur colloid scintiphotography. J. Nucl. Med., *12*:237, 1971.

Bragg, D. G., and Evans, J. A.: Roentgen aspects of liver and biliary tract diseases. *In* Schiff, L. (ed.): Diseases of the Liver, 4th ed. Philadelphia, J. B. Lippincott, 1975, pp. 1246–1277.

Brill, A. B., and Palton, D. D.: Radioisotope methods in diagnosis and assessment of liver metabolism. Int. J. Radiation Oncology Biol. Phys., *1*:981, 1976.

Cantor, R. E., Cohn, E. M., Park, C. H., and Shapiro, B.: Comparative liver scanning: Technetium sulfide Tc^{99m} vs. gold Au^{198}. J.A.M.A., *211*:1677, 1970.

Edmonson, H. A., and Schiff, L.: Needle biopsy of the liver. *In* Schiff, L. (ed.): Diseases of the Liver, 4th ed. Philadelphia, J. B. Lippincott, 1975, pp. 247–271.

Ghadimi, H., and Sakk-Kortusk, A.: Evaluation of the radioactive rose-bengal test for the differential diagnosis of obstructive jaundice in infants. N. Engl. J. Med., *96*:351, 1961.

Malini, S., and Sobel, J.: Ultrasonography in obstructive jaundice. Radiology, *123*:429, 1977.

Parks, S. N., Blaisdell, F. W., and Lim, R. C.: Special diagnostic tests for the evaluation of liver and biliary tract disorders. Surg. Clin. North Am., *57*:295, 1977.

Rossi, P., and Gould, H. R.: Angiography and scanning in liver disease. Radiology, *96*:553, 1970.

Vicary, F. R.: Progress report: Ultrasound and gastroenterology. Gut, *18*:386, 1977.

Virologic and other serologic tests for diagnosis of hepatic disease

Glynn, L. E.: Immunopathology of liver disease. *In* Popper, H., and Schaffner, F. (eds.): Progress in Liver Diseases, vol. V. New York, Grune & Stratton, 1976, pp. 311–325.

Hoofnagle, J. H.: Viral hepatitis. *In* Hook, E. W., Mandell, G., Gwaltney, J., and Sande, M. (eds.): Current Concepts of Infectious Disease. New York, John Wiley & Sons, Inc., 1977, pp. 243–261.

Husby, G., Skrede, S., Blomboff, J. P., Jacobsen, C. D., Berg, K., and Gjone, E.: Serum immunoglobulins and organ non-specific antibodies in diseases of the liver. Scand. J. Gastroenterol., *12*:297, 1977.

Vitamin B$_{12}$ levels in liver disease

Rachmilewitz, M., and Eliakim, M.: Serum B$_{12}$—a diagnostic test in liver disease. Israel J. Med. Sci., *4*:47, 1968.

Serum enzymes in liver disease

Karmen, A.: A note on the spectrophotometric assay of glutamic-oxaloacetic transaminase activity in human blood serum. J. Clin. Invest., *34*:131, 1955.

Kontinnen, A.: Serum enzymes as indicators of hepatic disease. Scand. J. Gastroenterol., *6*:667, 1971.

Skrede, S., Blomboff, J. P., and Gjone, E.: Biochemical features of acute and chronic hepatitis. Ann. Clin. Res., *8*:182, 1976.

Zimmerman, H. J., and Seeff, L. B.: Enzymes in hepatic disease. *In* Coodley, E. L. (ed.): Diagnostic Enzymology. Philadelphia, Lea & Febiger, 1970, pp. 1–38.

Also see references for Chapter 12.

12

CLINICAL ENZYMOLOGY

Hyman J. Zimmerman, M.D.,
and John Bernard Henry, M.D.

Enzymes, organic catalysts that are responsible for most of the chemical reactions of the body, are found in all tissues. Some have been identified in the plasma (or serum), to which they gain access from injured cells or even perhaps from intact cells. Interest of clinicians in serum enzymes began about five decades ago with the demonstration of the usefulness of alkaline phosphatase levels in the diagnosis of osseous and hepatobiliary disease, of acid phosphatase levels in the diagnosis of carcinoma of prostate, and of amylase and lipase levels for the diagnosis of pancreatic disease. Despite the clinical usefulness of these parameters of disease and the demonstration, during the next 25 years, of a number of other enzymes in the serum, clinical interest in serum enzymology remained relatively dormant until 1953. The demonstration in that year of glutamate oxalacetate transaminase (GOT) or aspartate aminotransferase (AST) in the serum of normals and the subsequent observations that increased levels of this enzyme were helpful in the diagnosis of cardiac and hepatic disease led to a marked intensification of interest in serum enzymology.

By now, well over 50 enzymes have been identified in the serum (Zimmerman, 1970). Table 12-1 lists many of these. The levels of many enzymes have been studied extensively in a variety of conditions (Table 12-1). Some serum enzyme tests have been applied so widely to clinical problems as to be considered routine laboratory procedures (Table 12-2, Group A). Others (Table 12-2, Group B), though clearly shown also to reflect various diseases reliably, are performed in relatively few clinical laboratories because the assay is technically difficult or because the information provided is considered to add too little to that

Table 12–1. CLASSIFICATION OF ENZYMES DEMONSTRATED IN SERUM WITH TYPE AND DEGREE* OF ABNORMALITY IN DISEASE

	CONDITION†								
TYPE OF ENZYME	Hepa-titis	Inf. Mono.	Cirrho-sis	Met. Ca.	Obst. Jaundice	Heart Failure	Myocard. Infarct.	Prog. Musc. Dyst.	Comments or Other Abnor-malities
I. Carbohydrate metabolism									
A. Glycolytic									
1. Phosphoglucomutase	↑↑		N	↑	↑				
2. Phosphohexoisomerase (PHI)	↑↑↑	↑↑	↑	↑	↑	↑	↑↑	↑	Fig. 12–7
3. Fructose 1,6-diphosphate aldolase (ALS.)	↑↑↑	↑	↑	↑	N or ↑	↑	↑↑	↑↑↑	Fig. 12–7
4. Fructose-P-aldolase	↑↑↑			N	N		N	N	
5. Lactate dehydrogenase (LD)	↑	↑↑	↑	↑↑	N or ↑	↑	↑↑	↑↑	Table 12–11
6. Pyruvate kinase (PK)	↑↑			↑↑					
7. Enolase	↑						↑		Fig. 12–7
8. Triose-P-isomerase				↑					
9. Glyceraldehyde 3-P-dehydrogenase	↑	↑							
B. Hexose monophosphate shunt									
(pentose phosphate pathway)									
1. Glucose-6-phosphate dehydrogenase (GPD)	N		N		N		↑↑		Fig. 12–10
2. 6-P-Gluconate dehydrogenase (6-P-GD)	↑	↑							
3. 5-Phosphoriboisomerase	N		↑↑	↑↑	↑				
4. Transketolase	↑								
C. Citric acid cycle									
1. Malate dehydrogenase (MD)	↑↑↑	↑	↑	↑	↑	↑	↑↑		Fig. 12–9
2. Isocitrate dehydrogenase (ICD)	↑↑↑	↑	N or ↑	↑↑	N or ↑	↑	N	N	
3. Fumarase	↑		↑						
D. Other									
1. Amylase (AMS)	N	N	N or ↓	N	N	N	N	N	Chapter 23
2. β-Glucuronidase	↑↑						N or ↑		Ca, Pregnancy
3. Iditol dehydrogenase (ID)	↑↑↑	↑	↑	N or ↑	N or ↑		N	N	Fig. 12–13
II. Esterases									
A. Lipid									
1. Lipase (LPS)	N	N	N	N	N	N	N	N	Chapter 23
2. Aliesterase	N	N	N	N	N	N	N	N	Acute pancreatitis
3. Cholesterol esterase	↓		↓	N or ↓	N				
4. Lipoprotein lipase (LPL)	↑↑		↑↑		↓				
5. Lecithinase	N		N	N	N				Acute pancreatitis
B. Nonlipid									
1. Cholinesterase (pseudo)	↓	↓	↓		N or ↑	N or ↑		N	Fig. 12–11
2. Phosphatases									Increase in
a. Alkaline phosphatase (ALP)	↑	↑	↑	↑↑	↑↑↑	↑	N	N	bone disease Table 12–7
b. Acid phosphatase (ACP)	N	N	N	N	N	N	N	N	Ca. of prostate
c. 5′-Nucleotidase (5′-N)	↑		↑	↑↑	↑↑↑				Normal in bone disease
d. Adenosine triphosphatase									Elevated in
(ATPase)	↑		↑	↑	↑↑				bone disease
3. Deoxyribonuclease I									Acute hem-orrhagic
(DNAse)	↑	+			N			N	pancreatitis
4. Ribonuclease (RNase)	N		N	N	N	↑	↑		Uremia, myeloma
5. Adenosine deaminase	↑↑	↑↑↑	↑↑	↑↑↑			↑↑	N	Leukemia
III. Protein and amino acid enzymes									
A. Proteolytic enzymes (trypsin)									Acute pan-creatitis
B. Peptidases									
1. Leucine aminopeptidase									Pregnancy
(LAP)	↑	↑↑↑	↑	↑↑	↑↑↑	↑↑	N	N	Ca. of pancreas
2. Aminotripeptidase	↑↑	↑↑	↑	↑↑	↑↑				Pancreatitis
3. γ-Glutamyl transpeptidase (GGTP)									
(γ-Glutamyl transferase (GGT))	↑		↑	↑↑↑	↑↑		↑↑		
C. Pepsinogen									Duod. ulcer
D. Amino acid substrate									
1. Aminotransferases (Transaminases)									
a. Aspartate aminotransferase (AST)									
(Glutamate oxalacetate transaminase (GOT))	↑↑↑	↑↑	↑	↑	↑	↑	↑↑	↑↑	Table 12–10 Fig. 12–6
b. Alanine aminotransferase (ALT)									
(Glutamate pyruvate transaminase (GPT))	↑↑↑	↑↑	↑	↑	↑	↑	N or ↑	↑↑	Chapter 11
c. Glutamate dehydrogenase (GD)	↑↑	N	N or ↑	N	N	N	N	N	
2. Urea cycle									
a. Ornithine carbamoyl									Acute cho-lecystitis.
transferase (OCT)	↑↑↑		↑	↑↑					
b. Arginase	↑↑		↑						Fig. 12–12

Table 12–1. CLASSIFICATION OF ENZYMES DEMONSTRATED IN SERUM WITH TYPE AND DEGREE* OF ABNORMALITY IN DISEASE (*Continued*)

TYPE OF ENZYME	Hepatitis	Inf. Mono.	Cirrhosis	Met. Ca.	Obst. Jaundice	Heart Failure	Myocard. Infarct.	Prog. Musc. Dyst.	Comments or Other Abnormalities
V. Other enzymes									
A. Glutathione reductase (GR)	↑↑		↑	↑↑			↑		
B. Ceruloplasmin	↑↑	↑	↑	↑↑	↑↑				Wilson's disease
C. Creatine kinase (CK) (Creatine phosphokinase (CPK))	N		N	N	N	N	↑↑↑	↑↑↑	Dermatomyositis
D. Benzidine oxidase	↑		↑	↑↑↑	↑↑	↑	↑↑↑		Fig. 12–13
E. Hydroxybutyrate dehydrogenase (HBD)	↑	↑	±	↑	±	↑	↑↑↑	±	Isoenzyme of LD.
F. Guanase	↑↑↑	↑	↑	↑	↑				

* ↑—slight increase
↑↑—moderate increase
↑↑↑—marked increase
N—no change
†Inf. Mono.—infectious mononucleosis
Met. Ca.—metastatic carcinoma
Obst. Jaundice—obstructive jaundice
Prog. Musc. Dyst.—progressive muscular dystrophy
Myocard. Infarct.—myocardial infarction

provided by the enzymes in Group A. Others are of investigative rather than regular clinical interest (Group C) or of importance only in special clinical situations (Group D). A fifth group (Group E) includes enzymes that have not been studied sufficiently to assess their clinical usefulness. In Table 12–1 are shown the main conditions in which abnormal values of the enzymes listed are found.

The usefulness of several serum enzymes (alkaline phosphatase, glutamate oxalacetate transaminase (GOT)—now called aspartate aminotransferase (AST), glutamate pyruvate transaminase (GPT)—now called alanine aminotransferase (ALT)) in the diagnosis of hepatic disease and of several other enzymes (amylase, lipase) in the diagnosis of pancreatic disease is considered in the chapters devoted to liver (Chapter 11) and pancreas (Chapter 23). In this chapter the more general aspects of serum enzymology are considered. The principles of the methods for measuring enzyme activity are discussed, the possible factors responsible for abnormal values are ana-

Table 12–2. CATEGORIZATION OF SERUM ENZYMES ACCORDING TO CLINICAL USEFULNESS

GROUP	ENZYMES*
A. Routinely employed in most hospitals	ALP, ACP, lipase, amylase, AST (GOT), ALT (GPT), LD, CPK (CK)
B. Clinically useful, but employed much less widely than enzymes in Group A	Pseudocholinesterase, LAP, 5′N, GGT, ALS, PHI, ICD, OCT, HBD, ID, LPS
C. Primarily of investigative interest; employed for routine clinical purposes in few or no hospitals	α-Lecithinase, LPL, aliesterase, fructose-6-P aldolase, MD, β-glucuronidase, GD, guanase, GR
D. Employed only in special circumstances	Ceruloplasmin (for diagnosis of Wilson's disease): pseudocholinesterase (to study patients with insecticide poisoning and patients with prolonged apnea after muscle relaxants), muramidase in patients with leukemia
E. Data too scanty to evaluate prospective usefulness or indicative of no clinical utility	ATPases (alk. and acid), heroin esterase, procaine esterase; DNAses (I and II), cholesterol esterase, glucokinase, phosphoglucomutase, triose-P-isomerase, glyceraldehyde-3-P dehydrogenase, phosphoglycerate dehydrogenase, enolase, 3-P-glyceric acid kinase, pyruvate kinase, malic enzyme, fumarase, succinic dehydrogenase, G-6-PD, 6-PGD, 5-P-riboisomerase, transketolase, tripeptidase, dipeptidases, oxytocinase, amine oxidases, arginase, adenosine deaminase, benzidine oxidase

*See Table 12–1 for meaning of abbreviations.

lyzed, and special attention is devoted to a few of the enzymes found in the serum. Brief reference is made to enzymes of other body fluids and to the clinical significance of enzymes in the formed elements of the blood.

PRINCIPLES OF ENZYME ACTIVITY DETERMINATIONS

Because they exist in very small amounts in biologic fluids and are so similar chemically, enzymes are measured by their activity rather than their concentration. Enzyme activity is expressed in units that usually represent one

Table 12-3. CLASSIFICATION OF ENZYMES: SIX CLASSES WHICH REFLECT SUBCLASSES AND SUB-SUBCLASSES

I. Oxidoreductases
   Oxidases
      Cytochrome oxidase
   Dehydrogenases
      Iditol dehydrogenase (ID)
      Lactate dehydrogenase (LD)
      Malate dehydrogenase (MD)
      Isocitrate dehydrogenase (ICD)
      Glucose-6-phosphate dehydrogenase (GPD)
      Hydroxybutyrate dehydrogenase (HBD)
II. Transferases
   Aspartate aminotransferase (AST) or
      Glutamate oxalacetate transferase (GOT)
   Alanine aminotransferase (ALT) or
      Glutamate pyruvate transaminase (GPT)
   Creatine kinase (CK) or
      Creatine phosphokinase (CPK)
   Gamma glutamyl transferase (GGT)
   Ornithine carbamoyl transferase (OCT)
III. Hydrolases
   Esterases
      Phosphatase, acid (ACP)
      Phosphatase, alkaline (ALP)
      Cholinesterase (CHS)
      Lipase (LPS)
   Peptidases
      Leucine aminopeptidase (LAP)
      Trypsin (PTS)
      Pepsin (PPS)
   Glycosidases
      Amylase (AMS)
      Amylo-1-6-glycosidase
      Glucoside
      Galactosidase
IV. Lyases
   Aldolase (ALS)
   Glutamate decarboxylase
   Pyruvate decarboxylase
   Tryptophan decarboxylase
V. Isomerases
   Glucose phosphate isomerase
   Ribose phosphate isomerase
VI. Ligases

of the following: (1) increase in concentration of one of the products, (2) decrease in concentration of substrate, or (3) rate of change in concentration of coenzyme as a measure of rate of reaction.

Although a great deal of confusion has resulted from the lack of uniform terminology in the expression of units, attention has been directed to this problem and recommendations have been made by the Commission on Enzymes of the International Union of Biochemistry. (Tables 12-3 and 12-4).

Immunochemical methods for the measurement of enzyme levels have not found clinical application. Assays of levels of isoenzymes of LD, CPK, ALP, and pepsinogen employing specific antisera have thus far been of mainly research interest. It is likely, however, that advances in purification of enzymes for the

Table 12-4. UNITS FOR EXPRESSING ENZYME ACTIVITY

International unit (U)

1 unit (U) = the amount of enzyme that catalyzes the conversion of 1 micromole (microequivalent) of substrate or coenzyme per minute under the defined conditions of the test (temperature with optimal pH and substrate concentration). Activity may be expressed in units, milliunits, microunits, etc., per milliliter of sample. Concentration should be expressed in terms of U/ml or mU/ml = (U/l), whichever gives the more convenient minimal value.

$$1 \text{ unit} = 1 \text{ micromole per minute} \\ (\mu \text{ mol/min})$$

$$1 \text{ milliunit (mU)} = 1 \text{ millimicromole per minute} \\ (\text{m}\mu\text{mol/min})$$

$$1 \text{ microunit } (\mu U) = 1 \text{ micromicromole per minute} \\ (\mu\mu\text{mol/min})$$

Example:
Lactate dehydrogenase 25°C.

$$\text{O. D. unit} = \text{O. D. of } (.001)/\text{min/ml}$$

$$\text{Standard unit} = \frac{\text{O.D.}}{6.25} \times \frac{3.0}{0.2} = \text{O.D./min} \times 2.4$$

$$\text{Standard unit} = \text{difference of 5 min lines on graph} \\ = \text{O.D.}_5 \times 0.48 \\ = \text{O.D.} \times \tfrac{1}{2}$$

Example:

Test gave O.D. = 0.020/min for 0.2 ml sample
Old method: O.D. = 20 × 5 = 100 O.D. units
Standard method: 0.020 × 2.4 = 0.048 units, or 48 mU

Normal range:
80 to 120 O.D. units
40 to 60 standard milliunits (mU)/ml

Recently, the katal has been recommended. One unit (U) is equal to one micromole catalyzed per minute. One katal is equal to one mole catalyzed per second. Thus, one U is equal to 16.67 nanokatals.

development of antisera and employment of radioimmunoassay will yield clinically useful methods for quantitation of amounts of circulating enzyme protein. At that time enzyme levels would be expressed in concentration of enzyme rather than catalytic activity.

The numerical designation for each enzyme consists of four numbers separated by periods, e.g., E.C. 1.1.1.27 for lactate dehydrogenase. EC stands for "Enzyme Commission," the first number defines class (one of six reactions) to which enzyme belongs while the next two numbers indicate subclass and sub-subclass to which the enzyme is assigned (Table 12–3). An amino transferring subclass can thus be separated from a phosphate transferring group. A specific serial number is the last number given each enzyme in its sub-subclass.

An enzyme may be considered as follows:

$$\text{Holoenzyme} = \text{apoenzyme} + \text{coenzyme}$$

Apoenzyme is the protein portion subject to denaturation, as are all proteins. This denaturation, due to physical and chemical agents, is associated with a loss of enzyme activity.

Coenzyme is the dialyzable portion and is essential for catalytic activity. It is tightly bound to enzyme and is not a protein. An example of a coenzyme is NAD (nicotinamide adenine dinucleotide). Another coenzyme (organic co-factor) is pyridoxine as pyridoxamine phosphate; it is essential for aminotransferase (transaminase) activity.

Activators are substances which modify reactions catalyzed—metal ions such as zinc and magnesium, for example.

Enzymes display specificity with regard to substrate (substance which is acted on) and effect (chemical action). Lactate dehydrogenase catalyzes the following reaction:

$$\text{Lactate} + \text{NADH} \rightleftharpoons \text{Pyruvate} + \text{NADH}_2$$

It catalyzes both the forward and reverse reactions as indicated. It acts virtually only on L-lactic acid and pyruvic acid as substrates and catalyzes the reversible transfer of hydrogen ion (H^+) between lactate and NAD. Other enzymes are required for the decarboxylation or amination of pyruvic acid.

Many chemical and physical agents exert a marked influence on enzymes. Temperature and hydrogen ion concentration are probably the two best-studied agents. Inactivation of

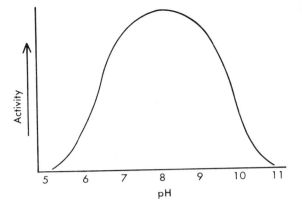

Figure 12–1. Typical curve of activity versus pH for an enzymatic reaction. (From Henry, J. B.: Postgrad. Med., *33*:A-66, 1963.)

most enzymes will occur in the neighborhood of 65°C. Freezing, however, does not usually destroy enzymes. For each 10°C. rise in temperature (Q_{10}), several enzymes will demonstrate a twofold increase in activity, but the increase in denaturation is even greater. Hence, the temperature activity curve for an enzyme will show a maximum, depending on the opposed activating and denaturing effects of rising temperature. Although there is not complete agreement, 37°C. appears to be the best single choice of reaction temperature, followed by 30°C. for the majority of clinical serum enzyme assays. Statland (1977) has reviewed the arguments regarding one temperature versus another. These fall into chemical, technical, and economic categories.

A bell-shaped curve will also often describe the optimum pH for an enzyme (Fig. 12–1). This may also reflect the cumulative effects of hydrogen ion concentration on activation and denaturation of enzyme protein.

Although an enzyme reaction represents very complex mechanisms that are not fully understood, it can be stated that an enzyme reversibly forms a transitory complex with its substrate. Functional groups of coenzymes or prosthetic groups or both may play a role in the formation of the enzyme-substrate complex. The enzyme-substrate complex decomposes to enzyme and product. The enzyme is not altered in the overall reaction. The

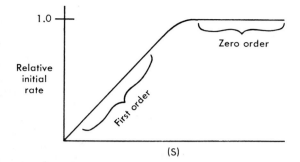

Figure 12–2. Relative rate of reaction expressed as function of substrate concentration (*S*). (From Henry, J. B.: Postgrad. Med., *33*:A-66, 1963.)

Michaelis-Menten hypothesis describes this sequence of events, as shown at the bottom of this page.

In addition to a high substrate concentration, with the important assumption of an intermediate enzyme-substrate complex, this theory further states that the rate of conversion of the substrate to the products of the reaction is determined by the rate of conversion of the enzyme-substrate complex to reaction products and the enzyme.

Units of enzyme activity are best expressed in terms of rate of the catalyzed reaction. The rate of reaction can be considered graphically (Figs. 12–2 and 12–3). In Figure 12–2, the relative rate of reaction is expressed as a function of substrate concentration [S]. At low concentration, the rate is first order* with respect to [S]. The rate is zero order,* independent of [S], at a high concentration. In measuring enzyme activity, one should use this part of the curve.

In an enzyme assay, one may measure activity as ΔP (increase in product) or ΔS (decrease in substrate) depending on which is more convenient analytically (Fig. 12–3). Often the product or substrate may be colored and, if so, may be quantitatively determined by colorimetry or spectrophotometry. The concentration of coenzyme (e.g., NAD with virtually no absorption at 340 nm; NADH [DPNH$_2$] with maximal absorption at 340 nm, can be measured spectrophotometrically as in the lactate dehydrogenase assay.

An enzyme exerts maximal influence when substrate concentration is highest and product concentration nil. This is most likely to be the case at the beginning of the reaction, when the rate is described as zero order with respect to substrate, followed by a progressive decrease in reaction velocity as equilibrium is reached. Zero-order reaction rate simply means in this case that the rate is constant and independent of substrate and product concentrations. If reaction is zero order, concentration of product will rise linearly with respect to time (Fig. 12–3a). Ideally, enzyme assays are performed under conditions which permit reaction to approach zero order with respect to product and substrate during the entire measuring period. Multiple or serial determinations of substrate or product concentration against time are recorded in the assay.

To be valid, an enzyme assay must be so designed that the enzyme concentration is the only limiting factor; i.e., the result reflects the amount of enzyme and is not influenced by other substances present. This is illustrated graphically in Figure 12–4. The rate of product formation increases proportionately with enzyme concentration, e.g., one unit of product formed per minute per each 0.1 ml of serum. Ultimately, the concentration of enzyme exceeds the amount of substrate available; i.e., substrate concentration becomes a limiting factor and proportionality is no longer present. At this point, the assay is no longer a reflection of enzyme activity.

Figure 12–5 illustrates potential hazards of utilizing a single determination. With a single or one-point (E) measuring system, three dif-

---

* A first-order enzyme reaction is one in which the rate of reaction is determined by the concentration of substrate as well as of enzyme. Accordingly, the reaction rate changes continuously with time as the substrate is consumed, and measurement of enzyme activity is difficult. In zero-order enzyme reaction, the rate of reaction is linear with time, independent of the concentration of substrate and directly proportional to the concentration of enzyme (Fig. 12–4). The greater ease of measuring enzyme activity in a zero order, than in a first-order reaction, is shown in Figure 12–5.

$$\text{Enzyme (E) + substrate (S)} \underset{k_2}{\overset{k_1}{\rightleftarrows}} \text{enzyme-substrate complex (ES)}$$

$$\downarrow \ k_3$$

$$(k_1, k_2, k_3 = \text{rate constants}) \qquad \text{products (P) + enzyme (E)}$$

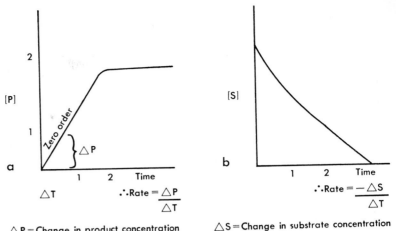

Figure 12–3. Rate of product formation (*a*) and substrate disappearance
(*b*). (From Henry, J. B.: Postgrad. Med.,
33:A-68, 1963.)

$$\therefore Rate = \frac{\triangle P}{\triangle T}$$

$$\therefore Rate = \frac{-\triangle S}{\triangle T}$$

$\triangle P$ = Change in product concentration $\triangle S$ = Change in substrate concentration

$\triangle T$ = Change in time

[P] = Product concentration   [S] = Substrate concentration

ferent reaction rates would have given the same apparent activity.

An assay system must progress in a zero-order reaction during its entire period of observation if the measurement is to reflect true enzyme activity. Performance of multiple determinations has the advantage of permitting assessment of kinetics and confirmation of zero-order reaction.

Multiple-point or serial measurements of the concentration of products per unit time permit the recognition of rapid attainment of equilibrium and substrate exhaustion with samples of biologic fluids containing very high concentrations of enzyme. In such instances it is preferable to use a smaller volume of sample rather than to make dilutions of sample in repeat assays. In the lactate dehydrogenase assay, the volume ratio, i.e., volume of sample to volume of total assay, should be reduced when very high concentrations of enzyme activity are suspected. Inhibition of enzyme may be suspected when the enzymatic reaction is proceeding at a rate less than expected (Fig. 12–5, curve D). Partial, total, reversible, or irreversible inhibition may occur. Competitive reversible inhibition occurs when the inhibitor resembles the substrate sufficiently to com-

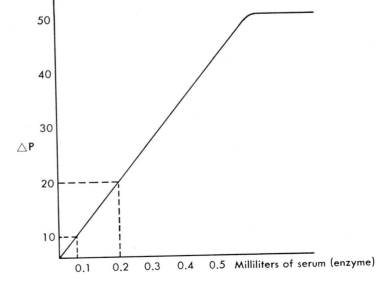

Figure 12–4. Change in product concentration ($\triangle P$) as a function of enzyme concentration. The abscissa represents increments of serum added to reaction mixture. (From Henry, J. B.: Postgrad. Med., *33*:A-70, 1963.)

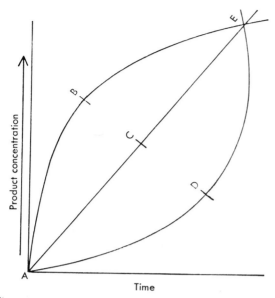

Figure 12–5. Illustration of potential hazards of using a single determination in enzyme assays. Line *ACE* is a zero-order reaction that permits accurate determination of enzyme activity for the entire reaction time. Curve *ABE* shows initial zero-order reaction of high rate followed by falling off of rate of reaction. This is possibly due to exhaustion of substrate prior to termination of assay at point *E*. Curve *ADE* reveals an initial lag phase which masks true activity. (From Henry, J. B.: Postgrad. Med., *33*:A-72, 1963.)

bine with it and form a complex (E.I.); this complex does not break down to form products. A higher substrate concentration may overcome such inhibition.

Numerous pitfalls are encountered in enzyme assays in the clinical laboratory. Hemolysis may be associated with the release of enzymes from red blood cells into the serum, causing falsely high serum values. Because of the adverse effects on enzyme activity of various anticoagulants, serum rather than plasma is the preferred specimen for clinical enzyme assays. Lactescence, or milky serum, may result in variable absorbance readings in spectrophotometric assays. Most enzymes in biologic fluids are quite stable at 6°C. for at least 24 hours and at room temperature for lesser periods. For prolonged storage, temperatures of −20°C. or lower* must be used in order to assure preservation of enzyme activity. Heat

lability must be considered with respect to each enzyme to be assayed as well as other components in the entire enzyme system, especially coenzymes and substrates. Accuracy in timing each assay and use of meticulously clean glassware are essential.

Enzyme assays requiring kinetic measurements in the ultraviolet wavelength region pose new problems for many clinical laboratories. Most of these procedures depend on the changes in absorption at 340 nm of pyridine nucleotides $(NAD \rightarrow NADH_2)$. Owing to the increasing number of nucleotide-dependent enzymes of clinical importance, the ability to work in the 340 nm range is more important. Indeed, a spectrophotometer which measures accurately in the ultraviolet range is virtually essential in clinical enzymology.

A review of the lactate dehydrogenase determination underscores salient features of clinical enzyme assays. In the pH range 7 to 8, the equilibrium favors reduction of pyruvate to lactate, whereas the reverse reaction is favored in the pH range 9 to 10. Wacker (1956) has reported a lactate dehydrogenase assay incorporating a buffer at pH 8.8, lactate as the substrate, and NAD as the coenzyme. The addition of serum provides enzyme, and the assay is conducted at 25°C. Spectrophotometric measurements of absorbance (optical density) are made each minute for 5 minutes at wavelength 340 nm. Lactate is oxidized to pyruvate with conversion of coenzyme (NAD) to reduced coenzyme $(NADH_2)$. The multiple measurements at 1-minute intervals provide an assessment of adherence to zero-order reaction. One unit of activity represents a change in absorbance of 0.001 optical density units per ml of serum per minute at 25°C. This in turn can be converted to International Units (U/1) as shown in Table 12–4.

Cabaud (1958) reported a colorimetric assay for lactate dehydrogenase in which the substrate pyruvate is converted to lactate at 37°C. Pyruvic acid reacts with 2,4-dinitrophenylhydrazine to form a colored hydrazone. The amount of pyruvate remaining after the incubation is inversely proportional to the amount of lactate dehydrogenase present in the reaction.

To insure accuracy and precision in clinical enzyme determinations, one must be aware of the pitfalls and informed regarding the principles of enzyme assays. A quality control program for clinical enzyme assays should include the following: (1) adherence to zero-order ki-

*Some enzymes (e.g., CPK) do not remain reliably preserved at −20°C. and must be kept at −70°C. to retain activity. A few enzymes are inactivated at refrigerator temperatures, e.g., lactate dehydrogenase (liver isoenzymes, LD4 and LD5) is least stable at lower temperatures. Hence, sera for LD assays should not be refrigerated.

netics, (2) proportionality studies with increments of sample, (3) use of pooled frozen serum or stable reference materials (lyophilized) as control solutions, and (4) replicate measurements to evaluate precision of assay.

PRINCIPLES OF DIAGNOSTIC SERUM ENZYMOLOGY

All the serum enzymes have their origin in cells. Some enzymes are found in many tissues (e.g., lactate dehydrogenase (LD), aldolase (ALS), phosphohexoisomerase (PHI), malate dehydrogenase (MD)). Other enzymes are uniquely concentrated in one or two tissues. For example, ornithine carbamoyl transferase (OCT) and iditol dehydrogenase (ID) are found almost exclusively in the liver; significant amounts of creatine phosphokinase (CPK)* are found only in skeletal muscle, myocardium, and brain. Increase in the serum levels of an enzyme which is ubiquitous in its distribution, however, is a less specific biochemical clue to the site of injury than increased levels of an enzyme normally found in only one or two tissues. In order to enhance the diagnostic value of serum enzymology, attention has been directed to the different molecular forms of a given enzyme (isoenzyme) that may be found in different tissues. Some of the enzymes for which multiple molecular forms have been identified are listed in Table 12-5. Isoenzymes of amylase, alkaline phosphatase (ALP), acid phosphatase, glutamate oxalacetate transaminase (GOT)—now called aspartate aminotransferase (AST)—leucine aminopeptidase (LAP), LD, MD, isocitric dehydrogenase (ICD), creatine phosphokinase (CPK), cholinesterase, and other enzymes have been demonstrated in different tissues and are of interest to the biochemist, physiologist, geneticist, and clinical investigator. Only the isoenzymes of the LD, CK, and ALP, however, have been of important clinical relevance. These are discussed and the types of methods available for their demonstration are listed in a subsequent portion of this chapter. Some enzymes are found in the cytoplasm of cells and reach the plasma with relatively slight injury (LD, ALS). Enzymes that are found only in mitochondria (e.g., glutamate dehydrogenase) gain entry to the serum as the result of sufficient injury to those organelles. At present, the efforts to define the organelle injury by corre-

*Preferred name—creatine kinase (CK).

Table 12-5. SOME ENZYMES* FOR WHICH ISOENZYME FORMS HAVE BEEN DEMONSTRATED

α-Glycerophosphate dehydrogenase
LD
MD
ICD
GPD
6-PGD
Peroxidase
AST (GOT)
CK (CPK)
Phosphoglucomutase (PGM)
Esterases
Acetylcholinesterase
Cholinesterase (CHS)
ALP
ACP
5'-N
LAP
Ceruloplasmin
RNAse
Amylase (AMS)
γ-Glutamyl transferase (GGT)

*See Table 12-1 for meaning of abbreviations.

lation of the intracellular source of the enzyme with the serum levels are of investigative rather than clinical relevance.

The use of serum enzymes as diagnostic aids has been largely empirical; but the values observed in clinical and experimental circumstances permit speculative analysis of the factors that lead to abnormal levels in diseased subjects (Table 12-6). The serum levels of a particular enzyme may be increased in diseases that lead to increased rates of release from tissue, increased amount available for release, or decreased rate of disposition. The levels of an enzyme may be decreased in disease that interferes with its production.

Increased rate of release is clearly responsible for the high serum levels of hepatic, pancreatic, and myocardial enzymes in diseases that produce necrosis of the respective tissue. The pattern of abnormality of serum enzyme values that results depends on the normal enzyme content of the tissue involved, on the extent and type of necrosis, and on other poorly understood factors. Thus, high serum levels of a number of digestive enzymes are found in acute pancreatitis, and a number of enzymes of intermediary metabolism are found in myocardial infarction or acute hepatitis. Although these enzymes are richly concentrated in both liver and myocardium, higher levels are produced by hepatitis than

Table 12-6. HYPOTHETICAL MECHANISMS FOR ABNORMAL SERUM ENZYME LEVELS

MECHANISM	EXAMPLE	ENZYMES	COMMENTS
I. Increased serum levels			
A. Increased release			
1. Necrosis	Myocardial infarction	AST (GOT), LD, ALS, MD, GR, CK, HBD, RNase, and others	
	Acute hepatitis	AST (GOT), ALT (GPT), OCT, ICD, ID, GD, LD, ALS, PHI, MD, ALP, LAP, and others	Increased levels of some enzymes (ALP) may represent increased production as well as release from necrotic cells and decreased excretion
	Acute pancreatitis	Amylase, lipase, lecithinase, trypsin, DNase I	
2. Increased permeability; cell membranes without necrosis	Progressive muscular dystrophy, delirium tremens, dermatomyositis	CK, ALS, LD, PHI, MD, AST (GOT), ALT (GPT)	
B. Increased tissue source of enzymes; Increased release from tissue or both	Neoplastic disease (carcinoma, lymphoma), granulocytic leukemia	LD, ALS, PHI, MD, GR, glucuronidase	
	Megaloblastic Anemia	LD, ALS, PHI, MD	May be result of increased numbers of megaloblasts, increased intramedullary destruction, or both
	Osteoblastic lesions (Paget's disease, osteogenic sarcoma, healing fractures, rickets, etc.)	ALP, ATPase	
	Peptic ulcer	Pepsinogen	
C. Impaired excretion of enzyme	Uremia	Amylase	Elevated amylase levels secondary to renal failure rare and of uncertain origin
	Obstructive jaundice	ALP, LAP, 5-N, GGT	Increased production main factor in increased levels of ALP in obstructive jaundice.
II. Decreased serum levels			
A. Decreased formation			
1. Genetic	Hypophosphatasia	ALP	
	Wilson's disease	Ceruloplasmin	
	Acholinesterasemia	Pseudocholinesterase	
2. Acquired	Hepatitis	Pseudocholinesterase	
	Starvation	Amylase (AMS)	
B. Enzyme inhibition	Insecticide poisoning	Pseudocholinesterase	
C. Lack of cofactors	Pregnancy?	AST	
	Cirrhosis?		? Pyridoxine deficiency or defective pyridoxine metabolism

by myocardial infarction, presumably because the necrosis and degeneration of hepatitis are diffuse and those of infarction, discrete.

High serum levels of enzymes* in which

liver is uniquely rich (ALT or GPT, OCT, ID) are produced almost exclusively by acute hepatic disease. The minimal degree of elevation of serum ICD levels in myocardial infarction, despite the rich myocardial content of this enzyme, has been attributed to the rapid re-

*See Table 12-1 for meaning of abbreviations.

moval of this enzyme from the circulation. The relatively slight increase of LD levels in hepatic necrosis, despite the high hepatic content of this enzyme, remains to be explained adequately. Conceivably, it may relate to the simultaneous release of an inhibitor of LD.

Increased rate of release of enzyme into the circulation may occur even without apparent tissue necrosis. Increased permeability of cell membranes seems to account for the elevated serum levels of aldolase, CK, and other enzymes in progressive muscular dystrophy. The high serum levels of CPK, GOT, ALS, PHI, LD, and MD in patients with delirium tremens or alcoholic myopathy, but without recognizable liver disease, also may depend upon increased permeability of skeletal muscle membrane.

An increase in the tissue source of enzymes because of increased rate of production per cell or increase in the number of cells may be responsible for increased serum levels. This seems to be the mechanism for the increased levels of pepsinogen, ALP, and acid phosphatase in patients with peptic ulcer, osteoblastic bone lesions, and prostatic carcinoma, respectively. The serum levels of glycolytic and other enzymes associated with neoplastic diseases seem to reflect the total mass of tumor. There is evidence that the increased ALP levels of the serum in obstructive jaundice are primarily the result of increased hepatic production of the enzyme, although decreased biliary excretion may play a role.

Impaired disposition of serum enzymes has been considered to contribute to the increased levels of ALP and AST (GOT) in biliary obstruction and for increased amylase levels in renal failure. Evidence for this thesis is lacking. Experimental studies with the "LDH" agent suggest that the mechanism by which this virus causes increased serum levels of LD in mice is by interfering with the uptake of the enzyme by the reticuloendothelial system (Zimmerman, 1970).

Abnormally low levels of some serum enzymes are also observed, presumably as the result of decreased synthesis. Levels of cholinesterase and cholesterol esterase may be low in hepatic disease; levels of amylase are low in chronic hepatic or pancreatic disease or in starvation; levels of pepsinogen are low in gastric mucosal atrophy; levels of ALP are low in hypophosphatasia; and levels of ceruloplasmin are low in Wilson's disease.

The selection of serum enzyme tests for clinical use has depended on historical circumstance, the experience gained in correlating the values with other measures of disease, and the technical ease of performing the respective procedure. A serum enzyme, the diagnostic value of which has been established for a clinical setting, is not likely to be supplanted by a subsequently discovered one, unless the diagnostic usefulness of the more recent candidate is far superior to that of its predecessor. Alkaline phosphatase, a time-honored aid for the diagnosis of hepatobiliary disease, has not been replaced by leucine aminopeptidase,[*] or 5′-nucleotidase,[*] despite recent reports of the diagnostic advantages of the latter two enzymes. Ornithine carbamoyl transferase[*] and iditol dehydrogenase,[*] more recent arrivals than ALT (GPT) to the serum enzyme scene, have not replaced the latter as measures of hepatic disease, despite reports of somewhat greater specificity.

The serum enzymes discussed in detail in this chapter are those which have been of the greatest clinical usefulness or interest in the past or which hold the most promise. Particular attention is given to the phosphatases, transaminases (aminotransferases), lactate dehydrogenase and its isoenzymes, and cholinesterase. Many of the other serum enzymes are described, and their clinical relevance is discussed briefly.

PHOSPHATASES

The phosphatases of the blood, more properly called phosphomonoesterases or orthophosphoric ester monohydrolases, include two main types. The "alkaline phosphatase" has a pH optimum of approximately 9, while the "acid phosphatase" has its optimal activity at a pH of approximately 5. Although there is evidence that alkaline and acid phosphatases each include several different enzymes (isoenzymes), it has been convenient for clinical purposes to consider each a single enzyme.

Alkaline Phosphatase (EC 3.1.3.1). The application of ALP determination to the study of hepatic disease is discussed in Chapter 11. The demonstration that bone is rich in alkaline phosphatase and that normal plasma (or serum) contains the same or a similar enzyme led to the study of serum ALP levels in patients with diseases of bone. Elevated levels of

---

[*]See later section of chapter for description of these enzymes.

Table 12–7. CONDITIONS IN WHICH THE SERUM ALKALINE
PHOSPHATASE LEVEL IS INCREASED*

HEPATOBILIARY DISEASE		BONE DISEASE		OTHER CONDITIONS	
Obstructive jaundice	↑↑↑	Osteitis deformans	↑↑↑	Healing fractures	↑
Biliary cirrhosis	↑↑↑	Rickets	↑↑	Normal growth	↑
Intrahepatic cholestasis	↑↑↑	Osteomalacia	↑↑	Pregnancy (last trimester)	↑
Space-occupying lesions	↑↑	Hyperparathyroidism	↑↑		
(granuloma, abscess, metastatic		Metastatic bone disease	↑↑		
carcinoma)		Osteogenic sarcoma	↑↑↑		
Viral hepatitis	↑				
Infectious mononucleosis	↑↑				
Cirrhosis (alcoholic)	↑				

*Degree of increase indicated by number of arrows.
Depressed values: hypophosphatasia, malnutrition.

the enzyme occur in patients with bone diseases characterized by increased osteoblastic activity (Table 12-7). These include osteitis deformans, rickets, osteomalacia, hyperparathyroidism, healing fractures, and osteoblastic bone tumors, both primary and secondary. Growing children and pregnant women in the third trimester have "physiologically" elevated serum ALP levels.

Lower than normal levels are observed in patients with hypophosphatasia (an inborn error of metabolism), and in malnourished patients.

The alkaline phosphatase determination is useful in the recognition of diseases of bone, especially osteitis deformans, hyperparathyroidism, and bone neoplasms. Hepatic disease as a cause of serum ALP elevation usually can be distinguished by other laboratory procedures and clinical features. The increased levels of this enzyme in normal, growing children should be kept in mind when attempting to apply the serum alkaline phosphatase levels to diagnosis.

ISOENZYMES OF ALKALINE PHOSPHATASE. Studies of the properties of ALP isolated from various tissues (liver, bone, spleen, kidney, intestine) indicate that each differs from the others. Total serum ALP in normals consists of isoenzymes contributed by liver, bone, and, in some individuals, intestine. During the last trimester of pregnancy 40 to 65 per cent of the serum ALP derives from placenta. Isoenzymes from these four sources have been distinguished from each other by electrophoretic analysis, differential inhibition by chemicals and heat, and immunochemically, although there are also differences in substrate dependence and reaction kinetics.

The degrees of inhibition of isoenzymes of hepatic, osseous, intestinal, and placental origin produced by heating to 56°C. for 15 minutes, exposure to 3 M urea for 18 minutes, incubation with 5×10^{-3} M L-phenylalanine, and the relative electrophoretic migration of these isoenzymes are shown in Table 12-8. (Note that the Regan isoenzyme, found in the serum of about 5 per cent of patients with

Table 12–8. CHARACTERISTICS OF ISOENZYME OF ALKALINE PHOSPHATASE

SOURCE OF ENZYME	INHIBITION* BY		ORDER ANODAL MIGRATION
	L-Phenylalanine§ (%)	Heat† or Urea‡ (%)	
Liver	10	60	1
Bone	10	90	2
Intestine	75	60	4
Placenta	80	0	3
Regan (carcinoma)	80	0	3

*Approximate figures.
†56°C for 15 minutes.
‡3M concentration
§L-Phenylalanine (5×10^{-3} M)

carcinomas of various types, resembles the placental ALP). These properties are helpful in identifying placental and intestinal ALP (both phenylalanine-inhibited) and in distinguishing them from hepatic and bone isoenzymes. Distinction of hepatic from osseous ALP is aided by heat or urea inhibition, but the overlapping effects lead to imprecision. Nevertheless, the susceptibility of the osseous isoenzyme to heat inactivation has been applied quite widely to distinguish it from hepatic isoenzyme. Electrophoretic analysis of ALP isoenzymes employing acrylamide gel will also, in most instances, permit identification of the main isoenzyme contributing to an elevated level. Quantitation of the fractions, however, is prevented by the lack of distinct separation of the two rapidly moving isoenzymes (hepatic and osseous). None of the physicochemical methods employed is reliable in distinguishing between hepatocellular and posthepatic jaundice as a cause of elevated ALP levels, although an isoenzyme which migrates more slowly than any of the others has been described in the serum of patients with posthepatic jaundice. Regular clinical application of ALP isoenzymology, however, must await improved means of quantitation of the individual isoenzymes and extensive testing of quantitative values in clinical circumstances (Gorman, 1977).

As discussed in Chapter 11, the probable hepatic origin of an elevated serum ALP level can be recognized by assay of LAP, 5'-N, or GGT activity. Values for these enzymes are high in patients whose hepatobiliary disease leads to high ALP levels but not in those with bone disease responsible for this increased phosphatase value.

Study of placental ALP has yielded interesting data. It appears in plasma at the beginning of the second trimester of pregnancy, rises to a maximum during the third trimester, when it contributes 40 to 65 per cent of ALP activity, and then declines to normal during the first postpartum month.

Acid Phosphatase (ACP) (EC 3.1.3.2). This enzyme, first demonstrated in the urine in 1925, was found to be much more prevalent in male than in female urine. It was soon shown that prostatic tissue contains this enzyme in high concentration. Another acid phosphatase, which differs from that found in the prostate (Table 12-9), is present in erythrocytes and platelets. The methods used for determination of acid phosphatase are similar

Table 12-9. EFFECT OF INHIBITORS ON ACID PHOSPHATASE OF PROSTATE AND OTHER TISSUES*

INHIBITOR	INHIBITION OF PROSTATIC PHOSPHATASE	INHIBITION OF ERYTHROCYTE PHOSPHATASE
L(+)—Tartaric acid acid 0.02 M	+	−
Formaldehyde 2%	−	+
Cupric sulfate 0.001 M	−	+

* + represents marked inhibition
  − represents minimal inhibition

to and include the same substrates as those used for alkaline phosphatase assay.

Elevated serum levels of acid phosphatase (ACP) are seen in patients with prostatic carcinoma that has metastasized. One half to three fourths of patients with carcinoma of the prostate that has extended beyond the capsule have elevated acid phosphatase levels. Patients with prostatic carcinoma still confined within the capsule usually have normal serum levels of this enzyme. However, patients with benign prostatic hypertrophy may have slight elevations of the serum ACP level after vigorous prostatic "massage." Since other tissues, such as erythrocytes, may also release acid phosphatase into the serum, minor elevations of enzyme levels may reflect such an origin rather than the prostate. Accordingly, efforts have been made to distinguish "prostatic" ACP from the isoenzymes that are of erythrocyte and other origin. The efforts to distinguish "prostatic" acid phosphatase from erythrocyte acid phosphatase have been based on the differential effect of various substrates and various inhibitors on enzymes from these two sources (Table 12-9). The inhibition of prostatic acid phosphatase by tartrate and the lack of inhibition by cupric ion, compared with the lack of inhibition of erythrocyte ACP by tartrate and the inhibition by cupric ion, are the properties most commonly utilized (Table 12-9). Acid phosphatase (ACP) released from platelets, however, resembles prostatic enzyme in its response to inhibitors (Wilkinson, 1976).

Elevations of the serum ACP using the method of Bodansky (β-glycerophosphate as substrate) usually reflect carcinoma of the prostate (as discussed previously), especially if the levels exceed 5 Bodansky units. When the method of Gutman (phenylphosphate as substrate) or the King-Armstrong method is used, other diseases may yield abnormal levels occasionally. Such elevations are frequent in Gaucher's disease and occasional in osteitis deformans.

Acid phosphatase (ACP) determination has been useful in detecting metastases from carcinoma of the prostate. As a diagnostic clue to the presence of resectable carcinoma of the prostate, however, it is of no value.

Schumann (1976) has confirmed that quantitative ACP determination of vaginal specimens may substantiate the allegation of rape with respect to time.

Leucine Aminopeptidase (LAP)
(EC 3.4.1.1)

A number of peptidases have been identified in the serum of patients with various diseases. One of these, leucine aminopeptidase (LAP, naphthylamidase*), has been studied more extensively than the others. Elevated levels of this serum enzyme have been reported in most types of hepatobiliary disease. These include hepatitis, cirrhosis, obstructive jaundice, metastatic carcinoma of the liver, and pancreatitis. Patients with carcinoma of the pancreas have increased levels only if obstructive jaundice or metastases of the liver have developed. The elevated values observed during the last trimester of pregnancy appear to be of placental origin. Although several isoenzymes of LAP have been identified, there has been no clinical application of LAP isoenzymology.

The serum values for this enzyme in patients with hepatobiliary disease appear to parallel those of alkaline phosphatase, with the highest levels in obstructive biliary disease and only moderately elevated levels in hepatocellular injury. Values for LAP, however, are normal in patients with bone disease. This has led to the suggestion that distinction between osseous and hepatobiliary disease as a cause of elevated alkaline phosphatase levels can be provided by assay of LAP activity. Differentiation between the high alkaline phosphatase levels of hepatobiliary disease and those of osseous disease, however, can usually be re-

solved by clinical and other criteria; LAP determination has enjoyed a limited popularity.

5'-Nucleotidase (5'-N)
(EC 3.1.3.5)

A serum esterase that has been the subject of a number of recent reports is 5'-nucleotidase. Introduced as a measure for the differentiation of obstructive from hepatocellular jaundice and of hepatobiliary from osseous disease, 5'-N has been the subject of a number of studies. The effects of disease on serum levels of 5'-N are similar to those on LAP. The highest values are observed in patients with posthepatic jaundice, intrahepatic cholestasis, and infiltrative lesions of the liver. Relatively slightly elevated levels are observed in patients with hepatocellular disease. Values in patients with osseous disease, like those of LAP, are normal. Measurement of 5'-N also has been proposed as a diagnostic aid, more specific than alkaline phosphatase, in patients with hepatobiliary disease. In our experience this enzyme test has been less sensitive than alkaline phosphatase as a measure of obstructive biliary disease. Other workers have found it of more value in this clinical setting.

Gamma-glutamyl transferase
(gamma-glutamyl
transpeptidase, GGT)
(EC 2.3.2.1)

This enzyme catalyzes the transfer of a γ-glutamyl group from a γ-glutamyl peptide to another peptide or an amino acid. Kidney, and to a lesser extent, liver and pancreas, are rich in GGT. A number of other tissues contain small amounts. Although several isoenzymes of GGT have been demonstrated, the isoenzymology of this enzyme has found no clinical application.

The chief clinical value of measuring GGT is in the study of hepatobiliary disease. Values parallel those of ALP, LAP, and 5'-N in obstructive (posthepatic) jaundice and infiltrative disease of the liver. Accordingly, assay of GGT, like that of 5'-N and LAP, serves as an estimate of the level of the hepatic isoenzyme of ALP. Since GGT is a microsomial enzyme, its tissue levels increase in response to microsomal enzyme induction. This phenomenon may explain the elevated serum levels in chronic alcoholics and in patients taking drugs (e.g., phenytoin) known to induce the microsomal enzyme system (Rosalki, 1975).

---

* Recent usage has favored the term "naphthylamidase" rather than LAP, since the enzyme is usually assayed by employing an acyl-β-naphthylamide as substrate.

Serum GGT has thus been advocated in the evaluation of patients with alcoholism.

AMINOTRANSFERASES (TRANSAMINASES)

The application of serum aminotransferases (transaminases) to the study of hepatic disease and the principles of assay for these enzymes are discussed in Chapter 11. Aspartate aminotransferase (AST) or glutamate oxalacetate transaminase (GOT) levels of the serum are elevated in patients with hepatobiliary disease, cardiovascular disease, muscle disease, and some miscellaneous conditions. Alanine aminotransferase (ALT), formerly known as glutamate pyruvate transaminase (GPT), levels are elevated in the serum of patients with hepatic disease. In other conditions elevations are negligible unless there is hepatic involvement.

Aspartate Aminotransferase (AST) or Glutamate Oxalacetate Transaminase (EC 2.6.1.1).* This enzyme is elevated in diseases involving the tissues that are rich in it. In Table 12–10 are also shown the tissues with the highest AST concentration, the categories of disease that may show abnormal levels, and the range of values seen in many of these conditions. The AST levels in patients with liver disease are discussed in Chapter 11.

Extensive studies have shown that many patients with acute myocardial infarction have elevated serum AST (GOT) levels, if measured at the proper interval after infarction. (West, 1966). The values are usually 4 to 10 times the upper limit of normal. These usually develop within 12 hours of the time of infarction and reach the peak by the second day; the levels usually return to normal by the fifth day after infarction (Fig. 12–6). Secondary rises may reflect extension or recurrence of myocardial infarction. Experimental work with animals suggests that the degree of rise of serum AST (GOT) is related to the extent of myocardial necrosis.

Our experience confirms that of Galen (1975a); in the laboratory diagnosis of myocardial infarction, creatine phosphokinase (CPK), CPK isoenzymes, lactate dehydrogenase (LD), and LD isoenzyme determinations are suffi-

cient and reliable indicators of myocardial necrosis. Indeed, the combined sensitivity and specificity have resulted in the AST (GOT) being labeled as a redundant cardiac enzyme (Galen, 1975b). Thus, AST (GOT) assays have

Table 12–10. TISSUES RICH IN AST (GOT) AND CONDITIONS IN WHICH THE SERUM ENZYME IS ABNORMAL*

A. Tissue content of AST (GOT) (descending order of concentration)

1. cardiac
2. hepatic
3. skeletal muscle
4. kidney
5. brain
6. pancreas
7. spleen
8. lung
9. serum

	Usual Values U/l
B. Conditions in which serum AST (GOT) is elevated	
1. *Cardiac disease*	
myocardial infarction	20–200
pericarditis	<100
cardiac arrhythmias	<200
acute rheumatic fever (?)	<100
postcardiac surgery and catheterization	<100
heart failure	<100
2. *Hepatic disease*	
acute hepatitis (viral, toxic)	500–4000
infectious mononucleosis	50–800
cirrhosis	<100
hepatic congestion	<100
space-occupying lesions (granuloma, metastatic carcinoma)	<200
obstructive jaundice	<200
3. *Other diseases*	
shock	20–1000
pulmonary infarction	<50
acute pancreatitis	20–1000
renal infarction (experimental animals)	<200
cerebral necrosis	<50
dermatomyositis	<200
progressive muscular dystrophy	<100
delirium tremens	<100
hemolysis (slight)	<50
gangrene (slight)	<50
C. Conditions in which serum AST (GOT) is depressed	
1. Pregnancy	0–6

*In acute hepatitis, values above 300 U/l are usual and above 500 are frequent. In all the other conditions shown the levels are usually below this value, although higher values are occasionally observed in infectious mononucleosis and shock. Almost all patients with acute myocardial infarction have elevated values during the first few days. In the other cardiac diseases listed, elevations are less frequent and usually are slight.

---

*Currently accepted nomenclature for the glutamate oxalacetate transaminase (GOT) is *aspartate transaminase* or *aspartate aminotransferase* (AST). The term GOT is used interchangeably, since it is still the one that is understood most widely in the U.S.A.

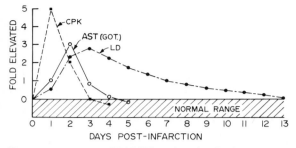

Figure 12–6. CPK, AST (GOT), and LD levels after myocardial infarction (means of values for 200 patients). Note that the CPK rise is earliest, the LD rise is latest, and the LD elevations are present longer than those of CPK and AST (GOT).

been discontinued in our hospital for the laboratory diagnosis of myocardial infarction.

In patients with electrocardiographic and clinical criteria of "coronary insufficiency" rather than myocardial infarction, elevated serum AST (GOT) levels may occur. It is not clear whether this phenomenon represents myocardial necrosis which has not been recognized by other means or "leakage" of the enzyme into the serum even without frank myocardial necrosis.

Mild elevations of the serum AST (GOT) levels have been reported in some patients with pulmonary infarction. The incidence has varied from 0 to 30 per cent, and the elevations are slight to moderate. Animal studies have also yielded inconclusive results on the occurrence of elevated serum AST (GOT) levels in experimental pulmonary infarction. The incidence of increased values in humans is low, the degree of abnormality slight, and the rise delayed for three to five days after the onset of pain.

In patients with congestive heart failure and in those with marked tachycardia, mild to moderate degrees of AST (GOT) elevation may occur. These have been attributed to the hepatic necrosis secondary to hepatic congestion. Patients with pericarditis have also been reported to have a 50 per cent incidence of slightly elevated AST (GOT) levels. The incidence and mechanism of occurrence of elevated enzyme levels in patients with rheumatic fever are not clear. Slight serum AST (GOT) elevations have been reported after cardiac catheterization and mitral commissurotomy (Galen, 1975a).

Determination of AST (GOT) or other enzyme levels is not necessary for the diagnosis of myocardial infarction in most patients with classic clinical and electrocardiographic evidence of this condition. Enzyme determinations are of value in patients whose electrocardiographic changes are insufficiently helpful, e.g., those with left bundle branch block or Wolff-Parkinson-White syndrome or in those with electrocardiographic abnormalities remaining from previous infarction, which may obscure acute changes. Measurement of serum enzymes is also of value in recognizing the recurrence or extension of an infarction during convalescence. Normal values obtained at the proper time are of value in excluding a diagnosis of myocardial infarction.

Patients with disease or injury producing inflammation or destruction of skeletal muscle may also have elevated serum AST (GOT) levels. Patients with progressive muscular dystrophy, dermatomyositis, and trichinosis may have elevated levels, while those with amyotrophic lateral sclerosis, myasthenia gravis, and nerve section do not. Gangrene of the extremities and surgical or other trauma may produce slight AST elevations. In less than 50 per cent of patients with cerebrovascular accidents serum AST elevations may be found.

Elevated serum AST levels in patients with hepatic disease are discussed in Chapter 11. In acute pancreatitis, levels may be elevated. It has been suggested that obstruction of the biliary tree by the edematous pancreas and the presence of associated hepatic disease or of delirium tremens may contribute to the elevated AST levels in these patients.

Alanine Aminotransferase (ALT) or Glutamate Pyruvate Transaminase (E.C. 2.6.1.2). * This enzyme is also discussed in Chapter 11. In patients with myocardial infarction, elevations of the serum levels of ALT (GPT) are slight or absent. Heart failure or shock with the attendant hepatic necrosis, however, may lead to elevated ALT (GPT) levels. The chief application of determination of this serum enzyme is in the diagnosis of hepatocellular destruction.

GLYCOLYTIC ENZYMES

The glycolytic pathway, which is found in virtually all tissues, includes a number of enzymes (Fig. 12–7). Almost all of these have been demonstrated in the serum. In patients

---

*The currently accepted term for glutamate pyruvate transaminase is *alanine aminotransferase* (ALT).

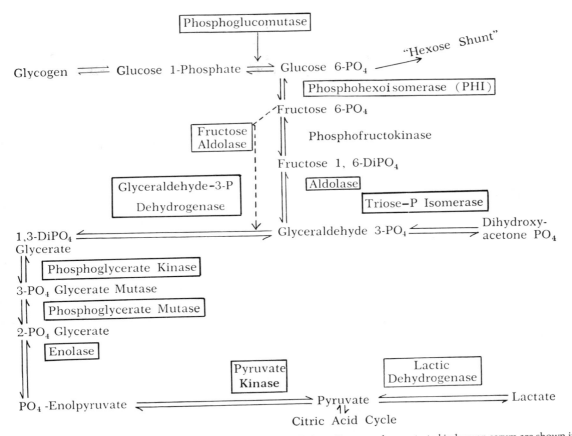

Figure 12–7. Scheme of glycolytic pathway of carbohydrate metabolism. Enzymes demonstrated in human serum are shown in boxes.

with extensive carcinoma, elevated levels of several of these enzymes (phosphohexo-isomerase, aldolase, and lactate dehydrogenase) have been observed. These elevations have served as a guide to chemotherapy, particularly in carcinoma of the breast and prostate.

Elevated levels of these enzymes also have been observed in patients with megaloblastic and hemolytic anemias and in granulocytic and acute leukemias but not in patients with chronic lymphocytic leukemia, aplastic anemia, or iron deficiency anemia. The most extensively studied of the glycolytic enzymes in the serum are lactate dehydrogenase (LD), aldolase ALS, and phosphohexoisomerase (PHI). The serum levels of all three are elevated to approximately the same degree in patients with extensive carcinomatosis, megaloblastic anemia, granulocytic leukemia, infectious mononucleosis, hemolytic states, and myocardial infarction (Table 12–11). Levels of

PHI seem to reflect carcinomatosis more sensitively, and those of LD seem to be a more sensitive reflection of megaloblastic anemia than are those of the other two. Aldolase is the most sensitive of the three as a reflector of

Table 12–11. RELATIVE SENSITIVITY OF GLYCOLYTIC ENZYME LEVELS TO VARIOUS TYPES OF DISEASES

	LD	ALS	PHI
Myocardial infarction	↑↑	↑↑	↑↑
Pulmonary infarction	↑	↑	↑
Carcinoma, granulocytic leukemia	↑↑	↑↑	↑↑↑
Megaloblastic anemia	↑↑↑	↑↑	↑↑
Hepatic necrosis	↑ or N	↑↑↑	↑↑↑
Muscle disease	↑↑	↑↑↑↑	↑↑

muscle diseases (progressive muscular dystrophy, trichinosis, and dermatomyositis). Levels of ALS and PHI are much more strikingly elevated than those of LD in patients with hepatic necrosis. Indeed, the very insensitivity of the serum LD level to parenchymal hepatic damage coupled with its sensitivity as a measure of carcinomatosis enhances its usefulness for the recognition of metastatic or primary carcinoma of the liver. Other glycolytic enzymes have not been studied sufficiently to delineate their value in clinical circumstances.

Phosphohexoisomerase (PHI) (EC 5.3.1.9). This glycolytic enzyme catalyzes the conversion of glucose-6-phosphate to fructose-6-phosphate (Fig. 12–7). First studied in the serum of tumorous rats by Warburg and Christian, PHI levels of the serum have been investigated in patients with carcinoma and other diseases during the past few years.

The activity of PHI is assayed by using glucose-6-phosphate as substrate. The rate of formation of fructose-6-phosphate using the Seliwanoff reaction (resorcinol) is a measure of PHI activity.

Phosphohexoisomerase levels have been used as an index of metastases in patients with carcinoma of the breast and prostate and to monitor the response to therapy. Other diseases in which elevations are observed are

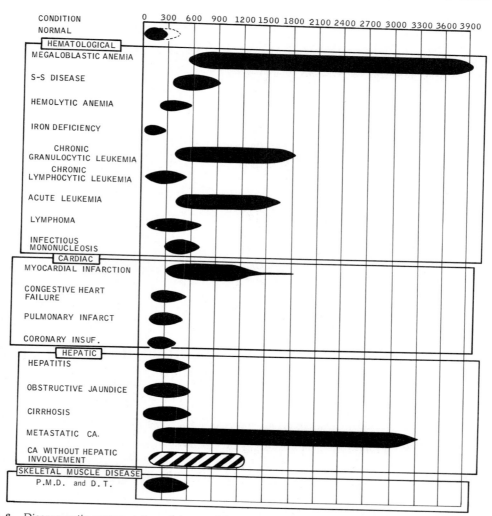

Figure 12–8. Diagrammatic representation of lactate dehydrogenase values (U/l or Units/liter) in normals (dotted line represents higher values in children) and in various diseases. Equivalent degrees of elevation of ALS and PHI occur in all these conditions with the exceptions of megaloblastic anemia, in which levels of LD are relatively higher, and acute hepatitis, in which levels of LD are relatively lower than those of PHI and ALS. Values for ALS are higher than those of PHI and LD in muscle disease.

listed in Tables 12-1 and 12-11. Determination of this serum enzyme, however, has not been applied extensively to clinical medicine.

Aldolase (EC 4.1.2.13). This glycolytic enzyme catalyzes the cleavage of fructose-1-6-diphosphate into two triose molecules (glyceraldehyde phosphate and dihydroxyacetone phosphate) (Fig. 12-7). Several methods have been devised for this assay, based on the rate at which the trioses are formed. One involves measuring the colored dinitrophenylhydrazone.

Serum aldolase (ALS) levels are elevated in skeletal muscle disease, carcinomatosis, granulocytic leukemia, megaloblastic anemia, hepatitis, other types of hepatic necrosis, and the other conditions that are listed in Figure 12-8 and Tables 12-1 and 12-11. The aldolase levels reflect particularly sensitively progressive muscular dystrophy and inflammatory muscle disease (dermatomyositis, trichinosis), in which strikingly elevated values can be seen. Patients destined to develop progressive muscular dystrophy usually have elevated aldolase levels before any overt clinical manifestation of muscle disease. The chief clinical application of aldolase assay in the United States has been in the study of muscle disease. In other parts of the world and in a few laboratories in the United States, aldolase levels are employed as sensitive measures of hepatic disease and in the study of neoplastic disease.

LACTATE DEHYDROGENASE (LD) (EC 1.1.1.27)

This enzyme catalyzes the reversible oxidation of lactate to pyruvate (Fig. 12-7). It is widely distributed in mammalian tissues, being rich in myocardium, kidney, liver, and muscle.

METHODS. Spectrophotometric, fluorometric, and colorimetric methods have been applied to the assay of this enzyme. In the spectrophotometric method, the rate of change in concentration of NADH (DPNH) is determined. The reaction may be measured by following the disappearance of NADH (pyruvate + NADH $\xrightarrow{\text{LD}}$ lactate + NAD) at a pH of 7.4 or by following the appearance of NADH (lactate + NAD $\xrightarrow{\text{LD}}$ pyruvate + NADH) at a pH of 8.8 or higher. The results should be expressed as U/l, that is, μmoles/minute of NADH reacting per liter of specimen assayed (Table 12-4).

Elevated serum levels of LD are observed in a variety of conditions (Fig. 12-8). The highest values (two- to fortyfold elevations) are seen in patients with megaloblastic anemia, in those with extensive carcinomatosis, and in those with severe shock and hypoxia. Moderate elevations (two- to fourfold) occur in patients with myocardial infarction, pulmonary infarction, granulocytic or acute leukemia, hemolytic anemia, infectious mononucleosis, and in patients with progressive muscular dystrophy. Relatively slight elevations occur in patients with hepatitis, obstructive jaundice, or cirrhosis, but higher values occur in those with delirium tremens. Patients with chronic renal disease, especially those with nephrotic syndrome or hemolytic anemia, also have increased values. In patients with myxedema, the LD values are also regularly elevated.

The pattern of elevated serum LD levels in patients with myocardial infarction is quite characteristic. High levels are observed in almost all patients within 24 hours of the apparent onset of infarction. Although the degree of elevation is not so striking as that of AST (GOT), the elevated levels persist longer (10 to 14 days). The characteristically prolonged period of elevated LD values with an increase of LD isoenzymes, i.e., LD_1 higher than LD_2 ("flipped" LD), yields a pattern that is useful in the laboratory diagnosis of myocardial infarction (Galen, 1975a). The "flipped" LD pattern usually appears within 12 to 24 hours and is present within 48 hours in sera of 80 per cent of patients with a myocardial infarction (Galen, 1975a) (Fig. 12-6).

Most patients with pulmonary infarction have elevated levels of LD, usually within 24 hours of the onset of pain. The pattern of normal AST (GOT) and elevated LD levels within one to two days after an episode of chest pain provides suggestive evidence for pulmonary infarction.

Almost all patients with megaloblastic anemia have elevated LD levels. Often the values are strikingly increased. Possible factors in the production of the high values include the large number of megaloblasts, presumably rich in LD, and the intramedullary destruction of these cells. As the anemia responds to treatment, the LD levels return to normal. Hemolytic anemias yield slightly elevated levels. Patients with aplastic and iron deficiency anemias usually have normal values.

Patients with granulocytic and acute leukemia have moderately elevated LD levels. In lymphocytic leukemia, the values are usually normal, unless there is an associated hemolytic state. In patients with lymphosarcoma and Hodgkin's disease, LD levels are normal or moderately elevated, depending on the total mass of tumor and the presence of hemolysis.

Patients and animals with small, localized carcinomas usually have normal serum levels of LD, while those with distant metastases or even local extension have increased levels. The highest values occur in patients with metastases to the liver, although increased levels are also found in some patients with only extrahepatic metastases or extension.

The serum LD level does not provide a sensitive measure of hepatic disease. Patients with viral hepatitis have slightly elevated (one- to twofold) values. In patients with infectious mononucleosis, LD levels are usually somewhat higher, perhaps released from the aggregates of immature mononuclear cells throughout the body. Only slightly increased values are seen in patients with obstructive jaundice and in those with cirrhosis. Interestingly, almost all patients with delirium tremens have increased values, perhaps of skeletal muscle origin, since, like the elevated LD levels of progressive muscular dystrophy, they are accompanied by increased serum levels of creatine phosphokinase (see later).

The large number of conditions in which elevated LD levels are seen detracts somewhat from the diagnostic usefulness of its measurement. The LD level is clinically useful in the recognition of myocardial infarction and pulmonary infarction. It is often a somewhat superfluous clue to extensive carcinomatosis, but it may be used to monitor the course of cancer chemotherapy, since response to therapy is often mirrored by decreasing serum levels. Other clinical applications entail analysis of the clinical problem in the light of conditions known to cause elevated LD levels.

Isoenzymes of Lactate Dehydrogenase. The LD of normal human serum has been found to be separable into five different com-

Table 12–12. PRINCIPLES OF SOME OF THE TECHNIQUES EMPLOYED TO MEASURE ISOENZYMES OF LACTATE DEHYDROGENASE

METHOD	COMMENT	CLINICAL APPLICABILITY
I. Physical		
A. Electrophoretic	Demonstrates the five isoenzymes	Somewhat cumbersome and not sufficiently quantitative, but clinically useful
B. Selective absorption on DEAE cellulose	Selective absorption of fast ($LD_{1,2}$) isoenzymes, leaving slow ($LD_{3,4,5}$)	Remains to be demonstrated
C. Solvent precipitation techniques in which acetone or chloroform is used	Selective precipitation of slow isoenzymes, leaving fast in supernatant	Remains to be demonstrated
D. Heat denaturation at 65° C. for 30 minutes	Destroys activity of all isoenzymes except most rapid (LD_1)	Useful in the diagnosis of myocardial infarction
II. Chemical		
A. Substrate-product relationship		
1. Measurement of ability to dehydrogenate α-hydroxybutyrate dehydrogenase (HBD) activity	1. HBD activity is largely equivalent to LD_1 activity	1. Suitable for demonstrations of approximate LD_1 activity
2. Relative inhibition by various concentrations of pyruvate or lactate	2. Individual isoenzymes show different degrees of inhibition by high pyruvate concentration	2. Of theoretical interest, but no clinical applicability as yet
B. Coenzyme affinity Measurement of relative activity isoenzymes with DPN and its analogues	Each isoenzyme shows characteristic rates of activity with various analogues of NAD	Extremely useful research tool. Remains to be clinically applicable
C. Differential chemical inhibition of LD activity	Individual isoenzymes are characteristically and differentially inhibited by several chemical agents (urea, sulfate, oxamate, chloroform)	No clinical application as yet
III. Immunologic	Specific antibody to LD_1 and another to LD_5	Evolving

ponents by appropriate electrophoretic techniques. Each of these isoenzymes is distinguishable from the others by serologic, electrophoretic, and various other chemical procedures (Table 12-12). Indeed, the great current interest in isoenzymology derives from the observations on the multiple molecular forms of LD. The isoenzymes of LD are designated according to their electrophoretic mobility. The fraction with the greatest mobility (anodic) is called LD_1, the one with least anodic mobility is called LD_5, and the other three are designated accordingly as LD_2, LD_3, and LD_4, respectively.

The five LD isoenzymes have the same molecular weight (135,000) but differ in the charge that they carry. Each isoenzyme is a tetramer made up of four subunits, each of 34,000 molecular weight. There are two types of these subunits, designated H and M, respectively, for heart polypeptide chain (H) and skeletal muscle chain (M). The five isoenzymes of LD consist of the five possible combinations of monomers H and M (Table 12-13). Hence there are two homotetramers (LD_1 and LD_5) and three hybrids. The H and M chains differ significantly in their amino acid composition and thus in their structural and kinetic properties; they are probably under the control of two distinct genes.

Tissue LD consists of the five isoenzymes in varying proportions, and the LD activity of each tissue has a characteristic isoenzyme composition (Table 12-13). Thus, the LD of myocardium and erythrocytes consists largely of the fastest moving isoenzymes (LD_1 and LD_2).

In liver and skeletal muscle, the principal isoenzymes are LD_4 and LD_5. In general, tissues exhibiting aerobic metabolism demonstrate predominantly faster moving isoenzymes (LD_1) with more H subunits, while tissues exhibiting anaerobic metabolism demonstrate predominantly slower moving isoenzymes (LD_5) with more M units. A number of tissues (lung, spleen, pancreas, thyroid, adrenals, and lymph nodes) consist mainly of LD_3. The relative concentration of the several isoenzymes in normal serum is LD_2, LD_1, LD_3, LD_4, and LD_5 in descending order. Normal serum LD has been presumed to derive mainly from erythrocytes with LD_2 higher than LD_1.

Studies of the isoenzyme composition of the elevated serum LD levels of various diseases have revealed abnormal patterns that reflect the tissues involved (Table 12-14). In acute myocardial infarction, the elevated serum LD levels consist largely of LD_1 and LD_2 (classically $LD_1 > LD_2$ or "flipped" LD), the isoenzymes in which myocardium is particularly rich. When lactate dehydrogenase is elevated and the ratio of LD_1 : LD_2 is greater than 1, (LD_1 greater than LD_2 is called "flipped" LDH) three diagnostic possibilities emerge: it is seen after acute myocardial infarction, acute renal infarction, and in hemolysis such as hemolytic anemia. Following acute myocardial infarction, the LD isoenzymes assume the "flip" profile within 12 to 24 hours with LD_1 greater than LD_2. "Flipped LD" is present in 80 per cent of patients with myocardial infarction within 48 hours after the acute episode. It is not necessarily maintained, since it is present in less than half of such patients (who earlier had a flipped LD) at the end of a week even though the serum LD is elevated (Galen, 1975a). Likewise, an increased LD_5 indicates other hepatic or skeletal muscle injury. LD patterns with intermediate hybrid fractions are found in several pathologic

Table 12-13. NOMENCLATURE, COMPOSITION, ISOENZYMES, AND TISSUE SOURCE OF LACTATE DEHYDROGENASE FOUND IN HUMAN SERUM BY ELECTROPHORETIC TECHNIQUES

NOMENCLATURE OF ISOENZYME STARTING WITH MOST ANODIC	COMPOSITION PROPORTION OF MONOMERS* IN EACH ISOENZYME	RELATIVE CONTENT† OF ISOENZYME					
		Myocardium	Liver	Skeletal Muscle	Brain	Kidney	RBC
1	HHHH	+ + + +	±	±	+ +	+	+ + +
2	HHHM	+ + + +	±	±	+ +	+	+ + +
3	HHMM	+	+	+	+ +	+ +	+
4	HMMM	±	+ +	+ +	+ +	+ +	±
5	MMMM	±	+ + + +	+ + + +	±	+ +	±

*Monomer H (myocardial). Monomer M (skeletal muscle).
†Content graded from ±, which represents almost no activity, to + + + +, which represents high activity.

Table 12–14. RELATIVE DEGREE OF INCREASE OF LACTATE DEHYDROGENASE AND PATTERN OF ABNORMALITY OF ISOENZYME IN VARIOUS DISEASES

| DISEASE | RELATIVE DEGREE INCREASE TOTAL LD ACTIVITY | ISOENZYME FRACTION MOST ABNORMAL | | | | |
| | | MOST ANODIC (+) | | | | (−) |
		LD_1	LD_2	LD_3	LD_4	LD_5
Myocardial infarction	↑↑	X	X			
Pulmonary infarction*	↑				X	X
Congestive heart failure	↑				X	X
Viral hepatitis	↑				X	X
Toxic hepatitis	↑				X	X
Cirrhosis	↑				X	X
Leukemia, granulocytic	↑↑		X	X		
Pancreatitis	↑		X	X		
Carcinomatosis (extensive)	↑↑↑		X	X		
Megaloblastic anemia	↑↑↑↑	X	X			
Hemolytic anemia	↑	X	X			
Muscular dystrophy†	↑	X	X			

*In pulmonary infarction, LD_3 may be elevated.

†In muscular dystrophy, LD_1 and LD_2 are elevated only in a relative sense because LD_4 and LD_5 are depressed.

conditions but are less specific than the homotetramer elevations and, thus, are less diagnostic in value. Such patterns are seen in pulmonary embolism as well as in disease states in which levels of all five isoenzymes are increased but their relationship to one another is virtually unchanged (isomorphic elevation). In acute viral hepatitis, the serum LD shows a higher proportion of LD_4 and LD_5 than does the normal. Some of the isoenzyme patterns observed in other diseases are indicated in Table 12–14. The determination of the LD isoenzyme "profile" for the analysis of clinical problems, however, has been employed to only a limited degree. Quantitation of the isoenzymes is difficult and the techniques are too awkward for use in the study of large numbers of sera. Approximations of LD_1, the myocardial isoenzyme, however, may be accomplished by techniques that are as simple as the measurement of total LD activity. Isoenzyme LD_1 resists denaturation at 65°C. for 30 minutes, while the activity of the other four isoenzymes is destroyed under these conditions. Accordingly, the relative amounts of LD_1 can be esti-

mated by comparing the heat-stable LD to the total LD activity. A number of clinical laboratories determine "heat-stable" LD as a relatively routine aid in the diagnosis of acute myocardial infarction. An estimate of the serum level of LD_1 can also be obtained by measuring the level of α-hydroxybutyrate dehydrogenase (HBD). At one time considered to be the activity of a separate enzyme, HBD activity is now recognized to represent that of isoenzymes of LD (largely LD_1 with smaller amounts of other isoenzymes). The measurement of HBD activity is accomplished by a technique similar to that for measuring LD. Measurement of HBD is much less widely employed than that of heat-stable LD for clinical purposes. Electrophoresis employing cellulose acetate or agarose is the best way to determine LD isoenzymes. Fluorescent excitation or tetrazolium reduction by NADH permit visual display and measurement of LD isoenzymes by scanning. Indeed, this has made possible application of LD isoenzymology to clinical problems, especially in evaluation of patients with ischemic heart disease.

THE TRICARBOXYLIC ACID CYCLE

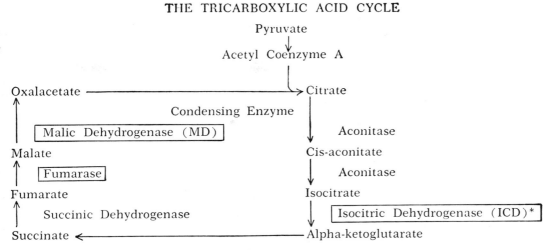

*Strictly speaking, the ICD of the serum differs from that of the citric acid cycle. The ICD demonstrated in the serum is TPN-linked, while that of the citric acid cycle is DPN-linked.

Figure 12–9. The tricarboxylic acid cycle. Scheme of citric acid cycle pathway of carbohydrate metabolism. Enzymes demonstrated in human serum are shown in boxes.

"CITRIC ACID CYCLE" ENZYMES

Several of the enzymes identified in the serum have been considered to be citric acid cycle enzymes (Fig. 12–9) released into the blood. Although they are shown as such in this discussion, this is an oversimplification for convenience. Enzymes of the citric acid cycle are located in the mitochondria, and are less likely to enter the blood than the cytoplasmic enzymes. Furthermore, the isocitrate dehydrogenase (ICD) found in the serum requires NADP as the coenzyme, while the mitochondrial ICD is a NAD-linked enzyme. Malate dehydrogenase activity has been demonstrated in the cytoplasm and mitochondria. Fumarase appears to be a mitochondrial enzyme.

Isocitrate Dehydrogenase (ICD) (EC 1.1.1.42). ICD catalyzes the conversion of isocitric acid to alpha-ketoglutarate. The serum levels have been reported to be increased up to fortyfold in patients with viral hepatitis. Values are moderately elevated in patients with cirrhosis, obstructive jaundice, and metastatic carcinoma of the liver. Carcinoma, even without metastatic involvement, megaloblastic anemia, and congestive heart failure are also associated with mildly elevated levels of this enzyme. Levels have been reported to be normal in patients with myocardial infarction despite the rich content of ICD in the myocardium. Apparently, the myocar-

dial isoenzyme of ICD loses its activity shortly after release into the blood. While ICD levels are sensitive reflections of acute hepatic necrosis, this serum enzyme test has not been widely adopted. It is not so sensitive and is no more specific a test of acute hepatic injury than is GPT. It is likely that this procedure will continue to be of investigative interest rather than a clinical tool.

Malate Dehydrogenase (MD) (EC 1.1.1.37). This enzyme catalyzes the reversible oxidation of malate to oxaloacetate. Elevated values have been observed in patients with myocardial infarction, hepatic necrosis, hemolytic syndromes, megaloblastic anemia, and neoplastic disease. In general, the abnormalities of this enzyme appear to parallel those observed with the glycolytic enzymes, but the degree of abnormality is usually less. This enzyme test is also of investigative rather than clinical usefulness.

HEXOSE "SHUNT" ENZYMES

Several of the enzymes of the hexose monophosphate shunt have been demonstrated in the serum (Fig. 12–10). Reports have appeared on the occurrence of elevated serum levels of glucose-6-phosphate dehydrogenase and of 6-phosphogluconic dehydrogenase in patients with hepatic disease. 5-P-ribose isomerase and transketolase have also been reported to be

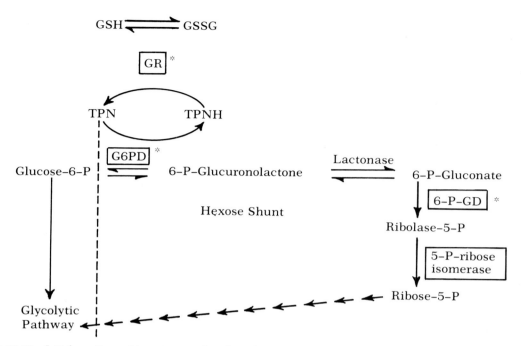

Figure 12-10. Initial reactions of hexose monophosphate shunt showing the rate of generation of TPNH in maintaining reduced glutathione. Enzymes in boxes (GR, G6PD, 6-P-GD, 5-P-ribose isomerase) may be found in serum. Transketolase (not shown) also reported in serum. *Assays performed most frequently on hemolysates of erythrocytes. (After Carson and Frischer, 1966.)

found in the serum; but the clinical significance and applicability of assay of these serum enzymes remain to be established. See Tables 12-1 and 12-2.

CHOLINESTERASE (CHS)

The cholinesterase of the serum (CHS) (EC 3.1.1.8) has been referred to as pseudocholinesterase to distinguish it from the true cholinesterase (AcCHS) (EC 3.1.1.7) of the erythrocytes and nerve tissue. The tissue enzyme acts optimally on acetylcholine and on acetylbetamethyl choline, while the serum enzyme hydrolyzes acetylcholine and other cholinesters even more rapidly (Fig. 12-11; Table 12-15).

Alkylphosphates are potent inhibitors of both serum and tissue cholinesterases. Simplified electrometric, manometric, and colorimetric methods have been devised for cholinesterase assay.

Serum CHS values are characteristically depressed in patients with parenchymatous liver disease, including viral hepatitis, cirrhosis, metastatic carcinoma, the hepatic congestion of heart failure, and amebic hepatitis and abscess. In acute hepatitis, levels of the enzyme are lowest at the peak of the disease. Since, with recovery, the CHS level returns to normal, it has been suggested that the enzyme level may serve as an index of recovery and prognosis. In cirrhosis with jaundice, ascites,

Table 12-15.   SUBSTRATE RELATIONSHIP OF BLOOD CHOLINESTERASES

ENZYME	SOURCE IN BLOOD	SUBSTRATES HYDROLYZED				KINETICS WITH ACETYLCHOLINE	
		Acetyl-choline	Acetylbeta-methylcholine	Butyryl-choline	Benzoyl-choline	Optimal concentration	Inhibition by excess
Acetylcholinesterase (true cholinesterase)	RBC	+	+	−	−	3×10^{-3}	+
Cholinesterase (pseudocholinesterase)	Plasma or serum	+	−	+	+	2×10^{-2}	−

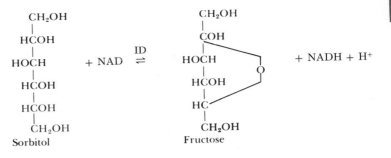

Figure 12–13. Reaction catalyzed by iditol dehydrogenase (ID), principle of method of assay, and conditions in which abnormal values are found.

Method of assay depends on measuring the rate of reduction of coenzyme (NAD), which is measured spectrophotometrically.

Abnormal levels
Acute hepatitis $\uparrow \uparrow \; \uparrow$
Cirrhosis $\uparrow$ or N
Obstructive jaundice $\uparrow$

not completely specific adjunct in the diagnosis of myocardial and muscle disease. Specificity of CPK assay is enhanced by measurement of its isoenzymes.

Isoenzymes (Roberts, 1976). The physiochemical properties of creatine kinase (CK) found in extracts of the human heart, brain, and skeletal muscle (CK_1 or BB) differ. Enzyme in the brain moves most rapidly toward the anode; that in skeletal muscle (CK_3 or MM) moves most slowly. The CK found in myocardium has two components, one moving as slowly as the muscle isoenzyme and the other somewhat faster. The isoenzyme is a dimer; the form found in the brain consists of two similar units, termed accordingly BB or CK_1. The CK found in the muscle consists of two other identical subunits and is called the MM (CK_3) isoenzyme. Myocardial extracts consist mainly of the MM isoenzyme and of another which is the MB (CK_2) isoenzyme. Normal

$$\text{Creatine-P} + \text{ADP} \underset{}{\overset{CK}{\rightleftharpoons}} \text{Creatine} + \text{ATP}$$

Method of assay: Several are available. One depends on measuring creatine-P formed by measuring phosphorus after liberating it. Another involves several coupled reactions in which ADP formed is utilized to convert phosphoenolpyruvate to pyruvate in the presence of pyruvate kinase. Pyruvate formed is measured by following disappearance of NADH (at 340 mμ) under influence of added lactate dehydrogenase.
    Conditions characterized by increased levels:
Progressive muscular dystrophy
Dermatomyosis
Myocardial infarction
Delirium tremens
Crush syndrome
Hypothyroidism

Figure 12–14. Reaction catalyzed by creatine phosphokinase (CK), principle of assay, and significance of abnormal serum levels.

serum CK is virtually 100 per cent CK_3 or MM as is skeletal muscle. Heart yields about 40 per cent CK_2 (MB) and 60 per cent CK_3 (MM). Brain tissue yields about 90 per cent CK_1 or BB and 10 per cent CK_3 or MM. The brain fraction CK_1 (BB) is almost never observed in sera even after cerebrovascular accidents, since the enzyme does not appear to cross the blood-brain barrier (Galen, 1975a). However, CK (BB) has been noted in sera of patients with carcinoma of prostate, colon, lung, and esophagus.

The presence of CK_2 (MB) in sera indicates damage to the myocardium; it is found during the 48-hour period following acute myocardial infarction in all patients (Galen, 1975a). However, it is also found to a lesser degree in patients with severe angina and coronary insufficiency without evidence of infarction. CK_3 (MM) is found in sera of patients with muscle trauma, including intramuscular injections, shock, and postoperatively following major surgical procedures. After acute myocardial infarction, CK_2 (MB) appears within approximately four to eight hours and peaks at 24 hours; it may persist throughout the remainder of the initial 72-hour period. CK_2 (MB) activity never exceeds 40 per cent of the total CK serum activity, with the remainder being CK_3 (MM) (Galen, 1975a). However, CK_3 (MM) level of serum remains elevated for four to five days following the onset of chest pain (Galen, 1975a). CK isoenzyme determinations performed subsequent to day four even with an elevated CK level will reveal only CK_3 (MM) activity, and its origin in heart or muscle cannot be established.

The presence of CK_2 (MB) in the serum is

not 100 per cent specific for myocardium because CK_2 is found in patients with certain muscular dystrophies, polymyositis, and significant myoglobinuria. We emphasize CK_2 (MB) presence qualitatively following electrophoretic separation; the precision leaves much to be desired. Griffiths has recently compared CK isoenzyme MB methods (1977).

At best, electrophoresis is a semiquantitative procedure in which the presence or absence of CK_2 (MB) should suffice. We have found the Corning ACI (agarose film) electrophoresis of CK isoenzyme (catalog No. 470114, Palo Alto, Cal. 94306) acceptable. Interpretation using appropriate fluorometric equipment yields adequate visualization for noting presence or absence of CK_2 (MB).

OTHER SERUM ENZYMES

Many other enzymes have been demonstrated in the serum (Table 12-1). These are too numerous for individual description in this discussion, but there are a few that warrant special mention. These include guanase, an enzyme that has been reported to reflect, sensitively and specifically, hepatic disease; beta glucuronidase, considered a biochemical clue to neoplastic, hepatic, and other diseases; alcohol dehydrogenase, proposed as a measure of hepatic disease; plasma pepsinogen, an enzyme precursor that reflects function and disease of the stomach (high levels in patients with peptic ulcer, low levels in patients with pernicious anemia); and ceruloplasmin, a copper-carrying protein that is also an enzyme and the serum levels of which are depressed in patients with hepatolenticular degeneration (Wilson's disease). Ceruloplasmin measurement is useful in the diagnosis of Wilson's disease. The practical role that the other enzymes cited and others listed in Tables 12-1 and 12-2 may play in clinical medicine remains to be demonstrated.

CLINICAL APPLICATION OF SERUM ENZYME ASSAYS

Serum enzymology provides aid in making the diagnosis, monitoring the course, and demonstrating subclinical evidence of disease. Diseases that are characterized by distinctly abnormal values of one or more enzymes (Table 12-16) can be readily distinguished from clinically similar states in which abnormal values for the respective enzymes do not occur. The diagnostic circumstances that are most clearly aided by serum enzymology are the distinction of myocardial infarction from other causes of chest pain, the differential diagnosis of hepatobiliary and muscle disease, the diagnosis of pancreatitis, and the recognition of metastases of neoplastic disease to bone or liver (Table 12-17).

The diagnostic application of serum enzyme assays is based on the accumulated clinical experience and experimental data that permit formulation of factors that lead to abnormal enzyme levels (Table 12-6) and correlation of particular serum enzymes with the nature of the pathologic process and the organ involved (Table 12-16). This type of assessment serves to epitomize most of the foregoing material. It permits selection of the enzyme tests most likely to be of diagnostic value and of the clinical circumstances most likely to be benefited by current knowledge of serum enzymology. Some disease processes are characterized by abnormal values of one or more enzymes (Table 12-16). Thus, osteoblastic lesions lead to elevations of ALP values that range from slight to marked. Obstruction of the biliary tree (or intrahepatic cholestasis) leads to markedly elevated values of ALP, LAP, 5'-N, and GGT; relatively slightly elevated values of transaminases, OCT, ID, ICD, LD, HBD, MD, ALS, and PHI; and normal values for CK. Hepatic necrosis leads to lesser values of ALP, LAP, 5'-N, and GGT, but very high values of AST (GOT), ALT (GPT), OCT, ID, ICD, MD, ALS, and PHI; and normal values for CK. In myocardial necrosis, moderately elevated levels of AST, LD, HBD, MD, ALS, PHI, and CK are noted. Skeletal muscle disease of the progressively degenerative or inflammatory type (progressive muscular dystrophy, dermatomyositis, trichinosis) leads to striking elevations of CK and LD levels; moderate elevations of LD, ALS, PHI, and MD, with the increase the AST (GOT) level and even lesser values of ALT (GPT) and normal levels of the other enzymes listed in Table 12-16. Neoplastic disease is characterized by increased values of LD, ALS, PHI, and MD, with the increase seemingly dependent on the tumor having reached sufficient total mass. Reports of GGT suggest that this enzyme is also increased in the serum of patients with carcinomatosis. Metastatic carcinoma of the liver leads to moderate or marked elevations of ALP, LAP, 5'-N, and GGT and to slightly or moderately elevated values of AST (GOT) and ALT (GPT).

Table 12–16.   ABNORMAL VALUES OF SOME SERUM ENZYMES IN VARIOUS PATHOLOGIC PROCESSES*

| ENZYME | OSTEO-BLASTIC ACTIVITY | BILIARY OBSTRUCTION | NECROSIS OF | | | | NEOPLASTIC DISEASE† | |
			Liver	Heart	Skeletal Muscle	Pancreas	Neoplastic Growth	Hepatic Metastases
ALP	1-4+	4+	+	−	−	−	−	1-4+
ACP	−	−	−	−	−	−	+(prostate)	
LAP	−	4+	+	−	−	−	−	1-4+
5′-N	−	4+	+	−	−	−	−	1-4+
Gl. TP	−	4+	+	+	−	−	+	1-4+
AST (GOT)	−	+	4+	2+	1+	±	−	2+
ALT (GPT)	−	+	4+	±	±	±	−	1+
ID	−	+	4+	−	−	−	−	1+
ICD	−	+	4+	−	−	−	−	1+
LD	−	+	+	2+	2+	±	3+	3+
HBD	−	±	±	2+	±	±	+	+
MD	−	+	2+	2+	2+	±	2+	2+
ALS	−	+	3+	2+	4+	±	3+	3+
PHI	−	+	3+	2+	2+	±	3+	3+
CPK	−	−	−	4+	4+	−	−	−
Amylase	−	±	−	−	−	4+	−	−
Lipase	−	±	−	−	−	4+	−	−

*1-4+ represents grades of elevated values; − represents values within the expected reference interval.
†Includes granulocytic leukemia.

These abnormalities are also seen with other "space-occupying" lesions of the liver (granuloma, abscess, amyloidosis). The pattern of serum enzyme abnormality of hepatic metastases also includes increased values of enzymes that reflect neoplastic growth. Metastases to various sites from prostatic carcinoma lead to high acid phosphatase levels. Metastases of carcinoma to the bone, if osteoblastic, lead to high alkaline phosphatase levels but to normal values of AST (GOT) and ALT (GPT).

Monitoring the course of disease by serial determinations of serum enzyme levels is useful in the management of hepatitis, in the chemotherapy of neoplastic disease, and in the recognition of recurrent infarction or other complications during the convalescence from acute myocardial infarction. Detection of sub-clinical disease by serum enzyme assay is exemplified by the use of serum aldolase or CK levels to recognize individuals destined to develop progressive muscular dystrophy, or the employment of AST, ALT, and alkaline phosphatase to monitor patients exposed to known or potentially hepatotoxic agents. In Table 12–17 are shown the patterns of abnormality obtained in various clinical circumstances utilizing a small panel of enzyme tests.

SERUM ENZYMES IN MYOCARDIAL INFARCTION

Serum enzyme analysis has become as routine a measure as electrocardiography in the diagnostic approach to patients suspected of having sustained a myocardial infarction. Dis-

Table 12-17. PATTERNS OF ABNORMAL SERUM ENZYME VALUES IN SEVERAL CLINICAL SETTINGS*

		AST (GOT)	ALT (GPT)	LD	LD₁ (HEAT STABLE) (HBD)	CK or CPK	ALS	AL
CHEST PAIN AND RELATED CIRCUMSTANCES	Myocardial infarction	↑↑	±	↑↑	↑↑	↑↑↑	↑↑	N
	Pulmonary infarction	±	±	↑↑	±	±	↑↑	N
	Heart failure	±	±		±	±	↑	↑
	Shock	↑↑	↑	↑↑	±	±	↑↑	N
MUSCLE DISEASE	Progressive muscular dystrophy / Trichinosis / Dermatomyositis / Polymyositis / Delirium tremens	↑↑	↑	↑↑	↑	↑↑↑	↑↑↑	N
	Neurogenic muscle disease	N	N	N	N	N	N	N
JAUNDICE (SEE CHAPTER 13)	Acute hepatitis	↑↑↑↑	↑↑↑↑	↑	±	N	↑↑	↑
	Cirrhosis (Laennec's)	↑	±	±	±	±	±	↑
	Obstructive jaundice	↑↑	↑↑	↑	±	±	↑	↑↑↑
NEOPLASTIC DISEASE	Localized carcinoma of small size	N	N	N	N	N	N	N
	Extensive carcinoma without hepatic or bone metastases	N	N	↑↑	±	±	↑↑	N
	Carcinoma with metastases to liver or hepatoma	↑↑	↑	↑↑	±	±	↑↑	↑↑↑
	Carcinoma with osteoblastic metastases to bone	N	N	↑↑	±	±	↑↑	↑↑↑
	Leukemia (granulocytic or acute)	N	N	↑↑	±	±	↑↑	N
	Leukemia (chronic lymphatic)	N	N	N	N	N	N	N
ANEMIA	Megaloblastic	N	N	↑↑↑↑	↑	N	↑↑↑	N
	Iron deficiency	N	N	N	N	N	N	N
	Hemolytic	N	N	↑↑	↑	N	↑↑	N

*Number of arrows indicates magnitude of increase; N indicates no change.

tinction is usually readily made from pulmonary infarction, which is characterized by elevated LD levels and usually by normal AST values. In a small proportion of patients with pulmonary embolism, slightly elevated values for AST occur by three or four days after the bout of chest pain.

The complication of myocardial infarction by shock leads to higher values of AST and LD and to abnormal levels of enzymes that reflect hepatic injury (ALT, ICD). Indeed, shock of any origin, or severe hypoxia, leads to high levels of a large number of enzymes presumably released from the liver and perhaps from other tissues.

Of the large number of enzymes released to the blood from infarcted myocardium (Tables 12-6 and 12-16), only a few have been regularly applied to the diagnosis of infarction (Table 12-17). Most extensively employed are the total serum activity of CK and LD, each of which yields abnormal values in almost all patients with proven infarction. The degree, onset, and duration of rise of each enzyme are characteristic. CK values increase within four to six hours following myocardial infarction, with a peak value up to 12 times greater than normal CK value occurring at approximately 24 hours. A return of CK to normal activity is found usually by the third day. Within the first 48 hours CK_2 (MB) is present in virtually all patients with myocardial infarction, as well as in some cases of severe coronary insufficiency (Galen, 1975). The determination of CK isoenzymes with demonstration of a CK_2 (MB) isoenzyme during this period is virtually diagnostic of myocardial infarction. At 72 hours only 66 per cent of patients with myocardial infarction exhibit MB (CK_2 fraction) with significantly lower levels of activity. CK_2 (MB) then disappears rapidly, although the serum CK_3 (MM) fraction may still be elevated.

Serum LD activity increases two- to fourfold following myocardial infarction, with persistence of elevation considerably longer (10 to 14 days). The measurement of LD isoenzymes, as noted previously (p. 367), provides a further refinement in laboratory assessment of patients with myocardial infarction. However, the "flipped LDH" ($LD_1 > LD_2$) is a more variable phenomenon which may become evident at 12 hours and be present in approximately 80 per cent of patients with myocardial infarction within the first 48 hours (Galen, 1975a). It is not necessarily maintained, since in less than half of the patients with myocardial infarctions there may not be a "flipped LDH" at the end of one week, even though serum LD level may still be elevated.

COMBINED CRITERIA
ISOENZYME ANALYSIS

The simultaneous use of CK and LD isoenzyme determinations combines the high degree of sensitivity offered by CK with the high degree of specificity offered by LD (Galen, 1975a) (Table 12-18). Combined criteria are met when there is a "flipped LDH" pattern ($LD_1 > LD_2$) present in a patient exhibiting CK_2 (MB) in specimens drawn during the first 48 hours following an acute episode of suspected myocardial infarction (Galen, 1975a).

Ideally, three separate specimens are collected; first on admission, a second at 24 hours, and a third at 48 hours. Both CK and LD serum assays are measured. If total enzyme activity is elevated, isoenzyme analyses are performed. The "flipped LD" comes after the appearance of CK_2 (MB). Galen has also emphasized that the criteria do not have to be demonstrated in a single specimen. Indeed, they are frequently met by examining serum patterns in 24- and 48-hour specimens together. Table 12-8 displays the format for interpreting combined isoenzyme data during the initial 48 hour period (Galen, 1975a).

To be used most efficiently the combined criteria must be evaluated during the initial 48 hours of suspected onset of ischemic heart disease. Once diagnostic criteria are met, there is no need for further determinations to document the diagnosis. Indeed, if at 24 hours both criteria are met the diagnosis is affirmative (Galen, 1975a). A CK_2 (MB) determination may then be done to estimate the infarct size or detect extension or reinfarction (Roberts, 1976). If combined criteria are not met by 48 hours, the diagnosis is then presumptively not myocardial infarction (Table 12-18). It should be emphasized, however, that the combined criteria after a 48-hour interval do not rule out myocardial infarction with the same high degree of certainty present during the acute phase (initial 48-hour period) of potential ischemic injury. Indeed, it is possible that a myocardial infarction may reveal CK_2 (MB) and the usual LD profile on day four.

Galen has also emphasized the application of combined isoenzyme analysis to special conditions in which confirmation of acute myocardial infarction is hampered by non-specific enzyme elevation. In electroshock cardioversion, there is no CK_2 (MB); furthermore, with intramuscular drugs, serum total CK elevation

Table 12-18. COMBINED ISOENZYME ANALYSIS: RULE OUT MYOCARDIAL INFARCTION (MI)*

CK-MB absent	CK-MB present Usual LDH	CK-MB present Flipped-LDH
↓	↓	↓
100 per cent predictive value that there is no MI	Both MI and non-MI cases†	100 per cent predictive value that there is MI

*During acute 48 hour period following episode.

†Non-MI cases reflect clinical and electrocardiographic evidence of ischemia.

From Galen, R. S.: The enzyme diagnosis of myocardial infarction. Hum. Pathol., 6:2, 1975. With permission of R. S. Galen, M.D.

reflects only CK_3 (MM). In major operative procedures, there is no CK_2 (MB) but only MM. Pre- and postoperative total serum LD and CK, however, are not helpful in the postoperative period. Then evaluation of myocardial infarction requires the combined isoenzymes "flipped LD" and CK_2 (MB). With cardiopulmonary bypass, patients undoubtedly have a high risk of myocardial infarction; with manipulation of heart, etc., ischemic injury probably takes place during surgery. Hence, discrimination between myocardial infarction and non-myocardial infarction following open-heart surgery is extremely difficult. Indeed, Galen (1975a) has noted, as we have, that an overlap is present between the two groups. However, it is still useful, although not a definitive adjunct procedure. There is also myocardial injury with cardiac valve replacement and aneurysmectomy surgery. Hence, LD and CK isoenzymes are less specific and must be interpreted with caution. Furthermore, a "flipped LDH" pattern may appear in 25 per cent of non-myocardial infarction patients secondary to hemolysis from extracorporeal circulation (Galen, 1975a).

SERUM ENZYMES IN LIVER DISEASE

The enzymologic approach to liver disease is discussed in Chapter 11. It remains to be proved that employment of the apparently liver-specific OCT, ID, or guanase or of the isoenzymes of LD will add a significant measure of sensitivity or specificity to that provided by the simple panel of AST and ALT. Similarly, the distinction of the elevated ALP levels of hepatobiliary disease from those caused by osteoblastic lesions offers little difficulty if consideration is given to other laboratory measurements and clinical features of hepatic and biliary tract disease. This distinction may be aided by assay of the LAP, GGT, or 5'-N, the levels of which parallel those of ALP in hepatobiliary disease but are normal in diseases of bone. Studies of isoenzymes of ALP by electrophoretic, kinetic, or other techniques for the purpose of distinguishing bone from hepatic phosphatase seem at present to be of greater theoretical interest than clinical benefit. Cholinesterase levels, at one time considered a valuable enzymologic tool for the management of hepatic disease, have been supplanted by the more readily measurable, more sensitive, and more specific transaminases.

Enzyme analysis in hepatobiliary disease is useful in differential diagnosis, as discussed in Chapter 11. Monitoring the course of serum enzyme levels is helpful in following the course of acute or chronic hepatitis or of active postnecrotic cirrhosis. For this purpose AST and ALT assays may be employed. Monitoring of patients exposed to possible hepatotoxins is usefully accomplished by a simple panel consisting of ALP, AST, and ALT. If evidence of mitochondrial injury is sought, glutamate dehydrogenase levels also may be measured.

SERUM ENZYMES IN MUSCLE DISEASE

Measurement of serum enzyme levels has become a major component of the diagnostic approach to muscle disease. The enzymes that have been studied most extensively are ALS, AST, LD, and CK. The last named is the most reliable measure of skeletal muscle disease, since, as discussed previously, elevated values are relatively specific for disease of striated muscle (skeletal muscle and myocardium). Aldolase levels appear to be as sensitive to disease of muscle, although somewhat less specific.

Elevated levels of these enzymes occur in patients with dystrophic or myositic processes. In the progressive muscular dystrophies, especially the Duchenne type, the values are particularly high. Moderate or marked elevations are seen in dermatomyositis, in polymyositis, in scleroderma with an associated myositis, and in trichinosis. Slightly or moderately increased levels of these enzymes are also observed in myotonic dystrophy, in myotonia congenita, in the crush syndrome, and in McArdle's disease. High values of these and other enzymes occur in patients with delirium tremens, irrespective of associated hepatic disease, and may arise in muscle (LD_5 and CK_3). The muscle involvement of myxedema appears to be responsible for the elevated serum enzyme levels seen in this condition. Strenuous muscle activity in untrained individuals also leads to increased levels of these enzymes. Serum enzyme levels are normal in patients with neurogenic muscle disease. Disease of the upper motor neuron, the anterior horn cell, or the peripheral nerve does not lead to elevated values.

For the clinical application to the diagnosis of muscle disease, both aldolase (ALS) and CK should be measured. If values for both are abnormal, the results can be interpreted with greater confidence. These tests are of help in recognizing early muscular dystrophy before clinical manifestations appear and may be useful clues to the carrier female. They are also of value in the differential diagnosis of the other muscular diseases cited and in following the course of inflammatory disease of the muscle.

Isoenzymes of CK (MM) and LD (LD_5) also reflect skeletal muscle injury. In Duchenne's muscular dystrophy, CK_2 (MB) appears in sera as well as in heart disease with LD_1.

SERUM ENZYMES IN NEOPLASTIC DISEASE

A large number of studies have demonstrated high serum levels of glycolytic and other enzymes (Table 12-16) in the serum of animals and humans with a variety of carcinomas and other neoplastic lesions. In general, the levels of enzymes studied are normal in patients with small localized tumors; increased values are seen when the local tumor has become large, has extended to surrounding tissue, or has reached distant metastatic sites. Data from several laboratories indicate that the serum levels of these enzymes reflect and are proportional to the total mass of tumor rather than the involvement of tissue at specific metastatic sites. Measurement of levels of any of the glycolytic or other enzymes that are elevated in patients with carcinomatosis fails to provide a means of detecting early neoplasms that are resectable; however, perhaps the search for such an enzymologic clue should continue to be pursued. Patterns of serum enzyme abnormality are of value in supporting the diagnosis of carcinomatosis, and the monitoring of serum enzyme levels is useful in following the response to chemotherapy of patients with inoperable neoplasms.

Increased levels of the same enzymes are observed in patients with Hodgkin's disease, lymphosarcoma, and granulocytic and acute leukemia. Adequate response to chemotherapy is reflected in decreasing values. The values are normal in patients with chronic lymphocytic leukemia and in most patients with multiple myeloma.

The enzymes that have been most extensively studied in neoplastic states and that can be used to monitor the course of widespread neoplastic disease are lactate dehydrogenase, phosphohexoisomerase, and aldolase; however, the others listed in Table 12-17 also reflect the process.

ENZYMES OF THE FORMED ELEMENTS OF THE BLOOD

During the past few years, considerable attention has been devoted to the metabolic activity and enzyme content of erythrocytes and leukocytes. The extensive studies related to the employment of these elements as *in vitro* metabolic models and to the factors involved in blood preservation are beyond the scope of this discussion. This section attempts to summarize some of the studies of erythrocyte enzymes that have unraveled several genetic hemolytic syndromes (Table 12-19) and the studies of erythrocyte and leukocyte enzymes that have been useful in the diagnosis of several genetic and acquired systemic conditions (Table 12-20).

HEMOLYTIC ANEMIA ASSOCIATED WITH DEFICIENCY OF ERYTHROCYTE ENZYMES

Genetic defects in erythrocyte metabolism have been found or suspected to be responsible for well over a dozen forms of hemolytic anemia (Table 12-19). Some of the demonstrated or assumed enzymatic defects relate to the hexose monophosphate shunt (G-6-PD, 6-PGD, GR, GSH-synthetase, GSH-peroxidase), and some of the enzymatic defects relate to the anaerobic glycolytic pathway (HK, PHI, PFK, ALS, TPI, 2-3DPGM, PGK, PK, and ATP-ase). The hemolytic syndromes associated with enzymatic defects are listed in Table 12-19.

Hemolytic Anemia Secondary to G-6-PD Deficiency. Deficiency of erythrocyte G-6-PD activity has been estimated to involve 2 to 3 per cent of the world population and to be responsible for almost one third of the cases of chronic or recurrent non-spherocytic hemolytic anemia. The defect is sex-linked and appears in a number of genetic variants. The first to be recognized is the relatively mild condition observed almost exclusively in blacks and characterized by deficient concentration of G-6-PD in erythrocytes but normal concentration in leukocytes and platelets. These individuals develop hemolysis on exposure to a number of drugs, including primaquine, sulfonamides, and other agents, and to other stresses, including various infections. A more severe form of G-6-PD deficiency, characterized by G-6-PD deficiency in leukocytes and erythrocytes, by more severe anemia, and by sensitivity to fava beans and to various drugs, is seen in Cauca-

Table 12-19. TYPES OF HEREDITARY NON-SPHEROCYTIC HEMOLYTIC ANEMIA (HNHA) WHICH ARE KNOWN OR SUSPECTED TO BE DUE TO ENZYMATIC DEFECTS OF ERYTHROCYTES*

Condition (Names indicate missing enzymes)

Most important and frequent conditions
1. Glucose-6-phosphate dehydrogenase (G-6-PD) deficiency.
2. Pyruvate kinase (PK) deficiency.
3. Phosphohexoisomerase (PHI) (Glucose phosphate isomerase) deficiency.

Rare conditions
4. Hexokinase (HK) deficiency.
5. Phosphofructokinase (PFK) deficiency.
6. Triosephosphate isomerase (TPI) deficiency.
7. Phosphoglycerate kinase (PGK) deficiency.

Very rare conditions
8. Pyrimidine-5'-P-nucleotidase (5-5'-PN) deficiency.
9. Aldolase deficiency.†
10. GSH synthetase deficiency.
11. GSH peroxidase deficiency.

Very rare or equivocal conditions
12. Glutathione reductase (GR) deficiency.
13. Glyceraldehyde phosphate dehydrogenase deficiency.
14. 6-Phosphoglycerate dehydrogenase (6-PGD) deficiency.
15. 2-3 Diphosphoglycerate mutase (2-3 DPGM) deficiency.
16. ATPase deficiency.
17. Adenylate kinase (AK) deficiency.
18. Diphosphoglycerate phosphatase (DPGP) deficiency.
19. Enolase deficiency.

*See Beutler, 1976.

†At one time aldolase deficiency was considered to be responsible for familial spherocytic anemia; now known not to be true.

sians, particularly Sephardic Jews, other ethnic groups of the Mediterranean littoral, American Indians, and Orientals. Studies of the various forms of G-6-PD deficiency have shown not only differences in the severity of the clinical illness and the degree of depression of enzyme levels of erythrocytes and leukocytes, but also that there are different molecular variants (isoenzymes) of G-6-PD. The mechanism whereby G-6-PD deficiency permits drug-induced hemolysis remains incompletely understood but is indirectly related to the inability to maintain adequate levels of reduced glutathione in the erythrocyte on exposure to offending agents.

Assay of G-6-PD activity has become a routine procedure in patients with hemolytic anemia, especially if it occurs after administration of a drug or during an acute illness. A precise assay of G-6-PD activity of hemolysate involves measuring the rate at which NADP is reduced in the presence of glucose-6-phosphate. Simplified assays suitable for screening large populations are available.

Deficiency of 6-PGD. Decreased erythrocyte levels of 6-PGD have been reported, but the role of this abnormality in inducing susceptibility to hemolysis remains to be proved.

The principle of assay of 6-PGD activity of erythrocytes is similar to that of G-6-PD.

HEMOLYTIC ANEMIA SECONDARY TO DEFICIENCY OF GLUTATHIONE REDUCTASE (GR), GLUTATHIONE PEROXIDASE (GSH-Px), OR GLUTATHIONE SYNTHETASE

A few instances of mild hemolytic anemia have been reported in patients with genetic deficiency in erythrocyte levels of GR. Some have been instances of chronic hemolysis and others of hemolytic anemia after exposure to drugs (primaquine). Thus far, the condition appears to be rare and primarily of genetic interest. Almost complete absence of glutathione from erythrocytes as a genetic abnormality has been found to occur in several genera. The deficiency of glutathione in these individuals appears to be transmitted as an autosomal recessive and presumably results from subnormal glutathione synthetase activity. The erythrocytes of patients with GSH deficiency, like those of patients with G-6-PD and GR deficiency, are susceptible to drug-induced hemolysis. A similar syndrome has been attributed to deficiency of GSH-Px, the enzyme presumed to be mainly responsible for destroying H_2O_2 in human erythrocytes.

HEMOLYTIC ANEMIAS SECONDARY TO DEFICIENCY IN GLYCOLYTIC ENZYMES

Pyruvate kinase (PK) deficiency is the most frequent and important form of hemolytic anemia due to deficiency of glycolytic enzymes in the erythrocyte. It is transmitted as an autosomal recessive and characterized by a non-spherocytic, chronic hemolytic anemia. The hemolysis is attributable to the inability of the PK-deficient erythrocyte to maintain normal ATP levels and the resulting membrane defect. Enzyme activity of the erythrocyte can be assayed by measuring the ability of hemolysate to form pyruvate from ADP and phosphoenol pyruvate.

Similar syndromes appear to result from deficient erythrocyte content of hexokinase, phosphohexoisomerase, phosphofructokinase, triose phosphate isomerase, 2-3 diphosphoglycerate mutase, phosphoglycerate kinase, and ATPase and other enzymes. These are rare and, at present, of little clinical importance (see Chapter 29 for further discussion).

SYSTEMIC DISEASES REFLECTED IN ABNORMAL ERYTHROCYTE AND LEUKOCYTE ENZYMES

Several genetic diseases are reflected by abnormal levels of enzymes in the erythrocytes (Table 12–20). Acatalasia, also called Takahara's disease or oral gangrene, is a condition characterized by marked deficiency in the concentration of catalase in the tissues and in the erythrocytes. Deficiency of catalase, an enzyme which destroys hydrogen peroxide ($2 H_2O_2 \xrightarrow{catalase} 2 H_2O + O_2$), leads to the accumulation of hydrogen peroxide when it is produced in excess. This is often asymptomatic and becomes of clinical importance only in some patients with oral sepsis, in whose oral cavities peroxide formed by bacteria can accumulate and lead to gangrene. It is a self-limiting state which disappears after the teeth are lost. Transmitted as an autosomal recessive, the condition is of greater genetic interest than clinical importance. Homozygous abnormals who have almost no catalase in the erythrocytes can be distinguished from the heterozygotes whose values are midway between the homozygote abnormal and normal. Hereditary methemoglobinemia secondary to deficiency of erythrocyte diaphorase is a rare oligosymptomatic condition which is transmitted as an autosomal recessive. The methemoglobinemia, which leads to cyanosis, is the result of deficiency of NADH-methemoglobin reductase (diaphorase).

Glycogenosis of types III, IV, and VII and hypophosphatasia can be identified by measuring the leukocyte content of the relevant enzyme. Confirmation of the diagnosis of type IV glycogenosis, which is due to *hepatophosphorylase* deficiency, can be obtained by measuring the phosphorylase activity of leukocytes.

Table 12–20. SYSTEMIC DISEASES IN WHICH DIAGNOSIS CAN BE ESTABLISHED BY ANALYSIS OF ENZYME ACTIVITY OF FORMED ELEMENT OF BLOOD

CONDITION	FORMED ELEMENT	ENZYME ASSAY
Genetic		
Methemoglobinemia	RBC	NADH-methemoglobin reductase
Acatalasemia	RBC	Catalase
Galactosemia		Gal-1-P-uridyl transferase
Glycogenosis (Type III)	WBC	Amylo-1-6-glucosidase
(Type IV)	WBC	Phosphorylase
(Type VII)	RBC	Phosphofructokinase
Hypophosphatasia	WBC	Alkaline phosphatase
Lipid storage diseases		
Gaucher's	WBC	β-Glucosidase
Niemann-Pick	WBC	Sphingomyelinase
Krabbes' leukodystrophy (globoid)	WBC	β-Galactosidase
Metachromatic leukodystrophy	WBC	Sulfatidase
Fabry's disease	WBC	α-Galactosidase
Tay-Sachs disease	WBC	Hexosaminidase
Acquired		
Thiamine deficiency	RBC	Transketolase
Pyridoxine deficiency	RBC	Alanine aminotransferase
Hyperthyroidism	RBC	Carbonic anhydrase
Leukemia, granulocytic	WBC	Alkaline phosphatase
Lead poisoning	RBC	δ-Aminolevulinic acid dehydrase

Type III glycogenosis, which is a manifestation of deficiency of the glycogen *debrancher* enzyme (amylo-1-6-glucosidase), can also be diagnosed by measuring the leukocyte content of that enzyme. Type VII glycogenosis, which is associated with a hemolytic anemia, can be identified by demonstrating deficient phosphofructokinase activity in the erythrocytes. *Hypophosphatasia* is characterized by a genetic deficiency of alkaline phosphatase content of tissues and blood. Measurement of alkaline phosphatase levels of the leukocytes can in the proper clinical setting assist in establishing the diagnosis.

Galactosemia is an inborn error of metabolism characterized by a specific defect in the utilization of galactose which results in widespread tissue damage. The defect has been found to be deficiency of the enzyme phosphogalactose-uridyl-transferase. The resulting accumulation of galactose-1-phosphate is considered responsible for the development of cataracts, liver disease, renal disease, and other abnormalities. The hereditary enzyme deficiency can be demonstrated by studying the erythrocyte. The ability of hemolysate to catalyze the conversion of galactose-1-phosphate to UDP-galactose in the presence of UDP-glucose is measured by following the disappearance of UDP-glucose. The test, which can be readily performed, yields very low values in patients with galactosemia, who are homozygous for the abnormal gene. Heterozygote carriers can usually be identified by this test, which yields values intermediate between the normal and the homozygous abnormal.

A number of lipid storage diseases can be identified by demonstrating deficient activity of the related enzyme in circulating leukocytes (Table 12-20). Several acquired diseases can also be identified by studying enzyme activity of the formed elements. Thiamine deficiency can be confirmed by demonstrating depressed transketolase activity of hemolysate. Pyridoxine deficiency can be demonstrated by measuring the ALT activity of erythrocytes before and after incubation with pyridoxal-5-phosphate. Abnormal levels of cholinesterase, carbonic anhydrase and several other enzymes have been demonstrated in the erythrocytes of patients with a variety of acquired systemic diseases, but these are of pathophysiologic rather than diagnostic importance. The recent description of depressed erythrocyte levels of δ-aminolevulinic acid dehydrase as a measure

of blood levels of lead suggests that measurement of this enzyme may be useful in the diagnosis of lead poisoning. Measurement of leukocyte alkaline phosphatase helps in distinguishing granulocytic leukemia from leukemoid states. Alkaline phosphatase levels are very low in the leukocytes of granulocytic leukemia, but they are normal or elevated in patients with non-leukemic leukocytosis.

ENZYME CONCENTRATIONS IN OTHER BODY FLUIDS

Measurement of enzyme activity in serous effusions, gastrointestinal juices, cerebrospinal fluid, and urine has been applied to the diagnosis of various diseases. Localized release of enzyme from neoplastic cells has been considered responsible for the high levels of LD (and other glycolytic enzymes) in malignant pleural and peritoneal effusions, in the gastric juice of patients with carcinoma of the stomach, and in the urine of patients with renal carcinoma. The glucuronidase in the urine of patients with carcinoma of the bladder and in the vaginal fluid of patients with carcinoma of the cervix may also be considered to be enzyme shed by neoplastic cells.

Determination of levels of LD in serous cavity effusions has been proposed as a method of demonstrating neoplastic involvement of serosal surfaces (Chap. 18). In such circumstances, the serous fluid usually shows higher levels of LD than does the serum. High levels of LD, however, are also found in patients with inflammatory and hemorrhagic effusions (p. 668). Accordingly, measurements of enzyme content of serous effusions appear to be of limited clinical value. Measurement of LD levels of gastric juice or urine to detect renal or gastric carcinoma, respectively, or of glucuronidase in the urine or vaginal fluid to detect carcinoma of the bladder or cervix, respectively, remains to be proven of clinical value.

The demonstration of a high amylase value in pleural or ascitic fluid is useful in making the diagnosis of pancreatitis. The demonstration of increased levels of amylase in the urine is also a useful supplement to the measurement of serum levels of the enzyme in the diagnosis of pancreatitis (Chap. 24).

Measurement of urinary levels of lactate dehydrogenase, alkaline phosphatase, muramidase (lysozyme), catalase, β-glucuronidase, and pepsinogen has been proposed for the diagnosis or monitoring of a number of conditions. Increased levels of lactate dehydrogenase, alkaline phosphatase, and β-glucuronidase are frequent in patients with carcinoma of the urinary tract but may also be caused by hematuria, urinary tract infection, or glomerulonephritis and are, accordingly, too non-specific to be clinically useful. Catalase may be found in the urine when there is bacteriuria, pyuria, or hematuria. Muramidase activity of the urine may be very high in patients with monocytic or monomyelocytic leukemia. For monitoring the course of the disease, however, serum levels of this enzyme are probably more useful. Urinary (and plasma) pepsinogen values are increased in patients with peptic ulcer and low in those with pernicious anemia. These observations are of pathophysiologic interest rather than clinical value.

Increased levels of β-glucuronidase and 6-phosphogluconate dehydrogenase have been demonstrated in the vaginal fluid of a high proportion of patients with carcinoma of the uterus, especially the cervix. However, the normal values found in some patients with cancer and the elevated values found in some patients with benign conditions prevent useful application of assay of vaginal fluid enzyme activity for the recognition of carcinoma. Measurement of tartrate inhibitable acid phosphatase in vaginal fluid is a useful procedure for the diagnosis of rape, since this isoenzyme is of prostatic origin and therefore high in semen.

Cerebrospinal fluid enzyme levels are relatively independent of the serum levels. Increased spinal fluid levels of glutamate oxaloacetate transaminase, lactate dehydrogenase, ribonuclease, and glutathione reductase have been described in patients with various diseases of the central nervous system. The levels of one or more of these enzymes are increased in patients with cerebrovascular hemorrhage, thrombosis or embolism, meningitis, and neoplasms of the central nervous system. The clinical application and value of spinal fluid enzyme determinations remain to be established. (Also see Chapter 18, p. 652.)

REFERENCES

General

Abderhalden, R.: Clinical Enzymology. Princeton, N.J., D. Van Nostrand Co., 1961.

Baron, D. N.: The clinical significance of serum enzyme estimations. Abstr. Wrld. Med., *40*:377, 1967.

Bergmeyer, H. U. (ed.): Methods of Enzymatic Analysis. New York, Academic Press, Inc., 1963.

Bodansky, O.: Diagnostic applications of enzyme in medicine: General enzymological aspects. Am. J. Med., *27*:861, 1959.

Cabaud, P. G., and Wroblewski, F.: Colorimetric measurement of lactic dehydrogenase activity of body fluids. Am. J. Clin. Pathol., *30*:234, 1958.

Cohen, L.: Serum enzyme determinations: Their reliability and value. Med. Clin. North Am., *53*:115, 1969.

Coodley, E. L. (ed.): Diagnostic Enzymology. Philadelphia, Lea & Febiger, 1970.

Henley, K. S., Schmidt, E., and Schmidt, F. W.: Enzymes in Serum. Springfield, Ill., Charles C Thomas, Publisher, 1966.

Henry, J. B. (ed.): Clinical Enzymology: Pre-Workshop and Technical Manuals. Chicago, American Society of Clinical Pathologists, 1964.

King, J.: Practical Clinical Enzymology. London, D. Van Nostrand Co., 1965.

Konttinen, A.: Serum enzymes as indicators of hepatic disease. Scand. J. Gastroenterol., *6*:667, 1971.

Latner, A. L., and Skillen, A. W.: Isoenzymes in Biology and Medicine. New York, Academic Press, Inc., 1968.

Shugar, D.: Enzymes and Isoenzymes, Structure, Properties and Function, vol. 18. New York, Academic Press, Inc., 1970.

Statland, B. E.: The case for standardizing enzyme assays. Lab. Manage., *15*:46, 1977.

Warburg, O., and Christian, W.: Gärunofermente im blutserum von tumorratten. Biochem. Ztschr., *314*:399, 1943.

White, L. (ed.): Enzymes in blood. Ann. N.Y. Acad. Med., *75*:1, 1958.

Wilkinson, J. H.: Isoenzymes. Philadelphia, J. B. Lippincott Co., 1966.

Wilkinson, J. H.: The Principles and Practice of Diagnostic Enzymology. London, Edward Arnold, 1976.

Wolf, P. L., Williams, D., and Von der Muehle, E.: Practical Clinical Enzymology. New York, John Wiley & Sons, Inc., 1973.

Wroblewski, F.: Increasing clinical significance of alterations in enzymes of body fluids. Ann. Intern. Med., *50*:62, 1959.

Serum enzyme levels in liver disease

Hutterer, F.: Recent progress in clinical enzymology for the diagnosis of liver disease. *In* Schaffner, F., Sherlock, S., and Leevy, C. M. (eds.): The Liver and Its Diseases. New York, International Universities Press, 1974, p. 876.

Konttinen, A., Hupli, V., and Sulmenkivi, K.: The diagnosis of hepatobiliary disease by serum enzyme analysis. Acta Med. Scand., *189*:529, 1971.

Patel, S., and O'Gorman, P. O.: Serum enzyme levels in alcoholism and drug dependency. J. Clin. Pathol., *28*:714, 1975.

Skreder, S., Blomkoff, J. P., and Gjone, E.: Biochemical features of acute and chronic hepatitis. Am. Clin. Res., *8*:182, 1976.

Wacker, W. E. C., Ulmer, D. D., and Vallee, B. L.: Metalloenzymes and myocardial infarction. N. Engl. J. Med., *255*:449, 1956.

Zimmerman, H. J., and Seeff, L. B.: Enzymes in hepatic disease. *In* Coodley, E. L. (ed.): Diagnostic Enzymology. Philadelphia, Lea & Febiger, 1970, p. 1.

Creatine phosphokinase and other enzymes in myocardial infarction and muscle disease

Auvinen, S.: Evaluation of serum enzyme tests in the diagnosis of acute myocardial infarction. Acta Med. Scand. [Suppl. 539], 1972.

Cohen, L., and Morgan, J.: The enzymatic and immunologic detection of myocardial injury. Med. Clin. North Am., *57*:105, 1973.

Doran, G. R., and Wilkinson, J. H.: The origin of the elevated activity of creatine kinase and other enzymes in the sera of patients with myxoedema. Clin. Chim. Acta, *62*:203, 1975.

Galen, R. S.: The enzyme diagnosis of myocardial infarction. Hum. Pathol., *6*:141, 1975a.

Galen, R. S., Reiffel, J. A., and Gambino, S. R.: Diagnosis of acute myocardial infarction: Relative efficiency of serum enzyme and isoenzyme measurement. J.A.M.A., *232*:145, 1975b.

Griffiths, J., and Handschuh, G.: Creatine kinase isoenzyme MB in myocardial infarction: Methods compared. Clin. Chem., *23*:567, 1977.

Konttinen, A., and Somer, H.: Specificity of serum creatine kinase isoenzymes in diagnosis of acute myocardial infarction. Br. Med. J., *1*:386, 1973.

Roberts, R., and Sobel, B. E.: CPK isoenzymes in evaluation of myocardial ischemic injury. Hosp. Pract., *11*:55, 1976.

Roe, C. R., Limbird, L. E., Wagner, G. S., and Nerenberg, S. T.: Combined isoenzyme analysis in the diagnosis of myocardial injury: Application of electrophoretic methods for the detection and quantitation of the creatine phosphokinase MB isoenzyme. J. Lab. Clin. Med., *80*:557, 1972.

West, M., Eshchar, J., and Zimmerman, H. J.: Serum enzymology in the diagnosis of myocardial infarction and related cardiovascular conditions. Med. Clin. North Am., *50*:171, 1966.

Phosphatases

Angellis, D., Ingles, N. R., and Fishman, W. H.: Isoelectric forming of alkaline phosphatase isoenzymes in polyacrylamide gels: Use of Triton x-100 and improved staining technique. Am. J. Clin. Pathol., *66*:929, 1976.

Bromhult, J., Fridell, E., and Sunblad, L.: Studies in alkaline phosphatase isoenzymes. Relation to γ-glutamyltransferase and lactate dehydrogenase isoenzymes. Clin. Chim. Acta, *76*:205, 1977.

Fishman, W. H.: Perspectives on alkaline phosphatase isoenzymes. Am. J. Med., *56*:617, 1974.

Fishman, W. H. (ed.): The Phosphohydrolases: Their Biology, Biochemistry, and Clinical Enzymology. New York, N.Y. Academy of Science, 1969.

Gorman, L., and Statland, B. E.: Clinical usefulness of alkaline phosphatase isoenzyme determinations. Clin. Biochem., *10*:171, 1977.

Gutman, A. B.: Serum alkaline phosphatase activity in diseases of the skeletal and hepatobiliary systems. Am. J. Med., *27*:875, 1959.

Kaplan, M. M.: Alkaline phosphatase. N. Engl. J. Med., *286*:200, 1972.

Marshall, G., and Amador, E.: Diagnostic usefulness of serum and β-glycerophosphatase activities in prostate disease. Am. J. Clin. Pathol., *32*:83, 1969.

Schumann, G. B., Badawy, S., Peglow, A., and Henry, J. B.: Prostatic acid phosphatase. Current assessment in vaginal fluid of alleged rape victims. Am. J. Clin. Pathol., *66*:6, 1976.

Warnes, T. W.: Alkaline phosphatase. Gut, *13*:926, 1972.

Woodard, H. Q.: The clinical significance of serum acid phosphatase. Am. J. Med., *27*:902, 1959.

γ-Glutamyltransferase

Davidson, D. C., McIntosh, W. B., and Forg, J. A.: Assessment of plasma glutamyl transpeptidase activity and urinary D-glucaric acid excretion as values of enzyme induction. Clin. Sci. Mol. Med., *47*:279, 1974.

Rosalki, S.B.: Enzyme tests in diseases of the liver and hepatobiliary tract. *In* Wilkinson, J.H. (ed.): The Principles and Practice of Diagnostic Enzymology. 1975 London. Edward Arnold Publication, p. 303.

Cholinesterase

Juul, P., and Leopold, I. H.: Human plasma cholinesterase isoenzymes. Clin. Chim. Acta, *19*:205, 1968.

Vorhaus, L. J., and Kark, R. M.: Serum cholinesterase in health and disease. Am. J. Med., *14*:707, 1953.

Aminotransferases (Transaminases)

Clermont, R. J., and Chalmers, T. C.: The transaminase tests in liver disease. Medicine, *46*:197, 1967.

DeRitis, F., Coltori, M., and Giusti, C.: Diagnostic value and pathogenic significance of transaminase activity changes in viral hepatitis. Minerva Med., *47*:101, 1956.

Wroblewski, F.: Clinical significance of alterations in transaminase activities of serum and other body fluids. Adv. Clin. Chem., *1*:313, 1958.

Enzymes of erythrocytes and leukocytes

Beutler, E.: Enzyme tests in hematological diseases. *In* Wilkinson, J. H. (ed.): The Principles and Practice of Diagnostic Enzymology. Chicago, Year Book Medical Publishers, 1976, pp. 423–454.

Brady, R. O., Johnson, W. G., and Uhlendorf, B. W.: Identification of heterozygous carriers of lipid storage diseases: Current status and clinical applications. Am. J. Med., *51*:423, 1971.

Carson, P. E., and Frischer, H.: Glucose-6-phosphate dehydrogenase deficiency and related disorders of the pentose phosphate pathway. Am. J. Med., *41*:744, 1966.

Jaffe, E. R.: Hereditary hemolytic disorders and enzymatic deficiencies of human erythrocytes. Blood, *35*:116, 1970.

Stanbury, J. B., Wyngaarden, J. B., and Fredrickson, D. S.: The Metabolic Basis of Inherited Disease, 3rd ed. New York, McGraw-Hill Book Co., Inc., 1972.

Weisberg, J. B., Lipschutz, F., and Oski, F. A.: δ-Aminolevulinic acid dehydratase activity in circulating blood cells: A sensitive laboratory test for the detection of childhood lead poisoning. N. Engl. J. Med., *284*:565, 197

13

RADIOIMMUNOASSAY AND RELATED TECHNIQUES

Joan H. Howanitz, M.D.,
and Peter J. Howanitz, M.D.

Development of the technique of radioimmunoassay has made an immense impact on many areas of medicine. Its sensitivity and specificity allow accurate quantitation of a wide variety of biologically important compounds, such as peptides, hormones, vitamins, and drugs, which may occur in biologic fluids or tissues at low concentrations. The technique or variations of the technique based on the same principles have been used to measure hundreds of different substances, some of which occur in the blood in ng/ml or pg/ml amounts. Before the development of radioimmunoassay, many of these substances could be assayed only with great difficulty, and in some cases no practical assay was available.

The diversity of terminology used to describe these methods may lead to confusion; some of the expressions such as *saturation analysis* or *displacement analysis* relate to the general principle, while other terms such as radioimmunoassay, radioassay, radioligand, and radioreceptor assay refer to the specific reagents used in a given assay system. The term *competitive protein binding assay* has been used as well, but neither this nor the other designations have gained wide acceptance for the group of assays as a whole.

In the 1950's Berson and Yalow, while studying the behavior of ^{131}I-labeled insulin, made several observations that led to the development of the radioimmunoassay for plasma insulin. They found that when patients with diabetes mellitus were treated with insulin, insulin-binding antibodies were formed to this injected insulin. Subsequently, Berson and Yalow succeeded in producing an insulin antibody in animals. In addition, they observed, using an *in vitro* system, that unlabeled insulin displaced radioactively labeled insulin from insulin antibody. They found that when the antibody concentration was kept fixed, the binding of label was a quantitative function of the amount of unlabeled insulin present (Yalow, 1971b). This work formed the basis of radioimmunoassay, the principle of which is summarized in Figure 13-1.

The reagents necessary to perform an assay for a given substance or antigen include an antibody specific for the antigen, labeled antigen, a standard preparation of the antigen, and a system to separate the fraction which is

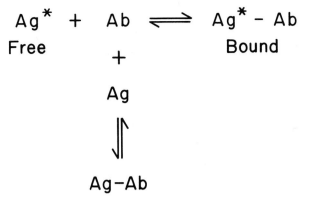

Figure 13–1. Principle of radioimmunoassay. Ag* represents the labeled antigen; Ab, the antibody; Ag, the unknown antigen or standard; Ag*-Ab and Ag-Ab, the complexes formed.

bound to the antibody from that which is unbound or free. An assay for plasma insulin thus would require (1) an antibody to insulin, (2) labeled insulin, (3) a preparation of insulin for use as a standard, (4) buffer, and (5) a separation system. The assay is performed by using a series of tubes containing a fixed concentration of antibody, fixed amount of label, appropriate amounts of buffer, and an aliquot of either standard or unknown. A number of standards and controls are determined with each assay, along with certain parameters of antibody binding and completeness of separation. The substance to be measured (unlabeled antigen) in the patient specimen competes with the labeled antigen for the antibody binding sites. The percentage of antigen bound to the antibody is related to the total antigen present and is reflected by the distribution of the radioactive label. With increasing amounts of unlabeled antigen, a corresponding decreased amount of labeled antigen will be bound to antibody. The percentage of the total radioactive label which is bound to the antibody and that which is free can be monitored after the two fractions are separated. By comparing the distribution of label obtained with the unknown to that observed with the standards, the concentration of unknown can be determined. The distribution of the radioactive label can be expressed in a number of ways, such as the percentage of total counts that are bound (%B) or free (%F) or the ratio of the counts of the two fractions (B/F). A curve then is prepared by plotting the percentage or ratio obtained with the

standard against the concentration of standard; unknown values then are determined using this standard curve (Fig. 13–2).

Radioimmunoassay and related techniques are dependent on the degree of similarity of behavior of the standard and the unknown but they do not fundamentally rely on the use of antibodies or a radioactive label. In general terms, the principle involves partitioning of the substance to be measured into two moieties by the reaction with a specific binding reagent of limited capacity (Ekins, 1974). The ratio of the two moieties depends on the amount of unknown or standard in the system. For example, the assay of thyroxine which was described by Ekins at about the same time as the insulin assay was developed was based on principles identical to those governing the insulin method (Ekins, 1974). However, this assay relied on a naturally occurring protein, thyroxine binding globulin, rather than on an antibody as a specific binding reagent in the system. Since this type of assay uses a binding protein instead of an antibody it is referred to as a radioassay rather than a radioimmunoassay. Although superficially different, the fundamental principle on which all these assays is based depends on the use of a limited amount of specific binding reagent which is held constant in the system. The binder may be antibody, as in the insulin assay; specific binding proteins, as in the thyroxine assay; cellular receptors; or even an enzyme, as in the assay of methotrexate. A requirement of the technique is that there must be a means of separating or identifying the bound and free components.

SPECIFIC BINDING REAGENTS

The specific binding reagent is an extremely important component of the assay system. Antibodies, receptors, and certain naturally occurring proteins have been used, each having its advantages and disadvantages (Table 13–1). Two important characteristics of the binder are its specificity and affinity. Specificity denotes the degree of uniqueness with which the substance being assayed is bound. The association constant or K is a measure of the affinity or strength of binding. High affinity binders form a relatively stable complex with limited dissociation.

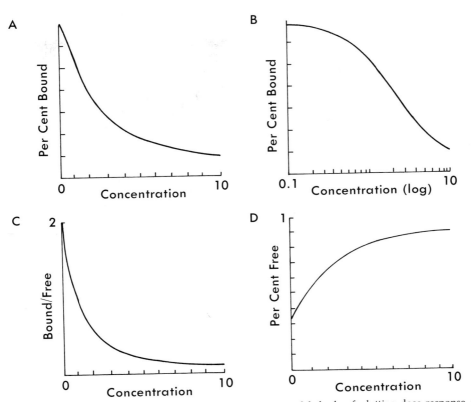

Figure 13–2. Examples of standard curves for radioimmunoassays. Methods of plotting dose-response curves.

A, Percentage or fraction bound versus concentration.
B, Percentage or fraction bound versus log concentration.
C, Bound to free ratio versus concentration.
D, Percentage (or fraction) free versus concentration.

ANTIBODIES

Antibodies are the most widely used binding reagents, since they can be readily produced to a large variety of compounds, including proteins, hormones, drugs, and intracellular metabolites. Many of these compounds have molecular weights below 1000 and are not immunogenic unless they are attached to a carrier such as a protein. The production of antibody suitable for use is dependent on many factors such as carrier protein, purity of antigen, animal species, method and route of injections, and time of bleeding (Parker, 1976.)

Table 13–1. PROPERTIES OF SPECIFIC BINDING REAGENTS

PROPERTY	ANTIBODY	RECEPTORS	BINDING PROTEINS
Stability	Stable	Unstable	Stable
Source	Immunized animals	Cells	Naturally occurring proteins
Specificity	Immunologic	Biologic	Biologic
*Association Constant or K (liters/mole)	10^{10} to 10^{12}	10^{8} to 10^{11}	10^{8} to 10^{10}

*A measure of affinity of strength of binding; large K values reflect strong bonds, and high affinity binders form a relatively stable complex with limited dissociation.

Specificity of an antiserum may be assessed by reacting it with a number of compounds, with which it may be expected to cross-react. Cross-reactivity occurs because of structural similarity of the compounds: for example, antibody to digitoxin may cross-react with digoxin and antibodies to L-thyroxine may cross-react with D-thyroxine. The chains of various glycoprotein hormones are very similar; thus, antibody to TSH may cross-react with LH, FSH, or HCG. One approach has been to select the most specific antiserum and to absorb out the cross-reacting antigens. This can be accomplished if only a proportion of the antibodies cross-react or if the cross-reacting substance differs in affinity for the antibody.

Immunologic activity may have little to do with biologic activity. For example, an inactive precursor or degradation product of an antigen may be relatively inactive biologically but react with the antibody. In addition to assessment of cross-reactivity, the identity of the behavior of the unknown and standard must be evaluated and tested: a necessary but not totally acceptable condition for identical reactivities is that the concentration of the unknown falls linearly with dilution or that a dilution curve of unknown is superimposable on a dilution curve of the standard over a wide range of concentrations. When the concentration does not fall linearly with dilution, a number of factors must be considered, such as damaged label or pH (Yalow, 1971b).

The sensitivity of an immunoassay depends predominantly on the affinity of the antibody employed. The term *affinity* is used to denote the energy of the antigen-antibody reaction and is discussed on page 1185 in Chapter 35.

The advantages of using antibodies as the binding agent include versatility and potential for obtaining highly specific and sensitive assays. Some of the disadvantages are that it may be difficult to make antibody to a given substance, immunologic rather than biologic activity is measured, and there may be serious problems with cross-reactivity. In addition, the variability of antibodies made to the same substance makes it necessary to characterize antisera individually.

no preparation and of having uniform characteristics. The binding proteins, in general, have a lower affinity constant than do antibodies and may or may not show good specificity. For example, cortisol binding protein may react with a number of steroids, while thyroxine binding globulin (TBG) is fairly specific for T4, although it also binds T3. Serum contains binding proteins for cortisol, thyroid hormones, testosterone, and vitamin B_{12}, but the binding proteins may be from a number of sources. Binding proteins from one species may be used to measure compounds from another species, and sources of binding proteins other than serum may be used. For example, vitamin B_{12} radioassays have been developed using various binders, including hog intrinsic factor, chicken serum, or serum of oyster toad fish (Kubiatowicz, 1977). Milk-binding proteins commonly are used to measure serum folate (Rothenberg, 1976). In the binding protein assays, it is important to eliminate any interferences from endogenous binding proteins prior to the assay. In order to measure thyroxine using TBG, interference of the patient's TBG must be eliminated by such techniques as alcohol extraction. Heating of the sample commonly is employed to eliminate interference with endogenous binding proteins in the case of vitamin B_{12}. Characterization of the naturally occurring binding proteins is carried out in essentially the same manner as for antibody assessment.

Disadvantages of using naturally occurring binding proteins are that they are available only for a limited number of compounds, they may not show good specificity, and their affinity is relatively low. Thus, assays with a high degree of sensitivity are difficult to obtain. The naturally occurring binding proteins do have the advantage of being stable, relatively inexpensive, and easy to prepare. They have the added advantage of being consistent from preparation to preparation.

Enzymes also have been used in competitive protein-binding assays; an assay was developed for methotrexate based on the binding of the drug to the enzyme dihydrofolate reductase (Myers, 1975).

BINDING PROTEINS

Naturally occurring *binding proteins* also have been used as specific binding agents. They have the advantage of requiring little or

RECEPTORS

Another source of specific binder is membrane, cytoplasmic, or nuclear receptors. In general, the term *receptor* refers to a molecule or a molecular complex which is capable of recognizing and selectively interacting with a substance such as a hormone, neurotransmitter, or drug. A receptor has a specificity directed toward the biologically active portion of the molecule.

Receptors tend to be rather unstable, and they must be obtained by isolation from tissue where they exist in low concentrations. The source of receptor preparations may include intact cells and particulate or other cell fractions. Isolated cell preparations are obtained from blood and tissue culture as well as by enzymatic or mechanical disruption of tissues. The techniques employed to isolate cells can profoundly affect the concentration or affinity of receptors (Kahn, 1976). Receptor assays have been developed for a number of substances such as hormones and neurotransmitters. Receptors from bovine adrenal cortex, bovine skeletal muscle, or calf uterus, for example, have been used to assay cyclic AMP (Parker, 1976). Advantages of receptor assays include measurement of biologic rather than immunologic activity and uniformity among the preparations. However, in practice, uniformity among preparations may not always be achieved for a number of reasons, including problems in making the preparation and source variation in concentration or affinity of receptors. Broken cell preparations may have high concentrations of receptor-degrading activity (Roth, 1975). Disadvantages include the instability of the receptor, and non-specific binding in receptor assays may be a difficult problem to overcome. Receptors may be more sensitive than the other binders in distinguishing changes in a molecule introduced by labeling. Since the equilibrium constant is in the range of 10^8 to 10^{11} liters per mole, receptor assays may show lower sensitivity than a corresponding immunoassay employing an avid antibody (Parker, 1976).

LABELS

The indicator molecule employed in the assay system may be labeled in a number of ways, including with radioactivity, enzyme activity, or fluorescence. In order to have a valid assay, it is not necessary that the labeled molecule behave identically with the unlabeled unknown: however, the unlabeled unknown and the standard must show identical behavior in the assay system. Since the validity of the assay does not depend on the identical affinity of the labeled and the unlabeled material, provided both react at the same binding site, some difference in affinity may be acceptable. If the affinity of the label is less than that of the unknown, maximal assay sensitivity cannot be achieved. In addition, labeled material that has different properties than the unknown may give rise to unexpected effects such as interaction with the incubation constituents in an unpredictable manner (Hunter, 1974).

RADIOACTIVE LABELS

Although they have several disadvantages, radioactive labels have been employed widely because of their flexibility and sensitivity. Disadvantages of radioactive labels include potential health hazards, instability of the label, and expense of the detection equipment. Radioassay isotopes employed generally fall into two groups: (1) beta-emitting isotopes such as tritium (^{3}H) and (2) gamma emitting isotopes such as iodine-125 (^{125}I).

Each element has a unique number of extranuclear electrons and intranuclear protons. Atoms that have the same number of protons but different number of neutrons in the nucleus are termed isotopes. Isotopes that are unstable and undergo radioactive decay are termed radioisotopes. The decay may occur in various ways with the emitted radiation of three kinds; alpha particles, beta particles, and gamma rays. The alpha particle is identical with the helium nucleus and consists of two neutrons and two protons with the charge of $+2$; the beta particle has a mass equal to an electron and carries a negative or positive charge; and the gamma emission is electromagnetic radiation. The half-life of the population of radioactive atoms is the time interval in which half of the original number of atoms will have decayed. Table 13-2 shows the half-life and the type of emission of some radioisotopes that are commonly used in the clinical laboratory. The term *specific activity* refers to the activity expressed in millicuries per mass of the element. In addition, the term is employed for the activity divided by the mass of the compound of which the element forms a part (Veall, 1971). One curie is equal to 3.7×10^{10} disintegrations per second. It requires approximately 10,000 atoms of ^{14}C or 100 atoms of ^{3}H to produce the same number of disintegrations per minute as one atom of ^{125}I (Landon, 1976). When a radioactive marker of low specific activity is used, rela-

Table 13–2. SELECTED CHARACTERISTICS OF COMMONLY EMPLOYED RADIOISOTOPES

ISOTOPE	HALF-LIFE	EMISSION
^{14}C	5730 years	β
^{3}H	12.26 years	β
^{125}I	60.2 days	γ
^{131}I	8.1 days	γ, β
^{75}Se	120 days	γ
^{57}Co	270 days	γ

tively high concentrations are required to obtain a practical level of radioactivity in the immunoassay. The radioactivity is usually counted to 10,000 counts to ensure a high degree of precision in counting (Ekins, 1974). If an attempt is made to increase marker specific activity by maximizing the number of radioactive atoms incorporated per molecule, rapid decomposition sometimes occurs.

Compounds labeled with beta-emitting isotopes have several advantages and disadvantages. The replacement of hydrogen by tritium, for example, does not cause marked steric alterations or other changes and therefore seldom influences antigenicity. The resultant label is stable, and since tritium has a half-life of 12.3 years, the reagent has a relatively long shelf life. Beta emittors are detected by using liquid scintillation counting systems. As radioactive isotopes decay, emitting radiation, excitation of the scintillation fluid or fluor occurs. As the fluor returns to ground state, light is emitted. Interference with the emission of light (that is, quenching) results in decreased counts detected by the liquid scintillation counter. Chemical quenching, for example, occurs when the scintillation solution absorbs the beta energy without emission of detectable light. Techniques to correct for quenching include internal standardization, external standardization, and channel ratio methods (Dalrymple, 1976). Disadvantages of liquid scintillation counting include the necessity of expensive scintillation fluids or fluors and considerable time in sample preparation.

There are a number of advantages to employing material labeled with gamma-emitting isotopes. Counting is done directly in a gamma counter without need for quench correction. The counting time may be reduced because of the higher specific activity obtainable.

Cobalt-57 (^{57}Co) is utilized to label vitamin B_{12}, and selenium-75 (^{75}Se) has been employed

to directly label steroids (Eckert, 1976). Iodine-125 (^{125}I) has replaced iodine-131 (^{131}I) and now is the most commonly employed gamma-emitting isotope. Although it has a lower specific activity than ^{131}I, ^{125}I has several advantages compared with ^{131}I, including its greater isotope abundance, better counting efficiency, and longer half-life. In addition, the gamma radiation given off by ^{125}I is less energenic than ^{131}I and thus there is less radiation hazard. Since ^{125}I is a weak emitter, there is about a 20 per cent loss of counts if glass rather than plastic tubes are employed (Walker, 1977). Compounds containing ^{125}I tend to be more stable than those of ^{131}I. The shelf life of preparations of ^{125}I depends on a number of factors. As the specific activity of the labeled antigen is increased, it is more likely that the preparation will have decreased immunoreactivity and increased susceptibility to radioactive damage. As the specific activity is increased, a significant number of molecules will have a label at two sites, and these preparations thus may have a decreased shelf life. Decay catastrophy refers to the phenomenon in which two radioactive atoms are present at different sites in one molecule. When radioactive disintegration occurs from one atom, it disrupts part of the molecule, resulting in the production of labeled molecular fragments or free iodide; therefore, the remaining portion with the other radioactive iodine can expect to have decreased immunoreactivity (Yalow, 1978).

A variety of methods have been used to introduce iodine into compounds for use as labels. In the 1960's, Hunter (1962) showed that low concentrations of chloramine-T promoted a highly effective incorporation of inorganic iodine into protein. The mechanism of the reaction probably involves the generation of ionic iodine, which is a potent oxidizing agent. Introduction of radioactive iodine atoms into proteins occurs through a substitution in the tyrosyl residue, although substitution of iodine in other groups such as histidyl also is possible. Other iodination techniques include lactoperoxidase (Marchalonis, 1969), electrolytic iodination (Rosa, 1964), and the introduction of iodinated acyl group in a method described by Bolten (1973). The lactoperoxidase method is useful for proteins that are subject to damage during the chloramine-T iodination. The Bolten-Hunter method involves iodination of an ester by chloramine-T and subsequent condensation at a free amino group in the material to be iodinated. The advantage of this method is that it provides an alternative procedure to reduce iodination damage, and it may be used to label proteins that contain no tyrosine.

There are a number of causes of iodination damage, including partial degradation of the antigen during labeling, introduction of isotope into the antigenic determinant, and damage caused by radiation during or after iodination. Following labeling it is necessary to assess its suitability. A variety of physiochemical techniques, such as gel chromatography, have been employed for purification of the label, and several methods have been used to assess the suitability of the iodinated compound. Incubation of the label with excess antibody has been used to indicate the suitability of the label; a satisfactorily labeled preparation will be bound to the extent of 90 to 98 per cent when incubated with excess high avidity antibody (Hunter, 1974). In addition, the sensitivity of the assay calibration curve obtained with the tracer should be checked.

Immunoradiometric assay

In attempting to improve assay systems with respect to sensitivity and precision, the immunoradiometric assay technique was developed. Immunoradiometric assay differs from conventional radioimmunoassay systems in that the compound to be measured combines directly with radioactively labeled antibodies. In one variation of this type of assay, the standards or samples are reacted with excess labeled antibody: an immunoadsorbent consisting of antigen coupled to a solid phase (see below) is then added to bind the unreacted antibody, which then is removed by centrifugation (Fig. 13–3A). Labeled antibody has several advantages, especially in the assay of certain compounds. For example, it may be difficult to iodinate the antigen, or when iodinated, the antigen may lose immunologic reactivity or may be unstable (Woodhead, 1974). Disadvantages of the technique are that it requires large amounts of antibody and the preparation of reagents is demanding. An immunoadsorbent is prepared by binding purified antigen to a solid phase system, and this is used to isolate specific antibodies. Iodination is carried out with the antibody linked to immunoadsorbent in order to protect the antigenic binding site from damage. This also allows rapid separation of iodine that is not

incorporated and of damaged material (Addison, 1971).

A so-called two-site immunoradiometric assay (or the "sandwich" technique) also may be used. The method involves coupling of unlabeled antibody to insoluble matrix, which then can be reacted with antigen. Provided that the antigen has more than one immunologically reactive group, its uptake to the immunoadsorbent can be measured by subsequent reaction with antibody that has been labeled (Figure 13–3B). The amount of radioactivity taken up during the second incubation is proportional to the concentration of antigen in the first reaction. In addition, a labeled double antibody reagent has been prepared for use in either the immunoradiometric or two-site assay (Woodhead, 1974).

Enzyme Labels

Enzymes may be used in place of selected radioactive isotopes to label either the antigen or the antibody. Disadvantages of enzyme labels include steric hindrance due to presence of the enzyme, which can lead to decreased sensitivity. In addition, enzyme labels are technically more difficult to prepare and interference with enzyme activity may occur (Yalow, 1978).

In a method analogous to radioimmunoassay, enzyme-labeled antigen is employed (Engvall, 1971). Antibody is attached to a solid phase system (see below); thus, bound and free can be separated by centrifugation after incubation. The enzyme activity then is determined in the bound or free fraction. The antibody can be labeled with enzyme (Engvall, 1972) and employed in assays that are analogous to the immunoradiometric or two-site "sandwich" technique. These techniques are referred to as enzyme-linked immunosorbent assays (ELISA).

Immunoassays that require no separation steps are known as "homogeneous assays." Homogeneous enzyme assays have been developed in which labels are made by covalently linking antigen to enzyme (Rubenstein, 1972). When the enzyme molecule that is covalently bound to antigen reacts with antibody to that antigen, the enzymatic activity is inhibited. Inhibition of enzyme activity by antibody is probably caused by either conformational change induced by the antibody binding to the active group or by prevention of the conformation changes necessary for catalytic activ-

A. Labeled antibody and solid-phase antigen

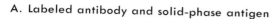

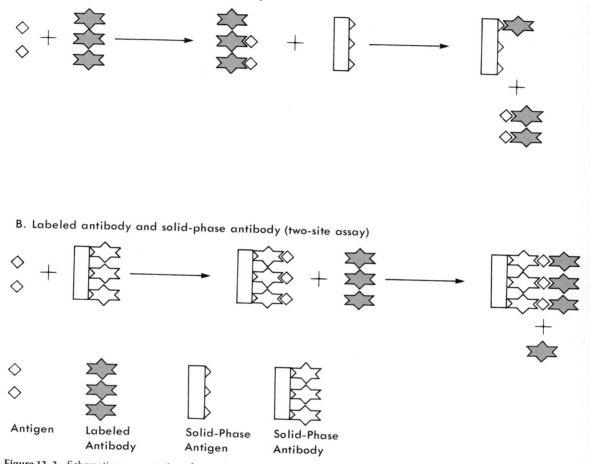

B. Labeled antibody and solid-phase antibody (two-site assay)

| Antigen | Labeled Antibody | Solid-Phase Antigen | Solid-Phase Antibody |

Figure 13–3. Schematic representation of assays employing labeled antibody. (Modified from Woodhead, J. S., Addison, G. M., and Hales, C. N.: The immunoradiometric assay and related techniques. Br. Med. Bull., *30*:44, 1974.)

ity (Rowley, 1975). Enzyme-labeled antigen and unknown antigen compete for antibody binding sites: the enzyme-labeled antigen that remains free is enzymatically active and can be determined in the presence of the bound label (Fig. 13–4). This technique is commercially available as the enzyme-multiplied immunoassay technique (EMIT—Palo Alto, Cal.)

A number of enzymes, including alkaline phosphatase and lysozyme, have been used for labels. It is important that the enzymes employed not be subject to large interferences by the presence of tissue or serum and that convenient, rapid means of measuring the reaction are available. Several methods have been used to link enzymes to antibodies and protein antigens, including glutaraldehyde linkage and dimaleimide linkage (Wisdom, 1976).

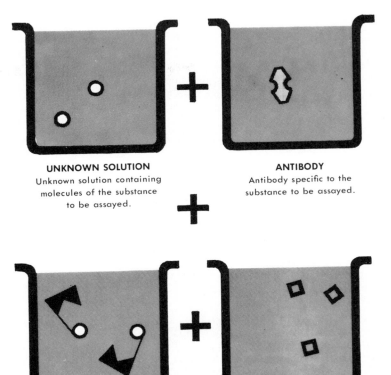

UNKNOWN SOLUTION
Unknown solution containing
molecules of the substance
to be assayed.

ANTIBODY
Antibody specific to the
substance to be assayed.

ENZYME LABEL
Molecules to be assayed
are labelled with an enzyme.

SUBSTRATE
Substrate sensitive
to the enzyme.

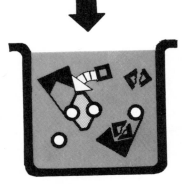

EMIT ENZYME IMMUNOASSAY
Competition for antibody binding sites
causes enzyme-labelled molecules to remain
unbound. The resultant enzyme activity
is directly related to the concentration
of free molecules in the unknown solution.

Figure 13–4. Homogeneous enzyme immunoassay. (From the Syva Company, Palo Alto, Cal.)

OTHER NON-RADIOACTIVE INDICATOR MOLECULES

Although other approaches to non-radioactive indicator molecules have been developed, such as fluorescence, bacteriophage, and spin labels, for the most part they have not been used widely. In these systems, the free and bound labels show differences such that the fractions can be detected in the presence of one another. If an antigen of low molecular weight is conjugated to fluorescein or some other fluorescent molecule and reacted with antibody, a change in fluorescence polarization is observed (Parker, 1976). Spin-labeled molecules—that is, those containing a free radical—have also been used. The spin of the unpaired electron produces a magnetic moment that can be detected and measured by an electron spin resonance spectrometer. Differences in the signal occur as spin label is immobilized by reaction with antibody (Leute, 1972). When bacteriophage is incubated with antiphage serum, neutralization occurs and the phage cannot form plaques. Bacteriophage that has been conjugated to an antigen can be specifically neutralized with antibodies against a convalently linked antigen (Andrieu, 1974).

STANDARDS

In order to have a valid assay, standards and specimens must behave in the same manner in the system. Standardization, especially for those substances that have not been well characterized, is a complex problem. Some of the difficulties that may be encountered in preparation of a suitable standard include natural variations of the substances in question, such as differences among species, heterogeneity of forms, and precursor or degradation products. Synthetic peptides, especially those with more than 20 amino acids, are likely to contain error peptides and racemized residues (Bangham, 1974). In addition, there may be artifacts produced in the standard during its preparation or storage; for example, alterations may occur with freezing or thawing. Any differences in the binding sites of the standard as compared with the unknown may yield differences in affinity for the binder: differences in affinity thus are likely to affect assay results. The stability of the standard is important, since it ideally will be used over a long period of time. Loss of activity may be due to a number of causes, including adsorption to surfaces, contamination with bacterial or tissue enzymes, or oxidation (Bangham, 1971). Assay validity also depends on the control non-specific factors which may influence the reaction, including salt concentration, pH, buffer, and protein concentration of incubation medium. Often it is desirable to prepare standard solutions in serum or plasma devoid of the unknown substance in order to control effects of the assay medium.

Even if a standard which is pure, well-defined, uniform, and stable is available, different results may be obtained using different assay reagents. For example, antibodies vary in their cross-reactivity to substances in the specimen and composition of the specimen may or may not influence a given separation system.

SEPARATION SYSTEMS

The assay endpoint involves determining the relative proportion of antigen which is free (unbound) or bound to specific, saturable binding reagent (bound). In order to determine this distribution, the bound or free fraction is quantitated, usually after physical separation of the two components. The separation step is not essential, however, if one of the components is detectable in the presence of the other, as in homogeneous enzyme immunoassay systems. Commonly, radioactive labels such as ^{125}I are used and the fraction bound to antibody does not spontaneously precipitate: separation of the bound and free is necessary before the fractions are counted. Various systems have been developed taking advantage of the differences in the properties of the bound and free fractions. The choice of method for separating the two moieties depends on a number of factors, such as the adsorption properties of the label and requirements of the assay in terms of speed and susceptibility of the complexes to dissociation during separation.

There are a number of characteristics or criteria of an ideal separation system, including the following: (1) the separating agent does not interfer with the equilibrium state of the completed reaction; (2) the complete separation of the bound and free moieties is obtained; (3) the separation system is reproducible from assay to assay and is uniform within the assay; (4) the separation has a wide mar-

Table 13-3. METHODS OF SEPARATING FREE AND BOUND TRACER

CLASSIFICATION	PRINCIPLE	EXAMPLE
1. Differential migration of bound and free	a. mainly due to differences in charge b. mainly due to differences in molecular weight	a. electrophoresis b. gel filtration

2. Adsorption	a. non-specific adsorption of free moiety	a. 1. charcoal
		   2. silicates—Quso G-32, talc, Florisil, Fuller's earth
		   3. resins (Amberlite)
		b. resins (DEAE-cellulose)

3. Precipitation of bound	b. adsorption of bound
	a. non-specific precipitation
		a. 1. ammonium sulfate
		   2. polyethylene glycol (PEG)
		   3. ethanol
		b. double (second) antibody

4. Solid phase	b. immunologic usually antibody attached to solid material	a. antibody-coated tubes or discs b. antibody coupled to dextran or cellulose particles
5. Combination	more than one of the above	a. mixture of PEG and second antibody b. second antibody linked to a solid phase

gin of error in the conditions used; (5) the separation is fast, simple, inexpensive, and performed with readily available equipment and reagents; (6) it is not influenced by non-specific substances in the samples. Other characteristics that may be helpful include wide applicability to a variety of systems and the ability to distinguish between damaged and undamaged label (Ratcliffe, 1974). For each new assay, a separation system must be tested carefully before it is employed. Important considerations include the amount of separation material used, the reaction time employed, and the conditions of the centrifugation.

A wide variety of separation systems are available (see Table 13-3). Some of the first separation methods used, such as electrophoresis, generally are not employed for routine assays because of certain technical disadvantages.

Methods that involve adsorption, usually of the free fraction, commonly have been employed in assays for steroids, small peptides, and drugs such as digoxin. Generally the adsorption methods are most satisfactory for antigens with a molecular weight of 30,000 or less (Yalow, 1978). Separations can be performed rapidly, but several factors, including timing of the separation and amount of adsorbent added to each tube, must be carefully controlled. Adsorption is determined by many factors, including relative surface area of the

adsorbent, size and charge of the antigen, protein in the system, temperature, ionic strength, and pH (Ratcliffe, 1974). Certain types of charcoal such as Norit A have satisfactory characteristics for adsorption of the free fraction. Charcoal, which usually is pretreated with dextran or protein, has a high affinity for a wide variety of substances. However, it may adsorb the bound as well as free fractions: the affinity of charcoal for the free fraction may be so high as to disturb the equilibrium of the reaction. The effects of this stripping phenomenon on the assay system can be minimized by keeping the temperature of the incubation mixture low during the period of charcoal addition and by insuring that the time of exposure to charcoal is identical in all tubes (Ekins, 1976). A number of steps for systemically optimizing conditions of the separation, such as varying the amounts of charcoal and the reaction times, have been suggested by Binoux (1973). Other substances may be used to adsorb the free fraction, including various silicates such as talc, Florisil, and Quso G-32.

The bound fraction may be precipitated, leaving the free fraction in solution. This may be accomplished by a non-specific precipitating system employing ammonium sulfate, ethanol, polyethylene glycol, or a number of other substances. The double antibody or second antibody, which also precipitates the bound fraction, is a commonly used system that depends on the ability of anti-immuno-globulin antibodies to bind the soluble anti-gen-antibody complex and cause precipitation. For example, if the antibody against the un-known antigen (first antibody) is made in a rabbit, the antibody for the separation (second antibody) is made to rabbit gamma globulin. This technique requires that the antigenic determinants of the gamma globulin are distinct from the antigen-combining sites and that the relative concentration of the reagents in the system favors precipitin formation. This type of separation system often is em-ployed in the assay of polypeptide hormones such as prolactin and growth hormone. The second antibody must be carefully screened for cross-reactivity with human gamma glob-ulin before use. The double antibody system may be used in several ways. Commonly the so-called post-precipitation method is em-ployed: in this method the second antibody and carrier serum or non-immune gamma globulin is added after the first antibody reac-tion is completed. Major factors affecting the separation include conditions of the second antibody incubation, centrifugation, carrier protein concentration, and characteristics and concentration of the second antibody, as well as non-specific effects due to serum and anti-coagulants. In general interfering factors may be minimized by using a prolonged incubation of 24 to 48 hours in the precipitation step (Ratcliffe, 1974). In the pre-precipitation method, the first antibody is precipitated by the second before the reaction is carried out. The double antibody system may also be com-bined with the solid phase system (vide infra). In addition, separation systems have been de-vised in which sub-precipitating concentra-tions of materials such as ammonium sulfate are used in combination with the second anti-body.

Antibody can be insolubilized through cova-lent or non-covalent bonding to solid supports such as tubes, discs, or other materials. These so-called solid phase systems provide a rapid, versatile, and efficient separation of fractions. In general, the disadvantages of the solid phase system include relatively large amounts of antibody required, and it may be difficult to insure uniformity of the system.

For each assay which is developed, the exact conditions of the separation procedure must be worked out, including the amount of mate-rial used, the reaction times, and centrifuga-tion step. In addition, there are several practi-cal problems associated with the separation procedures. Exact timing of the separation step is critical with some systems, for exam-ple, charcoal. The effects of and variations in total protein concentration are very impor-tant. Adsorption systems, for example, are particularly sensitive to total protein, and precipitating systems such as ammonium sul-fate may be markedly dependent on protein as the carrier. Approximately the same protein concentration thus must be employed in all tubes, including the standard. It sometimes may be difficult to obtain serum free of the substance to be assayed for use in establishing a standard curve. Substitutions, for example, animal serum or serum treated with charcoal to remove the substance in question, have been employed. These manuevers, however, may not be entirely satisfactory. Anticoagu-lants also may affect the separation system. For example, complement may reduce the rate of precipitin formation in the second antibody system. Iodination or incubation damage may alter the behavior of the label in the separa-tion systems (see p. 394). Damaged tracer may affect an assay in different ways. In double antibody methods, generally there is a reduc-tion in the bound fraction; however, if the damaged tracer aggregates or adsorbs to the precipitate more than the intact label, the apparent bound fraction will increase (Hunter, 1971). Adsorption systems tend to be sensitive to alterations in label.

ASSAY DEVELOPMENT AND VALIDATION

Even if facilities for generation and evalua-tion of the binding reagents and labels are available, for many laboratories it is more efficient to purchase reagents in assay kit or component form. Periodically product direc-tories or buyers' guides listing available kits or components are published. For example, in the September, 1977, issue of Lab World (North American Publishing Co., Philadel-phia), over 30 thyroxine kits and more than 20 digoxin kits were listed. In addition, kits with enzyme rather than radioactive labels are available for thyroxine (Jaklitsch, 1976) and digoxin (Rosenthal, 1976). In selecting assay kits many aspects should be considered, in-cluding cost, separation technique, type of label, and cross-reacting substances. For ex-ample, rapid turn-around time may be partic-ularly important for a determination; thus, a separation step such as a double antibody procedure with a long incubation would not be appropriate.

Not only do kits provide the reagents necessary for the assay, but some steps involved in assay development, such as assessment of antibody binding, have already been performed. After proper preparation of the reagents according to the manufacturer's directions, the assay can be performed following the instructions provided. However, the kit performance must be evaluated before it is used routinely. Although in general the principles of assay development, validation, and quality control are the same as for other types of determinations, certain aspects warrent special emphasis.

Sensitivity is defined as the minimum amount of antigen that can be measured with acceptable precision (Ekins, 1971). The limits of sensitivity are determined by the affinity of the specific binding reagent employed. The antibody dilution usually is chosen so that 20 to 70 per cent of the label is antibody-bound in the absence of unlabeled antigen. With excess antibody, loss of sensitivity occurs (Hurn, 1971). Other measures designed to increase sensitivity of radioimmunoassays include prolongation of the incubation period, use of small quantities of label, and delayed addition of label (Chard, 1971). Although the sensitivity can be increased by delayed addition of label, that is, with "non-equilibrium" assays, failure to reach equilibrium may lead to loss of precision (Rodbard, 1971). If the label affinity differs from that of the unlabeled material, the full sensitivity of the assay cannot be achieved. Another approach is to extract and concentrate the specimen. In general, attempts to employ assays at the extreme limits of sensitivity can introduce problems.

Parameters of assay validity include quantitative recovery of added antigen and demonstration that the assay reads zero in the absence of antigen. It is essential to demonstrate that the apparent antigen content in the unknown is independent of the dilution at which it is assayed. This requires that the concentration in the unknown decrease linearly with dilution or that a dilution curve of unknown sample be superimposed on a dilution curve of standard (Yalow, 1978).

Two types of "blanks" should be included with every assay: one containing labeled antigen, antibody, and antigen-free serum or plasma; the other, labeled antigen and anti-gen-free serum or plasma but no antibody. The first check provides information on the reaction of label and antibody and the completeness of the separation step (Challand, 1974). The second yields information regarding the non-specific binding of the label.

Other considerations when using a radioactive label include counting error, adsorption of the label to glassware, and the possibility of radioactive contamination of the specimen.

To have a valid assay, cross-reactivity studies using appropriate substances should be performed, and non-specific factors such as pH and protein content of media must be controlled. Because of their variability, it is necessary to characterize each antibody individually. When the antibody lot used in a particular assay is changed, it is important that this antibody be recharacterized. Assay values must show appropriate response under various physiologic conditions. This is particularly important to demonstrate with the use of antibody as the specific binding reagent. Since antibody measures immunologic rather than biologic activity, it should be understood that measurements by immunoassay may not always reflect the true *in vivo* activity. For example, proinsulin, which is relatively inactive, may cross-react with antibody to insulin.

Generally, it is recommended that assay samples be measured in duplicate and, if a wide variety of concentrations is expected, the duplicates be assayed at more than one dilution (Challand, 1974). In some cases each sample is run singly at two dilutions (Walker, 1977).

The precision of radioimmunoassay is less than that achieved with most routine chemical assays: the coefficient of variation of between-batch replicates is usually not less than 6 per cent (Challand, 1974). The precision is not the same in each portion of the standard curve: the phenomenon of changes in precision is called non-uniformity of variance or heteroscedasticity.

Plots of the dose-response curve, such as percentage bound vs. log dose, yield a sigmoidal curve. Attempts have been made to linearize data: the most commonly employed technique is that of logit transformation in which the logit B/Bo is plotted versus the log dose. The logit $B/Bo = \log (B/Bo)/(1-B/Bo)$, where B equals the fraction of tracer bound and Bo equals the value of B with no unlabeled antigen in the system. The linearization by this method is an empirical finding (Rodbard, 1968). The method has the disadvantage of resulting in marked heteroscedasticity, necessitating use of weighted regression (Rodbard, 1974). These calculations, however, can be done automatically by a computer or desk-top calculator. In general, three quality control samples should be run, and these should be at widely different concentrations.

Quality control systems have been developed in which various assay parameters are recorded, such as specific activity of tracer, amount of tracer, total counts per minute, within-assay variance, and between-assay variance. For further details see Rodbard (1968) and Rodbard (1974).

RECEPTOR ASSAYS

In addition to their use as specific binding reagents, receptors have a growing importance in the clinical laboratory. For example, there are a number of conditions in which receptor dysfunction appears to have a pathogenic role. Tentative classification of these disorders has been proposed: (1) inherited abnormalities of receptor function, such as occur in some androgen-resistant states; (2) receptors as targets for autoantibodies, for example, in myasthenia gravis and Graves' disease and in a small group of patients with insulin-resistant diabetes; (3) tolerance and hypersensitivity (Jacobs, 1977). In addition, receptor assays may be useful in evaluating certain treatment modalities; for example, the hormonal responsiveness of prostatic cancer may be related to the presence of cytoplasmic receptor proteins that bind androgen. Menon (1977) has reviewed the methods of measurements of androgen receptors in human prostatic tissue.

The most important practical application of receptor assays at present, however, is the quantitation of estrogen receptors in breast cancer tissue. Breast carcinoma is often responsive to endocrine therapies that have been employed for its treatment. Approximately one third of patients with metastatic breast carcinoma respond with objective remissions of disease either to ablative or additive endocrine therapy. Therapeutic modalities include ovariectomy, adrenalectomy, hypophysectomy (ablative therapy), as well as treatment with antiestrogens, pharmacologic doses of estrogens, androgens, progestin, or glucocorticoids (additive ther-

apy). Regardless of the type of endocrine therapy employed, objective tumor regression occurs in approximately 20 to 40 per cent of patients (McGuire, 1977a).

Studies of classic estrogen-dependent tissue such as the uterus have lead to the discovery of a cytoplasmic protein that binds estrogen with high affinity and specificity. The interaction of the estrogen molecule with its cytoplasmic protein is believed to be the initial event leading to a complex series of responses characteristic of estrogen stimulation. An extension of these studies was the search for estrogen receptors in breast tumor tissue. Subsequently the relationship of the presence of estrogen receptor and response of the tumor to endocrine therapy was studied.

Many assay methods have been used to measure estrogen receptors, including sucrose gradient ultracentrifugation and a dextran-coated charcoal method. Although estrogen receptors cannot be readily detected in the non-lactating human breast, the amount of estrogen receptor in primary malignant breast tumors ranges up to 1000 femtomoles/mg of cytosol protein (McGuire, 1977a). If a patient is found to have an estrogen-positive tumor (greater than 3 femtomoles/mg of cytosol protein with the dextran-coated charcoal method), response to endocrine therapy occurs in about 60 per cent of patients; there is some suggestion that the higher the estrogen receptor value the more likely the patient is to respond (McGuire, 1975b). In general the highest tumor estrogen receptor levels are found in post-menopausal patients, possibly due at least in part to the amount of endogenous estrogen secreted by the patient. If a patient has a tumor with very little or no estrogen, that is, less than 3 femtomoles/mg of cytosol protein, the chances of tumor regression with endocrine therapy are minimal (McGuire, 1975a). Some workers recommend that receptor content be expressed in other ways, for example, in terms of tissue weight, μg DNA (Jensen, 1975), or tissue protein correcting for serum protein (Heuson, 1975). Jensen (1977), using a sucrose gradient ultracentrifugation, regards the following levels as positive: greater than 750 femtomoles/g of tumor in the post-menopausal or castrated patient and greater than 250 femtomoles/g in the pre-menopausal patient. In addition, absence of estrogen receptor in a primary breast carcinoma specimen may be a prognostic indicator of early recurrence. In patients whose tumors lack significant estrogen binding, the response to hormonal manipulations is only about 5 per cent (Young, 1977).

Several reasons have been proposed why all patients with estrogen-positive tumors do not respond to therapy. It is known, for example, that tumors that have progesterone receptors in addition to estrogen receptors respond to hormonal therapy better than tumors that are progesterone-receptor negative and estrogen-receptor positive. Progesterone receptors are found in 9 per cent of estrogen-negative metastatic breast tumors but are present in over 70 per cent of estrogen-positive tumors (McGuire, 1977a). If metastatic tumor tissue contains both estrogen receptor and progesterone receptor, the response rate to endocrine therapy has been reported to be 92 per cent (McGuire, 1977b). Receptor measurements for other hormones, including prolactin and androgens, may also be of value in making a prediction of management with a favorable outcome. Tumors may contain a heterogeneous population of hormone-dependent cells and, therefore, display a mixed response to hormonal therapy. Other reasons proposed for the non-responsiveness of estrogen-positive tumors include possibility of defective cytoplasmic receptor proteins; these may prevent the induction of the sequence of biochemical events that ultimately lead to tumor regression with hormonal therapy. Also, there may be absent or defective specific nuclear receptors. Results of assay of estrogen receptors from a group of breast carcinoma patients show that 17 per cent had cytoplasmic but no nuclear estrogen receptors (Laing, 1977).

One of the most important aspects of receptor assays is the handling of the tumor tissue. Since estrogen receptors are very labile at room temperature, tissue must be kept cold and frozen in liquid nitrogen immediately after excision. It has been suggested that dextran-coated charcoal assay or some modification is the most practical method for routine assay of estrogen receptors in breast tissues. In this method, non-receptor-bound titrated estradiol is removed from the specific receptors in the tissue preparation by charcoal. The frozen tissue is pulverized, homogenized, and centrifuged at 4°C. at greater than 100,000 g to obtain the supernatant cytosol fraction. Binding data are obtained from incubating aliquots of cytosol preparation with increasing concentrations of labeled hormone. After addition of charcoal and centrifugation, the amount of receptor-bound hormone remaining in solution is plotted against the ratio of bound to free. In this Scatchard plot, the slope of the line gives a measure of the affinity constant. Scatchard plots of binding usually reveal a single class of receptor sites with high affinity binding.

With the charcoal method non-specific binding may not be recognized as readily as with the sucrose gradient method, nor does it distinguish receptor that sediments at 8S and 4S, a distinction considered important by some workers (Jensen, 1977). If cytoplasmic estrogen receptor is transferred to nuclear sites, it is inaccessible for assay using conventional techniques (McGuire, 1977a).

Detection and measurement of specific progesterone receptors has been difficult, because of instability of the progesterone-receptor complex and interferences by plasma binding proteins. The use of a highly potent synthetic progestin R5020 has helped resolve this problem (Raynaud, 1977).

REFERENCES

Addison, G. M., and Hales, C. N.: The immunoradiometric assay. *In* Kirkham, K. E., and Hunter, W. M. (eds.): Radioimmunoassay Methods. Edinburgh, Churchill Livingstone, 1971.

Andrieu, J. M., Mamas, S., and Dray, F.: Viroimmunoassay of 17β-oestradiol. Radioimmunoassay and related procedures. *In* Medicine, vol. 2. Vienna, International Atomic Energy Agency, 1974.

Bangham, D. R., and Cotes, P. M.: Reference standards for radioimmunoassay. *In* Kirkham, K. E., and Hunter, W. M. (eds.): Radioimmunoassay Methods. Edinburgh, Churchill Livingstone, 1971.

Bangham, D. R., and Cotes, P. M.: Standardization and standards. Br. Med. Bull., *30*:12, 1974.

Binoux, M. A., and Odell, W. D.: Use of dextran-coated charcoal to separate antibody-bound from free hormone: A critique. J. Clin. Endocrinol., Metabol., *36*:303, 1973.

Bolton, A. E., and Hunter, W. M.: The labelling of proteins to high specific radioactivities by conjugation to a 125 containing acylating agent. Biochem. J., *133*:529, 1973.

Butler, V. P.: Assays of digitalis in the blood. Prog. Cardiovasc. Dis., *14*:571, 1972.

Challand, G., Goldie, D., and Landon, J.: Immunoassay in the diagnostic laboratory. Br. Med. J., *30*:38, 1974.

Chard, T.: Observations on the uses of a mathematical model in radioimmunoassay. *In* Kirkham, K. E., and Hunter, W. M. (eds.): Radioimmunoassay Methods. Edinburgh, Churchill Livingstone, 1971.

Dalrymple, G. V., Baker, M. L., Vandergrift, J. F., and Walaski, S. L.: The measurement of radiations emitted by radioactive isotopes used in RIA procedures. *In* Moss, A. J., Jr., Dalrymple, G. V., and Boyd, C. M. (eds.): Practical Radioimmunoassay. Saint Louis, The C. V. Mosby Co., 1976.

Eckert, H. G.: Radioimmunoassay. Agnew Chem. Int. Ed. Engl., *15*:525, 1976.

Ekins, R. P.: General principles of hormone assay. *In* Loraine, J. A., and Bell, E. T. (eds.): Hormone Assays and Their Clinical Application. Edinburgh, Churchill Livingstone, 1976.

Ekins, R. P.: Mathematical treatment of data. *In* Kirkham, K. E., and Hunter, W. M. (eds.): Radioimmunoassay Methods. Edinburgh, Churchill Livingstone, 1971.

Ekins, R. P.: Basic principles and theory. Br. Med. Bull., *30*:3, 1974.

Engvall, E., Jonsson, K., and Perlmann, P.: Enzyme-linked immunosorbent assay II. Quantitative assay of protein antigen, immunoglobulin by means of enzyme labelled antigen and antibody coated tubes. Biochim. Biophys. Acta, *251*:427, 1971.

Engvall, E., and Perlmann, P.: Enzyme-linked immunosorbent assay (ELISA)III. Quantitation of specific antibodies by enzyme-labeled anti-immunoglobulin in antigen-coated tubes. J. Immunol., *109*:129, 1972.

Heuson, J. C., Leclercq, G., Longeval, E., Deboel, C., Mattheien, W. H., and Heimann, R.: Estrogen receptors: Prognostic significance in breast cancer. *In* McGuire, W. L., Carbone, P. P., and Vollmer, E. P.: Estrogen Receptors in Human Breast Cancer. New York, Raven Press, 1975.

Hunter, W. M., and Ganguli, P. C.: The separation of antibody bound from free antigen. *In* Kirkham, K. E., and Hunter, W. M. (eds.): Radioimmunoassay Methods. Edinburgh, Churchill Livingstone, 1971.

Hunter, W. M., and Greenwood, F. C.: Preparation of iodine-131 labelled human growth hormone of high specific activity. Nature, *194*:495, 1962.

Hunter, W. M.: Preparation and assessment of radioactive tracers. Br. Med. Bull., *30*:18, 1974.

Hurn, B. A. L., and Landon, J.: Antisera for radioimmunoassay. *In* Kirkham, K. E., and Hunter, W. M. (eds.): Radioimmunoassay Methods. Edinburgh, Churchill Livingstone, 1971.

Jacobs, S., and Cuatrecasas, P.: Cell receptors in disease. N. Engl. J. Med., *297*:1383, 1977.

Jaklitsch, A. P., Schneider, R. S., Johannes, R. J., Lavine, J. E., and Rosenberg, G. L.: Homogeneous enzyme immunoassay for T-4 in serum. Clin. Chem., *22*:1185, 1976.

Jensen, E. V., and DeSombre, E. R.: The diagnostic implications of steroid binding in malignant tissues. Adv. Clin. Chem., *19*:57, 1977.

Jensen, E. V., Polley, T. Z., Smith, S., Block, G. E., Ferguson, D. J., and DeSombre, E. R.: Prediction of hormone dependency in human breast cancer. *In* McGuire, W. L., Carbone, P. P., and Vollmer, E. P.: Estrogen Receptors in Human Breast Cancer. New York, Raven Press, 1975.

Kahn, C. R.: Membrane receptors for hormones and neurotransmitters. J. Cell Biol., *70*:261, 1976.

Kubiatowicz, D. O., Ithakissios, D. S., and Windorski, D. C.: Vitamin B-12 radioassay with oyster toad fish (*Opsanus tau*) serum as binder. Clin. Chem., *23*:1037, 1977.

Laing, L., Calman, K. C., Smith, M. G., Smith, D. C., and Leake, R. E.: Nuclear estrogen receptors and treatment of breast cancer. Lancet, *2*:168, 1977.

Landon, J.: The radioimmunoassay of drugs. Analyst, *101*:225, 1976.

Leute, R., Ullman, E. F., and Goldstein, A.: Spin immunoassay of opiate narcotics in urine and saliva. J.A.M.A., *221*:1231, 1972.

McGuire, W. L., Carbone, P. P., Sears, M. E., and Escher, G. C.: Estrogen receptors in human breast cancer: An overview. *In* McGuire. W. L., Carbone, P. P., and Vollmer, E. P.: Estrogen Receptors in Human Breast Cancer. New York, Raven Press, 1975a.

McGuire, W. L., Horwitz, K. B., Pearson, O. H., and Segaloff, A.: Current status of estrogen and progesterone receptors in breast cancer. Cancer, *39*:2934, 1977a.

McGuire, W. L., Pearson, O. H., and Segaloff, A.: Predicting hormone responsiveness in human breast cancer. *In* McGuire, W. L., Carbone, P. P., and Vollmer, E. P. (eds.): Estrogen Receptors in Human Breast Cancer. New York, Raven Press, 1975b.

McGuire, W. L., Raynaud, J. P., and Baulieu, E. E.: Progesterone receptors: Introduction and overview. *In* McGuire, W. L., Raynaud, J. P., and Baulieu, E. E.: Progesterone Receptors in Normal and Neoplastic Tissues. New York, Raven Press, 1977b.

Marchalonis, J. J.: An enzymatic method for the trace iodination of immunoglobulins and other proteins. Biochem. J., *113*:299, 1969.

Menon, M., Tananis, C. E., McLoughlin, M. G., and Walsh, P. C.: Androgen receptors in human prostatic tissue: A review. Cancer Treat. Rep., *61*:265, 1977.

Myers, C. E., Lippman, M. E., Eliot, H. M., and Crabner, B. A.: Competitive protein binding assay for methotrexate. Proc. Natl. Acad. Sci. U.S.A. *72*:3683, 1975.

Parker, C. W.: Radioimmunoassay of Biologically Active Compounds. Englewood Cliffs, N.J., Prentice-Hall, Inc., 1976.

Playfair, J. H. L., Hurn, B. A. L., and Schulster, D.: Production of antibodies and binding reagents. Br. Med. Bull., *30*:24, 1974.

Ratcliffe, J. G.: Separation techniques in saturation analysis. Br. Med. Bull., *30*:32, 1974.

Raynaud, J. P., Ojasoo, T., Delarue, J. C., Magdelenat, H., Martin, P., and Philibert, D.: Estrogen and progestin receptors in human breast cancer. *In* McGuire, W. L., Raynaud, J. P., and Baulieu, E. E.: Progesterone Receptors in Normal and Neoplastic Tissues. New York, Raven Press, 1977.

Rodbard, D.: Statistical quality control and routine data processing for radioimmunoassays and immunoradiometric assays. Clin. Chem., *20*:1255, 1974.

Rodbard, D., Rayford, P. L., Cooper, J. A., and Ross, G. T.: Statistical quality control of radioimmunoassays. J. Clin. Endocrinol. Metabol., *28*:1412, 1968.

Rodbard, D., Ruder, H. J., Vaitukaitis, and Jacobs, H. S.: Mathematical analysis of kinetics of radioligand assays: Improved sensitivity obtained by delayed addition of labeled ligand. J. Clin. Endocrinol. Metabol., *33*:343, 1971.

Rosa, U., Scassellati, G. A., and Pennisi, F.: Labelling of human fibrinogen with 131-I by electrolytic iodination. Biochim. Biophys. Acta, *86*:519, 1964.

Rosenthal, A. F., Vargas, M. G., and Klass, C. S.: Evaluation of enzyme-multiplied immunoassay technique (EMIT) for determination of serum digoxin. Clin. Chem., *22*:1899, 1976.

Roth, J.: Assay of peptide hormones using cell receptors: Application to insulin and to human growth hormone.

In Colowick, S. P., and Kaplan, N. O. (eds.): Methods of Enzymology, vol. 37. New York, Academic Press, Inc., 1975.

Rothenberg, S. P., and daCosta, M.: Folate binding proteins and radioassay for folate. Clin. Hematol., *5*:569, 1976.

Rowley, G. L., Rubenstein, K. E., Huisjen, J., and Ullman, E. F.: Mechanism by which antibodies inhibit hapten-malate dehydrogenase conjugates. J. Biol. Chem., *250*:3759, 1975.

Rubenstein, K. E., Schneider, R. S., and Ullman, E. F.: "Homogeneous" enzyme immunoassay. A new immunochemical technique. Biochem. Biophys. Res. Comm., *47*:846, 1972.

Skelley, D. S., Brown, L. P., and Besch, P. K.: Radioimmunoassay. Clin. Chem., *19*:146, 1973.

Vaitukaitis, J., Robbins, J. B., Nieschlag, E., and Ross, G. T.: A method for producing specific antisera with small doses of immunogen. J. Clin. Endocrinol. Metabol., *33*:988, 1971.

Veall, N.: Radioisotopes and their radiations. *In* Belcher, E. H., and Vetter, H. (eds.): Radioisotopes in Medical Diagnosis. London, Appleton-Century-Crofts, 1971.

Walker, W. H. C.: An approach to immunoassay. Clin. Chem., *23*:384, 1977.

Wisdom, G. B.: Enzyme immunoassay. Clin. Chem., *22*:1243, 1976.

Woodhead, J. S., Addison, G. M., and Hales, C. N.: The immunoradiometric assay and related techniques. Br. Med. J., *30*:44, 1974.

Yalow, R. S.: Heterogeneity of peptide hormones: Its relevance in clinical radioimmunoassay. Adv. Clin. Chem., *20*:1, 1978.

Yalow, R. S., and Berson, S. A.: Problems of validation of radioimmunoassay. *In* Odell, W. D., and Daughaday, W. H. (eds.): Competitive Protein Binding Assays. Philadelphia, J. B. Lippincott Company, 1971a.

Yalow, R. S., and Berson, S. A.: Problems of validation of considerations. *In* Odell, W. D., and Daughaday, W. H. (eds.): Competitive Protein Binding Assays. Philadelphia, J. B. Lippincott Company, 1971b.

Young, R. C., Lippman, M., DeVita, V. T., Bull, J., and Tormey, D.: Perspectives in the treatment of breast cancer: 1976. Ann. Intern. Med., *86*:784, 1977.

14

EVALUATION OF ENDOCRINE FUNCTION

Peter J. Howanitz, M.D.,
and Joan H. Howanitz, M.D.

Not all of the hormones will be presented in this chapter. Other sections which have information relating to the endocrine system include Chapters 23 and 24, pancreatic and gastrointestinal hormones; Chapter 10, calcium metabolism (parathyroid hormone and calcitonin); Chapter 19, placental hormones; and Chapter 7, hormones associated with glucose metabolism.

FUNDAMENTAL PRINCIPLES

CLASSIFICATION OF HORMONES

The endocrine system produces its regulatory effect by elaborating hormones which stimulate or inhibit the function of cells. The hormones produced have an important role in controlling the metabolic function of the body; for example, they play a central role in reproduction, growth and differentiation, and adaptation to the environment. Most hormones are secreted directly into the blood and then are carried to responsive cells where they exert their effects, while others exert their influence by acting locally. Although their chemical structures vary widely, most of the hormones can be grouped into (1) polypeptides or small proteins, including adrenocorticotropic hormone (ACTH), vasopressin, and growth hormone; (2) those derived from amino acids such as epinephrine and thyroxine; and (3) steroids such as cortisol.

THEORIES OF ACTION

The mode of action of the hormones at the cellular and molecular levels has undergone intensive investigation. The effects of the peptides and protein hormones on their target cells now are recognized to be mediated by a series of biochemical events which involve the ability of these hormones to combine with specific high affinity sites—that is, *receptors*—on the *plasma membranes* of their target cells. After binding to the receptor, there is a rapid activation of cellular responses, many of which are mediated by the action of cyclic AMP (adenosine 3′,5′ monophosphate). Cyclic AMP thus acts as the so-called second messenger. After the initial event of cyclic AMP formation from adenosine triphosphate (ATP) by the action of the enzyme adenyl cyclase, target cell responses are activated via stimulation of protein kinase. Protein kinase, which appears to be universally present in mammalian cells, mediates the effects of cyclic AMP by phosphorylation of specific substrates, which in turn regulate cell function (Figs. 14-1 and 14-2). There is evidence that cyclic GMP (cyclic guanosine 3′,5′ monophosphate) also may affect phosphorylation of specific proteins. Certain actions of a number of hormones, including epinephrine and norepinephrine, may be mediated or modulated via cyclic GMP (Greengard, 1978). The

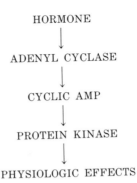

HORMONE

↓

ADENYL CYCLASE

↓

CYCLIC AMP

↓

PROTEIN KINASE

↓

PHYSIOLOGIC EFFECTS

Figure 14-1. Schematic representation of the role of cyclic AMP as a second messenger.

pathway of biochemical degradation for cAMP and cGMP is hydrolysis to the corresponding 5′ nucleoside monophosphate by phosphodiesterase enzymes. As shown in Figure 14-2, in some tissues, particularly those which respond by contractile and secretory activity, calcium seems to play a role in mediating cellular response (Catt, 1976). It is thought that some of the substances which modulate hormonal function may assert their effects by influencing the cyclic AMP concentration in cells; for example, the prostaglandins may act through this mechanism (Fig. 14-2). Some of the hormones derived from amino acids also act through stimulation of formation of cyclic AMP. The steroid and thyroid hormones, however, act predominantly through increased transcription of messenger RNA within the target cell nucleus. The hormone enters the target tissue by diffusion through the cellular membrane and combines with the *cytoplasmic receptor* to form a receptor complex. The complex then is transferred to the nucleus, where it stimulates gene transcription. Messenger RNA is formed, and subsequent synthesis of specific proteins occurs (Fig. 14-3).

HORMONE CONTROL MECHANISMS

In studying patients with endocrine disorders, it is important to understand the feedback mechanisms controlling hormone function. The endocrine glands secrete hormones in response to physiologic requirements. In general these secretions are controlled by mechanisms whereby the production of a hormone is stimulated when its action is required and inhibited when the effect has been attained. Secretion of the trophic hormones of the anterior pituitary is governed largely by the hormones produced in their target glands. For example, when thyroid hormone secretion decreases, the pituitary normally responds by producing an increased amount of thyroid stimulating hormone (TSH), and when thyroid hormones increase, TSH decreases.

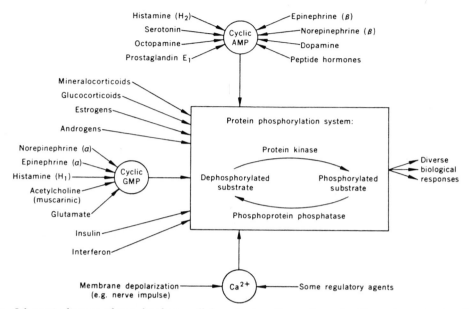

Figure 14-2. Schematic diagram of postulated intracellular role played by cyclic nucleotides and protein phosphorylation in mediating some of the biologic effects of a variety of regulatory agents. (From Greengard, P.: Phosphorylated proteins as physiological effectors. Science, *199*:146, 1978. Copyright © 1978 American Association for the Advancement of Science.)

These reciprocal changes are an example of a *negative feedback system.* The anterior pituitary is regulated by the hypothalamus and the thyroid hormones in turn may influence the hypothalamic hormone thyroid releasing hormone (TRH). *Positive feedback* occurs when an elevation in hormone concentration stimulates release of another hormone. In addition to this type of control, a hormone may influence its own secretion. There are other regulatory mechanisms controlling the secretion of endocrine glands, such as direct influence by the physical or chemical processes which they regulate. There is evidence that the sympathetic and parasympathetic nervous systems play a role in the regulation of hormonal secretion.

CHARACTERISTICS AND PATTERNS OF SECRETION

Hormones circulate in low concentrations, permeating most of the tissues of the body but influencing only those target glands and organs which are capable of responding to them. The protein and peptide hormones generally are water soluble and exist in sera without demonstrable interaction with serum proteins. These hormones generally have a rapid metabolic turnover with half-life in minutes and undergo striking fluctuations in blood concentrations within a short time. The blood concentrations of hormones such as the catecholamines may fluctuate within a few seconds. In contrast, the steroid hormones, such as cortisol or testosterone, and thyroxine are relatively hydrophobic and exist in aqueous solution by virtue of their firm binding to one or more serum protein carriers (Sterling, 1977). These and other factors should be kept in mind when studying patients with possible abnormalities in hormonal secretion. The peptide hormones may exhibit heterogeneity; that is, hormonal forms of varying molecular weight such as larger

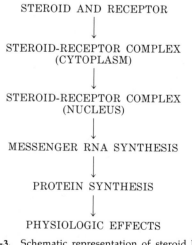

Figure 14-3. Schematic representation of steroid hormone action.

precursor forms and smaller degradation products may exist in the circulation. Many of the hormones show a diurnal variation; that is, the pattern of secretion varies throughout the day. For example, growth hormone secretion increases during sleep. In addition, some hormones show other patterns of secretion, such as the cyclic pattern of follicle stimulating hormone (FSH) and luteinizing hormone (LH).

STIMULATION AND SUPPRESSION TESTS

Stress, nutritional state, and drug therapy also may influence hormonal secretion. In evaluating patients, often it is helpful to use stimulatory and suppressive tests in addition to baseline hormone levels. Stimulation tests may be useful in determining reserve capacity; for example, an ACTH stimulation test can be performed in a patient presenting with symptoms of adrenal hypofunction. This test may help determine if the hypofunction is primary in the adrenal itself or if it is secondary to a pituitary lesion. In cases of endocrine hyperfunction, suppression tests may be helpful in revealing abnormalities in physiologic function and control. For example, glucose normally suppresses growth hormone (GH) levels; thus, the lack of suppression of GH after a glucose load may indicate an abnormality in growth hormone secretion such as occurs in acromegaly.

PITUITARY GLAND AND HYPOTHALAMUS

HORMONES OF THE PITUITARY

The pituitary gland is divided into an anterior lobe, a rudimentary intermediate lobe, and the posterior or neural lobe. The anterior lobe secretes growth hormone (GH), adrenocorticotropic hormone (ACTH), thyroid stimulating hormone (TSH), follicle stimulating hormone (FSH), luteinizing hormone (LH), and prolactin. The pituitary also synthesizes a lipolytic polypeptide of 91 amino acids, beta lipotropic hormone (beta LPH). The intermediate lobe of the pituitary is thought to contain most of the beta LPH, although it has been found in the anterior lobe as well (Chrétien, 1977). The intermediate lobe hormone, beta melanocyte stimulating hormone (beta MSH), is a peptide which is believed to control pigmentation in humans. It has been reported that beta MSH appears not to exist as a separate entity in humans but may be an artifact formed from beta LPH (Bachelot, 1977). The posterior pituitary secretes vasopressin, also called antidiuretic hormone (ADH), and oxytocin.

Depending on the presence and staining characteristics of intracellular granules, the cells of the anterior pituitary classically have been divided into three types: acidophils, basophils, and chromophils. Numerous staining techniques have been employed in order to obtain morphologic separation of the cells into distinct subtypes, and recently immunologic methods have also been applied to the study of this question. These techniques have been used to confirm the existence of separate growth hormone and prolactin acidophils (Doniach, 1977).

HYPOTHALAMIC CONTROL

After the hormones of the anterior pituitary reach their target organs and tissues, they regulate various processes, as indicated in Figure 14-4. For further details on ACTH, TSH, LH, and FSH, refer to the appropriate subsequent sections on the adrenal cortex, thyroid gland, and gonads. The release and synthesis of the anterior and intermediate lobe pituitary hormones are influenced by hypothalamic substances known as hypothalamic releasing factors or hormones. The hypothalamic substances that are under investigation for a role in controlling pituitary function commonly are referred to as factors and those that have been definitely characterized are termed hormones. The releasing factors probably are transported by a process of axonal flow to the median eminence of the hypothalamus in response to certain stimuli. They pass into the portal venous system and down the pituitary stalk to the pituitary gland, where they effect the synthesis and release of the pituitary hormones. The hypothalamic releasing hormone, thyrotropin releasing hormone (TRH), and somatostatin have been well characterized. Thyrotropin releasing hormone, which is a tripeptide, stimulates the synthesis and release of TSH as well as the release of prolactin (see p. 429). Somatostatin and TRH, which have been found in the hypothalamus as well as in other areas of the brain, are thought to serve as central neurotransmitters. Somatostatin has been found in locations other than the brain, including parts of the gastrointestinal tract and pancreas. In addition to its effect as an inhibitor of growth hormone secretion, somatostatin has also been found to inhibit secretion of other substances, including TSH, glucagon, insulin, gastrin, secretin, and pepsin (Gomez-Pan, 1977). Gonadotropin releasing hormone (GnRH), which is also termed luteinizing hormone releasing hormone (LH-RH or LRH) or LH/FSH releasing hormone (LH/FSH-RH), also has been well characterized. Although separate gonadotropin releasing hormones may be found, the decapeptide GnRH has been shown to be capable of stimulating the secretion of both FSH and LH from the pituitary. There is physiologic and chemical evidence for the existence of a number of other hypothalamic-adenohypophyseal factors. Although these substances have not been fully characterized, putative releasing factors include a growth hormone releasing factor (GRF), a corticotropin releasing factor (CRF), a prolactin releasing factor (PRF), and a prolactin inhibiting factor (PIF) (Vale, 1977). Growth hormone and prolactin thus are apparently under a dual system of hypothalamic control, one system that is

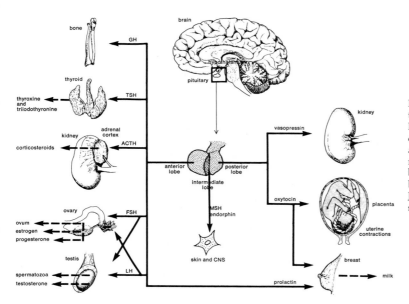

Figure 14–4. Target organs for the pituitary hormones GH, TSH, ACTH, FSH, LH, MSH, vasopressin and oxytocin. (From Schally, A. V., Kastin, A. J., and Arimura, A.: Hypothalamic hormones: The link between brain and body. Am. Sci., 65:712, 1977. Reprinted by permission of American Scientist, Journal of Sigma Xi, The Scientific Research Society of North America.)

inhibitory and one that is stimulatory. Prolactin is unique among the anterior pituitary hormones in that its secretion is under the tonic inhibitory control of the hypothalamus. If there is a disruption in the connection between the hypothalamus and the pituitary, the secretion of all the anterior pituitary hormones is decreased with the exception of prolactin, which is secreted in excess.

BETA-LIPOTROPIC HORMONE

Beta lipotropic hormone (beta LPH) contains within its structure amino acid sequences that have several distinct physiologic functions. The peptide as a whole induces fat metabolism as does its amino acid segment 1-58, which is designated gamma lipotropic hormone (gamma LPH). It now appears that beta MSH, which was the peptide hormone believed to control pigmentation in humans, is a fragment of beta lipotropic hormone. Amino acid sequences of beta lipotropic hormone have been identified as having morphine-like biologic properties and are

thought to play a role as neurotransmitters (Guillemin, 1977). Beta endorphin or C-fragment, largest of these compounds, is amino acid sequence 61-91 (Fig. 14–5). During fetal life and in pregnancy, when a distinct pars intermedia of the human pituitary gland is present, alpha melanocyte stimulating hormone (alpha MSH) and corticotropin-like intermediate lobe peptide (CLIP) have been demonstrated. The significance of these observations is unclear (Rees, 1977).

DISORDERS OF PITUITARY FUNCTION

Hypopituitarism is a term employed for the decreased function of the anterior pituitary; it refers to a wide spectrum of entities ranging from isolated lack of one trophic hormone to complete absence of all hormones. Some of these syndromes are not due to lack of hormone-producing cells in the pituitary gland, but are caused by deficiency of the hypothalamic releasing hormones. The clinical presentation of the patient depends on the patient's age and the nature of the deficiency; for example, growth hormone deficiency in children or gonadotropin deficiency in females in the childbearing age leads to easily recognized clinical manifestations. Growth hormone deficiency in adults and gonadotropin deficiency in some age groups, however, may not give rise to any distinctive clinical picture. Primary hypopituitarism may result from pituitary ablation by surgery or radiation, pituitary tu-

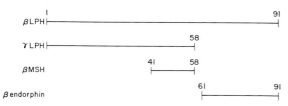

Figure 14–5. Relationship of the amino acid sequence of beta lipotropic hormone (βLPH) to gamma lipotropic hormone (γLPH), beta melanocyte stimulating hormone (βMSH), and beta endorphin.

mors, metastatic tumors, infarction, and infiltrative granulomatous processes. The endocrinologic investigation of hypopituitarism can be divided into the assessment of the adrenal function, thyroid function, and gonadal function as well as growth hormone and prolactin release. Posterior pituitary function is discussed on page 412. In the past, it was thought that features of hypogonadism secondary to failure in secretion of FSH and LH were the first endocrine disorders to be manifested in patients with pituitary tumors. However, assay of the pituitary hormones in serum in conjunction with stimulatory tests of pituitary function has shown that the order in which deficiency of the pituitary hormones occurs is variable from patient to patient.

The term *empty sella syndrome* is used to refer to two clinical entities. Idiopathic empty sella syndrome results from an anatomic variation in the diaphragm sellae which leads to sellar remodeling. This is a benign condition associated with few if any clinical signs. Whether or not compromise in pituitary function occurs in association with the idiopathic empty sella syndrome is unclear. The occasional instances of endocrine dysfunction which occur are thought to be unrelated to sellar enlargement or to extension of the subarachnoid space into the sellar cavity (Neelon, 1973). The secondary variety results from surgery and/or irradiation for an intrasellar lesion and may cause visual impairment in the post-treatment period (Hodgson, 1972).

Clinical syndromes of *hypersecretion of pituitary hormones* occur in association with pituitary and hypothalamic disorders.

GROWTH HORMONE

Growth hormone, or somatotrophic hormone, a polypeptide with a molecular weight of 21,700, is made up of a single chain of 190 amino acids (Franchimont, 1975). Evidence indicates that there is more than one circulating species; i.e., a moiety with a molecular weight of 40,000 to 45,000, so-called "big growth" hormone, has been identified (Hunter, 1976). Although this accounts for some growth hormone (GH) activity in normals as well as in patients with disorders of GH secretion, the majority of circulating GH is thought to be of the smaller form.

Although a number of hormones are necessary for growth, growth hormone is the most important hormonal regulator, and in its absence growth in children proceeds at one third to one half the normal rate (Daughaday, 1977). The importance of human growth hormone has been confirmed by the finding that children of small stature who lack measurable blood levels of the hormone can be stimulated to grow at rates approaching those of normal children by administration of growth hormone (Hunter, 1976). The normal function of growth hormone in the adult has not been fully clarified.

The secretion of growth hormone by the anterior pituitary appears to be regulated by the hypothalamus via releasing and inhibitory factors: growth hormone releasing factor (GRF) and growth hormone release inhibiting hormone, which is also called somatostatin.

Growth hormone probably exerts its major effects on target tissues by controlling the hepatic production of somatomedin. The designation *sulfation factor* has been replaced with the term *somatomedin*, which encompasses all growth hormone-dependent substances in plasma that stimulate growth in responsive tissues. The somatomedins are a group of small, single-chain peptides with similar biologic actions which are transported in the plasma bound by a carrier protein. Differences, such as amino acid composition and immunologic reactivity, indicate that several molecular species exist, but the exact relationship between the molecular forms is unknown (Daughaday, 1977). Although immunologically distinct from insulin, members of the somatomedin family show many insulin-like metabolic activities *in vitro*. Less than 10 per cent of the plasma insulin-like activity measured by bioassay can be neutralized by antibodies against insulin; the remainder is called non-suppressible insulin-like activity (NSILA). It has been suggested that one portion of NSILA, termed NSILA-s because of its solubility in acid ethanol, is closely related to the somatomedins. Low basal levels of NSILA-s in patients with hypopituitarism may be increased by growth hormone infusion. In addition, other factors apparently influence the regulation of NSILA-s; levels are not increased in patients with acromegaly or anorexia nervosa in spite of the elevated GH levels in these conditions (Kahn, 1977). The major site of somatomedin production probably is the liver, but there is some evidence that muscle and kidney may also be sites of somatomedin generation (Van Wyk, 1975).

Growth hormone levels usually are measured by radioimmunoassay (see Chap. 13), with comparable values obtained using serum or plasma (Gleispach, 1977). In general, antisera with suitable specificity for GH can be readily obtained; however, cross-reactivity with the closely related placental hormone, human placental lactogen, may be a problem. Normal fasting serum values are within the range of 0 to 10 ng/ml for adults. For most of a given 24-hour period in normal non-stressed subjects, serum growth hormone values are undetectable or at very low concentrations, with most values less than 3 ng/ml (Weitzman, 1976). The secretion of growth hormone is intermittent in nature, with a rise in concentrations occurring in association with a number of events, including sleep. During the first two hours of sleep, growth hormone is secreted in substantial amounts, usually with the peak secretion occurring between the first and second hour. Following this major spike in growth hormone secretion, the concentration rapidly falls to low levels. There sometimes is a second and perhaps a third secretory peak during the remaining hours of the sleep period. The sleep onset-related growth hormone peak may be delayed or prevented for many hours when sleep is delayed (Weitzman, 1976). In adults over 50 years of age, sleep-associated GH release may be absent. During the day short bursts of growth hormone secretion occur in no consistent temporal pattern; however, the day-to-day pattern appears to be fairly constant in a given individual. Bursts of growth hormone secretion also may occur with exercise, especially in the fasting state. In premature and newborn infants, basal GH levels are elevated. During childhood, the pattern of growth hormone secretion may show more activity than in adulthood. In the normal adult, hyperglycemia abolishes GH secretion; after a glucose load, growth hormone remains undetectable in the absorptive phase, then shows a secondary rise. The sleep-onset GH peak cannot be suppressed by glucose infusion. Protein ingestion and the infusion of certain amino acids are associated with increased serum GH. Growth hormone is frequently, but not reproducibly, secreted following stress; major surgery can produce an increase in levels despite hyperglycemia (Franchimont, 1975). In addition, the secretion or administration of a number of hormones including insulin, glucagon, catecholamines, glucocorticoids, estrogen, progesterone, thyroid hormone, and vasopressin can alter basal growth hormone concentrations or the response to stimulation tests. For example, estrogen therapy can elevate basal GH levels and augment the response to insulin hypoglycemia and arginine; with pharmacologic doses of glucocorticoids, the GH response to insulin hypoglycemia is blunted (Cohen, 1977). Growth hormone release also may be stimulated by L-dopa; administration of this drug has been used to test GH function, sometimes in conjunction with propranolol, which enhances its effect (Neelon, 1978). Although the function of changes in growth hormone secretion is unknown, there is evidence that GH serves to mobilize free fatty acids and thus may have a protein sparing effect.

HYPOSECRETION

The determination of growth hormone hyposecretion in adults is important in the evaluation of patients with pituitary tumors as a sensitive indicator of pituitary dysfunction. In children GH deficiency is a relatively uncommon but important cause of short stature. The term *ateliotic dwarf* has been used to describe

those patients with monotrophic growth hormone deficiency, defects in generation of somatomedin, or decreased ability of the body to respond to GH (end organ unresponsiveness). Monotrophic growth hormone deficiency may be secondary to a deficiency in a hypothalamic releasing factor or a pituitary lesion. Ateliotic dwarfs do not have obvious physical abnormalities other than small size, and some may attain sexual maturity (sexual ateliosis). The birth weight of patients with GH deficiency is normal, but decreased growth rate occurs within the first few months of life (Merimee, 1974). Acquired pituitary dwarfism may be caused by any of the lesions known to cause hypopituitarism, with many of these children having defects in other trophic hormones as well as in growth hormone. Laron (1966) described a familial form of dwarfism with clinical features of GH deficiency in the presence of high serum GH levels. These patients, called Laron dwarfs, respond to growth hormone stimulation with increases in already elevated GH levels; however, they have low somatomedin levels which do not respond to growth hormone therapy. Patients with Turner's syndrome are thought to have peripheral nonresponsiveness to growth hormone (Edwards, 1974). Although infants with the psychosocial deprivation syndrome may have elevated GH levels, older children with the syndrome show decreased GH response to appropriate stimuli (Daughaday, 1975).

Provocative tests of GH function

Laboratory diagnosis of deficiency of GH levels may be made by measuring serum growth hormone levels in the fasting state, during sleep, after exercise, and following stimulation tests. Undetectable fasting levels of GH occur frequently in normal subjects and thus are not diagnostic of hypofunction. Elevated fasting levels and rises associated with sleep are helpful in excluding the diagnosis of GH deficiency. The assessment of GH response to exercise has been used in the evaluation of children with short stature. An insulin tolerance test (ITT) may be used to assess growth hormone as well as ACTH reserve in both childen and adults. Performance of an ITT is contraindicated in certain individuals, including those with a history of ischemic heart disease and those with evidence of myocardial infarction, cerebrovascular disease, epilepsy, and low basal plasma cortisol levels. The test is performed by injecting insulin intravenously. Often 0.15 unit insulin/kg body weight is used, but the amount of insulin recommended varies depending on the clinical situation. For example, children with growth hormone deficiency may become severely hypoglycemic when 0.1 unit insulin/kg of body weight is given intravenously; therefore, less is used if this diagnosis is suspected. For further specific details on insulin tolerance testing, see Neelon (1978) and Edwards (1974). Blood samples are drawn before the start of the test and at least at 30-minute intervals for two hours after the insulin is given. Usually specimens are collected every 15 minutes for the first hour.

An essential feature of the insulin tolerance test is that an adequate degree of hypoglycemia must be obtained. This usually is defined as a drop in blood glucose concentration to less than 40 mg/dl (2.2 mmol/l) or a depression to less than 50 per cent of the fasting glucose level. The patient must be under constant supervision during the entire procedure, and glucose must be available for immediate intravenous administration. The test should be terminated by giving glucose if the patient has serious signs and symptoms such as chest pain or loss of consciousness. Glucose, cortisol, and growth hormone are determined on each of the specimens, and prolactin may be measured as well (Fig. 14–6). In normal subjects, adequate hypoglycemia results in a consistent rise in growth hormone to levels over 20 ng/ml (Edwards, 1974). Normal adults consistently show a rise in serum GH levels after insulin hypoglycemia, whereas some normal children may not respond. Arginine infusion may also be used. Normal response is a rise in GH concentration of 7 ng/ml (Edwards, 1974), but normal adults as well as normal children may fail to respond. Arginine, 30 g in adults, and in children, 0.5 g/kg body weight (up to 30 g), is infused over a 30-minute period. GH levels are drawn before the start of the infusion and then at 30-minute intervals for two hours. The ITT may not cause GH release, while arginine infusion can cause a response, or vice versa; this dissociation may occur in normal children and less commonly in normal adults. In children the combination of arginine infusion and insulin hypoglycemia is probably the most satisfactory definitive test for growth hormone deficiency. Other stimulation tests have been employed, including use of vasopressin, glucagon, and L-dopa. The absolute value of serum GH which must be exceeded in order to

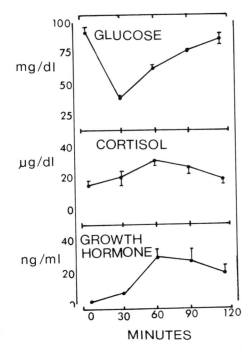

Figure 14–6. Normal response of glucose, cortisol, and growth hormone during an insulin tolerance test with 0.12 unit insulin/kg given intravenously at time zero. (Modified from Franchimont, 1975.)

be classified as normal is defined differently by various investigators, but usually ranges between about 6 and 10 ng/ml (Franchimont, 1975). Failure of GH levels to rise above the set limit after at least two provocative tests is indicative of growth hormone deficiency (Hunter, 1976).

The results of pituitary function tests can be altered by numerous factors. Hypothyroidism and also hyperthyroidism may cause impaired GH response to stimulatory tests. Hypothyroidism often is associated with short stature; such patients must be maintained in the euthyroid state for a considerable period before their true growth hormone status can be assessed properly. Obesity has an inhibitory effect on GH dynamics; a significant serum GH elevation does not occur in half the patients with the stimulus of an insulin tolerance test, and similar results are reported using arginine, L-dopa, and glucagon. Abnormal GH dynamics have also been reported in patients with diabetes mellitus, starvation, and cirrhosis, and in patients taking certain drugs. Starvation, for example, may cause hyper-responsiveness to arginine stimulation (Cohen, 1977).

HYPERSECRETION

Acromegaly and gigantism are clinical expressions of growth hormone hypersecretion.* If excess GH secretion occurs before puberty, gigantism results, while in adults, acromegaly occurs. Gigantism is a rare disorder characterized by generalized overgrowth of the skeleton and soft tissues. Acromegaly is usually first manifested by overgrowth of the head, hands, and feet, resulting in facial changes and changes in hat, glove, or shoe size. Headache and visual disturbances may result from the local effects of the tumor. The disease is associated with a number of other disturbances, including impaired glucose tolerance or frank diabetes mellitus and occasionally hyperthyroidism. Acromegaly is characterized by measurable growth hormone levels throughout the day and failure of GH to be suppressed following a glucose load. In some patients with acromegaly, fasting GH levels may be within normal limits; however, diagnosis of acromegaly may be confirmed by procedures that demonstrate the loss of normal growth hormone responsiveness (Mims, 1974). Because growth hormone release occurs in pulsatile bursts or in response to stress, the measurement of GH in a single specimen may reflect these peaks and thus be misleading. The growth hormone levels may not correlate with the severity of acromegalic manifestations in all cases, and it has been suggested that somatomedin measurements may be a better index of activity (Daughaday, 1975). Somatomedin determinations, however, are not readily available. With an oral glucose load, growth hormone levels normally are suppressed. This suppression is followed by a secondary rise occurring several hours later and related in magnitude to the amount of the glucose ingested (Hunter, 1976). Little or no suppression occurs in patients with acromegaly or gigantism. A glucose tolerance test with growth hormone levels thus is used to study patients with suspected GH hypersecretion. In the normal unstressed subject, growth hormone levels at the beginning of the test period are usually less than 10 ng/ml and suppress to less than 5 ng/ml at some time during the procedure. In patients with active acromegaly, basal levels usually are greater than 5 ng/ml and do not suppress to less than 5 ng/ml during the test; often growth hormone levels do not fall below 10 ng/ml (Ontjes, 1972). In some patients with acromegaly a paradoxical rise in growth hormone may occur, and in some patients partial

*Associated with pituitary tumor.

suppression of growth hormone has been reported.

Failure to suppress growth hormone with a glucose load may also occur in certain other conditions, including renal failure, cirrhosis, and starvation. In kwashiorkor, the elevated GH levels are associated with decreased somatomedin. It has been reported that somatomedin levels by bioassay may be spuriously low in these patients owing to the presence of inhibitory substances. Somatomedin levels also have been found to be low in renal insufficiency (VanWyk, 1975).

L-Dopa, which stimulates GH secretion in normal individuals, can produce a paradoxical fall of GH in acromegalic patients. TRH stimulation of GH occurs in acromegaly, but not in normal subjects. TRH infusion also may cause increased GH in patients with renal failure (Cohen, 1977). Patients with gigantism or acromegaly may develop partial or complete hypopituitarism during the course of their disease. Pituitary function, therefore, should be evaluated at the time of initial diagnosis and at a follow-up after therapy.

PROLACTIN

Prolactin is an anterior pituitary polypeptide hormone consisting of approximately 200 amino acids and having a molecular weight of about 22,000 (L'Hermite, 1976). There are several hormonal forms of prolactin including "big" and "little." The nature of big prolactin and its possible role as a prohormone remains in question. In some cases a "big, big" form of prolactin, which has little biologic activity, may be found in the serum as well (Friesen, 1977). Prolactin is under the inhibitory control of the hypothalamus. Evidence exists that the main prolactin inhibiting factor (PIF) may be dopamine. Prolactin secretion also is influenced by prolactin releasing factor (PRF). Although thyrotropin releasing hormone (TRH) releases prolactin, it seems unlikely that TRH acts as the sole physiologic PRF. Although many functions for prolactin in man have been suggested, there is evidence only for a role in lactation and in the control of gonadal function. Prolactin is essential for the initiation and maintenance of lactation. The physiologic hyperprolactinemia that occurs with lactation following parturition is associated with the delay in restoration of cyclic ovarian function (Thorner, 1977).

NORMAL SECRETORY PATTERNS

In clinical situations, prolactin is rarely deficient; deficiency is most commonly seen after pituitary necrosis or infarction. Serum prolactin levels are increased in a number of physiologic states, in patients treated with certain drugs, and in some

Table 14–1. CAUSES OF ELEVATED PROLACTIN LEVELS

PHYSIOLOGIC	PHARMACOLOGIC	PATHOLOGIC
Pregnancy	Phenothiazines	Prolactin secreting pituitary tumors
Nursing	Estrogens	
Newborn	Reserpine	Acromegaly
Stress	Alpha-methyldopa	Hypothalamic disorders
Exercise	Haloperidol	Pituitary stalk section
Sleep	Benzamides	Hypothyroidism
	Pimozide	Nelson's syndrome
	Thyrotropin releasing hormone (TRH)	Renal failure
		Ectopic production by malignant tumors
	Meprobamate	
	Tricyclic anti-depressants	

pathologic conditions (Table 14–1). Prolactin, which is measured by radioimmunoassay, has a normal range in serum of about 1 to 25 ng/ml for females and 1 to 20 ng/ml for males (Frantz, 1978).

Serial measurements of prolactin throughout the day reveal diurnal variation. Prolactin levels begin to rise 60 to 90 minutes after the onset of sleep, with the levels reaching their highest values four to five hours later. Prolactin levels fall with awakening but rise again during daytime naps. Alteration in the timing of the sleep period results in changes in the prolactin secretory pattern, indicating that this is not inherent neural rhythm. In addition to the diurnal variation, prolactin levels also show marked random fluctuations of a brief episodic variety (L'Hermite, 1976). Prolactin levels also rise after stress: for example, increase in prolactin levels is associated with exercise and the hypoglycemia which occurs with insulin tolerance testing. In pregnancy, maternal prolactin levels rise progressively to term but fall to basal levels within about three weeks after delivery in mothers who do not breast feed. In nursing mothers, basal levels remain somewhat elevated and breast feeding frequently but not uniformly causes a dramatic increase in prolactin concentration (Friesen, 1973). From about the twenty-fifth week of gestation to term, prolactin levels increase in the fetus and after birth decline in the infant, reaching normal adult levels within about a six-week period (Thorner, 1977).

CAUSES OF ELEVATED PROLACTIN LEVELS

There are many drugs that cause hypersecretion of prolactin. Dopamine receptor blocking drugs, such as the phenothiazine psychotropic agents, and dopamine depleting drugs, such as the antihypertensive agent reserpine, cause elevation of prolactin levels by interfering with the actions of prolactin inhibiting factor (PIF), while estrogens and TRH act directly on the pituitary (Thorner, 1977). L-Dopa and ergot derivatives such as bromergocryptine (bromocriptine; CB-154, Sandoz) lower prolactin levels and have been used in the treatment of hyperprolactinemic states.

Persistent hyperprolactinemia in the absence of obvious causes such as drug ingestion suggests a hypothalamic or pituitary lesion. Prolactin-secreting pituitary tumors are thought to be the most common of all pituitary tumors, with about 70 per cent of chromophobe adenomas associated with hyperprolactinemia (Jacobs, 1976). There is increased prolactin secretion in 20 to 40 per cent of patients with active acromegaly. The overproduction of prolactin by pituitary adenomas is not always accompanied by galactorrhea. Galactorrhea is more common in women than men with pituitary tumors; however, galactorrhea may fail to occur in some women even when serum levels of prolactin are very high. The height of serum prolactin levels has been correlated with the likelihood of the presence of a pituitary tumor. In the series of Kleinberg (1977), patients with galactorrhea who had prolactin levels above 100 ng/ml, 57 per cent had pituitary tumors; in those with levels above 300 ng/ml, all patients had tumors. In this series only one patient with an untreated pituitary tumor and without acromegaly had a normal serum prolactin level.

Gonadal dysfunction frequently is associated with elevated serum prolactin levels in both men and women. In hyperprolactinemic males, about one third have galactorrhea; and gynecomastia, if present, is slight (Thorner, 1977). Most men with gynecomastia do not have elevated prolactin levels. About 15 to 20 per cent of women with amenorrhea have elevated prolactin levels (Jacobs, 1976). When galactorrhea occurs in association with amenorrhea, there is usually an associated hyperprolactinemia. Several eponyms have been used in conjunction with the syndrome of amenorrhea and galactorrhea: Argonz del Castillo or Ahumada del Castillo to describe spontaneous lactation, Chiari-Frommel for persistent postpartum lactation, and Forbes-Albright for the association of galactorrhea with a pituitary tumor. It has been suggested that these syndromes may be a spectrum of the same disorder and that the eponyms should be abandoned. In patients with the amenorrhea-galactorrhea syndrome, the elevated prolactin levels can be inhibited by L-dopa or bromoergocryptine if the hypersecretion is functional or due to a pituitary tumor (Franchimont, 1974). It is important to make certain that pituitary tumors have been ruled out in these patients. With the induction of ovulation and subsequent pregnancy, pituitary tumors may expand rapidly, causing complications which necessitate neurosurgical intervention. In general, prolactin stimulation and suppression tests using a variety of agents including chlorpromazine, TRH, and L-dopa have not been helpful in making a definite diagnosis of the cause of galactorrhea in a given individual. Although the mechanism is uncertain, galactorrhea may occur with the use or discontinuation of oral contraceptives. A wide range of prolactin levels (4.8 to 180 ng/ml) has been reported in a series of patients in whom galactorrhea appeared to be related to taking oral contraceptives (Kleinberg, 1977). In some patients with primary hypothyroidism, marked hyperprolactinemia may occur. With thyroid hormone replacement, the prolactin levels return to normal in the majority of patients. Ectopic prolactin secretion has been reported in association with undifferentiated bronchogenic carcinoma and hypernephroma (Turkington, 1971).

VASOPRESSIN

ACTION

The posterior pituitary peptide hormone vasopressin, which is also called antidiuretic hormone (ADH), plays a major physiologic role in the control of water reabsorption by the distal convoluted and collecting tubules of the kidney. Vasopressin increases water permeability, allowing hypotonic fluid in the distal tubules to equilibrate with hypertonic fluid in the interstitial spaces of the medulla of the kidney. Water reabsorption occurs, leading to concentration of the urine. Three major stimuli control release of ADH: (1) changes in the osmolality of the blood, (2) alterations in blood volume, and (3) psychogenic stimuli. Under ordinary circumstances the osmotic factors probably predominate in regulating ADH secretion. Neurophysins are peptides which are released from the posterior pituitary in association with vasopressin. Vasopressin and neurophysin are synthesized in the hypothalamus. Once synthesized, they are held together loosely in neurosecretory granules which are transferred to the posterior pituitary where they are stored. It is thought that there may be a specific vasopressin neurophysin and a specific oxytocin neurophysin, but the biologic activity of these compounds is unknown (Robinson, 1977). In general, although radioimmunoassays for vasopressin have been developed, they are not widely available. In most studies, basal levels of plasma vasopressin have been found to lie between about 1 and 5 pg/ml (Robertson, 1977). The methods used to delineate and identify patients with abnormalities in ADH depend principally on accurate measurement of plasma and urine osmolality (see Chaps. 6 and 17).

DIABETES INSIPIDUS

Diabetes insipidus (DI) is a condition which is characterized by polyuria and polydipsia resulting from inadequate ADH secretion or inability of the renal tubules to respond to the hormone. The causes of decreased vasopressin secretion include head trauma, pituitary lesions, and an inherited form of the disorder. Nephrogenic diabetes insipidus (renal resistance to vasopressin) may be inherited or may be associated with such entities as hypercalcemia, hypokalemia, renal disease, and lithium therapy. In order to diagnose the various polyuric states, many different types of water deprivation tests have been proposed. For example, an overnight dehydration may be performed. At the end of eight hours of water deprivation, normal subjects generally have a urine osmolality greater than 800 mOsm/kg with normal plasma osmolality. In patients with DI, the urine osmolality is usually less than that of plasma, with the plasma osmolality greater than about 300 mOsm/kg (Edwards, 1977). With water deprivation, the osmolality of urine collected hourly usually reaches a plateau: this is defined as two and preferably three consecutive hourly samples with about equal osmolality. In normal subjects, approximately 16 to 18 hours are necessary to reach a plateau, but in patients with polyuria exceeding 5 liters per day, usually

Table 14–2. INTERPRETATION OF RESPONSES TO
THE WATER DEPRIVATION TEST*

CONDITION	SERUM OSMOLALITY	URINE OSMOLALITY	
	At Plateau	At Plateau	After Vasopressin
Normal	Usually < 300	>serum	<5% ↑
Primary polydipsia	Usually < 300	>serum	<5% ↑
Severe diabetes insipidus	Often > 300	<serum	>50% ↑
Nephrogenic diabetes insipidus	Often > 300	<serum	<50% ↑
Partial diabetes insipidus	Usually < 300	>serum	> 9% ↑

*From Neelon, F.A., and Sydnor, C.F.: The assessment of pituitary function. In Dowling, H.F., et al. (eds.): DISEASE-A-MONTH. Copyright © 1978 by Year Book Medical Publishers, Inc., Chicago. Used by permission.

only 4 to 8 hours is necessary. The subsequent response of the patient to subcutaneous injection of 5 units of aqueous vasopressin allows differentiation of the polyuric states (Table 14-2). Patients with severe or partial DI show increased urine osmolality with vasopressin injection. Before the dehydration test is undertaken, various conditions such as diabetes mellitus, hypercalcemia, and hypokalemia must be ruled out. Patients who excrete large volumes of urine must be closely observed during the test period for signs of vascular collapse (Moses, 1972).

INAPPROPRIATE ADH SECRETION

The syndrome of inappropriate ADH (SIADH) is the other important entity associated with abnormalities of vasopressin secretion. The diagnosis should be suspected in any patient with hyponatremia and low plasma osmolality who excretes urine that is not maximally dilute. The characteristic features of the syndrome of inappropriate antidiuretic hormone (SIADH) are (1) hyponatremia, (2) continued renal excretion of sodium, (3) absence of clinical evidence of volume depletion, (4) urine less than maximally dilute, (5) normal renal function, and (6) normal adrenal function (Bartter, 1967). Urinary sodium concentrations greater than 20 mEq/l (20 mmol/l) provide support of the diagnosis of SIADH. Water loading studies, with the measurement of plasma and urine osmolality and calculation of free water clearance, may be useful in the diagnosis of the syndrome (see Chap. 6, p. 142). Water loading is dangerous unless the patient

is free of symptoms of hyponatremia and has received appropriate treatment to raise the serum sodium to a safe level, generally above 125 mEq/l (125 mmol/l) (Moses, 1976). The syndrome of inappropriate ADH has been associated with a wide variety of disorders, including ectopic production of vasopressin, cerebral and pulmonary disorders, as well as the ingestion of certain drugs (Table 14-3). Moses (1974) has reviewed the causes of drug-induced hyponatremia. A number of drugs have been reported to affect various aspects of water metabolism but clinically have not produced significant problems. Clofibrate, which has been reported to inhibit excretion of a water load in normal subjects, possibly by releasing endogenous ADH, is an example of such a drug (Moses, 1973).

Table 14–3. POSTULATED CAUSES OF SYNDROME OF INAPPROPRIATE ANTIDIURETIC HORMONE

CONDITION	EXAMPLE
1. Ectopic production by tumors	a. Oat cell carcinoma of bronchus
	b. Pancreatic carcinoma
2. Pulmonary disorders	a. Tuberculosis
	b. Pneumonia
3. Cerebral disorders	a. Trauma
	b. Neoplasms
4. Drugs	a. Chlorpropamide
	b. Vincristine
	c. Cyclophosphamide
	d. Diuretics
5. Miscellaneous	a. Adrenal insufficiency
	b. Acute intermittent porphyria

OXYTOCIN

Little is known about the physiology or pathophysiology of oxytocin. In the male oxytocin has no known function and in the pregnant female it is unclear whether or not it plays important roles in either the initiation or maintenance of labor. In patients with neurohypophyseal disease who may have oxytocin deficiency, there appears to be no evidence that this has any deleterious effects. Oxytocin has been reported to be secreted ectopically by certain tumors such as oat cell carcinoma of the lung and adenocarcinoma of the pancreas. It is unclear, however, if the hypersecretion of oxytocin has any pathologic effects (Edwards, 1977).

THYROID GLAND

THYROID HORMONE SYNTHESIS AND RELEASE

The normal thyroid gland is composed of numerous follicles, each of which consists of a single layer of epithelial cells surrounding a central lumen containing colloid. The main constituent of colloid is thyroglobulin, a glycoprotein with a molecular weight of approximately 660,000. Thyroglobulin is the site of storage of thyroid hormones within the thyroid gland. Steps in the biosynthesis of thyroid hormones include:

1. trapping of iodine and conversion to an activated form
2. synthesis of thyroglobulin
3. uniting the activated form of iodine with tyrosine present in thyroglobulin to form iodotyrosine (termed organification)
4. coupling of iodotyrosyl residues to form the iodothyronines, thyroxine (T4), and triiodothyronine (T3)
5. proteolysis of thyroglobulin with release of T4 and T3 into the circulation.

Although a continuous supply of iodine is essential for normal thyroid hormone function and secretion, administration of iodine in large doses has been shown to have antithyroid effects (see p. 415). The usual intake of iodine varies widely, but normally is between 50 and 500 μg daily. In addition to iodide from food and water which is absorbed by the gastrointestinal tract, iodide is made available in the body from the peripheral deiodination of thyroxine. Under normal physiologic circumstances, iodide is actively taken up by the thyroid cells. This so-called iodine trap is believed to be a metabolically driven pump similar to other ion transport systems in the body. Thiocyanate (SCN^-) and perchlorate (ClO_4^-) inhibit operation of the

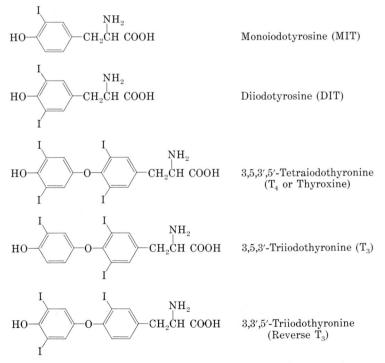

Monoiodotyrosine (MIT)

Diiodotyrosine (DIT)

3,5,3′,5′-Tetraiodothyronine
(T_4 or Thyroxine)

3,5,3′-Triiodothyronine (T_3)

3,3′,5′-Triiodothyronine
(Reverse T_3)

Figure 14–7. Structure of the thyroid hormones and related compounds.

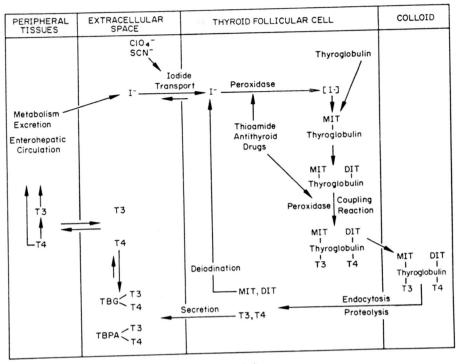

The major pathways of iodine metabolism.

Abbreviations are as follows: *T3* = triiodothyronine; *T4* = thyroxine; *MIT* = monoiodotyrosine; *DIT* = diiodotyrosine; *TBG* = thyroxine-binding globulin; *TBPA* = thyroxine-binding prealbumin.

Figure 14–8. Outline of iodine metabolism in relation to thyroid function (Used with permission from Gilman, A. G., and Murad, F.: Thyroid and antithyroid drugs. In Goodman, L. S., and Gilman, A. (eds.): The Pharmacological Basis of Therapeutics. New York, Macmillan Publishing Co., Inc., Copyright, 1975.)

iodine trap. The thyroidal iodine trapping mechanism is regulated by thyroid stimulating hormone (TSH) and intrathyroidal iodine concentration. TSH, which exerts its effect by binding to a specific receptor on the thyroid cell membrane and activating adenyl cyclase, accelerates almost all aspects of thyroid gland metabolism. After iodide is trapped by the thyroid gland, it probably is oxidized to a free radical form in a peroxidase-mediated reaction and united to tyrosine. Iodination of tyrosine residues in thyroglobulin results in the formation of monoiodotyrosine (MIT) and diiodotyrosine (DIT). Organification is blocked by large doses of iodide (Wolff-Chaikoff effect) and by the thioamide antithyroid drugs such as propylthiouracil. When two DIT residues couple, thyroxine (T4) is formed; and when one residue of DIT couples with one MIT residue, triiodothyronine (T3) is formed (Figs. 14–7 and 14–8). Thyroglobulin is thought to be iodinated within the apical secretory vesicles at the cell border just prior to liberation, or perhaps, after liberation into colloid (De Groot, 1977). When required,

the iodinated amino acids stored in the colloid are absorbed into the cell by pinocytosis, and proteolysis of the small fragments of thyroglobulin results in intracellular release of MIT, DIT, T3, and T4. The MIT and DIT are normally broken down by intracellular deiodinases, with most of the liberated iodine reutilized. The T4 and T3 rapidly diffuse into the blood where they are bound firmly by circulating plasma proteins. Figure 14–8 summarizes the major steps in iodine metabolism. Under normal physiologic circumstances the thyroid predominantly secretes T4; however, T3 secretion may predominate in certain situations such as iodine deficiency and hyperthyroidism. An important antithyroid action of iodide is the inhibition of the release of stored thyroid hormone.

SERUM TRANSPORT OF THYROID HORMONES

Serum normally contains 0.2 to 1.0 μg/dl inorganic iodine, and small amounts (less than 0.2 μg/dl) of non-hormonal iodine compounds, including MIT, DIT, thyroglobulin, and iodinated serum albumin (Sterling, 1975). The iodothyronines, thyroxine (T4) and triiodothyronine (T3), are considered to be the physiologically important iodinated hormones. The major fraction of organic iodine in the circulation is in the form of thyroxine (Fig. 14-7).

Approximately 70 per cent of T4 is bound to thyroxine-binding globulin (TBG), 20 per cent to thyroxine-binding prealbumin (TBPA), and 10 per cent to albumin. Most T3 is bound to TBG; however, binding to albumin and probably to TBPA also occurs. The affinity of T3 for TBG and TBPA is substantially less than that of T4. The biologic half-time or turnover for T4 in normal man is approximately one week, as compared to one day for T3. This difference in biologic half-life has been attributed largely to the firmer binding of T4 to plasma proteins. Total T4 concentration in serum is approximately 5.5 to 12.5 μg/dl (72 to 163 nmol/l), while total serum T3 concentration is only about 100 to 220 ng/dl (1.5 to 3.4 nmol/l). A small percentage of thyroid hormone remains unbound to plasma proteins, with about 0.02 to 0.04 per cent of T4 and approximately 0.2 to 0.4 per cent of T3 remaining free. It is this free fraction that is presumably active in stimulating metabolism. It has been estimated that 65 to 75 per cent of the total metabolic effect in man is due to T3. Although some investigators believe that T4 is really an inactive prohormone which must be converted to T3 before it can exert its physiologic effects, there is evidence that T4 does have intrinsic hormonal activity, (Schimmel, 1977). The majority of the circulating T3 arises by peripheral deiodination, with the liver and kidneys having an important role in this transformation. It has been estimated that 33 to 40 per cent of the circulating thyroxine is monodeiodinated to T3, with 15 to 20 per cent of the T4 changed to tetraiodothyroacetic acid ("Tetrac") or conjugated and excreted in the urine or bile. The remainder of the T4 is deiodinated to 3,3',5'-triiodothyronine (reverse T3 or rT3), which has little or no calorigenic activity (Sterling, 1977). It is thought that thyroxine deiodination may occur in many different organs and that alterations in this extrathyroidal deiodination profoundly affect the availability of biologically active hormone (Schimmel, 1977). Nearly all of the rT3 normally produced is from the extrathyroidal conversion of T4 (Chopra, 1975). There is evidence that 3,3'-L-diiodothyronine (T2) is a metabolite of both T3 and rT3 (Burger, 1977).

PERIPHERAL ACTIONS OF THYROID HORMONE

The precise manner in which thyroid hormones exert their effects is unknown. Postulated models for thyroid hormone action involve nuclear localization of the hormones after binding by a cytoplasmic receptor. Evidence has accumulated that the nucleus is the site of initiation of hormone action, possibly through derepression of information encoded in DNA (Oppenheimer, 1973). In addition, the concept of a direct thyroid hormone action on mitochondria has been supported by numerous observations of immediate effects on oxidative phosphorylation. A model has been proposed for the actions of thyroid hormone at the cellular level, which includes direct effects on mitochondria in addition to stimulation of nucleic acid and protein synthesis by way of receptors in the nuclear chromatin (Sterling, 1977). Some effects of thyroid hormone deficiency and excess are listed in Table 14-4.

HYPOTHALAMIC AND PITUITARY CONTROL OF THYROID SECRETION

Biosynthesis of thyroglobulin and release of thyroid hormone from thyroglobulin are controlled by thyroid stimulating hormone (TSH). TSH, which is synthesized in the anterior pituitary gland, is a glycoprotein hormone composed of two dissimilar subunits designated alpha and beta. There is general agreement that the thyroid hormones exert feedback inhibition of pituitary TSH secretion. This response is modulated by the hypothalamus. When the level of circulating thyroid hormone falls below a critical value, the feedback mechanism operating at the pituitary level causes an increase in secretion of TSH. The increased production of TSH accelerates the activity of the thyroid, including the production and secretion of the thyroid hormones. A rise in the level of circulating thyroid hormones leads to TSH suppression. Evidence suggests that thyroid hormones act on the pituitary to produce a protein intermediate which interferes with the TSH response to TRH. The details of thyroid hormone action at the pituitary level and the relative importance of T4 and T3 in suppressing TSH secretion, however, are unclear. The hypothalamus regulates the activity of TSH through the secretion of thyrotropin releasing hormone (TRH) and possibly of somatostatin (Fig. 14-9). Elucidation of the structure and subsequent synthesis of TRH has established its nature as the tripeptide, proglutamyl-histidyl-proline amide (Hall, 1976) (Fig. 14-10). TRH, which is stored in the median eminence and secreted into the venous portal system, causes the release of TSH from the anterior pituitary, probably by activating adenyl cyclase. TRH consistently releases prolactin in normal adults; however, the physiologic function of this is unknown. Somatostatin, which is a tetradecapeptide, has been shown to reduce the TSH response to TRH, and evidence suggests it may play a role in the regulation of TSH secretion (Sterling, 1977). Both TRH and somatostatin are found over a wide area of the hypothalamus and in extrahypothalamic sites; they are thought to have neurotransmitter functions in the central nervous system. The effects of thyroid hormones on the control of hypothalamic hormones are controversial.

Table 14-4. EFFECTS OF THYROID DEFICIENCY AND EXCESS OBSERVED AT DIFFERENT LEVELS OF ORGANIZATION*

LEVEL OF ORGANIZATION	HYPOTHYROID	HYPERTHYROID
Behavior	Mental retardataion Mentally and physically sluggish Somnolent Sensitive to cold	Often quick mentally Restless, irritable, anxious, hyperkinetic Wakeful Sensitive to heat
Whole individual	Deficient growth Low BMR Hypercholesterolemia Myxedema	Negative nitrogen balance High BMR Hypocholesterolemia Exophthalmos
Organ systems Cardiovascular	↓ Cardiac output ↑ BP, pulse pressure Weak heart beat ↑ Circulation time	↑ Cardiac output ↑ Systolic BP, pulse pressure Tachycardia, palpitations ↓ Circulation time
G.I.	Hypophagia Constipation Low glucose absorption rate	Hyperphagia Diarrhea High glucose absorption rate
Muscle	Weakness Hypotonia	Weakness Fibrillary twitchings, tremors
Immune mechanism	Infection-susceptible Subnormal phagocytic capacity of leukocytes?	Infection-susceptible (? related to excess protein catabolism)
Tissues	↓ QO$_2$ of liver, kidney muscle, etc. *in vitro* Normal QO$_2$ of brain, testis, retina, etc. Decreased sensitivity of some tissues to epinephrine	↑ QO$_2$ of same tissues Normal QO$_2$ of brain and same tissues Potentiation of epinephrine effect on intest. smooth muscle by thyronines
Organelle	Increased no. of mitochondria per cell. No change in P/O ratio	Increased no. of mitochondria per cell. P/O ratio ↓ (uncoupling of phosphorylation from oxidation)
Organelle component	———	Mitochondrial swelling (action on mitochondrial membrane?)
Enzymes	↓Oxidative enzymes	↑Oxidative enzymes in chronically treated animals

*From Tepperman, J.: Metabolic and Endocrine Physiology, 3rd ed. Copyright © 1973, by Year Book Medical Publishers, Inc., Chicago. Used by permission.

CLASSIFICATION OF THYROID DISEASE

Thyroid disease may be classified primarily on a functional basis into hyperthyroidism, euthyroidism, and hypothyroidism (Table 14-5).

Hyperthyroidism

The term *hyperthyroidism* is used to denote the physiologic and biochemical disturbances that result when tissues are exposed to excessive quantities of thyroid hormones (see Table 14-4). Signs and symptoms of hyperthyroidism include heat intolerance, tachycardia, palpitations, weight loss, weakness, emotional lability, tremor, and increased systolic blood pressure. In some patients, however, the clinical picture may not be striking and the underlying hyperthyroidism difficult to diagnose. The possibility of hyperthyroidism should be considered carefully in patients with unexplained cardiac failure and in those with supraventricular tachycardia.

Graves' disease, which is the most common clinical syndrome associated with hyperthyroidism, may be defined as a multisystem disorder consisting of one, two, or all of the following characteristic features: hyperthyroidism with diffuse goiter, infiltrative ophthalmopathy, and infiltrative dermopathy (pretibial myxedema). The disease, which is approximately five times more common in women than in men, usually becomes manifest between the third and fourth decades of life,

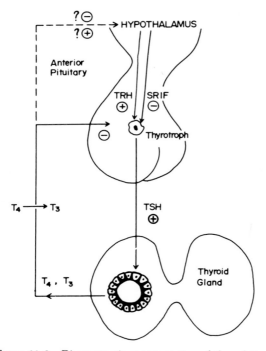

Figure 14-9. Diagrammatic representation of the relationships between the hypothalamus, pituitary, and thyroid. The effects of the thyroid hormones on the hypothalamus are controversial, but they inhibit the response of the pituitary thyrotroph to TRH.

TRH = thyrotropin releasing hormone
SRIF = somatotropin release inhibiting factor (somatostatin)
TSH = thyroid stimulating hormone

+ indicates stimulation, − indicates suppression

(Used with permission from Burger, H. G., and Patel, Y. C.: Thyrotropin releasing hormone—TSH. Clin. Endocrinol. Metabol., 6:83, 1977.)

but may occur at any age. The patient usually has signs and symptoms of hyperthyroidism with thyroid gland enlargement. When the infiltrative ophthalmopathy occurs in the absence of hyperthyroidism, the syndrome has been termed euthyroid Graves' disease. The ophthalmopathy of Graves' disease may occur

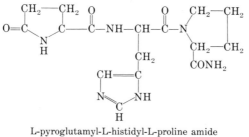

L-pyroglutamyl-L-histidyl-L-proline amide
Thyrotropin Releasing Hormone (TRH)

Figure 14-10. Structure of thyrotropin releasing hormone (TRH).

before, simultaneously with, or after the onset of hyperthyroidism, but in about 40 per cent of patients with Graves' disease there is no exophthalmos at any time (Volpe, 1977). Graves' disease is associated with circulating immunoglobulins that are thought to be an antibody to the TSH receptor. It appears that long acting thyroid stimulator (LATS), LATS-protector and human thyroid stimulator are all antibodies to the human thyroid TSH receptor (see p. 429). There are several techniques that are available for demonstrating the presence of human thyroid stimulator using human thyroid cells, slices, or cell membranes. Although the determinations are not widely available, it has been reported that these human thyroid stimulating immunoglobulins are present in the majority of patients with untreated Graves' disease, and determination of these immunoglobulins may be valuable in certain clinical situations such as following Graves' disease patients treated with antithyroid drugs (Volpe, 1977).

Other much less common causes of hyperthyroidism include TSH secreting pituitary tumors, thyroid carcinoma, choriocarcinoma, and hydatidiform mole. In some patients with choriocarcinoma or hydatidiform mole, it has been suggested that human chorionic gonadotropin (HCG) is the substance which is responsible for thyroid stimulating activity (Morley, 1976). A syndrome of TSH-induced hyperthyroidism, possibly due to abnormalities in pituitary feedback mechanisms, has been reported (Gershengorn, 1975). Hyperthyroidism also may be caused by toxic multinodular goiter or by a solitary functioning thyroid nodule (Plummer's disease, toxic adenoma). Iodine administration may result in hypothyroidism as well as hyperthyroidism. The normal thyroid gland is insensitive to antithyroid effects of iodide, since it has the ability to prevent the maintenance of intracellular iodide concentrations high enough to produce inhibitory effects. In patients with an abnormal thyroid gland, this adaptation phenomenon does not occur and hypothyroidism can be produced. Iodide thus may have a beneficial effect in the treatment of hyperthyroidism (Utiger, 1972). Iodide administration, however, also has been reported to induce hyperthyroidism; this is referred to as the Jod-Basedow phenomenon and has been reported in patients with nontoxic as well as iodine-deficient goiter (Vagenakis, 1972).

Subacute thyroiditis may be associated with

Table 14-5.   CLASSIFICATION OF THYROID DISEASE

Diseases Primarily Characterized by Euthyroidism
1. Diffuse goiter
    a. Sporadic—idiopathic
    b. Sporadic—known cause (congenital defect in hormone synthesis; chemical goitrogen; iodine deficiency)
    c. Endemic—idiopathic
    d. Endemic—known cause (iodine deficiency; dietary goitrogens)
2. Uninodular goiter
    a. Functional (hot nodule)
    b. Non-functional (cold nodule)
3. Multinodular goiter
    a. Sporadic—idiopathic
    b. Sporadic—known cause (similar to diffuse goiter above)
    c. Endemic—idiopathic
    d. Endemic—known cause (similar to diffuse goiter above)
4. Tumors
    a. Benign—follicular adenoma, atypical adenoma, teratoma
    b. Malignant—follicular adenocarcinoma, papillary adenocarcinoma, medullary carcinoma, undifferentiated carcinoma, miscellaneous
5. Thyroiditis
    a. Acute
    b. Subacute
    c. Chronic
        1. Hashimoto's and variants
        2. Riedel's
        3. Non-suppurative
        4. Suppurative
6. Congenital anomaly

Diseases Primarily Characterized by Hyperthyroidism
1. Diffuse toxic goiter (Graves' disease)
2. Toxic goiter
    a. Uninodular
    b. Multinodular
3. Exogenous thyroid hormone excess
4. Tumors
    a. Follicular adenoma
    b. Follicular carcinoma
    c. Secretion of TSH-like substance (choriocarcinoma, hydatidiform mole, embryonal carcinoma of testis)

Diseases Primarily Characterized by Hypothyroidism
1. Idiopathic
    a. Adult
    b. Childhood, including congenital aplasia
2. Loss of thyroid mass
    a. Surgery
    b. Radioiodine
    c. Other
3. Biochemical lesions
    a. Iodide deficiency
    b. Goitrogens
    c. Inborn error of metabolism
4. TSH deficiency
    a. Isolated
    b. Panhypopituitarism
5. TRH deficiency due to hypothalamic injury or disease

symptoms of hyperthyroidism; in addition, the patients classically present with malaise, slight elevation of temperature, difficulty swallowing, and usually, but not always, with thyroid tenderness. Excess thyroid medication such as T3, T4, or desiccated thyroid, surreptitiously taken by the patient may cause hyperthyroidism (thyrotoxicosis factitia). This syndrome may be confused with subacute thyroiditis, since in both conditions the patients will have symptoms of hyperthyroidism and a marked suppression of radioactive iodine uptake by the thyroid gland (see p. 430.)

In the majority of patients with hyperthyroidism, serum concentrations of the total T4, free T4, and total T3 levels are elevated, with serum TSH values within normal limits.

Hypothyroidism

Hypothyroidism is the systemic disorder which results from the lack of thyroid hormone action on tissues (see Table 14-4). Signs and symptoms of hypothyroidism may include hoarseness, cold sensitivity, dry skin, and muscular weakness. The signs and symptoms vary with the severity of the hypothyroidism, and such non-specific complaints as weakness, muscle cramps, or weight gain may be the only indication of the condition. Myxedema coma is the advanced stage of thyroid hormone deficiency and is characterized by progressive stupor, hypothermia, and hypoventilation. It is associated with respiratory acidosis, hyponatremia, and hypoglycemia. *Cretinism* is the term employed for the functional failure of the thyroid in the newborn period. The prompt diagnosis and treatment of these patients is essential to avoid or minimize retardation of mental development. Because the usual signs and symptoms associated with neonatal hypothyroidism may be absent or difficult to recognize, the diagnosis generally depends on the detection of abnormally low circulating thyroid hormones, and, in patients with primary hypothyroidism, elevated TSH. It is felt that delay in the diagnosis and treatment of neonatal hypothyroidism until classic features of infantile hypothyroidism occur is unjustified, since this may lead to irreparable damage to the nervous system (Hayles, 1972). Screening programs have been developed for newborns to detect neonatal hypothyroidism, which is estimated to occur in 1 in 4,000 to 1 in 10,000 births. The goal of early detection and treatment of hypothyroid infants is to eliminate the severe mental retardation associated with thyroid hormone deficiency in early infancy.

The most common cause of hypothyroidism is so-called primary hypothyroidism, which results from the failure of the thyroid itself to secrete adequate amounts of thyroid hormone. Although primary hypothyroidism has a number of causes, including ablation of the thyroid gland by surgery or radioactive iodine, it is most commonly associated with idiopathic atrophy of the gland. The majority of cases of idiopathic myxedema are thought to represent a variant of Hashimoto's thyroiditis, in which the thyroid gland is atrophied (Volpe, 1975). Secondary hypothyroidism, a relatively rare disorder that results when the release of TSH is diminished, often is due to a destructive lesion of the pituitary. Hypothalamic disease leading to impaired TSH release also may cause hypothyroidism.

Serum TSH is the most sensitive index of thyroid gland failure. Elevated values of serum TSH are helpful in diagnosing primary hypothyroidism, especially in patients with borderline low total T4 or low free T4 values (Vagenakis, 1976). In patients with anterior pituitary or hypothalamic failure, serum TSH concentrations characteristically are not elevated.

Thyroiditis

The term *thyroiditis* refers to a group of inflammatory disorders of the thyroid which may be classified into acute and chronic forms. Although thyroiditis is usually characterized by euthyroidism, it may be associated with hyperthyroidism and, in some cases, may lead to hypothyroidism. Acute suppurative thyroiditis is a severe bacterial infection of the thyroid, usually recognized by signs of acute inflammation and pain. Subacute thyroiditis, in which the thyroid gland may be enlarged and tender, seems to be related to viral infection. A variety of synonyms have been applied to this disorder, including DeQuervain's thyroiditis, giant cell thyroiditis, granulomatous thyroiditis, and non-suppurative thyroiditis. Although the characteristic feature of the disease is the gradual or sudden appearance of pain in the region of the thyroid, some patients have painless subacute thyroiditis. The disorder runs a variable course of several weeks to several months and usually subsides spontaneously without sequelae. In the early phase of subacute thyroiditis, inflammatory destruction of the gland results in leakage of stored thyroid hormones, colloid, and a variety of iodinated materials into the circulation. The circulating iodinated proteins, peptides, and amino acids lead to a disproportionate increase in serum PBI levels as compared with total T4 determined by methods such as radioimmunoassay. The damaged thyroid gland becomes unable to trap iodine, and consequently radioactive iodine uptake is usually decreased. As recovery occurs, the radioactive iodine uptake may rise above the normal range, gradually subsiding to normal. The elevated serum thyroid hormone levels fall as the colloid is depleted and may reach hypothyroid levels before restoration of normal values occurs. Some patients may become permanently hypothyroid following subacute thyroiditis (Volpe, 1975).

There are two types of chronic thyroiditis: Riedel's struma, a rare type of chronic sclerosing thyroiditis, and Hashimoto's thyroiditis, also known as lymphocytic thyroiditis. Patients with Hashimoto's thyroiditis usually present with an enlarged thyroid but few if any other symptoms. Hashimoto's thyroiditis, which is characterized by diffuse lymphocytic infiltration of the thyroid gland, sometimes may be associated with hypothyroidism. A close relationship seems to exist between Graves' disease and Hashimoto's thyroiditis; the two disorders may occur in the same family and may exist within the same thyroid gland (Volpe, 1977). The diagnosis of Hashimoto's thyroiditis may be confirmed by the demonstration of antithyroglobulin antibodies circulating in the serum at high titer. In addition, other antibodies have been identified in this condition, including antibodies to the microsomes of the thyroid cell, a nuclear component, and a colloid component other than thyroglobulin (Sterling, 1975). For further information on the thyroid antibodies, see Chapter 38.

Goiter

Goiter is the term employed for abnormal enlargement of the thyroid gland. Although the assessment of thyroid gland size is difficult, it is usually accepted that a goiter is thyroid enlargement to twice its normal size or to an estimated weight of 40 g or more. A patient with an enlarged thyroid may be euthyroid, hyperthyroid, or hypothyroid. Simple non-toxic goiter is a designation widely used for a non-malignant thyroid enlargement not associated with increased thyroid hormone production. The patient may be euthyroid or hypothyroid with diffuse or nodular thyroid enlargement. The most common cause of non-toxic goiter is dietary iodide deficiency. Other causes of non-toxic goiter include Hashimoto's thyroiditis, goitrogen ingestion, and dyshormonogenesis. Potentially goitrogenic substances include lithium, sulfonamides, and even certain foods. Hereditary or dyshormonogenic goiter is a rare condition caused by abnormalities in the various steps of thyroid hormone synthesis, such as defects in the iodine trap, impaired thyroglobulin synthesis, and inability to couple MIT and DIT (Lissitzky, 1973). Pendred's syndrome is the combination of goiter and deafness secondary to a defect in organification of iodide in the thyroid. Patients with disorders of thyroid hormone synthesis may present with goitrous cretinism.

Thyroid tumors

A common presentation of thyroid tumors is the incidental discovery of a lump in the neck. Although there are a large number of individuals who have nodular thyroids, only a small portion of these individuals have thyroid carcinoma. Thyroid cancer is a significant problem, however, since it must be differentiated from the much more frequent adenomas and multinodular goiters. Occasionally, the patient with thyroid carcinoma may present with signs and symptoms which include an enlarging, painful neck mass, metastatic nodules in the neck, or pathologic fractures. Only rarely does the patient with thyroid carcinoma exhibit signs and symptoms of hyperthyroidism caused by excess functioning of the cancer. Papillary thyroid cancer is the most common form of thyroid malignancy, accounting for greater than half of all adult thyroid cancers. In general, the patients have a good prognosis, since the majority of papillary carcinomas grow at a relatively slow rate. Follicular carcinoma, which makes up about one fourth of all cases of thyroid malignancy, is also a relatively slow growing lesion. However, the patient's prognosis is not favorable if the disease is discovered after metastasis has occurred. Follicular carcinoma and its metastatic lesions often are able to concentrate iodine, and thus it is possible to employ radioactive iodine therapy in these patients (DeGroot, 1975). Undifferentiated carcinoma accounts for less than 15 to 20 per cent of the cases of thyroid malignancy. Medullary carcinoma of the thyroid, which accounts for less than 10 per cent of cases of thyroid malignancy, may occur as part of the syndrome of multiple endocrine adenomatosis, type II (MEA II) (Sterling, 1975) (see p. 468). These tumors are derived from the calcitonin-secreting cells of the thyroid, which are called the "C" or "parafollicular" cells. Although the serum calcium is usually normal in these patients, medullary thyroid carcinoma has been demonstrated to secrete calcitonin. An exaggerated serum calcitonin response to such stimuli as calcium infusion or pentagastrin injection has been of value in the early diagnosis of occult medullary thyroid carcinoma in high risk persons (Hennessy, 1974). In addition, these tumors have been reported to secrete a number of other substances such as ACTH, serotonin, and prostaglandins (DeGroot, 1975).

In patients with thyroid adenoma or thyroid carcinoma, the serum T3, T4, free T4, and TSH are usually within the expected reference interval.

MEASUREMENT OF THYROID
HORMONES

Thyroxine

Before methods for determining circulating thyroid hormone concentrations became available, assessment of thyroid function was based on physiologic parameters. The relatively non-specific methods such as the basal metabolism rate (BMR) and relaxation time of

the Achilles tendon reflex largely have been replaced by measurement of thyroid hormones in blood. The estimation of circulating levels of thyroid hormone became possible when, in the 1940's, the protein bound iodine (PBI) method was developed. Small amounts of non-hormonal iodine are present in serum of normal subjects; under most clinical circumstances 80 to 90 per cent of the PBI is derived from thyroxine. The PBI, which has a normal range of 4 to 8 μg/dl, is largely a reflection of the total T4 concentration, since normal total T3 serum concentration expressed in terms of iodine is only about 0.10 μg/dl (Fig. 14–11). The PBI procedure involves conversion of organically bound iodine to inorganic iodine by acid digestion or alkaline ash incineration and subsequent quantitation of inorganic iodine. The liberated iodine catalyzes reduction of an acid cerate solution by trivalent arsenic with the rate of decolorization of the solution proportional to the amount of iodine present. The major problem with PBI is spurious elevations

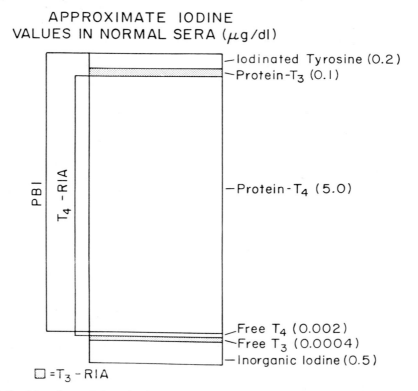

Figure 14–11. Relationships of protein bound iodine (PBI), thryoxine (free and protein bound), triiodothyronine (free and protein bound), and inorganic iodine.

Table 14-6.   IODINE-CONTAINING COMPOUNDS WHICH MAY CAUSE DECREASED RAI UPTAKE AND INCREASED PBI

COMPOUND	APPROXIMATE DURATION OF EFFECT*	COMPOUND	APPROXIMATE DURATION OF EFFECT*
Iodine antiseptics		Amebicides	
Tincture of iodine	1-4 weeks	Diodoquin	2- 4 weeks
Betadine	1-4 weeks	Entero-Vioform	2- 4 months
Topical preparations		*Iodinated radioisotopes used for diagnosis*	
Cosmetics	1-4 weeks	RISA	1- 8 weeks
Suntan preparations	1-4 weeks	Rose bengal [131]I	1- 8 weeks
Antidandruff medications	1-4 weeks	*Radiographic contrast media*	
Proprietary medications		Cholecystography	
Cough syrups and lozenges	1-4 weeks	Biligrafin	3 weeks
Cod liver oil products	1-4 weeks	Orabilex	8 weeks
Toothpastes containing iodine	1-4 weeks	Oragrafin	8 weeks
Multivitamin preparations	1-4 weeks	Cholegrafin	1- 4 months
Miscellaneous		Telepaque	1- 4 months
Potassium iodide (large doses)	1-6 weeks	Priodax	4-12 months
Foods or drugs colored red with erythrosine (tetraiodo-fluorescein)	1-4 weeks	Teridax	1-30 years
		Pyelography	
		Hypaque	1 week
Iodinated penicillin	1-4 weeks	Diodrast	2 weeks
Iodothiouracil (antithyroid drug)	1-4 weeks	Hippuran	2 weeks
DOPA (used in treatment of Parkinson's disease)	1-4 weeks	Miokon	2 weeks
		Neo-Iopax	2 weeks
BSP (some lots)	1-4 weeks	Pyelombrine	2 weeks
Metrecal	1-4 weeks	Renografin	2 weeks
Choloxin (dextrothyroxine)	1-4 weeks	Skiodan	2 weeks
Indwelling venous or arterial catheters	1-4 weeks	Urokon	4 weeks
		Bronchography-myelography	
Bromides	1-4 weeks	Dionosil	1- 5 months
Barium (used for gastro-intestinal radiography)	0-6 days	Lipiodol (myelogram)	1-30 years
		Lipiodol (bronchogram)	1- 5 years
Antiparasitic drugs		Pantopaque	1-30 years
Trichomonacides (vaginal suppositories)		Salpingography	
Vioform	1-3 weeks	Salpix	1- 5 months
Floraquin	1-2 weeks		

*Varies in different patients

due to inorganic or organic iodine contamination, as shown in Table 14-6. In such circumstances the PBI becomes invalid as an estimate of circulating thyroxine. Although the PBI procedure has been abandoned for most purposes, it still may be useful in certain clinical situations such as thyroiditis. The butanol extractable iodine (BEI) and the T4 by column, (thyroxine (chromatographic), T4 (C)) which are both based on iodometry, employ a step to remove iodine contamination. They do not completely eliminate the problem, however, since they are susceptible to contamination with certain organic iodine-containing compounds (Wellby, 1976).

Total T4 by competitive protein binding or displacement analysis (T4 (D)), described by Murphy (1964), is based on the specific binding properties of TBG, thus allowing determination of T4 independent of its iodine content. The technique involves the extraction of T4 from the serum with ethanol to eliminate interference of thyroxine binding proteins and an incubation step employing TBG and radioactively labeled thyroxine. The method of total T4 by competitive protein binding is subject to a number of limitations, including variability in the extraction step. T4 by radioimmunoassay (T4 (RIA)), which is also unaffected by iodine, employs an antibody to thyroxine which is specifically induced in animals for use in the assay. In general, antisera to T4 can be readily produced and have satisfactory specificity for L-thyroxine, although commonly they do cross-react with D-thyroxine. The *in vitro* interference by serum binding proteins must be eliminated; this may be accomplished by the use of blocking agents such as thiomerisol,

Table 14–7. REVISED NOMENCLATURE OF THYROID HORMONES IN SERUM*

NAME OF TEST	ABBREVI-ATION	ACTUALLY MEASURED	UNITS	COMMENTS
A. Iodine concentration				
1. Protein-bound iodine	PBI	I	μg/dl	1. Only use now is to establish non-thyroxine PBI.
2. Butanol-extractable iodine	BEI	I	μg/dl	2. Rarely used now.
3. Thyroxine iodine (chromatographic)	$T_4I(C)$	I	μg/dl	
B. Hormone concentration				
4. Thyroxine (chromatographic)	$T_4(C)$	I	μg/dl	4. Calculated as $T_4I/0.65$.
5. Thyroxine (displacement)	$T_4(D)$	T_4	μg/dl	5. Often called "Thyroxine (Murphy-Pattee)." Displacement refers to the group of methods which have been described as displacement analysis, isotope displacement assays, saturation analysis, competitive protein-binding, and radioligand binding.
6. Thyroxine (radioimmunoassay)	$T_4(RIA)$	T_4	μg/dl	6. Although radioimmunoassay is clearly a subtype of displacement assay, it is given a separate designation and abbreviation (RIA) because of its unique characteristics and importance.
7. Triiodothyronine (radioimmunoassay)	$T_3(RIA)$	T_3	ng/dl	
8. Free thyroxine	FT_4	$T_4(C)$, $T_4(D)$ or $T_4(RIA)$ and % FT_4	ng/dl	8. Equal to $[10 \times (T_4) \times (\% FT_4)]$. The % FT_4 is usually estimated by equilibrium dialysis.
9. Free triiodothyronine	FT_3	$T_3(RIA)$ and % FT_3	ng/dl	9. Equal to $[(T_3) \times (\% FT_3)/100]$. The % FT_3 is usually estimated by equilibrium dialysis.
C. Estimate of free hormone fraction†				
10. Triiodothyronine uptake	T_3U	Uptake of ^{131}I-T_3 on a solid phase	%	10. T_3U tests include use of a variety of non-cellular absorbing media, such as resins, charcoal, Sephadex, etc.
11. Triiodothyronine uptake ratio	T_3U	Uptake of ^{131}I-T_3 on a solid phase	Fraction of normal	11. The ratio is the T_3U of the patient divided by the T_3U of a pool of normal standard reference serum included in the same assay run. This form is strongly preferred over No. 10 and is the only form which should be used in calculating a free thyroxine index. The normal range, although centered on 1.0, is not necessarily identical for each method. The inverted fraction has been used at times. This leads to extreme confusion and should be stopped. As long as tests reported as the inverted fraction remain in use, the result must be *divided into* the T_4 to calculate a free thyroxine index.
D. Indirect estimates of free hormone concentration				

† Per cent free thyroxine and per cent free triiodothyronine, measured by equilibrium dialysis, would be listed under this heading, as they were in the first presentation of the Nomenclature. They are omitted this time because these tests are not now used in ordinary clinical practice.

Table 14-7. REVISED NOMENCLATURE OF THYROID HORMONES IN SERUM* (*Continued*)

NAME OF TEST	ABBREVI-ATION	ACTUALLY MEASURED	UNITS	COMMENTS
12. Free thyroxine index	FT$_4$ index	T$_4$(D) or T$_4$(RIA) and T$_3$U ratio	None	12. Calculated as (T$_4$) × (T$_3$U ratio) or estimated by the sequential performance of two competitive protein-binding maneuvers. If desired, the use of the latter procedure may be indicated by the designation, "Free thyroxine index (sequential)," abbreviated FT$_4$ index (S). A welter of commercial brand names have been employed, but are confusing and should be discarded. Since the calculated index is the product of T$_4$ concentration and a ratio, it theoretically has units of concentration (μg/dl). However, to avoid confusion with measurements of T$_4$ itself, units should be omitted.
13. Free triiodothyronine index	FT$_3$ index	T$_3$(RIA) and T$_3$U ratio	None	13. See comment No. 12. The FT$_3$ index is coming into use, but the precise significance of correcting T$_3$(RIA) for variations of TBG by means of the T$_3$U ratio is uncertain at this time.
E. Thyroxine-binding proteins				
14. Thyroxine-binding globulin capacity	TBG cap	Maximal binding capacity for T$_4$	μg/dl	14. Capacity expressed in terms of T$_4$, never T$_4$I.
15. Thyroxine-binding globulin concentration	TBG	Concentration of TBG	mg/dl	15. Measured by RIA or competitive ligand-binding assay.
F. Miscellaneous				
16. Thyroglobulin	Tg(RIA)	Tg(RIA)	μg/dl	

*Reproduced with permission from Solomon, D. H., et al.: J. Clin. Endocrinol. Metabol., 43:395, 1976.

salicylate, 8-anilino-1-naphthalene sulfonic acid (ANS), or heat denaturation. For example, in the method of Chopra (1972), ANS is used to block T4 binding to TBG, while barbital buffer is used to inhibit binding of T4 to TBPA. The advantages of the T4 (RIA) include its sensitivity and elimination of the extraction step. The reference interval of T4 (RIA) in adults is approximately 5.5 to 12.5 μg/dl (72 to 163 nmol/l) as thyroxine.

Confusion has arisen concerning the values for the reference interval of thyroxine. As procedures such as the Murphy-Pattee competitive binding assay for thyroxine were introduced, results were expressed in terms of the whole thyroxine molecule rather than the thyroxine iodine (T4I), as had been done previously. About 65 per cent of the weight of thyroxine is contributed by iodine; the reference value expressed as iodine thus is approximately two thirds as great as that expressed

as thyroxine. Further confusion arose when the determinations based on iodine were recalculated to correspond to the whole thyroxine molecule by dividing the T4I by 0.65. For example, thyroxine (chromatographic) expressed as iodine has a normal range of about 4 to 8 μg/dl, but when calculated as thyroxine by dividing T4I by 0.65, the reference interval is approximately 6.2 to 12.3 μg/dl (Table 14-7). Since assays based on iodine are falling rapidly into disuse, these difficulties should disappear. To avoid any confusion in the interpretation of T4 determinations, it is recommended that any thyroxine values reported as iodine be clearly designated as such (Solomon, 1976).

Total thyroxine by any of these methods is affected by changes in the serum thyroxine binding proteins. In situations in which drugs or other factors cause increased protein binding, there is an increased total T4 level, and

Table 14–8. CAUSES OF ABNORMALITIES OF THYROID
BINDING GLOBULIN (TBG) AND THYROID BINDING
PREALBUMIN (TBPA)

		INCREASED BINDING CAPACITY	DECREASED BINDING CAPACITY
TBG		Estrogens	Androgens
		Oral contraceptives	Prednisone
		Pregnancy	Active acromegaly
		Newborn infants	Nephrotic syndrome
		Acute intermittent porphyria	Hepatic disease
		Hepatic disease	Acute illness or surgical stress
		Perphenazine (Trilafon)	Phenytoin (diphenylhydantoin, Dilantin)
		Hypothyroidism	
		Genetic	Genetic
TBPA		Androgens	Acute illness or surgical stress
		Prednisone	Hyperthyroidism
		Active acromegaly	Nephrotic syndrome
			Salicylates

when decreased binding capacity occurs, there is a decreased total T4. These effects, however, are not reflected at the physiologic level, and in these situations the free or unbound concentration of thyroxine correlates better than total T4 with thyroid status. It is presumably the free fraction which is the active form of thyroxine and the moiety which is homeostatically controlled. Increased TBG occurs in pregnant subjects, patients treated with estrogens, and patients with acute liver disease. Hereditary increases in TBG are relatively rare. The administration of testosterone or anabolic steroids causes a lowering of TBG concentration and a consequent decrease in serum total T4. Genetic decrease or absence of TBG may occur, also causing low total T4 values. Drugs such as salicylates and phenytoin (diphenylhydantoin) interfere with binding. In these situations, as well as others listed in Table 14-8, the changes in the total T4 level are not accompanied by corresponding alterations in clinical thyroid state.

Provided there are no abnormalities in the serum binding proteins, serum T4 is useful in following most patients with hyperthyroidism and has been used to screen for thyroid dysfunction. Most patients with hyperthyroidism have both elevated total T4 and total T3 values. Hyperthyroidism has been reported in patients with normal T4 and elevated T3, so-called "T3 thyrotoxicosis" (see p. 428). Patients with elevated T4 values with low to normal T3 have been regarded by some workers as having a form of hyperthyroidism

termed "T4 thyrotoxicosis" (Irvine, 1976). Although some workers have reported a slight but not significant reduction in total T4 levels in euthyroid patients with a variety of illnesses (Burger, 1976), others have found that T4 levels may be slightly elevated under these circumstances (Cavalieri, 1977). Some patients who present with non-thyroidal intercurrent disease but with increased serum T4 and normal serum T3 may develop hyperthyroidism; in the study of Birkhäuser (1977), this occurred in 45 per cent of these patients. Patients treated with T4 preparations have serum levels of total T4 which do not show an increase following oral administration of the medication (Saberi, 1974). Patients treated with T3 preparations have very low or undetectable total T4 levels. Evaluation of total T4 values in infants is complicated by TBG elevations in the neonatal period and a TSH surge occurring at the time of birth, both of which lead to increased total T4 levels that may remain elevated for a number of weeks (Larsen, 1975). At birth, normal infants have been reported to have serum T4 concentrations in the range of 7.8 to 16 μg/dl (101 to 208 nmol/l) (Burman, 1976).

Free thyroxine index (FTI) and free thyroxine

With changes in thyroxine binding proteins as shown in Table 14–8, high or low levels of total serum thyroxine occur which are not reflected in the corresponding alterations in clinical state. In these situations the free or unbound thyroxine is more closely correlated with the patient's thyroid status. The free thyroxine (FT4) may be estimated using the T3 uptake (T_3U) or determined by such techniques as equilibrium dialysis.

The T3 uptake essentially provides information about the free binding sites of TBG. When used in this context, the term T3 refers to the radioactive label used in the determination and not to the measurement of triiodothyronine (T3). In performance of the T3 uptake, radioactively labeled T3 is added to the plasma sample and equilibrated with certain inert materials such as resins, which non-specifically adsorb the label. The radioactive labeled T3 is partitioned between the sample and the adsorbent, depending on the number of unoccupied binding sites present (thyroid binding protein). The uptake of T3 by the adsorbent material, therefore, is inversely proportional to the number of free binding sites of TBG. There are a large variety of methods based on this principle, which differ mainly in the nature of the substance used to adsorb the labeled T3 (Wahner, 1972). The reference interval varies not only with the individual laboratory, but also with the test procedure employed. In hyperthyroidism, increased thyroid hormone secretion leads to a greater than normal degree of saturation of the binding proteins and fewer available serum binding sites. Greater binding of the labeled T3 to the adsorbent thus occurs. In hypothyroidism, there is a decrease in saturation of the binding sites and increased binding of the labeled T3 to the serum binding proteins. This leads to a decreased uptake of radioactivity by the adsorbent. The T3 uptake is useful as an indirect test for evaluating thyroid status. With pronounced alterations in total T4 binding capacity or in the presence of substances in the circulation which compete for T4 binding, the T3 uptake does not accurately reflect the thyroid status. In conjunction with the total T4, the T3 uptake can be used to calculate the free thyroxine index. The advantage of the free thyroxine index or measurement of free thyroxine concentration is a better correlation with thyroid status in the presence of thyroid binding protein abnormalities. The values for the T3 uptake may be expressed in a number of ways, such as the per cent of radioactivity bound by the absorbent. This has lead to confusion in calculating the free thyroxine index and the reference intervals for the determination. The Committee on Nomenclature of the American Thyroid Association recommends that T3 uptake be expressed as a ratio and considers this mandatory when calculating the free thyroxine index (Solomon, 1976). The problem is further complicated by the bewildering array of synonyms for the free thyroxine index (see Table 14-7).

Various methods have been developed for the quantitation of free thyroxine, including gel filtration, ultrafiltration, and equilibrium dialysis. In the equilibrium dialysis technique, radioactively labeled T4 in tracer quantities is added to serum. The assumption is made that the radioactive thyroxine and endogenous thyroxine behave in the same manner. The free T4 is separated from the bound by dialysis and the radioactivity in the dialysate, the so-called dialyzable fraction, is determined. The product of the total T4 concentration, which has been determined by standard techniques, and the dialyzable fraction yield the free thyroxine concentration (Sterling, 1976). In hyperthyroid patients, the free T4 is elevated and in hypothyroidism, the free T4 concentrations are decreased. The free T4 concentration is not altered by variations in TBG, despite the change this causes in total hormone concentration. Elevated or decreased concentrations of free thyroxine (or free thyroxine index) have been reported in certain clinical situations without concomitant changes in metabolic state. A significant number of individuals with non-thyroidal systemic illness (for example, fever, terminal illness, malignancy), have elevated free thyroxine values. Various drugs have been reported to cause changes as well; heparin has been reported to increase free thyroxine levels *in vivo* (Schatz, 1969) and phenytoin (diphenylhydantoin) decreases the levels (Hansen, 1974).

In certain patients it may be helpful to measure the TBG more directly (Table 14-8). Several methods have been developed for the assay of TBG, including radioimmunoassay and the determination of maximal binding capacity of TBG by electrophoretic techniques (Wahner, 1972).

Triiodothyronine

Serum triiodothyronine (T3) values are much lower than serum thyroxine concentrations. In most laboratories the reference interval for serum total T3 (T3 by radioimmunoassay (T3RIA)) is approximately 100 to 220 ng/dl (1.5 to 3.4 nmol/l). Since T3 is much less tightly bound to the proteins TBG, TBPA, and albumin, a relatively greater proportion of T3 than T4 exists in the free, diffusible state. It is estimated that approximately 0.4 per cent of total T3 is free or non-protein bound. Changes in the binding capacity of the serum carrier proteins are reflected by concomitant changes in total T3 levels. By analogy to the T4 concept, it is the free moiety that may be the determining factor in the rate of T3 delivery to the tissues. Total T3 usually is measured by radioimmunoassay (see Chap. 13). The assays employ highly specific T3 antisera with little cross-reactivity to thyroxine and a blocking agent, such as 8-anilino-1-naphthalene sulfonic acid (ANS) or sodium salicylate to eliminate endogeneous protein binding. Free T3 has been measured by methods similar to those used for free T4 (Sterling, 1976).

In over 90 per cent of patients with hyperthyroidism both T3 and T4 values are increased in parallel with the increase in T3 greater than the increase in T4. This disproportionate increase in serum T3 in hyperthyroidism is thought to occur as the result of enhanced secretion of T3 from the thyroid and greater peripheral production of T3 due to the increased T4 availability (Utiger, 1974). Hyperthyroidism with elevated T3 levels in the presence of a normal total T4 and normal free T4 is termed T3 thyrotoxicosis (Sterling, 1970). Patients with this syndrome are a heterogeneous group with no distinctive or unusual signs or symptoms of hyperthyroidism. Although most of the patients have Graves' disease, T3 thyrotoxicosis may occur in patients with other causes of hyperthyroidism such as toxic nodular goiter or toxic adenoma. The prevalence of T3 hyperthyroidism in hyperthyroid patients is about 4 per cent except in regions of iodine deficiency where it is more common (Schimmel, 1977). Hyperthyroidism with elevated T3 levels and normal T4 levels may also occur in patients early in the course of hyperthyroidism and in those relapsing after a course of antithyroid drugs for hyperthyroidism. Patients receiving thyroid preparations containing T3, such as desiccated thyroid and synthetic T3 and T4 combinations, or those patients treated with T3 alone will have uninterpretable serum T3 results unless the time of the hormone administration is known. Administration of T3 results in a rise in serum T3 concentrations with peak values at two to four hours. Patients treated with T3 alone have very low or undetectable serum T4 levels. In patients treated with daily doses of T4 alone, the serum T3 levels do not show a peak after ingestion of the medication. Stable levels of T3 from the peripheral conversion of the T4 are reached only after weeks of treatment (Utiger, 1974).

In clinically euthyroid patients, there are a number of situations in which serum T3 concentrations are elevated in the presence of increased TSH levels. This is seen in patients with mild thyroid failure in whom serum T4 values are within the normal range and in some cases of endemic iodine deficiency in the presence of low serum T4 concentrations (Ingbar, 1975).

Low values of T3 in patients who are presumably euthyroid may occur in certain clinical situations. Serum total T3 concentrations are low in cord blood but increase rapidly in the infant during the first few hours of life, attaining values higher than those in normal adults (Abuid, 1974). A significant number of hospitalized patients suffering from non-thyroidal diseases have low serum total T3 concentrations (Bermudez, 1975). These findings are thought to reflect impaired T4 to T3 conversion. In the majority of the patients with low serum T3 levels associated with systemic illness, the TSH values are within normal limits. Serum T3 levels are often low in patients with cirrhosis and may be profoundly low with normal or slightly elevated total and free T4 values. It has been reported that there is a progressive decrease in T3 concentrations with advancing age (Rubenstein, 1973).

Reverse T3,* which is thought to be metabolically inactive, is quantitatively a major metabolite of thyroxine. Although the mechanisms controlling the pathways of thyroxine deiodinization are unknown, they seem to be determined by the metabolic needs of the body. Reverse T3, which is measured by radioimmunoassay, has been reported to have a mean value in the range of 18 to 60 ng/dl in normal human subjects (Kaplan, 1977). In general, the specificity of the radioimmunoassay for reverse T3 is such that cross-reactivity with T3 assays is not significant. In many clinical situations, T3 and reverse T3 have been found to vary reciprocally. In normal newborns, reverse T3 has been reported to be increased. Serum reverse T3 is elevated in some but not all the patients with non-thyroidal disease in whom T3 concentrations are decreased. It is uncertain if the elevated re-

---

*rT3.

verse T3 concentration reflects increased production from T4 or decreased rT3 clearance (Cavalieri, 1977). Reverse T3 concentrations are increased in hyperthyroidism.

In addition to evaluating patients suspected of having T3 thyrotoxicosis, serum T3 measurement may be helpful in confirming the diagnosis of hyperthyroidism in patients with minimal elevations of serum T4 or ambiguous clinical manifestations. Although serum T3 concentrations characteristically are decreased in hypothyroidism, up to 30 per cent of clinically hypothyroid patients may have T3 concentrations in the expected normal range. Measurements of serum T3 thus generally are not valuable in hypothyroid states. Assay of reverse T3 is not widely available.

Thyroid stimulating hormone (TSH)

Thyroid stimulating hormone (TSH) accelerates nearly all aspects of metabolism of the thyroid gland, including the production and secretion of thyroid hormones. TSH, which is an anterior pituitary hormone consisting of an alpha and beta subunit, is a glycoprotein with a molecular weight of about 28,000 (Tunbridge, 1976). The alpha subunit of the glycoprotein hormones TSH, LH, FSH, and HCG are similar if not identical; however, the beta subunits differ significantly. The beta subunit confers biologic specificity to the glycoproteins and is the major determinant of immunologic specificity. Bioassay of TSH has largely been replaced by radioimmunoassay. TSH antibody preparations used in the radioimmunoassay may cross-react with the glycoprotein hormones, giving falsely elevated values for TSH in such clinical situations as pregnancy (elevated HCG levels) and postmenopausal states (elevated FSH, LH). Methods which have been developed to avoid this difficulty include adsorption of TSH antisera with HCG prior to use or addition of a standard amount of HCG to all TSH radioimmunoassay tubes in order to adsorb the cross-reacting antibodies. These techniques, however, do not completely solve the problem (DeGroot, 1975). Although normal or reference values for TSH vary from laboratory to laboratory, they are usually less than 10 μU/ml. Few TSH assays can readily distinguish subnormal TSH values from normal levels; thus, basal TSH values are not helpful in distinguishing hyperthyroid from euthyroid indi-

viduals. The major value of serum TSH levels is in the diagnosis of primary thyroid failure and as a useful guide to therapy in such patients. In primary hypothyroidism, serum TSH levels are markedly elevated. In hypothyroidism secondary to hypothalamic or pituitary disease, characteristically basal TSH levels are not elevated.

TSH values may be elevated in newborn infants during the first few days of life and may be increased in certain other euthyroid individuals. Elevated levels of TSH in euthyroid patients may occur in a number of clinical conditions, including lymphocytic thyroiditis and post-treatment with radioactive iodine for hyperthyroidism, and in individuals residing in areas of severe iodine deficiency (Carlson, 1975).

TSH values following the administration of thyroid releasing hormone (TRH) may be used as a test of thyroid function. A TRH test may be performed in a number of ways which vary as to the dose and route of administration of the TRH, as well as the parameter measured. Usually a single bolus of TRH is administered intravenously after a baseline serum TSH has been drawn. Another serum TSH level is obtained 30 minutes after the TRH has been given, or TSH levels may be drawn at 20 and 60 minutes. Intravenous administration of TRH is associated with a high incidence of side effects, but most of them are minor. Intravenous TRH administration causes a rapid rise in serum TSH, within about 5 minutes, reaching a peak in 20 to 30 minutes and returning to baseline in two to four hours (Fig. 14-12). The normal response of subjects to the intravenous injection of 500 μg of TRH is a prompt rise in serum TSH, peaking within 15 to 30 minutes to a concentration of about 16 to 26 μU/ml in women (slightly lower in men) from the basal mean value of about 6 μU/ml (Sterling, 1977). In euthyroid subjects, serum T3 increases to about 70 per cent above baseline levels one to four hours after administration of TRH, while there is an increase in serum T4 but to a lesser extent; serum T3 and T4 levels usually are not measured during a TRH test. TRH normally stimulates the secretion of prolactin from the pituitary as well.

The TSH response to TRH may be affected by a number of conditions and drugs. There is a significant time interval following withdrawal of long-term thyroid hormone therapy before the normal response to TRH is restored

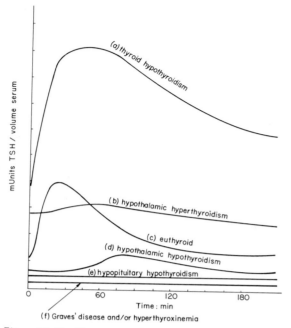

Figure 14-12. Response to TRH in thyroid disease. (Used with permission from Bartuska, D. G., and Dratman, M. B.: Evolving concepts of thyroid function. Med. Clin. North Am., 57:1117, 1973.)

(Burger, 1977). It is blunted by pharmacologic doses of the corticosteroids and by therapy with L-dopa. The TRH test is unreliable in patients with poor renal function (Hall, 1976).

Occasionally normal subjects may fail to respond to TRH on one occasion yet respond normally on subsequent occasions. In hyperthyroid patients, the response of TSH to TRH is suppressed. Although the presence of an impaired response to TRH is commonly due to hyperthyroidism, it may occur in a number of other conditions, including multinodular goiter and in Graves' disease patients who are euthyroid after therapy. The TRH test has been used as a reliable index of TSH suppression in patients treated with thyroxine for such disorders as thyroid carcinoma and thyroid nodules (Hoffman, 1977). Until recently, thyroid autonomy was demonstrated by inadequate suppression of thyroidal radioactive iodine uptake by exogenous administration of T3. In order to perform the T3 suppression test, the patient underwent a radioactive iodine uptake before and after a course of oral administration of T3. Normally T3 ingestion reduces the uptake almost to background level. The TRH test has been shown to correlate well

with the T3 suppression test; a normal TRH test is correlated with normal T3 suppressibility, and absent or impaired TSH response to TRH correlates with impaired or absent suppression of T3. The TRH test has been recommended as a replacement for the T3 suppression test (Evered, 1974), since it avoids the administration of T3, which may be dangerous, especially in patients who already have high circulating levels of thyroid hormone.

Patients with primary hypothyroidism have a high basal TSH level and an exaggerated TSH response to TRH. In patients with hypothyroidism secondary to pituitary or hypothalamic disease, basal TSH levels usually are within normal limits; however, some patients with hypothalamic hypothyroidism may have slightly elevated basal TSH values. With hypothalamic hypothyroidism, the peak TSH secretion after TRH administration may be delayed, occurring at 45 to 90 minutes rather than 30 minutes (Fig. 14-12). Absent TSH response to TRH in a patient who does not have primary hyperthyroidism suggests a pituitary rather than hypothalamic lesion; however, intact response of TSH to TRH may be seen in patients with pituitary disease (Burger, 1977). Some hypothyroid patients with pituitary lesions have a delay in TSH peak after TRH; this pattern suggests hypothalamic involvement (Reichlin, 1978).

Radioactive uptake and scan

The radioactive iodine (RAI) uptake reflects the ability of the thyroid to accumulate iodine (Fig. 14-13). A tracer dose of isotope is given and the percentage which accumulates in the thyroid is determined by gamma scintillation counting at some fixed interval such as 24 hours. The test can be performed using ^{131}I or other isotopes such as [125]I. The radioactive uptake results are affected by alterations in the iodine pool and by drugs which interfere with the trapping and retention of iodine (see Table 14-6). Abnormally high radioactive iodine uptakes are consistent with hyperthyroidism but also may occur in certain patients with goiter. An abnormally low thyroid uptake is characteristic of hypothyroidism. It is not specific, however, since low uptakes may occur with subacute thyroiditis and with administration of thyroid hormones, antithyroid drugs, or large doses of iodide (Rosenberg, 1972). In general, the T3 suppression test has been replaced by other determinations (see p.

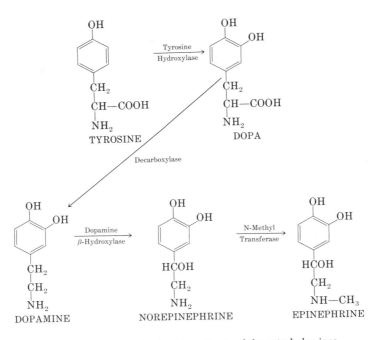

Figure 14–14. Pathway for the biosynthesis of the catecholamines.

amino acid precursor of the catecholamines is tyrosine. The enzyme required for conversion of norepinephrine to epinephrine is present predominantly within the adrenal medulla. In the chromaffin cells of the adrenal medulla and in neurons, the catecholamines are stored within membrane-bound vesicles. They probably are released from these vesicles by a process of exocytosis in which the vesicle fuses with the cell wall and the contents are expelled to the exterior. The storage of catecholamines in vesicles serves to inactivate them as well as to protect them from the degradative action of monoamine oxidase, which is present in the cell cytoplasm. When catecholamines are released from sympathetic tissues other than the adrenal medulla, the primary means of physiologic inactivation is an active transport mechanism which returns the unaltered catecholamines into the nerve endings. The residual hormone may then be metabolized or excreted unchanged by the kidney. The adrenal medulla contains very large quantities of both norepinephrine and epinephrine, which upon release appear directly in the circulation. Two enzymes are important for catecholamine metabolism: monoamine oxidase (MAO), which is responsible for oxidative deamination, and catechol-o-methyltransferase (COMT), which is responsible for o-methylation. Methylation may precede the deamination or vice versa. COMT is principally responsible for inactivating circulating catecholamine, with MAO probably playing a major role in disposing of excessive stores by deamination *in situ.* In either case, the initial metabolic product is pharmacologically inactive and the major end product 3-methoxy-4-hydroxymandelic acid (vanillylmandelic acid, VMA). The other major urinary metabolites of the catecholamines include metanephrine and normetanephrine (Fig. 14–15). Derivatives of dopamine give rise to the metabolites 3,4-dihydroxyphenyl-acetic acid (DOPAc) and 3-methoxy-4-hydroxyphenylacetic acid (homovanillic acid, HVA) (Pullar, 1976). The metabolite, 3-methoxy-4-hydroxyphenylethylene glycol (MHPG), which appears in urine as well, is apparently derived mainly from the brain (Kopin, 1977). In addition, small amounts of epinephrine and norepinephrine are excreted in the urine, some in the free form and some conjugated and excreted as sulfates or glucuronides. The major urinary metabolite of epinephrine and norepinephrine is VMA (Fig. 14–15).

CATECHOLAMINE-PRODUCING TUMORS

Pheochromocytoma is a catecholamine-producing tumor which may arise at the same locations in the body where chromaffin tissue has been found to occur. Although pheochromocytoma is rare, its diagnosis and successful treatment are of great importance, since it causes a potentially curable form of hypertension and, if left untreated, may be fatal. Approximately 60 per cent of pheochromocytomas occur within the adrenal medulla, and greater than 90 per cent of the tumors lie between the diaphragm and the pelvic floor (Page, 1968). In less than 10 per cent of patients, the tumors are malignant, as evidenced by metatasis to non-chromaffin tissue. Multiple primary tumors occur in about 20 per cent of patients.

The most characteristic, but not the most common manifestation of pheochromocytoma is paroxysmal hypertension. The attacks may occur several times a day or at infrequent intervals only; they may last for only a minute or for as long as a week. Accompanying signs and symptoms may include headache, tachycardia, palpitations, sweating, nervousness, and tremor. Clinical manifestations of pheochromocytoma, however, are variable, and the patient may present simply with sustained hypertension. Important physical findings in pheochromocytoma patients are excessive perspiration and orthostatic hypotension. About two thirds of untreated pheochromocytoma patients show orthostatic hypotension, which appears to be related to a type of autonomic dysfunction simulating ganglionic blockade (Engelman, 1977). Approximately 10 per cent of the patients with pheochromocytoma have associated inherited disorders of neuroectodermal origin, including von Recklinghausen's syndrome (neurofibromatosis), Von Hippel-Lindau disease, and Sturge-Weber disease. In Sipple's syndrome (multiple endocrinopathy, type II), bilateral pheochromocytoma may be associated with medullary carcinoma of the thyroid and hyperparathyroidism.

Other disorders of the adrenal medulla which are associated with increased catecholamines and their metabolites include neuroblastoma and ganglioneuroma. Neuroblastoma is one of the most common malignant soft tissue tumors of infancy and early childhood, with about three fourths of the patients under five years of age. A frequent mode of presentation is that of a mass which may cause symptoms secondary to invasion or compression of surrounding tissues. With neuroblastoma, the course is primarily that of metastatic malignancy, and hypertension is often modest or absent. It has been suggested that neuroblastomas lack the ability to store catecholamines, and thus catecholamines are released from the tumor cells and inactivated soon after their formation. It has been postulated that this inactivation may account for the paucity of sympathetic nervous system symptoms in patients with neuroblastoma. Ganglioneuromas are well-differentiated tumors of the sympathetic nervous system which rarely metastasize. They occur in older children and young adults (Moskowitz, 1977).

LABORATORY DETERMINATIONS

Pharmacologic procedures are no longer commonly used for the evaluation of patients suspected of having pheochromocytomas. They yield a large percentage of false positive and negative responses and are associated with serious adverse side effects (Engelman, 1977). The diagnosis of pheochromocytoma can be confirmed by demonstrating increases in catecholamines or their metabolites. These biochemical determinations are usually performed using an aliquot of a 24-hour urine specimen which has been collected in acid. In less than 1 per cent of the total group of patients with pheochromocytoma, the excretion of the catecholamines and their metabolites is normal between attacks. In such cases, carefully timed urine collections over the period associated with the attack may be useful in confirming the diagnosis. Plasma catecholamines can be measured by a fluorometric or a radioenzymatic procedure. For normal subjects, not under stress, plasma norepinephrine values are in the range of 0.2 to 0.4 ng/ml and plasma epinephrine values 0.02 to 0.4 ng/ml (Kopin, 1977). Plasma catecholamine values increase with a change in posture from reclining to standing and increase even further with exertion. In addition, plasma norepinephrine levels have been shown to increase with age (Kopin, 1977). Although plasma concentrations of norepinephrine and/or epinephrine are increased in most patients with pheochromocytoma, the variability and range of values in normals are such that levels diagnostic for pheochromocytoma cannot readily be established (Engelman, 1977).

Many non-specific assay procedures for urinary catecholamines or their metabolites have been introduced for screening patients with pheochromocytoma. These assays do not reliably differentiate the rare patient with pheochromocytoma from the patient with more common disorders. Even some of the more specific methods show significant interference by a number of substances. For example, some drugs such as alpha methyldopa interfere with certain assay procedures. In addition, catecholamine-containing drugs or drugs which influence catecholamine metabolism may affect the determinations. Another consideration is that various forms of stress cause increases in catecholamines and their metabolites.

The three most common determinations used for confirmation of the diagnosis of phe-

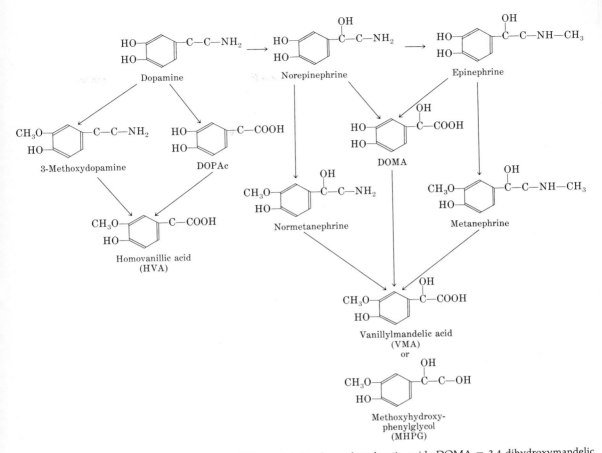

Figure 14–15.   Catecholamine metabolism. DOPAc = 3,4-dihydroxyphenylacetic acid. DOMA = 3,4-dihydroxymandelic acid.

ochromocytoma are urinary VMA, metanephrine, and catecholamines.

VMA

The most widely used assay for VMA involves its oxidation to vanillin with subsequent determination of this compound. Vanillin may be determined directly by UV spectrophotometry (Pisano, 1962) or coupled with indole to form a colored product. Gas chromatography and high pressure liquid chromatography also have been employed (Felice, 1977). Certain screening techniques such as those employing diazotized *p*-nitroaniline are interfered with by phenolic acids of dietary origin, such as those that occur in coffee, vanilla, and certain vegetables and fruits. It has been reported that diet does not significantly change the determination of VMA excretion by the Pisano technique (Rayfield, 1972). Certain

drugs such as methyldopa and monoamine oxidase inhibitors have been reported to decrease urinary excretion of VMA. VMA results may vary considerably with the technique employed for measurement; for example, L-dopa has been reported to both increase and decrease VMA excretion. In studies in which VMA was reported decreased, the Pisano technique was employed, while those studies in which increased values occurred, VMA was purified and quantitated by gas chromatography or thin layer chromatography (Feldman, 1974). Patients with a pheochromocytoma secreting primarily epinephrine will excrete relatively little VMA (Fig. 14-15).

Metanephrines, total

Metanephrines may be measured by a method involving extraction and subsequent oxidation to vanillin (Pisano, 1960) or by a fluorometric technique (Taniguchi, 1964). In addition, a high performance liquid chromatographic procedure has been developed (Shoup, 1977). Because of the overall reliability and ease of performance, the assay of total metanephrines has been recommended for the screening of hypertensive patients for pheochromocytoma. The major drawback of the total urinary metanephrine assay is the variability of excretion during illness. Patients subjected to severe stress, including hemorrhagic shock, sepsis, and widespread metastatic disease, may have elevated values (Gitlow, 1970). Monoamine oxidase inhibitors have been reported to increase metanephrines. Various drugs have been reported to interfere with the total urinary metanephrine determinations, some apparently dependent on the technique employed. Alpha-methyldopa, for example, has been reported to increase metanephrines as measured by a fluorometric method (Freier, 1973), although other workers using a modification of the Pisano technique have found it does not significantly affect the determinations (Gitlow, 1970).

Catecholamines

Urinary free catecholamines may be assayed by a modification of the trihydroxyindole fluorometric technique. The method also may be used to assay epinephrine and norepinephrine separately as well as to measure total catecholamines. Total catecholamines include those that are excreted in the urine in the conjugated form as glucuronides or sulfates as well as those that are free. Total catecholamines are measured by hydrolyzing the urine samples prior to assay. There are several disadvantages in measuring the total catecholamines; for example, the large range of normal may obscure the diagnosis of a minimally secreting tumor. The majority of dietary catecholamines occur in the conjugated form and may interfere with total catecholamine determinations. The determination of urinary free catecholamines is the preferred determination (Page, 1968). Urinary free catecholamines usually represent approximately 2 to 4 per cent of the total catecholamines produced by the sympathetic nervous system and the adrenal medulla. In those patients with rare intermittent attacks, it may be useful to measure catecholamine output fractionated into norepinephrine and epinephrine in carefully timed urine collections from the period associated with the attack (Engelman, 1977).

Catecholamine-containing medication can cause high urinary levels and determinations by some techniques may be interfered with by drugs, including alpha-methyldopa (Mell, 1977). Stress may increase urinary free catecholamines.

INTERPRETATION

In general, the following amounts of catecholamines and their metabolites are excreted under usual circumstances in a 24-hour period: less than 0.1 mg free catecholamines, less than 1.3 mg metanephrines, and less than 6.8 mg of VMA (Engelman, 1977). Gitlow (1968) recommends expression of values in terms of urinary creatinine; normal adult subjects have a mean of 1.4 μg VMA per mg creatinine and 0.42 μg metanephrine per mg creatinine. Values in children differ from those of adults. Levels of urinary VMA, HVA, and metanephrines, for example, tend to be higher and more variable in children, not reaching adult levels until about age 15 (Gitlow, 1968).

Most patients with pheochromocytoma will have elevated urinary VMA, metanephrines, and free catecholamines. In some patients with pheochromocytoma, however, one or more of these determinations may be within normal limits. For example, in the series of Gitlow (1970), about 3 per cent of patients with pheochromocytoma had normal VMA excretion. Although some false negatives do occur, urinary metanephrines have been recommended as the most accurate screening method for the diagnosis of pheochromocytoma (Remine, 1974). In evaluating the biochemical determinations used in the diagnosis of pheochromocytoma, the possibility of false negative and positive interferences from drugs should be considered. Stress may cause increases in urinary catecholamines and their metabolites. In addition, in some patients the urinary excretion of the catecholamines and their metabolites may be normal between attacks.

Excessive urinary excretion of 3-methoxy-4-hydroxy-phenyl ethylene glycol (MHPG) has been commonly observed in association with pheochromocytoma; in some patients, excessive urinary excretion of dopamine and HVA may occur as well. Concentrations of plasma catecholamines may be very high in patients with pheochromocytoma. There is, however, a significant overlap of values from patients without the disease; for example, elevated plasma catecholamines have been reported in about 15 per cent of hypertensive patients without pheochromocytoma. Plasma levels are elevated in patients with increased intracranial pressure and uremia (Amery, 1967).

In patients with neuroblastoma or ganglioneuroma, the excretion of catecholamines and their metabolites in urine may be increased. Elevated urinary VMA is the most common abnormal laboratory finding in patients with neuroblastoma. About 20 per cent of patients will not show an elevated urinary VMA but may have elevated urinary MHPG, HVA, metanephrine, or dopamine. In patients with neuroblastoma about 95 per cent have an increase in either urinary VMA or HVA (Knight, 1975). Since local tumor recurrences and distant metastases may secrete catecholamines, elevated levels of catecholamine metabolites have been used not only to assist in the diagnosis of neuroblastoma, but also to follow the course of tumor treatment. In following patients with neuroblastoma, it has been recommended that 24-hour urines be used for determinations. Excessive urinary excretion of catecholamines or their metabolites occasionally is detected in patients with ganglioneuroma or ganglioneuroblastomas. The most consistent abnormal finding in these patients is elevated urinary VMA (Moskowitz, 1977).

THE ADRENAL CORTEX

STEROID BIOCHEMISTRY

Structure

Structurally, steroids are derived from the cyclopentanoperhydrophenanthrene skeleton. This nucleus consists of a five-member carbon ring (labeled D) fused to a phenanthrene nucleus (rings A, B, and C).

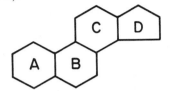

The major precursor of the steroids, if not the only one, is cholesterol. The 27 carbons of cholesterol are numbered by a standard system of nomenclature, as seen below.

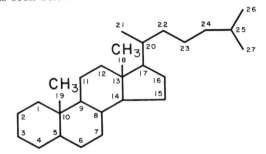

Table 14–10. SUFFIXES AND PREFIXES FOR STEROIDS*

SUFFIX OR PREFIX	MEANING
Suffix	
-ane	Saturated hydrocarbon
-ene	Unsaturated hydrocarbon
-ol	Hydroxyl group, as in an alcohol or phenol
-one	Ketone group
Prefix	
hydroxy- (oxy-)	Hydroxyl group
keto- (oxo-)	Ketone group
deoxy-	Loss of an oxygen atom
dehydro-	Loss of two hydrogen atoms
dihydro-	Gain of two hydrogen atoms
cis-	Refers to spatial arrangement of two groups on the same side of the molecule
trans-	Refers to spatial arrangement of two groups on opposite sides of the molecule
α-	Refers to group which is *trans* to the methyl at C-10
β-	Refers to group which is *cis* to the methyl at C-10
epi-	Isomeric in configuration to a reference compound; specifically α at location C-3
iso-	Similar to epi-, but not restricted to C-3
allo-	Differing from reference compound in having 5α instead of 5β configuration; rings A and B in *trans* instead of *cis* relation to each other
etio-	Refers to final degradation product of a more complex molecule which still retains the essential chemical character of the original molecule
nor-	Refers to compound similar chemically to reference substance, but having one less carbon atom in side-chain
Δ	Indicates position of unsaturated linkage

*From Cantarow, A. and Schepartz, B.: Biochemistry, 4th ed. Philadelphia, W. B. Saunders Company, 1967.

Steroid hormones differ in the degree of saturation of ring A or B, or the types and spatial orientation of a number of side chains. Side chains are designated α or β according to their orientation or relation to the plane of the ring structure. If the ring is parallel to the plane of the paper, those side chains which are below the plane are designated β and those above are α. Those above the plane are designated by a solid line while those below the plane utilize a dotted line. For example, in the cholesterol molecule, the C-17, C-18, and C-19 are designated α (above the plane).

Those steroids which have 21 carbons (C-21) are called pregnanes and include adrenal steroids and progestins; C-19 steroids are androstanes and include male sex hormones; and C-18 steroids with a benzene structure in ring A are called estranes and are the female sex hormones. An example of each is seen below.

ADRENAL STEROIDS <u>C-21</u>

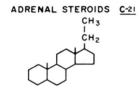

ANDROSTANE (ANDROGENS) <u>C-19</u>

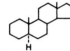

ESTRANE (ESTROGENS) <u>C-18</u>

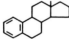

Most steroids isolated from the adrenal cortex, other than estrogens, are unsaturated between the two adjacent carbon atoms 4 and 5, or 5 and 6.

The suffix *-one* designates the existence of ketones in the molecule and *-ol* a hydroxyl steroid. Thus, corti*sone* designates a ketone and corti*sol* a hydroxyl group (Table 14-10).

Biosynthesis

The cortex of the adrenal gland is divided into three distinct zones; the zona fasciculata, the zona glomerulosa, and the zona reticularis, each of which produces a different group of steroid hormones. The zona fasciculata is responsible for the formation of glucocorticoids; the glomerulosa and reticularis are mainly responsible for mineralocorticoids and sex hormones, respectively. The synthetic pathway for these groups of hormones is seen in Figure 14-16. For the sake of simplicity, many of the minor pathways involving interconversion of the various adrenal hormones are not shown.

The enzymes involved in the formation of steroids are of four general types: (1) hydroxylases;

(2) dehydrogenases; (3) desmolases; and (4) isomerases. These enzymes are named depending on the carbon atom transformed. Since most of the inborn errors of metabolism affecting the adrenal cortex involve the hydroxylases, clinically they comprise the most important group. Examples of these enzymes, which involve the transfer of a hydroxyl group, are 11-hydroxylase (transfers a hydroxyl on to carbon 11), 21-hydroxylase, and 17-hydroxylase. The dehydrogenases catalyze the transfer of hydrogen from NADP to NADPH; one of the important inborn errors of metabolism involves the absence of 3-β-ol-dehydrogenase. Desmolases involve degradation of side chains. Two are of importance; one is a 20-22 desmolase which converts cholesterol (a 27-carbon compound) into pregnenolone (a 21-carbon compound). Isomerases catalyze the change in position of a double bond; an important isomerase is involved in the conversion of pregnenolone to progesterone.

The end product of the glucocorticoid pathway is cortisol, which has a negative feedback on the pituitary regulating ACTH (adrenocorticotropic hormone) secretion (Table 14-11). The glucocorticoid pathway from pregnenolone to cortisol involves four enzymes, a dehydrogenase and three hydroxylases, which act in sequence at carbons 3, 17, 21, and 11. Thus, the end product of the glucocorticoid pathway, cortisol, is a 21-carbon steroid with a ketone group at position 3 and a hydroxyl group at positions 17, 21, and 11. Absence of any of these four enzymes leads to a syndrome of congenital adrenal hyperplasia. This is discussed on page 445. Intermediates in the glucocorticoid pathway are first pregnenolone, then progesterone, 17-hydroxyprogesterone, 11-desoxycortisol, and finally cortisol. Although cortisol is the most important glucocorticoid, corticosterone (mineralocorticoid pathway) also has glucocorticoid activity.

A similar pathway occurs in the zona glomerulosa and involves a dehydrogenase (at position 3) and three hydroxylases; it is responsible for the formation of aldosterone, the principal mineralocorticoid. In this sequence, reactions involve carbon atoms 3, 21, 11, and finally 18. The mineralocorticoid pathway differs from the glucocorticoids in that the 17-hydroxylase enzyme is absent and there is a final step involving hydroxylation at position 18. Compounds formed (from pregnenolone) in this sequence are progesterone, then desoxycorticosterone (DOC), corticosterone, and aldosterone. The most important mineralocorticoid is aldosterone, but desoxycorticosterone (DOC) and 11-desoxycortisol (glucocorticoid pathway) have some mineralocorticoid activity. These two minor mineralocorticoids are responsible for hypertension in some of the congenital adrenal hyperplasia syndromes.

The zona reticularis is responsible for the synthesis of the sex hormones: steroids containing either 17 or 18 carbons and an hydroxyl at position 17. Those 17-carbon compounds which have an un-

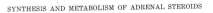

SYNTHESIS AND METABOLISM OF ADRENAL STEROIDS

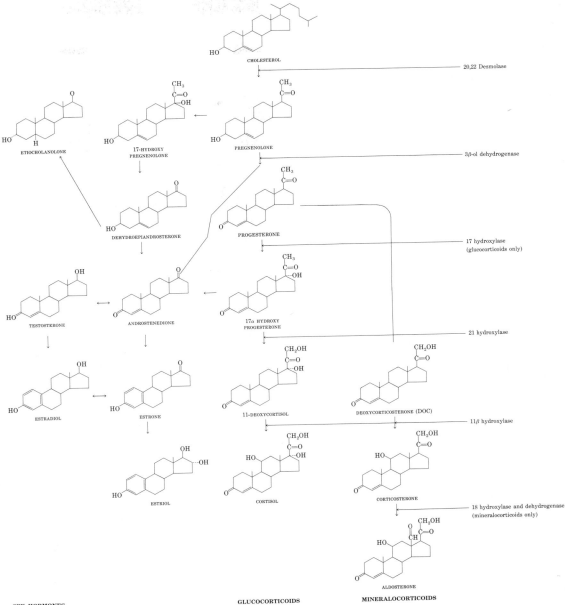

Figure 14–16. Simplified pathways of adrenocortical hormone synthesis and metabolism.

saturated A ring are estrogens, while the C-18 carbon steroids are androgenic and do not have an unsaturated A ring. The discussion of the sex hormones is found on page 459.

Metabolism

Plasma transport and protein binding are discussed under serum cortisol (p. 448). The degradation system for steroids is widespread throughout most tissues, with the liver the most active. The reduction of the A ring with the attachment of hydrogen at position 5 can be either α or β; this step is controlled to a large extent by the structure of the steroid substrate. Cortisol metabolism favors 5β reduction, while corticosterone is primarily metabolized to a 5α compound.

The 3-ketone group is metabolized to a 3α hydroxyl compound, which in some instances is called a tetrahydro derivative. The major urinary metabolites of cortisol and cortisone are tetrahydrocortisol and tetrahydrocortisone. There are also tetra-

Table 14–11. ADRENOCORTICAL HORMONES: EFFECTS AND DIAGNOSTIC APPROACH

REPRESENTATIVE HORMONE	BIOLOGIC EFFECTS	DIAGNOSTIC PROCEDURES

Cortisol (compound F or hydrocortisone) as a representative glucocorticoid	Gluconeogenesis
	Protein nitrogen catabolism increase and anabolism decrease
	    Increased blood glucose concentration
	    Decreased glucose tolerance
	    Increased liver glycogen
	    Increased liver glycogenolysis
	    Decreased peripheral uptake and utilization of glucose
	Decreased synthesis of acid sulfated mucopolysaccharides
	Fat synthesis and redistribution
	Cellular or tissue effects
	    Anti-inflammatory (retardation of inflammatory reactions)
	    Dissolution of lymphoid tissue
	    Lymphopenia
	    Eosinopenia
	    Increased erythropoiesis
	    Alteration of cellular permeability, especially decreased membrane permeability to water
	    Increased gastric (HCl and pepsin) secretion
		Carbohydrate (glucose tolerance) function test
		
		Eosinophil count
		
		Water load test
		
		Urine calcium with low calcium intake
		Plasma and urinary hydroxycorticoids plus ACTH stimulation or specific suppressive tests

Aldosterone as a representative mineralocorticoid	Electrolyte regulation
	    Sodium (Na) retention
	    Potassium (K) excretion
	    Retention of water and expansion of extracellular fluid volume
	Hypertension
		Na:K ratio in saliva and sweat
		Plasma electrolytes
		Urine electrolytes (Na, K) with low sodium intake
		EKG for K effect
		Urinary aldosterone
		Plasma aldosterone and renin

Androgens (C-19 compounds, adrenosterone) as representative sex hormones	Protein nitrogen anabolism Growth and maturation—osseous and muscular Body hair (pubic and axillary) Seborrhea	Urinary 17-ketosteroids Dehydroepiandrosterone (DHEA) Plasma testosterone

hydro derivatives of aldosterone, 11-desoxycortisol, corticosterone, and 11-desoxycorticosterone.

Those compounds which have a 5α group are conjugated with glucuronic acid or sulfuric acid and excreted in the urine. A 20-ketone group is reduced to a 20-hydroxyl, which gives rise to a more polar urinary metabolite. Reduction of the A ring and the 20-ketone group of progesterone or 17-hydroxyprogesterone gives rise to two important metabolites: pregnanediol and pregnanetriol. Cleavage of C-19 side chains occurs with some 17α hydroxylated C-21 compounds, e.g., cortisol.

REGULATION OF CORTISOL SECRETION

Secretion of cortisol by the adrenal cortex occurs in response to three identifiable influences: ACTH, a diurnal rhythm, and stress.

Adrenocorticotropic hormone (ACTH) consists of 39 amino acid residues with the amino terminal end of 1 to 24 amino acid residues possessing full steroidogenic activity. Other forms of ACTH also occur, including "big" ACTH, a form with a mass of 20,000 daltons or greater which has little biologic activity, "little" ACTH, and an "intermediate" variety. These forms may predominate under certain conditions, for example, "big" ACTH in primary or metastatic lung carcinoma and "little" ACTH or the "intermediate" form in some patients with Nelson's syndrome (Orth, 1977). Nelson's syndrome is the occurrence of a pituitary tumor and skin pigmentation following bilateral adrenalectomy for adrenal hyperplasia.

Although several substances which have ACTH releasing capacity are known, corticotropic releasing factor (CRF) itself has not been identified (Saffran, 1977). Cortisol by direct action on the pituitary inhibits ACTH directly and probably inhibits the release of CRF as well (Liddle, 1977). Vasopressin (ADH), which has been found to release ACTH, has been used in the study of patients with Cushing's syndrome (Table 14–12).

The interaction of ACTH with a specific membrane receptor, leading to activation of membrane adenylate cyclase, is thought to be the earliest event that occurs in response of the adrenal to ACTH. Adenylate cyclase then catalyzes the for-

Table 14–12. SERUM CORTICOSTEROID RESPONSES TO DIAGNOSTIC MANEUVERS DESIGNED TO DEMONSTRATE NON-AUTONOMY OR AUTONOMY OF ADRENAL FUNCTION*

			SERUM CORTISOL CONCENTRATIONS			
CONDITION	Basal (8 A.M.)	Circadian Variation	Response to Dexamethasone (1 mg at 11 P.M.)	Response to Aqueous Pitressin (10 units IM)	Response to Cortrosyn	8 A.M. ACTH
Normal	10–25 μg/dl	A.M. greater than P.M.	<6 μg/dl (166 nmol/l)	Increased 15 μg/dl above baseline	Doubling of baseline value	20–100 pg/ml
Adrenal hyperplasia	Normal or increased	Absent	>6 μg/dl (166 nmol/l)	Increased	Increased	Normal or increased
Adrenal adenoma	Normal or increased	Absent	>6 μg/dl (166 nmol/l)	Absent	None or normal	Decreased
Adrenal carcinoma	Increased	Absent	>6 μg/dl (166 nmol/l)	Absent	None	Decreased
Pituitary	Increased	Absent	>6 μg/dl (166 nmol/l)	Absent	None to slight	Markedly increased
Ectopic ACTH syndrome	Increased	Absent	>6 μg/dl (166 nmol/l)	Absent	Usually none	Markedly increased

*Modified from Krieger, 1976.

mation of adenosine cyclic 3′,5′-monophosphate within the cell. ACTH thereby acutely stimulates steroidogenesis, leading to formation of cortisol, the predominant glucocorticoid. The rate-limiting step in the formation of glucocorticoids is the conversion of cholesterol to pregnenolone. This conversion is under the direct control of ACTH, so that when ACTH rises there is an increase in the amount of cholesterol which is converted to pregnenolone and finally to cortisol. When plasma cortisol becomes elevated, it suppresses the release of ACTH (and probably corticotropin releasing factor, CRF), thereby ultimately lowering cortisol. Conversely, when cortisol levels reach a low level, the pituitary responds with increased ACTH production, resulting in stimulation of cortisol secretion. By this mechanism, ACTH and cortisol control the concentration of each other within a very narrow range, and a small change in one results in a concomitant change in the other. When the adrenal is unable to respond to ACTH because of damage or disease, cortisol levels are low and ACTH levels high. In those conditions in which the pituitary is destroyed, ACTH is not formed and cortisol levels tend to be low. If the pituitary-adrenal axis is interrupted by administration of large amounts of exogenous glucocorticoids, these glucocorticoids feed back on the hypothalamus and pituitary, suppressing ACTH production. If this suppression is continued, the pituitary may become permanently unable to respond to stress or may respond in an inadequate manner.

The second influence on plasma cortisol levels is the diurnal pattern. Evidence has indicated that there is a circadian pattern of ACTH release, with a major increase in secretion occurring between 4 and 8 A.M. in subjects with a normal sleep-wake schedule (Krieger, 1971) and with the lowest ACTH concentrations from 9 P.M. to the early morning (Fig. 14–17). Sudden changes in the sleep-wake

patterns have little effect on the diurnal pattern, but permanent changes in daily sleeping habits will result in the gradual change in diurnal pattern. Superimposed on the circadian periodicity is an ultradien rhythm of 5 to 10 secretory bursts. The level of plasma cortisol gradually falls from its highest concentration (up to 25 μg/dl) in the early morning to a 9 P.M. level that is about one half of the 8 A.M. level. The level of cortisol from 9 P.M. to about 4 A.M. is relatively constant. Although cortisol generally follows ACTH, it cannot be assumed that plasma cortisol concentration exactly mirrors that of the ACTH. Krieger (1977) points out that corti-

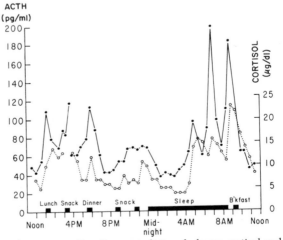

Figure 14–17. Circadian periodicity of plasma cortisol and plasma ACTH levels over a 24 hour period as determined by half-hourly sampling. ACTH and cortisol are lowest at about 4 a.m. and rise to highest level when awakening. Solid line indicates ACTH; dotted line indicates cortisol. (Modified from Krieger, D. T., Allen, W., Rizzo, F., and Krieger, H. P.: Characterization of the normal temporal pattern of plasma corticosteroid levels. J. Clin. Endocrinol. Metabol., 32:266, 1971.)

sol levels do not necessarily reflect ACTH levels because of episodic secretion of ACTH and the lag of cortisol secretion, differences in half-lives (the half-life of ACTH is exceedingly short, i.e., about 5 minutes; for cortisol, about 65 minutes) and an occasional ACTH surge may not result in a rise of cortisol.

The third important influence on cortisol secretion is stress. Stimuli such as surgical trauma, pyrogens, hypoglycemia, and hemorrhage are capable of bringing about an acute increase in ACTH and cortisol secretion. Response to stress may be absent or decreased in magnitude in patients in whom large doses of steroids have been administered for some time. The initiation of any stressful response also is dependent on an intact nervous system. For example, trauma results in the acute release of ACTH and cortisol; however, in patients with spinal cord transections, the same trauma applied to an extremity will not elicit any ACTH or cortisol response. There is evidence that the stress-response of cortisol is mediated through excitatory and inhibitory inputs which become integrated at the level of the hypothalamus and modulate corticotropin releasing factor (CRF).

HYPERCORTISOLISM: CUSHING'S SYNDROME

Cushing's syndrome is a clinical and metabolic entity characterized by adrenal cortical hyperfunction; it is associated with excessive production of glucocorticoids, or glucocorticoids and androgens. The lesion responsible for excessive adrenal cortical secretion may reside in the adrenal, the pituitary, or the hypothalamus, or the glucocorticoids may be produced in response to an ectopic tumor. Most frequently, the lesion appears to be hypothalamic in origin. Since the therapeutic modality employed and prognosis differ depending on the location of the lesion, it is important that a specific diagnosis be reached. Adrenal adenomas and carcinomas account for about 25 per cent of the cases of Cushing's syndrome, adrenal hyperplasia about 60 per cent, and pituitary adenomas about 10 per cent. Although many patients with ectopic ACTH producing tumors may have elevated ACTH and glucocorticoids, this remains a rare cause of the clinical presentation of Cushing's syndrome. Because of the rapid growth of these tumors, the patient's demise may occur before the clinical signs of the syndrome become evident. The most common tumors associated with ectopic ACTH production include lung, thymic, and pancreatic carcinomas (see p. 466).

Hallmarks of Cushing's syndrome are (1) excessive production of cortisol measured as elevated serum cortisol; increased urinary free cortisol, or cortisol metabolites; (2) loss of normal circadian rhythm of ACTH and cortisol; (3) loss of suppression of the adrenal production of cortisol by the administration of a synthetic glucocorticoid, dexamethasone, in a dosage of 2 mg per day; this dose is equivalent to about twice the normal maximum secretory rate of cortisol. Of the findings that suggest Cushing's syndrome, the most common are obesity, hypertension, and diabetes mellitus. To differentiate those patients with Cushing's syndrome from normal patients or those with obesity and hypertension may be extremely difficult.

Before diagnosis of Cushing's syndrome can be substantiated, a group of suppressive or stimulatory testing procedures is necessary. Suppressive testing usually involves oral administration of dexamethasone, a steroid that has about 25 times more glucocorticoid potency than cortisol. It is administered in small quantities to suppress ACTH but provoke little interference with glucocorticoid measurements by any of the commonly used methods. Suppressive testing procedures are divided into two groups: those in which only a serum cortisol reponse to a single dose of dexamethasone is quantitated and those in which serum cortisol and a 24-hour urine are collected and the response of the glucocorticoids is evaluated. Because of difficulty in collection of a complete 24-hour urine and in administration of dexamethasone on a regularly scheduled basis, those groups of tests which involve urine collection are usually reserved for hospitalized patients. In contrast, a suppressive test using serum specimens alone lends itself to outpatient testing. The response of serum and urine determinations to suppressive maneuvers is shown in Tables 14-12 and 14-13).

Although urinary 17-hydroxycorticosteroids may be elevated in obesity, urinary free cortisol and serum cortisol are normal and suppress in response to overnight dexamethasone (vide infra). This response and normal circadian variation of plasma cortisol make it possible to differentiate obese normals from patients with Cushing's syndrome.

A simple screening test is the overnight dexamethasone suppression test; it is especially valuable for differentiating those patients with normal pituitary-adrenal axis from those with Cushing's syndrome. One mg of dexamethasone is ingested by the patient at 11 P.M., and at 8 A.M., a serum cortisol level is obtained. Normally, a serum cortisol of less than 5 μg/dl (138 nmol/l) is observed, but in patients with Cushing's syndrome there rarely is suppression to less than 10 μg/dl (276 nmol/l) (Melby, 1971). Psychiatric disease and stress can cause non-suppressibility in patients without Cushing's syndrome. Since

Table 14–13.   URINARY CORTICOSTEROID RESPONSES TO DIAGNOSTIC MANEUVERS DESIGNED TO DEMONSTRATE NON-AUTONOMY OR AUTONOMY OF ADRENAL FUNCTION*

| | URINARY 17-HYDROXYCORTICOSTEROIDS | | | | URINARY 17-KETOSTEROIDS |
| | | Suppression with Dexamethasone | | ACTH Stimulation | Basal |
CONDITION	Basal	2 mg	8 mg		
Normal	3–10 mg/24 hr	<3 mg/24 hr	<50% initial value	2-to-3-fold baseline increase	Female: 5–15 mg/24 hr Male: 8–20 mg/24 hr
Adrenal hyperplasia	Increased	Not suppressed	<50% initial value, occasional "para-doxical response"	Hyper-responsive	Normal or increased
Adrenal adenoma	Increase	Not suppressed	Not suppressed	None or normal response	Decreased or normal
Adrenal carcinoma	Markedly increased	Not suppressed	Not suppressed (rare exceptions)	No response (rare exceptions)	Markedly increased
Pituitary tumor	Markedly increased	Not suppressed	Not suppressed	No to slight response	Increased
Ectopic ACTH syndrome	Markedly increased	Not suppressed	Usually not suppressed	Usually no response	Increased

*Modified from Krieger, 1976.

phenytoin (diphenylhydantoin) causes increased metabolism of dexamethasone, a high 8 A.M. cortisol level may be found in normal patients taking this drug. Drugs such as estrogens cause increased transcortin (serum transport protein for cortisol); this results in a higher than normal 8 A.M. cortisol level. Although this test is relatively easy to perform, perhaps 10 per cent of "normal" patients fail to exhibit adequate suppression. At least one patient has been described with Cushing's syndrome who suppressed using this test (Meikle, 1975).

"Low dose" dexamethasone is utilized to differentiate normal patients from those with Cushing's syndrome. For two days, 0.5 mg of dexamethasone is given orally every six hours and the response of urinary 17-hydroxycorticosteroids (or urinary free cortisol) is measured. On the second day of dexamethasone, a reference group of patients will suppress their urinary 17-hydroxycorticosteroids to less than 3 mg/24 hours (urinary free cortisol to less than 20 μg (552 nmol) per 24 hours), while patients with Cushing's syndrome fail to suppress to this level. However, since the introduction of this procedure, a number of patients with Cushing's syndrome have been described whose response is within normal limits.

"High dose" dexamethasone suppression test (2 mg given orally every six hours for two days) is used to differentiate patients with adrenal hyperplasia from those with adrenal adenomas, carcinomas, pituitary tumors, or ectopic ACTH syndrome. A reference population and those with adrenal hyperplasia will show urinary 17-hydroxycorticosteroid levels which are less than 50 per cent of the initial value (urinary free cortisol is less than 20 per cent of baseline value). However, occasionally a "paradoxical" response of non-suppression will occur in patients with adrenal hyperplasia. Most patients with adrenal adenomas, carcinoma, pituitary tumors, or ectopic ACTH syndromes will not show this suppression. Patients with adrenal carcinoma usually have elevated 17-ketosteroids and signs of virilization; those with adrenal adenomas present without these findings. Pituitary and ectopic tumors can be identified by appropriate radiographic procedures. The laboratory findings are summarized in Tables 14-12 and 14-13.

Vasopressin (ADH) has been found to release ACTH, probably because its structure is so similar to CRF (Saffran, 1977). This CRF-like material has been of value in the diagnosis of adrenal and pituitary disease. A normal response following the administration of 10 units of ADH (Pitressin) intramuscularly is a doubling of ACTH levels and an increase in serum cortisol of 15 μg/dl (414 nmol/l) over baseline values. In instances where there is an adrenal carcinoma, adenoma, or pituitary tumor, the high circulating levels of cortisol from this autonomously secreting lesion suppress the intact pituitary-adrenal axis so that a normal response is not seen. Another aid to the localization of the lesion responsible for Cushing's syndrome is the cortisol response to stimulatory testing. Those patients whose Cushing's syndrome occurs from adrenal hyperplasia will have an increased response of serum cortisol to Pitressin and Cortrosyn, a synthetic ACTH analog, while patients with other forms of the syndrome have little or no response to these stimuli (Table 14-12).

Two modifications of the dexamethasone suppression test by Streeten (1969) have resulted in improved accuracy in the diagnosis of Cushing's syndrome. When the dose of dexamethasone is administered in terms of body weight (i.e., 5 µg/kg/6 hr for the low dose) and the excretion of 17-OH corticosteroids is expressed in mg/g creatinine, better discrimination between Cushing's syndrome and a reference population is observed (Streeten, 1976).

Plasma ACTH levels are markedly elevated in hypercortisolism of hypothalamic, pituitary, or ectopic origin and suppressed in patients with adrenal tumors.

HYPOCORTISOLISM: ADDISON'S DISEASE AND PITUITARY INSUFFICIENCY

Primary adrenal cortical insufficiency (Addison's disease), which usually occurs from an autoimmune process (Chap. 38), tuberculosis, and other granulomatous diseases, or is idiopathic, can be demonstrated by the failure of the adrenal to respond to ACTH. When hypocortisolism results from a pituitary lesion, it is termed *secondary adrenal insufficiency*.

The most convenient procedure for studying patients suspected of having Addison's disease is the injection of a commercially available ACTH analogue, Cortrosyn. This peptide is the biologically active amino terminal end of the ACTH molecule which contains amino acids 1-24. Serum specimens for cortisol determination are drawn as a baseline and 30 and 60 minutes after Cortrosyn injection. A normal response is a doubling of the plasma cortisol, but a more stringent criterion such as a baseline of 5 µg/dl (138 nmol/l), with an increase of at least 7 µg/dl (195 nmol/l) at 30 minutes, and 11µg/dl (304 nmol/l) at 60 minutes or the 30 minute level exceeding 18 µg/dl (Dluhy, 1976) has been applied. This procedure assumes that the adrenal rather than the pituitary is the source of the insufficiency, and normal response serves to rule out primary adrenal insufficiency.

Other stimulatory testing involves infusion of ACTH or its analogues for two to five days, with the response of 17-hydroxysteroids (or urinary free cortisol) measured. Patients with either primary or secondary adrenal insufficiency may present with low serum cortisol and not respond to Cortrosyn. Exposure of the adrenal to ACTH over an extended period of time is essential not only in making the diagnosis of adrenal insufficiency, but also in localizing the insufficiency as primary or secondary. An intravenous infusion of ACTH for two days, as proposed by Rose (1970), appears to be the most advantageous in this regard. In this procedure a normal adrenal cortical response is shown by an elevation of urinary 17-hydroxycorticoids from three to five times the baseline value, whereas patients with primary adrenal insufficiency have extremely low baseline values which fail to exhibit this degree of stimulation. Patients with secondary adrenal cortical insufficiency (hypopituitarism) or patients receiving suppressive doses of steroids for any protracted period of time usually have an inadequate or absent response in urinary 17-hydroxycorticosteroids the first day of testing and a slight response to about 10 mg/24 hours on the second day. The diagnosis of pituitary insufficiency is more easily made by the insulin tolerance test. This is described in the section on the pituitary on page 408. It should be noted that the ACTH infusion test can be performed on patients presenting with signs of acute adrenal insufficiency, a medical emergency. If this diagnosis is suspected, a baseline cortisol and ACTH should be obtained and a stimulation test performed over two days, with dexamethasone used to provide the patient with an immediate source of glucocorticoids.

Metyrapone has been utilized to indicate pituitary reserve. For the performance of this test, metyrapone is given orally in divided doses over two days and the urinary excretion of glucocorticoids is measured. Since metyrapone is an inhibitor of the 11-hydroxylase enzyme, it blocks the formation of cortisol from 11-deoxycortisol. With the administration of this compound, cortisol levels fall, resulting in an increase in ACTH secretion. If metyrapone is continued for a period of time, the blockade is overcome and glucocorticoids rise. Patients with reduced pituitary reserve, such as those with pituitary tumors, are unable to increase the ACTH secretion to maintain the cortisol levels. If glucocorticoids are not provided during testing in those with decreased pituitary reserve, acute adrenal insufficiency may be precipitated. This provocative test also has gained disfavor because the length of time required to perform it is three days and a more rapid evaluation of pituitary reserve by insulin tolerance testing is available. Metyrapone, however, can be used as a single dose in an overnight procedure (Spiger, 1975). A dose of 30 mg/kg body weight is given at bedtime; plasma 11-desoxycortisol and ACTH are measured the following morning. In a reference population 11-desoxycortisol increases to greater than 7 μg/dl and ACTH to greater than 100 pg/ml, while those patients with secondary adrenal insufficiency are unable to respond as well (West, 1977).

As the use of steroids for the treatment of many malignant and immunologic disorders increases, iatrogenic adrenal insufficiency is becoming more common. The use of glucocorticoids for the treatment of systemic diseases results in adrenal suppression of variable duration after withdrawal of steroids. The degree of adrenal suppression is dependent upon the specific glucocorticoid dose, as well as the duration, frequency, and route of administration. A protocol has been derived by Byyny (1976) for tapering steroids and testing for adrenal insufficiency; at various intervals the morning exogenous hydrocortisone is omitted and the 8 A.M. serum cortisol is measured. If it is above 10 μg/dl (276 nmol/l), routine supplementation of steroids can be ended. Since the adrenal cortex lags behind the pituitary in recovery for steroid suppression, recovery can be assessed to be complete when an 8 A.M. Cortrosyn infusion results in an appropriate serum cortisol increase.

CONGENITAL ENZYME DISORDERS OF THE ADRENAL

Six different metabolic defects in the synthesis of cortisol and aldosterone have been described; each is recognized by a deficiency of a specific adrenal enzyme. These enzymatic deficiencies are all inherited as autosomal recessive traits with a variable degree of penetrance. Depending on the severity and location of the enzymatic defect, deficiencies of glucocorticoids, mineralocorticoids, or sex hormones occur, resulting in shock, salt wasting, or anomalous sexual development. Other findings such as hypertension, which occurs from the accumulation of mineralocorticoids, or virilization, which occurs from the shunting of metabolism toward the sex hormone pathway, are clinically useful in differentiating the various enzyme deficiencies. Since the normal

integrity of the pituitary-adrenal axis is interrupted in these syndromes and cortisol is formed in decreased amounts, there is a compensatory increase in ACTH, the magnitude of which may be sufficient to avoid adrenal insufficiency. This occurs only at the expense of continued hypersecretion of precursors and is responsible for the development of hyperplastic adrenal glands. These syndromes are summarized in Table 14-14.

The *21-hydroxylase* deficiency is the most common, occurring in about 90 per cent of the cases and involving the enzyme which converts 17-α-hydroxyprogesterone (17-OH progesterone) to 11-deoxycortisol. If the deficiency is mild, as is commonly seen, patients may have normal or increased aldosterone secretion and conserve sodium normally. An affected female may have a mild defect at birth, which does not manifest itself until early childhood or adolescence. This diagnosis can be confirmed by demonstrating elevated levels of 17-ketosteroids or pregnantriol in the urine, or elevated levels of 17-hydroxyprogesterone in the serum. Normally serum 17-α-hydroxyprogesterone is less than 100 ng/dl, but in affected patients it may be greater than 1000 ng/dl. The severe form of the 21-hydroxylase deficiency results in impairment of cortisol and aldosterone secretion, and patients may manifest salt wasting and adrenal collapse in the first few weeks of life. Females have ambiguous genitalia, while males may appear normal. The diagnosis is made by finding elevated 17-ketosteroids in the urine (greater than 5 mg/24 hours in the first two weeks of life) and an elevated plasma 17-hydroxyprogesterone level. Early in life, the plasma 17-hydroxyprogesterone may be the only abnormality (Youssefnejadian, 1975). Identification of heterozygotes by measuring plasma 17-OH progesterone following Cortrosyn infusion has been only mildly successful (Krensky, 1977; Gutai, 1977). With replacement, Hughes (1978) has found that when 17-OH progesterone levels were less than 200 ng/dl, normal adrenal secretion of the sex hormones occurred.

The *11-hydroxylase* deficiency is probably the second most common defect and results in hypertension from increased deoxycorticosterone (DOC) and 11-deoxycortisol levels. Virilization occurs as well. The finding of elevated 11-deoxycortisol concentrations in the plasma and urine is diagnostic.

The *3-beta-ol-dehydrogenase* defect is involved in the conversion of the delta-5-steroids

Table 14-14. CLINICAL AND BIOCHEMICAL FEATURES

ENZYME DEFICIENT	ADRENAL HYPERPLASIA	VIRILIZATION	ADRENOCORTICAL INSUFFICIENCY (salt losers)	HYPERTEN-SION	ANOMALOUS SEXUAL DEVELOPMENT	ALDOSTERONE PRODUCTION	LABORATORY FINDINGS
1. 21-Hydroxy-lase	Present	Present	Present in less than one third	Absent	Female virilized	Deficient (salt losers)	Greatly increased urinary pregnanetriol and 17-ketosteroids; increased plasma 17-OH progesterone
2. 11-Hydroxy-lase	Present	Present	Absent	Present in majority	Female virilized	Normal	Increased plasma 11-desoxycortisol
3. 20,22-Desmo-lase	Present	Absent	Present	Absent	Lack of masculinization	Deficient	All urine and plasma steroids decreased
4. 3-Beta-hydrox-ysteroid de-hydrogenase	Present	Slight (in female)	Present	Absent	Female normal or slight virilization	Deficient	Increased dehydroepiandrosterone; increased 17-ketosteroids
5. 17-Hydroxy-lase	Present	Absent	Absent	Present	Absent secondary sex characteristics	Deficient	Metabolites of corticosterone and 11-desoxycorticosterone increased
6. 18-Hydroxy-lase and 18-hydroxyster-oid dehy-drogenase	Absent	Absent	Present	Absent	Normal	Absent	Metabolites of corticosterone and 11-desoxycorticosterone increased; 17-hydroxycorticosteroids increased in 18-dehydrogenase defect

to delta-4-steroids. It is extremely rare and invariably results in neonatal death. Males are born without complete masculinization and females with clitoromegaly. These patients have adrenal insufficiency in the neonatal period. The diagnosis is confirmed by the finding of elevated 17-ketosteroids and dehydroepiandrosterone values in the urine.

The *17-hydroxylase* enzyme is not required for mineralocorticoid synthesis; hence, patients with this defect have an intact mineralocorticoid axis. However, they cannot convert delta-5-pregnenolone or progesterone to their 17-hydroxy derivatives. Consequently, affected individuals present with hypertension and exceedingly high DOC levels plus hypokalemic alkalosis. Lack of sex hormone synthesis results in the absence of secondary sexual characteristics in the female and incomplete masculinization in the male.

Desmolase deficiency also is rare and involves the inability to convert cholesterol to delta-5-pregnenolone in the adrenal and testes. Consequently, affected males will present with complete lack of masculinization and marked adrenal insufficiency. The absence of steroids in the urine and plasma of a male with incomplete masculinization suggests this diagnosis.

Deficiency of *18-hydroxysteroid dehydrogenase and hydroxylase* results in the impaired production of aldosterone, but there is neither virilization nor adrenal hyperplasia. However, these patients are salt losers, and metabolites of corticosterone and 11-deoxycorticosterone are found in the urine.

LABORATORY MEASUREMENTS OF GLUCOCORTICOID FUNCTION

ACTH

Although the first peptide hormone to be measured by radioimmunoassay was ACTH (Yalow, 1964), widespread popularity and utility of ACTH measurements in clinical medicine has not yet occurred. Although ACTH by radioimmunoassay has been found to be diagnostically useful, technical and practical limitations as well as expense involved have restricted its use. The instability of ACTH in plasma probably has been the greatest limitation of its use. ACTH appears to be rapidly deactivated by proteolytic enzymes in plasma, and even the addition of the usual proteolytic enzyme inhibitor (Trasylol) has lit-

tle effect on its preservation. An inhibitor of SH-peptidases, N-ethyl maleimide (NEM), has been utilized in Great Britain. It has been reported to inhibit degradation of plasma ACTH for up to 72 hours (Jubiz, 1978). Although no current method completely arrests the destruction of ACTH, a temperature of 4°C. greatly reduces its enzymatic degradation. Thus, it is recommended that blood specimens for ACTH be collected in plastic syringes, transferred to plastic tubes, and transported on ice to the laboratory where plasma should be rapidly separated from the blood cells at 4°C. (Rees, 1976). Timing of specimen collection is important because of the circadian variation in ACTH. If plasma cannot be analyzed immediately, it should be stored at −20°C. or colder. Other problems associated with the measurement of ACTH are adsorption to glass, incubation damage during the assay, and poor sensitivity and precision of the assay at low concentrations.

West (1977) has presented evidence that ACTH levels are useful in differentiating primary from secondary adrenal insufficiency. Primary adrenal insufficiency results in low cortisol concentrations; because of the negative feedback mechanisms and an intact functioning pituitary, high ACTH levels are expected. In secondary adrenal insufficiency (pituitary insufficiency), normal to low ACTH levels are the rule. Although in the past stimulatory tests such as Cortrosyn and ACTH infusions have been utilized, a single ACTH level will distinguish between primary and secondary adrenal insufficiency. In the primary disorder, ACTH levels are usually found to be greater than 200 pg/ml, while in pituitary insufficiency ACTH concentrations are usually less than 75 pg/ml. Best discrimination of normal individuals from those with adrenal insufficiency can be obtained if the specimens for ACTH are collected between 8 and 10 A.M.

Undoubtedly ACTH concentrations may be of greatest value in establishing the differential diagnosis of patients with Cushing's syndrome. The majority of patients with ectopic ACTH production have oat cell carcinoma of the lung, and although this diagnosis may be obvious, ACTH measurements can be helpful when tissue confirmation is not available. Occasionally neoplasms may be occult and because of diagnostic difficulties, ACTH measurements on blood specimens obtained by selective catheterization of the venous system may be useful in localization or identification of the lesion (Rees, 1977). Those patients with ectopic ACTH secreting tumors characteristically have an elevated plasma ACTH (usually greater than 200 pg/ml) and an elevated serum cortisol.

In patients with increased levels of circulating glucocorticoids due to adrenal adenomas or carcinomas, ACTH secretion is inhibited; hence, circulating ACTH levels are low or undetectable. In patients with adrenal hyperplasia, plasma ACTH may be at or above the upper limit at 9 A.M., but fail to show the expected fall near midnight. It should be emphasized that in patients with suspected Cushing's syndrome, the best discrimination from a reference population is obtained if the blood specimen for ACTH is drawn between 9 and 12 P.M. (midnight).

Another use of ACTH assays is the determination of the adequacy of cortisol replacement in the congenital adrenal hyperplasia syndromes. When replacement therapy is optimal in these patients, ACTH values should be similar to those seen in a reference population.

Serum cortisol

About 90 per cent of the cortisol circulates bound to serum protein, while the remainder is unbound or free. It is estimated that 10 to 20 per cent is loosely attached to albumin, while the remainder is bound to the glycoprotein transcortin (cortisol binding globulin), an alpha-1-globulin. It is believed that only free cortisol is active and that the protein bound fraction is metabolically inert. The protein bound fraction probably serves as a reservoir of free cortisol. Protein binding also may protect cortisol from deactivation by the liver or filtration by the kidney.

One of the earliest and simplest methods to determine serum cortisol is the method of Mattingly (1962). Cortisol simply is extracted from the serum with dichloromethane and after the addition of an ethanol–sulfuric acid mixture, the fluorescence is measured. Corticosterone is the most important interference (about 4 μg/dl), while other adrenal steroids such as dihydroepiandrosterone, testosterone, and 11-desoxycortisol contribute about 2 μg/dl (Scriba, 1976). Spironolactone, tetracycline, and birth control pills containing estrogen lead to spuriously high cortisol levels by this method.

Cortisol can be determined by competitive protein binding (CPB) (Murphy, 1967). Although there have been many modifications, this technique still lacks specificity. Competitive protein binding (CPB) assays make use of transcortin, the naturally occurring cortisol binding protein. The specificity of the method depends on the binding specificity of transcortin; cortisone and 11-desoxycortisol, for example, compete equally well. Progesterone, which is present in increased amounts in pregnancy, also competes with cortisol for transcortin. The CPB method has a major advantage in that 11-deoxycortisol can be extracted with carbon tetrachloride and subsequently measured in the assay. The competitive protein binding technique gives results which are about 25 per cent lower than those of the Porter-Silber reaction (vide infra) and 25 to 50 per cent lower than the fluorometric procedure.

The most specific method for cortisol estimation is radioimmunoassay. Other advantages of RIA include small specimen volume and rapid turnaround time. Some of the antibodies used show a large amount of cross-reactivity with steroids such as 11-deoxycortisol, desoxycorticosterone, and some synthetic steroids such as dexamethasone. Although the cross-reactivity does not pose a problem with baseline testing, in stimulatory and suppressive maneuvers such as metyrapone or dexamethasone suppression this can lead to spuriously high values. The major disadvantage of cortisol assays continues to be lack of specificity; however, the specificity of the radioimmunoassay is better than that of either the fluorometric or the CPB method.

Reference values for serum cortisol are in the range of 5 to 25 μg/dl (138 to 690 nmol/l) at 8 to 10 A.M. and by 8 P.M. are about 2 to 12 μg/dl (55 to 331 nmol/l).

Estimation of glucocorticoids in urine

One of the first procedures for the estimation of glucocorticoids in urine was the method described by Porter (1950). Phenylhydrazine and sulfuric acid are added to urine; those steroids which contain 21 carbons and have a characteristic dihydroxyacetone side chain produced a color with a peak absorption at 410 nm (Porter-Silber chromogens). Since most of the glucocorticoids are excreted in the urine as conjugates, hydrolysis with a glucuronidase is performed prior to the measurement. The principal glucocorticoids which

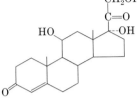

CH$_2$OH
C=O
--OH

11-DESOXYCORTISOL

CH$_2$OH
C=O
HO --OH

CORTISOL

CH$_2$OH
C=O
O --OH

CORTISONE

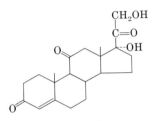

CH$_2$OH
CO
HO --OH

HO   H

TETRAHYDROCORTISOL

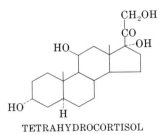

CH$_2$OH
CO
O --OH

HO   H

TETRAHYDROCORTISONE

Figure 14–18. Principal glucocorticoids which have a dihydroxyacetone side chain (Porter-Silber chromagens).

are measured are 11-deoxycortisol, cortisol, and cortisone (a metabolite of cortisol) (Fig. 14–18). Other metabolites of cortisol and cortisone, such as the tetrahydro derivatives (saturated A ring), also are measured. Although

this method has been used to measure 17-OH corticosteroids in urine, in certain pathologic states it does not measure all the 17-OH corticosteroids which are excreted. For example, such compounds as pregnanetriol (a metabolite of 17-OH progesterone) and certain 20-OH compounds may be strikingly increased, but are not measured by this technique. Reference intervals for urine measurements are 5 to 15 mg/24 hours for males and 5 to 13 mg/24 hours for females. The Porter-Silber methodology usually is not used for the glucocorticoid estimations in serum because of its lack of specificity and the need for a prior extraction step.

Urinary free cortisol

Only 1 per cent of the total adrenal secretion appears in the urine as cortisol, but it is this fraction which provides a valuable aid in diagnosis of adrenal disease. In the kidney, the glomerular filtration of free cortisol is followed by passive tubular reabsorption without a demonstrable reabsorption maximum (see p. 137).

At serum cortisol levels of about 20 to 25 μg/dl (552 to 690 nmol/l) (the A.M. upper normal reference values), the binding capacity of transcortin is exceeded; this leads to a very rapid and disproportionate increase in the unbound fraction compared to the total serum cortisol. For example, a doubling of the cortisol from 20 to 40 μg/dl (552 to 1104 nmol/l) results in at least a fivefold increase in the unbound cortisol in serum. At these levels, free cortisol clearance by the kidneys is directly proportional to the unbound serum cortisol concentration and leads to a steep rise in cortisol clearance. Thus, when urinary free cortisol excretion rather than serum cortisol is used, it is easier to discriminate between patients with adrenal hyperfunction and a reference population.

Urinary free cortisol levels are unaffected by alterations of hepatic metabolism of cortisol. Hepatic metabolism of cortisol is increased in obese individuals. Although total cortisol production and urinary 17-hydroxy corticosteroids are increased, the serum cortisol and the urinary free cortisol remain normal. In pregnancy and estrogen therapy, as a result of the increased serum concentration of transcortin, serum cortisol is increased. This increase is not reflected by an elevation of cortisol metabolites in the urine, but urinary free cortisol may be increased. Since the renal clearance of cortisol is dependent on normal kidney function, it is not surprising that patients with renal disease may have low values (Sederberg-Olsen, 1975). Conditions in which spuriously elevated values occur include starvation (Galvao-Teles, 1976), application of topical steroids (Cave, 1973), and perhaps hydration in the form of water loading (Baum, 1975).

In Addison's disease, a urinary free cortisol of less than 20 μg/24 hours is suggestive of adrenal hypofunction, but the overlap with the normal range is great. The greatest value of urinary free cortisol determinations, however, is for states of adrenal hyperfunction, such as Cushing's syndrome. In an extensive study, Burke (1973) found that patients with Cushing's syndrome have a urinary free cortisol of greater than 90 μg/24 hours, whereas the urinary free cortisol values of healthy individuals are 20 to 90 μg/24 hours.

The techniques used for urinary free cortisol measurement include competitive protein binding (CPB) and radioimmunoassay. The specificity of the competitive protein technique is limited by the specificity of the transcortin used as the binding protein. The measurement of urinary free cortisol using radioimmunoassay is the most specific procedure for the estimation of cortisol in the urine.

However, specificity is dependent upon the antibody used. Following extraction, the radioimmunoassay is performed as in the serum specimens. Reference intervals, which are similar to those of urinary free cortisol by CPB, are 20 to 90 μg/24 hours.

THE RENIN-ALDOSTERONE AXIS

Hypertension is a major affliction of modern society, affecting at least 10 to 15 per cent of the adult population of the industrialized nations of the world (National Center for Health Statistics, 1966). At least 20 million people in the United States have hypertension, with 90 to 98 per cent of the cases classified as essential hypertension. Because of the mortality and morbidity from associated myocardial and cerebrovascular complications, the necessity of treating this disorder has become obvious (Veterans Administration Cooperative Study, 1970). Investigation of the etiology of hypertension has indicated the importance of the renin-angiotensin-aldosterone system, not only in the origin and maintenance of hypertension but also as a guide to treatment.

Renin is a proteolytic enzyme formed and stored by juxtaglomerular cells of the kidney and released into the lymph and the renal

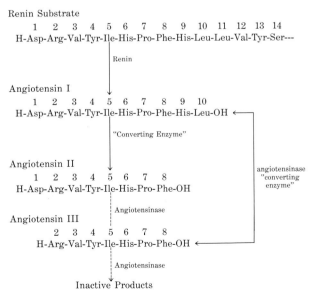

Figure 14–19. The renin-angiotensin system. Angiotensin II is thought to modulate vasoconstriction and is formed from Angiotensin I by "converting enzyme." Angiotensin III is formed from Angiotensin II; however, it can also be formed from the action of an angiotensinase and converting enzyme without being converted to Angiotensin II. (Modified from Oparil, S.: Theoretical approaches to estimation of plasma renin activity: A review and some original observations. Clin. Chem., *22*:583, 1976.)

venous blood. Renin acts with its substrate (renin substrate or angiotensinogen), an α_2 globulin made by the liver, to split off a decapeptide angiotensin-I. Angiotensin-I is converted within the circulation to an octapeptide, angiotensin-II, by an enzyme (converting enzyme) system found mainly in the lung. It is believed that angiotensin-II is the peptide responsible for the physiologic effects on target tissues. Evidence indicates that the octapeptide angiotensin-II is further split to a heptapeptide, angiotensin-III, or angiotensin-I may be changed directly to angiotensin-III without being converted to angiotensin-II. Although the functions of angiotensin-III are speculative, it appears to modulate aldosterone secretion (Bumpus, 1977). The active angiotensins are rapidly cleared by various peptidases (angioteninases) within the circulation and while in transit through the tissues. These relationships are shown in Figure 14–19. Renin is synthesized in a larger form (prorenin or big renin) and converted to its active form. Circulating prorenin has been associated with some renal tumors, (Day, 1974) and has been found to increase in parallel with renin in patients undergoing various diagnostic and therapeutic maneuvers (Atlas, 1977).

Regulation of renin secretion

The renin-angiotensin-aldosterone system regulates sodium and potassium balance, fluid volume, and blood pressure, as seen in Figure 14–20. Aldosterone stimulates sodium conservation and potassium wasting.

Renin, through its product, angiotensin-II, directly stimulates the synthesis and secretion of aldosterone by the adrenal zona glomerulosa. Renin release is dependent on changes in "effective" plasma volume, which in turn is dependent on tubular reabsorption of serum sodium by the kidney. Low plasma volume and low serum sodium stimulate the secretion of renin, resulting in aldosterone release which causes sodium retention with an increase in plasma volume, and elevated blood pressure and potassium loss. Conversely, increased "effective" blood volume or acute elevation in blood pressure results in low renin, low angiotensin-II, low aldosterone, and subsequent sodium loss. Potassium loss suppresses aldosterone secretion and stimulates renin release, while elevated potassium has the opposite effect. Although a number of studies have demonstrated that ACTH stimulates aldosterone secretion, it has been found to be less important than potassium and the renin-angiotensin system in the control of aldosterone production.

RENIN-ALDOSTERONE PROFILE

The work of Laragh (1972) has indicated that essential hypertension can be classified on the basis of renin measurement as either (1) high renin, (2) low renin, or (3) normal renin. A classification of these groups, based on specific derangements of the renin-angiotensin-aldosterone system, assumes that chronic hypertension is maintained by three

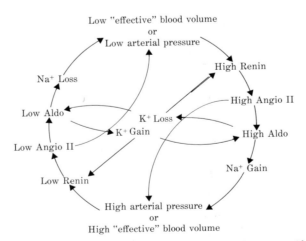

Figure 14–20.   Interaction of renin-angiotensin-aldosterone in maintaining blood pressure. Aldo = aldosterone; Angio II = angiotensin II. (Modified from Laragh, J. H.: Vasoconstriction—volume analysis for understanding and treating hypertension: The use of renin and aldosterone profiles. Am. J. Med., 55:261, 1973.)

dominant patterns: (1) arterial constriction without increased volume (vasoconstriction hypertension); (2) arterial overfilling (volume hypertension); (3) an interaction of both (1) and (2) (volume and vasoconstriction hypertension) (Laragh, 1973). Initial data indicated that based on this classification of essential hypertension, those patients with low renin hypertension had a better prognosis than those with high renin hypertension. While not entirely refuted, most work appears to contradict this initial hypothesis (Kaplan, 1977).

High renin hypertension

Patients with vasoconstriction hypertension exhibit increased plasma renin levels and, when treated with propranolol, respond with a decrease in renin and a reduction in blood pressure. About 15 per cent of patients with essential hypertension have high renin hypertension; this excessive renin, which is secondary to lesions found in the kidney or its vascular supply, ultimately leads to increased aldosterone production and subsequent changes in sodium and potassium excretion. The increased aldosterone (secondary aldosteronism) may contribute significantly to the symptomatology and course of high renin hypertension. Some of the causes of high renin hypertension are listed in Table 14–15.

Renin secreting tumors are an extremely rare finding; markedly elevated plasma renin and hyperaldosteronism with hypokalemia in the absence of a renovascular lesion are almost pathognomonic of this lesion. Malignant hypertension is associated with an elevated plasma renin and plasma aldosterone; when these patients are given antihypertensive therapy, the increased activity of renin usually can be normalized. In unilateral renal disease, both plasma renin and aldosterone are elevated. The most firmly established clinical application of the renin assay occurs in these patients. Asymmetry in the renin levels obtained during renal vein catheterization offers one of the best prognostic measurements to judge the likelihood of the blood pressure response to corrective surgery (Juncos, 1974). It has been established that when the ratio of plasma renin in the renal vein of the affected to non-affected side is at least 1.5 to 1, surgery may lead to improvement. Suppression of renin release from the non-affected side also indicates the likelihood of curative surgery (Brown, 1975). In patients with renovascular hypertension and a ratio of at least 1.5 to 1, almost 40 per cent have a normal peripheral plasma renin (Streeten, 1975). Consequently, in these patients peripheral plasma renin has been judged not to be a useful index of surgical prognosis. Other attempts at using renin values obtained during renal vein catheterization have involved sampling from a segmental lesion and comparing levels obtained with those from areas of the kidney.

Where there is an acceleration of hypertension, renin is usually markedly increased. With chronic renal failure, almost any renin level can be expected. A small number of hypertensive patients on dialysis have intractable, accelerated hypertension. In these patients dialysis cannot control the hypertension, but plasma renin that is markedly elevated is lowered by nephrectomy. In those renal transplant patients with rejection, elevated plasma renin may be indicative of renal ischemia. Systemic hypertension has been found to be present in patients with Cushing's syndrome. In some patients, plasma renin and renin substrate are increased (Krakoff, 1975). In other patients with Cushing's syndrome and hypokalemia, it has been found that the secretion of a minor mineralocorticoid such as DOC or corticosterone is responsible for the hypertension. A suppressed plasma renin in a patient with Cushing's syndrome is presumptive evidence that a mineralocorticoid is present in excess. Other causes of a high renin hypertension include treatment with medications such as diuretics, vasodilators, or antihypertensives. Hormonal agents such as glucocorticoids

Table 14–15. SYNDROME OF HYPERTENSION ASSOCIATED WITH HIGH LEVELS OF PLASMA RENIN

A. Renin secreting tumor
B. Malignant/accelerated hypertension
C. Renovascular hypertension
  1. Major arterial lesions
  2. Segmental lesions
  3. Other types of possibly renin-dependent hypertension
D. Chronic renal failure
  1. Parenchymal
  2. Accelerated phase, end stage
  3. Transplant rejection
E. Cushing's syndrome
F. Iatrogenic
  1. Volume depleting agents
  2. Vasodilating agents
  3. Glucocorticoids
  4. Estrogens

as well as some estrogen-containing oral contraceptives have been found to increase renin substrate activity.

Normal renin hypertension

Although plasma renin, aldosterone, and urinary sodium excretion may be normal in 60 per cent of hypertension patients, evidence has accumulated which indicates that the renin-angiotensin system plays a significant part in normal renin hypertension. The use of saralasin, the angiotensin-II antagonist (Streeten, 1975b), and a converting enzyme inhibitor (Garvas, 1974) have implicated an absolute or relative excess of renin and angiotensin-II as being involved at least in part in sustaining the hypertension in those patients with normal plasma renin.

Low renin hypertension

It was found that low renin essential hypertension, which involves chronic expansion of plasma and extracellular fluid volume, is characterized by aldosterone oversecretion and responds to diuretic therapy. At least 25 per cent of patients with essential hypertension are found to have "low renin hypertension." Most investigators have characterized this state as "hyporesponsive," meaning low renin hypertension patients fail to stimulate as vigorously as normals with upright posture, sodium restriction, diuretics, vasodilators, or a combination of these. It has been found that renin suppression increases with age, appears to be more common in women, and is more frequently found in older black people.

Listed in Table 14–16 is a group of syndromes associated with low levels of plasma renin. These have been divided into a group

Table 14–16. SYNDROME OF HYPERTENSION ASSOCIATED WITH LOW LEVELS OF PLASMA RENIN*

I. "Primary" excess of mineralocorticoids
   A. Primary aldosteronism
   B. Pseudoprimary aldosteronism
   C. 11-Deoxycorticosterone excess
   D. 18-Hydroxy-11-deoxycorticosterone excess
II. "Secondary" excess of mineralocorticoids
   A. Licorice ingestion
   B. Excess unsupervised sodium intake
   C. Low renin, low aldosterone syndrome
      1. Longstanding essential hypertension
      2. Diabetes mellitus

*Primary aldosteronism.

that is of adrenal origin (primary) and a group that is non-adrenal or "secondary" in origin. Primary aldosteronism is characterized by (1) arterial hypertension caused by an oversecretion of aldosterone by an adrenal adenoma; (2) low renin; (3) potassium wastage; and (4) sodium retention. Removal of the adenoma is curative. Pseudoprimary aldosteronism is bilateral adrenal hyperplasia which microscopically has been described as micronodular. Since removal of micronodules has not been found to be curative, it has been postulated that perhaps there may be some unknown extraadrenal stimulus. Aldosterone is markedly elevated and renin usually suppressed in patients with these lesions. Other causes of renin suppression include excess secretion of mineralocorticoids, 18-hydroxy-11-deoxycorticosterone (18-hydroxy-DOC) (Melby, 1977), and 11-deoxycorticosterone, but the significance of these findings is now in doubt. In addition, suppressed renin may occur in situations such as ingestion of licorice, which has a high content of glycyrrhizic acid, (Conn, 1968); excess, unsupervised sodium intake; and a syndrome of low renin, low aldosterone which is most commonly seen in patients with diabetes mellitus (Perez, 1976) and renal disease (Weidmann, 1973).

Secondary aldosteronism results from nonadrenal disease in which both adrenal glands are stimulated, producing increased aldosterone secretion. Typically, these patients are not hypertensive. Such conditions as nephrosis, cirrhosis, and heart failure are the usual causes. In all these, renin and aldosterone are increased. Especially noteworthy is Bartter's syndrome with decreased growth, normal or low blood pressure, hyponatremia, hypokalemia, and increased renin and aldosterone. Etiology of this disorder remains obscure, but the renin system and other vasoactive hormones may play a role (McGiff, 1977). The response of the renin-aldosterone system in pregnancy is especially complex; there appear to be increased renin, renin substrate, angiotensin-II, and aldosterone.

ALDOSTERONE MEASUREMENTS

Since the concentration of aldosterone in plasma is low (1000-fold lower when compared with cortisol), it has been quite difficult to measure. Techniques such as the double isotope dilution have been used to measure urine aldosterone; however, the complexity of the method precluded its use for routine purposes. Some radioimmunoassay methods have been developed which give analytical sensitivity similar to that of the double isotope technique (Drewes, 1972), but these procedures require chromatography. Urine aldosterone assays using ^{125}I are now available without chromatography in the kit form. In a reference population urinary aldosterone usually is 6 to 25 $\mu g/24$ hours.

The cross-reactivity of aldosterone antibody with related steroids depends on the particular antibody employed in the radioimmunoassay. Because some steroids occur in much higher concentrations than aldosterone, even a small percentage of antibody cross-reactivity can lead to a problem with assay specificity. A rapid, direct, sensitive, and highly specific technique for plasma aldosterone using ^{125}I which does not require extraction has been reported (Al-Dujaili, 1978).

Low salt diet (<2 g/day), stress, upright posture, and diuretics will all increase aldosterone, whereas a high salt diet and lying in a supine position suppress aldosterone secretion in a healthy subject. On a high salt diet a person lying in the supine position should have a plasma aldosterone level by RIA of less than 10 ng/dl. Plasma aldosterone values in a reference population in the supine position are 1 to 9 ng/dl (Horton, 1972). After one hour in the upright position aldosterone levels in patients with Addison's disease are less than 5 ng/dl.

Appropriate maneuvers to demonstrate the relative autonomy of the aldosterone secretion are of two types. One approach has been the administration of large amounts of sodium chloride—in one procedure, two liters of isotonic saline infused over a four-hour period. A reference population or those with other types of hypertension will suppress their plasma aldosterone to below 5 ng/dl, while those with primary aldosteronism do not show this degree of suppression (Kem, 1971). An alternative maneuver is the administration of 200 ng of synthetic mineralocorticoid, Florinef, three times a day for three days, and the demonstration of non-suppressibility of plasma aldosterone (Horton, 1973). A reference population suppresses plasma aldosterone to less than 4 ng/dl.

Renin Measurements

There are important technical differences in the determination of renin utilizing current methodology. Renin measurements are of two types: plasma renin activity and plasma renin concentration. In the past bioassays of the precursor activity of angiotensin were used, but now radioimmunoassay of the generated angiotensin-I is commonly employed (Fukuchi, 1973). A plasma specimen containing renin is allowed to react with its substrate; then, after a specified period of time, the reaction is terminated. Then, as in any radioimmunoassay, a small amount of labeled antigen (angiotensin-I) and specific antibody are incubated with plasma: separation of bound and free fractions is then performed by the usual techniques. To insure stability of the angiotensin-I which is generated, angiotensinases are inhibited by prior acid inactivation, chelation, or specific enzyme inhibitors. For the estimation of what has become known as plasma renin activity (PRA), angiotensinase activity in the sample is inhibited but the substrate is not eliminated. Therefore, the rate of generation of angiotensin-I is influenced by both the concentration of endogeneous renin and its substrate. Comparison of results among laboratories is an impossibility because of procedural differences such as variations of pH, ionic strength, the length of the assay, the angiotensinase inhibitor, lack of a specific reference preparation, and the conditions under which the specimen was obtained. In addition, literature on renin assays reveals a hopeless confusion regarding units of measurement employed, and even when an attempt is made to express the many arbitrary units in the same terms (nanograms of angiotensin liberated/ ml/hour) there is a wide range of values reported for normal human plasma renin activity (Mendelson, 1971). A list of some of the reference intervals and assay conditions is reviewed by Oparil (1974). This type of assay is the most widely used method for the determination of renin.

When measuring renin concentration rather than plasma renin activity (PRA), the effect of substrate is eliminated. To accomplish this, the specimen may be treated in a number of ways; for example, the plasma may be incubated at a low pH, denaturing the substrate. The angiotensinases and highly active ovine substrate then are added (Stockigt, 1971). Since the substrate is in excess, angiotensin-I generation occurs linearly with increasing renin concentrations. Under these conditions, angiotensin generation is independent of substrate concentration and proportional to renin concentration (zero order kinetics). An international reference standard has been developed for this method, and plasma renin activity, which is expressed in Goldblatt units/dl (GU/dl) can be compared among different laboratories (Beevers, 1975).

Assays of plasma renin activity and plasma renin concentration provide similar information except in a few clinical situations. With oral contraceptive administration, plasma renin concentration remains normal, while plasma renin activity increases owing to the increase in substrate which occurs. Other procedures such as freezing, thawing, and acidification have been found to convert prorenin to renin and thereby increase values in the plasma renin concentration assays.

The direct measurement of renin substrate, angiotensin-I, or angiotensin-II is not widely utilized in clinical practice, because of tedious extraction or concentration steps as well as difficulty in eliminating the formation or degradation of these compounds by proteases and other enzymes involved in the renin system.

Since renin release is controlled by many physiologic and pharmacologic variables, it is extremely important to know the conditions under which the specimen was obtained. Such conditions as upright posture, the administration of diuretics, or low sodium diets are potent stimuli of renin release and should be adequately controlled prior to the measurement of plasma renin. Renin also appears to be extremely labile so that the variables involved in specimen processing should be vigorously controlled. Blood should be drawn into iced tubes containing chelating agents or enzyme inhibitors to slow converting enzyme angiotensinases, centrifuged in the cold, and the plasma frozen to avoid substantial losses from angiotensinase activity (Oparil, 1976); with this technique, the specimen is stable for several months at $-20°C$.

Plasma renin has been interpreted in individuals relative to a simultaneous 24-hour urine sodium excretion after several days on a stable sodium intake and off diuretics. With normal kidney function, the urinary sodium excretion is related to the extracellular or fluid volume and inversely related to the plasma concentration of renin (Fig. 14–21). From this nomogram it should be possible to distinguish low, normal, and high plasma renin groups.

Because this test is quite cumbersome and involves a 24-hour urine collection, various stimuli for renin release have been used. One

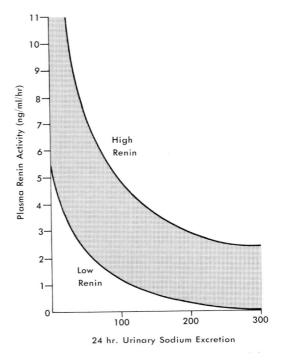

Figure 14–21. Plasma renin activity as a function of the 24 hour urinary sodium excretion. (Modified from Brunner, H. R., Laragh, J. H., Baer, L., Newton, M. A., Goodwin, F. T., Krakoff, L. R., Band, R. H., and Buhler, F. R.: Essential hypertension: Renin and aldosterone, heart attack and stroke. N. Engl. J. Med., *286*:441, 1972.)

of the simplest is the procedure described by Kaplan (1976): plasma renin is determined in fasting subjects after 30 minutes in an upright position following 40 mg of furosemide (Lasix) given intravenously. This test does not require hospitalization, a special diet, or prolonged standing. In this study, a reference population of whites and blacks had plasma renin activities > 1.0 and 0.5 ng/ml/hr respectively, while low renin hypertensive patients were unable to respond as well. This test correlates well with other procedures being used to identify low renin hypertensives.

GONADOTROPINS AND THE SEX HORMONES

LH AND FSH

Evidence has accumulated which suggests that the hypothalamus secretes a single peptide releasing hormone that controls the secretion of the gonadotropins, luteinizing hormone (LH) and follicle stimulating hormone (FSH) from the anterior pituitary (Schally, 1976). This hormone, which is a decapeptide, releases both LH and FSH. It has been called luteinizing releasing hormone (LRH), since LH is released to a greater extent than FSH, but is known also as LH/FSH RH or gonadotropin releasing hormone (GnRH). LRH acts on the pituitary by binding to specific high affinity receptors and activating adenyl cyclase. Rabinowitz (1975) has reported that a single population of pituitary cells secretes both LH and FSH. Both LH and FSH consist of a glycopeptide framework to which carbohydrate side chains are attached.

There appears to be no general agreement as to the molecular weight of the gonadotropin hormones; estimates of the mass range from 32,600 to 52,500 daltons for FSH and 26,000 to 41,700 daltons for LH (Klopper, 1976). These wide ranges may be due to the heterogeneity of these hormones or to separation artifacts which occur during purification.

Structurally LH and FSH are related to the other glycoprotein hormones, thyroid stimulating hormones (TSH), and human chorionic gonadotropin (HCG); they are made up of two non-identical, non-covalently bound, biologically inactive subunits designated alpha and beta. It has been found that alpha and beta subunits can be separated and then recombined to give an active hormone. The alpha subunit is nearly identical for all glycoproteins, but the beta unit is different for each hormone, i.e., this subunit is responsible for hormone specificity. Stimulation with LRH causes the release of large amounts of free alpha chains in addition to LH and FSH hormones. Free α chains are found in excess in the pituitary gonadotrophs, serum, and urine (Prentice, 1975). LH and FSH are secreted from the pituitary and are carried in the blood stream to their site of action, the testes or ovary. Secretion of LH and FSH from the pituitary occurs in a pulsatile manner (Yen, 1972).

The serum values of both gonadotropins are low and relatively non-pulsatile during infancy. During this period, FSH is greater than LH in children of both sexes and the FSH response to LRH is greater than LH. During puberty, both gonadotropins increase, with FSH reaching a plateau during mid-puberty and LH reaching a maximum at the end of puberty. In pubertal children a major increment in plasma LH concentrations first occurs

in an episodic pattern during the nocturnal sleep pattern (Boyar, 1974). In general, these episodes closely follow the onset of non-REM (Rapid Eye Movement) sleep and terminate in relation to REM sleep. As puberty proceeds, daytime secretory episodes also begin to occur so that by the completion of puberty, the sleeping and waking patterns are equivalent.

In the adult male the secretion of LH and to a lesser degree FSH is episodic, with 9 to 14 such secretory surges of LH per 24 hours, corresponding to a 200 to 300 per cent increase over the mean value. FSH also is secreted in a pulsatile manner, but the oscillations are of such low levels that they represent only 25 per cent of the mean.

In adult females, all cycles that are ovulatory have a pattern similar to that seen in Figure 14-22. The female menstrual cycle is divided by a mid-cycle surge of the pituitary gonadotropins into a follicular phase and a luteal phase. There is a single major sharp peak in luteinizing hormone (LH) concentration at about mid-cycle near the time of ovulation. A peak of FSH occurs coincident with the peak of LH but is of lesser magnitude and briefer duration. The gonadotropin levels are generally higher during the preovulatory period than during the luteal phase; however, there is a fall in FSH concentration antecedent to the mid-cycle surge. FSH levels are higher during the first few days that precede ovulation. Following the mid-cycle of LH and FSH, there is a drop in the concentration of both hormones to lower, more irregular levels with occasional "spikes" of LH unaccompanied by "spikes" of FSH. At and after menopause, the gonadotropins continue to be secreted in episodic fashion. FSH levels are higher than those seen during the course of the menstrual cycle, probably because of the lack of inhibition of an ovarian substance similar to inhibin, which is responsible for the feedback suppression of FSH. Evidence suggests that inhibin is a protein produced by the ovary which selectively inhibits FSH secretion (Franchimont, 1977). Serum LH levels after menopause may be similar to or slightly higher than those during the menstrual cycle; this may be a reflection of the persistance of the episodic pattern of release as well as a suppressive effect of estradiol, which is secreted from the adrenal.

In men, at about the sixth decade there is a gradual increase in LH and FSH in response to decreasing testosterone and probably in-

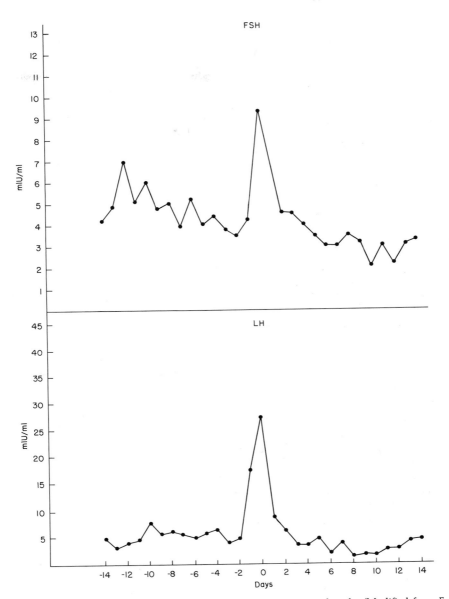

Figure 14–22. Evolution of FSH and LH levels during the course of the menstrual cycle. (Modified from Franchimont, P., Valcke, J. C., and Lambotte, R.: Female gonadal dysfunction. Clin. Endocrinol. Metabol., 3:533, 1974.)

hibin (Rubens, 1974). However, there are great individual variations among individuals older than 50 years.

FSH and LH can be measured by radioimmunoassay. Since the glycoprotein hormones are structurally similar, antibody cross-reactivity may be a problem. In addition, because of the cyclic pattern of gonadotropin release it is possible to obtain an isolated sample at either the peak or the valley of secretion. For these reasons some workers have advocated obtaining at least six specimens for LH over a six-hour period; the specimens may be assayed individually or pooled. However, in those patients in whom gonadotropins are high, such as those with anorchia, testicular failure, or menopause, only one determination may be necessary. Reference values for LH are up to

Table 14–17. BASAL HORMONE LEVELS IN DISORDERS OF THE HYPOTHALAMIC-PITUITARY-GONADAL AXIS IN MALES*

DIAGNOSIS	LH	FSH	TESTOS-TERONE	ESTRA-DIOL
Hypothalamus and pituitary				
Hypopituitarism	↓ or N	↓ or N	↓ or N	↓ or N
Kallmann's syndrome	↓ or N	↓ or N	↓ or N	↓ or N
Isolated gonadotrophin deficiency	↓ or N	↓ or N	↓ or N	↓ or N
Simple delayed puberty	↓ or N	↓ or N	↓	↓
Gonad				
Primary testicular failure	↑	↑	↓	↓ or N
Anorchia	↑	↑	↓	↓ or N
Cryptorchidism	N	N or ↑	N	N
Azoospermia and oligospermia	N or ↑	N or ↑	N	N
Varicocele	N	N	N	N
Klinefelter's syndrome	↑ or N	↑	↓ or N	N or ↑
Complete testicular feminization syndrome	↑	↑ or N	N or ↑	↑
Precocious puberty				
Idiopathic or CNS lesion	↑	↑	↑	↑
Adrenal tumors or congenital adrenal hyperplasia	↓	↓	↑	↑ or N

*Modified from Marshall, J.C.: Investigative Procedures. Clin. Endocrinol. Metabol., 4:545, 1975.

12 mIU/ml in children, up to 15 mIU/ml in adult males, and between 30 and 200 mIU/ml in castrates. In menstruating females LH values are up to 10 mIU/ml except during the mid-cycle peak when they may reach 80 mIU/ml. Reference values for FSH in children are up to 12 mIU/ml; in adult males, up to 15 mIU/ml; and in postmenopausal patients up to 200 mIU/ml. Menstruating females have FSH values which are up to 10 mIU/ml except during the mid-cycle peak when FSH values may extend up to 20 mIU/ml.

LH and FSH measurements have also been used for the diagnosis of ectopic tumor production. This is discussed on page 466.

Those patients who have a lesion in the hypothalamus or pituitary will have low gonadotropins and low sex hormones; those with a primary lesion in the gonads will have low sex hormones and elevated gonadotropins. The findings in some disorders of the hypothalamic-pituitary-gonadal axis are summarized in Table 14-17.

Clomiphene testing

Clomiphene, an anti-estrogen which is used as a diagnostic or therapeutic agent, has achieved widespread clinical use. It competes with estrogens at the hypothalamic-pituitary level by blocking the uptake of estrogens at these sites. Thus the feedback of estrogens on the hypothalamic-pituitary system is interrupted, resulting in secretion of larger amounts of LH and FSH which, in turn, induce follicular maturation and initiate an ovulatory cycle.

Since a functioning hypothalamic-pituitary-ovarian axis is essential for successful therapy, clomiphene is indicated in anovulatory patients in whom there is evidence of follicular function, estrogen production is adequate (in that they bleed after administration of progesterone), and the gonadotropins are within the normal range or slightly diminished.

Clomiphene citrate is given in a dosage of 50 to 100 mg daily for 5 to 10 days. A convenient starting point is the fifth day of menstrual bleeding induced by progesterone. Although induction of bleeding prior to the administration of clomiphene is not essential, it gives the advantage of simulating a normal menstrual cycle.

A reference population (those with adequate pituitary gonadotropin reserve) will have a 50 per cent increase of LH over baseline, and an 85 per cent increase of FSH over baseline on the last day of clomiphene testing. With the seven-day test, ovulation, if it results, will occur about 11 days after beginning clomiphene. Although only a single LH determination as a baseline and on the sixth day is considered adequate by some; others recommend two baseline samples and a sample on days four, five, six, and seven for LH and FSH (Franchimont, 1974).

Ovulation may be induced in 70 per cent of anovulatory patients, while the pregnancy rate in several large series ranges from 27 to 40 per cent (Jewelewicz, 1976). Clomiphene also can be used in males who have signs and symptoms of androgen deficiency but in whom the measurement of gonadotropins and testosterone has not lead to a diagnosis. The minimum normal response has been defined as an increase over baseline of 30 per cent for LH and 22 per cent for FSH (Walsh, 1977).

ESTROGENS

All estrogens have an A ring which has three unsaturated double bonds. Although over 30 estrogens have been identified, measurements of only three estrogens—estradiol, estrone, and estriol—are utilized in clinical practice. The structure of the three common ones and their interrelationships are seen below.

Estradiol is secreted almost entirely by the ovary, while most estrone is derived from the peripheral conversion of androstenedione and from estradiol metabolism. During the follicular phase of the menstrual cycle, ovarian secretion represents only one third of the total estrogen production. The ovary, as well as the testes and adrenal, have the capacity to synthesize estrogens from androstenedione and testosterone. In normal postmenopausal women, the ovaries do not secrete significant quantities of steroids, and virtually all estrogen produced is from the peripheral conversion of androstenedione made by the adrenal.

In men, the testes secrete significant quantities of estradiol and small amounts of estrone. However, the testicular secretion probably accounts for only one third of the total production of estradiol in men, the remainder arising by extraglandular conversion from testosterone and estrone. Thus, the testes are indirectly responsible for most of the estrogen production in men.

Estradiol, estriol, and estrone are bound to sex hormone binding globulin (SHBG), the same carrier protein which also binds testosterone. However, there are differences in the state of estrogens circulating in blood. Estradiol is largely in the unconjugated form and is bound to sex hormone binding globulin (SHBG). In contrast, most of estrone in plasma circulates as estrone sulfate. Almost all estriol is excreted as conjugates of sulfuric or glucuronic acid or both (Baird, 1976). Estriol glucuronide is filtered and also secreted by the renal tubule.

A wide range of organs in the body, including skin, fat, red blood cells, uterus, and liver, have the enzymatic ability to perform some of the reactions involved in the metabolism of estrogens, but liver plays a most important role. The metabolic pattern or rate of estrogen metabolism apparently does not change during various disease states.

Estradiol and estrone are converted in the liver to estrogenic metabolites, which are then conjugated and excreted as sulfates and glucuronates. The clearance of the conjugates from the circulation is relatively slow so that the concentration in peripheral plasma usually exceeds that of free estrogen. Estrone sulfate and other estrogen conjugates are excreted in the bile and then hydrolyzed in the gut and reabsorbed into the peripheral circulation.

The method of Brown (1968) has been used to estimate total estrogens in urine (also see Chap. 20). This endpoint reaction depends on the ability of the phenolic group of estrogens to react with Kober reagent (a mixture of

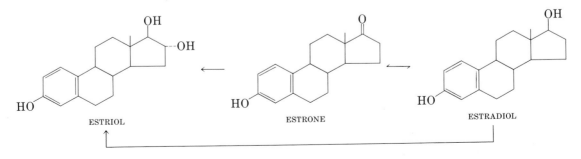

ESTRIOL   ESTRONE   ESTRADIOL

phenol and sulfuric acid) to produce a pink color. This can be measured colorimetrically or the colored product can be extracted and measured fluorometrically. Before the urinary estrogens, which are in the form of water soluble conjugates, can be measured, the glucuronate or sulfate derivatives must be hydrolyzed prior to extraction with organic solvents. Hydrolysis is performed with strong acid or enzymatic preparations.

For the estimation of estrogens in the plasma, the method of Brown is too insensitive and often radioimmunoassay is used. When the hapten estradiol was conjugated with protein at the 3 or 17 position and injected into animals for preparation of an antibody, antibody cross-reaction with other estrogens of 30 to 50 per cent was found. Antibodies produced by methods which employ conjugation at the C-6 position are more specific.

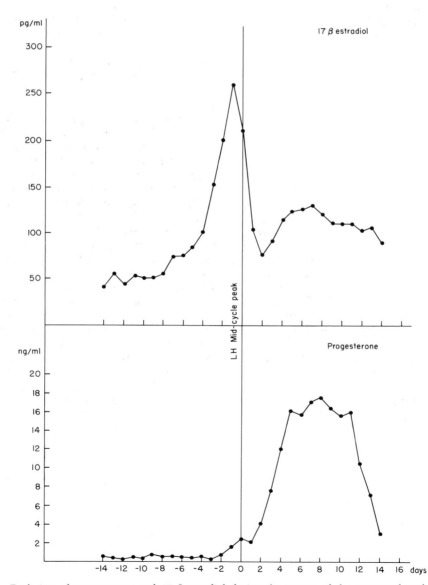

Figure 14–23. Evolution of progesterone and 17-β-estradiol during the course of the menstrual cycle. (Modified from Franchimont, P., Valcke, J. C., and Lambotte, R.: Female gonadal dysfunction. Clin. Endocrinol. Metabol., 3:533, 1974.)

Estradiol is the most potent of the ovarian estrogens and is present in low concentrations (less than 50 pg/ml) in the preovulatory period. Concentrations rise during the second half of the follicular phase and reach a peak of 150 to 500 pg/ml the day prior to or the day of the LH peak. It is this rising estrogen, present for appropriate duration, which may be related to the mid-cycle surge of LH. Following the LH surge, plasma estradiol drops precipitously, almost to preovulatory levels, but then rises slightly to 100 to 200 pg/ml during the luteal phase (Fig. 14-23).

When Block (1974) compared estradiol in plasma with total estrogens in urine, the plasma estradiol assay was found to be a more accurate monitor of ovarian function than urinary excretion of total estrogens. When ovarian secretion of estradiol is high the correlation between plasma and urinary levels is good; but if the ovarian secretion is low, correlation is poor. In prepubertal children, reference values for estradiol by RIA are 20 pg/ml, while in adult males they are usually 10 to 80 pg/ml.

The use of estriol assay in the assessment of the fetoplacental unit is discussed in Chapter 20.

PROGESTERONE

Progesterone concentrations are low prior to the mid-cycle gonadotropin surge. Progesterone concentrations begin to rise rapidly shortly after the gonadotropin surge and reach peak levels during the middle of the luteal phase. Thereafter there is a progressive fall with barely detectable levels reached prior to menses (Fig. 14-23).

Progesterone production by the corpus luteum can be indirectly assessed by the measurement of the basal body temperature. There is about a 0.5°C. rise in body temperature which lasts about 10 to 12 days and parallels the increase in progesterone concentration during the luteal phase.

Progesterone can be monitored by the measurement of urinary pregnanediol, usually by colorimetry or gas chromatography (Wotiz, 1976). Reference values for urinary pregnanediol excretion are less than 1 mg/24 hr during the preovulatory phase, rising to between 2.5 and 6 mg/24 hr during the luteal phase.

Plasma progesterone concentration is a more direct measurement of corpus luteal function. With radioimmunoassay (Abraham, 1971), the method of choice, a progesterone concentration of less than 1 ng/ml is found during the preovulatory phase. At the time of the LH surge, plasma progesterone levels begin to rise and reach a peak of about 10 to 20 ng/ml at about four to six days. After remaining more or less stable for about one week, progesterone concentrations drop rapidly a short time before the onset of menstruation. In the adult male, progesterone originates predominately from the adrenal gland. In this group plasma progesterone concentrations are fairly constant and lower than levels in the female during the follicular phase of the menstrual cycle.

Function of the corpus luteum can be assessed with the use of human chorionic gonadotropin (HCG). During the luteal phase starting on the third day of the hypothermic phase, 3 mg dexamethasone is given daily for six consecutive days. On the first, third, and fifth days, 5000 units of HCG are injected intramuscularly. Urinary or plasma steroids are measured as a baseline: plasma estradiol or progesterone, urinary estrogens, or pregnanediol may be used. The normal response is a doubling of the baseline value on the sixth day.

TESTOSTERONE

In the male, LH has been found to bind Leydig cell receptors in the testes. By working through cyclic AMP (Catt, 1976) it enhances the conversion of pregnenolone to testosterone (Fig. 14-24). Once testosterone is formed in the Leydig cell, capillaries and veins carry it to the periphery or it traverses the myoid cell to the seminiferous tubules, where it is involved in spermatogenesis. In addition to testosterone, the testes also secrete dihydrotestosterone, 17-hydroxyprogesterone, pregnenolone, and 4-androstenedione.

In the male, the testes have two main functions; spermatogenesis, the production of germ cells, and steroidogenesis, the synthesis and subsequent secretion of the steroid hormones.

The androgens have widespread effects on sexual and non-sexual tissue. These effects involve growth of the seminal vesicles, prostate, penis, scrotum, vas deferens, and epididymis. Growth in general also is stimulated, and there is an increase in total body mass with such tissues as muscle, bones, kidney, and larynx relatively sensitive to the effects of

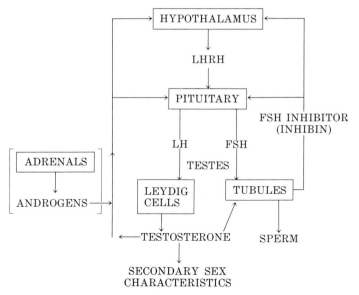

Figure 14-24. Physiologic considerations in the male reproductive process.

testosterone. The androgens also have specific effects on hair growth. All areas except scalp and eyebrows in the newborn are covered with soft, light colored hair (vellus hair). Later in life the hairs at specific sites, under the influence of the androgens, become replaced with longer, coarser, and darker terminal hair. The amount of androgen necessary for the change depends on the race, sex, and age of the individual as well as the site of the follicle on the body.

FSH has been shown to activate the seminiferous tubules and through this mechanism is responsible for the production of sperm (see Chap. 21). A product formed by the Sertoli cells, named inhibin, is responsible for the feedback on FSH. This substance is poorly characterized and its mechanism of action is not completely understood. The testosterone in the seminiferous tubules is bound to a protein; its concentration is 20 times that which occurs in the peripheral circulation. The testosterone which has been secreted locally has been found to stimulate primary spermatocytes to form secondary spermatocytes and finally young spermatocytes.

About 60 per cent of the circulating testosterone binds strongly to sex hormone binding globulin (SHBG), a β globulin which also binds estradiol and other steroids containing a 17-β hydroxy substitution. Almost 40 per cent of the testosterone is loosely bound to albumin and about 2 per cent is free (unbound) (Ruder, 1971). Hormones such as estradiol which affect testosterone binding are important because they may lead to changes in free testosterone. The administration of androgens decreases and estrogens increases the concentration of SHBG. Thyroid and growth hormones also decrease the concentration of sex hormone binding globulin. Those mechanisms which decrease the sex hormone binding globulin increase the concentration of free hormone, while those that increase the binding protein decrease free hormone concentration. It has been postulated that free testosterone feeds back on LH at the level of the pituitary and hypothalamus, and testosterone metabolites may have similar feedback effects. Reference intervals in prepubertal children are less than 100 ng/dl in males and less than 40 ng/dl in females. In adults, male reference values are greater than 300 ng/dl, and female reference values, less than 80 ng/dl. In the adult female, testosterone values above 160 ng/dl are reflected in virilization (see p. 464). Low values in a male are suggestive of hypogonadism and warrant further evaluation with gonadotropin measurements to localize the cause of hypogonadism.

SEMINAL FLUID

The evaluation of the functional aspects of the seminiferous tubules can be achieved by the examination of the seminal fluid (see

Chap. 21). It contains spermatozoa which are suspended in epididymal secretions together with the fluids secreted by the prostate and seminal vesicles. The epididymal secretions are characterized by high content of glycerol-phosphorylcholine; the prostate secretion, by acid phosphatase and citrate; and the seminal vesical secretion, by fructose. Absence of these substances can be used to localize the defect of spermatogenesis; however, each of these is under the influence of testosterone for their development and functional integrity. Lack of testosterone leads either to a failure of pubertal development or, after puberty, to marked involution of these glands.

The volume of the ejaculate varies between 1.5 and 5 ml, the normal sperm count is in excess of 40 million/ml, with 60 per cent or more of the spermatozoa having high grade motility and morphology (Amelar, 1977) (see p. 715). The volume, the ejaculate, and the number, motility, and morphology of the spermatozoa all determine fertility. The important parameters of sperm analysis are discussed in Chapter 21.

Since sperm concentrations vary tremendously within the same individual, several (as many as six or more) separate specimens should be examined before drawing conclusions as to the status of the patient (Paulsen, 1976).

17-KETOSTEROIDS

17-Ketosteroids (17-KS) comprise a group of steroid compounds which have a ketone at position C-17 of the steroid nucleus. These compounds are secreted almost entirely by the adrenals in women, while in men, the adrenals are responsible for two thirds and the testes the remainder. Quantitation of these compounds is important because of their androgenic properties. However, not all of the 17-ketosteroids measured are androgens nor are the most important androgens measured as 17-KS. For example, androsterone and dehydroepiandrosterone both have androgenic properties and are measured, while etiocholanolone, although measured, does not have these properties. The structures of these compounds are shown below. Both etiocholanolone and androsterone have saturated B rings and are derived from dehydroepiandrosterone (unsaturated B ring) but differ in that the hydrogen on position 5 is oriented in different planes. The most potent androgens, testosterone and dihydrotestosterone, are not measured as 17-KS. Other compounds such as the

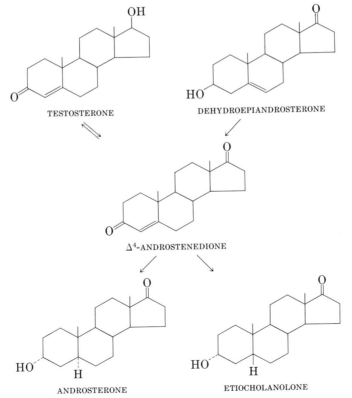

TESTOSTERONE

DEHYDROEPIANDROSTERONE

Δ^4-ANDROSTENEDIONE

ANDROSTERONE

ETIOCHOLANOLONE

estrogens, although possessing a ketone group at C-17, are not measured as 17-ketosteroids, since they are removed during the extraction procedure. Most of the 17-ketosteroids are excreted as sulfate or glucuronide conjugates. Measurements of the 17-ketosteroids involve a cleavage of the conjugates with acid prior to extraction, and reaction with *m*-dinitrobenzene and alcoholic alkali to produce a reddish purple color with an absorption of 520 nm (Zimmermann reaction). This reaction is pictured below.

When a keto group occurs on another carbon such as the 3-keto group in progesterone, a less intense color with a different absorption maximum occurs with the Zimmerman reaction.

Because of the interference by brown chromogens, a variety of approaches have been used to improve the specificity of the 17-KS determination. Extractions which remove the interfering chromogens have been utilized, but a more common approach has been the use of a mathematical formula relating to the different wavelengths near the absorption peak (Allen correction) to eliminate this problem. A detailed procedure has been described by Henry (1969).

The reference values for 17-KS are 6 to 15 mg/24 hours and 8 to 20 mg/24 hours in women and men, respectively. In children who have not undergone puberty, reference values are much lower, usually less than 3 mg/24 hours and gradually increasing until puberty. Elevated urine 17-KS are associated with some adrenal, testicular, and ovarian tumors, Cushing's syndrome, some of the congenital adrenal hyperplasia syndromes (see p. 445), and pregnancy. Decreased 17-KS occur after adrenalectomy or castration and in Addison's disease, the nephrotic syndrome, and hypothyroidism (Table 14–18).

HIRSUTISM

Hyperandrogenism is one of the most common endocrinopathies occurring in women; 5 to 10 per cent of American women are hirsute and most (greater than 90 per cent) hirsute women are hyperandrogenic. Hirsutism is defined as an excessive growth of hormone-dependent hair in females, and is most noticeable when located on the chin, upper lip, and sides of the face, but excess pubic, axillary, and chest hair may also occur. In healthy women, testosterone, androstenedione, and dehydroepiandrosterone (DHEA) are the major androgens produced and secreted into the circulation. In non-hirsute women, these compounds are present in the peripheral blood in a concentration of about 40 ng/dl, 175 ng/dl, and 375 ng/dl, respectively (Givens, 1976). Testosterone, the most active of the androgens, is 5 to 10 times more potent than androstenedione and 20 times more potent than dehydroepiandrosterone. In healthy women, 5 to 20 per cent of circulating testosterone is derived from the ovaries and 1 to 30 per cent from the adrenals. Approximately 50 per cent of the testosterone is derived from the peripheral conversion of androstenedione to testosterone in the liver, blood, skin, and skeletal muscle. In the normal female approximately 50 per cent of the circulating androstenedione comes from the adrenals and 50 per cent from the ovaries, except at mid-cycle when the ovarian contribution is twice that of the adrenals. Androstenedione shows a circadian rhythm which follows cortisol and results in a 50 per cent change in plasma concentration. The adrenal contributes about 80 per cent of the circulating DHEA.

Most hirsute women have elevated production rates and plasma levels of androstenedione and testosterone (Kirschner, 1972). Whereas in a reference population 50 per cent of the plasma testosterone is derived from the peripheral conversion of androstenedione, only 25 per cent of plasma testosterone in hirsute women is derived from peripheral conversion of androstenedione. Thus, most of the testosterone in the plasma of hirsute women is secreted as testosterone directly into the circulation. Since there are small swings in

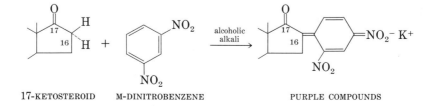

17-KETOSTEROID   M-DINITROBENZENE   PURPLE COMPOUNDS

Table 14–18. CLINICAL CORRELATIONS: URINARY
17-KETOSTEROIDS

INCREASED VALUES	DECREASED VALUES
Adrenocortical carcinoma	Addison's disease
Adrenocortical adenoma	Panhypopituitarism
Adrenocortical hyperplasia	Myxedema
Acromegaly (vary from low, normal to high)	Nephrotic syndrome
Arrhenoblastoma and luteal cell tumor of ovary	Chronic illness with debility
Interstitial cell (Leydig) tumor of testes	Gout
Pregnancy—last trimester	Castration of male or eunuchoidism
Hirsutism, occasionally	Thyrotoxicosis
ACTH therapy	Female hypogonadism
Stress, severe	Diabetes mellitus
	Prepubertal children

plasma testosterone but large swings in androstenedione concentration in response to ACTH, it is recommended that samples for androstenedione be obtained sometime distant to the ACTH-dependent morning peak.

The laboratory work-up of a hirsute female should begin with a determination of urinary 17-KS. Urinary 17-KS are useful as a screening test for ovarian and adrenal tumors, but most hirsute women have normal values. However, if greater than twice normal (with or without the elevation of 17-hydroxycorticosteroids), then a dexamethesone suppression test should be done to rule out adrenal tumors (see p. 422). Congenital adrenal hyperplasia also should be considered; over 90 per cent of these patients can be identified by elevated plasma 17-hydroxycorticosteroid progesterone levels.

If the 17-KS are normal or mildly elevated, then plasma testosterone and androstenedione should be measured; if both of these are normal, then a testosterone binding globulin deficit is suggested. If plasma testosterone and androstenedione are elevated, then suppression with a combination type oral contraceptive can be used as a further diagnostic maneuver. Androgens from ovarian or adrenal tumors do not suppress to normal with this diagnostic maneuver, while in gonadotropin-dependent syndromes such as polycystic ovarian disease they do suppress. In contrast to the pituitary adrenal axis, the pituitary ovarian axis is much slower to suppress, sometimes

requiring up to three weeks. In the majority of women with hirsutism, the ovary rather than adrenal is the source of the increase in secretion.

One of the most common causes is polycystic ovarian disease, which is characterized by increased androstenedione, testosterone, and serum LH, while serum FSH is either low or low normal (Greenblatt, 1976). Because the eponym Stein-Leventhal syndrome refers to only a portion of the spectrum of polycystic ovarian disease, this term should be abandoned to avoid confusion. Polycystic ovarian disease syndrome may be secondary to androgen production outside the ovary: for example, polycystic ovaries are observed in females with congenital adrenal hyperplasia. Ovarian causes of the syndrome include ovarian stromal hyperplasia. Hyperplasia of hilus of the ovary, as well as ovarian tumors including arrhenoblastoma, luteomas, hilus cell, and Krukenberg tumors are associated with hirsutism. Adrenal hyperandrogenism from congenital adrenal hyperplasia, adrenal tumors such as carcinomas and adenomas, and ectopic ACTH syndromes are frequent causes of hirsutism.

In some hirsute women, the urinary 17-KS are normal or minimally elevated, the ovaries are not enlarged, and the patient has a normal cortisol and no evidence of ovarian, adrenal, or ectopic tumor. These who are said to have idiopathic hirsutism, account for about 40 per cent of all hirsute patients (Rose, 1976). They usually have slightly elevated plasma androstenedione levels and testosterone levels and may have a depressed testosterone binding globulin capacity.

MISCELLANEOUS

ECTOPIC HORMONES

Benign and malignant tumors, derived from tissues which usually are not considered to be endocrine in nature, may produce hormonal substances. The so-called ectopic hormone syndromes which are produced were first described over 50 years ago but until recently were thought to be a clinical rarity. The availability of radioimmunoassay for the measurement of small amounts of circulating hormones, however, has made possible the documentation of a large number of these syndromes. Odell (1977) has suggested that malignant cell replication is commonly or perhaps universally associated with ectopic hormone production. The ectopic hormone produced may be indistinguishable from the native hormone or may be a fragment or a larger molecular weight form such as a prohormone. Although the ectopic hormone produced may not be chemically identical to the native hormone and may not have full biologic activity, it may be measured as the hormone by a given radioimmunoassay. Rarely syndromes have been described in which a substance is produced which has the biologic activity of a certain hormone but bears no structural relationship to it. The activity of these substances can be demonstrated only by tedious bioassays; this probably accounts in part for the description of only a few of these syndromes.

Ectopic hormone production is important, since it may lead to confusion in making the correct diagnosis or instituting proper treatment in certain endocrine disorders. In other situations, ectopic hormone production can be taken advantage of to provide a biochemical marker for screening of certain malignancies and for monitoring patients with documented or suspected tumors. To establish hormone production as ectopic, Vaitukaitis (1976) has recommended documentation of the following points:

1. Hormonal concentration greater in tumor than in surrounding normal tissue.

Table 14-19. COMMON ECTOPIC HORMONE SYNDROMES

HORMONE	TYPE OF NEOPLASM
Adrenocorticotropic hormone (ACTH)	Lung (oat cell, bronchial adenoma) Thymus Pancreatic islets
Parathyroid hormone (PTH)	Kidney Lung (squamous cell) Pancreas Ovary
Antidiuretic hormone (ADH)	Lung (oat cell)
Human chorionic gonadotropin (HCG)	Testicle (embryonal, choriocarcinoma) Liver
Growth hormone (GH)	Lung (bronchogenic) Stomach
Human placental lactogen (HPL)	Lung
Erythropoietin	Cerebellar (hemangioblastoma) Pheochromocytoma Hepatoma
Renin	Lung (oat cell)
Thyrocalcitonin (TCT)	Lung Stomach
Enteroglucogen	Kidney
Prolactin	Lung Kidney
Thyroid stimulating hormone (TSH)	Lung Breast

2. Hormonal location in tissue by immunologic or histochemical techniques.
3. After tumor removal, disappearance of the ectopic hormone.
4. Arteriovenous difference of tumor concentration across tumor bed.
5. *In vitro* hormonal production by the tumor.

Of the ectopic hormones isolated, most have been peptides and none have been steroid or thyroid hormones (Table 14-19). Many theories have been proposed for the occurrence of these syndromes. The one most widely held is the derepression of the DNA code and subsequent *m*-RNA production, leading to synthesis of polypeptides at an unregulated rate. Hormones such as thyroid or steroids require a number of enzymatic steps for their formation; for these to be produced by a tumor, a series of ectopically produced enzymes located in a specific compartment presumably would be essential. Obviously, this is a much more complex requirement than the production of a simple polypeptide chain and may possibly account for the type of hormone produced. When enzymes are ectopically produced, only a single enzyme may be formed. An example is the production of the Regan isoenzyme of alkaline phosphatase by a variety of tumors (Stolbach, 1969).

Another popular theory, the "endocrine cell" hypothesis, suggests a gene function change in a cell that already possesses structural and biochemical characteristics of polypeptide secreting cells. Evidence supporting this theory has been accumulated by Pearse (1974) for a group of potential endocrine cells with their origin in the neural crest. These cells, which migrate to various locations in the embryo, have been called APUD cells (*A*mine content, amine *P*recursor *U*ptake, amino acid *D*ecarboxylase) based on the cytochemical properties. The ectopic secretion of ACTH by pheochromocytomas, medullary carcinoma of the thyroid, pancreatic islet cell neoplasias, and carcinoid tumors clearly can be comprehended as a change in the role of the APUD cell.

Cushing's syndrome, associated with an ACTH-producing tumor, was the first description of ectopic polypeptide hormone production. Although features of Cushing's syndrome initially may not be apparent in these patients, they become obvious within a short period. The syndrome develops rapidly and as it progresses, extreme muscle wasting, abnormal glucose tolerance, hypertension, and a marked hypokalemic alkalosis occur. Serum cortisol measurements are often greater than 40 μg/dl (104 nm/l) and ACTH greater than 200 pg/ml. Usually neither ACTH nor cortisol is suppressed by the administration of dexamethasone. In approximately two thirds of the patients, ectopic ACTH production is associated with oat cell carcinoma of the lung, while tumors such as bronchial adenomas and pancreatic and thymic tumors account for the other cases. In about half the patients with bronchial adenomas, dexamethasone suppression may occur (Jones, 1969). A large number of these tumors produce an ACTH with a molecular weight that is greater than that of the native hormone but similar to the weight of pro-ACTH (big ACTH) (Yalow, 1973; Gewirtz, 1974). In addition, small ACTH, CLIP (corticotrophin-like intermediate lobe peptide) and fragments of ACTH also have been reported to occur (Rees, 1977).

Hypercalcemia, perhaps the most common biochemical abnormality, is associated with a variety of malignant lesions. It may be clinically manifested in subtle ways, such as anorexia, nausea, vomiting, constipation, and weakness, or may be the cause of life-threatening arrhythmias or coma. Since treatment is effective and relatively benign, all patients with tumors should have serum calcium determinations (see Chap. 10). Hypercalcemia may result from bony metastasis or may be secondary to ectopic production of parathyroid (PTH). When hypercalcemia, hypophosphatemia, and decreased tubular reabsorption of phosphorus occur in patients with tumors in the absence of bony lesions, ectopic PTH production should be suspected. Clinically this syndrome is different from primary hyperparathyroidism in that weight loss and constitutional symptoms are profound, hypercalcemia tends to be greater, and hyperchloremic metabolic alkalosis is less frequent. Bony lesions of hyperparathyroidism are uncommon; renal stones and peptic ulceration are absent. Renal cell carcinoma and squamous cell carcinoma of the lung make up about two thirds of these ectopic PTH producing tumors, with the remainder originating in a variety of sites. Because of the development of sophisticated radioimmunoassays of PTH, it has become apparent that several different fragments as well as prohormones of PTH occur. Depending on the assay system utilized, ectopic PTH production has been found to be associated with 30 to 90 per cent of all squamous cell carcinomas of the lung. Other cases have been described in which hypercalcemia and hypophosphatemia occur without increased circulating levels of PTH or without an increased arteriovenous gradient across the tumor bed; however, removal of the tumor did result in the normalization of the calcium and phosphorus (Powell, 1973). In some cases where hypercalcemia and no increase in PTH concentrations have been found, the cause has been ascribed to prostaglandins (Demers, 1977) or in the hematopoietic malignancies, to osteocyte activating factor (OAF) (Mundy, 1974).

Tumors responsible for the production of antidiuretic hormone (ADH) are manifested by the cardinal signs of hyponatremia, depressed serum osmolality, and inappropriately elevated urine osmolality. To fulfill the criteria for the diagnosis of inappropriate ADH secretion, renal and adrenal function must be normal. The detailed diagnostic criteria for the inappropriate ADH syndrome may be found in a discussion of the posterior pituitary (p. 413). Lung tumors and pancreatic tumors are most often responsible for this syndrome. Hamilton (1972, 1975), has reported that neurophysin, the normal protein carrier for ADH, also has been found in some of the tumors that have ectopic ADH synthesizing ability. Patients with the syndrome of water intoxication may present virtually asymptomatic or comatose depending on the level of serum sodium. Mild symptoms of water intoxication are most often characterized by lethargy, weakness, or confusion.

Of the gonadotropins, only the ectopic production of luteinizing hormone (LH) and human chorionic gonadotropin (HCG) is likely to lead to clinically recognizable syndromes. Manifestations include precocious puberty occurring in prepubertal boys or gynecomastia occurring in men. Since HCG is not present in the peripheral blood except during pregnancy, its presence under any other conditions strongly suggests the presence of a tumor. Adenocarcinomas of the stomach, ovary, and pancreas and hepatomas are tumors most commonly associated with ectopic HCG secretion. Braunstein (1973) reported that 7 to 14 per cent of patients with a variety of cancers have elevated concentrations of HCG. The glycoprotein hormones are made up of nearly identical alpha chains but differ in beta chain structure; it is entirely possible that only one chain may be produced by a particular tumor. A few lung or pancreatic tumors have been reported to produce free alpha chains (Rosen, 1974), but more frequently the beta subunit is formed (Rosen, 1975). In a group of patients with islet cell tumors, some of the malignant lesions were found to secrete alpha chains, some beta chains, and still others HCG, while non-malignant islet tumors failed to secrete these markers (Kahn, 1977). Trophoblastic tumors have been reported to secrete HCG, but these tumors are not ectopic, since the secretion of this hormone is the normal physiologic function of the trophoblast.

Growth hormone (GH) production rarely has been reported and only in association with a few tumors, most commonly bronchogenic and gastric carcinoma (Beck, 1972). In bronchogenic carcinoma, human placental lactogen (HPL) as a tumor marker has been frequently observed. HPL has an amino acid sequence very similar to that of growth hormone but in a group of patients reported by Rosen (1975) clinical features of GH or HPL excess were not found.

Erythropoietin has been found in association with neoplastic renal disease, but since the kidney is normally responsible for its production, these tumors are not ectopic syndromes. However, erythropoietin has been secreted by hepatomas, pheochromocytomas, and 10 to 20 per cent of cerebellar hemangioblastomas, with lung tumors conspicuous by their absence in the production of this hormone. Other ectopic hormones such as thyrocalcitonin (TCT), prolactin, and thyroid stimulating hormone (TSH) have been found in a few cases, each from a variety of human neoplasms (Table 14-19).

MULTIPLE ENDOCRINE ADENOPATHY SYNDROME

A number of syndromes are produced by hyperplastic or neoplastic changes which occur in one or a number of glands in the endocrine system. These syndromes tend to be familial with both sexes affected equally. They are not considered to be ectopic hormone syndromes because the tumors produce hormones that the glands ordinarily make.

Two different types of syndromes have been classically described: Type I (Wermer's syndrome) and Type II (Sipple's syndrome). Type I

Table 14-20. COMMON FINDINGS IN MULTIPLE ENDOCRINE ADENOPATHY

Type I (Wermer's syndrome)
  1. *Parathyroid hyperplasia
  2. *Pancreatic islet cell adenoma
  3. *Pituitary adenoma
  4. Adrenal corticoid hyperplasia
  5. Goiter
  6. Carcinoid tumors

Type II (Sipple's syndrome)
  1. Pheochromocytoma
  2. Medullary carcinoma of the thyroid
  3. Parathyroid hyperplasia

* Most common in Wermer's syndrome.

(Wermer's) commonly includes pituitary adenomas, pancreatic adenomas (beta cell and non-beta cell), and parathyroid chief cell hyperplasia; adrenal adenomas, goiters, and bronchial carcinoids occasionally occur. Manifestations of the endocrinopathy may occur in any combination or in any order (Table 14-20). The most common presenting features usually are from gastrointestinal ulceration, hypoglycemia, hypoparathyroidism, pituitary tumors, or diarrhea with associated weight loss. A combination of these clinical features, especially in those patients with relevant family history, should suggest the possibility of multiple endocrine adenomatosis and lead to appropriate investigation.

Type II (Sipple's syndrome) consists of parathyroid chief cell hyperplasia, medullary carcinoma of the thyroid, and pheochromocytoma (Table 14-20). Although the most common variety of the syndrome is medullary thyroid carcinoma with pheochromocytoma in one or both adrenals, a few patients have hyperparathyroidism as well. Variants of the syndrome may occur: for example, one includes medullary carcinoma, pheochromocytoma, and multiple small neuromas of the eyelids and buccal mucosa with diffuse hypertrophy of the lips (Montgomery, 1975).

When a diagnosis of endocrine disease is made, it is important to consider these syndromes especially if more than one gland or system is involved. If one of these syndromes is identified, the family members should be evaluated for a similar syndrome.

PINEAL

The pineal is a small conical organ of about 120 g located at the base of the brain. The cells of the pineal secrete a ground substance that serves as a matrix for pineal calcification which begins at puberty. Although this calcification is a ubiquitous finding in any large autopsy series, it does not interfere with the endocrine function of the pineal. From serotonin (5-hydroxytryptamine) the pineal synthesizes a group of biologically active compounds called methoxyindoles, of which melatonin (5-methoxy-*N*-acetyltryptamine) is the most important. Darkness stimulates melatonin synthesis, while light inhibits its formation (Vaughan, 1976). Sympathetic nerve endings which terminate in the pineal release the neurotransmitter, norepinephrine, in response to impulses originating in the retina. Through this pathway, enzymes involved in the synthesis of melatonin are regulated. These synthetic enzymes show the same diurnal pattern as melatonin.

Melatonin is concentrated in the pineal but is also found in cerebrospinal fluid and plasma. It also is present in high concentrations in the hypothalamus, the pituitary, and the ovaries. Although its precise role is not known, there is some evidence that it is important in sexual development, perhaps by modulating the release of LH at the pituitary level. Tumors of the pineal usually are associated with precocious puberty; however, rarely delayed puberty may occur.

Melatonin has been measured by bioassay, by gas chromatography-mass spectrometry (Wilson, 1977), and by radioimmunoassay (Arendt, 1977), but its determination remains a research tool. Wurtman (1977a and b) provides additional information regarding melatonin assays.

PROSTAGLANDINS

Prostaglandins are a large family of compounds which are derived from prostanoic acid, a 20-carbon fatty acid which consists of a cyclopentane ring with two attached hydrocarbon side chains (Fig. 14-25). The naturally occurring prostaglandins are divided into four series, E, F, A, and B, depending on the arrangement of the constituents on the cyclopentane ring. The main groups are then further subdivided according to the number of double bonds occurring in the side chains. In the F series, alpha and beta are used to designate the position of the hydroxyl group at carbon 9.

Many tissues appear to have the ability to

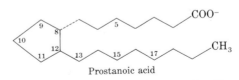

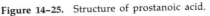

Figure 14-25. Structure of prostanoic acid.

Table 14–21. SOME EFFECTS OF
PROSTAGLANDINS*

TISSUE	EFFECT
Lung	Bronchodilation
Gastrointestinal tract	Contraction
Gastric mucosa	Inhibition of acid secretion
Blood vessels	Vasodilation
Platelets	Inhibits aggregation
Uterus	Contraction
Corpus luteum	Stimulation of steroidogenesis
Kidney	Natriuresis and increased free water clearance
Adipocyte	Inhibits lipolysis

*Modified from Tepperman, J.: Metabolic and Endocrine Physiology, 3rd ed. Chicago, Year Book Medical Publishers, Inc., 1973.

synthesize prostaglandins from essential fatty acid precursors. They have been isolated from tissues such as kidney, lung, spleen, gastrointestinal tract, thyroid, skin, and brain. Prostaglandins are apparently not stored by tissues but are synthesized immediately before release. It has been postulated that the prostaglandins may be regulators of physiologic activities which mediate or modulate a wide variety of functions. For example, prostaglandins are thought to play a role in reproduction and blood pressure control and to act as mediators of inflammation. In addition, they have been reported to have a number of other effects (Table 14–21). For example, prostaglandins possess many pharmacologic actions and have been used therapeutically to induce abortion via uterine smooth muscle contraction.

Although a number of methods are available for the measurement of prostaglandins, including radioassay and gas chromatography, assays are not widely available for clinical use. Kelly (1973) has reviewed methods for prostaglandin measurement. Prostaglandins have been reported to be increased in a number of conditions: for example, urinary prostaglandins have been found to be increased in patients with Bartter's syndrome (Gill, 1976). Prostaglandins also have been implicated as mediators of hypercalcemia caused by certain tumors (Seyberth, 1975).

REFERENCES

Hypothalamus and Pituitary

Bachelot, I., Wolfsen, A. R., and Odell, W. D.: Pituitary and plasma lipotropins: Demonstration of the artifactual nature of βMSH. J. Clin. Endocrinol. Metabol. *44*:939, 1977.

Bartter, F. C., and Schwartz, W. B.: The syndrome of inappropriate secretion of antidiuretic hormone. Am. J. Med., *42*:790, 1967.

Catt, K. J., and Dufau, M. L.: Basic concepts of the mechanism of action of peptide hormones. Biol. Reprod., *14*:1, 1976.

Chrétien, M., Seidah, N. G., Benjannet, S., Dragon, N., Routhier, R., Motomatsu, T., Crine, P., and Lis, M.: A βLPH precursor model: Recent developments concerning morphine-like substances. Ann. N.Y. Acad. Sci., *297*:84, 1977.

Cohen, K. L.: Metabolic, endocrine and drug-induced interference with pituitary function tests: A review. Metabolism, *26*:1165, 1977.

Daughaday, W. H.: Hormonal regulation of growth by somatomedin and other tissue growth factors. Clin. Endocrinol. Metabol., *6*:117, 1977.

Daughaday, W. H., Herington, A. C., and Phillips, L. S.: The regulation of growth by endocrines. Annu. Rev. Physiol., *37*:211, 1975.

Doniach, I.: Histopathology of the anterior pituitary. Clin. Endocrinol. Metabol., *6*:21, 1977.

Edwards, C. R. W.: Vasopressin and oxytocin in health and disease. Clin. Endocrinol. Metabol., *6*:223, 1977.

Edwards, C. R. W., and Besser, G. M.: Diseases of the hypothalamus and pituitary gland. Clin. Endocrinol. Metabol., *3*:475, 1974.

Franchimont, P., and Burger, H.: Human Growth Hormone and Gonadotrophins in Health and Disease. Amsterdam, North-Holland Publishing Company, 1975.

Franchimont, P., Valcke, J. C., and Lambotte, R.: Female gonadal dysfunction. Clin. Endocrinol. Metabol., *3*:533, 1974.

Frantz, A. G.: Prolactin. N. Engl. J. Med., *298*:201, 1978.

Friesen, H., and Hwang, P.: Human prolactin. Annu. Rev. Med., *24*:251, 1973.

Frieson, H. G.: Prolactin and prolactin secreting tumors. *In* Syllabus. Twenty-ninth Annual Postgraduate Assembly of the Endocrine Society, 1977.

Gleispach, H., Kreutzer, B., Fellier, H., and Borkenstein, M.: How to collect blood for measurement of HGH, LH, FSH, cyclic AMP, folic acid, cortisol and testosterone. Clin. Chim. Acta, *80*:381, 1977.

Gomez-Pan, A., and Hall, R.: Somatostatin (growth hormone-releasing inhibiting hormone). Clin. Endocrinol. Metabol., *6*:181, 1977.

Greengard, P.: Phosphorylated proteins as physiological effectors. Science, *199*:146, 1978.

Guillemin, R.: Endorphins, brain peptides that act like opiates. N. Engl. J. Med., *296*:226, 1977.

Hodgson, S. F., Randall, R. V., Holman, C. B., and MacCarty, C. S.: Empty sella syndrome. Med. Clin. North Am., *56*:897, 1972.

Hunter, W. M.: Growth hormone. In Loraine, J. A., and Bell, E. T. (eds.): Hormone Assays and their Clinical Application. Edinburgh, Churchill-Livingstone, 1976.

Jacobs, H. S.: Prolactin and amenorrhea. N. Engl. J. Med., *295*:954, 1976.

Kahn, R., Megyesi, K., Bar, R. S., Eastman, R. C., and

Flier, J. S.: Receptors for peptide hormones. Ann. Intern. Med., *86*:205, 1977.

Kleinberg, D. L., Noel, G. L., and Frantz, A. G.: Galactorrhea: A study of 235 cases, including 48 with pituitary tumors. N. Engl. J. Med., *296*:589, 1977.

Laron, Z., Pertzelon, A., and Mannheimer, A.: Genetic pituitary dwarfism with high serum concentration of growth hormone: A new inborn error of metabolism? Isr. J. Med. Sci., *2*:152, 1966.

L'Hermite, M.: Prolactin. *In* Loraine, J. A., and Bell, E. T. (eds.): Hormone Assays and Their Clinical Applications. Edinburgh, Churchill-Livingstone, 1976.

Merimee, T. J.: Isolated growth hormone deficiency and related disorders. Annu. Rev. Med., *25*:137, 1974.

Mims, R. B., and Bethune, J. E.: Acromegaly with normal fasting growth hormone concentrations but abnormal growth hormone regulation. Ann. Intern. Med., *81*:781, 1974.

Moses, A. M., Howanitz, J., vanGemert, M., and Miller, M.: Clofibrate induced antidiuresis. J. Clin. Invest., *52*:535, 1973.

Moses, A. M., and Miller, M.: Drug-induced dilutional hyponatremia. N. Engl. J. Med., *291*:1234, 1974.

Moses, A. M., and Miller, M.: Urine and plasma osmolality in differentiation of polyuric states. Postgrad. Med., *52*:187, 1972.

Moses, A. M., Miller, M., and Streeten, D. H. P.: Pathophysiologic and pharmacologic alterations in the release and action of ADH. Metabolism, *25*:697, 1976.

Neelon, F. A., Goree, J. A., and Lebovitz, H. E.: The primary empty sella: Clinical and radiographic characteristics and endocrine function. Medicine, *52*:73, 1973.

Neelon, F. A., and Sydnor, C. F.: The assessment of pituitary function. DM, *24*:6, 1978.

Ontjes, D. A., and Ney, R. L.: Tests of anterior pituitary function. Metabolism, *21*:159, 1972.

Rees, L. H.: ACTH, lipotrophin and MSH in health and disease. Clin. Endocrinol. Metabol., *6*:137, 1977.

Robertson, G. L.: The regulation of vasopressin function in health and disease. Rec. Prog. Horm. Res., *33*:333, 1977.

Robinson, A. G.: The neurophysins in health and disease. Clin. Endocrinol. Metabol., *6*:261, 1977.

Schally, A. V., Kastin, A. J., and Arimura, A.: Hypothalamic hormones: The link between brain and body. Am. Sci., *65*:712, 1977.

Sterling, K., and Lazarus, J. H.: The thyroid and its control. Annu. Rev. Physiol., *39*:349, 1977.

Thorner, M. O.: Prolactin. Clin. Endocrinol. Metabol., *6*:201, 1977.

Turkington, R. W.: Ectopic production of prolactin. N. Engl. J. Med., *285*:1455, 1971.

Vale, W., Rivier, C., and Brown, M.: Regulatory peptides of the hypothalamus. Annu. Rev. Physiol., *39*:473, 1977.

VanWyk, J. J., and Underwood, L. E.: Relation between growth hormone and somatomedin. Annu. Rev. Med., *26*:427, 1975.

Weitzman, E. D.: Circadian rhythms and episodic hormone secretion in man. Annu. Rev. Med., *27*:225, 1976.

Thyroid

Abuid, J., Klein, A. H., Foley, T. P., and Larsen, P. R.: Total and free triiodothyronine and thyroxine in early infancy. J. Clin. Endocrinol. Metabol., *39*:263, 1974.

Bartuska, D. G., and Dratman, M. B.: Evolving concepts of thyroid function. Med. Clin. North Am., *57*:1117, 1973.

Bermudez, F., Surks, M. I., and Oppenheimer, J. H.: High incidence of decreased serum triiodothyronine concentration in patients with nonthyroidal disease. J. Clin. Endocrinol. Metabol., *41*:27, 1975.

Besser, G. M., and Mortimer, C. H.: Hypothalamic regulatory hormones: A review. J. Clin. Pathol., *27*:173, 1974.

Birkhäuser, M., Busset, R., Burer, T., and Burger, A.: Diagnosis of hyperthyroidism when serum thyroxine alone is raised. Lancet, *2*:53, 1977.

Burger, A., and Sakoloff, C.: Serum 3, 3'-diiodothyronine, a direct radioimmunoassay in human serum: Method and clinical results. J. Clin. Endocrinol. Metabol., *45*:384, 1977.

Burger, A., Suter, P., Nicod, P., Vallotton, M. B., Vagenakis, A., and Braverman, L.: Reduced active thyroid hormone levels in acute illness. Lancet, *1*:653, 1976.

Burger, H. G., and Patel, Y. C.: Thyrotrophin releasing hormone—TSH. Clin. Endocrinol. Metabol., *6*:83, 1977.

Burman, K. D., Read, J., Dimond, R. C., Strum, D., Wright, F. D., Patow, W., Earll, J. M., and Wartofsky, L.: Measurement of 3, 3', 5'-triiodothyronine (reverse T3), 3, 3¹-L-diiodothyronine, T3 and T4 in human amniotic fluid and in cord and maternal serum. J. Clin. Endocrinol. Metabol., *43*:1351, 1976.

Burrows, A. W., Shakespear, R. A., Hesch, R. D., Cooper, E., Aickin, C. M., and Burke, C. W.: Thyroid hormones in the elderly sick: "T4 euthyroidism". Br. Med. J., *4*:437, 1975.

Carlson, H. E., and Hershman, J. M.: The hypothalamic-pituitary-thyroid axis. Med. Clin. North Am., *59*:1045, 1975.

Cavalieri, R. R., and Rapoport, B.: Impaired peripheral conversion of thyroxine to triiodothyronine. Annu. Rev. Med., *28*:57, 1977.

Chopra, I. J.: A radioimmunoassay for measurement of thyroxine in unextracted serum. J. Clin. Endocrinol. Metabol., *34*:938, 1972.

Chopra, I. J., Chopra, U., Smith, S. R., Reza, M., and Solomon, D. H.: Reciprocal changes in serum concentrations of 3,3',5'-triiodothyronine (reverse T3) and 3, 3',5'-triiodothyronine (T3) in systemic illnesses. J. Clin. Endocrinol. Metabol., *41*:1043, 1975.

DeGroot, L. J.: Thyroid carcinoma. Med. Clin. North Am., *59*:1233, 1975.

DeGroot, L. J., and Niepomniszcze, H.: Biosynthesis of thyroid hormone: Basic and clinical aspects. Metabolism, *26*:665, 1977.

DeGroot, L. J., and Stanbury, J. B.: The Thyroid and its Diseases. New York, John Wiley and Sons, Inc., 1975.

Evered, D.: Diseases of the thyroid gland. Clin. Endocrinol. Metabol., *3*:425, 1974.

Gershengorn, M. C., and Weintraub, B. D.: Thyrotropin-induced hyperthyroidism caused by selective pituitary resistance to thyroid hormone. J. Clin. Invest., *56*:633, 1975.

Hall, R., and Gomez-Pan, A.: The hypothalamic regulatory hormones and their clinical applications. Adv. Clin. Chem., *18*:173, 1976.

Hansen, J. M., Skovsted, L., Lauridsen, U. B., Kirkegaard, C., and Siersbaek-Neilsen, K.: The effect of diphenylhydantoin on thyroid function. J. Clin. Endocrinol. Metabol., *39*:785, 1974.

Hayles, A. B., and Cloutier, M. D.: Clinical hypothyroidism in the young—a second look. Med. Clin. North Am., *56*:871, 1972.

Hennessy, J. F., Wells, S. A., Ontjes, D. A., and Cooper, C. W.: A comparison of pentagastin injection and calcium infusion as provocative agents for the detection of medullary carcinoma of the thyroid. J. Clin. Endocrinol. Metabol., *39*:487, 1974.

Hoffman, D. P., Surks, M. I., Oppenheimer, J. H., and Weitzman, E. D.: Response to thyrotropin releasing hormone: An objective criterion for the adequacy of thyrotropin suppression therapy. J. Clin. Endocrin. Metabol., *44*:892, 1977.

Ingbar, S. H., and Braverman, L. E.: Active form of the thyroid hormone. Annu. Rev. Med., *26*:443, 1975.

Irvine, W. J., and Toft, A. D.: The diagnosis and treatment of thyrotoxicosis. Clin. Endocrinol., *5*:687, 1976.

Kaplan, M. M., Schimmel, M., and Utiger, R. D.: Changes in serum 3,3′,5′-triiodothyronine (reverse T3) concentrations with altered thyroid hormone secretion and metabolism. J. Clin. Endocrinol. Metabol., *45*:447, 1977.

Larsen, P. R.: Hyperthyroidism. D.M., *22*:3, 1976.

Larsen, P. R.: Tests of thyroid function. Med. Clin. North Am., *59*:1063, 1975.

Lissitzky, S., Bismuth, J., Jaquet, P., Castay, M., Michel-Béchet, M., Koutras, D. A., Pharmakiotis, A. D., Moschos, A., Psarras, A., and Malamos, B.: Congenital goiter with impaired thyroglobulin synthesis. J. Clin. Endocrinol. Metabol., *36*:17, 1973.

Morley, J. E., Jacobson, R. J., Melamed, J., and Hershman, J. M.: Choriocarcinoma as a cause of thyrotoxicosis. Am. J. Med., *60*:1036, 1976.

Murphy, B. E. P., and Pattee, C. J.: Determination of thyroxine utilizing the property of protein-binding. J. Clin. Endocrinol. Metabol., *24*:187, 1964.

Oppenheimer, J. H.: Interaction of drugs with thyroid hormone binding sites. Ann. N.Y. Acad. Sci., *226*:333, 1973.

Reichlin, S.: Regulation of the hypothalamic-pituitary-thyroid axis. Med. Clin. North Am., *62*:305, 1978.

Rosenberg, I. N.: Evaluation of thyroid function. N. Engl. J. Med., *286*:924, 1972.

Rubenstein, H. A., Butler, V. P., and Werner, S. C.: Progressive decrease in serum triiodothyronine concentrations in human aging: Radioimmunoassay following extraction of serum. J. Clin. Endocrinol. Metabol., *37*:247, 1973.

Saberi, M., and Utiger, R. D.: Serum thyroid hormone and thyrotropin concentrations during thyroxine and triiodothyronine therapy. J. Clin. Endocrinol. Metabol., *39*:923, 1974.

Schatz, D. L., Sheppard, R. H., Steiner, G., Chandarlapaty, C. S., and DeVeber, G. A.: Influence of heparin on serum free thyroxine. J. Clin. Endocrinol. Metabol., *29*:1015, 1969.

Schimmel, M., and Utiger, R. D.: Thyroidal and peripheral production of thyroid hormones. Ann. Intern. Med., *87*:760, 1977.

Solomon, D. H., Benotti, J., DeGroot, L. J., Greer, M. A., Oppenheimer, J. H., Pileggi, V. J., Robbins, J., Selenkow, H. A., Sterling, K., and Volpe, R.: Letter to the editor: Revised nomenclature for tests of thyroid hormones in serum. J. Clin. Endocrinol. Metabol., *42*:595, 1976.

Sterling, K.: Determinations of free thyroxine and free triiodothyronine in serum by equilibrium dialysis. *In* Breuer, H., Hamel, D., and Krüskemper, H. L. (eds.): Methods of Hormone Analysis. New York, John Wiley and Sons, Inc., 1976.

Sterling, K.: Diagnosis and Treatment of Thyroid Diseases. Cleveland, CRC Press Inc., 1975.

Sterling, K., and Lazarus, J. H.: The thyroid and its control. Annu. Rev. Physiol., *39*:349, 1977.

Sterling, K., Milch, P. O., Brenner, M. A., and Lazarus, J. H.: Thyroid hormone action: The mitochondria pathway. Science, *197*:996, 1977.

Sterling, K., Refetoff, S., and Selenkow, H. A.: T3 thyro-toxicosis. Thyrotoxicosis due to elevated serum triiodothyronine levels. J.A.M.A., *213*:571, 1970.

Tunbridge, W. M. G., and Hall, R.: Thyroid stimulating hormone. *In* Loraine, J. A., and Bell, E. T. (eds.): Hormone Assays and their Clinical Application. Edinburgh, Churchill-Livingstone, 1976.

Utiger, R. D.: The diverse effects of iodide on thyroid function. N. Engl. J. Med., *287*:562, 1972.

Utiger, R. D.: Serum triiodothyronine in man. Annu. Rev. Med., *25*:289, 1974.

Vagenakis, A. G., and Braverman, L. E.: Thyroid function tests—which one? Ann. Intern. Med., *84*:607, 1976.

Vagenakis, A. G., Wang, C., Burger, A., Maloof, F., Braverman, L. E., and Ingbar, S. H.: Iodide-induced thyrotoxicosis in Boston. N. Engl. J. Med., *287*:523, 1972.

Volpé, R.: The role of autoimmunity in hypoendocrine and hyperendocrine function. Ann. Intern. Med., *87*:86, 1977.

Volpé, R.: Thyroiditis: Current views of pathogenesis. Med. Clin. North Am., *59*:1163, 1975.

Wahner, H. W., and Walser, A. H.: Measurements of thyroxine-plasma protein interactions. Med. Clin. North Am., *56*:849, 1972.

Wellby, M. L.: The laboratory diagnosis of thyroid disorders. Adv. Clin. Chem., *18*:103, 1976.

Adrenal Medulla

Amery, A., and Conway, J.: A critical review of diagnostic tests for pheochromocytoma. Am. Heart J., *73*:129, 1967.

Engelman, K.: Pheochromocytoma. Clin. Endocrinol. Metabol., *6*:769, 1977.

Feldman, J. M., Butler, S. S., and Chapman, B. A.: Interference with measurement of 3-methoxy-4-hydroxyl-mandelic acid and 5-hydroxyindoleacetic acid by reducing metabolites. Clin. Chem., *20*:607, 1974.

Felice, L. J., and Kissinger, P. T.: A modification of the Pisano method for vanilmandelic acid using high pressure liquid chromatography. Clin. Chim. Acta, *76*:317, 1977.

Freier, D. T., and Harrison, T. S.: Rigorous biochemical criteria for the diagnosis of pheochromocytoma. J. Surg. Res., *14*:177, 1973.

Gitlow, S. E., Mendlowitz, M., and Bertani, L. M.: The biochemical techniques for detecting and establishing the presence of a pheochromocytoma. Am. J. Cardiol., *26*:270, 1970.

Gitlow, S. E., Mendlowitz, M., Wilk, E. K., Wilk, S., Wolf, R. L., and Bertani, L. M.: Excretion of catecholamine catabolites by normal children. J. Lab. Clin. Med., *72*:612, 1968.

Knight, J. A., Fronk, S., and Haymond, R. E.: Chemical basis and specificity of chemical screening tests for urinary vanilmandelic acid. Clin. Chem., *21*:130, 1975.

Kopin, I. J.: Catecholamine metabolism. Clin. Endocrinol. Metabol., *6*:525, 1977.

Mell, L. D., and Gustafson, A. B.: Urinary free norepinephrine and dopamine determined by reverse-phase high-pressure liquid chromatography. Clin. Chem., *23*:473, 1977.

Moskowitz, M. A.: Diseases of the autonomic nervous system. Clin. Endocrinol. Metabol., *6*:745, 1977.

Pisano, J. J.: A simple analysis for normetanephrine and metanephrine in urine. Clin. Chem. Acta, *5*:406, 1960.

Pisano, J. J., Crout, J. R., and Abraham, D.: Determination of 3-methoxy-4-hydroxymandelic acid in urine. Clin. Chem. Acta, *7*:285, 1962.

Pullar, I. A.: Catecholamines. *In* Loraine, J. A., and Bell, E. T. (eds.): Hormone Assays and Their Clinical Application. Edinburgh, Churchill-Livingstone, 1976.

Rayfield, E. J., Cain, J. P., Casey, M. P., Williams, G. H., and Sullivan, J. M.: Influence of diet on urinary VMA excretion. J.A.M.A., *221*:704, 1972.

Remine, W. H., Chang, G. C., Van Heerdan, J. A., Sheps, S. G., and Harrison, E. G.: Current management of pheochromocytoma. Ann. Surg., *179*:740, 1974.

Shou, R. E., and Kissinger, P. T.: Determination of urinary normetanephrine, metanephrine and 3-methoxy-tyramine by liquid chromatography, with amperometric detection. Clin. Chem., *23*:1268, 1977.

Steer, M. L.: Adrenergic receptors. Clin. Endocrinol. Metabol., *6*:577, 1977.

Taniguchi, K., Kakimoto, Y., and Armstrong, M. D.: Quantitative determination of metanephrine and normetanephrine in urine. J. Lab. Clin. Med., *64*:469, 1964.

Young, J. B., and Landsberg, L.: Catecholamines and intermediary metabolism. Clin. Endocrinol. Metabol., *6*:599, 1977.

Adrenal Cortex

Al-Dujaili, E. A. S., and Edwards, C. R. W.: The development and application of a direct radioimmunoassay for plasma aldosterone using ^{125}I-labeled ligand—comparison of three methods. J. Clin. Endocrinol. Metabol., *46*:105, 1978.

Atlas, S. A., Laragh, J. H., Sealey, J. E., and Moon, C.: Plasma renin and "prorenin" in essential hypertension during sodium depletion, beta-blockade, and reduced arterial pressure. Lancet, *2*:785, 1977.

Baum, C. K., Davison, M. J., and Landon, J.: Urinary free cortisol excretion by normal subjects. Proc. Soc. Endocrinol., *3*:47P, 1975.

Beevers, D. G., Brown, J. J., Fraser, R., Lever, A. F., Morton, J. J., Robertson, J. I. S., Semple, P. F., and Tree, M.: The clinical value of renin and angiotensin estimations. Kidney Int., 8:S-181, 1975.

Brown, J. J., Fraser, R., Lever, A. F., and Robertson, J. I. S.: Renovascular and other renal hypertension. Hosp. Pract., *9*:105, 1975.

Brunner, H. R., Laragh, J. H., Baer, L., Newton, M. A., Goodwin, F. T., Krakoff, L. R., Band, R. H., and Buhler, F. R.: Essential hypertension: Renin and aldosterone, heart attack and stroke. N. Engl. J. Med., *286*:441, 1972.

Bumpus, F. M., and Khosla, M. C.: Pathologic factors involved in renovascular hypertension: State of the art. Mayo Clin. Proc., *52*:417, 1977.

Burke, C. W., and Beardwell, C. G.: Cushing's syndrome. Q. J. Med., *42*:175, 1973.

Byyny, R. L.: Withdrawal from glucocorticoid therapy. N. Engl. J. Med., *295*:30, 1976.

Cave, W. T., Gaskin, J. H., and Owen, J. A.: Artifactual elevation of free cortisol. N. Engl. J. Med., *289*:870, 1973.

Conn, J. W., Rovner, D. R., and Cohen, E. L.: Licorice-induced pseudoaldosteronism. J.A.M.A., *205*:80, 1968.

Day, R. P., and Luetscher, J. A.: Big renin: A possible prohormone in kidney and plasma of patient with Wilms' tumor. J. Clin. Endocrinol. Metabol., *38*:923, 1974.

Dluhy, R. G.: Diagnosis and treatment of adrenocortical insufficiency. *In* Rose, L. I., and Lavine, R. L. (eds): The Thirty-ninth Hahnemann Endocrinology-Metabolism Symposium. New York, Grune and Stratton, Inc., 1976.

Drewes, P. A., Demetriou, J. A., and Pileggi, V. J.: Measurement of urinary aldosterone by a simplified radioimmunoassay procedure. Clin. Biochem., *6*:88, 1973.

Fukuchi, S., Takeuchi, T., and Torikai, T.: Determination of plasma renin activity by radioimmunoassay of angiotension I. Clin. Sci., *44*:43, 1973.

Galvao-Teles, A., Graves, L., Burke, C. W., Fotherby, K., and Fraser, R.: Free cortisol in obesity; effect of fasting. Acta Endocrinol., *81*:321, 1976.

Gavras, H., Brunner, H. R., Laragh, J. H., Sealey, J. E., Gavras, I., and Vukovich, R. A.: An angiotensin converting-enzyme inhibitor to identify and treat vasoconstrictor and volume factors in hypertensive patients. N. Engl. J. Med., *291*:817, 1974.

Gutai, J. P., Kowarski, A. A., and Migeon, C. J.: The detection of the heterozygous carrier for congenital virilizing adrenal hyperplasia. J. Pediatr., *90*:924, 1977.

Horton, R.: Aldosterone: Review of its physiology and diagnostic aspects of primary aldosteronism. Metabolism, *22*:1525, 1973.

Horton, R., and Finck, E.: Diagnosis and localization in primary aldosteronism. Ann. Intern. Med., *76*:885, 1972.

Hughes, I. A., and Winter, J. S. T.: The relationship between serum concentrations of 17-OH progesterone and other serum and urinary steroids in patients with congenital adrenal hyperplasia. J. Clin. Endocrinol. Metabol., *46*:98, 1978.

Jubiz, W., and Nolan, G.: N-Ethylmaleimide prevents destruction of corticotropin (ACTH) in plasma. Clin. Chem., *24*:826, 1978.

Juncos, L. I., Stong, C. G., and Hunt, J. C.: Prediction of results of surgery for renal and renovascular hypertension. Arch. Intern. Med., *134*:655, 1974.

Kaplan, N. M.: The prognostic implications of plasma renin in essential hypertension. J.A.M.A., *231*:167, 1975.

Kaplan, N. M., Kem, D. C., Holand, O. B., Kramer, N. J., Higgins, J., and Gomez-Sanchez, C.: Intravenous furosemide test: Simple way to evaluate renin responsiveness. Ann. Intern. Med., *84*:639, 1976.

Kem, D., Weinberger, M., and Mayes, D.: Saline suppression of plasma aldosterone in hypertension. Arch. Intern. Med., *128*:380, 1971.

Krakoff, L., Nicolis, G., and Amsel, B.: Pathogenesis of hypertension in Cushing's syndrome. Am. J. Med. *58*:216, 1975.

Krensky, A. M., Bonagiovanni, A. M., Marino, J. Parks, J., and Tenore, A.: Identification of heterozygote carriers of congenital adrenal hyperplasia by radioimmunoassay of serum 17-hydroxyprogesterone. J. Pediatr., *90*:930, 1977.

Krieger, D. T.: Diagnosis management of Cushing's syndrome. 28th Postgraduate Assembly of the Endocrine Society. Syllabus. Bethesda, Maryland, 1976.

Krieger, D. T.: Regulation of circadian periodicity of plasma ACTH levels. Ann. N.Y. Acad. Sci., *297*:561, 1977.

Krieger, D. T., Allen, W., Rizzo, F., and Krieger, H. P.: Characterization of the normal temporal pattern of plasma corticosteroid levels. J. Clin. Endocrinol. Metabol., *32*:266, 1971.

Laragh, J. H.: Vasoconstriction-volume analysis for understanding and treating hypertension: The use of renin and aldosterone profiles. Am. J. Med., *55*:261, 1973.

Laragh, J. H., Baer, L., Brunner, H. R., Buhler, F. R., Sealey, J. E., and Vaughan, E. D.: Renin, angiotensin and aldosterone system in pathogenesis and management of hypertensive vascular disease. Am. J. Med., *52*:633, 1972.

Liddle, U. G. W.: Cushing's syndrome. Ann. N.Y. Acad. Sci., *297*:594, 1977.

Mattingly, D.: A simple fluorimetric method for the estimation of free 11-hydroxycorticoids in human plasma. J. Clin. Pathol., *15*:374, 1962.

McGiff, J. C.: Bartter's syndrome results from an imbalance of vasoactive hormones. Ann. Intern. Med., *87*:369, 1977.

Meikle, A. W., Lagerquist, L. G., and Tyler, F. H.: Apparently normal pituitary-adrenal suppressibility in Cushing's syndrome: dexamethasone metabolism of plasma levels. J. Lab. Clin. Med., *86*:472, 1975.

Melby, J. C.: Assessment of adrenocortical function. N. Engl. J. Med., *285*:735, 1971.

Melby, J. C., and Dale, S. L.: Role of 18-hydroxy-11-deoxycorticosterone and 16α, 18-dihydroxy-11-deoxycorticosterone in hypertension. Mayo Clin. Proc., *52*:317, 1977.

Mendelsohn, F., Hutchinson, J., and Johnston, C. I.: A review of plasma renin measurements and their clinical significance. Aust. N.Z. J. Med., *1*:86, 1971.

Murphy, B. E. P.: Some studies on the protein binding of steroids and their applications to the routine micro and ultramicro measurement of various steroids in body fluids by competitive protein-binding radioassay. J. Clin. Endocrinol. Metabol., *27*:973, 1967.

National Center for Health Statistics: Hypertension and hypertensive heart disease in adults: United States. *In* Vital and Health Statistics, Series II, No. 13. Washington, D.C., U.S. Government Printing Office, May, 1966.

Oparil, S.: Theoretical approaches to estimation of plasma renin activity: A review and some original observations. Clin. Chem., *22*:583, 1976.

Oparil, S., and Haber, E.: The renin-angiotensin system (first of two parts). N. Engl. J. Med., *291*:389, 1974.

Orth, D. N., and Nicholson, W. E.: Different molecular forms of ACTH. Ann. N.Y. Acad. Sci., *297*:27, 1977.

Perez, G., Lespier, L., Jacobi, J., Oster, J., Katz, F., Vaamonde, C., and Fishman, L.: Hyporeninemic hypoaldosteronism in diabetes mellitus. Clin. Res., *24*:367, 1976.

Porter, C. C., and Silber, R. H.: A quantitative color reaction for cortisone and related 17,21, dihydroxy-20-ketosteroids. J. Biol. Chem., *185*:201, 1950.

Rees, L. H., Bloomfield, G. A., Gilkes, J. J. H., Jeffcoate, W. J., and Besser, G. M.: ACTH as a tumor marker. Ann. N.Y. Acad. Sci., *297*:603, 1977.

Rees, R. H., and Landon, J.: Adrenocorticotrophic hormone. *In* Loraine, J. A., and Bell, E. T.: Hormone Assays and Their Clinical Application. Edinburgh, Churchill Livingstone, 1976.

Rose, L. I., Williams, G. H., Jagger, P. I., and Lauler, D. P.: The 48-hour adrenocorticotrophin infusion test for adrenocorticol insufficiency. Ann. Intern. Med., *73*:49, 1970.

Saffran, M., and Schally, A. V.: Corticotropin-releasing factor isolation and chemical properties. Ann. N.Y. Acad. Sci., *297*:395, 1977.

Scriba, T. C., and Müller, O. A.: Determination of cortisol in serum by fluorimetry. *In* Brewer, H., Hamel, D., and Krüskemper, H. L. (eds.): Methods of hormone analysis. New York, John Wiley and Sons, Inc., 1976.

Sederberg-Olsen, P., Binder, C., and Kehlet, H.: Urinary excretion of free cortisol in impaired renal function. Acta Endocrinol., *78*:86, 1975.

Spiger, M., Jubiz, W., Meikle, A. W., West, C. D., and Tyler, F. H.: Single dose metyrapone test. Arch. Intern. Med., *136*:698, 1975.

Streeten, D. H. P., Anderson, G. H., Freiberg, J. M., and Dalakos, T. G.: Angiotensin II blockade in the hypertensive patient. Hosp Pract., *10*:83, 1975a.

Streeten, D. H. P., Anderson, G. H., Freiberg, J. M., and Dalakos, T. G.: Use of an angiotensin II antagonist (Saralasin) in the recognition of "angiotensinogenic" hypertension. N. Engl. J. Med., *292*:657, 1975b.

Streeten, D. H. P., Dalakos, T. G., and Anderson, G. H.: Diagnosis and treatment of Cushing's syndrome. *In* Rose, L. I., and Lavine, R. L. (eds.): The Thirty-ninth Hahnemann Endocrinology-Metabolism Symposium. New York, Grune and Stratton, Inc., 1976.

Streeten, D. H. P., Stevenson, C. T., Dalakos, T. G., Nicholas, J. J., Dennick, L. G., and Fellerman, H.: The diagnosis of hypercortisolism. Biochemical criteria differentiating patients from lean and obese normal subjects and from females on oral contraceptives. J. Clin. Endocrinol. Metabol., *29*:1191, 1969.

Stockigt, J. R., Collins, R. D., and Biglieri, E. G.: Determination of plasma renin concentration by angiotensin I immunoassay. Circ. Res., *28* (Suppl. 175), 1971.

Veteran's Administration Cooperative Study Group on Anti-hypertensive Agents. Effects of treatment on morbidity in hypertension II. Results in patients with diastolic blood pressure averaging 90 through 114 mm Hg. J.A.M.A., *213*:1143, 1970.

Weidmann, P., Reinhart, R., Maxwell, M. H., Rowe, P., Coburn, J. W., and Massry, S. G.: Syndrome of hyporeninemic hypoaldosteronism and hyperkalemia in renal disease. J. Clin. Endocrinol. Metabol., *36*:965, 1973.

West, C. D., and Dolman, L. I.: Plasma ACTH radioimmunoassays in the diagnosis of pituitary-adrenal dysfunction. Ann. N.Y. Acad. Sci., *297*:205, 1977.

Yalow, R. S., Glick, S. M., Roth, J., and Berson, S. A.: Radioimmunoassay of human plasma ACTH. J. Clin. Endocrinol. Metabol., 24:1219, 1964.

Youssefnejadian, E., and David, R.: Early diagnosis of congenital adrenal hyperplasia by measurement of 17-hydroxyprogesterone. Clin. Endocrinol., *4*:451, 1975.

Gonadotropins and the Sex Hormones

Abraham, G. E., Swerdloff, R., Tulchinsky, D., and Odell, W. B.: Radioimmunoassay of plasma progesterone. J. Clin. Endocrinol. Metabol., *32*:619, 1971.

Amelar, R. D., and Dubin, L.: Semen analysis. *In* Amelar, R. D., Dubin, L., and Walsh, P. C.: Male Infertility. Philadelphia, W. B. Saunders Company, 1977.

Baird, D. T.: Oestrogens in clinical practice. *In* Loraine, J. A., and Bell, E. T. (eds.): Hormone Assays and Their Clinical Application. Edinburgh, Churchill Livingstone, 1976.

Boyar, R. M., Rosenfeld, R. S., Kapen, S., Finkelstein, J. W., Roffwarg, H. P., Weitzman, E. D., and Hellman, L.: Human puberty. Simultaneous augmented secretion of luteinizing hormone and testosterone during sleep. J. Clin. Invest., *54*:609, 1974.

Brown, J. B., MacLeod, S. C., MacNaughtan, C., Smith, M. A., and Symyth, B.: A rapid method for estimating oestrogens in urine using semi-automatic extractor. J. Endocrinol., *42*:5, 1968.

Catt, K. J., and Dufau, M. L.: Basic concepts of the mechanism of action of peptide hormones. Biol. Reprod., *14*:1, 1976.

Franchimont, P.: Pituitary gonadotrophins. Clin. Endocrinol. Metabol., *6*:101, 1977.

Franchimont, P., Valcke, J. C., and Lambotte, R.: Female gonadal dysfunction. Clin. Endocrinol. Metabol., *3*:533, 1974.

Givens, J. R.: Hirsuitism and hyperandrogenism, Adv. Intern. Med., *21*:221, 1976.

Greenblatt, R. B., and Mahesh, V. B.: The androgenic polycystic ovary. Am. J. Obstet. Gynecol., *125*:712, 1976.

Henry, J. B., and Krieg, A. F.: Endocrine measurements. *In* Davidsohn, I., and Henry, J. B. (eds): Clinical Diagnosis by Laboratory Methods, 14th ed. Philadelphia, W. B. Saunders Company, 1969.

Jewelewicz, R.: Induction of ovulation: Current practice and prospects. Bull. N.Y. Acad. Med., *4*:466, 1976.

Kirschner, M. A., and Bardin, C. W.: Androgen production and metabolism in normal and virilized women. Metabolism *21*:667, 1972.

Marshall, J. C.: Investigative procedures. Clin. Endocrinol. Metabol., *4*:545, 1975.

Paulsen, C. A.: Diagnosis and management of male infertility. Twenty-eighth Annual Postgraduate Assembly of the Endocrine Society. Syllabus. Bethesda, Md., The Endocrine Society, 1976.

Prentice, L. G., and Ryan, R. J.: LH and its subunits in human pituitary, serum and urine. J. Clin. Endocrinol. Metabol., *40*:303, 1975.

Rabinowitz, D., and Spitz, I. M.: Isolated gonadotropin deficiency and related disorders. Isr. J. Med. Sci., *11*:1011, 1975.

Rose, L. I.: Evaluation and therapy of the hirsute female. *In* Rose, L. I., and Laven, R. L. (eds.): The Thirty-ninth Hahnemann Endocrinology Metabolism Symposium. New York, Grune and Stratton, Inc., 1976.

Rubens, R., Dhant, M., and Vermeulen, A.: Further studies on Leydig cell function in old age. J. Clin. Endocrinol. Metabol., *39*:40, 1974.

Ruder, H., Corvol, P., Mahoudeau, J. A., Ross, G. T., and Lipsett, M. B.: Effects of induced hyperthyroidism on steroid metabolism in man. J. Clin. Endocrinol. Metabol., *33*:382, 1971.

Schally, A. V., Kastin, A. J., and Coy, D. H.: LH-releasing hormone and its analogues: Recent basic and clinical investigations. Int. J. Fertil., *21*:1, 1976.

Walsh, P. C.: Endocrine evaluation of the infertile male. *In* Amelar, R. D., Dubin, L., and Walsh, P. C. (eds.): Male Infertility. Philadelphia, W. B. Saunders Company, 1977.

Wide, L.: Human pituitary gonadotropins. *In* Loraine, J. A., and Bell, E. T. (eds.): Hormone Assays and Their Clinical Application. Edinburgh, Churchill Livingstone, 1976.

Wotiz, H. H.: Determination of pregnanediol in urine by gas-liquid chromatography. *In* Breuer, H., Hamel, D., and Krüskemper, H. L.: Methods of Hormone Analysis. New York, John Wiley and Sons, Inc., 1976.

Yen, S. S. C., Tsai, C. C., Naftolin, F., Vandenberg, G., and Ajabor, L.: Pulsatile patterns of gonadotropin release in subjects with and without ovarian function. J. Clin. Endocrinol. Metabol., *34*:671, 1972.

Miscellaneous

Arendt, J., Wetterberg, L., Heyden, T., Sizonenko, P. C., and Paunier, L.: Radioimmunoassay of melatonin: Human serum and cerebrospinal fluid. Hormone Res., *8*:65, 1977.

Beck, C., and Burger, H. G.: Evidence for the presence of immunoreactive growth hormone in cancers of the lung and stomach. Cancer, *30*:75, 1972.

Braunstein, G. D., Vaitukaitis, J. L., Carbone, P. P., and Ross, G. T.: Ectopic production of human chorionic gonadotrophin by neoplasms. Ann. Intern. Med., *78*:39, 1973.

Demers, L. M., Allegra, J. C., Harvey, H. A., Lipton, A., Luderer, J. R., Mortel, R., and Brenner, D. E.: Plasma prostaglandins in hypercalcemic patients with neoplastic disease. Cancer, *39*:1559, 1977.

Gewirtz, G., Schneider, B., Krieger, D. T., and Yalow, R. S.: Big ACTH: Conversion to biologically active ACTH by trypsin. J. Clin. Endocrinol. Metabol., *38*:227, 1974.

Gill, J. R., Frölich, J. C., Bowden, R. E., Taylor, A. A., Keiser, H. R., Seyberth, H. W., Oates, J. A., and Bartter, F. C.: Bartter's syndrome: A disorder characterized by high urinary prostaglandins and a dependence of hyperreninemia on prostaglandin synthesis. Am. J. Med., *61*:43, 1976.

Hamilton, B. P.: Presence of neurophysin proteins in tumors associated with the syndrome of inappropriate ADH secretion. Ann. N.Y. Acad. Sci., *248*:153, 1975.

Hamilton, B. P. M., Upton, G. V., and Amatruda, T. T.: Evidence for the presence of neurophysin in tumors producing the syndrome of inappropriate antidiuresis. J. Clin. Endocrinol. Metabol., *35*:764, 1972.

Jones, J. E., Shane, S. R., Gilbert, E., and Flunk, E. B.: Cushing's syndrome induced by the ectopic production of ACTH by bronchial carcinoid. J. Clin. Endocrinol. Metabol., *29*:1, 1969.

Kahn, C. R., Rosen, S. W., and Weintraub, B. D.: Ectopic production of chorionic gonadotropin and its subunits by islet-cell tumors. N. Engl. J. Med., *297*:565, 1977.

Kelly, R. W.: Physical methods of measurement of prostaglandins. Clin. Endocrinol. Metabol., *2*:375, 1973.

Montgomery, D. A. D., and Welbourn, R. B.: Medical and Surgical Endocrinology. London, Edward Arnold Ltd., 1975.

Mundy, G. R., Raisz, L. G., Cooper, R. A., Schechter, G. P., and Salmon, S. E.: Evidence for the secretion of an osteoclast stimulation factor in myeloma. N. Engl. J. Med., *291*:1041, 1974.

Odell, W.: Glycopeptide hormones and neoplasms. N. Engl. J. Med., *297*:609, 1977.

Pearse, A. G.: The APUD cell concept and its implications in pathology. *In* Summers, S. C. (ed.): Pathology Annual. New York, Appleton-Century-Crofts, 1974.

Powell, D., Singer, F. R., Murray, T. M., Minkin, C., and Potts, J. T.: Nonparathyroid humoral hypercalcemia in patients with neoplastic diseases. N. Engl. J. Med., *289*:176, 1973.

Rees, L. H., Bloomfield, G. A., Gilkes, J. J. H., Jeffcoate, W. J., and Besser, G. M.: ACTH as a tumor marker. Ann. N.Y. Acad. Sci., *297*:605, 1977.

Rosen, S. W., and Weintraub, B. D.: Ectopic production of the isolated alpha subunit of the glycoprotein hormones. N. Engl. J. Med., *290*:1441, 1974.

Rosen, S. W., Weintraub, B. D., Vaitukaitis, J. L., Sussman, J. M., Hershman, J. M., and Muggia, F. M.: Placental proteins and their subunits as tumor markers. Ann. Intern. Med., *82*:71, 1975.

Seyberth, H. W., Segre, G. V., Morgan, J. L., Sweetman, B. J., Potts, J. T., and Oates, J. A.: Prostaglandins as mediators of hypercalcemia associated with cancer. N. Engl. J. Med., *293*:1278, 1975.

Stolbach, L. L., Krant, M. J., and Fishman, W. H.: Ectopic production of an alkaline phosphatase isoenzyme in patients with cancer. N. Engl. J. Med., *281*:757, 1969.

Tepperman, J.: Metabolic and Endocrine Physiology, 3rd ed. Chicago, Year Book Medical Publishers, Inc., 1973.

Vaitukaitis, J. L.: Peptide hormones as tumor markers. Cancer, *37*:557, 1976.

Vaughn, G. M., Pelham, R. W., Pang, S. F., Loughlin, L. L.,

Wilson, K. M., Sandock, K. L., Vaughn, M. K., Koslow, S. H., and Reiter, R. J.: Nocturnal elevation of plasma melatonin and urinary 5-hydroxyindoleacetic acid in young men: Attempts at modification by brief changes in environmental lighting and sleep and by automatic drugs. J. Clin. Endocrinol Metabol., *42*:752, 1976.

Wilson, B. W., Snedden, W., Silman, R. E., Smith, I., and Mullen, P.: A gas chromatography-mass spectrometry method for the quantitative analysis of melatonin in plasma and cerebrospinal fluid. Anal. Biochem., *81*:285 1977.

Wurtman, R. J., and Moskowitz, M. A.: The pineal organ (first of two parts). N. Engl. J. Med., *296*:1329, 1977a.

Wurtman, R. J., and Moskowitz, M. A.: The pineal organ (second of two parts). N. Engl. J. Med., *296*: 1977b.

Yalow, R. S., and Berson, S. A.: Characteristics of "big" ACTH in human plasma and pituitary extracts. J. Clin. Endocrinol. Metabol., *36*:415, 1973.

15

THERAPEUTIC DRUG MONITORING AND TOXICOLOGY

Joan H. Howanitz, M.D., Peter J. Howanitz, M.D., and
John Bernard Henry, M.D.

FUNDAMENTAL CONCEPTS

TYPES OF SERVICES

Clinical laboratory toxicology services may include overdose or emergency toxicology, drug abuse screening, and therapeutic drug monitoring. A toxicology laboratory may also contribute to public health screening or forensic toxicology. Drug analyses are used to establish or exclude drug overdose as a cause of selected clinical conditions, including coma; they may be helpful in establishing treatment regimens such as if and when dialysis should be employed.

Several problems are attendant with these services. Results must be made available rapidly so that therapy can be instituted promptly or, if necessary, further diagnostic steps taken. Since specimens arrive unpredictably, batch analysis is usually not possible. In addition, trained personnel must be available at all times. Because of the large variety of drugs that may be involved in acute poisonings, compromises must be made in terms of which determinations are offered. Information is available about the frequency with which drugs may lead to hospitalization and/or death, and attempts have been made to assess the clinical importance of the ability to identify and quantitate a particular agent. Choices are often based on the importance of the analyses, in terms of both the frequency of the poisoning and the clinical value of the results. Local factors must be taken into account; for example, in some areas of the nation certain abused drugs or industrial problems may be more common than in others (Done, 1977). The availability of the following determinations will suffice for about 80 per cent of acute intoxications: blood analysis of alcohol, salicylates, barbiturates, chlordiazepoxide, diazepam, and glutethimide, and the detection of phenothiazines and imipramine in urine (Jatlow, 1977). However, as the pattern of drugs involved in acute intoxications changes and as new treatment modalities become available, it becomes necessary to constantly re-evaluate the laboratory determinations that are made available.

Drug screening is used by drug treatment facilities to diagnose addiction, select patients for admission to treatment programs, and assess drug use patterns. In addition, patients are monitored in their progress toward discontinuation of drug use, and the success of such a program is evaluated. Frings (1977) offers further information on the role of the laboratory and its relationship to drug abuse treatment facilities. The special problems and demands of the laboratory in its role in forensic toxicology are reviewed by Sunshine (1977).

THERAPEUTIC DRUG MONITORING

Perhaps the most important and rapidly growing portion of clinical laboratory toxicology service is the area of therapeutic drug monitoring. After a diagnosis is made and an appropriate drug selected, one of the remaining problems for the clinician is identifying a dosage schedule which gives optimal drug concentration for the individual patient. If the drug concentration is too low, therapeutic failure may occur, and if it is too high, side effects may ensue. Drug dosage regimens necessary for optimal therapeutic effect differ widely among individual patients. Depending on the individual treated, the usual drug dosage may lead to toxicity or lack of efficacy. With some therapeutic agents, such as antihypertensives, the drug dosage may be adjusted depending on the patient's response. In many clinical situations, the best dosage schedule of a drug for an individual patient may be difficult to determine because the pharmacologic response cannot be readily quantitated. For some drugs, the intensity of the pharmacologic action and the severity of the side effects correlate better with the steady-state concentration in blood than with the daily dosage (Marks, 1973). Blood levels of certain drugs thus may be useful in determining the optimal drug dosage for a given individual.

For a drug to be therapeutically effective, it must reach the site of its intended pharmacologic activity within the body at a sufficient rate and in sufficient amounts to yield an effective concentration. Individual differences in absorption, distribution, metabolism, and excretion of drugs, as well as factors such as intercurrent disease and interaction with other therapeutic agents, account for differences in concentrations of drugs at the receptor sites and variation in response to a given concentration. In addition, the drug formulation used to treat a patient is important.

Bioavailability

Bioavailability describes the extent to which and the rate at which an active drug reaches the systemic circulation and ultimately the receptors or sites of action. Because a drug must cross several membranes, exist in numerous physiologic environments, and be subject to tissue uptake, biotransformation, and excretion, most of the administered dose never reaches the receptors. Different dosage forms of a drug may provide varying amounts of drug for absorption and thereby cause differences in the onset, extent, and duration of pharmacologic effects. In addition, excessive variation in tablet content of drugs has been reported; this problem is exemplified by digoxin. When a large batch of digoxin tablets is prepared, it is a challenge to be certain that every tablet has the same content of active glycoside and that it will be effectively and predictably released. Figure 15–1 is a schematic presentation of a 0.25 mg digoxin tablet: only about 1 part in 500 by weight is digoxin. The remainder of the tablet is made up of a variety of excipients (Butler, 1975). Dosage

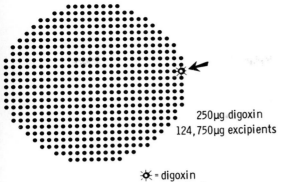

250μg digoxin
124,750μg excipients

☀ = digoxin
• = excipients

Figure 15–1. Schematic representation of a typical 0.25 mg digoxin tablet. Tablet weighs 125 mg (125,000 μg). White circle depicts 0.25 mg (250 μg) digoxin. Black circles represent various excipients. (With permission: Butler, V.P. and Lindenbaum, J.: Serum digitalis measurements in the assessment of digitalis resistance and sensitivity. Am. J. Med. 58:460, 1975.)

form variation of a drug due to manufacturing methods or physicochemical properties of the drug may modify the bioavailability.

Absorption

Absorption of drugs from the gastrointestinal tract is a complex process that is subject to many variables, such as pH, gastric emptying time, intestinal transit time, and mesenteric blood flow. When taken with food, drugs usually are absorbed more slowly and the total amount of absorption may be decreased. The presence of other drugs in the gastrointestinal tract may enhance or decrease absorption. Drug absorption may be altered in patients with gastrointestinal disease, and even under well-controlled conditions in healthy volunteers, wide individual differences occur in rates of absorption (Prescott, 1974). Even when drugs are administered by intramuscular or subcutaneous injection, the rate of absorption varies not only from individual to individual, but from site to site in the same patient (Marks, 1973). Orally administered drugs traverse the hepatic portal system before reaching the systemic circulation; thus if a drug is extensively cleared by the liver, only a small fraction of it will reach the systemic circulation. This so-called first pass elimination occurs with a number of therapeutic agents in common use and is one explanation why an intravenous dose of a drug may give a greater response than an equipotent oral dose. Propranolol is an example of a drug which is ex-

tensively removed on the first passage through the liver.

Distribution

After absorption, distribution of a drug will depend largely on its physicochemical properties, including lipid solubility, the extent to which it is ionized, and its molecular size. The property of lipid solubility allows drugs to cross biologic membranes, such as the blood-brain barrier and cell membranes. Highly ionized water-soluble drugs will cross such membranes only if they are of small molecular size. Drugs are transported to receptor sites via the blood, with serum albumin being an important carrier of many types of therapeutic agents. Interaction between proteins and drugs are reversible, with many drugs existing in the blood in two forms—protein-bound and free. Presumably only unbound drugs can diffuse into tissues because the drug-protein complex is unable to cross cell membranes. Drugs may be divided into water-soluble or polar compounds and lipid-soluble compounds. Water-soluble drugs are excreted mainly unchanged through the kidney, whereas lipid-soluble drugs initially are filtered by the glomerulus, but may be fully reabsorbed in the distal nephron. The lipid-soluble drugs are metabolized to more polar compounds before they are excreted in the urine. Metabolites that are formed usually, but not always, are less active than the parent compound. The liver is an active site of drug metabolism, but other tissues such as the kidney and intestine are also important.

Metabolism

A wide variety of biochemical reactions take place during the metabolism of a drug. These reactions may be divided into phase 1 and phase 2 reactions. In phase 1 reactions, polar compounds are introduced into the drug molecule by oxidation, reduction, or hydrolysis. Many of the phase 1 reactions are catalyzed by enzymes in the smooth endoplasmic reticulum of hepatic cells. Phase 2 reactions are synthetic and involve conjugation with glucuronic acid, sulfate, glycine, or other groups. Phenytoin (diphenylhydantoin), for example, is initially hydroxylated and then conjugated with glucuronic acid (Sjöqvist, 1976). Some drugs may pass through both types of reactions before being excreted, while others pass through only one or the other.

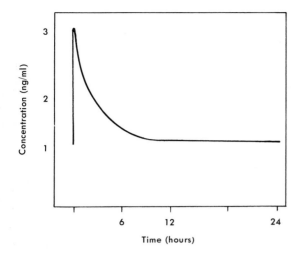

Figure 15–2. Serum digoxin concentrations following a single oral dose at steady state.

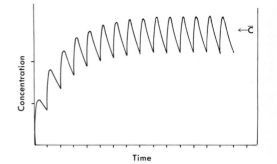

Figure 15–3. Serum drug concentrations when dosage interval is equal to serum half-life of drug. Four to seven doses are required to reach 95 per cent of the steady-state concentration.

Different kinetic variables have been used to assess rates of drug metabolism. When the fraction of drug that is eliminated from the body after a given time period is constant, it is meaningful to speak about the biologic half-life. With continuous administration of a drug by intravenous infusion, serum drug concentration gradually increases and eventually reaches a plateau or steady state. Following a period of infusion equal to four times the biologic half-life of the drug, the plasma concentration reaches about 90 per cent of steady-state levels. In the case of repetitive oral administration of the same dose of drug at regular intervals, concentrations in serum during the dosing interval first will increase and then decrease (Fig. 15-2). These changes result from absorption, distribution, and elimination with the magnitude in difference depending on the rate at which these events occur (Gibaldi, 1976). When the dosage interval of a drug is equal to the half-life of the drug, four to seven doses are required to reach 95 per cent of steady state (Fig. 15-3). In clinical practice, the measurement of steady-state serum concentrations may give an accurate index of drug metabolism. For some drugs, the rate of metabolism proceeds at a constant rate independent of the concentration of drug in the body. For others, the time required for an initial drug concentration to decrease by 50 per cent increases with increasing dose. This type of kinetics has been documented for a number of drugs, including phenytoin and salicylates. The clinical use of such drugs may be difficult, since small incre-ments of dose may result in a disproportionate increase in serum levels resulting in toxicity (Sjöqvist, 1976).

Influence of disease states

With disease states the absorption, distribution, metabolism, and excretion of drugs may be affected. Protein binding of drugs may be altered in certain clinical states; for example, in renal failure the percentage of binding of some acidic drugs to albumin is less than with normal renal function. This increase in free drug is a potential cause of toxicity. In uremia, drug metabolites may accumulate to toxic levels; even if non-toxic, metabolites may displace the bioactive parent drug from binding sites (Dettli, 1974). Uremic patients also show a slowing of certain pathways of drug metabolism and a decreased excretion of drugs and their metabolites. The existence of hepatic disease in a patient may significantly influence the efficacy or potential toxicity of a therapeutic regimen (Black, 1974). Diseases that induce disturbances in cardiac, renal, and hepatic function may result in variation of biologic half-lives of the drugs.

Usefulness of drug monitoring

A number of prerequisites are necessary if drug concentrations are to be useful in patient management. Drug concentrations must be interpreted in the context of the clinical data as well as with certain pharmacologic and methodologic factors in mind. There must be a reasonably good correlation between the concentration of drug and the therapeutic effect or toxicity. Although it may be a difficult task, determining serum levels of drugs is of most value when the therapeutically effective range of serum concentration is known with certainty. This effective range has been defined by clinical studies for a number of different drugs. Drug levels below the therapeutic range can exert beneficial effects but are inadequate in most patients, and some patients require high levels for a fully satisfactory response. In general, as the serum concentrations exceed the therapeutic range, the frequency and severity of toxic effects increase (Koch-Weser, 1972). There are a number of instances when there is a dissociation between the blood level and pharmacologic effect. Certain drugs, for example, may continue to exert their effect after they are no longer measurable in serum, and others localize in certain tissues, giving deceptively low serum levels. The serum half-life of the drug must be sufficiently long that minor differences in timing of specimen collection have only a small effect on interpretation of the value. Even with drugs having a relatively long half-life, the timing of the specimen collection is critical in the interpretation of concentrations. Generally, it is preferable to obtain the speciman at the end of the dosage interval or after an overnight fast (Marks, 1973). In certain clinical situations other times are preferable, for example, after a seizure in a patient receiving anticonvulsant drugs. It is important, however, to measure the concentration when the absorption and distribution are complete or nearly complete. Following the oral administration of digoxin, for example, serum levels peak at well above the usual therapeutic range. Toxic effects are not associated with these levels, since presumably myocardial levels are not correspondingly high. Serum digoxin levels reflect myocardial levels only at equilibrium, which generally occurs six to eight hours after the last oral dose. During intravenous infusions, blood specimens for drug levels are drawn after the steady state is reached. With intravenous administration of a drug, correlation between serum concentration and intensity of action is the least immediately after the dose is given (Koch-Weser, 1975). Although free drug is probably the active component, total drug concentrations are usually measured. In most therapeutic situations this is not a serious problem, since the free drug concentration is a fairly constant percentage of the total.

Serum levels are particularly useful if a drug is not readily monitored by clinical observations or if there is a wide pharmacokinetic variation among patients. Serum drug measurements are helpful when there is only a small difference between median toxic and effective concentrations; that is, if the therapeutic index of the drug is low. In addition, therapeutic monitoring is useful in patients with cardiac, renal, and hepatic dysfunction and when there is unexpected ineffectiveness or toxic manifestations. Drug level determinations may be helpful in a patient who does not comply with taking medications as directed. The percentage of noncompliant patients has been reported to vary in different clinical situations depending on such factors as the condition treated and the method of measuring adherence to the regimen. About 25 to 50 per cent of outpatients fail to take their medication. Although various methods have been developed to study compliance, one of the more accurate ways appears to be measurement of the drug or its metabolites in blood or urine (Komaroff, 1976). When many drugs are given concomitantly, some of which may alter the metabolism of others, it is also helpful to determine drug levels.

Salivary and cerebrospinal fluid levels have also been used to monitor drug therapy. For a number of therapeutic agents, it has been found that drug transfer from serum to saliva appears to be a passive, pH-dependent process, with salivary levels proportional to concentration of the compound in serum. It has been found that for several drugs, the concentration in saliva provides a good estimate of the free form of drug in serum without correction for pH (Dvorchik, 1976). Urine samples commonly are used to determine drug elimination and to screen for drug abuse.

The practical problem of which drug assays a laboratory should provide involves many considerations. One approach has been the development of a scoring system for the selection of the drugs. Dangerous toxicity without well-defined clinical endpoints and the width of the therapeutic range are two of the important considerations taken into account in the system proposed by Werner (1975).

Laboratory methods must be available which will yield accurate as well as precise results within a reasonable amount of time. In order for a laboratory to evaluate its performance, survey quality control programs are available, such as the College of American Pathologists toxicology series and the Antiepileptic Drug Level Quality Control Program (Pippenger, 1978). A number of techniques have been developed, such as immunoassay, gas chromatography, and high performance liquid chromatography, which are sensitive enough for the measurements of drugs at low serum concentrations. The given technique employed depends on many factors, including such practical considerations as availability of equipment and trained technical personnel. The results must be available rapidly and economically enough to be practical.

Therapeutic drug levels, in spite of their clinical value, cannot substitute for careful clinical observation and judgment. Drug levels must always be interpreted in the context of all clinical data.

CARDIAC GLYCOSIDES: DIGOXIN AND DIGITOXIN

The term *digitalis* is often used to designate the entire group of cardiac glycosides. These drugs have the ability to increase the force as well as the velocity of myocardial contraction. They are used in the treatment of congestive heart failure and arrhythmias such as atrial fibrillation and atrial flutter. Gastrointestinal manifestations are among the earliest symptoms of cardiac glycoside toxicity. Cardiac manifestations of digitalis toxicity include increasing severity of congestive heart failure and alterations in cardiac rate and rhythm. A wide variety of arrhythmias may occur, including extrasystole, atrioventricular dissociation, paroxysmal atrial tachycardia, and ventricular fibrillation.

Each cardiac glycoside is a combination of one or more sugars and an aglycone, which is the pharmacologically active residue (Fig. 15–4). Table 15–1 shows a comparison of two of the commonly prescribed cardiac glycoside preparations, digoxin and digitoxin. Digoxin differs from digitoxin by a hydroxyl group at carbon 12; this results in increased polarity and decreased lipid solubility. Absorption of digoxin tends to be enhanced by drugs that decrease gastrointestinal motility and decreased by drugs that increase motility.

Table 15–1. COMPARISON OF TWO CARDIAC GLYCOSIDE PREPARATIONS

	DIGOXIN	DIGITOXIN
Absorption (%)	60–75	90–100
Serum protein binding (%)	23	97
Metabolism in liver (%)	10	90
Elimination	90% excreted unchanged in urine	Metabolites excreted in urine, bile
Half-life (average)	35–40 hours	4–6 days
Usual therapeutic range (adults) in serum	0.5–2.0 ng/ml	9–25 ng/ml

In addition, compounds such as cholestyramine, kaopectate, and antacids can interfere with gastrointestinal absorption of digoxin. Cardiac glycosides circulate bound to serum proteins; approximately 23 per cent of digoxin and about 97 per cent of digitoxin is bound to serum proteins (Smith, 1973). The distribution of digoxin between heart and serum is approximately 29 to 1 even in the face of large differences in stores (Butler, 1972). The major site of digoxin deposition in the body is skeletal muscle, with lower concentrations found in fat (Marcus, 1975). Since digoxin is bound to tissues to a high degree, it is not effectively removed by dialysis; in addition, it has been shown that cardiopulmonary bypass and exchange transfusion remove only small amounts from the body (Smith, 1973). The half-life of digoxin in adults in the absence of renal failure is in the range of 35 hours, with shorter times reported in infants. The majority of digoxin is excreted in the urine unchanged, with only about 10 per cent of an orally administered dose metabolized. Digitoxin, which has a half-life of approximately 4.5 days, is metabolized in the liver and excreted mainly in altered forms with varying degrees of cardiac activity. Although some digitoxin is converted to digoxin, this is not a major metabolic pathway. Microsomal enzyme induction by various drugs may lead to increased metabolism of digitoxin, resulting in increased dosage requirements. In severe renal failure, the half-life of digoxin and digitoxin is about the same (Finkelstein, 1975). In renal failure, more digitoxin is metabolized to digoxin (Doherty, 1975).

Immunoassay usually is employed to deter-

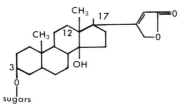

Figure 15–4. Structure of digitoxin. Digoxin differs from digitoxin by a hydroxyl group at carbon 12.

mine serum concentrations of the cardiac glycosides (see Chap. 13). Most assay procedures employ antiserum with specificity for the aglycone portion of the digitalis molecule. The metabolic breakdown products of the cardiac glycosides containing intact aglycone thus will react. In addition, antisera to one digitalis compound may cross-react to some extent with other cardiac glycosides and aglycones. Because of this cross-reactivity, digitalis immunoassays are meaningful only if it is known with certainty which glycoside the patient is receiving. Since digitoxin has a relatively high serum concentration and long half-life, it may interfere with the assay of digoxin for several weeks after it has been discontinued.

Following the administration of digitalis, the serum concentration rises, reflecting the entry of the glycoside into the circulation. The magnitude and rapidity of the increase reflects the dosage and route of administration. For example, when 0.5 mg of digoxin is given intravenously to a normal person receiving no digoxin, serum concentrations a few minutes later may be greater than 10 ng/ml. After the same oral dose, it may require an hour or more to reach peak serum concentrations which are in the range of 2 to 3 ng/ml (Butler, 1972). The rise in serum digitalis concentration is followed by a decrease reflecting the equilibrium phase that occurs as the glycoside is taken up by binding sites of the heart and other tissues. After equilibrium is completed, the serum digitalis concentration tends to stabilize and decline very slowly until the next dose is administered. Serum digitalis concentrations are meaningful only if the specimen is obtained during this plateau phase under steady-state conditions (see p. 480). After oral administration of digoxin, although the maximum serum concentration is usually obtained within one to two hours, in some individuals this takes three to four hours and tissue equilibrium may not be completed until four to six hours. It is recommended that blood specimens for serum digoxin levels be collected at least six and preferably at least eight hours after the last oral dose. Serum plateau levels of digoxin occur 10 to 12 hours after intramuscular (IM) administration and two to four hours after intravenous (IV) administration (Doherty, 1975). If serum levels are measured before equilibrium, very high values may be obtained; these levels do not result in toxicity because presumably these levels do not reflect myocardial drug levels. In order to interpret serum

digoxin values after IM or IV administration, serum samples must be obtained after appropriate time has elapsed; that is, when plateau levels have been reached.

The usual therapeutic range for digoxin in adults is 0.5 to 2 ng/ml, but a significant number of non-toxic patients have serum concentrations greater than 2 ng/ml, usually in the 2 to 4 ng/ml range. In most adult patients with evidence of digoxin toxicity, serum concentrations are in excess of 2 ng/ml, but some patients have levels in the range of 1.4 to 2 ng/ml (Butler, 1975). In the presence of supraventricular arrhythmias, some patients require high doses of digitalis to control their cardiac rate; these patients may have serum digoxin concentrations in the range of 2 to 4 ng/ml without evidence of clinical toxicity. A number of factors such as hypokalemia, hypothyroidism, severe heart disease, and renal function abnormalities may predispose a patient to digitalis toxicity.* Although elevated serum calcium may potentiate the toxic effects of the cardiac glycosides, this has not been a consistent finding in all studies (Smith, 1975). A number of workers have reported relatively high serum digoxin levels in infants; in digoxin-treated children more than two years of age, serum digoxin levels more closely resemble adult values (Butler, 1972). An overlap between toxic and therapeutic range also occurs in patients receiving digitoxin. Serum digitoxin concentrations in patients without toxicity usually are between 5 and 40 ng/ml, whereas in patients with toxicity, serum levels are usually greater than 25 ng/ml (Butler, 1975). Patients taking digitalis leaf have serum digitoxin concentrations comparable to those taking crystalline digitoxin (Smith, 1975). It has been recommended that blood specimens for serum digitoxin levels be collected at least six to eight hours after the last oral or parenteral dose. Because of the long half-life, differences in serum concentration after various routes of administration are not significant (Doherty, 1975).

ANTIARRHYTHMIC AGENTS

PROCAINAMIDE

Procainamide, a p-aminobenzamide, is used in the treatment of ventricular and atrial cardiac arrhythmias. Serious toxic manifestations such as hypotension and cardiac disturbances

---

*The relationship of red cell electrolyte concentration and digoxin has been reviewed (Loes, 1978).

including ventricular asystole or fibrillation may occur, especially after intravenous administration. With procainamide, there is a wide variation in the ratio of the daily dose to plasma concentration due to individual differences in absorption, apparent volume of distribution, and rate of elimination of the drug. Although absorption from the gastrointestinal tract is 75 to 95 per cent complete in most subjects, some patients absorb less than half of the oral dose. About 15 per cent of plasma procainamide is bound to protein.

The mean biologic half-life of procainamide in subjects without major abnormalities in renal function is 3.5 hours; however, there is wide variation among individuals. The apparent volume of distribution is decreased in the presence of low cardiac output, and renal insufficiency markedly prolongs the biologic half-life (Koch-Weser, 1971). A major pathway of procainamide elimination is excretion of the unchanged drug in the urine. The major metabolite of procainamide is *N*-acetyl procainamide (NAPA) which is almost equally active and may exceed the plasma concentration of the parent drug. It has been shown that there is considerable individual difference in the ratio of NAPA and procainamide in plasma (Elson, 1975). Some of the procainamide also may be hydrolyzed to para-amino-benzoic acid.

Procainamide and NAPA can be measured simultaneously by gas chromatography or high performance liquid chromatography (Carr, 1976). Procainamide and NAPA can each be determined fluorometrically (Matusik, 1975). The usual effective antiarrhythmic concentration of procainamide has been reported as 4 to 8 $\mu g/ml$, with only an occasional patient showing a better therapeutic effect at 8 to 12 $\mu g/ml$. Toxic manifestations commonly occur at concentrations greater than 16 $\mu g/ml$; they are rare with concentrations less than 12 $\mu g/ml$ (Koch-Weser, 1971).

QUINIDINE

Quinidine, a cinchona alkaloid, is used in the treatment of atrial fibrillation and certain other cardiac arrhythmias. Although the most common toxic reactions are gastrointestinal, sudden death and serious manifestations including cardiac arrhythmias may occur. In addition, quinidine is associated with idiosyncratic and hypersensitivity reactions. After oral administration, quinidine is well absorbed from the gastrointestinal tract, with maxi-

mum effects occurring within one to three hours. The biologic half-life is about five hours. Quinidine is approximately 85 per cent bound to plasma protein; however, the protein binding may vary in individuals and has been reported to be impaired in some patients with renal disease. The major pathway of quinidine elimination in man is metabolism to hydroxyl derivatives, with a minor pathway the renal excretion of unchanged quinidine (Kessler, 1974a). Dihydroquinidine, which has been found in commercial quinidine preparations, has been shown to have antiarrhythmic activity equal to or greater than quinidine.

Most methods for the quantitative determination are based on the ability of quinidine to fluoresce in acid. Fluorometric determinations of quinidine generally fall into two categories: direct methods involving protein precipitation and extraction methods involving the use of organic solvents to extract the quinidine (Osinga, 1976). Most methods measure both quinidine and dihydroquinidine. In general, protein precipitation methods measure quinidine as well as its metabolites, which are considered to be remarkably lower in toxicity and antiarrhythmic activity than the parent drug. The apparent prolongation of plasma quinidine half-life in patients with poor renal function is thought to be due to fluorescent metabolites that are excreted slowly by these patients. Kessler (1974b), using a double extraction technique, found quinidine elimination to be grossly normal in patients with poor renal function or with congestive heart failure.

The use of certain blood collection tubes may cause small decreases in plasma quinidine levels (Shand, 1976). Therapeutic effectiveness has been reported to be associated with steady-state plasma quinidine concentrations of 2.3 to 5 $\mu g/ml$ at the end of the dosage interval (Kessler, 1974a).

LIDOCAINE

Intravenous (IV) administration of lidocaine is commonly used in the treatment of ventricular arrhythmias. Usually the drug is administered in one to three intravenous boluses given 5 to 10 minutes apart until the arrhythmia stops or toxicity occurs. To sustain plasma concentrations, an intravenous infusion of lidocaine is started, ranging from 20 to 50 $\mu g/min/kg$ (1.4 to 3.5 mg/min) in a 70 kilogram patient (Melmon, 1973). Plasma levels, however, will vary with individual variations in lidocaine clearance; conservative doses may be necessary in certain patients such as those with severe heart failure. It is metabolized mainly in the liver to N-dealkylated metabolites, such as monoethylglycinexylidide and glycinexylidide, which are pharmacologically active. The elimination half-life of lidocaine is approximately two hours; however, the plasma clearance may be reduced in patients with congestive heart failure and liver disease. In patients with poor renal function, the active lidocaine metabolite glycinexylidide may accumulate (Collinsworth, 1975).

Several methods are available for the measurement of lidocaine, including gas chromatography (Adjepon-Yamoah, 1974) and homogeneous enzyme immunoassay (Cobb, 1977). The usual therapeutic range of lidocaine is 1.2 to 5.5 µg/ml; at levels greater than 9 µg/ml, convulsions, central nervous system depression, and hypotension may occur. Similar toxic manifestations occasionally may be seen at lower plasma levels. Measurement of plasma lidocaine may be useful in patients with heart failure or renal disease: in interpreting values, the time lag in reaching a plateau must be taken into consideration. When infusion rates are changed, the time to reach plateau plasma concentrations in normal subjects is about five to eight hours; however, in patients with heart failure or liver disease this may take an even longer period (Thomson, 1973).

PROPRANOLOL

Propranolol (Inderal) is a beta-adrenergic blocking agent that is used in the treatment of a number of clinical conditions including cardiac arrhythmias, angina pectoris, and hypertension. Although there is controversy regarding the mechanism of its antihypertensive activity, it has been suggested that propranolol lowers blood pressure in essential hypertension via renin-dependent and renin-independent effects (Hollifield, 1976). Propranolol produces most of its important effects, both beneficial and adverse, by blocking the beta effects of the catecholamines. Adverse effects of propranolol include precipitation of heart failure, bronchospasm, bradycardia, and hypoglycemia.

After an oral dose, propranolol is well absorbed from the gastrointestinal tract. It has a half-life of about three hours and is metabolized mainly in the liver. One of the active propranolol metabolites, 4-hydroxypropranolol, is known to contribute to beta blockade after oral administration of the drug. The contribution to therapy of this and the other propranolol metabolites is unclear. It has been suggested that six hours after oral administration, effects are largely due to propranolol itself. Although in an individual plasma levels of propranolol after oral administration are relatively consistent, there is a wide variation in concentrations attained among individuals given the same dose (Shand, 1970). These large differences, which may be up to 20-fold, are due to individual differences in the ability of the liver to extract propranolol from blood (Shand, 1975).

Commonly, fluorometric techniques have been used to measure propranolol (Shand, 1970; Ambler, 1974), but gas chromatographic procedures have been developed as well (DiSalle, 1973). Spuriously low propranolol values have been reported with the use of certain blood collection tubes. Substances in the stopper reduce plasma propranolol binding and results in redistribution of the drug such that greater amounts are present in the blood cells and less in the plasma (Cotham, 1975).

Plasma propranolol levels of 50 to 100 ng/ml at the end of the dosage interval confer a high degree of beta blockage in most patients. These levels also have been associated with alleviation of angina, antiarrhythmic activity, and lowering of plasma renin activity (Shand, 1975).

ANTICONVULSANTS

PHENYTOIN

Phenytoin (diphenylhydantoin or Dilantin) is the drug of choice for tonic-clonic (grand mal) seizures. It appears to inhibit the spread of seizure activity in the motor cortex by stabilizing neurons against hyperexcitability by promoting sodium efflux. Its general usefulness results from its ability to limit the development of seizure activity and to stop the spread of seizures from an active focus. It exerts these effects without causing generalized central nervous system depression. Phenytoin also exerts stabilizing effects on membranes, which may underlie its effectiveness in the relief of pain in neuralgias and its reduction of ventricular ectopic activity in digitalis intoxication.

Table 15-2. PHARMACOLOGIC PROPERTIES OF SIX ANTIEPILEPTIC DRUGS

DRUG	DOSAGE mg/kg	mg/day	EXPECTED SERUM LEVEL, μg/ml RANGE	DAYS TO ACHIEVE STEADY-STATE BLOOD LEVEL	SERUM HALF-LIFE (hours)	SERUM LEVELS THERA-PEUTIC μg/ml	TOXIC μg/ml	ACTIVE METABOLITES
Phenytoin	1	–	1–3	5–10	24 ± 12	10–20	20	HPPH
	–	300–400	5–20					
Phenobarbital	1	–	5–15	14–21	96 ± 12	10–30	40	Parahydroxy phenylbarbital
	–	180	10–30					
Primidone	1	–	0.5–3	4–7	12 ± 6	5–12	15	PEMA
	–	750	5–15					
Phenobarbital	Derived		5–32	14–21	–	–	–	
Ethosuximide	1	–	1–4	8–10	60	40–80	100	–
	–	1000	40–100		(30 ±)*			
Carbamazepine	1	–	0.1–0.5	2–4	12 ± 3	3–10	8	10, 11 epoxide
	–	1200	3–12					
Valproic Acid	20–30	1500			8–15	50–100		–

*In children and adolescents.
Modified from Kutt, H.: Arch. Neurol., *31*:283, 1974.

Absorption of phenytoin from the gastrointestinal tract usually occurs within 3 to 12 hours, but it may be decreased by food or antacids. Since neonates cannot absorb phenytoin for the first few months of life, other anticonvulsants are used in this age group. The usual maintenance dose is 300 to 400 mg/day or 1 mg/kg (Table 15-2). Because blood levels rise slowly after the ingestion of phenytoin, it usually is given in one dose to increase patient compliance (Strandjord, 1974). However, others believe that giving the drug in divided doses throughout the day is more appropriate. Phenytoin also can be given by the intramuscular route; however, its absorption can be erratic and slow. This slow absorption is probably a consequence of its precipitation in muscle; it has been shown that absorption may occur for up to four or five days after a single intramuscular dose. For those patients who cannot take oral medication, therapeutic phenytoin levels can be maintained by using the intravenous route, but close supervision of the patient is necessary because of potential adverse cardiovascular effects. For this reason Perrier (1976) has developed a protocol to maintain therapeutic levels utilizing intramuscular injections. Intracellular level in the brain approaches two to three times that of serum.

Although phenytoin is one of the most thoroughly investigated anticonvulsants, its metabolism is still not fully elucidated. Less than 5 per cent is excreted unchanged in the urine, while the remainder is metabolized primarily by the hepatic microsomal enzyme system. About two thirds of the administered dose is metabolized to para-hydroxyphenylhydantoin (HPPH), which then is conjugated to glucuronide and eliminated in the urinary and biliary tracts. The presence of liver disease results in reduced capacity to metabolize phenytoin, and thus toxicity may occur at the usual doses. The rate of hydroxylation of phenytoin is dose-dependent at low concentrations, and as the concentration increases, the hydroxylation increases. At serum concentrations in the therapeutic range (15 to 20 μg/ml) the metabolism becomes independent of serum concentration, because the hydroxylating system for the metabolism of phenytoin is saturated. Thus, small increases in the dose result in much greater increases in serum levels than they do at lower levels (Richens, 1975).

About 90 to 95 per cent of phenytoin is bound to serum albumin with the remainder free or unbound. In uremia, serum protein binding is decreased, resulting in reduced total drug concentration and an increased percentage of free drug. Acetylsalicylic acid (aspirin), sulfisoxazole, phenylbutazone, and chlorthiazide also reduce the amount of binding of phenytoin to albumin, but other drugs known to bind albumin, such as penicillin G or phenobarbital, have little effect on this binding (Porter, 1975). Isoniazide (INH) is recognized to change phenytoin levels. In about 10 per cent of patients, INH has been reported to inhibit the degradation of phenytoin to HPPH, thereby raising the phenytoin concen-

Table 15–3. DRUGS THAT ELEVATE
SERUM PHENYTOIN LEVELS

DRUG	PROBABILITY OF SIGNIFICANT ELEVATIONS OF PHENYTOIN LEVEL
Disulfiram	High
Isoniazid	Moderate
Dicumarol	Low
Chloramphenicol	Low
Chlordiazepoxide hydrochloride or diazepam	Low
Sulfamethizole	–
Phenylbutazone	Low
Sulfaphenazole	?Low
Ethosuximide	Low
Chloropromazine hydrochloride	Low
Chlordiazepoxide	Low
Propoxyphene	Low
Phenobarbital	Low

Modified from Kutt, H.: Arch. Neurol., *31*:283, 1974.

tration and producing toxic manifestations. Patients who genetically are slow inactivators of INH are most susceptible. In addition, elevations of serum phenytoin concentrations occur when disulfuram is taken. The decreased amount of HPPH in the urine with this drug suggests that it inhibits the hydroxylating system from forming HPPH. Other drugs that may increase serum levels of phenytoin by increasing the half-life are dicumarol and chloramphenicol. Several of these are shown in Table 15–3. Some drugs, including carbamazepine, ethanol, and folate, decrease phenytoin concentration, presumably by stimulation of its metabolism. Phenobarbital may have one of three effects on phenytoin: it has been reported to stimulate the metabolizing enzyme system, to compete with phenytoin for these enzymes, or to have no effect on its metabolism. Thus, administration of phenobarbital to a patient receiving phenytoin can decrease, increase, or have no effect on phenytoin concentrations. Phenytoin also increases phenobarbital concentrations while decreasing digitoxin, dicumarol, metyrapone, dexamethasone, cortisol, 25-OH-calciferol (25-OH-D$_3$), and folate. Its effects on thyroid hormone assays are reviewed in Chapter 14.

Current methods of phenytoin analysis include gas chromatography, radioimmunoassay, homogeneous enzyme immunoassay, and spectrophotometry. A comparison of these methods was reported by Spiehler (1976). With a method developed for high-performance liquid chromatography, the simultaneous analysis of phenytoin and four other commonly used anticonvulsants can be accomplished (Kabra, 1977).

The therapeutic range of phenytoin is usually recognized to be from 10 to 20 μg/ml. Occasionally, levels of 14 to 20 μg/ml result in nystagmus on a lateral gaze, but this is usually observed when levels exceed 20 μg/ml. Other signs of intoxication, such as slurred speech and ataxia, develop when blood concentrations approach 30 μg/ml (Lund, 1974); mental changes such as somnolence occur at 40 μg/ml. Elderly patients show greater mental changes at a given serum concentration of phenytoin than do younger patients. At higher levels, such as above 60 μg/ml, some patients are unable even to sit up (Plaa, 1975). Paradoxical intoxication has been described by Troupin (1975), who noted increased seizure activity as the serum level of phenytoin was increased in the toxic range. This study emphasizes the necessity of obtaining serum levels rather than empirically changing the dose.

The therapeutic range for the antiarrhythmic effects of phenytoin appears to be about the same as a therapeutic range for the anticonvulsant effects (Karlsson, 1975). About three fourths of the responsive arrhythmias were abolished at serum levels of 10 to 18 μg/ml (Bigger, 1968).

Although there is a direct relationship between phenytoin serum concentrations and clinical toxicity, there are frequent exceptions. With decreased serum proteins, differences in the protein-bound and free phenytoin affect the relationship between total serum concentrations and the degree of clinical intoxication. However, attempts at measuring free serum phenytoin concentrations are tedious (Booker, 1973), making them of little clinical utility. Such specimens as saliva or cerebrospinal fluid are utilized because these represent sources of relatively free material (Horning, 1977). Although not widely utilized at this time, these approaches represent areas for future investigation.

BARBITURATES

Barbiturates are a group of sedative-hypnotic drugs which are frequently the cause of accidental and intentional poisonings, i.e. suicide and homicide.

Barbituric acid

Over 100 years ago, Von Baeyer prepared barbituric acid from the condensation of urea and malonic acid. Barbituric acid is a six-member ring with a ketone group at C2, C4, and C6 (see Fig. 15-5).

To obtain barbiturates with hypnotic action, both hydrogens on the carbon atom in position 5 must be replaced with alkyl or aryl groups. Some barbiturates, such as thiopental, have a sulfur instead of a carbonyl oxygen at position 2 and are used as anesthetic agents. If the nitrogen at position 3 is methylated, the affinity for lipids increases, and the duration of action tends to be decreased. Mephobarbital is the only one of the clinically important barbiturates that contains a methyl group at this location; however, it is metabolized to phenobarbital. In general, structural changes that increase lipid solubility increase rate of absorption, decrease the duration of activity, and tend to increase degradation. A phenyl group at C-5, such as is present in phenobarbital, confers selective anticonvulsive activity. Changes in the acetyl side chain at C-5 also affect activity. If the chain is too long, hypnotic activity decreases and anticonvulsant properties may disappear.

Barbiturates are divided into long-acting (six hours or more), intermediate-acting (three to six hours), short-acting (less than three hours), and ultrashort-acting (10 to 15 minutes) (Table 15-4). The ultrashort-acting agents are used as intravenous anesthetics, the short- and intermediate-acting agents as sedative hypnotics, and long-acting barbiturates used as antiepileptic agents. The anticonvulsant and hypnotic activities are independent variables and dependent on the individual barbiturate.

Barbiturates reversibly depress the activity of all excitable tissue in the central nervous system, but not all tissues are affected by the same dose or concentration. All degrees of depression of the central nervous system are seen—from mild sedation to coma—with the degree of depression depending on the dose, the route of administration, and the particular barbiturate. Absorption of short-acting barbiturates is much more rapid than the long-acting barbiturates, with peak levels obtained within 30 minutes. Long-acting barbiturates such as phenobarbital peak in 12 to 18 hours or longer, with a serum half-life in adults of about four to six days (Glazko, 1975).

Phenobarbital is one of the least toxic and most effective of the anticonvulsants. Since phenobarbital has the greatest anticonvulsant potency of all barbiturates, there is generally no reason to use any of the other barbiturates for this indication. It is particularly useful for treating tonic-clonic (grand mal) and complex partial seizures. When tonic-clonic seizures are incompletely suppressed by phenytoin alone, phenobarbital may be added. The drug may be used alone for tonic-clonic seizures in infants and preschool children for whom it is the drug of choice because of adverse effects with phenytoin. Phenobarbital is considered one of the least toxic drugs with the major side effect drowsiness; at low serum levels tolerance oc-

Table 15-4. CLASSIFICATION OF SELECTED BARBITURATES ON THE BASIS OF DURATION OF HYPNOTIC ACTION AFTER AVERAGE ORAL DOSE

GENERIC NAME	TRADE NAME	R_1	R_2	R_3	X
Long-acting (6 or more hours)					
Phenobarbital	Luminal	ethyl	phenyl	H	O
Mephobarbital	Mebaral	ethyl	phenyl	CH_3	O
Barbital	Veronal	ethyl	ethyl	H	O
Short-acting (less than 3 hours) to intermediate-acting (3 to 6 hours)					
Amobarbital	Amytal	ethyl	isopentyl	H	O
Butabarbital	Butisol	ethyl	isopentyl	H	O
Secobarbital	Seconal	allyl	1-methylbutyl	H	O
Pentobarbital	Nembutal	ethyl	1-methylbutyl	H	O
Ultra short-acting (intravenous anesthetic)					
Thiopental	Pentothal	ethyl	1-methylbutyl	H	S

H = Hydrogen
O = Oxygen
S = Sulfur

curs within a few weeks and the drowsiness disappears. In the elderly, phenobarbital may cause stimulation of the central nervous system, with confusion and delirium, while in young children irritability may occur. Nystagmus and ataxia also occur acutely, but diminish as sedation decreases.

About 25 per cent of the phenobarbital is excreted unchanged in the urine. The major metabolite is parahydroxyphenylbarbital, a compound with weak anticonvulsant activity of its own. Since this metabolite is rapidly removed from the blood by conjugation and renal filtration, it does not contribute significantly to the anticonvulsant activity of phenobarbital. The metabolite appears in the urine mainly as a glucuronide or sulfate conjugate.

Analysis of phenobarbital is readily accomplished by gas chromatography, which is quite specific and sensitive (Kupferberg, 1970). Other procedures, such as homogeneous enzyme immunoassay and high performance chromatography (Kabra, 1977), have been used. Each of these methods is specific and quite sensitive.

A serum concentration of 10 to 30 μg/ml, which can be reached in about 2 to 3 weeks of therapy, is effective in the control of seizures (Table 15-2). Higher doses are required in children, as the rate of elimination appears to be greater. Serum levels of phenobarbital below 15 μg/ml are frequently ineffective in controlling seizures, while those between 40 and 60 μg/ml may be associated with somnolence (Kutt, 1974). Withdrawal of phenobarbital in patients taking high doses can lead to the precipitation of status epilepticus. Adverse effects are not observed with chronic therapy when serum concentrations are less than 30 μg/ml. Although about 20 per cent of those taking phenobarbital have a depressed serum calcium and elevated alkaline phosphatase, osteomalacia due to increased vitamin D_3 metabolism occurs rarely (Anast, 1975). Phenobarbital also decreases the absorption and increases the metabolism of hydroxycoumarin. Phenobarbital may enhance the metabolism of digitoxin, presumably by induction of hepatic microsomal enzymes, resulting in decreased serum digitoxin levels and hence underdigitalization.

Barbiturate poisoning is a common problem which remains one of the leading causes of coma secondary to drug ingestion. Phenobarbital, pentobarbital, and secobarbital are the most commonly abused barbiturates. A method commonly used for barbiturate identification is a barbiturate screen, which is based on the differential absorption of the barbiturate in the ultraviolet range (Goldbaum, 1952). In acid solution, barbiturate is ionized with almost no absorption from 230 to 270 nm. At pH 10, one ionized group with absorption maximum of 240 occurs and at a pH of 14, a second form with absorption maximum of 252 and minimum of 235 is found (Fig. 15-5). However, if a barbiturate has a methyl group on C-3, such as mephrobarbital, it is capable of having only one ionized form and one maximal absorption at 245 nm. A di-

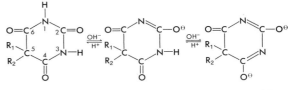

Acid form
Non-ionized acid pH

First ionized form
pH 10

Second ionized form
pH 14

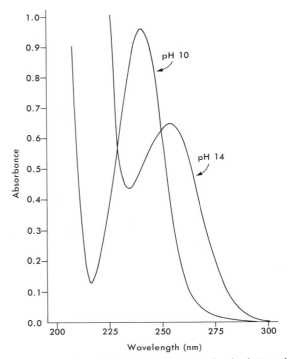

Wavelength (nm)

Figure 15-5. A typical absorption curve of a disubstituted barbiturate. Because of the distinguishing absorption characteristics two ionizable forms at pH 10 and 14, a differential scan can be used to identify the presence of barbiturates.

rect comparison of the aliquots at pH 14 and pH 10 can be made with a single scan in a double-beam spectrophotometer or in a single-beam instrument by using the pH 10 aliquot as a blank. For a drug to interfere with this assay, it must be extracted with chloroform and show a spectral shift upon changing the pH from 10 to 14. Salicylates and sulfonamides are the most commonly cited drugs which interfere but with the modifications of Jatlow (1973), the interference of these drugs as well as others is minimal. The barbiturate can be identified as a member of its respective group by heat treatment of an alkali extract. Fast-acting barbiturates are more resistant to this treatment, while slow- and intermediate-acting are more likely to be hydrolyzed to barbituric acid and urea. This ultraviolet analysis for barbiturates is sensitive, accurate, and specific but does not indicate which particular barbiturate is present. Other methods of barbiturate identification include thin layer chromatography, gas chromatography, and radioimmunoassay. These have been compared by Roerig (1975). A homogeneous enzyme immunoassay is available (Walberg, 1974) as is a procedure for the simultaneous identification of six individual barbiturates using high performance liquid chromatography (Tjaden, 1977).

The serum barbiturate level in an overdose is an unreliable guide to therapy. Patients who have used barbiturates habitually, particularly those who are addicted to such agents, may tolerate far larger dosages than persons who are not habitual users. For example, a secobarbital addict may be alert with serum secobarbital level of 20 μg/ml, while a person who has not developed a tolerance to secobarbital would probably be comatose with a similar serum level. The clinical implication of any given concentration is more serious for the shorter-acting barbiturates than for phenobarbital. In general, a serious reaction is likely to occur when the amount ingested is more than 10 times the oral hypnotic dose. Potentially lethal serum levels are those in excess of 80 μg/ml for phenobarbital, 50 μg/ml for amobarbital and butabarbital, and approximately 30 μg/ml for secobarbital. It should be noted that such levels represent those in which a patient takes an acute dose. Because of wide individual variations in tolerance, serum barbiturate determinations are useful primarily to establish the identity of the agent. If a barbiturate is found in a seriously ill patient, a

determination of the barbiturate as long-, medium-, or short-acting should be made, since this may influence treatment. Although there appears to be no correlation between barbiturate levels and the length of coma (Matthew, 1975), a clear-cut correlation between length of coma and the depth of coma has been observed (Arieff, 1973).

Since the majority of deaths are due to respiratory causes, close observation of the unconscious patient for apnea is necessary. With the longer-acting barbiturates, there is some evidence that an osmotic diuresis is helpful in the renal elimination of the barbiturates, but with an intermediate- and a short-acting barbiturate, diuresis is of little value. Forced alkaline diuresis will remove long-acting barbiturates and should be used when a patient is severely intoxicated by such a preparation. Hemodialysis is capable of removing large quantities of long-acting barbiturates from the body with the reduction in serum concentration parallelling clinical improvement. Since short-acting barbiturates are lipid-soluble and have low serum protein binding and high tissue binding, lipid hemodialysis has been successful in limited clinical trials.

PRIMIDONE

Primidone (Mysoline) is a desoxy derivitive of phenobarbital. It is converted in the body to phenobarbital by oxidation and then to phenylethylmalonamide (PEMA) by ring cleavage. Both metabolites have anticonvulsant activity. Primidone has been found to elevate the threshold for seizures: PEMA shows antiepileptic properties itself and has synergistic action with phenobarbital. Primidone alone or combined with phenytoin are the agents of choice in partial seizures (temporal lobe epilepsy). The ratio of phenobarbital to the parent drug during steady-state equilibrium in blood of patients taking primidone alone is usually about 1 to 1. Fincham (1974) has reported that this ratio was over 4:1 in patients receiving phenytoin and primidone. A possible cause for this increase of phenobarbital to primidone ratio is thought to be the induction of the enzyme system responsible for the conversion of primidone to phenobarbital. In some patients, primidone levels are increased after administration of carbamazepine.

Primidone is rapidly absorbed in the gastrointestinal tract, with a mean half-life of about 12 to 14 hours. The half-life of its active metabolites phenobarbital and PEMA are 96 hours and 24 to 48 hours, respectively. Primidone and PEMA are poorly bound to protein, while phenobarbital is about 60 per cent protein bound. In patients who ingest the usual therapeutic dose of primidone, neither phenobarbital or PEMA are produced in the first 24 hours. However, in patients on phenytoin who acutely ingest toxic levels of primidone, phenobarbital has been found to occur within the first 12 hours.

The method of choice for measurement has been gas chromatography (GC). Kupferberg (1970) has reported a GC method in which multiple anticonvulsants can be estimated simultaneously using a single injection. Development of a homogeneous enzyme immunoassay has provided a method of convenient quantitation. There appears to be no cross-reactivity with PEMA, although phenytoin and phenobarbital react to a small extent in this assay. In a comparison of the GC and enzyme immunoassay, a good correlation was found by Sun (1976). High performance liquid chromatography also has been used (Kabra, 1977).

The maintenance levels of primidone are 5 to 12 μg/ml serum, although effective control in some patients may require serum concentrations outside this range (Table 15-2). Toxic effects may occur with levels over 15 μg/ml, but data are still incomplete. The major side effect is profound sedation, while ataxia may or may not occur. Sedation is usually observed on initiation of treatment and may persist for several days. However, the patient usually adapts to this and other acute side effects such as vertigo, dizziness, nausea, diplopia, and nystagmus. Chronic side effects are very similar to those of phenobarbital.

Although the relationship of serum levels of primidone, phenobarbital, and PEMA in acute toxicity have not been delineated, Brillman (1974) has suggested that toxicity correlates best with primidone levels. In his study, when coma was rapidly disappearing, primidone levels were falling from toxic to therapeutic levels. At the same time, phenobarbital and PEMA were increasing. In some patients with acute primidone intoxication, hexagonal primidone crystals have been identified in the urine (Cate, 1975).

ETHOSUXIMIDE

Ethosuximide (Zarontin) is considered to be the drug of choice for absence seizures (petit mal epilepsy). The frequency of seizures is reduced by the depression of the motor cortex and elevation of the threshold to convulsive stimulation. It also depresses the paroxysmal spike and wave seizure pattern.

Ethosuximide is absorbed almost completely from the gastrointestinal tract. Peak serum levels are found within four hours after ingesting a dose. The half-life is about 60 hours in adults and 30 hours in children: an 8 to 10 day period is required to obtain a steady-state concentration. Serum concentrations are the same whether the dose is given once a day or in divided doses (Goulet, 1976). Although once a day dosage maintains therapeutic levels (Buchanan, 1976), this regimen is more likely to produce gastrointestinal upset by direct gastric irritation. There appears to be very little protein binding, and cerebrospinal fluid concentrations are quite similar to serum levels. While about 30 per cent of ethosuximide appears unchanged in the urine, at least five hydroxylated derivatives, some of them conjugated to glucuronide, are also found.

Gas chromatography has been used for measurement of ethosuxide since it was introduced for clinical use, and more recently homogeneous enzyme immunoassay has been developed. These two methods have been shown to compare favorably (Sun, 1977). Desmethylmethsuximide, the active metabolite of methsuximide (Celantin), has been reported to cross-react in the homogeneous enzyme immunoassay for ethosuximide (Pippenger, 1978). A method has been described using high performance liquid chromatography in which all five commonly used anticonvulsants are determined simultaneously after one extraction (Kabra, 1977).

Clinical control of seizures occurs when serum levels are from 40 to 80 μg/ml (Penry, 1972) (Table 15-2), although a few patients cannot be controlled even when serum levels reach 120 to 150 μg/ml (Baird, 1977). In children levels as high as 170 to 190 μg/ml may be tolerated without evidence of toxic effects. The relationship of serum concentration to adverse affects has not been completely established. In some studies adverse reactions did not occur, while in others almost half the patients had side effects. Most common side effects that have been reported are gastric distress, loss of appetite, fatigue, lethargy, headaches, and dizziness; these appear to be related to the dose. Side effects that are not dose-related include skin rashes and hematologic manifestations such as eosinophilia, leukopenia, and thrombocytopenia, and systemic lupus erythematosis. Rarely, psychotic episodes have been described in adolescents. There are no reports indicating that serum levels of ethosuximide are altered by other drugs (Kutt, 1975b). In general, adverse reactions to ethosuximide are usually of a minor nature and can be minimized by careful adjustments of the dose over a period of time (Schottelius, 1978).

Carbamazepine

Carbamazepine (Tegretol) is used for tonic-clonic (grand mal) seizures, psychomotor seizures, and trigeminal neuralgia, alone or in combination with other drugs. It has pharmacologic properties similar to those of phenytoin, but the mechanism of action is still unknown. It depresses convulsive activity, alleviates paroxysms of trigeminal neuralgia, and depresses digitalis-induced cardiac arrhythmias. Gastrointestinal absorption is extremely slow, with peak levels occurring between 6 and 24 hours after an oral dose (Morselli, 1975). About 24 per cent of the carbamazepine is found in the unbound form in serum, while the rest is bound to serum proteins, mainly albumin. Its half-life is 8 to 20 hours.

Carbamazepine is almost completely metabolized, with less than 1 per cent occurring unchanged in the urine. The major pathway is thought to be metabolism to the 10,11 epoxide, which then is converted to a 10,11 dihydroxide compound. The epoxide, which has a concentration in serum of about 10 per cent of the parent drug, is important because it has anticonvulsant activity (Frigerio, 1975). The metabolism of carbamazepine to the 10,11 epoxide can be enhanced by other antiepileptic drugs. About 20 per cent of the administered dose of the parent drug is excreted in the urine as the dihydroxide, two thirds of this metabolite in the free form and one third conjugated, probably to glucuronide.

Methods of measurement of carbamazepine include ultraviolet and visual spectrophotometry, gas-liquid chromatography, and high performance liquid chromatography. These have been reviewed by Kutt, 1975a. High performance liquid chromatography methods are available which measure carbamazepine and four of the commonly used anticonvulsants simultaneously (Kabra, 1977). Homogeneous enzyme immunoassay methods also are available and are quite specific.

The side effects of carbamazepine include drowsiness, blurring of vision, and paresthesias (Livingston, 1974). With massive overdosage of carbamazepine, seizures have been reported, but the role of the drug has not been established with certainty (Cereghino, 1975). Other side effects are rare and have recently been reviewed by Pisciotta (1975). Carbamazepine may cause nystagmus at serum levels from 1.5 to 6 μg/ml, and headache, feelings of inhibition, and disturbances of vision occur at levels of 8.5 to 10 μg/ml or greater. Serum concentrations greater than 10 μg/ml often are associated with unsteadiness of gait, but data are still incomplete (Kutt, 1974). Although the therapeutic range is not known with certainty, 3 to 10 μg/ml currently is accepted (Table 15–2). Some workers, however, have suggested a lower range. The serum concentration is decreased by the concurrent administration of phenytoin, phenobarbital, or primidone. Idiosyncratic reactions such as leukopenia, thrombocytopenia, and pancytopenia have been found to occur rarely (Pisciotta, 1975).

Valproic Acid

Valproic acid (Depakene) has found increasing use in the treatment of tonic-clonic seizures (grand mal epilepsy) and absence seizures (petit mal epilepsy) in children, both alone and in combination with other anticonvulsants (Simon, 1975). It was released by the FDA in mid 1977 and probably will be used with increasing frequency for seizures refractory to other drugs. The main side effect is fatigue, often associated with hypersalivation, but sedation and alopecia occur occasionally.

Valproic acid was first used as an antiepileptic drug in 1963. However, its mode of action still remains to be defined. It is absorbed rapidly after oral administration, with the peak concentration occurring within four hours after ingestion. Since its biologic half-life is between 8 and 15 hours, it is given in three divided doses during the day. Because of the relatively short half-life and the relatively rapid absorption, the daily fluctuations in serum concentration of valproic acid are marked (Loiseau, 1975). About 90 per cent of the drug in serum is bound to proteins (Wulff, 1977). Although metabolic pathways of degradation still have not been elucidated, it appears that very little of the drug is metabolized, and most appears in the urine unchanged. To keep phenobarbital levels in the therapeutic range when administered with valproic acid, phenobarbital dosage must be reduced by approximately one third.

The most widely used method of determination is gas-liquid chromatography (Löscher, 1977). Therapeutic range is between 50 to 100 μg/ml (Table 15-2). In some studies a correlation between concentrations of valproic acid in serum and clinical effects, including the adverse reactions, have not been demonstrable (Wulff, 1977; Loiseau, 1975).

BENZODIAZEPINES

Benzodiazepines are the most commonly prescribed drugs in the United States. They are used mainly for the treatment of anxiety; however, other uses include the treatment of status epilepticus and alcohol withdrawal. In addition, they are used in the induction of amnesia during minor surgical procedures.

DIAZEPAM

The most widely prescribed of the benzodiazipines is diazepam (Valium). When given by the intravenous route, peak serum diazepam levels occur in 15 minutes, while by the intramuscular or oral route, peak levels occur in 30 and 60 minutes, respectively. Diazepam, which is about 95 per cent bound to albumin, has a biologic half-life of 54 hours. Diazepam is metabolized to desmethyldiazepam, which is active and has a half-life of 92 hours. A hydroxylated metabolite of desmethyldiazepam, oxazepam, is also active. Oxazepam, marketed commercially as Serax, has a much shorter half-life than diazepam and shows very little accumulation in serum with chronic dosing. A urine glucuronide conjugate of oxazepam is its major metabolite.

Methods for diazepam analysis include gas chromatography (Rey, 1977), but with this method the active metabolites are not measured. With ultraviolet spectrophotometric methods, values are found that are higher than those obtained by gas chromatography, probably because the active metabolites are measured (Rejent, 1976). A high performance liquid chromatographic technique has been developed (Harzer, 1977) which separates chlordiazepoxide, diazepam, oxazepam, and a fourth commonly used benzodiazepine, flurazepam (Dalmane), with one injection. This method is especially useful for the detection of benzodiazepines in suicide attempts.

Serum diazepam concentrations associated with clinical efficacy or toxicity have not been clearly established. The concentration of diazepam and its metabolite are between 0.1 and 1.0 μg/ml with chronic therapy, while after a single oral dose of 10 to 15 mg, peak levels range from 0.2 to 0.3 μg/ml within two hours. Nearly all subjects show signs of drowsiness with this range of serum concentrations. With chronic diazepam administration, tolerance develops. Whereas the acute administration of diazepam may cause profound symptoms when serum levels are above 0.4 μg/ml, with chronic dosage these levels result in few symptoms (Hillestad, 1974a; 1974b). When diazepam is given acutely, desmethyldiazepam is in lower concentration than the parent drug (Kaplan, 1973), but after discontinuance of diazepam or with chronic therapy, this metabolite may be found in higher concentrations.

Patients who have ingested a toxic dose in a suicide attempt may present with lethargy, stupor, or coma which can progress to frank respiratory depression. When ethanol and diazepam are ingested together, diazepam concentrations are significantly higher than when diazepam was ingested alone (Hayes, 1977). It was concluded that ethanol enhanced diazepam absorption; this may account for the enhanced sedation and respiratory insufficiency which occurs when they are ingested together. In a large series, about 15 per cent of those attempting suicide with drugs used diazepam, and about half of these took ethanol in addition (Rejent, 1976). Many similar studies indicate the importance and significance of ingesting this combination of ethanol and diazepam.

CHLORDIAZEPOXIDE

Chlordiazepoxide (Librium) is a benzodiazepine which is used as an antianxiety agent, as a hypnotic, and for the treatment of acute alcohol withdrawal. In suicide attempts, it is one of the most common agents used, either alone or in combination with other drugs. It is slowly absorbed from the gastrointestinal tract and may take several hours to reach peak concentrations. When given by the intramuscular route, peak serum chlordiazepoxide levels occur much later and are much lower than when given by the oral route (Greenblatt, 1974b). This is important when treating alcohol withdrawal and rapid therapy is needed. About 90 per cent of the drug is bound to serum proteins, and its half-life is one to two days. Two active metabolites, a lactam and demethylated derivative, occur. Small amounts of free and conjugated chlordiazepoxide are found in the urine.

After overdoses of chlordiazepoxide, qualitative identification can be performed using thin layer chromatography. The usual methods of quantitation of chlordiazepoxide are those employing ultraviolet spectrophotometry (Jatlow, 1972), fluorimetry (Schwartz, 1966), gas chromatography, or high performance liquid chromatography (Harzer, 1977).

After chronic oral therapy with total daily doses of 75 to 150 mg, serum levels are in the range of 3.2 to 6.9 $\mu g/ml$ (Greenblatt, 1974a), and at this level patients are profoundly sedated. A large series of patients have been reported who had serum determinations performed after ingesting up to 2 grams of chlordiazepoxide (Cate, 1973). With serum levels greater than 20 $\mu g/ml$, drowsiness or stupor occurred, but even at levels of about 60 $\mu g/ml$, coma did not ensue.

Regardless of the level, if a patient is in coma following chlordiazepoxide overdose, another drug or cause of the coma should be suspected. When combined with other central nervous system depressants, an additive effect with chlordiazepoxide occurs. Since about three fourths of all cases of overdosage with chlordiazepoxide involve a second drug, the additive central nervous system depressant effects are exceedingly important.

TRICYCLIC ANTIDEPRESSANTS

Amitriptyline, imipramine, and related compounds are tricyclic drugs that are widely used for the treatment of depression. The most frequent side effects caused by amitriptyline and imipramine are those attributable to anticholinergic effects, including dry mouth, constipation, dizziness, palpitations, and urinary retention. Acute toxicity due to overdosage of the tricyclic antidepressants may lead to coma, cardiac arrhythmias, tachycardia, and blood pressure changes. Electrocardiographic changes, which include prolongation of PR and QRS intervals and changes in the ST-T waves, may occur as well. Children and the elderly may require conservative dosage schedules for the tricyclic antidepressants. It has been suggested that elderly patients may show severe adverse effects from high doses owing at least in part to decreased drug metabolism, decreased protein binding, and increased receptor sensitivity (Hollister, 1977).

Tricyclic antidepressants are metabolized by the liver; the tertiary amine compounds such as amitriptyline and imipramine are desmethylated to secondary amines which are pharmacologically active. Amitriptyline is metabolized to nortriptyline, imipramine to desimipramine. The metabolites nortriptyline and desimipramine also have been used as tricyclic antidepressants, however, they appear to be no more effective and perhaps less effective than the parent compounds. Over 90 per cent of amitriptyline and nortriptyline are bound to plasma proteins.

The tricyclic antidepressants can be measured by gas chromatography with the use of a nitrogen detector (Dorrity, 1977). They show a wide variation in steady-state plasma concentration among patients, with this variation thought to be genetically determined. Plasma concentrations of tricyclic antidepressants can be increased by concomitant administration of drugs that inhibit oxidative phosphorylation in the liver. Several clinical trials have found a correlation between the plasma level and the clinical response. Therapeutic range for nortriptyline has been reported to be about 50 to 140 ng/ml (Åsberg, 1974). In patients treated with amitriptyline, Ziegler (1976) reported an optimal range of total tricyclic levels (amitriptyline and nortriptyline) of 160 to 240 ng/ml. Others have found no other important correlations between therapeutic outcome and the steady-state plasma levels of amitriptyline and its active metabolite nortriptyline (Coppen, 1978).

Serious tricyclic overdose has been reported when total plasma levels are equal to or greater than 1000 ng/ml (Spiker, 1975). In this study total plasma tricyclic levels were determined by GC-mass spectrometry, a technique which allowed quantitation of all available tricyclic antidepressants and their metabolites. Plasma levels may remain elevated for several days after the acute ingestion, particularly if the patient has ingested a tertiary tricyclic antidepressant. Occasionally patients have maintained toxic drug levels for five to six days. The prolonged elevation of the tricyclic antidepressant plasma levels following an overdose has several clinical implications. It has been suggested that sustained drug levels may play a role in unexpected cardiac death, which has been reported in some patients three to six days after the overdose. If a serious overdose is suspected, it has been recommended that patients have continuous cardiac monitoring for five to six days (Spiker, 1976). In patients with total tricyclic antidepressant levels greater than 1000 ng/ml, the QRS interval of the ECG has been reported to be equal to or greater than the upper limit of normal (100 milliseconds). As the total plasma tricyclic level falls, a decrease in the duration of the QRS may be used to assist in the clinical evaluation of patients with serious tricyclic overdose (Spiker, 1975).

GLUTETHIMIDE

Glutethimide (Doriden) is an orally effective non-barbiturate hypnotic which is no longer used widely. Severe glutethimide poisoning results in a mortality of almost 15 per cent (Holland, 1975); this was reported to be the highest mortality of all drug-induced comas (Arieff, 1973). Glutethimide is absorbed erratically from the gastrointestinal tract, with blood levels varying about twofold and plateau values about sixfold. This has been attributed to its very low aqueous solubility and its extreme solubility in lipoidal tissue. After absorption, it is concentrated in adipose tissue and subsequently released into the blood. About 2 per cent of ingested drug in the body is present in the blood with about 50 per cent of that in blood bound to serum proteins. Hepatic degradation yields inactive glucuronide metabolites that are excreted in both the urine and the bile, while less than 2 per cent is excreted in the urine unchanged. An active metabolite 4-HG (4-hydroxy-2-ethyl-2-phenylglutarimide) has been identified that is in higher concentration than glutethimide itself and may even be more potent. The average serum half-life of glutethimide is 10 hours, but in acute intoxication it may be as long as 105 hours.

Glutethimide has been measured by gas chromatography; a method has been described which simultaneously measures the parent drug and 4-HG (Hansen, 1974). Therapeutic serum levels of glutethimide are about 5.0 μg/ml, but there is great individual variation.

In contrast to severe barbiturate intoxication, coma may be of unusually long duration, but the respiratory depression and hypotension are probably no more frequent. Pulmonary edema, cerebral edema, convulsions, and sudden apnea are encountered at an extremely high frequency with overdoses. A dose of 5 g is sufficient to produce severe intoxication, while the lethal dose is between 10 and 20 g. Deep unconsciousness or coma usually occurs when glutethimide levels approach 30 μg/ml, and when serum levels range from 30 to 200 μg/ml death may occur. Hemodialysis has been recommended for intoxication or serum levels greater than 30 μg/ml (Schreiner, 1971), but the benefit of dialysis remains controversial. If serum levels of glutethimide are followed during hemodialysis, they are misleading, since serum glutethimide may be efficiently cleared without removing glutethimide which is in tissues. As a result, the management of glutethimide overdoses is complicated by poor correlation between glutethimide serum levels and the clinical course.

When the clinical course of a patient ingesting an overdose was related to the sum of the serum levels of glutethimide and 4-HG, adjusted for their relative potency, a good correlation was seen (Hansen, 1975). If these data are confirmed in a large series of patients, then quantitative serum levels may prove useful.

PHENOTHIAZINES

Chlorpromazine and related phenothiazine derivatives are among the most widely used drugs. They are employed in the treatment of psychoses, but they have other important uses, such as the control of nausea and vomiting. Side effects include weakness, orthostatic hypotension, and palpitations. A number of neurologic manifestations also may occur; these include a parkinsonian syndrome and acute dystonic reactions such as torticollis. Although phenothiazines have a high therapeutic index, occasionally they may cause serious overdose. There is a wide range of plasma levels achieved among patients. The main metabolic pathway is hydroxylation and subsequent conjugation with glucuronic acid; however, formation of sulfoxides also occurs (Cimbera, 1972). Although chlorpromazine has a half-life of about six hours, metabolites may be excreted in the urine for months after cessation of the drug.

Analysis is complicated by the fact that there are many phenothiazine derivatives employed therapeutically, and phenothiazines undergo extensive metabolism in the body. Screening methods are available for detection of phenothiazines in urine; the main difficulty is lack of specificity. One commonly used procedure employs FPN reagent (mixture of ferric chloride, perchloric, and nitric acids); this reagent is mixed with urine and the color observed immediately (Forrest, 1961). A pink, red, or purple color indicates that phenothiazines may be present. Since false positives may occur, confirmatory tests are required for positive identification. False negatives are uncommon after ingestion of relatively large amounts of phenothiazines.

For a review of phenothiazine methods, see Cimbera (1972). A high performance liquid chromatographic method has been reported by Williams (1977).

SALICYLATES

Salicylates are non-addictive analgesics which also have remarkable antipyretic, anti-inflammatory, and antirheumatic effects in man. The first description of salicylates was by Hippocrates, but it was not until 100 years ago that their toxicity was recognized. One out of every four cases of childhood poisoning is due to the ingestion of salicylates (Andrews, 1973). Despite the use of safety containers since 1970, the accidental ingestion of salicylates remains the single most common cause of drug toxicity in preschool children (Pierce, 1974). Toxicity has also been observed in chronic users, both children and adults, but these may not always be obvious. In a study by Anderson (1976), 30 per cent of adult salicylate intoxication went unrecognized for up to 72 hours and occurred in patients on chronic salicylate therapy. Salicylates are also one of the drugs most commonly ingested in suicide attempts.

Salts of salicylic acid are rapidly absorbed, mainly from the small intestine, with peak levels achieved in two to four hours. However, this absorption is quite variable and dependent on tablet dissolution. The salicylic acid salts, such as acetylsalicylic acid (aspirin), are rapidly hydrolyzed in the circulation to free salicylic acid, which then is bound principally to albumin. Although up to 90 per cent of the salicylic acid may be bound to serum proteins, at toxic serum levels protein binding is exceeded and an increased percentage of the salicylate remains unbound. Salicylates are metabolized to salicyluric acid and a phenolic glucuronide through the two major pathways, which become saturated when the concentration of salicylate is in the therapeutic range. The contribution of the metabolism of salicyluric acid and the glucuronide to the elimination of salicylate is in the therapeutic range. the therapeutic range, with the renal excretion attaining more importance as salicylate levels rise. This results in a more than proportional increase in serum salicylate levels with increases in dosage (Levy, 1972). Renal excretion of salicylic acid, a weak acid, is dependent upon hydrogen ion concentration, with a more alkaline environment favoring salicylic acid dissociation and promoting its more rapid excretion. This mechanism is exceedingly sensitive to even small changes in urine pH, and increased excretion can be promoted by infusions of bicarbonate. Such decreases in urine pH can markedly decrease the excretion, resulting in toxicity. The use of certain antacids to prevent gastric irritation also results in an increased urinary pH. In a group of children who had a therapeutic salicylate level, when antacids which contained aluminum and magnesium hydroxide were added to the regimen, serum salicylate levels fell below the therapeutic range (Levy, 1975).

Major toxic effects are those of gastrointestinal irritation, vomiting, epigastric discomfort, and hemorrhage, but frank bleeding is uncommon. The hemorrhage may be related to the decreased levels of clotting factors, the impairment of platelet function, and perhaps an increased capillary fragility. Other symptoms of toxicity include tinnitus, irritability, and irrationality similar to the alcoholic intoxication but without the euphoria. Toxicity may progress to coma and death. One of the most important side effects of salicylates is the direct stimulatory effect on the central nervous system. Early in the course of intoxication, hyperpnea may occur, lowering the Pco_2 and causing a respiratory alkalosis. A metabolic acidosis soon intervenes from the renal compensation for the respiratory alkalosis and from an accumulation of salicylic acid itself. Other metabolic acids also accumulate because salicylate interferes with intermediary metabolism and increases lipid metabolism, producing an accumulation of fatty acids and ketones. Salicylates also act to uncouple oxidative phosphorylation, causing an increased metabolic rate and producing mild hyperglycemia which rarely exceeds 200 mg/dl (11.0 mmol/l). Patients on chronic salicylate therapy for acute rheumatic fever, juvenile rheumatoid arthritis, rheumatoid arthritis, systemic lupus erythematosus, or Reiter's syndrome (Ricks, 1976), as well as normal subjects (O'Gorman, 1977), have been reported to develop hepatotoxicity. Non-cardiogenic pulmonary edema has been recognized as a compli-

cation of salicylate intoxication (Temple, 1976). If this side effect occurs, modalities of treatment other than large amounts of alkaline fluids are necessary.

A screening test for salicylates involves the addition of ferric chloride in acid to urine resulting in a purple color. Even if a small amount of salicylate, such as one tablet, is ingested, a color develops. This color reaction is non-specific in that many substances, such as amino acids, keto acids, and certain drugs also react to produce a colored product (see Chap. 19) (Chiou, 1973). A commonly used procedure for measuring serum salicylate is the

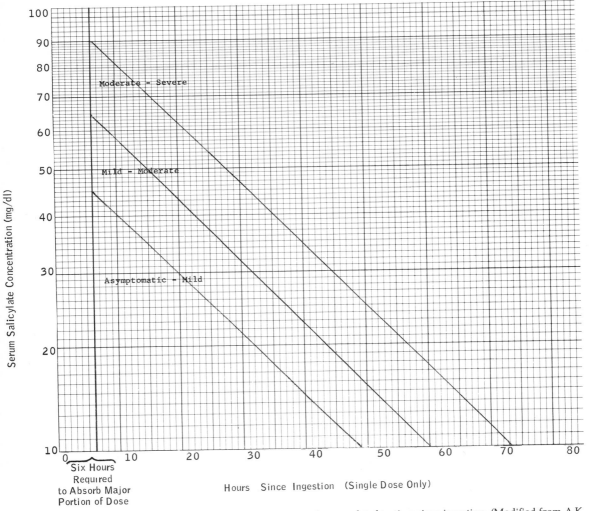

Figure 15-6. Toxicity in children (salicylism) vs. serum concentration as related to time since ingestion. (Modified from A.K. Done: Pediatrics *26:*800, 1960).

ferric nitrate technique, described by Natelson (1961), which has been modified for the large automated clinical analyzers, e.g., DuPont *aca*. Single doses of salicylates yield serum concentrations of less than 60 μg/ml (0.5 mmol/l).

Toxicity is associated with serum salicylate levels of about 300 μg/ml (2.2 mmol/l), but severe toxic effects occur when serum levels reach 500 μg/ml (3.6 mmol/l). In a series reported by Irey (1974), the lethal range was from 550 to 1400 μg/ml (4.0 to 10.1 mmol/l). Older children and adults showed good correlation between serum salicylate levels and severity of the toxic state, but young children displayed a variable susceptibility to salicylate levels. For toxicity in children, a nomogram by Done (Fig. 15–6) relates the serum concentration following a single dose and the time of ingestion to the severity of the effect. If the time of salicylate ingestion is known, the nomogram can help the physician to predict symptoms and alter therapy accordingly.

Dialysis, plasmapheresis, or exchange transfusion is an effective means of achieving a reduction in serum salicylate concentration and clinical improvement; these modalities should be used when levels in excess of 1000 μg/ml (7.0 mmol/l) have failed to respond to more conservative therapy. The mean lethal dose of salicylate lies between 20 and 30 g in an adult; however, 1 g of aspirin has been fatal and 130 g tolerated without death. Methyl salicylate (oil of wintergreen) is perhaps the most toxic member of the salicylate family, and the mortality from overdoses is close to 60 per cent (Trapnell, 1976). When salicylates are used in rheumatoid arthritis, the optimum therapeutic effect occurs with serum levels of 150 to 300 μg/ml (1.1 to 2.1 mmol/l). In a group of patients with rheumatoid arthritis, tinnitus, the most common side effect, was found to occur with salicylate levels between about 200 and 450 μg/ml (1.4 to 3.4 mmol/l), while hyperventilation usually occurred at levels greater than 350 μg/ml (2.6 mmol/l) (Mongan, 1973). Acidosis and other side effects were seen at concentrations greater than 460 μg/ml (3.4 mmol/l). When levels approach 300 μg/ml (2.1 mmol/l) a reversible bilateral hearing loss of 20 to 30 decibels at all frequencies was found to occur (Myers, 1965). However, in those patients who have a pre-existing hearing loss, tinnitus did not occur at levels of about 440 μg/ml (3.3 mmol/l); thus, in patients with pre-existing hearing deficits, tinnitus cannot be used as a guide to toxicity.

ACETAMINOPHEN

Acetaminophen (*N*-acetyl-para-amino-phenol) which is known abroad as paracetamol, is an antipyretic and an analgesic. The mechanism of its therapeutic action appears to be related to inhibition of the enzymatic mechanism for synthesis of prostaglandins. In the United States it is available without prescription and marketed under at least 200 formulations, of which the most common are Tylenol, Datril, Tempra, and Liquiprin. A comprehensive list of these formulations has been prepared by Ameer (1977). Phenacetin, an analgesic which is used with salicylates in a common formulation, is metabolized to acetaminophen. The major adverse reaction to acetaminophen is hepatotoxicity.

Acetaminophen is absorbed rapidly from the gastrointestinal tract, with peak concentrations occurring one to two hours after ingestion. The drug may be up to 50 per cent bound to plasma proteins, but there appear to be no major sites of tissue binding.

Approximately 80 per cent of an administered dose is conjugated by the hepatic enzymes to glucuronic and sulfuric acids, and these metabolites are excreted into the urine. The remainder is eliminated via other pathways such as hydroxylation and deacylation, which can be increased by the microsomal-inducing drugs such as phenobarbital and diphenhydramine.

Although the hydroxylation pathway accounts for very little of the acetaminophen metabolized, the hydroxylated compound, by covalently binding to hepatocellular macromolecules, causes hepatic necrosis. Normally the hydroxylated metabolite is detoxified by conjugation with hepatic glutathione and subsequently excreted into the urine. When large amounts of acetaminophen are ingested, hepatic glutathione may become depleted and the macromolecular structure of the liver arylated, thereby causing hepatic necrosis.

Ultraviolet spectrophotometry is the most common method of measurement of acetaminophen but is relatively insensitive. A modification by Love (1977) shows no interference with aspirin or the sulfate and glucuronide conjugates of acetaminophen. Phenacetin and acetaminophen have been measured simultaneously by a procedure which uses high performance liquid chromatography (Gotelli, 1977).

For analgesia in adults, doses of 325 to 650 mg usually are given every three to four hours. With this dose, essentially no side effects are seen. A serum concentration of 5 to 20 μg/ml is necessary to achieve an analgesic response, but no good correlation between serum concentration and the intensity of the analgesic action has been shown (Koch-Weser, 1976).

Hepatotoxicity may occur when large amounts of the drug are ingested accidentally or in suicide attempts. Initially nausea, vomiting, and abdominal pain may result, and within the first two days liver function tests become abnormal. These hepatic abnormalities, however, may not occur until four to six days after ingestion. With a single dose as small as 10 grams, hepatotoxicity may occur. Prescott (1971) has suggested a definite correlation between serum acetaminophen levels and subsequent liver damage. At four hours post-ingestion, patients with levels of less than 120 μg/ml do not develop hepatic insufficiency. Of those with levels of 120 to 300 μg/ml, 50 per cent develop hepatic necrosis, while levels greater than 300 μg/ml are associated with hepatic necrosis. The relationship of the half-life to prognosis is seen in Figure 15-7. The serum acetaminophen half-life is probably the best guide to the extent of hepatic injury and should be determined especially in those patients who have

achieved a serum level in the intermediate group, i.e., 120 to 300 μg/ml (Rumack, 1975). It has been shown that hepatic necrosis may occur when the serum half-life exceeds four hours, and hepatic coma is very likely if the half-life exceeds 12 hours. Since patients with acetaminophen half-lives of less than four hours are able to metabolize the toxic products, usually they do not develop hepatic insufficiency. However, patients taking enzyme-inducing drugs such as phenobarbital are at a greater risk of developing hepatic toxicity, probably from increased formation of the hydroxylated metabolite.

The determination of acetaminophen may be important for prognosis and even more important for treatment. Although there are some studies that appear to be contradictory, Peterson, (1977) found that sulfhydryl-containing compounds such as acetylcysteine may reduce hepatic toxicity. These agents are being evaluated to determine their applicability in altering the outcome of patients who have ingested a toxic dose of acetaminophen. The toxic side effects include nausea, drowsiness, and vomiting. Furthermore, since they represent an additional protein and ammonia load for a liver which may have already suffered a fatal insult, it is extremely important to predict if they are necessary. Therefore,

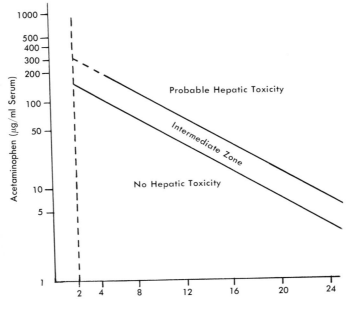

Figure 15–7. Semilogarithmic plot of serum acetaminophen levels vs time. The serum half-life can be estimated using two specimens obtained several hours apart. (Modified from Krenzelok, E. P., Best, L., and Manoguerra, A. S.: Am. J. Hosp. Pharm. 34:391, 1977.)

before treatment is begun in cases of acetaminophen overdosage, it is important to determine the quantity ingested, the initial serum level, the half-life, and the history regarding microsomal-inducing drugs.

Chronic acetaminophen therapy for analgesia has been reported to be associated with the development of liver injury in some patients (Barker, 1977; Johnson, 1977).

PROPOXYPHENE

Propoxyphene, as the hydrochloride (Darvon) or napsylate (Darvon-N) salt, is an analgesic that is one of the five most commonly prescribed drugs in the United States. It is also dispensed in a common formulation with other analgesics such as aspirin and acetaminophen. Propoxyphene is a congener of the narcotic methadone, but is classified as non-narcotic. Accidental or intentional ingestion of large amounts of propoxyphene may cause death; dependence and parenteral abuse are additional problems associated with the drug.

Following ingestion as the hydrochloride salt, propoxyphene reaches a peak level in one to two hours, but as the napsylate salt, the peak occurs in three to four hours. Most propoxyphene is metabolized on the first pass through the liver, with only about 20 per cent reaching systemic circulation unchanged. It has a half-life of about 12 hours. The major route of biotransformation is N-demethylation to norpropoxyphene, a compound with a half-life of about 37 hours. The pharmacologic activity and significance of this compound are unknown. At least seven other intermediates have been identified, but none appears to be important (McMahon, 1973).

Rapid tissue binding of propoxyphene occurs, resulting in the immediate and almost complete disappearance of the drug from the blood stream and relatively high concentrations in the brain, lung, liver, and kidney. In a controlled clinical trial, analgesia and serum concentrations of propoxyphene did not show significant correlation (Wolen, 1971); however, others accept a therapeutic level of about 0.3 µg/ml (Feinberg, 1973).

After the ingestion of a lethal dose, convulsions, cardiovascular collapse and respiratory depression usually occur in about one hour (Miller, 1977). Following the ingestion of a toxic dose of propoxyphene, symptoms of nausea, vomiting, and drowsiness, which can progress to a central nervous system depression, occur within 30 minutes. The finding of miotic pupils serves to differentiate intoxication with propoxyphene from that with non-narcotic drugs. A combined drug overdose with alcohol is more lethal than an overdose of propoxyphene alone, probably because of the additive depressive effect on the central nervous system. Although death in an adult has been reported with a propoxyphene dose as low as 800 mg, McBay (1975) concluded that about 1000 mg of the hydrochloride salt or 1500 mg of the napsylate preparation may cause death. The minimal fatal propoxyphene level is thought to be 1.0 µg/ml (McBay, 1976).

A spectrophotometric method has been used (Wallace, 1965), but it is relatively insensitive. Work by McBay (1974) has indicated that both norpropoxyphene and propoxyphene are measured by this procedure. Since norpropoxyphene may reach higher concentration than propoxyphene, non-specific methods may lead to falsely elevated propoxyphene values. With gas chromatographic methods such as developed by Nash (1975), both propoxyphene and norpropoxyphene can be quantitated individually. Methods for tissue propoxyphene measurements have been developed and applied in a series of fatal poisonings (Worm, 1971). The usual modalities of treatment for overdose, such as dialysis or diuresis, have been of very little benefit in overdoses of propoxyphene, probably because the tissue levels are about 10 to 20 times greater than serum concentrations. However, the toxic respiratory effects can be neutralized by the administration of morphine antagonists (Lovejoy, 1974).

MISCELLANEOUS

THEOPHYLLINE

Theophylline (1,3 dimethyl xanthine) exhibits many pharmacologic actions, including stimulation of respiration, augmentation of cardiac function, diuresis, and relaxation of smooth muscle. The symptoms of asthma often result from constriction of bronchial smooth muscle, and it is the relaxation of this musculature which is the basis for the therapeutic effectiveness of theophylline. The postulated mechanism of action of theophylline appears to be through cyclic AMP. It is thought to increase cyclic 3'5' AMP levels by causing inhibition of phosphodiesterase, the enzyme which is responsible for the degrada-

THEOPHYLLINE

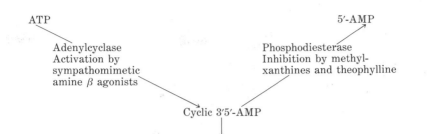

Figure 15–8. Postulated mechanism of bronchodilator activity. Cyclic 3′5′-AMP is believed to be the mediator for bronchial smooth muscle relaxation. Sympathomimetic bronchodilators increase its formation by stimulating adenylcyclase, while theophylline inhibits the enzyme phosphodiesterase, which increases cyclic 3′5′-AMP levels by decreasing its degradation to the inactive 5′-AMP.

tion of cyclic 3′5′ AMP to inactive 5′ AMP (Fig. 15–8). For symptoms of asthma, theophylline may be given by intravenous infusion, while for chronic disease, an oral preparation usually is given every four to six hours. Most of the commonly used oral preparations of theophylline are combination drugs which also may contain ephedrine, various barbiturates, or other drugs in a common formulation. Bioavailability and variability in tablet theophylline is bound to serum proteins, while the preparations (Webb-Johnson, 1977). Following absorption, theophylline is distributed widely in extracellular fluid and tissues, but does not enter erythrocytes. About 60 per cent of theophylline is bound to plasma proteins, while the other 40 per cent is free. Degradation of theophylline involves oxidation and methylation by the liver, mainly to inactive metabolites 3-methyl xanthine, 1-methyluric acid, and 1,3 dimethyl uric acid. About 10 per cent of the administered dose of theophylline is excreted into the urine in an unchanged form.

Methods of theophylline measurement include ultraviolet spectrophotometry, homogeneous enzyme immunoassay, gas chromatography, and high performance liquid chromatography (HPLC). For many years ultraviolet spectrophotometry was the most commonly used method (Schack, 1949), but this method is subject to interferences by furosemide, barbiturates, and xanthines (Jenne, 1977). Such xanthines as caffeine, commonly found in tea and coffee, and theobromine, a major constituent of chocolate, co-extract and are measured as theophylline. Jatlow (1975) improved this method by altering the pH of extraction, thereby removing the interfer-

ences of phenobarbital. A homogeneous enzyme immunoassay technique has been introduced which is also subject to minor interferences by urea, xanthine, and theophylline metabolites. In gas chromatographic procedures for theophylline measurements, interfering xanthines are separated from theophylline, but this technique requires considerable sample preparations (Johnson, 1975). A HPLC method has been described which requires very little sample preparation and in which the dietary xanthines and other interferences are eliminated (Orcutt, 1977).

A serum level should not be obtained until plateau is reached. When oral theophylline is administered, serum samples should be obtained just prior to the next dose. With intravenous preparations a slow infusion will not produce a therapeutic effect in two hours.

Normal therapeutic levels are 10 to 20 μg/ml, although at 5 to 10 μg/ml a therapeutic effect does occur (Mitenko, 1973). Theophylline toxicity is to a large extent correlated with the serum concentration (Jacobs, 1976). At concentrations higher than 20 μg/ml, side effects invariably occur, while patients with serum theophylline values in the range of 15 to 20 μg/ml occasionally experience some adverse effects. Common side effects observed include anorexia, nausea, vomiting, and abdominal discomfort. In most patients with gastrointestinal symptoms, serum theophylline concentrations usually are greater than 25 μg/ml. Since oral theophylline is a direct irritant of the gastric mucosa, with chronic ingestion of oral preparations, gastrointestinal symptoms may not reflect systemic toxicity. Severe toxicity, manifested by cardiac arrhythmias, seizures, respiratory arrest, and cardiac arrest, occurs in the range of 30 to 60 μg/ml. Zwillich (1975) determined that usually gastrointestinal symptoms did not precede the onset of seizures. Oral theophylline preparations commonly are administered three or four times daily. This dosage schedule, which is less than 10 mg/kg for most adults, may produce low serum theophylline concentrations in many individuals (Jacobs, 1976).

The half-life of theophylline is about 3.5 hours in children and about 4.5 hours in adults. In patients with ventricular failure, acute pulmonary edema, liver dysfunction, or chronic obstructive pulmonary disease and in those ingesting macrolide antibiotics (troleandomycin and erythromycin), the half-life tends to be significantly longer. Jenne (1977) has found that in young cigarette smokers the half-life is significantly shorter than in non-smokers; he has theorized that non-smokers require less theophylline for bronchodilation than do smokers.

Recent evidence has indicated that patients who are ill have prolonged metabolic degradation rates and this leads, in turn, to toxicity in a large number of patients (Hendeles, 1977; Kordash, 1977). A nomogram has been employed to reduce the maintenance dose by one third in patients over the age of 50 and by half in patients with congestive heart failure or liver dysfunction (Jusko, 1977). Use of salivary specimens has been suggested as a source of free (non–protein-bound) drug levels (Koysooko, 1974). Although not widely utilized at this time for theophylline, it is likely that this technique will be of value in the future.

METHOTREXATE

Methotrexate, a folic acid antagonist, has been used in the treatment of psoriasis for 25 years. The occasional occurrence of hepatotoxicity is the only major side effect associated with low dose chronic oral methotrexate therapy for dermatologic disease (Weinstein, 1977). It also has been used clinically for its antitumor activity in acute leukemia and other neoplastic diseases. When given orally over an extended period of time, it has been found to be quite toxic. Methotrexate inhibits the enzyme dihydrofolate reductase, thereby reducing the pool of folates available as methyl donors for production of thymidylate,

one of the four precursors of DNA. The lethal effect occurs when the available thymidylate is reduced, resulting in the inhibition of DNA synthesis, RNA synthesis, and cell division. The most rapidly proliferating cells, such as those of the bone marrow, gastrointestinal tract, and hair roots, are affected.

Since 1973, large doses of methotrexate administered as intravenous infusions lasting from six hours to almost two days have been used for the treatment of osteogenic sarcomas, childhood leukemias, and many other highly malignant tumors. The high dose methotrexate is followed within a few hours by the administration of leucovorin (5-formyl tetrahydrofolate, also called citrovorum factor). By administering the product of the enzyme inhibited by methotrexate, the block is circumvented, and cellular functions are allowed to continue. Differences in normal and neoplastic cells allow leucovorin to penetrate and "rescue" the normal cells, leaving the neoplastic ones unprotected against the lethal effects of high and persistant methotrexate concentrations. The use of leucovorin permits about 100 times more methotrexate to be administered than when the drug is given alone. Unfortunately, leucovorin cannot "rescue" normal cells if the rescue is delayed, nor will tumor cells be killed if serum methotrexate levels are too low. Thus, the cytotoxic action of methotrexate on the target tissue requires the intracellular presence of the drug above a specific threshold for an extended period of time.

Methotrexate exhibits a triphasic serum disappearance with extensive intrahepatic circulation and probably enteric bacterial metabolism (Chabner, 1975); however, most is excreted within the first eight hours, mainly unchanged in the urine. If serum concentrations are in the toxic range and urine pH less than 5.5, methotrexate may precipitate in the kidney, causing direct tubular toxicity. For this reason, patients treated with high dose therapy must not only have their urine alkalinized, but must also have adequate urine production.

Methods of measurement include radioimmunoassay (Raso, 1975), radioassay using dihydrofolate reductase as the binding protein (Kamen, 1976), and an enzymatic method using the inhibition of the dihydrofolate reductase as the endpoint (Falk, 1976). High performance liquid chromatography with fluorescence detection (Nelson, 1977), as well as fluorimetry, also have been utilized. The specificity of these assays in the presence of the folates and their analogues has not been characterized completely. All appear to have sensitivity sufficient to measure methotrexate during high dose infusion protocols.

Following high level methotrexate infusion, serum levels are obtained that range from 1×10^{-4} M (45.4 μg/ml) to 1×10^{-8} M (0.00454 μg/ml), depending on the time after the infusion at which the level is measured. The serum concentration of methotrexate during this infusion also has been shown to correlate not only with hematologic, gastrointestinal, and hepatic toxicity, but also with the efficacy of treatment. At levels less than 4.5×10^{-6} M (2.1 μg/ml) at 48 hours after the start of an infusion, severe toxicity is unlikely (Wang, 1976). Methotrexate determinations also have been used to adjust the dose of leucovorin used in the "rescue" (Frei, 1975).

It has been reported that methotrexate falsely elevates cerebrospinal fluid (CSF) protein by most methods (Zwieg, 1976). Since methotrexate is given intrathecally for a number of tumors, including meningeal leukemias and lymphomas, this should be considered when interpreting CSF protein values (see Chap. 18).

NITROPRUSSIDE

Nitroprusside (Nipride) is an antihypertensive agent that is utilized in a wide variety of clinical situations. It has been employed as a hypotensive agent in surgical procedures, renal angiography, and hypertensive crisis, and to facilitate correction of abnormal hemodynamics in acute myocardial infarction and congestive heart failure. It is available only for intravenous therapy and is initially infused at an average rate of 3 μg/kg/minute with careful monitoring of the blood pressure. The structure of nitroprusside is unusual in that it is a hydrated nitrosyl pentacyanoferrate compound (Fig. 15-9).

Although it is known to cause vasodilation of vascular smooth muscle, little is understood about the mechanism of action at the cellular level. Nitroprusside initially reacts with sulfhydryl groups in either erythrocytes or other tissues, yielding cyanogen (CN^-). This cyanide group is rapidly detoxified to thiocyanate (SCN^-) in the presence of a sulfur donor, thiosulfate, in a reaction catalyzed by the hepatic enzyme rhodanase. In individuals with normal renal function, thiocyanate is removed almost

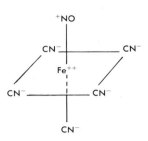

Figure 15-9. Schematic representation of the iron coordination complex of nitroprusside. In sodium nitroprusside, the overall complex has a net negative charge and must be associated with cations such as the two sodiums.

entirely by the kidney, with a half-life of approximately one week (Palmer, 1975).

The manifestations of toxicity are anorexia and nausea followed by vomiting, disorientation, psychotic behavior, trembling, labored respiration, rigidity, convulsions, and finally death. Rare toxic symptoms may include headache, skin rash, and, in one patient, hypothyroidism after extended use of nitroprusside (Nourok, 1964). In some of the fatal cases reported, high doses of nitroprusside were used (greater than 10 μg/mg/kg/minute); in several of these cases, because a resistance was noted 5 to 10 minutes after beginning the infusion, the drug was rapidly increased to maintain hypotension. In others, tachyphylaxis occurred from 30 to 60 minutes after beginning the infusion (Greiss, 1976). Of the patients treated, young adults and children are most susceptible to tachyphylaxis. In all fatalities, an associated severe metabolic acidosis and an increasing mixed venous oxygen content have been found. In one patient who was treated for a massive myocardial infarction, methemoglobinemia was noted during sodium nitroprusside therapy (Bower, 1975).

Because of the rapid decomposition of nitroprusside in the presence of erythrocytes, serum thiocyanate levels are used to monitor therapy. They are usually determined by a modification of the spectrophotometric method of Barker (1936). In an early report, Page (1955), indicated that the therapeutic range of thiocyanate after chronic oral administration was 80 to 120 μg/ml. However, since symptoms of thiocyanate toxicity begin at serum levels of about 100 μg/ml, Tuzel (1975) recommended that when thiocyanate levels are over 100 μg/ml, nitroprusside be temporarily discontinued. Death has been reported at a level of 200 μg/ml.

In a case report of death from oral ingestion of sodium nitroprusside, the "burnt almond" odor of cyanide was noted in some tissues from the postmortem examination (Hill, 1942). This led Perschau (1977) to theorize that the fatalities involving nitroprusside were attributable to cyanide poisoning. They successfully treated with thiosulfate a hypotensive, acidotic patient who they felt was critically ill from iatrogenic nitroprusside intoxication. Vesey's group (1976) has measured cyanide and thiocyanate concentrations in patients receiving nitroprusside and found cyanide to be elevated. Their data indicate that blood cyanide concentrations are a better indicator of nitroprusside toxicity than thiocyanate levels; however, the potential dangers and the safety requirements of cyanide measurements have made this assay impractical for the routine clinical laboratory. For further information, see the section on cyanide on page 511.

LITHIUM

Lithium, as the carbonate salt, is employed in the control of manic-depressive disorders and also has been used in the treatment of other psychological disturbances. Although lithium probably has some effects of its own, it resembles sodium, potassium, magnesium, and calcium in many respects. The partial similarity of lithium to these four biologically important cations may account for some of its effects (Schou, 1976).

Lithium is absorbed well by the gastrointestinal tract, with peak levels after the ingestion of lithium carbonate reached in one to four hours. Lithium is not bound to serum proteins and is not metabolized; its distribution in the body is complicated and occurs slowly. It is eliminated from the body almost entirely by renal excretion and also is secreted into saliva and breast milk. Plateau levels of lithium are reached 12 to 24 hours after ingestion of the drug. For practical purposes, lithium can be considered to have a serum half-life between 24 and 48 hours, which is decreased by salt feeding and increased by salt deprivation or renal damage (Marks, 1973). In man, lithium poisoning primarily affects the central nervous system and the kidneys. Protracted coma, anuria, or circulatory failure may ensue before death occurs. Acute intoxication is characterized by vomiting, diarrhea, ataxia, coma, and convulsions. Chronic toxic manifestations include nausea, vomiting, abdominal pain, diarrhea, and sedation, as well as tremors, seizures, focal neurologic signs, and arrhythmias. Lithium therapy has been reported to cause goiter, with or without hypothyroidism, leukocytosis, polyuria, and polydipsia. Lithium has been shown to inhibit renal response to antidiuretic hormone (Schou, 1976).

Atomic absorption spectrophotometry and emission flame photometry may be used to determine serum lithium levels (Levy, 1970).[*] Lithium levels usually are measured just before the morning dose. The usual therapeutic range for lithium is approximately 0.6 to 1.3 mEq/l (0.6 to 1.3 mmol/l). Although toxic side effects can occur at almost any serum level, they are seldom serious below 1.5 mEq/l (1.5 mmol/l). Steady-state lithium levels above 3.0 mEq/l (3.0 mmol/l) are life threatening and levels greater than 4.5 mEq/l (4.5 mmol/l) are almost invariably fatal (Marks, 1973).

It has been claimed that the ratio of the erythrocyte lithium to serum lithium may be related to a clinical state and the response to therapy, but such correlation has not been reported by all investigators. The ratio exhibits considerable variation among subjects but has been shown to be relatively stable in individual patients (Rybakowski, 1977). Erythrocyte lithium concentrations, which can be determined by atomic absorption spectrophotometry, appear to reflect impending neurotoxicity and may prove useful in monitoring patients on lithium therapy (Hisayasu, 1977).

BROMIDE

Bromides, which were used as anticonvulsants and sedatives, are still available in certain non-prescription products in low doses. Although there is a declining availability of proprietary bromide-containing compounds, certain nerve tonics and headache remedies

---

[*]These methods yield similar results, although the flame photometry method appears to be more sensitive but slightly less precise than atomic absorption spectrophotometry.

continue to be a source of bromide. The main reason for the continued interest in bromide is the occasional occurrence of chronic bromide intoxication from the indiscriminate use of these preparations. Acute bromide intoxication is rare; the drug tends to cause gastrointestinal irritation, and thus it is difficult to ingest and retain an amount sufficient to attain toxic levels without vomiting. Chronic ingestion of bromide may lead to toxic levels, since bromides are excreted slowly by the kidney and thus may accumulate. The features that may suggest the presence of bromide intoxication include fever, neurologic disturbances, skin rash, and a history of ingesting proprietary bromide-containing drugs (Trump, 1976). Toxic manifestations which frequently appear are irritability, agitation, and delirium. Neurologic disturbances may include tremors and motor incoordination. Chronic bromide intoxication may be associated with elevated cerebrospinal fluid pressure, as well as elevated CSF protein. In some patients, mental or neurological disorders may persist for some time after the drug is eliminated from the body. Distribution of bromide in the body is similar to that of chloride. Since the tissues do not readily distinguish between chloride and bromide, ingestion of either halide results in the displacement of the other.

Serum bromide concentration is determined by using a protein-free filtrate of serum or plasma and reacting it with gold chloride to form a red-orange color which is proportional to bromide concentrations (Wuth, 1927). A good correlation between the severity of bromide intoxication and serum bromide levels does not always exist: some patients may show signs of severe intoxication when the drug is present in relatively low concentration. Bromide intoxication should be considered as the possible cause of mental or neurologic symptoms when the level exceeds 9 mEq/l (9 mmol/l). Most patients show unmistakable signs of poisoning with serum bromide levels in the range of 19 to 25 mEq/l (19 to 25 mmol/l) (Sharpless, 1965).

Mercuric thiocyanate methods for chloride yield elevated values in the presence of bromide; the apparent chloride results are elevated because bromide has a greater affinity for the mercuric ion. It is not possible, however, to predict concentration of the interfering bromide accurately from the elevated chloride values (Blume, 1968).

Ethanol

Alcoholism is one of the major health problems of this country. It has been estimated that in the United States 95 million people drink ethyl alcohol (ethanol), and 9 million are classified as chronic abusers. One in 25 hospital admissions is associated with ethanol abuse, and 50 per cent of all drivers involved in fatal automobile accidents have been reported to be drinking. Similar to many other drugs of abuse, alcohol influences an individual's physical, social, mental, and economic status in myriad ways. Combined effects of alcohol are believed to constitute a third or fourth leading cause of death of adults, with an annual economic impact in the United States placed at 15 to 25 billion dollars (Lundberg, 1976).

The overall effect of ethyl alcohol on central nervous system function is that of a depressant and an anesthetic. The initial effect is loss of inhibition, followed by loss of judgment and personality change, impairment of memory, and loss of coordination. Additional ingestion leads to disorientation and then stupor, followed by coma and death. When the performance of an individual under the influence of ethanol puts others at risk, he becomes a threat to society. For this reason laws have been adopted which legislate against those who drink heavily and operate a motor vehicle. In addition to the need for blood ethanol levels as legal evidence, ethanol measurements commonly are used in cases of coma due to drug overdosage. In a study by a large laboratory, almost 20 per cent of specimens sent by the emergency room staff for toxicologic analyses other than ethanol contained ethanol (Hirsch, 1973).

Metabolism. Ethanol usually is ingested in beer (2 to 6 per cent), in wine (10 to 20 per cent), or in whiskey (40 to 50 per cent). Proof is twice the per cent of ethanol content; i.e., 100 proof whiskey is 50 per cent ethanol. The amount of ethanol in one ounce of whiskey is about the same as in one bottle of beer or in four ounces of wine. On an empty stomach the absorption is so rapid that at least half of the ingested load is absorbed and the peak level is reached in 40 to 70 minutes. Ethanol is unique in that it is one of the few substances that is absorbed in the stomach. Approximately 20 to 25 per cent of that ingested will pass through the stomach wall with absorption affected by factors such as stomach emptying time, as well as concentration and volume of ethanol ingested. Eating immediately prior to ethanol intake is associated with prolonging the peak blood level by one or two hours and reducing the peak level attained. Absorption from the skin, bladder, and inspired air contribute little to blood alcohol levels.

About 10 per cent of the ingested ethanol is excreted in the urine, sweat, and breath, while 90 per cent is metabolized in the liver first to acetaldehyde, and then to CO_2 and water. Alcohol dehydrogenase, which is the first enzyme in this pathway, is the rate-limiting step of metabolism and becomes saturated at a blood ethanol concentration of 16 mg/dl (3.5 mmol/l). At levels higher than this, the rate of metabolism remains constant. A 70 kg person metabolizes about 7 to 10 g of ethanol per hour, which is equivalent to an average of about 20 to 30 ml of 90 proof spirits (two-thirds to one ounce), 8 to 12 ounces of beer, or 3 to 4 ounces of wine. Very little can be done acutely to increase this metabolism.

Another pathway of ethanol metabolism is the microsomal system, which metabolizes not only ethanol but also such drugs as barbiturates and other sedatives. Drugs that are capable of inducing activity of the microsomal enzyme system increase the capacity for the degradation of ethanol. The interaction of various drugs and ethanol with this enzyme system is responsible for the increased mortality of combined ethanol and barbiturate ingestion (see p. 508).

Alcohol Methodology. There are three different groups of analytical procedures that are used for the determination of ethanol: (1) dichromate reduction, (2) alcohol dehydrogenase, and (3) gas chromatography.

Dichromate methodology is dependent on the reduction of dichromate in acid solution by ethanol. The amount of dichromate reduced is proportional to the concentration of alcohol.

$$2\,Cr_2O_7^{-2} + 16\,H^+ + 3\,C_2H_5OH \longrightarrow$$
$$4\,Cr^{+3} + 3\,CH_3COOH + 11\,H_2O$$

However, this reaction is not specific in that other alcohols, ketones, and aldehydes also reduce dichromate. From the clinical point of view, two alcohols of importance besides ethanol are methanol and isopropanol. At ethanol

levels of 100 mg/dl (21.7 mmol/l), which is the level required for the legal definition of intoxication, methanol is lethal. Isopropanol is more intoxicating than ethanol; a patient who appears intoxicated and has an "ethanol level" less than 100 mg/dl (21.7 mmol/l), should be suspected of isopropanol ingestion. Since acetone is the end product of isopropanol metabolism, a urine acetone determination can be used to help confirm the ingestion of isopropranol. Paraldehyde, a drug used in the treatment of agitation, is metabolized to acetaldehyde, which also is capable of reducing dichromate; therefore, it results in a positive test for ethanol. Adaptation of this methodology is used in the Conway diffusion plate, in which dichromate and a patient's specimen are placed in different wells. If ethanol is present, it diffuses and reacts with dichromate to form a green color. This method can be performed fairly quickly and is a semiquantitative estimate of ethanol when read at 30 minutes. When diffusion is allowed to continue for 16 to 18 hours, the results are quite precise.

The alcohol dehydrogenase (ADH) method is simple, accurate, and fairly specific; for many clinical laboratories it appears to be the method of choice for diagnostic purposes. Ethanol is converted to acetaldehyde by alcohol dehydrogenase, and NADH is generated. NADH can be quantitated by its increased absorbance at 340 nm in the following reaction:

$$C_2H_5OH + NAD^+ \underset{\longleftarrow}{\overset{ADH}{\longrightarrow}} CH_3CHO + NADH + H^+$$

Since the equilibrium of this reaction lies far to the left, to drive the reaction to the right, acetaldehyde is removed by coupling it with a semicarbazide.

This methodology is not specific, since other alcohols such as isopropanol react. A favorable comparison of the kit forms of this methodology recently has been reported (Redetzki, 1976). A similar methodology is available on large automated clinical analyzers, e.g., DuPont *aca.*

Chromatography of the alcohols has been the method of choice for forensic and toxicologic laboratories. This methodology is qualitative as well as quantitative and because of its specificity, it has become quite popular. Samples can be either directly injected, extracted, distilled, or a vapor phase (head space) prepared and injected. The advantages of each of these techniques of sample preparations are presented by Butler (1976).

Breath Analysis. Breath analysis (Breatholizer) is utilized in some states as a portable method of alcohol detection. The subject blows through a mouth piece, forcing his breath into an ampule containing potassium dichromate in acid solution. Ethanol is oxidized and the reduction of dichromate can be quantitated. This method is subject to interferences by other alcohols, as well as recently ingested alcohol remaining in the mouth. With vomiting of alcohol, the Breatholizer also may become positive. Some subjects confronted by the law, and intoxicated from illegal drugs, wash their mouths with ethanol, giving a positive Breatholizer test in an attempt to avoid a much more serious charge of drug abuse. If the subject washes his mouth with water before performing a breath analysis or if the breath analysis is repeated during the hour, it is possible to overcome this limitation.

Specimen. Blood is the only specimen required for analysis for medicolegal reasons in the United States, since systemic effects of ethanol are well correlated with blood concentrations. Arterial, venous, or capillary blood properly collected in a closed system is the preferred specimen.* The specimen tube should be completely filled and must be kept tightly stoppered for centrifugation and storage to avoid loss of volatile constituents. Serum should be removed from the blood cells

*Serum or plasma may be used, but values average 1.18 times the whole blood values.

and either analyzed promptly or stored under refrigeration in a stoppered tube. Cleaning of the puncture site should be performed with a non-alcoholic solution. Müller (1976) reported the effect on ethanol levels using a chlorahexidine/ethyl alcohol gauze to cleanse the skin and to control bleeding from the puncture site. In their study, with retraction of the needle, alcohol from the gauze was aspirated into the blood collection tube, artifactually raising serum levels up to 3420 mg/dl (744 mmol/l). For this reason, it is imperative that a disinfectant other than alcohol be used.

The relationship between blood and urine alcohol is ordinarily quite constant and can be a reliable index to blood ethanol concentrations. Kidneys do not have the ability to concentrate ethanol, and in a group of volunteers given ethanol, the average urine to blood ratio was found to be 1.35 (Lundquist, 1961). However, the assumptions which are necessary to utilize urine determinations are that the peak blood alcohol content has been passed and that the bladder has been emptied in the preceding 30 minutes. Thus, if a urine level is obtained, a serum level of at least 1.35 times the urine level must have occurred in the past. The determination of ethanol in urine is accepted as legal evidence in some European countries.

In Table 15-5 are presented the concentration of blood ethanol and its influence on the subject. One shot of whiskey (1 ounce) will raise the blood ethanol level to about 25 to 35 mg/dl (5.4 to 7.5 mmol/l). At 100 mg/dl (21.7 mmol/l), a driver is legally under the

Table 15-5. INFLUENCE OF ACUTE ETHANOL INGESTION ON ETHANOL LEVELS AND BEHAVIOR

WHISKEY (ounces)	BLOOD CONCENTRATION	INFLUENCE
1-2	10-50 mg/dl (2.2-10.9 mmol/l)	None to mild euphoria
3-4	50-100 mg/dl (10.9-21.7 mmol/l) or greater	Mild influence on stereoscopic vision and dark adaptation
	100 mg/dl (21.7 mmol/l)	Legally intoxicated
4-6	100-150 mg/dl (21.7-32.6 mmol/l)	Euphoria; disappearance of inhibition; prolonged reaction time
6-7	150-200 mg/dl (32.6-43.4 mmol/l)	Moderately severe poisoning; reaction time greatly prolonged; loss of inhibition and slight disturbances in equilibrium and coordination
8-9	200-250 mg/dl (43.4-54.3 mmol/l)	Severe degree of poisoning; disturbances of equilibrium and coordination; retardation of the thought processes and clouding of consciousness
10-15	250-400 mg/dl (54.3-86.8 mmol/l)	Deep, possibly fatal coma

influence of ethanol, and at 150 mg/dl (32.6 mmol/l), most persons appear intoxicated. At 350 to 400 mg/dl (76 to 87 mmol/l), coma is a common finding. Lethal levels require large alcohol ingestions of between 250 and 500 g. These values apply only to the patients who are acutely ingesting alcohol. In a group of chronic alcoholics, Lindblad (1976) demonstrated a remarkable degree of tolerance to potentially lethal ethanol levels, ranging from 500 to 780 mg/dl (108.7 to 169.3 mmol/l). These patients not only were able to survive, but tolerated the alcohol so well that they were not obtunded. Ethanol can be metabolized almost twice as fast in an alcoholic as in a nonalcoholic subject. In alcoholics, the increased acetaldehyde formed by both of the metabolic pathways is postulated to cause liver damage (Korsten, 1975).

Interactions with Other Drugs. The hepatic degradation system located in the microsomes is a focal point for the interaction of ethanol and other drugs. Examples of these are widely prescribed drugs, such as chlordiazepoxide, diazepam, meprobamate, phenytoin, guanethidine, and isoniazid. The drugs, when metabolized by this system in the presence of alcohol, have increased half-lives and their effects are prolonged. Interactions with this enzyme system are responsible for the increased mortality of combined alcohol and barbiturate ingestion. Since the microsomal enzymes metabolize both ethanol and barbiturate, when they are taken together, dangerously high levels may be reached, causing coma.

Disulfuran, which is used to treat chronic alcoholism, results in symptoms so unpleasant that the patient is unlikely to imbibe any ethanol-containing beverages while on a maintenance dose. This drug is thought to inhibit the metabolism of acetaldehyde.

Although elevations of glucose and urea are well recognized as causing increases in serum osmolality, ethanol is thought to be the most common cause of this increase (Robinson, 1971). At ethanol levels of 100 mg/dl (21.7 mmol/l), the serum osmolality is increased by 22 mOsmol/kg (Beard, 1974). The finding of an elevated serum osmolality in a patient should at least raise suspicion of alcohol ingestion (Rawnsley, 1976).

Methanol

Methanol, also called wood alcohol or methyl alcohol, is utilized in a number of industrial processes and as an adulterant of ethyl alcohol to make it impotable. Although single cases occur, poisoning involving methanol tends to occur in clusters. For example, in an incident reported by Bennett (1953), an epidemic involving over 300 patients with 41 deaths occurred when bootleggers delivered whiskey that was 40 per cent methanol. The toxicity which develops appears not to be directly related to the dose ingested. Although fatal doses usually occur from the ingestion of 30 to 100 g, a dose as small as 6 g has been fatal and one as high as 200 g was not lethal.

Following absorption, methanol is widely distributed in the body with the concentration in cerebrospinal fluid exceeding that of serum. Probably very little ingested methanol is eliminated in expired air or excreted in the urine. Most is oxidized by the liver to formaldehyde and formic acid by the enzyme alcohol dehydrogenase at a rate independent of the plasma level. Since methanol is metabolized at about one seventh the rate of ethyl alcohol, complete oxidation of a toxic dose may take several days.

Usually there is a latent period of about 24 hours between ingestion and the toxic symptoms. Patients complain of nausea, vomiting, headache, blurring of vision which then progresses to blindness, stupor, coma, convulsions, and respiratory arrest (Morgan, 1974). Formic acid and other metabolites that accumulate are probably responsible for the blindness and the metabolic acidosis that occurs. In those patients without the metabolic acidosis, any loss of vision is extremely unlikely.

Methanol can best be identified by gas chromatography (Baker, 1969). Other techniques utilizing oxidation of methanol to formaldehyde and the photometric determination after reaction with chromotrophic acid (Hindberg, 1963) have proved to be unsatisfactory as emergency procedures.

Potentially toxic ingestion of alcohols has been predicted by the use of the serum osmolality. For example, a potentially lethal methanol level of 800 μg/ml (24.2 mmol/l), theoretically would increase the serum osmolality by 27 mOsmol/kg (Glasser, 1973). In a case report, Stern (1974) not only found an increased osmolality extremely helpful in suggesting the diagnosis of methanol ingestion, but used the osmolality to calculate a methanol value which agreed remarkably well with the measured level.

In order to retard the formation of toxic

methanol intermediates, the treatment of methanol ingestion should include the administration of ethanol to compete with the enzyme alcohol dehydrogenase. Dialysis has proved to be of benefit in the treatment of patients who have ingested methanol (Humphery, 1974). In a small group of patients requiring dialysis, methanol concentrations ranged from 1500 to 2000 μg/ml (46.8 to 62.4 mmol/l) 24 hours after ingestion. Eight hours later, a reduction to about 85 per cent of admission levels was found in those patients treated by peritoneal dialysis while those undergoing hemodialysis showed a decrease to 15 per cent of initial levels. No complications were seen in those on hemodialysis; in the peritoneal dialysis group, one died, another became blind, and the third had no serious complications (Keyvan-Larijarni, 1974). The rapidity of the serum methanol reduction appeared to be critical in preventing severe permanent complications in the hemodialysis group.

Isopropanol

Isopropanol (isopropyl alcohol) has been utilized as a disinfectant for several decades. It has gained considerable popularity because of its known antiseptic properties, its non-potability, and the lack of legal restrictions for its use. Although slightly more toxic than ethanol when ingested, it has no noticeable harmful effect on the human skin. Strengths varying from 30 to 99.9 per cent have been recommended, but a preparation of 70 per cent isopropyl alcohol, also known as rubbing alcohol, is widely used. When ingested, isopropanol may result in symptoms similar to those of ethanol ingestion.

Isopropyl alcohol reacts in methods utilizing alcohol dehydrogenase with a cross-reactivity of about 40 per cent (Vasiliades, 1977). Gas chromatographic methods are available which are precise and specific.

Diagnosis of isopropanol ingestion is suggested by the presence of an elevated osmolality. About 15 per cent of isopropanol is metabolized to acetone, and the presence of acetone further substantiates the diagnosis of isopropanol ingestion. When the intake of isopropanol is small, acetone may be found only in the urine, but when large amounts are ingested, it can be found both in the blood and urine. Serum isopropanol levels of 1.5 mg/ml have

been found in fatal poisonings (Adelson, 1962). Isopropanol is twice as potent as ethyl alcohol. It readily produces coma and other effects similar to ethanol, but even after ingestion of large amounts, the only other sequela is that of gastritis. Although usually only supportive treatment is necessary, dialysis may be of value in selected cases (Dwa, 1974).

CARBON MONOXIDE

Carbon monoxide (CO) is a colorless, nonirritating, almost odorless gas which is generated by incomplete combustion of organic matter. It is present in the products of many industrial processes and in tobacco smoke, fumes from fires, and the exhaust of gasoline engines. Carbon monoxide combines with hemoglobin to form carboxyhemoglobin, which impairs oxygen transport in the blood through two mechanisms. The affinity of hemoglobin is over 200 times greater for carbon monoxide than it is for oxygen; exposure to even low concentrations of CO can reversibly inactivate a significant percentage of the oxygen-carrying capacity of blood. In addition, the presence of carboxyhemoglobin interfers with the release of the oxygen carried by the hemoglobin molecule (Goldsmith, 1968). The tissue oxygen tensions thus must fall to lower levels before oxyhemoglobin gives up its oxygen.

The toxic manifestation of carbon monoxide are primarily the result of hypoxia caused by the inability of the blood to carry oxygen; these include headache, vertigo, weakness, nausea, confusion, ataxia, convulsions, and coma. The signs and symptoms of acute CO toxicity depend on the proportion of hemoglobin which is combined with CO; this is a function of the concentration of CO in the inhaled air and the volume of the inspired air (Goldsmith, 1968). Toxicity also is governed by a number of other factors, including the patient's cardiac output, hemoglobin concentration in blood, and oxygen demand of the tissue. Since these factors affect an individual's response to a given concentration of carbon monoxide, the patient may present with variable clinical findings. The intensity of the symptoms also may vary, and when high concentrations of CO are inhaled, loss of consciousness may occur without the classic symptoms of headache, nausea, and vomiting (Stewart, 1975).

A number of methods are available for the measurement of carbon monoxide in blood, including highly sensitive gas chromatographic techniques. Automated differential spectrophotometry is a rapid and convenient technique for the measurement of carbon monoxide. The concentrations of reduced hemoglobin, oxyhemoglobin, and carboxyhemoglobin can be calculated from the measured absorbances at three suitable wavelengths and the solving of a simultaneous equation. Methemoglobin may be converted to reduced hemoglobin to eliminate interference in this system (Dubowski, 1973). Automated instruments which process specimens and compute results as per cent oxyhemoglobin, per cent carboxyhemoglobin, and total hemoglobin are available, e.g., CO-Oximeter I.L. 282 (Instrumentation Laboratory, Lexington, Mass.).

Carbon monoxide is produced endogenously from the metabolism of heme pigments, and the concentration may be increased in a number of conditions including hemolytic disease. In normal non-smokers living in cities, 0.25 to 2.1 per cent carboxyhemoglobin saturations have been found, while the levels in smokers have been reported in the order of 0.7 to 6.5 per cent (Dubowski, 1973). In a national survey it has been reported that 45 per cent of non-smoking blood donors in 18 sections of the country had carboxyhemoglobin saturations greater than 1.5 per cent (Stewart, 1975). In a group of patients who smoked excessively and had elevated hematocrits, carboxyhemoglobin values were found to vary from 4.2 to 21.3 per cent with a mean of 11.6 per cent. In this study, the mean carboxyhemoglobin level in the normal non-smoking control group was 0.6 per cent (Smith, 1978).

Symptoms of acute carbon monoxide poisoning generally occur at about 20 per cent carboxyhemoglobin and become severe at about 30 per cent. In fatal poisoning, the carboxyhemoglobin usually ranges from 60 to 80 per cent but death sometimes may occur at lower levels (Dubowski, 1973).

METHEMOGLOBIN AND SULFHEMOGLOBIN

Methemoglobin, a derivative of hemoglobin in which the ferrous ion has been oxidized to the ferric form, does not transport oxygen. Normally less than about 1 per cent of the total hemoglobin is in the form of methemoglobin; amounts exceeding this are termed methemoglobinemia. Although the major clinical feature is cyanosis, severe acute methemoglobinemia may produce symptoms of anemia, and blood concentrations exceeding 60 to 70 per cent may be associated with vascular collapse and death. Ordinarily the small amounts of methemoglobin which are produced in the body are reduced back to hemoglobin. Reduction of methemoglobin in the normal red cell is achieved mainly through a NADH-linked enzyme system. Hereditary deficiency of methemoglobin reductase (NADH diaphorase), the enzyme which catalyzes a step in the major pathway of methemoglobin reduction, may result in congenital methemoglobinemia. Other enzyme deficiencies and certain hemoglobinopathies also may be associated with methemoglobinemia. Oxidation of hemoglobin may be accelerated by many chemicals and drugs, including nitrites, sulfonamides, acetanilid, and phenacetin.

The term sulfhemoglobin refers to a poorly characterized hemoglobin derivative which can be produced *in vitro* from the action of hydrogen sulfide on hemoglobin. Sulfhemoglobinemia may occur in association with the administration of various drugs, including phenacetin and acetanilid, but also has been reported in the absence of drug administration or exposure to toxins. Although sulfhemoglobin usually produces few symptoms, the cyanosis produced is intense. Once formed, the sulfhemoglobin is stable; it disappears as the red cells become senescent and are destroyed.

Methemoglobin and sulfhemoglobin may be determined by differences in their differential absorption spectra. In dilute acid, methemoglobin has an absorption band at 630 nm, which almost completely disappears when it is converted to cyanomethemoglobin by the addition of sodium cyanide. The change in absorbance is proportional to the concentration of methemoglobin. A band in the 620 nm range occurs with sulfhemoglobin; this band does not disappear with the addition of cyanide (see Fig. 15-10). Since methemoglobin if present interferes, the concentration of sulfhemoglobin is determined after methemoglobin is converted to cyanomethemoglobin. For details of the quantitative determination of methemoglobin and sulfhemoglobin, the

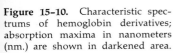

Red   Orange Yellow   Green   Blue

700   600   575   550   525   500

Oxyhemoglobin — narrow absorptive bands at 540 and 575 nm.

Reduced hemoglobin — single absorption band at 565 nm.

Figure 15–10. Characteristic spectrums of hemoglobin derivatives; absorption maxima in nanometers (nm.) are shown in darkened area.

Carboxyhemoglobin — absorption bands at 535 and 572 nm.

Methemoglobin — absorption band at 630 to 634 nm.

Sulfhemoglobin — absorption band at 618 to 620 nm.

700   600   575   550   525   500

Cyanmethemoglobin — absorption band at 550 nm.

reader should consult Dubowski (1964) and Chapter 27 for further discussion.

CYANIDE

Cyanide poisoning may result from the inhalation or ingestion of compounds that release the cyanide ion. In addition, prolonged contact with cyanide solutions may result in absorption of toxic amounts through the skin. Cyanides are used extensively in certain industries and have been employed as insecticides and rodenticides. Sporadic cases of cyanide poisoning have been reported after ingestion of certain kinds of fruit seeds. Most cases of serious cyanide intoxication, however, are the result of suicide attempts. Acute cyanide poisoning may be manifest by headache, excitement, vomiting, hypotension, cyanosis, convulsions, and coma. The scent of bitter almonds is a classic sign; however, many individuals are unable to recognize this smell. Cyanide inhibits the cytochrome oxidase system, thus blocking cellular respiration. Cyanide is metabolized rapidly within the body and up to about 50 per cent of absorbed cyanide may be inactivated within one hour after exposure. It is converted by the liver rhodanase system to thiocyanate, which is a relatively non-toxic compound that is excreted in the urine.

Sodium nitrite has been used to treat cyanide poisoning; the nitrites produce methemoglobin, which then presumably traps and inactivates free cyanide by forming the stable complex, cyanomethemoglobin. Sodium thiosulfate also is given to furnish a sulfur for the rhodanase-mediated reaction in which cyanide is converted to thiocyanate. Several recent reports have pointed out the importance of supportive therapy in the treatment of cyanide poisoning (Graham, 1977; Edwards, 1978). For a review of the treatment of acute cyanide poisoning, see Graham (1977).

Many spot tests are available for the rapid detection of cyanide, and quantitative techniques are available as well (Free, 1970). An automated fluorometric method for blood cyanide levels has been reported with the sensitivity of 0.5 μg/ml (Groff, 1977). Normally there is no significant level of cyanide in blood or urine. Fatal cyanide poisoning has been reported with blood levels greater than 3 μg/ml (Graham, 1977). Serious poisonings, however, may occur with only modestly elevated blood levels several hours after the poisoning (Berlin, 1977). Thiocyanate levels may be of use if chronic cyanide intoxication is suspected.

HEAVY METALS

Arsenic

Inorganic arsenicals are employed as insecticides, herbicides, and rodenticides. These and arsine (arsenous hydride), which is a colorless, non-irritating gas, can cause arsenic poisoning. Most cases of arsine poisoning have been associated with the use, in various industrial processes, of acid and crude metals, one or both of which contain arsenic as an impurity (Fowler, 1974). The toxic action of arsenic occurs through its ability to inhibit the sulfhydral enzyme systems of the body. Acute toxicity may be manifested by gastrointestinal symptoms, such as severe gastric pain, vomiting, and diarrhea. In severe poisoning, convulsions, coma, and death may occur. In some patients, nervous system symptoms such as irritability, stupor, and coma predominate. Characteristic of arsine poisoning is the triad of abdominal pain, hematuria, and jaundice. It may also cause a hemolytic anemia and may lead to renal failure. Chronic arsenic poisoning has an insidious onset and is manifested by many signs and symptoms including diarrhea, skin pigmentation, hyperkeratosis, hepatomegaly, renal tubular damage, and hair loss. As toxicity advances, central nervous system symptoms may predominate and blood dyscrasias may occur. Arsenic is stored mainly in the liver, kidney, walls of the gastrointestinal tract, spleen, and lung. Since it has a high affinity for keratin, the concentration of arsenic in hair and nails is higher than in other tissues. Several weeks after exposure, transverse white stria may appear in the fingernails which are called Mees lines. Arsenic is excreted mainly in the urine (Giberson, 1976).

Arsenic may be determined by screening techniques in which it forms a dull black deposit on copper strips under acid conditions (Kaye, 1971). A quantitative procedure, the silver diethyldithiocarbamate method, also is available (Sunshine, 1971). In acute poisoning, confirmation of the diagnosis is made by finding increased arsenic in urine, stomach contents, vomitus, or gastric lavage. In chronic exposure, urine, hair, or nail clippings are preferred specimens. Arsenic may be found in hair as soon as 30 hours after ingestion. Normal arsenic levels range from 3 to 7 μg/dl (0.4 to 0.9 μmol/l) in blood, up to 200 μg/l (2.6 μmol/l) in urine, and 20 to 60 μg/100 g of hair or nails (Sunshine, 1971). Normally no arsenic is detectable in gastric contents. Some overlap in urinary levels may occur between normal individuals and those with arsenic intoxication. Blood or urine arsenic levels may be measured periodically during the treatment period as a parameter of the effectiveness of therapy (Kaye, 1970).

Iron toxicity

Although large doses of iron may be well tolerated by adults, a relatively small number of iron tablets may cause death in children. Iron tablets vary considerably in the amount of elemental iron they contain: an iron dose of 150 mg/kg is considered dangerous (Dreisbach, 1977). Signs and symptoms of toxicity, which may occur within 30 minutes after ingestion or may be delayed several hours, include gastrointestinal irritation and abdominal pain, often accompanied by vomiting and bloody diarrhea. Iron toxicity also may be associated with cyanosis, drowsiness, lethargy, convulsions, coma, and death. If death does not occur in the first few hours, a transient, nearly asymptomatic period may occur before death ensues. If recovery occurs, corrosive injury to the gastrointestinal tract may result in severe scarring.

The toxic effects of iron salts result from the presence of unbound serum iron; normally the serum iron binding capacity is 250 to 400 μg/dl (44.8 to 71.6 μmol/l). Shock and coma may occur in up to 50 per cent of patients with serum iron levels above 700 μg/dl (125 μmol/l) (Dreisbach, 1977). Serum iron levels greater than 500 μg/dl (89.5 μmol/l) indicate serious poisoning (Callender, 1974). For discussion of iron metabolism and methods of analysis, see Chapter 10.

Lead

Lead is a heavy metal without any known function in the human body. Since the sources of lead are ubiquitous, lead poisoning is a serious public health problem. The most common cause of clinical lead intoxication in children is ingestion of lead-containing paints. A single paint chip may contain 10,000 μg of lead (Fielding, 1977). As paint on walls may crack and chip or as old houses are renovated with extensive scraping and sanding of the old paint layers, the risk of lead poisoning increases. For children with a tendency to pica, the risk is further increased. Other sources of lead include automobile emissions, fumes from burning storage batteries, and some types of ceramic tableware. Considerable amounts of lead occur in certain decorative decals and glazes used on the exterior of glasses.

Lead is absorbed slowly and incompletely from the gastrointestinal tract and can be absorbed from the respiratory tract after inhalation. In adults about 8 per cent of dietary lead is absorbed, but in infants and young children absorption has been found to be approximately 50 per cent, although the accuracy of this estimate has been questioned (Hammond, 1977).

The distribution of lead in the body is primarily in two pools, an active pool in the blood and soft tissues and a storage pool in bones. In the blood, nearly all circulating inorganic lead is associated with the erythyrocytes. Following absorption, lead is distributed in the soft tissues, with the highest concentrations reached in the kidney. Over a period of time, the lead is redistributed and accumulates in bone, teeth, and hair, with a small quantity of inorganic lead becoming deposited in the brain. Since the rate of excretion of lead is very slow, it tends to accumulate in the body. Lead is excreted mainly by the kidneys.

Signs and symptoms of lead poisoning may include malaise, anorexia, abdominal pain, vomiting, irritability, and apathy. Manifestations of lead poisoning include effects on the hematopoietic, renal, and central nervous systems. Lead poisoning commonly is associated with anemia (see p. 984). Fanconi's syndrome, characterized by aminoaciduria, glucosuria, and phosphoturia, may occur but is reversible with chelation therapy. Lead encephalopathy is characterized by sudden onset of cerebral edema, coma, and convulsions. Sequelae may include mental retardation, seizure disorders, behavior abnormalities, and occasionally blindness, aphasia, and hemiparesis (Chisolm, 1977). Neurologic damage, especially in children, is often irreversible, and acute neurologic toxicity may develop without previous symptoms. Therefore, it is important to detect and treat lead poisoning before symptoms become obvious. The limits between normal lead levels and excessive exposure are ill-defined. Because the symptoms of lead poisoning are variable, and lead encephalopathy so catastrophic, many clinicians have questioned if low lead levels may produce a subtle form of brain injury. Some studies have reported, in fact, that asymptomatic lead poisoning may cause significant and permanent impairment in nervous system function (Fielding, 1977).

The heme biosynthetic pathway is affected by lead at several different sites. Enzymes in the heme pathway that are sensitive to lead include the enzyme delta-aminolevulinic dehydratase, which is responsible for condensation of two molecules of delta-aminolevulinic acid (ALA) to form porphobilinogen. The enzyme ferrochelatase, which inserts iron into protoporphyrin IX to form heme, also is affected. Interference with the incorporation of iron into the tetrapyrole ring results in its replacement by zinc.

Analysis of blood lead is associated with certain problems, such as the necessity of scrupulous care in order to avoid contamination of the specimen by environmental lead. Efforts to screen for lead poisoning, therefore, have been directed toward measurement of effects of lead on heme synthesis. Toxic effects of lead may be manifested by increased excretion of delta-aminolevulinic acid and coproporphyrin, increased erythyrocyte protoporphyrin, and decreased delta-aminolevulinic dehydratase. Although coproporphyrinuria is used as a diagnostic determination, it occurs as a delayed response to lead ingestion, is not very sensitive, and is not specific (Labbé, 1977). The enzyme delta-aminolevulinic dehydratase, which may be assayed in whole blood, is an indicator of acute exposure to lead, since it is affected by the lead level at the time of the determination (Granick, 1978). Delta-aminolevulinic acid in urine has been used as a parameter of excess lead burden; however, difficulties in collecting a 24-hour urine specimen are encountered. Increased levels of zinc protoporphyrin or its extraction product, free erythrocyte protoporphyrin, occurs in individuals with increased blood lead concentrations and is a sensitive index of toxicity. Free erythyrocyte protoporphyrin or zinc protoporphyrin reflects chronic lead exposure (Granick, 1978). Several methods of erythyrocyte protoporphyrin detection have been developed. In the method of Piomelli (1973), free erythyrocyte protoporphyrin is extracted and measured fluorometrically. Protoporphyrin accounts for the majority of the porphyrin extracted. Zinc protoporphyrin can be determined in whole blood by direct measurement of its fluorescence (Lamola, 1975). A portable filter fluorometer has been specifically designed for rapid assay of erythyrocyte zinc protoporphyrin in whole blood (Blumberg, 1977). Erythrocyte protoporphyrin (EP) values may be expressed as $\mu g/dl$ of erythrocytes, $\mu g/dl$ of whole blood, or $\mu g/g$ of hemoglobin. For uniformity the Center for Disease Control (CDC) recommends that the erythyrocyte protoporphyrin be expressed as equivalents of free erythyrocyte protoporphyrin in $\mu g/dl$ in whole blood. Normal values have been reported equal to or less than 59 $\mu g/dl$ of whole blood (= or < 5 $\mu g/g$ hemoglobin) with moderately elevated values in the range of 60 to 189 $\mu g/dl$ (5 to 17 $\mu g/g$ hemoglobin) (Piomelli, 1977). Erythyrocyte protoporphyrin levels may be increased in diseases other than lead poisoning, including iron deficiency anemia and erythropoietic protoporphyria. Extremely elevated values, that is, 190 $\mu g/dl$ whole blood or greater, are almost always due to lead intoxication (Center for Disease Control, 1975). In erythropoietic protoporphyria the levels also are very high, but this disorder has a number of distinguishing clinical features, including prominent photosensitivity.

About 90 per cent of circulating lead is associated with erythrocytes, and thus whole blood or red cells are used in lead determinations. Lead determinations may be performed using venous or capillary blood specimens. The difficulty with the capillary method is that the skin contamination may lead to falsely elevated values, (Klein, 1977). Christian, (1976) has reviewed methods for lead analysis. Flameless atomic absorption and polarography in the anodic stripping analysis mode are sensitive and possess a high degree of specificity. Clinical toxicity does not always relate precisely to blood lead levels. Some children may be asymptomatic at levels as high as 250 $\mu g/dl$ (12.07 $\mu mol/l$), while lead encephalopathy may occur at levels of 100 $\mu g/dl$ (4.83 $\mu mol/l$) (Zarkowsky, 1976). The Center for Disease Control has established normal values as up to 29 $\mu g/dl$ (1.40 $\mu mol/l$), with two successive blood levels between 30 and 49 $\mu g/dl$ (1.45 to 2.36 $\mu mol/l$) considered mildly elevated. For intermediate lead levels, treatment is given on the basis of additional testing. The use of provocative chelation tests, in which urinary lead concentration is measured after injection of edathamil calcium disodium (EDTA), is one procedure which may be used. There are several modifications of these provocative chelation or mobilization tests which may vary as to the amount of EDTA used and the timing of the urine specimens (Zarkowsky, 1976). The mobilization tests are good indicators of the body burden of lead but should be reserved for asymptomatic patients. It has been suggested that the ideal method is the determination of the 24-hour excretion of lead after administration of 50 mg/kg of calcium disodium EDTA. The results are expressed as the ratio of micrograms of lead excretion per milligram EDTA, with values greater than 1 considered indicative of lead poisoning (Center for Disease Control, 1975). In a statement by the Center for Disease Control (1975) lead poisoning is said to exist when (1) two successive blood lead determinations are equal to or greater than 80 $\mu g/dl$ (3.86 $\mu mol/l$) whole blood with or without symptoms; (2) erythrocyte protoporphyrin levels are equal to or greater than 190 $\mu g/dl$ (9.17 $\mu mol/l$) whole blood, with or without symptoms; (3) confirmed blood lead level is 50 to 79 $\mu g/dl$ (2.41 to 3.81 $\mu mol/l$) with compatible symptoms or associated with abnormal erythrocyte protoporphyrin, aminolevulinic acid, urinary coproporphyrin, or abnormal calcium disodium EDTA mobilization; or (4) erythyrocyte protoporphyrin (EP) levels are 110 to 189 $\mu g/dl$ whole blood, compatible with symptoms.

Both erythrocyte protoporphyrin and blood lead are acceptable as primary screening tests, since negative results usually exclude lead intoxication (Center for Disease Control, 1975). A positive result by either measurement does not establish the risk of lead poisoning, since EP may be increased by other diseases and elevated blood lead may be due to specimen contamination. Because of the problems of contamination, elevated blood lead levels should be confirmed on a repeat specimen. Both EP and blood lead are necessary for full evaluation and monitoring of those individuals positive on screening by either method. The Center for Disease Control (1975) recommends EP determinations for screening for lead poisoning because of the greater ease and reproducibility of EP measurement. In addition there is the benefit of detecting those children who may have iron deficiency. A blood lead level is recommended for all children with positive EP.

Mercury

Since medicinal uses of mercury have markedly decreased, the mercurial compounds are mainly of toxicologic importance. Compounds containing mercury are widely used in agriculture and industry. Methyl mercury compounds are the most toxic and the most important of the environmental mercury contaminants. Methyl mercury is known to be highly resistant to biodegradation and can be synthesized from any other form of mercury and concentrated in the aquatic food chain. Most of the biologic properties of mercury are due to its ability to form covalent bonds with sulfur; mercurials even in low concentrations are capable of inactivating sulfhydryl enzymes.

The absorption, distribution, and excretion of mercury vary with the form of the metal. Depending on its chemical state, mercury in toxic concentration causes a wide variety of clinical manifestations. After inhalation of mercury vapors, elementary mercury passes into the blood stream, penetrates the blood-brain barrier, and then accumulates in the central nervous system (Gerstner, 1977). After ingestion and absorption of inorganic mercu-

rials, mercury may be deposited in many organs, including the kidney, liver, heart, skeletal muscle, bone marrow, brain, and lung. The absorption, distribution, and excretion of the organic mercurials are determined by the physiologic properties of a given compound and the extent of the *in vivo* conversion to inorganic mercury. Although most of the organic mercurials are excreted quickly, urinary excretion of methyl mercury is slow owing to its low decomposition to inorganic mercury, its complete reabsorption when excreted in bile, and its low urinary excretion compared with inorganic mercury (Magos, 1975). Methyl mercury crosses the blood-brain barrier quite easily and causes irreversible damage to the nervous system. Mercury is excreted mainly by the kidney and gastrointestinal tract.

Mercury poisoning can be divided into acute and chronic. Acute poisoning usually results from the oral ingestion of inorganic mercury, although it may result from the inhalation of mercury vapors or from organic mercurials. Inhalation of mercury vapors leads to pneumonitis, fever, cough, chest pain, and other pulmonary symptoms. Ingestion of inorganic mercury is characterized by gastrointestinal symptoms such as vomiting and bloody diarrhea; shock and death may occur. The signs and symptoms of chronic poisoning from inorganic mercurials include stomatitis, colitis, progressive renal damage, anemia, and peripheral neuritis. Many central nervous system manifestations occur, including behavioral changes, irritability, tremors, and drowsiness. The methyl mercuric compounds cause mainly neurologic signs and symptoms, including ataxia, tremor, and dysarthria. Severe poisoning may lead to blindness, coma, and death.

Another type of toxic reaction occurs in children and is called acrodynia or pink disease. It is characterized by a pinkish discoloration of the skin and evidence of central nervous system involvement leading to marked hypotonia. The syndrome is thought to represent sensitization to mercury.

Techniques such as the Reinsch test or one of its modifications, which depend on the deposition of heavy metals on a copper strip, can be used to screen for mercury (Kaye, 1970). Mercury can be quantitated by flameless atomic absorption (Richardson, 1976).

Although the correlation between urinary mercury excretion and symptoms of mercury poisoning is considered poor, it is the most reliable way available to assess exposure to inorganic mercury (Littlejohn, 1977). Exposure to organic mercury compounds, however, probably is not reliably reflected by urinary levels. In contrast to inorganic mercury, methyl mercury is mainly located in the red blood cells, and thus estimation of levels must be made using red cells or whole blood. Analysis of hair also has been used, and this has been reported to help recapitulate the history of exposure (Magos, 1975).

In normal subjects mercury concentrations range from 0 to 20 μg per liter of urine (Kaye, 1971). Exposure to 0.05 mg mercury vapor/cu m of air has been suggested as the maximum allowable concentration for industrial atmosphere. This level of mercury exposure is likely to result in urinary mercury concentration of 150 μg/l (Magos, 1975).

DRUG ABUSE

One of the distinguishing features of recent drug use patterns is the variety of drugs abused. In a review of drug trends, Smith, in 1974 commented that the only constant in the American drug abuse scene "is that it will change." The drugs abused vary with such factors as geographic location, availability of the substance, and fads. In many cases, two or more drugs are combined to enhance the state of intoxication. In general, abused drugs, excluding alcohol and nicotine, can be placed in the categories of narcotic analgesics, central nervous system stimulants and depressants, cannabinoids, and psychedelics or hallucinogens. The metabolism and physiologic effects of the drugs of abuse, including amphetamines, morphine, cocaine, cannabinoids (marihuana), and lysergic acid diethylamide (LSD), have been reviewed by Lemberger (1976).

Although a number of screening techniques are available, thin layer chromatography is probably the most widely employed method. Urine specimens usually are used to screen for the drugs of abuse. Many drugs, such as cocaine, barbiturates, glutethimide, morphine, and amphetamines, may be detected using this technique. Confirmatory methods are necessary because of interferences and metabolites. Although some drugs may be excreted in the urine unchanged, others may be partially or almost completely metabolized. The use of some drugs may be indicated only

by the presence of their metabolites. For example, cocaine is extensively metabolized to benzoylecgonine and ecgonine with little free cocaine available for detection in the urine (Bastos, 1973).

For further discussion of the role of the laboratory in the analysis of the drugs of abuse, see Frings (1977).

DRUG OVERDOSE

Evaluation of a patient in coma with a suspected overdose should include the exclusion of a number of entities, such as diabetic ketoacidosis, hyperosmolar non-ketotic coma, hypoglycemia, myxedema, hyponatremia, uremia, stroke syndrome, hepatic coma, trauma, and the encephalidities. However, finding a specific cause for the coma through the investigative procedures does not exclude a drug overdose as a precipitating or associated cause of coma. In addition, the presence of an elevated drug level does not rule out a second drug or a metabolic cause of the coma.

The pattern of drug overdose is dependent on the popularity of a particular drug in a given locality and varies from time to time. For example, acetaminophen was abused in Great Britain in the early 1970's but rarely abused in the United States at that time. Phencyclidine (PCP or angel dust) apparently was not a major problem in 1972, but by 1976 was commonly abused (Walberg, 1978). Other factors such as instrumentation, the technical expertise available, and the turnaround time are considerations in determining which drug assays are made available. In several large studies, alcohol, barbiturates, and salicylates account for more than half of the overdoses. However, since there are almost 2500 drug products listed in the 1977 edition of the Physicians' Desk Reference (PDR) and since abused substances include not only these but many chemicals, it is an impossibility for even the largest laboratory specializing in toxicologic analyses to screen for all available compounds.

Techniques that are available for screening specimens from comatose patients for drugs include spectrophotometry, paper chromatography, thin layer chromatography, gas chromatography, gas chromatography-mass spectrophotometry, radioimmunoassay, enzyme immunoassay, and high performance liquid chromatography. Many of these procedures are time consuming, lack specificity and sensitivity, and are only applicable to the measurement of a single drug. Some single determinations are available on large automated instruments. For example, the salicylate and ethanol assays on the DuPont *aca*, which have a turnaround time of less than 10 minutes, are suitable for rapid detection of these substances. Other procedures such as radioimmunoassay are less suitable for use on an emergency basis, since turnaround time is relatively long. However, homogeneous enzyme immunoassay is useful as a screening technique and may be employed for barbiturates and narcotics. Techniques in which multiple drug estimations are made are convenient for screening procedures: these include thin layer chromatography, gas chromatography, and high pressure liquid chromatography. Procedures such as that of Kabra (1978), in which 12 sedatives and hypnotics can be qualitated and quantitated within 30 minutes by high performance liquid chromatography, are particularly well suited for this purpose.

For most drug overdoses, the treatment is mainly supportive, with close monitoring for the appearance of apnea. With salicylates and long-acting barbiturates, alkalinization of the urine is an additional therapeutic modality. With some drugs, such as narcotics and propoxyphene, treatment with morphine antagonists may be of benefit. In patients with stage 3 or 4 coma with an unknown intoxicant, hemodialysis may be initiated if improvement is not noted within 24 hours or if methyl alcohol intoxication is suspected (Arieff, 1973). When the identity of the intoxicant is known, hemodialysis usually is indicated when criteria outlined by Schreiner (1972) are met.

In conclusion, many factors determine which drugs should be screened for in a comatose patient. At a minimum, ethanol, salicylates, and barbiturates should be determined, and depending on the resources available, other screens for the alcohols, hypnotics, opiates, and phenothiazines are recommended as appropriate.

Methods

Ethanol. Modification of the microdiffusion technique (Conway-Feldstein-Klendshoj).

Procedure

1. Sealer: 2 ml of potassium carbonate (saturated) is placed in the small groove of rim of the microdiffusion cell.

2. Reactant: 2 ml of Ansties reagent is placed in the center chamber. Ansties: Dissolve 3.70 g of potassium dichromate c.p. in 150 ml of distilled water. Add slowly, with constant stirring, 280 ml of sulfuric acid c.p. Finally dilute to 500 ml with distilled water.

3. One ml of blood or urine is spread in the outer chamber.

4. Spread 1 ml of potassium carbonate (saturated) on top of the blood and quickly seal with the lid.

5. Put the lid in place and gently twist to obtain a liquid seal. Then gently swirl entire unit to mix specimen and liberating agent. Diffusion is started.

6. Allow to diffuse at least 1 hour at room temperature (30°C.).

7. Ethanol standards may be used: 1 ml of 95 per cent ethanol in 250 ml of water makes a stock solution.

STOCK SOLUTION		APPROX. G/100 ML OF BLOOD	COLOR OF ANSTIES SOLUTION
0.00 ml	0	0.00	yellow-canary
0.25	+	0.08	yellow-yellow-green
0.50	+ +	0.15	yellow-green
0.75	+ + +	0.23	yellow-green-green
1.00	+ + + +	0.30 (dangerous) (above 0.40 is dangerous to life)	green blue

8. Terminal blood-alcohol levels may sometimes be low if survival time permitted metabolism and elimination or presence of other depressant drugs acting synergistically.

9. Methanol and isopropanol also give this reaction: 0.05 per cent methanol or 0.22 per cent isopropanol will give readings equivalent to 0.09 per cent using ethanol standards. Differentiation should therefore be made, because treatment is quite different.

Salicylates

SALICYLATES: URINE

Materials and Reagents

1. Ten per cent ferric chloride.

2. Test tubes and rack, graduated cylinder.

Procedure. To 3 ml of urine add 1 ml of 10 per cent ferric chloride. If salicylate is present, a purple color will appear and persist. This test is very sensitive and is positive in urine after the ingestion of only one 0.3 g (5 gr) aspirin tablet. This test is positive for aspirin, sodium, phenyl, or methyl salicylates, or phenol derivatives.

Paper strip test (Phenistix) may also be used. Whereas a positive test is suggestive, a negative test is certain.

SALICYLATES: SERUM (NATELSON, 1961)

Reagents

1. Ferric nitrate: 1 per cent in 0.07 N nitric acid.

2. Nitric acid: 0.07 N (4.69 ml of nitric acid sp. gr. 1.42 and 70.5 per cent; made up to 1 liter).

3. Salicylate standard: 25 mg/100 ml: 29 mg of

sodium salicylate; or 25 mg of salicylic acid/100 ml H$_2$O.

Procedure

Qualitative. Serum or urine, 0.01 ml, is placed in a small white evaporating dish; then add 1 drop 1 per cent nitrate (in 0.07 N nitric acid). A purple color is positive for salicylates.

Report amount present as: Negative, faint, moderate, or large.

Barbiturates*

Procedure

1. To three 50 ml screw cap, round-bottom glass tubes, labeled Positive, Negative, and Test, add 3 ml positive control, 3 ml negative control, and patient serum or urine, respectively.

2. Dispense 2.0 ml 0.5 M phosphate buffer, pH 7.4, into each tube.

3. Dispense 30 ml chloroform into each tube.

4. Shake each tube on a mechanical shaker for 5 minutes.

5. Centrifuge each tube for 3 minutes at 1000 rpm.

6. Aspirate and discard the upper aqueous phase. Be careful not to aspirate too much of the lower organic phase.

7. Filter the organic phase with Whatman No. 1 filter paper into a 100 ml graduated cylinder. Collect 25 ml of the organic phase and transfer it into a properly labeled 50 ml screw cap, round-bottom glass tube.

_____

*From Jatlow, 1973.

8. Pipette 5 ml of 0.45 N NaOH into each tube. Shake each tube and centrifuge as noted in steps 4 and 5.

9. Pipette 2.0 ml of the upper aqueous phase and transfer it to a cuvette identified as pH 10. Pipette another 2.0 ml aliquot of the aqueous phase and transfer it to another cuvette identified as pH 14. (A 1.0 ml Biopipette may be used.)

10. Pipette 0.5 ml of 10.7 per cent NH$_4$Cl and transfer it to the cuvette identified as pH 10.

11. Pipette 0.5 ml of 0.45 N NaOH and transfer it to the cuvette identified as pH 14.

12. Mix both cuvettes by inversion.

13. Place the cuvette identified as pH 10 in the reference side of the spectrophotometer. The cuvette identified as pH 14 is placed in the sample side.

14. Set baseline at 50. Scan from 280 nm to 220 nm. Label the tracing with the date and patient's name or number.

15. Scan the positive and negative controls first. Label the absorption peaks for the positive control with the corresponding wavelengths. A positive scan (differential scan) should give absorption peaks at 255 nm and 240 nm.

16. Scan the patient's sample(s) and label any absorption peaks. Report the results as positive screen for barbiturates or negative screen for barbiturates. The barbiturate in a positive barbiturate screen must be identified as long-acting or as short- to intermediate-acting.

REFERENCES

Adelson, L.: Fatal intoxication with isopropyl alcohol (rubbing alcohol). Am. J. Clin. Pathol., 33:144, 1962.

Adjepon-Yamoah, K. K., and Prescott, L. F.: Gas-liquid chromatographic estimation of lignocaine, ethylglycyl-xylidide, glycylxylidide, and 4-hydroxyxylidine in plasma and urine. J. Pharm. Pharmacol., 26:889, 1974.

Ambler, P. K., Singh, B. N., and Lever, M.: A simple and rapid fluorometric method for the estimation of 1-(2-hydroxy-3-isopropyl-amino-propoxy)-naphthalene hydrochloride, propranolol, in blood. Clin. Chim. Acta, 54:373, 1974.

Ameer, B., and Greenblatt, D. J.: Acetaminophen. Ann. Intern. Med., 87:202, 1977.

Anast, C. S.: Anticonvulsant drugs and calcium metabolism. N. Engl. J. Med., 292:587, 1975.

Anderson, R. J., Potts, D. E., Gabow, P. A., Rumack, B. H., and Schrier, R. W.: Unrecognized adult salicylate intoxication. Ann. Intern. Med., 85:745, 1976.

Andrews, H. B.: Salicylate poisoning. Am. Fam. Physician, 8:102, 1973.

Arieff, A. I., and Friedman, E. A.: Coma following nonnarcotic drug overdosage: Management of 208 patients. Am. J. Med. Sci., 266:405, 1973.

Åsberg, M.: Individualization of treatment with tricyclic compounds. Med. Clin. North. Am., 58:1083, 1974.

Baird, H. W., Carter, S., Lombroso, C., McFarland, H. R., Penry, J. K., and Pippenger, C.: Getting to know the epilepsies. Patient Care, 11:102, 1977.

Baker, R. N., Alenty, A. L., and Zack, J. F.: Simultaneous determination of lower alcohols, acetone and acetaldehyde in blood by gas chromatography. J. Chromatogr. Sci., 7:312, 1969.

Barker, J. D., deCarle, D. J., and Anuras, S.: Chronic excessive acetaminophen use and liver damage. Ann. Intern. Med., 87:299, 1977.

Barker, M. H.: The blood cyanates in the treatment of hypertension. J.A.M.A., 106:762, 1936.

Bastos, M. L., Jukofsky, D., and Mulé, S. J.: Routine identification of cocaine metabolites in human urine. J. Chromatogr., 89:335, 1974.

Beard, J. D., Knott, D. H., and Fink, R. D.: The use of plasma and urine osmolality in evaluating the acute phase of alcohol abuse. South. Med. J., 67:271, 1974.

Bennett, I. L., Cary, F. H., Mitchell, G. L., and Cooper, M. N.: Acute methyl alcohol poisoning: A review based on experiences in an outbreak of 323 cases. Medicine, 32:431, 1953.

Berlin, C.: Cyanide poisoning—a challenge. Arch. Intern. Med., 137:993, 1977.

Bigger, J. T., Schmidt, D. H., and Kutt, H.: Relationships between the plasma level of diphenylhydantoin sodium and its cardiac antiarrhythmic effects. Circulation, 38:363, 1968.

Black, M.: Liver disease and drug therapy. Med. Clin. North Am., 58:1051, 1974.

Blumberg, W. E., Eisinger, J., Lamola, A. A., and Zuckerman, D. M.: The hematofluorometer. Clin. Chem., *23*:270, 1977.

Blume, R. S., MacLowry, J. D., and Wolff, S. M.: Limitations of chloride determination in the diagnosis of bromism. N. Engl. J. Med., *279*:593, 1968.

Booker, H. E., and Darcy, B.: Serum concentrations of free diphenylhydantoin and their relationship to clinical intoxication. Epilepsia, *14*:177, 1973.

Bower, P. J., and Peterson, J. N.: Methemoglobinemia after sodium nitroprusside therapy. N. Engl. J. Med., *294*:865, 1975.

Brillman, J., Gallagher, B. B., and Mattson, R. H.: Acute primidone intoxication. Arch. Neurol., *30*:255, 1974.

Buchanan, R. A., Kinkel, A. W., Turner, J. L., and Heffelfinger, J. C.: Ethosuximide dosage regimens. Clin. Pharmacol. Ther., *19*:143, 1976.

Butler, T. J.: Analytic approaches and problems in blood alcohol analysis. *In* Lundberg, G. D. (ed.): The Professional and Community Role of the Pathologist in Alcohol Abuse. Washington, D.C., U.S. Department of Transportation. National Highway Traffic Safety Administration, 1976.

Butler, V. P.: Assays of digitalis in blood. Prog. Cardiovasc. Dis., *14*:571, 1972.

Butler, V. P., and Lindenbaum, J.: Serum digitalis measurements in the assessment of digitalis resistance and sensitivity. Am. J. Med., *58*:460, 1975.

Callender, S. T.: Treatment of iron deficiency, *In* Jacobs, A., and Worwood, M. (eds.): Iron in Biochemistry and Medicine. London, Academic Press, 1974.

Carr, K., Woosley, R. L., and Oates, J. A.: Simultaneous quantification of procainamide and N-acetylprocainamide with high-performance liquid chromatography. J. Chromatogr., *129*:363, 1976.

Cate, J. C., and Jatlow, P. I.: Chlordiazepoxide overdose: Interpretations of serum drug concentrations. Clin. Toxicol., *6*:553, 1973.

Cate, J. C., and Tenser, R.: Acute primidone overdosage with massive crystalluria. Clin. Toxicol., *8*:385, 1975.

Center for Disease Control: Increased lead absorption and lead poisoning in young children. J. Pediatr., *87*:824, 1975.

Cereghino, J. J.: Serum carbamazepine concentration and clinical control. Adv. Neurol., *11*:309, 1975.

Chabner, B. A., Myers, C. E., Coleman, C. N., and Johns, D. G.: The clinical pharmacology of antineoplastic agents (first of two parts). N. Engl. J. Med., *292*:1107, 1975.

Chiou, W. L., and Onyemelukwe, I.: Possible errors and role of mercuric chloride in using Trinder's reagent for assay of salicylates in urine specimens. J. Pharm. Sci., *62*:1742, 1973.

Chisolm, J. J.: Is lead poisoning still a problem? Clin. Chem., *23*:252, 1977.

Christian, G. D.: The biochemistry and analysis of lead. Adv. Clin. Chem., *18*:289, 1976.

Cimbera, G.: Review of methods of analysis for phenothiazine drugs. J. Chromatogr. Sci., *10*:287, 1972.

Cobb, M. E., Buckley, N., Hu, M. W., Miller, J. G., Singh, P., and Schneider, R. S.: Homogeneous enzyme immunoassay for lidocaine in serum. Clin. Chem., *23*:1161, 1977.

Collinsworth, K. A., Strong, J. M., Atkinson, A. J., Winkle, R. A., Perlroth, F., and Harrison, D. C.: Pharmacokinetics and metabolism of lidocaine in patients with renal failure. Clin. Pharmacol. Ther., *18*:59, 1975.

Coppen, A., Montgomery, S., Ghose, K., RamaRao, V. A., Bailey, J., Christiansen, J., Mikkleson, P. L., van Praag, H. M., van de Poel, F., Minsker, E. J., Kozulja, V. G.,

Matussek, N., Kungkunz, G., and Jorgensen, A.: Amitriptyline plasma concentration and clinical effect. A World Health Organization collaborative study. Lancet, *1*:63, 1978.

Cotham, R. H., and Shand, D.: Spuriously low plasma propranolol concentrations resulting from blood collection methods. Clin. Pharmacol. Ther., *18*:535, 1975.

Dettli, L.: Individualization of drug dosage in patients with renal disease. Med. Clin. North Am., *58*:977, 1974.

DiSalle, D., Baker, K. M., Bareggi, S. R., Watkins, W. D., Chidsey, C. A., Frigerio, A., and Morselli, P. L.: A sensitive gas chromatographic method for the determination of propranolol in human plasma. J. Chromatogr., *84*:347, 1973.

Doherty, J. E., and Kane, J. J.: Clinical pharmacology of digitalis glycosides. Ann. Rev. Med., *26*:159, 1975.

Done, A. K.: Role of the physician—hospital emergencies. *In* Thoma, J. J., Bondo, P. B., and Sunshine, I. (eds.): Guidelines for Analytical Toxicology Programs, vol. I. Cleveland, CRC Press, Inc., 1977.

Done A. K.: Salicylate intoxication, significance of measurements of salicylate in blood in cases of acute ingestion. Pediatrics, *26*:800, 1960.

Dorrity, F., Linnoila, M., and Habig, R. L.: Therapeutic monitoring of tricyclic antidepressants in plasma by gas chromatography. Clin. Chem., *23*:1326, 1977.

Dreisbach, R. H.: Handbook of Poisoning. Diagnosis and Treatment. Los Altos, Cal., Lange Medical Publications, 1977.

Dubowski, K. M., and Luke, J. L.: Measurement of carboxyhemoglobin and carbon monoxide in blood. Ann. Clin. Lab. Sci., *3*:53, 1973.

Dubowski, K. M.: Measurement of hemoglobin derivatives. *In* Sunderman, F. W., and Sunderman, F. W., Jr. (eds.): Hemoglobin. Its Precursors and Metabolites. Philadelphia, J. P. Lippincott Co., 1964.

Dvorchik, B. H., and Vesell, E. S.: Pharmacokinetic interpretation of data gathered during therapeutic drug monitoring. Clin. Chem., *22*:868, 1976.

Dwa, S. L.: Peritoneal dialysis for isopropyl alcohol poisoning. J.A.M.A., *230*:35, 1974.

Edwards, A. C., and Thomas, I. D.: Cyanide poisoning. Lancet, *1*:92, 1978.

Elson, J., Strong, J. M., Lee, W., and Atkinson, A. J.: Antiarrhythmic potency of N-acetylprocainamide. Clin. Pharmacol. Ther., *17*:134, 1975.

Falk, L. C., Clark, D. R., Kalman, S. M., and Long, T. F.: Enzymatic assay for methotrexate in serum and cerebrospinal fluid. Clin. Chem., *22*:785, 1976.

Feinberg, A.: Propoxyphene hydrochloride (Darvon) poisoning. A report of two cases. Clin. Pediatr., *12*:402, 1973.

Fielding, J. E., and Russo, P. K.: Exposure to lead: Sources and effects. N. Engl. J. Med., *297*:943, 1977.

Fincham, R. W., Schottelius, D. D., and Sahs, A. L.: The influence of diphenylhydantoin on primidone metabolism. Arch. Neurol., *30*:259, 1974.

Finkelstein, F. O., Goffinet, J. A., Hendler, E. D., and Lindenbaum, J.: Pharmocokinetics of digoxin and digitoxin in patients undergoing hemodialysis. Am. J. Med., *58*:525, 1975.

Forrest, F. M., Forrest, I. F., and Mason, A. S.: Review of rapid urine tests for phenothiazine and related drugs. Am. J. Psychiatry, *118*:300, 1961.

Fowler, B. A., and Weissberg, J. B.: Arsine poisoning. N. Engl. J. Med., *291*:1171, 1974.

Free, A. H., and Free, H. M.: Laboratory detection of cyanide poisoning. *In* Sunderman, F. W., and Sunderman, F. W., Jr. (eds.): Laboratory Diagnosis of Diseases Caused by Toxic Agents. St. Louis, Warren H. Green, Inc., 1970.

Frei, E., Jaffe, N., Tattersall, M. H. N., Pitman, S., and Parker, L.: New approaches to cancer chemotherapy with methotrexate. N. Engl. J. Med., *292*:846, 1975.

Frigerio, A., and Morselli, P. L.: Carbamazepine: Biotransformation. Adv. Neurol., *11*:295, 1975.

Frings, C. S.: Role of the laboratory with regard to drug-abuse treatment facilities. *In* Thomas, J. J., Bondo, P. B., and Sunshine, I. (eds.): Guidelines for Analytical Toxicology Programs, vol. I. Cleveland, CRC Press, Inc., 1977.

Gerstner, H. B., and Huff, J. E.: Selected case histories and epidemiologic examples of human mercury poisoning. Clin. Toxicol., *11*:131, 1977.

Gibaldi, M., and Levy, G.: Pharmacokinetics in clinical practice. J.A.M.A., *235*:1987, 1976.

Giberson, A., Vaziri, N. D., Mirahamadi, K., and Rosen, S. M.: Hemodialysis of acute arsenic intoxication with transient renal failure. Arch. Intern. Med., *136*:1303, 1976.

Glasser, L., Sternglanz, P. D., Combie, J., and Robinson, A.: Serum osmolality and its applicability to drug overdose. Am. J. Clin. Pathol., *60*:695, 1973.

Glazko, A. J.: Antiepileptic drugs: Biotransformation, metabolism, and serum half-life. Epilepsia, *16*:367, 1975.

Goldbaum, L. R.: Determination of barbiturates. Analyt. Chem., *10*:1604, 1952.

Goldsmith, J. R., and Landaw, S. A.: Carbon monoxide and human health. Science, *162*:1352, 1968.

Gotelli, G. R., Kabra, P. M., and Marton, L. J.: Determination of acetaminophen and phenacetin in plasma by high-pressure liquid chromatography. Clin. Chem., *23*:957, 1977.

Goulet, J. R., Kinkel, A. W., and Smith, T. C.: Metabolism of ethosuximide. Clin. Pharmacol. Ther., *20*:213, 1976.

Graham, D. L., Laman, D., Theodore, J., and Robin, E. D.: Acute cyanide poisoning complicated by lactic acidosis and pulmonary edema. Arch. Intern. Med., *137*:1051, 1977.

Granick, J. L., Sassa, S., and Kappas, A.: Some biochemical and clinical aspects of lead intoxication. Adv. Clin. Chem., *20*:287, 1978.

Greenblatt, D. J., and Shader, R. I.: Detection and quantitation. *In* Greenblatt, D. J., and Shader, R. I. (eds.): Benzodiazepines in Clinical Practice. New York, Raven Press, 1974.

Greenblatt, D. J., Shader, R. I., and Koch-Weser, J.: Slow absorption of intramuscular chlordiazepoxide. N. Engl. J. Med., *291*:1116, 1974.

Greiss, L., Tremblay, N. A. G., and Davies, D. W.: The toxicity of sodium nitroprusside. Can. Anaesth. Soc. J., *23*:480, 1976.

Groff, W. A., Cucinell, S. A., Vicario, P., and Kaminskis, A.: A completely automated fluorometric blood cyanide method: A specific assay incorporating dialysis and distillation. Clin. Toxicol., *11*:159, 1977.

Hammond, P. B.: Exposure of humans to lead. Ann. Rev. Pharmacol. Toxicol., *17*:197, 1977.

Hansen, A. R., and Fischer, L. J.: Gas-chromatographic simultaneous analysis for glutethimide and an active hydroxylated metabolite in tissues, plasma and urine. Clin. Chem., *20*:236, 1974.

Hansen, A. R., Kennedy, K. A., Ambre, J. J., and Fischer, L. J.: Glutethimide poisoning. A metabolite contributes to morbidity and mortality. N. Engl. J. Med., *292*:250,

1975.

Harzer, K., and Barchet, R.: Analyse von benzodiazepinen und deren hydrolysenprodukte, den benzophenonen, durch hochdruckflussigkeitschromatographie in umgekehrter phase und ihre anwendung auf biologisches material. J. Chromatogr., *132*:83, 1977.

Hayes, S. L., Pablo, G., Radomski, T., and Palmer, R. F.: Ethanol and oral diazepam absorption. N. Engl. J. Med., *296*:186, 1977.

Hendeles, L., Bighley, L., Richardson, R. H., Hepler, C. D., and Carmichael, J.: Frequent toxicity from IV aminophylline infusions in critically ill patients. Drug Intell. Clin. Pharm., *11*:12, 1977.

Hill, H. E.: A contribution to the toxicology of sodium nitroprusside. I. The decomposition and determination of sodium nitroprusside. Am. J. Cardiol., *9*:89, 1942.

Hillestad, L., Hansen, T., and Melsom, H.: Diazepam metabolism in normal man. II. Serum concentration and clinical effect after oral administration and cumulation. Clin. Pharmacol. Ther., *16*:485, 1974a.

Hillestad, L., Hansen, T., Melsom, H., and Drivenes, A.: Diazepam metabolism in normal man. I. Serum concentrations and clinical effects after intravenous, intramuscular, and oral administration. Clin. Pharmacol. Ther., *16*:479, 1974b.

Hindberg, J., and Wieth, J. O.: Quantitative determination of methanol in biologic fluids. J. Lab. Clin. Med., *61*:355, 1963.

Hirsch, C. S., Valentour, J. C., Adelson, L., and Sunshine, I.: Unexpected ethanol in drug-intoxicated persons. Postgrad. Med., *54*:53, 1973.

Hisayasu, G. H., Cohen, J. L., and Nelson, R. W.: Determination of plasma and erythrocyte lithium concentrations by atomic absorption spectrophotometry. Clin. Chem., *23*:41, 1977.

Holland, J., Massie, M. J., Grant, C., and Plumb, M. M.: Drugs ingested in suicide attempts and fatal outcome. N.Y. State J. Med., *75*:2343, 1975.

Hollifield, J. W., Sherman, K., Vander Zwagg, R., and Shand, D. G.: Proposed mechanisms of propranolol's antihypertensive effect in essential hypertension. N. Engl. J. Med., *295*:68, 1976.

Hollister, L. E.: Individualized dosage of tricyclic antidepressants. Drugs, *14*:161, 1977.

Horning, M. J., Brown, L., Nowlin, J., Lertratanangkoon, K., Kellaway, P., and Zion, T. E.: Use of saliva in therapeutic drug monitoring. Clin. Chem., *23*:157, 1977.

Humphery, T. J.: Methanol poisoning: Management of acidosis with combined haemodialysis and peritoneal dialysis. Med. J. Aust., *1*:833, 1974.

Irey, N. S.: Blood and tissue concentrations of drugs associated with fatalities. Med. Clin. North Am., *58*:1093, 1974.

Jacobs, M. H., Senior, R. M., and Kessler, G.: Clinical experience with theophylline. Relationships between dosage, serum concentration, and toxicity. J.A.M.A., *235*:1983, 1976.

Jatlow, P.: Ultraviolet spectrophotometry of theophylline in plasma in the presence of barbiturates. Clin. Chem., *21*:1518, 1975.

Jatlow, P.: Ultraviolet spectrophotometric analysis of barbiturates: Evaluation of potential interferences. Am. J. Clin. Pathol., *59*:167, 1973.

Jatlow, P.: Ultraviolet spectrophotometric determination of chlordiazepoxide in plasma. Clin. Chem., *18*:516, 1972.

Jatlow, P. I.: Analytical toxicology in the clinical laboratory—an overview. *In* Thoma, J. J., Bondo, P. B., and

Sunshine, I. (eds.): Guidelines for Analytical Toxicology Programs, vol. I. Cleveland, CRC Press, Inc., 1977.

Jenne, J. W., Chick, T. W., Miller, B. A., and Strickland, R.D.: Apparent theophylline half-life fluctuations during treatment of acute left ventricular failure. Am. J. Hosp. Pharm., *34*:408, 1977.

Johnson, G. F., Dechtiaruk, W. A., and Soloman, H. M.: Gas-chromatographic determination of theophylline in human serum and saliva. Clin. Chem., *21*:144, 1975.

Johnson, G. K., and Tolman, K. G.: Chronic liver disease and acetaminophen. Ann. Intern. Med., *87*:302, 1977.

Jusko, W. J., Koup, J. R., Vance, J. W., Schentag, J. J., and Kuritzky, P.: Intravenous theophylline therapy: Nomogram guidelines. Ann. Intern. Med., *86*:400, 1977.

Kabra, P. M., Koo, H. Y., and Marton, T. J.: Simultaneous liquid-chromatographic determination of 12 common sedatives and hypnotics in serum. Clin. Chem., *24*:657, 1978.

Kabra, P. M., Stafford, B. E., and Marton, L. J.: Simultaneous measurement of phenobarbital, phenytoin, primidone, ethosuximide, and carbamazepine in serum by high-pressure liquid chromatography. Clin. Chem., *23*:1284, 1977.

Kamen, B. A., Takach, P. L., Vatev, R., and Caston, J. D.: A rapid radiochemical–ligand binding assay for methotrexate. Anal. Biochem., *70*:54, 1976.

Kaplan, S. A., Jack, M. L., Alexander, K., and Weinfeld, R. E.: Pharmacokinetic profile of diazepam in man following single intravenous and oral and chronic oral administrations. J. Pharm. Sci., *62*:1789, 1973.

Karlsson, E.: Procainamide and phenytoin. Comparative study of their antiarrhythmic effects at apparent therapeutic plasma levels. Br. Heart J., *37*:731, 1975.

Kaye, S.: Arsenic type A procedure. *In* Sunshine, I (ed.): Manual of Analytical Toxicology. Cleveland, the Chemical Rubber Company, 1971.

Kaye, S.: Handbook of Emergency Toxicology. Springfield. Ill. Charles C Thomas, Publisher, 1970.

Kessler, K. M.: Individualization of dosage of antiarrhythmic drugs. Med. Clin. North Am., *58*:1019, 1974a.

Kessler, K. M., Lowenthal, D. T., Warner, H., Gibson, T., Briggs, W., and Reidenberg, M. M.: Quinidine elimination in patients with congestive heart failure or poor renal function. N. Engl. J. Med., *290*:706, 1974b.

Keyvan-Larijarni, H., and Tannenberg, A. M.: Methanol intoxication. Comparison of peritoneal dialysis and hemodialysis treatment. Arch. Intern. Med., *134*:293, 1974.

Klein, R.: Lead poisoning. Adv. Pediatr., *24*:103, 1977.

Koch-Weser, J.: Acetaminophen. N. Engl. J. Med., *295*:1297, 1976.

Koch-Weser, J.: Drug therapy. Serum drug concentrations as therapeutic guides. N. Engl. J. Med., *287*:227, 1972.

Koch-Weser, J.: The serum level approach to individualization of drug dosage. Eur. J. Clin. Pharmacol., *9*:1, 1975.

Koch-Weser, J., and Klein, S. W.: Procainamide dosage schedules, plasma concentrations and clinical effects. J.A.M.A., *215*:1454, 1971.

Komaroff, A. L.: The practitioner and the compliant patient. Am. J. Public Health. *66*:833, 1976.

Kordash, T. R., Van Dellen, R. G., and McCall, J. T.: Theophylline concentrations in asthmatic patients after administration of theophylline. J.A.M.A., *238*:139, 1977.

Korsten, M. A., Matsuzaki, S., Feinman, L., and Lieber, C. S.: High blood acetaldehyde levels after ethanol administration. N. Engl. J. Med., *292*:386, 1975.

Koysooko, R., Ellis, E. F., and Levy G.: Relationship between theophylline concentration in plasma and saliva of man. Clin. Pharmacol. Ther., *15*:454, 1974.

Krenzelok, E. P., Best, L., and Manoguerra, A. S.: Acetaminophen toxicity. Am. J. Hosp. Pharm., *34*:391, 1977.

Kupferberg, H. J.: Quantitative estimation of diphenylhydantoin, primidone, and phenobarbital in plasma by gas-liquid chromatography. Clin. Chim. Acta, *29*:283, 1970.

Kutt, H.: Carbamazepine: Chemistry and methods of determination. Adv. Neurol., *11*:249, 1975a.

Kutt, H.: Interactions of antiepileptic drugs. Epilepsia, *16*:393, 1975b.

Kutt, H., and Penry, J. K.: Usefulness of blood levels of antiepileptic drugs. Arch. Neurol., *31*:283, 1974.

Labbé, R. F.: History and background of protoporphyrin testing. Clin. Chem., *23*:256, 1977.

Lamola, A. A., Joselow, M., and Yamane T.: Zinc protoporphyrin (ZPP): A simple, sensitive, fluorometric screening test for lead poisoning. Clin. Chem., *21*:93, 1975.

Lemberger, L., and Rubin, A.: Physiologic Deposition of Drugs of Abuse. New York, Spectrum Publications, Inc., 1976.

Levy, A. L., and Katz, E. M.: Comparison of serum lithium determinations by flame photometry and atomic absorption spectrophotometry. Clin. Chem., *16*:840, 1970.

Levy, G., and Tsuchiya, T.: Salicylate accumulation kinetics in man. N. Engl. J. Med., *287*:430, 1972.

Levy, G., Lampman, T., Kamath, B. L., and Garrettson, L. K.: Decreased serum salicylate concentrations in children with rheumatic fever treated with antacid. N. Engl. J. Med., *293*:323, 1975.

Littlejohn, D., Fell, G. S., and Ottaway, J. M.: Modified determination of total and inorganic mercury in urine by cold vapor atomic absorption spectrometry. Clin. Chem., *22*:1719, 1976.

Lindblad, B., and Olsson, R.: Unusually high levels of blood alcohol? J.A.M.A., *236*:1600, 1976.

Livingston, S., Paul, L. L., and Berman, W.: Carbamazepine (Tegretol R) in epilepsy. Dis. Nerv. Syst., *35*:103, 1974.

Loes, M. W., Singh, S., Lock, J. E., and Mirkin, B. L.: Relation between plasma and red-cell electrolyte concentrations and digoxin levels in children. N. Engl. J. Med., *299*:501, 1978.

Loiseau, P., Brachet, A., and Henry, P.: Concentration of dipropylacetate in plasma. Epilepsia, *16*:609, 1975.

Löscher, W.: Rapid determination of valproate sodium in serum by gas-liquid chromatography. Epilepsia, *18*:225, 1977.

Love, E. B.: Measuring plasma paracetamol. Lancet, *1*:195, 1977.

Lovejoy, F. H., Mitchell, A. A., and Goldman, P.: The management of propoxyphene poisoning. J. Pediatr., *85*:98, 1974.

Lund, L.: Anticonvulsant effect of diphenylhydantoin relative to plasma levels. Arch. Neurol., *31*:289, 1974.

Lundberg, G. D.: Concepts of substance abuse and addiction. *In* Lundberg, G. D. (ed.): Professional and Community Role of the Pathologist in Alcohol Abuse. Washington, D.C., U.S. Department of Transportation. National Highway Traffic Safety Administration, 1976.

Lundquist, F.: The urinary excretion of ethanol by man. Acta Pharmacol. Toxicol., *18*:231, 1961.

Magos, L.: Mercury and mercurials. Br. Med. Bull., *31*:241, 1975.

Marcus, F. I.: Digitalis pharmacokinetics and metabolism. Am. J. Med., *58*:452, 1975.

Marks, V., Lindup, W. E., and Baylis, E. M.: Measurement of therapeutic agents in blood. Adv. Clin. Chem., *16*:47, 1973.

Matthew, H.: Barbiturates. Clin. Toxicol., *8*:495, 1975.

Matusik, E., and Gibson, T. P.: Fluorometric assay for N-acetylprocainamide. Clin. Chem., *21*:1899, 1975.

McBay, A. J.: Propoxyphene and norpropoxyphene concentrations in blood and tissues in cases of fatal overdose. Clin. Chem., *22*:1319, 1976.

McBay, A. J., and Hudson, P.: Propoxyphene overdose deaths. J.A.M.A., *233*:1257, 1975.

McBay, A. J., Turk, R. F., Corbett, B. W., and Hudson, P.: Determination of propoxyphene in biological materials. J. Forensic Sci., *19*:81, 1974.

McMahon, R. E., Sullivan, H. R., Due, S. L., and Marshall, F. J.: The metabolite pattern of d-propoxyphene in man. The use of heavy isotopes in drug disposition studies. Life Sci., *12*:463, 1973.

Melmon, K. L., Rowland, M., Sheiner, L., and Trager, W.: Clinical implications of the deposition of lidocaine in man: A multidisciplinary study. *In* Davies, D. S., and Prichard, B. N. C. (eds.): Biological Effects of Drugs in Relation to Their Plasma Concentrations. Baltimore, University Park Press, 1973.

Miller, R. R.: Propoxyphene: A review. Am. J. Hosp. Pharm., *34*:413, 1977.

Mitenko, P. A., and Ogilvie, R. I.: Rational intravenous doses of theophylline. N. Engl. J. Med., *289*:600, 1973.

Mongan, E., Kelly, P., Nies, K., Porter, W. W., and Pamlus, H. E.: Tinnitus as an indication of therapeutic serum salicylate levels. J.A.M.A., *226*:142, 1973.

Morgan, R., and Cagan, E. J.: Acute alcohol intoxication, the disulfiram reaction, and methyl alcohol intoxication. *In* Kissin, B., and Begleiter, H. (eds.): The Biology of Alcoholism. vol. 3. Clinical Pathology. New York, Plenum Press, 1974.

Morselli, P. L.: Carbamazepine: Absorption, distribution and excretion. Adv. Neurol., *11*:279, 1975.

Müller, F. O., and Hundt, H. K. L.: Ethyl alcohol; contamination of blood specimens. S. Afr. Med. J., *50*:91, 1976.

Myers, E. M., Bernstein, J. M., and Fastiropolous, G.: Salicylate ototoxicity. N. Engl. J. Med., *273*:587, 1965.

Nash, J. F., Bennett, I. F., Bopp, R. J., Brunson, M. K., and Sullivan, H. R.: Quantitation of propoxyphene and its major metabolites in heroin addict plasma after large dose administration of propoxyphene napsylate. J. Pharm. Sci., *64*:429, 1975.

Natelson, S.: Microtechniques of Clinical Chemistry for the Routine Laboratory, 2nd ed. Springfield, Ill., Charles C Thomas, Publisher, 1961.

Nelson, J. A., Harris, B. A., Decker, W. J., and Farquhar, D.: Analysis of methotrexate in human plasma by high pressure liquid chromatography with fluorescence detection. Cancer Res., *37*:3970, 1977.

Nourok, D. S., Glassock, R. J., Solomon, D. H., and Maxwell, N. H.: Hyperthyroidism following prolonged sodium nitroprusside therapy. Am. J. Med. Sci., *248*:129, 1964.

O'Gorman, T., and Koff, R. S.: Salicylate hepatitis. Gastroenterology, *72*:726, 1977.

Orcutt, J. J., Kozak, P, P., Gillman, S. A., and Cummins, L. H.: Microscale method for theophylline in body fluids by reversed-phase, high-pressure liquid chromatography. Clin. Chem., *23*:599, 1977.

Osinga, A., and DeWolff, F. A.: Determination of quinidine in human serum in the presence of diuretics. Clin. Chim. Acta, *73*:505, 1976.

Page, I. H., Corcoran, A. C., Dustan, H. P., and Koppanyi, T.: Cardiovascular actions of sodium nitroprus-side in animals and hypertensive patients. Circulation, *11*:188, 1955.

Palmer, R. F., and Lasseter, K. C.: Sodium nitroprusside. N. Engl. J. Med., *292*:294, 1975.

Penry J. K., Porter, R. J., and Dreifuss, F. E.: Ethosuximide: Relation of plasma levels to clinical control. *In* Woodbury, D. M., Penry, J. K., and Schmidt, R. P. (eds.): Antiepileptic Drugs. New York, Raven Press, 1972.

Perrier, D., Rapp, R., Young, B., Kostenbauder, H., Cady, W., Pancorbo, S., and Hackman, J.: Maintenance of therapeutic phenytoin plasma levels via intramuscular administration. Ann. Intern. Med., *85*:318, 1976.

Perschau, R. A., Modell, J. H., Bright, R. W., and Shirley, P. D.: Suspected sodium nitroprusside-induced cyanide intoxication. Anesth. Analg. (Cleve.), *56*:533, 1977.

Peterson, R. F., and Rumack, B. H.: Treating acute acetaminophen poisoning with acetylcysteine. J.A.M.A., *237*:2406, 1977.

Physicians' Desk Reference. Oradell, N.J., Medical Economics Company, 1977.

Piafsky, K. M., and Ogilvie, R. I.: Dosage of theophylline in bronchial asthma. N. Engl. J. Med., *292*:1218, 1975.

Pierce, A. W.: Salicylate poisoning. Pediatrics, *54*:342, 1974.

Piomelli, S.: Free erythrocyte porphyrins in the detection of undue absorption of Pb and of Fe deficiency. Clin. Chem., *23*:264, 1977.

Piomelli, S.: A micromethod for free erythrocyte porphyrins: The FEP test. J. Lab. Clin. Med., *81*:932, 1973.

Pippenger, C. E., and Kutt, H.: Common errors in the analysis of antiepileptic drugs. *In* Pippenger, C. E., Penry, J. K., and Kutt, H. (eds.): Antiepileptic Drugs in Quantitative Analysis. New York, Raven Press, 1978.

Pisciotta, A. V.: Hematologic toxicity of carbamazepine. Adv. Neurol., *11*:355, 1975.

Plaa, G. L.: Acute toxicity of antiepileptic drugs. Epilepsia, *16*:183, 1975.

Porter, R. J., Robert, B., and Lazer, R. B.: Plasma albumin concentrations and diphenylhydantoin binding in man. Arch. Neurol., *32*:298, 1975.

Prescott, L. F.: Gastrointestinal absorption of drugs. Med. Clin. North Am., *58*:907, 1974.

Prescott, L. F., Roscoe, P., Wright, N., and Brown, S. S.: Plasma-paracetamol half-life and hepatic necrosis in patients with paracetamol overdosage. Lancet, *1*:519, 1971.

Raso, V., and Schreiber, R.: A rapid and specific radioimmunoassay for methotrexate. Cancer Res., *35*:1407, 1975.

Rawnsley, H. M.: Nontoxicologic clinical laboratory aspects. *In* Lundberg, G. E. (ed.): The Professional and Community Role of the Pathologist in Alcohol Abuse. Washington, D.C., U.S. Department of Transportation. National Highway Traffic Safety Administration, 1976.

Redetzki, H. M., and Dees, W. L.: Comparison of four kits for enzymatic determination of ethanol in blood. Clin. Chem., *22*:83, 1976.

Rejent, T. A., and Wahl, K. C.: Diazepam abuse: Incidence, rapid screening, and confirming methods. Clin. Chem., *22*:889, 1976.

Rey, E., Turquais, J-M., and Olive, G.: Micromethod for determination of diazepam by electron-capture gas-liquid chromatography. Clin. Chem., *23*:1338, 1977.

Richardson, R. A.: Automated method for determinations of mercury in urine. Clin. Chem., *22*:1604, 1976.

Richens, A.: A study of the pharmacokinetics of phenytoin

(diphenylhydantoin) in epileptic patients, and the development of a nomogram for making dose increments. Epilepsia, *16*:627, 1975.

Ricks, W. B.: Salicylate hepatoxicity in Reiter's syndrome. Ann. Intern. Med., *84*:52, 1976.

Robinson, A. G., and Loeb, J. N.: Ethanol ingestion—commonest cause of elevated plasma osmolality? N. Engl. J. Med., *284*:1253, 1971.

Roerig, D. L., Lavand, D. L., Mueller, M. A., and Wang, R. I. H.: Comparison of radioimmunoassay with thin layer chromatographic method of barbiturate detection in human urine. Clin. Chem., *21*:672, 1975.

Rumack, B. H., and Matthew, H.: Acetaminophen poisoning and toxicity. Pediatrics, *55*:871, 1975.

Rybakowski, J., Frazer, A., Mendels, J., and Ramsey, T. A.: Prediction of the lithium ratio in man by means of an *in vitro* test. Clin. Pharmacol. Ther., *22*:465, 1977.

Schack, J. A., and Waxler, S. H.: An ultraviolet spectrophotometric method for the determination of theophylline and theobromide in blood and tissues. J. Pharmacol. Exp. Ther., *97*:283, 1949.

Schottelius, D. D., and Fincham, R. W.: Clinical application of serum primidone levels. *In* Pippenger, C. E., Penry, J. K., and Kutt, H.: Antiepileptic Drugs: Quantitative Analysis and Interpretation. New York, Raven Press, 1978.

Schou, M.: Pharmacology and toxicity of lithium. Annu. Rev. Pharmacol. Toxicol., *16*:231, 1976.

Schreiner, G. E., and Teehan, B. P.: Dialysis of poisons and drugs: Annual review. Trans. Am. Soc. Artif. Intern. Organs, *17*:513, 1971.

Schreiner, G. E., and Teehan, B. P.: Dialysis of poisons and drugs: Annual review. Trans. Am. Soc. Artif. Intern. Organs, *18*:563, 1972.

Schwartz, M. A., and Postmas, E.: Metabolic N demethylation of chlordiazepoxide. J. Pharm. Sci., *55*:1358, 1966.

Shand, D. G.: Propranolol. N. Engl. J. Med., *293*:280, 1975.

Shand, D. G.: Reduced binding of quinidine in plasma from Vacutainers. (Letter) Clin. Pharmacol. Ther., *20*:120, 1976.

Shand, D. G., Nuckolls, E. M., and Oates, J. A.: Plasma propranolol levels in adults. Clin. Pharmacol. Ther., *11*:112, 1970.

Sharpless, S. K.: Hypnotics and sedatives. II. Miscellaneous agents. *In* Goodman, L. S., and Gilman, A. (eds.): The Pharmacological Basis of Therapeutics. 3rd ed. New York, The Macmillan Company, 1965.

Simon, D., and Penry, J. K.: Sodium di-N-propylacetate (DPA) in the treatment of epilepsy. A review. Epilepsia, *16*:549, 1975.

Sjöqvist, F., Borgå, O., and Orme, M. L'E.: Fundamentals tals of clinical pharmacology. *In* Avery, G. S. (ed.): Drug Treatment: Principles and Practice of Clinical Pharmacology and Therapeutics. Sidney, ADIS Press, 1976.

Smith, D. E., and Wesson, D. R.: Drugs of abuse 1973: Trends and developments. Ann. Rev. Pharmacol. Toxicol., *14*:513, 1974.

Smith, J. R., and Landaw, S. A.: Smokers' polycythemia. N. Engl. J. Med., *298*:6, 1978.

Smith, T. W., and Haber, E.: Digitalis (third of four parts). N. Engl. J. Med., *289*:1063, 1973.

Smith, T. W.: Digitalis toxicity: Epidemiology and clinical use of serum concentration measurements. Am. J. Med., *58*:470, 1975.

Spiehler, V., Sun, L., Miyada, D. S., Sarandis, S. G., Walwick, E. R., Klein, M. W., Jordan, D. B. and Jessen, B.: Radioimmunoassay, enzyme immunoassay, spectrophotometry, and gas-liquid chromatography compared for determination of phenobarbital and diphenylhydantoin. Clin. Chem., *22*:749, 1976.

Spiker, D. G., and Biggs, J. T.: Tricyclic antidepressants. Prolonged plasma levels after overdose. J.A.M.A., *236*:1711, 1976.

Spiker, D. G., Weiss, A. N., Chang, S. S., Ruwitch, J. F., and Biggs, J. T.: Tricyclic antidepressant overdose: Clinical presentation and plasma levels. Clin. Pharmacol. Ther., *18*:539, 1975.

Stern, E. L.: Serum osmolality in cases of poisoning. N. Engl. J. Med., *290*:1026, 1974.

Stewart, R. D.: The effect of carbon monoxide on humans. Annu. Rev. Pharmacol. Toxicol., *15*:409, 1975.

Strandjord, R. E., and Johannessen, S. I.: One daily dose of diphenylhydantoin for patients with epilepsy. Epilepsia, *15*:317, 1974.

Sun, L., and Szafir, I.: Comparison of enzyme immunoassay and gas chromatography for determination of carbamazepine and ethosuximide in human serum. Clin. Chem., *23*:1753, 1977.

Sun, L., and Walwick, E. R.: Primidone analyses: Correlation of gas-chromatographic assay with enzyme immunoassay. Clin. Chem., *22*:901, 1976.

Sunshine, I.: Arsenic type B procedure. *In* Sunshine, I. (ed.): Manual of Analytical Toxicology. Cleveland, The Chemical Rubber Company, 1971.

Sunshine, I.: Forensic toxicology: Role of the laboratory. *In* Thoma, J. J., Bondo, P. B., and Sunshine, I.: Guidelines for Analytical Toxicology Programs, vol. I. CRC Press, Inc., 1977.

Temple, A. R., George, D. J., Done, A. K., and Thompson, J. A.: Salicylate poisoning complicated by fluid retention. Clin. Toxicol., *9*:61, 1976.

Tjaden, U. R., Kraak, J. C., and Huber, J. F. K.: Rapid trace analysis of barbiturates in blood and saliva by high-pressure liquid chromatography. J. Chromatogr., *143*:183, 1977.

Thomson, P. D., Melmon, K. L., Richardson, J. A., Cohn, K., Steinbrunn, W., Cudihee, R., and Rowland, M.: Lidocaine pharmacokinetics in advanced heart failure, liver disease and renal failure in humans. Ann. Intern. Med., *78*:499, 1973.

Trapnell, K.: Salicyate intoxication. J. Am. Pharm. Assoc., *16*:147, 1976.

Troupin, A. S., and Moretti, L., and Ojemann, L. M.: Paradoxical intoxication a complication of anticonvulsant administration. Epilepsia, *16*:753, 1975.

Trump, D. L., and Hockberg, M. C.: Bromide intoxication. Johns Hopkins Med. J., *138*:119, 1976.

Tuzel, I., Limjuco, R., and Kahn, D.: Sodium nitroprusside in hypertensive emergencies. Curr. Ther. Res., *17*:95, 1975.

Vasiliades, J.: Emergency toxicology. The evaluation of three analytical methods for the determination of misused alcohols. Clin. Toxicol., *10*:339, 1977.

Vesey, C. J., Cole, P. V., and Simpson, P. J.: Cyanide and thiocyanate concentrations following sodium nitroprusside infusion in man. Br. J. Anaesth., *48*:651, 1976.

Walberg, C. B., Pantlik, U. A., and Lundberg, G. D.: Toxicology test-ordering patterns in a large urban general hospital during five years: An update. Clin. Chem., *24*:507, 1978.

Wallace, J. E., Biggs, J. D., and Dohl, E. V.: A rapid and specific spectrophotometric method for determining propoxyphene. J. Forensic Sci., *10*:179, 1965.

Wang, Y., Lantin, E., and Sutow, W. W.: Methotrexate in blood, urine and cerebrospinal fluid of children receiving high doses by infusion. Clin. Chem., *22*:1053, 1976.

1

Webb-Johnson, D. C., and Andrews, J. L.: Bronchodilator therapy (second of two parts). N. Engl. J. Med., *297*:758, 1977.

Weinstein, G. D.: Methotrexate. Ann. Intern. Med., *86*:199, 1977.

Werner, M., Sutherland, E. W., and Abramson, F. P.: Concepts for the rational selection of assays to be used in monitoring therapeutic drugs. Clin. Chem., *21*:1368, 1975.

Williams, D. C., and Burnett, R. W.: A reverse phase liquid chromatographic method for the determination of therapeutic levels of phenothiazines in serum. Clin. Chem., *23*:1139, 1977.

Wolen, R. L., Gruber, C. M., Kiplinger, G. F., and Scholz, N. E.: Concentration of propoxyphene in human plasma following repeated oral doses. Toxicol. Appl. Pharmacol., *19*:493, 1971.

Worm, K.: Determination of dextropropoxyphene in organs from fatal poisoning. Acta Pharmacol. Toxicol., *30*:330, 1971.

Wulff, K., Flachs, H., Würtz-Jorgensen, and Gram, L.: Clinical pharmacological aspects of valproate sodium. Epilepsia, *18*:149, 1977.

Wuth, O.: Rational bromide treatment: New methods for its control. J.A.M.A., *88*:2013, 1927.

Zarkowsky, H. S.: The lead problem in children: Dictum and polemic. Curr. Probl. Pediatr., *6*:3, 1976.

Ziegler, V. E., Co, B. T., Taylor, J. R., Clayton, P. J., and Biggs, J. T.: Amitriptyline plasma levels and therapeutic response. Clin. Pharmacol. Ther., *19*:795, 1976.

Zweig, M.: Methotrexate in cerebrospinal fluid. N. Engl. J. Med., *295*:52, 1976.

Zwillich, C. W., Sutton, F. D., Neff, T. A., Cohn, W. M., Matthay, R. A., and Weinberger, M. M.: Theophylline-induced seizures in adults, correlation with serum concentrations. Ann. Intern. Med., *82*:784, 1975.

16

QUANTITATIVE APPROACHES USED IN EVALUATING LABORATORY MEASUREMENTS AND OTHER CLINICAL DATA

Bernard E. Statland, M.D., Ph.D.,
Per Winkel, M.D., Doc. Med. Sci.,
M. Desmond Burke, M.D., and
Robert S. Galen, M.D., M.P.H.

FUNDAMENTAL DEFINITIONS

The clinician relies greatly upon the clinical laboratory to provide him with information to make judgments regarding his patients. The laboratory produces a steadily increasing number of values on an ever-expanding array of assays. These values are considered in conjunction with other clinical data in order to aid in clinical decision making. In this chapter we will introduce some quantitative approaches which can be used to optimize the utilization of laboratory data already present and to assist in ordering additional laboratory measurements.

CLINICAL CLASSES

Although each patient and each patient's clinical presentation are unique, the clinician attempts to classify the patient into some clinical entity which has previously been described and characterized. This process is necessary so that a reasonable treatment program and/or additional diagnostic work-up can be instituted on the basis of guidelines known to be appropriate for most of the members of the clinical entity so selected. These entities are called *clinical classes*. A *clinical class* may be defined explicitly on the basis of the following: (1) a set of *common validated pathologic findings* (e.g., the various classes of patients distinguished on the basis of demonstrated autopsy findings); (2) the *established prognosis* after some predefined point in time of the disease (e.g., the class of patients *alive* two years after suffering a myocardial infarction and the class of patients *not* alive two years after a myocardial infarction); or (3) the documented *response to a stated therapy* (e.g., the class of hypercholesterolemic patients whose serum cholesterol dropped more than 30 per cent after instituting some therapeutic maneuver and the class of hypercholesterolemic patients who did not so respond).

It should be noted that a clinical class should be defined with certainty; however, such definitions may be made only retrospectively (survival rates or therapeutic responses) or by invasive techniques having a high risk to the patient, such as an exploratory laparotomy. In the clinical setting, the physician often uses *other* evidence to assess the probability that his patient is actually a member of a particular clinical class. It should be obvious that if a clinical class is adequately defined on available information (e.g., the class of patients with a measured serum potassium concentration above 7.0 mmol/l), the probability that a given patient belongs to the class will be either 1.0 or 0.0, given that the information is obtained. For this type of diagnostic problem the clinician relies on the definitions of classes and logical reasoning (Boolean algebra). For a more extensive exposition of the potentials and the pitfalls of this approach, the interested reader is referred to the reviews by Ledley (1959) and by Feinstein (1973, 1974).

Throughout this chapter we will refer to a particular class by the letter "D" and a numerical subscript, e.g., D_1. If we wish to consider the class of all subjects not members of class D_1 but belonging to the Universe of patients considered, we will use the notation "$\overline{D}_1$." Thus, for any class D_1, an individual *must* be a member of either D_1 or $\overline{D}_1$ but *cannot* be a member of both D_1 and $\overline{D}_1$. This is called the rule of mutual exclusivity.

VARIATES

The word *variate* is used here as defined in Chapter 2 (see p. 44). Although our concern will be related mainly to clinical chemistry variates, the same logic and quantitative approaches can be (and should be) applied to other clinical variates.

We distinguish two types of variates: *continuous* and *discrete*. A continuous variate, strictly, is one that can take on *all* values in a certain interval of real values. Data, of course, can never be continuous in this sense, since there is always some degree of rounding off. Clinical chemistry variates such as plasma potassium, serum triglycerides, etc., are generally considered to be continuous. A discrete variate is a variate which can take on only a limited number of values. In the simplest case, the discrete variate can take on only two possible values. This type of variate is called *binary*. It should be noted that in the clinical setting a continuous variate is often transformed into a discrete one. For example, all values of a clinical chemistry quantity which are equal to or less than a certain cutoff value may be transformed to the value "0" and all values greater than the cutoff value to the value "1." In the following we will assume that each clinical variate has been divided by its unit. We will denote such variates by the letter "S" and a numerical subscript, e.g., S_1. The value of the variate will be presented after the "equals sign" following the variate name, e.g., $S_1 = 142$.

In this chapter, we will discuss the assignment of a patient to a clinical class based on a single laboratory result (univariate analysis) as well as the assignment of a patient to a clinical class using more than one laboratory result (multivariate analysis). Finally, we will present methods used to form new clinical classes, i.e., classifying patients based on available laboratory and clinical data. The following sections will introduce the various ways in which the clinician transforms the observations obtained on his patient into an estimated probability that his patient is a member of a clinical class. We will begin with the simplest case, i.e., the case of one discrete binary variate and two possible clinical classes.

ASSESSMENT OF A SINGLE VARIATE VALUE

BAYESIAN MODEL FOR ONE BINARY VARIATE

The foundation for much of the probabilistic approach used for the evaluation of test results can be traced to a theorem presented in the treatise of Reverend Bayes published in 1763. Bayes formulated an equation which relates the probability of an item being a member of a particular group, given the presence of an attribute, to the probability of known group members having the attribute and the probability of obtaining a group member when picking at random an item from the total number of items considered (the Universe). If we were to substitute "patient" for

item, "clinical class" for group, "positive test result" for attribute, and "prevalence of the clinical class" for the probability of obtaining a group member when picking at random an item from the Universe, we will easily begin to appreciate the Bayesian model in our model of diagnostic sensitivity and specificity.

Table 16-1 defines the terms used in the Bayesian model for our purposes. All subjects are either members of class D_1 or members of class $\bar{D}_1$ (they must be a member of one and only one class). D_1 could signify the class of patients known to have suffered a myocardial infarction. The *prevalence* of any class, i.e., $P(D_1)$, is the probability of finding a subject who is a member of the stated class. The single variate S_1 is binary, a positive test result being denoted by "1" and a negative test result by "0."

A *conditional probability* is the probability of the occurrence of a second event given knowledge of the presence of a prior event. The conditional probability is written as $P(b|a)$, which is read as the probability of "b" occurring given the fact that "a" has occurred, the vertical bar being read as "given the fact

Table 16-1. BASIC DEFINITIONS FOR THE CASE OF ONE BINARY VARIATE "S_1" AND THE UNIVERSE: D_1 AND $\bar{D}_1$, WHERE D_1 SIGNIFIES THE CLASS OF SUBJECTS SUFFERING FROM A GIVEN DISEASE

	NOTATION	DEFINITION	SYNONYM
(1)	n_{D_1}	Number of subjects suffering from the disease	–
(2)	$n_{\bar{D}_1}$	Number of subjects not suffering from the disease	–
(3)	$P(D_1)$	$\left(\dfrac{n_{D_1}}{n_{D_1} + n_{\bar{D}_1}}\right)$ or number fraction of subjects suffering from the disease	Prevalence
(4)	$S_1 = 1$	Signifies the presence of the attribute in question	Positive test result
(5)	$S_1 = 0$	Signifies the absence of the attribute in question	Negative test result
(6)	$P(S_1 = 1 | D_1)$	Probability that a subject suffering from the disease will present the attribute	Diagnostic sensitivity
(7)	$P(S_1 = 0 | \bar{D}_1)$	Probability that a subject not suffering from the disease will *not* present the attribute	Diagnostic specificity
(8)	$P(S_1 = 1 | \bar{D}_1)$	Probability that a subject not suffering from the disease will present the attribute	–
(9)	$P(S_1 = 0 | D_1)$	Probability that a subject suffering from the disease will *not* present the attribute	–
(10)	$P(D_1 | S_1 = 1)$	Probability that a subject suffers from the disease given that he presents the attribute	Predictive value of a positive test result
(11)	$P(\bar{D}_1 | S_1 = 0)$	Probability that a subject does *not* suffer from the disease given that he does *not* present the attribute	Predictive value of a negative test result

Table 16–2. NOMENCLATURE USUALLY USED WHEN BAYES THEOREM FOR ONE VARIATE IS APPLIED IN CLINICAL MEDICINE

	NUMBER OF SUBJECTS WITH POSITIVE TEST RESULT	NUMBER OF SUBJECTS WITH NEGATIVE TEST RESULT	TOTALS
Number of subjects with disease	TP	FN	TP + FN
Number of subjects without disease	FP	TN	FP + TN
Totals	TP + FP	FN + TN	TP + FP + TN + FN

Definitions:

TP = True positives *or* number of diseased patients correctly classified by the test.

FP = False positives *or* number of patients without the disease misclassified by the test.

FN = False negatives *or* number of diseased patients misclassified by the test.

TN = True negatives *or* number of patients without the disease correctly classified by the test.

Diagnostic sensitivity $= \dfrac{\text{TP}}{\text{TP} + \text{FN}} = P(S_1 = 1 | D_1)$

Diagnostic specificity $= \dfrac{\text{TN}}{\text{FP} + \text{TN}} = P(S_1 = 0 | \bar{D}_1)$

Predictive value of positive test $= \dfrac{\text{TP}}{\text{TP} + \text{FP}} = P(D_1 | S_1 = 1)$

Predictive value of negative test $= \dfrac{\text{TN}}{\text{TN} + \text{FN}} = P(\bar{D}_1 | S_1 = 0)$

Efficiency of the test (number fraction of patients correctly classified), that is, $\dfrac{\text{TP} + \text{TN}}{\text{TP} + \text{FP} + \text{FN} + \text{TN}}$

that." Medical textbooks, journal reports, and annual reviews supply the clinician with the conditional probability of a patient's presenting a symptom given the fact that he has a particular disease, e.g., 90 per cent of patients with hepatic metastases have an elevated serum alkaline phosphatase value. The probability of obtaining a positive test result given the fact that a patient is a member of a particular class, i.e., $P(S_1 = 1 | D_1)$, has been referred to as the *diagnostic sensitivity* of the test. Note that this is very different from the *analytical sensitivity* of an analytical procedure, the latter being a property of the method to detect very low amounts of an analyte in biologic material. *Diagnostic specificity*, i.e., $P(S_1 = 0 | \bar{D}_1)$, is the probability of finding a negative result given the fact that the subject is not a member of class D_1. The definitions of *false positive test results* and *false negative test results* can be noted in Table 16–2.

In the clinical setting we do not know if a patient is a member of a particular clinical class, for that question is the critical issue of the diagnostic process. The conditional probability that a patient is a member of a particular clinical class given the finding of a positive test result, i.e., $P(D_1 | S_1 = 1)$ has been referred to as the *predictive value of a positive test result*. In an analogous manner, $P(\bar{D}_1 | S_1 = 0)$ is defined as the *predictive value of a negative test result*. The importance of determining the predictive values of both positive and negative test results has been presented by Vecchio (1966) and more recently by Galen (1975b). As will be demonstrated, the predictive value of either a positive or a negative test result is a function of three other units of information—the diagnostic sensitivity of the test, the diagnostic specificity of the test, and the prevalence of the clinical class in the population of patients considered.

Table 16–2 presents the 2 × 2 table demonstrating the four possible combinations of test values and the presence or absence of disease: true positives (TP), true negatives (TN), false positives (FP), and false negatives (FN). The relative occurrences of these four events in turn are used to define the diagnostic sensi-

Table 16-3. DERIVATION OF THE EQUATION RELATING THE PREDICTIVE VALUE OF A POSITIVE TEST RESULT ($PV_{\oplus}$) TO PREVALENCE, SENSITIVITY, AND SPECIFICITY

Assumptions:

(1) $P(D_1) + P(\bar{D}_1) = 1.0$

(2) $P(S_1 = 1 | D_1) + P(S_1 = 0 | D_1) = 1.0$

(3) $P(S_1 = 1 | \bar{D}_1) + P(S_1 = 0 | \bar{D}_1) = 1.0$

Definitions:

(4) Number fraction of TP $= P(D_1) \cdot P(S_1 = 1 | D_1)$

(5) Number fraction of FP $= P(\bar{D}_1) \cdot P(S_1 = 1 | \bar{D}_1)$

(6) $P(D_1 | S_1 = 1) = \dfrac{\text{Number fraction of TP}}{\text{Number fraction of TP} + \text{Number fraction of FP}}$

By substitution:

(7) $P(D_1 | S_1 = 1) = \dfrac{P(D_1) \cdot P(S_1 = 1 | D_1)}{[P(D_1) \cdot P(S_1 = 1 | D_1)] + [P(\bar{D}_1) \cdot P(S_1 = 1 | \bar{D}_1)]}$

(8) $P(D_1 | S_1 = 1) = \dfrac{P(D_1) \cdot P(S_1 = 1 | D_1)}{[P(D_1) \cdot P(S_1 = 1 | D_1)] + \{[1 - P(D_1)] \cdot [1 - P(S_1 = 0 | \bar{D}_1)]\}}$

Stated in words:

(9) $PV_{\oplus} = \dfrac{(\text{Prevalence}) \cdot (\text{Sensitivity})}{[(\text{Prevalence}) \cdot (\text{Sensitivity})] + [(1 - \text{Prevalence}) \cdot (1 - \text{Specificity})]}$

tivity and diagnostic specificity of a test. Table 16-3 presents the derivation of Bayes theorem for one discrete binary variate and for two clinical classes (D_1 and $\bar{D}_1$), with D_1 being the group of diseased subjects whom we wish to identify by means of a positive test result.

EFFECT OF PREVALENCE ON THE PREDICTIVE VALUE OF A POSITIVE TEST RESULT

A critical question in the clinical setting is the following: Of the total number of subjects having a positive test result, how many will actually be found to have the disease (clinical class) which the test supposedly identifies? Stated alternatively, what is the predictive value of a positive test result? (Unless otherwise indicated, "predictive value" will be used to refer to the predictive value of a positive test result.) The importance of noting the predictive value of a positive test result should be apparent in that a positive test result will usually point to the need for a detailed diagnostic work-up and perhaps the initiation of a treatment plan.

As noted by its definition stated in Table 16-3, the predictive value is very dependent upon the prevalence of disease in the population under study. This contention can be supported by a typical example, as illustrated in Table 16-4. We will assume that we are evalu-

ating the predictive value of a test which has a diagnostic sensitivity of 95 per cent and a diagnostic specificity of 95 per cent. We now apply the formula of the predictive value for various prevalences of the disease. With a prevalence of 50 per cent, the predictive value is 95 per cent; with a prevalence of 5 per cent, the predictive value is 50 per cent; and for a disease with a prevalence of 1 per cent, the predictive value of a positive test result is only 16.1 per cent in spite of the test's having a diagnostic sensitivity of 95 per cent and a diagnostic specificity of 95 per cent (Table 16-4).

The examples cited above should explain why a good *diagnostic* test frequently fails as a *screening* test when the prevalence of the disease in the general population is very low. Let us compare two clinical situations: (1) classifying patients suspected of having a myocardial infarction who enter the Coronary Care Unit (CCU) with a history of recent chest pain, and (2) classifying patients who enter the outpatient screening clinic with a history of chest pain. We will assume that the prevalence of myocardial infarction among the patients admitted to the CCU is 50 per cent, while the prevalence of myocardial infarction in the defined clinical population is only 5 per cent. Given a serum enzyme test with a 95 per cent diagnostic sensitivity, i.e., $P(S_1 = 1 | D_1) = 0.95$, and with a diagnostic

Table 16–4. PREDICTIVE VALUE OF A POSITIVE TEST RESULT AS A FUNCTION OF DISEASE PREVALENCE*

PREVALENCE OF DISEASE (per cent)		PREDICTIVE VALUE OF A POSITIVE TEST † (per cent)
(a)*	1	16.1
(b)	2	27.9
(c)*	5	50.0
(d)	10	67.9
(e)	15	77.0
(f)	20	82.6
(g)	25	86.4
(h)*	50	95.0

Calculations of the Predictive Value of a Positive Test Result $(\text{PV}_{\oplus})$:

$$\text{PV}_{\oplus} = \frac{(\text{Prevalence}) \cdot (\text{Sensitivity})}{[(\text{Prevalence}) \cdot (\text{Sensitivity})] + [(1 - \text{Prevalence}) \cdot (1 - \text{Specificity})]}$$

(a) $\quad \text{PV}_{\oplus} = \dfrac{(0.01)(0.95)}{(0.01)(0.95) + (0.99)(0.05)} = 0.161$

(c) $\quad \text{PV}_{\oplus} = \dfrac{(0.05)(0.95)}{(0.05)(0.95) + (0.95)(0.05)} = 0.500$

(h) $\quad \text{PV}_{\oplus} = \dfrac{(0.50)(0.95)}{(0.50)(0.95) + (0.50)(0.05)} = 0.950$

†Assuming $P(S_1 = 1 | D_1) = 0.95$ (95% sensitivity), and $P(S_1 = 0 | \bar{D}_1) = 0.95$ (95% specificity).

specificity of 95 per cent, i.e., $P(S_1 = 0 | \bar{D}_1) = 0.95$, the predictive value of the enzyme test would be 95 per cent when used on the CCU population (i.e., 95 per cent of patients with positive tests should have a myocardial infarction); alternatively, the predictive value of the enzyme test for the patients seen in the screening clinic would be 50 per cent. (See Table 16–4 for calculations.) For additional worked-through clinical examples of computing predictive values of positive test results, the interested reader is referred to the textbook by Galen (1975b).

DIAGNOSTIC SENSITIVITY AND SPECIFICITY AS A FUNCTION OF THE CUTOFF VALUE

Figure 16–1 presents the distributions of enzyme test results for the total population of patients admitted to the coronary care unit: 50 per cent of the patients are assumed to suffer from a "myocardial infarction," i.e., $P(D_1) = 0.50$. The identification with 100 per cent certainty of subjects with a myocardial infarction is very difficult, since the diagnosis is founded on histopathology; however, we usually base the independent definition on history and electrocardiographic findings. As

shown in Figure 16–1, patients with myocardial infarctions tend to have higher serum enzyme activities; however, there is an overlap of the two clinical classes for this variate. If

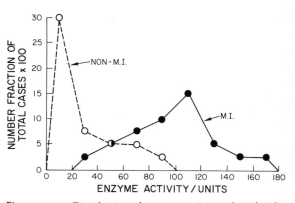

Figure 16–1. Distribution of enzyme activity values for the class of patients independently known to have suffered a myocardial infarction (MI) presented as closed circles and for the class of patients independently known *not* to have suffered a myocardial infarction (non-MI) presented as open circles. It is assumed that the prevalence of myocardial infarction in the total population is 50 per cent. The mean enzyme activity in the class of patients with MI is 97 units. The mean enzyme activity in the class of patients with non-MI is 27 units. However, the overlap of the two groups is very apparent.

Table 16-5. THE DIAGNOSTIC SENSITIVITY, DIAGNOSTIC SPECIFICITY, PREDICTIVE VALUE OF A POSITIVE TEST RESULT, AND PREDICTIVE VALUE OF A NEGATIVE TEST RESULT OF AN ENZYME ACTIVITY ASSAY FOR THE DIAGNOSIS OF A MYOCARDIAL INFARCTION GIVEN A PREVALENCE OF 50 PER CENT*

CUTOFF VALUE	DIAGNOSTIC SENSITIVITY (per cent)	DIAGNOSTIC SPECIFICITY (per cent)	PREDICTIVE VALUE OF A POSITIVE TEST (per cent)	PREDICTIVE VALUE OF A NEGATIVE TEST (per cent)
20	100.0	60.0	71.4	100.0
40	95.0	75.0	79.2	93.8
50	90.0	80.0	81.8	88.9
60	85.0	85.0	85.0	85.0
80	70.0	95.0	93.3	76.0
100	50.0	100.0	100.0	66.7

*See Figure 16-1 for pertinent data base.

we wish to report the enzyme test as a binary discrete variate, that is, a positive (elevated) result or a negative (not elevated) result, we must select a cutoff value such that all values which are equal to or less than that value are reported as "negative," whereas values which are greater than the value are reported as "positive." The diagnostic sensitivity and specificity are dependent upon the cutoff value selected. Table 16-5 presents various possible cutoff values based on the results depicted in Figure 16-1, along with the computed diagnostic sensitivity, diagnostic specificity, and predictive value of the test for each cutoff value chosen. At a relatively low cutoff value, e.g., 20 units, the diagnostic sensitivity is 100 per cent. However, using a cutoff value of 20 units, the diagnostic specificity is only 60 per cent; i.e., 40 per cent of patients *not* having a myocardial infarction would be misclassified. On the other hand, by selecting a cutoff value of 100 units, the diagnostic specificity improves to 100 per cent; however, the enzyme test has lost much of its sensitivity. For this constructed example (and for most actual clinical examples), it is impossible to select a cutoff value for a single variate that affords complete discrimination between two clinical classes. Whenever we change the cutoff value, we are sacrificing the diagnostic sensitivity of a test for the diagnostic specificity or vice versa. Since the predictive value of a test is a function of the diagnostic sensitivity and diagnostic specificity of the test, the predictive value is obviously a function of the cutoff value. Later in this chapter we will discuss a rational approach used for selecting the optimum cutoff value.

ASSESSING THE RELATIVE DIAGNOSTIC VALUE OF A SINGLE TEST

The prevalence of a clinical class is often very difficult to determine. Furthermore, the prevalence will vary from population to population. For these reasons, clinicians very seldom report on the predictive value of a test result, but rather present the diagnostic sensitivity and the diagnostic specificity of the considered test. Clinicians frequently compare the predictive value of laboratory tests to that obtained by flipping a coin. This analogy is not as straightforward as it might appear. The most common error made is to equate a 50 per cent predictive value with that obtained by flipping a coin. It is possible to achieve a 50 per cent predictive value with a coin, but only if disease prevalence equals 50 per cent. Flipping a coin has a sensitivity of 50 per cent and a specificity of 50 per cent. The predictive value, therefore, depends entirely on and is equal to disease prevalence. Any time sensitivity and specificity add to 100 per cent or less, the test under evaluation does *not* perform better than chance. That this must be so may be realized from the following reasoning: If a test is positive with the same frequency in healthy subjects as in diseased subjects, obviously it is *not* working better than chance. Assume that in this case the fraction of positive test results is 30 per cent; then the sensitivity of the test is 30 per cent (fraction of positive among diseased) and the specificity is 70 per cent (fraction of negative in healthy subjects). Thus the sum of the sensitivity and the specificity of the test is 100 per cent. The dangers of developing laboratory tests and reporting only clinical trials in diseased patients are obvious. When such a report describes a test with 90 per cent sensitivity, there is no way of knowing whether the specificity is better than 10 per cent.

The sum of the sensitivity and specificity can be considered the "diagnostic index" of the test; and thus a "perfect test" would have a diagnostic index of 200 per cent (i.e., 100 per cent + 100 per cent), while a test performing at the level of chance alone would have a diagnostic index of 100 per cent.

Table 16-6 lists nine separate tests and the clinical class which each test should diagnose.

Table 16–6. SENSITIVITY AND SPECIFICITY OF SELECTED VARIATES BASED ON HISTORY, PHYSICAL EXAMINATION, RADIOLOGIC, AND LABORATORY STUDIES RANKED ACCORDING TO THE DIAGNOSTIC INDEX*

TEST†	CLINICAL CLASS DIAGNOSED BY THE TEST	DIAGNOSTIC SENSITIVITY (per cent)	DIAGNOSTIC SPECIFICITY (per cent)	DIAGNOSTIC INDEX (per cent)
(a) Physical exam	Hepatomegaly	50	47	97
(b) Blood alcohol assay	Biopsy-proven alcoholic liver disease	40	99	139
(c) Plasma carcino-embryonal antigen	Colorectal carcinoma	72	80	152
(d) Hepatic scintigraphy	Biopsy-proven hepatic pathology	90	63	153
(e) Clinical exam and mammography	Breast carcinoma	67	98	165
(f) History of "heavy drinking"	Biopsy-proven alcoholic liver disease	76	99	175
(g) Serum lactate dehydrogenase isoenzyme pattern	Myocardial infarction	78	98	176
(h) Serum creatine kinase isoenzymes	Myocardial infarction	100	85	185
(i) History of diarrhea after lactose ingestion	Biopsy-proven lactase deficiency	100	88	188

*Sum of diagnostic sensitivity and diagnostic specificity.

†*References:*
(a) Blendis, L. M., McNeilly, W. J., Sheppard, L., et al.: Br. Med. J., *1*:727, 1970.
(b) Hamlyn, A. N., Sherlock, S., Brown, A. J., and Baron, D. N.: Lancet, *2*:345, 1975.
(c) Hansen, H. J., Snyder, J. J., Miller, E., et al.: Hum. Pathol., *5*:139, 1974.
(d) Drum, D. E., and Christacopoulos, J. S.: J. Nucl. Med., *13*:908, 1972.
(e) Shapiro, S., Strax, P., and Venet, L.: J.A.M.A., *215*:1777, 1971.
(f) Hamlyn, A. N., Sherlock, S., Brown, A. J., and Baron, D. N.: Lancet, *2*:345, 1975.
(g) Galen, R. S.: N. Eng. J. Med., *292*:433, 1975.
(h) Galen, R. S.: N. Eng. J. Med., *292*:433, 1975.
(i) Newcomer, A. D., McGill, D. B., Thomas, P. J., and Hoffman, A. F.: N. Engl. J. Med., *293*:1232, 1975.

The diagnostic sensitivity and specificity for each test-class combination have been extracted from the reports in the literature which are referenced in the table. Finally, the diagnostic index (sum of sensitivity and specificity) is listed. The tests included in the table are based on history taking, physical examination, and laboratory studies. A test with a very low diagnostic index is the physical exam for hepatomegaly—it performs no better than chance (Blendis, 1970). Hamlyn reported that a random blood alcohol assay had a diagnostic sensitivity of 40 per cent in identifying patients with biopsy-proven alcoholic liver disease (example *b*, Table 16–6); however, they also noted that 76 per cent of their patients with alcoholic liver disease did admit to heavy drinking (example *f*, Table 16–6). The specificity of either test can be considered to be 99 per cent. Thus, the diagnostic index of a random

blood alcohol assay would be 139 per cent, while the diagnostic index of the history of heavy drinking would be 175 per cent. Thus it appears that questioning the patient about his alcohol intake could replace the laboratory test, since the sensitivity of the history was superior to that of the laboratory test. However, before discarding the laboratory test, one should ask the following question: Is the information obtained by the laboratory test completely redundant as compared with the information obtained by the history taking? The present discussion, however, pertains to the simplified problem of choosing one test or other kind of clinical information among a number of possible tests or other kinds of clinical information.

For those variates which are continuous in nature and cover a large interval of values, the magnitudes of the sensitivity and specificity can be altered by changing the cutoff value (see earlier discussion); however, at some point, the diagnostic index (sum of sensitivity and specificity) reaches a maximum value. Given the choice of a test with a relatively high diagnostic sensitivity and a relatively low diagnostic specificity versus another test with a relatively low sensitivity but higher specificity, which test should one prefer? The answer is dependent upon the clinical situation. Tests with relatively high diagnostic sensitivity (preferably 100 per cent) are desirable for detecting diseases which are serious and treatable. An example of such a disease state is pheochromocytoma. This disease may certainly be fatal if not detected; however, if found early enough, it is nearly always curable. For detecting a pheochromocytoma, we desire a test with the highest sensitivity possible. A "false positive" result will usually be identified in that repeated tests as well as additional assays are performed on the urine specimens prior to making the decision to perform surgery. By performing additional tests, we gain the needed diagnostic specificity so as to rule out a pheochromocytoma. Other examples of clinical classes which should be initially detected by tests of high sensitivity include hypothyroidism, venereal disease, and treatable infectious diseases.

Clinical classes for which we should demand tests of highest specificity (preferably 100 per cent) include diseases which are serious but are not treatable or curable. In these cases, false positive results may lead to serious psychological trauma or economic harm to the patient. Conversely, a true negative result (knowledge that the disease is not present) may have psychological value to the community. An example of such a disease is multiple sclerosis. This disease is serious, but not curable. If a case of multiple sclerosis is missed, there is no need for undue concern, because the patient will return. On the other hand, a false positive diagnosis can cause serious psychological harm. Other examples include some occult cancers and any other serious but untreatable disease. As an example, a test for occult cancer of the lung must have a specificity of 100 per cent. The only treatment available at present is lobectomy or radiation, and treatment of a false positive would have serious consequences.

Tests with equally high sensitivity and specificity are desired in the following situations: the disease is serious but treatable, and false positive results and false negative results are essentially equally costly or serious.

ASSESSING THE RISKS AND BENEFITS OF VARIOUS COURSES OF ACTION

A clinician relies upon laboratory results obtained on his patient in order to make certain managerial decisions. There are three general types of managerial decisions: (1) whether one should perform additional diagnostic examinations on the patient, (2) whether one should begin (or discontinue) a specific therapeutic regimen, and (3) whether one should make a statement pertaining to the prognosis (e.g., the expected life span) of the patient. The decision process involves two elements: *first*, the clinician must assess the likelihood that a patient is a member of a particular clinical class, and *second*, the clinician must know the risks and benefits involved in pursuing various courses of action. In the previous section we have discussed how the probability that a patient belongs to a given clinical class may be estimated, based on the value of a binary variate; in this section, we will explore the consequences of various actions undertaken by the clinician. The considerations and computations involved in this section form the domain called "decision analysis."

MINIMIZING THE COSTS OF MISCLASSIFICATIONS

When a quantitative measurement is actually continuous in nature but is transformed into a discrete binary variate, the choice of the cutoff value will affect the number of false positive and false negative results in the total population. We will use the data presented in Figure 16-1 and Table 16-5 to illustrate the manner of selecting the best cutoff value. In the clinical setting the consequences of a false negative may be more serious (i.e., greater loss) than those of a false positive, e.g., at least for the case of myocardial infarction (MI); that is, it may cause less harm to classify a patient without an MI as having an MI rather than to assign a patient with an MI to the class of patients without MI. It is very difficult to assign costs in terms of dollars and cents to such errors. However, by convention, one can give a relative value to false positive and false negative results. In our example we will assign a

Table 16–7. TOTAL COSTS OF MISCLASSIFYING PATIENTS SUSPECTED
OF HAVING A MYOCARDIAL INFARCTION: RELATIONSHIP OF "CUTOFF VALUE"
TO THE COSTS OF "FALSE NEGATIVES" AND "FALSE POSITIVES" ASSUMING
A PREVALENCE OF 50 PER CENT FOR MYOCARDIAL INFARCTION*

| | A | B | |
CUTOFF VALUE	COST OF FALSE NEGATIVES (ASSUMING A COST OF 200 UNITS PER CASE)†	COST OF FALSE POSITIVES (ASSUMING A COST OF 100 UNITS PER CASE)‡	TOTAL COST (A + B)
20	$(0.5) \cdot (0.00) \cdot (200) = 0.0$	$(0.5) \cdot (0.40) \cdot (100) = 20.0$	20.0
40	$(0.5) \cdot (0.05) \cdot (200) = 5.0$	$(0.5) \cdot (0.25) \cdot (100) = 12.5$	17.5
50	$(0.5) \cdot (0.10) \cdot (200) = 10.0$	$(0.5) \cdot (0.20) \cdot (100) = 10.0$	20.0
60	$(0.5) \cdot (0.15) \cdot (200) = 15.0$	$(0.5) \cdot (0.15) \cdot (100) = 7.5$	22.5
80	$(0.5) \cdot (0.30) \cdot (200) = 30.0$	$(0.5) \cdot (0.05) \cdot (100) = 2.5$	32.5
100	$(0.5) \cdot (0.50) \cdot (200) = 50.0$	$(0.5) \cdot (0.00) \cdot (100) = 0.0$	50.0

*Based on information presented in Table 16–5.
†Cost FN = $P(D_1) \cdot (1 - \text{Sensitivity}) \cdot (200)$
‡Cost FP = $P(\bar{D}_1) \cdot (1 - \text{Specificity}) \cdot (100)$

cost of 100 units for a false positive result and 200 units for a false negative result. Our objective can now be stated as finding the optimal cutoff value such that the total cost of misclassification is minimal. Table 16–7 shows the computed cost of misclassification at cutoff values of 20, 40, 50, 60, 80, and 100 units of enzyme activity. (See Figure 16–1 and Table 16–5 for the data base.) The prevalence of an MI is assumed to be 50 per cent. The number fraction of false negative results is equal to $P(D_1) \cdot (1 - \text{sensitivity})$, while the number fraction of false positive results is equal to $P(\bar{D}_1) \cdot (1 - \text{specificity})$. The number fraction of false negative results is multiplied by 200 units to give the cost due to false negatives, while the number fraction of false positive results is multiplied by 100 units to give the cost due to false positives. As noted in Table 16–7, the lowest total cost is at a cutoff value of 40. The cutoff value of 40 will result in more false positive than false negative results; however, owing to the greater cost of a false negative result, the total cost of misclassification at this value is the lowest, compared with the other possibilities considered in this illustrative example.

DECISION ANALYSIS

In optimizing the cutoff value for discrete variates, the clinician may evaluate not only the relative risks but also the benefits of his actions based on such information. Decision analysis is a practical strategy for considering the risks and benefits of decision making in a quantitative rather than in a qualitative fashion. Decision analysis quantitates outcome probabilities and their usefulness and combines both factors to provide an *expected value* for a particular decision. Thus, decisions can be compared and the best course of action can be followed.

A decision analysis can be depicted in flow chart form as a decision tree. At one point, a decision *must* be made. Subsequent outcomes either occur as a consequence of chance or are dictated on the basis of the combined effects of chance and the results of previous actions. Each possible outcome must be considered. As in the previous problem of minimizing the costs of misclassification, the decision maker wishes to maximize the value of his action. Each possible outcome is assigned some relative worth or value; the probability of each outcome (i.e., within each course of action taken) is computed; and the expected value of each outcome is defined as the probability of the outcome times the assigned value of the outcome. The expected values are added for all outcomes resulting from each course of action. The course of action (at the decision point) having the highest total expected value should be followed (Sisson, 1976).

A relatively simple example of decision analysis involving the use of a laboratory measurement, i.e., serum alkaline phosphatase, is presented in Figure 16–2. The decision here deals with the detection of hepatic metastases. The patient is assumed to have colorectal carcinoma. If it were known that the patient also has hepatic metastases, the ma-

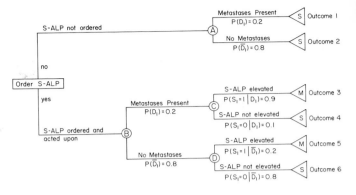

Figure 16–2. Flow diagram illustrating the consequences of two courses of action: ordering and acting upon a serum-alkaline phosphatase (S–ALP) determination versus *not* ordering a S–ALP for the detection of hepatic metastases in the patient with primary colorectal carcinoma. The treatment plan is either surgery (S) or medical symptomatic therapy (M). Outcomes 1 and 2 follow *not* ordering a S–ALP, while outcomes 3 to 6 result from ordering and acting upon a S–ALP. (See text and Table 16–8 for computation of the "expected value" for each course of action.)

lignancy would be treated only with symptomatic medical care. If it were known that there are no metastatic deposits in the liver, the primary tumor would be removed surgically. It is further assumed that the patient has no clinical evidence of hepatic metastases.

Will a serum alkaline phosphatase test result improve the decision making? If the physician decides to forego testing, he is relying on negative clinical findings and assumes that metastases are absent. Let us assume that the probability of hepatic metastases $P(D_1)$ in the preoperative phase of colorectal cancer is 0.2. This figure for the prevalence of hepatic metastases is well-documented (Read, 1977). This means that the probability of no metastases $P(\bar{D}_1)$ is 0.8. Therefore, in choosing not to order a serum alkaline phosphatase (S–ALP), the physician can exclude metastases with a probability of 0.8 and confirm metastases with a probability of 0.2. Obviously, under these circumstances, he chooses to exclude metastases and treats the patient surgically (Outcomes 1 and 2 in Figure 16–2). On the other hand, if the physician chooses to order *and* act upon a serum alkaline phosphatase, he does so to improve upon the prior probabilities of metastases or no metastases. The prior probabilities of metastases and no metastases are shown as outcome branches of chance node B. Whether the patient has hepatic metastases or not, the test results may be positive or negative. We assume that the probability that the S–ALP is elevated in cases of hepatic metastases is 0.9, i.e., $P(S_1 = 1 | D_1) = 0.9$, and thus the probability that the S–ALP is not elevated in hepatic metastases $P(S_1 = 0 | D_1)$ is 0.1. These are the outcome probabilities for chance node C (Fig. 16–2). Thus, if S–ALP is elevated, the patient would be treated medically (Outcome 3); and if the S–ALP is not elevated, the

patient would be treated surgically (Outcome 4). We also assume that the diagnostic specificity $[P(S_1 = 0 | \bar{D}_1)]$ of S–ALP is 0.8; i.e., in 80 per cent of patients without hepatic metastases, the S–ALP will not be elevated (Read, 1977). Thus, for the patient without hepatic metastases, the probability that the test result will be negative is 0.8 and the probability that the test result will be positive is 0.2. In the latter case, the patient would be treated medically (Outcome 5) and in the former case, the patient would undergo surgery (Outcome 6).

The next step is to assign numerical values to various outcomes. To do this we must make value judgments. The outcomes and assigned numerical values are presented in Table 16–8. The outcomes of surgery + no hepatic metastases (Outcomes 2 and 6) and medical treatment + hepatic metastases (Outcome 3) are considered *appropriate* and thus each is assigned a numerical value of +100. The outcome of medical treatment + no metastases (Outcome 5) is *inappropriate* and carries a very great risk to the patient and therefore is assigned a numerical value of −100. Finally, the outcome of surgery + hepatic metastases (Outcomes 1 and 4) is also *inappropriate;* however, it does not constitute as much *added* harm to the patient as in Outcome 5. Outcomes 1 and 4 are assigned numerical values of −20.

Next we calculate the expected value (EV) for each outcome by multiplying the probability of the outcome with the appropriate numerical value. Outcomes 1 and 2 would come about if the physician decided not to rely on the results of the S–ALP; the EV of O_1 and O_2 is +76. (see Table 16–8). Outcomes 3 through 6 occur if the physician orders and acts upon the S–ALP result; the EV of $O_3 - O_6$ is +65.6 (see Table 16–8). Thus, according to the theory of decision analysis and the assumptions made,

Table 16–8. EVALUATION OF VARIOUS OUTCOMES FOR THE "NET WORTH" OF ORDERING AND ACTING UPON A SERUM ALKALINE PHOSPHATASE MEASUREMENT*

OUTCOME (O)	CONDITION	ASSIGNED VALUE (V)
1	Surgery + metastases present	−20
2	Surgery + no metastases	+100
3	Medical treatment + metastases present	+100
4	Surgery + metastases present	−20
5	Medical treatment + no metastases	−100
6	Surgery + no metastases	+100

Expected value (EV) of not ordering S-ALP: (Outcomes: $O_1 + O_2$) = +76

$$EV_{O_1} = P(D_1) \cdot V_{O_1} = (0.2) \cdot (-20) = -4$$
$$EV_{O_2} = P(\overline{D}_1) \cdot V_{O_2} = (0.8) \cdot (100) = \underline{+80}$$
$$SUM = +76$$

Expected value (EV) of ordering and acting upon S-ALP: (Outcomes: O_3 through O_6) = +65.6

$$EV_{O_3} = P(D_1) \cdot P(S_1 = 1 | D_1) \cdot V_{O_3} = (0.2) \cdot (0.9) \cdot (100) = +18.0$$
$$EV_{O_4} = P(D_1) \cdot P(S_1 = 0 | D_1) \cdot V_{O_4} = (0.2) \cdot (0.1) \cdot (-20) = -0.4$$
$$EV_{O_5} = P(\overline{D}_1) \cdot P(S_1 = 1 | \overline{D}_1) \cdot V_{O_5} = (0.8) \cdot (0.2) \cdot (-100) = -16.0$$
$$EV_{O_6} = P(\overline{D}_1) \cdot P(S_1 = 0 | \overline{D}_1) \cdot V_{O_6} = (0.8) \cdot (0.8) \cdot (100) = \underline{+64.0}$$
$$SUM = +65.6$$

*Based on information presented in Figure 16-2.

the physician should not rely solely on the S-ALP result to decide whether to operate. However, if the physician changed the cutoff value of S-ALP to optimize the outcome value of decision node B, the conclusion might be another one. Furthermore, valuable information is lost by transforming S-ALP to a binary variate. The foregoing is a simple example; moreover, one might question the numerical values assigned.

Although decision analysis has been applied to various managerial decisions for years, its introduction to clinical medicine is relatively recent (Schwartz, 1973; Pauker, 1975; Patrick, 1977). It has been applied in relation to the following subject matter: screening programs (Bay, 1976), the prevention of deep vein thrombosis following myocardial infarction (Emerson, 1974), gastroenterologic decision making (deDombal, 1975), case finding in hypertensive renovascular disease (McNeil, 1975b), computer-aided management of acute renal failure (Gorry, 1973), the evaluation of coronary artery surgery (Pauker, 1976), and the evaluation of lymphangiography in the management of patients with Hodgkin's disease (Safran, 1977).

Decision analysis has been met with both skepticism (Ingelfinger, 1975) and criticism (Ransohoff, 1976; Feinstein, 1977) from the medical profession. There are difficulties in assigning probability values to various outcomes, simply because information is lacking. However, the real difficulty lies in trying to place a value on outcome. Apart from the obvious difficulties of trying to quantitate intangible benefits and risks, e.g., human gratification or loss of employment, values differ depending upon who makes the decision; society's view of what constitutes the value of a particular outcome is not always that of the individual concerned or his relatives. "Society as a decision maker might place a small utility on trying to save the life of a cirrhotic patient in coma with gastrointestinal bleeding. To this patient's family, however, the utility might be great" (Ransohoff, 1976).

SEQUENTIAL ASSESSMENT OF MULTIPLE VARIATE VALUES

In the clinical setting the physician has available a large number of laboratory and other clinical data. Thus, based on the available data the clinician may use various multivariate methods to estimate the probability that a patient is a member of a particular clinical class. In this section we present two general methods used in evaluating the results

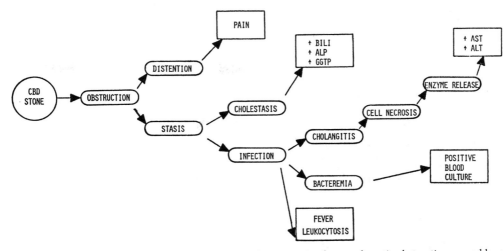

Figure 16–3. Illustrations of pathogenetic reasoning. Cause-effect reasoning for extrahepatic obstruction caused by a common bile duct stone. Abbreviations used include: CBD = common bile duct; BILI = concentration of total bilirubins in serum; ALP = alkaline phosphatase activity in serum; GGTP = gamma-glutamyl transferase activity in serum; AST = aspartate aminotransferase activity in serum; and ALT = alanine aminotransferase activity in serum.

of multiple variates: (1) sequential assessment (clinical algorithms), and (2) simultaneous assessment (pattern recognition).

PATHOGENETIC VERSUS DIAGNOSTIC REASONING

In the *diagnostic* process, the clinician proceeds from *effect* (e.g., laboratory measurement) to the likely *cause* (e.g., pathologic lesion). This is contrasted to the manner in which "disease" is presented in most textbooks of pathology; that is, the reasoning is *pathogenetic*, proceeding from *cause* to *effect*. Before presenting the strategy used in the diagnostic process, let us first examine the nature of pathogenetic reasoning.

An example of pathogenetic reasoning is shown in Figure 16-3. Common duct stone causes obstruction; obstruction causes duct distention and stasis of duct contents; distention causes pain, stasis causes cholestasis, etc. Intermediate effects are the causes of later effects. The ultimate effects are the clinical and laboratory manifestations of common duct stone, for example, the increased concentration of total bilirubins in serum. The physician must take these relatively non-specific clinical and laboratory observations and reverse the reasoning process if he is to reach the correct pathogenetic endpoint. Thus, in the example given in Figure 16-3, the clinician elicits a complaint of right upper quadrant

abdominal pain of a colicky nature and notes the laboratory findings of increased concentration of total bilirubins and activity values of alkaline phosphatase and gamma-glutamyl transferase in the serum of his patient and clinical findings and finally that one of the pathologic entities causing cholestasis and distention would be a common bile duct stone. According to Feinstein (1973, 1974), the *purpose of diagnostic reasoning* is to provide satisfactory explanations for the observed evidence, and that *clinical diagnosis* is the process of converting clinical and laboratory data to the names of diseases. The *format of diagnostic reasoning* consists of branching series of logical decisions, each of which produces intermediate conclusions during the progressive transformation of input (clinical and laboratory data) to output (assigning the patient to a particular clinical class).

CLINICAL ALGORITHMS OR SEQUENTIAL ASSESSMENT OF MULTIPLE VARIATE VALUES

"An algorithm is a set of rules for getting a specific output from a specific input" (Knuth, 1977). In simpler terms, an algorithm is a recipe or strategy for solving a problem. The sequence of logic in algorithms is illustrated in flow chart form with graphic symbols for each act of reasoning and strategy. The symbols used are depicted in Figure 16-4. The symbols

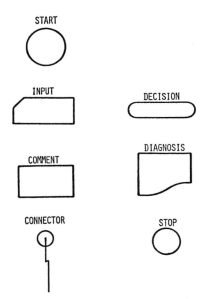

Figure 16–4. Selected, conventional symbols used in algorithms.

are not sacrosanct; frequently diamond- or hexagon-shaped decision boxes are used instead of ovals. The decision box is the most important component of the algorithm. It must have at least two outlet branches (usually yes and no), but other branches (such as maybe, unknown, etc.) can also be used.

Only a minority of the clinical algorithms reported so far have been designed for computer execution; the majority have been constructed to facilitate the diagnostic work-up of relatively common clinical problems that can be followed easily without the aid of a computer. Examples include the following: the diagnosis of anemia (Wallerstein, 1976); recognition and management of cardiac tamponade (Shoemaker, 1975); management of critically injured patients (Bietz, 1977); jaundice (Katon, 1975; Ostrow, 1975); urinary tract infection (Kunin, 1975); obesity (Bray, 1976); chest pain (Hurst, 1976); hypertension (Maronde, 1975; Grim, 1977). Algorithms can be used to train paraclinical personnel (Charles, 1977) and to allow such personnel to conduct early routine phases of the diagnostic process (Greenfield, 1975). Algorithms for computer execution have been reported for the assessment of acid-base disorders (Bleich, 1969); the diagnosis of congenital heart disease (Johnson, 1975); hypercalcemia (Briccetti, 1975); and pulmonary function testing (Ellis, 1975).

Although largely unexploited, algorithms are useful in the teaching of laboratory medicine to students and residents (Ward, 1976). They may also be useful to the practicing pathologist in his role as a laboratory consultant.

An Algorithm Used to Evaluate a Combination of Laboratory Variates Related to Hepatic Disease. A profile of laboratory test results may often supply the first evidence that a patient is suffering from a disease. The advent of multichannel instruments has made such profiles of test results easily available. Profiles can be interpreted in a qualitative fashion by noting visually displayed patterns (Ward, 1973), or by formulating a simplified analytical approach (Cole, 1975). Generally, symptoms and signs generate hypotheses. Early hypotheses are modified by profile (or organ panel) results that facilitate exclusion of less likely diseases and confirmation of more likely diagnostic candidates (Henry, 1977). The certainty required to exclude a particular disease is a function of its severity and prevalence. A rare but relatively harmless disease can be easily dismissed, but a dangerous disease demands further laboratory testing before it can be safely excluded. Similarly, subsequent confirmation of likely diagnostic candidates requires further laboratory testing when therapeutic risk is great.

We will now present an example of an algorithm used for the interpretation of the "hepatic profile" of chemical measurements. It should be understood that the following algorithm and the other two algorithms to be subsequently presented are given merely as illustrations as to possible approaches to be used in evaluating laboratory data. They should *not* be construed as specific recommendations. Most assuredly many readers of this text may use somewhat different strategies in interpreting the same variate values and/or may rely on a different set of variates for evaluation of hepatic disorders. Eight laboratory-based variates and 15 potential clinical classes are presented in Table 16-9. Our clinical experience indicates that the combination of the eight assays (Table 16-9) are most efficient in identifying and sorting patients with liver disease. The algorithm presented in Figure 16-5*A* and *B* is intended as a recommended procedure to find the cause of the abnormal results. Certain investigators may disagree with the logic, the order of the stepwise analysis, and/or the cutoff values used in the decision steps; however, the reader is exposed to this algorithm

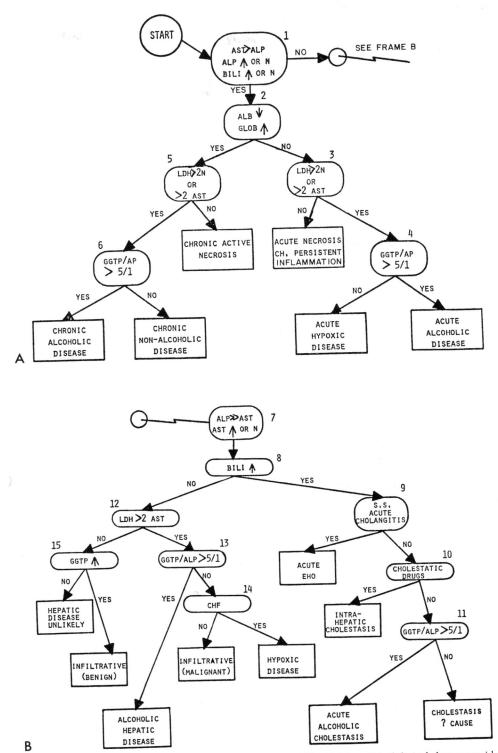

Figure 16-5. Algorithm for the interpretation of a hepatic panel. See Table 16-9 for a list of clinical classes considered, variates used, and abbreviations of variate names. Non-standard abbreviations include: CH = chronic; CHF = congestive heart failure; EHO = extrahepatic obstruction; N = normal (i.e., within the reference interval for "healthy" subjects); 2N = twice the upper limit of the reference interval; and S.S. = symptoms and signs.

Table 16–9. VARIATES PRESENT IN THE HEPATIC PANEL AND A LIST OF VARIOUS CLINICAL CLASSES IN WHICH PATIENTS SHOW ONE OR MORE ABERRATIONS IN THE VARIATE VALUES

VARIATES	CLINICAL CLASSES
1. S-Alanine aminotransferase (ALT)	1. Acute alcoholic cholestasis
2. S-Aspartate aminotransferase (AST)	2. Acute alcoholic disease
3. S-Alkaline phosphatase (ALP)	3. Acute extrahepatic obstruction
4. S-Total bilirubin (BILI)	4. Alcoholic hepatic disease
5. S-Albumin (ALB)	5. Acute hypoxic disease
6. S-Globulin (GLOB)	6. Acute necrosis
7. S-Lactate dehydrogenase (LDH)	7. Cholestasis of unknown cause
8. S-Gamma-glutamyl transferase (GGTP)	8. Chronic active necrosis
	9. Chronic alcoholic disease
	10. Chronic non-alcoholic disease
	11. Chronic persistent inflammation
	12. Infiltrative benign disease
	13. Infiltrative malignant disease
	14. Intrahepatic cholestasis
	15. Hepatic disease unlikely

mainly as an example of one way to narrow the number of diagnostic possibilities. It should be emphasized that the algorithm employs no more than a crude transformation of continuous variates to discrete variates as a basis for its decision making. The decision boxes are numbered 1 to 14 (see Table 16–9 for appropriate abbreviations). The justification for those decisions is as follows:

Decision 1. Whether S-ALP or S-bilirubin is elevated or not, if S-AST in U/l is greater than S-ALP in U/l, the serum concentrations of albumin and globulin should be examined (Fig. 16–5A).

Decisions 2 to 6. The remainder of the reasoning process depicted in Figure 16–5A depends primarily upon S-albumin and S-globulin values and secondarily on S-LDH/S-AST and S-GGTP/S-ALP ratios. Low S-albumin and high S-globulin imply chronic active hepatic disease; normal S-albumin and normal or high S-globulin imply acute disease or chronic persistent inflammation. S-LDH greater than twice normal or greater than twice S-AST (in terms of actual units, i.e., U/l), in the face of normal S-albumin and S-globulin, points to acute hypoxic or acute alcoholic disease. Lower S-LDH/S-AST ratios favor acute necrosis or chronic persistent inflammation. S-GGTP/S-ALP (each value is first divided by upper reference limit) ratio greater than 5/1 favors acute alcoholic disease.

Similarly, when S-albumin is low and S-globulin high, a low S-LDH/S-AST value favors chronic active necrosis and a high value indicates either chronic alcoholic or some variety of chronic active non-alcoholic disease. Again, a high S-GGTP/S-ALP value favors alcoholism (Fig. 16–5A).

Decision 7. Whether S-AST is elevated or not, when the value of S-ALP is relatively more elevated than is the value of S-AST, the S-bilirubin value should be inspected (Fig. 16–5B).

Decisions 8 to 15. The S-bilirubin value is central to the remainder of the sequence. An elevated S-bilirubin implies either extrahepatic obstruction or intrahepatic cholestasis; a normal S-bilirubin indicates focal intrahepatic cholestasis only. When bilirubin is elevated, symptoms and signs of acute cholangitis indicate acute extrahepatic obstruction. A history of cholestatic drug ingestion indicates intrahepatic cholestasis, and a high S-GGTP/S-ALP value is found with acute alcoholic cholestasis. Without clinical evidence of cholangitis or a drug history, and in the absence of any indication of alcoholism, a cholestatic picture deserves further work-up. On the other hand, when S-bilirubin is normal and S-LDH/S-AST ratio is low, a normal S-GGTP makes any diagnosis of hepatic disease very unlikely. Under these circumstances, with a low S-LDH/S-AST, an elevated S-GGTP implies benign infiltrative disease such as sarcoidosis, tuberculosis, or a non-specific chronic pericholangitis. On the other hand, when the S-LDH/S-AST ratio is elevated, a high S-GGTP/S-ALP ratio favors alcoholic hepatic disease, while a lesser ratio, in the absence of congestive cardiac failure, points at infiltrative malignant disease, notably metastases (Fig. 16–5B).

Similar algorithms can be developed for the interpretation of other test profiles, e.g., profiles pertaining to electrolyte balance and renal function. However, algorithmic approaches to the interpretation of comprehensive biochemical profiles, e.g., SMA 12/60 profiles, are difficult because of the number of quantities involved, and pattern recognition approaches are preferable (Ward, 1973).

Diagnostic Search Algorithms. Previously we considered the use of an algorithm for a profile or panel of laboratory results, all of which were readily available. In the clinical setting the clinician often begins the sequential assessment of laboratory and other clinical data with only one datum, i.e., the presenting reason to begin a diagnostic work-up. Examples of such problems include hypertension of uncertain etiology, failure to thrive owing to uncertain etiology, or one grossly abnormal clinical chemistry quantity. It is in these cases that subsequent clinical and laboratory evidence not at hand must be sought. Since additional testing procedures may be very costly and/or may place the patient at some added risk, the optimal choice of particular tests and the sequence of ordering such data must be well thought out. It is here that diagnostic search algorithms are most useful. We will consider two such problems: (1) the patient who presents with Cushingoid clinical features, and (2) the patient who presents with hypercalcemia. As stated above in relationship to the example of the algorithm for the hepatic profile of tests, the following two diagnostic search algorithms are presented mainly for illustrative purposes.

EVALUATION OF A PATIENT WITH CUSHINGOID

CLINICAL FEATURES. An example of a diagnostic search algorithm for the evaluation of Cushingoid clinical features is shown in Figure 16-6. Many issues can be presented concerning the proposed illustrative algorithm for evaluating Cushingoid syndrome. First, the term "Cushingoid" describes a myriad of clinical presentations. Second, although the reasoning sequence in an algorithm must, by definition, be depicted sequentially, many of the clinical and laboratory tests used may be determined simultaneously. Third, although there is justification for much of the algorithm presented (Eddy, 1973), there are dissenting views as well. The illustrated algorithm contains six decision boxes, and the reasoning proceeds as follows:

Decision 1. If the patient appears Cushingoid, a determination of the excretion in urine of free cortisol during 24 hours should be ordered.

Decision 2. If the excretion in urine of free cortisol is elevated, a 1 mg dexamethasone test should be performed.

Decision 3. If the excretion in urine of free cortisol is within the expected reference interval for healthy subjects and the 24-hour urine collec-

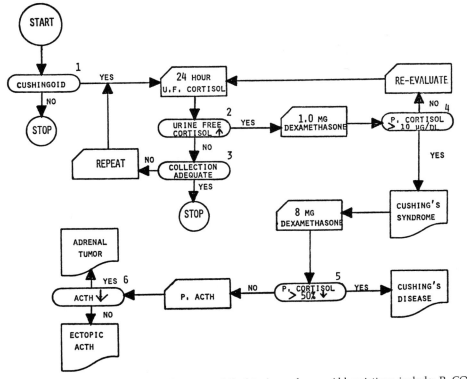

Figure 16-6. Algorithm for the detection and diagnosis of Cushing's syndrome. Abbreviations include: P. CORTISOL = plasma cortisol concentration and U.F. CORTISOL = the excretion in urine of free cortisol during 24 hours.

tion is deemed adequate, the diagnosis can be excluded. If the 24-hour collection is inadequate or questionable, the test should be repeated.

Decision 4. A plasma cortisol concentration greater than 10 μg/dl at 8 A.M. on the morning following a 1.0 mg dexamethasone dose is presumptive evidence of Cushing's syndrome. A value less than that demands re-evaluation.

Decision 5. Following presumptive evidence of Cushing's syndrome, investigation must be directed to determining specific etiology. The first step is to perform a high-dose dexamethasone suppression test using a total dose of 8.0 mg. If plasma cortisol concentration following this dose falls more than 50 per cent of baseline values, the diagnosis is bilateral adrenocortical hyperplasia or "Cushing's disease." If the degree of suppression is less than 50 per cent, plasma ACTH concentration can be determined.

Decision 6. If the plasma ACTH concentration is suppressed, the likelihood is that Cushing's syndrome is due to adrenal tumor. On the other hand, if the plasma ACTH concentration is not suppressed, ectopic ACTH production should be considered.

It is important to note that small cell bronchogenic carcinoma, the most common source of ectopic ACTH production, rarely results in Cushingoid features. Patients with this syndrome are more likely to present with severe hypokalemia and muscle weakness.

The recent widespread application of biochemical profiling has itself created a need for diagnostic search algorithms. Frequently, the cause of an isolated biochemical abnormality is readily apparent on clinical grounds. However, there are occasions when persistent hypercalcemia or hyponatremia, for example, requires a fairly extensive work-up.

EVALUATION OF A PATIENT WITH HYPERCALCEMIA. An example of a diagnostic search algorithm for hypercalcemia is shown in Figure 16–7. Decision boxes are numbered 1 to 8. Reasoning proceeds as follows:

Decision 1. Hypercalcemia, in the presence of severe chronic renal disease, indicates the development of autonomous hyperparathyroidism superimposed on the usual secondary hyperparathyroidism characterizing this disease. The term used for this development is "tertiary hyperparathyroidism."

Decision 2. If serum albumin is elevated, the

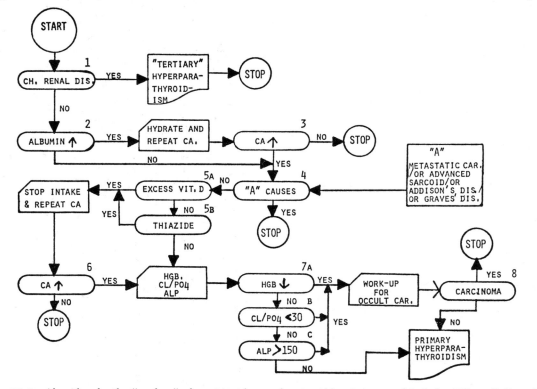

Figure 16–7. Algorithm for the "workup" of persistent hypercalcemia. Abbreviations used include: ALP = alkaline phosphatase activity in serum; CA = total serum calcium; CAR = carcinoma; CH = chronic; CL/PO$_4$ = ratio of the serum chloride concentration to the serum phosphate concentration where chloride is presented in mmol/l and where phosphate is expressed as mg/dl of "phosphorus"; and DIS = disease.

patient should be hydrated and serum calcium determination repeated.

Decision 3. If serum calcium is now normal, further investigation is unnecessary. If serum albumin is not elevated or serum calcium does not return to normal following hydration, further investigation is required.

Decision 4. The causes listed in comment box A should be considered. If any one of these conditions is present, further investigation is unnecessary.

Decision 5. The patient should be questioned about possibilities of excess vitamin D intake or thiazide therapy. If evidence for either is found, intake should be stopped and the serum calcium determination repeated.

Decision 6. If serum calcium is now normal, further investigation is unnecessary. If not and if there is no evidence of excess vitamin D intake or thiazide therapy taking place, blood hemoglobin, serum chloride, serum phosphate, and serum ALP should be ordered.

Decision 7. Anemia, a chloride-phosphate ratio less than 30, or an ALP activity greater than 150 U/l justifies an extensive work-up for an occult carcinoma. On the other hand, if there is no evidence of anemia, if the chloride-phosphate ratio is greater than 30, and if the serum alkaline phosphatase is within the reference interval, or elevated to only a minor degree, a provisional diagnosis of primary hyperparathyroidism should be made. (See legend of Figure 16-7.)

Decision 8. If an occult carcinoma is found, further investigation should stop and the patient should be treated.

Note that parathormone estimations are not included. The decision-making value of parathormone assay for the diagnosis of primary hyperparathyroidism is controversial. In practice, persistent hypercalcemia in the absence of an identifiable cause usually requires neck exploration irrespective of parathormone test results. This is particularly true when renal or skeletal complications are present. Hypercalcemia is the subject of several recent reviews (Singer, 1977; Bone, 1977).

At each decision step of the clinical algorithm, the clinician intuitively relies upon a high probability that a positive test (or conversely that a negative test) implies that a patient is a member of one or more clinical classes. Thus, in an algorithm which involves n decision steps, there are n probability distributions to consider. Obviously, the nature of the probability distributions as well as the number of decision steps greatly influences the confidence that one has in the final assignment of a patient to a particular clinical class. Furthermore, continuous variates are transformed to discrete variates with a subsequent reduction of available information. Since algorithms are usually based on anecdotal experience rather than on large prospective studies, they should be subjected to continuous re-evaluation in terms of choice of cutoff values and sequence of decision steps, to minimize the possibility of missing a diagnosis.

SIMULTANEOUS ASSESSMENT OF MULTIPLE VARIATE VALUES: PATTERN RECOGNITION

BAYES THEOREM FOR MORE THAN ONE DISCRETE VARIATE

Previously, we considered the Bayesian conditional probability model for one discrete binary variate, S_1, and two clinical classes: D_1 and $\bar{D}_1$. The Bayesian theorem can be applied to a diagnostic problem where one evaluates a very large number of variates and many possible clinical classes such that the patient with certainty belongs to one and only one of these. For illustrative purposes, we will consider two binary variates: S_1 and S_2, and three clinical classes: D_1, D_2, and D_3. The notation applied for this problem is presented in Table 16-10.

Figure 16-8 presents the values of S_1 and S_2

	CONDITIONAL PROBABILITY $P(S_1=a_1, S_2=a_2 \mid D_j)$			CONDITIONAL PROBABILITY $P(D_j \mid S_1=a_1, S_2=a_2)$ *		
$(S_1=a_1, S_2=a_2)$	D_1	D_2	D_3	D_1	D_2	D_3
$(S_1=0, S_2=0)$	0.24	0.36	0.04	0.249	0.746	0.005
$(S_1=1, S_2=0)$	0.36	0.24	0.16	0.419	0.558	0.023
$(S_1=0, S_2=1)$	0.16	0.04	0.16	0.615	0.308	0.077
$(S_1=1, S_2=1)$	0.24	0.36	0.64	0.231	0.692	0.077

$$*P(D_j \mid S_1=a_1, S_2=a_2) = \frac{P(S_1=a_1, S_2=a_2 \mid D_j) \times P(D_j)}{\sum_{j=1}^{3} P(D_j) \times P(S_1=a_1, S_2=a_2 \mid D_j)}$$

Figure 16-8. The values of two discrete binary variates (S_1 and S_2) in each of 25 randomly selected patients from each of three clinical classes (D_1, D_2, and D_3). The subjects are depicted as squares with a diagonal; $S_1 = 1$ is depicted by a solid shading in the upper left portion of the squares, and $S_2 = 1$ is depicted by lines drawn in the lower right portion of the square; when either of the variate values is zero, the appropriate portion of the square is left open. The prevalences, the conditional probabilities, and Bayes formula for computing the posterior probability are presented in this figure. (See text for explanation of the various symbols used in this figure.)

Table 16–10. SOME DEFINITIONS FOR THE CASE OF TWO BINARY VARIATES, "S_1" AND "S_2", AND THREE CLINICAL CLASSES, "D_1", "D_2", AND "D_3"

NOTATION	DEFINITION
(1) $P(D_1)$	Prevalence of Class D_1
(2) $P(D_2)$	Prevalence of Class D_2
(3) $P(D_3)$	Prevalence of Class D_3
(4) $S_1 = 1$	Signifies the presence of attribute #1
(5) $S_1 = 0$	Signifies the absence of attribute #1
(6) $S_2 = 1$	Signifies the presence of attribute #2
(7) $S_2 = 0$	Signifies the absence of attribute #2
(8) $P(S_1 = 1, S_2 = 1 \mid D_1)$	Probability that a member of class D_1 will present attribute #1 and attribute #2
(9) $P(S_1 = 1, S_2 = 0 \mid D_2)$	Probability that a member of class D_2 will present attribute #1 but not attribute #2
(10) $P(S_1 = 0, S_2 = 1 \mid D_3)$	Probability that a member of class D_3 will not present attribute #1 but will present attribute #2
(11) $P(D_2 \mid S_1 = 1, S_2 = 0)$	Probability that a subject is a member of class D_2 given that he presents attribute #1 but not attribute #2
(12) $P(D_3 \mid S_1 = 0, S_2 = 0)$	Probability that a subject is a member of class D_3 given that he presents neither attribute #1 nor attribute #2

for a randomly selected subset of 25 patients from each of the three clinical classes. It is assumed that the distribution of values of S_1 and S_2 among these patients is identical with that of the total population. As a consequence, various conditional probabilities can be computed from the information presented in Figure 16–8, i.e., the probability that a patient will present certain values of S_1 and S_2, given that he is a member of a particular clinical class.

One other critical type of information is needed, i.e., the prior probabilities (prevalences) of obtaining a member of each clinical class when a patient is picked at random from the universe of patients, i.e., $P(D_1)$, $P(D_2)$, and $P(D_3)$. This information is also presented in Figure 16–8. As mentioned above, it is assumed that there are only three clinical classes: D_1, D_2, and D_3, and that a patient must be a member of one and only one of these classes. This is an example of the principle of the exhaustive and mutually exclusive nature of the classes. Given the prevalences of the clinical classes and the prior conditional probabilities presented in the figure, we can proceed to compute the posterior probabilities. The *posterior probability* can be symbolized as $P(D_j \mid S_1 = a_1, S_2 = a_2)$, that is, the probability of a patient being a member of class D_j, given that he presents the values a_1 and a_2 for the variates S_1 and S_2. In our example, a_1 and a_2 can be only "0" or "1."

Independency versus Dependency of the Variates. Two binary variates are considered to be *independent* when knowing the value of one variate does not affect the probability of the value that the other variate may assume. The variates S_1 and S_2 are considered to be independent within a given clinical class D_j if the following condition can be met for all possible values of a_1 and a_2:

$$P(S_1 = a_1, S_2 = a_2 \mid D_j)$$
$$= [P(S_1 = a_1 \mid D_j)] \cdot [P(S_2 = a_2 \mid D_j)]$$

where (in this case) a_1 and a_2 can take on the values "0" or "1." The constructed examples in Figure 16–8 illustrate independency for variates S_1 and S_2 as observed in members of class D_1 and class D_3. Using $S_1 = 1$ and $S_2 = 1$ as one pattern, we note for example for class D_1:

$$P(S_1 = 1, S_2 = 1 \mid D_1)$$
$$= [P(S_1 = 1 \mid D_1)] \cdot [P(S_2 = 1 \mid D_1)]$$

is a correct statement, in that, $0.24 = (0.60) \cdot (0.40)$, and also for class D_3:

$$P(S_1 = 1, S_2 = 1 \mid D_3)$$
$$= [P(S_1 = 1 \mid D_3)] \cdot [P(S_2 = 1 \mid D_3)]$$

is a correct statement, in that $0.64 = (0.80) \cdot (0.80)$. However, as observed among the members of class D_2, there is a *dependency* of the variates; i.e.,

$$P(S_1 = a_1, S_2 = a_2 \mid D_2)$$
$$\neq [P(S_1 = a_1 \mid D_2)] \cdot [P(S_2 = a_2 \mid D_2)]$$

for, as can be noted in Figure 16–8, the probability of finding a patient for whom $S_1 = 1$ and $S_2 = 1$ is greater than the product of the probability of finding a patient for whom $S_1 = 1$ and the probability of finding a patient for whom $S_2 = 1$. Specifically, based on the constructed example,

$$P(S_1 = 1, S_2 = 1 | D_2)$$
$$> [P(S_1 = 1 | D_2)] \cdot [P(S_2 = 1 | D_2)]$$

i.e., $0.36 > [(0.60) \cdot (0.40)]$.

Computing the Desired Conditional Probabilities.

Because of the possible dependency of the variates, we must determine the probabilities of each combination of variate values separately. For illustrative purposes, let us examine the case when we observe a pattern of $S_1 = 1$ and $S_2 = 1$ in a patient who must be a member of either D_1 or D_3. The Bayes theorem used here is an extension of the theorem originally applied for the case of one binary variate and two clinical classes discussed earlier in this chapter. Thus, instead of using the value of one binary variate, we insert the stated values for both variates. Rather than summing the products of prevalence and the corresponding conditional probability for two clinical classes, we sum the products for three clinical classes and enter the sum in the denominator of the equation:

$$P(D_j | S_1 = 1, S_2 = 1)$$
$$= \frac{P(S_1 = 1, S_2 = 1 | D_j) \cdot P(D_j)}{\sum\limits_{i=1}^{3} [P(D_i) \cdot P(S_1 = 1, S_2 = 1 | D_i)]}$$

We then compute the various desired conditional probabilities for each clinical class given the combination $S_1 = 1$ and $S_2 = 1$. These results, as well as the results for each of the four possible combinations, can be noted in Figure 16-8. The three clinical classes are ranked in decreasing order of probability for $S_1 = 1$, $S_2 = 1$. The importance of prevalence can be appreciated in this example. If the prevalences of each of the classes were equal, the rank order (in descending order of probability) would have been D_3, D_2, D_1 as:

$$P(D_3 | S_1 = 1, S_2 = 1)$$
$$> P(D_2 | S_1 = 1, S_2 = 1)$$
$$> P(D_1 | S_1 = 1, S_2 = 1)$$

However, with the stated prevalences given for this example, the actual rank order (in descending order of probability) is D_2, D_1, D_3 as:

$$[P(D_2 | S_1 = 1, S_2 = 1)] \cdot [P(D_2)]$$
$$> [P(D_1 | S_1 = 1, S_2 = 1)] \cdot [P(D_1)]$$
$$> [P(D_3 | S_1 = 1, S_2 = 1)] \cdot [P(D_3)]$$

Bayesian Model for Multiple Binary Variates.

A model postulating independency among variates within clinical classes was originally applied for automating the diagnosis of congenital heart diseases (Warner, 1961). The advantage of this model is that in addition to the prior probabilities, we need estimate only as many probabilities for each disease as there are variates. From these probabilities all other probabilities may be computed. If we do not postulate independency, we must estimate the probability for each combination of variate values; i.e., we would estimate the probability as the number of patients with the disease who present the pattern of variate values divided by the total number of patients with the disease. In general, for a given disease, if we have "n" binary variates, there are 2^n possible patterns and therefore $2^n - 1$ probabilities to estimate when we do *not* assume independency among variates. Often times, however, symptoms are strongly related and this information may be of diagnostic importance. Therefore in some cases the model assuming independency of variates may represent too crude an approximation and alternative models have to be formulated. The reader is referred to Norusis (1975) for a discussion of models allowing for various degrees of dependency among variates.

Bayesian Model for Two Discrete Variates in General.

Thus far we have considered only discrete variates where each variate can attain one of two possible values. We will now begin to investigate the case of discrete variates which can attain one of multiple possible values by way of a constructed example. Figure 16-9A to D depicts the bivariate 99 per cent tolerance regions (see Chapter 2 for definition of tolerance intervals) of two continuous variates: V_1 and V_2, for each of three clinical classes: D_1, D_2, and D_3. We assume that V_1 or V_2 can take on any value in the interval 0,600. However, V_1 and V_2 are transformed to obtain two discrete variates, S_1 and S_2. This form of data reduction will decrease the information content originally present in the values of the continuous variates. However, by increasing the possible discrete values which S_1 and S_2 can take on, we retain more and

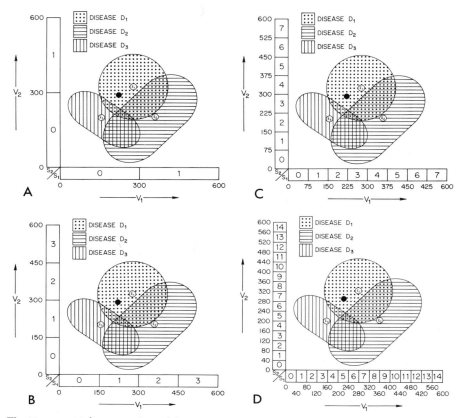

Figure 16–9. The 99 per cent tolerance regions of the two continuous variates V_1 and V_2 are depicted for three clinical classes: D_1, D_2, and D_3. The circled values of $\bar{X}_1$, $\bar{X}_2$, and $\bar{X}_3$ are the sets of mean values of the classes D_1, D_2, and D_3, respectively. The closed circle corresponds to the case where $V_1 = 220$ and $V_2 = 290$. In each of the four figures in this series the continuous variates V_1 and V_2 are transformed to the discrete variates S_1 and S_2. In A, the total number of possible values that each discrete variate can obtain is two; in B, the number is four; in C, the number is eight; and in D, the number is fifteen.

more of the information present in the original variates, V_1 and V_2. We can apply Bayes theorem to discrete variates having more than two values; however, the computations are more cumbersome and we usually need a large population sample so that all (or most) of the possible combinations of the discrete values are covered. Figure 16-9A to D presents the bivariate tolerance regions for the three classes: D_1, D_2, and D_3; with each successive frame the total number of possible discrete values for S_1 and S_2 increases. In Figure 16-9A, S_1 and S_2 can take on only the values 0 and 1; in Figure 16-9B, they can take on the values 0, 1, 2, and 3; in Figure 16-9C the possible values are any real integer between 0 and 7 inclusive; and in Figure 16-9D, any real integer between 0 and 14 inclusive. The discrete variates (S_1 and S_2) are functions of the con-

tinuous variates (V_1 and V_2). The cutoff values are values at which this function is discontinuous and the function value increases by one. For example, in Case A, the cutoff value is 300; that is, $S_1 = 0$ for all V_1 less than or equal to 300, and $S_1 = 1$ for all V_1 greater than 300.

In each case (Figure 16-9A to D), the solid circle corresponds to the same set of observations: $V_1 = 220$ and $V_2 = 290$. In all of the four cases, the points labeled $\bar{X}_1$, $\bar{X}_2$, and $\bar{X}_3$ are the set of mean values of the clinical classes: D_1, D_2, and D_3, respectively. The solid circle represents the values of a patient whom we wish to classify into one of the three classes. It is assumed that sets of observations from patients belonging to a given clinical class are more likely to fall in the immediate neighborhood of the mean values of the particular clinical class than anywhere else. Thus, the probability that a patient presenting the mentioned values belongs to clinical class D_1 is quite high, since the set of observations is close to the mean of this class. In case A, S_1 and S_2 each can attain two values, "0" and "1." Obviously much of the original information is lost during this transformation. Thus, the values of the discrete variates S_1 and S_2 corresponding to the solid circle are (0,0). Given that $S_1 = 0$ and $S_2 = 0$ and that the original values of V_1 and V_2 are not available, and assuming that the prevalence of D_3 is of reasonable magnitude, we would conclude that the patient in all likelihood belongs to clinical class D_3. In case B the number of possible values that the discrete variates may attain is four. In this case, the set of discrete values corresponding to the solid circle is (1,1). In case C, S_1, S_2 would be equal to (2,3) and in case D (5,7). In case C, there are a total of 64 possible combinations and in case D, a total of 225 possible combinations. In the latter case (case D) we conclude that the patient is most likely a member of class D_3, knowing that $S_1 = 5$ and $S_2 = 7$ for this patient. The larger the number of values per discrete variate, the more of the original information is retained. In each case (Figure 16-9A to D), the Bayesian model for discrete variates may be applied. However, we would have to estimate the probabilities corresponding to each square area formed, and the number of observations necessary to estimate the probabilities would very soon be prohibitively large. For two variates, the number of squares would be n^2 where "n" is the number of discrete values of each variate; e.g., for n = 20, the number of squares would be $(20)^2$ or 400.

BAYES THEOREM FOR CONTINUOUS VARIATES

Theory of Linear Discriminant Analysis. An alternative approach for computing probabilities for continuous variates is based on the "probability density function." Mathematically this is done by defining a function, i.e., a probability density function (in this case a function in two variates S_1 and S_2) which has the property that when integrated over all possible sets of values, the result is equal to 1.0; and when integrated over any particular region (in the example above, any particular area, e.g., the area defined by $b_1 \leq V_1 \leq c_1$ and $b_2 \leq V_2 \leq c_2$), the result is equal to the probability that a subject picked at random from the population in question will have a set of values falling within the region. The Bayesian formula for continuous data then is derived from that of discrete data by replacing probabilities with density function values.

As in the discrete case, we must make simplifying assumptions regarding the relationships among the variates in order to solve the estimation problem. This is done by postulating a general algebraic formula according to which the value of the density function can be computed for all combinations of variate values. The formula includes a number of constants (parameters) which characterize the distribution of the data and which, therefore, have to be estimated from the data. Thus, instead of estimating all the probabilities directly, we may estimate the parameters of the density functions once and for all and then use these functions to calculate any desired probability, according to Bayes formula for continuous data. For a discussion of the various models which may be used for this purpose the reader is referred to Lachenbruch (1975). Here we shall consider only the model most commonly used, that implied in the technique of linear discriminant analysis. Linear discriminant analysis was originally proposed by Fisher (1936) as a means of deriving a linear function which could best discriminate between two groups of items on which multiple observations were made. He derived a linear combination of the measurements called the linear discriminant function "Z," which has the property that the univariate distributions of "Z" in the two groups are maximally separated. In the particular model of linear discriminant analysis that we are going to present it is assumed that the values from each of the classes follow a multivariate Gaussian distribution. Furthermore, it is assumed that the distributions differ only with regard to location, i.e., differ with regard to mean values.

The statistical technique of linear discriminant analysis was first applied for clinical problems by Zieve (1955). In principle, linear discriminant analysis amounts to the computation of density function values. If prior probabilities are known or estimated, Bayes formula may be applied subsequently. Owing to the assumptions made, the computations become very simple. Here we shall illustrate the example for two classes: D_{10} and D_{20}, and for "p" variates: $S_1, S_2, \ldots, S_p$. Essentially, the p variates involved in this linear discriminant analysis are weighted (multiplied) by (b_1, $b_2, \ldots, b_p$) and expressed mathematically as

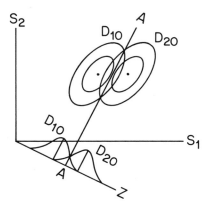

Figure 16–10. Tolerance regions (90 and 95 per cent) of two continuous variates S_1 and S_2 for two clinical classes D_{10} and D_{20}. The classes have equal prevalences, and the corresponding bivariate distributions have equal variances and correlation coefficients. For further explanation of symbols, see text.

$Z = b_1S_1 + b_2S_2 + \cdots + b_pS_p$. This linear function "Z," a weighted sum, is termed the discriminant function. When the discriminant function is evaluated for a patient, the resulting number "z" is the discriminant score for that patient. We can then use the Z value to classify patients into various groups. We will assume that "A" is the critical value of Z used to assign the patients into either class D_{10} or D_{20} (see Figs. 16–10 and 16–11). In the case of two classes, D_{10} and D_{20}, if $Z \leq A$, the patient is allocated to D_{10}, and if $Z > A$, the patient is

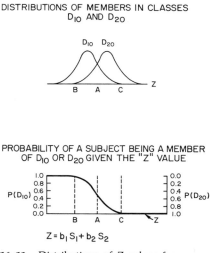

Figure 16–11. Distributions of Z values from members in classes D_{10} and D_{20}. For further explanation, see text.

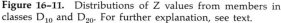

allocated to D_{20}, where A is the discriminant score when $P(\hat{D}_{10}|(Z = A)) = P(D_{20}|(Z = A))$, that is, when there is equal probability that a patient could be a member of either class. This approach, then, attempts to minimize the number of misclassifications.

Where there is an overlap of the distributions, we may convert the actual value of "Z" to a probability value that a patient is a member of a particular class. We will use this latter approach in illustrating a constructed example of the use of linear discriminant analysis (Fig. 16–10). For didactic purposes only, let us examine a geometric interpretation of the discriminant analysis where we have two classes, D_{10} and D_{20}, and two variates, S_1 and S_2. The two variates S_1 and S_2 are positively correlated as illustrated. Each ellipse in the diagram is the focus of points of equal probability density for a particular class. For example, the outer ellipse for class D_{10} might define the region within which 95 per cent of class D_{10} lies. These ellipses are called centours (centile contours). The two points at which corresponding centours intersect define the discriminator "A," the line of equal probability density values for the two classes. If a second line Z is constructed perpendicular to line A, and if the points in the two-dimensional space are projected onto Z, the overlap between the two groups will be smaller than for any other possible line. The linear function used for this projection is the discriminant function. It is noted that the discriminant function follows a univariate Gaussian distribution for each of the two populations. The two distributions have identical variances and their intersection falls on the line of equal density function values in the original two-dimensional distributions. The technique of linear discriminant analysis may be generalized to more than two groups (see textbooks by Anderson, 1958, and Lachenbruch, 1975).

Figure 16–11 presents the frequency distribution of the Z values for each clinical class, D_{10} and D_{20}. We will assume that the prior probabilities are equal; i.e., $P(D_{10}) = P(D_{20})$. As an example of two clinical groups, D_{10} could be the patients *not* alive two years after the first myocardial infarction and D_{20} the patients alive two years after the first myocardial infarction. The Z values can be transformed to probability values, e.g., the probability that a patient will be alive two years after the insult of myocardial infarction. In Figure 16–11, it is noted that when Z = B, the probability of a patient being in group D_{20} is approximately 0.0; when Z = A (discriminator value), the probability of a patient being in group D_{20} is 0.50; and when Z = C, the probability of being in D_{20} is approximately 1.0. When the prior probabilities (prevalences) are not identical, the discriminator value is changed to adjust for this fact. Thus, if $P(D_{10}) > P(D_{20})$ the discriminator value is shifted to the right, and if $P(D_{10}) < P(D_{20})$ it is shifted to the left.

The net effect of transforming the bivariate data (Figs. 16–10 and 16–11) to Z values (linear transformation) is to reduce the multivariate problem to a univariate one with the new variate being "Z." As presented earlier (Fig. 16–1), we attempt to assign patients into one of two classes (D_{10} or D_{20}) according to the relative probabilities of finding a member in one of the two classes at a particular value of Z. As in the case for the univariate classification problem, we also should consider the relative costs of misclassification as well as be certain of the *a priori* prevalences of the two classes. A linear transformation which results in no overlap between the two classes should afford perfect discrimination. Unfortunately, this is a very rare occurrence in clinical medicine.

Choosing the Variates to Use in the Discriminant Function. The purpose of using linear discriminant analysis in clinical medicine is to utilize the discriminatory ability of the variates which is due to their interrelationships. However, often times a multitude of variates is available, and one must therefore choose from among the variates those which discriminate the best. In the clinical setting, we are faced with the problem of selecting the smallest subset of variates which contains all the discriminatory information from the total number of variates available. One approach might be to perform a univariate test for each of the variates (t-test in the case in which we are considering two clinical classes or an F-test in the case in which we are discriminating among more than two clinical classes) and then eliminate all variates for which the t-test (or F-test) is insignificant according to some predefined level of significance. Figure 16–12 is an illustration of the fallacy of this approach. This figure is modified from Johnson (1974). It shows the joint distribution of two laboratory tests, S_1 and S_2, for each of two clinical classes, D_1 and D_2, for two cases. Evaluating the variates S_1 and S_2 univariately, we

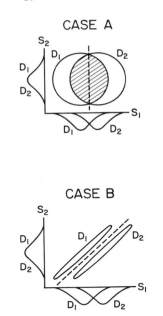

Figure 16–12. Bivariate tolerance regions of two continuous variates S_1 and S_2 for two clinical classes D_1 and D_2. In both A and B, the univariate distributions of S_1 and of S_2 are the same for both classes. There is a definite separation of values for S_1, but the univariate distributions for S_2 are identical. In Case A, there is no correlation between S_1 and S_2 and thus there is much overlap of the two tolerance regions. In Case B, there is a very strong (positive) correlation between S_1 and S_2 such that there is much less overlap of the two tolerance regions.

note that the univariate distributions for classes D_1 and D_2 are comparable in both cases. Specifically, the two classes differ in their values for S_1 (D_2 being greater on the average than D_1); however, there is some degree of overlap. In both cases (A and B) the univariate distributions of S_2 are identical for the two clinical classes. We would expect that the group t-test would be statistically significant for variate S_1 (mean of D_1 significantly different from mean of D_2) but be insignificant for variate S_2 (means of D_1 and D_2 not significantly different).

Let us now examine the bivariate distributions for classes D_1 and D_2 in each of the cases. In case A, there is a high degree of overlap for the two classes using the values of S_1 and S_2; however, in case B there is minimal overlap of the two clinical classes. The difference between the two cases is that in case A there is zero correlation between the two variates, while in case B the two variates are strongly and positively correlated. As a matter of fact, in case A, using the values of S_1 only, the degree of overlap in the two clinical classes is identical with the degree of overlap based on the value of both S_1 and S_2 (Fig. 16-12, see upper frame). Thus, had we decided to ignore S_2 as one of the variates on the basis of a non-significant t-test, the discrimination in case A would have been unchanged. However, the discrimination in case B would have decreased dramatically.

Applications of Linear Discriminant Analysis. Linear discriminant analysis has been applied in searching for the "best" test combination to discriminate among clinical classes defined on the basis of pathology in patients presenting with hypercalcemia (Amenta, 1971), in subjects with suspected hepatobiliary disease (Burbank, 1969; Ramsoe, 1970; Winkel, 1975; Solberg, 1975; Sher, 1977), and in patients with chronic renal failure for predicting peripheral neuropathy (Nielsen, 1971). The diagnostic effectiveness of biochemical liver tests (activities of alkaline phosphatase (ALP), alanine aminotransferase (ALT), aspartate aminotransferase (AST), lactate dehydrogenase, concentrations of bilirubins, albumin, globulins, and quantities relating to coagulation) has been evaluated by several investigators. In these studies, the definitive diagnosis was made by liver biopsy and/or exploratory laparotomy. In general, it was found that the diagnostic effectiveness was no better than 60 to 70 per cent using the biochemical tests and that the most significant information for discrimination was obtained from combining either ALP and AST, or ALP and ALT. It should be noted that in most studies the diagnostic effectiveness is examined using the same cases that were used in deriving the discriminant functions. Thus, the discriminatory effectiveness is probably somewhat overestimated (Sher, 1977). Frazer (1971) applied linear discriminant analysis in the differential diagnosis of hypercalcemia. A simple, single test is not readily available for this differential diagnosis. Therefore, they used the admission values of total calcium, inorganic phosphate, alkaline phosphatase, sodium, potassium, chloride, bicarbonate, and urea, all in serum, to derive discriminant functions to distinguish most clearly among the following four categories: (1) hyperparathyroidism with normal alkaline phosphatase, (2) hyperparathyroidism with raised alkaline phosphatase, (3) non-parathyroid disease with moderate increases in urea and phosphate, and (4) non-parathyroid disease with striking increases in urea and phosphate. The analysis showed that sodium and potassium made little

contribution to the discrimination, and these tests were therefore deleted from the discriminant functions. The derivation of the discriminant functions was based on 103 retrospective cases. They proceeded to classify 65 additional retrospective cases using the discriminant function previously derived. Of these, 59 cases were correctly placed in the two groups: hypercalcemia due to hyperparathyroidism, and hypercalcemia due to other causes. In a prospective study, they were able to classify correctly 34 out of 39 patients with primary hyperparathyroidism and 6 out of 9 patients with hypercalcemia due to other causes (Frazer, 1971).

Testing for Possible Redundancy of Laboratory Tests. The redundancy of laboratory tests, i.e., the lack of improved "diagnostic effectiveness" when adding more assays to the clinical chemistry laboratory repertoire of tests, has been evaluated using the same discriminant analysis programs. Werner (1972) computed the diagnostic effectiveness of the results obtained from paper electrophoresis of serum proteins (five fractions: albumin, alpha 1-, alpha 2-, beta-, and gamma-globulins) versus the results of 12 specific protein determinations in discriminating among patients with documented cirrhosis, hepatitis, IgG myeloma, IgA myeloma, systemic lupus erythematosus, nephritis, and no known disease. They concluded that the results obtained from paper electrophoresis of the proteins provide the same discriminatory separation as a battery of specific assays for individual proteins in terms of the diseases evaluated.

Computer Programs Available for Linear Discriminant Analysis. Because of the correlations among variates, ideally one should examine *all* possible combinations of variates even if by univariate tests the variates are poor discriminators (Zieve, 1955). In theory one could evaluate all possible combinations of the variates; but unless the number of variates is relatively small, this approach requires a very large amount of computer time. One approach which has been commonly used is the *stepwise procedure*. By this procedure the single variate which gives the best discrimination (smallest number of misclassifications) is first selected (Efroymsen, 1960). At each of the following steps a new variate is selected, namely the variate which, combined with the previously selected variate, gives the best discrimination. After each step, the previously selected variates are reevaluated and if a variate no longer contributes significantly to the discrimination, it is eliminated. The discriminatory ability of each variate combination may be compared with that of all the variates when used in combination (Ramsoe, 1970). When this difference is no longer significant (at some predefined level of statistical significance), the variates not yet entered in the analysis are declared redundant. If the problem is to decide whether or not a particular test is redundant, the discriminatory ability of all tests is computed and compared with that obtained when the test in question is excluded. This procedure and other similar ones are available through the BMDP (Bio Medical Data Processing) computer program package, which has three discriminant analysis programs: BMDP4M, BMDP5M, and BMDP7M. The latter (BMDP7M) is the stepwise discriminant analysis program (Dixon, 1975). Techniques alternative to the stepwise discriminant analysis are available, and the recent trend among statisticians has been away from stepwise discriminant analysis. A presentation of these techniques is beyond the scope of this book.

Non-linear Discriminant Analysis. Discriminant methods other than linear discriminant analysis have been introduced for those cases in which linear discriminant analysis is inappropriate. For instance, when the classes have unequal variances and different correlation values, a quadratic discriminant function is used. The geometric representation in this case is a curved surface. For additional information on approaches alternative to the linear discriminant analysis described here, the reader is referred to Lachenbruch (1975).

BAYES THEOREM FOR A MIXTURE OF CONTINUOUS AND DISCRETE VARIATES

Luria (1976) used a linear discriminant function model with five variates to estimate the probability of surviving two years after a myocardial infarction (MI), i.e., assignment into one of two classes based on prognosis: the class of patients surviving two years after MI, and the class of patients not surviving two years after MI. They found that 110 of the 137 patients were alive after two years. They used five variates, S_1 to S_5, to discriminate the two classes. The linear discriminant function was

$$Z = 0.023(S_1) + 0.047(S_2)$$
$$+ 1.46(S_3) + 1.55(S_4) + 1.48(S_5)$$

where S_1 is the admission systolic blood pressure value in mm Hg; S_2 is the highest blood urea nitrogen value in mg/dl that the patient had while in the Coronary Care Unit; S_3 to S_5 are attributes of atrial arrhythmias, longstanding angina, and ventricular ectopic beats, respectively. S_3 to S_5 were treated as binary discrete variates (attribute present coded as "1" and attribute absent coded as "0"). The Z-value was converted to a probability of two-year survival. The smallest number of misclassifications occurred with a discriminator (A-value as in Figures 16–10 and 16–11) of 8.6; in this case, only 23 of the 137 patients were incorrectly classified. The classification rule was: If the Z-value is ≤ 8.6, the patient is assigned to the "surviving group"; and if the Z-value is > 8.6, the patient is assigned to the "non-surviving group."

Clinical problems such as that presented in the example above usually involve a mixture of continuous and discrete variates. In this situation, one may transform the continuous variates to discrete variates and use a discrete model; or, alternatively, treat the discrete data as continuous data and use a continuous model, as was done in the example above; or, finally, formulate a model which may accommodate a mixture of discrete and continuous data, usually subject to some simplifying assumptions such as conditional independency in each disease between continuous and discrete data. A discussion of the various approaches is beyond the scope of this chapter and the interested reader is referred to Starmer (1976).

CONSIDERATIONS WHEN USING DISCRIMINANT ANALYSIS

The use of discriminant analysis demands an independent and valid means of determining the clinical classes to which the patients are assigned. If not, the reasoning becomes circular. The importance of performing *prospective* studies using the previously derived discriminant function should be emphasized. If not, we are never certain if the function derived from past data is also valid for future cases.

One of the problems in most applications of discriminant analysis is that the duration of the disease is not adequately taken into consideration. Therefore, there is usually a large variability among the patients within a given clinical class because they are at different stages of their disease. This variability could be reduced if the clinical class were subdivided into subclasses representing various stages of the same disease (Winkel, 1972, 1973).

Another source of variability within clinical classes is the lack of information about the baseline values of the quantities as measured in the subjects prior to the contraction of disease. If this information were available, the effect of the interindividual differences among the subjects' values prior to the development of disease could be eliminated by studying the *changes* from baseline values rather than the actual values (Winkel, 1977).

CONSTRUCTING NEW CLINICAL CLASSES

The probabilistic approach used to assign a given patient to a particular clinical class is based in part upon well-accepted definitions of the various clinical classes. These definitions are made by clinicians or pathologists who have studied the consistent observations present in a number of patients. Clinical classifications are of two types, "monothetic" and "polythetic." A monothetic class includes *only* members that share the same attribute or attributes implied by the definition of the clinical class; for example, all patients with nephrotic syndrome must demonstrate peripheral edema, hypoalbuminemia, and proteinuria. By contrast, a polythetic class is a class for which it is not required that any one attribute (symptom, sign, or laboratory result) be shared by all patients making up the class. Consider four patients possessing the following attributes respectively: $S_1S_3S_4$, $S_1S_2S_4$, $S_1S_2S_3$, and $S_2S_3S_4$. Although none of the attributes is shared by all four patients, each patient is similar to the other three by having two attributes in common. According to the definition of polythetic classes, these four patients *may* very well fall into one clinical class (cluster). This section will present various techniques of automated polythetic classifications (techniques of numerical taxonomy) and the criteria used to test their validity. The clinical meaningfulness of the classes formed by these techniques will be discussed. The interested reader is referred to Jardin (1971) and Hartigan (1975) for extensive reviews of the theoretical and computational problems of numerical taxonomy and to Winkel (1973) for a review of the applications in clinical medicine.

The main steps of a numerical taxonomic classification of patients based on similarity measures include the following: first, a quantitative measure of the similarity between all possible pairs of patients—a similarity coefficient—is defined. This measure is obtained on the basis of multiple comparisons. Based on the computed values of the similarity coefficient, the patients are sorted into groups or clusters of patients being most similar to each other.

A similarity coefficient is a function the range of which is 0,1. The value of this function increases as the degree of sameness between the two patients also increases. All kinds of clinical data can be used in computing similarity measures; however, because a meaningful strategy for assigning weights to quantitative data is not available, there are as yet unsolved problems relating to the construction of a similarity coefficient. A very simple similarity coefficient has been used for most medical applications. For each pair of patients these are compared with respect to binary variates (attribute present or absent) observed. The number of matches divided by the total number of comparisons is then defined as the coefficient of similarity between the two patients.

When the values of the similarity coefficient, i.e., the similarity of all possible pairs of patients, have been computed, the sorting of the patients into groups (clusters) can take place. Only the hierarchic methods will be mentioned here. A hierarchic classification proceeds in the following steps. At the first step each patient is considered a single member cluster. Clusters are then joined in successive fusion steps by combining at each step those two clusters which have the highest similarity. The various methods differ with respect to the definition of the similarity between two clusters. In the single linkage method (Sneath, 1957), the similarity between two clusters is defined as the highest value of the similarity coefficient between two patients, each belonging to different clusters.

The techniques of cluster analysis may also be used for the classification of variates rather than patients. All possible pairs of variates are examined for the degree of similarity, e.g., defined as the number of patients having the same value for both variates divided by the total number of patients in the population. The clusters formed in this case would be equivalent to new syndromes and would be evaluated subsequently for clinical meaningfulness.

Applications of Cluster Analysis. Numerical taxonomy has been used to demarcate subgroups of patients suffering from such ailments as acute leukemia (Hayhoe, 1964), chronic liver disease (Baron, 1968), non-specific colitis (Jones, 1972), heart disease (Manning, 1966), thyroid disease (Bouchaert, 1971), pyelonephritis (Zinsser, 1962), and hepatic cirrhosis (Winkel, 1976). In the latter study numerical taxonomy was applied to construction of classes from a group of 442 cirrhotic patients entering a controlled trial of prednisone treatment. The data analyzed were data obtained prior to treatment with prednisone or placebo. Using the single-linkage method, Winkel (1976) discovered that the patients formed two clusters based on clinical data; however, 68 per cent of the patients were unclassifiable. The merit of this cluster analysis was obvious when evaluating the response to prednisone therapy. Patients in "Cluster 2" (104 patients) had a significantly better prognosis with prednisone therapy than without prednisone treatment (five year survival rates were 63 per cent versus 41 per cent), whereas there was no significant effect of prednisone treatment in "Cluster 1" (26 patients) or in the patients not classified into either cluster. This example demonstrates that the result of such a classification may be clinically meaningful in that the classification was related to differential response to therapy (Winkel, 1976).

CONSIDERATIONS WHEN USING CLUSTER ANALYSIS

Table 16-11 summarizes the conditions which should be fulfilled before the results of a

Table 16-11. CONDITIONS TO BE FULFILLED BEFORE THE RESULTS OF A CLUSTER ANALYSIS CAN BE USED

I. Classification should be clinically relevant; i.e., classes should be heterogeneous with regard to one or more of the following qualities:
   A. Predominance of patients with characteristics of possible etiologic importance
   B. Prognosis
   C. Response to treatment
II. Results should be reproducible
   A. Ideally, patients to be classified should be a simple randomly selected subset obtained from a well-defined population
   B. Classification should be reproduced in other patients

cluster analysis can be used. For a clinical classification to be meaningful, it must segregate the various classes on the basis of different etiologies, prognoses, and/or responses to therapy. If the classification does not allow such a distinction, the classes formed by numerical taxonomy will be of no immediate value to the clinician. It is also important that a classification can be reproduced by others. A necessary condition for this is that the population to be classified is demarcated according to well-defined criteria.

SUMMARY

In this chapter we have examined various quantitative approaches used in evaluating laboratory measurements and other types of clinical data. Many of the methods discussed have at least one principle in common. These methods present the clinician with likelihood values, e.g., the probability that his patient is a member of a clinical class, or the probability of one outcome occurring, given a certain course of action. Probabilistic reasoning makes more demands on the clinician than does categorical reasoning. The clinician must be aware of the various assumptions, conditions, and considerations as enumerated in this chapter concerning probabilistic reasoning.

The limitations as well as the potential of the quantitative approaches presented in this chapter should be clearly understood. In addition to meeting the theoretical demands of any of the proposed methods, the user of these approaches must be assured that he has the necessary data to apply the various formulae, e.g., an accurate estimate of the prevalence of a particular clinical class, knowledge of relevant prior conditional probabilities, etc. Most often, such data are not readily available; and when available, their accuracy may be suspect. The worked-through examples presented in this chapter represent only illustrations so that the reader can better understand the theory and practice of these various quantitative approaches. Given different assumptions, assuming different prior probabilities, and accepting different values for certain outcomes may each lead to an alternative conclusion.

At this time, many conflicting forces in our society are asking the clinical pathologist to increase or to decrease the number of assays performed in the clinical laboratory. Rather than react emotionally or intuitively, we should rationally evaluate the effects of increasing or decreasing the number of assays offered. Various techniques presented in this chapter should be of great benefit to the laboratorian who wishes to approach such issues on a logical and on a quantitative basis.

REFERENCES

Amenta, J. S., and Harkins, M. D.: The use of discriminant functions in laboratory medicine. Evaluation of phosphate clearance studies in the diagnosis of hyperparathyroidism. Am. J. Clin. Pathol., 55:330, 1971.

Anderson, T. W.: Introduction of multivariate statistical analysis. New York, John Wiley & Sons, Inc., 1958.

Baron, D. N., and Frazer, P. M.: Medical applications of taxonomic methods. Br. Med. Bull., 24:236, 1968.

Bay, K. S., Flatham, D., and Nestman, L.: The worth of a screening program: An application of a statistical decision model for the benefit evaluation of screening projects. Am. J. Pub. Health, 66:145, 1976.

Bayes, T.: An essay toward solving a problem in the doctrine of chance. Phil. Trans. R. Soc., 53:370, 1763.

Bietz, D. S.: Algorithm for critically injured patients. J. Trauma, 17:55, 1977.

Bleich, H. L.: Computer evaluation of acid-base disorders. J. Clin. Invest., 48:1689, 1969.

Blendis, L. M., McNeilly, W. J., Sheppard, L., et al.: Observer variation in the clinical and radiological assessment of hepatosplenomegaly. Br. Med. J., 1:727, 1970.

Bone, H. G., Snyder, W. H., and Pak, C. Y.: Diagnosis of hyperparathyroidism. Ann. Rev. Med., 28:111, 1977.

Bouchaert, A.: Computer diagnosis of goiters: I. Classification and differential diagnosis. J. Chron. Dis., 24:299, 1971.

Bray, G. A., Jordan, H. A., and Sims, E. A. H.: Evaluation of the obese patient. I. An algorithm. J.A.M.A., 235:1487, 1976.

Briccetti, A. B., and Bleich, H. L.: A computer program that evaluates patients with hypercalcemia. J. Clin. Endocrinol. Metab., 41:365, 1975.

Burbank, F.: A computer diagnostic system for the diagnosis of prolonged undifferentiating liver disease. Am. J. Med., 46:401, 1969.

Charles, G., Stinson, D. H., and Maurier, M. D.: A physician extender training program based on clinical algorithms. West. J. Med., 127:63, 1977.

Cole, G. W., and Bradley, W.: Hospital admission laboratory profile interpretation. The SGOT and SLDH-SGOT ratio used in the diagnosis of hepatic disease. Hum. Pathol., 4:85, 1975.

deDombal, F. T., Horrocks, J. C., and Staniland, J. R.: The computer as an aid to gastroenterological decision making. Scand. J. Gastroenterol., 10:225, 1975.

Dixon, W. J.: BMD Biomedical Computer Programs. Berkeley and Los Angeles, Cal., University of California Press, 1975.

Drum, D. E., and Christacopoulos, J. S.: Hepatic scintigraphy in clinical decision making. J. Nucl. Med., 13:908, 1972.

Eddy, R. L., Jones, A. L., Gilland, P. F., Ibarra, J. D., Thompson, J. Q., and McMurray, J. T.: Cushing's syndrome: A prospective study of diagnostic methods. Am. J. Med., 55:621, 1973.

Efroymsen, M. A.: Multiple regression analysis. In Ralston, A., and Wilf, H. S. (eds.): Mathematical Methods for Digital Computers. New York, John Wiley & Sons, Inc., 1960.

Ellis, J. H., Perera, S. P., and Leven, D. C.: A computer program for calculation and interpretation of pulmonary functions studies. Chest, 68:209, 1975.

Emerson, P. A., Teather, D., and Handley, A. J.: The application of decision theory to the prevention of deep vein thrombosis following myocardial infarction. Q. J. Med., 43:389, 1974.

Feinstein, A. R.: Analysis of diagnostic reasoning. Yale J. Biol. Med., 46:212, 264, 1973; 47:5, 1974.

Feinstein, A. R.: Clinical biostatistics. XXXIX. The haze of Bayes, the aerial palaces of decision analysis, and the computerized Ouija board. Clin. Pharmacol. Therap., 21:483, 1977.

Fisher, R. A.: The use of multiple measurements in taxonomic problems. Ann. Eugenics, 7:179, 1936.

Frazer, P., Healy, M., Rose, N., and Watson, L.: Discriminant functions in differential diagnosis of hypercalcemia. Lancet, 1:1314, 1974.

Galen, R. S.: Interpretation of laboratory tests. N. Engl. J. Med., 292:433, 1975a.

Galen, R. S., and Gambino, S. R.: Beyond normality: The predictive value and efficiency of medical diagnosis. New York, John Wiley & Sons, Inc., 1975b.

Galen, R. S., Reiffel, J. A., and Gambino, S. R.: Diagnosis of acute myocardial infarction: Relative efficiency of serum enzyme and isoenzyme measurements. J.A.M.A., 232:145, 1975c.

Gorry, G. A., Kassirer, J. P., Essing, A., and Schwartz, W. B.: Decision analysis as the basis for computer-aided management of acute renal failure. Am. J. Med., 55:473, 1973.

Greenfield, S., Bragg, F. E., McCraith, D. L., and Blackburn, J.: Upper-respiratory tract complaint protocol for physician extenders. J. Fam. Pract., 2:13, 1975.

Grim, C. E., Winberger, M. H., Higgins, J. T., and Kramer, N. J.: Diagnosis of secondary forms of hypertension: A comprehensive protocol. J.A.M.A., 237:1331, 1977.

Hamlyn, A. N., Sherlock, S., Brown, A. J., and Baron, D. N.: Casual blood-ethanol estimations in patients with chronic liver disease. Lancet, 2:345, 1975.

Hansen, H. J., Snyder, J. J., Miller, E., et al.: Carcinoembryonic antigen (CEA) assay. Hum. Pathol., 5:139, 1974.

Hartigan, J. A.: Clustering algorithms. New York, John Wiley & Sons, Inc., 1975.

Hayhoe, F. G. J., Quaglino, D., and Doll, R.: The cytology and cytochemistry of acute leukemias: A study of 140 cases. Medical Research Council Special Report Series 304, London, 1964.

Henry, J. B.: Introduction to organ panels. In Henry, J. B., and Giegel, J. L. (eds.): Quality Control in Laboratory Medicine. New York, Masson, 1977.

Hurst, J. W., and King, S. B.: The problem of chest pain. J.A.M.A., 236:2100, 1976.

Ingelfinger, F. J.: Decision in medicine. N. Engl. J. Med., 293:254, 1975.

Jardine, N., and Sibson, R: The construction of hierarchic and non-hierarchic classification. Comput. J., 11:117, 1968.

Jardine, N., and Sibson, R.: Mathematical Taxonomy. New York, John Wiley & Sons, Inc., 1971.

Johnson, E. A.: Multivariate clustering. In Blume, P., and Frier, E. (eds.): Enzymology in the Practice of Laboratory Medicine. New York, Academic Press, Inc., 1974.

Johnson, P. E., Moller, J. H., and Bass, G. M.: Analysis of

expert diagnosis of a computer simulation of congenital heart disease. J. Med. Educ., *50*:466, 1975.

Jones, J. H.: The application of numerical taxonomy to the separation of colonic inflammatory disease. *In* Rose, J. (ed.): Computers in Medicine. Dorchester, John Wright & Sons, 1972.

Katon, R. M., Bilbao, M. K., and Rösch, J.: Algorithm for an aggressive diagnostic approach to obstructive jaundice. West. J. Med., *122*:206, 1975.

Knuth, D. E.: Algorithms. Sci. Am., *236*:63, 1977.

Kunin, C. M.: Urinary tract infections: Flow charts (algorithms) for detection and treatment. J.A.M.A., *233*:458, 1975.

Lachenbruch, P. A.: Discriminant Analysis. New York, Hafner Press, 1975.

Ledley, R. A., and Lusted, L. B.: Reasoning foundation of medical diagnosis. Science, *130*:9, 1959.

Luria, M. H., Knoke, J. D., Margolis, R. M., Hendricks, F. H., and Kuplic, J. B.: Acute myocardial infarction: Prognosis after recovery. Ann. Intern. Med., *85*:561, 1976.

Manning, R. T., and Watson, L.: Signs, symptoms and systematics. J.A.M.A., *198*:1180, 1966.

Maronde, R. F.: The hypertensive patient: An algorithm for diagnostic work-up. J.A.M.A., *233*:997, 1975.

McNeil, B. J., Keeler, E., and Adelstein, S. J.: Primer on certain elements of medical decision making. N. Engl. J. Med., *293*:211, 1975a.

McNeil, B. J., and Adelstein, S. J.: Value of case finding in hypertensive renovascular disease. N. Engl. J. Med., *293*:221, 1975b.

Newcomer, A. D., McGill, D. B., Thomas, P. J., and Hoffmann, A. F.: Prospective comparison of indirect methods for detecting lactase deficiency. N. Engl. J. Med., *293*:1232, 1975.

Nielsen, V. K., and Winkel, P.: The peripheral nerve function in chronic renal failure. III. A multivariate statistical analysis of factors presumed to affect the development of clinical neuropathy. Acta Med. Scand., *190*:119, 1971.

Norusis, M. J., and Jacquez, J. A.: Diagnosis. I. Symptom nonindependence in mathematical models for diagnosis. Comput. Biomed. Res., *8*:156, 1975.

Ostrow, J. D.: Jaundice in older children and adults: Algorithms for diagnosis. J.A.M.A., *234*:522, 1975.

Patrick, E. A.: Expected outcome loss to evaluate medical diagnosis and treatments. Comput. Biol. Med., *7*:1, 1977.

Pauker, S. G.: Coronary artery surgery: The use of decision analysis. Ann. Intern Med., *85*:8, 1976.

Pauker, S. G., and Kassirer, J. P.: Therapeutic decision-making: A cost-benefit analysis. N. Engl. J. Med., *293*:229, 1975.

Ramsoe, K., Tygstrup, N., and Winkel, P.: The redundancy of liver tests in the diagnosis of cirrhosis estimated by multivariate statistics. Scand. J. Clin. Lab. Invest., *26*:307, 1970.

Ransohoff, D. F., and Feinstein, A. R.: Is decision analysis useful in clinical medicine? Yale J. Biol. Med., *49*:165, 1976.

Read, D. R., Hambrical, E., Abcarian, H., and Levine, H.: The preoperative diagnosis of hepatic metastases in cases of colorectal carcinoma. Dis. Col. Rect., *20*:101, 1977.

Safran, C., Desforges, J. F., Tsichlis, P. N., and Bluming, A. Z.: Decision analysis to evaluate lymphangiography in the management of patients with Hodgkin's disease. N. Engl. J. Med., *296*:1088, 1977.

Schwartz, W. B., Gorry, G. A., Kassirer, J. P., and Essig, A.: Decision analysis and clinical judgment. Am. J. Med., *55*:459, 1973.

Shapiro, S., Strax, P., and Venet, L.: Periodic breast cancer screening in reducing mortality from breast cancer. J.A.M.A., *215*:1777, 1971.

Sher, P. P.: Diagnostic effectiveness of biochemical liver-function tests as evaluated by discriminant function analysis. Clin. Chem., *23*:627, 1977.

Singer, F. R., Bethune, J. E., and Massry, S. G.: Hypercalcemia and hypocalcemia. Clin. Nephrol., *7*:154, 1977.

Sisson, J. C., Schoomaker, E. B., and Ross, J. C.: Clinical decision analysis. J.A.M.A., *236*:1259, 1976.

Sneath, P. H. A.: The application of computers to taxonomy. J. Gen. Microbiol., *17*:201, 1957.

Solberg, H. E., Skrede, S., and Blomhoff, J. P.: Diagnosis of liver disease by laboratory results and discriminant analysis: Identification of best combination of laboratory tests. Scand. J. Clin. Lab. Invest., *35*:713, 1975.

Starmer, C. F., and Lee, K. L.: A mathematical approach to medical decisions: Application of Bayes rule to a mixture of continuous and discrete clinical variates. Comput. Biomed. Res., *9*:531, 1976.

Vecchio, T. J., Predictive value of a single diagnostic test in unselected populations. N. Engl. J. Med., *274*:1171, 1966.

Wallerstein, R.: Role of the laboratory in the diagnosis of anemia. J.A.M.A., *236*:490, 1976.

Ward, P. C. J.: Chemical profiles of disease. Hum. Pathol., *4*:47, 1973.

Ward, P. C. J., Harris, I. B., Burke, M. D., and Horwitz, C. A.: An approach to systematic instruction in laboratory medicine. J. Med. Educ., *51*:648, 1976.

Warner, H. R., Toronto, A. F., Veasey, L. G., and Stephenson, R.: A mathematical approach to medical diagnosis. J.A.M.A., *177*:177, 1961.

Werner, M., Brooks, S. H., and Cohen, G.: Diagnostic effectiveness of electrophoresis and specific protein assays evaluated by discriminant analysis. Clin. Chem., *18*:116, 1972.

Winkel, P., Lyngborg, K., Olesen, K. H., Meibom, J., and Fritz Hansen, P.: A method for systematic assessment of the relative prognostic significance of symptoms and signs in patients with a chronic disease. Comput. Biomed. Res., *5*:576, 1972; *6*:457, 1973.

Winkel, P., Ramsoe, K., Lyngbye, J., and Tygstrup, N.: Diagnostic value of routine liver tests. Clin. Chem., *21*:71, 1975.

Winkel, P., Juhl, E., Tygstrup, N., & the Copenhagen Study Group for Liver Diseases (CSL): The clinical significance of classifications of cirrhosis. A comparison between conventional criteria and numerical taxonomy. Scand. J. Gastroenterol., *11*:33, 1976.

Winkel, P.: Patterns and clusters—Multivariate approach for interpreting clinical chemistry results. Clin. Chem., *19*:1329, 1973.

Winkel, P., and Statland, B. E.: Using the subject as his own referent in assessing day-to-day changes of laboratory test results. Contemp. Top. Analyt. Clin. Chem., *1*:287, 1977.

Zieve, L., and Hill, E.: An evaluation of factors influencing the discriminative effectiveness of a group of liver function tests. III. Relative effectiveness of hepatic tests in cirrhosis. Gastroenterology, *28*:785, 1955.

Zinsser, H., Bonner, R., Lemlich. A., and Roots, L.: Pyelonephritis: A study of a disease in depth. *In* Proceedings of the Fourth IBM Medical Symposium. New York, 1962.

Part 2

MEDICAL MICROSCOPY AND EXAMINATION OF OTHER BODY FLUIDS

Edited by John Bernard Henry, M.D.

17

EXAMINATION OF URINE

Mary Bradley, M.D.,
G. Berry Schumann, M.D.,
and Patrick C. J. Ward, M.D.

2

The urine specimen has been referred to as a liquid tissue biopsy of the urinary tract—painlessly obtained. It yields a great deal of information quickly and economically. Like any other laboratory procedure, urine tests need to be carefully performed and properly controlled.

The use of simple tests such as those for proteinuria, sugars, and the examination of the urinary sediment will provide the physician with helpful information concerning the diagnosis and management of renal disease, urinary tract disease, and many systemic diseases. With the introduction of simple techniques in which reagent strips and tablets are used, tests that previously required more complex chemical analysis may now be accomplished with ease. A physician should be able to perform the necessary screening tests himself and know how to interpret them in relation to the health and management of his patient.

Examination of the urine may be considered from two general standpoints—diagnosis and management of renal or urinary tract disease, and the detection of metabolic or systemic diseases not directly related to the kidney.

Among the most important conditions readily detected by chemical means are proteinuria, glycosuria, ketonuria, and the presence of the pigments bilirubin, urobilinogen, hemoglobin, and the porphyrins. The urine may also be screened for metabolites of drugs such as phenothiazines, abnormal amino acid metabolites, calcium, and other substances present in abnormal amounts or not normally present.

Proteinuria is probably the most common indication of renal disease. It is, for example, an early indication of latent glomerulonephritis, toxemia of pregnancy, and diabetic nephropathy. The finding of proteinuria may strongly suggest the presence of renal disease as opposed to lower urinary tract disease. When considered with the clinical findings, confirmation of the presence of renal disease can be made by finding casts in the microscopic examination of the urine sediment.

Microscopic examination of the sediment in a properly collected sample of urine may not only provide evidence of renal disease but also indicate the kind of lesion present or the state of activity of a known lesion. It should be included in every complete medical examination because it provides important information concerning the kidneys and urinary tract not readily obtainable in any other way. For a more detailed discussion of urinary findings in renal disease, the reader is referred to Lippman (1957) and Strauss (1971).

The usefulness of qualitative examination of urine has been discussed in detail by Free (1975), but has also been questioned in terms of cost and significant yield when it is used as a required screening procedure (Fraser, 1977).

COMPOSITION OF URINE

Nutritional status, the state of metabolic processes, and the ability of the kidney to handle selectively the material presented to it are three principal factors affecting the composition of the urine.

In the normal adult, about 1200 ml of blood passes through the kidney each minute, exposing the plasma to the semipermeable membrane of each functioning glomerulus. The ultrafiltrate that collects in Bowman's capsule contains all of the substances of the plasma capable of passing through the membrane. The pH of the filtrate (7.4) and its osmolality (about 285 mOsm/kg water) are the same as in plasma. Modification of this filtrate to produce excreted urine occurs in the tubules and collecting duct of the nephron. Glucose, amino acids, and other threshold substances are reabsorbed in the proximal tubules, leaving urea, uric acid, phosphates, and other materials in the filtrate. By the time the fluid reaches Henle's loop in the medulla, the original rate of flow of 130 ml/min has been reduced to about 16 ml/min because of the absorption of most of the water and electrolytes. In the distal tubule, more water may be absorbed and acidification of urine occurs. Further absorption of water may take place in the collecting duct. The filtrate is now reduced to a flow rate of about 1 ml/min, has a pH of about 6, and an osmolality of about 800 to 1200 mOsm/kg water. This is urine, and its formation is reviewed in more detail in Chapter 6.

Urine Solute. A large proportion of the urine solute is made up of urea and sodium chloride. On an ordinary diet of about 1 g of protein per kg, an average adult excretes in the urine about 10 g/day of nitrogen, most of which will be in the form of urea. Other substances, such as uric acid, creatinine, amino acids, ammonia, and traces of proteins, glycoproteins, enzymes, and purines, account for the remaining nitrogen excreted. There is a continuous excretion of uric acid, for example, even when purine intake is absent. Creatinine excretion is higher in children than in adults and higher in males than in females and is not related to dietary protein unless the intake is very high.

Excretions of sodium and chloride are directly related to dietary intake, principally from salt added to food. Since individual intake is quite variable, output may vary from about 5 to about 20 g as sodium chloride in a 24-hour period. Potassium is quite ubiquitous in the diet and is found in meats and vegetables. Normally about 70 mEq of potassium is excreted in a 24-hour period. Sulfate is excreted as inorganic sulfate, organic sulfate, and other sulfur-containing substances, such as sulfides, cysteine, and mercaptan. Urinary inorganic sulfate is derived from the metabolism of cystine and methionine and is thus related to protein intake. Organic sulfates are generally conjugates of steroids and phenols. Phosphate excretion is variable and is derived chiefly from nucleic acid in food, casein, and other organic and inorganic phosphates. About 1 g of phosphate is excreted as organic phosphate in 24 hours. Phosphate and sulfate are partly responsible for the acidity of urine.

Other than the nitrogenous material and salts already mentioned, normal urine contains small amounts of sugars, which, for example, like pentoses, will vary in amount with dietary intake. Intermediary metabolites, such as oxalic acid, citric acid, and pyruvate, are present. Free fatty acids and trace amounts of cholesterol are also found, as are trace amounts of metals.

Hormones such as the ketosteroids, estrogens, aldosterone and pituitary gonadotropins, and the biogenic amines—the catecholamines and serotonin metabolites—are normally found in urine and reflect metabolic and endocrine status. Vitamins such as ascorbic acid are excreted in the urine in amounts that depend on the sufficiency of dietary intake. While hemoglobin and heme pigments are not normally present, trace amounts of porphyrins and related compounds such as delta aminolevulinic acid are found.

Details on these values are available in the Biology Data Book, 1974.

In a concentrated normal urine, uric acid (at an acid pH) and phosphates (alkaline pH) will commonly crystallize out at room temperature and are, therefore, frequently found in routine examination of the urine. Urea and sodium chloride crystals are not seen, although these substances are present in high concentration.

Normal urine also contains "formed" elements—these are red blood cells and leukocytes, renal tubular epithelial cells, transitional epithelial cells, and squamous epithelial cells. The source of the erythrocytes and leukocytes is not known. Because of problems associated with the collection of random specimens and different methods of microscopic examination, there is no good agreement on reference values for routine evaluation. Quantitative counts have been done in 12 to 24 hour specimens (Addis, 1948; Prescott, 1965).

In general, the composition of the urine reflects the ability of the normal kidney to retain and reabsorb those substances essential to basic metabolism and homeostasis and to excrete the excess materials from the diet together with the end products of endocrine and metabolic processes.

Reference values for physical properties and cellular constituents of urine are shown in Appendix 1 (p. 2069).

Identification of Urine. Occasionally, following abdominal or pelvic surgery, drainage fluid is submitted to the laboratory for identification as urine. After centrifugation, the supernatant may be tested for urea, creatinine, sodium, and chloride. These levels are usually sufficiently concentrated in urine (even when diluted with wound site effusion) to separate probable urine from plasma or serous exudate.

Amniotic Fluid. Occasionally it is necessary to distinguish between maternal urine and fetal amniotic fluid. The pH of amniotic fluid is usually 7 or more, the specific gravity is usually high, and the protein level is significantly elevated (0.2 to 1.0 g/dl) compared with normal urine. Urea and creatinine levels in amniotic fluid are similar to blood levels, whereas the maternal urine will have high levels of these substances.

It should be noted that amniotic fluid constituents vary with the age of the fetus; in late pregnancy, with the addition of fetal urine, the level of urea and creatinine will be approximately two to three times the maternal blood level.

Protein and albumin decrease with fetal age from about 1/10 serum level to 1/20 near term (see Chap. 20 and Appendix 1).

COLLECTION OF URINE

There are certain important considerations to be borne in mind relative to the collection of urine specimens for examination. If these are followed, one is less apt to commit serious errors in the interpretation of results obtained.

Containers. Glass urine specimen bottles of about 6-oz. capacity are available. These should be washed with detergent and rinsed well with water and dried.

Disposable wax-coated paper specimen bottles and disposable plastic containers with lids are available in several sizes and are preferred by many for routine screening urinalysis. Conical containers are less likely to tip over.

A sterile kit for collection of urine for bacteriologic examination is available. It contains a disposable plastic bottle, detergent-impregnated pad, and dry pad. A sterile tray may be prepared for clean-voided specimens for hospital use. Sterile wrapped bedpans should always be available.

Pediatric urine collectors of clear pliable polyethylene are available for male and female infants. These are more comfortable than rigid tube containers. With these containers, an estimate of the volume excreted may be made. The bag may be folded and self-sealed for transportation. For a 24-hour collection, a tube is attached to the bag and can be connected to a collection bottle. Sterile and non-sterile plastic bags are available.

Large one-gallon glass jars with wide mouths and screw caps are used for 24-hour collections, usually with added preservative or refrigeration between voidings (Chap. 3, p. 59). Pliable plastic containers are also available and are less cumbersome for the patient. Bedpans used to collect voiding urine should be scrupulously clean.

Deterioration of Specimens. The urine sample must be collected in a clean, dry container and should be examined when freshly voided. Red blood cells and leukocytes, which may be present, are affected adversely and will eventually be destroyed by the hypotonicity of the urine. Casts also decompose in urine that has been allowed to stand for several hours. Bacterial contamination regularly occurs, resulting in alkalinization of the urine owing to the conversion of urea to ammonia and also in an increase in nitrite. pH will increase as CO_2 is lost. Occasionally pH will decrease. Bilirubin and urobilinogen will decrease, as will glucose and ketones. Turbidity develops, the color will change (usually darken), and the odor will eventually become offensive.

Collection of Urine for Screening Purposes. For *chemical* and *microscopic* examination, a voided specimen is usually suitable. If the specimen is likely to be contaminated by vaginal discharge or hemorrhage, a clean-voided specimen is collected. It may be necessary to pack the vagina or use a tampon in some cases, especially when examination of the urinary sediment is critical.

For most routine examinations, a fairly concentrated specimen is preferable to a dilute one. This is true of examinations for protein and also for the microscopic examination of the sediment. The concentration of solutes and formed elements in the urine varies throughout the patient's waking hours, depending upon his water intake. Ordinarily the first morning specimen of urine, voided on rising, is the most concentrated specimen, since the patient has not been drinking water during the hours of sleep. Therefore, this specimen is the best one to examine for nitrite and protein and the contents of the sediment. (An ambulatory person will excrete larger amounts of protein, but for comparison the night specimens are probably better.) Valuable information may also be gained from determinations of the volume and specific gravity of this specimen. On the other hand, the first morning specimen is not the best one to examine for glucose; this is best obtained after eating (postprandial). A randomly collected specimen is often more convenient for the patient and will be suitable for most screening purposes.

Storage. Random specimens should be examined fresh, or refrigerated and examined as soon as possible. Preservatives with refrigeration are occasionally useful for specimens that need to be saved (p. 59). One crystal of thymol/10 to 15 ml urine is useful; it will help preserve sediments but will interfere with the acid precipitation test for protein. Formalin (40 per cent v/v) 1 drop/10 ml urine will preserve sediments. Freezing is useful for bilirubin, urobilinogen, or ketones, but losses will still occur and irreversible turbidity may ensue.

Preservative tablets* for routine screening urinalysis (for transportation to insurance companies, for example) preserve glucose and other constituents by releasing formaldehyde; they also contain benzoate and mercury and have an acid reaction. One tablet is used with 30 ml urine. In this concentration formaldehyde will not react with the copper reduction test (tablet form). The specific gravity will be slightly increased (0.005/one tablet/30 ml).

Collection of Urine for Quantitative Analysis. A 24-hour specimen is collected for many assays; 2- to 12-hour timed collections are also made, e.g., for urobilinogen, xylose, Addis count.

Because substances like hormones, protein, and electrolytes are variably excreted during a 24-hour period, a better comparison of day-to-day values can be made with 24-hour collections than with random specimens (Schwartz,

---

*Metropolitan Preservative Tablet, Cargille.

1973). Errors in the results of quantitative urine tests are most often related to collection problems: loss of a voided specimen, too many voidings (usually the first voiding has not been discarded), poor preservation, or inadequate refrigeration. The adequacy of a 24-hour collection has been related to the creatinine excretion, which is fairly constant in an individual; however, this method for checking on the completion of a collection has been disputed (Edwards, 1969).

When possible, fluids should be moderately restricted during the 24-hour collection period and alcohol, certain foods, and drugs may need to be withheld. Specifications relating to each assay are available from central or reference laboratories for the more unusual substances to be tested.

Patients should be given *printed instructions* for the collection of timed specimens.

The patient is carefully instructed to empty his bladder at 8:00 A.M. (this presumably being before breakfast) and discard this urine. He collects all subsequent urine up to and including that at 8:00 A.M. the following morning. The total volume of this sample is measured and recorded and the urine thoroughly mixed before a measured sample is withdrawn for analysis.

Preservatives used for urine collections will depend on the substance to be tested and the method used (see Chap. 3, p. 59). Chemical preservatives usually act as antibacterial and anti-yeast agents. However, refrigeration or the acidification of urine is a preferable method.

All specimens should be refrigerated between voidings. Collections for protein and creatinine are satisfactory with refrigeration. Sodium fluoride and/or thymol have been used to preserve glucose. Thymol (antibacterial) crystals or thymol (10 per cent in isopropanol) 5 to 10 ml for a 24-hour collection, is generally acceptable and will interfere only with the acid precipitation test for proteins. Very large amounts (1 mg/ml) will interfere with the *o*-toluidine glucose test color. Sodium fluoride,* which inhibits cellular glycolysis, will inhibit the reagent strip test for glucose (if this is used for screening) but at low levels does not interfere with the hexokinase or other quantitative tests (Onstad, 1975). Approximately 0.5 g/gallon jar has been useful.

---

*Sodium fluoride. Urine preservative tablet. Cambridge Chemical Products.

Toluol and chloroform are usually not desirable. Toluol, to be effective, is layered on the surface and clings to pipettes; chloroform at greater than saturation levels will sink and may contaminate the sediment. For many hormones and other substances, boric acid 0.8 per cent or in tablet form has been found useful for mailing aliquots of urine to reference laboratories.

A very low pH (<3) will prevent bacterial growth and stabilize substances like catecholamines or VMA. For a pH of 1 to 2, 30 ml of 6N HCl (equal parts of concentrated HCl and water) is placed in a one gallon (3 to 4 liter) dark glass container and appropriately labeled. For amino acid assay, a pH of 3 is desirable. Before transporting or mailing aliquots of acidified urine specimens, a narrow range pH indicator paper should be used to check the pH.

Alkaline urine is preferred for porphyrins and urobilinogen. Porphyrins are stabilized by adding 5 g sodium bicarbonate to a 3 to 4 liter dark brown container before starting the collection. To retard oxidation, urobilinogen may be collected under a layer of petroleum ether in a dark bottle; it should be protected from light. Porphobilinogen and delta aminolevulinic acid are preserved by acidifying (pH < 7) and freezing.

Cells and casts for quantitation may be preserved by "rinsing" the empty container with formalin prior to use or by adding 10 ml of 40 per cent formalin to a one-gallon container.

Some labile materials require low temperatures for preservation, and some assay methods preclude the use of preservatives or acids. Frozen aliquots may be mailed in Styrofoam containers in Dry Ice. Freezing will also retard loss of urobilinogen and bilirubin, but not completely.

Thawing after freezing may reveal some turbidity that does not redissolve (possibly colloidal protein) and may cause assay problems. Freeze-drying is not as suitable for preservation as freezing for the recovery of certain hormones and other constituents in urine (Leach, 1975).

For *bacteriologic examination*, collection of a clean-voided midstream specimen is desirable; but catheterization or suprapubic aspiration of the bladder is sometimes necessary. Bacteriologic culture should be done immediately. When this is not possible, the urine should be refrigerated at 4°C. until cultured—for a period of not more than 12 hours as a rule, although specimens have been cultured without detriment after four days of adequate refrigeration (Ryan, 1963).

In the male the glans should be exposed adequately, thoroughly cleaned with a mild antiseptic solution, and dried. The midstream urine should be collected in a sterile container after the initial flow has been allowed to escape.

The female patient should be instructed to kneel or squat over a bedpan or to stand astride a toilet bowl. Using sterile gloves, the nurse should separate the labia minora widely to expose the urethral orifice and to keep the labia separated throughout the procedure. With sterile, soapy cotton balls, cleanse on each side of urinary meatus; then cleanse the meatus. Rinse the cleansed area with sterile, water-saturated cotton balls. Instruct the patient to void forcibly, and allow the initial stream of urine to drain into the bedpan or toilet, continuing to keep the labia separated. Catch the subsequent midstream specimen in a sterile container, and do not touch any portion of perineum with the container. About 30 to 100 ml of urine should be collected. After obtaining the urine specimen, allow the labia to close. The patient then continues to void into the bedpan or toilet.

QUALITY CONTROL

Precision and accuracy are essential elements in the conduct of any test. Difficulties arise in the implementation of quality control programs in urinalysis because of the subjective or qualitative nature of many of the tests. This is especially true of the microscopic sediment examination (Winkel, 1974). As seen in other areas of the clinical laboratory, the best results are obtained from better qualified personnel who are performing tests on a regular basis (Free, 1973b). Surveys have revealed large numbers of false negative results and some false positive results when poorly trained personnel are assigned the task of routine urinalysis (Simpson, 1977). With adequate training, improvement in test results will be seen (Becker, 1973). With the implementation of quality control programs and the proper selection of test methods, results should be comparable to those expected in other areas of clinical chemistry (Assa, 1977).

Urinalysis Controls. Urinalysis controls

are used as a check on urinalysis reagents and procedures, and as a means of evaluating the laboratory personnel's ability to perform tests correctly and to interpret the results.

Controls are used to monitor reagent strip tests *daily* and all qualitative wet chemical tests. Where possible, both positive and negative controls should be used. For some procedures, e.g., Bence Jones protein, known positive urine samples can be saved and refrigerated for use as controls. Samples of urobilinogen and porphobilinogen should be kept frozen and in the dark. In other tests, e.g., for cystine, sugars, and calculi, known chemical solutions are used as positive controls. In addition to chemical tests, it is important to check *daily* the calibration of specific gravity instruments—urinometer or refractometer. Other equipment used in the laboratory should be routinely checked, including refrigerator-freezer temperatures, centrifuge speed, balance, spectrophotometer (daily check), etc.

All reagents should be properly labeled, dated, and stored. Lot numbers and expiration dates for reagent strips are recorded and periodically checked for outdating, e.g., monthly for infrequently used tests.

Precautions in Use of Reagent Strips. Protect reagent strips from moisture and excessive heat to prevent loss of sensitivity. Discoloration may indicate significant loss of reactivity; reagent strips with such discoloration should not be used. This also applies to test tablets. Store strips in a cool, dry area but not in a refrigerator. Remove only enough strips for immediate use, and recap tightly immediately. Urine should be at room temperature when tested with reagent strips.

Avoid contamination of reagent strip. Do not touch test areas with fingers. Do not lay reagent strip on table surface—use clean sheet of paper. Do not use strips in the presence of volatile acid or alkaline fumes.

Properly moisten reagent strip in well-mixed urine when testing specimen. Avoid incomplete dipping; all test areas must be completely moistened. Avoid prolonged dipping; excessive dipping may cause leaching of test reagents.

Exercise care in reading reagent strips. Observe time elements indicated in the directions for their use. Hold the reagent strip close to the appropriate color chart when reading. Read only under good lighting conditions.

Table 17–1. QUALITY CONTROL REAGENTS

REAGENT	LOW CONTROL		HIGH CONTROL	
	1 liter	concn.	1 liter	concn.
Sodium chloride AR	5.0 g	500 mg/dl	10.0 g	1000 mg/dl
Urea AR	5.0 g	500 mg/dl	10.0 g	1000 mg/dl
Creatinine AR	0.5 g	50 mg/dl	0.5 g	50 mg/dl
Glucose AR	3.0 g	300 mg/dl	15.0 g	1500 mg/dl
30% Bovine albumin	5.0 ml	150 mg/dl	35 ml	1050 mg/dl
Whole normal blood (with Hct. 40-45) (Hbg. 13-15 g/dl)	100 μl	1.3-1.5 mg/dl	–	–
Acetone AR	–	–	2 ml	160 mg/dl
Chloroform AR	5 ml	0.5 ml/dl	5 ml	0.5 mg/dl
Distilled water qs	to 1 liter		to 1 liter	

QUALITY CONTROL RAGENTS FOR ROUTINE URINALYSIS

Lyophilized, tablet, or liquid control preparations are available with varying concentrations of the constituents sought in routine urinalysis. Among these are Kova-Trol (ICL Scientific), QC-U (General Diagnostics), Tek-Chek (Ames), and Urintrol (Harleco). These should be reconstituted with the appropriate diluent as directed. Special attention should be given to storage time, temperature, and expiration dates. Controls for sediment examination with stabilized red cells and particles simulating leukocytes in size need to be properly mixed before use.

The solutions in Table 17–1 have the advantage of being considerably less expensive than commercially available preparations.

To facilitate dissolution, pulverize all dry reagents with a mortar and pestle. Dilute to volume with distilled water. Store controls in stock bottle at room temperature. Remove 50 to 100 ml aliquots periodically to working control bottle. Solutions are stable for six to nine months.

Chloroform is used as a preservative and allows the reagent to be at room temperature. It should be noted that chloroform may interfere with the specific gravity test, which uses the falling drop method (Clinilab[a]). Since chloroform is hepatotoxic, another suitable preservative may be substituted, or vials may be frozen and stored without preservative.

Expected Result

Low Control. Multiple Reagent strip[a]: pH 6, protein 2+, glucose +, ketone neg., blood sm. to mod. protein ppt. 2+, Benedict's 1+, Clinitest[a] trace, Tes-tape[b] 2+, Acetest[a] neg., specific gravity 1.006, osmolality 305 mOsm/kg water.

High Control. Multiple Reagent Strip: pH 6,

protein 4+, glucose + + +, ketone small, blood neg., protein ppt. 3-4+, Benedict's 3+, Clinitest 3+, Tes-tape 3+, Acetest small, specific gravity 1.020, osmolality 660 mOsm/kg water.

Bilirubin and urobilinogen are negative for each control.

Negative Control. A salt solution containing sodium chloride and urea in distilled water is used as a negative control.

Note. For teaching purposes, solutions may be made in advance (without chloroform) with varying amounts of reactants, frozen in 10 ml amounts, and stored. Bile or bilirubin may be added. A positive Erhlich's reaction is possible with p' aminosalicylic acid.

Normal hepatitis-free plasma may be substituted for bovine albumin in an appropriate concentration. It is important to include creatinine to obtain good copper reduction test results (Benedict's test). Food coloring may be added to simulate the color of urine. Specimens should be thoroughly thawed before use.

When to use controls

Check all previously opened bottles of reagent strips daily.

Check each new bottle upon opening and record lot number.

New personnel should run reagent strip controls (and confirmatory tests) and check results with a supervisor. It is also useful to have part-time or night staff who do these tests infrequently check controls periodically.

Controls (positive and negative) are run with all qualitative tests whenever feasible.

When new reagents are made, positive and neg-

---

[a] Ames Company, Elkhart, Ind.
[b] Lilly Company, Indianapolis, Ind.
[c] Bio-Dynamics/bmc, Indianapolis, Ind.
Superscripts a, b, and c throughout the chapter refer to these companies.

ative controls are performed—indicate check on bottle label.

Daily procedure

Positive and negative control solutions are treated as routine urine specimens:

Measure specific gravity.

Test with a multiple reagent strip (or routine test strips) and record results.

Do an acid precipitation test for protein. Record results.

Do a copper reduction test and record results.

If the control used has red cells or "leukocytes," centrifuge and examine the sediment—unstained and stained.

Records

Record daily test results of positive and negative "routine" controls.

Record daily results of urinometer or refractometer check.

Record results of new reagent strips (with lot numbers and expiration dates).

Record disposition of outdated reagent strips and tablets.

Separate records or charts may be used for other equipment or instruments.

Proficiency testing

All laboratories (office, clinic, hospital, etc.) should participate in proficiency testing programs. The small cost involved is more than compensated by the experience and benefit gained (Free, 1973b).

Each laboratory will have to establish its own acceptable range of performance. This is difficult when so much of routine urinalysis involves subjective interpretation of colors, precipitates, or microscopic elements (Becker, 1973). Even in the best hands, there may be as much as ±1 color block difference in the interpretation of positive reagent strip results. However, in most instances one should not expect clearly negative specimens to be called positive or a positive result negative. Laboratory supervisors may wish to introduce positive and negative controls with the daily work load as unknown routine specimens.

Each person should be aware of the principle involved in each test, its sensitivity and specificity, the necessity for quality specimens, the likelihood of interference, and the patterns of expected results for common diseases. This awareness will ensure quality control in the urinalysis laboratory.

PROCEDURE FOR ROUTINE SCREENING URINALYSIS

Before any tests are performed, a quality control check should be made as described on page 565.

The Urine Specimen. The volume of urine necessary depends on the number of tests to be performed. As little as 2 ml will suffice; however, 15 ml or more is preferable for routine work (see below).

Specimens must be refrigerated if not examined immediately, but should be brought to room temperature before using enzymatic reagent strips. All specimens should be free from fecal and vaginal contamination.

Screening for Bacteriuria. If only one specimen is available for complete urinalysis, screening for bacteriuria should be done first. Alternative procedures include a Gram's stain of the uncentrifuged, well-mixed specimen and the quantitative loop culture method or a miniculture method, all of which require a drop or two of urine.

Specific Gravity. At this point, a drop may be used for refractometer estimation of specific gravity.

Chemical Screening (Basic). Using multiple reagent strips, dip and read for all or some of the following:*

pH	blood
protein	bilirubin
glucose	urobilinogen
ketone	nitrite

If a multiple reagent strip is not used, Ictotest[a], a tablet test for bilirubin, is simple, more sensitive, and easier to interpret. The use of reagent strips makes it more certain that tests will be done because of the ease of operation.

Test for Copper-reducing Substances. It is most important that this test be performed on all specimens from infants by either Benedict's or the Clinitest[a] tablet method.

At this point, the specimen should be centrifuged in a disposable centrifuge tube, and the clear supernatant separated from the sediment and refrigerated.

The Sediment. A drop of the concentrated sediment is examined under a coverslip for red

---

*Any positive reaction for protein or glucose should be confirmed with a method that employs a different principle.

blood cells, leukocytes, renal epithelial cells, casts, and excessive numbers of crystals. These are usually graded as to number of cells in an average of 10 high-power fields.

Alternatively, the uncentrifuged, well-mixed specimen may be examined in a counting chamber and reported as cells per cubic millimeter.

The Supernatant. The supernatant is used for the following tests:

1. A confirmatory protein test, Bence Jones test, and electrophoresis.
2. Separation of sugars carried out by chromatography when a copper reduction test is positive and the glucose oxidase test is negative.
3. Check for ascorbic acid when erythrocytes are present and the reagent strip test for blood is negative.
4. Confirmation of cystine crystals by a qualitative test.

The Result. Before any specimen is discarded, the entire report should be examined to determine whether the sediment results match the chemical screen and whether all abnormal findings have been followed up through appropriate confirmation.

Volume Needed. More than 10 ml is required for routine urinalysis. However, most tests can be accomplished on a smaller volume when necessary. For volumes between 3 and 10 ml, for example, a multiple reagent strip test, specific gravity (refractometer), copper reducing substances (2 to 5 drops), bilirubin (tablet), and dilution for "large" ketones are possible. Then either 2.5 ml is centrifuged to produce a 0.25 ml sediment or 5 ml is centrifuged to produce 0.5 ml for sediment examination. When the volume is less than 2.5 ml, usually a multiple reagent strip, specific gravity, copper reducing test, and bilirubin test are feasible. The urine may be examined microscopically and the findings reported as uncentrifuged. Occasionally volumes of 0.5 ml or less are tested for specific constituents at the request of the physician.

CLINICAL CORRELATION OF ROUTINE SCREENING URINALYSIS

Some of the most common findings are summarized here, with some practical comments regarding the tests. Details of each determination are presented later in this chapter.

Appearance. Cloudy urine, due to phosphates (alkaline) or urates (acid), is usually normal. Occasionally, cloudiness is due to blood (pink, red, or brown), leukocytes, and mucus. Dark amber usually represents normal concentrated urine, but may indicate the presence of urobilin or conjugated bilirubin. Bright orange urine is seen when azo dye compounds are given therapeutically, and bright yellow with riboflavin.

Specific Gravity (SG). This correlates roughly with osmolality. Concentrated urine is seen with dehydration; high specific gravity is recorded with x-ray dye (>1.035), with high concentration of glucose, and to a lesser extent with protein. Dilute urine is present with high fluid intake and when the kidney is unable to concentrate urine owing to kidney disease. Polyuria (excretion of too much urine, e.g., 2.5 liters or greater per day) occurs with diabetes insipidus and with diabetes mellitus; the urine in diabetes mellitus is pale but has a high SG when much glucose is excreted (osmotic diuresis).

NOTE. A very dilute urine may negate findings of proteinuria or lower the bacterial count on culture, i.e., produce false negative results.

pH. A very alkaline pH usually indicates a stale ammoniacal specimen not worth testing. Ammonia is produced by urea splitting bacteria, and this is confirmed by the nose test. The pH of the urine indicates the acid-base status: acidosis (starvation diets, severe diarrhea, diabetes mellitus, and respiratory disease) and alkalosis (excess alkali, severe vomiting, respiratory hyperventilation). However, a urinary tract infection associated with urea-splitting organisms, e.g., *Proteus* or *Pseudomonas*, may also cause an alkaline urine. Paradoxical aciduria (less than pH 7) occurs in potassium-depleted, chloride-depleted alkalosis.

NOTE. The pH is very helpful in identifying crystals in urine.

Protein. Proteinuria is indicative of renal disease. Indeed, it is probably the single most sensitive indicator of renal disease, and quantitative measurement often correlates with severity of renal disease. Large amounts are lost in urine in the nephrotic syndrome. Small amounts accompany hematuria and acute urinary tract infection. With chronic renal disease, proteinuria may be intermittent. More protein is excreted by ambulatory persons than by those in bed. The greater relative sensitivity of reagent strips to albumin than to globulin or Bence Jones protein is noteworthy. Normally, small amounts of protein are excreted and may show as a trace result in a concentrated specimen; conversely, proteinuria may be missed in a dilute specimen.

Glucose. Reagent strip tests are specific for glucose. Although glucose appears in urine in diabetes mellitus, it is not a sensitive test for detection of diabetes mellitus. In renal glucosuria, in which there is a low renal threshold, glucose loss is most commonly due to an inherited, isolated proximal tubular defect and is harmless, or it may be associated with diseases of the proximal tubule. Glucosuria is occasionally seen with rapid intestinal absorption and massive glucose intake.

NOTE. The glucose oxidase enzyme test may be inhibited or delayed by large amounts of ascorbic acid. The same ascorbic acid will give a positive copper reduction test, adding to the confusion. Reducing sugars other than glucose may be present when the copper reduction test is positive and the glucose oxidase test negative, e.g., with galactosemia or lactosuria. The glucose oxidase test is more sensitive to glucose than the reduction test.

Ketones. Ketonuria occurs with starvation, weight reducing diets, and often in febrile children not eating. It is also found with diabetes mellitus. A tablet or powder reagent is also used on serum or plasma to estimate ketonemia semiquantitatively in diabetic acidosis; drops of serum are diluted, if necessary, with drops of water, and the degree of dilution for a given result will indicate the severity of or quantity of ketones in the ketosis.

Blood. Hematuria is relatively common, hemoglobinuria uncommon, and myoglobinuria rare. Any pink, red, or brown urine is bloody until proven otherwise. When casts are present with significant proteinuria, the red cells are probably emanating from the kidney and associated with diseases such as acute glomerulonephritis or lupus nephritis. Red cells and smaller amounts of protein are seen with lower urinary tract bleeding and inflammation.

Glomerulitis associated with several renal diseases (e.g., lupus erythematosus, polyarteritis nodosa, malignant hypertension, subacute bacterial endocarditis, glomerulonephritis, etc.) may yield hematuria of renal rather than lower urinary tract origin. Hemoglobinuria reflects intravascular hemolysis. Urine specific gravity of 1.010 or higher is necessary to preclude lysis of erythrocytes in hematuria, which might otherwise be misinterpreted as hemoglobinuria.

NOTE. The reagent strip test is inhibited by ascorbic acid, so that a test for blood may be negative while the sediment reveals many red cells. This finding underscores the importance of the sediment examination.

Bilirubin. The urine may be dark with yellow foam if much bilirubin is present. Bilirubin in urine is in the conjugated form and is seen when there is obstruction to the outflow of bile, either extrahepatic or intrahepatic. It may stain sediment elements.

Urobilinogen. Excessive urobilinogen appears in hemolytic states and in some liver diseases. It will not show a colored foam. The combination of tests for urinary bilirubin and urobilinogen helps separate obstructive jaundice from jaundice associated with hemolytic anemia.

Nitrite. Bacteria will convert normal urinary nitrite in bladder urine, provided there is sufficient incubation time. A first morning specimen is, therefore, required for an indication of significant bacteriuria. False negative results may occur.

Urinary Sediment. Examination of the urinary sediment is an essential part of the routine urinalysis (see Tables 17-15 (p. 613) and 17-16 (p. 615)).

REAGENT STRIP METHODOLOGY

Since reagent strips and multiple reagent strips are so commonly used, their chemical reactants, sensitivities, and specificities are summarized below, followed by similar data for the most commonly used additional or confirmatory tests. It should be noted that reagent strip methods are changed periodically, sensitivities and color reactions altered, and new tests added. Manufacturers supply tables of common interfering substances and these should be consulted. In practice, ascorbic acid and drugs producing colored urines like phenazopyridine (Pyridium), other azo compounds, and those containing methylene blue are most frequently encountered. More detailed information on drug interference is listed in Hansten (1975) and Young (1975). For a comparison of multitest reagent strips, see Smith (1977).

pH

CHEMISTRY. Indicators impregnated with methyl red and bromthymol blue (and phenolphthalein[c]).

SENSITIVITY. Permits differentiation of pH values to half a unit within the range 5 to 9. Should be read immediately.

SPECIFICITY. pH is not affected by the urinary buffer concentration. Bacterial growth in a specimen may cause a marked alkaline shift and render it unsuitable for testing, usually because of urea conversion to ammonia.

Protein. Based on "protein error of pH indicators."

CHEMISTRY. Impregnated with tetrabromphenol blue[a] buffered to an acid pH of 3. (Chemstrip[c] has tetrachlorophenol and tetrabromsulfophthalein). This area is yellow in the absence of protein but, at the same pH, changes to a shade of green depending on type and concentration of protein present.

SENSITIVITY. Five to 20 mg of albumin/dl of urine may be detected. The test area is more sensitive to albumin than to globulin, Bence Jones protein, or mucoprotein. High salt levels will lower results. Read at 30 to 60 seconds.

SPECIFICITY. Although buffered adequately for most urines, exceptionally alkaline and/or highly buffered urines may give positive results in the absence of significant proteinuria, e.g., with patients on alkaline medication, bacterial contamination, contamination of specimen container, stale urine. The test is unaffected by urine turbidity, x-ray contrast media, most drugs or their metabolites, or urine preservatives which occasionally affect other protein tests, such as thymol. False positive results occur with quaternary ammonium compounds.

Glucose. Glucose oxidase/peroxidase method—a double sequential enzyme reaction. Reagent strips differ in the chromogen used.

CHEMISTRY.

$$\text{glucose} + O_2 \xrightarrow{\text{glucose oxidase}} \text{gluconic acid} + H_2O_2$$

$$H_2O_2 + \text{chromogen} \xrightarrow{\text{peroxidase}} \text{oxidized chromogen} + H_2O$$

Older Formulation Reagent Strip[a]—*o*-tolidine. Color changes from pink to purple.

N-Multistix[a]—potassium iodide chromogen. Color changes from blue to brown.

Chemstrip[c*]—*o*-tolidine. Color changes from yellow to green.

Tes-Tape[b]—*o*-tolidine. Color changes from yellow to blue.

SENSITIVITY. Older Formulation Reagent Strips—approximately 100 mg/dl urine is detectable. Report as positive or negative at 10 seconds. Sensitivity is decreased by inhibiting substances, homogentisic acid, massive doses of aspirin, or a large urinary concentration of ascorbic acid from therapeutic doses of vitamin C or from parenteral solutions using it as a stabilizing agent. A delayed positive may be seen with ascorbic acid. Tes-Tape—report as positive or negative at 30 seconds.

N-Multistix—50 to 100 mg/dl urine is detectable. Report as positive or negative at 10 seconds and semiquantitate at 30 seconds up to 2 g/dl, eliminating the need for a second confirmatory test on *adults*, unless moderate or large numbers of ketones are present. If so, confirm with Clinitest[a]. High specific gravity will decrease sensitivity. Large amounts of ketone bodies may decrease color development, but this test is less affected by ascorbic acid than the above test.

Chemstrip*—40 mg/dl urine is detectable. Report as positive or negative at 30 to 60 seconds. Sensitivity is influenced by large amounts of ascorbic acid.

SPECIFICITY. The test is specific for glucose; it does not react with lactose, galactose, fructose, or reducing metabolites of drugs. False positive readings may be produced by strongly oxidizing cleaning agents in the urine container.

Ketones. Based on a nitroprusside (sodium nitroferricyanide) reaction.

CHEMISTRY. Impregnated with sodium nitroferricyanide, glycine, and buffer. Sodium nitroferricyanide and glycine react with acetoacetic acid in an alkaline medium to form a violet dye. A positive result is indicated by a color change from beige to violet. The sensitivity and reaction of the reagent strip is similar to that of the tablet (Acetest[a]).

Chemstrip[c]—read at 60 seconds. N-Multistix[a]—read at 15 seconds.

SENSITIVITY. The reagent area detects 5 to 10 mg acetoacetic acid/dl of urine. It is much less sensitive to acetone and does not react with beta-hydroxybutyric acid. With large or 3+ results, urine may be diluted and retested.

SPECIFICITY. This test reacts with acetoacetic acid and acetone in urine. Color reactions (false positives) may be obtained from patients after phthaleins (B.S.P. or P.S.P.) or in the presence of extremely large amounts of phenylketones, and the preservative 8-hydroxyquinoline, or L-dopa metabolites. Acetylcysteine (aerosol) produces a strong red color.

Blood. Based on the liberation of oxygen from peroxide by the peroxidase-like activity of heme from free hemoglobin or lysed red cells in well-mixed urine.

---

*New formulation with semi-quantitation available late 1978.

CHEMISTRY. Impregnated with a buffered mixture of organic peroxide and *o*-tolidine.

$$H_2O_2 + chromogen \xrightarrow[\substack{peroxidase \\ activity}]{hemoglobin}$$

oxidized chromogen + H_2O
(highly colored)

Heme catalyzes the oxidation of *o*-tolidine, producing a blue color. With Chemstrip[c] the test zone is yellow in the absence of blood and green in the presence of blood. Timing is important.

SENSITIVITY. The test is sensitive to hemoglobin and myoglobin but less so to intact erythrocytes. It complements the microscopic examination for red cells. False negative readings may be obtained in the presence of high urinary concentrations of ascorbic acid or with formaldehyde. Large amounts of nitrite may delay reactions. Sensitivity is reduced in urines with high specific gravity.

Old formulation[a] detects 0.1 mg/dl urine. N-Multistix[a] and Chemstrip[c] detect 0.05 to 0.3 mg hemoglobin/dl urine. Read at 30 and 60 seconds, respectively. Sensitivity decreases with age of the reagent strip. Sensitivities shown are those seen in practice. Note that 0.3 mg hemoglobin/dl is equivalent to that from 10 lysed red blood cells per μl. These are assumed to be normal erythrocytes containing approximately 30 picograms of hemoglobin per cell.

SPECIFICITY. Hemoglobin, myoglobin, and erythrocytes give a positive reaction; however, certain oxidizing contaminants such as hypochlorites may produce a false positive result, e.g., when bleach is used for cleaning bed pans or urinals.

Bilirubin. Based on a diazo reaction. Tests differ in the diazonium salt used. Urine must be fresh.

CHEMISTRY. Reaction is based on the coupling reaction of bilirubin with a diazonium salt in an acid medium.

N-Multistix[a]—diazotized 2,4-dichloroaniline. Color changes from buff to tannish purple; with older formulas, yellow to brown. Read at 20 seconds.

Chemstrip[c] — 2,6-dichlorobenzene-diazonium tetrafluoroborate. Color changes from buff to tan. Read at 30 to 60 seconds.

SENSITIVITY. With N-Multistix the reagent detects 0.2 to 0.4 mg/dl urine. Chemstrip detects 0.5 mg/dl urine. Large amounts of ascorbic acid and nitrite (in urinary tract infections) may lower bilirubin results.

SPECIFICITY. False positive reactions may occur with urine from patients receiving very large doses of chlorpromazine. Metabolites of drugs such as phenazopyridine may give a reddish color and mask the result.

Urobilinogen. Based on the Ehrlich aldehyde reaction or the formation of a red azo dye. Urine must be fresh.

CHEMISTRY. N-Multistix[a]—impregnated with *p*-dimethyl-amino-benzaldehyde, which produces a reddish brown color with urobilinogen. The test is read in Ehrlich units/dl. Color varies from light yellow to shades of brown. Color blocks representing 0.1 to 12 Ehrlich units/dl are provided.

Chemstrip[c]—impregnated with 4-methoxybenzene-diazonium-tetrafluoroborate, which couples with urobilinogen in an acid medium to form a red azo dye. Values are read at 10 to 30 seconds.

SENSITIVITY. N-Multistix—will detect urobilinogen in concentrations of approximately 0.1 Ehrlich unit/dl urine. Normally 1 U/dl may be present.

Chemstrip—detects approximately 0.4 mg/dl. Values up to 1 mg/dl are considered normal. Nitrite or formalin may reduce the color reaction. Urobilinogen is very labile in an acid urine and with light; a negative result is not significant.

SPECIFICITY. N-Multistix—not specific for urobilinogen. The test area will react with the substances known to react with the Ehrlich's reagent in the Watson-Schwartz method of urobilinogen assay. These substances include porphobilinogen, sulfisoxazole, and *p*-aminosalicylic acid. Indole will also react. Azo compounds may cause a golden color.

Chemstrip—urine from patients receiving phenazopyridine may show a false positive reaction.

Bilirubin may occasionally cause a green color.

Nitrite. Azo dye formed from nitrite.

CHEMISTRY. The test depends upon the conversion of nitrate to nitrite by certain bacterial action in the urine. The test requires an overnight (minimum of four hours) bladder bacterial population to convert urinary nitrate to nitrite; a first morning specimen is best. At an acid pH, nitrite, if present, reacts with *p*-arsanilic acid to give a diazonium salt, which by coupling with N-(1-naphthyl) ethylenediamine forms a pink-violet azo dye, specific for nitrite.

SENSITIVITY. N-Multistix[a]—detects 0.075

mg of nitrite/dl in solution. High ascorbic acid levels and high specific gravity reduce sensitivity. Read at 30 seconds.

Chemstrip[c]—detects 0.05 mg of nitrite/dl. Read at 30 seconds.

SPECIFICITY. False positive readings may be produced by medication that colors the urine red or turns red in an acid medium (e.g., phenazopyridine). Bacterial growth in an "old" specimen may give a false positive result. A negative result does not rule out significant bacteriuria.

CONFIRMATORY TESTS

Protein. Sulfosalicylic acid. Used to confirm reagent strip; when globulin is suspected; with colored or alkaline urine. May be used as a primary test (see p. 604).

CHEMISTRY. Acid precipitation of protein.

SENSITIVITY. 5 to 10 mg of protein/dl of urine.

SPECIFICITY. Specific for albumin, globulins, glucoproteins, and Bence Jones protein. May give false positive results with compounds used for diagnostic radiographic procedures when a contrast dye is present; specific gravity is usually over 1.035 and precipitate will increase upon standing.

Glucose. Clinitest[a]—used when reagent strip for glucose is positive in the presence of moderate or large amount of ketones and for pediatric specimens, for some diabetics with marked glucosuria, and for patients on parenteral nutrition with fructose. Benedict's qualitative test is not as convenient but may be preferred. (see p. 590).

CHEMISTRY. Sugars reduce cupric to cuprous oxide (red).

SENSITIVITY. $\simeq 0.25$ g glucose/dl urine.

5-drop test—color blocks range from 0.25 g per cent (trace) to 2 g per cent (4+ orange). Greater than 2 g per dl may cause reversion of color.

2-drop test—color blocks range from trace (green) to 5 g per cent (orange-brown). See page 589 for details of 2- and 5-drop tests.

SPECIFICITY. Not specific for glucose and will react with sufficient quantities of any reducing substance, e.g., non-glucose reducing sugars—fructose, pentose, lactose, galactose; non-sugar reducing substances—creatinine, uric acid. Large amount of ascorbic acid may cause false positive results. Tablets deteriorate rapidly with moisture or heat.

Bilirubin. Ictotest[a] (diazo reaction) tablet test is easier to read and more sensitive than the reagent strip tests. Useful when reagent strip has questionable result. The tablet test is useful in early hepatitis detection before jaundice appears (see p. 584).

Blood. Check for presence of *ascorbic acid* with C-Stix[a] if microscopic analysis shows 1+ or more erythrocytes and result of reagent strip is negative. See chemistry and specificity of test for ascorbic acid (p. 583).

Urobilinogen. Watson-Schwartz test. When the Ehrlich aldehyde reagent strip is positive or inconclusive, the test will separate urobilinogen and other reactive substances. For chemistry and specificity, see procedure for urobilinogen and porphobilinogen (p. 608).

AUTOMATED REAGENT STRIP METHOD

An *automated* system, Clinilab[a] measures specific gravity and six reagent strip tests—pH, protein, glucose, ketones, bilirubin, and blood.

The specific gravity is measured by a falling drop method and is related to the time it takes for a drop of urine to pass between two sets of photo cells; the high specific gravity (heavier) drop falls more quickly than a low specific gravity drop. The reagent strip tests are similar to those in common use.

Urine is automatically aspirated and deposited as drops for specific gravity measurement and then on each reagent strip. The strips issue automatically from a cassette, each reel having the capacity for 400 tests. Colors are read by reflectance, and the results are printed out. The instrument can be interfaced with a computer system.

The system is useful for high volume laboratories, and with strict attention to cleaning, especially of the specific gravity module, performance is satisfactory.

The advantages of the instrument are its speed and objectivity (Wert, 1973). It is possible, although not necessary, to centrifuge a second, properly labeled tube of a specimen and have sediments prepared while the chemistry screening is being done automatically. The original "automated" tube is available for any indicated additional tests after the routine examination is completed. A rapid flow of work and faster reporting is then possible.

Calibration is made daily with standard high and low content solutions.

Controls are used daily. These are Tek-Chek[a]

and QC-U (General Diagnostics) or other suitable control solutions.

Bloody or colored specimens are not satisfactory and should be tested by hand; otherwise false positive results will be recorded owing to pigmentation of the reagent areas.

Specific gravity measurements of 1.035 or more are duplicated and checked with a refractometer.

A *semi-automated* instrument, Clini-Tek,[a] is available to read out hand-dipped reagent strips. Color changes are read by reflectance, the amount of light reflected being inversely related to the depth of the color reaction and, in turn, to the concentration of substance being measured. Results are displayed on a display panel.

The instrument is calibrated with a reference strip. The tests performed are the same as those on the multiple reagent strip and include pH, protein, glucose, ketone, bilirubin, blood, nitrite, and urobilinogen.

Controls are similar to those used daily for manual reading. Positive (high and low) and negative controls should be used.

Intensely colored urine specimens may cause false positive results. With these specimens color reactions should be estimated visually.

The advantages of the instrument are those of reproducibility between operators (Peele, 1977).

URINARY SCREENING FOR INBORN ERRORS

Urine has been used for many years to screen for metabolic diseases, including those determined by genetic inheritance. In these diseases an abnormal metabolite or a larger than normal amount of a normal metabolite is often excreted in the urine, although the kidney itself is not always involved. Many of these diseases are associated with mental deficiency, degeneration of the nervous system, and "failure to thrive." Early detection is useful in galactosemia, for example, and may be helpful in other diseases and for genetic counseling. Amniotic fluid testing is available for many of the same diseases. Very careful laboratory and clinical interpretation of screening tests is required because of the number of false positives, e.g., transient tyrosinuria of the newborn. On the other hand, false negative results will occur if the newborn has not

had several days to ingest appropriate food or because urine is not the best test material for testing; e.g., in phenylketonuria blood tests are preferable for screening purposes. Mass screening will provide a very low yield; screening of infants at risk and those with slow development will provide higher levels of positive results.

Because of the rarity of these disorders, testing is best performed by state or regional public health laboratories. Newborn filter-paper blood specimens are used to screen for phenylketonuria, galactosemia, homocystinuria, maple syrup urine disease, and hypothyroidism. Urine specimens may be tested at three to four weeks of age to follow-up phenylketonuria or for other amino acid disorders (Bennett, 1977).

Genetic disease of the kidney is uncommon, and many patients are diagnosed from history and clinical findings; however, in some instances urinary screening may indicate the presence of a specific disease. Functional genetic abnormalities are usually associated with a transport defect of proximal renal tubular epithelial cell, including renal glucosuria, cystinuria, and the Fanconi syndrome. Polyuria and low specific gravity are found in vasopressin-resistant diabetes insipidus. Urinary pH measurement is helpful in diagnosis of distal renal tubular acidosis. With structural abnormalities such as polycystic disease and various genetic nephrites, proteinuria, hematuria, increased leukocytes, and renal epithelial cells are found. Frequently there is a urinary tract infection associated with a structural defect in the urinary tract. Urinary findings associated with genetic disease of the kidney may appear on a careful routine examination. For other metabolic diseases, additional screening tests are needed.

A laboratory offering these screening procedures should have the capability of further investigation or access to a reference laboratory. Amino acids can be separated by chromatography and if necessary later quantitated. Sugars can be separated by thin-layer chromatography after a positive copper reduction and negative glucose oxidase test are found.

Specimen Requirements.   About 20 ml of a fresh or refrigerated specimen is required. In older children a concentrated specimen is usually available. The following tests are simple screening procedures:

1. Copper reduction test for sugars (p. 588).

2. Cyanide-nitroprusside test for cystine and homocystine (p. 586).
3. Ferric chloride test for several amino acids (p. 597).
4. Nitroso naphthol test for tyrosine (p. 607).
5. Berry spot test for mucopolysaccharides (p. 596).

General references are Stanbury (1972), Shih (1973), Stuber (1972), and Thomas (1973) for tests; and Boggs (1971) for a review.

PHYSICOCHEMICAL TESTS

Possibly because an unwarranted amount of attention was given for many centuries to the appearance of urine, and because the yield in terms of positive results is small, simple gross examination of the urine has been too often ignored by the physician and the medical student. There are certain characteristics of the gross urine specimen, however, which provide useful diagnostic information and should not be overlooked.

Appearance of Normal Urine. The amber yellow color of urine is due largely to the pigment urochrome and to small amounts of urobilin and uroerythrin. Urochrome excretion is thought to be proportional to the metabolic rate and is increased during fever, thyrotoxicosis, and starvation. The pink pigment (uroerythrin) may be deposited on uric acid or urate crystals (brick dust deposit), and these should not be confused with blood. Pale urine in a normal person follows high fluid intake. Darker urines may be seen when fluids are withheld. Thus, the color roughly indicates the degree of concentration, but the latter, of course, should always be checked. For example, pale urine of high specific gravity may be found in diabetes mellitus.

Normal urine may show a sedimentary deposit if allowed to stand after cooling from body temperature. Precipitation will occur *in vivo* or *in vitro* with changes of pH. This deposit is usually a compact white crystalline precipitate composed largely of inorganic phosphate; in acid urine it may be due to orange urate crystals and amorphous urate material. Mucus from the urinary and genital tracts may appear in sediment as small, cloudy patches (nubeculae) in normal urine.

Appearance of the Urine in Abnormal States. When a patient's urine has an unusual color or appearance, a detailed history of dietary intake of food, candies, and drugs should be obtained. Certain food and candy dyes will color urine, as will drugs used for investigation and therapy. The family history may be important in the investigation of the autosomal recessive inheritance of alcaptonuria, which is associated with black or brown urine. Red urine associated with ingestion of beets is seen in genetically susceptible persons.

Some of the more important changes in the gross appearance of the urine are described below. A comprehensive listing is given in Table 17-2.

Cloudy Urine. Cloudy urine is most often normal and due to *phosphate* precipitation (and occasionally carbonate) in alkaline urine; the phosphates and carbonates redissolve when acetic acid is added. *Urates* cause a white or pink cloud in acid urine and redissolve on warming to 60° C. *Leukocytes* may form a white cloud similar to that caused by phosphates, but in this case the cloud remains after the addition of dilute acetic acid; the presence of leukocytes is confirmed by microscopic examination of the sediment. *Bacterial growth* will cause a uniform opalescence which is not removed by acidification or by filtering through paper; the odor of these specimens is unpleasant and usually ammoniacal because of the splitting of urea by the bacterial organisms. When the turbid urine is examined microscopically, rod-shaped bacteria, sometimes motile, are most commonly seen, e.g., *E. coli* and *Proteus. Enterococcus*, a coccal form, is also common.

Turbidity or smokiness may be due to *red blood cells*—hematuria. This turbidity does not clear on acidification or warming, and the presence of erythrocytes may be confirmed microscopically. *Spermatozoa and prostatic fluid* may cause turbidity not cleared by acidification or heating. Prostatic fluid normally contains a few leukocytes and other formed elements. *Mucin* from the urinary passages may cause a fluffy, bulky deposit; this is increased in inflammatory states of the lower urinary tract or genital tract. Turbidity due to blood clots, menstrual discharge, and other particulate material such as pieces of tissue, small calculi, clumps of pus, and fecal material is sometimes seen. Contamination with powders or with antiseptics which become opaque with water (phenols) will also cause a turbid urine.

CHYLURIA. The urine contains lymph and is

Table 17-2.   APPEARANCE AND COLOR OF URINE

APPEARANCE	CAUSE	REMARKS
Colorless	Very dilute urine	Polyuria, diabetes insipidus
Cloudy	Phosphates, carbonates	Soluble in dilute acetic acid
	Urates, uric acid	Dissolve at 60°C.
	Leukocytes	Insoluble in dilute acetic acid
	Red cells ("smoky")	Lyse in dilute acetic acid
	Bacteria, yeasts	Insoluble in dilute acetic acid
	Spermatozoa	Insoluble in dilute acetic acid
	Prostatic fluid	
	Mucin, mucous threads	May be flocculent
	Calculi "gravel"	Phosphates, oxalates
	Clumps, pus, tissue	Rectovesical fistula
	Fecal contamination	In acid urine
	X-ray media	
Milky	Many PMN (pyuria)	Insoluble in dilute acetic acid
	Fat	
	Lipuria, opalescent	Nephrosis, crush injury— soluble in ether
	Chyluria, milky	Lymphatic obstruction— soluble in ether
Yellow	Acriflavine	Green fluorescence
	Mepacrine	
	Nitrofurantoin	
	Riboflavin	
Yellow-orange	Concentrated urine	Dehydration, fever
	Urobilin in excess	No yellow foam
	Bilirubin	Yellow foam
	Pyridium	Color increases with HCl
Yellow-green	Bilirubin-biliverdin	Yellow foam
Yellow-brown	Bilirubin-biliverdin	"Beer" brown, yellow foam
	Senna, rhubarb, cascara	In acid urine
Red	Hemoglobin	o-Tolidine pos.
	Red blood cells	o-Tolidine pos.
	Myoglobin	o-Tolidine pos.
	Porphyrin	o-Tolidine neg., may be colorless
	Phenindione	Anticoagulant
	Amidopyrine	
	Fuscin, aniline dye	Foods, candy
	Beets	Yellow alkaline, genetic
	Menstrual contamination	Clots, mucus
Red-pink	Phenolsulfonphthalein	In alkaline urine
	Phenolphthalein	In alkaline urine
	Sulfobromophthalein	In alkaline urine
	Santonin	In alkaline urine
	Rhubarb, senna, cascara	In alkaline urine
Red-purple	Porphyrin	May be colorless
Red-brown	Red blood cells	
	Hemoglobin on standing	
	Methemoglobin	
	Myoglobin	
Brown-black	Methemoglobin	On standing, alkaline
	Homogentisic acid	Alkaptonuria
	Melanin, methyldopa	On standing
	Phenols	Reduce Benedict's
Blue-green	Methylene blue	In drugs
	Indigo-carmine	Decolorize with alkali
	Indicans	Intestinal putrefaction
	Pseudomonas infection	
Dark brown	Levodopa	Large dose

associated with obstruction to lymph flow and rupture of lymphatic vessels into the renal pelvis, ureters, bladder, or urethra. Filariasis (late in the disease), abdominal lymph node enlargement, and tumors have been associated with chyluria. Even with filariasis this is a rare event.

The appearance of the urine varies with the amount of lymph present. It may appear normal, opalescent, or milky. Clots may form. If sufficient lymph is present after a meal, the urine may layer, showing the chylomicrons on top and fibrin and cells beneath. Large numbers of red cells may cause a pink color. Chylomicrons may not be apparent microscopically unless they have coalesced as microglobules. The fat can be extracted from urine using an equal volume of ether or chloroform, and if urine is turbid due to phosphates, for example, it will not clear. The protein test is positive; leukocytes and red blood cells are present (Sanjurjo, 1970).

LIPIDURIA. Fat globules appear in urine in degenerative tubular disease, with the nephrotic syndrome, and from contamination. Embolism from bone marrow fat can occur with fractures of large bones or trauma to fatty tissue. With renal infarction, fat may enter the urine. Fat microglobules from coalesced chylomicrons also cause fat embolization. Neutral fat (triglyceride) droplets do not polarize, but stain with Sudan III and IV and oil red O. Cholesterol esters polarize and do not stain. Paraffin does not stain.

Red Urine. The most common abnormal color is red or red-brown. When seen in the female, contamination with menstrual flow should be considered. The urine in *hematuria* (presence of red blood cells) may appear cloudy, smoky, pink, red, or brown. The urine in *hemoglobinuria* may be clear red, clear red-brown, or dark brown. *Methemoglobin* has a dark brown color and may develop in bladder urine of acid pH or in acid urine on standing. Blood and blood pigments are easily detected by means of a reagent strip or tablet containing orthotolidine. A positive test will indicate the presence of hemoglobin or myoglobin. In order to distinguish hematuria from hemoglobinuria, sediment from a fresh urine specimen should be examined microscopically for red blood cells. A markedly hypotonic urine may cause lysis of erythrocytes, and therefore the specific gravity of the specimen should also be checked. *Myoglobin* in urine has a red-brown color and will give a positive orthotolidine or

Table 17-3. TYPES AND CAUSES OF MYOGLOBINURIA

Familial myoglobinuria
Hyperthermia
Infarction of muscle
Infection: Acute polymyositis
"March" myoglobinuria: Excessive unaccustomed exercise, anterior tibial syndrome
Paroxysmal myoglobinuria: Muscle cramps with myoglobinuria for 72 hours after attack
Toxin: Fish poisoning (Haff's disease), sea snake bite
Trauma: Beating, bullet, crush injury

guaiac test. In myoglobinuria brown pigment casts and an occasional red cell may be found. For causes of myoglobinuria, see Table 17-3.

In the porphyrias, the urine may be normal, red, or purple. It is usually red in congenital erythropoietic porphyria and the cutanea tarda form of porphyria. In acute intermittent hepatic porphyria, it is normal but darkens on standing. In lead porphyrinuria, the urine color is normal. Tests for porphyria are given on page 601. Red urine also may be associated with the use of drugs and dyes in diagnostic tests; for example, phenolsulfonphthalein, which is used in testing renal function, will cause a red color in alkaline urine (Table 17-4).

YELLOW-BROWN OR GREEN-BROWN URINE. Yellow-brown or green-brown urine is most often associated with bile pigments, chiefly bilirubin. Bilirubin becomes oxidized to green biliverdin on standing. In severe obstructive jaundice, the urine may be dark green. On shaking the urine specimen, a yellow foam may be seen which distinguishes bilirubin from a normal, dark, concentrated urine, which will have white foam. See tests for bilirubin on p. 584.

ORANGE-RED OR ORANGE-BROWN URINE. Urine containing large amounts of urobilin may resemble a dark, concentrated normal urine. Excreted urobilinogen is colorless but is converted in the presence of light and acid pH to urobilin which is dark yellow or orange. Urobilin will not color the foam on shaking a urine sample. See test for urobilinogen on pp. 607–608. Urinary analgesics (phenazopyridines) will cause an orange color and will color any foam present.

DARK BROWN OR BLACK URINE. An acid urine containing hemoglobin will darken on standing because of the formation of methemoglobin. Other rarer causes of dark brown urine are homogentisic acid (alcaptonuria) and melanin. In both cases the urine turns darker

Table 17-4. URINE COLOR CHANGES WITH COMMONLY USED DRUGS *

DRUG	COLOR	DRUG	COLOR
Alcohol, ethyl	Pale, diuresis	Levodopa (L-DOPA) (for Parkinsonism)	Red then brown, alkaline
Anthraquinone laxatives	Reddish, in alkaline	Methyldopa (Aldomet) (antihypertensive)	Darken, if oxidizing agents present red to brown
Azuresin (Diagnex Blue) (gastric acid test)	Blue, blue-green for several days after the test	Metronidazole (Flagyl) (for *Trichomonas* infection)	Darkening, reddish brown
Chlorzoxazone (Paraflex) (muscle relaxant)	Red	Methylene blue (in many urinary tract related drugs)	Blue, blue-green
Deferoxamine mesylate (Desferal) (chelates iron)	Red	Nitrofurantoin (Furadantin) (antibacterial)	Brown
Ethoxazene (Serenium)	Orange, red	Phenazopyridine (Pyridium) also compounded with sulfonamides (Azo-Gantrisin, etc.)	Orange-red, in acid
Fluorescein sodium (given I.V.)	Yellow		
Furazolidone (Furoxone) (an antibacterial nitrofuran)	Brown	Phenolphthalein	Red-purple, in alkaline
Inandione (Phenindione) anticoagulants (Miradon, Hedulin) (important to distinguish from hematuria; color disappears on acidifying)	Orange, in alkaline	Phenolsulfonphthalein (PSP also BSP)	Pink-red, in alkaline
		Quinacrine (Atabrine)	Yellow, in acid
		Rifampin (Rifadin, Rimactone) (tuberculosis therapy)	Bright orange-red
Iron sorbitex (Jectofer) (possibly other iron compounds forming iron sulfide in urine)	Brown on standing	Riboflavin	Bright yellow
		Sulfasalazine (Azulfidine) (for ulcerative colitis)	Orange-yellow, in alkaline

* Other commonly used drugs have been noted to produce color change once or occasionally: Amitriptyline (Elavil)—blue-green; phenytoin (Dilantin)—red; phenothiazines—red; triamterene (Dyrenium)—pale blue. An extensive list may be found in Young et al.: Clin. Chem., *21*:379-380, 1975.

on standing; urine containing homogentisic acid will darken more rapidly when alkaline (see p. 592). In patients with extensive malignant melanoma, a colorless pigment called melanogen is excreted. The addition of a few drops of 10 per cent ferric chloride will produce a gray precipitate that darkens to black. Occasionally melanuria is seen in patients with Addison's disease and in highly pigmented persons with chronic intestinal obstruction. For tests for melanuria, see page 597. Dark brown urine is seen in the urine of some patients taking levodopa. See Table 17-2 for causes of colored urines and Table 17-4 for a list of common drugs causing colored urines.

Odor. Normal urine has a faint, aromatic odor of undetermined source. Odor is chiefly important in the recognition of specimens that, due to bacterial contamination on standing, are ammoniacal, fetid, and unsuitable for laboratory examination.

Characteristic urine odors are produced after ingestion of asparagus or thymol. In maple syrup urine disease, a congenital metabolic disorder in amino acid metabolism, the urine smells like maple syrup. In phenylketonuria, a mousy odor has been noted. In Oasthouse disease, also a congenital metabolic disorder, the urine has a distinctive odor due to excessive alpha-hydroxybutyric acid.

Urine Volume. Measurement of the urine volume during timed intervals may be a valuable aid in clinical diagnosis. The average daily volume in the normal adult is 1200 to 1500 ml, the range of normal being from 600 to 2000 ml. The night urine is generally not in excess of 400 ml, which is to say that the ratio of day to night urine is better that 2:1 and often more than 3:1. Young children excrete about three to four times as much urine per kilogram of body weight as do adults (Table 17-5).

Table 17–5. URINARY SPECIFIC GRAVITY AND
URINE VOLUME-AGE RELATED REFERENCE VALUES

	REFERENCE VALUES	REFERENCE
Specific gravity		
Newborn (first few days)	1.012	Rubin, 1964
Infants	1.002–1.006	
Adults	1.001–1.035	
Adult normal fluid intake	1.016–1.022	
Volume		
Newborn (1–2 days old)	30–60 ml/24 h	
Infants		
3–10 days	100–300 ml/24 h	
10–60 days	250–450 ml/24 h	
60–365 days	400–500 ml/24 h	
Children		
1–3 years	500–600 ml/24 h	
3–5 years	600–700 ml/24 h	
5–8 years	650–1000 ml/24 h	
8–14 years	800–1400 ml/24 h	
Adults	600–1600 ml/24 h	
Older adults	250–2400 ml/24 h	Howell, 1956

A volume of more than 2000 ml is termed *polyuria*. Any increase in urine volume, even though transitory, is called *diuresis*. By definition, *oliguria* is the excretion of less than 500 ml of urine daily, and *anuria* is virtually complete suppression of urine formation. *Nocturia* is arbitrarily defined as the excretion by an adult of more than 500 ml of urine with a specific gravity of less than 1.018 at night. This is characteristic of chronic glomerulonephritis and is due to the kidney's inability to concentrate the urine. It occurs also in other polyuric states. Under ordinary physiologic conditions, the chief determinant of urine volume is the intake of water. Water is excreted extrarenally by the lungs, skin, and large bowel. These are not particularly sensitive to the body's needs either to conserve or to excrete water. It falls upon the kidney to control the body's state of hydration in the face of variations of water intake.

INCREASES IN URINE VOLUME. Excessive intake of water (polydipsia), such as may occur occasionally in neurotic states, will result in polyuria that may be confused with diabetes insipidus. Increased salt intake and high protein diets will also require more water for excretion.

Certain pharmacologic preparations exert a diuretic effect. Among these are caffein, alcohol, thiazides, and mercurial diuretics. Intravenous saline or glucose solutions may increase the urine output.

Classic pathologic states characterized by a continuous polyuria are *diabetes insipidus* and *diabetes mellitus*. In both conditions polyuria is frequently so marked as to be quite noticeable to the patient; it results in excessive thirst and in excessive water intake. In diabetes insipidus there is a deficiency of antidiuretic hormone. In diabetes mellitus there is an excessive amount of glucose, causing a solute diuresis.

In *chronic progressive renal failure*, functioning renal tissue is lost and the kidney gradually loses its ability to concentrate urine. In order to excrete the daily renal load, an increase in urine volume is inevitable. The urine eventually becomes isosmotic with the plasma ultrafiltrate; the normal day and night volume ratio of urine is lost. Polyuria may also result when there is *tubular damage*. With impairment of the countercurrent mechanism, urine will have low specific gravity. Increased output of urine is observed in primary *aldosteronism* due to tumor of the adrenal cortex and may occur in any condition in which prolonged and severe *potassium depletion* leads to renal tubular injury. In Addison's disease, secondary adrenal insufficiency, and adrenalectomy, deficiency of adrenocortical hormones is responsible for the relative inability of the kidneys to reabsorb sodium and therefore water. In a high percentage of cases, hyperparathyroidism is associated with polyuria.

DECREASES IN URINE VOLUME. Water deprivation will cause a decrease in urine volume even before signs of dehydration appear. Excessive loss of water by extrarenal routes has the same effect. This latter commonly occurs in hot weather when excessive sweating takes place.

Decreases in urine volume to oliguric levels occur also under pathologic circumstances such as the following:

Dehydration. In prolonged vomiting, diarrhea, or excessive sweating, such as may occur in febrile states, loss of body water without adequate replacement results in dehydration and hemoconcentration. Oliguria occurs, and there may even be retention of nitrogenous waste products due to a decrease in the glomerular filtration rate. Specific gravity is elevated to about 1.030. Oliguria will also occur when water is shifted from intravascular to extravascular compartments with edema.

Renal ischemia. In *shock* from any cause, with its characteristic low blood pressure and reduced blood volume, oliguria occurs even to the point of anuria. The urine has an elevated specific gravity and low sodium level. Anuria (or oliguria) also follows major hemolytic *transfusion reactions* and also accompanies the "crush" syndrome. Anuria in these conditions is thought to be related to loss of functioning renal mass. Renal ischemia is a likely etiologic factor.

Renal disease due to exposure to certain toxic agents, such as mercury bichloride, carbon tetrachloride, diethylene glycol, and the sulfonamides, may result in anuria due to acute tubular necrosis. Pyelonephritis will cause predominantly tubular dysfunction with polyuria early in the disease, but later oliguria of chronic renal failure. In acute glomerulonephritis, there is frequently oliguria, and there may be anuria. This is apparently due to blockage of glomerular capillary tufts, which results in decreased renal blood flow and decreased glomerular filtration. With *glomerular dysfunction*, oliguria is accompanied by high specific gravity and urea and low sodium. When there is oliguria with *uremia* due to progressive renal disease, urinary specific gravity is low, sodium concentration is elevated, and proteinuria, casts, and cells may be evident. This is in contrast to oliguria due to inadequate renal blood flow.

Obstruction. Bilateral hydronephrosis, resulting as it does from high-grade or longstanding obstruction of the urinary tract, may be associated with a marked decrease in urine flow and even anuria. The anuria associated with sulfonamide intoxication appears, at times, to be at least partially due to obstruction caused by the precipitation of crystals in the renal tubules or in the intramural portion of the ureter. Uric acid crystals and urates may precipitate after therapy with uricosuric agents or leukemia therapy. On the other hand, retention of urine in the bladder is not synonymous with oliguria or anuria, because there may be no decrease in urine formation by the kidney. Catheterization, of course, permits one to distinguish such retention from true oliguria.

Specific Gravity and Osmolality. The volume of excreted urine and its concentration of solute is varied by the kidney to maintain homeostasis of body fluid and electrolytes. In order to achieve this, the kidneys produce a urine much more concentrated than the plasma from which it is derived. The solute concentration of the urine varies with water and solute ingestion, the state of the tubular cells, and the influence of antidiuretic hormone (ADH) on water reabsorption in the distal tubules. Final concentration of urine takes place in the collecting system of the medulla. The inability to concentrate or dilute urine is an indication of renal disease or hormonal deficiency (ADH). See Chapter 6 for a discussion of the concentrating ability of the kidney.

Urines of low specific gravity are called *hyposthenuric*, the specific gravity being less than 1.007. Urines of fixed specific gravity of about 1.010 are known as *isosthenuric*. The specific gravity of the protein-free glomerular filtrate is about 1.007. Its osmolal concentration is about 285 mOsm., or the osmolality of protein-free plasma (the plasma protein makes little contribution to the total osmolality of the plasma, only about 2 mOsm.).

The measurement of specific gravity or osmolality should give an indication of the urinary total solute concentration. The measurement of osmolality of urine and plasma is preferred to the measurement of specific gravity, although it may be well to measure both properties. The reader should refer to Chapter 6 for a discussion of osmolality versus specific gravity of urine.

SPECIFIC GRAVITY. Useful clinical information can be obtained from the measurement of maximal specific gravity, although the usual methods are technically not as precise as the measurement of osmolality. Urea (20 per cent), chloride (25 per cent), and sulfate and phosphate contribute most to the specific gravity of normal urine.

Reference Values. Normal adults with normal diets and normal fluid intake will produce urine of specific gravity 1.016 to 1.022 during a 24-hour period. If a random specimen of urine has a specific gravity of 1.023 or more, concentrating ability can be considered normal.

Urinary specific gravity after taking no fluids for 12 hours overnight should be about 1.022, and after 24 hours without fluid, 1.026. For values in children, see Table 17-5. After vasopressin (5 units), urinary specific gravity should reach at least 1.020.

Minimum specific gravity after a standard water load should be less than 1.003. For details of concentration and dilution tests, see Chapter 6.

OSMOLALITY (NORMAL VALUES). The normal adult on a normal diet with a normal fluid intake will produce a urine of about 500 to 850 mOsm/kg water. The normal kidney is able to produce urine of osmolality in the range of 800 to 1400 mOsm/kg water in dehydration and a minimal osmolality of 40 to 80 mOsm/kg water during water diuresis. After a period of dehydration, the osmolality of the urine should be three to four times that of the plasma (e.g., with a normal plasma osmolality of 285 mOsm/kg water, the urine osmolality should be at least 855 mOsm/kg water).

Methods for Measuring Osmolality. The freezing point depression method is commonly employed. A solution containing 1 osmol or 1000 mOsm/kg water depresses the freezing point 1.86°C. below that of water (take as 0°C.). For method, see Chapters 4 and 6.

Measurement of Specific Gravity. In the measurement of specific gravity, the hydrometer (urinometer) is used. There are certain technical limitations in the method, but careful attention to detail will provide a reasonably accurate measurement. Measurements of concentrating ability are useless in the presence of diuresis, solute diuresis (glucose, urea), and radiographic dyes. Corrections should be made for protein and for glucose; however, since glucose produces a solute diuresis, it is debatable whether corrections for it are of value. If a high specific gravity is found in a pale urine, the presence of glucose should be suspected.

The *urinometer* is a hydrometer adapted to measure the specific gravity of urine at room temperature. It should be checked each day by measuring the specific gravity of distilled water, which has a specific gravity of 1.000. If the urinometer does not give a reading of 1.000, an appropriate correction must be applied to all readings taken with that urinometer.

Procedure. The urinometer vessel is filled three-fourths full with urine (minimum volume of urine required is about 15 ml.). The urinometer is inserted with a spinning motion to make sure that it is floating freely. (When reading the urinometer, be sure that it is not touching the sides or the bottom of the cylinder. Avoid surface bubbles which obscure the meniscus.) Read the bottom of the meniscus.

Because temperature influences the specific gravity, urines should be allowed to come to room temperature before a reading is made, or a correction of 0.001 should be made for each 3°C. above or below the calibration temperature indicated on the urinometer, usually 15.6°C. (60°F.).

For accurate determinations of specific gravity in concentration-dilution tests, correction must be made for protein or sugar present. Subtract 0.003 for every 1 g/100 ml of either glucose or protein.

The accuracy of a urinometer may be further checked in solutions of known specific gravity; e.g., a solution of potassium sulfate with a specific gravity of 1.015 may be prepared by diluting 20.29 g potassium sulfate to 1 liter with distilled water.

Specific Gravity of Small Volumes. When only a small amount of urine is available, specific gravity may be measured by using a small volume urinometer, by weighing the urine, by a falling-drop technique in organic solvent solution, e.g., chloroform and benzene in a graded series of mixtures, or by measuring the refractive index.

The refractive index of a solution is related to the content of dissolved solids present. It is the ratio of the velocity of light in air to the velocity of light in a solution. This ratio varies directly with the number of dissolved particles in solution. The refractive index varies with, but is not identical to, the specific gravity of a urine specimen. Measurement of refractive index of urine has become feasible and convenient with the development of a clinical refractometer. This device requires only a few drops of urine (unlike the minimum 15 ml of urine necessary with the urinometer), and results generally correlate well with urinometer readings. The specific gravity reading on the refractometer is generally slightly lower than a urinometer reading on the same specimen by about 0.002. Although the refractometer measures refractive index of solution, scale readings of the instrument have been calibrated in terms of specific gravity, refractive index, and total solid content (Rubini 1957; Wolfe 1962).

Refractometer. A temperature-compensated hand model is available.[*] The instrument is temperature-compensated between 60° and 100°F. It is damaged by heat above 150°F. and by immer-

---

[*]TS meter. American Optical Company, Buffalo, N.Y.

sion of the eye-piece and focusing ring in water. It should read zero with distilled water; the zero reading can be reset if necessary by breaking the seal over the setscrew, turning it with a small screwdriver, and resealing. To prevent dropping and lens damage, a stand is recommended to support the refractometer.

Always check calibration daily. If the zero reading is correct for distilled water, it is probably not necessary to check the instrument with high and low specific gravity salt solutions. However, some laboratories may prefer to do this.

To make a specific gravity determination of urine, first clean the surfaces of the cover and prism with a drop of distilled water and a damp cloth and then dry. Close the cover. Apply a drop of urine at the notched bottom of the cover so that it flows over the prism surface by capillary action.

Point the instrument toward a light source at an angle that gives optimum contrast. Rotate the eye-piece until the scale is in focus. Read directly on the specific gravity scale the *sharp* dividing line between light and dark contrast.

The entire procedure should be repeated with a second drop of urine from the same sample.

The pH of Urine. The pH of urine is a reflection of the ability of the kidney to maintain normal hydrogen ion concentration in plasma and extracellular fluid. The metabolic activity of the body produces non-volatile acids which cannot be extracted by the lungs—principally sulfuric, phosphoric, and hydrochloric acids, but also small amounts of pyruvic, lactic, and citric acids and some ketone bodies. These acids are excreted by the glomerulus with cations, chiefly sodium. The distal tubular cells exchange hydrogen ions for sodium of the glomerular filtrate, and the urine becomes acid in reaction. For a discussion of this exchange process, see Chapter 6.

Normal pH. The average adult on a normal diet excretes urine about pH 6. In health, urine pH may vary from pH 4.6 to pH 8. When protein intake is high, more phosphates and sulfates are produced; this results in more acid urine. On a predominantly vegetable diet, as in many non-western countries, the urine may have a pH higher than 6. The urine becomes less acid following a meal as a result of secretion of acid into the stomach (the so-called alkaline tide). At night, during the mild respiratory acidosis of sleep, a more acid urine may be formed.

Interpretation of Urine pH in Pathologic States. The capacity to exchange hydrogen ion for cation and the formation of ammonia is decreased when tubular function is impaired. In *renal tubular acidosis*, glomerular filtration is normal, but tubular ability to form ammonia and exchange hydrogen ions for cations is defective. The urine is relatively alkaline, and the pH cannot be lowered below pH of 6 to 6.5, even with the administration of an acid loading substance. Titratable acidity and the concentration of ammonium are decreased.

In metabolic acid-base disturbances, the pH of the urine may reflect attempts at compensation by the kidneys. In *metabolic acidosis* an acid urine is produced and titratable acidity and ammonium ion concentrations are increased. In *metabolic alkalosis* an alkaline urine is produced and ammonia production is decreased. In *respiratory acidosis* an acid urine is formed and the amount of ammonium excreted is increased; in *respiratory alkalosis* an alkaline urine is produced which is associated with increased excretion of bicarbonate. In *potassium depletion* such as in hypokalemic alkalosis of prolonged vomiting or in hypercorticism, there may be paradoxical aciduria with slightly acid urine in the presence of a metabolic alkalosis. Potassium and hydrogen ions are excreted and bicarbonate is reabsorbed.

Acid urine may be produced by a diet high in meat protein and in some fruits such as cranberries. Ammonium chloride, methionine, methenamine mandelate, or acid phosphate is used to produce an acid urine in treatment of calculi. Acid phosphates with or without antibacterials help keep calcium in solution. Acidifiers are useful for ammonium magnesium stone prevention, since these form in an alkaline urine.

Alkaline urine may be induced by use of a diet high in certain fruits and vegetables, especially citrus fruits. Sodium bicarbonate, potassium citrate, and acetazolamide may be used to induce alkaline urines in the treatment of calculi, since uric acid, calcium oxalate, and cystine precipitate in acid urine. They may also be used in some urinary tract infections (the antibiotics neomycin, kanamycin, and streptomycin are more active in alkaline urine), in sulfonamide therapy in which sulfadiazine or sulfamerazine is used (sulfisoxizole is more soluble in the tubular lumina), and in the treatment of salicylate poisoning.

Measurement of Urine pH. Measurement of urine pH and acidity must always be made on freshly voided specimens. If precise measurements are required, the urine should be covered tightly and the container filled in order to minimize the amount of dead space. On standing, the pH tends to rise because of loss of carbon dioxide (the PCO_2 of freshly voided urine is approximately 40 mm Hg, that of normal plasma) and because bacterial growth produces ammonia from urea.

A rough estimate of the pH is usually sufficient and may be made with indicator paper. In patients with disturbances of acid-base balance, urinary pH may be accurately measured with a pH meter with a glass electrode. In measuring titratable acidity, the specimen should be fresh, or if a 24-hour urine collection is made, the pooled urine should be refrigerated from the onset of collection.

DETERMINATION OF pH IN URINE. Urinary pH may be measured by means of a closed glass electrode and read directly from the scale of a pH meter. Since the pH meter may tend to drift, it must be standardized with a buffer of known pH immediately prior to use. After standardization, spray the electrodes with distilled water, clean, and dry with tissue. Immerse the electrodes in the urine sample. Report the pH of urine at the temperature of measurement.

TITRATABLE ACIDITY OF URINE. The pH of the urine is largely dependent on the amount of mono- and dibasic phosphate present. Titratable acidity is measured by titrating a fresh or preserved (toluol) specimen of urine with 0.1 N NaOH with pH 7.4 as an endpoint. If phenolphthalein is used as an indicator, the endpoint is pH 8.3. The test may be used together with urinary ammonia determination in patients with chronic acidosis of obscure origin.

Procedure. To 25 ml of urine in a flask, add 10 g of powdered potassium oxalate (to precipitate calcium). Mix well. Titrate to pH 7.4 using 0.1 N NaOH. If phenolphthalein is used as the indicator, titrate to a pale pink color (pH 8.3).

Titratable acidity is usually reported as number of milliliters of 0.1 N NaOH required to neutralize a 24-hour specimen.

$$= \frac{\text{ml NaOH} \times 24\text{-hour volume}}{25}$$

Normal titratable acidity is in the range of 200 to 500 ml 0.1 N NaOH (or 6 ml 0.1 N NaOH per kg body weight).

CHEMICAL TESTS

AMINOACIDURIA

Aminoacidurias may be classified into two general types—overflow and renal.

Overflow Type. Abnormal metabolism of amino acids results in the abnormal accumulation of an amino acid or amino acids in plasma

Table 17–6. PRIMARY OVERFLOW AMINOACIDURIAS*

DISEASE	AMINO ACIDS INCREASED IN BLOOD AND URINE	ABNORMAL ENZYME
Phenylketonuria	Phenylalanine	Phenylalanine hydroxylase
Tyrosinosis	Tyrosine	p-Hydroxyphenylpyruvic acid oxidase
Histidinemia	Histidine	Histidase
Maple-syrup urine disease	Valine, leucine, and isoleucine	Branched chain keto acid decarboxylase
Hypervalinemia	Valine	Probably valine transaminase
Hyperglycinemia	Glycine (lysine on high protein diet)	Associated with CP synthetase deficiency and other disorders
Hyperprolinemia Type I Type II	Proline	Proline oxidase Δ^1pyrrolin-5-carboxylate dehydrogenase
Hydroxyprolinemia	Hydroxyproline	Hydroxyproline oxidase
Homocystinuria	Methionine, homocystine	Cystathionine synthetase
Hyperlysinemia	Lysine	Lysine-alpha-ketoglutarate reductase†
Citrullinemia	Citrulline	Argininosuccinic acid synthetase
Alcaptonuria	Homogentisic acid (2:5 dihydroxyphenyl-acetic acid). No abnormal amino acid.	Homogentisic acid oxidase
Oasthouse urine disease	Methionine, phenylalanine, valine, leucine, isoleucine, and tyrosine, and also alpha-hydroxybutyric acid in urine.	Possibly methionine malabsorption syndrome

*From Efron, M. L.: Aminoaciduria. N. Engl. J. Med., *272*:1060, 1965.

†Gardner, L. I.: Endocrine and genetic diseases of childhood and adolescence, 2nd ed. Philadelphia, W. B. Saunders Company, 1975, p. 1049.

Table 17-7. NO-THRESHOLD AMINOACIDURIAS*

DISEASE	AMINO ACIDS IN URINE	ABNORMAL ENZYME
Argininosuccinic aciduria	Argininosuccinic acid (also citrulline)	Argininosuccinase
Cystathioninuria	Cystathionine	Cystathioninase
Homocystinuria	Homocystine	Cystathionine synthetase
Hypophosphatasia	Phosphoethanolamine	Serum alkaline phosphatase

*Modified from Efron, M. L.: Aminoaciduria. N. Engl. J. Med., *272*:1060, 1965.

and their excretion in the urine. The kidney is normal, but the amount of amino acids excreted in the glomerular filtrate exceeds the threshold value for reabsorption. Examples of this type of aminoaciduria include phenylketonuria, tyrosinosis, alkaptonuria, maple syrup urine disease, and the generalized aminoaciduria of liver disease. In a few instances (e.g., homocystinuria), the substrate does not accumulate in the blood because there is no reabsorption in the kidney; therefore, blood levels are low but urine levels are increased. This is known as the "no-threshold" type of aminoaciduria (Tables 17-6 and 17-7).

Patients receiving protein hydrolysates show gross aminoaciduria, since the D-amino acids of the DL mixture are poorly metabolized and are excreted. Cachectic patients excrete excess beta-amino-isobutyric acid, as is also seen in starvation. In severe liver disease, such as massive hepatic necrosis, and in hepatic coma, breakdown of amino acids by the liver is reduced and a generalized aminoaciduria is seen with cystine and methionine present. Leucine and tyrosine crystals are sometimes observed in the urine sediment. In hepatic coma, glutamine is often the dominant amino acid excreted. In acute hepatitis the patterns

are normal if the disease is not severe, but in more severe cases, a generalized aminoaciduria with the appearance of cystine is seen.

Renal Type. A renal tubular defect is the cause of aminoaciduria. The plasma level of amino acids is normal. Examples are congenital disorders (e.g., the Fanconi syndrome, cystinosis, Hartnup disease, and cystinelysinuria) and the secondary renal tubular disorders seen in Wilson's disease, galactosemia, rickets, scurvy, and occasionally the nephrotic syndrome. Heavy metal poisoning, oxalic acid poisoning, phenol poisoning, and occasionally burns may also produce renal tubular defects resulting in aminoaciduria (Tables 17-8 and 17-9).

The aminoaciduria seen in the Fanconi syndrome, hepatolenticular degeneration (Wilson's), and infantile galactosemia is generalized: all amino acids appear in the urine in increased amounts. In cystinosis the aminoaciduria and other findings are similar to those of Fanconi syndrome, but cystine crystals accumulate in the tissues.

Normal Values. In the normal adult, urinary excretion of amino acids is fairly constant, averaging 200 mg of alpha-amino nitrogen excreted in a 24-hour period. Al-

Table 17-8. RENAL TRANSPORT AMINOACIDURIAS*

DISEASE	AMINO ACIDS IN URINE	ABNORMALITY
Cystinuria (cystine stones)	Cystine; lysine; arginine, ornithine (basic amino acids)	Incomplete absorption of cystine, lysine, arginine and ornithine
Hartnup disease	Monoaminomonocarboxylic (neutral) amino acids (proline, glycine, hydroxyproline, and methionine not increased)	Incomplete absorption of monoaminomonocarboxylic amino acids
Glycinuria—renal type Familial Iminoglycinuria	Glycine—proline, hydroxyproline	Membrane transport defect

*Modified from Efron, M. L.: Aminoaciduria, N. Engl. J. Med., *272*:1060, 1965.

Table 17-9. SECONDARY AMINOACIDURIA*

PRIMARY DISORDER	AMINO ACIDS IN URINE	ABNORMAL ENZYME
Wilson's disease	Generalized (cystine and threonine often most prominent)	Ceruloplasmin
Galactosemia	Generalized aminoaciduria	Galactose-1-phosphate-uridyl-transferase
Cystinosis	All plasma amino acids (also loss of glucose, phosphate, potassium, and water, and Fanconi syndrome)	Unknown

*Modified from Efron, M. L.: Aminoaciduria. N. Engl. J. Med., *272*:1060, 1965.

though most amino acids found in normal humans have been detected in normal urine, usually not more than about 6 to 8 are detected by paper chromatography or column chromatography in more than trace amounts. In the normal urine, amino acid chromatogram *glycine* is usually most prominent. This is followed by *alanine, serine*, and *glutamine* and then by *taurine, histidine*, and *methylhistidine*. With a high-protein (meat) diet, histidine and methylhistidine are excreted in larger amounts. Other amino acids which may be demonstrated in normal urine, depending on the technique used, are glutamic acid, threonine, tyrosine, and lysine and a trace of arginine; beta-amino-isobutyric acid may also be seen.

In infants the pattern may vary with feeding. The level of amino acid excretion is relatively higher in infants, and increased amounts of cystine, asparagine, glutamine, glutamic acid, and occasionally proline are seen. Relatively large amounts of taurine are present in the urine at birth, but adult levels are seen at six months of age. Children show the same pattern as adults (Smith, 1960).

Screening Tests for Aminoaciduria. The overflow aminoacidurias, including phenylketonuria, are probably best diagnosed by examining the amino acid composition of plasma. Examination of urine should also be performed, since in renal aminoaciduria of the no-threshold type, where the mechanism of reabsorption of amino acids is abnormal, blood levels of amino acids will be normal or only slightly increased, but urine levels may greatly increase.

A bacterial inhibition assay with dried blood has been successfully used in screening programs (Efron, 1965; Guthrie, 1963; Bennett, 1977).

A number of simple screening tests have been described for the diagnosis of inborn errors of metabolism (Buist, 1968; Renuart, 1966; Shih, 1973). Scriver (1973) has reviewed the screening, diagnosis, and investigation of hereditary aminoacidopathies, a study which is especially helpful from a laboratory approach.

Identification of amino acids can be made by chromatography, high voltage electrophoresis, and column amino acid analysis.

For qualitative tests see page 592 for alkaptonuria (homogentisic acid), page 586 for cystine, page 599 for phenylketonuria, page 607 for tyrosine, and page 597 for the ferric chloride test.

ASCORBIC ACID

A large urinary concentration of ascorbic acid from therapeutic doses of vitamin C* or preparations containing ascorbic acid may inhibit the glucose oxidase-peroxidase reactions for glucose and also the tests for occult blood based upon the peroxidase activity of hemoglobin. It is useful to check for the presence of ascorbic acid when the microscopic examination of a urine sediment shows 1+ or more red blood cells and the screening test for blood on the uncentrifuged urine specimen is negative. The test has also been used as an indication of adequate ascorbic acid therapy.

C-Stix reagent strips[a] have a reagent-impregnated area consisting of phosphomolybdates buffered in an acid medium. Phosphomolybdates are reduced by ascorbic acid to "molybdenum blue."

Procedure. Dip the test end of the strip into the specimen. Ten seconds later compare the color

* L-ascorbic acid, $C_6H_8O_6$, is usually made from dextrose, $C_6H_{12}O_6$ by removing 4 hydrogens. It is a strong reducing agent and is readily converted into dehydroascorbic acid, $C_6H_8O_6$, by oxidizing agents. This is a reversible reaction, allowing oxidation and reduction reactions *in vivo*.

of the reagent area of the strip with the color chart supplied by the manufacturer, and report as indicated on the chart.

SENSITIVITY. 5 mg ascorbic acid/dl urine.

SPECIFICITY. May show false positives with gentisic acid and L-dopa. Will not show false positives with urates, salicylates, or creatinine.

Ascorbic acid interference with tests

Blood Test. Normal reaction of hemoglobin with orthotolidine.

hemoglobin
(peroxidase + H_2O_2 + orthotolidine $\longrightarrow$ reduced
activity)

$$\text{oxidized orthotolidine} + H_2O$$
$$(\text{blue})$$

Effect of Ascorbic Acid

$$H_2O_2 + \begin{array}{c}\text{ascorbic acid}\\\text{(reduced form)}\end{array} \longrightarrow$$

$$\begin{array}{c}\text{oxidized}\\\text{ascorbic acid}\end{array} + H_2O$$

BILIRUBIN

Bilirubin is a breakdown product of hemoglobin formed in the reticuloendothelial cells of the spleen and bone marrow and carried in the blood by protein. Free or unconjugated bilirubin is not able to pass through the glomerular barrier of the kidney. When free bilirubin is conjugated in the liver with glucuronic acid, it becomes water soluble and is able to pass through the glomerulus of the kidney. Conjugated bilirubin is normally excreted in the bile. In patients with obstructive jaundice, bilirubin is found in the urine; urine with yellow foam may accompany pale acholic stools. Bilirubin is also found in the urine when intracanalicular pressure rises because of periportal inflammation or fibrosis and from swelling of liver cells. Bilirubin may, for example, appear in the urine in hepatitis before the appearance of jaundice. A positive test for urinary bilirubin with a negative test for urobilinogen in urine is indicative of intra- or extrahepatic biliary obstruction.

In congenital hyperbilirubinemias, bilirubin will appear in the urine in the Dubin-Johnson type and the Rotor type. It does not appear with Gilbert's disease or Crigler-Najjar disease.

Excretion of bilirubin is enhanced by alkalosis.

Normal adult urine contains about 0.02 mg of bilirubin/dl (With, 1954).

A *screening test* for bilirubin in urine may be used to detect latent or unsuspected liver disease. It should be performed when the color of the urine indicates the possibility of bilirubin. The screening test is also of value in the differential diagnosis of jaundice, since bilirubinuria is not found with hemolytic jaundice, but accompanying obstructive and parenchymatous jaundice. It is helpful in diagnosis and in following the course of infectious hepatitis. In persons exposed to toxins and ingesting certain drugs, a positive test for bilirubinuria may be an early indication of liver damage.

Two tests are commonly used: the diazo method, in which bilirubin is coupled to *p*-nitrobenzene diazonium *p*-toluene sulfonate to form a blue or purple color (this is in the form of a tablet or reagent strip) and one which employs a ferric chloride reagent to oxidize bilirubin to a green biliverdin.

The reagent strip (diazo test) is not as sensitive as the tablet (diazo) test. The diazo test may give a false negative reaction, while the oxidation test is positive due to biliverdin. In severe jaundice, biliverdin may be excreted in the urine (Bryant, 1955).

Bilirubin glucuronide will hydrolyse on standing, and bilirubin will oxidize to biliverdin, which is not reactive. Hence, urine should be protected from light and examined as quickly as possible.

Tests will detect levels of bilirubin in urine of 0.05 to 0.1 mg/dl.

Diazo method (Free, 1953)

Reagents. Tablets containing *p*-nitrobenzene diazonium *p*-toluene are used. The tablets also contain sulfosalicylic acid and sodium bicarbonate to provide an acid medium for the reaction and an effervescent mixture that will insure the solution of a portion of the tablet when water is added. (Ictotest kit, including asbestos-cellulose mats and reagent tablets, is available through Ames Company, Elkhart, Ind.)

Procedure

1. Place 5 drops of specimen on an asbestos-cellulose mat provided with the kit. Bilirubin, if present, will be adsorbed onto the mat surface.

2. Place a reagent tablet on the moistened area of the mat.

3. Allow 2 drops of water to flow over the tablet. If bilirubin is present, there will be a coupling of bilirubin with *p*-nitrobenzene diazonium *p*-toluene sulfonate from the tablet, as shown by the formation of a blue to purple color within 30 seconds. A pink or red color is negative.

SPECIFICITY. The diazo test reacts positively to

bilirubin. There is no purple reaction with urobilin or other pigments or with any other known constituent of normal urine. High levels of urobilin or indican will give a red color; salicylates may give an orange to red color (Bryant, 1955). Ascorbic acid may interfere with the test. Azo compounds cause an atypical color.

SENSITIVITY. The diazo test has a sensitivity ranging between 0.1 and 0.05 mg of bilirubin/dl of urine (Giordano, 1953).

STABILITY OF REAGENT. Ictotest[a] reagent tablets are effervescent and somewhat hygroscopic, and, accordingly, they should be protected from moisture or high humidity. The tablets are packed in a brown bottle, since prolonged direct exposure to strong light results in decomposition of the stabilized diazonium compound. Prolonged exposure of several weeks to temperatures of 100°F. or more may also result in deterioration of the tablets.

Reagent strip.

See reagent strip method (p. 570).

Oxidation method (Watson, 1946).

Reagents

1. Thick filter paper (Schleicher and Schuell, No. 470) that has been soaked in saturated barium chloride, dried, and cut into small strips.

2. Fouchet's reagent. Dissolve 25 g trichloroacetic acid in 100 ml distilled water. Add 10 ml of 10 per cent $FeCl_3$ solution.

Procedure

1. Hold the strip of $BaCl_2$ paper perpendicularly in the urine for a few seconds so that it is about one half inch below the surface. Remove.

2. Drop 1 to 2 drops of Fouchet's reagent on the saturated area. A green color, usually deepening on standing because of the formation of biliverdin, represents a positive test.

High levels of urobilin or indican may cause a brown-purple color; salicylates give a purple color; high levels of urobilinogen may cause a red color over the green of biliverdin.

CALCIUM

The urinary output of calcium depends upon dietary intake of calcium, skeletal weight, and endocrine factors.

Estimation of calcium excretion may be useful if a 24-hour collection of urine is made and the dietary intake of calcium is known. The Albright-Reifenstein diet (1948), for example, contains about 130 mg calcium per day. The patient is placed on the diet for three days before urine collections are started and continues on the diet for the next three days while urine is collected.

High levels of calcium are seen in urine in hyperparathyroidism; hence, if more than 400 mg per day is excreted on a normal diet, hyperparathyroidism should be suspected. In osteolytic bone diseases, in osteoporosis, especially after immobilization, and in hyperthyroidism, there is increased excretion of calcium. Hypercalciuria occurs in renal tubular acidosis when there is excessive loss of base and in vitamin D intoxication from increased intestinal absorption (see Chap. 10).

Urinary calcium levels are low when serum calcium levels are low, except in renal disease; low serum levels occur in hypoparathyroidism due to defective mobilization of calcium from bone and with reduced calcium absorption, steatorrhea, or vitamin D deficiency (see Chap. 10).

Methods for measuring calcium include ethylenediaminetetra-acetic acid (EDTA) titration, titration of oxalate precipitate, and by atomic absorption spectrophotometry, polarography, and glass electrodes sensitive to divalent cations (Henry, 1974).

Screening Test for Urinary Calcium (Barney, 1937). The normal serum calcium level is above the renal threshold for calcium, which is about 7 mg/dl. If the serum level is below this, no calcium is excreted. The test may be useful as a rapid screening test for hypoparathyroidism. See Ritter (1960) for criticisms of the test. Results will be affected by concentration of the urine and calcium intake (Albright, 1948).

Principle. Calcium is precipitated as calcium oxalate at a pH at which the calcium and magnesium phosphates are soluble. The degree of precipitation is noted visually.

Reagents

1. Glacial acetic acid.

2. Calcium solution, 25 mg/dl. Dissolve 69 mg anhydrous $CaCl_2$ in water and dilute to 100 ml with water.

3. Sulkowitch reagent:

    2.5 g oxalic acid.

    2.5 g ammonium oxalate.

    5.0 ml glacial acetic acid.

    150.0 ml distilled water.

Procedure

1. Adjust the pH of the urine sample to 5 with acetic acid. If the urine specimen is cloudy, it may be centrifuged after the pH has been adjusted to 5. If the centrifugate is still cloudy, a blank should be made with 5 ml of urine and 5 ml of water. Compare with the test to see if turbidity has increased.

2. Pipette 5 ml of urine into a test tube. Add 5 ml of Sulkowitch reagent and mix by inversion. Also carry out the test on 5 ml of solution containing 25 mg/dl calcium.

3. Wait 2 minutes and observe the turbidity. Report as *decreased* (little or no precipitate) and

serum calcium probably less than 8.5 mg per cent (4.3 mEq/l), *moderate* (turbidity seen but less than that produced by the 25 mg/dl calcium solution), or *increased* (turbidity equal to or greater than that produced by the 25 mg/dl calcium solution) and serum calcium probably above 12 mg per cent (6 mEq/l).

CYSTINURIA

The defective transport of cystine by the epithelial cells of the renal tubules and gut is transmitted as an autosomal recessive trait (Dent 1951; Milne, 1961). While large amounts of the dibasic acids—ornithine, lysine, and arginine—are also excreted in this disease, cystine is the only one that crystallizes out.

Cystinuria occurs equally in both sexes, with an incidence estimated at 1 per 20,000 (homozygous) and in larger numbers for heterozygotes (Crawhall, 1969). Calculus formation in the urinary tract is related to the amount of cystine excreted and the acid pH of the urine. Cystine stones are radiopaque, yellow-brown, and often multiple.

Increased amounts of cystine are also found in the urine in renal tubular disease, heavy metal poisoning, renal tubular acidosis, and generalized aminoaciduria.

Procedure. Examine a first morning urine specimen for colorless, hexagonal crystals. Urine will be at an acid pH. Note that the solubility of cystine is less in water and that cystine may not always crystallize in a concentrated urine although present in large amounts (Ettinger, 1971).

Cyanide-nitroprusside test

This test is Brand's modification of the Legal nitroprusside reaction (Brand, 1930; Legal, 1883). Cystine is reduced to cysteine by sodium cyanide, and the sulfhydryl groups then react with nitroprusside to produce a red-purple color. A positive control urine should be tested.

Place 3 to 5 ml urine (and control) in a test tube and add 2.0 ml fresh sodium cyanide solution (5 g/dl water*) and allow to stand for 5 to 10 minutes.

Add fresh aqueous sodium nitroprusside solution (5 g/dl) dropwise (about 5 drops) and mix. A stable red-purple color will develop with cystine. Normal specimens may develop a faint color.

Further identification of cystine is made by chromatography, high voltage electrophoresis, or quantitative chemical tests.

CONTROL. A positive control with cystine added

Poisonous—discard remaining solution in sink, flushing with large amounts of water.

to normal urine is used. Use 5 mg cystine dissolved in 10 ml 0.1 N HCl, diluted to 100 ml with normal *urine*. Freeze aliquots.

POSITIVE SPECIMENS. To save these, acidify with 0.1 N HCl to pH 1 to 2 and freeze.

SENSITIVITY. Control urine contains 50 mg/l. Normal adults excrete up to about 100 mg/24 hr. A concentrated normal specimen could give a weak positive result. Homozygous stone formers usually excrete more than 250 mg/g creatinine and will be detected, but not all heterozygotes will.

SPECIFICITY. Cysteine, cystine, homocystine, and ketones (dark red) will give positive reactions.

NORMAL VALUES. About 1 to 2 mg/kg/day of cystine is excreted. The output increases with the amount of protein in the diet.

Nitroprusside tablet test (Acetest[a])

One tablet is placed in a spot-plate depression. Add one large drop of fresh 10 per cent sodium cyanide in 1 N sodium hydroxide, then one large drop of urine. Positive will show a cherry red color. A few false negatives may occur (Hambraeus, 1963).

Sodium borohydride–nitroprusside test

This test substitutes a less toxic reagent for the sodium cyanide and eliminates ketone interference (Henry, 1974).

Cystinosis, a recessively inherited disorder, is characterized by cystine crystal deposition in cells. With renal involvement, the Fanconi syndrome develops and there is a generalized aminoaciduria, glucosuria, etc. Unlike cystinuria, the cystine loss in cystinosis parallels the loss of other amino acids in the urine, and the urine is relatively alkaline because of tubular damage.

Homocystinuria, a rare disorder, is the result of an inborn error of methionine metabolism inherited as an autosomal recessive. There is a defect in cystathionine synthetase activity. Urinary excretion of homocystine and homocysteine are increased. The sodium cyanide-nitroprusside test is positive for homocystinuria. The silver nitroprusside test will detect homocystine in the presence of cystine (Spaeth, 1967).

FRUCTOSURIA

Essential fructosuria is a rare benign condition due to a deficiency of fructokinase. Blood levels become elevated after ingestion of fructose, and it appears in the urine. Glucose levels are normal.

Hereditary fructose intolerance, on the

other hand, leads to failure to thrive, liver and renal involvement, aminoaciduria, and proteinuria. Hepatic fructose-1-phosphate aldolase is deficient and fructose-1-phosphate accumulates in cells. Fructosuria is inherited as an autosomal recessive trait. Hypoglycemia and severe reactions occur soon after ingestion of fructose or sucrose. With dietary restriction, the patients remain healthy.

Fructosuria has also been noted in patients receiving fructose parenterally. Fructosuria is suspected when there is a negative glucose oxidase test and a positive copper reduction test. It will reduce Benedict's copper reagent at low temperatures (50°C. water bath) or at room temperature. The time taken will depend on the amount of sugar present; e.g., 1 ml of 1 per cent fructose will cause a yellow precipitate in 10 minutes at 50°C. when mixed with 5 ml Benedict's reagent. Fructose will ferment yeast and give a positive Seliwanoff test.

Positive identification is made by paper or thin-layer chromatography.

Resorcinol Test. (Seliwanoff, 1887). Boil 5 ml of urine with 5 ml of 25 per cent HCl. Add about 5 mg resorcinol and boil for 10 seconds. Fructose will cause the formation of a heavy red precipitate. Separate the precipitate by filtration and dissolve it in ethanol. The precipitate should form a red solution in ethanol for the test to be positive. The fructose is converted to hydroxymethyl furfural; this condenses with resorcinol to form a red color. Use a positive control. Sensitivity is about 100 mg/dl urine.

Note. Fructose will form from glucose in alkaline urine, so the specimen should be fresh.

QUANTITATIVE TEST. Glucose is removed with glucose oxidase and a method for inulin (a polyfructose) is used (e.g., Froesch, 1957—a resorcinol method).

REFERENCE VALUE. Fructose—about 60 mg/24 hours in urine.

GALACTOSURIA (GALACTOSEMIA)

Galactose is found in the urine in genetic disorders of galactose metabolism associated with either a deficiency of galactokinase or of galactose-1-phosphate uridyl transferase. These diseases are transmitted as autosomal recessives with an incidence for transferase deficiency ranging up from 1/100,000 births.

Because of the enzyme deficiencies, galactose, which is derived from lactose in the diet, is not converted to glucose in the liver. With galactokinase deficiency, a milder disease ensues: galactose accumulates and is reduced to galactitol in the lens of the eye where cataracts are formed. Transferase deficiency causes an accumulation of galactose and galactose-1-phosphate. Clinically there is diarrhea with failure to thrive from early infancy. Liver dysfunction and jaundice occur early, and renal toxicity is followed by generalized aminoaciduria, proteinuria, and cataract formation. A lactose (galactose)-free diet will cause regression of symptoms.

Heterozygotes and Duarte variant carriers have half-normal transferase activity and do not have the disease. The disease may be diagnosed by means of enzyme studies on cultured cells obtained by amniocentesis (see Chap. 20).

Screening. Mass screening tests on newborn blood are carried out in some regional or state public health laboratories (Bennett, 1977). A copper reducing test on neonate urines has been recommended for infants on the day of discharge or at the time of checkup. Galactose oxidase reagent strips have been tried (Dahlquist, 1968).

Identification. A reducing substance in urine that does not react with glucose oxidase reagent strips may be galactose, lactose, fructose, or pentose (or a number of other substances). In an infant with failure to thrive, the sugar should be identified by chromatography (thin-layer or paper) followed by an assay for red cell enzyme activity.

Reference Value. Normal newborns, premature infants, and some children with high milk consumption may have galactosuria (Dahlquist, 1969; Hall, 1970). Reference values are about 14 mg/24 hours.

GLYCOSURIA

Diabetes Mellitus. The level and duration of hyperglycemia required to make a diagnosis of diabetes mellitus is variously interpreted by groups in different parts of the world. Although hyperglycemia alone is not necessarily indicative of diabetes mellitus, the appearance of glucose in the urine is regarded as a hallmark of the disease and requires that the patient receive a work-up for diabetes mellitus.

Those at risk are early or latent diabetics whose usually normal glucose tolerance curve becomes abnormal with stress, pregnancy, or obesity. Asymptomatic or chemical diabetes may be defined as hyperglycemia with no significant glycosuria or symptoms (see Chap. 7).

The patient diagnosed as having diabetes mellitus has hyperglycemia which results in glycosuria when the renal threshold for glucose is exceeded. With glycosuria there are polyuria and thirst. With the need to metabolize protein and then fats, ketone levels rise in the blood and urine, and with the excretion of ketones and the accompanying base, metabolic acidosis ensues.

Glycosuria (glucosuria) *with hyperglycemia* is also seen in *endocrine disorders* other than diabetes mellitus, e.g., in pituitary and adrenal disorders such as acromegaly and in the Cushing's syndrome or hyperadrenocorticism, and with functioning alpha- or beta-cell pancreatic tumors, hyperthyroidism, and pheochromocytoma. Pancreatic disease with loss of functioning islets is also associated with glycosuria, e.g., hemochromatosis, carcinoma, pancreatitis, and cystic fibrosis.

Glycosuria and hyperglycemia may be seen with central nervous system disorders: brain tumor or hemorrhage, hypothalamic disease, and asphyxia, and with disturbances of metabolism associated with burns, infection, fractures, myocardial infarction, and uremia. Liver disease, glycogen storage diseases, obesity, and feeding after starvation are also associated with glycosuria, as are certain drugs, e.g., thiazides, corticosteroids and ACTH, and birth control pills. Glycosuria may occur in late pregnancy and care should be taken to rule out diabetes.

Glycosuria *without hyperglycemia* is usually associated with renal tubular dysfunction and relates to the inability to reabsorb glucose. This may be due to drugs or poisons or endogenous "toxins," e.g., in the Fanconi syndrome, galactosuria, and amino acid disorders.

Renal glycosuria is benign and is characterized by repeated glycosuria with blood levels of glucose below 100 mg/dl. Some persons may have thresholds that are exceeded only after meals. With aging, this variety of glycosuria may decrease.

QUALITATIVE TESTS FOR GLUCOSE IN URINE. Two methods are used, one in which glucose reduces alkaline copper sulfate to cuprous sulfate and one in which glucose is oxidized to gluconic acid by glucose oxidase. The second method is specific for glucose, since, with the exception of ascorbic acid, non-glucose reducing agents do not interfere with it.

The simplest, most specific test is the *glucose oxidase paper strip* method (Free, 1957a). It is more sensitive than copper reduction methods and will detect levels of 10 to 12 mg/dl of urine glucose. It is not affected over a pH range of 5 to 9 or by the addition of significant amounts of uric acid (200 mg/dl), creatinine (100 mg/dl), or protein. Ascorbic acid, however, will inhibit the test for at least 2 minutes when the ascorbic acid level is about twice as great as the glucose level (Nakamura, 1965). With newer formulation reagent strips, ascorbic acid interference is not as great (Free, 1973). It is important to remember that ascorbic acid is added to many antibiotic preparations as a stabilizer. As a screening test, the glucose oxidase test will not detect increased levels of galactose or other sugars in urine. It is therefore important that a copper reduction test such as Benedict's be routinely used for pediatric patients.

Of the copper reduction tests used for screening purposes, the qualitative Benedict's test (1909) is more sensitive to reducing substances in urine than the single-tablet copper reduction test (Clinitest—Cook, 1953). Benedict's test becomes positive at levels of 50 to 80 mg/dl of reducing substance (Henry, 1974). Urines containing non-glucose reducing substances may give positive results in healthy persons. Many substances in urine, metabolites, or drug-related metabolites will influence urinary glucose tests. Strong reducing substances like ascorbic acid, gentisic acid, or homogentisic acid may inhibit the enzyme test while contributing to the positivity of the copper test. Oxidizing bleaches (in containers) may give false positive reagent strip tests. Many drug metabolites have reducing properties, and a comprehensive listing of these is given by Young (1975). They include many of the penicillins and other antibiotics, sulfonamides, salicylates, and other analgesics and many other commonly prescribed drugs. In these instances, when the copper test is positive and the glucose oxidase test is negative, glycosuria is ruled out; but before investigating for other sugars the clinical findings and drug history should be evaluated.

GLUCOSE OXIDASE TEST. See reagent strip method (p. 569). This is a specific test for glucose in which glucose oxidase reacts with glucose in the urine to remove two hydrogen ions and forms gluconolactone, which is promptly hydrated to gluconic acid. The removed hydrogen ion is then combined with atmospheric oxygen to form hydrogen peroxide. The hydrogen peroxide, in the presence of peroxidase, oxidizes orthotolidine, which in its oxidized state turns blue (Comer, 1956; Free, 1957a).

COPPER REDUCTION TESTS. Benedict's qualitative test and a tablet version of it are commonly used.

COPPER REDUCTION TABLET TEST. Clinitest[a] tablets, like Benedict's test, will react with sufficient quantities of any reducing substances in the urine, including other reducing sugars such as lactose, fructose, galactose, maltose, and the pentoses. Since it is a reducing substance, large amounts of ascorbic acid may cause false positive results.

Both a 5-drop and a 2-drop Clinitest method have been described (Belmonte, 1967), and corresponding color charts are available for both. The 2-drop method was developed in response to a so-called "pass-through" phenomenon, which may occur if more than 2 g/dl of sugar is present in the urine. In the "pass-through" phenomenon, the solution that results after addition of the Clinitest tablet goes through the entire range of colors and back to a dark greenish-brown. This final color does not compare with any section of the color chart; however, it corresponds most closely to a significantly lower result. It is important to observe the entire reaction and 15 seconds after so that the reversion to a different color is not missed and a falsely low result reported.

Chemistry. Copper sulfate, sodium hydroxide, sodium carbonate, and citric acid are incorporated into a tablet. Copper sulfate reacts with reducing substances in the urine, converting cupric sulfate to cuprous oxide. Based on Benedict's copper reduction reaction,

$$Cu^{++} \xrightarrow{\text{hot alkaline solution}} Cu^{+}$$

$$Cu^{+} + OH^{-} \longrightarrow CuOH \text{ (yellow)}$$

$$2\,CuOH \xrightarrow{\text{heat}} Cu_2O \text{ (red)} + H_2O$$

Heat is caused by the reaction of sodium hydroxide with water and citric acid.

Procedure

5-drop Method. Place 5 drops of urine in a test tube and add 10 drops of water. Add one Clinitest tablet. Watch while boiling takes place, but do not shake. Wait 15 seconds after boiling stops, then shake the tube *gently,* and compare the color of the solution with the color scale. Grade results as negative, trace, $1+$, $2+$, $3+$, or $4+$. These results correspond to the following concentrations: trace $= 0.25$ g/dl; $1+ = 0.5$ g/dl; $2+ = 0.75$ g/dl; $3+ = 1.0$ g/dl; $4+ = 2.0$ g/dl. It is important to watch the solution carefully while it is boiling. If at this time the solution passes through orange to a dark shade of greenish brown, it indicates that more than $4+$ sugar is present, and this should be recorded as $4+$ without reference to the color scale. Urines showing this "pass-through" phenomenon should be retested with the 2-drop method.

2-drop Method. Place 2 drops of urine in a test tube and add 10 drops of water. Add one Clinitest tablet. Watch while boiling takes place, but do not shake. Wait 15 seconds after boiling stops, then shake the tube gently, and compare the color of the solution with the color scale supplied for the 2-drop method. The "pass-through" phenomenon may also occur with the 2-drop test with large concentrations of sugar, over 10 g/dl. Therefore, it is important to watch the test throughout the entire reaction and waiting period. Report results as negative, trace, 0.5 g/dl, 1 g/dl, 2g/dl, 3 g/dl, 5 g/dl, and over 10 g/dl if a "pass-through" reaction occurs.

Sensitivity. Clinitest reagent tablets will detect 150 to 250 mg glucose/dl of urine.

Specificity. Specificity is described in Table 17-10.

Precautions. Observe the precautions in the literature supplied with the Clinitest tablets. The bottle must be kept tightly closed at all times to prevent absorption of moisture and kept away

Table 17-10. REACTIONS OF SUBSTANCES FOUND IN URINE TO TESTS FOR GLUCOSURIA

CONSTITUENTS	GLUCOSE OXIDASE REAGENT STRIP	COPPER REDUCTION
Glucose	Positive	Positive
Sugars other than glucose		
Fructose		
Galactose		
Lactose	No effect	Positive
Maltose		
Pentose		
Sucrose	No effect	No effect
Urine constituents		
Creatinine	No effect	May cause false positive*
Uric acid		
Homogentisic acid (alcaptonuria)	No effect	Positive
Drug or contaminants in urine		
Ascorbic acid (therapy or in antibiotic prep.)	Large quantities may delay color	May cause false positive*
Hydrogen peroxide	False positive	
Hypochlorite (bleach)	False positive	

* Also amino acids, caronamide, cephalothin, chloral, chloroform, chloramphenicol, L-Dopa, x-ray dye, formaldehyde, hippuric acid, homogentisic acid, isoniazid, ketone bodies, nalidixic acid, thiazides, oxytetracycline, *p*-aminosalicylic acid, penicillin, phenols, protein, salicylates, streptomycin, phenothiazine, and sulfonamides. Data from Caraway, 1962; Wirth, 1965; Young, 1975.

from direct heat and sunlight, in a cool, dry place. The tablets normally have a spotted bluish white color. If not stored properly they will absorb moisture or deteriorate from heat, turning dark blue or brown. In this condition they will not give reliable results. They are also available individually packaged in aluminum foil to help prevent this absorption of moisture. Although more expensive, such packaging is useful when a limited number of tests are performed.

QUALITATIVE BENEDICT'S METHOD (1911)

Principle. Glucose in urine reduces blue alkaline copper sulfate reagent (Benedict's reagent) to red cuprous oxide precipitate. A green, yellow, or orange color and precipitate is formed, depending upon the amount of glucose and other reducing substances present.

Reagent

1. Dissolve 17.3 g $CuSO_4 \cdot 5H_2O$ in 100 ml hot water in large beaker.

2. Dissolve 173 g sodium citrate and 100 g anhydrous sodium carbonate in 800 ml water with heat. Cool and pour into first reagent and dilute to 1 liter with water.

Procedure. Place 5 ml of Benedict's qualitative reagent in a test tube. Add 0.5 ml of urine (8 drops). Mix by shaking. Place rack into pan of boiling water for 5 minutes (or over flame for 2 minutes). Remove from boiling water and read immediately.

Interpretation

REACTION	REPORT AS	APPROXIMATE GLUCOSE CONCENTRATION (MG/DL)
Clear blue or green opacity, no precipitate	0 or trace	0 to 100
Green with yellow precipitate	1+	100 to 500
Yellow to green with yellow precipitate	2+	500 to 1400
Muddy orange with yellow precipitate	3+	1400 to 2000
Orange to red precipitate—clear supernatant	4+	2000 or more

The sensitivity of the test is approximately 50 to 80 mg glucose/dl (Henry, 1974). According to Apthorp (1957), a negative Benedict's test corresponds to a blue, blue-green, or green color with gray precipitate and is usually equivalent to less than 50 mg/dl of reducing sugar. The green-with-yellow precipitate is equivalent to 50 mg/dl. Specimens showing green-with-a-dull-yellow precipitate are "doubtful." Bickel (1961) found that green-yellow reactions were equivalent to 115 to 550 mg/dl of reducing sugars, but specimens showing the opaque green reaction could contain from less than 50 mg/dl to 290 mg/dl of reducing sugars. The interpretation of the opaque green reaction is therefore difficult (Wright, 1956), and it is recommended that it be reported as trace.

The bulk of the precipitate is the index of positivity of the reaction according to Benedict (1909) and is associated with the presence of cuprous creatinine. A dilute urine with low creatinine levels of less than 0.03 mg/dl may therefore appear negative, even when glucose is present (Samson, 1939). False negative reactions may be associated with inadequate heating (Cook, 1953). False positive results may be due to prolonged boiling.

Reference Values. The urine of normal children and adults is negative. Normal neonatal infants during the first 10 to 14 days of life may excrete urine giving a positive reaction due to glucose, galactose, fructose, and lactose (Bickel, 1961). Normal pregnant and postpartum women may give positive reactions to tests for lactose.

NON-GLUCOSE MELITURIA
(Table 17-11)

1. A negative glucose oxidase reagent strip test and positive copper reduction test (Clinitest[a] or Benedict's) are usually the first findings. Rule out interfering substances with the glucose oxidase reagent before proceeding, e.g., ascorbic acid. The possibility of reducing drug metabolites should also be evaluated (Table 17-10).

2. Chromatography, thin-layer or paper, is the best way to identify the sugars.

Table 17-11. IDENTIFICATION OF URINARY SUGARS

SUGAR	COPPER REDUCTION	FERMENTABLE	CONFIRMATORY TEST
Glucose	+	+	Glucose oxidase
Lactose	+	−	Chromatography (Rubner's test)
Fructose	+	+	Chromatography (resorcinol test)
Galactose	+	−	Chromatography (red cell enzyme test)
Maltose	+	+	Chromatography
Mannose	+	+	Chromatography
Pentose	+	−	Chromatography
Sucrose	−	+	Chromatography

3. Other qualitative tests are available but are not as satisfactory.

   a. Benedict's test at 50°C. or room temperature for fructose or pentose (see p. 599).
   b. Seliwanoff (resorcinol) test for fructose (see p. 587).
   c. Fermentation test with baker's yeast. Pentose does not ferment but glucose and fructose will. Galactose and lactose have little activity. See page 58 of Davidsohn (1974) for yeast fermentation test procedure.

Thin-layer chromatography is faster than paper chromatography for the separation of urinary sugars, but paper can be left overnight for development.

For thin-layer chromatography (TLC), silica gel chromatography sheets are available prepared for use (Eastman Silica gel G) or a silica gel layer of $250\,\mu$ on glass may be preferred (Brinkman). A kit is available from Kodak with chromatography sheets, development gel and stain, and standard solutions (Chromato/Screen).

A single-pass ascending migration takes about 30 to 40 minutes with most methods. A double-pass method is recommended for better separation (Henry, 1974). After the sheets or plate is spotted with the unknown and standard sugar solutions, it is allowed to develop in the solvent, a pyridine or ethyl acetate mixture. When the solvent front has reached the desired height, the plate is dried, sprayed with a "stain" (aniline or other reagent), heated briefly, and the spots visualized.

Migration of the sugars varies in different preparations, so there are no standard R_f values. Sugars are identified by their R_f values compared to the known sugars on the plate.

$$R_f = \frac{\text{distance traveled by sugar}}{\text{distance traveled by solvent front}}$$

Sugars may also be related to the distance traveled by glucose:

$$R_g = \frac{\text{unknown distance}}{\text{glucose distance}} \times 100$$

With thin layer chromatography (TLC), xylulose, ribose (arabinose), fructose, glucose, galactose, and lactose are commonly separated. Maltose, raffinose, sucrose, and xylose can be added to the standards if necessary. Galactose and glucose are sometimes difficult to separate and glucose may be removed beforehand with glucose oxidase if this is necessary.

Urine specimens should be tested for positive reducing substance before starting. Urine may need pretreating to elicit the disaccharides (Henry, 1974). Different methods are described by several authors (Smith, 1969; Becker, 1968; Young, 1970).

Hemoglobin in Urine

The presence of an abnormal number of red blood cells in urine is known as *hematuria*, whereas the term *hemoglobinuria* indicates the presence of hemoglobin in solution in urine.

Because of the diagnostic importance of small amounts of hematuria, and because of the tendency of red blood cells to undergo lysis in urine, a screening test for hemoglobinuria is a useful adjunct to the microscopic examination of the sediment.

The combination of a positive test for hemoglobin and normal urinary sediment suggests that a fresh urine sample should be examined for red blood cells. The microscopic examination for red cells should not be omitted, because red cells that do not react to the usual screening test may be present. Inhibition of the reagent strip test is frequently due to the presence of ascorbic acid.

Reference values cited for red blood cells in urine are quite variable. This reflects the technique and care used in the assessment as well as the problems inherent in random specimens.

Wright (1959) indicated that normal urine averaged about 1000 red blood cells/ml. However, it has been suggested that an upper level of normal of 20,000/ml be used. This would include 95 per cent of the study group, most of whom had only occasional cells per high power field, depending on the method used (Freni, 1977). Reagents strips will detect between 10,000 and 50,000 red cells/ml and would probably not miss levels near the upper limit. On the other hand, positive results could be found in apparently healthy persons, again depending on the reference intervals established.

Hematuria.

See causes under erythrocytes (p. 614).

Hemoglobinuria

The presence of hemoglobinuria indicates significant intravascular hemolysis. Free hemoglobin binds to plasma haptoglobin, and once this binding capacity is saturated, hemoglobin will pass through the glomerulus. Some hemoglobin is reabsorbed by proximal tubular cells, and the remaining hemoglobin is excreted. Hemoglobin is metabolized in the tubular cells into ferritin and to hemosiderin, which can later be detected in the urinary sediment with Prussian blue stain.

Hemoglobinuria may follow severe exertion in which there is *direct trauma* to small blood vessels, e.g., marching, jogging, karate, or bongo drum playing. Myoglobin may also be excreted owing to some muscle damage.

With artificial *heart valves*, hemolysis can be marked, especially with aortic valves. Hemoglobinuria is often observed after hemotherapy with frozen-thawed red blood cells, and more frequently in children. Hemolytic uremic syndrome and thrombotic thrombocytopenic purpura are also associated with red cell destruction and hemolysis.

Paroxysmal cold hemoglobinuria is caused by an IgG antibody directed against the red cell. Attacks are precipitated by cold. It occurs with viral infections and syphilis.

Paroxysmal nocturnal hemoglobinuria is caused by an acquired defect of the red cell, causing it to be sensitized to complement. It is usually seen in young adults. Intermittent gross hemoglobinuria occurs, but hemosiderinuria is usually present.

Other causes of hemoglobinuria are hemolytic transfusion reaction, hemolysis due to bacterial toxins or snake and spider venom, malaria, and severe burns.

Screening Test for Hemoglobin in Urine. The orthotolidine and benzidine tests are sensitive to a hemoglobin level of about 0.0003 mg/ml, equivalent to 10 million red blood cells per liter (10,000 per ml). Because of the carcinogenic effect of benzidine, the orthotolidine test is recommended. Either a wet chemical test or a reagent strip or tablet may be used. In this test, hemoglobin and other iron porphyrin derivatives including myoglobin catalyze the oxidation of orthotolidine to a blue product by oxygen release from hydrogen peroxide. (See reagent strip method, p. 569.)

HOMOGENTISIC ACIDURIA

Homogentisic acid (dihydroxyphenylacetic acid) is excreted in urine in large quantities in a rare hereditary disease, alcaptonuria (alkali lover). Normally, phenylalanine and tyrosine are metabolized to homogentisic acid, which is then oxidized to maleyl acetoacetic acid. With a deficiency of homogentisic acid oxidase, there is an accumulation of homogentisic acid. This can be quantitated in serum and urine (Seegmiller, 1961).

Patients with alcaptonuria develop dark blue to black pigmentation in cartilage and connective tissue. The disease may not be diagnosed until arthritis develops.

Screening. If the urine is allowed to stand it will very slowly oxidize and darken at the surface. Urine at an acid pH is not colored; the addition of alkali will hasten darkening when homogentisic acid is present. If ascorbic acid is present it will inhibit the oxidation.

Homogentisic acid reduces the copper reagent in Benedict's test and, because of the alkaline reagent, it will also darken to produce a yellow precipitate in an orange to brown solution. This reaction will also take place (more slowly) at room temperature. Glucose oxidase reagent strip is negative, so that the reducing substance should not be confused with glucose.

FERRIC CHLORIDE TEST. A transient very dark blue color is seen as drops of 10 per cent $FeCl_3$ solution are added (Table 17-12).

SILVER NITRATE TEST. Add 4 ml 3 per cent silver nitrate solution to 0.5 ml urine. Mix, then add several drops of 10 per cent NH_4OH. Homogentisic acid will cause the development of a black color.

Identification is made by using paper (Knox, 1951) or thin-layer chromatography. Normally, there is no homogentisic acid present in urine.

INDICAN (INDOXYL SULFATE)

Indole is produced by bacterial action on tryptophan in the intestine. Most is eliminated in the feces, the remainder is absorbed and detoxified to be excreted as *indican* in the urine.

$$Indole \xrightarrow{oxidized} indoxyl + H_2SO_4 \longrightarrow$$

$$indoxyl\ sulfuric\ acid \xrightarrow{K^+}$$

$$indican\ (indoxyl\ potassium\ sulfate)$$

In normal urine the amount of indican excreted is small; it is increased with high-protein diets. In disease it originates from bacterial growth, often in the small intestine, and is increased with intestinal obstruction, gastric cancer, hypochlorhydria, biliary obstruction, and malabsorptive syndromes like sprue and blind loop syndrome.

In the rare Hartnup disease, amino acids are poorly absorbed from the intestine, and this allows bacterial decomposition to take place. Indoxyl sulfate and other indoxyl compounds are formed from tryptophan and excreted in the urine in large quantities.

Evidence of bacterial growth in the small intestine is probably most reliably detected by identifying bacterial deconjugation of bile salts with the ^{14}C-glycocholic acid breath test.

Detection of indoxyl potassium sulfate depends upon its decomposition and subsequent oxidation of the indoxyl to indigo blue and its absorption by chloroform.

Procedure. To 5 ml of fresh urine in a test tube, add 5 ml ferric chloride reagent (0.2 per cent in concentrated HCl). Mix. Add 2 ml chloroform and invert several times. Allow the chloroform to settle and observe. When indican is present, the chloroform layer shows a deep violet to blue color. Normal urine may give a faint blue color. Report as positive or negative.

Comment. Indigo red may form occasionally because of slow oxidation. If iodides are present, iodine will be formed by oxidation and cause a violet color; thymol will also cause a violet color. These are removed by adding a crystal of sodium thiosulfate.

Bile pigments interfere with the reaction and should be removed by shaking the urine with barium chloride and filtering. Formalin will also interfere with the reaction.

Urine from cows and horses will usually give positive reactions and may be used for comparison.

Normally less than 100 mg is excreted in 24 hours.

5-Hydroxy Indoleacetic Acid

Serotonin (5-hydroxytryptamine) is produced by the argentaffin cells of the intestines from tryptophan and is carried in the blood by platelets.

Tryptophan $\longrightarrow$ 5-OH tryptophan $\longrightarrow$

5-OH tryptamine $\xrightarrow[\text{monoamine oxidase}]{}$

5-OH indole acetaldehyde $\xrightarrow[\text{oxidase}]{}$

5-OH indoleacetic acid

Carcinoid tumors (argentaffinoma) arising from the argentaffin cells produce excessive amounts of serotonin, especially when metastatic. Serotonin causes intestinal disturbances, vasomotor disturbances, and bronchoconstriction. Edema, right-side valvular heart disease, and neurologic symptoms are seen. The screening test (Sjoerdsma, 1955) is useful for the detection of the serotonin metabolite 5-hydroxy indoleacetic acid in the urine if it appears in fairly large amounts. The quantitative method is more sensitive, since it eliminates the interfering ketoacids and indoleacetic acid (Udenfriend, 1955).

Normal excretion of 5-hydroxy indoleacetic acid in 24 hours is 1 to 5 mg. A random specimen of urine is usually sufficient for screening purposes; if a 24-hour collection is made, it should be acidified with HCl or acetic acid. Patients should not take any drugs for 72 hours before the test; phenothiazines or acetanilid drugs will interfere with this test.

The principle of the test is based on the development of a purple color specific for 5-hydroxy indoles with nitrous acid and 1-nitroso-2-naphthol. Ethylene dichloride is used to remove interfering chromogens.

Reagents. 1-nitroso-2-naphthol, 0.1 per cent in 95 per cent ethanol. Nitrous acid prepared fresh by adding 0.2 ml of 2.5 per cent sodium nitrite solution to 5 ml 2 N H_2SO_4 ethylene dichloride.

Procedure. Pipette into a test tube 0.2 ml urine, 0.8 ml distilled water, 0.5 ml 1-nitroso-2-naphthol solution. Mix well. Add 0.5 ml fresh nitrous acid and mix. Allow to stand at room temperature for 10 minutes. Shake with 5.0 ml ethylene dichloride and allow the two layers to separate. A positive test shows a purple color in the upper aqueous layer. Always use positive and negative controls. Control solutions may be kept frozen.

Interpretation. A purple color may appear with as little as 40 mg 5-hydroxy indoleacetic acid in 24 hours. Patients with malignant carcinoid tumors may excrete up to 350 mg 5-hydroxy indoleacetic acid per day, and the test will show a black color. Positive findings should be checked with a quantitative method. For interfering substances, see Young, 1975.

Ketones

Ketonuria. In ketonuria the three ketone bodies present in the urine are acetoacetic acid (20 per cent), acetone (2 per cent), and beta-hydroxybutyric acid (about 78 per cent) (Henry, 1974). Acetone is formed by non-reversible acid. Beta-hydroxybutyric acid forms reversibly from acetoacetic acid.

Acetoacetic acid $\xrightarrow{-CO_2}$ acetone

Acetoacetic acid $\underset{-2H}{\rightleftharpoons}$ hydroxybutyric acid

Ketone bodies are the products of incomplete fat metabolism, and their presence is indicative of acidosis. Ketonuria is commonly seen in uncontrolled diabetes mellitus.

Non-diabetic Ketonuria. In infants and children, ketonuria commonly occurs in a variety of conditions, such as acute febrile diseases and toxic states accompanied by vomiting or diarrhea (Riekers, 1958). Ketonuria is also present in vomiting of pregnancy, cachexia, and following anesthesia. In these cases, it is related most probably to increased tissue, especially fat, catabolism in the face of limited food intake. The use of the ketogenic diet for weight reduction and in treatment of seizures in children will produce ketonuria. Occasionally ketonuria is seen following exposure to cold or severe exercise.

Severe neonatal ketoacidosis results from a deficiency of propionyl CoA carboxylase. In this genetic disease, propionic acid is not converted to methyl malonate. Other causes of genetically determined ketoacidosis in infancy are glycogen storage disease, branched-chain ketonuria, and methyl malonic aciduria.

Examination of the urine for ketone bodies is not a necessary part of the routine urine examination except in specimens from young children. However, in the presence of any of the above conditions, or whenever acidosis or ketosis is suspected clinically, urine should be examined for ketones.

Diabetic Ketonuria. The presence of ketonuria indicates the presence of ketoacidosis (ketosis) and may provide a warning of impending coma. Up to 50 mg of acetoacetic acid per dl may be present without clinical evidence of ketosis (Killander, 1962). Diabetic children and young adults are more prone to episodes of ketosis, often associated with infection as well as other problems in management. It is the usual practice in the management of diabetes to test for ketonuria when the urine, on qualitative examination, displays more than a 2+ glycosuria. It is suggested that the urine of diabetic patients controlled with oral hypoglycemic agents should be tested regularly for ketone bodies as well as glucose, especially in the presence of infection, since insulin may then be required for control. Ketonuria should also be checked when changes in diabetic therapy are prescribed.

While there are large amounts of ketones and glucose in urine in diabetic ketoacidosis, ketonuria is not found with the hyperosmolar hyperglycemia coma sometimes occurring in older diabetics.

Lactic acidosis. Lactic acidosis occurs with shock and with diabetes mellitus, renal failure, liver disease, and infections, and in response to certain drugs, especially phenformin and salicylate poisoning.

Acetoacetate and β-hydroxybutyrate may both be highly elevated in lactic acidosis, but usually the butyrate is high and the acetoacetate will not be detected by the nitroprusside test (Cohen, 1976; Hansen, 1978).

Methods for Testing Ketonuria. Since it seems that the three ketone bodies have equal significance (Rickers, 1958), there is no need to attempt separation. The Gerhardt *ferric chloride* test has been used for many years as a test for acetoacetic acid (see Fig. 17–8); however, ferric chloride tests are not very specific and the sensitivity is low—about 25 to 50 mg/dl.

Acetone and acetoacetic acid react with sodium nitroprusside in the presence of alkali to produce a purple colored complex. This reaction was described by Legal (1883) in diabetic urines. In the simplest form of the nitroprusside test, reagent strips impregnated with sodium nitroprusside and alkali are used. A tablet form of the same test is available with similar sensitivity. The blood level of ketone bodies may also be estimated by the nitroprusside test; this is especially helpful in determining the severity of ketosis in the treatment of diabetic acidosis.

REAGENT STRIP METHOD. Sodium nitroprusside, glycine, and buffer are the reagents used (see p. 569).

TABLET TEST METHOD. The Acetest[a] tablet contains sodium nitroprusside (nitroferricyanide), glycine, and a strongly alkaline buffer. It can be used to test whole blood, plasma, serum, or urine.

Procedure. Place the tablet on a clean surface, preferably a piece of white paper. Place one drop of urine, serum, plasma, or whole blood on the tablet. For *urine* testing, compare color of tablet to color chart at 30 seconds after application of the specimen. For *serum* or *plasma* testing, compare color of tablet to color chart at 2 minutes after application of specimen. For *whole blood* testing, 10 minutes after application of the specimen remove clotted blood from tablet and compare color of tablet to color chart.

If acetone and acetoacetic acid are present, the tablet will show a color varying from lavender to deep purple. Report the results as negative, small, moderate, or large. If large, a dilution may be made (see below).

Sensitivity. Acetest[a] will detect 5 to 10 mg of acetoacetic acid/dl of urine and 20 to 25 mg acetone/dl of urine.

Dilution. In urine, reagent strips react to 10 mg of acetoacetic acid/dl and are less sensitive to acetone. When a patient is being followed with repeated determinations of acetone and diacetic acid in plasma, the concentrations of these compounds may start at a high level and fall but still give "large" results. Therefore, repeated reports of "large" would not reflect the change taking place. In such an instance, semiquantitative results can be obtained with either the reagent strip or Rothera's test by testing several different dilutions of each specimen. Report these analyses in a form such as this: undiluted "large," 1:2 dilution "large," 1:4 dilution "moderate," etc.

Specificity. This is similar for the reagent strip (p. 569), tablet, and Rothera's tube test (vide infra).

ROTHERA'S TEST—URINE (1908)

Reagents

1. Pulverize and mix 7.5 g sodium nitroprusside and 200 g ammonium sulfate.

2. Concentrated ammonium hydroxide.

Procedure

1. To 5 ml of urine in a test tube, add approximately 1 g of Rothera's reagent. Mix well.

2. Overlay with about 1 ml of concentrated ammonium hydroxide. A positive test is the appearance of a reddish purple ring at the interface within 1 minute and 30 seconds. A brown ring is not a positive reaction.

3. Report as follows: *Negative*—No ring, or a brown ring. *Trace*—A faint pinkish purple ring appearing slowly. *2+*—Narrow dark purple ring. *4+*—Wide dark purple ring appearing very rapidly.

The nitroprusside test of Rothera is sensitive to acetoacetic acid, about 1 to 5 mg/dl, and acetone with a sensitivity of 10 to 25 mg/dl.

Specificity. The reagents react with both acetoacetic acid and acetone in urine, plasma, or serum. They do not react with salicylates. Levodopa may cause a false positive result. Urine containing Bromsulphalein and phenylketones will cause color reactions with the reagent similar to that produced by acetoacetic acid and acetone. Bromsulphalein reacts with the aklaline buffers of the reagent strips to form a colored complex. If the level of phenylketones is 100 mg/dl or greater, a color may develop; however, such high levels of phenylketones are uncommon and are seldom present in patients with phenylketonuria.

Stability of Ketones. In urine, bacterial action will cause loss of acetoacetic acid. This may happen *in vivo* as well as *in vitro*. Acetone is lost at room temperature but not if kept in a closed container in a refrigerator. If a sample cannot be tested immediately, it should be refrigerated.

Reference or Normal Values

Depending on the methods used, total ketone bodies (as acetone) range from 1.7 to 42 mg/dl (Henry, 1964). According to Killander (1962), up to 2 mg acetoacetic acid/dl is normal.

LACTOSURIA

Lactose may appear in the urine late in normal pregnancy or during lactation.

Intestinal *lactase deficiency* is present in a large number of the population, particularly in Africa and Asia. Intolerance increases with age through childhood to adolescence.

In *intestinal disease*, lactase activity may be depressed earlier than the activity of other disaccharidases, e.g., maltase and sucrase. Patients with celiac disease, tropical sprue, and kwashiorkor are most affected.

Lactose intolerance in infancy may by associated with lactase deficiency and variable lactosuria or can occur as a result of a toxic effect of lactose when lactase is not deficient. In these children there are high levels of lactose in the urine associated with damage to the intestine. Renal tubular dysfunction and aminoaciduria are present.

Small amounts of disaccharides are normally excreted in the urine—about 50 mg in 24 hours. With intestinal damage the level will rise to 250 mg or more; and with high levels of sugars in the gut as in lactase deficiency, lactose will be absorbed and excreted unchanged in the urine.

Patients with malabsorption of carbohydrate have symptoms relative to the osmotic activity of the sugars in the gut. Cramping pain and fullness occur shortly after ingestion, and watery diarrhea follows. Bacteria metabolize the carbohydrate to form fatty acids, and the stool pH is lowered to less than 6.

Screening. Urine is tested with the glucose oxidase reagent strip and a copper reduction test. Lactosuria is not always present with lactose intolerance. A qualitative test (Rubner) may also be used.

Feces from infants and children is usually watery; if not, it is suspended in a small amount of water. A Clinitest[a] tablet test for reducing sugar is done using the supernatant of the centrifuged specimen. The watery specimen is smeared onto pH paper and the pH read. With lactose intolerance, reducing sugars may be present and the pH will be low (acid). The same results will be found when there is rapid intestinal transit time associated with infectious or other diarrheas.

The diagnosis of lactose intolerance is made by withdrawing lactose-containing foods. Lactase deficiency may be established by means of oral lactose tolerance tests with analysis of blood glucose levels (lactose splits to form glucose and galactose) at half hour intervals. Capillary blood may be used. Normal persons may give flat results with lactose loading.

An enzyme assay of a biopsy of the small intestine will provide a definitive diagnosis when necessary by measuring the amount of glucose released per gram wet weight from a 5 to 10 mg sample.

LACTOSE TEST (RUBNER, 1884). To 15 ml urine in a test tube, add 3 g lead acetate. Shake and filter. Boil filtrate, add 2 ml concentrated NH_4OH, and boil. Lactose will cause the formation of a brick red solution and then a red precipitate with clear supernatant. Glucose will cause a yellow solution and yellow precipitate.

Lactose should be confirmed by thin-layer chromatography.

MAPLE SYRUP URINE DISEASE

Branched-chain ketonuria is an extremely rare, inherited disease with early neurologic manifestations and episodes of hypoglycemia. Leucine, isoleucine, valine, and their corresponding keto-acids are elevated in the plasma and are excreted in the urine. The urine has an odor resembling maple syrup or caramelized sugar. The urinary keto-acids are demonstrable by the first week of life whereas with phenylketonuria the metabolites appear later. A screening test with dinitrophenyl hydrazine demonstrates keto-acids and their transformation into keto-acid phenylhydrazones. They are then separated by thin-layer (or paper) chromatography. A microbiologic blood screening test for the elevated amino acids is also available.

Dinitrophenylhydrazine Test. This test indicates the presence of keto amino acids in the urine. A positive result is, therefore, likely in phenylketonuria (phenylpyruvic acid); histidinemia (imidazole pyruvic acid); methionine malabsorption (Oasthouse syndrome) (α-ketobutyric acid). The test is positive with acetone (hyperglycinemia, isovaleric acidemia, and glycogen storage diseases Type 1, 3, 5, and 6) and with ketonuria due to other causes. A preliminary screening test for ketonuria should be done.

Reagents
1. 100 mg of 2-4-dinitrophenylhydrazine in 100 ml of 2 N HCl. The reagent should be stored in a brown bottle in the refrigerator.

Procedure
1. Reagents should be at room temperature.
2. Add 10 drops of reagent to 1 ml of clear urine.
3. After or within 10 minutes look for a yellow or chalky white precipitate to indicate a positive reaction.

MUCOPOLYSACCHARIDOSES

These are a diverse group of heritable diseases generally characterized by the storage in tissues of dermatan (a chondroitin) sulfate and heparin sulfate. These are mucopolysaccharides derived from fibroblasts and mast cells, respectively, located in connective tissue. In some of the diseases there is increased deposition of gangliosides in the brain (Dorfman, 1972).

The prototype of these diseases is Hurler's disease; the others have been classified into two to seven groups based on clinical and biochemical findings. In Hurler's disease large amounts of these mucopolysaccharides are excreted in urine; keratan sulfate is excreted in several of the other disorders.

In Hurler's disease, metachromatic staining of large granules of acid mucopolysaccharides in neutrophils, lymphocytes, and histiocytes, especially from the bone marrow, are demonstrated with toluidine blue.

Screening. The toluidine blue spot test and turbidity tests have been used. With the spot test, false negative results of 32 per cent were found by Carter (1968) when known patients were tested. The false positive rate in non-Hurler patients was 1.5 per cent.

A turbidity test using cetylpyridium chloride has been found reliable by Pennock (1970).

The acid albumin turbidity test of Dorfman (1958) may be used as a qualitative or semi-quantitative test. In this test, dialysed, buffered urine is mixed with albumin at an acid pH; a uniform turbidity is seen when acid mucopolysaccharides are present. This test has been more reliable than the spot test in detecting Hurler's disease (Carter, 1968; Pennock, 1970).

None of the screening tests will detect the keratosulfate excreted in Morquio's disease—group IV or in generalized gangliosidosis.

Reference Values. In adults, small amounts of chondroitin sulfates and heparin sulfates are excreted in the range of 10 mg/24 hours. Levels increase with rapid growth.

Procedure. (Berry and Spinlanger, 1960). The test is based on the metachromasia produced with the basic groups of the toluidine blue dye in the presence of large amounts of acid mucopolysaccharide. Further separation and identification of the mucopolysaccharide should be made by paper chromatography.

Equipment
1. Whatman filter paper No. 1. Micropipettes.
2. Control solution of chondroitin sulfate containing 0.1 mg/ml in distilled water.
3. Toluidine blue, 0.04 per cent in 1 M sodium acetate at pH 2. Use a certified buffer tablet.

Method
1. 5, 10, and 25 μl of urine are placed in separate spots on a piece of filter paper. Each spot should be allowed to dry before the next is made. A normal urine may be spotted for comparison.
2. 5 μl of the standard chondroitin sulfate solution is applied separately and dried.
3. The dry paper is dipped into the toluidine blue solution for 1 minute.
4. Rinse the paper in 95 per cent alcohol 2 or 3 times. Dry, then examine.

Result. Urine from children with Hurler's syndrome will show a purple spot against a blue background, as will the standard chondroitin sulfate. Normal urine is blue.

Comment. The pH of 2 is important in achieving a good result. Control must be run for comparison. False positive results were obtained in most newborn infants, but after 2 weeks of age, only 0.2 per cent of the normal infants gave positive results (Berry, 1960). Heparin may give false positive results.

MELANIN

Melanin is a pigment derived from tyrosine, which is normally present in hair and skin and in the eye.

Patients with widespread melanotic tumors excrete in the urine a colorless precursor, a conjugate of 5,6-dihydroxyindole, which pol-

Table 17–12. FERRIC CHLORIDE TEST IN URINE*

SUBSTANCE OR DISEASE	COLOR CHANGE
Acetoacetic acid	Red or red-brown
Bilirubin	Blue-green
Homogentisic acid	Blue or green; fades quickly
o-Hydroxyphenylacetic acid	Mauve
o-Hydroxyphenylpyruvic acid	Red-brown; turns to green or blue then fades to mauve
p-Hydroxyphenylpyruvic acid	Green; fades in seconds
Imidazolepyruvic acid	Green or blue-green
α-Ketobutyric acid	Purple; fades to red-brown
Maple-syrup urine disease	Blue
Melanin	Gray precipitate; turns black
Phenylpyruvic acid	Green or blue-green; fades to yellow
Pyruvic acid	Deep gold-yellow or green
Xanthurenic acid	Deep green; later brown
Drugs	
Aminosalicylic acid	red-brown
Antipyrines and acetophenetidines	Red
Cyanates	Red
Phenol derivatives	Violet
Phenothiazine derivatives	Purple-pink
Salicylates	Stable purple

*Modified from Henry, R. J.: Clinical Chemistry: Principles and Techniques. New York, Harper & Row, Publishers, 1964.

ymerizes into a dark pigment after about 24 hours at room temperature.

Screening tests for melanin should be made on fresh specimens of urine. If a small amount of melanogen is present, it may be extracted by evaporation of the urine over a water bath followed by repeated washings until clear with absolute methyl alcohol. Melanin is left in the residue and is then extracted with acidified (2 drops concentrated HCl per 100 ml) methyl alcohol. Melanin is then precipitated by ether and may be recovered after centrifugation.

Ferric chloride, Ehrlich's aldehyde reagent, and nitroprusside will give non-specific color reactions with melanin; chromatography has been used to separate out and identify melanin.

Ferric Chloride Test for Melanin

Procedure. To 5 ml urine in a test tube, add 1 ml 10 per cent $FeCl_3$ in 10 per cent HCl. A gray or black precipitate will form if positive. The HCl prevents phosphate precipitation. Melanogen is oxidized to melanin. Homogentisic acid, which also causes a dark color in urine, gives a transient blue-green color with ferric chloride (see Table 17–12).

Nitroprusside Test for Melanin

Procedure. To 2 ml urine in a test tube, add 3 to 4 drops fresh solution of sodium nitroprusside (shake a few crystals in 10 ml water). Add 2 drops of 10 per cent NaOH to make the solution alkaline. Shake. A red color will develop if acetone, creatinine, or melanin is present. Acidify with 2 drops of glacial acetic acid. Small amounts of melanogen cause a green color; larger amounts cause blue, then black. Acetone causes a purple color and creatinine an amber color (Beeler, 1961).

MYOGLOBINURIA

When there is acute destruction of muscle fibers, myoglobin is released, rapidly cleared from the blood, and excreted in the urine. If large amounts of myoglobin are presented to the kidney, anuria may result from renal damage (see Table 17–3, p. 575).

Trauma to muscle, such as crushing or excessive exertion, will release myoglobin. This may occur with convulsions (see Table 17–3).

Familial myoglobinuria (Meyer-Betz disease) in which exertion or infection precipitates muscle fiber damage, polymyositis, alcoholic polymyopathy, and McArdle's disease cause myoglobinemia and myoglobinuria.

Hyperthermia and malignant hyperthermia

Table 17-13. PORPHYRIAS: URINARY FINDINGS AND OTHER SPECIAL DETERMINATIONS*

| PORPHYRIAS | URINARY FINDINGS | | SPECIAL DETERMINATIONS |
	Elevated	Normal	
Congenital Erythropoietic porphyria, Extreme photosensitivity Hemolytic anemia	UP↑↑CP Pink-brown, fluctuates	PBG ALA	Red cell UP↑↑CP, PP (fluoresce) Feces CP↑
Erythropoietic protoporphyria Skin lesions		PBG ALA UP CP	Red cell PP↑fluoresce Feces PP↑↑may fluoresce
Hepatic—inherited Acute intermittent porphyria Abdominal pain, drug induced No skin lesions	PBG↑ALA PBG→UP on standing→ dark color	UP CP var.	
Porphyria variegata (cutanea tarda, S. African) Photosensitivity, skin lesions Acute abdominal pain, drug ppt.	PBG ALA with acute attack CP	variable	Feces UP CP↑, PP↑↑
Hereditary coproporphyria Photosensitivity Acute abdominal pain, drug ppt.	CP PBG ALA in acute attack	PBG ALA var.	Feces CP↑↑ UP↑
Hepatic—acquired (cutaneous, toxic) Liver disease, etc. Photosensitivity	UP↑CP Pink-brown	PBG ALA var.	Feces UP, CP↑
Lead poisoning	CP ALA	PBG UP var.	Red cell PP↑↑ CP↑

*CP = Coproporphyrin   PP = Protoporphyrin
UP = Uroporphyrin   var. = Variable
PBG = Porphobilinogen   ↑ = Degree increase
ALA = Delta-aminolevulinic acid

with anesthesia in susceptible persons cause destruction of muscle fibers. Infarction of muscle will also cause myoglobinuria, and this has been shown with large skeletal muscles and with cardiac muscle.

Hemoglobin and myoglobin

The distinction between hemoglobinuria and myoglobinuria is difficult to make on examination of the urine. In both cases, the urine is dark red or brown and red cells are seen in the sediment.

Screening. The reagent strip test for blood is positive with hemoglobin and myoglobin. If serum can be examined, it will often be pink with hemoglobinemia but a normal color with myoglobinemia because this pigment is cleared so rapidly. None of the qualitative

tests have been satisfactory in separating myoglobin and hemoglobin. The salt precipitation method of Blondheim has been used, as have spectroscopic methods.

Immunochemical tests with antisera to human myoglobin appear to be promising. These require a human myoglobin standard from muscle or from urine containing myoglobin and an antiserum that does not cross-react with hemoglobin (Kagen, 1967).

Procedure (Blondheim, 1958)

1. Use a fresh morning urine specimen or one voided after exercise. Observe the color of urine. Characteristically, urine with myoglobinuria is red when fresh and turns brown on standing.

2. Mix 1 ml of urine and 3 ml of 3 per cent sulfosalicylic acid. Filter. If the pigment is precipitated, it is a protein. If the filtrate is a normal color, no abnormal non-protein pigment is present. (*Note:*

the heat + acetic acid test does not precipitate myoglobin or hemoglobin.)

3. To 5 ml of urine in a test tube, add 2.8 g of ammonium sulfate. Dissolve by mixing. The urine is now 80 per cent saturated with ammonium sulfate. This is optimum for precipitation of hemoglobin. Filter or centrifuge. If the supernatant shows a normal color, the precipitated pigment is hemoglobin. If the supernatant fluid is colored, this is presumptive evidence of myoglobin.

PENTOSURIA

Essential pentosuria is a rare benign disorder resulting from reduced activity of xylitol dehydrogenase. This results in the excretion of large amounts of L-xylulose in the urine, with losses in the range of 1 to 4 g in 24 hours. The constant excretion of xylulose will give a persistent positive copper reduction test and patients may mistakenly be labeled as diabetic.

Alimentary pentosuria can occur following the ingestion of large amounts of certain fruits; L-xylose and L-arabinose are excreted in small amounts.

Benedict's copper reduction test is positive and the glucose oxidase test negative in pentosuria. At concentrations of 250 to 300 mg/dl, L-xylulose will reduce Benedict's qualitative reagent at 50° C. (water bath) within 10 minutes or at room temperature in several hours. Use 1 ml urine and 5 ml Benedict's solution. Like fructose, it is a stronger reducing agent than glucose or lactose, but the time for reduction depends on the amount of sugar present. Known control sugar solutions should be run.

L-xylulose can be readily separated from other sugars by paper or thin-layer chromatography. Red blood cells are used to measure the activity of xylitol dehydrogenase.

Reference Values. About 60 mg of L-xylulose in 24 hours is excreted.

PHENOTHIAZINE DRUGS IN URINE

Screening Test. Phenothiazine drugs are used in the treatment of psychiatric disorders. The average daily urinary excretion is about one-half of the daily intake; some continues to be excreted over a period of time after therapy has ceased. The screening test has been used to monitor the amount of drug ingested (or not ingested) by the patient. For identification of the drug, spectrophotometric methods are used. Refer to Chapter 15, p. 495.

Procedure (Forrest, 1961). Mix 1 ml urine in a test tube with 1 ml of ferric chloride reagent (5 ml $FeCl_3$ 5 per cent in water, 45 ml perchloric acid 20 per cent, and 50 ml nitric acid 50 per cent).

Read immediately. Disregard colors appearing after 10 seconds.

Interpretation. Shades of pink to purple indicate dosage levels of 20 to 2000 mg/day. False negative results of up to 25 per cent have been reported (Brownstein, 1966). These may be due to low dose levels, overhydration, and the lack of sensitivity of some related drugs. Prochlorperazine, trifluoperazine, perphenazine, and thioridazine (Mellaril) are not as sensitive as chlorpromazine.

False positive results may be seen when high doses of para-aminosalicylic acid are ingested or with estrogens or phenylketonuria. Indican may cause a purple color. Aspirin does not produce false positive reactions. (Phenothiazine drugs may cause positive reactions in other urine tests—for urobilinogen, ferric chloride test, etc. (Young, 1975).

PHENYLKETONURIA

Phenylketonuria is an autosomal recessive inherited disease associated with an absence of active liver enzyme, phenylalanine hydroxylase. Because dietary L-phenylalanine is not converted to tyrosine, phenylalanine and other metabolites accumulate. Both sexes are affected equally, with an incidence of about 1 in 20,000 with most cases stemming from Northern European stock. There is a higher incidence in Celtic populations. In this disease there is an accumulation of normal metabolites in abnormal amounts. Plasma phenylalanine and phenylpyruvic acid levels are elevated; urinary phenylpyruvic acid (highest), phenylacetic acid, and phenylalanine are increased. Urinary indole acetic acid and other indoles arising from altered tryptophan metabolism and indican (an indole) are also increased. The excretion of 5-hydroxy indoleacetic acid is diminished, paralleling the low level of serum 5-hydroxytryptamine.

Ferric Chloride Test. The ferric chloride test is non-specific. It will give color reactions with several amino acid disorders, with other metabolites, and with drugs. The ferric ion chelates with the enol grouping and will produce color formation with keto acids from corresponding amino acids. Alcaptonuria (homogentisic acid), histidinemia, tyrosinosis, oasthouse urine disease, and maple syrup urine disease may cause color reaction in urine.

Procedure. Add 1 drop of 1 N H_2SO_4 to 1 ml of urine in a test tube (also to a positive control). Add 2 drops of $FeCl_3 \cdot 6H_2O$ solution (10 g/100 ml water) and mix. Observe the color. A green or grey-green color should be observed over a period of 2 minutes. It will fade slowly. The ferric chloride solution is kept in a brown bottle and refrigerated.

Controls. Positive specimens can be frozen in aliquots. Positive controls are available, e.g., QC-U (General Diagnostics).

Sensitivity. The test is positive for phenylpyruvic acid when the plasma level of phenylalanine exceeds 15 mg/100 ml. About 10 mg/100 ml phenylpyruvic acid is detected. Urine must be fresh.

Specificity. Since colored compounds occur with many urinary metabolites, this test should be regarded as a preliminary screening procedure. Phosphate in urine may interfere with the test and a modified test using a phosphate precipitating reagent (magnesium) has been advocated (Henry, 1964). Rapidly fading blue-green colors may be seen with homogentisic acid or *p*-hydroxy phenylpyruvic acid (tyrosinosis). Imidazole pyruvic acid will give a green color (histidinemia), but this is very rare. Bilirubin, if present, may cause a blue-green color. Ketones, as acetoacetate, will form a red to red brown color. It is unlikely that drugs would be present in specimens used for screening for inherited disease, but salicylates (red-purple), phenothiazines, and levo-dopa (brown) are known to interfere with the test (Hansten, 1975; Wirth, 1965). (Table 17-12, p. 597.)

Reagent Strip Test. Phenistix[a] reagent strips contain ferric ammonium sulfate, magnesium sulfate, and cyclohexylsulfamic acid. The cyclohexylsulfamic acid provides optimum acidity for the reaction.

Procedure. Dip the reagent-impregnated portion of the strip into the urine and remove immediately or press it against a wet diaper. At 30 seconds compare the color of the dipped end of the strip with the color chart provided. A positive test is a gray to gray-green color. Report as positive or negative.

Sensitivity. 5 to 10 mg per 100 ml.

Specificity. Beta-imidazolepyruvic acid is the only substance other than phenylpyruvic acid that gives the gray-green with reagent strip at 30 seconds. It is excreted in the urine in a rare disorder of children—deficiency of the enzyme histidine alpha-deaminase.

Salicylates and metabolites of phenothiazine derivatives may cause a pink to purple color. High concentrations of bilirubin in the urine may alter the color reaction with phenylpyruvic acid.

Alkaline urines which are old and decomposed will interfere with the color reactions. Fresh or refrigerated specimens should be used.

PORPHYRINS

A description of the chemistry and synthesis of porphyrins with clinical pathologic correlation and analytical techniques is given in Chapter 10. A classification of the disorders of porphyrin metabolism is shown on page 274 (Table 10-1). However, a *summary of the synthesis of porphyrins* with disease correlations is shown below and in Figure 10-9, p. 273.

1. ALA = delta amino levulinic acid.
2. PBG = porphobilinogen.
3. URO'GEN = uroporphyrinogen; URO (UP) = uroporphyrin.
4. COPRO'GEN = coproporphyrinogen; COPRO (CP) = coproporphyrin.
5. PROTO (PP) = protoporphyrin.

Hepatic Porphyrias {
1 & 2 increase in acute intermittent porphyria.
3 & 4 increase in acute attack in acquired porphyria cutanea tarda.
1, 2, 3, & 4 increase in acute attack in hereditary coproporphyria.
1, 2, 3, 4, & 5 increase in acute attack in porphyria variegata.

Erythroid Porphyrias {
3 & 4 increase in congenital erythropoietic porphyria.
5 increases in erythropoietic protoporphyria in feces and red cells.

The patterns of excretion of the various porphyrins vary with the different diseases (Table 17-13 and Table 10-2, p. 276). These and the clinical findings help establish the diagnosis. Skin photosensitivity and skin lesions fre-

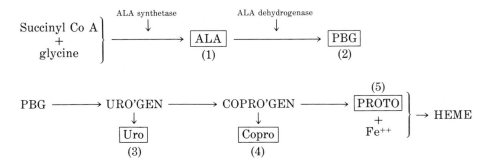

quently accompany high levels of porphyrins. The one entity without skin lesions is acute intermittent porphyria. In patients presenting with neurologic disease and acute abdominal pain—the hepatic group—there is increased production and excretion of amino levulinic acid (ALA) and porphobilinogen during the acute porphyric attack. There is probably increased activity of ALA synthetase and subsequent increased production of the precursors. Exacerbations of the hepatic diseases are precipitated by drugs known to induce liver enzyme activity, e.g., barbiturates and certain steroids.

Screening tests. In the patient suspected of having an acute porphyric attack, porphobilinogen is sought in a urine specimen using the Watson-Schwartz test (p. 602). Porphobilinogen is insoluble in chloroform or butanol and remains in the aqueous phase of the separation. The Hoesch test is used as a confirmatory test. During the acute attack, high levels of porphobilinogen are excreted, but the urine is not always colored because about 500 μg/l of porphyrins can be present without causing a red-purple color (Henry, 1974).

Uroporphyrin and coproporphyrin are detected by fluorescence. An orange-red fluorescence is seen if the specimen is placed near an ultraviolet light source. The porphyrins are excreted in most of the porphyrias and in lead poisoning (Table 17-13 and Table 10-2, p. 276). Coproporphyrin and uroporphyrin can also be separated by thin-layer chromatography or by extraction and fluorometry.

Screening tests together with the clinical findings will indicate whether quantitative tests should be done. These are usually performed by reference or research laboratories.

The urine specimen for *porphobilinogen* should be kept at a near neutral pH (between 6 and 7) and protected from light. Hydrochloric acid may be used to acidify the specimen. Frozen specimens are fairly stable. *Delta amino levulinic acid* is not stable unless the urine is acidic. Acidification with HCl is effective. These substances are detected by eluting from different columns and reacting with Ehrlich's reagent.

Porphyrins (uro- and coproporphyrin) can be quantitated if necessary. Urine specimens are collected in a dark container containing 5 g sodium carbonate for a 24-hour specimen to give a concentration of 0.1 per cent sodium carbonate. Porphyrins are separated by column elution and quantitated fluorometrically. Note that 24-hour urine collections for the porphy-

rins are not suitable for porphobilinogen or ALA because of the alkalinity.

Fecal porphyrins can be qualitatively estimated by acid extraction and UV light or quantitated. In erythropoietic protoporphyria, the fecal specimen may fluoresce owing to high protoporphyrin levels.

Red cells may show fluorescence when an unstained smear is examined microscopically. The nucleated bone marrow red cells give greater fluorescence. Total porphyrins or protoporphyrins and coproporphyrins can be quantitated by acid extraction of the cells and fluorometry. For details of methods, see Henry (1974).

In *lead poisoning*, blood and urinary lead levels, delta amino levulinic acid levels in serum and urine, and coproporphyrin levels in urine are all used to help make a diagnosis. The level of ALA dehydrogenase in red cells is decreased and it is possible to measure this by determining the conversion of ALA to porphobilinogen.

Reference Values

ALA (amino levulinic acid)	1.5–7.5 mg/24 hr (11.2–55.2 mol/24 hr)
PBG (porphobilinogen)	<1.0 mg/24 hr (<4.4 mol/24 hr)
Coproporphyrin	50–160 μg/24 hr (0.075–0.24 mol/24 hr)
Uroporphyrin	10–30 μg/24 hr (10–30 μg/24 hr)

Procedure

The urine is acidified and the extracted porphyrin exposed to ultraviolet light.

1. Place 5 ml urine in a glass centrifuge tube. Add 3 ml of a mixture of glacial acetic acid 1 part with 4 parts of ethyl acetate.

2. Shake and allow to separate. Centrifuging will accelerate the separation.

3. Using a Wood's lamp, observe the upper layer for fluorescence. Inspect the tube in a dark room with ultraviolet reflected light. A lavender to violet color indicates the presence of porphyrins; pink to red fluorescence indicates higher levels of porphyrin. Pale blue with no pink color is negative. Normal urine may fluoresce blue.

To increase the sensitivity of the test and remove interfering drug metabolites, transfer the upper layer to a glass tube and acidify with 0.5 ml of 3 M HCl (25 ml concentrated HCl diluted to 100 ml with water). Shake. Porphyrins are extracted into the lower aqueous layer and will give a red-orange fluorescence (Haining, 1969).

An alternative screening method utilizes an anion exchange resin column (Dowex column available from Bio Rad Laboratories, Richmond, Cal.). Porphyrins are adsorbed, eluted, and exposed to fluorescent light. This method removes interfering substances and is similar in principle to quantitative methods.

A qualitative screening procedure for porphobilinogen is described with concurrent method for urobilinogen on page 607.

Porphobilinogen in Urine—Hoesch Test. The Hoesch test is based on the inverse Ehrlich's reaction (i.e., of maintaining an acid solution by adding a small urine volume to a relatively large reagent volume) eliminating the problem of urobilinogen reaction. The sensitivity is similar to the Watson-Schwartz test and the reaction is specific for porphobilinogen (see Lamon, 1974; Hoesch, 1947).

REAGENT

20 g para-dimethylaminobenzaldehyde diluted to 1000 ml with HCl, 6 mol/liter (50 per cent—1:2 dilution of the concentrated HCl). It is stable for nine months on shelf in a clear glass container.

PROCEDURE

Pour approximately 2 ml of the reagent in a test tube. Add 2 drops of fresh urine to the reagent. Examine for an instantaneous cherry red color predominantly on the top of the solution, but throughout the tube on brief agitation. Report as positive or negative for porphobilinogen.

PROTEINURIA

Normally there is a scant amount of protein in urine up to about 150 mg/24 hr or 20 mg/dl.

Healthy persons may exceed these levels during exercise or with dehydration. Proteinuria can occur in the absence of urinary tract disease with hemorrhage or salt depletion and in febrile illnesses. These may be related to dehydration and relative renal ischemia.

In renal disease, the protein lost in greatest amount is usually albumin. In glomerular damage, larger proteins tend to appear in the filtrate and are not reabsorbed by tubules. Globulins are excreted with macroglobulinemia and multiple myeloma and amyloidosis and, depending on the amount of renal damage, may be present without much albumin.

With tubular damage, low molecular weight proteins like lysozyme that are normally reabsorbed are lost in the urine along with globulins. This is called tubular proteinuria. The amount of protein lost is usually less than 2 g/24 hr, and it occurs with renal tubular acidosis, the Fanconi syndrome, pyelonephritis, and medullary cystic disease. Tubular proteinuria may be missed by the reagent strip test because of the absence of albumin but will be detected by acid precipitation tests.

Nephrotic syndrome is diagnosed when the protein excretion is greater than 3.5 g/sq m/day. The type of protein excreted may help elucidate the cause. When only albumin or smaller proteins are present, the proteinuria is called selective. This occurs with lipoid nephrosis and generally has a better prognosis. As larger proteins appear, the proteinuria is non-selective, indicating greater morphologic changes.

Heavy Proteinuria (>4 g/day). Heavy proteinuria is characteristically seen with the nephrotic syndrome. It may also be found in acute and chronic glomerulonephritis, lupus nephritis, amyloid disease, and severe venous congestion of the kidney.

Moderate Proteinuria (0.5 to 4 g/day). Moderate proteinuria may be found in a large number of renal diseases, including those mentioned above and nephrosclerosis, pyelonephritis with hypertension (also multiple myeloma, diabetic nephropathy, pre-eclampsia of pregnancy, and a variety of toxic nephropathies, including radiation nephritis).

Minimal Proteinuria (<0.5 g/day). Minimal proteinuria may be noted in chronic pyelonephritis, in which it may be intermittent, and in relatively inactive phases of glomerular diseases. It is also seen with polycystic kidney disease and in renal tubular diseases. Minimal proteinuria is present in "benign" postural proteinurias.

Proteinuria may be *absent* in phases of acute pyelonephritis, in chronic pyelonephritis, and in the presence of obstructive nephropathy, kidney stones, kidney tumors, and congenital malformations.

Postural Proteinuria. Postural proteinuria (orthostatic) occurs in 3 to 5 per cent of healthy young adults. In these persons, proteinuria is found during the day but not at night when a recumbent position is assumed. Persistent proteinuria may develop in some of these healthy subjects at a later date, and renal biopsies have shown abnormalities of the glomerulus in a few cases (Robinson, 1961). Proteinuria is apparently related to an exaggerated lordotic position and may result from renal congestion or ischemia. The total daily excretion of protein rarely exceeds 1 g. In most instances, no other evidence of renal disease develops.

To evaluate the possibility of postural proteinuria, the patient is instructed to empty his bladder upon going to bed in the evening and to discard the specimen. Immediately upon rising in the morning, the patient voids and saves this specimen. After 2 hours of standing and walking about, the patient voids again and saves the specimen. The two urine specimens are tested for protein. If the first is negative and the second positive, the patient may have postural proteinuria. Frequent examination of the patient should be made to re-evaluate this condition.

Functional Proteinuria. Functional proteinuria may be associated with fever, exposure to cold, emotional stress, or severe and unaccustomed exercise. Proteinuria of this type is transient and apparently benign, although it may persist for up to three days after severe exercise.

Measurement of Proteinuria. Qualitative, semiquantitative, and quantitative methods are available for analysis of protein in urine. Since the positive result of a screening test may have grave significance, it is important to be able to confirm it by a second different method.

Screening Tests for Proteinuria. Screening tests should not be too sensitive, as they are required to differentiate normal protein excretion from abnormal and therefore should not detect less than about 8 to 10 mg/dl in a normal adult with a normal rate of urine flow. It should be noted that a very dilute random specimen of urine may have a falsely low protein value. Cells and casts can be found in the urine in significant numbers when the protein screening test is negative. In an analysis of 3152 urine specimens submitted for routine analysis in a tertiary care institution (approximately one third outpatient), 67 per cent had negative protein and 81.1 per cent had negative and trace protein results. Of the *negative protein* specimens, 2.4 per cent had 3 to 6 rbc/hpf and 2.2 per cent 6 to 30 rbc/hpf; 5 per cent had 4 to 15 wbc/hpf, and 1.5 per cent had 15 to 50 wbc/hpf; 4 per cent had positive casts (Bradley, 1978).

In the simplest screening test a reagent strip is used. This is a colorimetric test that employs the principle of protein error of a pH indicator: bromphenol blue is yellow at pH 3, but with protein present, the color becomes green-blue. The sensitivity of the test is about 20 to 30 mg/dl of albumin (Free, 1957b), and the results are graded as trace and 1 through 4+. The test material is not as sensitive to globulins as to albumin. Binding of the indicator dyes to proteins is highly pH-dependent. Only albumin binds bromphenol blue and tetrabromophenol-phthalein between pH 5 and 7. At a lower pH 3, albumin predominates in binding bromphenol blue. Gamma globulin and Bence Jones protein are not detected (Bowie, 1977).

A comparison of reagent strips and the sulfosalicylic acid method shows that with reagent strips accurate results are obtained only when albumin is measured. Changes in urinary concentration affect the reagent strip results but not the sulfosalicylic acid method. High salt levels lower the reagent strip result (Gyure, 1977).

Although not as sensitive as precipitation tests, the reagent strip has the advantage of avoiding false positive reactions with organic iodides such as those used in renal pyelography and tolbutamides or other drugs (Table 17-14).

Most other qualitative screening tests rely on a protein precipitation, e.g., with heat and acetic acid, with nitric acid, and with sulfosalicylic and trichloroacetic acids. Probably the best standard test for routine screening of proteinuria is the acetic acid test. This test is based on the heat coagulation properties of albumin and globulin at pH 4 to 5 in the presence of inorganic salt. Acetic acid is used to produce the required pH, and in Purdy's modification (Purdy, 1900), sodium chloride provides the ionic strength needed to dilute urines. This method will also precipitate globulins and proteoses and has a sensitivity of 5 to 10 mg/dl (Davidsohn, 1974).

Sulfosalicylic and trichloroacetic acids are used to precipitate protein in the cold and are used as satisfactory and convenient screening tests. The sensitivity may be as low as 0.25 mg/dl, depending on the techniques used.

Because of a lack of sensitivity of the reagent

Table 17-14. FALSE POSITIVE AND FALSE NEGATIVE REACTIONS IN TESTS FOR PROTEINURIA

URINARY CONSTITUENTS	BROMPHENOL REAGENT STRIP	SULFOSALICYLIC ACID	HEAT AND ACETIC ACID
Radiographic contrast media (Diatrizoate)	No effect	May cause false pos.	May cause false pos.
Tolbutamide metabolities	No effect	May cause false pos.	May cause false pos.
Penicillins (massive doses)	No effect	May cause false pos.	May cause false pos.
Sulfisoxazole metabolites (sulfonamide)	No effect	May cause false pos.	May cause false pos.
Highly buffered alkaline urine	May cause false pos.	May cause false neg.	May cause false neg.
Quaternary ammonium compounds (alters pH)	May cause false pos.	No effect	No effect
Detergents (Tergitol) (high concentration)	May cause false	False neg.	–
High salt concentration	May cause false neg.	No effect	No effect

strip to globulins, it may be necessary to use an acid precipitation test for screening purposes. This will depend on the patient population and the diseases being screened.

SULFOSALICYLIC ACID METHOD—QUALITATIVE. Several acids have been used to precipitate protein: nitric, trichloroacetic, acetic (with heat), and sulfosalicylic. All produce a turbidity. The sulfosalicylic acid method is also used for quantitative protein in 24-hour specimens. Different concentrations and proportions of sulfosalicylic acid have been used in the qualitative test and provide different ranges of results. Using 1 ml of urine and 3 ml of 3 per cent sulfosalicylic acid solution, a lower range of protein may be quantitatively differentiated, about 10 to 500 mg/dl.

Specimens should be clear and centrifuged before use.

Procedure. To approximately 3 ml of urine aliquot (about 1 inch) in a 16 by 125 mm test tube, add an equal amount of 3 per cent sulfosalicylic acid (SSA). Invert to mix. Let stand exactly 10 minutes. Invert again. Using ordinary room light (not a lamp), observe the degree of precipitation and grade the results according to the following descriptions:

Negative	No turbidity, or no increase in turbidity (approximately 0.005 g/dl or less)*
Trace	Barely perceptible turbidity (approximately 0.010 g/dl)
1+	Distinct turbidity, but no discrete granulation (approximately 0.050 g/dl)
2+	Turbidity with granulation, but no flocculation (approximately 0.20 g/dl)
3+	Turbidity with granulation and flocculation (approximately 0.5 g/dl)
4+	Clumps of precipitated protein, or solid precipitate (approximately 1.0 g/dl or more)

Sensitivity. About 0.005 to 0.010 g/dl (5 to 10 mg/dl). High levels of detergents may decrease the result.

Specificity. Specific for albumin, globulins, glucoproteins, and Bence Jones protein. When *radiographic dye* is present, the specific gravity is usually >1.035 and the precipitate will increase on standing. Another specimen should be tested. However, the effects of the media may persist up to 3 days. A reagent strip test may be substituted or the heat and acetic acid test used. In the acetic acid test, radiographic contrast media will clear with heat, whereas protein will increase.

SULFOSALICYLIC ACID TABLET TEST REAGENT (BUMINTEST[a]). The tablets contain sulfosalicylic acid and sodium bicarbonate. These are dissolved

in deionized water to make a 5 per cent stable solution.

Semiquantitative and Quantitative Methods. Often more useful information may be obtained by quantitatively analyzing the amount of protein excreted over a 24-hour period than is available from a random specimen of urine.

In 1874 Esbach developed a method of urinary protein precipitation in which picric acid was used and by which the amount of precipitated protein could be estimated by volume. The Esbach method, even with modifications, is much less precise and accurate than the turbidimetric methods (Lewis, 1961). It should be used only in a semiquantitative fashion to give an estimate of protein present; and even in this case, unless the urine is acidified before precipitation, results will often be erroneous.

Sulfosalicylic acid and trichloroacetic acid are commonly used as precipitants; the resultant turbidity is measured by a photometer or nephelometer, or by eye, and compared with known standards. With sulfosalicylic acid, the turbidity produced with albumin is 2.4 times that produced with globulin (Henry, 1956). Polypeptides, proteoses, and Bence Jones proteins are also precipitated. Exton's reagent contains sulfosalicylic acid, sodium sulfate, and an indicator—bromphenol blue. This produces a yellow turbidity that is usually compared with a set of standard tubes and provides an estimate of the amount of protein present (Exton, 1925). Trichloroacetic acid is a protein precipitant that causes gamma globulin to be precipitated with greater turbidity than albumin. However, the difference is not marked (Henry, 1956). More precise measurements especially suitable for small amounts of protein are available. In these tests the trichloroacetic acid precipitate may be dissolved in sodium hydroxide and measured by use of the biuret reaction (Kibrick, 1958). The biuret test as used for serum proteins is not sensitive enough to use as a test for proteinuria.

In routine clinical practice, quantitative measurement of protein by the turbidimetric procedure with sulfosalicylic acid as the precipitant is satisfactory as follows:

SULFOSALICYLIC ACID TURBIDITY METHOD

Principle. Sulfosalicylic acid precipitates protein in urine with a turbidity that is approximately proportional to the concentration of protein in a solution. The turbidity may be measured with a photometer.

Reagents

1. Sulfosalicylic acid solution 3 per cent w/v in distilled water.

---

*These values were quantitated by TCA (trichloracetic acid) biuret method with bovine albumin standard solutions.

2. 1.25 per cent HCl.

Procedure

1. Centrifuge an aliquot of a well-mixed measured 24-hour collection of urine, and use the supernatant for determination.

2. Pipette into Coleman cuvettes:

Unknown	*Blank*
	(for *each* patient)
2 ml urine	2 ml urine
8 ml sulfosalicylic	
acid solution	8 ml HCl

3. Mix by inversion and let stand 5 minutes before reading.

4. Read in a spectrophotometer at 500 mμ, using the blank to set the transmittance at 100 per cent.

5. Read the values from a calibration chart. If greater than 140 mg/dl, repeat with 1:10 dilution with normal saline.

Preparation of Standard Curve. A standard solution with a known amount of protein (Versatol, 7 gm/dl or a Bovine Albumin Standard) is used in several dilutions. A normal serum of known protein concentration may be used.

1. Add 5 ml distilled water to a vial of protein standard and swirl gently until well mixed. Let stand 30 minutes, then dilute 1:50 with 0.85 per cent NaCl to make a solution containing 140 mg/dl.

2. Set up a series of test tubes numbered 1 through 7 and add the following:

TUBE NO.	PROTEIN SOLUTION	0.85% NACL	PROTEIN (MG/DL)
1	4.5 ml	1.5 ml	105
2	3.0 ml	3.0 ml	70
3	2.4 ml	3.6 ml	56
4	1.5 ml	4.5 ml	35
5	0.9 ml	5.1 ml	21
6	0.3 ml	5.7 ml	7
7	0.0 ml	6.0 ml	0

3. Read each tube as an unknown, using tube 7 as blank, and plot results on semilog paper.

Interpretation. Report result as mg/dl of urine, or mg or g/24-hour volume of urine. Average normal excretion of protein is about 2 to 8 mg/dl, or up to 150 mg in 24 hours (see p. 602).

Comment. Each acidified urine is used as its own blank to offset the effects of urinary pigments. Sulfosalicylic acid precipitates urinary proteose, polypeptides, and Bence Jones protein in addition to albumin and globulin.

Bence Jones Proteinuria (Bence Jones, 1848).

The presence of Bence Jones globulin is indicated by a single sharp peak in the globulin region on paper electrophoresis. Bence Jones globulin represents either the kappa or lambda immunoglobulin light chain. Bence Jones proteinuria is associated with multiple myeloma, macroglobulinemia, and malignant lymphomas. The incidence of Bence Jones proteinuria in multiple myeloma has been estimated as 50 to 80 per cent; however, its demonstration depends greatly on the technique used.

Excretion of Bence Jones protein in large amounts causes the tubular cells to become degenerated because of the high levels of protein reabsorbed. Inclusions may form in the cells. Desquamated cells form casts in the tubular lumen. With renal failure, less protein is reabsorbed and more Bence Jones protein and other proteins appear in the urine. The damaged kidney is sometimes called a myeloma kidney.

MEASUREMENT OF BENCE JONES PROTEIN. Globulins are not sensitive to the reagent strip test for protein, which screens predominantly for albumin (Bowie, 1977). Many techniques have been proposed, most of them based on the unusual heat solubility properties of Bence Jones protein. This protein precipitates at temperatures between 40° and 60°C. and redissolves again near 100°C. Other tests depend on precipitation in the cold with salts, ammonium sulfate, and acids.

In the presence of marked Bence Jones proteinuria, most tests yield positive results. When only a small amount of Bence Jones protein is present, or when other globulins are also present, results may be doubtful. With proper pH control and salt concentration, precipitation may be achieved at levels of about 30 mg/dl (Putnam, 1959). False positive reactions are seen when other globulins are precipitated by acetic acid in the heat precipitation method or because of clearing due to acid hydrolysis in the sulfosalicylic acid heat test. A false negative reaction may occur if the Bence Jones protein is too concentrated and the precipitate does not redissolve on boiling (Naumann, 1965).

The best method for detection of Bence Jones protein in urine is by protein electrophoresis, when a homogeneous band in the globulin region is seen on paper or cellulose acetate. For electrophoretic analysis, urine needs to be concentrated; this is usually accomplished by dialysis in cellophane tubing or by vacuum dialysis.

BENCE JONES PROTEIN—THERMAL METHOD. The qualitative sulfosalicylic acid test for urine protein is performed first; it is negative if no detectable Bence Jones protein is present.

Reagent. Acetate buffer, pH 4.9, 2 M. Place 17.5 g sodium acetate trihydrate in a 100 ml volumetric flask, add 4.1 ml glacial acetic acid, and add water to 100 ml.

Procedure

1. Place 4 ml clear urine in a test tube (centrifuge or filter urine if turbid). Add 1 ml acetate buffer and mix. Final pH should be 4.9 ± 0.1.

2. Heat for 15 minutes in a 56°C. water bath. Any precipitation is indicative of Bence Jones protein.

3. If there is a turbidity or precipitate, heat the same tube in a boiling water bath for 3 minutes and observe for any *decrease* in the amount of

precipitate or turbidity. Bence Jones protein will redissolve at 100°C.

4. An increase in turbidity or precipitate on boiling indicates the presence of albumin and globulin. This will mask any dissolving Bence Jones protein. Filter the contents of the tube taken directly from the boiling water, and observe the filtrate. If it is clear, becomes cloudy as it cools, and then becomes clear again at room temperature, the test is positive for Bence Jones protein.

Comment. A heavy precipitate of Bence Jones protein at 56°C. may not redissolve on boiling; the test should be repeated with diluted urine. The urine specimen should be fresh or refrigerated, since heat-coagulable protein will denature or decompose if the urine is left at room temperature and give false positive reactions.

SALICYLATES

Ferric ions react with metabolites of aspirin or other salicylates in weakly acid solutions to form a deep wine-red color (Bordeaux red), which is heat stable. This reaction provides a simple method for the detection of salicylates in cases of suspected overdosage, or in monitoring patients receiving high dosage therapy.

Ferric Chloride Test. To 5 ml urine in test tube, add 10 per cent ferric chloride drop by drop until the precipitate of ferric phosphate redissolves. A red-brown or deep Bordeaux red color develops in the presence of salicylates. This test is also positive if acetoacetic acid is present (Table 17-12).

To confirm a positive reaction for salicylates, divide the test solution in half and boil half for five minutes, or boil 5 ml urine and repeat the test. If the boiled or retested sample still shows the Bordeaux red color, the test is positive for salicylates, which are not changed by heating. If the boiled solution becomes lighter, or if the test after boiling is negative, the reaction was due to acetoacetic acid.

Reagents. Phenistix[a] reagent strips contain a ferric salt, magnesium sulfate, and cyclohexylsulfamic acid.

Procedure. Dip the reagent-impregnated portion of the strip into the urine. Immediately compare the color of the dipped end of the strip with a special color chart available from the manufacturer. Metabolites of aspirin or other salicylates will give a pink to Bordeaux red color with Phenistix. (Phenylpyruvic acid in urine, in cases of phenylketonuria, produces a gray to blue-gray color.) (Johnson, 1953)

SUCROSURIA

Sucrose may appear in the urine after the ingestion of very large amounts of sucrose. Sucrose intolerance is a rare disorder associated with sucrase and alpha dextrinase (isomaltase) deficiencies. Symptoms are similar to those seen with lactase deficiency.

Factitious sucrosuria may create a high specific gravity urine with negative glucose oxidase and negative copper reduction tests. Sucrose will ferment yeast and can be separated by chromatography but needs to be stained with a substance not dependent on reducing properties.

SULFONAMIDE

Sulfonamides are conjugated in the body by acetylation. Both free and acetylated forms can be found in the blood and urine.

Sulfonamides, such as sulfisoxazole, are less likely to form crystals in the urine than the older sulfanilamide, sulfapyridine, or sulfathiazole. Acetylated sulfadiazine is more soluble in urine than free sulfadiazine.

The sulfonamides contain a sulfonamide group and a free amino group. The sulfonamide is diazotized with nitrous acid and coupled with N-(1-naphthyl)-ethylenediamine to produce a colored compound. Since acetylation blocks the amino group, the conjugated form cannot be diazotized. To measure total sulfonamide, the sample is first hydrolyzed with HCl. A protein-free specimen of urine is used.

Procedure. See Bratton and Marshall, 1939; Gershenfeld, 1943.

Reagents

1. 15 per cent aqueous solution of trichloroacetic acid.

2. 0.1 per cent aqueous solution of sodium nitrate.

3. 0.5 per cent aqueous solution of ammonium sulfamate.

4. 0.4 N hydrochloric acid solution (dilute 3.8 ml concentrated HCl with 100 ml).

5. 0.1 per cent aqueous solution of N-(1-naphthyl)-ethylenediamine dihydrochloride (Eastman Organic Chemicals, Division of Eastman Kodak Co., Rochester, New York). Keep in a dark bottle in the refrigerator.

Standards

Stock Standard. A 0.2 per cent aqueous solution of a sulfonamide. It is desirable to use as a standard the identical form of the sulfa drug that is administered. Keep in a dark bottle in the refrigerator. Stable for several weeks.

Dilute Standards. Into three 100 ml flasks containing 18 ml of the 15 per cent trichloroacetic acid solution, add the following amounts of the *stock standard* and dilute to the mark:

No. 1: 1.0 ml (10 ml contains 0.02 mg).
No. 2: 2.5 ml (10 ml contains 0.05 mg).
No. 3: 5.0 ml (10 ml contains 0.10 mg).

Technique

Free Sulfanilamide. Protein-free urine is diluted by mixing 1 ml with sufficient distilled water to 250 ml.

If the urine contains proteins, mix 1 ml of urine

with 1 ml of 15 per cent trichloroacetic acid, dilute to 10 ml, and filter. Dilute a portion of the filtrate 1 to 25.

To 5 ml of either of the above final dilutions, add 5 ml of 0.4 N HCl. To the 10 ml of this mixture and to 10 ml of each of the three dilute standards, add 1 ml of the sodium nitrite solution, mix, and after allowing it to stand 3 minutes, add 1 ml of the ammonium sulfamate solution. Allow to stand 2 minutes and add 1 ml of the ethylenediamine reagent. Compare in a colorimeter with the dilute standard (which matches closest) within 1 hour.

Total Sulfanilamide. Five ml of diluted protein-free urine (freed of protein if necessary and diluted as above) is mixed with 5 ml 0.1 N HCl and kept for 1 hour in a boiling water-bath. Cool and adjust to 10 ml to replace evaporated water. Proceed as above.

TYROSINE
(*p*-HYDROXYPHENYLALANINE)

Tyrosinemia with tyrosinuria occurs when there is abnormal metabolism of tyrosine derived from the diet or from phenylalanine. This may be part of a generalized amino acid disorder associated with liver disease, or a transitory tyrosinemia seen in premature or low weight infants, or, rarely, with the syndrome of hereditary tyrosinemia. The genetic disease tyrosinosis is extremely rare.

Transitory hypertyrosinemia occurs in infants of low birth weight and in about 2 per cent of infants tested in screening programs (Levy, 1969). There is no liver or renal disease present, and the entity is benign. The elevated tyrosine levels may on occasion be accompanied by transiently elevated phenylalanine levels. Tyrosine and the phenolic acids *p*-hydroxyphenyllactic and *p*-hydroxyphenlpyruvic are excreted in larger than normal amounts in the urine.

Hereditary tyrosinemia is accompanied by a generalized aminoacidemia with a marked loss of *p*-hydroxyphenyllactic acid, glucosuria, proteinuria, and loss of phosphate. Cirrhosis of the liver, renal dysfunction, and rickets are the principal findings. The clinical entity in some respects resembles those of hereditary fructosemia and galactosemia in which there is liver and kidney involvement and a generalized aminoaciduria.

Tyrosine crystals

Very fine, silky crystals are seen in the urinary sediment in severe liver disease. They are scattered in the field or aggregated to form sheaves. The crystals appear brown to black while focusing. Leucine crystals may accompany the tyrosine. The crystals precipitate at an acid pH and are soluble in alkali.

Nitrosonaphthol Test for Tyrosine. This is a non-specific screening test and should be confirmed by chromatography or quantitative serum assay of tyrosine.

Reagents. One volume of concentrated 2.63 N nitric acid in five volumes of water. Nitrosonaphthol—100 mg 1-nitroso-2-naphthol in 100 ml 95 per cent ethanol. All reagents are refrigerated.

Procedure. Mix the following reagent in a test tube: To 1 ml of 2.63 N nitric acid add one drop of 2.5 aqueous sodium nitrite solution and 10 drops of nitrosonaphthol reagent. Add 3 drops of urine and mix. Let stand for 3 to 5 minutes. An orange-red color will develop. A positive control is tested at the same time.

Control. 50 mg tyrosine in 100 ml water. Refrigerate. The control can be a mixture of amino acids in aqueous solution used for qualitative tests.

The Millon reaction is due to the hydroxyphenol group, and tyrosine and other phenols will be positive. For urine, the inorganic salts interfere with the test and a modification is needed (Hawk, 1954).

UROBILINOGEN

After bile is excreted into the intestine, conjugated bilirubin is reduced by bacterial action to mesobilirubin, stercobilinogen, and urobilinogen. Stercobilinogen and urobilinogen are colorless and are oxidized to the colored pigments urobilin and stercobilin.

The reduced products of bilirubin are normally reabsorbed into the portal circulation to be re-excreted by the liver. Part of the reabsorbed urobilinogen and stercobilinogen is excreted in the urine together with mesobilirubinogen. Urobilin, the oxidized form of urobilinogen, is also found in normal urine.

Normal adult urine contains from about 0.5 to 2.5 mg of urobilinogen in a 24-hour collection; less than 1 Ehrlich unit in 2 hours is excreted as measured by a semiquantitative method (Balikov, 1957). Urinary and fecal urobilinogen is increased when there is hemolysis of red cells, as in hemolytic anemia. Raised levels of urinary urobilinogen may also be present in liver disease because the liver cells may not be able to reabsorb or re-excrete circulating urobilinogen, thus causing more to appear in the urine. Urobilinogen may be absent from the urine (and decreased in feces) in patients with complete obstruction of the bile duct, as in carcinoma of the head of the pancreas.

Quantitative 2-Hour Urine Urobilinogen

Collection. A 1 to 3 P.M. urine specimen is collected. The patient voids at 1 P.M. and the urine is discarded. The patient voids again at 3 P.M. and the total specimen is collected and sent to the laboratory immediately. Because urobilinogen is rapidly oxidized to urobilin, the determination should be done within one half hour of collection of the specimen. Protect from light.

Procedure

1. Measure and record the total 2 hour volume.*†
2. Use two 25 by 150 mm test tubes for each specimen. One is the blank; the other is for color development. The same solutions will be added to both but in different order. The order of addition of the first two solutions may be interchanged, but the solution listed last below must be added last. Mix well after *each* addition.

In the color development tube add the sodium acetate *immediately* after mixing the urine with Ehrlich's reagent. (When Ehrlich's reagent is added directly to urine, the color produced increases with time owing to slower reacting non-urobilinogen substances. The addition of saturated sodium acetate stops these slower reactions.)

	Blank	*Color Development*
	3 ml Ehrlich's reagent	3 ml Ehrlich's reagent
	6 ml sodium acetate	3 ml urine
Add last	3 ml urine	6 ml sodium acetate

The blank should be colorless. Colored blanks may be due to the use of sodium acetate that is not saturated or to inadequate mixing of the Ehrlich's reagent and sodium acetate before adding the urine.

3. Read immediately at 565 nm in a spectrophotometer. (Color development is not stable; in addition, color may develop slowly in blanks from unknowns with very high concentrations.) Any "test" solution which reads below the last standard on the prepared calibration curve should be diluted.

4. If the color is too intense, dilute both "blank" and "test" with reagents; e.g., "diluted blank"—mix 2 ml Ehrlich's reagent with 6 ml saturated sodium acetate, then add 2 ml "blank" solution from above; "diluted test"—mix 2 ml "test" solution with 2 ml Ehrlich's reagent, then add 6 ml saturated sodium acetate. Record the volumes used in making these extra dilutions. Read the diluted test against the diluted blank.

5. Using the calibration curve which has been obtained from pontacyl dyes or urobilinogen standards, determine the concentration in mg/dl or use the PSP standard method. See below.

---

*Because bilirubin will be oxidized to the green color biliverdin in the reaction, a test should be done before proceeding. If positive, remove by adsorbing onto barium chloride and filtering.

†Ascorbic acid 100 mg/10 ml urine is used to prevent oxidation of urobilinogen. This is dissolved in the urine (centrifuged if needed) before pipetting the urine into the test tubes for testing.

Note that 1 Ehrlich Unit = 1 mg urobilinogen. Results are given as Ehrlich units excreted in 2 hours.

Standardization

Standards of pure crystalline stercobilin hydrochloride are preferred for the calibration of spectrophotometers. Watson (1941) proposed an alternate standard using a mixture of pontacyl dyes that, in a stated combination and concentration, had an absorbance equivalent to certain concentrations of urobilinogen reacting with Ehrlich's reagent and sodium acetate. It is applicable to the Coleman Junior II spectrophotometer at 565 nm. (See Davidsohn, 1974, p. 62.)

Another standard has been proposed which may be preferable for use with narrow-band spectrophotometers; this is phenolsulfonphthalein (PSP) (Henry, 1961).

PSP Standard. A single standard solution of phenolsulfonphthalein is used.

Stock Standard. Dissolve 20 mg PSP-phenol red-acidic form in 100 ml 0.05 per cent NaOH.

Working Standard. Dilute stock standard 1:100 with 0.05 per cent NaOH to make a solution containing 0.20 mg/100 ml. This is equivalent to urobilinogen 0.35 mg/100 ml (0.346 mg/100 ml (Henry, 1974)). The absorbance of this PSP solution* at 565 nm is measured against water set at zero.

Calculation

Ehrlich U/100 ml =

$$\frac{\text{Absorbance of unknown} - \text{Absorbance of blank}}{\text{Absorbance of standard}}$$

$$\times \ 0.35 \times \frac{12 (\text{ml tube vol.})}{3 (\text{ml urine})}$$

Ehrlich U/2 hr = above $\times \dfrac{\text{2-hr volume in ml}}{100}$

Reference Values. 0 to 1.1 Ehrlich unit/2 hr for females, 0.3 to 2.1 U/2 hr for males (Henry, 1974). Output is higher in alkaline urines; this may account for the rise noted in afternoon specimens collected following a meal.

Urobilinogen and porphobilinogen

(Qualitative Ehrlich's Aldehyde Reaction) (Watson-Schwartz, 1941). Methods for measuring urobilinogen and porphobilinogen in urine measure the total chromogens in the urine. Ehrlich's reagent, *p*-dimethyl amino benzaldehyde in concentrated hydrochloric acid, reacts with urobilinogen and porphobilinogen to form a colored aldehyde. The addition of sodium acetate intensifies the red color of the aldehyde and inhibits color formation by skatoles and indoles. Extractions of the colored complex using butanol and chloroform

---

*Dye lots will vary and the solution should be checked for absorbance (see Henry, 1961).

are employed to separate urobilinogen and porphobilinogen from other Ehrlich's-reactive compounds.

Reagents

1. Ehrlich's reagent: Combine 0.7 g *p*-dimethyl amino benzaldehyde, 150 ml concentrated hydrochloric acid, and 100 ml deionized water. Store in brown bottle. Stable for 3 to 6 months.
2. Saturated sodium acetate in deionized water.
3. Chloroform.
4. Butanol.

Procedure

1. To one volume (approximately 3 ml) of urine in a test tube, add an equal volume of Ehrlich's reagent. Mix well by inversion.
2. Immediately add two volumes of saturated sodium acetate and mix well by inversion. (When Ehrlich's reagent is added directly to urine, the color produced increases with time owing to slower reacting *non-urobilinogen* substances. The addition of saturated sodium acetate stops these slower reactions.) The color of a positive reaction ranges from a definite light pink to a deep cherry red. Pale peach and light orange colors are often seen, but these are *not* positive reactions. If the test is positive at this stage, split the colored solution into two parts and continue with the next two steps.
3. Add a few milliliters of chloroform to one portion of the colored solution and shake vigorously. Allow layers to separate. Observe whether or not the color is completely extracted into the *lower* chloroform layer. Extract more than once if necessary. Color due to urobilinogen will be extracted into chloroform; that due to porphobilinogen and other Ehrlich's-reactive compounds will not be.
4. If the pink color is not extracted by the chloroform, suggesting the presence of porphobilinogen or other Ehrlich's-reactive compounds, add a few milliliters of butanol to the other portion of the colored solution. Shake vigorously, then allow layers to separate. Observe whether or not the color is completely extracted into the *upper* butanol layer. If color still remains in the urine-acetate layer, re-extract with more butanol. As with chloroform, color due to urobilinogen will be extracted into the solvent. Color due to other Ehrlich's-reactive compounds will also be extracted into butanol; that due to porphobilinogen will not be.
5. Report as negative, positive for urobilinogen, positive for porphobilinogen, or positive for both urobilinogen and porphobilinogen (rare). The finding of Ehrlich's-reactive compounds that are neither urobilinogen nor porphobilinogen is due to interfering substances such as sulfonamides, procaine, 5-hydroxy indole acetic acid, and other compounds that react with Ehrlich's reagent.

NOTE. Fresh urine should be cooled to room temperature before the Ehrlich test is carried out. Normal urine contains a chromogen (probably indoxyl) which gives a weak Ehrlich reaction at body temperature—the so-called "warm aldehyde" reaction.

Interpretation of the Watson-Schwartz Test for Urobilinogen and Porphobilinogen

Ehrlich's reagent and saturated sodium acetate are added to a portion of urine in a test tube. A red or definite pink color is a positive result and indicates the presence of urobilinogen, porphobilinogen, and/or other Ehrlich's-reactive compounds. Extraction of these compounds by butanol and chloroform is done for further identification (Fig. 17-1), p. 610.

Urobilinogen is soluble in both chloroform and butanol. *Porphobilinogen* is not soluble in either chloroform or butanol, always remaining in the urine-acetate layer. It is the only one of these Ehrlich's-reactive compounds which is not soluble in either one of the solvents. Other Ehrlich's-reactive compounds are soluble in butanol but not in chloroform. The following sets correspond to the results shown in Figure 17-1.

Set No. 1	*Set No. 2*
+ Urobilinogen	+ Porphobilinogen
0 Porphobilinogen	0 Urobilinogen
0 Other Ehrlich's-reactive compounds	0 Other Ehrlich's-reactive compounds

Set No. 3	*Set No. 4*
+ Other Ehrlich's-reactive compounds	+ Urobilinogen
0 Urobilinogen	+ Other Ehrlich's-reactive compounds
0 Porphobilinogen	0 Porphobilinogen

*Set No. 5**	*Set No. 6†*
+ Porphobilinogen	+ Urobilinogen
+ Other Ehrlich's-reactive compounds	? Porphobilinogen
0 Urobilinogen	? Excess urobilinogen

*When the deeper color is in the urine-acetate mixture, and the butanol layer is a lighter shade, results can be reported without further extraction.

† In this instance, the tube containing butanol is never left with color in both layers. Further extraction of the urine-acetate layer is done with more butanol. If all the color is extracted into the butanol layer, there is no porphobilinogen present (6-a). However, if the color after the re-extraction with the butanol remains in the urine-acetate layer and the butanol layer is colorless, the test is positive for porphobilinogen (6-b). Extract the urine-acetate layer until color remains in only one layer.

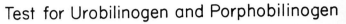

Test for Urobilinogen and Porphobilinogen

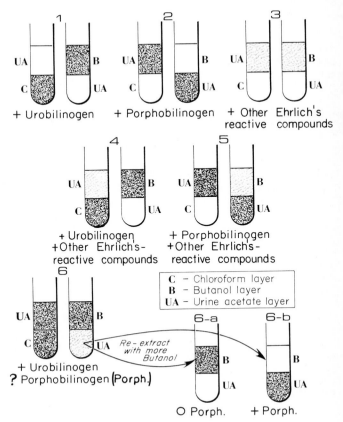

Figure 17-1. Interpretation of the screening method for urine urobilinogen and porphobilinogen (Watson-Schwartz test).

URINARY CALCULI

Analysis of the constituents of urinary calculi may be of help in the management of patients with calculous disease.

Calcium oxalate is the most commonly found constituent of urinary calculi. It precipitates at an acid or neutral pH. Calcium phosphate (hydroxy apatite $Ca_{10}(PO)_6(OH)_2$) forms calculi at the normal urinary pH of 6.0 to 6.5, whereas magnesium ammonium phosphate forms calculi in an alkaline urine probably associated with bacterial infection.

In Prien's series (1963), calcium oxalate or a mixture of oxalate and calcium phosphate were most often found in stones (80 to 84 per cent). Mixed calcium phosphate, magnesium ammonium phosphate, and uric acid were the next most common constituents (3 to 10 per cent each), and these were followed by cystine (1 to 2 per cent). Uric acid, cystine and xanthine precipitate in acid urines at pH less than 6. Rarely, calculi containing sulfonamides are found, and silica calculi have been reported in patients ingesting silica gel over a long period

of time (Lagergren, 1962). Carbonate, which is frequently detected in chemical analysis, probably results from adsorption of carbon dioxide to the calcium phosphate crystal. Supersaturation of the urine with oxalate, phosphate, uric acid, and calcium may lead to stone formation, depending on urinary pH. Calculi are commonly seen in hyperparathyroidism, since calcium excretion is high in this condition. Stasis in any part of the urinary tract will cause crystalline precipitation, usually phosphate.

The origin of oxalate in the urine is not entirely understood. When oxalates are ingested, they are eliminated, at least in part, unchanged in the urine. Common articles of diet which contain oxalate are asparagus, apples, cabbage, grapes, lettuce, rhubarb, spinach, and tomatoes, and these are probably the source of unmetabolized oxalic acid. Part of the oxalic acid of the body is formed, however, in the course of the metabolism of protein, fat, and carbohydrate.

Primary hyperoxaluria is a genetic disorder

in which excessive excretion of oxalate leads to nephrolithiasis. Calcium oxalate is found in the tissues. Oxalic acid excretion exceeds the upper limit of normal—about 60 mg/1.73 m^2/24 hr. There is stone formation and excessive oxalate excretion with pyridoxine deficiency, in diseases of the small bowel, and in some individuals after ingesting large doses of ascorbic acid.

Uric acid stones are radiolucent and form as a complication of gout and in association with chemotherapy for leukemia, with polycythemia, and in patients with ileostomies or chronic diarrhea. However, uric acid stones may form without evidence of hyperuricemia.

Xanthine stones are uncommon and may be associated with a genetic disorder with an absence of liver xanthine oxidase.

The finding of clusters of calcium oxalate (or of uric acid) crystals in freshly voided urine suggests that conditions in the urinary passages are favorable for calculus formation but, of course, does not prove that calculi are present.

The passage of stones down the ureter produces renal colic, which is characterized by severe pain in the back radiating to the groin. Stones may also be passed through the urethra with great pain. Hematuria is a common urinary finding when symptoms of stone are present. If stones obstruct the pelvis of the kidney or ureter, hydronephrosis will result with pyelonephritis as a probable consequence.

Calculi may be of various sizes, commonly described as sand, gravel, and stone. Large round stones are characteristic of those found in the bladder. The physical characteristics of the various calculi rarely will suffice for their identification, but a few points are worth noting. Uric acid and urate stones are always colored yellow to brownish red and are moderately hard. Phosphate stones are usually pale and friable. Calcium oxalate stones are very hard, often of a dark color, and typically have a rough surface.

Several methods are available for the analysis of calculi, such as optical crystallography, x-ray diffraction, and infrared spectroscopy. A review of chemical methods is presented by Beeler (1974).

Qualitative analysis of urinary calculi*

GROSS EXAMINATION OF CALCULI
1. If not done previously, wash stone free from blood, mucus, preservative solution, etc. Place

stone(s) in a beaker, cover with several thicknesses of gauze held firmly in place with rubber bands and wash under cold running water. Drain, remove gauze carefully and dry beaker and stone(s) in oven. Rinse tiny stone(s) with water from a squeeze bottle (not running water).
2. Obtain measurements of stone's (stones') dimensions in centimeters.
3. Describe briefly the color and texture of the stone's (stones') exterior surface.
4. Cut, saw, or break the stone(s) so as to examine the interior. Note whether there is a foreign body which may have acted as a nucleus for its formation. Describe the color and texture of the interior.
5. Reduce stone(s) to a fine powder by pulverizing with a mortar and pestle.
6. If possible, where there is a very large stone, it may be advisable to make separate analyses of layers which appear to have different constituents.

Reagents. Some of these are for the rarer stones and are not routinely used. Reagent kits are available.*
1. 20 per cent Na_2CO_3
2. 20 per cent NaOH
3. 10 per cent HN_4OH
4. Nessler's reagent: Prepare commercially available Nessler's compound, reagent brand, Koch-McMeekin formula, according to instructions on label. Store at room temperature.
5. Uric acid reagent (phosphotungstic acid): Harleco Item No. 3030. Add 40 g $Li_2SO_4 \cdot H_2O$ to each liter.
6. H_2SO_4-ammonium molybdate reagent (Fiske and Subbarow phosphorus method): Dissolve 2.5 g ammonium molybdate in 50 ml of 10 N H_2SO_4 and make up to 100 ml with distilled water.
7. Amino naphthol sulfonic acid reagent (Fiske and Subbarow phosphorus method): Store this reagent in a dark bottle. Prepare commercially available product according to directions on the label, heating slightly to aid solution.
8. Mg reagent: 0.001 per cent *p*-nitro benzene azoresorcinol in 2 N NaOH. Store in a polyethylene bottle in a dark place.
9. 5 per cent NaCN (preserved with 1 ml 28 per cent NH_4OH per 500 ml solution).
10. 5 per cent sodium nitroferricyanide (nitroprusside): This solution is quite unstable so we find it satisfactory to dissolve a few crystals in a small test tube of distilled water. If stored, use a brown glass bottle.
11. 10 per cent HCl
12. Saturated ammonium oxalate
13. MnO_2 powder (native powder, not reagent grade)

* Oxford Laboratories, San Mateo, Calif. and C. W. Allen, Co., St. Louis, Mo.

*Adapted from Winer, 1943, 1959.

For Rare Stones

1. 0 to 1 per cent sodium nitrate ($NaNO_2$) (Sulfa determination—prepared fresh on alternate days)
2. 0.5 per cent ammonium sulfamate (sulfonimide)
3. Sulfa dye reagent: 0.1 per cent (w/v) N-(1-naphthyl)ethylenediamine dihydrochloride. The dye is more soluble in warm water. Store this solution in a dark bottle. Refrigerate.
4. Concentrated HNO_3—xanthine test
5. Concentrated H_2SO_4—cholesterol
6. Acetic anhydride—cholesterol
7. Chloroform—cholesterol

Sequence of Chemical Determinations in Urinary Calculi

Since most small calculi consist of calcium oxalate, the best way to analyze them is to put all available powder in one test tube. (If the stone is very tiny, it may be placed directly in the test tube, and crushed with a spatula). Add HCl, pour off the supernatant for the calcium, and add MnO_2 to the residue for the oxalate. If the stone is a little larger, then some of the powder could be used to test for phosphates. Perform tests in the following sequence when there is a sufficient amount of stone for all of the analyses (see Appendix 3, p. 2080).

EXAMINATION OF THE URINE SEDIMENT

Interpretation of urine sediment requires time, skill, and experience acquired through constant use of various microscopic methods and continuous pathophysiologic correlation of the sediment findings with the clinical status of the patient. Important formed elements such as cells, casts, organisms, etc. must clearly be identified to achieve early diagnosis of renal parenchymal and/or urinary tract disease. Crystals and amorphous materials commonly found in the urinary sediment are generally of less significance but occasionally may provide useful information.

Formed Elements of Urine

Centrifuged urine sediment contains all the insoluble materials (commonly referred to as formed elements) that have accumulated in the urine in the process of glomerular filtration and during passage of fluid through the tubules of the kidney and lower urinary tract. Cells found in urine come from two sources: (1) desquamation or spontaneous exfoliation of epithelial cells lining the upper and lower urinary tract and adjacent structures, and (2) cells of the circulating blood (leukocytes and erythrocytes). Casts formed in the renal tubules and collecting ducts are the other formed elements frequently seen.

Organisms (bacteria, fungi, viral inclusion cells, parasites, etc.) and neoplastic cells represent elements foreign to the urinary system, and proper identification of these elements may provide important diagnostic clues as to the etiology of certain urinary system disorders.

"Normal" or reference values for formed elements will vary from one laboratory to another. Because of (1) the variation in concentration of random urine specimens, (2) the different methods used to concentrate the sediment (1:10, 1:20, complete, or none), and (3) different centrifuge speeds, there are no valid qualitative reference values.

Methods for Examining Urine Sediment

Brightfield microscopy of unstained urine

Subdued light is needed to delineate the more translucent formed elements of the urine such as hyaline casts, crystals, and mucous threads. Identification of leukocytes (neutrophils, lymphocytes, etc.), histiocytes, renal epithelial cells, viral inclusion cells, neoplastic cells, and cellular casts may be very difficult in unstained preparations.

Procedure. The urine specimen must be examined while fresh, since cells and casts begin to lyse within 1 to 3 hours. Each specimen is concentrated tenfold. (Twenty-fold concentrations may also be used).

1. Mix the specimen well (casts tend to settle). Pour exactly 10 ml of urine into a graduated disposable centrifuge tube. Centrifuge at 2000 rpm for 5 minutes. Remove the supernate by decanting into another tube and resuspend the sediment in exactly 1 ml of urine. A disposable pipette with rubber bulb is convenient for this purpose.

2. Place a drop of resuspended sediment on one area of a slide and coverslip with a 22-mm square coverslip, avoiding bubbles. Too much fluid will cause the coverslip to float. (Some workers prefer to examine the sediment in a counting chamber to assure even depth).

3. Examine with both low and high power fields. Examine with low power ($\times 100$) and subdued light. The fine focus should be varied continuously while scanning. Systematically progress around all four sides of the coverslip. Either the stained or unstained mount may be used, depending on the kind of specimen and the experience of the examiner.

Casts are often found along the edge of the

Table 17–15. A COMPARISON OF ADDIS COUNTS AND ROUTINE EXAMINATION OF THE SEDIMENT*

FORMED ELEMENT	ADDIS COUNT TOTAL EXCRETION PER 12 HOURS	ROUTINE SCREENING EXAMINATION (PER HIGH-POWER FIELD)
Casts	6,700 to 79,000	0 or 1 to 2
	122,000 to 1,000,000	1 to 2
	6,000,000 to 15,000,000	10 to 20
Red cells	220,000 to 2,400,000	0 to 10
	2,500,000 to 8,200,000	1 to 20
	190,000,000 to 570,000,000	5 to 60
Leukocytes and epithelial cells	Less than 1,000,000	0 (occasionally) 3 to 5 (usually)
	1,000,000 to 10,000,000	5 to 10
	10,000,000 to 75,000,000	10 to 20 (clumped)

*From R. M. Kark *et al.*: A Primer of Urinalysis. 2nd edition. New York, Hoeber Medical Division, Harper & Row, Publishers, 1963.

coverslip. Count the number of casts per low power field in 10 fields. Switch to high power (×440) and identify casts present.

Erythrocytes, leukocytes, and epithelial cells are identified with the high power objective and counted in 10 fields. Squamous epithelial cells are noted if a large number of them are present. Bacteria and yeasts should be noted.

Crystals are reported if the number is unusually large or they are abnormal; these are counted under low power. The identity of certain abnormal crystals should be confirmed chemically (see cystine and sulfonamide tests).

Report. After averaging the contents of 10 representative fields, the results may be compared with the quantitative data of Kark (1963) (see Table 17–15). A scale for reporting results of examination of urinary sediment is shown below:

Addis Count. The Addis count (Addis, 1948), although a more accurate method of assessing quantitative changes in the sediment, is no longer in general use. Its chief value (where still in use) lies in following the progress of active renal disease, notably acute glomerulonephritis. (For diagnostic purposes, careful examination of the sediment from a random fresh urine sample is usually sufficient). For details of methodology, see page 39 of Davidsohn (1974).

Brightfield microscopy with supravital staining

Cellular detail is best seen with stained sediments. A crystal-violet safranin stain (Sternheimer, 1951) may be used to aid in the identification of cellular elements.

Reagent

Solution I.	Crystal violet	3.0 g
	Ethyl alcohol (95%)	20.0 ml
	Ammonium oxalate	0.8 g
	Distilled water	80.0 ml
Solution II.	Safranin O	1.0 g
	Ethyl alcohol (95%)	40.0 ml
	Distilled water	400.0 ml

Three parts of Solution I and 97 parts of Solution II are mixed and filtered. The mixture should be clarified by filtering every two weeks: discard after three months. Separately, Solutions I and II keep indefinitely at room temperature. In highly alkaline urines, the stain will precipitate.

Procedure. Add one or two drops of crystal-violet safranin stain to approximately 1 ml of precentrifuged, concentrated urine sediment. Mix with a pipette and place a drop of this suspension on a slide under a coverslip.

Methylene blue and toluidine blue may also be used as simple, quick supravital stains. An improved supravital stain which facilitates identification of cells, casts, and their inclusions has recently been recommended (Sternheimer, 1975).

Phase and interference microscopy

Many laboratories prefer to use phase microscopy for the detection of more translucent formed elements of the urinary sediment. Such elements, notably hyaline casts (but also mucous threads and bacilli), may escape detec-

SEDIMENT— CONCENTRATION 1:10	NEG.	OCCASIONAL	1+	2+	3+	4+
Erythrocytes (high power field) × 440	0	less than 4	4–8	8–30	greater than 30, less than packed	packed field
White cells (high power field) × 440	0	less than 5	5–20	20–50	greater than 50, less than packed	packed field
Casts and abnormal crystals (low power field) × 100	0	less than 1	1–5	5–10	10–30	greater than 30

tion using ordinary brightfield microscopy, especially when the iris diaphragm is insufficiently constricted. Phase microscopy has the advantage of hardening the outlines of even the most ephemeral formed elements, making detection simple (see Fig. 17–11*A* and *B*) (Brody, 1968). Even greater morphologic detail of formed elements (notably casts and cells) is afforded by interference contrast microscopy (Haber, 1972). This technology, however, is not in common use at the present time, in part due to cost.

Combined cytocentrifugation and Papanicolaou stain method

A combined cytocentrifugation (Cytospin, Shandon Southern Instruments, Sewickley, Pa.) and Papanicolaou staining method has been used to evaluate changes in the urine sediment in renal allograft recipients during acute rejection (Schumann, 1977). Use of cytocentrifugation permits a simple, rapid, reproducible, and semiquantitative method for preparing urine sediments. Cellular casts, mononuclear cells, (plasma cells, lymphocytes, histiocytes, etc.), tissue fragments, and neoplastic cells may be clearly demonstrated with this method.

Procedure. When possible, early morning urine (volumes ranging from 10 to 30 ml) is collected. The container is placed in an ice bath and immediately carried to the cytopathology laboratory with an accompanying requisition noting history of transplantation, radiation, and chemotherapy. A 10-ml sample of urine is immediately spun in a standard centrifuge at 1500 rpm for 10 minutes. The supernatant is then discarded by hand-pipetting to 1 ml and the sediment resuspended. Using a cytocentrifuge, four slides are prepared using four drops of resuspended specimen per chamber and spinning at 900 rpm for 3 minutes. After the filter is discarded, one to two drops of Parlodion* are applied to the cellular area of a horizontally held slide. The slide is then fixed for 15 minutes in acetic acid-alcohol† and stained by the Papanicolaou technique.‡ All four slides are screened, noting background pattern, cellularity, erythrocytes, viral inclusions, and abnormal cells. Ten high power fields are counted on the most cellular slide, differentiating between neutrophils, lymphocytes, renal tubular cells, and casts. All specimens are counted separately by at least two cytotechnologists.

---

*200 ml 95% EtOH, 200 ml anhydrous ether, 1 g Parlodion (Mallinckrodt).

†One part glacial acetic acid to nine parts 95% ethanol.

‡Aqueous alum hematoxylin, OG-6, EA-36.

Standardized slide method

The KOVA system (ICL Scientific, Fountain Valley, Cal.) offers a standardized procedure that is more reproducible than conventional brightfield microscopy. The complete system includes a clear, accurately graduated centrifuge tube, a transfer pipette, supravital staining system, and a 1 by 3 inch patented, optically clear plastic microscopic slide with four individual, covered examination chambers. The system offers a measure of standardization (and hence reproducibility) apparently superior to usual methods.

In some laboratories the hemocytometer is used with random, uncentrifuged specimens to quantitate cells and to evaluate pyuria.

MICROSCOPIC CHARACTERISTICS OF URINE SEDIMENT

CELLS

Erythrocytes

Under high power, unstained erythrocytes or red blood cells appear as pale discs. They vary somewhat in size but are usually about $7\,\mu$ in diameter. If the specimen is not fresh when it is examined, the cells will appear as faint, colorless circles or "shadow cells," since the hemoglobin has "dissolved" out. Red blood cells may become crenated in hypertonic urine and appear as small, rough cells with "crinkly" edges (Fig. 17–2). Smooth, folded, and crenated cells may be seen in the same specimen. On occasion, red blood cells may be confused with oil droplets or yeast cells. Oil droplets, however, exhibit a great variation in size, are highly refractile, and will not "tumble" when the coverglass is touched with a pencil to set the fluid in motion. Yeast cells usually show budding. If there is doubt about identification, two preparations may be made and a few drops of acetic acid added to one. Red blood cells are lysed in the acidified preparation.

Both erythrocytes and leukocytes are found in small numbers in normal urine. How these cells enter the urine is not known. The proportion of leukocytes to erythrocytes is much greater in urine than in blood; thus diapedesis of leukocytes through the glomerular membrane or tubular wall may be postulated.

In normal males and females, occasional (1

Table 17-16. CELLS AND CASTS

	RANGE	MEAN	REFERENCE
Erythrocytes	to 1 million/day	130,000/day	Addis, 1948
	0-473,000/hr., female	29,000/hr., female	Prescott, 1965
	0-915,000/hr., male	38,000/hr., male	
Casts—hyaline and occasional granular	to 5,000/day	2,000/day	Addis, 1948
Leukocytes and nonsquamous epithelial cells	to 2 million/day	650,000/day	
Differential			
Renal tubular cells	5,000-243,000/hr., female	68,000/hr., female	Prescott, 1965
	12,000-262,000/hr., male	78,000/hr., male	
Leukocytes (PMN)	0-5,042,000/hr., female	108,000/hr., female	
	0-956,000/hr., male	28,000/hr., male	
Squamous epithelial	variable		

to 2/hpf) red cells may be seen on microscopic examination of the sediment. (See discussion under hemoglobinuria, p. 591). Smoking appears to be related to microhematuria (Freni, 1977). Exercise and lordosis may transiently increase the rate of excretion of erythrocytes (Goldring, 1931). The normal ranges for both cells and casts are shown in Table 17-16.

When increased numbers of red cells are found in the urine in conjunction with red blood cell casts, bleeding may be assumed to be renal in origin. In the absence of casts or proteinuria, increased red blood cells suggest a bleeding site distal to the kidney.

Increased numbers of red blood cells in the urine may be present in (1) renal disease—including glomerulonephritis, lupus nephritis, calculus, tumor, acute infection, tuberculosis, infarction, renal vein thrombosis, trauma (including renal biopsy), hydronephrosis, polycystic kidney, and occasionally acute tubular necrosis and malignant nephrosclerosis; (2) lower urinary tract disease—including acute and chronic infection, calculus, tumor, and stricture; (3) extrarenal disease—including acute appendicitis, salpingitis, diverticulitis, and tumors of the colon, rectum, and pelvis.

Hematuria may occur during acute febrile episodes, malaria, subacute bacterial endocarditis, polyarteritis nodosa, malignant hypertension, blood dyscrasias, and scurvy. Hematuria may also reflect toxic reactions to drugs such as sulfonamides, salicylates, methena-

mine, and anticoagulant therapy. Hemorrhagic cystitis is occasionally noted following cyclophosphamide therapy.

Leukocytes

Under high power, neutrophilic leukocytes appear as granular spheres about $12\,\mu$ in diameter. In freshly voided urine, nuclear detail is fairly well defined even with brightfield microscopy. Nuclear segments appear as small round discrete nuclei. When stasis has occurred and cellular degeneration has begun, nuclear detail may be lost. Neutrophils may then become difficult to distinguish from renal tubular epithelial cells. By allowing a small drop of dilute acetic acid to run under the coverslip, one may enhance nuclear detail so that definition may still be possible (Fig. 17-3). Ultimately, however, with continued degeneration, neutrophilic nuclear segments fuse, making distinction from tubular cells difficult or impossible.

Supravital staining may also be helpful in emphasizing nuclear detail. With crystal-violet safranin, neutrophilic nuclei appear reddish purple and cytoplasmic granules violet. Cytochemical definition of neutrophils using the peroxidase reaction has been found especially useful in distinguishing neutrophils (Fig. 17-4) from tubular cells (Bradley, 1968).

In dilute or hypotonic urine, neutrophils swell and cytoplasmic granules exhibit Brownian movement. Because of the refrac-

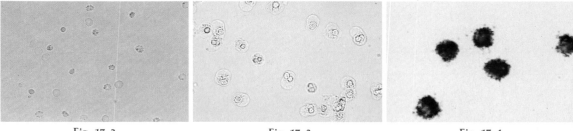

Fig. 17-2 Fig. 17-3 Fig. 17-4

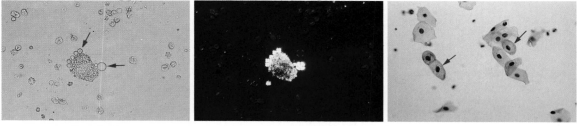

Fig. 17-5 Fig. 17-6 Fig. 17-7

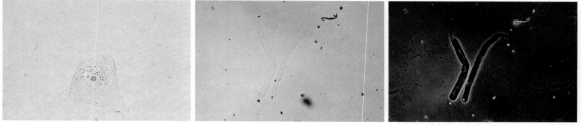

Fig. 17-8A Fig. 17-8B Fig. 17-9

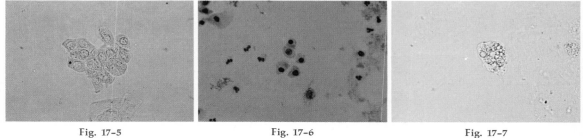

Fig. 17-10 Fig. 17-11A Fig. 17-11B

Figure 17-2. Red cells, some crenated (×160).

Figure 17-3. Neutrophils with dilute acetic acid (×200).

Figure 17-4. Neutrophils, peroxidase positive (×500).

Figure 17-5. Renal tubular epithelial cells (×200).

Figure 17-6. Renal tubular epithelial cells and neutrophils. Papanicolaou stain (×430).

Figure 17-7. Oval fat body (×160).

Figure 17-8. Oval fat body with attached fat droplets (×160): *A*, brightfield and, *B*, polarized (×160).

Figure 17-9. Transitional epithelial cells. Papanicolaou stain (×430).

Figure 17-10. Squamous epithelial cell, pyridium stained (×200).

Figure 17-11. Hyaline casts: *A*, brightfield and, *B*, phase contrast microscopy (×100).

616

tility of the moving granules, neutrophils in this setting are known as "glitter cells." These cells take supravital stains poorly, if at all. Papanicolaou staining also reflects the swelling of neutrophils in hypotonic urine. In addition, the neutrophils show loss of nuclear segmentation (Palmieri, 1977).

Increased numbers of leukocytes in the urine, principally neutrophils, are seen in almost all renal diseases and diseases of the urinary tract. They may also be transiently increased during fevers and following strenuous exercise (Goldring, 1931). When accompanied by leukocyte casts or mixed leukocyte-epithelial cell casts, increased urinary leukocytes are considered to be renal in origin.

The presence of many leukocytes (more than 50/hpf) and/or clumps of leukocytes in the sediment is strongly suggestive of acute infection. Repeatedly sterile cultures in this setting may indicate tuberculosis or lupus nephritis. Gross pyuria may reflect rupture of a renal or urinary tract abscess.

Moderate numbers of leukocytes in conjunction with leukocyte casts may reflect either bacterial (chronic pyelonephritis) or non-bacterial (acute glomerulonephritis, lupus nephritis) renal disease. They are frequently absent, however, in chronic pyelonephritis. Calculous disease at any level may give rise to increased numbers of urinary leukocytes because of either stasis-induced ascending infection or localized mucosal inflammatory response. Bladder tumors, as well as a variety of acute or chronic localized inflammatory processes, may also cause leukocytes to be increased in the urine. The latter disorders include cystitis, prostatitis, urethritis, and balanitis. It should be recognized that even in normal circumstances, some leukocytes are found in the secretions of the male and female genital tracts.

Some success has recently been reported in separating mononuclear from polynuclear leukocytes and both from renal tubular epithelial cells using phase contrast microscopy (Lindqvist, 1975). When mononuclear cells (histiocytes, lymphocytes, or plasma cells) constitute 30 per cent or more of a differential count, lupus nephritis (or in Scandinavia, Balkan nephropathy) may be the underlying disease process.

Finally, leukocytes are rapidly lysed in hypotonic or alkaline urine. Approximately 50 per cent are lost following 2 to 3 hours of standing at room temperature (Triger, 1966). This dramatizes the need for prompt examination of the urinary sediment following collection.

Renal tubular epithelial cells

Unstained renal tubular cells are slightly larger than leukocytes but usually less than 15 µ in diameter. They contain single relatively large round nuclei which are frequently eccentric (Fig. 17-5). With most special stains, the cytoplasm is smooth and devoid of organelles. Tubular cells may be flat, cuboidal, or columnar. Brush borders, indicating origin in proximal convoluted tubules, are rarely seen. Small numbers of tubular cells may be seen in normal urine, reflecting the normal sloughing of aging cells (Table 17-16). They are present in somewhat larger numbers in the urine of normal newborns (Cruikshank, 1967).

The Papanicolaou stain has been shown to be especially useful in distinguishing renal tubular cells from other mononuclear cells in the urine (Fig. 17-6) (Schumann, 1977). The stain readily distinguishes renal tubular cells from transitional cells, histiocytes, and lymphocytes. The presence of more than 15 renal tubular cells per 10 high power fields provides strong evidence of impending allograft rejection following renal transplantation. However, these criteria may only be applied three days after transplantation. (In the immediate postoperative period, deteriorating renal function may be due to acute tubular necrosis. Hence, since desquamation of renal tubular cells might be expected in this setting, these cells cannot be used as evidence for rejection. More than 50 lymphocytes per 10 high power fields is therefore considered a more reliable—though substitute—criterion for rejection in the first three days following transplantation). The tubular cells most commonly found during episodes of impending rejection are of the cuboidal type and measure from 10 to 14 µ. They are believed to originate in small collecting ducts (Schumann, 1977). With the Papanicolaou stain, nuclei are sharply defined and dark purple. The cytoplasm is orange-purple and forms a narrow rim about the nucleus.

Apart from the special circumstance of transplantation, *increased numbers of renal tubular epithelial cells* (or casts containing these cells) suggest acute tubular damage.

They might therefore be expected in pyelonephritis and in the diuretic phase of acute tubular necrosis. They are also found in increased numbers in malignant nephrosclerosis, as well as in some cases of acute glomerulonephritis accompanied by tubular damage. Ingestion of various drugs and chemicals may also cause significant tubular desquamation. Tubular cells are easily found in the urine following salicylate intoxication. Finally, clumps of tubular cells may be seen in acute tubular necrosis, necrotizing papillitis, and acute renal allograft rejection.

In the final analysis, it must be admitted that much of the foregoing information on the clinical significance of renal tubular cells is predicated on the premise that they can be identified with certainty in the urinary sediment. The Papanicolaou stain appears to be especially useful in identifying these cells. With the much more commonly used brightfield microscopy, considerable difficulties remain in distinguishing renal tubular (epithelial) cells (RTC's) from degenerating neutrophils, mononuclear cells, histiocytes, or even transitional epithelial cells (Kern, 1971). Slightly smaller size and obvious nuclear segmentation identify polymorphonuclear neutrophils. Larger size and evidence of phagocytic activity (notably of red blood cells) help identify histiocytes. Transitional cells are considered below.

LIPIDS. Certain tubular cells may be identified with some degree of confidence using brightfield microscopy. These are *oval fat bodies*, i.e., tubular cells which have apparently absorbed lipids (cholesterol, triglycerides) leaked from nephrotic glomeruli (Fig. 17-7). Oval fat bodies therefore constitute one form of lipiduria. Lipids may also appear in the urine as free fatty droplets. These, though morphologically similar to red cells, vary considerably in size and do not tumble when pressure is applied to the coverslip. Histiocytes may also ingest lipids and become impossible to distinguish from oval fat bodies. Their clinical significance, however, is similar. Finally, lipids may become incorporated into cast matrices as free fatty droplets or oval fat bodies. Resulting casts are described as fatty (see below). The presence of any or all of these lipid forms is characteristic of the nephrotic syndrome (Zimmer, 1961).

Positive identification of lipid is required for reporting lipiduria. When free or incorporated droplets contain large amounts of cholesterol, they exhibit Maltese cross formation under polarized light (Fig. 17-8). When they contain large amounts of triglycerides, fat stains (oil red O or Sudan III) are required for lipid identification, since triglycerides do not polarize.

Lipiduria is also present in a significant number of patients who have sustained major skeletal trauma with one or more fractures to major long bones or pelvis. Presumably the source of lipid is exposed fatty marrow. Although in the past the demonstration of fat droplets in the urine has been used as a sign of post-traumatic fat embolism, there is recent evidence which negates the diagnostic significance of this finding. Quantitative estimations of urinary fat in trauma patients reveal no significant differences between those with fat embolism and those without (Hansen, 1973).

Transitional epithelial cells

These cells line the urinary tract from the renal pelvis to the trigone of the female and to the distal urethra in the male. In the urine, they are two to four times as large as renal epithelial cells and have round or pear-shaped contours. The nuclei are round and central. Occasionally these cells may be binucleate. A few are present in normal urine, reflecting normal desquamation. The presence of large clumps or sheets of these cells suggests the need for full cytologic examination with the Papanicolaou stain because of possible transitional cell carcinoma anywhere from renal pelvis to bladder.

Caudate cells are merely variants of transitional cells in which one or two long cytoplasmic tails are present. These cells derive from either the renal pelvis or the bladder trigone, and have no special diagnostic significance per se.

When stained, transitional cells have dark blue nuclei with variable amounts of pale blue cytoplasm (Fig. 17-9). Occasional cytoplasmic inclusions may be seen.

Squamous epithelial cells

Much of the female urethra and the terminal 0.5 to 1.0 cm of the male urethra are lined by squamous epithelial cells. In the urine these cells are large and flat, with abundant cytoplasm and small round central nuclei (Fig. 17–10). Their margins are often folded. Occasionally the cells are rolled into cylinders. Many of the squamous cells present in female urine may derive from the vagina or vulva. When stained with crystal-violet safranin, nuclei are purple and cytoplasm pink to violet. By and large, squamous cells in female urine have little diagnostic significance.

CASTS

Casts form when proteins precipitate and gel in tubular lumina. When they appear in the urine, they reflect the shapes and diameters of the lumina of origin. In normal individuals, very few casts are seen, i.e., no more than one per low power field. This relates to the small amounts of protein present in normal urine (less than 150 mg/24 hrs). Such proteins as are normally present derive in part from glomerular leakage (e.g., albumin) and in part from the secretions of the cells lining the ascending limb of Henle's loop and distal convoluted tubule (Tamm-Horsfall mucoprotein). Thus the proteins of urinary casts derive from plasma, tubular cells, or both. It is generally held that Tamm-Horsfall mucoproteins form the basic matrix of all casts, whether or not plasma proteins are present. An increased number of casts in the urine is known as cylindruria.

Hyaline casts (Fig. 17–11)

Basic protein casts are described as hyaline. They form in either distal convoluted tubules or collecting ducts. Presumably, broader casts form in collecting ducts. Increased numbers of hyaline casts do not necessarily imply renal disease. Transient cylindruria may be noted during fevers or postural proteinuria. It may also follow strenuous exercise or diuretic therapy (Imhof, 1972). The hyaline casts which follow ethacrynic acid or furosemide therapy are composed of Tamm-Horsfall mucoprotein. There is no concomitant proteinuria. The casts which follow strenuous exertion are of essentially the same composition. In general, the casts produced by patients with renal disease contain blood proteins in addition to renal proteins (Imhof, 1972).

Factors favoring cast formation include: (1) decreased urine flow (stasis), (2) low pH, (3) high solute concentration, and (4) high protein concentration. The suggestion has been made that increased numbers of hyaline casts in urine from patients at rest may presage future cardiovascular or renal diease as much as 10 years in advance of clinical manifestations (Schreiner, 1957). Hyaline casts are increased in acute glomerulonephritis, acute pyelonephritis, malignant hypertension, chronic renal disease, congestive heart failure, and diabetic nephropathy.

When stasis is prolonged, as in severe renal disease, changes in the nephron include tubular dilatation and epithelial atrophy. Casts forming and released from such lumina are likely to be broad. Breadth therefore adds a measure of gravity to the diagnostic significance of hyaline casts.

The presence of various particulate or cellular inclusions in the basic protein matrix of hyaline casts further increases the likelihood of intrinsic renal disease. Further, the type of inclusion may give valuable information as to the presence of specific groups of diseases. Previous theories as to the method of incorporation of cells into cast matrices have recently come under close scrutiny with the application of scanning electron microscopic techniques to the examination of the urinary sediment (Haber, 1977). Rather than becoming entrapped in protein during the process of gelation, cells appear to be bound to a cast surface by delicate fibrillar processes which arise from the underlying hyaline matrix. Whatever the pathophysiologic significance of these observations, clinical decisions continue to be made on light microscopic findings (Fig. 17–11). An improved method for examining casts using Papanicolaou stain has been described (Schumann, 1978).

Red blood cell casts

Red blood cell casts in the urine are of singular importance. By and large they are diagnostic of glomerular disease. Glomerular damage (most frequently due to immune injury) allows red blood cells to escape into the tubule. If there is concomitant proteinuria and conditions are optimal for cast formation, red cell casts form in the distal nephron. In urine, these casts appear yellow under the low power objective. A prerequisite for the identification of a red blood cell cast is that red blood cell outlines be sharply defined in at least part of the cast (Fig. 17-12). If many red cells are present, the matrix may not be visible. With supravital staining, the red blood cells are colorless or lavender in a pink matrix. When stasis has occurred in the nephron, a red cell cast may degenerate and appear in the urine as a reddish brown, coarsely granular cast. Such a cast is known as a blood (Fig. 17-13) or hemoglobin cast. In the absence of concomitant bilirubinuria or pyridium therapy (both of which spontaneously color formed elements in the urine), a pigmented, coarsely granular cast should raise the suspicion of a blood cast. The clinical significance of such a cast is the same as that of an intact red blood cell cast.

Disorders reflected in the presence of red blood cell casts in the sediment include acute glomerulonephritis, lupus nephritis, subacute bacterial endocarditis, Goodpasture's syndrome, and renal infarction. Rarely, tubulo-interstitial disease may allow transtubular entry of red blood cells with subsequent incorporation into a cast. This may occur in severe pyelonephritis (Haber, 1975).

White blood cell casts

White blood cells usually enter tubular lumina from the interstitium. They enter through and between tubular epithelial cells (Haber, 1975). Hence, diseases which might be expected to be associated with white blood cell casts (Fig. 17-14) in the urine are those in which neutrophilic exudates and interstitial inflammation are present in the kidney. The most common disease satisfying these criteria is pyelonephritis. Although it is also true that white blood cell casts may be present in glomerular disease, this is by no means a common finding. By and large white blood cell casts reflect tubulo-interstitial disease.

With brightfield microscopy, leukocyte casts (Fig. 17-15) may be difficult to identify as such, particularly if stasis and nuclear fragmentation or fusion have occurred. Phase microscopy may be helpful in delineating nuclear segments.

In addition to acute pyelonephritis, white blood cell casts may be found in the urine of patients with lupus nephritis. In this setting, urine cultures are sterile. Finally, these casts have been reported in acute glomerulonephritis, interstitial nephritis, and even in the nephrotic syndrome (Schreiner, 1957).

Tubular epithelial cell casts

The difficulties encountered in distinguishing free polymorphonuclear cells from tubular cells are amplified when trying to identify casts in which either or both of these cell types occur. When well preserved, tubular casts contain two parallel rows of cells. This appearance implies origin in one segment of a damaged tubule. When the tubular cells are randomly distributed throughout a cast, origin of the cells in different parts of the tubule may be postulated. Supravital staining, phase contrast microscopy, and Papanicolaou staining (Fig. 17-16) may be helpful in separating tubular epithelial casts from white blood cell casts.

Renal tubular epithelial cell casts are among the rarest casts seen in urine. This relates to the rarity of pure tubular necrosis, viral disease (e.g., cytomegalovirus disease), or exposure to a variety of drugs. Heavy metal poisoning and ethylene glycol and salicylate intoxication may cause tubular cells and casts to appear in the urine. In transplant units, these casts constitute one of the more reliable criteria for detecting acute allograft rejection after the third postoperative day (see above). Rarely, epithelial cells may be seen in eclampsia and amyloidosis (Schumann, 1977).

Mixed and cellular casts

When tubular cells and white blood cells are identified with certainty in a cast, the resulting hybrid is called a mixed cast (Fig. 17-17). This hybrid form implies tubulo-interstitial disease. When the cell type cannot be established with certainty, the resulting cast is known as a cellular cast (Fig. 17-18). Some inferences as to cell type may be drawn from the dominant population of free cells in the surrounding sediment. If not, the differential diagnosis is additive, i.e., that of white blood cell casts and tubular epithelial cell casts.

Granular casts

The basic matrix of all casts is Tamm-Horsfall mucoprotein. When granules are present in a basic cast matrix, the cast is described as granular (Fig. 17-19). The granules derive either from plasma proteins which have aggregated in a Tamm-Horsfall matrix (Rutecki, 1971) or from the breakdown products of contained degenerating cells. Using

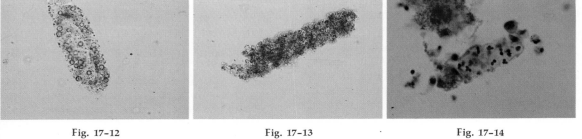

Fig. 17-12   Fig. 17-13   Fig. 17-14

2

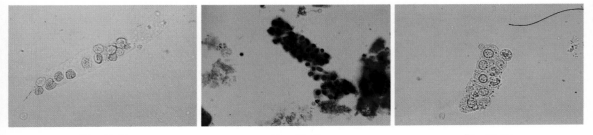

Fig. 17-15   Fig. 17-16   Fig. 17-17

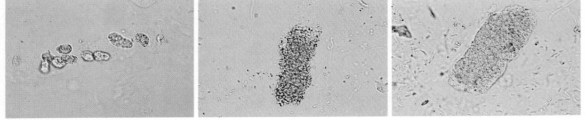

Fig. 17-18   Fig. 17-19   Fig. 17-20

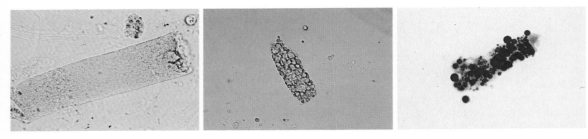

Fig. 17-21   Fig. 17-22   Fig. 17-23

Figure 17-12. Red blood cell cast ($\times$200). **Figure 17-13.** Blood or hemoglobin cast ($\times$200).

Figure 17-14. White cell cast. Papanicolaou stain ($\times$430). **Figure 17-15.** White blood cell cast ($\times$200).

Figure 17-16. Tubular epithelial cast. Papanicolaou stain ($\times$430).

Figure 17-17. Mixed white cell and tubular epithelial cast ($\times$200).

Figure 17-18. Cellular cast ($\times$200). **Figure 17-19.** Granular cast ($\times$200).

Figure 17-20. Finely granular cast becoming waxy ($\times$200).

Figure 17-21. Waxy cast ($\times$200).

Figure 17-22. Fatty cast, non-polarizing ($\times$160).

Figure 17-23. Fatty cast, non-polarizing but positive oil red O ($\times$200).

fluoroscein-tagged antibodies to plasma proteins, many granules in granular casts have been shown to be composed of plasma proteins. Initially most granules are large and coarse. With prolonged intrarenal stasis, these granules ultimately break down to fine granules. There is no clinical advantage, however, to separating coarsely granular from finely granular casts in reporting cylindruria. Because of the possible sources of these granules (glomerular or tubulo-interstitial), granular casts almost always indicate significant renal disease. Exceptions include the brief showers of granular casts which may follow strenuous exercise or those which appear during adherence to a pure carbohydrate diet. The mechanism of granular cast formation in the latter circumstances is not understood. Occasionally, red cell detritus may contribute to cast granularity.

Granular casts may be present in pyelonephritis, viral disease, and chronic lead intoxication. They are intermittently seen in acute allograft rejection.

Waxy casts

These smooth-appearing blunt-ended casts differ from hyaline casts in that they are easily visualized because of their high refractive index even with brightfield microscopy. Early waxy casts are believed to reflect the final phase of dissolution of the fine granules of granular casts (Fig. 17-20). Since time is required for granules to undergo lysis, waxy casts imply localized nephron obstruction and oliguria.

With brightfield microscopy, later forms are homogeneously smooth in appearance (see Fig. 17-21). Their margins are sharp even in subdued light. Their ends are blunt, and cracks or convolutions are frequently seen along the lateral margins, indicating a measure of brittleness while negotiating the distal nephron. Waxy casts are most commonly associated with tubular inflammation and degeneration. They are observed most frequently in patients with chronic renal failure. They are also occasionally found during acute and chronic renal allograft rejection. When waxy casts are unusually broad, they are known as renal failure casts. These casts carry the implication of advanced tubular atrophy and/or dilatation, in turn reflecting end-stage renal disease. Broad waxy casts are therefore the most ominous of all casts found in the urinary sediment.

Fatty casts

Fatty casts are best defined as cylindroids containing fatty droplets or oval fat bodies (Fig. 17-22). The clinical significance of fatty casts is essentially the same as that of fatty droplets or oval fat bodies themselves. If the droplets are anisotropic, polarization results in Maltese cross formation, reflecting the presence of cholesterol. Isotropic droplets, however, do not polarize. Fat stains are then required to demonstrate the presence of triglycerides (Fig. 17-23). Sudan III and oil red O stains are equally effective in staining triglycerides, whether free, in tubular cells, or in casts.

Crystal casts

Casts containing urates and oxalates are occasionally noted in the urinary sediment. Apart from the possible significance of these crystals per se, the clinical significance of these casts remains that of cylindruria in general. Caution must be exercised in identifying crystal casts, since they polarize rather brightly and may be mistaken for fatty casts. Neither urates nor oxalates polarize as Maltese crosses however. The only particles polarizing as Maltese crosses other than lipids are starch granules. These may be free or attached to cast surfaces. They always reflect specimen contamination.

Other miscellaneous casts or cast-like structures

Bacteria on rare occasions may be embedded in cast matrices. On supravital staining, they appear dark purple in a pale pink matrix. Mucous threads are commonly confused with casts. However, they are long and ribbon-like, with poorly defined edges and pointed or split ends. Occasionally they appear to have longitudinal striations.

THE TELESCOPED SEDIMENT

This term is used to describe the simultaneous occurrence of elements of acute and chronic glomerulonephritis as well as those of the nephrotic syndrome in the same urine. A telescoped sediment might therefore include red cells, red cell casts, cellular casts, broad waxy casts, lipid droplets, oval fat bodies, and fatty casts. Such sediment may be found in

Table 17–17. URINALYSIS ABNORMALITIES FOUND IN VARIOUS URINARY SYSTEM DISEASES

DISEASES	MACROSCOPIC URINALYSIS	MICROSCOPIC URINALYSIS
Acute glomerulonephritis	Gross hematuria "Smoky" turbidity Proteinuria	Erythrocyte and blood casts Epithelial casts Hyaline and granular casts Waxy casts Neutrophils Erythrocytes
Chronic glomerulonephritis	Hematuria Proteinuria	Granular and waxy casts Occasional blood casts Erythrocytes Leukocytes Epithelial casts Lipid droplets
Acute pyelonephritis	Turbid Occasional "odor" Occasional proteinuria	Numerous neutrophils (many in clumps) Few lymphocytes and histiocytes Leukocyte casts Epithelial casts Renal epithelial cells Erythrocytes Granular and waxy casts Bacteria
Chronic pyelonephritis	Occasional proteinuria	Leukocytes Broad waxy casts Granular and epithelial casts Occasional leukocyte cast Bacteria Erythrocytes
Nephrotic syndrome	Proteinuria Fat droplets	Fatty and waxy casts Cellular and granular casts Oval fat bodies and/or vacuolated renal epithelial cells occurring singly or as cellular clusters
Acute tubular necrosis	Hematuria	Necrotic or degenerated renal epithelial cells Neutrophils and erythrocytes Granular and epithelial casts Waxy casts Broad casts Epithelial tissue fragments
Cystitis	Hematuria	Numerous leukocytes Erythrocytes Transitional epithelial cells occurring singly or as fragments Histiocytes and giant cells Bacteria Absence of casts
Acute renal allograft rejection (lower nephrosis)	Hematuria Occasional proteinuria	Renal epithelial cells Lymphocytes and plasma cells Neutrophils Epithelial casts Epithelial fragments Granular, bloody, and waxy casts
Urinary tract neoplasia	Hematuria	Atypical mononuclear cells with enlarged, irregular hyperchromatic nuclei and sometimes containing prominent nucleoli that occur singly or as tissue fragments Neutrophils Erythrocytes Transitional epithelial cells
Viral infection	Hematuria Occasional proteinuria	Enlarged mononuclear cells and/or multinucleated cells with prominent intranuclear and/or cytoplasmic inclusions Neutrophils Lymphocytes and plasma cells Erythrocytes

2

Table 17-18. CHARACTERISTICS OF AMORPHOUS AND CRYSTALLINE URINARY SEDIMENTS

SUBSTANCE	DESCRIPTION	URINE pH WHERE FOUND			SOLUBILITY CHARACTERISTICS
		Acid	Neutral	Alkaline	
Bilirubin	Reddish brown; amorphous needles, rhombic plates, or cubes. May color uric acid crystals	+	−	−	Soluble in alkali, acid, acetone, chloroform
Cholesterol	Rare; flat, colorless plates with corner notch	+	+	−	Very soluble in chlorform, ether, hot alcohol
Calcium carbonate	Small, colorless dumbbells or spheres; rarely needles	−	+	+	Soluble in acetic acid with effervescence
Calcium oxalate	Small, colorless octahedron common; dumbbell, ring form	+	+	Slight	Soluble in dilute HCl
Cystine	Colorless, hexagonal, flat; rapidly destroyed by bacteria. May be confused with uric acid	+	−	−	Soluble in alkali, especially ammonia, and dilute hydrochloric acid. Insoluble in boiling water, acetic acid, alcohol, ether
Hematin	Small, biconvex whetstone seen with hemoglobinuria	+	−	−	
Hemosiderin	Clumps of golden brown granules	+	+	−	Blue with Prussian blue
Hippuric acid	Rare; colorless needles, rhombic plates, and four-sided prisms. Distinguish from phosphates	+	+	+	Soluble with hot water, alkali. Not soluble in acetic acid
Indigotin	Rare; amorphous blue or small crystals. Colors other crystals	+	+	+	Very soluble in chloroform. Soluble in ether. Insoluble in acetone
Leucine	Yellow spheroids with radial striations. Seen with tyrosine. Probably not pure	+	−	−	Soluble in hot alcohol, alkali. Slightly soluble in hot water. Crystallizes out as hexagonal plates in pure form
Phosphates					
Ammonium magnesium (triple phosphate)	Common form. Colorless, three- to six-sided prisms, "coffin lid." Sometimes fern leaf	−	+	+	Soluble in dilute acetic acid
Calcium hydrogen	Less common. Star-shaped or long, thin prisms; needles or occasional plates	Slight	+	+	Soluble in dilute acetic acid
Sulfonamides					
Sulfadiazine	Dense, greenish globules	+	+	−	Soluble in acetone
Acetylsulfadiazine	Wheat sheaves, eccentric binding	+	+	−	
Tyrosine	Colorless or yellow, fine silky needles in sheaves or rosettes	+	−	−	Soluble in alkali, dilute mineral acid, relatively heat soluble. Insoluble in alcohol, ether
Urates	Yellow, calcium, magnesium, and potassium, mostly amorphous	+	−	−	Soluble in alkali, soluble at 60°C.
	Ammonium—thorn apple, brown	−	+	+	Soluble at 60°C. with acetic acid; soluble strong alkali
	Potassium—small, spherical, brown Sodium acid urate—colorless, needles or amorphous	+	−	−	Soluble at 60°C.
Uric acid	Yellow, red-brown, large variety of crystals—rhombic, four-sided plates, rosettes. Colorless, smaller crystals	+	−	−	Soluble in alkali. Insoluble in alcohol, acids
Xanthine	Rare, colorless, rhombic plates	+	+	−	Soluble in alkali, soluble with heat. Insoluble in acetic acid
Radiographic media (Diatrizoate)	Colorless, thin, rhombic, some with notch	+	−	−	Soluble in 10% NaOH. Insoluble in ether, chloroform

collagen vascular disease (notably lupus nephritis) and subacute bacterial endocarditis.

SUMMARY

The cells and casts encountered in common
renal diseases are summarized in Table 17–17.
Further details of the urinary sediment in
these and other renal diseases may be found
in Lippman (1957), Strauss (1971), and Kurtzman (1974).

CRYSTALS

By and large, crystals in the urine are of
limited clinical significance. Phosphates,
urates, and oxalates are especially common
and occur in normal urine sediment. Their
presence often deflects attention from more
important formed elements. A few crystals,
however, are important. For the purpose of
separating these from more commonly occurring "nuisance" crystals, a summary of crystal
morphology is presented (Table 17–18).

A prerequisite for the positive identification
of crystals is a knowledge of the pH. This
helps to separate more ambiguous forms from
each other, e.g., amorphous phosphates from
amorphous urates.

Crystals found in normal acid urine

1. *Amorphous urates:* yellow-red granular
   precipitate.
2. *Sodium acid urates:* brown spheres. Revert to uric acid plates on acidification
   with acetic acid (Fig. 17–24).
3. *Uric acid:* yellow or red-brown, irregular
   but usually "whetstone" crystals or
   rhomboids (Figs. 17–26 and 17–27).
   Rarely hexagonal, like cystine.
4. *Calcium oxalate:* refractile, octahedral
   "envelopes" (Fig. 17–28). Rarely oval (see
   Fig. 17–25).

Crystals found in normal alkaline urine

1. *Amorphous phosphates:* fine granular
   precipitate.
2. *Triple phosphates:* colorless, three- to
   six-sided prisms. Occasionally fern leaf.
3. *Ammonium biurate:* yellow-brown,
   thorny spheres (Fig. 17–29).
4. *Calcium phosphate:* stellate prisms; occasionally sheaves like sulfonamide or large
   clear plates (Figs. 17–30 and 17–31).

5. *Calcium carbonate:* colorless spheres or
   dumbbells, always tiny.

Crystals found in abnormal urine

1. *Cystine:* colorless, refractile, hexagonal
   plates (Fig. 17–32).
2. *Tyrosine:* fine needles arranged in
   sheaves or clumps, usually yellow, silky
   (Fig. 17–33).
3. *Leucine:* yellow, oily-appearing spheres
   with radial and concentric striations.
   Leucine and tyrosine crystals may occur
   together.
4. *Sulfonamides:* yellow-brown asymmetrical, striated sheaves (Fig. 17–34) or round
   forms with radial striations (Fig. 17–35).
5. *Renografin (meglumine diatrizoate):*
   found briefly after radiographic studies
   of the urinary tract; flat, clear, colorless
   rhombic plates, easily polarized, inter-
   secting at 80 degrees (Fig. 17–36).
6. *Ampicillin (high dosage):* long, fine colorless crystals (Fig. 17–37).

Clinical significance

Little significance can be attached to crystals detected in urine standing at room
temperature. When heated to 37°C., most
crystals disappear. Those still present at 37°C.
might have some significance when correlated
with clinical symptoms.

Phosphate crystals have little if any clinical
significance. Large numbers of uric acid crystals may reflect increased nucleoprotein turnover, especially during chemotherapy of leukemias or lymphoma. They may provide
circumstantial evidence for the nature of
small stones lodged in the ureters, especially
when found in conjunction with raised serum
uric acid levels. Urates in large amounts may
have similar connotations but may herald the
urate nephropathy of gout. Oxalate crystals in
large numbers may reflect severe chronic renal
disease, ethylene glycol or methoxyflurane
toxicity. Oxaluria has recently come into
prominence as a reflection of the increased
absorption of oxalates from food following
small bowel resection, notably for Crohn's disease (Earnest, 1974; Dobbins, 1977). Cystine
crystals are colorless hexagonal plates (Berman, 1974) which are frequently laminated
(see Fig. 17–32). They may, however, be confused with hexagonal forms of uric acid (Fig.

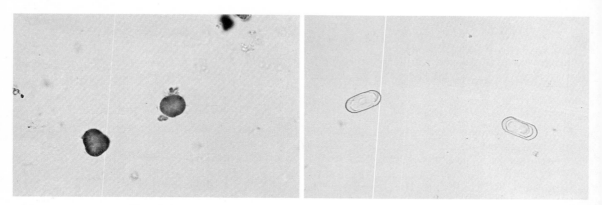

Fig. 17-24   Fig. 17-25

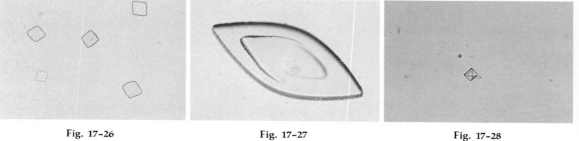

Fig. 17-26   Fig. 17-27   Fig. 17-28

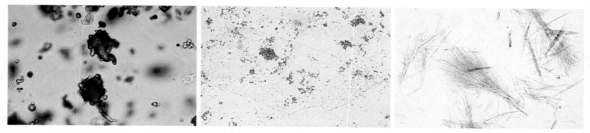

Fig. 17-29   Fig. 17-30   Fig. 17-31

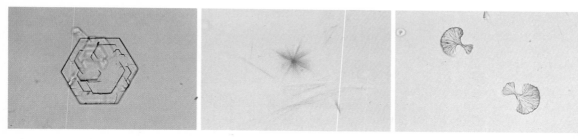

Fig. 17-32   Fig. 17-33   Fig. 17-34

Figure 17-24. Sodium acid urates ($\times 160$). **Figure 17-25.** Unusual oval forms of calcium oxalate ($\times 200$).

Figure 17-26. Uric acid ($\times 160$). **Figure 17-27.** Large uric acid plate, laminated ($\times 160$).

Figure 17-28. Calcium oxalate ($\times 200$). **Figure 17-29.** Ammonium biurate ($\times 160$).

Figure 17-30. Large clear plate of calcium phosphate; also amorphous phosphates ($\times 64$).

Figure 17-31. Rare fine sheaves of calcium phosphate ($\times 160$).

Figure 17-32. Hexagonal cystine, non-polarizing and laminated ($\times 200$).

Figure 17-33. Tyrosine ($\times 160$). **Figure 17-34.** Sulfadiazine ($\times 160$).

17–38*A*). Whereas uric acid crystals polarize (Fig. 17–38*B*), cystine crystals do not. Cystine crystals are among the most important found in the urine. They occur in patients with congenital cystinosis or cystinuria and may be associated with cystine calculi. Tyrosine and leucine crystals are occasionally seen in the urine of patients with severe liver disease. With the advent of more soluble sulfa drugs, sulfa crystals (see Fig. 17–34) are no longer frequently found in urine, especially when the urine is examined at 37°C. (Alfthan, 1972). Renograffin crystals (see Fig. 17–36) frequently follow radiographic examinations of the urinary tract. Ampicillin may crystallize in the urine under conditions of high dosage (see Fig. 17–37). Other drugs are occasionally reported to cause crystalluria when administered in high dosage schedules or following overdosage. Examples include high dosage 6-mercaptopurine therapy (Duttera, 1972) and primidone overdosage (Bailey, 1972).

ABNORMAL CELLS AND OTHER FORMED ELEMENTS

Viral Inclusion and Tumor Cells. Malignant tumor cells exfoliated from renal pelvis, ureter, bladder wall, and urethra may be identified (Tweeddale, 1977). Kidney tumor cells are rarely diagnosed in a urine sediment.

Epithelioid cells with inclusion bodies may be found in the urine in viral diseases (Dewall, 1966). Occasionally syncytial giant cells containing nuclear inclusions are seen in the urine in measles. In children or immunosuppressed patients with cytomegalic inclusion disease, epithelioid cells with nuclear inclusion bodies are found in the urine.

For cytologic study, the urine should be collected into an equal volume of 70 per cent alcohol. A fixed film of centrifuged sediment may be stained with Papanicolaou stain or a special stain for inclusion bodies (Lippman, 1957).

Bacteria, Fungi, and Parasites. Bacteria may or may not be significant, depending on the method of urine collection and how soon after collection of the specimen the examination takes place. A dry film may be made by spreading a drop or two of the urine sediment on a glass slide. It may then be fixed and stained with Gram's stain. The uncentrifuged urine may be examined in the same manner. If bacteria are identified in the uncentrifuged

specimen under an oil-immersion lens, it suggests that more than 100,000 organisms per ml are present, i.e., significant bacteriuria. Most commonly, rod-shaped bacteria are seen, since the enteric organisms are most often found in urinary tract infection. If urinary tract infection is indeed present, usually many leukocytes also will be seen in the sediment.

Using direct immunofluorescence as a means of visualizing antibody complexed with the bacteria in the urine, Thomas (1974) found a significant correlation between the presence or absence of antibody-coated bacteria and the localization of the infection in the kidney or the bladder, respectively.

Acid-fast staining of the urine sediment may reveal tubercle bacilli, but since smegma contains non-pathogenic acid-fast organisms, the presence of tubercle bacilli in urine must be substantiated by culture. An early morning catheterized specimen is preferred for culture purposes.

Yeast cells (*Candida*) may be found in urinary tract infection (e.g., in diabetes mellitus), but yeasts are also common contaminants from skin and air. They may be confused with red blood cells; budding is usually seen and helps to identify them as yeast cells (Fig. 17–39). Pseudomycelial forms of *Candida* are occasionally found (Fig. 17–40).

Parasites and parasitic ova may be seen in urine sediments as a result of fecal or vaginal contamination. When these are noted, the examination should be repeated on a fresh, clean-voided urine specimen. In patients with schistosomiasis due to *Schistosoma haematobium*, typical ova may be found in the urine accompanied by red blood cells from the urinary bladder. *Trichomonads* may be present in urine as a result of vaginal contamination. When urethral or bladder infection is suspected, the protozoa should be searched for immediately in a wet preparation of the sediment; the motility of the organism is helpful in making the appropriate identification. Ameba are rarely seen in the urine; these may reach the bladder from lymphatics or more likely from fecal contamination of the urethra. The pathogenic *Entamoeba histolytica* is usually accompanied by erythrocytes and leukocytes.

Contaminants and Artifacts. The vinegar eel, fly larvae, and other parasites may be found in urine as a result of dirty or contami-

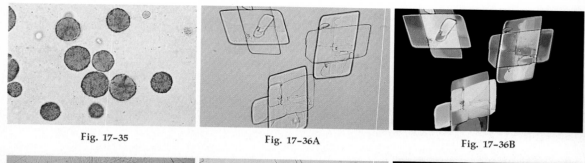

Fig. 17–35   Fig. 17–36A   Fig. 17–36B

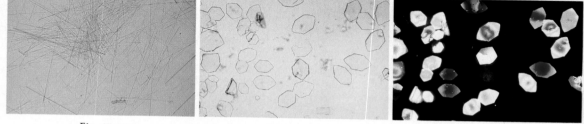

Fig. 17–37   Fig. 17–38A   Fig. 17–38B

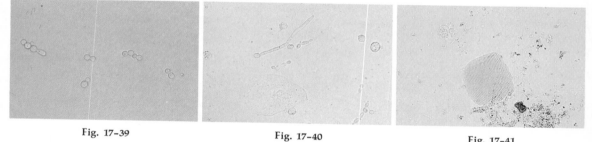

Fig. 17–39   Fig. 17–40   Fig. 17–41

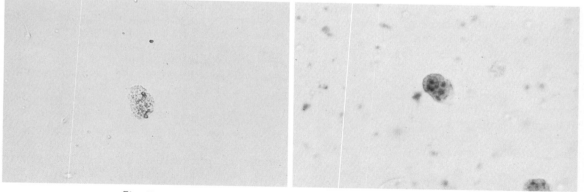

Fig. 17–42   Fig. 17–43

Figure 17–35. Sulfasalazine (Azulfidine).

Figure 17–36. *A,* Renografin, unpolarized ($\times$160); *B,* Renografin, polarized ($\times$160).

Figure 17–37. Ampicillin ($\times$40).

Figure 17–38. *A,* Hexagonal uric acid, unpolarized ($\times$50); *B,* Hexagonal uric acid, polarized ($\times$50).

Figure 17–39. Candida: budding spores ($\times$200). **Figure 17–40.** Candida: pseudohyphae ($\times$160, unstained).

Figure 17–41. Muscle fiber: patient with rectovesical fistula ($\times$200).

Figure 17–42. Tubular cell containing brown pigment; iron, unstained ($\times$260).

Figure 17–43. Tubular cell positive with Prussian blue stain (hemosiderinuria) ($\times$260).

nated containers. Partly digested muscle fibers or vegetable cells may be found when there is fecal contamination (Fig. 17–41).

Spermatozoa are generally present in the urine of men after nocturnal emissions. They are easily recognized.

Cotton, hair, and other fibers may be seen and are easily identified. Wood fibers, from applicator sticks may be found if sticks are used to mix the sediment. Oil droplets from lubricants may be confused with cells, especially red cells, but are structureless. Granules of starch appear bright and striated and should not be confused with cells.

SPECIAL METHODS FOR EXAMINING URINE SEDIMENT

Method for Examining Refractile Bodies in Urine. *Lipid droplets containing choles-terol are anisotropic in polarized light, show up brightly against a dark field,* and appear to be divided into four quadrants. This appearance resembles a *Maltese cross*. Visible evidence of anisotropy depends on the orientation of the crystal in the field; not all will be seen. Crystals, hair, and clothing fibers also show up brightly, but do not exhibit Maltese cross forms. Neutral fat, triglyceride, does not show anisotropy.

A polarizing microscope with rotating stage may be used in this examination. If one is not available, an ordinary light microscope can be easily made usable by the addition of suitable filters. Polaroid filters, consisting of an analyzer circle and a polarizer circle, are used. Install the analyzer disc in the ocular lens of a microscope by unscrewing the eye lens assembly. Insert the polarizer disc in the slotted opening under the substage condenser.

Sediment from a fresh urine sample is examined. Using a high power magnification and bright illumination, turn the polarizing filter in the eyepiece by turning the ocular itself until a maximum darkening of the field is produced. The refractile bodies will have the typical Maltese cross form.

Method for Examining Fat Droplets in Urine
Reagent. Saturated solution of Sudan III in 70 per cent alcohol.

Procedure
1. Urine specimen must be collected in clean, fat-free container (glass, Pyrex, or polyethylene). Waxed cardboard containers are not suitable.

2. Centrifuge about 15 ml of the urine in a clean centrifuge tube for 15 minutes.

3. With a clean medicine dropper, carefully take a drop of urine from the surface of the centrifuged specimen and transfer to a slide, making two deposits. Add a drop of Sudan III to one and coverslip. Coverslip the unstained deposit.

4. Look at unstained specimen for fat. Examine the stained deposit microscopically for round droplets of fat which are colored red-orange with Sudan III. Use the low power objective with subdued light and then the high power objective. The staining reaction may take some minutes.

Leukocyte Peroxidase Stain (Kaplow, 1965). This is a stain for localizing peroxidase activity in which *benzidine dihydrochloride* is used as the indicator compound in a single, stable, reusable staining solution. The method is a rapid and highly sensitive one. The cells are fixed, thereby preserving cell morphology. A method for staining cells in the wet sediment has also been proposed (Prescott, 1964). By this technique, renal epithelial cells and neutrophilic leukocytes are easily differentiated.

Procedure
1. Use fresh smears of the urinary sediment. The urine should be at acid pH. Smears are made by placing a drop of the sediment on a glass slide and making a short smear with another slide edge as for peripheral blood smears. Dry the preparation by waving it rapidly in the air. Thicker smears are made by placing a drop or two of the sediment on a slide and tilting to spread. Allow these to dry in air. Satisfactory smears have been made from refrigerated sediments up to 24 hours old providing the pH of the specimen is acid. An adhesive is not needed. Cytocentrifuged smears may also be used.

2. After proper drying of the smear, fix slides for 60 seconds at room temperature in 10 per cent formol-ethanol (made by adding 10 ml of 37 per cent formaldehyde to 90 ml of absolute ethyl alcohol in a Coplin jar). Wash for 15 to 30 seconds under very gently running tap water. Shake off excess water.

3. Place *wet* slides in incubation mixture in a Coplin jar for 30 seconds at room temperature. The *incubation* mixture is made as follows:

30 per cent ethyl alcohol	100 ml
Benzidine dihydrochloride	0.3 g
0.132 M (3.8 per cent w/v) $ZnSO_4 \cdot 7 H_2O$	1.0 ml
Sodium acetate $(NaC_2H_3O_2 \cdot 3 H_2O)$	1.0 g
3 per cent hydrogen peroxide (must be fresh)	0.7 ml

1.0 N sodium hydroxide	1.5 ml
Safranine O	0.2 g

The reagents should be added in the order listed and be mixed well with each addition. The benzidine salt may contain a small amount of inert residue which will not go into solution. A precipitate forms upon addition of the zinc sulfate; this dissolves upon addition of the remaining reagents. The final pH is 6.00 ± 0.05. The solution should be filtered and stored in a capped Coplin jar or bottle at room temperature. The same solution has been used satisfactorily for as long as six months.

4. Wash briefly (5 to 10 seconds) in running tap water, dry, and examine.

5. If greater nuclear detail is desired, the stained preparations may be counterstained in 1 per cent aqueous cresyl violet acetate for 1 minute.

6. After drying, the slides may be rinsed with xylol and mounted with Permount and a coverslip. The stained preparation is stable for at least 12 months.

Peroxidase activity is represented by discrete dark blue granules in the cytoplasm of granulocytes and monocytes. The cytoplasm of neutrophils is filled with blue granules. Rarely, a neutrophil is observed that is weakly stained or unstained. Renal epithelial cells, squamous epithelial cells, and bacteria stain only with the safranine counterstain.

Hemosiderin in Urine (Rous, 1918). *Hemosiderin appears in the urine sediment in diseases involving a true siderosis of kidney parenchyma (e.g., pernicious anemia, chronic hemolytic anemia, microangiopathic hemolytic anemia, multiple transfusions, paroxysmal nocturnal hemoglobinuria, and hemochromatosis). It may be found as yellow-brown granules that are free or in epithelial cells and occasionally in casts (Fig. 17–42). The Prussian blue reaction is used to demonstrate hemosiderin (Fig. 17–43).*

Procedure

1. Centrifuge a complete morning specimen or random urine sample and pool the sediment. Examine several drops of sediment microscopically, searching for coarse brown granules, especially within epithelial cells.

2. If such granules are seen, suspend the rest of the sediment in a fresh mixture of 5 ml of 2 per cent potassium ferrocyanide and 5 ml of 1 per cent HCl and allow to stand for 10 minutes.

3. Centrifuge, and discard the supernatant. Examine the sediment microscopically. Coarse granules of hemosiderin appear blue in this preparation (Fig. 17–43). If granules do not stain, re-examine after 30 minutes (occasionally, the reaction is delayed).

Metachromatic Staining of Urine Sediment in Metachromatic Leukoencephalopathy (Austin, 1957). Large quantities of metachromatic staining granules are accumulated free in tissues (liver, renal tubules) or within the glial cells of the brain in a demyelinating disease in young children known as metachromatic leukoencephalopathy. The material is a sulfuric acid ester of a cerebroside and results from deficiency of a sulfatase.

Metachromatic staining is seen when the tissue dye complex has an absorption spectrum different from the original dye. The change is caused by polymerization of the dye induced by the negative charge of the sulfatides.

Procedure

A sample of fresh urine (10 ml) is centrifuged for 5 minutes at 2000 rpm. Decant the supernatant. One drop of sediment is placed on a slide. Add 1 to 2 drops of 2 per cent toluidine blue solution to the remaining sediment and stir gently. Transfer one drop of the stained sediment to the slide, place coverslip over it, and examine microscopically.

The abnormal material stains golden brown and is found as free granules or in casts. A negative sediment will remain blue.

REFERENCES

Addis, T.: Glomerular Nephritis. New York, The Macmillan Company, 1948.

Alfthan, O. S., and Liewendahl, K.: Investigation of sulfonamide crystalluria in man. Scand. J. Urol. Nephrol., 6:44, 1972.

Albright, F., and Reifenstein, E. C., Jr.: The Parathyroid Glands and Metabolic Bone Diseases. Baltimore, The Williams & Wilkins Co., 1948.

Altman, P., and Dittmer, D. S.: Biology Data Book, 2nd ed., vol. 111. Bethesda, Md., Federation of American Societies of Experimental Biology, 1974.

Apthorp, G. H.: Investigation of the sugar content of urine from normal subjects and patients with renal and hepatic diseases by paper chromatography. J. Clin. Pathol., 10:84, 1957.

Assa, S.: Evaluation of urinalysis methods in 35 Israeli laboratories. Clin. Chem., 23:126, 1977.

Austin, J. H.: Metachromatic form of diffuse sclerosis: Diagnosis during life by urine sediment examination. Neurology, 7:415, 1957.

Bailey, D. N., and Jatlow, P. I.: Chemical analysis of massive crystalluria following primidone overdose. Am. J. Clin. Pathol., 58:583, 1972.

Balikov, B.: Urobilinogen excretion in normal adults, results of assays with notes on methodology. Clin. Chem., 3:145, 1957.

Barney, J. D., and Sulkowitch, H. W.: Progress in the management of urinary calculi. J. Urol., *27*:746, 1937.

Becker, S., and May, P.: Chromatography of urine sugars. Am. J. Clin. Pathol., *49*:436, 1968.

Becker, S. M., Ramirez, G., Pribor, H. C., and Gillen, A. L.: A quality control product for urinalysis. Am. J. Clin. Pathol., *59*:185, 1973.

Beeler, M., and Henry, J.: Melanogenuria—Evaluation of several commonly used laboratory procedures. J.A.M.A., *176*:136, 1961.

Beeler, M., Veeth, D., Morriss, R., and Biskind, G.: Analysis of urinary calculus comparison of methods. Am. J. Clin. Pathol., *41*:553, 1964.

Belmonte, M. M., Sarkozy, E., and Harpur, E.: Urine sugar determination by the two drop clinitest method. Diabetes, *16*:557, 1967.

Bence Jones, H.: On a new substance occurring in the urine of a patient with mollities ossium. Phil. Tr. Roy. Soc. (London) *138*:55, 1848.

Benedict, S. R.: A reagent for the detection of reducing sugars. J. Biol. Chem., *5*:485, 1909.

Bennett, A. J. E.: New England regional newborn screening programs. N. Engl. J. Med., *297*:1178, 1977.

Berman, L. B.: Urinary hexagons. J.A.M.A., *229*:827, 1974.

Berry, H. K., and Spinlanger, J.: A paper spot test useful in the study of Hurler's syndrome. J. Lab. Clin. Med., *55*:136, 1960.

Bickel, H.: Mellituria, a paper chromatographic study. J. Pediatr., *59*:641, 1961.

Blondheim, S. H., Margoliash, E., and Shafur, E.: A simple test for myohemoglobinuria (myoglobinuria). J.A.M.A., *167*:453, 1958.

Boggs, D. E.: Detection of inborn errors of metabolism. CRC Crit. Rev. Clin. Lab. Sci., *2*:529, 1971.

Bowie, L., Smith, S., and Gochman, N.: Characteristics of binding between reagent-strip indicators and urinary proteins. Clin. Chem., *23*:128, 1977.

Bradley, G. M.: Differentiating epithelial cells from leukocytes in urine. Postgrad. Med., *43*:245, 1968.

Bradley, P. W.: University of Minnesota Clinical Laboratories: Utilization Study, 1978.

Brand, E., Harris, M. M., and Biloon, S.: Cystinuria: The excretion of cystine complex which decomposes in the urine with the liberation of free cystine. J. Biol. Chem., *86*:315, 1930.

Bratton, A. C., and Marshall, E. K., Jr.: A new coupling component for sulfanilamide determination. J. Biol. Chem., *128*:537, 1939.

Brody, L. H., Webster, M. C., and Kark, R. M.: Identification of elements of urinary sediment with phase-contrast microscopy. J.A.M.A., *206*:1977, 1968.

Brownstein, H., and Roberge, A. R.: Detection of phenothiazine derivatives in urine. Clin. Chem., *12*:844, 1966.

Bryant, D., and Flynn, F. V.: An assessment of new tests for detecting bilirubin in urine. J. Clin. Pathol., *8*:163, 1955.

Buist, N. R. M.: Set of simple side room tests for detection of inborn errors of metabolism. Br. Med. J., *2*:745, 1968.

Caraway, W. T.: Chemical and diagnostic specificity of laboratory tests. Am. J. Clin. Pathol., *37*:445, 1962.

Carter, C. H., Wan, A. T., and Carpenter, D. G.: Commonly used tests in the detection of Hurler's syndrome. J. Pediatr., *73*:47, 1968.

Cohen, R. D., and Woods, H. F.: Clinical and biochemical aspects of lactic acidosis. London, Blackwell Scientific Publications, 1976.

Comer, J. P.: Semi-quantitative specific test paper for glucose in urine. Anal. Chem., *28*:48, 1956.

Cook, M. H., Free, A. H., and Giordano, A. S.: The accuracy of urine sugar tests. Am. J. Med. Technol., *19*:283, 1953.

Crawhall, J. C., Purkiss, P., Watts, R. W., and Young, E. P.: The excretion of amino acids by cystinuric patients and their relatives. Am. Hum. Genet., *33*:149, 1969.

Cruikshank, G., and Edmond, E.: "Clean catch" urine in the newborn—bacteriology and cell excretion patterns in the first week of life. Br. Med. J., *4*:704, 1967.

Dahlquist, A.: A test paper for galactose in urine. Scand. J. Clin. Lab. Invest., *22*:87, 1968.

Dahlquist, A., and Svenningsen, N. W.: Galactose in the urine of newborn infants. J. Pediatr., *75*:454, 1969.

Davidsohn, I., and Henry, J. B., (eds.): Todd-Sanford Clinical Diagnosis by Laboratory Methods, 15th ed., Philadelphia, W. B. Saunders Company, 1974.

Dent, C. E., and Rose, G. A.: Amino acid metabolism in cystinuria. Q. J. Med., *20*:205, 1951.

Dewall, C. P., Casazza, A. R., Grimley, P. M., Carbone, P. P., and Rowe, W. P.: Recovery of cytomegalovirus from adults with neoplastic disease. Ann. Intern. Med., *64*:531, 1966.

Dobbins, J. W., and Binder, H. J.: Importance of the colon in enteric hyperoxaluria. N. Engl. J. Med., *296*:298, 1977.

Dorfman, A.: Studies in the biochemistry of connective tissue. Pediatrics, *22*:576, 1958.

Dorfman, A., and Matalon, R.: *In* Stanbury, J. B., Wyngaarden, J. B., and Fredrikson, D. S.: Metabolic Basis of Inherited Disease. New York, McGraw-Hill Book Co., 1972.

Duttera, M. J., et al.: Hematuria and crystalluria after high-dose 6-mercaptopurine administration. N. Engl. J. Med., *287*:292, 1972.

Earnest, D. L., et al.: Hyperoxaluria in patients with ileal resection: An abnormality in dietary oxalate absorption. Gastroenterology, *66*:1114, 1974.

Edwards, O. M., Bayliss, R. I. S., and Millan, S.: Urinary creatinine excretion as an index of the completeness of 24 hour collections. Lancet, *2*:1165, 1969.

Efron, M. L.: Aminoaciduria. N. Engl. J. Med., *272*:1058, 1965.

Esbach, G.: Dosage pratique de l'albumine: Tris méthodes. C. R. Soc. Biol. (Paris) *1*:33, 1874.

Ettinger, B., and Kolb, F. O.: Factors involved in crystal formation in cystinuria in vivo and in vitro crystallization dynamics and a simple quantitative colorimetric assay for cystine. J. Urol., *106*:106, 1971.

Exton, W. G.: A simple and rapid quantitative test for albumin in urine. J. Lab. Clin. Med., *10*:722, 1925.

Forrest, F. M., Forrest, I. S., and Mason, A. S.: Review of rapid urine tests for phenothiazine and related drugs. Am. J. Psychiatr., *118*:300, 1961.

Fraser, C. G., Smith, B. C., and Peake, M. J.: Effectiveness of an outpatient urine screening program. Clin. Chem., *23*:2216, 1977.

Free, A. H., and Free, H. M.: A simple test for urine bilirubin. Gastroenterology, *24*:414, 1953.

Free, A. H., and Free, H. M.: Influence of ascorbic acid on urinary glucose tests. Clin. Chem., *19*:662, 1973a.

Free, A. H., and Free, H. M.: Urinalysis in Clinical Laboratory Practice. Cleveland, CRC Press, 1975.

Free, A. H., Adams, E. C., Kercher, M. L., Free, H. M., and Cook, M. H.: Simple specific test for urine glucose. Clin. Chem., *3*:163, 1957a.

Free, A. H., Rupe, C. O., and Metzler, L.: Studies with a new colorimetric test for proteinuria. Clin. Chem., *3*:716, 1957b.

Free, H. M., and Free, A. H.: Quality control of urinalysis in large hospital and in small laboratories. *In* Anido, G.,

Van Kampen, E., and Rosalki, S. B. (eds.): Progress in Quality Control in Clinical Chemistry, Translations of the 5th International Symposium. Bern, Switzerland, Hans Huber, Publisher, 1973b.

Freni, S. C., and Freni, L. W.: Microhematuria found by mass screening of apparently healthy males. Acta Cytol., *21*:421, 1977.

Freni, S. C., Heederik, G. J., and Hol, C.: Centrifugation techniques and reagent strips in the assessment of microhaematuria. J. Clin. Pathol., *30*:336, 1977.

Froesch, E. R., Reardon, J. B., and Renold, A. E.: The determination of inulin in blood and urine using glucose oxidase for the removal of interfering glucose. J. Lab. Clin. Med., *50*:918, 1957.

Gershenfeld, L.: Urine and urinalysis, 2nd ed. Philadelphia, Lea & Febiger, 1943.

Giordano, A. S., and Winstead, M.: A tablet test for bilirubin in urine. Am. J. Clin. Pathol., *23*:610, 1953.

Goldring, W.: Studies of the kidney in acute infection. J. Clin. Invest., *10*:355, 1931.

Guthrie, R., and Susi, A.: Simple phenylalanine method for detecting phenylketonuria in large populations of newborn infants. Pediatrics, *32*:338, 1963.

Gyure, W. L.: Comparison of several methods for semi-quantitative determination of urinary protein. Clin. Chem., *23*:876, 1977.

Haber, M. H.: Interference contrast microscopy for identification of urinary sediments. Am. J. Clin. Pathol., *57*:316, 1977.

Haber, M. H.: Urine Casts, Their Microscopy and Clinical Significance. Chicago, Am. Soc. Clin. Pathol., 1975.

Haining, R., Hulse, T., and Labbé, R.: Rapid porphyrin screening of urine, stool and blood. Clin. Chem., *15*:400, 1969.

Hall, W. K., Cravey, C. E., Chen, P. T., et al.: An evaluation of galactosuria. J. Pediatr., *77*:625, 1970.

Hambraeus, L.: Comparative studies of the value of two cyanide-nitroprusside methods in the diagnosis of cystinuria. Scand. J. Clin. Lab. Invest., *15*:657, 1963.

Hansen, J. L., and Freier, E. F.: Direct assays of lactate, pyruvate, β-hydroxybutyrate and acetoacetate with a centrifugal analyzer. Clin. Chem., *24*:475, 1978.

Hansen, O. H., et al.: The relationship of lipuria to the fat embolism syndrome. Acta Chir. Scand., *139*:421, 1973.

Hansten, P. D.: Drug Interactions, 3rd ed. Philadelphia, Lea and Febiger, 1975.

Hawk, P. B., Oser, B. L., and Summerson, W. H.: Practical Physiological Chemistry. New York, Blakiston, 1954.

Henry, R. J.: Clinical Chemistry: Principles and Techniques. New York, Harper & Row, Publishers, 1964.

Henry, R. J., et al.: Clinical Chemistry: Principles and Techniques. 2nd ed. New York, Harper & Row, Publishers, 1974.

Henry, R. J., Jacobs, S. L., and Berkman, S.: Studies on the determination of bile pigments. III. Standardization of the determination of urobilinogen as urobilinogenaldehyde. Clin. Chem., *7*:231, 1961.

Henry, R. J., Sobel, C., and Segalove, M.: Turbido metric determination of proteins with sulfosalicylic and trichloroacetic acids. Proc. Soc. Exp. Biol. Med., *92*:748, 1956.

Hoesch, K.: Über die Auswertung der Urobilinogenurie und die umgekehrte Urobilinogenreaktion. Dtsch. Med. Wochenschr., *72*:704, 1947.

Howell, T. H.: Urinary excretion after the age of ninety. J. Gerontol., *11*:61, 1956.

Imhof, P. R., et al.: Excretion of urinary casts after the administration of diuretics. Br. Med. J., *2*:199, 1972.

Johnson, P. K., Free, H. M., and Free, A. H.: A simplified urine and serum screening test for salicylate intoxication. J. Pediatr., *63*:949, 1963.

Kagen, L. J.: Immunologic detection of myoglobinuria after cardiac surgery. Ann. Int. Med., *67*:1183, 1967.

Kaplow, L. S.: Simplified myeloperoxidase stain using benzidine dihydrochloride. Blood, *26*:215, 1965.

Kark, R. M., Lawrence, J. R., Pollak, V. E., Pirani, C. L., Muehrcke, R. C., and Silva, H.: A Primer of Urinalysis, 2nd ed. New York, Harper & Row, Publishers, 1963.

Kern, W. H.: Epithelial cells in urine sediment. Am. J. Clin. Pathol., *56*:67, 1971.

Killander, J., Sjolin, S., and Zaar, B.: Rapid tests for ketonuria. Scand. J. Clin. Lab. Invest., *14*:311, 1962.

Kibrick, A. C.: Extended use of the Kingsley biuret reagent. Clin. Chem., *4*:232, 1958.

Knox, W. E., Le May-Knox, M.: The oxidation in liver of L-tyrosine to acetoacetate through p-hydroxyphenylpyruvate and homogentisic acid. Biochem. J., *49*:686, 1951.

Kurtzman, N. A., and Rogers, P. W.: A Handbook of Urinalysis and Urinary Sediment. Springfield, Ill., Charles C Thomas, Publisher, 1974.

Lagergren, C.: Development of silica calculi after oral administration of magnesium trisilicate. J. Urol., *87*:994, 1962.

Lamon, J., Torben, K., and Realker, A.: The Hoesch test: Bedside screening for urinary porphobilinogen in patients with suspected porphyria. Clin. Chem., *20*:1438, 1974.

Leach, C., Rambault, P. C., and Fischer, C. L.: A comparative study of two methods of urine preservation. Clin. Biochem., *8*:108, 1975.

Legal, E.: Regarding a new acetone reaction and its use in urinalysis. Chemisches Zentralblatt., *13*:652, 1883.

Levy, H. L., Shih, V. E., Madigan, P. M., and MacCready, R. A.: Transient tyrosinemia in full term infants, J.A.M.A., *209*:249, 1969.

Lewis, B., and Richards, P.: Measurement of urinary protein. Lancet, *1*:1141, 1961.

Lindqvist, B., and Wahlin, A.: Differential count of urinary leucocytes and renal epithelial cells by phase contrast microscopy. Acta Med. Scand., *198*:505, 1975.

Lippman, R. W.: Urine and the Urinary Sediment, 2nd ed. Springfield, Ill. Charles C Thomas, Publisher, 1957.

Milne, M. D., Asatoor, A. M., Edwards, K. D. G., and Loughridge, L. W.: The intestinal absorption defect in cystinuria. Gut, *2*:323, 1961.

Nakamura, R. M., Reilly, E. B., Fujita, K., Brown, J., and Kunitake, G. M.: False negative reactions and sensitivity in the urine glucose oxidase test. Diabetes, *14*:224, 1965.

Naumann, H. N.: Differentiation of Bence Jones protein from uroglobulins. Am. J. Clin. Pathol., *44*:413, 1965.

Nakao, K., Wada, O., and Yamo, Y.: Delta-aminoleoulinic acid dehydratase activity in erythrocytes for the evaluation of lead poisoning. Clin. Chim. Acta, *19*:319, 1968.

Onstad, J., Hancock, D., and Wolf, P.: Inhibitory effect of fluoride on glucose tests with glucose oxidase strips. Clin. Chem., *21*:898, 1975.

Palmer, W. W., and Henderson, L. J.: Clinical studies on acid base equilibrium and the nature of acidosis. Arch. Intern. Med., *12*:151, 1973.

Palmieri, L. J., and Schumann, G. B.: Osmotic effects on neutrophil segmentation. An in vitro phenomenon. Acta Cytol., *21*:2, 1977.

Peele, J. D., Gadsden, R. H., and Crews, R.: Evaluation of Ames' "Clini-Tek." Clin. Chem., *23*:2238, 1977.

Peele, J. D., Gadsden, R. H., and Crews, R.: Semi-automated versus visual reading of urinalysis dipsticks. Clin. Chem., 23:2242, 1977.

Pennock, C. A., Most, M. G., and Batstone, G. F.: Screening for mucopolysaccharidoses. Clin. Chem. Acta, 27:93, 1970.

Prescott, L. F.: Urinary white cell excretion patterns. Lancet, 2:238, 1965.

Prescott, L. F., and Brodie, D. G.: A simple differential stain for urinary sediment. Lancet, 2:940, 1964.

Prien, E. L.: Crystallographic analysis of urinary calculi: A 23 year survey study. J. Urol., 89:917, 1963.

Purdy, C. W.: Practical Urinalysis and Urinary Diagnosis. Philadelphia, F. A. Davis Co., 1900.

Putnam, F. W., Easley, C. W., Lynn, L. T., Ritchie, A. E., and Phelps, R. A.: The heat precipitation of Bence Jones proteins. I. Optimum conditions. Arch. Biochem. Biophys., 83:115, 1959.

Renuart, A.: Screening for inborn errors of metabolism associated with mental deficiency or neurologic disorders or both. N. Engl. J. Med., 274:384, 1966.

Riekers, H., and Miale, J. B.: Ketonuria. An evaluation of tests and some clinical implications. Am. J. Clin. Pathol., 30:530, 1958.

Ritter, S., Spencer, H., and Samachson, J.: The Sulkowich test and quantitative urinary calcium excretion. J. Lab. Clin. Med., 56:314, 1960.

Robinson, R. R., Glover, S. N., Phillippi, P. J., Lecocq, F. R., and Langelier, P. R.: Fixed and reproducible orthostatic proteinuria. Am. J. Pathol., 39:291, 1961.

Rous, P.: Urinary siderosis. J. Exper. Med., 28:645, 1918.

Rothera, A. C. H.: Note on the sodium nitro-prusside reaction for acetone. J. Physiol., 37:491, 1908.

Rubin, M. I.: Urine and urination. In Nelson, W. E. (ed.): Textbook of Pediatrics. Philadelphia, W. B. Saunders Company, 1964.

Rubini, H. E., and Wolfe, A. V.: Refractometric determination of total solids and water of serum and urine. J. Biol. Chem., 225:869, 1957.

Rubner, M.: Über die Einwirkung von Bleiacetat auf Trauben-und Milchzucker. Z. Biol., 20:397, 1884.

Rutecki, G. J., et al.: Characterization of proteins in urinary casts. N. Engl. J. Med., 284:1049, 1971.

Ryan, W. L., and Mills, R. D.: Bacterial multiplication in urine during refrigeration. Am. J. Med. Tech., 29:175, 1963.

Samson, M.: The relation of cuprous creatinine to tests for sugar in urine. J. Am. Chem. Soc., 61:2389, 1939.

Sanjurjo, L. A.: Parasitic diseases of the genitourinary system. In Campbell, M. F., and Harrison, J. H.: Urology, 3rd ed., vol. 1. Philadelphia, W. B. Saunders Company, 1970.

Schreiner, G. E.: Identification and significance of casts. A.M.A. Arch. Intern. Med., 99:356, 1957.

Schumann, G. B., Burleson, R. L., Henry, J. B., and Jones, D. B.: Urinary cytodiagnosis of acute renal allograft rejection using the centrifuge. Am. J. Clin. Pathol., 67:2, 1977.

Schumann, G. B., Harris, S., and Henry, J. B.: An improved technique for examining urinary casts and a review of their significance. Am. J. Clin. Pathol., 69:18, 1978.

Schumann, G. B., Palmieri, L. J., and Jones, D. B.: Differentiation of renal epithelium in renal transplantation cytology. Am. J. Clin. Pathol., 67:6, 1977.

Schwartz, M. K.: Interferences in Diagnostic Biochemical Procedures. Adv. Clin. Chem., 16:1, 1973.

Scriver, C. R., Clow, C. L., and Lamm, P.: On the screening, diagnosis and investigation of hereditary aminoacidopathies. Clin. Biochem., 6:142, 1973.

Seegmiller, J. E., Zannoni, V. G., Laster, L., and LaDu, B. N.: An enzymatic spectrophotometric method for the determination of homogentisic acid in plasma and urine. J. Biol. Chem., 236:774, 1961.

Selivanoff, S.: Ber. d. deutch. chem. Gesellsch, 20:181, 1887. In Silber, S., and Reiner, M.: Essential fructosuria. Report of three cases with metabolic studies. Arch. Intern. Med., 54:412, 1934.

Shih, V. E.: Laboratory Techniques for the Detection of Hereditary Metabolic Disorders. Cleveland, CRC Press, 1973.

Simpson, E., and Thompson, D.: Routine urinalysis. Lancet, 2:361, 1977.

Sjoerdsma, A., Weissbach, H., and Udenfriend, S.: Simple test for diagnosis of metastatic carcinoid. J.A.M.A., 159:397, 1955.

Smith, I. (ed.): Chromatographic and Electrophoretic Techniques, 3rd ed., vol. I. London, Heinemann, 1969.

Smith, B. C., Peake, M. J., and Fraser, C. G.: Urinalysis by use of multitest reagent strips: Two dipsticks compared. Clin. Chem., 23:2337, 1977.

Spaeth, G. L., and Barber, G. W.: Prevalence of homocystinuria among the mentally retarded: Evaluation of a specific screening test. Pediatrics, 40:586, 1967.

Stanbury, J. B., Wyngaarden, J. B., and Fredrikson, D. S.: Metabolic basis of inherited disease. New York, McGraw-Hill Book Co., 1972.

Sternheimer, R.: A supravital cytodiagnostic stain for urinary sediments. J.A.M.A., 231:8, 1975.

Sternheimer, R., and Malbin, B.: Clinical recognition of pyelonephritis with a new stain for urinary sediments. Am. J. Med., 11:312, 1951.

Strauss, M. B., and Welt, L. G. (eds.): Diseases of the Kidney, vols. 1 and 2. Boston, Little, Brown & Co., 1971.

Stuber, A.: Screening tests and chromatography for the detection of inborn errors of metabolism. Clin. Chim. Acta, 36:309, 1972.

Thomas, G. H., and Howell, R. R.: Selected Screening Tests for Genetic Metabolic Diseases. Chicago, Year Book Publishers, Inc., 1973.

Thomas, V., Shelokov, A., and Forland, M.: Antibody-coated bacteria in the urine and the site of urinary-tract infection. N. Engl. J. Med., 290:11, 1974.

Triger, D. R., and Smith, J. W. C.: Survival of urinary leucocytes. J. Clin. Pathol., 19:443, 1966.

Tweeddale, D. N.: Urinary Cytology. Boston, Little, Brown & Co., 1977.

Udenfriend, S., Titus, E., and Weissbach, H.: The identification of 5-hydroxy-3-indoleacetic acid in normal urine and a method for its assay. J. Biol. Chem., 216:499, 1955.

Watson, C. J., and Hawkinson, V.: Semiquantitative estimation of bilirubin in the urine by means of the barium strip modification of Harrison's test. J. Lab. Clin. Med., 31:914, 1946.

Watson, C. J., and Schwartz, S.: A simple test for urinary porphobilinogen. Proc. Soc. Exp. Biol. Med., 47:393, 1941.

Wert, E. B.: The Clinilab automated urinalysis system; Six months experience in a community hospital. Ann. Clin. Lab. Sci., 3:319, 1973.

Winer, J.: Practical value of analysis of urinary calculi. J.A.M.A., 169:1715, 1959.

Winer, J., and Mattice, M. R.: Routine analysis of urinary calculi: Rapid, simple method using spot tests. J. Lab. Clin. Med., 28:898, 1943.

Winkel, P., Statland, B., and Jorgenson, J.: Urine microscopy, an ill-defined method examined by multifactorial technique. Clin. Chem., 20:436, 1974.

Wirth, W. A., and Thompson, R. L.: The effect of various conditions and substances on the results of laboratory procedures. Am. J. Clin. Pathol., 43:579, 1965.

With, T. K.: Biology of Bile Pigments, Including a Review of Their Chemistry and a Discussion of analytical Methods. Copenhagen, Arne Frost-Hansen, 1954.

Wolfe, A. V.: Urinary concentrative powers. Am. J. Med., *32*:329, 1962.

Wright, W. T.: Cell counts in urine. Arch. Intern. Med., *103*:76, 1959.

Wright, W. T.: Significance of an opaque green Benedict reaction. N. Engl. J. Med., *254*:570, 1956.

Young, D., and Jackson, A.: Thin layer chromatography of urinary carbohydrates: A comparative evaluation of procedures. Clin. Chem., *16*:954, 1970.

Young, D. S., Pestaner, L. C., and Gibberman, V.: Effects of drugs on clinical laboratory tests. Clin. Chem., *21*:386 D, 1975.

Zimmer, J. G., Dewey, R., Waterhouse, C., and Terry, R.: The origin and nature of anisotropic urinary lipids in the nephrotic syndrome. Ann. Intern. Med., *54*:205, 1961.

18

CEREBROSPINAL FLUID AND OTHER BODY FLUIDS

Arthur F. Krieg, M.D.

CEREBROSPINAL FLUID

FORMATION, CIRCULATION, AND COMPOSITION

About 70 per cent of cerebrospinal fluid (CSF) is formed in the ventricular choroid plexuses by a combined process of active transport and ultrafiltration (Hammock, 1976). About 30 per cent of CSF is formed at other sites, which apparently include the ependymal lining of the ventricles and the cerebral subarachnoid space.

Modern studies support the classic view that CSF (1) is formed within the ventricles, (2) exits from the foramina of Lushka and Magendie in the fourth ventricle, (3) circulates upward over the cerebral hemispheres as well as downward over the spinal cord and nerve roots, and (4) is resorbed through arachnoid villi in dural sinuses as well as at dural reflections over cranial and spinal nerves. The arachnoid villi may also function as unidirectional valves capable of clearing particles 4 to 12 μ in diameter from CSF (e.g., cellular debris from leukocytes and erythrocytes) (Plum, 1975).

The concept of a *blood-CSF barrier* accounts for different concentrations of solutes in plasma and CSF. Anatomically, the blood-CSF barrier is represented by the choroid plexus epithelium and the endothelium of all capillaries in contact with the CSF.

CSF also is in equilibrium with interstitial fluid of the central nervous system (CNS) across a *CSF-brain barrier*. Anatomically, the CSF-brain barrier is represented by the pia mater of the CNS (Dunn, 1972).

A third barrier, the *blood-brain barrier*, anatomically is represented by capillary endothelium in contact with astrocyte foot processes.

Total volume of CSF in adults is approximately 150 ml: about 20 ml in the ventricles, about 60 ml in the subarachnoid cisterns, and about 70 ml in the spinal canal. Total volume of CSF in neonates is approximately 10 to 60 ml. Rate of formation is about 500 ml/day, or 21 ml/hr. Rate of formation is independent of pressure, while rate of resorption depends on the pressure gradient between CSF and venous blood in the dural sinuses (about 60 to 80 mm water). In most cases, hydrocephalus appears related to defects in absorption rather than to increased formation of CSF; usually the difficulty is in blockage of the flow of CSF rather than any

clearly demonstrated abnormality in the absorption apparatus itself (Collins, 1978).

The CSF concentrations of some substances are regulated within narrow limits, notably the ions K^+, H^+, Mg^{++}, and Ca^{++} (Table 18-1). Regulation of these ions probably depends on (1) active transport across the blood-CSF barrier and (2) exchanges between CSF and CNS interstitial fluid. Water and chloride diffuse rapidly across the blood-CSF barrier. Lipid-soluble drugs, including anesthetics and ethyl alcohol, diffuse from plasma to CSF in proportion to their lipid solubility. Glucose, urea, and creatinine diffuse freely but require several hours for equilibration. Other substances, e.g., drugs such as penicillin and streptomycin, do not normally enter CSF from plasma. Proteins

Table 18-1. REFERENCE VALUES FOR LUMBAR CEREBROSPINAL FLUID IN ADULTS*

	CEREBROSPINAL FLUID	SERUM
Protein**	15–45 mg/dl	6.0–7.8 g/dl
prealbumin	2– 7%	–
albumin	56–76%	52–67%
α_1 globulin	2– 7%	2– 5%
α_2 globulin	4–12%	6–14%
β globulin	8–18%	8–16%
γ globulin	3–12%	10–22%
Electrolytes and acid-base		
measurements		
osmolality	280–295 mOsm/l	280–295 mOsm/l
sodium	136–150 mEq/l	136–150 mEq/l
potassium		
lumbar fluid	2.6–3.0 mEq/l	3.0–4.5 mEq/l
cisternal fluid	2.3–2.7 mEq/l	
chloride	118–130 mEq/l	96–104 mEq/l
bicarbonate	20–25 mEq/l	21–26 mEq/l
calcium	2.1–2.7 mEq/l	4.6–5.4 mEq/l
magnesium	2.4–3.0 mEq/l	1.5–2.4 mEq/l
lactate	10–22 mg/dl	3–7 mg/dl
	(0.2–0.4 mmol/l)	(arterial)
pH		
lumbar fluid	7.28–7.32	7.38–7.42
cisternal fluid	7.32–7.34	(arterial)
Pco_2		
lumbar fluid	44–50 mmHg	36–40 mmHg
cisternal	40–46 mmHg	(arterial)
Po_2	40–44 mmHg	95–100 mmHg
		(arterial)
Other constituents		
ammonia	0.5–1.0 μg/ml	1.0–2.0 μg/ml
		(arterial)
creatinine	0.5–1.2 mg/dl	0.5–1.2 mg/dl
glucose	50–80 mg/dl	70–100 mg/dl
		(fasting)
iron	1–2 μg/dl	50–150 μg/dl
phosphorus	1.2–2.0 mg/dl	3.0–4.5 mg/dl
urea	6–16 mg/dl	8–20 mg/dl
uric acid	0.5–3.0 mg/dl	2.0–8.0 mg/dl
zinc	2–6 μg/dl	50–150 μg/dl

*Data from various sources including Millen (1962), Plum (1973), Kalin (1975), Woodbury (1968), and Jaiken (1969).
**See also Table 18-7.

apparently diffuse slowly across a concentration gradient from plasma to CSF, at rates which decrease with increasing hydrodynamic radii (Felgenhauer, 1974).

Recent studies indicate that the blood-CSF barrier can be reversibly opened by several mechanisms, including acute hypertension, seizures, hypercapnea, and injections of radiographic dyes (Plum, 1975). Functionally as well as anatomically, the blood-CSF barrier is a complex structure not yet fully understood.

Lumbar Puncture

Indications for lumbar puncture may include:

1. Suspected meningitis, encephalitis (including neurosyphilis), brain abscess, subarachnoid hemorrhage, leukemia involving the central nervous system, multiple sclerosis, Guillain-Barré syndrome, and spinal cord tumor.

2. Differential diagnosis of cerebral infarct vs. intracerebral hemorrhage (xanthochromic CSF found in about 80 per cent of patients with the latter condition).

3. Introduction of anesthetics, radiographic contrast media, or certain drugs (methotrexate in meningeal leukemia and amphotericin in fungal meningitis).

4. Treatment of selected patients with benign intracranial hypertension (the effectiveness of this therapy is not established). Emergency lumbar puncture may be indicated in patients with suspected meningitis, subarachnoid hemorrhage, or leukemia involving the central nervous system. In most other situations, lumbar puncture is an elective procedure. Elective lumbar puncture should be performed in the morning, with the patient fasting overnight: (a) prompt evaluation by trained laboratory staff may be unavailable during the second and third shifts; (b) glucose levels in CSF can be best evaluated by comparison with blood glucose under fasting conditions; (c) consultants are more likely to be available in event of unexpected problems.

Potential problems and complications of lumbar puncture include:

1. Herniation of the uncus through the tentorium, or the cerebellar tonsils through the foramen magnum, in patients with increased intracranial pressure. In the presence of papilledema, mortality rate from lumbar puncture may be about 0.3 per cent (Marshall, 1970). Papilledema probably is not a contraindication, provided (a) the information sought is not available by other methods (e.g., brain scan); (b) there is a high probability that CSF findings will significantly influence both treatment and outcome; (c) neurosurgical consultation is available.

2. With spinal cord tumor, progression of paresis to paralysis may follow lumbar puncture with removal of CSF. If spinal cord tumor is suspected, it is best to combine lumbar puncture with myelography, and to follow these with surgical exploration, if needed.

3. Extradural or subdural hematoma with resultant paraplegia may follow lumbar puncture in patients who have clotting defects (e.g., thrombocytopenia) or who are receiving anticoagulant drugs (Messer, 1976). Although these conditions are not absolute contraindications, potential benefits should be carefully weighed against risk.

4. In the presence of sepsis, perforation of the meninges enhances development of meningitis (Fischer, 1975). If sepsis is suspected, blood cultures should be obtained prior to lumbar puncture, and repeat examination of CSF performed if the clinical condition warrants.

5. In infants, death may occur from asphyxiation caused by (a) excessive restraint (Campbell, 1968) or (b) tracheal obstruction caused by pushing the head forward (Hintenbuchner, 1968).

6. If no stylet is used, epidermoid tumors may develop after a period of two to ten years (Shaywitz, 1972).

7. Introduction of infection by passing the needle through superficial or deep sepsis in the lumbar regions (e.g., superficial skin infection, cellulitis, or epidural abscess). Indeed, lumbar puncture is contraindicated if there is any infection in the region of the puncture site. If epidural abscess is suspected, aspiration should be performed as the needle is introduced (Alexander, 1967).

8. Postpuncture headache resulting from leakage of CSF has been reported in 13 to 32 per cent of patients (Fishman, 1971). The use of a small needle with stylet (22 gauge) may decrease incidence of postpuncture headache.

Lumbar puncture is performed at L3-L4 or lower to avoid damage to the spinal cord. In small children and infants, the cord may extend as low as L3-L4, so puncture should be performed at L4-L5 or lower.

Pressure and Dynamics

Before any fluid is withdrawn, the pressure should be measured by allowing CSF to rise in a sterile, graduated manometer tube. Normal pressure varies between 50 and 180 mm of CSF, measured with the patient in the lateral recumbent position. Should opening pressure exceed 180, reassure the patient, straighten the legs, back, and neck, and ensure that there is no breath holding, jugular compression, or abdominal compression. If pressure then falls to normal, it is probable that the initial elevation was artifactual. When the needle is correctly placed, minor variations in pressure (5 to 10 mm) occur with respiration. Absence of these minor variations may be due to incorrect placement of the needle or to a block between the needle and the dural sinuses.

CSF pressure is directly related to pressure in the jugular and vertebral veins, which communicate with the intracranial venous sinuses. Measured CSF pressure may be decreased with (1) circulatory collapse; (2) severe dehydration; (3) acute hyperosmolality (causes decrease in brain volume owing to passage of water from CNS to systemic circulation); (4) leakage of CSF (e.g., tear in dura following injury to low back, CSF rhinorrhea, previous lumbar puncture); (5) complete spinal subarachnoid block (lumbar fluid does not communicate with fluid at levels above the block). Measured CSF pressure may be increased with (1) congestive heart failure; (2) inflammation of the meninges (interferes with return of fluid through arachnoid granulations); (3) acute obstruction of superior vena cava (before collateral drainage has developed); (4) obstruction of intracranial venous sinuses owing to thrombosis; (5) acute hyposmolality owing to hemodialysis (causes increase in brain volume owing to passage of water from systemic circulation to CNS); (6) impaired resorption of CSF owing to elevated CSF protein, or subarachnoid hemorrhage; (7) mass lesions (e.g., tumor, abscess, or intracerebral hemorrhage); (8) cerebral edema. If initial pressure is over 200 mm, only 1 to 2 ml of fluid should be removed. A 25 to 50 per cent fall in pressure after removing 1 to 2 ml suggests cerebellar herniation or spinal cord compression above the puncture site. In such cases, *no* additional fluid should be removed, and the patient should be observed closely for several hours. Provided initial pressure is not elevated, and there is no marked fall in pressure when fluid is removed, from 10 to 20 ml of CSF may be obtained without danger to the patient. Ordinarily, three 2 to 4 ml samples are taken in sterile tubes, labeled sequentially as No. 1 (chemistry and serology studies), No. 2 (bacteriologic studies), and No. 3 (cell count).

If the initial pressure is normal and there is clinical suspicion of subarachnoid block or spinal cord tumor, jugular compression (Queckenstedt test) may be performed. This test is contraindicated in suspected intracranial disease, particularly in the presence of increased intracranial pressure! It should *not* be performed as a "routine procedure!"

Normally, if both jugular veins are compressed, CSF pressure increases rapidly to over 300 mm, then rapidly returns to normal when compression ceases. This effect depends on rapid transmission of pressure from the jugular veins, through dural sinuses and arachnoid villi, to intracranial CSF. With sinus thrombosis, obstruction at the foramen magnum, or a mass lesion in the spinal canal, the rise in CSF pressure may be decreased or delayed (a "positive test"). In such cases, normal variations in pressure owing to respiration will be decreased or absent, but straining or abdominal compression results in increased CSF pressure owing to vertebral vein congestion.

About 80 per cent of patients with cord compression have a positive Queckenstedt test. Lesions may include herniated intervertebral disc, vertebral fracture, extradural abscess, adhesions owing to pachymeningitis, and neoplasms.

GROSS EVALUATION AND EXAMINATION FOR XANTHOCHROMIA

Normal CSF is crystal clear, with viscosity comparable to water. However, abnormal CSF may appear "cloudy," "smoky," "hazy," opalescent, turbid, or grossly bloody. Turbidity may be graded from 0 to 4+:

0 = crystal clear fluid
1+ = faintly "cloudy," "smoky," or "hazy," with slight (barely visible) turbidity
2+ = turbidity clearly present, but newsprint easily read through tube
3+ = newsprint not easily read through tube
4+ = newsprint cannot be seen through tube

Turbidity may be caused by:
leukocytes—at least 200 cells/μl required to cause slight turbidity (Fishman, 1971)
erythrocytes—at least 400 cells/μl required to cause slight turbidity (Gooch, 1976; Patten, 1968)
microorganisms (bacteria, fungi, amebas)
contrast media

aspiration of epidural fat during lumbar puncture (Mealey, 1962)

Clotting due to elevated CSF protein may occur with Froin's syndrome, which includes (a) subarachnoid block; (b) very high levels of protein in lumbar CSF; (c) xanthochromia due to elevated protein in lumbar CSF; (d) gel formation in CSF after standing. Clot formation is fairly common with protein levels over 1000 mg/dl but also may occur at lower levels. Very fine clots or "pellicles" may be detected by observing the surface of CSF after 12 to 24 hrs at refrigerator temperature.

Clot formation is abnormal, and indicates increased amounts of fibrinogen in CSF. This may be due to traumatic tap or to increased protein owing to subarachnoid block, suppurative meningitis, tuberculous meningitis, neurosyphilis, etc.

Increased viscosity of CSF has been reported with metastatic mucinous adenocarcinoma to the meninges (Fishman, 1971).

Gross blood (or red cells on microscopic examination) presents the problem of differentiating traumatic tap from pathologic bleeding owing to spontaneous subarachnoid hemorrhage, intracerebral hemorrhage, or trauma. Crenation of erythrocytes is *not* useful in differential diagnosis of traumatic tap vs. subarachnoid hemorrhage. Differential diagnosis of traumatic tap vs. subarachnoid hemorrhage is based on the following: (1) Findings at the bedside. A traumatic tap usually shows nonhomogenous mixing in the manometer, and gradual clearing as several samples are taken. (2) Gross appearance of CSF. Visible clearing of blood between the first and third tubes (or a significant drop in erythrocyte count) is evidence of traumatic tap. (3) Clotting. A very bloody specimen (over 200,000 erythrocytes per μl) due to traumatic tap will clot on standing (Calabrese, 1976), while blood from subarachnoid bleeding will not clot in vitro. (4) Xanthochromia.

Xanthochromia refers to a pale pink to orange or yellow color in the supernatant of centrifuged CSF. In traumatic samples, the supernatant typically is crystal clear, while in subarachnoid hemorrhage, the supernatant usually is xanthochromic, provided erythrocytes have been present in CSF sufficiently long to cause lysis. Initial lysis of erythrocytes in CSF begins after about one to four hours (Calabrese, 1976). This rapid lysis of erythrocytes in CSF is not caused by an osmotic difference between plasma and CSF, since osmolality of both fluids is essentially the same (Table 18-1). Probably, lysis of erythrocytes in CSF is due to lack of plasma proteins and lipids needed to stabilize the erythrocyte membrane. Thus, examination for xanthochromia requires that CSF be centrifuged *within one hour or less* after collection, to avoid false positives.

A variety of pigments may contribute to xanthochromia as observed visually:
1. Oxyhemoglobin
   a. from lysed erythrocytes present in CSF before lumbar puncture
   b. traumatic tap with lysis of erythrocytes after lumbar puncture:
      (1) detergent in lumbar puncture needle and/or sample tube
      (2) greater than one hour delay prior to centrifuging CSF
2. Methemoglobin
3. Bilirubin
   a. from lysed erythrocytes in CSF
   b. from plasma, due to:
      (1) increased levels of direct bilirubin (e.g., 5 to 10 mg/dl) with normal blood-CSF barrier
      (2) increased levels of indirect bilirubin associated with increased permeability of the blood-CSF barrier
4. Increased concentration of CSF protein
   a. levels of CSF protein over 150 mg/dl
   b. traumatic tap with sufficient plasma in "CSF" sample to produce protein concentration over 150 mg/dl
5. Contamination of CSF by merthiolate used to disinfect the skin
6. Carotenoids in CSF due to systemic hypercarotenemia
7. Melanin in CSF due to meningeal melanosarcoma

Xanthochromia occurs in CSF of normal premature infants owing to combined effects of (a) immaturity of the blood-CSF barrier; (b) elevated bilirubin in blood; (c) elevated protein in CSF (see Total Protein, p. 645).

About 2 to 4 hours after subarachnoid hemorrhage, pale pink to pale orange xanthochromia due to oxyhemoglobin appears in CSF, reaching a peak at about 24 to 36 hours, and gradually disappearing at about four to eight days. About 12 hours after subarachnoid hemorrhage, yellow xanthochromia due to bilirubin appears in CSF, reaching a peak at about 2 to 4 days, and gradually disappearing at about two to four weeks (Walton, 1956).

Since the early 1960's, there has been increasing interest in spectrophotometric evaluation of xanthochromia. At least two methods have been described:

1. Qualitative estimates of oxyhemoglobin, methemoglobin, and bilirubin based on spectrophotometric scans (Kjellin, 1974).

2. Calculations based on absorbance at specific wavelengths (Kronholm, 1960; Van Der Meulen, 1966).

Spectrophotometric estimates of xanthochromia may be more sensitive and more specific than visual estimates: (1) methemoglobin may be detected in patients with subdural hematomas (one to two weeks duration or longer) despite clear CSF on visual examination; (2) xanthochromia due to bilirubin can be distinguished from xanthochromia due to increased protein. There is evidence that a higher percentage of patients with clinical central nervous system (CNS) hemorrhage have spectrophotometric xanthochromia as compared with visually detected xanthochromia. Although further studies are needed, spectrophotometric evaluation of xanthochromia may well provide a useful supplement to visual evaluation.

CELL COUNTS AND MICROSCOPIC EXAMINATION

TOTAL LEUKOCYTE COUNT

The generally accepted reference interval or normal range for CSF leukocyte counts in adults is 0 to 5 mononuclear cells (lymphocytes and monocytes) per μl. The reference interval for neonates is somewhat higher: about 0 to 30 mononuclear cells per μl (Dryken, 1975; Sarff, 1976). According to Kolmel (1977), if more than a few milliliters of CSF is taken, the count may rise to 20 or even 30/μl.

Leukocyte counts usually are performed in a Fuchs-Rosenthal counting chamber (depth 0.2 mm), either with undiluted CSF and phase microscopy, or with a small amount of acidified crystal violet added to CSF (Skeel, 1968). Using nine large squares on each side of the chamber, a total of $18 \times \frac{1}{5} \mu$l (3.6 μl) is examined. If there are 5 cells per μl, then 18 cells will be counted in 3.6 μl.

Assuming a Poisson distribution, the coefficient of variation is given by:

$$CV = \frac{100}{\sqrt{\text{no. of cells counted}}}$$

$$= \frac{100}{\sqrt{18}} = \frac{100}{4.2} = 24\%$$

Thus, at the upper limit of the reference interval (5 leukocytes per μl), we may expect ±2 CV of about ±48 per cent.

CSF cell counts should be performed promptly, since leukocytes, like erythrocytes, begin to lyse within about one hour. For this reason, physicians should be prepared to personally perform CSF cell counts when these cannot be done within one hour by available technical staff.

Increased precision of CSF leukocyte counts is possible by counting larger numbers of cells. Electronic cell counters are not yet practical, since variable background counts cause poor precision in the normal range. However, leukocytes can be collected from 1.0 ml of CSF on a membrane filter, using a Swinney cartridge (Burechailo, 1974). By this method, the upper limit of normal is reported as 2 leukocytes per μl.

Erythrocyte counts on CSF are sometimes used to "correct" CSF leukocyte counts or CSF protein measurements for contamination by peripheral blood associated with traumatic tap. Use of such corrections requires (1) that all measurements (RBC, WBC, and/or total protein) be performed on the same tube; (2) an assumption that *all* RBC present are due to traumatic tap, with *no* contribution from subarachnoid or intracerebral hemorrhage; (3) an appreciation that accuracy of the "corrected" CSF WBC and protein is limited by precision of the CSF erythrocyte count. This last limitation may be appreciated in reference to the following examples. If serum protein is 7.0 gm/dl, hematocrit is 45 per cent, CSF RBC is 10,000 per μl, and peripheral RBC is 4.6 million per μl, added protein due to traumatic tap is:

$$= \frac{(7,000 \times 0.55) \text{ mg/dl} \times 10,000 \text{ RBC}/\mu\text{l}}{4,600,000 \text{ RBC}/\mu\text{l}}$$

$$= 8.4 \text{ mg/dl}$$

Therefore, 8 mg/dl should be subtracted from measured CSF protein to obtain a "corrected" value. Some authorities suggest "correction factors" of 15 mg/dl/10,000 RBC/μl (or 1 mg/dl for every 700 RBC/μl). However, as seen from the foregoing example, these formulas do not take into account the fact that whole blood total protein is about 55 per cent that of plasma protein. A more accurate "correction factor" might be 8 mg/dl/10,000 RBC/μl (or 1 mg/dl for every 1200 RBC/μl), assuming normal hematocrit and normal serum protein.

With a high CSF erythrocyte count, inherent errors of chamber RBC counting become important. If 400 erythrocytes are counted in the hemocytometer,

$$CV = \frac{100}{\sqrt{400}} = \frac{100}{20} = 5\%$$

Thus, 2 CV represents a 10 per cent error owing to inherent limitations of the counting procedure. If serum protein is 7.0 gm/dl, hematocrit is 40 per cent, CSF RBC is 1.0 million/μl, and peripheral RBC is 4.6 million/μl, added protein due to traumatic tap is:

$$= \frac{(7,000 \times 0.6) \text{ mg/dl} \times 1 \times 10^6 \text{ RBC}/\mu\text{l}}{4.6 \times 10^6 \text{ RBC}/\mu\text{l}}$$

$$= 913 \text{ mg/dl}$$

However, if there is a 10 per cent error in CSF erythrocyte count, the "true" added protein due to traumatic tap is:

$$= \frac{(7,000 \times 0.6) \text{ mg/dl} \times 0.9 \times 10^6 \text{ RBC}/\mu\text{l}}{4.6 \times 10^6 \text{ RBC}/\mu\text{l}}$$

$$= 822 \text{ mg/dl}$$

Thus in this case, the "correction" is accurate only within a range of ± 10 per cent or ± 90 mg/dl.

Similar calculations can be used to correct CSF WBC for traumatic tap:

$$WBC_{added} = \frac{WBC_B \times RBC_{CSF}}{RBC_B}$$

where
WBC_{added} = leukocytes added to CSF for traumatic tap
WBC_B = leukocyte count in peripheral blood
RBC_{CSF} = erythrocyte count in CSF
RBC_B = erythrocyte count in peripheral blood

With normal peripheral blood, this amounts to 1 to 2 leukocytes per 1000 RBC.

DIFFERENTIAL COUNT

Methods

A "chamber differential" may be performed using either a small amount of acidified crystal violet added to CSF (Skeel, 1968) or phase microscopy with unstained fluid (Sornas, 1967, 1971). However, since only a few cells are observed, the "chamber differential" has relatively poor precision. Concentration of leukocytes prior to the differential count can provide larger numbers of cells for improved precision and better staining for more accurate cell identification. Methods for concentrating CSF leukocytes prior to differential counting include:

1. Centrifugation, with Wright's stain of resuspended sediment (Skeel, 1968)
2. Millipore or Nucleopore filter techniques (Gondos, 1976)
3. Sedimentation methods (Kolmel, 1977; Chu, 1977)
4. Cytocentrifuge and related methods (Woodruff, 1973; Ito, 1972).

Centrifugation is relatively rapid (under 1/2 hr) and requires no special equipment. Also, the supernatant fluid is available for further analysis (e.g., total protein, glucose, electrophoresis). Disadvantages include (a) variable and incomplete recovery of sedimented cells; (b) distortion and damage to cells during high-speed centrifugation; (c) the need for careful attention to technique to prepare a high quality film from the sediment. Because of these disadvantages, other methods are now replacing ordinary centrifugation in the United States as well as in Europe.

Millipore (Millipore Corporation, Bedford, Mass.) or Nucleopore (General Electric, Pleasanten, Cal.) filtration, like centrifugation, allows use of supernatant fluid for further analysis. With proper technique, recovery of cells exceeds 90 per cent, so that CSF leukocyte count can be determined from the total number of cells collected (Burechailo, 1974). Although tumor cells are well preserved (Gondos, 1976), other cellular elements are better studied by sedimentation or cytocentrifuge (Sornas, 1967; Krentz, 1972; Hansen, 1974; Castleberry, 1975; Kolmel, 1977). The principal disadvantages of filter techniques include more technical time required than for simple centrifugation, sedimentation, or cytocentrifuge and more technical skill required to cope with problems (e.g., clogging of membranes, staining and clearing techniques).

Sedimentation methods provide better preservation of cellular morphology than filter techniques or cytocentrifuge (Kolmel, 1977; Chu, 1977). The procedure is rapid (1/2 to 1 hour) and technically simple. Disadvantages include loss of cells in the range of 70 per cent owing to absorption on filter paper (Kolmel, 1977); more time required than for cytocentrifuge; and unavailability of the supernatant fluid for chemical analysis.

The cytocentrifuge and related methods provide the following advantages: (a) speed and simplicity superior to other concentration methods, (b) excellent cell preservation, comparable to sedimentation methods, and (c) recovery of cells comparable to sedimentation (though inferior to filtration techniques). Disadvantages include (a) cell recovery inferior to filtration techniques, (b) supernatant fluid unavailable for chemical analysis, and (c) need for special equipment.

For many laboratories, the cytocentrifuge provides an excellent "compromise." The method is rapid, easy to learn, and provides good cytologic detail. Cost of equipment is modest; alternatively, special adapters can be used with an ordinary centrifuge (Ito, 1972). And numerous cells are available for microscopic examination from 0.5 ml CSF.

NOTE: If we assume a "normal" CSF leukocyte count of 1 per μl, a 10 per cent recovery from 0.5 ml would produce 50 cells for study. In actual practice, about 30 to 50 cells are obtained by sedimentation or cytocentrifuge from 0.5 ml of "normal" CSF (Dyken, 1975; Sheth, 1977).

Clinical Correlation

At this time, there is no general agreement on nomenclature for cytologic elements in normal CSF. Sheth (1977) identifies lymphocytes, pia arachnoid mesothelial (PAM) cells, monocytes, and neutrophils (rare) as normally present (Table 18-2). Kolmel (1977) identifies lymphocytes, monocytes, "monocytoid" cells (morphologically similar to the PAM cells described by Sheth), neutrophils (rare), and ependymal cells (rare) as normally present. Dryken (1975) identifies lymphocytes and monocytes in adults, plus a few neutrophils

and macrophages also present in normal neonates. The PAM cells described by Sheth appear similar to young monocytes: relatively large nuclei which are round rather than indented; cytoplasm which is more basophilic and less abundant than mature monocytes. These pia arachnoid mesothelial cells have functional similarities to monocytes of peripheral blood (Oechmichen, 1976; Guseo, 1977).

Suggested reference intervals for differential count in CSF (sedimentation or cytocentrifuge technique) are outlined in Table 18-2. These are based on reports by Dryken (1975) and Sheth (1977), as well as on unpublished data from our own laboratory. However, reported normal ranges from the older literature usually specify a lower percentage of monocytes and a higher percentage of lymphocytes (about 14 per cent and 86 per cent, respectively). One possible explanation has been suggested by Kolmel (1977): after the first few milliliters of CSF, the percentage of monocytes increases while the percentage of lymphocytes decreases. A second explanation is that with sedimentation or cytocentrifuge, monocytes are easily recognized, while with other methods, monocytes which are not "spread out" may be classified as lymphocytes. A third explanation is loss of small lymphocytes by sedimentation or cytocentrifuge.

There has been considerable discussion on whether neutrophils are present in "normal" CSF. Some authors consider even one neutrophil as abnormal (Cole, 1969) while others suggest that up to 10 per cent neutrophils (e.g., 5 out of 50 cells counted) are within normal limits (Sheth, 1977). According to Kolmel (1977), neutrophils in CSF probably come from contamination by peripheral blood owing to traumatic tap. At this time, there is no general agreement on the "upper limit of normal." Significance of small numbers of neutrophils should be evaluated in reference to (a) clinical and laboratory evidence of traumatic tap; (b) findings on neurologic examination; (c) other laboratory findings (e.g., Gram's stain).

Increased numbers of neutrophils may be found in infections, including bacterial meningitis, early viral meningoencephalitis (first one to two days; rarely may persist), early tuberculous or mycotic meningitis, amebic encephalomyelitis, early stages of meningovascular syphilis, and aseptic meningitis owing to septic focus adjacent to the meninges (e.g.,

Table 18-2. REFERENCE INTERVALS FOR CSF DIFFERENTIAL COUNTS BY SEDIMENTATION OR CYTOCENTRIFUGE

CELL TYPE	ADULTS	NEONATES
Lymphocytes	62% ± 34	20% ± 18
PAM cells* and monocytes	36% ± 20	72% ± 22
Neutrophils	2% ± 5	3% ± 5†
Histiocytes	Rare	5% ± 4
Ependymal Cells	Rare	Rare
Eosinophils	Rare	Rare

NOTE: Ordinarily the absolute numbers of cells counted are reported as well as percentages. Since recovery is *not* 100%, the absolute number for each cell type does *not* represent total number for the volume of fluid examined. The CV for a given count can be estimated using the formula $CV = \dfrac{100}{\sqrt{n}}$ where n = number of cells counted.

*PAM = Pia-arachnoid mesothelial cells.
†Some authors report higher upper limit of normal (McCracken, 1976).

septic emboli due to bacterial endocarditis; osteomyelitis of skull or spine; subdural empyema; cerebral abscess; phlebitis of dural sinuses or cortical veins). Noninfectious causes include reaction to CNS hemorrhage (e.g., three to four days after hemorrhagic infarct, subarachnoid hemorrhage, or intracerebral hematoma) (Sornas, 1972), reaction to repeated lumbar puncture (possibly related to hemorrhage caused by traumatic tap), the injection of foreign materials into subarachnoid space (e.g., RISA, xylocaine, methotrexate, or contrast media) (Dramov, 1971; Swartz, 1965), pneumoencephalogram, chronic granulocytic leukemia involving the CNS, lumbar puncture with needles contaminated by detergent, metastatic tumor (necrotic and in contact with CSF, and infarct (hemorrhagic or pale and in contact with CSF).

A neutrophilic reaction classically suggests meningitis owing to pyogenic organisms. During the early acute stage, CSF leukocyte counts frequently exceed 1,000/μl and may reach 20,000/μl, with 90 per cent neutrophils. Other neutrophilic reactions (see above) usually are less marked. In viral meningoencephalitis, the cell count seldom exceeds 1000/μl, and usually changes to a lymphocytic response within two to three days. In bacterial meningitis, successful treatment is associated with rapid disappearance of granulocytes. Unsuccessful treatment, with progression to chronic meningitis or cerebral abscess, is characterized by a mixed reaction, i.e., monocytes, lymphocytes, and granulocytes (Kolmel, 1977).

Increased numbers of lymphocytes have been reported in infections, including (a) viral meningoencephalitis (plasma cells and some macrophages also may be present); (b) tuberculous meningitis (the combination of lymphocytes, granulocytes, and plasma cells is characteristic; multinucleate giant cells may be present); (c) fungal meningitis, e.g., cryptococcosis, coccidioides (a mixed reaction with lymphocytes, granulocytes, and plasma cells is characteristic); (d) syphilitic meningoencephalitis (lymphocytes, plasma cells, and monocytes usually predominate); (e) leptospiral meningitis (this may present a mixed reaction with up to 50 per cent granulocytes); (f) partially treated bacterial meningitis (according to Converse (1973), perhaps 10 per cent of patients revert to a lymphocytic reaction following partial treatment with antibiotics); (g) bacterial meningitis due to uncommon organisms (e.g., *Listeria monocytogenes* in infants) (Hyslop, 1975); (h) parasitic disease (e.g., cysticercosis, trichinosis, toxoplasmosis); (i) aseptic meningitis due to septic focus adjacent to the meninges (see above); and (j) subacute sclerosing panencephalitis (SSPE) due to measles virus (cytologic findings similar to multiple sclerosis). Non-infectious causes include (a) multiple sclerosis (about 50 per cent of cases show increased total cell count with lymphocytes and plasma cells); (b) encephalopathy owing to drug abuse (Sheth, 1977); (c) Guillain-Barré syndrome (about 15 per cent of cases may show lymphocytic pleocytosis) (Fishman, 1971); (d) acute disseminated encephalomyelitis; (e) sarcoidosis of meninges; (f) polyneuritis (lymphocytes, plasma cells, and macrophages present during the recovery stage); and (g) periarteritis involving the central nervous system.

Increased numbers of plasma cells may occur in association with lymphocytic reactions. In some cases, e.g., multiple sclerosis, CSF plasma cells may be the only abnormality. Normally, plasma cells are absent from CSF. Morphologic evidence suggests that lymphocytes undergo transformation to plasma cells within the central nervous system (Glasser, 1977). Transitional forms between lymphocytes, "reactive lymphocytes," "plasmacytoid lymphocytes," and classical plasma cells have been described by various observers (Spriggs, 1968; Kolmel, 1977; Glasser, 1977).

Increased numbers of eosinophils (over 5 per cent of total leukocytes) have been reported in the following infections: (a) bacterial meningitis (e.g., some cases of pneumococcal meningitis), (b) tuberculous meningitis (a few cases), (c) fungal meningitis (e.g., coccidioidomycosis), (d) syphilitic meningoencephalitis (a few cases), (e) some cases of viral meningoencephalitis (Sheth, 1977), and (f) parasitic infestation (e.g., cysticercosis, hydatid disease). Non-infectious causes include (a) intrathecal injections of foreign protein (e.g., RISA (radioactive serum albumin), radiographic contrast media), (b) rabies vaccination, (c) intracranial shunts (reaction to rubber catheter), (d) periarteritis nodosa, (e) acute polyneuritis, (f) drug reactions, (g) food allergies, (h) urticaria, (i) allergic bronchial asthma, and (j) lymphocytic leukemia with spread to CNS. Persistent eosinophilia in CNS suggests the possibility of parasitic infestation, including ascariosis, paragonimiasis, or animal parasites which do not ordinarily affect humans.

Increased numbers of basophils may be seen in chronic granulocytic leukemia involving the meninges.

Increased numbers of ependymal cells may be seen following pneumoencephalography, in hydrocephalus, in specimens obtained by cisternal or ventricular puncture, or following intrathecal administration of chemotherapeutic agents.

Increased numbers of pia arachnoid mesothelial (PAM) cells and/or monocytes usually are seen as part of a "mixed reaction," along with (a) neutrophils, lymphocytes, and plasma cells, or (b) lymphocytes and plasma cells. A "mixed reaction" with neutrophils, lymphocytes, plasma cells, and monocytes is characteristic of tuberculous meningitis, fungal meningitis, chronic bacterial meningitis, rupture of brain abscess, leptospiral meningitis, and amebic encephalomyelitis. A "mixed reaction" with lymphocytes, plasma cells, and monocytes is characteristic of viral meningo-encephalitis, syphilitic meningoencephalitis, some cases of partially treated bacterial meningitis, some cases of bacterial meningitis due to uncommon organisms (e.g., *Listeria monocytogenes*), leptospiral meningitis, some cases of parasitic infestation (e.g., cysticercosis), some cases of aseptic meningitis due to septic focus adjacent to the meninges (e.g., encapsulation of brain abscess), subacute sclerosing panencephalitis (SSPE), and non-infectious conditions including multiple sclerosis and polyneuritis. None of these patterns is "diagnostic." The foregoing "lists" of conditions should serve as "reminders" rather than as absolute criteria.

Increased numbers of macrophages, including giant cells, may be associated with tuberculous or mycotic meningitis, reaction to erythrocytes in CSF (following brain surgery, trauma, or subarachnoid hemorrhage) (hemosiderin granules may appear after about four days), reaction to foreign substances in CSF, e.g., contrast media or ventricular drains, and reaction to lipid in CSF derived from CNS injury (e.g., contusion, infarction, brain abscess).

Lupus erythematosus (LE) cells have been described in CSF (Nosanchuk, 1976); however, this finding is rare.

Leukemic cells in CSF are of special importance and have received increasing attention in recent years. Leukemic infiltration of the meninges is related to special characteristics of the blood-CSF barrier, which is almost impermeable to present chemotherapeutic agents. Thus, leukemic cells which enter CSF from blood or from meningeal infiltrates can undergo uninhibited proliferation.

An initial finding of leukemic cells in CSF is uncommon. More often, leukemic cells appear in CSF after the illness has become established, e.g., after several remissions have been achieved by chemotherapy. Indeed, leukemic cells may appear in CSF during apparent remission, and after chemotherapy has been discontinued.

Leukemic cell counts in CSF vary between only a few leukemic cells, and more than $1000/\mu l$. Morphologic appearance is similar to peripheral blood or bone marrow. Meningeal spread is common in lymphoblastic leukemia, acute myeloblastic leukemia, and promyelocytic leukemia (perhaps 30 to 40 per cent of all cases). Meningeal spread is unusual in chronic myeloid and chronic lymphocytic leukemia. Malignant lymphomas may infiltrate the meninges, with appearance of lymphoma cells in CSF. Morphologically these may be difficult or impossible to distinguish from leukemic infiltrates.

Leukemoid reactions in CSF may be associated with coma, which can mimic chronic granulocytic leukemia with promyelocytes present in CSF (Sheth, 1977).

Tumor cells in CSF may be derived from primary or metastatic neoplasms. Primary intracranial tumors include medulloblastoma, retinoblastoma, astrocytoma, ependymoma, pinealoma, oligodendroglioma, meningioma, schwannoma, and pituitary adenoma. Metastatic tumors to CNS include lung, breast, gastrointestinal tract, and melanoma. Examination for "malignant tumor cells" usually is performed in a special tumor cytology laboratory using Papanicolaou stains. The appearance of tumor cells on Wright's stain is well illustrated in Kolmel's atlas (1977).

IDENTIFICATION OF MICRO-ORGANISMS ON MICROSCOPIC EXAMINATION

In bacterial meningitis, the most valuable single examination is a carefully examined Gram's stain of CSF. Reported sensitivity of this procedure ranges from 70 per cent (Hyslop, 1975) to 80 per cent (McCracken, 1976) to 90 per cent (Carpenter, 1962). Specificity is less well documented, although false positives may occur from (a) gram-positive

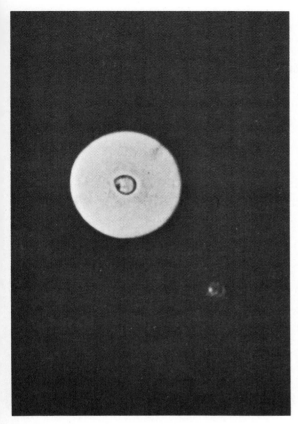

Figure 18–1. *Cryptococcus neoformans* in cerebrospinal fluid. India ink preparation; ×200. (From Anderson: The Clinical Practice of Bacteriology. Philadelphia, F. A. Davis, 1966.)

artifacts in staining solutions; (b) dead bacteria in tubes used for collection or processing CSF specimens (Musher, 1973; Weinstein, 1975). According to Smith (1973), a positive Gram's stain occurs at bacterial concentrations of 10^5/ml; other authors suggest that concentrations over 10^6/ml are required for a positive Gram's stain (Smith, 1976). Additional studies are needed to establish the concentration of bacteria needed for a positive Gram's stain and optimal methods for concentrating CSF prior to Gram's stain.

In fungal meningitis, the classic examination is India ink preparation using centrifuged sediment for detection of *Cryptococcus neoformans* (Fig. 18-1). However, the India ink preparation is positive in only about 50 per cent of cases (Butler, 1964). About 80 per cent of cases can be detected by special stains (PAS, mucicarmine, methenamine silver) on specimens prepared by Millipore filter or cytocentrifuge (Jequier, 1972; Jameson, 1972; Saigo, 1977). Without special stains, crypto-

cocci may be mistaken for small lymphocytes in "routine" preparations (Sheth, 1977). If initial preparations are negative, fungi sometimes may be detected on cisternal puncture (Gonyea, 1973), or on culture of 10 to 30 ml CSF.

Primary amebic meningoencephalitis, as distinguished from infections by *Entamoeba histolytica*, is a rapidly fatal disease which is uncommon but not rare (Hecht, 1972). The organisms (e.g., *Acanthameba* and *Nagleria*) are difficult to detect and identify on Gram's stain or Wright's stain of CSF (Aspock, 1977): frequently the condition is first recognized at autopsy. Motile trophozoites may be recognized by their active movement using a CSF wet mount examined by phase microscopy with a warmed stage or prewarmed counting chamber. However, experience is needed to distinguish amebas from the motility of macrophages and monocytes (Sornas, 1967, 1971).

Acid-fast stains for tuberculous meningitis are frequently performed on CSF. We have found the fluorescent rhodamine stain more sensitive than the Ziehl-Neelsen's method. Concentration of 10 ml CSF may further improve sensitivity. In some cases of tuberculous meningitis, a fine clot or pellicle will form over the surface of CSF after standing for 12 to 24 hours in the refrigerator: this pellicle should be carefully examined for organisms with appropriate stain and culture. We have occasionally found false positive stains for tuberculosis due to saprophytic acid-fast organisms in deionized water; these can be eliminated by preparing reagents using sterile water for intravenous infusion.

TOTAL PROTEIN

Protein normally diffuses from plasma to CSF across the blood-CSF barrier. Most of the serum proteins are present in CSF, including fibrinogen and beta lipoprotein in low concentrations (Table 18-3). The concentration ratios between plasma and CSF correlate moderately well with hydrodynamic radii, and somewhat less well with molecular weights. It is apparent from Table 18-3 that the IgM level in CSF is about five times higher than expected: this may be due to IgM monomers in addition to the pentamer. The prealbumin level in CSF is about twelve times higher than expected, and the transferrin level is about two times higher than expected. Reasons for these apparent discrepancies are unknown; selective transport

Table 18-3. CONCENTRATIONS OF PROTEINS IN PLASMA AND CEREBROSPINAL FLUID*

PROTEIN	MOLECULAR WEIGHT	HYDRODYNAMIC RADIUS (Å)	PLASMA CONCENTRATION (mg/l)	CSF CONCENTRATION (mg/l)	PLASMA/CSF RATIO
Prealbumin	61,000	32.5	238	17.3	14
Albumin	69,000	35.8	36,600	155.0	236
Transferrin	81,000	36.7	2,040	14.4	142
Ceruloplasmin	152,000	46.8	366	1.0	366
IgG	150,000	53.4	9,870	12.3	802
IgA	150,000	56.8	1,750	1.3	1346
α_2 macroglobulin	798,000	93.5	2,220	2.0	1111
Fibrinogen	340,000	108.0	2.964	0.6	4940
IgM	800,000	121.0	700	0.6	1167
β lipoprotein	2,239,000	124.0	3,728	0.6	6213

*Adapted from Felgenhauer, K.: Protein size and cerebrospinal fluid composition. Klin. Wochenschr., *52*:1158–1164, 1974.

may be involved. The tau protein of CSF, which migrates in the beta-gamma region, represents an altered form of transferrin, which apparently lacks neuraminic acid due to the action of neuraminidase (Bock, 1975).

Methods

Methods used to measure total protein in CSF can be classified in six categories:
1. Turbidimetric procedures
   a. Sulfosalicylic acid plus sodium sulfate
   b. Trichloracetic acid (TCA)
2. Ultraviolet spectrophotometry at 210 nm following:
   a. Column chromatography
   b. Ultrafiltration
3. Lowry method using Folin-Ciocalteau reagent
   a. Blanked
   b. Unblanked
4. Modified biuret procedures with measurement at 330 nm
5. Dye binding
   a. Ponceau S
   b. Other dyes
6. Immunologic methods

Turbidimetric methods are widely used in the United States. There is a linear relationship between turbidity and temperature, and accurate temperature control is essential for reproducible results (Schriever, 1965; Pennock, 1968). Sulfosalicylic acid gives greater turbidity with albumin than with globulin; however, variations in the albumin/globulin ratio have no significant effect on the SSA/SS (3 per cent sulfosalicylic acid in 7 per cent sodium sulfate) method of Meulmans or the TCA method of Meulmans (3 per cent trichloracetic acid). Because of variations in reactivity with albumin and globulin, albumin should *not* be used as a standard for turbidimetric methods (Schriever, 1965). Advantages of turbidimetric methods include its simplicity and the fact that some drugs

which interfere with the unblanked Lowry and biuret procedures do not cause turbidity with SSA or trichloracetic acid (TCA). Disadvantages include the fact that about 500 μl CSF is required, compared with 25 to 200 μl for other methods, and that interference may occur from xanthochromia as well as from intrathecal methotrexate.

Ultraviolet (UV) spectrophotometry at 210 nm is based on the principle that protein solutions exhibit strong absorbance at 210 to 220 nm, reflecting presence of the peptide bond. Interference due to short-chain polypeptides and drugs may be removed by column chromatography (Igou, 1967) or a "blank" prepared by ultrafiltration (Werner, 1969). Disturbances of the albumin/globulin ratio have no effect, since albumin and globulin have comparable absorbance at 210 nm. UV spectrophotometry requires only 100 to 200 μl of CSF, and precision appears somewhat superior to turbidimetric methods. On the other hand, it is more time consuming and difficult than turbidimetric methods; the upper limit of the reference interval by this method is somewhat higher (60 mg/dl) than for other techniques, and instrumentation is not available in all laboratories.

The Lowry method using Folin-Ciocalteau reagent is widely used in Europe. Two reactions are involved: (a) an initial reaction of protein and copper related to the biuret reaction; (b) a second reduction of phosphotungstic and phosphomolybdic acids with the copper-protein complex as well as with tyrosine and tryptophan. The Lowry method requires only 100 to 200 μl of CSF. However, it is more time consuming and difficult than turbidimetric methods, and it experiences variable interference from endogenously produced phenols and drugs (salicylates, chlorpromazine, tetracyclines, and sulfa drugs).

Modified biuret methods have been reported by several authors, including Burgi (1967). However, these seem less widely used than turbidimetric procedures, ultraviolet spectrophotometry, or the

Lowry method. Only 100 to 200 μl of CSF is required. Biuret methods are more time consuming and difficult than turbidimetric methods and experience interference from short chain polypeptides (can be compensated by blank using protein-free filtrate).

Dye binding methods have been reported (Salo, 1974), but experience to date appears limited. Potential advantages include technical simplicity and the fact that only 50 to 100 μl of CSF are required. However, limited experience in comparison with other CSF protein methods is a disadvantage.

Immunologic methods for CSF total protein have also been reported (Heintges, 1973). A major advantage is that only small amounts of CSF (25 to 50 μl) are required. After reaction conditions are established and reagents standardized, the technique is relatively simple and comparable to turbidimetric methods. Disadvantages are that different proteins may give different precipitin curves as well as different light scattering responses when bound to their specific antibodies. Also, variation between different lots of antisera may occur. Although immunologic methods offer significant advantages for CSF total protein, widespread use will require further experience, as well as reliable antisera which react in a uniform manner with all CSF proteins (Bock, 1975).

REFERENCE INTERVALS AND CLINICAL CORRELATION

As noted above, there may be some variation in reference intervals for different methods: UV spectrophotometry apparently gives a somewhat higher upper limit of normal than other procedures (Igou, 1967).

Reference intervals for CSF total protein vary slightly with age. During the neonatal period, reported reference intervals for CSF total protein vary from 30 to 140 mg/dl (Kluge, 1968) to 20 to 170 mg/dl (Sarff, 1976). This relatively high "upper limit" of normal has been attributed to immaturity of the blood-CSF barrier. By age six months, reference intervals fall below normal adult levels, to about 10 to 30 mg/dl (Fishman, 1971), then gradually increase to normal young adult levels of 15 to 45 mg/dl. After age 40, there appears to be a gradual increase with age (Tibbling, 1977). A summary of reference intervals for CSF protein, based on reports in the literature plus our own experience, is outlined in Table 18-4.

Reference intervals for CSF total protein are affected by source of CSF: cisternal and ventricular fluids have lower levels of total protein than lumbar fluid (Table 18-4). Thus, if several tubes of CSF are collected, the final

Table 18-4. REFERENCE INTERVALS FOR TOTAL PROTEIN IN CSF*

AGE	REFERENCE INTERVAL (mg/dl)
1–30 days	20–150
30–90 days	20–100
3–6 months	15–50
½–10 years	10–30
10–40 years	15–45
10–40 years	15–25 (cisternal fluid)
10–40 years	5–15 (ventricular fluid)
40–50 years	20–50
50–60 years	25–55
60 years and over	30–60

NOTE: These ranges represent a summary of personal experience plus reports in the literature; individual laboratories should establish their own reference intervals before using results for patient care.

*Lumbar fluid unless otherwise specified.

tubes will have a lower protein concentration than the initial tubes (Bock, 1975). In young children, concentrations of protein are reported as comparable in lumbar and cisternal fluid, possibly owing to (a) increased activity which causes more rapid circulation of CSF; (b) comparable permeability of lumbar and cisternal blood-CSF barriers; (c) smaller volumes of CSF, so that some cisternal fluid is obtained on lumbar puncture.

Decreased concentration of protein in lumbar CSF (15 mg/dl or less) may be due to (1) leakage of CSF from a dural tear caused by trauma or previous lumbar puncture, or to CSF rhinorrhea or otorrhea; (2) removal of large volumes of CSF (e.g., pneumoencephalography); (3) increased intracranial pressure (may cause increased filtration of CSF through arachnoid granulations of dural sinuses); (4) hyperthyroidism (mechanism not known). Of the foregoing conditions, leakage of CSF is especially important. A history of repeated meningitis in a patient with normal immunologic function and low CSF protein should suggest the possibility of nasal or aural CSF leakage.

Increased concentration of protein in lumbar CSF may be caused by (1) traumatic tap, with admixture of peripheral blood in CSF, (2) increased permeability of the blood-CSF barrier, (3) obstruction to circulation of CSF, (4) increased synthesis of protein within the central nervous system, or (5) tissue degeneration. Traumatic tap may cause increased CSF protein owing to the marked difference between plasma and CSF protein (ratio about 250:1). If

Table 18–5. DISORDERS ASSOCIATED WITH INCREASED CSF TOTAL PROTEIN

CONDITION	COMMENTS
Increased plasma protein	Slightly increased CSF protein due to diffusion across blood-CSF barrier
Traumatic tap	Normal pressure; CSF initially streaked with blood, clearing in subsequent tubes
Increased permeability of blood-CSF barrier	
Infectious	
Bacterial meningitis	CSF protein 100-500 mg/dl; Gram's stain usually positive; culture may be negative if antibiotics administered
Tuberculous meningitis	CSF protein 50-300 mg/dl; mixed cellular reaction typical
Fungal meningitis	CSF protein 50-300 mg/dl; special stains helpful
Viral meningoencephalitis	CSF protein usually under 100 mg/dl
Non-infectious	
Subarachnoid hemorrhage	Xanthochromia 2-4 hrs after onset
Intracerebral hemorrhage	CSF protein 20-200 mg/dl; marked fall in pressure after removing small amounts of CSF; xanthochromic fluid in 80%
Cerebral thrombosis	Slightly increased CSF protein in 40% of cases (usually under 100 mg/dl)
Endocrine, metabolic, and toxic	
Endocrine conditions: diabetic neuropathy, myxedema, hyperadrenalism, hypoparathyroidism	CSF protein 50-150 mg/dl in about 50% of cases
Metabolic conditions: uremia, hypercalcemia, hypercapnea, dehydration	CSF protein slightly elevated (usually under 100 mg/dl)
Toxic conditions: ethanol, isopropanol, heavy metals, phenytoin	CSF protein slightly elevated in about 40% of cases (usually under 200 mg/dl)
Obstruction to circulation of CSF	
Mechanical obstruction (tumor, abscess, etc.)	Rapid fall in pressure on removal of CSF; Froin's syndrome may be present
Loculated effusion of CSF	Repeated taps may show progressive increase in "CSF" protein; diagnosis by myelography
Increased CNS synthesis of IgG plus increased permeability of blood-CSF barrier	
Meningitis (see above)	About 20% of patients with viral meningoencephalitis have increased CSF IgG as well as increased CSF protein
Guillain-Barré syndrome (infectious polyneuritis)	CSF protein usually 100-400 mg/dl
Collagen diseases (e.g., periarteritis, lupus)	CSF protein usually under 400 mg/dl
Increased CNS synthesis of IgG	
Multiple sclerosis	CSF protein slightly increased in about 40% (usually under 100 mg/dl); CSF IgG elevated in about 80%
Subacute sclerosing panencephalitis (SSPE)	CSF IgG almost invariably increased
Neurosyphilis	CSF protein normal or slightly increased (usually under 100 mg/dl); about 20% have elevated IgG

1 ml of CSF contains 0.1 ml of blood due to traumatic tap, we may expect a CSF RBC of about 0.5 million, and a CSF protein of about 400 mg/dl. Although "corrections" for traumatic tap can be performed based on RBC, these may be inaccurate in some cases (p. 641).

Increased permeability of the blood-CSF barrier is a common cause for pathologic increases in CSF total protein (Table 18–5). In meningitis there is damage to the blood-CSF barrier, plus decreased removal of protein molecules at the arachnoid villi (Fishman, 1971). Various endocrine, metabolic, and toxic conditions may cause reversible changes in permeability of the brain-CSF barrier; however, the exact mechanisms are not known.

Obstruction to circulation of CSF classically is related to mechanical blockage between the site of lumbar puncture and the foramen magnum, e.g., cord compression due to tumor, herniated disc, adhesions, or extradural abscess. Owing to the obstruction, resorption of water (and/or leakage of plasma proteins) produces xanthochromic CSF of high protein content, which may clot spontaneously (Froin's syndrome). A similar syndrome may be caused by leakage of CSF after lumbar puncture to form loculated epidural and/or subdural effusions: subsequent punctures reveal "CSF" protein of progressively higher concentration (Derakhshan, 1973).

Synthesis of immunoglobulins apparently

occurs under normal conditions within lymphocytes and plasma cells of the central nervous system (Tourtellotte, 1975). However, no albumin is produced within the CNS. Daily synthesis of IgG in normal humans is minimal: about 3 mg/day (Tourtellotte, 1975). Increased synthesis of IgG within the CNS can occur with lymphocytic and plasmacytic infiltrates involving the central nervous system (Table 18-5).

In some degenerative conditions such as Parkinson's disease, Friedrich's ataxia, amyotrophic lateral sclerosis (ALS), etc., there is an increase in CSF protein; it is possible that tissue degeneration contributes to such protein elevation (Collins, 1978).

PROTEIN FRACTIONATION

Immunologic measurements

CSF protein may be derived from two sources: diffusion across the blood-CSF barrier, and synthesis within the central nervous system (CNS). Diffusion across the blood-CSF barrier occurs along concentration gradients between plasma and CSF. Rate of diffusion across these gradients (and plasma-CSF ratios) appears related to hydrodynamic radii for most proteins (Felgenhauer, 1974). The normal plasma:CSF ratio for albumin is generally accepted as about 230. Reported "normal" plasma:CSF ratios for IgG vary from about 370 (Tourtellotte, 1975) to about 500 (Tibbling, 1977) to about 800 (Felgenhauer, 1974). This variation probably is related to different antisera and different standards, which can cause errors in the range of 200 per cent (Bock, 1975; Thompson, 1977). Despite these problems related to standardization, immunologic measurement of CSF albumin and IgG have be- come widely accepted as methods for evaluating integrity of the blood-CSF barrier and synthesis of IgG within the CNS.

Because albumin is not produced within the CNS, the CSF/plasma albumin ratio is considered to reflect functional integrity of the blood-CSF barrier (Tibbling, 1977; Tourtellotte, 1975). An increased ratio may be due to traumatic tap, increased permeability of the blood-CSF barrier, or impaired resorption of CSF protein caused by subarachnoid block or meningitis (impaired resorption of CSF protein at arachnoid villi). Although variations in plasma albumin may affect the CSF albumin concentration, such variations do not affect the CSF/plasma albumin ratio, which accurately reflects permeability of the blood-CSF barrier. Immediately after birth, the CSF/plasma albumin ratio is relatively high, reflecting immaturity of the blood-CSF barrier (Table 18-6). By age six months, the value falls to adult levels, then gradually increases after age 30 to 40 years (Table 18-6).

The CSF/plasma IgG ratio reflects (1) permeability of the blood-CSF barrier; (2) synthesis of IgG within the CNS. Absolute levels of CSF IgG are relatively high during the first month of life, reflecting an increased permeability of the blood-CSF barrier as well as high levels of plasma IgG (Table 18-6). After age 30 days, CSF IgG falls rapidly, owing to decreasing levels of plasma IgG and increasing maturity of the blood-CSF barrier. The CSF/plasma IgG ratio shows changes with age comparable to the CSF/plasma albumin ratio (Table 18-6).

From a clinical point of view, CSF IgG measurements can provide an estimate of IgG synthesis within the CNS. Three methods have been used to "correct" CSF IgG measurements for variation in

Table 18-6. CEREBROSPINAL FLUID (CSF): PLASMA PROTEIN RATIOS WITH RESPECT TO AGE[*]

AGE	CSF/PLASMA ALBUMIN RATIO × 1000	CSF ALBUMIN (mg/l)	CSF/PLASMA IgG RATIO × 1000	CSF IgG (mg/l)	CSF IgG × 1000 / CSF ALBUMIN	CSF IgG INDEX
1–30 days	14†	450†	5 ± 3	10–100		
30–90 days	8†	300†	3 ± 1	3–15		
3–6 months	6†	220†	1 ± 0.5	3–6		
½–4 years	4†	160†	1.5 ± 1	3–12		
4–30 years	3.7 ± 1.0	120–220	1.7 ± 0.5	10–20	80–130	0.34–0.58
30–40 years	4.0 ± 1.1	130–230	1.9 ± 0.5	15–30	90–140	0.34–0.58
40–50 years	4.6 ± 1.3	140–260	2.1 ± 0.7	15–35	90–140	0.34–0.58
50–60 years	5.5 ± 1.7	160–320	2.5 ± 0.7	20–40	90–140	0.34–0.58
60 years and over	5.6 ± 1.7	160–320	2.6 ± 0.9	20–40	90–140	0.34–0.58

[*] Adapted from Tibbling, G., Link, H., and Ohman, S.: Principles of albumin and IgG analyses in neurological disorders. Scand. J. Clin. Lab. Invest., *37*:385–401, 1977; Olsson, J. E., and Pettersson, B.: A comparison between agar gel electrophoresis and CSF serum quotients of IgG and albumin in neurological diseases. Acta Neurol. Scand., *53*:308–322, 1976; Harms, D.: Comparative quantitation of immunoglobulin G(IgG) in cerebrospinal fluid and serum of children. Eur. Neurol., *13*:54–64, 1975.

† Estimated from total protein measurements (Harms, 1975).

plasma IgG and permeability of the blood-CSF barrier: (1) CSF IgG expressed as a percentage of CSF total protein or CSF albumin; (2) the CSF IgG/albumin index, with CSF IgG expressed as a ratio to plasma IgG, compared with CSF albumin expressed as a ratio to plasma albumin:

$$\frac{CSF/plasma\ IgG}{CSF/plasma\ albumin}$$

(Olsson, 1976; Tibbling, 1977); (3) calculation of IgG synthesis within central nervous system (Tourtellotte, 1975). For CSF IgG expressed as a percentage of CSF albumin, the upper limit of normal is about 12 per cent (Thompson, 1977). For CSF IgG expressed as a percentage of CSF total protein, the upper limit of normal is about 8 per cent (Tibbling, 1977). If we assume that increased permeability of the blood-CSF barrier causes increased CSF IgG proportional to increased CSF albumin, then expressing CSF IgG as a percentage of CSF albumin will compensate for increased CSF IgG due to increased permeability of the blood-CSF barrier. Of course, in some cases, damage to the blood-CSF barrier may change the CSF/plasma IgG ratio more than the CSF/plasma albumin ratio. However, in actual practice, this "correction" appears useful.

The IgG/albumin index

$$\frac{CSF\ IgG/plasma\ IgG}{CSF\ albumin/plasma\ albumin}$$

is sometimes used to "correct" for changes in plasma proteins as well as for increased permeability of the blood-CSF barrier. Since CSF IgG and CSF albumin are expressed as ratios to plasma levels, variations in plasma protein have little effect on the index. To obtain adequate precision, all four protein measurements should be performed simultaneously. Of course, this index will fail to "correct" for damage to the blood-CSF barrier which changes the CSF/plasma IgG ratio more than the CSF/plasma albumin ratio.

If the "normal" ratios of plasma:CSF albumin and IgG are known, we can calculate daily synthesis of IgG within the CNS (Tourtellotte, 1975). Although this approach appears promising, it is not yet widely used. Accuracy of such calculations is highly dependent upon accurate "normal values" for CSF/plasma ratios of albumin and IgG. And at this time, different authorities report different reference values or "normal values" for the ratio of CSF/plasma IgG.

In addition to albumin and IgG, other immunologic studies performed on CSF include IgA and IgM measurements, immunoelectrophoresis, evaluation of kappa-lambda ratio, subtyping of IgG (Vandvik, 1976; Palmer, 1976), and immunofixation (Cawley, 1976). At present these techniques are primarily of research interest rather than established clinical value.

Table 18–7. REFERENCE INTERVALS FOR CEREBROSPINAL FLUID (CSF) PROTEIN ELECTROPHORESIS

	CSF (Kaplan, 1967)*	CSF (Windisch, 1970)†	SERUM
Prealbumin	3.7- 6.1%	2.2- 7.1%	–
Albumin	56.2-66.8%	56.8-76.4%	52.2-67.0%
α_1 globulin	3.1- 5.9%	1.1- 6.6%	2.4- 4.6%
α_2 globulin	4.9- 8.5%	3.0-12.6%	6.6-13.6%
β globulin	10.1-17.3%	7.3-17.9%	9.1-14.7%
γ globulin:‡	6.2-11.4%	3.0-13.0%	9.0-20.6%

* Concentration by vacuum ultrafiltration.
† Concentration by Amicon membrane.
‡ Children have lower values for CSF and serum γ globulin.

Electrophoresis

Three support media are used for CSF protein electrophoresis: cellulose acetate, agarose (agar gel), and polyacrylamide gel. In the United States, cellulose acetate is the most popular technique. This separates CSF into six fractions: prealbumin, albumin, α_1 globulin, α_2 globulin, β globulin, and γ globulin. Concentration of CSF may be performed by vacuum ultrafiltration (Schleicher and Schell, Keene, N. H.) or by Amicon membrane (Amicon Corp., Lexington, Mass.). Reference intervals reported in two different studies are outlined in Table 18–7. Compared with serum, CSF has proportionally less gamma globulin and more albumin. The upper limit of normal for gamma globulin in adults is about 12 per cent of total CSF protein. For children, the upper limit is somewhat less.

In Europe, and in specialized laboratories within the United States, agar gel electrophoresis is preferred over cellulose acetate for CSF (Link, 1971). On agar gel electrophoresis, over 90 per cent of patients with multiple sclerosis have two or more discrete bands in the gamma globulin region, with no corresponding bands on serum electrophoresis (oligoclonal IgG). Recent studies suggest that these bands represent IgG1 (Vandvik, 1976; Palmer, 1976). At present, agar gel electrophoresis is probably the most sensitive single method available to the "routine" clinical laboratory for detection of multiple sclerosis. The technique has been described by several authors, including Johnson (1977).

Polyacrylamide gel electrophoresis (PAGE) provides even greater resolution than agar gel (Epstein, 1976). Although PAGE can demonstrate oligoclonal bands in multiple sclerosis (MS) (Thompson, 1977), PAGE is not now widely used for study of CSF.

Isoelectric focusing of CSF proteins also permits demonstration of oligoclonal bands (Thompson, 1977), but further experience is needed before this technique becomes generally accepted.

Qualitative tests

Lange's colloidal gold test is an empirical method for evaluating CSF protein. In this procedure, progressive dilutions of CSF are added to 10 test tubes containing colloidal gold solutions. Precipitation causes the brilliant red colloidal gold color (0) to change to reddish blue (1+), purple (2+), deep blue (3+), pale blue (4+), or colorless (5+). The highest CSF concentration is reported on the left, with progressively decreasing concentrations to the right.

Normal CSF causes either no reaction or only slight precipitation in the middle dilutions, e.g., 0001210000.

A "first zone curve" is found in about 50 per cent of patients with multiple sclerosis, as well as in neurosyphilis, SSPE, CNS hemorrhage, meningitis, polyneuritis, and other conditions. A typical series would be 5554210000. In general, a first zone curve is associated with increased gamma globulin as detected by electrophoresis (Thompson, 1977).

The "mid zone" and "end zone" curves are nonspecific and may be found in any CSF with high protein concentration.

The Pandy test requires that one drop of CSF be added to saturated aqueous solution of phenol: turbidity is read as 0 to 3+. Increased concentrations of CSF globulin are associated with increased turbidity.

Since the 1960's, there has been a trend to replacement of these methods by cellulose acetate electrophoresis, agar gel electrophoresis, and immunologic measurements. However, the colloidal gold and Pandy tests are still used for evaluation of CSF in some laboratories.

Clinical correlation

The most important clinical application of CSF protein fractionation is detection and diagnosis of multiple sclerosis (MS). About 90 to 95 per cent of patients with MS have multiple discrete gamma bands on agar gel electrophoresis (Olsson, 1973; Tibbling, 1977; Johnson, 1977). However, this finding may also occur in about 90 per cent of patients with subacute sclerosing panencephalitis (SSPE) (Johnson, 1977), about 60 per cent of patients with neurosyphilis (Link, 1971), about 40 per cent of patients with bacterial or viral meningoencephalitis (Olsson, 1976), and some patients with acute necrotizing encephalitis (van Welsum, 1970), Guillain-Barré syndrome (Link, 1975), meningeal carcinomatosis, toxoplasmosis involving the CNS, herpes zoster encephalitis, herpes simplex encephalitis, progressive multifocal leukoencephalopathy, and other neurologic conditions (Johnson, 1977).

Distinct immunoglobulin bands may occur on agar gel electrophoresis of serum and CSF of patients with infections outside the CNS. For this reason, it is advisable simultaneously to perform agar gel electrophoresis on CSF and serum. An oligoclonal pattern in CSF does not necessarily suggest MS if similar bands are present in serum.

About 75 per cent of patients with multiple sclerosis (MS) have increased CSF gamma globulin on cellulose acetate electrophoresis, when gamma globulin is expressed as a per cent of CSF total protein or CSF albumin. Measurement of CSF gamma globulin on electrophoresis is more sensitive and more specific than older semiquantitative methods such as the Pandy test and colloidal gold curve (Ivers, 1961).

About 75 per cent of patients with MS have increased CSF IgG, when IgG is expressed as a per cent of CSF total protein or CSF albumin.

About 85 per cent of patients with MS apparently have an increased IgG/albumin index (Tibbling, 1977):

$$\frac{\text{CSF IgG/plasma IgG}}{\text{CSF albumin/plasma albumin}}$$

There is suggestive evidence that the IgG/albumin index also may provide improved specificity (Tibbling, 1977).

Increased CSF, gamma globulin (IgG), and/or IgG/albumin index also may occur in about 95 per cent of patients with subacute sclerosing panencephalitis, about 50 per cent of patients with neurosyphilis, about 40 to 50 per cent of patients with meningitis, and some patients with Guillain-Barré syndrome, systemic lupus erythematosus involving the CNS, viral meningoencephalitis, and other neurologic conditions. Among Japanese patients with MS only about 40 per cent have elevated IgG in CSF (Iwashita, 1976). The reason for this relatively low percentage is not known.

Although CSF protein studies currently are of considerable value in the diagnosis of MS, in the future, other approaches may supplement or even supplant evaluation of CSF proteins (Levy, 1976; Cohen, 1976).

At this time, the following procedures are of established value in detection and diagnosis of MS: agar gel electrophoresis of CSF (and serum), immunologic measurements of CSF (and serum) IgG and albumin, and cellulose acetate electrophoresis of CSF (as a method for calculating per cent gamma globulin if the foregoing methods are unavailable).

GLUCOSE

Normal CSF glucose in adults is about 60 to 70 per cent of blood levels, or about 50 to 80 mg/dl in fasting patients with plasma glucose of 80 to 110 mg/dl. Glucose enters CSF from plasma by at least two mechanisms: active transport and passive diffusion. Active transport increases up to plasma levels of about 300 mg/dl, after which the transport system reaches a maximum with CSF glucose in the range of 200 mg/dl (Calabrese, 1976). Thus with plasma glucose in the range of 1000 mg/dl, CSF glucose may be under 300 mg/dl, or less than 30 per cent of plasma levels.

Passive diffusion of glucose from plasma to CSF is influenced by level and duration of elevated plasma glucose. Following a change in plasma glucose, CSF glucose rises or falls slowly over about two hours. Thus accurate evaluations of CSF glucose require a relatively constant level of plasma glucose.

According to Fishman (1971), the CSF/ plasma glucose ratio approaches 1.0 during the neonatal period. Although this observation needs further confirmation, immaturity of the blood-CSF barrier might account for such findings.

Elevated CSF glucose (absolute or relative to plasma glucose) is evidence of hyperglycemia 2 to 4 hours prior to lumbar puncture.

Decreased CSF glucose is considered present when CSF glucose is under 40 mg/dl in a fasting patient with normal plasma glucose. Decreased CSF glucose may be due to impairment of active transport; to increased utilization of glucose (by CNS, tissue, leukocytes, erythrocytes, and/or microorganisms); or to hypoglycemia. CSF glucose is decreased in about 50 per cent of patients with bacterial meningitis (Swartz, 1965). At least two mechanisms are believed involved: (a) impaired transport of glucose from plasma to CSF; (b) increased utilization of glucose by central nervous system, leukocytes, and microorganisms.

Although CSF glucose is usually considered normal in viral meningoencephalitis, low CSF glucose may occur in about 25 per cent of patients with mumps meningoencephalitis (Azimi, 1975). Impaired transport of glucose has been suggested as a possible mechanism.

Other reported causes of decreased CSF glucose include tuberculous meningitis, fungal meningitis, amebic meningoencephalitis, subarachnoid hemorrhage (decreased CSF glucose typically appears 4 to 8 days after onset), intrathecal administration of radioiodinated serum albumin, viral meningitis including lymphocytic choriomeningitis, herpes simplex meningoencephalitis, herpes zoster meningitis (Wolf, 1974), neurosyphilis (most cases have normal CSF glucose), sarcoidosis involving the meninges, and neoplasms involving the meninges (e.g., leukemia, lymphoma, melanoma, metastatic carcinoma, glioma). In some of these conditions, several different mechanisms probably operate simultaneously to cause decreased CSF glucose. For example, in bacterial meningitis there is evidence of (1) impaired glucose transport; (b) increased CNS utilization of glucose; (c) increased utilization of glucose by leukocytes in CSF.

CEREBROSPINAL FLUID RHINORRHEA AND OTORRHEA

Occasionally the question arises whether small amounts of clear fluid draining from nose or ear represent cerebrospinal fluid. This question is of especial importance in patients with recurrent meningitis and no evidence of immunologic impairment. Trauma is the most common cause of CSF rhinorrhea, which usually begins within 48 hours, but may not develop for several months.

Glucose oxidase test strips are of *no* clinical value for distinguishing CSF from nasal secretions (Hull, 1975). Diagnosis of CSF rhinorrhea and otorrhea must be made by other means: e.g., intrathecal ^{131}I serum albumin, with cotton pledgets in nose (or ear) counted for radioactivity.

ENZYMES

Many different enzymes have been measured in CSF; however, only lactate dehydrogenase (LDH) appears clinically useful at this time.

One source of LDH in normal CSF may be diffusion across the blood-CSF barrier. Normal CSF LDH activity is about 5 to 10 per cent of plasma activity (Mullan, 1969; Morrison, 1971). The "normal range" for the ratio of CSF/ serum LDH is not yet well established. And it is not yet customary simultaneously to measure activities in serum as well as in CSF. Indeed, some reports of CSF enzyme activity fail to specify one or more of the following: (a) normal range for enzyme activity in CSF; (b) normal range for enzyme activity in serum;

(c) reaction conditions, including assay temperature and source of reagents; (d) results of simultaneous measurements on serum and CSF.

A second source of CSF LDH is from CNS by diffusion across the brain-CSF barrier. Brain tissue is rich in LDH, and damaged CNS tissue can cause increased levels of CSF LDH.

A third source of CSF LDH activity is cellular elements in CSF: leukocytes, bacteria, and tumor cells.

Based on these considerations, it might seem reasonable to report CSF LDH as a percentage of CSF albumin or total protein, analogous to gamma globulin. However, few reports include CSF LDH activity expressed as a ratio to other proteins.

Increased CSF LDH activity has been reported in many different conditions: about 90 per cent of patients with bacterial meningitis (Beaty, 1969; Nelson, 1975; Feldman, 1975); about 10 per cent of patients with viral meningitis (Beaty, 1969; Feldman, 1975); subarachnoid hemorrhage; leukemia, lymphoma, or metastatic carcinoma involving the CNS.

Measurements of CSF LDH have been used for differential diagnosis of bacterial vs. viral meningitis. High levels of CSF LDH in the latter condition appear associated with encephalitis and a poor prognosis (Beaty, 1969).

LDH isozymes (p. 366) have been used to improve the specificity of LDH measurements in CSF:

Granulocytes—LDH 5 and 4 predominate
Lymphocytes—LDH 3 and 2 predominate
Brain tissue—LDH 2 and 1 predominate

With viral meningitis, the LDH isozyme pattern reflects a combined CNS-lymphocytic reaction, with LDH 1-2-3 present. With bacterial meningitis, the LDH isozyme pattern reflects a granulocytic reaction with LDH 4-5 present. In either viral or bacterial meningitis, high levels of LDH 1 and 2 suggest extensive CNS damage and appear associated with a poor prognosis.

Although reports to date appear promising, the value of CSF LDH and LDH isozymes is not yet well established.

Increased CSF creatine kinase (CK) activity has been reported in a wide variety of neurologic disorders, including subarachnoid hemorrhage, cerebral thrombosis, multiple sclerosis and other demyelinating disorders, Guillain-Barré syndrome, following epileptic seizures, primary CNS tumors, metastatic tumors involving CNS, viral meningoencephalitis, and bacterial meningitis. Elevated CSF

CK appears to be a sensitive but non-specific index of CNS disease. Owing to poor specificity, the clinical value of CSF CK measurements is not established.

Increased CSF aspartate aminotransferase (AST or GOT) has been reported in a variety of neurologic disorders: bacterial meningitis (elevated levels appear associated with a poor prognosis), intracerebral hemorrhage, subarachnoid hemorrhage, and primary or metastatic malignancy involving the CNS. The clinical value of CSF AST measurements is not established.

LACTIC ACID

Lactic acid in CSF may vary independently of blood levels: apparently diffusion across the blood-CSF barrier is very slow (Bland, 1974). The source of lactic acid in CSF probably is CNS anaerobic metabolism: CSF lactate appears to be a reliable indicator of brain lactate content (Bland, 1974; Siesjo, 1972).

Reported reference intervals for CSF lactate vary from 10 to 22 mg/dl (0.11 to 0.24 mmol/l) (Pryce, 1970) to 12 to 16 mg/dl (0.13 to 0.18 mmol/l) (Bland, 1974). About 25 mg/dl (0.28 mmol/l) has been suggested as an "upper limit" for clinical purposes (Controni, 1977). These levels are slightly higher than reference intervals for arterial and venous lactate in adults (3 to 7 mg/dl and 5 to 20 mg/dl), but slightly lower than reference intervals for venous lactate in children (Meites, 1977).

Any condition associated with reduced cerebral blood flow, reduced oxygenation of the brain, or increased intracranial pressure can cause elevated lactate in CSF (Controni, 1977). Conditions associated with increased CSF lactate include traumatic brain injury (Cold, 1975), idiopathic seizures (Brooks, 1975), respiratory alkalosis (hypocapnea), intracranial hemorrhage, hydrocephalus, brain abscess, cerebral ischemia due to arteriosclerosis, low blood pressure, low arterial Po_2, cerebral infarct, multiple sclerosis (less than 50 per cent of patients), and primary or metastatic carcinoma involving CNS. Several reports suggest that CSF lactate may aid in differential diagnosis of bacterial meningitis vs. viral meningitis if other conditions can be excluded (Bland, 1974; Controni, 1977). Over 90 per cent of patients with bacterial meningitis apparently have CSF lactate elevated above 25 mg/dl, while less than 15 per cent of patients with aseptic meningitis have a CSF lactate above this level (Bland, 1974; Controni, 1977). Measurements of CSF lactate may be useful as a "screening test" to detect CNS disease and as an aid in differential diagnosis of meningitis if other causes for elevated levels can be excluded. With additional experience, it seems likely that CSF lactate may become accepted as a "routine" laboratory procedure.

SEROLOGIC TESTS

TESTS FOR SYPHILIS

In patients with neurosyphilis, the CSF cell count, CSF total protein, and CSF gamma globulin all may be within normal limits (Hooshmand, 1977; John, 1977). The recommended serologic test for CSF, the VDRL procedure, also may be negative in 40 to 50 per cent of patients with neurosyphilis (Escobar, 1970; Hooshmand, 1972) (see Fluorescent Treponemal Antibody in Chapter 54, p. 1889).

The CSF FTA (fluorescent treponemal antibody) and FTA-ABS (fluorescent treponemal antibody absorption test) have much greater sensitivity, and apparently are positive in 80 to 90 per cent of patients with neurosyphilis (Hooshmand, 1972; McCracken, 1974). However, this increased sensitivity is accompanied by increased false positives: according to Jaffe (1975), the false positive rate may be as high as 4 to 5 per cent.

Some authorities (Jaffe, 1975) regard the CSF FTA and FTA-ABS as still experimental, owing to the high incidence of false positives. However, in patients with clinical findings consistent with early neurosyphilis but a negative CSF VDRL, the CSF FTA may aid in deciding whether to initiate treatment (John, 1977).

OTHER SEROLOGIC TESTS FOR INFECTIOUS DISEASE INVOLVING CNS

Serologic tests on CSF are of established value in diagnosis of cryptococcal meningitis (Kaufman, 1976). The India ink preparation is positive in only about 50 per cent of patients. However, the latex agglutination test for cryptococcal antigen in CSF is positive in about 90 per cent of patients with cryptococcal meningitis. False positives are infrequent.

During the past few years, there has devel-

oped increasing interest in diagnosis of bacterial meningitis by countercurrent immunoelectrophoresis (CIE). Sensitivity depends on potency of the antiserum and varies from about 50 per cent to over 90 per cent (McCracken, 1976; Denis, 1977; Feldman, 1977). Specific antisera are needed for each organism suspected: thus "false negatives" occur with meningitis owing to unusual organisms such as *Listeria monocytogenes*, *Salmonella*, or diphtheroids (Schlesinger, 1977). Although CIE appears highly promising, it is not yet generally accepted as a "routine" procedure for the "average" laboratory.

LIMULUS LYSATE TEST FOR ENDOTOXIN

In 1965, Levin and Bang described gel formation of lysate from *Limulus polyphemus* (horseshoe crab) due to endotoxin produced by gram-negative bacteria. There is considerable interest in the CSF limulus lysate assay for rapid diagnosis of gram-negative bacterial meningitis (Nachum, 1973; Ross, 1975; Berman, 1976). Positive limulus assays have been reported in CSF of almost all patients with gram-negative meningitis, e.g., *Hemophilus influenzae*, *Escherichia coli*, *Neisseria meningitidis*, *Acinetobacter calcoaceticus*, *Proteus morganii*, *Citrobacter freundii*, *Eikenella corrodens*, etc. Negative limulus assays have been reported in CSF of patients with gram-positive meningitis. "False negative" results may occur in some patients with gram-negative bacterial meningitis; false negatives also may be caused by misinterpretation of the gel endpoint (McCracken, 1976). "False positive" results may occur owing to endotoxin contamination of glassware (McCracken, 1976).

If additional experience confirms present reports of excellent sensitivity and specificity for gram-negative meningitis, the limulus assay may become widely accepted as a routine method.

OTHER MEASUREMENTS AND EXAMINATIONS

Acid-base balance

Acid-base balance in CSF has been recently reviewed by Plum (1975) and by Wichser (1975). Since CSF has little capacity to buffer changes in P_{CO_2}, accurate measurements of CSF pH are difficult: anaerobic conditions must be strictly maintained during and after sampling. And since CO_2 diffuses rapidly across the blood-CSF barrier, reproducible measurements require that the patient be in a respiratory steady state.

Although CSF pH has been suggested as helpful in differential diagnosis of meningitis (Bland, 1974), additional studies are needed before this can be accepted as a "routine" laboratory service.

Alcohol

Increased CSF ethanol is no longer considered clinically useful in diagnosis of cryptococcal meningitis.

Ammonia

The concentration of ammonia in CSF is about one half arterial blood levels (Jaiken, 1969). With hepatic failure, ammonia levels increase in CSF as well as in blood: there appears to be a relation between CSF ammonia concentration and the degree of hepatic encephalopathy. Increased levels also may occur in hypercapnea (Wichser, 1975). At this time, measurements of CSF ammonia concentration appear of primarily research interest with selected clinical applications (Chap. 11, p. 328).

Biogenic amines

Each of the biogenic amines has its own distribution in the brain, and each may modulate the neuronal activity in a functionally distinct system: 5-hydroxytryptamine (5-HT) in limbic structures and dopamine in the extra pyramidal system (Moir, 1970). The major metabolites of 5-HT and dopamine are 5-hydroxyindoleacetic acid (5-HIAA) and homovanillic acid (HVA), respectively.

Reductions of HVA have been reported in CSF of patients with Parkinson's disease, depression, and head injuries. This difference is accentuated by administration of probenecid, which blocks excretion of biogenic amines from CSF.

Increased CSF 5-HIAA and HVA have been reported in hyperactive patients and possibly may be related to increased mixing of ventricular and lumbar CSF: levels in ventricular fluid are several times those in lumbar fluid (Jakupcevic, 1977). If multiple CSF samples are taken by lumbar puncture, initial samples have relatively low concentrations of 5-HIAA and HVA as compared with the second, third, and fourth tubes (Jakupcevic, 1977). At present, these measurements appear to be primarily of research interest, rather than practical clinical value.

Calcium

The calcium content of CSF is approximately equal to diffusible serum calcium. However, the exchange of calcium between plasma and CSF also depends on active transport mechanisms. Measurements of CSF calcium are not considered clinically useful at this time.

Chloride

The distribution of chloride between plasma and CSF is dependent on the Donnan equilibrium: since plasma proteins are negatively charged, to maintain electrical neutrality in the relatively protein-free CSF, there is a compensatory increase in chloride. Low CSF chloride levels have been noted in meningitis: this change is non-specific and reflects systemic hypochloremia often associated with meningeal infections. Routine measurement of CSF chloride is not useful in differential diagnosis of meningitis.

Creatinine

Creatinine concentration in CSF is similar to venous blood levels, and increases in patients with renal insufficiency.

Glutamine

Glutamine is formed by an enzymatic intracellular reaction between ammonia and glutamic acid. Thus production of glutamine provides a mechanism for removing ammonia from the CNS. Elevation of CSF glutamine has been described in hepatic encephalopathy and in some cases of Reye's syndrome (Hourani, 1971; Glasgow, 1974). Increased CSF glutamine also occurs as a compensatory response to CSF acidosis (may be caused by hypercapnia) (Jaiken, 1969; Wichser, 1975).

Although CSF glutamine measurements are technically simpler than older methods for blood ammonia, newer methods for blood ammonia are easier to perform than CSF glutamine (Chap. 11, p. 329).

Hormone measurements

Many different hormones have been measured in CSF:

Cortisol—normal plasma/CSF ratio approx. 25:1 (Rodriquez, 1976).

Triiodothyronine—normal plasma/CSF ratio approx. 10:1 (Hagen, 1973).

Thyroxine—normal plasma/CSF ratio approx. 40:1 (Hagen, 1973).

TSH—normal plasma/CSF ratio approx. 2:1 (Schaub, 1977).

Growth hormone—normal plasma/CSF ratio approx. 6:1 (Schaub, 1977).

Prolactin—normal plasma/CSF ratio approx. 20:1 (Jordan, 1976).

Insulin—normal plasma/CSF ratio approx. 4:1 (Rodriquez, 1976).

Antidiuretic hormone—normal plasma/CSF ratio approx. 2:1 (Rodriquez, 1976).

ACTH—normal plasma/CSF ratio approx. 1:1 (Jordan, 1976).

LH—normal plasma/CSF ratio approx. 10:1 (Jordan, 1976).

FSH—normal plasma/CSF ratio approx. 8:1 (Jordan, 1976).

Measurements of adenohypophyseal hormones in CSF may provide sensitive indicators for suprasellar extension of pituitary tumors and response of tumors to treatment (Jordan, 1972). However, additional studies are needed to establish normal ranges for plasma/CSF ratios of these hormones.

Measurements of human chorionic gonadotropin (hCG) in CSF have been used for detection and diagnosis of choriocarcinoma metastatic to the CNS. In the absence of CNS metastases, the plasma/CSF ratio for hCG exceeds 60:1 (Chen, 1977). When CNS metastases are present, concentration of CSF hCG rises, and the plasma/CSF ratio falls below 60:1 (Chen, 1977). Additional studies are needed to establish reference values for plasma/CSF ratio of hCG.

Magnesium

CSF magnesium is maintained at a level approximately 30 per cent greater than in serum, in contrast with calcium (CSF level approximately 50 per cent that of serum) and zinc (CSF level negligible as compared with serum). The ratio of CSF/serum magnesium remains relatively constant under normal conditions. However, with meningitis or ischemic brain disease, CSF magnesium levels tend to decrease toward plasma values (Woodbury, 1968).

Phosphorus

The concentration of phosphorus in CSF averages about 40 per cent of plasma levels (Fishman, 1971). However, this measurement has no established clinical value at present.

Potassium

The CSF potassium concentration is maintained within narrow limits of about 2.6 to 3.0 mmol/l, even in the presence of systemic hypokalemia, hyperkalemia, disturbances in acid-base balance (Sambrook, 1975), or subarachnoid hemorrhage with release of potassium from lysed erythrocytes (Fishman, 1971). Following cardiac arrest, potassium increases promptly in cisternal CSF, and more gradually in lumbar CSF (Siemkowicz, 1977). In patients not resuscitated after cardiac arrest, potassium levels rise to 7.0 mmol/l in cisternal CSF and 4.0 mmol/l in lumbar fluid (Siemkowicz). Following death, CSF potassium rises rapidly to about 20 mmol/l within 10 to 12 hours. Although postmortem CSF potassium has been suggested as an aid in estimating time of death, such estimates have limited accuracy (Coe, 1976).

Sodium

The concentration of CSF sodium tends to parallel plasma sodium, although these are not necessarily identical at any given time. According to Fishman (1971), the changes in CSF sodium associated with hyponatremia and hypernatremia are less marked than changes in plasma sodium. CSF sodium is not clinically useful in diagnosis of neurologic disease.

Urea

Changes in plasma urea are followed by parallel changes in CSF urea, after a period of about one hour. The time lag required for urea to reach equilibrium between plasma and CSF probably is responsible for the transient osmotic effects of renal dialysis: rapid fall in plasma urea may lead to coma caused by relative hyperosmolality of CNS interstitial fluid, and shift of water from plasma to CNS. Coma due to hyperglycemia (plasma glucose over 800 mg/dl) may have a similar etiology, based on shifts of water from CNS interstitial fluid to plasma; however, the exact mechanism is not understood.

Uric Acid

Changes in plasma uric acid are accompanied by similar changes in CSF uric acid. Increased CSF uric acid has been reported in progressive cerebral atrophy, uremia, eclampsia, and meningitis. However, this measurement has virtually no established clinical value at present.

SYNOVIAL FLUID

FORMATION

The synovial membrane lines joints, bursae, and synovial tendon sheaths, but not the articular cartilages or menisci. The synovial lining cells are loosely arranged in a layer one to three cells thick, over a mucopolysaccharide matrix. Unlike other body cavities, there is no basement membrane and no desmosomes joining adjacent synovial cells (Haselwood, 1977). Indeed, the lining presents a discontinuous surface, often with wide gaps between adjacent synovial cells.

The synovial lining cells are classified into three types: (1) A cells, which appear suited for phagocytosis, and morphologically resemble macrophages (numerous mitochondria, vacuoles, and lysosomes); (2) B cells, which appear suited for protein synthesis (abundant endoplasmic reticulum); (3) C cells, intermediate cells with characteristics of both A and B cells.

Synovial fluid (SF) is believed to be produced by dialysis of plasma across the synovial membrane and by secretion of a hyaluronate-protein complex by the synovial membrane. Thus, SF represents a plasma ultrafiltrate to which a hyaluronate-protein complex has been added (Table 18-8).

Hyaluronate is a polymer composed of repeating disaccharide units (glucuronic acid-glucosamine). Molecular weight varies from about 5 to 10 million, depending on the degree of polymerization (Jessar, 1972; Haselwood, 1977). This polymer is linked with about 2 per cent protein. Both hyaluronate and protein probably are produced by the synovial lining cells.

Functions of SF are to provide lubrication and nourishment for articular cartilage.

Table 18-8. REFERENCE INTERVALS FOR CONSTITUENTS OF SYNOVIAL FLUID

	SYNOVIAL FLUID	PLASMA
Protein	1-3 g/dl	6-8 g/dl
albumin	55-70%	50-65%
α_1 globulin	6-8%	3-5%
α_2 globulin	5-7%	7-13%
β globulin	8-10%	8-14%
γ globulin	10-14%	12-22%
Hyaluronate	0.3-0.4 g/dl	–
Glucose	70-110 mg/dl	70-110 mg/dl
Uric acid		
males	2-8 mg/dl	2-8 mg/dl
females	2-6 mg/dl	2-6 mg/dl
Lactate	10-20 mg/dl	3-7 mg/dl (arterial)
	(1-2 mmol/l)	5-20 mg/dl (venous)
pH	7.30-7.40	7.38-7.44 (arterial)
		7.36-7.42 (venous)
pCO_2	40-60 mm Hg	35-40 mm Hg (arterial)
		40-45 mm Hg (venous)
pO_2	40-80 mm Hg	75-100 mm Hg (arterial)
		40-50 mm Hg (venous)

Information compiled from Binette, 1965; Lund-Olesen, 1970; Falchuk, 1970; McCarty, 1974; Cohen, 1975; Haselwood, 1977; Kushner, 1977.

ARTHROCENTESIS AND SAMPLE COLLECTION

Joint aspiration should be performed *only* by an experienced operator under strictly sterile conditions. The technique has been described by various authors (Cohen, 1975; Currey, 1976). Almost any joint can be aspirated, provided an effusion is present. Since even large joints (e.g., knee) normally contain only 0.1 to 2.0 ml SF (Currey, 1976), a "dry tap" is common unless an effusion is present. Synovial fluid aspiration may provide useful information for diagnosis of the following conditions: suspected infection, e.g., acute suppurative arthritis; arthritis due to uric acid (gout) or calcium pyrophosphate (pseudogout); differential diagnosis of arthritis (Tables 18-9 and 18-10). In most cases, synovial fluid examination is not highly specific for any particular type of arthritis. Only in septic arthritis or crystal-induced arthritis is SF examination highly sensitive and specific for a single disease entity.

Synovial fluid should be collected using sterile disposable needles with a sterile disposable plastic syringe, to avoid contamination from exogenous birefringent material (Phelps, 1968). Ideally, the patient should be fasting for at least 6 and preferably 12 hours to allow equilibration of glucose between plasma and

Table 18-9. CLASSIFICATION OF SYNOVIAL FLUID FINDINGS*

	NORMAL	NON-INFLAMMATORY (GROUP I)	INFLAMMATORY MILD (GROUP IIa)	INFLAMMATORY SEVERE (GROUP IIb)	INFECTIOUS-SEPTIC (GROUP III)
Appearance	clear yellow	clear yellow	clear yellow to slightly turbid	turbid	turbid to purulent
Viscosity	high	high	decreased	decreased	decreased
Mucin clot	good	good	good to fair	fair to poor	poor
Leukocyte count (per μl)	0-200	0-5,000	0-10,000	500-50,000	500-200,000
Neutrophils (%)	0-25	0-25	0-50	0-90	40-100
Glucose (blood-synovial fluid difference in mg/dl)	0-10	0-10	0-20	0-40	20-100
Comments				MSU† crystals in gout; CPPD‡ crystals in pseudogout	Gram's stain and/or culture positive in about 50%

* Adapted from Cohen, 1975, and Ropes, 1953.
† MSU = Monosodium urate (p. 661).
‡ CPPD = Calcium pyrophosphate dihydrate (p. 661).

SF. If the patient is not fasting, SF glucose measurements are of little value, except when markedly decreased (under 40 mg/dl).

For routine examination, the syringe can be moistened with about 25 units of heparin per milliliter of synovial fluid as anticoagulant (Naib, 1973): powdered anticoagulants such as oxalate and EDTA should be avoided, since these can present confusing artifacts on microscopic examination (Phelps, 1968).

Detection of Trace Amounts of Synovial Fluid. Occasionally it is important to determine after aspiration whether the synovial space has been entered. In such cases, the material within the needle may be expelled directly into a test tube or flushed into the tube with a small amount of saline. As little as 0.5 μl of this synovial fluid can be identified by (1) turbidity or clot formation with 2 per cent acetic acid; (2) metachromasia with toluidine blue (Goldenberg, 1973). Although the latter method is more sensitive, false positives may result from contact with heparin.

Even if no SF is apparent within the syringe, a drop of SF may be present within the needle, and can be used for culture or microscopic examination. In such cases, the needle may be left on the syringe, and inserted into a sterile cork before transport to the laboratory.

GROSS EXAMINATION, VISCOSITY, AND MUCIN CLOT TEST

Appearance of normal SF is crystal clear and pale yellow. Turbid yellow fluid may occur with increased numbers of leukocytes due to septic or non-septic inflammation. Turbidity is

Table 18-10. SYNOVIAL FLUID ANALYSIS IN DISEASE*

	OSTEOARTHRITIS (DEGENERATIVE JOINT DISEASE)	TRAUMATIC ARTHRITIS	RHEUMATIC FEVER	SYSTEMIC LUPUS ERYTHEMATOSUS
Appearance	clear yellow	clear yellow (occasionally bloody)	slightly turbid	clear yellow to slightly turbid
Viscosity	variable	variable	variable	variable
Mucin clot	good-fair	good-fair	good-fair	good-fair
Leukocyte count (per μl)	700 (50-5,000)	1,000 (50-10,000)	14,000 (50-50,000)	2,000 (50-10,000)
Neutrophils (%)	15 (0-30)	25 (0-30)	50 (0-60)	30 (0-40)
Glucose (blood-synovial fluid difference in mg/dl)	0 (0-10)	5 (0-20)	5 (0-20)	20 (0-30)
Other Findings	Collagen fibrils and/or cartilage fragments usually present	Fat globules may be present		LE cells may be present in SF

* Adapted from Cohen, 1975; Jessar, 1972; Owen, 1970; Hollander, 1966; Ropes, 1953.

usually reported as 1+ to 4+ (see section on cerebrospinal fluid) (p. 638).

Milky or "pseudochylous" fluid may occur with tuberculous arthritis (Wallace, 1976), chronic rheumatoid arthritis, acute gouty arthritis (Cracchiolo, 1971), or systemic lupus erythematosus (Ryan, 1973).

Grossly purulent fluid may occur with acute septic arthritis, but is often absent, especially during the early stages of infection.

Greenish tinged fluid may occur with *H. influenzae* septic arthritis (Krauss, 1974), chronic rheumatoid arthritis (Jessar, 1972), and acute episodes of crystal synovitis due to gout or pseudogout (Currey, 1976).

Grossly bloody fluid may occur with fracture through the joint surface, tumor involving the joint, traumatic arthritis, neurogenic arthropathy, hemophilic arthritis, or pigmented villonodular synovitis. Occasionally, bloody fluid may be noted with septic arthritis, rheumatoid arthritis, or osteoarthritis (Jessar, 1972). Traumatic tap can be distinguished by (a) decreasing amounts of blood as aspiration is continued (rarely blood may appear as tissues are traumatized later during aspiration); (b) uneven distribution with streaking in the syringe; (c) clotting about blood streaks in the syringe; (d) lack of xanthochromic supernatant after centrifugation. Although xanthochromia is difficult to interpret, owing to the yellow appearance of normal synovial fluid, a dark red or dark brown supernatant in the presence of gross blood is suggestive evidence of hemarthrosis rather than traumatic tap.

Viscosity usually is estimated either by allowing synovial fluid to form a string by dropping from a syringe into a beaker or by placing a drop of SF on the thumb, touching this with a finger, and separating the finger to form a string (we prefer to use gloves, since some specimens may be contaminated). Normal SF forms a string 4 to 6 cm in length. If the string breaks before reaching a length of 3 cm, viscosity is lower than normal (Hollander, 1966).

Quantitative measurements of viscosity can be performed using an ordinary white blood cell diluting pipette (Hasselbacher, 1976). However, the additional information gained probably has little clinical significance.

Viscosity is related primarily to the concentration and polymerization of SF hyaluronate. Decreased viscosity may occur in a wide variety of inflammatory conditions including septic arthritis, gouty arthritis, and rheumatoid arthritis. Decreased viscosity also may occur if hyaluronate is diluted by rapid effusion after trauma (Jessar, 1972).

The mucin clot test (Ropes test) reflects the polymerization of SF hyaluronate. A few drops of SF are added to about 10 ml of 2 to 5 per cent acetic acid in a small beaker and allowed to stand for a few minutes (Hollander, 1966; Owen, 1970; Jessar, 1972). Normally, a firm clot will form, surrounded by a clear solution: this is graded as "good." A soft clot forming in a slightly turbid solution is graded as "fair." A friable clot, forming in a turbid solution and shredding on agitation, is graded as "poor." No clot formation, with flakes in a cloudy suspension, is graded as "very poor." Decreased polymerization of hyaluronate and an abnormal mucin clot test may occur in a

Table 18-10.   SYNOVIAL FLUID ANALYSIS IN DISEASE* (Continued)

RHEUMATOID ARTHRITIS	GOUT	PSEUDOGOUT	ACUTE BACTERIAL ARTHRITIS	TUBERCULOUS ARTHRITIS
turbid yellow, milky, or greenish	turbid yellow to milky	clear yellow to slightly turbid	turbid to purulent (occasionally bloody)	turbid
decreased	decreased	decreased	decreased	decreased
fair-poor	fair-poor	fair-poor	poor	poor
20,000 (200–80,000)	20,000 (100–100,000)	15,000 (50–75,000)	90,000 (200–200,000)	20,000 (2,000–100,000)
70 (0–90)	70 (0–90)	70 (0–90)	90 (50–100)	60 (20–95)
30 (0–60)	10 (0–80)	10 (0–20)	80 (40–100)	70 (0–100)
Leukocyte count occasionally exceeds 100,000; RA§ cells usually present	MSU† crystals in over 90% of patients with acute gouty arthritis	CPPD‡ crystals required for diagnosis	Gram's stain and culture positive in about 50%	Acid-fast stain and culture frequently negative; biopsy may be needed for diagnosis

†MSU = Monosodium urate (p. 661).
‡CPPD = Calcium pyrophosphate dihydrate (p. 661).
§RA = Rheumatoid arthritis (p. 661).

wide variety of inflammatory conditions including septic arthritis, gouty arthritis, and rheumatoid arthritis. Since both viscosity and clot formation reflect the polymerization of hyaluronate, fluids with poor viscosity usually form poor mucin clots. Exceptions may occur with acute effusions (e.g., rheumatic fever, sepsis, trauma, or overuse) in which viscosity has been decreased by dilution with plasma dialysate, but polymerization remains normal (Hollander, 1966).

MICROSCOPIC EXAMINATION

Cell count

The "upper limit of normal" or reference value for SF leukocyte count varies in different reports:

under 200/μl (Ropes, 1953)
under 200/μl (Owen, 1970)
under 300/μl (Jessar, 1972)
under 600/μl (Hollander, 1966)
under 750/μl (Currey, 1976)

However, most authorities accept 200/μl as the upper limit of normal (Cohen, 1975). In this discussion, we will consider 200/μl the "upper limit of normal."

Total leukocyte counts can be performed by examining undiluted fluid in a Fuchs-Rosenthal chamber or a hemocytometer (Currey, 1976). Alternatively, physiologic saline plus a small amount of 0.1 per cent methylene blue can be used as diluent (Cohen, 1975). It is essential that the fluid be thoroughly mixed before adding to the counting chamber. A standard bench vibratory mixer is satisfactory for this purpose. Highly viscous fluids may need to stand for over 30 minutes before the cells can be counted.

A phase contrast microscope provides accurate distinction between leukocytes and erythrocytes without the need for methylene blue as a diluent. If ordinary light microscopy is used, a diluent with 0.1 per cent methylene blue will aid in recognition of leukocytes. For high cell counts (over 50,000/μl), saline dilution may be needed even with phase microscopy.

If the fluid is grossly bloody, one of the following methods may be used to lyse erythrocytes prior to performing a leukocyte count: (a) dilution with 1 per cent saponin in saline (Donaldson, 1972); (b) dilution with 0.3 per cent saline (Jessar, 1972); (c) dilution with 0.1 N HCl (Blau, 1971). If erythrocytes are present, an effort should be made to judge whether these are derived from traumatic tap (see Gross Examination). The erythrocytes should be counted unless it is clear that they are due to traumatic tap.

A very high leukocyte count (over 100,000 leukocytes/μl) strongly suggests bacterial infection. However, in the early stages of a bacterial infection, the leukocyte count may be normal. Occasionally, active gout or rheumatoid arthritis may present with SF leukocyte counts over 100,000/μl; in such cases the differential diagnosis from septic arthritis may be difficult.

Differential count

The percentage of neutrophils can be estimated by (1) phase contrast microscopy at the time of leukocyte count; (2) Wright's stain of unconcentrated SF; (3) Wright's stain of centrifuged SF sediment. Hollander (1966) recommends that the sediment be washed by redilution with isotonic saline and recentrifuged to remove most of the mucin; (4) Wright's stain of SF concentrated by cytocentrifuge. We use 0.5 ml SF diluted with 2.5 ml 0.1 per cent methylene blue in saline; (5) SF concentrates prepared by centrifugation or filtration plus Papanicolaou stain (Naib, 1973; Broderick, 1976). Phase contrast is the most convenient method and is adequate for most purposes. However, it is not optimal for detailed morphologic study and does not provide a permanent record. Papanicolaou stain probably is optimal for careful morphologic study but requires considerably more time than the other methods.

The "routine" differential count usually is reported only as the percentage of neutrophils. The generally accepted upper limit is 25 per cent neutrophils (Ropes, 1956; Hollander, 1966; Owen, 1970; Jessar, 1972; Naib, 1973; Scott, 1975; Cohen, 1975), although others report a higher "upper limit of normal" (Currey, 1976). A very high percentage of neutrophils (over 90 per cent) is suggestive evidence of bacterial arthritis, even if the total cell count and other measurements are within normal limits.

Cellular morphology

Rheumatoid arthritis. In about 95 per cent of patients, both phase and ordinary light microscopy reveal small, dark cytoplasmic granules, from 0.5 to 2.0 μ diameter, within 5 to 100 per cent of neutrophils. Such neutrophils are called "RA cells." A given RA cell may contain from 1 to 20 of these granules in its cytoplasm (Hollander, 1965; Cohen, 1975). These granules can be clearly identified using phase contrast with oil immersion, and by immunofluorescent techniques can be shown to consist of immune complexes: IgG, IgM, complement, and rheumatoid factor. RA cells are *not* specific for rheumatoid arthritis, but also occur in other conditions such as gout and septic arthritis (Scott, 1975).

Lymphoblasts and Sezary cells have been reported in SF of rheumatoid arthritis (Traycoff, 1976; Van Leeuwen, 1976); additional studies are needed to confirm these findings and to establish their clinical significance.

Lupus Erythematosus. LE cell formation is a relatively common in vivo phenomenon in synovial fluid (Hunder, 1970). In some cases, LE cells are present in SF with a negative LE test on peripheral blood. A few patients with rheumatoid arthritis also may have "LE cells" in synovial fluid.

Reiter's Syndrome. Large histiocytic cells with intracytoplasmic inclusions have been described on Giemsa and Papanicolaou stains (Naib, 1973; Broderick, 1976). Other workers describe large phagocytic cells with ingested neutrophils visualized on Wright's stain (Pekin, 1967; Cracchiolo, 1971). Additional studies are needed to confirm these reports, and to establish their clinical significance.

Osteoarthritis. Multinucleated cartilagenous cells in SF are reported as characteristic (Naib, 1973; Broderick, 1976). Papanicolaou stain may be needed for definitive identification.

Pigmented Villonodular Synovitis. Foreign body giant cells with hemosiderin pigment, and papillary aggregates of synovial cells, are reported as characteristic (Naib, 1973; Broderick, 1976). Papanicolaou stain may be needed for definitive identification.

Septic Arthritis. Gram's stain is positive in about 50 per cent of patients with joint sepsis (Cooke, 1971; McCord, 1977). Depending upon the type of infection, culture may be positive in about 30 to 80 per cent of patients with septic arthritis. If sepsis is suspected but Gram's stain and culture are inconclusive, synovial biopsy may be needed to establish a diagnosis (Bayer, 1977). It is important to remember that septic arthritis can co-exist with other types of arthritis such as lupus, gout, and pseudogout.

Crystals

Five types of crystal-induced arthritis have been reported: (1) arthritis associated with apatite crystals (Schumacher, 1977); (2) gout caused by monosodium urate (MSU); (3) pseudogout caused by calcium pyrophosphate dihydrate (CPPD); (4) chronic arthritis caused by talcum crystals introduced during joint surgery (Naib, 1973); (5) acute synovitis caused by intra-articular injection of crystalline corticosteroid preparations (Schumacher, 1977). Arthritis associated with apatite crystals is uncommon and no specific treatment is available. The apatite crystals appear as shiny inclusions on wet preparations, or dark cytoplasmic inclusions on Wright's stain (Schumacher, 1977); definitive diagnosis requires electron microscopy.

The remaining four types of crystals can be detected and identified by compensated polarized light microscopy (p. 662). Synovial fluid for examination by polarized light should be collected either with no anticoagulant or with a small amount of heparin. EDTA and calcium oxalate crystals are birefringent and can be confused with MSU or CPPD.

Initial examination for crystals should be conducted on a wet preparation, using both plain and polarized light. The slide and coverslip should be cleaned with alcohol or acetone immediately prior to examination, then carefully dried with gauze or lens paper. A few drops of SF are placed on the slide, so that when the coverslip is gently added, the fluid margins barely reach the coverslip periphery. The preparation is promptly rimmed with clear nail polish to prevent drying. Allow the nail polish to dry for about 15 minutes before examination to prevent damage to the microscope objective.

Crystals of MSU appear as birefringent rods or needles under polarized light, varying from 1 to 20 μ in length (McCarty, 1965) (Fig. 18-2A). Certain crystalline corticosteroid preparations appear morphologically identical to MSU: e.g., betamethasone acetate (Celestone R), and triamcinolone hexacetonide (Kahn, 1970). Also, cholesterol crystals can appear as birefringent needles in chronic synovial effusions (Nye, 1968). Definitive identification of needle-like crystals may be aided by incubation with uricase (McCarty, 1961).

Crystals of CPPD appear as birefringent rods, rectangles, or rhomboids varying from 1 to 20 μ in length and up to about 4 μ in width

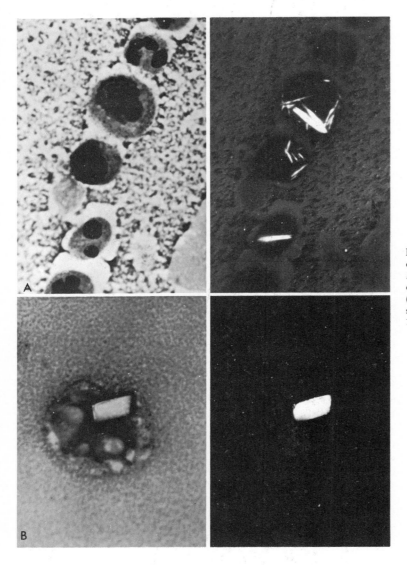

Figure 18-2. *A*, Leukocytes with uric aci crystals under normal and polarized ligh *B*, Leukocyte with calcium pyrophospha crystal under normal and polarized ligh (From Good and Frishette: Crystals in drie smears of synovial fluid. J.A.M.A., *198*:8 1966.)

(McCarty, 1965) (Fig. 18-2*B*). Some corticosteroids used for intra-articular injection can be confused with CPPD (Wild, 1975). Also, cholesterol crystals may appear as rhomboid forms in some chronic effusions (Nye, 1968).

Talcum crystals present a Maltese cross appearance and may be as small as 5 to 10 μ (Naib, 1973). Lipid droplets in SF, associated with chronic inflammation or traumatic arthritis, also may have a Maltese cross appearance under polarized light (Wild, 1975).

Crystalline corticosteroids may appear under polarized light as long needles or rhomboids identical in appearance to MSU or CPPD; they may also appear as short rods, plates, fragments, or clumps (Kahn, 1970).

Such crystals may persist in SF for a month or longer following intra-articular injection.

Collagen fibrils and fibrin strands vary from 2 to over 100 μ in length. Although these may resemble MSU crystals under ordinary light, they show little or no birefringence with polarized light (Kitridou, 1969). Electron microscopy is required to distinguish definitely collagen fibrils from fibrin (Kitridou, 1969).

Fragments of cartilage may appear birefringent under polarized light (Kitridou, 1969), but unlike MSU or CPPD do not have parallel margins. These fragments, as well as collagen fibrils, may be present in SF of osteoarthritis or traumatic arthritis.

Cholesterol crystals typically appear as irregular birefringent plates, often with notched margins. However, in chronic effusions, cholesterol crystals may appear either as long birefringent needles or as rhomboids, similar to MSU or CPPD (Nye, 1968). Cholesterol crystals may be present in any chronic effusion, e.g., tuberculous or rheumatoid arthritis.

Gout. MSU crystals can be demonstrated in SF of about 90 to 95 per cent of patients, during attacks of acute gouty arthritis (McCarty, 1965; Schumacher, 1975). Between attacks of acute gouty arthritis, MSU crystals can be demonstrated in about 75 per cent of patients. During attacks of acute gouty arthritis, the majority of crystals are intracellular, within neutrophils or macrophages; between attacks the majority of crystals are extracellular. However, in a few patients with acute gout, even careful examination with compensated polarized light fails to reveal MSU crystals (Abeles, 1975; Schumacher, 1975). Possible reasons for this failure to demonstrate MSU crystals may include crystals loculated within a joint and dissolution of crystals which initiated the acute attack. Occasionally, a 30 to 45 minute search may be required to find one or two MSU crystals in a patient with acute gouty arthritis (Schumacher, 1975). In such cases, there is an obvious need for the attending physician to communicate his clinical impression to the clinical microscopist, and to request a prolonged study of the specimen.

The report should note whether MSU crystals are lying free in SF or have been ingested by leukocytes. Phagocytosis of crystals suggests that these are responsible for acute arthritis. If only extracellular crystals are found, it is unlikely that these are responsible for acute symptoms (Wild, 1975).

Pseudogout. In this condition, clinical symptoms may mimic gout, rheumatoid arthritis, or osteoarthritis (Skinner, 1969). Diagnosis requires the demonstration of CPPD crystals. As in gout, the crystals may be either intracellular or extracellular (Figure 18–2B).

CHEMICAL EXAMINATION

Total protein in normal SF averages about 2 g/dl with a range of about 1 to 3 g/dl. Concentration of a specific protein in SF depends upon several factors, including plasma levels, molecular size, permeability of the synovial membrane, local synthesis, and local consumption. As plasma levels of a specific protein increase, levels in SF fluid also tend to increase. Thus, the concentration of a specific protein in SF frequently is expressed as SF:plasma ratio, to compensate for variations in plasma concentration.

For proteins which diffuse from plasma to synovial fluid, the SF:plasma ratio tends to decrease as molecular size increases (Kushner, 1971). Thus low molecular weight proteins from plasma tend to have higher SF:plasma ratios than larger proteins.

Certain proteins—notably haptoglobin and prothrombin—have lower SF:plasma ratios than expected from their molecular weights. Synovial membrane may be less permeable to these proteins, with rejection based on some property other than size.

Inflammation causes increased permeability of the synovial membrane, and increased SF:plasma ratios for all proteins in synovial fluid. This increase appears to be greater for large proteins (e.g., alpha-2-macroglobulin) than for small proteins (e.g., albumin). Reference intervals for proteins (and other constituents) in synovial fluid are outlined in Table 18–8. In comparison to plasma, SF is characterized by relatively high albumin, high α_1 globulin, low α_2 globulin, and low γ globulin. With inflammation, total protein of synovial fluid increases, and the electrophoretic pattern becomes more similar to that of plasma. Local synthesis of gamma globulins may occur within inflamed synovial tissue and contributes to increased gamma globulin. Local consumption of protein within synovial fluid is related to decreased levels of complement, observed in SF of rheumatoid arthritis and systemic lupus erythematosus.

For clinical purposes, increased SF total protein merely provides evidence of inflammation. Indeed, in most laboratories this measurement is not included as part of the "routine" synovial fluid examination (appearance, viscosity, mucin clot test, leukocyte count, per cent neutrophils, examination for crystals, and SF plus plasma glucose). Protein electrophoresis of SF is generally considered primarily of research interest rather than of practical clinical importance.

Glucose in SF normally is identical to or slightly less than plasma glucose. Since equilibration between blood and SF glucose is slow, samples of blood and SF should be obtained after the patient has been fasting for 6 to 12 hours.

In non-inflammatory arthritis, the blood-SF

glucose difference is about 10 mg/dl. With inflammatory arthritis (e.g., rheumatoid, septic, or tuberculous) the blood-SF glucose difference frequently exceeds 25 mg/dl or even 50 mg/dl. If fasting specimens are unavailable, a SF glucose under 40 mg/dl suggests decreased SF glucose; and a SF glucose under 20 mg/dl is considered definitely decreased.

Enzyme measurements in SF appear to have little clinical value, despite extensive investigations during the past 10 to 15 years. Enzymes which have been studied include the lysosomal enzymes (e.g., acid phosphatase and muramidase), alkaline phosphatase, LDH, and the transaminases (Cohen, 1975).

Uric acid measurements in SF (as opposed to microscopic examination for MSU crystals) appear to have little or no diagnostic value. Although some authors have suggested that measurement of SF uric acid might be useful in diagnosing acute gouty arthritis, most investigators feel that gouty effusions have a urate content essentially identical to that of serum (Cohen, 1975).

Lactate and pH measurements in SF may provide a useful but non-specific index of inflammation (McCarty, 1974). A lactate over 20 mg/dl (2/mmol/1) and/or a pH under 7.3 is suggestive evidence of septic or non-septic inflammation. Increased lactate and decreased pH appear to be associated with a rapid change from aerobic to anaerobic metabolism in synovial tissue as the Po_2 falls below 30 mm Hg (Falchuk, 1970). The clinical value of these measurements is not yet well established.

IMMUNOLOGIC STUDIES

Rheumatoid factor refers to a group of immunoglobulins reacting with the Fc regions of IgG molecules. About 80 per cent of patients with rheumatoid arthritis have rheumatoid factor in serum; about 60 per cent have rheumatoid factor in SF (Cracchiolo, 1972). In early rheumatoid arthritis, rheumatoid factor may appear in SF before becoming measurable in serum (Waxman, 1975). With suspected rheumatoid arthritis and a negative test for rheumatoid factor in serum, measurement of rheumatoid factor in SF may have some clinical value. However, a high incidence of false positive results has been reported (Huskisson, 1971).

Antinuclear antibodies have been demonstrated in SF of patients with systemic lupus erythematosus (about 70 per cent), as well as in SF of patients with rheumatoid arthritis (about 20 per cent) (Cracchiolo, 1972; Cohen, 1975). At present this finding is primarily of research interest rather than practical clinical value.

Complement measurements on SF have excited great interest, particularly over the past five years. The reference interval for SF complement varies with the concentration of SF protein so that SF complement should be expressed in relation to total protein (Bunch, 1974).

In rheumatoid arthritis, decreased SF complement is noted in about 60 to 80 per cent of seropositive patients (rheumatoid factor present in serum), and in about 30 to 40 per cent of seronegative patients (Bunch, 1974). Although measurements of total hemolytic complement (CH 50) are most widely used, measurement of C4 may provide a more sensitive index (Ruddy, 1975). Decreased SF complement is not specific for rheumatoid arthritis: about 80 per cent of patients with systemic lupus have low SF complement. Low levels of SF complement also are occasionally observed in rheumatic fever, bacterial arthritis, gout, pseudo-gout, and other types of inflammatory arthritis.

Simultaneous measurement of serum and SF complement may be helpful in patients with seronegative rheumatoid arthritis. In about 40 per cent of such patients, serum complement is normal or increased, while SF complement is decreased (Ruddy, 1975).

Although potentially useful, complement measurements on SF probably should not be considered a "routine" examination at this time.

CLINICAL CORRELATION

The "routine" synovial fluid examination includes appearance, viscosity, mucin clot test, microscopic study with compensated polarized light, Gram's stain, culture, and glucose. Except for Gram's stain and crystal identification, the synovial fluid examination is *not* highly specific for any single type of arthritis. Indeed, even Gram's stain and crystal identification do not exclude the possibility of two different diseases, since the following conditions may exist simultaneously in the same joint:

septic arthritis and lupus erythematosus
(Edelen, 1971)

septic arthritis and pseudogout (McConville, 1975)

septic arthritis and gout (Smith, 1972)

gout and rheumatoid arthritis (Owen, 1966)

gout and pseudogout (Jackson, 1965)

According to some authorities (Currey, 1976), small numbers of MSU or CPPD crystals may occur in conditions other than gout or pseudogout; however, this has not been confirmed, and as noted above, steroid or cholesterol crystals may have an appearance very similar to MSU or CPPD.

Even Gram's stain and crystal identification have less than 100 per cent sensitivity: about 50 per cent of patients with septic arthritis have negative Gram's stain, and about 5 to 10 per cent of patients with acute gouty arthritis (about 25 per cent of patients with inactive gouty arthritis) have a negative examination for crystals.

The finding of LE cells in synovial fluid is not specific, since these may also occur in rheumatoid arthritis. However, if rheumatoid arthritis can be excluded, the specificity of this finding probably exceeds 95 per cent.

To provide improved sensitivity and specificity, two approaches are commonly used for interpretation: classification of synovial fluids into "reaction types" based on multiple findings (Table 18-9), and evaluation of results with regard to "typical" patterns found in different diseases (Table 18-10).

Non-inflammatory effusions (Table 18-9) usually have leukocyte counts of about 1000/μl and seldom exceed 5000/μl (Cohen, 1975). The percentage of neutrophils is usually under 25 per cent, although some authors report higher levels (Currey, 1976). Non-inflammatory conditions associated with articular effusion include osteoarthritis; traumatic arthritis (may occasionally be hemorrhagic); and neurogenic joint disease. Occasionally, the inflammatory fluids of mild rheumatic fever, systemic lupus erythematosus, or bacterial infection may present similar findings. Under phase microscopy, collagen fibrils and/or cartilage fragments may be seen in osteoarthritis, traumatic arthritis, or neurogenic joint disease.

Mild inflammatory effusions may be associated with minimal inflammation and synovial fluid findings similar to Group I, e.g., early rheumatic fever; early systemic lupus erythematosus; early bacterial infection; and arthritis accompanying systemic disease such as ulcerative colitis, regional enteritis, psoriasis. In such cases, the SF leukocyte count seldom exceeds 10,000/μl and the percentage of neu-

trophils usually is under 50 per cent.

However, with severe *inflammatory effusions*, the synovial reaction may be moderate or severe, e.g., rheumatoid arthritis, gout, and pseudogout. The leukocyte count may exceed 50,000 or even 100,000/μl, with over 90 per cent neutrophils (Frischknecht, 1975; Cohen, 1975).

Infectious effusions owing to bacterial sepsis usually are associated with SF leukocyte counts over 50,000/μl and over 90 per cent neutrophils (Cohen, 1975). Counts of over 100,000 to 200,000/μl almost always indicate bacterial infection. However, SF leukocyte counts of under 1,000 may be observed in some patients with early infectious arthritis (Brandt, 1974).

Many of the common viral diseases are associated with arthritis and joint effusions. Indeed, arthritis may sometimes precede other manifestations of viral infection. In viral arthritis, the SF leukocyte count commonly is under 10,000/μl with a mononuclear cell response, although exceptions have been reported (Cohen, 1975).

In Reiter's syndrome, the SF leukocyte count tends to be higher than with viral arthritis and associated with increased neutrophils. However, the leukocyte count and neutrophil reaction usually are less marked than with typical bacterial sepsis.

Hemorrhagic effusions may be associated with trauma, fracture, neurogenic joint, tumor (especially hemangioma), pigmented villonodular synovitis, hemorrhagic diathesis (e.g., hemophilia, anticoagulant therapy), or septic arthritis (Hollander, 1966; Jessar, 1972; Cohen, 1975).

Typical SF findings in various diseases are outlined in Table 18-10. With monoarticular effusions, the possibility of bacterial infection (e.g., tuberculosis or gonococcal arthritis) should be considered even if clinical and laboratory findings are atypical. Repeated aspirations, repeated radiologic studies, or even synovial biopsy may be indicated if the diagnosis is in doubt, and there is clinical evidence of progression.

MICROSCOPIC EXAMINATION OF SF: COMPENSATED POLARIZED LIGHT MICROSCOPY

An ordinary microscope with mechanical stage can be modified for compensated polarized light microscopy (Fig. 18-3):

1. A 32 mm polarizing disc (called "the polarizer") is placed over the light source.

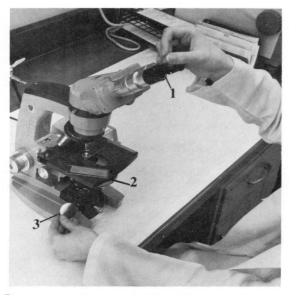

Figure 18-3. Adaptation of ordinary laboratory microscope for compensated polarized light microscopy: *1*, Polarizing disc for eyepiece; *2*, glass slide with two thicknesses of clear cellophane tape to be placed over No. 3; *3*, polarizing disc to be placed over light source.

2. A glass microscope slide (called "the compensator") is prepared with two thicknesses of clear cellophane or cellophane tape applied to one side (Fagan, 1974). Streaks in the two layers of cellophane tape must be parallel rather than crossed. Translucent tape is *not* satisfactory. The prepared slide is placed over the polarizer.

3. A second polarizing disc (called "the analyzer") is placed either in the barrel of the microscope or in the eyepiece.

The same components are available from most microscope manufacturers (Fig. 18-4):

1. A polarizer which fits over the light source (AO part No. K2108)

2. A compensator which fits over the polarizer (included with AO part No. K2108)

3. An analyzer which fits into the microscope barrel (AO part No. 1114)

A gliding circular stage with mechanical controls for positioning the specimen (AO part No. K2270) greatly facilitates crystal identification, especially for inexperienced observers (Fig. 18-4). An attached camera (AO part No. 668) is useful for preparing permanent records of interesting samples.

With the compensator removed, and the polarizers crossed, the field will appear dark, except for birefringent material such as MSU crystals, CPPD crystals, talc crystals, cholesterol crystals, certain corticosteroid crystals, and oval fat bodies.

With the compensator added, the field will appear red, and a given crystal (e.g., MSU) will appear either blue or yellow, depending upon its orientation (Fig. 18-5).

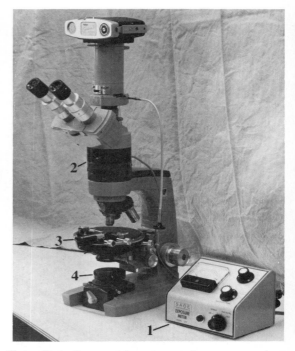

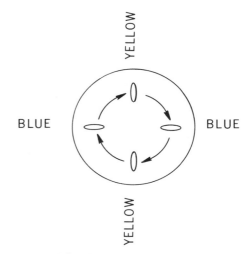

Figure 18-4. Commercial components for compensated polarized light microscopy: *1*, Exposure meter for camera; *2*, analyzer; *3*, circular stage with mechanical controls; *4*, polarizer with compensator.

With the compensator in a constant position, a birefringent crystal of MSU will change color (from blue to yellow or vice versa) as the crystal is rotated 90 degrees (Fig. 18-5).

If the crystal is kept in a constant position but

YELLOW

BLUE   BLUE

YELLOW

Figure 18-5. Color changes in birefringent crystal observed with compensated polarized light during rotation of microscope stage. (Colors in a given position vary according to setting of compensator and must be checked against a control.)

Table 18-11. CHYLOUS AND PSEUDOCHYLOUS EFFUSIONS

	CHYLOUS EFFUSION	PSEUDOCHYLOUS EFFUSION
Appearance	Milky: may form creamy top layer on standing	Milky to greenish—or "gold paint" appearance
Odor	Odorless	Variable from odorless to foul
pH	Alkaline	Variable
Extraction with ether after acidification with dilute HCl	Clearing and decrease in volume	Does not clear or decrease in volume
Microscopic examination	Lymphocytes plus fine fat droplets	Mixed cellular reaction with cholesterol crystals
Triglycerides	2x-8x serum triglycerides	Lower than serum triglycerides
Cholesterol	Lower than serum cholesterol	May be higher than serum cholesterol
Lipoprotein electrophoresis	Increased chylomicron band in relation to plasma	Chylomicrons scanty or absent
Effect of diet with no long-chain fatty acids	Decreased accumulation of lipid in effusion	No significant change in effusion
Ingestion of lipophilic dye	Dye appears in effusion	Dye does not appear in effusion
Culture	Always sterile	Usually sterile (check for tuberculosis or fungus)
Etiology	Damage or obstruction to thoracic duct	Chronic effusion of any cause (e.g., cyst fluid, rheumatoid disease, tuberculosis, myxedema)

the compensator rotated 90 degrees, a similar color change will be observed.

Control slides may be prepared from scrapings of a gouty tophus, a known specimen from acute gouty arthritis, a suspension of betamethasone acetate (appearance under compensated polarized light identical to uric acid crystals), or according to the procedure described by Bartlett (1978). In this last procedure, the control is prepared by adding 5 mg of uric acid to 15 ml of boiling distilled water. After the crystals are dissolved, the solution is cooled and 0.1 g/ml of sodium bicarbonate added until a pH of 7 is reached. This solution is then stored for several days at room temperature, allowing evaporation to dryness. The sediment contains crystals of uric acid which may be resuspended in distilled water for use as a control. The control slides should be rimmed with nail polish and saved for comparison with unknown specimens.

Immediately before examination of an unknown, use the control slide to sketch the colors of a uric acid crystal in different orientations, with the compensator in a fixed position. Prepare a sketch similar to Figure 18-5 by rotating the stage or by observing crystals lying in different positions. Then observe the unknown: rotate the stage as needed to bring the unknown crystals into the same positions as noted in your sketch. Crystals of MSU will appear identical to those in the control slide, while CPPD crystals will have opposite colors from MSU. Certain corticosteroids may have an appearance identical to MSU under compensated polarized light. Although Nye (1968) describes cholesterol crystals appearing identical to MSU, findings with compensated polarized light were not reported. Digestion with uricase as described by McCarty (1961) may be used to confirm crystal identification

in selected cases: (1) Add one part of a saline uricase suspension (minimal activity 0.75 units per ml) to 5 parts of SF (as little as 50 μl SF may be used). (2) Add one part of saline control to 5 parts of SF in a separate tube. (3) Incubate both tubes at 45° C. for 4 hours. (4) Place a drop of SF from each tube on a glass slide and examine by compensated polarized light microscopy.

PLEURAL, PERICARDIAL, AND PERITONEAL FLUIDS

TRANSUDATES AND EXUDATES

Effusions of fluid in the pleural, pericardial, or peritoneal cavity may form on the basis of plasma ultrafiltration. Such ultrafiltrates commonly are classified as transudates and exudates. A transudate is an effusion caused by mechanical factors influencing formation or resorption of fluid, e.g., decreased plasma albumin and/or increased venous pressure. An exudate is an effusion caused by damage to mesothelial linings, e.g., tuberculosis, bacterial or fungal infection, neoplasm, rheumatoid disease, or systemic lupus erythematosus. Effusions also may form owing to escape of chyle from the thoracic duct (chylous effusions, Table 18-11). Some causes for pleural, pericardial, and peritoneal effusions are outlined in Table 18-12.

In pleural fluid, a protein level of 3.0 g/dl classically is used to separate transudates

Table 18-12. CAUSES OF PLEURAL, PERICARDIAL, AND PERITONEAL EFFUSIONS

PLEURAL	PERICARDIAL (continued)
Transudates	*Exudates* (continued)
Congestive heart failure	Neoplasms
Hepatic cirrhosis	metastatic carcinoma or lymphoma
Hypoproteinemia (e.g., nephrotic syndrome)	Trauma (may be associated with hemorrhagic effusion)
Exudates	Myocardial infarct
Neoplasms	Hemorrhagic effusion
bronchogenic carcinoma	secondary to anticoagulant therapy
metastatic carcinoma	leakage of aortic aneurysm
lymphoma	Metabolic (uremia, myxedema)
mesothelioma (increased hyaluronate content of effusion fluid)	Rheumatoid disease
Infections	Systemic lupus erythematosus
tuberculosis (high percentage of lymphocytes with under 1% mesothelial cells)	**PERITONEAL**
bacterial pneumonia	*Transudates*
viral or mycoplasmal pneumonia	Congestive heart failure
Trauma (may be associated with hemorrhagic effusion)	Hepatic cirrhosis
Pulmonary infarct (may be associated with hemorrhagic effusion)	Hypoproteinemia (e.g., nephrotic syndrome)
Rheumatoid disease (low pleural fluid glucose in most cases)	*Exudates*
Systemic lupus erythematosus (LE cells occasionally present)	Neoplasms
Pancreatitis (elevated amylase activity in effusion fluid)	hepatoma
Ruptured esophagus (elevated amylase activity and low pH in effusion fluid)	metastatic carcinoma
Chylous effusion	lymphoma
Damage or obstruction to thoracic duct, e.g., trauma, lymphoma, carcinoma, tuberculosis	mesothelioma
	Infections
PERICARDIAL	tuberculosis
	primary bacterial peritonitis (may be superimposed on transudate)
Exudates	secondary bacterial peritonitis (e.g., appendicitis, intestinal infarct)
Infections	Trauma
bacterial pericarditis	Pancreatitis
tuberculosis	Bile peritonitis (secondary to ruptured gallbladder or needle perforation of bile duct)
fungal pericarditis	*Chylous effusion*
viral or mycoplasmal pericarditis	Damage or obstruction to thoracic duct, e.g., trauma, lymphoma, carcinoma, tuberculosis, parasitic infestation

from exudates: about 90 per cent of pleural exudates have a total protein over 3.0 g/dl, and about 80 per cent of pleural transudates have a total protein under 3.0 g/dl. An alternative classification has been suggested by Light (1972) based on three ratios: (1) pleural fluid protein to serum protein (ratio over 0.5 suggests exudate); (2) pleural fluid LDH to serum LDH (ratio over 0.6 suggests exudate); (3) pleural fluid LDH to serum LDH upper limit of normal (ratio over 0.67 suggests exudate). According to Light (1972), over 95 per cent of pleural exudates have at least one of these characteristics, while over 95 per cent of pleural transudates have none of these findings. Additional studies are needed to confirm the value of LDH measurements in laboratory classification of pleural effusions.

In pericardial fluid, the laboratory criteria for transudates are less clearly defined. Indeed, most pericardial effusions are caused by damage to mesothelial linings rather than mechanical factors (Table 18-12). At this time, the clinical validity of total protein measurements to separate pericardial "transudates" from "exudates" is not well established.

In peritoneal fluid, the recommended laboratory criteria for differentiating transudates from exudates vary. Some authorities (Ball, 1976) use a protein level of 2.0 g/dl to separate transudates from exudates, while others use 2.5 g/dl (McClement, 1975; Sabiston, 1974). Both of these recommended "cut-off points" are lower than the generally accepted cut-off of 3.0 g/dl for pleural fluid.

"Routine study" for pleural, pericardial, and or peritoneal effusion of unknown etiology usually includes gross appearance, total protein, erythrocyte count, leukocyte count, differential count and microscopic study of Wright's stained film, Gram's stain, culture, and cytologic study. Additional studies which may be useful in specific circumstances include glucose (suspected rheumatoid disease or infection), amylase (pleural fluid with suspected esophageal perforation; pleural or peritoneal fluid with suspected pancreatitis), LDH (differential diagnosis of pleural transudate vs. exudate), pH (pleural fluid with suspected esophageal perforation; parapneumonic effusion), ammonia (peritoneal fluid with suspected intestinal necrosis or perforation; differential diagnosis of effusion vs. urinary extravasation), creatinine (differential diagnosis of peritoneal effusion vs. urinary extravasation), alkaline phosphatase (peritoneal fluid with suspected infarction or perforation of small intestine), spot test for bile (peritoneal fluid of greenish appearance), hyaluronate (suspected mesothelioma), and biopsy (suspected tuberculosis with negative acid-fast stain and culture).

ASPIRATION OF PLEURAL FLUID

The usual indications for thoracentesis include effusion of unknown etiology, clinical symptoms (e.g., dyspnea) caused by fluid accumulation, intrapleural instillation of drugs for treating infection or malignancy, hemothorax, and empyema. Complications of thoracentesis may include hemothorax due to laceration of the lung and mediastinal shift after removing large amounts of fluid. These complications may be minimized by gradual drainage of fluid via a plastic cannula introduced at the time of thoracentesis (van Heerden, 1968; Wilson, 1975).

ASPIRATION OF PERICARDIAL FLUID

The usual indications for pericardial aspiration include pericardial effusion of unknown etiology and acute or chronic cardiac tamponade. Complications of aspiration include (1) cardiac arrhythmias; (2) infection of pleural spaces by purulent pericardial fluid; (3) laceration of atrium or a coronary artery; (4) inadvertent injection of air into a cardiac chamber. These complications may be minimized either by open biopsy (Kilpatrick, 1965) or by use of a soft catheter for drainage with EKG monitoring during pericardial tap.

ASPIRATION OF PERITONEAL FLUID

The usual indications for abdominal paracentesis include ascites of unknown etiology; clinical symptoms (e.g., dyspnea) caused by fluid accumulation; suspected intestinal infarct, intestinal perforation, or intra-abdominal hemorrhage; and instillation of cytotoxic drugs for treating malignancy. Combined aspiration and lavage have been described by a number of authors (McCoy, 1971; Olsen 1972; Perry, 1972; Parvin, 1975; Engrav, 1975; Jergens, 1977). A catheter is introduced through a trocar, and if aspiration is negative (no free blood, bile, feces, or urine), one liter of normal saline or Ringer's lactate (10 to 20 ml/kg body weight) is infused over 15 to 20 minutes. After manipulation of the abdomen, lavage fluid is siphoned back from the peritoneal cavity into the original container and examined.

GROSS EXAMINATION

PLEURAL FLUID

Normal pleural fluid is clear, pale yellow, and scanty in amount (under 20 ml). Increased amounts of normal appearing fluid commonly are found with congestive heart failure or chronic liver disease. Cloudy or turbid fluid usually is due to large numbers of leukocytes, associated with septic or non-septic inflammation (e.g., bacterial infection, tuberculosis, rheumatoid disease, rheumatic fever).

"Milky" fluid is characteristic of chylous or pseudochylous effusions. True chylous effusions are due to leakage of thoracic duct contents, while pseudochylous effusions are due to breakdown of cellular lipids in chronic effusions from any cause. Approaches to differential diagnosis are outlined in Table 18–11. With regard to ingestion of lipophilic dye: following oral or gastric tube administration of 1 g lipophilic dye (D and C Green No. 6 Lipophilic Dye, H. Kohnstamn, 161 Avenue of the Americas, New York, NY 10013) in one-fourth pound of margarine, the dye will appear in true chylous fluid after 12 to 24 hours, but will not appear in pseudochylous effusions (Klepser, 1954). With regard to lipoprotein electrophoresis, chylous fluid shows markedly elevated chylomicrons in comparison with plasma, while chylomicrons are scanty or absent in pseudochylous effusions (Seriff, 1977).

It is important to distinguish hemorrhagic

fluid from blood-tinged fluid due to traumatic tap. In traumatic tap, the blood typically is non-uniform in distribution and frequently clears with aspiration. Hemorrhagic fluids most often are caused by intrapleural malignancy, but may also occur in some effusions due to pneumonia, closed chest trauma, pulmonary infarct, pancreatitis, and postmyocardial infarction syndrome (Dressler's syndrome). Occasionally, pleural transudates due to congestive heart failure or hepatic cirrhosis may appear hemorrhagic for no apparent cause.

PERICARDIAL FLUID

Normal pericardial fluid is clear, pale yellow, and varies from about 10 to 50 ml in volume.

Interpretation of gross appearance is similar to that for pleural fluid. Hemorrhagic effusions may occur in a wide variety of conditions, including idiopathic hemorrhagic pericarditis, postmyocardial infarction syndrome, postpericardiectomy syndrome, tuberculosis, rheumatoid arthritis, systemic lupus erythematosus, metastatic carcinoma, bacterial pericarditis, or leaking aneurysm. Hemorrhagic pericardial effusion can be distinguished from inadvertant aspiration of blood from the cardiac cavity by observing clot formation: an effusion will not clot, since it has been defibrinated in vivo.

Milky fluid presents the problem of differential diagnosis between true chylous and pseudochylous effusion (Hudspeth, 1966). The latter condition may be associated with any chronic effusion of long duration (Table 18–11).

PERITONEAL FLUID

Normal peritoneal fluid is clear, pale yellow, and scanty in amount (under 50 ml).

Cloudy or turbid fluid suggests peritonitis due to appendicitis, pancreatitis, strangulated or infarcted intestine, ruptured bowel following trauma, or primary bacterial infection.

Greenish (bile-stained) fluid has been described with perforated duodenal ulcer, perforated intestine, cholecystitis, perforated gallbladder, and acute pancreatitis (McCoy, 1971). A spot test for bilirubin should be performed in such cases to confirm the presence of bile. Although ruptured gallbladder with bile in the peritoneal cavity can be rapidly fatal, sterile bile may be fairly well tolerated (Dinmonon, 1964).

Milky fluid is rare, and may be due to chylous, or pseudochylous effusion. These may be differentiated as outlined in Table 18–11. Causes for true chylous ascites include damage to or blockage of the thoracic duct due to lymphoma, carcinoma, tuberculosis, parasitic infestation, adhesions, or hepatic cirrhosis (Lesser, 1970).

Grossly bloody aspirate, or blood-tinged lavage, must be distinguished from traumatic tap. As with other body fluids, traumatic tap is characterized by clearing on continued aspiration.

For lavage fluid, visual quantitation of blood is outlined in Table 18–13. Greater than 25 ml of blood in one liter of lavage fluid produces bright red fluid sufficiently opaque that newsprint cannot be read through the lavage tubing (Olsen, 1972). This amount of blood (25 ml) corresponds to an erythrocyte count of over $100,000/\mu l$ in the lavage fluid. In the series reported by Olsen, 98 per cent of patients with 3+ to 4+ lavage fluid had significant intraabdominal injuries which required exploration, while only 32 per cent of patients with 1+ to 2+ lavage fluid had significant injuries requiring exploration. In the series reported by Engrav (1975), with 100,000 erythrocytes/μl

Table 18–13. VISUAL QUANTITATION OF BLOOD
IN PERITONEAL LAVAGE FLUID*

APPEARANCE OF LAVAGE FLUID IN TUBING	APPEARANCE OF LAVAGE FLUID IN BOTTLE	AMOUNT OF BLOOD NECESSARY TO PRODUCE GROSS APPEARANCE
Gross blood, opaque	gross blood (4+)	>100 ml/l
Bright red, opaque	bright red (3+)	>25 ml/l
Pink, clear	bright red (2+)	5–15 ml/l
Clear	pink (1+)	2 ml/l
Clear	pale pink (+ Race)	8 drops/l
Clear	clear	0

*Adapted from Olsen, W. R., Redman, H. C., and Hildreth, D. H.: Quantitative peritoneal lavage in blunt abdominal trauma. Arch. Surg., *104*:536–543, 1972. Copyright 1972, American Medical Association.

used as the criteria for a "positive" lavage and 50,000 to 100,000 considered "borderline," 85 per cent of patients with erythrocyte counts over 100,000/μl had significant intraperitoneal injury, while only 4 per cent of patients with erythrocyte counts under 50,000/μl had significant injuries requiring exploration.

MICROSCOPIC EXAMINATION

A leukocyte count, erythrocyte count, and differential count often are considered as part of the "routine" examination for pleural, pericardial, and peritoneal fluids. Undiluted fluid is ordinarily used; however, with grossly bloody pleural fluids it may be necessary to hemolyze the erythrocytes by dilution with 3 per cent acetic acid before performing a leukocyte count. An electronic cell counter should *not* be used, since debris may produce falsely elevated counts.

Cells for differential count may be concentrated by centrifugation and resuspension, by cytocentrifuge, or by Millipore filtration.

The percentage of mesothelial cells has clinical significance in pleural fluid and should be reported (Winckler, 1976). This percentage may be specified either as part of the differential count or as a percentage of total leukocytes (neutrophils, eosinophils, basophils, lymphocytes, monocytes, and macrophages).

In ascitic fluid, the percentage of mesothelial cells ordinarily is specified as a percentage of total leukocytes, rather than as part of the differential count (Kline, 1976).

PLEURAL FLUID

The value of pleural fluid erythrocyte counts, leukocyte counts, and differential counts has been questioned by some authorities (Storey, 1976).

Other workers suggest that careful leukocyte and differential counts are useful in detection and diagnosis of tuberculous effusions. About 90 per cent of such cases are characterized by (1) hypercellularity (leukocyte count over 1000/μl) and/or (2) lymphocytosis (over 50 per cent lymphocytes) and/or (3) scarcity of mesothelial cells (under 1 per cent) (Yam, 1967; Spriggs, 1968; Light, 1973; Winckler, 1976). However, these findings are not specific for tuberculosis, and may also occur with uremic effusions, carcinoma, or lymphoma involving the pleural cavity, chronic lymphatic leukemia, chylothorax, and postpneumonic effusions (Spriggs, 1968; Berger, 1975; Winckler, 1976). Some transudates (perhaps 10 per cent) may present findings similar to tuberculosis, with leukocyte counts over 1000/μl, over 50 per cent lymphocytes, and/or under 1 per cent mesothelial cells (Light, 1973). Tuberculous empyema is *not* associated with lymphocytosis, but is characterized by a change from lymphocytic to neutrophil predominance (Spriggs, 1968).

Pleural fluid leukocyte count and differential may be useful in diagnosis of parapneumonic effusions (effusions associated with pneumonia): about 50 per cent of these have a leukocyte count over 10,000/μl, and about 80 per cent have a predominance of neutrophils (Light, 1973). Less than 10 per cent of transudates have a leukocyte count over 10,000/μl and/or a predominance of neutrophils (Light, 1973).

Eosinophilic pleural effusions are considered by some authors to include cases with 10 per cent eosinophils, while others use this term only for effusions with over 50 per cent eosinophils (Spriggs, 1968). Recently, Askin (1977) described reactive eosinophilic pleuritis as frequently associated with pneumothorax and suggested that pleural eosinophilia is a nonspecific reaction to pleural injury. Pleural fluid eosinophilia may be associated with many different conditions, including pneumothorax; postoperative effusions; postpneumonic effusions; closed chest trauma (Kumor, 1976); pulmonary infarct; congestive heart failure; ventriculopleural shunt (Venes, 1974); fungal infections; parasitic disease (e.g., hydatid disease); hypersensitivity syndromes; systemic lupus erythematosus; polyarthritis; Hodgkin's disease; and mesothelioma (Ayvazian, 1977). Although some authors state that pleural eosinophilia is seldom present with tuberculous effusion, this has limited value for diagnosis, since pleural fluid eosinophilia is unusual and pneumothorax can cause a marked eosinophilic reaction in the presence of co-existing tuberculosis. Thus eosinophilia is quite non-specific and of little diagnostic value.

Rheumatoid arthritis (RA) cells may be seen in rheumatoid pleural effusions, but are nonspecific (Boddington, 1971).

LE cells are uncommon, but considered specific when present (Osamura, 1977).

Echinococcosis involving the pleural space may be diagnosed by toluidine blue-stained wet films; the scolices also may be identified on Papanicolaou or Wright's stain (Jacobson, 1973).

PERICARDIAL FLUID

Microscopic findings in tuberculous pericarditis are similar to those in pleural fluid, with a predominance of lymphocytes (Spriggs, 1968).

Increased leukocytes (over $1000/\mu l$) with a predominance of neutrophils are characteristic of bacterial pericarditis but may also be seen in viral pericarditis or postmyocardial infarction syndrome (Soloff, 1971).

Eosinophilia of pericardial fluid is rare: in 1968 Spriggs found no cases either in the literature or in his own experience.

LE cells have been described in pericardial fluid (Seaman, 1952), but this finding is unusual.

Amebic pericarditis has been described; however, the diagnosis is more likely to be made by serologic studies than by microscopic examination of pericardial fluid.

PERITONEAL FLUID

For lavage fluid, an erythrocyte count of over $100,000/\mu l$ in lavage fluid is considered "positive," consistent with over 20 to 25 μl whole blood in the peritoneal cavity. Counts in the 50,000 to 100,000 range are considered "borderline." Combined with a history of abdominal trauma, an elevated erythrocyte count may be an indication for celiotomy (Olsen, 1972; Engrav, 1975).

A leukocyte count of over $500/\mu l$ in lavage fluid is considered abnormal, but is not in itself diagnostic for peritonitis (Perry, 1972; Engrav, 1975; Parvin, 1975; Jergens, 1977).

For undiluted ascitic fluid, a leukocyte count of over $300/\mu l$ in undiluted sterile ascitic fluid is considered "abnormal" (Kline, 1976). Higher counts are seen in over 90 per cent of patients with spontaneous bacterial peritonitis, which may develop either from passage of bacteria from blood into ascitic fluid or from passage of bacteria through the bowel wall. However, about 50 per cent of cirrhotic patients with sterile ascitic fluid may have ascitic fluid leukocyte counts of over $300/\mu l$ (Kline, 1976). Although an ascitic fluid leukocyte count of over $300/\mu l$ has about 90 per cent sensitivity for spontaneous bacterial peritonitis, if we consider peritoneal transudates due to cirrhosis, specificity is only about 50 per cent. If $500/\mu l$ is used as a cut-off level, specificity is increased with a slight loss in sensi-

tivity (Kline, 1976).

A differential count with over 25 per cent neutrophils is considered increased for ascitic fluid. Higher percentages are seen in over 90 per cent of patients with spontaneous bacterial peritonitis (SBP); however, about 50 per cent of cirrhotic patients with sterile ascites due to cirrhosis also have over 25 per cent neutrophils. If 50 per cent is used as a cut-off level, specificity is increased with a slight loss in sensitivity (Kline, 1976).

The *absolute* granulocyte count with a cut-off level of $250/\mu l$ may provide both sensitivity (about 90 per cent of patients with SBP) and specificity (about 90 per cent in patients with sterile ascites due to cirrhosis have an ascitic fluid absolute granulocyte count under $250/\mu l$) (Jones, 1977).

Conn (1976) concludes that: "When the clinical picture is compatible [with SBP] and the ascitic fluid contains more than 500 WBC's per cu mm,* more than half of which are PMN's, it is in the patient's best interest to begin antibiotic therapy."

A high percentage of lymphocytes should suggest the possibility of tuberculous peritonitis, but also may be seen in chylous ascites. In contrast to pleural fluid, numerous mesothelial cells can occur with tuberculous effusions in the peritoneal cavity.

Eosinophilic ascites is uncommon, but has been reported in association with congestive heart failure, hypereosinophilic syndrome, eosinophilic gastroenteritis, chronic peritoneal dialysis, abdominal lymphoma, ruptured hydatid cyst, atopy, and vasculitis (Adams, 1977).

LE cells have been reported in peritoneal fluid (Metzger, 1974), but this finding is rare.

Rarely, a syndrome of fever and ascites, without infection, may occur several weeks after surgery, caused by talc (from surgical gloves) introduced into the peritoneum. Diagnosis may be made by paracentesis and identification of doubly refractile talc granules on examination with polarized light (Warshaw, 1972).

Rarely, microfilariae may occur in ascitic fluid in the absence of local or systemic symptoms (Figueroa, 1973).

MICROBIOLOGIC EXAMINATION

Acid-fast stain and culture are positive in only about 25 to 50 per cent of tuberculous

---

*1 mm^3 = 1 μl.

effusions. This incidence may be increased by special techniques which utilize the sediment from 100 to 500 ml of centrifuged fluid. With the addition of culture and histologic study on biopsy specimens, positive results may be obtained on 90 to 95 per cent of all cases (Levine, 1970).

CHEMICAL EXAMINATION

Normal glucose concentration in pleural, pericardial, and peritoneal fluid is approximately equal to whole blood glucose. Changes in blood glucose are reflected in these fluids after lag periods of two to four hours. Thus, systemic hypoglycemia or hyperglycemia may be associated with "false low" or "false high" results, respectively.

PLEURAL FLUID

Glucose under 60 mg/dl, or 40 mg/dl less than plasma glucose, is considered decreased (Light, 1973). Less than 1 per cent of transudates have decreased glucose, while about half of tuberculous effusions, about 10 per cent of neoplastic and septic effusions, and about 80 per cent of rheumatoid effusions are associated with decreased pleural fluid glucose (Light, 1973). Glucose measurements may be helpful in differential diagnosis of rheumatoid effusion vs. systemic lupus erythematosus, since in the latter condition, pleural fluid glucose usually is above 60 mg/dl (Carr, 1970).

Amylase activity is considered elevated in pleural effusions when this exceeds the upper limit of normal for serum or the amylase activity in a simultaneously obtained serum sample. Amylase activity is almost always elevated in pleural effusion associated with pancreatitis. Since pleural effusions are present in about 10 per cent of patients with pancreatitis (Light, 1973), amylase measurements can be helpful in differential diagnosis.

Elevated amylase also is characteristic of effusions associated with esophageal perforation: in these cases the amylase is of salivary origin (Light, 1973).

About 10 per cent of neoplastic effusions, and a smaller percentage of parapneumonic effusions, also may be associated with elevated pleural fluid amylase (Light, 1973).

Measurements of pH have been suggested as an aid in diagnosis of esophageal rupture (Dye, 1974). A pleural fluid pH under 6 is highly suggestive of esophageal rupture.

pH measurements also have been used to guide diagnosis and treatment of pleural effusions (Light, 1973; Potts, 1976). Perhaps 50 per cent of empyemas, loculated effusions, and tuberculous effusions have a pH under 7.30. In parapneumonic effusions with pH under 7.20, intercostal tube drainage usually is needed in addition to antibiotic therapy (Light, 1973).

Hyaluronate measurements in pleural fluid occasionally are helpful in diagnosis of pleural mesothelioma (Hellstrom, 1977).

PERICARDIAL FLUID

Glucose in pericardial fluid may be decreased in bacterial pericarditis, as well as in non-septic inflammation due to rheumatoid disease or malignancy.

PERITONEAL FLUID

Glucose levels in ascitic fluid may be reduced below 60 mg/dl in about 30 to 50 per cent of patients with tuberculous peritonitis (Brown, 1976), as well as in peritoneal carcinomatosis.

Amylase activity in peritoneal fluid is elevated above normal blood levels in about 90 per cent of patients with acute pancreatitis, pancreatic trauma, or pancreatic pseudocyst. Elevated peritoneal fluid amylase also may occur with intestinal strangulation or necrosis (Mansberger, 1964).

Ammonia levels in peritoneal fluid are markedly increased (two times the upper limit of normal for plasma) with perforated peptic ulcer, perforated appendix, or strangulation (with or without perforation) of small or large bowel (Mansberger, 1964). However, peritoneal fluid ammonia is normal in association with pancreatitis. Elevation in both ammonia and creatinine is characteristic of ruptured bladder with urinary extravasation (Mansberger, 1964).

Alkaline phosphatase activity in peritoneal fluid is markedly increased (over two times normal serum levels) in about 90 per cent of patients with strangulation or perforation of the small intestine (Lee, 1969; Delany, 1976). This elevation appears after about 2 to 3 hours and progressively increases during the next 3 to 4 hours (Rush, 1972). Although other enzymes in peritoneal fluid also increase following injury to the small intestine, these are less specific than alkaline phosphatase measurements.

Measurement of pH in peritoneal fluid has

little value in diagnosis of perforated peptic ulcer (Howard, 1963) and is not widely used at this time.

OTHER MEASUREMENTS AND EXAMINATIONS

Counterimmunoelectrophoresis for bacterial antigens has been used for detection and identification of bacteria in effusion fluids. However, this technique is not yet generally accepted as a "routine" procedure.

Limulus lysate assays have been used for diagnosis of effusions due to gram-negative organisms. Additional studies are needed to confirm the clinical value of this method.

Lysozyme measurements have been suggested as an aid in diagnosis of tuberculous effusions (Klockars, 1976). The transformation of monocytes into macrophages and epithelioid cells is accompanied by a corresponding increase in lysosomal enzymes, including lysozyme. However, the clinical value of this procedure is not yet established.

Cytologic examination for carcinoma is a highly accurate method for detection and diagnosis of malignant effusions. Sensitivity and specificity are in the range of 90 per cent.

REFERENCES

Cerebrospinal Fluid

Alexander, E.: Lumbar puncture. J.A.M.A. *201*:100, 1967.

Aspock, H.: Die Laboratoriumsdiagnostile der Amobeninfectioness des Menschen. Wien. Klin. Wochenschr., *89*:37, 1977.

Azimi, P. H., Shaban, S., Hilty, M.D., and Haynes, R. E.: Mumps meningoencephalitis. J.A.M.A. *234*:1161, 1975.

Beaty, H. N., and Oppenheimer, S.: Cerebrospinal fluid lactic dehydrogenase and its isoenzymes in infections of the central nervous system. N. Engl. J. Med., *279*:1197, 1968.

Berman, N. S., Siegel, S. E., Nachum, R., Lipsey, A., and Leedom, J.: Cerebrospinal fluid endotoxin concentrations in gram-negative bacterial meningitis. J. Pediatr., *88*:533, 1976.

Bland, R. D., Lister, R. C., and Ries, J. P.: Cerebrospinal fluid lactic acid level and pH in meningitis. Am. J. Dis. Child., *128*:151, 1974.

Bock, E.: Quantitation of plasma proteins in cerebrospinal fluid. *In* Axelsen, N. H., Kroll, J., and Wecke, B. (eds.): A Manual of Quantitative Immunoelectrophoresis. Oslo, Universitetsforlager, 1975, Chap. 14.

Bradbury, M. W. B., Stubbs, J., Hughes, I. E., and Parker, P.: The distribution of potassium, sodium, chloride and urea between lumbar cerebrospinal fluid and blood serum in normal human subjects. Clin. Sci., *25*:97, 1963.

Brooks, B. R.: Cerebrospinal fluid acid-base and lactate changes after seizures in unanesthetized man. Neurology, *25*:935, 1975.

Burechailo, F., and Cunningham, T. A.: Counting cells in cerebrospinal fluid collected directly on membrane filters. J. Clin. Pathol., *27*:101, 1974.

Burgi, W., Richterich, R., and Briner, M.: UV-photometric determination of total cerebrospinal fluid proteins with modified biuret reagent. Clin. Chim. Acta, *15*:181, 1967.

Butler, W. T., Alling, D. W., and Spickard, A.: Diagnostic and prognostic value of clinical and laboratory findings in cryptococcal meningitis. N. Engl. J. Med., *270*:59, 1964.

Calabrese, V. P.: The interpretation of routine CSF tests. Vir. Med. Month., *103*:207, 1976.

Campbell, R. A.: Lumbar puncture in the frail infant. J.A.M.A., *204*:180, 1968.

Carpenter, R. R., and Petersdorf, R. G.: The clinical spectrum of bacterial meningitis. Am. J. Med., *33*:262, 1962.

Castleberry, R. P., Moreno, H., and Wallace, L. S.: Cyto-logic analysis of cerebrospinal fluid. J. Pediatr., *86*:990, 1975.

Cawley, L. P., Minard B. J., Tourtellotte, W. W., Ma, B. I., and Chelle, C.: Immunofixation electrophoretic techniques applied to identification of proteins in serum and cerebrospinal fluid. Clin. Chem., *22*:1262, 1976.

Chen, J. H.: Measurement of gonadotropin in cerebrospinal fluid. N. Engl. J. Med., *297*:114, 1977.

Chu, J. Y., Freiling, P., and Wassilak, S.: Simple method for the cytological examination of cerebrospinal fluid. J. Clin. Pathol., *30*:486, 1977.

Coe, J. I.: Postmortem chemistry of blood, cerebrospinal fluid and vitreous humor. *In* Wecht, C. H. (ed.): Legal Medicine Annual 1976. New York, Appleton-Century-Crofts, 1976.

Cohen, S. R., Herndon, R. M., and McKann, G. M.: Radioimmunoassay of myelin basic protein in spinal fluid. N. Engl. J. Med., *295*:1455, 1976.

Cold, G., Enevoldsen, E., and Malmros, R.: Ventricular fluid lactate, pyruvate, bicarbonate and pH in unconscious brain-injured patients subjected to controlled ventilation. Acta Neurol. Scand., *52*:187, 1975.

Cole, M.: Pitfalls in cerebrospinal fluid examination. Hosp. Pract., *4*:47, 1969.

Collins, G.: Personal communication, 1978.

Controni, G., Rodriquez, W. J., Hicks, J. M., Ficke, M., Ross, S., Friedman, G., and Kahn, W.: Cerebrospinal fluid lactic acid levels in meningitis. J. Pediatr., *91*:379, 1977.

Converse, G. M., Gwaltney, J. M., Strassburg, D. A., and Hendley, J. O.: Alteration of cerebrospinal fluid findings by partial treatment of bacterial meningitis. J. Pediatr., *83*:220, 1973.

Denis, F., Samb, A., and Chiron, J. P.: Bacterial meningitis diagnosis by counterimmunoelectrophoresis. J.A.M.A., *238*:1248, 1977.

Derakhshen, I., and Kaufman, B.: Subdural effusion of cerebrospinal fluid after lumbar puncture. Arch. Neurol., *29*:127, 1973.

Dramov, B., and Dubou, R.: Aseptic meningitis following intrathecal radioiodinated serum albumin. Cal. Med., *115*:64, 1971.

Dryken, P. R.: Cerebrospinal fluid cytology: Practical clinical usefulness. Neurology, *25*:210, 1975.

Dunn, J. S., and Wyburn, E. M.: The anatomy of the blood brain barrier: A review. Scot. Med. J., *17*:21, 1972.

Epstein, E., Zak, B., Baginski, E. J., and Civin, H.: Interpretation of cerebrospinal fluid proteins by gel electrophoresis. Ann. Clin. Lab. Sci., 6:27, 1976.

Escobar, M. R., Dalton, H. P., and Allison, M. J.: Fluorescent antibody tests using cerebrospinal fluid. Am. J. Clin. Pathol., 53:886, 1970.

Feldman, W. E.: Cerebrospinal fluid lactic acid dehydrogenase activity. Am. J. Dis. Child., 129:77, 1975.

Feldman, W. E.: Relation of concentrations of bacteria and bacterial antigen cerebrospinal fluid to prognosis in patients with bacterial meningitis. N. Engl. J. Med., 296:433, 1977.

Felgenhauer, K.: Protein size and cerebrospinal fluid composition. Klin. Wochenschr. 52:1158, 1974.

Fischer, G. W., Brens, R. W., Alden, E. R., and Beckwith, J. B.: Lumbar punctures and meningitis. Am. J. Dis. Child., 199:590, 1975.

Fishman, R. A.: Cerebrospinal fluid. In Boher, A. B., and Baher, L. H. (eds.): Clinical Neurology. New York, Harper and Row, Publishers, Inc., 1971.

Glasgow, A. M., and Dhiensiri, K.: Improved assay for spinal fluid glutamine, and values for children with Reye's syndrome. Clin. Chem., 20:642, 1974.

Glasser, L., Payne, C., and Corrigan, J. J.: The in vivo development of plasma cells: A morphologic study of human cerebrospinal fluid. Neurology, 27:448, 1977.

Gondos, B., and King, E. B.: Cerebrospinal fluid cytology: Diagnostic accuracy and comparison of different techniques. Acta Cytol., 20:542, 1976.

Gonyea, E. F.: Cisternal puncture and cryptococcal meningitis. Arch. Neurol., 28:200, 1973.

Gooch, W. M., and Sotelo-Avila, C.: Meningitis in children: Laboratory diagnosis. J. Tenn. Med. Assn., 69:563, 1976.

Greenblatt, S. H.: Cerebrospinal fluid creatine phosphokinase in acute subarachnoid hemorrhage. J. Neurosurg., 44:50, 1976.

Guseo, A.: Classification of cells in the cerebrospinal fluid. Eur. Neurol., 15:169, 1977.

Hagen, G. A., and Elliott, W. J.: Transport of thyroid hormones in serum and cerebrospinal fluid. J. Clin. Endocrinol. Metab., 37:415, 1973.

Hammock, M. K., and Milhorat, T. H.: The cerebrospinal fluid: Current concepts of its formation. Ann. Clin. Lab. Sci., 6:22, 1976.

Hansen, H. H., Bender, R. A., and Shelton, B. J.: The cyto-centrifuge and cerebrospinal fluid cytology. Acta Cytol., 18:259, 1974.

Harms, D.: Comparative quantitation of immunoglobulin G (IgG) in cerebrospinal fluid and serum of children. Eur. Neurol., 13:54, 1975.

Hecht, R. H., Cohen, A. H., Stoner, J., and Irwin, C.: Primary amebic meningoencephalitis in California. Cal. Med., 117:69, 1972.

Heintges, M. G., Savory, J., and Killingsworth, L. M.: A micro-immunochemical procedure for the measurement of total protein in cerebrospinal fluid. Ann. Clin. Lab. Sci., 3:265, 1973.

Hinterbuchner, L. P.: Hazards of lumbar puncture in infants. J.A.M.A., 204:196, 1968.

Hochwald, G. M., Wallenstein, M. C., and Mathews, E. S.: Exchange of proteins between blood and spinal subarachnoid fluid. Am. J. Physiol., 217:348, 169.

Hooshmand, H., Escobar, M. R., and Kopf, W. C.: Neurosyphilis. J.A.M.A., 219:726, 1972.

Hourain, B. T., Hamlin, E. M., and Reynolds, T. B.: Cerebrospinal fluid glutamine as a measure of hepatic encephalopathy. Arch. Intern. Med., 127:1033, 1971.

Hull, H. F., and Morrow, G.: Glucorrhea revisited. J.A.M.A., 234:1052, 1975.

Hyslop, N. E., and Swartz, M. N.: Bacterial meningitis. Postgrad. Med., 58:120, 1975.

Igou, P. C.: An evaluation of a gel filtration-spectrophoto-metric method for spinal fluid protein. Am. J. Med. Tech., 33:354, 1967.

Ito, U., and Inaba, Y.: A simple sedimentation chamber adaptable to the laboratory centrifuge. Am. J. Clin. Pathol., 58:590, 1972.

Ivers, R. R., McKenzie, B. F., McGuckin, W. F., and Goldstein, N. P.: Spinal-fluid gamma globulin in multiple sclerosis and other neurologic diseases. J.A.M.A., 176:515, 1961.

Iwashita, H., Bauer, H., and Kuroiwa, Y.: Comparative studies of cerebrospinal fluid proteins of multiple sclerosis patients in Japan and Germany. Neurology, 26:37, 1976.

Jaffe, H. W.: The laboratory diagnosis of syphilis. Ann. Intern. Med., 83:846, 1975.

Jaiken, A., and Agrest, A.: Cerebrospinal fluid glutamine concentration in patients with chronic hypercapnea. Clin. Sci., 36:11, 1969.

Jakupcevic, M., Lackovic, Z., Stefoski, D., and Bulat, M.: Nonhomogenous distribution of 5-hydroxyindoleacetic acid and homovanillic acid in the lumbar cerebrospinal fluid. J. Neurol. Sci., 31:165, 1977.

Jameson, B., and Wells, D. G.: Cytologic diagnosis of cryptococcal meningitis. N. Engl. J. Med., 286:1267, 1972.

Jequier, M., and Dufrensue, J. J.: Diagnosis of cryptococcal meningitis. N. Engl. J. Med., 286:785, 1972.

John, J. F., and Cuetter, A. C.: Spinal syphilis: The problem of fluorescent treponemal antibody in the cerebrospinal fluid. South. Med. J., 70:309, 1977.

Johnson, K. P., Arrigo, S. C., and Nelson, B. J.: Agarose electrophoresis of cerebrospinal fluid in multiple sclerosis. Neurology, 27:273, 1977a.

Johnson, K. P., and Nelson, B. J.: Multiple sclerosis: Diagnostic usefulness of the cerebrospinal fluid. Ann. Neurol. 2:425, 1977b.

Jordan, R. M., Kendall, J. W., Seaich, L. J., Allen, J. P., Paulsen, C. A., Kerber, C. W., and Vanderlaan, W. P.: Cerebrospinal fluid hormone concentration in the evaluation of pituitary tumors. Ann. Intern. Med., 85:49, 1976.

Kalin, E. M., Tweed, W. A., Lee, J., and MacKeen, W. L.: Cerebrospinal-fluid acid-base and electrolyte changes resulting from cerebral anemia in man. N. Engl. J. Med., 293:1013, 1975.

Kaplan, A.: Electrophoresis of cerebrospinal fluid proteins. Am. J. Med. Sci., 253:549, 1967.

Kaufman, L.: Serodiagnosis of fungal diseases. In Rose, N. R., and Friedman, H. (eds.): Manual of Clinical Immunology. Washington, D.C., American Society for Microbiology, 1976.

Kjellin, K. G., and Soderstrom, C. E.: Diagnostic significance of CSF spectrophotometry in cerebrovascular diseases. J. Neurol. Sci., 23:359, 1974.

Kluge, H., Winkler, G., and Wieczorek, V.: Results of the comparison of different methods of total protein in CSF. Dtsch. Gesundh., 23:2039, 1968.

Kolmel, H. W.: Atlas of Cerebrospinal Fluid Cells. New York, Springer-Verlag, 1977.

Krentz, M. J., and Dyken, P. R.: Cerebrospinal fluid cytomorphology: Sedimentation vs filtration. Arch. Neurol., 26:253, 1972.

Kronholm, V., and Lintrup, J.: Spectrophotometric investigations of the cerebrospinal fluid in the near ultraviolet region. Acta Psychiatr. Neurol. Scand., 35:314, 1960.

Levy, N. L., Auerbach, P. S., and Hayes, E. C.: A blood test for multiple sclerosis based on the adherence of lymphocytes to measles-infected cells. N. Engl. J. Med., 294:1423, 1976.

Link, H.: Demonstration of oligoclonal immunoglobulin G

in Guillain-Barré syndrome. Acta Neurol. Scand., 52:111, 1975.

Link, H., and Miller, R.: Immunoglobulins in multiple sclerosis and infections of the nervous system. Arch. Neurol., 25:326, 1971.

Marshall, J.: Lumbar puncture. Br. J. Hosp. Med., 3:216, 1970.

McCracken, G. H.: Rapid identification of specific etiology in meningitis. J. Pediatr., 88:706, 1976a.

McCracken, G. H.: Neonatal septicemia and meningitis. Hosp. Pract., 11:89, 1976.

McCracken, G. H., and Kaplan, J. M.: Penicillin treatment for congenital syphilis. J.A.M.A., 228:855, 1974.

Mealey, J.: Fat emulsion as a cause of cloudy cerebrospinal fluid. J.A.M.A., 180:246, 1962.

Meites, S. (ed.): Pediatric Clinical Chemistry. Washington, D.C., American Association for Clinical Chemistry, 1977.

Messer, H. D., Forshan, V. R., Brust, J. C. M., and Hughes, J. E. O.: Transient paraplegia from hematoma after lumbar puncture. J.A.M.A., 235:529, 1976.

Miller, J. W., and Woolam, D. H. M.: The Anatomy of the Cerebrospinal Fluid. London, Oxford University Press, 1962.

Moir, A. T. B., Ashcroft, G. W., Crawford, T. B. B., Eccleston, D., and Guldberg, H. C.: Cerebral metabolites in cerebrospinal fluid as a biochemical approach to the brain. Brain, 93:357, 1970.

Morrison, J. C., Whybrew, D. W., Wiser, W. L., Bucovaz, E. T., and Fish, S. A.: Enzyme levels in the serum and cerebrospinal fluid in eclampsia. Am. J. Obstet. Gynecol., 110:619, 1971.

Mullan, D. P.: Studies in Clinical Enzymology. St. Louis, The C. V. Mosby Co., 1969.

Musher, D. M., and Schell, R. F.: False-positive gram stains of cerebrospinal fluid. Ann. Intern. Med., 79:603, 1973.

Nachum, R., Lippey, A., and Siegel, S.: Rapid detection of gram-negative bacterial meningitis by the limulus lysate test. N. Engl. J. Med., 289:931, 1973.

Nelson, P. U., Carey, W. F., and Pollard, A. C.: Diagnostic significance and source of lactate dehydrogenase and its isozymes in cerebrospinal fluid of children with a variety of neurological disorders. J. Clin. Pathol., 28:828, 1975.

Nosanchuk, J. S., and Kim, C. W.: Lupus erythematosus cells in CSF. J.A.M.A., 25:2883, 1976.

Oehmichen, M.: Characterization of mononuclear phagocytes in human CSF using membrane markers. Acta Cytol., 20:548, 1976.

Olsson, J. E., and Link, H.: Immunoglobulin abnormalities in multiple sclerosis. Arch. Neurol., 28:392, 1973.

Olsson, J. E., and Pettersson, B.: A comparison between agar gel electrophoresis and CSF serum quotients of IgG and albumin in neurological diseases. Acta Neurol. Scand., 53:308, 1976.

Palmer, D. L., Minard, B. J., and Cawley, L. P.: IgG subgroups in cerebrospinal fluid in multiple sclerosis. N. Engl. J. Med., 294:447, 1976.

Patten, B. M.: How much blood makes the cerebrospinal fluid bloody? J.A.M.A., 206:378, 1968.

Pennock, C. A., Passant, L. P., and Balton, F. G.: Estimation of cerebrospinal fluid protein. J. Clin. Pathol., 21:518, 1968.

Plum, F., and Price, R. W.: Acid-base balance of cisternal and lumbar cerebrospinal fluid in hospital patients. N. Engl. J. Med., 289:1346, 1973.

Plum, F., and Siesjo, B. K.: Recent advances in CSF physiology. Anesthesiology, 42:708, 1975.

Pryce, J. D., Gant, P. W., and Saul, K. J.: Normal concen-

trations of lactate, glucose, and protein in cerebrospinal fluid, and the diagnostic implications of abnormal concentrations. Clin. Chem., 16:562, 1970.

Rodriguez, E. M.: The cerebrospinal fluid as a pathway in neuroendocrine integration. J. Endocrinol., 71:407, 1976.

Ross, S., Rodriguez, W., Controni, G., Korengold, G., Watson, S., and Kahn, W.: Limulus lysate test for gram-negative bacterial meningitis. J.A.M.A., 233:1366, 1975.

Saigo, P., Rosen, P. P., Kaplan, N. H., Solan, G. and Melamed, M. R.: Identification of *Cryptococcus neoformans* in cytologic preparations of cerebrospinal fluid. Am. J. Clin. Pathol., 67:141, 1977.

Salo, E. J., and Honkavaara, E. L.: A linear single reagent method for determination of protein in cerebrospinal fluid. Scand. J. Clin. Lab. Invest., 34:283, 1974.

Sambrook, M. A.: The concentration of cerebrospinal fluid potassium during systemic disturbances of acid-base metabolism. J. Clin. Pathol., 28:418, 1975.

Sarff, L. D., Platt, L. H., and McCracken, G. H.: Cerebrospinal fluid evaluation in neonates: Comparison of high-risk infants with and without meningitis. J. Pediatr., 88:473, 1976.

Schaub, C., Bluet-Pajut, M. T., Szikla, G., Lornet, C., and Talairach, J.: Distribution of growth hormone and thyroid-stimulating hormone in cerebrospinal fluid and pathological compartments of the central nervous system. J. Neurol. Sci., 31:123, 1977.

Schlesinger, J. J., and Ross, A. L.: *Propionibacterium acnes* meningitis in a previously normal adult. Arch. Intern. Med., 137:921, 1977.

Shaywitz, B. A.: Epidermoid spinal cord tumors and previous lumbar punctures. J. Pediatr., 80:638, 1972.

Sheth, K. V.: Cerebrospinal and body fluids cell morphology. ASCP Workshop Manual. Chicago, American Society of Clinical Pathologists, 1977.

Shriever, H., and Gambino, S. R.: Protein turbidity produced by trichloracetic acid and sulfosalicylic acid at varying temperatures and varying ratios of albumin and globulin. Am. J. Clin. Pathol., 44:667, 1965.

Siemkowicz, E., Christiansen, I., and Sorsen, S. C.: Changes in cisternal fluid potassium following cardiac arrest. Acta Neurol. Scand., 55:137, 1977.

Siesjo, B. K.: The regulation of cerebrospinal fluid pH. Kidney Internat., 1:360, 1972.

Skeel, R. T., Yankee, R. A., and Henderson, E. S.: Meningeal leukemia. J.A.M.A., 205:155, 1968.

Smith, A. L.: Diagnosis of bacterial meningitis. Pediatrics, 52:589, 1973.

Smith, D. H.: The challenge of bacterial meningitis. Hosp. Pract., 11:71, 1976.

Sornas, R.: The cytology of the normal cerebrospinal fluid. Acta Neurol. Scand., 48:313, 1972.

Sornas, R.: A new method for the cytological examination of cerebrospinal fluid. J. Nuerol. Neurosurg. Psychiatr., 30:568, 1967.

Sornas, R.: Transformation of mononuclear cells in cerebrospinal fluid. Acta Cytol., 15:545, 1971.

Spriggs, A. L., and Boddington, M. M.: The Cytology of Effusions and of Cerebrospinal Fluid. London, Heinemann, 1968.

Swartz, M. N., and Dodge, P. R.: Bacterial meningitis—a review of selected aspects. N. Engl. J. Med., 272:725, 1965.

Thompson, E. J.: Laboratory diagnosis of multiple sclerosis: Immunological and biochemical aspects. Br. Med. Bull., 33:28, 1977.

Tibbling, G., Link, H., and Ohman, S.: Principles of albumin and IgG analyses in neurological disorders. Scand. J. Clin. Lab. Invest., 37:385, 1977.

Tourtellotte, W. W., Haerer, A. F., Fleming, J. O., Murthy,

K. N., Levy, J., and Brandes, D. W.: Cerebrospinal fluid (CSF) immunoglobulins-G (IgG) of extravascular origin in normals and patients with multiple sclerosis (MS): Clinical correlation. Trans. Am. Neurol. Assoc., 100:250, 1975.

Van Der Meulen, J. P.: Cerebrospinal fluid xanthochromia: An objective index. Neurology, 16:170, 1966.

Van Welsum, R. A., and Van der Helm, H. J.: The protein composition of the cerebrospinal fluid in acute necrotizing encephalitis. Neurology, 20:996, 1970.

Vandvik, B., Natvig, J. B., and Wiger, D.: IgG 1 subclass restriction of oligoclonal IgG from cerebrospinal fluids and brain extracts in patients with multiple sclerosis and subacute encephalitis. Scand. J. Immunol., 5:427, 1976.

Walton, J. N.: Subarachnoid Haemorrhage. Edinburgh, Livingstone, 1956.

Weinstein, R. A., Bauer, F. W., Hoffman, R. D., Tyler, P. G., Anderson, R. L., and Stamm, W. E.: Factitious meningitis. J.A.M.A., 233:878, 1975.

Werner, M.: A combined procedure for protein estimation and electrophoresis of cerebrospinal fluid. J. Lab. Clin. Med., 74:166, 1969.

Wichser, J., and Kazemi, H.: CSF bicarbonate regulation in respiratory acidosis and alkalosis. J. Appl. Physiol. 38:504, 1975.

Windisch, R. M., and Bracken, M. M.: Cerebrospinal fluid proteins: Concentration by membrane ultrafiltration and fractionation by electrophoresis on cellulose acetate. Clin. Chem., 16:416, 1970.

Wolf, S. M.: Decreased cerebrospinal fluid glucose in herpes zoster meningitis. Arch. Neurol., 30:109, 1974.

Woodbury, J., Lyons, K., Carretta, R., Hahn, A., and Sullivan, J. F.: Cerebrospinal fluid and serum levels of magnesium, zinc and calcium in man. Neurology, 18:700, 1968.

Woodruff, K. H.: Cerebrospinal fluid cytomorphology using cytocentrifugation. Am. J. Clin. Pathol., 60:621, 1973.

Synovial fluid

Abeles, M., and Urman, J. D.: Acute gouty arthritis: The importance of aspirating more than one involved joint. J.A.M.A., 238:2526, 1977.

Bartlett, R. C., et al.: *In* Inhorn, S. L. (ed.): Quality Assurance Practices for Health Laboratories. Washington, D.C., American Public Health Association, 1978.

Bayer, A. S., Chow, A. W., Louie, J. S., and Guze, L. B.: Sternoarticular pyoarthrosis due to gram-negative bacilli. Arch. Intern. Med., 137:1036, 1977.

Binette, J. P., and Schmid, K.: The proteins of synovial fluid: A study of α_1/α_2 globulin ratio. Arth. Rheum. 8:14, 1965.

Blau, S. P.: Leukocyte counts in synovial fluid. Ann. Intern. Med., 74:638, 1971.

Brandt, K. D., Cathcart, E. S., and Cohen, A. S.: Gonococcal arthritis. Arth. Rheum., 17:503, 1974.

Broderick, P. A., Corvese, N., Pierik, M. G., Pike, R. F., and Mariorenzi, A. L.: Exfoliative cytology interpretation of synovial fluid in joint disease. J. Bone Joint Surg., 58A:396, 1976.

Bunch, T. W., Hunder, G. G., McDuffie, F. C., O'Brien, P. C., and Markowitz, H.: Synovial fluid complement determinations as a diagnostic aid in inflammatory joint disease. Mayo Clin. Proc., 49:715, 1974.

Bunch, T. W., Hunder, G. G., Offord, K., and McDuffie, F. C.: Synovial fluid complement: Usefulness in diagnosis and classification of rheumatoid arthritis. Ann. Intern. Med., 81:32, 1974.

Cohen, A. S., Brandt, K. D., and Krey, P. R.: Synovial fluid. In Cohen, A. S. (ed.): Laboratory Diagnostic Procedures in the Rheumatic Diseases. Boston, Little, Brown & Co., 1975.

Cooke, C. L., Owen, D. S., Irby, R., and Toone, E.: Gonoccal arthritis. J.A.M.A., 217:204, 1971.

Cracchiolo, A.: Joint fluid analysis. Am. Fam. Physician, 4:87, 1971.

Cracchiolo, A., and Barnett, E. V.: The role of immunological tests in routine synovial fluid analysis. J. Bone Joint Surg., 54:828, 1972.

Currey, H. L. F., and Vernon-Roberts, B.: Examination of synovial fluid. Clin. Rheum. Dis., 2:149, 1976.

Donaldson, L. E. E.: Technique for performing white cell counts in joint fluids. Med. Lab. Technol., 29:1, 1972.

Edelen, J. S., Lockshin, M. D., and LeRoy, E. L.: Gonococcal arthritis in two patients with active lupus erythematosus. Arth. Rheum., 14:557, 1971.

Fagan, T. J., and Lidsky, M. D.: Compensated polarized light microscopy using cellophane adhesive tape. Arth. Rheum., 17:256, 1974.

Falchuk, K. H., Goetzl, E. J., and Kulka, J. P.: Respiratory gases of synovial fluids. Am. J. Med., 49:223, 1970.

Frischknecht, J., and Steigerwald, J. C.: High synovial fluid white blood cell counts in pseudogout. Arch. Intern. Med., 135:298, 1975.

Goldenberg, D. L., Brandt, K. D., and Cohen, A. S.: Rapid, simple detection of trace amounts of synovial fluid. Arth. Rheum., 16:487, 1973.

Haselwood, D. M., and Castles, J. J.: The biology of the rheumatoid synovial cell. Western J. Med., 127:204, 1977.

Hasselbacher, P.: Measuring synovial fluid viscosity with a white blood cell diluting pipette. Arth. Rheum., 19:1358, 1976.

Hollander, J. L., McCarty, D. J., Astorga, G., and Castro-Murillo, E.: Studies on the pathogenesis of rheumatoid joint inflammation. Ann. Intern. Med., 62:271, 1965.

Hollander, J. L., Reginato, A., and Torralba, T. P.: Examination of synovial fluid as a diagnostic aid in arthritis. Med., Clin. North Am., 50:1281, 1966.

Hunder, G. G., and Pierre, R. U.: In vivo LE cell formation in synovial fluid. Arth. Rheum., 13:448, 1970.

Huskisson, E. C., Hart, F. D., and Lacy, B. W.: Synovial fluid Waaler-Rose and latex tests. Ann. Rheum. Dis., 30:67, 1971.

Jackson, W. P. U., and Harris, F.: Gout with hyperparathyroidism. Br. Med. J., 2:211, 1965.

Jessar, R. A.: The study of synovial fluid. In Hollander, J. L., and McCarty, D. J. (eds.): Arthritis and Allied Conditions. Philadelphia, Lea and Febiger, 1972.

Kahn, C. B., Hollander, J. L., and Schumacher, H. R.: Corticosteroid crystals in synovial fluid. J.A.M.A., 211:807, 1970.

Kitridou, R., McCarty, D. J., Prockop, D. J., and Hummeler, K.: Identification of collagen in synovial fluid. Arth. Rheum., 12:580, 1969.

Krauss, D. S., Aronson, M. D., Gump, D. W., and Newcombe, D. S.: Hemophilus influenzae septic arthritis. Arth. Rheum., 17:261, 1974.

Kushner, I., and Somerville, J. A.: Permeability of human synovial membrane to plasma proteins. Arth. Rheum., 14:560, 1971.

Lund-Olesen, K.: Oxygen tension in synovial fluids. Arth. Rheum., 13:769, 1970.

McCarty, D. J.: Selected aspects of synovial membrane physiology. Arth. Rheum., 17:289, 1974.

McCarty, D. J., Gatter, R. A., Brill, J. M., and Hogan, J. M.: Crystal deposition diseases. J.A.M.A., 193:123, 1965.

McCarty, D. J., and Hollander, J. L.: Identification of

urate crystals in gouty synovial fluid. Ann. Intern. Med., *54*:452, 1961.

McConville, J. H., Pototsky, R. S., Calia, F. M., and Pachas, W. N.: Septic and crystalline joint disease. J.A.M.A., *231*:841, 1975.

McCord, W. C., Nies, K. M., and Louie, J. S.: Acute venereal arthritis. Arch Intern. Med., *137*:858, 1977.

Meyers, O. L., and Watermeyer, G. S.: Cholesterol-rich synovial effusions. South Afr. Med. J., *50*:973, 1976.

Naib, Z. M.: Cytology of synovial fluids. Acta Cytol., *17*:299, 1973.

Nye, W. H. R., Terry, R., and Rosenbaum, D. L.: Two forms of crystalline lipid in "cholesterol" effusions. Am. J. Clin. Pathol., *49*:718, 1968.

Owen, D. S., Cooke, C. L., and Toone, E.: Practical synovial fluid examination. Va. Med. Mon., *97*:88, 1970.

Owen, D. S., Toone, E., and Irby, R.: Coexistent rheumatoid arthritis and chronic tophaceous gout. J.A.M.A., *197*:123, 1966.

Pekin, T. J., Malinin, T. I., and Zvaifler, N. J.: Unusual synovial fluid findings in Reiter's syndrome. Ann. Intern. Med., *66*:677, 1967.

Phelps, P., Steele, A. D., and McCarty, D. J.: Compensated polarized light microscopy. J.A.M.A., *203*:166, 1968.

Ropes, M. W., and Bauer, W.: Synovial Fluid Changes in Joint Disease. Cambridge, Harvard University Press, 1953.

Ruddy, S., and Austen, K. F.: Complement and its components. *In* Cohen, A. S. (ed.): Laboratory Diagnostic Procedures in the the Rheumatic Diseases. Boston, Little, Brown & Co., 1975.

Ryan, W. E., Ellefson, R. D., and Ward, L. E.: Lipid synovial effusion. Arth. Rheum., *16*:759, 1973.

Schumacher, H. R., Jimenez, S. A., Gibson, T., Paseual, E., Tragcoff, R., Dorwart, B. B., and Reginato, A. J.: Acute gouty arthritis without urate crystals identified on initial examination of synovial fluid. Arth. Rheum. *18*:608, 1975.

Schumacher, H. R., Smolyo, A. P., Tse, R. L., and Maurer, K.: Arthritis associated with apatite crystals. Ann. Intern. Med., *87*:411, 1977.

Scott, J. T.: The analysis of joint fluids. Br. J. Hosp. Med., *14*:653, 1975.

Skinner, M., and Cohen, A. S.: Calcium pyrophosphate dihydrate crystal deposition disease. Arch. Intern. Med., *123*:636, 1969.

Smith, J. R., and Phelps, P.: Septic arthritis, gout, pseudogout and osteoarthritis in the knee of a patient with multiple myeloma. Arth. Rheum., *15*:89, 1972.

Traycoff, R. B., Pascual, E., and Schumacher, H. R.: Mononuclear cells in human synovial fluid: Identification of lymphoblasts in rheumatoid arthritis. Arth. Rheum., *19*:743, 1976.

Van Leeuwen, A. W. F. M., Meyer, C. J. L. M., Van de Putte, L. B. A., de Vries, E., and de Man, J. C. H.: Sezary type cells in rheumatoid synovial fluid. Lancet, *1*:248, 1976.

Wallace, R., and Cohen, A. S.: Tuberculous arthritis. Am. J. Med., *61*:277, 1976.

Waxman, J.: Immunology in rheumatology—1975. J. Louisiana State Med. Soc., *127*:203, 1975.

Wild, J. H., and Zvaifler, N. J.: An office technique for identifying crystals in synovial fluid. Am. Fam. Physician, *12*:72, 1975.

Pleural, pericardial, and peritoneal fluid

Adams, H. W., and Mainz, D. L.: Eosinophilic ascites. Am. J. Digest. Dis., *22*:40, 1977.

Askin, F. B., McCann, B. G., and Kuhn, C.: Reactive eosinophilic pleuritis. Arch. Pathol. Lab. Med., *101*:187, 1977.

Ball, W. C., Jr.: Pleural effusion. *In* Harvey A. M., Johns R. J., Owens A. H., Ross R. S.: The Principles and Practice of Medicine, 18th ed. New York, Appleton-Century-Crofts, 1976, p. 455.

Berger, H. W., Rammohan, G., Neff, M. S., and Buhain, W. J.: Uremic pleural effusion Ann. Intern. Med., *82*:362, 1975.

Boddington, M. M., Spriggs, A. I., Morton, J. A., and Mowat, A. G.: Cytodiagnosis of rheumatoid pleural effusions. J. Clin. Pathol., *24*:95, 1971.

Brown, J. D., and An, N. D.: Tuberculous peritonitis. Am. J. Gastroenterol., *66*:277, 1976.

Carr, D. T., Lillington, G. A., and Mayne, J. G.: Pleural fluid glucose in systemic lupus erythematosus. Mayo Clin. Proc., *45*:409, 1970.

Conn, H. O.: Spontaneous bacterial peritonitis. Gastroenterology, *70*:455, 1976.

Delany, H. M., Moss., C. M., and Carnevale, N.: The use of enzyme analysis of peritoneal blood in the clinical assessment of abdominal organ injury. Surg. Gynecol. Obstet., *142*:161, 1976.

Diamonon, J. S., and Barnes, J. P.: Choleperitoneum. Am. Surg., *30*:331, 1964.

Dye, R. A., and Laforet, E. G.: Esophageal rupture: Diagnosis by pleural fluid pH. Chest, *66*:454, 1974.

Engrav, L. H., Benjamin, C. I., Strate, R. G., and Perry, J. F.: Diagnostic peritoneal lavage in blunt abdominal trauma. J. Trauma, *15*:854, 1975.

Fiqueroa, J. M.: Presence of microfilariae of *Mansonella ozzardi* in ascitic fluid. Acta Cytol., *17*:73, 1973.

Hellstrom, P. E., Friman, C., and Teppo, L.: Malignant mesothelioma of 17 years duration with high pleural fluid concentration of hyaluronate. Scand. J. Resp. Dis., *58*:97, 1977.

Howard, J. M., and Singh, L. M.: Peritoneal fluid pH after perforation of peptic ulcers. Arch. Surg., *87*:483, 1963.

Hudspeth, A. S., and Miller, H. S.: Isolated (primary) chylopericardium. J. Thorac. Cardiovasc. Surg., *51*:528, 1966.

Jacobson, E. S.: A case of secondary echinococcosis diagnosed by cytologic examination of pleural fluid and needle biopsy of pleura. Acta Cytol., *17*:76, 1973.

Jergens, M. E.: Peritoneal lavage. Am. J. Surg., *133*:365, 1977.

Jones, S. R.: The absolute granulocyte count in ascitic fluid. West. J. Med., *126*:344, 1977.

Kilpatrick, Z. M., and Chapman, C. B: On pericardiocentesis. Am. J. Cardiol., *16*:722, 1965.

Klepser, R. G., and Berry, J. F.: The diagnosis and surgical management of chylothorax with the aid of lipophilic dyes. Dis. Chest, *25*:409, 1954.

Kline, M. M., McCallum, R. W., and Guth, P. H.: The clinical value of ascitic fluid culture and leukocyte count studies in alcoholic cirrhosis. Gastroenterology, *70*:408, 1976.

Klockars, M., Pettersson, T., Riska, H., and Hellstrom, P. E.: Pleural fluid lysozyme in tuberculous and nontuberculous pleurisy. Br. Med. J., *1*:1381, 1976.

Kumor, U. N., Varkey, B., and Mathai, G.: Post traumatic pleural fluid and blood eosinophilia. J.A.M.A., *234*:625, 1975.

Lee, Y. N.: Alkaline phosphatase in intestinal perforation. J.A.M.A., *208*:361, 1969.

Lesser, G. T., Bruno, M. S., and Enselberg, K.: Chylous ascites. Arch. Intern. Med., *125*:1073, 1970.

Levine, H., Metzger, W., Lacer, D., and Ludmillo, K.: Diagnosis of tuberculous pleurisy by culture of pleural biopsy specimen. Arch. Intern. Med., *126*:269, 1970.

Light, R. W., MacGregor, M. I., Luchsinger, P. C., and Ball, W. C.: Pleural effusions: The diagnostic separation of transudates and exudates. Ann. Intern. Med., 77:507, 1972.

Light, R. W., and Ball, W. C.: Glucose and amylase in pleural effusions. J.A.M.A., 225:257, 1973.

Light, R. W., Erozan, Y. S., and Ball, W. C.: Cells in pleural fluid: Their value in differential diagnosis. Arch. Intern. Med., 132:854, 1973.

Light, R. W., MacGregor, M. I., Ball, W. C., and Luchsinger, P. C.: Diagnostic significance of pleural fluid pH and PCO_2. Chest, 64:591, 1973.

Mansberger, A. R.: The diagnostic value of abdominal paracentesis with special reference to peritoneal fluid ammonia levels. Am. J. Gastorenterol., 42:150, 1964.

McClement, J. H.: Diseases of the pleura. In Beeson, P. B., and McDermott, W. (eds.): Textbook of Medicine, 14th ed., Philadelphia, W. B. Saunders Company, 1975.

McCoy, J., and Wolma, F. J.: Abdominal tap. Am. J. Surg., 122:693, 1971.

Metzger, A. L., Coyne, M., and Lee, S.: In vivo LE cell formation in peritonitis due to SLE. J. Rheumatol., 1:130, 1974.

Olsen, W. R., Redman, H. C., and Hildreth, D. H.: Quantitative peritoneal lavage in blunt abdominal trauma. Arch. Surg., 104:536, 1972.

Osamura, R. Y., Shioya, S., Handa, K., and Shimiza, K.: Lupus erythematosus cells in pleural fluid: Cytologic diagnosis in two patients. Acta Cytol., 21:215, 1977.

Parvin, S., Smith, D. E., Asher, W. M., and Virgilo, R. W.: Effectiveness of peritoneal lavage in blunt abdominal trauma. Ann. Surg., 181:255, 1975.

Perry, J. F., and Strate, R. G.: Diagnostic peritoneal lavage. Surgery, 71:898, 1972.

Potts, D. E.: Pleural fluid pH in parapneumonic effusions. Chest, 70:328, 1976.

Rush, B. F., Host, W. R., Fewel, J., and Hsieh, J.: Intestinal ischemia and some organic substances in serum and abdominal fluid. Arch. Surg., 105:151, 1972.

Sabiston, D. C., Jr.: Diseases of the pleura, mediastinum, and diaphragm. In Wintrobe, M. M., Thorn, G. W., Adams, R. D., Braunwald, E., Isselbacher, K. J., and Petersdorf, R. J.: Harrison's Principles of Internal Medicine, 7th ed. New York, McGraw-Hill Book Company, 1974, p. 1327.

Seaman, A. J., and Christerson, J. W.: Demonstration of LE cells in pericardial fluid. J.A.M.A., 149:145, 1952.

Seriff, N. S., Cohen, M. L., Samuel, P., and Schulster, P. L.: Chylothorax: Diagnosis by lipoprotein electrophoresis of serum and pleural fluid. Thorax, 32:98, 1977.

Soloff, L. A.: Pericardial cellular response during the post-myocardial infarction syndrome. Am. Heart J., 82:812, 1971.

Spriggs, A. I., and Boddington, M. M.: The Cytology of Effusions. London, Heinemann, 1968.

Storey, D. D., Dines, D. E., and Coles, D. T.: Pleural effusion: A diagnostic dilemma. J.A.M.A., 236:2183, 1976.

van Heerden, J. A., and Laufenberg, H. J.: Simplified thoracentesis. Mayo Clin. Proc., 43:311, 1968.

Venes, J. L.: Pleural fluid effusion and eosinophilia following ventriculopleural shunting. Den. Med. Child. Neurol., 16:72, 1974.

Warshaw, A. L.: Diagnosis of starch peritonitis by paracentesis. Lancet, 2:1054, 1972.

Wilson, T., and Lumb, P.: Improved method for aspiration of the pleural cavity. Br. Med. J., 2:70, 1975.

Winckler, C. F., and Yam, L. T.: Cytologic changes of pleural fluid in pulmonary embolism. Arch. Intern. Med., 136:1195, 1976.

Yam, L. T.: Diagnostic significance of lymphocytes in pleural effusions. Ann. Intern. Med., 66:972, 1967.

2

19

PREGNANCY TESTS AND EVALUATION OF PLACENTAL FUNCTION

Arthur F. Krieg, M.D.

The term "pregnancy test" is actually a misnomer. First, most "pregnancy tests" do not actually determine pregnancy, but human chorionic gonadotropin (hCG) produced by trophoblastic tissue. Second, measurement of hCG is used to diagnose conditions other than pregnancy. Clinical applications of "pregnancy tests" include confirmation of a clinical diagnosis of pregnancy early in the first trimester; identification of pregnant patients before ordering medications or radiographic examinations; diagnosis of ectopic pregnancy in patients with lower abdominal pain; evaluation of threatened abortion during the first trimester; guidance of diagnosis and treatment of trophoblastic tumors; and evaluation of selected non-trophoblastic tumors.

HUMAN CHORIONIC GONADOTROPIN

Human chorionic gonadotropin (hCG) is a glycoprotein consisting of an alpha polypep-

tide subunit (molecular weight 18,000) and a beta polypeptide subunit (molecular weight 32,000). Alpha subunits for the four human glycoprotein hormones (LH, FSH, TSH, hCG) are nearly identical (Ross, 1977). Beta subunits for these four hormones differ significantly. However, there are similarities between the beta subunits for LH and hCG: about 80 per cent of the first 115 amino terminal residues are identical (Ross, 1977). It is the beta chains that provide the distinctive characteristics of hCG, LH, FSH, and TSH. Under appropriate conditions, beta subunits from hCG can be reassociated with alpha chains from other glycoprotein hormones to reconstitute physiologically active hCG (Ross, 1977). However, the isolated alpha or beta subunits are by themselves physiologically inactive.

As "glycoproteins," the alpha and beta subunits are linked to carbohydrate side chains. These carbohydrate side chains include sialic acid, fucose, galactose, mannose, glucosamine, and galactosamine in varying combinations (Ross, 1977). Progressive removal of sialic acid causes decreased *in vivo* hCG activity, while *in vitro* hCG activity is not affected (Ross, 1977). This discrepancy between *in vivo* and *in vitro* activity is related to the decreased plasma half-life of hCG that accompanies progressive desialylation. The decrease in plasma half-life parallels decreased *in vivo* activity (Ross, 1977).

Since hCG is produced by trophoblastic tissue, it is first detected shortly after implantation (Catt, 1975). Four general methods are available to measure hCG activity: bioassay, immunoassay (hemagglutination inhibition, latex particle agglutination inhibition, direct agglutination of latex particles), radioimmunoassay, and radioreceptor assay.

BIOASSAY

The first clinically useful bioassay was introduced by *Aschheim and Zondek* (1928) based on corpus luteum formation induced by hCG in prepubertal female mice. The *Friedman test* (1931) was based on ovulation in mature female rabbits. The *Xenopus laevis* test (Bellerby, 1934) was based on ova release from the South African clawed toad. The *rat ovarian hyperemia* test (Frank, 1941) was based on ovarian hyperemia in prepubertal female rats. The *Rana pipiens frog test* (Wiltberger, 1948) and the *Galli-Mainini toad test* (1948) were based on sperm release using male frogs and toads, respectively.

Limitations of bioassays include interference from LH, high cost (Aschheim-Zondek test), technical difficulty (Friedman and ovarian hyperemia tests), and need for frequent restandardization (frog and toad tests). Although bioassays continue to be performed by some research laboratories (Lau, 1975), most "pregnancy tests" are now performed by immunoassay, radioimmunoassay, or radioreceptor assay.

IMMUNOASSAY

Immunoassays for hCG became available during the early 1960's (Wide, 1960; 1962) and have now largely replaced bioassays. Concentration of hCG may be expressed as:

IU/ml urine or serum
ng/ml urine or serum

The relationship between IU/ml and ng/ml is expressed as:

$$1 \text{ IU/ml} = 83.3 \text{ ng/ml}$$
$$1 \text{ mIU/ml} = 0.08 \text{ ng/ml}$$
$$1 \text{ ng/ml} = 12 \text{ M IU/ml}$$

The International Unit (IU) is related to gonadotropic activity of a powdered urinary gonadotropin standard maintained at the World Health Organization in London, England. Secondary standards are maintained by the National Institutes of Health in the United States.

Three basic types of immunoassay are available: hemagglutination inhibition, latex particle agglutination inhibition, and direct latex particle agglutination.

Hemagglutination inhibition (HAI) is based on the observation that non-agglutinated erythrocytes in low concentration settle in a test tube with a hemispheric bottom to form a sharply demarcated ring or "doughnut," while agglutinated erythrocytes form a uniform film. Progressively increasing agglutination causes the ring gradually to increase in size and decrease in clarity, until it "fades away" into a uniform film (Salk, 1944).

In the HAI procedure, anti-hCG serum and erythrocytes (RBC) coated with hCG are incubated with patient urine. If hCG is present, it will neutralize the antiserum, while if hCG is absent, the antiserum is unaffected. Unaffected antiserum will agglutinate the RBC, so that a diffuse mat of cells forms. However, if the antiserum is neutralized, the RBC will form a "doughnut" pattern or ring (Fig. 19–1).

By definition, HAI procedures are "tube tests." Between one and two hours is required for agglutination and settling to occur.

Latex particle agglutination inhibition (LAI) is similar in principle to HAI: anti-hCG serum is briefly mixed with patient urine and latex particles coated with hCG are added. If

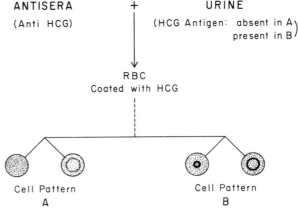

Figure 19–1. Immunoassay for hCG by hemagglutination inhibition.

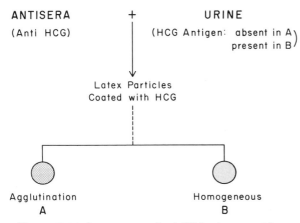

Figure 19-2. Immunoassay for hCG by latex particle agglutination inhibition.

hCG is present, it will neutralize the antiserum, while if hCG is absent, the antiserum is unaffected. Unaffected antiserum will cause visible agglutination of the latex particles. However, if the antiserum is neutralized, no visible agglutination occurs (Fig. 19-2).

Most LAI procedures are slide tests that require only a few minutes to perform. One tube test (Placentex) is commercially available; this is more sensitive than the slide tests but requires between one and two hours.

Direct latex particle agglutination utilizes anti-hCG, which is directly adsorbed on the latex particles. If hCG is present, agglutination occurs. In contrast to the LAI procedures, agglutination indicates presence of hCG, while lack of agglutination represents a "negative" result. One direct latex particle agglutination slide test is commercially available.

RADIOIMMUNOASSAY

Radioimmunoassays (RIA) for hCG are classified by the type of antiserum. The "beta subunit assays" utilize antisera against the beta subunit of hCG and are quite specific. At sensitivities of 5 mIU/ml hCG (0.4 ng/ml), the beta subunit assay described by Vaitukaitis (1972) is unaffected by elevated LH levels during midcycle or menopause. Present antisera for the beta subunit assay have only 1 to 2 per cent cross-reactivity against LH (Ross, 1977).

The "whole molecule" RIA for hCG (antibody against both alpha and beta subunits) is less specific, showing considerable cross-reaction with both LH and FSH.

Although early methods for the beta subunit RIA required 24 hours incubation, newer procedures require only 1 to 5 hours (Rasor, 1977) (Table 19-1).

RADIORECEPTOR ASSAY

Radioreceptor assays (RRA) for hCG utilize receptors from the ovaries of pregnant cows (Saxena, 1974). Compared with the beta subunit radioimmunoassay, RRA is more rapid (requires only one hour incubation) but less specific (shows cross-reaction with LH). Although sensitivity of RRA is about 5 to 10 mIU/ml (Landesman, 1976), "false positives" may occur owing to cross-reactions with LH. Elevated LH may be associated with midcycle peaks or premenopausal status. Two approaches are available to detect or eliminate such "false positives": repeated RRA on consecutive days to confirm "positive" results (early pregnancy is associated with rapidly increasing hCG, in contrast to midcycle LH peaks or premenopausal status), and use of a "cut off value" sufficiently high to avoid LH interference. The second approach is applied to commercial RRA kits, which are set at "cut off values" of 200 mIU/ml (Wampole Laboratories, Cranbury, N.J.). Although such kits can be used for quantitative hCG measurements with a sensitivity of 30 mIU/ml (Boyko, 1977), this increased sensitivity causes decreased specificity owing to cross-reactions with LH.

COMPARISON OF METHODS

Approximate sensitivities for various reagent systems are outlined in Table 19-1. In some cases, sensitivities specified by the manufacturer may vary from those reported in the literature.

It is difficult to assign "absolute" sensitivities with certainty. For HAI, LAI, and direct agglutination procedures, relative sensitivities for different reagents may vary for different urine specimens (Porres, 1975). This may be due to excretion of altered hCG molecules, which are detected with different sensitivities by different reagent systems.

A common approach to classification is "tube tests" and "slide tests." The classic "tube tests" are HAI procedures, with sensitivities in the range of 1.0 to 2.0 IU/ml, which require one to two hours for settling of RBC. Another "tube test," based on latex particle agglutination inhibition, has comparable sensitivity and

Table 19-1. "PREGNANCY TESTS" BASED ON hCG ASSAY

PRODUCT	INCUBATION TIME	SENSITIVITY IU/ml*	COMMENTS
Hemagglutination Inhibition (HAI) (Tube Tests)			
Pregnosticon (Organon)	1-2 hrs	0.6	Also available in lyophilized form as Pregnosticon Accuspheres
UCG (Wampole)	2 hrs	0.5	Also available in lyophilized form as UCG lyphotest
Gravindex (Ortho)	2 hrs	0.5	
Latex Particle Agglutination Inhibition (LAI) (Tube Test)			
Placentex (Roche)	1-2 hrs	1.0	Requires incubation at 37°C.
Latex Particle Agglutination Inhibition (LAI) (Slide Tests)			
Pregnosticon (Organon)	2 min	1.0-2.0	Also available in lyophilized form as Pregnosticon Dri Dot
UCG (Wampole)	2 min	2.0	
Gravindex (Ortho)	2 min	3.5	
Pregnosis (Roche)	2 min	1.5-2.5	
Direct Latex Agglutination (Slide Test)			
DAP test (Wampole)	1 min	2.0	May be used with serum as well as urine
Radioreceptor Assay (RRA)			
Biocept-G (Wampole)	1 hr	0.2	
Radioimmunoassay (RIA)			
beta-hCG (quantitative) (Monitor Science)	5 hrs	0.005	Continued improvements may provide shorter incubation times for RIA procedures
beta-hCG (qualitative) (Monitor Science)	1 hr	0.040	
beta-hCG (Radioassay Systems)	24 hrs	0.006	
beta-hCG (Serono)	18 hrs	0.005	
beta-hCG (Serono)	3 hrs	0.009	

*Estimates based on specifications published by manufacturers. Reports in literature suggest that under "routine" conditions tube tests may have sensitivity in the range of 1.0 to 2.0 IU/ml, while the most sensitive slide tests may have sensitivity in the range of 2.0 to 4.0 IU/ml.

time requirement (Table 19-1). The classic "slide tests" are LAI procedures, with sensitivities in the range of 2.0 to 5.0 IU/ml, which require only one to two minutes incubation at room temperature. Another "slide test," based on direct latex particle agglutination, has comparable sensitivity and time requirement (Table 19-1).

Although some slide tests may have slightly better specificity than some tube tests, the decreased sensitivity of slide tests is *not* necessarily associated with improved specificity (Cabrera, 1969; Kerber, 1970; Headden, 1972; Lamb, 1972; Arkin, 1972; Porres, 1975; Lewis, 1977; Roy, 1977).

False negative results in the HAI, LAI, and direct agglutination tests may occur with low hCG levels associated with early pregnancy, ectopic pregnancy, or threatened abortion. False negatives may also occur during the second and third trimesters, when hCG concentrations fall to about 5000 IU/l, close to the limit of sensitivity for LAI procedures (Kerber, 1970). With the direct agglutination slide test, prozoning may account for false negatives in some cases (Horwitz, 1971).

During the week after the first "missed period," or with ectopic pregnancy, the false negative rate is about 50 per cent for conventional immunoassays, but less than 10 per cent for the more sensitive beta subunit RIA or RRA procedures.

False positive results in the HAI, LAI and direct agglutination tests may be due to:

increased LH at midcycle peak.

increased LH in menopausal patients.

exogenous administration of hCG.

phenothiazine drugs, which may cause increased excretion of LH (Ravel, 1969).

promethazine (Phenergan), which may inhibit agglutination, causing false positive HAI or LAI but false negative direct agglutination (Tait, 1971).

methadone (Porres, 1975).

proteinuria in excess of 1.0 g/24 hrs (may cause non-specific inhibition of agglutination or cross-reactions with hCG antisera).

ectopic production of hCG and/or hCG-like substances by trophoblastic tumors.

ectopic production of hCG and/or hCG-like substances by non-trophoblastic neoplasms (e.g., carcinoma of the lung, ovarian cysts, testicular tumors).

tubo-ovarian abscess (Arkin, 1972).

deterioration of reagents (deterioration of hCG antiserum will cause "false positive" results in the HAI and LAI procedures, but "false negative" results in the direct agglutination procedure).

False positive results due to LH, drug interference, or proteinuria have not been reported with the beta subunit RIA method, which has less than 2 per cent cross-reactivity with LH. However, occasional false positives may occur with the RRA owing to cross-reactions with LH.

Reported accuracy of hCG assays is related to:

prevalence of causes for false negatives (early pregnancy, ectopic pregnancy, threatened abortion, etc.).

prevalence of causes for false positives (increased LH, etc.).

technical factors (improper shipment and storage of reagents, improper sample collection, quality control).

sensitivity and specificity of the assay procedure.

The incidence of "technical errors" under "normal working conditions" has been estimated to be between 1 and 4 per cent (Hardwick, 1974).

QUALITY CONTROL

Several authorities recommend that each assay be done in duplicate, using kits from two different manufacturers (Cabrera, 1969; Lau, 1975). According to Cabrera (1969): ". . . occasional bad lots of reagents are produced which can give very high proportions of false positives as well as false negatives . . . the degree of deficiency (may vary) within the same lot . . . some boxes of a particular lot (are) unusable, while others from the same lot (are) satisfactory . . . this unreliability . . . may result from damage . . . by extreme temperatures . . . (while) immunologic tests are fast and

easy to perform . . . many of these tests will go through periods of unreliability . . . we strongly recommend that two . . . immunologic tests be used together . . . one test checking on the other . . . anything less is fraught with danger."

In our opinion, it is desirable periodically to check sensitivities of kits against materials related to the International Standard. "Working Standards" may be provided through quantitative assay of aliquots from a *thoroughly mixed* pool of pregnancy urine by two or more reference laboratories. The remaining pool is frozen in tightly stoppered small aliquots at −70°C. (stable for at least one year).

Using this "working standard," quality control samples can be prepared by dilution to provide a "low positive" (2 to 4 times test sensitivity) and a "high negative" (one-fourth to one-half times test sensitivity) control. These two controls are checked each time a "pregnancy test" is run in order to detect altered sensitivity. If the "high negative" becomes positive, deterioration of HAI or LAI antisera is probable. If the "low positive" becomes negative, consultation with the manufacturer may be indicated.

Dilutions of "working standards" to prepare quality control pools may be performed by direct dilution or serial dilution. The diluent may be urine from males, urine from non-pregnant females, or phosphate buffered saline (pH 6.4) with 0.1 per cent bovine serum albumin. During dilution, reagents may be kept at either refrigerator temperature or room temperature.

Serial dilution tends to give lower values than direct dilutions, possibly owing to hCG adsorption on glass. Either normal urine or buffer with 0.1 per cent albumin tends to protect hCG from denaturation, which may occur in aqueous buffer or saline. The "protective effect" of normal urine seems to vary between different individuals (Tamada, 1969). Reagents should be kept at refrigerator temperature when dilutions are prepared: hCG may undergo slow denaturation at room temperature in dilute solutions (concentrated solutions deteriorate more slowly, possibly due to a "self-protective effect" of hCG).

DIAGNOSIS OF NORMAL PREGNANCY

Levels of hCG during pregnancy usually are expressed in relation to days (or weeks) after the last normal menstrual period (LNMP), as

EVALUATION OF
TESTICULAR TUMORS

Testicular choriocarcinomas are well known for their association with elevated plasma and urinary hCG. In most cases, hCG can be detected with the HAI or LAI assays. Using the beta subunit RIA, increased plasma hCG can be demonstrated in almost all testicular choriocarcinomas.

Other testicular tumors—notably seminomas, teratomas, and embryonal carcinomas—are well known for their association with elevated plasma and urinary hCG. About 10 to 20 per cent of such cases have elevated hCG by HAI or LAI; about 40 to 60 per cent have elevated hCG by beta subunit RIA. One hypothesis has been that hCG in such cases is produced by small foci of active or "burned-out" choriocarcinoma. However, there is evidence that other cell types also may produce hCG ectopically (Braunstein, 1973).

Sensitive hCG measurements (preferably the beta-subunit RIA) should be performed prior to treatment of testicular tumors; if hCG is found, this can be used as a "tumor marker" to evaluate treatment and/or suspected recurrence.

ECTOPIC hCG PRODUCTION IN
NON-TROPHOBLASTIC TUMORS

Ectopic hormone production by non-endocrine tumors is well known and has been studied extensively. Indeed, some non-endocrine neoplasms are capable of producing several hormones simultaneously. Also, some endocrine tumors may secrete both the "appropriate" hormone and an ectopic hormone; e.g., medullary carcinoma of the thyroid may produce ACTH as well as calcitonin. Such ectopic hormone production includes adrenocorticotropic hormone (ACTH), melanotropic-stimulating hormone (MSH), parathyroid hormone (PTH), calcitonin, luteinizing hormone (LH), antidiuretic hormone (ADH), insulin-like activity (ILA), vasoactive intestinal polypeptide (VIP), gastrin, erythropoeitin, and thyroid-stimulating hormone (TSH) in a variety of different tumors (Samaan, 1977).

Ectopic hCG production, as determined by beta-subunit RIA, has been described in up to 30 per cent of gastrointestinal neoplasms (especially gastric carcinoma, hepatoma, and pancreatic carcinoma); up to 2 per cent of patients with lymphoma/leukemia/myeloma; and occasional patients with retroperitoneal sarcoma, breast carcinoma, adrenocortical carcinoma, bronchogenic carcinoma, renal cell carcinoma, and melanoma (Braunstein, 1973; Rosen, 1975). In such cases, production of hCG may be as alpha subunits only, beta subunits only, or complete hCG, either alone or with subunits also present.

Ectopic production of the other placental proteins also may occur in association with various neoplasms, e.g., placental lactogen and placental alkaline phosphatase, either alone or in association with hCG (Braunstein, 1973).

OTHER "PREGNANCY TESTS"

PREGNANCY-ASSOCIATED
PLASMA PROTEINS

It is clear that the placenta produces, in addition to hCG, other proteins "specific" to pregnancy. Perhaps the best known is heat-stable alkaline phosphatase, which shows marked elevations in maternal serum during the third trimester. Although heat-stable alkaline phosphatase has been used as a "placental function test," in this role it has largely been replaced by plasma and urinary estriol (Watson, 1973). Like hCG, heat-stable alkaline phosphatase may serve as a useful "tumor marker" for a wide variety of neoplasms; however, its clinical value is not yet well established.

Recently, certain alpha and beta globulins known as "pregnancy-associated plasma proteins" (PAPP) have been identified (Lin, 1974; von Schoultz, 1974; Lin, 1975; Grudzinskas, 1977).

Although some of these proteins can be induced by exogenous estrogens or oral contraceptives (von Schoultz, 1974), others may have specificity comparable to hCG (Grudzinskas, 1977). Possible applications include (1) diagnosis of pregnancy during the first trimester and (2) evaluation of placental function (Masson, 1977).

Additional studies are needed to establish the clinical value of these measurements in comparison with measurements of hCG.

HORMONE WITHDRAWAL

The use of hormone withdrawal as a test for pregnancy was introduced following a report by Zondek (1942) that estrogen-progesterone preparations could induce uterine bleeding in patients with functional amenorrhea.

Administered progesterone is the key hormone: estrogen merely ensures priming of the endometrium. In a non-pregnant woman, these steroids hasten secretory maturation, so that hormone withdrawal is followed by bleeding. However, in pregnancy, endometrium is maintained by progesterone plus estrogen from the corpus luteum. After an appropriate dose of estrogen plus progesterone, about 90 per cent of non-pregnant women have bleeding within 5 to 10 days, while about 90 per cent of pregnant women have no evidence of bleeding.

Since the early 1970's, these "hormone-withdrawal pregnancy tests," have come under increasing criticism, based on suspected association with multiple congenital anomalies. These anomalies have been described by the acronym VACTEL (vertebral, anal, cardiac, tracheal, esophagel, limb) (Nora, 1973; Oakley, 1973; Harlap, 1975).

In 1973, oral "pregnancy test tablets" were withdrawn from sale in the United States on request of the FDA (United States Food and Drug Administration).

PLACENTAL FUNCTION TESTS

Human Placental Lactogen

Human placental lactogen (hPL) is a single chain polypeptide of about 21,000 molecular weight, similar in structure to pituitary growth hormone. Although hPL displays growth hormone effects which contribute to the metabolic changes of late pregnancy, its primary role is a lactogenic hormone functioning in combination with prolactin. An alternate name applied to hPL is human chorionic somatomammotropin (hCS).

Like hCG, hPL is produced by the syncytial trophoblast, starting shortly after implantation. During the first trimester, hPL appears in maternal plasma about 8 to 10 weeks after the LMP (last menstrual period) but is of no practical value for early pregnancy diagnosis, as compared with hCG.

Some reports suggest that hPL measurements may be used as a "placental function test." However, for this purpose, estriol measurements probably provide more useful clinical information than hPL (Watson, 1973; Josimovich, 1973). Possibly, hPL measurements may provide a useful supplement to estriol. At this time, the clinical value of hPL

as a "placental function test" is not yet well established.

In contrast to hCG, hPL is markedly decreased in association with hydatidiform mole and choriocarcinoma. Thus, the combination of high hCG and low hPL possibly may have some diagnostic value (Levitt, 1976). However, for monitoring treatment, measurement of hCG by beta subunit RIA is clearly superior to hPL measurements.

Some non-trophoblastic tumors are associated with increased hPL. Thus hPL, as well as hCG, may provide a useful "tumor marker" in some cases.

Estrogen Measurements

Although estrogen measurements have little value as "pregnancy tests" during the first trimester, in the third trimester, urinary and plasma estriol provide a valuable index of fetal-placental dysfunction (Watson, 1973; Bashore, 1977; Miller, 1977).

During pregnancy, estriol is synthesized in the placenta from dehydroepiandrosterone (DHEA) and 16-hydroxydehydroepiandrosterone (16-OHDHEA), which are produced as sulfates by the fetal zone of the adrenal cortex. Within the placenta, DHEA sulfate and 16-OHDHEA sulfate are (1) hydrolyzed to DHEA and 16-OHDHEA and (2) converted to estriol. Estriol then passes across the placenta to maternal plasma, where most of it is conjugated with glucuronic acid in maternal liver and excreted in maternal bile. Conjugated estriol also is excreted in maternal urine. In the intestine, conjugated estriol is split by bacterial enzymes, with reabsorption of unconjugated estriol into maternal plasma via the entero-hepatic circulation.

Production of DHEA and 16-OHDHEA in the fetal adrenal is stimulated by ACTH from the fetal pituitary, under feedback control of plasma cortisol.

In maternal plasma, about 85 to 90 per cent of estriol circulates as glucuronide and about 10 to 15 per cent as unconjugated or "free" estriol. The term "free estriol" is actually a misnomer; in plasma, about 70 per cent of conjugated and unconjugated estriol is bound to sex hormone binding globulin (SHBG). This protein (SHBG) also binds testosterone, dihydrotestosterone, estrone, and estradiol. Only the unbound hormones are physiologically active.

Decreased estriol in maternal plasma may reflect (a) decreased synthesis of ACTH by fetal pituitary (e.g., anencephaly, exogenous corticoids); (b) decreased synthesis of DHEA and/or 16-OHDHEA by fetal adrenals (e.g., adrenal hypoplasia, retarded fetal growth, fetal distress, intrauterine death); (c) decreased placental synthesis of estriol (e.g., placental insufficiency, placental infarcts, hydatidiform mole); (d) placental sulfatase deficiency (16-OHDHEA sulfate coming from fetal liver is normally hydrolyzed to 16-OHDHEA before conversion to estriol); or (e) disturbances of maternal enterohepatic circulation (e.g., antibiotic treatment or malabsorption, which prevent bacterial splitting or reabsorption of estriol). Measurements of urinary estriol may also be affected by incomplete urine collection (false low result), decreased maternal glomerular filtration rate (false low result), or decreased hepatic conjugation of estriol due to maternal liver disease (false low result).

There has been considerable discussion regarding the relative merits of measuring total plasma estriol, plasma unconjugated estriol (about 10 to 15 per cent of total plasma estriol), and urinary estriol. If plasma measurements are used, unconjugated estriol may be preferable to total estriol. Assay of unconjugated estriol does not require preliminary hydrolysis to separate estriol from glucuronide, and unconjugated estriol may more accurately reflect status of the feto-placental unit than total estriol (Crane, 1976; Klopper, 1977). Plasma estriol has significant advantages over urinary estriol: (a) plasma measurements do not require accurately timed urine collections; (b) plasma measurements are less affected by changes in glomerular filtration rate, which are common in patients with high-risk pregnancy (diabetes, toxemia, hypertension, etc.); and (c) plasma measurements are not affected by drugs, which may cause destruction of urinary estriol during acid hydrolysis (Trolle, 1977).

In order to avoid the need for accurately timed urine collections, some authors have recommended measurement of estrogen/creatinine ratios with random urine samples (Aubry, 1975; Rao, 1977). At this time, there is no general agreement regarding relative merits of plasma unconjugated estriol, plasma total estriol, and urinary estriol measurements.

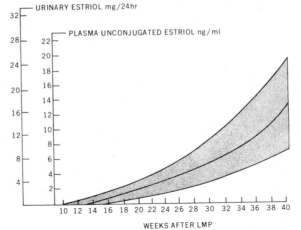

Figure 19-5. Normal ranges for plasma unconjugated estriol and urinary estriol. (Adapted from Bashore, R. A., and Westlake, J. R.: Plasma unconjugated estriol values in high-risk pregnancy. Am. J. Obstet. Gynecol., *128*:371–380, 1977, and Ansari, A. H., and Fuller, D. G.: Urinary estriol for assessment of fetoplacental function. Southern Med. J., *70*:142–146, 1977. Reprinted by permission.)

The relationship between plasma unconjugated estriol and 24-hour urinary estriol has been reported by Miller (1977). Urinary excretion of 1 mg/24 hr is approximately equivalent to 0.6 to 0.8 ng/ml of unconjugated plasma estriol. Normal ranges for plasma unconjugated estriol (Bashore, 1977) and urinary estriol (Ansari, 1977) are shown in Figure 19-5.

CLINICAL APPLICATIONS

An approach to management of high-risk pregnancies has been outlined by Crane (1976). Three basic patterns for plasma unconjugated estriol are described: normal pattern ("within normal limits"), chronically low results, and falling values. Chronically low estriol may be unrelated to fetal distress or placental failure. Possible causes include maternal steroid therapy, fetal adrenal insufficiency, congenital anomalies (e.g., anencephaly), and placental sulfatase deficiency.

A day-to-day decrease of 35 to 50 per cent is considered a significant fall in plasma or urinary estriol. Beyond the thirty-fourth week of gestation, values below 4 mg estriol/24 hr urine (3 ng estriol/ml plasma) indicate that fetal death has occurred or is imminent (Fig. 19-5). A single estriol measurement often has limited value; serial measurements in relation to the "normal pregnancy curve" (Fig. 19-5) provide greater sensitivity and specificity than isolated determinations.

About 60 per cent of molar pregnancies are associated with low serum estriol (Dawood, 1977a). However, in some cases, trophoblastic tissue may produce estriol in the absence of viable fetus.

SUMMARY

For most purposes, the term "pregnancy test" is equivalent to "hCG assay." Pregnancy tests may be indicated in a variety of situations, including (a) exclusion of pregnancy in women of childbearing age prior to surgery, drug treatment, rubella vaccination, or radio-graphic studies; (b) suspected ectopic pregnancy; (c) selection of patients for menstrual regulation; (d) evaluation of threatened abortion; (e) diagnosis and treatment of trophoblastic disease; (f) unexplained cases of gynecomastia or sexual precocity (tumors producing hCG may cause such symptoms in men and children); (g) regulation of treatment for non-trophoblastic neoplasms which produce hCG. Although other "pregnancy tests" have been described, their clinical value is not yet well established.

Of the various "placental function tests," measurements of urinary and/or plasma estriol appear most useful for evaluating the fetal-placental unit during the third trimester. The clinical value of other procedures, such as hPL and heat-stable alkaline phosphatase, is not yet established.

REFERENCES

Ansari, A. H., and Fuller, D. G.: Urinary estriol for assessment of fetoplacental function. South. Med. J., *70*:142, 1977.

Arkin, C., and Noto, T. A.: A false positive immunologic pregnancy test with tube-ovarian abscess. Am. J. Clin. Pathol., *58*:314, 1972.

Aschheim, S., and Zondek, B.: Pregnancy diagnosis with urine by the demonstration of the hormone. Klin. Wochenschr., *7*:8, 1928.

Aubry, R. H., Rouke, J. E., Cuenca, V. G., and Marshall, L. D.: The random urine estrogen/creatinine ratio. Obstet. Gynecol., *46*:64, 1975.

Bashore, R. A., and Westlake, J. R.: Plasma unconjugated estriol values in high-risk pregnancy. Am. J. Obstet. Gynecol., *128*:371, 1977.

Bellerby, C. W.: A rapid test for the diagnosis of pregnancy. Nature (London), *133*:494, 1934.

Boyko, W. L., and Russell, H. T.: Application of the radioreceptor assay for human chorionic gonadotropin in pregnancy testing and management of trophoblastic disease. Obstet. Gynecol., *50*:329, 1977.

Braunstein, G. D., Rasor, J., Adler, D., Danzer, H., and Wade, M. E.: Serum human chorionic gonadotropin levels throughout normal pregnancy. Am. J. Obstet. Gynecol., *126*:678, 1976.

Braunstein, G. D., Vaitukaitis, J. L., Carbone, P. P., and Ross, G. T.: Ectopic production of human chorionic gonadotropin by neoplasms. Ann. Intern. Med., *78*:39, 1973.

Brenner, W. E., Edelman, D. A., and Kessel, E.: Menstrual regulation in the United States: A preliminary report. Fertil. Steril., *26*:289, 1975.

Cabrera, H. A.: A comprehensive evaluation of pregnancy tests. Am. J. Obstet. Gynecol., *103*:32, 1969.

Catt, K. J., Dufau, M. L., and Vaitukaitis, J. L.: Appearance of hCG in pregnancy plasma following the initiation of implantation of the blastocyst. J. Clin. Endocrinol. Metab., *40*:537, 1975.

Crane, J. P., Sauvage, J. P., and Arias, F.: A high-risk pregnancy management protocol. Am. J. Obstet. Gynecol., *125*:227, 1976.

Dawood, M. Y., Brown, J. B., and Newman, K. L. H.: Serum free estriol and estriol glucuronide fractions in hydatidiform mole measured by radioimmunoassay. Obstet. Gynecol., *49*:303, 1977a.

Dawood, M. Y., Saxena, B. B., and Landesman, R.: Human chorionic gonadotropin and its subunits in hydatidiform mole and choriocarcinoma. Obstet. Gynecol., *50*:172, 1977b.

Frank, R. T., and Berman, R. L.: A twenty-four hour pregnancy test. Am. J. Obstet. Gynecol., *42*:492, 1941.

Friedman, M. H., and Lapham, M. E.: A simple rapid method for the laboratory diagnosis of early pregnancies. Am. J. Obstet. Gynecol., *21*:405, 1931.

Galli-Mainini, C.: Pregnancy test using the male batrachria. J.A.M.A., *138*:121, 1948.

Grudzinskas, J. C., Jeffrey, D., Gordon, Y. B., and Chard, T.: Specific and sensitive determination of pregnancy—specific B1-glycoprotein by radioimmunoassay. Lancet, *1*:333, 1977.

Harlap, S., Pryues, R., and Davies, A. M.: Birth defects and estrogens and progesterones in pregnancy. Lancet, *1*:682, 1975.

Hardwick, D. F., Brent, R., Burke, M. D., Cohen, H., Falkowski, F., Horwitz, C. A., Lazo-Wasem, E., Perrin, E. U., Poland, B. J., Reiss, A. M., Schenkel, B., Towell, M. E., and Vorherr, H.: Early diagnosis of pregnancy: An invitational symposium. J. Reprod. Med., *12*:1, 1974.

Headden, G. F.: An evaluation of immunological pregnancy tests. Med. Lab. Technol., *29*:332, 1972.

Horwitz, C. A., Polesky, H., Odenbrett, P., Gronli, M., Horowitz, A., Diamond, R., and Ward, P. C. J.: Clinical and immunologic study of a direct agglutination test for pregnancy. Am. J. Obstet. Gynecol., *111*:808, 1971.

Jones, W. B., Lewis, J. L., and Lehr, M.: Monitor of chemotherapy in gestational trophoblastic neoplasm by radioimmunoassay of the B-subunit of human chorionic gonadotropin. Am. J. Obstet. Gynecol., *121*:669, 1975.

Josimovich, J. B.: Placental protein hormones in pregnancy. Clin. Gynecol., *16*:46, 1973.

Kerber, I. J., Inclan, A. P., Fowler, E. A., David, K., and Fish, S. A.: Immunologic tests for pregnancy. Obstet. Gynecol., *36*:37, 1970.

Klopper, A. I., Wilson, G. R., and Masson, G. M.: Observations on the variability of plasma estriol. Obstet. Gynecol., *49*:459, 1977.

Kosasa, T. S., Levesque, L. A., Goldstein, D. P., and Taymor, M. L.: Clinical use of a solid-phase radioimmunoassay specific for human chorionic gonadotropin. Am. J. Obstet. Gynecol., *119*:784, 1974.

Kosasa, T. S., Pion, R. J., Hale, R. W., Goldstein, D. P., Taymor, M. L., Levesque, L. A., and Kobara, T. Y.: Rapid hCG-specific radioimmunoassay for menstrual aspiration. Obstet. Gynecol., *45*:566, 1975.

Kosasa, T. S., Taymor, M. L., Goldstein, D. P., and Levesque, L. A.: Use of a radioimmunoassay specific for human chorionic gonadotropin in the diagnosis of early ectopic pregnancy. Obstet. Gynecol., *42*:858, 1973.

Lamb, E. J.: Immunological pregnancy tests. Obstet. Gynecol., *39*:665, 1972.

Landesman, R., and Saxena, B. B.: Results of the first 1000 radioreceptor assays for the determination of human chorionic gonadotropin: A new, rapid, reliable, and sensitive pregnancy test. Fertil. Steril. *27*:357, 1976.

Lau, H.: Testing for pregnancy. *In* Tice, F., (ed.): Tice's Practice of Medicine, vol. II. Hagerstown, Md., Harper & Row, Publishers, Inc., 1975.

Levitt, M. J., and Josimovich, J. B.: Measurement of chorionic gonadotropin and placental lactogen in body fluids. *In* Rose, N. R., and Friedman, H. (eds.): Manual of Clinical Immunology. Washington, D.C., American Society for Microbiology, 1976.

Lewis, C.: Human chorionic gonadotrophin and its detection by immunochemical methods. Can. J. Med. Tech., *39*:58, 1977.

Lin, T. M., and Halbert, S. P.: Immunological comparison of various human pregnancy-associated plasma proteins. Int. Arch. Allergy Appl. Immunol., *48*:101, 1975.

Lin, T. M., Halbert, S. P., Kiefer, D., and Spellacy, W. N.: Three pregnancy-associated plasma proteins. Int. Arch. Allergy Appl. Immunol., *47*:35, 1974.

Masson, G. M., Klopper, A. I., and Wilson, G. R.: Plasma estrogens and pregnancy-associated plasma proteins. Obstet. Gynecol., *50*:435, 1977.

Milwidsky, A., Adoni, A., Palti, Z., Stark, M., and Segal., S.: The significance of human chorionic gonadotropin in blood serum for the early diagnosis of ectopic pregnancy. Acta Obstet. Gynecol. Scand., *56*:19, 1977a.

Milwidsky, A., Adoni, A., Segal., S., and Palti, Z.: Chorionic gonadotropin and progesterone levels in ectopic pregnancy. Obstet. Gynecol., *50*:145, 1977b.

Miller, C. A., Fetter, M. C., Bognslaski, R. C., and Heiser, E. W.: Maternal serum unconjugated estriol and urine estriol concentrations in normal and high-risk pregnancy. Obstet. Gynecol., *49*:287, 1977.

Morrow, C. P., Kletzky, O. A., Disaia, P. J., Townsend, D. E., Mishell, D. R., and Nakamura, R. M.: Clinical and laboratory correlates of molar pregnancy and trophoblastic disease. Am. J. Obstet. Gynecol., *128*:424, 1977.

Nora, J. J., and Nora, A. H.: Birth defects and oral contraceptives. Lancet, *1*:941, 1973.

Oakley, G. P., and Flynt, J. W.: Hormonal pregnancy tests and congenital malformations. Lancet, *2*:256, 1973.

Pastorfide, G. B., Goldstein, D. P., and Kosasa, T. S.: The use of a radioimmunoassay specific for human chorionic gonadotropin in patients with molar pregnancy and gestational trophoblastic disease. Obstet. Gynecol., *120*:1025, 1974.

Porres, J. M., D'Ambra, C., Lord, D., and Garrity, F.: Comparison of eight kits for the diagnosis of pregnancy. Am. J. Clin. Pathol., *64*:452, 1975.

Rao, L. G. S.: Predicting fetal death by measuring estrogen: Creatinine ratios on early morning samples of urine. Br. Med. J., *2*:874, 1977.

Rasor, J. L., and Braunstein, G. D.: A rapid modification of the beta-hCG radioimmunoassay. Obstet. Gynecol., *50*:553, 1977.

Ravel, R., Riekers, H. G., and Goldstein, B. J.: Effects of certain psychotropic drugs in immunologic pregnancy tests. Am. J Obstet. Gynecol., *105*:1227, 1969.

Rosal, T. P., Saxena, B. B., and Landesman, R.: Application of a radioreceptor assay of human chorionic gonadotropin in the diagnosis of early abortion. Fertil. Steril., *26*:1105, 1975.

Rosen, S. W., Weintraub, B. D., Vaitulcaitis, J. L., Sussman, H. H., Hershman, J. M., and Muggia, F. M.: Placental proteins and their subunits as tumor markers. Ann. Intern. Med., *82*:71, 1975.

Ross, G. T.: Clinical relevance of research on the structure of human chorionic gonadotropin. Am. J. Obstet. Gynecol., *129*:795, 1977.

Roy, S., Klein, T. A., Scott, J. Z., Kletzky, O. A., and Mishell, D. R.: Diagnosis of pregnancy with a radioreceptor assay for hCG. Obstet. Gynecol., *50*:401, 1977.

Salk, J. E.: A simplified procedure for titrating hemagglutination capacity of influenza virus and corresponding antibody. J. Immunol., *48*:87, 1944.

Salzberger, M., and Nelken, D.: The immunologic pregnancy test. Am. J. Obstet. Gynecol., *86*:899, 1963.

Samaan, N. A.: Hormone production in non-endocrine tumors. CA, *27*:148, 1977.

Saxena, B. B., Hasan, S. H., Haour, F., and Schmidt-Gullwitzer, M.: Radioreceptor assay of hCG: Detection of early pregnancy. Science, *184*:793, 1974.

Saxena, B. B., and Landesman, R.: The use of a radioreceptor assay of human chorionic gonadotropin for the diagnosis and management of ectopic pregnancy. Fertil. Steril., *26*:397, 1975.

Schreiber, J. R., Rebar, R. W., Chen, H. C., Hodgen, G. D., and Ross, G. T.: Limitation of the specific serum radioimmunoassay for human chorionic gonadotropin in the management of trophoblastic neoplasms. Am. J. Obstet. Gynecol., *125*:705, 1976.

Tait, B.: Interference in immunological methods of pregnancy testing by promethazine. Med. J. Aust., *2*:126, 1971.

Tamada, T., Tsukui, Y., and Matsumoto, S.: On diluent and dilution method in hemagglutination test for human chorionic gonadotropin. Endocrinol. Japan, *16*:399, 1969.

Trolle, D., Bock, J. E., and Gaede, P.: The prognostic and diagnostic value of total estriol in urine and in serum and of human placental lactogen hormone in serum in the last part of pregnancy. Am. J. Obstet. Gynecol., *126*:834, 1977.

United States Food and Drug Administration: Medroxyprogesterone acetate; norethindrone; norethindrone acetate; progesterone; dydrogesterone; and hydroxyprogesterone caproate. Fed. Reg., *38*:27947, 1973.

Vaitukaitis, J. L., Braunstein, G. D., and Ross, G. T.: A radioimmunoassay which specifically measures human chorionic gonadotropin in the presence of human luteinizing hormone. Am. J. Obstet. Gynecol., *113*:751, 1972.

von Schoultz, B.: A quantiative study of the pregnancy zone protein in the sera of pregnant and puerperal women. Am. J. Obstet. Gynecol., *119*:792, 1974.

Watson, D., Siddiqui, S. A., Stafford, J. E. H., Gibbard, S., and Hewitt, V.: A comparative study of five laboratory tests for faeto-placental dysfunction in late pregnancy. J. Clin. Pathol., *26*:294, 1973.

Wide, L.: An immunological method for the assay of human chorionic gonadotrophin. Acta Endocrinol., *41* (Suppl. 70):1, 1962.

Wide, L., and Gemzell, C. A.: An immunological pregnancy test. Acta Endocrinol., *35*:261, 1960.

Wiltberger, P. B., and Miller, D. F.: The male frog, rana pipiens, as a new test animal for early pregnancy. Science, *107*:198, 1948.

Yahia, C.: The quantitative toad test in normal and abnormal early gestation. Obstet. Gynecol., *23*:547, 1964.

Yuen, B. H., Cannon, W., Benedet, J. L., and Boyes, D. A.: Plasma B-subunit human chorionic gonadotropin assay in molar pregnancy and choriocarcinoma. Am. J. Obstet. Gynecol., *127*:711, 1977.

Zondek, B.: Simplified hormonal treatment of amenorrhea. J.A.M.A., *119*:705, 1942.

20

AMNIOTIC FLUID
AND ANTENATAL DIAGNOSIS

Robert E. Wenk, M.D.,
Jerald Rosenbaum, M.D., and
John Bernard Henry, M.D.

AMNIOTIC FLUID STUDY
    Anatomic and Physiologic
      Considerations
    Hemolytic Disease of Newborns
    Principles of Amniotic Fluid Analysis
      in Isoimmunization Syndrome
    Estimation of Fetal Pulmonary
      Maturity
    Assessment of Fetal Size and
      Gestational Age
    Fetal Hypothyroidism

    Diagnosis of Neural Tube Defects
    Intestinal Obstruction
    Genetic Disorders and Amniotic Fluid
    Amniotic Fluid and Fetal Infection
NON-AMNIOTIC LABORATORY TESTS OF
VALUE IN PERINATOLOGY
    Fetal Health and Fetoplacental
      Function
    Placental Function Tests
    Fetal Blood Sampling

AMNIOTIC FLUID STUDY

    Amniotic fluid was an untapped source of laboratory data until 1952 when Bevis suggested that it could yield information relating to hemolytic disease of the newborn (Bevis, 1952). Amniotic fluid analysis subsequently proved to be more useful than maternal serum antibody titration in the management of the Rh isoimmunization syndrome. More recently, amniotic fluid analyses have been used to define or characterize other fetal diseases including teratologic, genetic, endocrine, maturational, and infectious problems. Initially, amniocentesis was considered dangerous, but it is now regarded as underutilized in view of its demonstrated relative safety for both mother and fetus (Milunsky, 1975). Obviously, there are hazards (Table 20–1), particularly to the fetus, but these can be minimized if amni-

Table 20–1. REPORTED HAZARDS OF DIAGNOSTIC AMNIOCENTESIS

FETAL TRAUMA	MISSED DIAGNOSIS
Pneumothorax	Cell culture failure, maternal or fraternal twin's cells cultured
Splenic laceration	Specimen obtained not amniotic fluid (e.g., maternal urine)
Subdural hematoma	
Cardiac laceration-tamponade	
Arteriovenous fistula	**MATERNAL COMPLICATIONS**
Umbilical artery laceration	
Retroperitoneal hematoma	Amniotic fluid leakage
Laceration of extremity	Vaginal bleeding
Fetomaternal bleeding	Spontaneous abortion
Increased hemolysis following increased antibody titer	Amnionitis
Fetal exsanguination	Placenta abruptio

ocentesis is carried out safely by experienced persons. In selected cases, sonography is carried out to localize the placenta, ascertain fetal position, and help determine if there are twins or anomalies.

ANATOMIC AND PHYSIOLOGIC CONSIDERATIONS

The amniotic sac arises during the first week of gestation from embryonic tissues. It consists of an outer layer of mesoderm and an inner layer of ectoderm. The amniotic cavity enlarges, reflects over the embryo and its umbilical cord, and may be tapped (amniocentesis) by 14 weeks. At term (40 weeks), the sac contains 0.5 to 2.5 liters of fluid, which is apparently produced by cells of the fetal gastrointestinal system, respiratory tract, umbilical cord, amniotic membrane, and kidneys. In early gestation, fetal urine probably contributes little volume (Reynolds, 1969).

Normally, water exchanges between the amniotic fluid and mother, between mother and fetus, and between fetus and fluid. As pregnancy advances, the exchange between fetus and mother increases. In hydramnios, however, the fetomaternal exchange decreases, while the fetus increases its water contribution to fluid. The fluid, in turn, increases its contribution of water to the mother (Hutchinson, 1959).

In effect, in the first half of pregnancy, amniotic fluid volume can be regarded as an extension of the fetal extracellular fluid space (Lind, 1970). Rapidly developing fetal edema is, therefore, accompanied by acute hydramnios (excess amniotic fluid) in disorders such as recipient-twin transfusion syndrome, hydrops fetalis, and fetal heart failure. Chronic hydramnios may develop when the fetus fails to swallow fluid. It is associated with a 20 per cent incidence of fetal malformations such as anencephaly or esophageal atresia. Chronic hydramnios is also associated with maternal disease, commonly toxemia or diabetes mellitus. Oligohydramnios (less than 300 ml) may develop when chronically ill fetuses swallow more frequently than normal. There is often oligohydramnios in placental insufficiency or donor-twin transfusion syndrome.

In prolonged pregnancy, amniotic fluid may be obtained to determine if there is oligohydramnios (by hippurate dye dilution measurements). Oligohydramnios is associated with

Table 20–2. AN OUTLINE OF PERINATAL DISORDERS IDENTIFIABLE THROUGH AMNIOCENTESIS

Isoimmunization syndrome (Rh_o, other)
Immaturity (fetal size, pulmonary)
Neural tube defects (anencephaly, spina bifida, other)
Intestinal obstruction
Fetal infection (bacterial, viral, other)
Premature rupture of fetal membranes
Fetal hypoxia with meconium staining
Postmaturity syndrome
Metabolic diseases of:
  a. Amino acids (e.g., cystinosis)
  b. Mucopolysaccharides (e.g., Hurler's syndrome)
  c. Lipids (e.g., Tay-Sachs)
  d. Carbohydrates (e.g., galactosemia)
  e. Steroids (adrenogenital syndrome)
  f. Purines (Lesch-Nyhan syndrome)
  g. Thyroid hormones (cretinism)
Chromosomal abnormalities:
  a. Down's syndrome (translocation, trisomy, mosaic)
  b. Sex chromosomal disorders (Klinefelter's Turner's, other)
  c. Miscellaneous (trisomies, deletions, etc.)

fetal distress and calls for amniotomy, measurement of fetal blood pH, and determination of maternal estriol excretion (Beischer, 1969).

At term, amniotic water is exchanged at the high rate of 500 ml per hour; solutes in the water (1 per cent w/w) exchange at slower rates. A rapid rise in osmolality sometimes occurs in diabetic mothers and predicts a grave fetal outcome (Cassady, 1968).

The various solutes of amniotic fluid have been studied and a great variety of tests have been performed (Milunsky, 1976). This chapter is directed toward clinically relevant measurements (Table 20–2).

HEMOLYTIC DISEASE OF NEWBORNS

Sampling of amniotic fluid is now a common procedure in the isoimmunization syndrome. Although postpartum passive immunization of mothers with anti-Rh_o(D) can effectively prevent isoimmunization in many susceptible women, sporadic cases are expected to occur. Severe hemolytic disease may result when there are untreated mothers, iatrogenic failures, immunizations by transfusion, and abortions that are left untreated (Matthews, 1969). Fetomaternal bleeding at amniocentesis can produce maternal isoimmunization. Less likely, maternofetal bleeding at delivery can cause *infant* immunization (Beer, 1974). If these infants become mothers years later, they may transfer antibodies across the placenta, affecting the third generation. Most isoimmunizations will be directed against the $Rh_o(D)$ antigen, but others will involve other blood group antigens such as K, hr, and rh^w (Liley, 1970). The principles of management of these pregnancies are identical to those established for $Rh_o(D)$ isoimmunization.

When maternal IgG antibodies cross the placenta to react with fetal erythrocyte antigens, hemolysis is detectable as early as 16 weeks' gestation and may progress at an increasing rate until term. As fetal hemoglobin is catabolized to bilirubin, fetal plasma carries an increased concentration of unconjugated bilirubin to the placenta. The placenta excretes the pigment unless there is severe fetoplacental compromise. When unconjugated bilirubin increases in the fetal circulation, fetal hepatic glucuronyl transferase activity is induced earlier than usual so that conjugated bilirubin can be produced as early as 28 weeks (Brodersen, 1967). The conjugate is not cleared by the placenta and accounts for a variable fraction of the pigment (1 to 50 per cent) found in amniotic fluid. Much of the conjugated bilirubin is excreted via the fetal biliary tract and intestine, where a portion of it is hydrolyzed by intestinal epithelial beta-glucuronidase, reconverted to unconjugated bilirubin, and absorbed by the intestine. In the normal fetus or in one affected by mild hemolytic disease, there is no jaundice *in utero*, but following delivery, in the absence of the placenta, clinical jaundice may become evident (Poland, 1971). The severity of jaundice is related to increased pigment production found in isoimmunization syndrome. The majority of the pigment is unconjugated bilirubin (Brazie, 1966).

PRINCIPLES OF AMNIOTIC FLUID ANALYSIS IN ISOIMMUNIZATION SYNDROME

The examination of amniotic fluid in the maternal isoimmunization syndrome is based on the presence of the breakdown products of hemolysis, such as bilirubin or methemalbumin, in the fluid (Walker, 1957). It is unclear how these substances enter the amniotic sac.

Bilirubin pigment is bound to albumin; its concentration in the amniotic fluid is maintained at a fairly constant level despite the rapid turnover rate of amniotic fluid water, since the turnover of amniotic fluid protein is much slower.

A specimen of amniotic fluid may be aspirated, filtered, and examined with a double beam recording spectrophotometer. If the absorbance of the fluid is recorded continuously between 350 and 700 nm, the resulting curve can be used to (1) detect whether or not the fluid contains bilirubin and/or other pigmented products of hemolysis, and (2) quantitate the bilirubin pigment which is present.

Liley (1963) has shown that the net absorbance at 450 nm from isoimmunized patients who have unaffected babies always decreases as pregnancy progresses. This decreasing net absorbance at the 450 nm wavelength with increasing length of gestation parallels bilirubin pigment concentration and can be used to measure the severity of hemolytic disease. This is illustrated in Liley's prediction graph (Fig. 20-1). The greater the net absorbance at 450 nm, the more severe is the hemolysis and the lower the umbilical cord hemoglobin of a delivered newborn at any given age of gestation. The slope of the boundaries demarcating the three major zones of the graph indicates that there is a logarithmic decrease in pigment concentration in the amniotic fluid as pregnancy progresses. These decreases may be

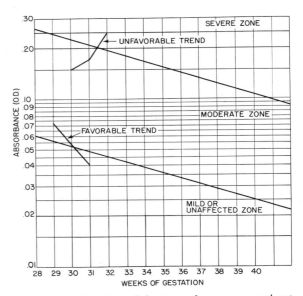

Figure 20-1. Relation of duration of pregnancy and net absorbance of amniotic fluid at 450 nm. Serial spectrophotometric scans at weekly intervals may show increasing, stationary, decreasing, or variable net absorbances.

the result of a physiologic dilution of bilirubin in the amniotic fluid in the last trimester of pregnancy. Thus, a measured net absorbance early in gestation predicts a better outcome than the same net absorbance value at a later date. Accurate dating of gestation is essential for proper interpretation.

Procedure. Approximately 5 ml of amniotic fluid is collected by the obstetrician when he considers the maternal Rh antibody titer critical, i.e., when a stillbirth or severely affected infant is anticipated (Freda, 1966a). "Critical" usually means an antibody titer of 1:16 ($\pm$1 dilution) or higher in the antiglobulin phase of the indirect antiglobulin Coomb's test. The specimen is sent in an opaque container (bilirubin is light sensitive) to a clinical pathology laboratory, where it is centrifuged in the dark at 4000 rpm for 10 minutes. An additional filtration (in the dark) through Whatman No. 4 filter paper is occasionally necessary to remove turbidity. If erythrocytes are present, the sediment can be submitted to the blood bank and hematology laboratories, where the cells are identified as maternal or fetal. Specimens may be mailed to reference laboratories for analysis provided they are sterile, centrifuged or filtered before shipment, and sent in opaque containers.

A spectral absorption curve of clear amniotic fluid is made with a calibrated narrow-band-width recording spectrophotometer against a distilled water blank. The absolute absorbance (optical density, or O.D.) is recorded from the scan at three points:

   1. 365 nm: O.D. = x
   2. 450 nm: O.D. = y
   3. 550 nm: O.D. = z

The absorbance values at 365 nm and 550 nm are transferred from the original linear scan recording (Fig. 20-2) to semilog scale (ordinate, O.D. in log scale; abscissa, wavelength in linear scale), and a straight line is drawn between x and z (Fig. 20-3). If the transfer of the linear scan points to semilog paper is not performed, results are inaccurate (Nelson, 1969). The "expected" O.D., or absorbance, is the point on the drawn line that intersects with the 450 nm wavelength. This drawn line represents

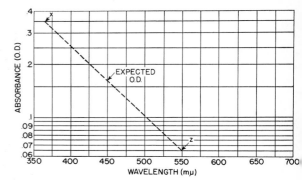

Figure 20-3. Scan shown in Figure 20-2 following transcription to semilog scale. Difference between point y (actual absorbance in Figure 20-2) and expected O.D. is the net absorbance at 450 nm.

the background absorbance of the normal (non-bilirubin-containing) amniotic fluid. Point y on the original scan is the "true O.D.," the sum of the absorbances of the amniotic fluid plus the absorbance contributed by bilirubin. Therefore, true O.D. at 450 nm − expected O.D. at 450 nm = net O.D. at 450 nm. The net O.D. is the absorbance contributed by bilirubin alone.

An assessment of fetal prognosis (based on net O.D.) is reported (Liley, 1963). A statement regarding current fetal well-being or jeopardy may also be reported (Freda, 1966b). A general discussion of both methods follows.

Interpretation of Spectrophotometric Tracings. The method of Liley is representative of a predictive type of interpretation. Its reliability and accuracy have been confirmed by considerable experience in many laboratories. Liley initially subdivided Rh-immunized mothers into three groups (Fig. 20-1):

1. Small net O.D. at 450 nm. These infants were either mildly affected or unaffected by hemolytic disease and required no transfusion.

2. Moderate net O.D. at 450 nm. These infants survived but often required one or more exchange transfusions.

3. Large net O.D. at 450 nm. These infants had grave prognoses. This zone included most stillbirths and neonatal deaths that occurred despite exchange transfusion.

Subsequently, Liley (1963) subdivided the moderate zone into two parts. A net O.D. at 450 nm within the upper half of the moderate zone usually is followed by equal or higher values on subsequent analyses. This indicates increasing hemolysis with lengthening gestation. Values in the lower half often decrease with time, indicating steady or decreasing hemolysis. The severe zone was also subdi-

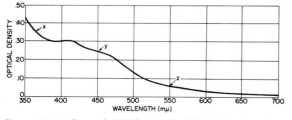

Figure 20-2. Scan of slightly jaundiced fluid showing three points used in determining net absorbance at 450 nm.

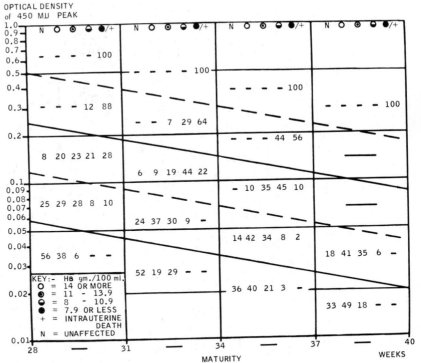

Figure 20-4. Liley prediction table showing the likelihood that a given net O.D. at a given week of gestation will estimate a cord hemoglobin concentration. (From Liley, A. W.: Am. J. Obstet. Gynecol., *86*:485, 1963.)

vided into a lower and upper (very severe) zone (Fig. 20-4).

Multiple scans beginning at 24 weeks are used to follow the trend of hemolytic disease. If an abnormal scan is obtained initially, subsequent scans may show a reduction in severity (below that which would be expected from the diagonally sloped lines of Liley's graph). Such a favorable trend is especially apt to occur when an infant is only mildly affected. An unfavorable (upward) or stationary (horizontal) trend is seen with increased hemolysis (Fig. 20-1). Trends are not always unidirectional. They may graphically change slope or even reverse direction. Trends are used to determine when to reassess the amniotic fluid scan or to decide when to induce labor. A clinical algorithm based on Liley's method has been developed by A.C.O.G. (*American College of Obstetrics and Gynecology*, 1972).

Predictions of the severity of anemia are valid if the infant is delivered within one week following amniocentesis. Prematurity complicates the predicted outcome of the pregnancy that is based on the severity of anemia. In other words, an infant that should do well on the basis of adequate cord blood hemoglobin could do poorly because of its immaturity at the time of delivery.

Thus, the Liley method does not incorporate the risk of prematurity in predicting fetal survival but simply distinguishes unaffected or mildly affected infants from those who are so severely affected that early delivery affords the only means of infant salvage, despite the risks of prematurity.

Instead of predicting the severity of the hemolytic disease of the newborn, it is possible to correlate spectrophotometric analysis of amniotic fluid with the general condition of the fetus, i.e., fetal well-being or jeopardy (Freda, 1965). This correlation acknowledges the dangers of early delivery and possible prematurity. Thus, spectrophotometric curves of amniotic fluid indicate the chances for survival of the fetus *in utero* for a given time period after amniocentesis at any age of gestation. Such curves permit the obstetrician to judge and compare the fetal status against chances for survival of the infant, if it is delivered during this time period. Survival is largely dependent on the maturity of the fetal lungs, which can be assessed by amniotic fluid phospholipid analysis (pp. 701-704).

Two shortcomings may be noted in using Freda's management method. First, repeated amniocenteses, with their small but definite obstetrical risks, are usually necessary, since

Grading of Abnormal Tracing	Optical Density Difference at 450 mμ
1+	0–0.2
2+	0.2 –0.35
3+	0.35–0.7
4+	0.7 and greater

Figure 20–5. Freda management table. 1+, Fetus unaffected or mildly affected with hemolysis at time of amniocentesis. 2+, Fetus affected but not in jeopardy. 3+, Fetus in distress. 4+, Impending fetal demise. (From Freda, V. J.: Antepartum management of the Rh problem. Progr. Hematol., 5:266, 1966.)

the given "safe" time periods are brief (one to two weeks). Second, despite the advantage of setting a parameter for obstetrical management (i.e., whether to deliver the child or allow the pregnancy to continue), Freda's method does not make a prediction of severity of disease in terms of cord hemoglobin or number of newborn transfusions required. It is quite disconcerting for the pediatrician caring for a severely jaundiced and anemic newborn requiring four or five exchange transfusions to recall a scan interpreted previously by the clinical pathologist or obstetrician as being only slightly to moderately abnormal (Robertson, 1969).

Liley's predictive and Freda's management methods of reporting may be used together, allowing for obstetric management *and* antenatal prediction of the severity of hemolytic disease in the newborn (Figs. 20–5 and 20–7). If the same amniotic fluid sample is also analyzed for lipid content, the state of fetal pulmonary maturity can be assessed, and the probability of respiratory distress can be predicted, if delivery is unavoidable.

A series of representative tracings is shown to illustrate various possible interpretations.

1. Normal filtered amniotic fluid is colorless to the naked eye. When a specimen is scanned on a recording spectrophotometer between 350 and 700 nm, a curve is obtained which relates a decrease in absorbance (O.D.) to increasing wavelength in the visible range. The curve is flat in the red (700 nm) range of the spectrum but then becomes steeper toward the violet (short, 350 nm) range (Fig. 20–6). A normal scan indicates either that the fetus is not afflicted with hemolytic disease or that it is mildly affected but is in no danger for the two weeks following the amniocentesis (Freda, 1966b). Cord hemoglobin, if the infant was delivered within a week, could be predicted according to the percentage probability given by Liley (Fig. 20–4).

2. A slightly abnormal tracing indicates a mildly affected fetus at the time of amniocentesis; this may regress to a normal curve or may progress to a more abnormal curve in 10 days' time. The curve is characterized by an increase in absorbance above the normal scan between 375 nm and 525 nm, with the peak of the increase occurring at approximately 450 nm.

3. Moderately abnormal tracings (Fig. 20–7) show greater increase in absorbance between 375 nm and 525 nm. As in the slightly abnormal tracing, peak absorbance occurs at 450 nm. The latter wavelength bisects the abnormal "bulge" in the curve. A moderately abnormal tracing usually indicates mild to moderate hemolytic disease, but severe disease is not uncommon. If the disease is severe, it is safe to allow the fetus to mature for up to one week (when the tracing is repeated), or the infant is delivered if it is sufficiently mature (i.e., pulmonary surfactants are sufficient to prevent atelectasis). If a repeat tracing in one week

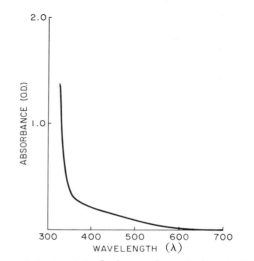

Figure 20–6. Amniotic fluid, normal scan (redrawn). Absolute (not net) absorbance vs. wavelength.

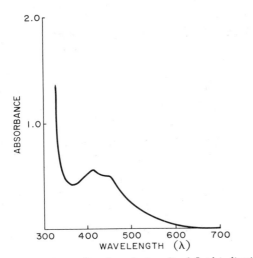

Figure 20-7. Scan of moderately jaundiced fluid indicative of hemolytic disease.

shows an unfavorable trend, either delivery or intrauterine transfusion may be warranted. Working criteria for fetal transfusion have been developed for the methods of Liley and Freda (Wade, 1969; A.C.O.G., 1972).

4. Markedly abnormal tracings show very large pigment "bulges" with net absorbances at 450 nm ranging from 0.35 to over 1.00 (3+ and 4+ of Freda). The most severely abnormal curves still retain the increased absorbance range of 375 nm to 525 nm, but the peak absorbance is shifted from 450 nm to a lower wavelength. This shift indicates a decrease in the pH of the amniotic fluid (normal pH 7.2), which is a sign of fetal death or impending death.

With markedly abnormal curves, owing either to bilirubin pigmentation or to staining by other pigments or meconium, the readings at 375 nm, 450 nm, and 550 nm may be off scale (i.e., absorbance is too high for the spectrophotometer to record). A several-fold dilution with distilled water may be necessary to obtain the net O.D. at 450 nm. Correction for this dilution is made by calculation.

5. Bloody amniotic fluid usually results from trauma to maternal tissues. Occasionally a placental vessel of the fetal circulation is lacerated. Erythrocytes that escape into the amniotic fluid may be identified as fetal by antiglobulin technique, Rh typing, and the Betke-Kleihauer blood film for detecting fetal hemoglobin (Betke, 1958). Identification of such fetal cells is important for three reasons. First, a second source of blood loss is established in a fetus that already has a compromising anemia. Anemia itself may be associated with hypoxic jaundice and kernicterus even with low bilirubin levels (Gartner, 1965). Secondly, it may also explain a sudden rise in maternal antibody response and increased rate of fetal hemolysis if the fetus bleeds into the maternal circulation. We have observed multiple additional antibodies arising during the third trimester. Therefore, it is wise to screen the maternal serum for qualitative (atypical) and quantitative (titer) changes in antibodies at the time of each amniocentesis. The value of this procedure is that it permits the blood bank to anticipate problems in finding compatible blood for exchange transfusion or obstetrical blood loss. Third, escape of fetal plasma into amniotic fluid augments abnormal tracings, since the circulating plasma bilirubin of even mildly affected infants is often high.

Maternal blood also distorts the normal tracing, but the scan may be interpreted unless the cell/total fluid-volume ratio of the specimen is 0.05 or more. If this ratio is exceeded, hemolysis is usually sufficient to obscure the bilirubin absorbance peak at 450 nm. (See supplementary techniques below.) The amniotic fluid curve is also distorted by maternal plasma contamination with moderate intra-amniotic maternal bleeding. A second clear sample can sometimes be obtained following minor bleeding, immediately after the bloody tap but before diffusion has occurred in

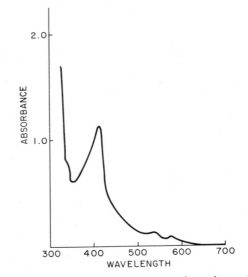

Figure 20-8. Bloody amniocentesis, moderate hemorrhage with hemolysis (no jaundice). Scan of filtered amniotic fluid.

the amniotic sac. A major hemorrhage requires about two weeks to clear the amniotic fluid. Major bleeding, with lysis of erythrocytes and release of hemoglobin, shows the three characteristic peaks of oxyhemoglobin at 415 nm, 540 nm, and 575 nm (Fig. 20-8). Minor bleeding may show only the Soret band at 415 nm. Generally the presence of these pigments decreases net absorbance at 450 nm, causing underestimation of fetal disease. (See supplementary techniques.)

6. Meconium staining of the amniotic fluid sample indicates fetal distress; it may accompany hemolytic disease, it may be related to complications of the anemia, or it may be associated with some other condition. In small quantities meconium may be identified spectrophotometrically; beginning at the red end of the spectrum, the tracing parallels that of normal amniotic fluid until about 525 nm, where it rises steadily above the baseline and reaches a peak absorbance at 405 to 410 nm. The absorbance then slowly recedes and does not return to the baseline at 350 to 375 nm (Fig. 20-9). Larger quantities of meconium are easily identified grossly by the turbid, dark green-black color; however, underlying hemolytic disease is obscured. The problem of distinguishing pigments is not easily solved in the laboratory because meconium contains bilirubin (conjugated and unconjugated). Chloroform extraction of fluid stained by pigment of either meconial or hemolytic origin shows bilirubin pigmentation (Fig. 20-10A). The resolution of the problem is obtained clinically: me-

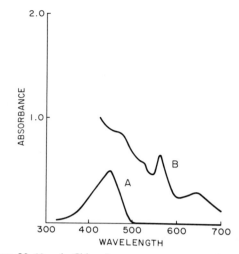

Figure 20-10. *A,* Chloroform extraction of amniotic fluid containing bilirubin. This curve may be observed after extracting amniotic fluid from a case of hemolytic disease or from fluid containing meconium. *B,* Hemochromogen complex of methemalbumin. Schumm test.

conium staining early in gestation is usually not caused by, or associated with, hemolytic disease and usually clears as term approaches. Staining near term, however, regardless of cause, is an indication for prompt delivery (Liley, 1963).

7. Occasionally, in a severely affected infant, in addition to a markedly abnormal tracing, an additional peak is observed at about 620 nm. This is the absorbance peak of methemalbumin. This pigment can be better identified by modification of Schumm's test (Fig. 20-10B).

Schumm's test involves overlaying 2.0 ml amniotic fluid with 2.0 ml ether, to which is added 0.2 ml saturated solution of $(NH_4)_2SO_4$. After mixing, the fluid layer is scanned with a recording spectrophotometer. In addition to the methemalbumin band at 620 nm, some of the methemalbumin is complexed, producing a hemochromogen peak at 558 nm. Presence of methemalbumin indicates massive hemolysis of long duration, depletion of haptoglobin, and a fetus that is either dead or dying.

8. The clinical pathologist should bear in mind that the obstetrician who performs amniocentesis may have technical problems in obtaining fluid when the placenta and fetus are difficult to localize or when the infant is hydropic. Under these circumstances, the fluid submitted to the laboratory may not be amniotic in origin. Thus, fetal ascitic fluid, fluid

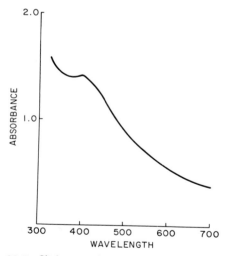

Figure 20-9. Slight to moderate meconium staining. Scan of amniotic fluid.

from the amnion of an unaffected or affected fraternal twin, amniotic cyst (chorionic bleb) fluid, and urine from the maternal urinary bladder may be aspirated. The most common non-amniotic fluid obtained is maternal urine. The spectrophotometric tracing is similar to normal amniotic fluid, except that there is a much steeper slope to the curve. Normal maternal urine may be distinguished from amniotic fluid by urea nitrogen measurement. Urine urea nitrogen should approximate a concentration of 300 mg/dl, or higher; amniotic fluid urea nitrogen averages about 30 mg/dl.

A simple bedside means of distinguishing maternal urine from amniotic fluid is as follows: a protein-glucose dipstick is positive for both solutes when wetted with amniotic fluid, but negative when wetted with urine unless there is maternal diabetes and renal disease (Pirani, 1976). Such testing should be confirmed by urea (or creatinine) analysis. (This dipstick test is also useful as a bedside procedure to determine whether a patient in labor has ruptured membranes or urinary incontinence.) Creatinine analysis is discussed subsequently.

Quality control of amniotic fluid spectrophotometry is achieved by regular wavelength and absorbance calibration of the spectrophotometer, matching of cuvettes, and rapid processing of properly stored, clear specimens. The instability of bilirubin solutions requires a control material to check instrumental response. An aqueous solution of 8-hydroxyquinoline has been suggested for this purpose (Hamlin, 1976).

SUPPLEMENTARY TECHNIQUES IN HEMOLYTIC DISEASE USING AMNIOTIC FLUID

Criteria have been suggested for obstetric decisions, e.g., when to perform first and subsequent amniocenteses, when to deliver, and when to attempt fetal transfusion. Management has usually been based on the concepts of Liley and Freda, which prove clinically satisfactory in over 95 per cent of patients (Robertson, 1969). As an alternative, a diazo chemical determination of bilirubin can be performed by the sensitive Jendrassik-Grof method (Gambino, 1966). Bilirubin concentration may be converted to net absorbance for use with the Liley prediction table (Kapitulnik, 1970). Bilirubin measurements by such

chemical methods yield less information (e.g., non-bilirubin pigments will not be detected), but can be used as a backup method or when recording spectrophotometry is not available.

A major difficulty in the laboratory is contamination of aspirated fluid by blood pigments which obscure the bilirubin peak on spectrophotometric scan. Methods that extract and measure bilirubin by direct spectrophotometry are less precise and may not yield 100 per cent recovery, but are sufficiently accurate to be of clinical value (Hochberg, 1976).

Extraction Procedure. To a 3.0 ml volume of clear amniotic fluid showing hemolysis, add an equal volume of chloroform. Vortex for 30 seconds. Centrifuge for five minutes at 3000 rpm and remove the chloroform (bottom) layer. Perform recording spectrophotometry against a chloroform blank and interpret as in direct amniotic spectrophotometry.

Admittedly, neither spectrophotometric nor chemical methods are completely satisfactory. Variation in laboratory technique can produce variable obstetric decisions. Specimens may be exposed to light, change in pH, or contain interfering pigments. There are differences in instruments, calibration, and methods. Varying dilution occurs in fluids of different patients at different gestational ages. The success of current methods is directly attributable to the coupling of vigorous clinical management and laboratory monitoring via repeated amniocenteses.

ESTIMATION OF FETAL PULMONARY MATURITY

Immature fetal lungs secrete the phospholipids lecithin and sphingomyelin in about equal concentrations. The major surfactant, dipalmitoyl lecithin (phosphatidyl choline) enables pulmonary alveoli to expand when the newborn first inspires air instead of fluid. If the fetus is immature, there is insufficient lecithin production via its major biochemical synthetic pathway (phosphocholine transferase). This normally matures at about 34 to 36 weeks (females about a week earlier than males). Maturation is thought to be partially dependent on glucocorticoid production by the fetus (Sharp-Cageorge, 1977). A hyperinsulinemic fetus responding to a hyperglycemic diabetic mother may inhibit its own cortisol production and thereby may delay adequate surfactant production (Robert, 1976). On the other hand, pregnant patients under stress and *some* diabetics cause *early* fetal pulmonary maturation. Fetal pulmonary maturation can also be induced early by administration of steroids to the mother (Liggins, 1972). Response often occurs within 2 to 4 days.

Low surfactant production is associated with the respiratory distress syndrome (RDS) of the newborn (Forman, 1973). *In utero*, there is continuity of the fluid in the unexpanded fetal pulmonary alveoli and the amniotic space. Lecithin and sphingomyelin diffuse from the lungs into the amniotic sac in about equal concentrations (1.0 ratio) when the lungs are immature. Some lecithin is produced via an alternate biochemical synthetic pathway (methyl transferase pathway produces phosphatidyl dimethylethanolamine). Both pathways are probably sensitive to endocrine imbalance and injury, resulting in a decrease in lecithin concentration.

Since the actual measurement of lecithin concentration in amniotic fluid involves a long, complicated procedure, a thin-layer chromatographic procedure was developed for clinical purposes (Gluck, 1971). This technique permits a rapid comparison of the *relative* amniotic fluid concentrations of lecithin and sphingomyelin. A mature pattern is a ratio of 2.0 or greater. Increased ratios result primarily from increased lecithin synthesis, while sphingomyelin concentration remains unchanged or slightly declines toward term, as normal dilution occurs in amniotic fluid in the last weeks of gestation. A mature pattern indicates that delivery may be accomplished with practically no risk of respiratory distress in the newborn. An intermediate ratio of greater than 1.5 but less than 2.0 usually indicates that the process of pulmonary maturation has begun; the process may be completed in a few days, but sometimes requires a week or more.

The lecithin/sphingomyelin (L/S) ratio analysis of amniotic fluid has become a common procedure. It helps determine the optimal time for early obstetrical intervention in cases of fetal jeopardy caused by isoimmunization syndrome, dysmaturity, toxemia, maternal diabetes, or other disease; it helps to determine when to carry out a planned Cesarean section; and it helps to estimate the age of gestation when historical information is questionable or unknown. Many variations of the original method of Gluck (1973) have been described. Gas chromatography, fluorescence polarization, surface tension, and chemical measurement of lecithin, palmitic acid, and other lipids have been reported. A bedside "shake test," in which bubble stability is related to surfactant presence is merited only when a more precise laboratory method is not available (Clements, 1972). Most tests can be used successfully, but all can suffer inaccuracy caused by the introduction of red blood cells into the fluid at amniocentesis and improper processing of the specimen. There is also an element of error in semiquantitative, poorly controlled, manual thin-layer chromatographic procedures.

Specimens with a hematocrit of over 1 per cent yield unreliable results and falsely lowered L/S values even when there is no visible hemolysis and when the red cells are removed (Badham, 1975). Hemolyzed samples should also be interpreted with great caution, particularly in borderline mature cases. This is because the L/S ratio of plasma is about 2.0. Obviously mature ratios of 3.0 or more may still be useful in the presence of small amounts of blood or hemolyzed blood contaminants.

Despite the problem of red cell contamination, large series of high-risk obstetric patients confirm that L/S ratios of over 2.0 are *not* associated with life-threatening RDS in 95 per cent of cases. Ratios of less than 2.0 *may* be associated with severe RDS in about 25 per cent of cases (Aubrey, 1976).

A second possible source of error is related to the recent observation that 75 to 90 per cent of fetal lecithin of pulmonary origin is found in the cell debris in the amniotic fluid (Abramovitch, 1975). Therefore, it is possible that extraction for L/S study is best carried out on uncentrifuged, unfiltered fluid. Until comprehensive clinical correlations of outcome and L/S ratios are detailed, it would seem prudent to follow Gluck's original recommendation of recentrifugation prior to analysis.

If spectrophotometric analysis is to be performed, removal of turbidity (which increases after 33 weeks gestation) *must* be accomplished first.

Another possible error is introduced by water-soluble dye used in amniography, a radiologic technique used to visualize the fetus. This dye will falsely increase the L/S ratio (Know, 1977). Finally, abnormal pregnancy reduces the accuracy of predicting maturity as well (Morrison, 1976).

Until the advent of fetal pulmonary maturity estimates in isoimmunization cases, the perinatologist was often faced with a dilemma: avoiding the potential complications of fetal disease (such as hemolysis and congestive heart failure) by deciding to deliver the infant vs. avoiding the risks of premature delivery (RDS of the newborn). The dilemma can now be resolved in most cases by decisions to deliver the fetus based on the L/S ratio.

PROCEDURE FOR L/S RATIO

Reference method (Gluck, 1971)

1. Centrifuge 2.0 ml of amniotic fluid at 6000 rpm for 5 minutes.
2. Separate the supernatant into a conical tube and mix with an equal volume of absolute methanol. Vortex.
3. Add a volume of chloroform equal to the volume of the mixture of liquids. Vortex. Centrifuge and remove the lower chloroform layer.
4. Evaporate to dryness under nitrogen at 60° C. Keep all residue at the tip of the conical tube. Dissolve residue in 10 μl. of chloroform.
5. Put the tube in an ice bath. Add dropwise 1.0 ml of anhydrous acetone. Wait 30 minutes. Centrifuge at 3000 rpm for 2 minutes.
6. Pour off the acetone and blot to remove all acetone. Dissolve the precipitate in 15 μl of chloroform and apply to Silica gel H plates along with standards and controls.
7. Develop using solvent containing 130 ml chloroform, 50 ml methanol, and 8 ml water.
8. Air dry, and spray under a hood with 50% H_2SO_4. Char on a hotplate. Lecithin migrates a greater distance than sphingomyelin; both appear as discrete spots.
9. Interpret cautiously by visual estimation, planimetry, or densitometry (Olson, 1974). See Figure 20–11A.

Rapid method (Gelman Instrument Company, Ann Arbor, Michigan. Modified by J. Lustgarten, Ph.D.)

1. Pipet 1.0 ml of centrifuged amniotic fluid into a 13 × 100 mm screw cap test tube.

2. Add 1.0 ml methanol, cap, mix well, but do not shake.
3. Add 2.0 ml chloroform, cap, invert 12 times *gently*.
4. Centrifuge at 2000 rpm for 10 minutes. Three layers form.
5. Transfer all of the chloroform extract (bottom layer) to a conical evaporating tube using a disposable Pasteur pipet. Avoid disturbing the upper aqueous and middle protein layers.
6. Evaporate to dryness using a 50° C. bath and air stream.
7. Cool the tube, add 30 μl of chloroform, swirl, and dissolve the residue.
8. Apply 10 μl of extract to Seprachrom silicic acid glass fiber (Gelman Instrument Company, Ann Arbor, Michigan).
9. Apply standards containing 1:1, 2:1, and 3:1 lecithin:sphingomyelin ratios. Dry in air for 10 minutes.
10. Develop the chromatogram using a solvent phase containing 79.1% dichloromethane, 18.6% ethanol, and 2.3% water (v/v). Development requires 3.5 minutes.
11. Remove the chromatogram; dry for 10 minutes in air. Under a hood, spray with phospholipid detection reagent (28.6% H_2SO_4, 1-5% molybdenum trioxide, and 0.05% molybdenum (w/v).
12. Visualization of spots shows blue phospholipids against a green-blue background. Air dry for 3 minutes and expose to acetone (450 ml in a 600 ml beaker) by standing the chromatogram upright. This diminishes background color.
13. Ratios are read by eye against the three standards. Control fluids should be run and the patient's sample may be run in duplicate (Fig. 20–11B).

Interpretation

Visual interpretation is usually sufficient when considered with other clinical information, but densitometric quantitation may be utilized (Olsen, 1974).

VISIBLE RESULT	QUANTITATIVE RESULT	INTERPRETATION
1. Sphingomyelin quantity equal to or greater than lecithin	L/S ratio equal to or less than 1.0	Immature lung; RDS (respiratory distress syndrome) probable, severe
2. Lecithin spot slightly larger than sphingomyelin	L/S 1.5 to 1.9	Intermediate lung; RDS probable; infant recovery probable
3. Lecithin spot clearly larger than sphingomyelin	L/S 2.0 to 3.4	Mature lung; no RDS expected
4. Lecithin spot large. Sphingomyelin barely visible or invisible	L/S 3.5	Mature lung a certainty
5. Lecithin spot very large with sphingomyelin spot invisible	L/S greater than 4.0	Postmature

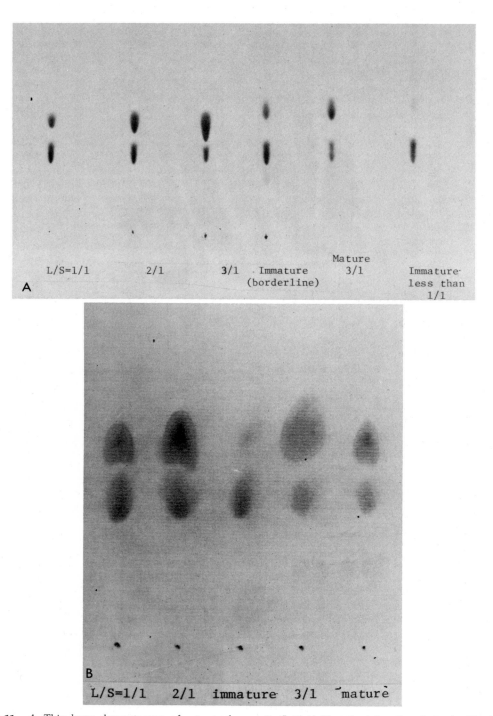

Figure 20–11. *A*, Thin layer chromatogram of extract of amniotic fluid (A.F.) stained for phospholipids. The lecithin/sphingomyelin (L/S) ratios (left to right) are: 1:1 (immature fetal lung), 2:1 (mature fetal lung), 3:1 (mature fetal lung), 0.5:1 (immature fetal lung), 3:1 (mature fetal lung), and less than 1:1 (immature fetal lung). *B*, Thin layer L/S chromatogram, rapid method (see text). Ratios read (left to right) 1:1 (standard), 2:1 (standard), less than 1:1 (immature A.F. pattern), 3:1 (standard), 2:1 (mature A.F. pattern).

ASSESSMENT OF FETAL SIZE AND GESTATIONAL AGE

During the first half of pregnancy, amniotic fluid volume is proportional to fetal weight and is comparable to fetal extracellular fluid in constitution. After 20 weeks, however, the fluid becomes dilute (Lind, 1969). Only a few amniotic metabolites consistently increase their concentrations for the duration of pregnancy. One measure of gestational age is creatinine, which increases in concentration to 1.8 mg/dl by 36 weeks (90th percentile) and to 2.0 mg/dl by 37 weeks. Creatinine concentration correlates with fetal muscle mass and fetal renal concentrating ability. Values less than 1.5 mg/dl are the rule when the fetus is immature; values greater than 2.0 mg/dl indicate definite maturity (Begneaud, 1969). Uric acid determinations may also be of value to assess fetal maturity (Wolf, 1970). Elevations of either uric acid or creatinine concentration in maternal plasma (renal disease, toxemia, hypertension) also increase amniotic fluid concentrations, and diminish the accuracy of the estimate.

The bilirubin scan according to Liley's method has also been correlated with fetal maturity. A net O.D. at 450 nm of 0.02 or less is associated with fetal gestation of more than 36 weeks, in normal pregnancies.

Amniotic cytology with Nile blue sulfate may be of some help in estimating gestational age. There is a rapid increase in the number of anucleate, orangeophilic cells after 35 weeks from a level of about 15 per cent or less to 30 per cent or more. Clumps of orangeophilic bodies indicate 38 weeks' gestation (White, 1969). Claims that cytologic evaluations are the most accurate tests of fetal maturity require further verification (Morrison, 1974).

FETAL HYPOTHYROIDISM

Fetal hypothyroidism (cretinism) is the result of biochemically defective synthesis of thyroxine (dyshormonogenesis). Separate enzymatic defects are recognized in iodide trapping, organification, coupling, iodoprotein release, and dehalogenase activity. Fetal cellular metabolism is regulated by reverse (R) triiodothyronine (T_3) rather than T_3 which is the adult product of T_4 (thyroxine) metabolism. The fetal hormone is 3,3',5'-triiodothyronine. RT_3 is found in very low concentrations in adult serum. Since maternal T_3 and T_4 do not readily cross the placenta, the amniotic fluid may serve as a convenient fluid from which fetal thyroid hormone can be sampled. RT_3 analysis may then serve to diagnose hyper- or hypothyroidism *in utero* (Chopra, 1975). Experience has shown that after 15 weeks of gestation, RT_3 measurement is sufficiently sensitive and accurate to diagnose hypothyroidism. Early diagnosis is important because development of the fetal brain during the last eight weeks of pregnancy is dependent on thyroid hormone. Prenatal treatment can be instituted and permanent psychophysical retardation may be prevented. Amniotic fluid RT_3 measurements are indicated in cases in which family histories suggest familial cretinism.* Screening of the population for decreased RT_3 in amniotic fluid appears to be cost effective if the incidence of sporadic cretinism is greater than one case in 5,000 or 10,000 births.

DIAGNOSIS OF NEURAL TUBE DEFECTS

Alpha-fetoprotein (AFP) is elevated in amniotic fluid when the fetus suffers failure of closure of the neural tube. AFP, which can be quantitated by immunoprecipitin and radioimmunoassay techniques, is abnormal after 14 weeks' gestation in cases of fetal myelocele, anencephaly (90 per cent positive), spina bifida (50 per cent positive), and similar neuro-ectodermal disorders (Brock, 1972; Allan, 1973). The more open the defect, the more likely the AFP will be abnormal. AFP is similarly increased in duodenal atresia, congenital nephrosis, omphalocele, tetralogy of Fallot, and Turner's syndrome. The association of each of these non-neural tube anomalies with increased AFP is not as well documented as the neural tube association. The normally low concentrations of amniotic AFP derive from low clearance of AFP from fetal serum via renal excretion into the fetal urine. Any trauma causing fetal bleeding into the amniotic space elevates AFP concentrations. (Bleeding may produce a false positive test for a fetal anomaly.) Suspected fetal bleeding into the amniotic fluid may be confirmed by Kleihauer staining, but is best avoided by carefully localizing the placenta. There is an additional 0.1 to 1.0 per cent false positive AFP test rate caused by twinning, various maternal diseases, and unknown factors. The non-specificity of the test indicates a cautious approach to diagnosis of possible abnormalities. Gross

---

*Reverse T3 (RT3), 3,3',5'-triiodothyronine measurement by radioimmunoassay of amniotic fluid serves as an estimate of fetal thyroid function. RT3 is probably manufactured by the fetal gland, is usually very low in concentration in maternal serum, and, like T3 and T4, probably does not cross the placenta. Therefore, amniotic fluid RT3 measurements reflect fetal thyroid output even though RT3 is not calorigenic.

anomalies, such as anencephaly, should be confirmed by ultrasound and amniographic procedures.

Because AFP has potential uncontrolled, widespread use as a tumor marker in cases of adult hepatomas and various germ cell tumors, the U.S. Food and Drug Administration will not license commercial AFP reagents until their efficacy is documented. Thus, AFP is not universally available as a test for fetal disease.

INTESTINAL OBSTRUCTION

Congenital lower intestinal obstruction, such as intestinal atresia or imperforate anus, may be detected antenatally by observing an absence of normal disaccharidases from amniotic fluid. Normally, maltase, lactase, sucrase, and other oligosaccharidases are excreted by the fetal intestine into the fluid up to 20 weeks of gestation. Therefore, amniocentesis is performed prior to 18 weeks; after that time, enzyme activity rapidly decreases (Potier, 1977).

GENETIC DISORDERS AND AMNIOTIC FLUID

Amniotic fluid can provide a sample of fetal cells from which fetal sex, blood group, karyotype, and biochemical information may be obtained. Despite the great promise of prenatal genetic diagnosis, a note of caution must be stated. For a variety of reasons, the prenatal search for hereditary diseases is often disappointing. The families at risk for some genetic disorder may be unavailable or they may refuse to cooperate; analytical methods are often complex, expensive, and sometimes inaccurate; few genetic diseases are treatable; and abortion may not be acceptable to the prospective parents.

For sex-linked disorders, determination of fetal sex may be performed by amniotic cytology. Cell study permits one to identify sex chromatin bodies (Barr bodies). A male fetus is presumed present when less than 25 cells in a count of 1000 possess the Barr body. The cells of amniotic fluid may be studied directly for sex chromatin without further culture (Fuchs, 1966), but confirmation should be obtained between 15 and 18 weeks' gestation if therapeutic abortion is to be safely undertaken by 24 weeks. Great care in techni-

cal methods is mandatory to prevent accidental culture of maternal cells (Littlefield, 1970).

Sex-linked disorders affect 50 per cent of male infants born to female carriers. Those which have been suspected *in utero* by amniotic cell analysis (and demonstrated following abortion and examination of the fetus) include Duchenne muscular dystrophy, Hunter's mucopolysaccharidosis, hemophilias A (factor VIII) and B (factor IX), Lesch-Nyhan hyperuricemia, Fabry's lipid storage disease, Lowe's nephropathic rickets, nephrogenic diabetes insipidus, Bruton's disease (hypogammaglobulinemia), and chronic granulomatous disease. It now appears possible to predict Duchenne muscular dystrophy by analysis of fetal blood obtained by placental sampling (see subsequent discussion).

Some chromosome abnormalities are identifiable by amniotic cell culture and karyotyping. These must be performed in laboratories which are highly proficient in these techniques. Pregnant women who are over 35 years old should be evaluated critically for trisomies 21, 13-15, and 18 and aneuploidies 47XO, 47XXY, 47XXX, and 47XYY. Screening should also be attempted when one parent is a carrier of translocations C/E, G/G, D/G, and 21/22-familial mongolisms (Milunsky, 1970). Viral and radiation-induced chromosome defects are also detectable antenatally in some cases (Nadler and Gerbie, 1970). The reader is referred to Chapter 26 for further information.

AMNIOTIC FLUID AND FETAL INFECTION

Rapid serologic methods for diagnosis of suspected fetal viral infection have not been fruitful when applied to amniotic fluid. However, cell culture of the fluid has allowed recovery and diagnosis of cytomegalovirus (David, 1971) and rubella (Levin, 1974) while radioimmunoassay (RIA) has produced occasional evidence of fetal infection with hepatitis B. False negatives are known to occur in both viral culture and RIA techniques. False positives have been reported for cell culture viral isolations. Much more development is necessary in the area of diagnosis of fetal viral disease from amniotic fluid analysis.

Bacterial infections commonly affect the amniotic space following rupture of membranes, but rarely before. Residual fluid may be examined microscopically for neutrophils and bacteria using Wright's and Gram's stains. More than one neutrophil per high power field ($450\times$) is considered a positive test, since such neutrophilia is associated with subsequent maternal fever and possible fetal infection, particularly when there is Cesarean section. Culture of such fluid yields a variety of aerobes and anaerobes, often in mixed culture. Gram-positive species commonly include *Streptococcus* and *Staphylococcus* and anaerobic cocci (*Peptococcus* and *Streptococcus*). Gram-negative organisms include coliforms and anaerobes of the *Bacteroides* and *Clostridium* groups (Larsen, 1976). Postpartum infection is increased in women who have ruptured membranes for over eight hours, prolonged labor, and multiple vaginal examinations during labor (Lewis, 1975).

Determining Amniotic Sac Rupture. Ruptured membranes increase the risk of infection, and it may be difficult to decide on clinical grounds if rupture has occurred. To identify released amniotic fluid, appropriate vaginal fluid specimens should be subjected to Papanicolaou staining and cytologic evaluation. If the Pap stain cannot be performed, a combination of history, alkaline pH (7.0 or greater), and positive crystallization test (amniotic fluid forms a treelike branching pattern when a glass slide smear is air dried) are sufficient (Friedman, 1969). A positive dipstick analysis for glucose and protein can also serve to identify amniotic fluid and differentiate it from urine (Pirani, 1976).

NON-AMNIOTIC LABORATORY TESTS OF VALUE IN PERINATOLOGY

FETAL HEALTH AND FETOPLACENTAL FUNCTION

Low maternal estriol is associated with fetoplacental depression. A similar decrease in estriol may be seen in amniotic fluid (Aleem, 1969), but this determination is not usually performed.

The placenta and fetus are interdependent in the production of estriol. For example, the placenta contributes the major synthesized portion of pregnenolone to the fetus for conversion to 16-hydroxydehydroepiandrosterone, since the placenta lacks 16-alpha hydroxylase. Estriol depression indicates early fetoplacen-

tal malfunction (Brown, 1974). Placental reserve may be evaluated by measuring estriol following stimulation by intra-amniotic injection of dehydroepiandrosterone (Hausknecht, 1969) or by its intravenous administration to the mother.

It should be emphasized that amniotic fluid constituent measurements constitute only part of the modern approach to assess fetal well-being or fetal distress and that a variety of clinical (e.g., stress tests) and other laboratory tests exist for this purpose. Current laboratory tests include maternal urinary estrogens, maternal serum placental lactogen (HPL), and the dehydroepiandrosterone sulfate loading test (Tulchinsky, 1976).

A maternal urinary estriol may be helpful in evaluation of the function of the fetoplacental unit because estriol is its major secreted estrogen and is not much affected by maternal hepatic or renal disease. It is a reflection of an intact biochemical pathway that requires functional tissues in both the fetus and the placenta. Depending on the stage of pregnancy, the mother may contribute only 10 per cent of the estriol. This pathway includes the conversion of dehydroepiandrosterone sulfate, a major steroid of the fetal adrenal, to 16-alpha-hydroxydehydroepiandrosterone sulfate by fetal adrenal and liver. The hydroxylate is converted to estriol by placental sulfatase and aromatizing enzymes. The secretory rate of estriol is steady. Because there is evidence that fetal health can be restored (e.g., by maternal bed rest and correction of nutritional deficiencies and anemia), measurement of estriol production appears to be of value to detect and monitor the high-risk pregnancy.

The collection of urine over 24 hours is an especially difficult and frustrating procedure during pregnancy when a decision must be made to intervene in a high fetal risk situation. Therefore, plasma estriol assays are preferable to urine. Plasma sampling can be repeated every three to six hours and yields rapid confirmatory information. Plasma specimens also provide more values per unit time than urine collections, allowing better monitoring of adverse or favorable trends (Brown, 1974). Estriol is only one of the estrogens in maternal plasma, so that highly specific and sensitive assays must be applied (e.g., radioimmunoassays). These methods are currently expensive and difficult to maintain as daily stand-by or emergency measurements.

Human placental lactogen (HPL) or its synonym, human chorionic somatomammotropin (HCS), is a short-lived, low molecular weight maternal peptide hormone constantly secreted by syncytiotrophoblastic cells of the placenta after five weeks of gestation. Serum values rise until about 38 weeks when they begin to decrease until term. HPL correlates with fetal or placental weight and is regarded primarily as a placental function test. Increased values are seen with twins. HPL measurements of less than 4 μg/ml of sera after the thirtieth week may be considered within a fetal danger zone, indicating a need for close monitoring of the pregnancy and possible obstetrical action (such as induction of labor). The sensitivity of the determination is poor if it is used as a screening test for neonatal compromise, and there are many false negative tests (Wenk, 1979). HPL is useful in predicting inevitable abortions. HPL is best measured by radioimmunoassay. Radial immunodiffusion procedures are not reliable.

PLACENTAL FUNCTION TESTS

Heat-stable alkaline phosphatase (HSAP) activity in maternal plasma has been advocated as a possible monitor of placental function. HSAP rises during pregnancy, particularly in the third trimester, and is produced by the syncytiotrophoblast. A very wide range of values in normal gestations and failure of values to correlate well with common placental disorders have not produced widespread confidence in this assay.

Slightly more promising is maternal plasma "oxytocinase" assay, which is reported to have better predictive value than HSAP; however, this aminopeptidase also shows great scatter of values in normal gestations. Increased values are noted in twinning. Decreased levels may indicate severe fetal growth retardation and postmaturity. Clinical value appears limited (Hensleigh, 1976).

FETAL BLOOD SAMPLING

Fetal tissues can now be sampled directly, allowing development of laboratory analyses for fetal disease. Perhaps the most promising development is the sampling of fetal blood for identification of qualitative hemoglobinopathies and thalassemias (Hobbins, 1974; A.C.O.G., 1976). Techniques have been re-

ported for approaching the fetus *in utero*, for *in vivo* identification of hemoglobin S, and for determining the synthesis rate of alpha and beta chains of hemoglobin (Kan, 1976).

Although it is less common than hemoglobinopathies, Duchenne muscular dystrophy also lends itself to effective prenatal diagnosis by virtue of its sex-linked, familial occurrence and the technique of fetal blood sampling. Fetal plasma creatine phosphokinase (CPK) activity appears to be markedly elevated in affected males. Thus, the combination of positive family history, determination of a male fetus by amniotic cell karyotyping (see above), and demonstration of increased fetal plasma CPK activity permits diagnosis. Fetal CPK estimation requires correction for maternal plasma and amniotic fluid enzyme activities and dilutions of the sample (Mahoney, 1977).

Currently the frequency of fetal loss secondary to blood sampling (fetoscopy or placental venipuncture) and false negative errors in diagnosis are too high to recommend such research procedures for routine clinical use (Alter, 1976).

On the other hand, during labor, capillaries of the presenting part (scalp) may be sampled to measure fetal pH and blood gases (Cohen, 1974). Measurements of pH and Po_2 give direct evidence of fetal acidosis and hypoxia (Saling, 1964). Hypoxia is a cause of late decelerations of the fetal heart (type II bradycardia) which is related, in time, to uterine con-

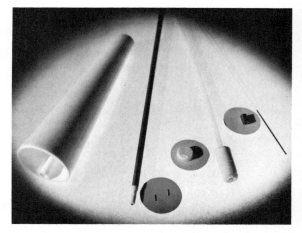

Figure 20–12. Intrapartum fetal blood sampling kit: *Left to right:* vaginal speculum, 2 mm deep safety scalpel for capillary sampling of presenting part, iron filings for mixing blood in capillary tube, putty sealant, tampon to stem bleeding following sampling, magnet for moving iron filing, long capillary tube partially filled with blood.

tractions and, in etiology, to placental insufficiency. The simple instrumentation required for obtaining such samples is shown in Figure 20–12.

RELATIONSHIP OF FETAL AND MATERNAL BLOOD pH AND GASES

The indications for intrapartum fetal capillary sampling are signs of fetal distress (passage of meconium, 30 seconds of bradycardia or tachycardia, late decelerations, repeated early decelerations of increasing depth and duration), maternal disease (toxemia, postmaturity, isoimmunization, diabetes, history of previous stillbirths, prolonged labor, dystocia), induction of labor, maternal use of alcohol or narcotics, and administration of anesthetics to the mothers.

Fetal capillary samples of blood are analyzed using ordinary micro pH, PCO_2, and PO_2 electrodes (Saling, 1964). The pH and PCO_2 measurements are the most useful clinically and are best interpreted when simultaneous maternal blood gas analysis is performed. Fetal PCO_2 is higher than maternal arterial blood by an average of 9 mm Hg. When maternal PCO_2 increases, fetal PCO_2 also increases. If the mother hyperventilates and decreases her PCO_2, fetal PCO_2 also decreases. Fetal reference values are 28 to 60 mm Hg, but values of less than 40 suggest admixture of blood with room air; i.e., invalid sampling. Despite wide fluctuations in maternal CO_2 tension, the difference between maternal and fetal levels tends to remain constant, provided that one recognizes a lag of about four minutes between maternal and fetal changes (Newman, 1967). Fetal capillary PCO_2 of over 60 mm Hg is abnormal. PCO_2 determinations permit calculation of base deficit when pH is known; the base deficit reflects fetal metabolic acidosis.

The pH is the single most critical measurement. Normal pH is 7.25 to 7.45. Values below 7.25 should be confirmed by repeat analysis (Lumley, 1971). Spurious results may occur owing to maternal acid-base imbalance, fetal scalp edema, specimen contamination with amniotic fluid, or improper instrument calibration. On verification, low pH is an indication for obstetrical intervention. Decrease in pH on repeat analysis to below 7.20 is a strong indication of fetal deterioration (James, 1976). Fetal blood sampling is increasing in popularity because of its clinical value and the few contraindications (maternal genital infection, potential bleeding disorder, laceration in face presentation) or complications (bleeding, infection).

REFERENCES

Abramovitch, D. R., Keeping, J. D., and Thom, H.: The origin of amniotic fluid lecithin. Br. J. Ob-Gyn, *82*:204, 1975.

Aleem, F., Neill, D., and Pinkerton, J.: A method for oestriol estimation in amniotic fluid and its use in the study of normal and abnormal pregnancy. Steroids, *13*:651, 1969.

Allan, L. D., Donald, I., Ferguson-Smith, M. A., Sweet, E. M., and Gibson, A. A. M.: Amniotic fluid alpha-fetoprotein in the antenatal diagnosis of spinal bifida. Lancet, *2*:522, 1973.

Alter, B. P., et al.: Prenatal diagnosis of hemoglobinopathies. N. Engl. J. Med., *295*:26, 1437, 1976.

A.C.O.G. Technical Bulletin No. 17: Management of erythroblastosis. Chicago, American College of Obstetricians and Gynecologists, 1972.

A.C.O.G. Technical Bulletin No. 42: Fetal blood sampling. Chicago, American College of Obstetricians and Gynecologists, 1976.

Aubrey, R. H., Rourke, J. E., Almanza, R., Cantor, R. M., and Vandoren, J. E.: The lecithin/sphingomyelin ratio in a high-risk obstetric population. Obstet. Gynecol., *47*:21, 1976.

Badham, L., and Worth, H. G. J.: Critical assessment of phospholipid measurement in amniotic fluid. Clin. Chem., *21*:1441, 1975.

Begneaud, W. P., Hawes, T. P., Mickal, A., and Samuels, M.: Amniotic fluid creatinine for prediction of fetal maturity. Obstet. Gynecol., *37*:7, 1969.

Beischer, N. A., Brown, J. B., and Townsend, L.: Studies in prolonged pregnancy. III Amniocentesis in prolonged pregnancy. Am. J. Obstet. Gynecol., *103*:496, 1969.

Betke, V. K., and Kleihauer, E.: Foetaler und bleibender Blutfarbstoff in Erythrocyten und Erythroblasten von menschlichen Feten und Neugeborenen. Blut Bank, *4*:241, 1958.

Bevis, D. C. A.: The antenatal prediction of hemolytic disease of the newborn. Lancet, *I*:395, 1952.

Brazie, J. V., Ibbott, F. A., and Bowes, W. A.: Identification of the pigment in amniotic fluid of erythroblastosis as bilirubin. J. Pediatr., *69*:354, 1966.

Brock, D. J. H., and Sutcliffe, R. G.: Alpha-fetoprotein in the antenatal diagnosis of anencephaly and spina bifida. Lancet, *2*:197, 1972.

Brodersen, R., Jacobsen, J., Hertz, H., Rebbe, H., and Sorensen, B.: Bilirubin conjugation in the human fetus. Scand. J. Clin. Lab. Invest., *20*:41, 1967.

Brown, J. B.: The value of plasma estrogen estimations in the management of pregnancy. Clin. Perinatol., *1*:2, 273, 1974.

Brown, R. C., and Beckfield, W. J.: Computer-assisted spectrophotometric analysis of amniotic fluid in erythroblastosis fetalis. Am. J. Clin. Pathol., *57*:649, 1972.

Cassady, G., and Barnett, R.: Amniotic fluid electrolytes and perinatal outcome. Biol. Neonatorum, *13*:155, 1968.

Clements, J. A., Platzker, A. C. G., Tierney, D. F., Hobel, C. J., Creasy, R. K., Margolis, A. J., Thibeault, D. W., Tooley, W. H., and Oh, W.: Assessment of the risk of the respiratory distress syndrome by a rapid test for surfactant in amniotic fluid. Obstet. Gynecol. Survey, 27:716, 1972.

Cohen, H.: Biochemical monitoring by fetal blood sampling. Clin. Anes., Parturition and Perint., Ed. by G. Marx, F. A. Davis, Phila., 1974.

Chopra, I. J., and Crandall, B. F.: Thyroid hormones and thyrotropin in amniotic fluid. New Engl. J. Med., 293:740, 1975.

Davis, L. E., Tweed, G. V., and Stewart, J. A.: Cytomegalovirus mononucleosis in a first trimester pregnant female with transmission to the fetus. Pediatrics, 48:200, 1971.

Forman, D. T., Biochemical basis of hyaline membrane disease. Ann. Clin. Lab. Sci., 3:242, 1973.

Freda, V. J.: Antepartum management of the Rh problem. Progr. Hematol., 5:266, 1966a.

Freda, V. J.: Recent obstetrical advances in the Rh problem. Bull. N. Y. Acad. Med., 42:474, 1966b.

Freda, V. J., and Robertson, J. G.: Antepartum management—amniocentesis and experience with hysterotomy and surgery in utero. Jewish Mem. Hosp. Bull (NYC), 10:47, 1965.

Friedman, M. L., and McElin, T. W.: Diagnosis of ruptured fetal membranes, clinical study and review of the literature. Am. J. Obstet. Gynecol., 104:544, 1969.

Fuchs, F.: Genetic information from amniotic fluid constituents. Clin. Obstet. Gynecol., 9:565, 1966.

Gambino, S. R., and Freda, V. J.: The measurement of amniotic fluid bilirubin by the method of Jendrassik and Grof, its correlation with spectrophotometric analysis. Am. J. Clin. Pathol., 46:198, 1966.

Gartner, L. H., and Bernstein, J.: Kernicterus and prematurity. Development of nuclear jaundice at relatively low serum concentrations of bilirubin. Jewish Mem. Hosp. Bull. (NYC), 10:125, 1965.

Gluck, L., Kulovich, M. V., Borer, R. C., Brenner, P. H., Anderson, G. G., and Spellacy, W. N.: Diagnosis of the respiratory distress syndrome by amniocentesis. Am. J. Obstet. Gynecol., 109:440, 1971.

Gluck, L., and Kulovich, M. V.: Lecithin/sphingomyelin ratios in amniotic fluid in normal and abnormal pregnancy. Am. J. Obstet. Gynecol., 115:539, 1973.

Hamlin, C. R., and Miller, K. M.: A quality control solution for use in the "ΔA_{450}" determination of amniotic fluid. Clin. Chem., 22:1935, 1976.

Hausknecht, R. U., and Mandelman, N.: The metabolism of intra-amniotically injected dehydroepiandrosterone as a placental function test. Am. J. Obstet. Gynecol., 104:433, 1969.

Hensleigh, P. A.: Enzymatic assessment of the high-risk pregnancy: Oxytocinase and placental phosphatase. In Spellacy, W. N. (Ed.): Management of the High-Risk Pregnancy. Baltimore, University Park Press, 1976, pp. 49-82.

Hobbins, J. C., and Mahoney, M. J.: In utero diagnosis of hemoglobinopathies: Technic for obtaining fetal blood. N. Engl. J. Med., 290:1065, 1974.

Hochberg, C. J., Witheiler, A. P., and Cook, H.: Accurate amniotic fluid bilirubin analysis from the "bloody tap." Am. J. Obstet. Gynecol., 126:531, 1976.

Hutchinson, D. L., Gray, M. J., Plentyl, A. A., Alvarez, H., Caldeyro-Barcia, R., Kaplan, B., and Lind, J.: The role of the fetus in the water exchange of the amniotic fluid of normal and hydramniotic patients. J. Clin. Invest., 38:971, 1959.

James, L. S.: Acid-base changes in the fetus and infant during the perinatal period. In Young, D. S., and Hicks, J. M. (Eds.): The Neonate: Current Topics in Clinical

Chemistry. New York, John Wiley and Sons, Inc., 1976, pp. 95-101.

Kan, Y. W., Golbus, M. S., and Trecortin, R.: Prenatal diagnosis of sickle cell anemia. N. Engl. J. Med., 294:1039, 1976.

Kapitulnik, J., Kaufmann, N. A., and Blondheim, S. H.: Chemical versus spectrophotometric determination of bilirubin in amniotic fluid and the influence of hemoglobin and methene pigments. Clin. Chem., 16:756, 1970.

Knox, E., Todd, K., and Cassady, G.: The effect of amniography on amniotic fluid L/S ratio. Obstet. Gynecol., 49:154, 1976.

Larsen, J. W., Weis, K. R., Lenichan, J. P., Crumrine, M., and Heggers, J. P.: Significance of neutrophils and bacteria in the amniotic fluid of patients in labor. Obstet. Gynecol., 47:143, 1976.

Levin, M. J., Oxman, M. N., Moore, M. G., Daniels, J. B., and Scheer, K.: Diagnosis of congenital rubella in utero. N. Engl. J. Med., 290:1187, 1974.

Lewis, J. F., Johnson, P., and Miller, P.: Evaluation of amniotic fluid for aerobic and anerobic bacteria. Am. J. Clin. Pathol., 65:58, 1976.

Liggins, G. C., and Howie, R. N.: A controlled trial of antepartum glucocorticoid treatment for prevention of the respiratory distress syndrome in premature infants. Pediatrics, 50:515, 1972.

Liley, A. W.: Errors in the assessment of hemolytic disease from amniotic fluid. Am. J. Obstet. Gynecol., 93:485, 1963.

Liley, A. W.: The epidemiology of severe haemolytic disease of the newborn. New Zealand Med. J., 71:76, 1970.

Lind, T., and Hytten, F. E.: Relation of amniotic fluid volume to fetal weight in the first half of pregnancy. Lancet, 1:1147, 1970.

Littlefield, J. W.: The pregnancy at risk for a genetic disorder. N. Engl. J. Med., 282:627, 1970.

Lumley, J., Potter, M., Newman, W., Talbot, J. M., Wakefield, E., and Wood, C.: The unreliability of a single estimation of fetal scalp blood pH. J. Lab. Clin. Med., 77:4, 535, 1971.

Mahoney, M. J., Haseltine, F. P., Hobbins, J. C., Banker, B. Q., Caskey, C. T., and Golbus, M. S.: Prenatal diagnosis of Duchenne's muscular dystrophy. N. Engl. J. Med., 297:968, 1977.

Matthews, C. D., Matthews, A. E. B., and Gilbey, B. E.: Antibody development in rhesus-negative patients following abortion. Lancet, 2:318, 1969.

Milunsky, A., Littlefield, J. W., Kanfer, J. N., Kolodny, E. H., Shih, V. E., and Atkins, L.: Prenatal genetic diagnosis. N. Engl. J. Med., 283:1370, 1441, 1498, 1970.

Milunsky, A.: Risk of amniocentesis for prenatal diagnosis. N. Engl. J. Med., 293:932, 1975.

Milunsky, A., Prenatal diagnosis of genetic disorders. N. Engl. J. Med., 295:377, 1976.

Morrison, J. C., Morrison, D. L., Lovett, F. A., Whybrew, W. D., Bucovaz, E. T., Wiser, W. L., and Fish, S. A.: Nile blue staining of cells in amniotic fluid for fetal maturity, a reappraisal. Obstet. Gynecol., 44:355, 1974.

Morrison, J. C., Whybrew, M. S., Bucovaz, E. T., Wiser, W. L., and Fish, S. A.: Amniotic fluid tests for fetal maturity in normal and abnormal pregnancies. Obstet. Gynecol., 49:20, 1976.

Nadler, H. L., and Gerbie, A. B.: Role of amniocentesis in the intrauterine detection of genetic disorders. N. Engl. J. Med., 282:596, 1970.

Nelson, G. H., and Talledo, O. E.: Amniotic fluid spectral analysis in the management of patients with rhesus sensitization. Am. J. Clin. Pathol., 39:363, 1969.

Newman, W., Braid, D., and Wood, C.: Fetal acid-base

status. (1) Relation between maternal and fetal Pco_2. Am. J. Obstet. Gynecol., *97*:1, 43, 1967.

Olsen, E. B., and Graven, S. N.: Comparison of visualization methods used to measure the lecithin/sphingomyelin ratio in amniotic fluid. Clin. Chem., *20*:1408, 1974.

Pirani, B. B. K., Doran, T. A., and Benzie, R. J.: Amniotic fluid or maternal urine? Lancet, *1*:303, 1976.

Poland, R. L., and Odell, G. B.: Physiologic jaundice: The enterohepatic circulation of bilirubin. N. Engl. J. Med., *284*:1, 1971.

Potier, M., Dallaire, L., and Melancon, S. B.: Prenatal detection of intestinal obstruction by disaccharidase assay in amniotic fluid. Lancet, *2*:982, 1977.

Reynolds, W. A., Pitkin, R. M., and Hodari, A. A.: Transfer of iodide into amniotic fluid by the normal and nephrectomized subhuman primate fetus. Am. J. Obstet. Gynecol., *104*:633, 1969.

Robert, M. F., Neff, R. K., Hubbell, J. P., Taeusch, H. W., and Avery, M. E.: Association between maternal diabetes and the respiratory-distress syndrome in the newborn. N. Engl. J. Med., *294*:357, 1976.

Robertson, J. G.: Management of patients with Rh isoimmunization based on amniotic fluid examination. Am. J. Obstet. Gynecol., *103*:713, 1969.

Saling, E.: Technik der endoskopischen miscroblutent-

nahme am feten. Geburtschilfe und Frauenheilkunde, *24*:464, 1964.

Sharp-Cageorge, S. M., Blicher, B. M., Gordon, E. R., and Murphy, B. E. P.: Amniotic fluid cortisol and human fetal lung maturation. N. Engl. J. Med., *296*:89, 1977.

Tulchinsky, D., Osathanondh, R., and Finn, A.: Dehydroepiandrosterone sulfate loading test in the diagnosis of complicated pregnancies. N. Engl. J. Med., *294*:517, 1976.

Wade, M. E., Ogden, J. A., and David, C. D.: Criteria for intrauterine fetal transfusion. Obstet. Gynecol., *34*:156, 1969.

Walker, A. H. C.: Liquor amnii studies in the prediction of haemolytic disease of the newborn. Br. Med. J., 376, August, 1957.

Wenk, R. E., London, R., Siegelbaum, M., Lustgarten, J. A., and Goldstein, P.: A prospective study of placental lactogen as a test for neonatal risk. Am. J. Clin. Pathol., vol. 71, 1979.

White, C. A., Doorenbos, D. E., and Bradbury, J. T.: Role of chemical and cytologic analysis of amniotic fluid in determination of fetal maturity. Am. J. Obstet. Gynecol., *104*:664, 1969.

Wolf, P. L., Block, D., and Tsudaka, T.: Biochemical profile of amniotic fluid to assess fetal maturity. Clin. Chem., *16*:610, 1970.

21

EXAMINATION OF SEMINAL FLUID

Donald C. Cannon, M.D., Ph.D.

PHYSIOLOGY OF SEMINAL FLUID
COLLECTION
GROSS EXAMINATION

MICROSCOPIC EXAMINATION
OTHER TESTS OF SEMEN
EXAMINATION FOR THE PRESENCE
    OF SEMEN

Examination of seminal fluid is usually performed as part of a comprehensive infertility investigation involving both partners of a barren marriage. As a result of its relative simplicity, semen examination is often requested before the more complicated and expensive examination of the female. It is now apparent that inadequacies on the part of the male contribute to a significant minority of infertility problems, estimated to be as high as 40 per cent by some investigators. Some cases of male infertility are now amenable to medical treatment.

In relation to the infertility investigation, it is important to recognize the proper scope of the semen examination. Most importantly, it is but one facet of the medical examination of the male, which must also include a detailed history and general physical examination. Such specialized procedures as studies of thyroid, adrenal, and pituitary functions or testicular biopsy may also be indicated. Not only must the results of the semen examination be interpreted in light of the remainder of the medical examination of the male; the female partner must be considered as well. Indeed, it has been suggested that for purposes of the infertility investigation the male and female involved should be considered not as individuals but as a reproductive unit. An inherent limitation of the semen examination is that the standards of semen quality are the result of population studies of males from fertile and infertile marriages. Consequently the standards of semen quality are relative, not absolute indications of fertility or sterility (with the single exception of complete aspermia). Furthermore, it is usually recommended that semen examination be repeated one or more times if an abnormal result is found.

In addition to infertility studies, the clinical pathology laboratory, particularly one actively engaged in forensic studies, may frequently be requested to examine vaginal secretions or clothing stains for the presence of semen in alleged or suspected rape. The semen examination can also be utilized to evaluate the effectiveness of vasectomy or to support or disprove a denial of paternity on the grounds of sterility.

PHYSIOLOGY OF SEMINAL FLUID

Semen is a composite solution formed by the testes as well as the accessory male reproductive organs and consists basically of spermatozoa suspended in the seminal plasma. The function of the seminal plasma is to provide a nutritive medium of proper osmolality and volume for conveying the spermatozoa to the endocervical mucus, whereupon its contribution to the fertilization process is ended. The seminal plasma also activates the spermatozoa to greater motility.

The components of semen are derived from the following organs:

Testis. Spermatozoa, which comprise less

than 5 per cent of the semen volume, are the only cell type present in normal semen in any appreciable number. Spermatozoa are largely stored in the ampullary portions of the vasa deferentia until released in the process of ejaculation. Spermatozoa stored in the ampullae are rather inactive metabolically because of the acid environment and diminished oxygen supply. In this location it has been estimated that spermatozoa can survive for periods of up to one month.

Seminal Vesicles. Approximately 60 per cent of the semen volume is derived from the seminal vesicles. This viscid, neutral, or slightly alkaline fluid is often yellow or even deeply pigmented as a result of its high flavin content, which is responsible for the fluorescence of semen in ultraviolet light. The seminal vesicles are the major source of the high fructose content of semen, which is the major nutrient for the spermatozoa. The importance of other components, such as the relatively high potassium and citric acid content and smaller amounts of ascorbic acid, ergothioneine, and phosphorylcholine, has not yet been established. The seminal vesicle secretion is also important in providing the substrate responsible for the coagulation of semen following ejaculation.

Prostate. The prostate contributes about 20 per cent of the volume of semen. This milky fluid is slightly acid, with a pH of about 6.5, largely as a result of its high content of citric acid, which constitutes the major anion in this component of semen. The prostatic secretion is also rich in proteolytic enzymes and acid phosphatase. These proteolytic enzymes are responsible for the coagulation and liquefaction of semen. Acid phosphatase can cleave phosphorylcholine present in the semen but the significance of this is not clear.

Epididymides, Vasa Deferentia, Bulbourethral Glands (Cowper's Glands), and Urethral Glands (Glands of Littré). Less than 10 to 15 per cent of the semen volume is contributed by these structures, and little is known of their biochemical significance in man.

Fractions of Semen. The process of ejaculation results in the mixing of three distinct fractions of semen, which enter the urethra individually in rapid succession. These fractions differ as to anatomic origin and therefore also in chemical composition. The first fraction, which is of relatively slight amount, consists of a clear viscid fluid believed to originate largely or perhaps exclusively from the urethral and bulbourethral glands. The function of this component is not known with certainty, but it may be to cleanse and lubricate the urethra in preparation for the bulk of the ejaculate which is to follow. The second fraction consists largely of prostatic secretion along with most of the spermatozoa and relatively small amounts of secretions from the epididymides and vasa deferentia which have been temporarily stored in the ampullae of the vasa deferentia. The final fraction consists almost entirely of a mucoid secretion resulting from emptying of the seminal vesicles.

An understanding of the temporal sequence of mixing of the various fractions in ejaculation is important to the proper conduct of the semen examination. For example, the use of semen samples obtained from the male urethra following coitus, as recommended by some investigators, will result in a specimen which is not only nonrepresentative of the semen as a whole but is also apt to be relatively sperm poor. Furthermore, samples obtained by coitus interruptus may result in loss of part of the sperm-rich middle fraction, although it represents only a minor part of the total volume of ejaculate.

COLLECTION

It is usually recommended that the semen sample be collected following a three-day period of continence. Others have suggested that a more meaningful specimen is one collected after a period of continence equal to the usual frequency of coitus for the couple involved. Prolonged continence prior to the semen collection is to be discouraged, since the quality of the semen, especially in regard to sperm motility, will actually diminish. Regardless of what method is employed for collection, the physician will be faced with occasional patients who will not comply because of religious or esthetic standards or who are unable to cooperate because of more complex psychologic considerations. The most satisfactory specimen is that collected in the physician's office or the clinical pathology laboratory by masturbation. This allows a complete examination of the semen, particularly of the process of coagulation and liquefaction, and also eliminates the possibility of cold shock. Acceptable but somewhat less satisfactory are specimens obtained in the patient's home by coitus interruptus or masturbation and delivered soon thereafter to the laboratory. With either method, the specimen may be collected in a wide-mouth clean glass jar supplied by the laboratory (to avoid the possibility of trace amounts of detergents or other harmful contaminants) or in suitable plastic or polyethylene containers such as those used for the collection of urine or sputum specimens. Specimens may be collected in condoms, which are then tied and placed in a clean glass jar. Valid objections to condom collection have been expressed because of the fact that powder or lubricants applied to the condoms or other material used in their manufacture may be actively spermicidal. If the condom is used, it must first be washed with soap and water, rinsed thoroughly, and then dried completely. Plastic sheaths* have been recommended as a means of avoiding the difficulties of condom collection.

In transporting specimens collected elsewhere to the laboratory, several precautions are necessary. First of all, the specimen must be received as soon as possible and in no case after more than two to three hours have elapsed following collection. It is essential that the semen specimen not be subjected to temperature extremes during delivery to the laboratory. Watson (1966) has emphasized the importance of the container temperature at the time of collection and recommends preliminary warming to body temperature. He found maintenance of the specimen at body temperature to be particularly important until liquefaction of the coagulum is complete (about 20 minutes).

GROSS EXAMINATION

Physical Characteristics. Freshly ejaculated semen is a highly viscid, opaque, white or gray-white coagulum which may have a distinct musty or acrid odor. Within 10 to 20 minutes the coagulum will spontaneously liquefy to form a translucent, turbid, viscous fluid which is mildly alkaline, with a pH of about 7.7. The pH usually does not vary greatly, although pH values of less than 7.0 are frequently associated with semen consisting largely of prostatic secretion due to congenital aplasia of the vasa deferentia and seminal vesicles (Raboch, 1965). Increased or decreased turbidity is of little significance except when increased turbidity is the result of leukocytes associated with an inflammatory process in

some part of the reproductive tract. With passage of time, colorless, needle-shaped crystals of spermine phosphate may form as a result of the reaction of spermine in the prostatic secretion with phosphoric acid formed from enzymatic cleavage of various organic phosphates.

Viscosity can be assessed while pouring the liquefied specimen from the collection container into the glass graduate for volume measurement. The specimen of normal viscosity can be poured drop by drop. Increased viscosity is of significance if sperm motility is thereby compromised. Upon occasion, increased viscosity has been shown to be associated with poor invasion of the cervical mucus in postcoital studies and may be the only demonstrable defect in an infertile couple.

Coagulation and Liquefaction. Coagulation and subsequent liquefaction is believed to be a three-stage process (Mann, 1964): (1) Coagulation results from the action of a prostatic clotting enzyme on a fibrinogen-like precursor formed by the seminal vesicles. (2) Liquefaction is initiated by enzymes of prostatic origin. (3) The protein fragments are degraded further to free amino acids and ammonia by the action of several poorly characterized proteolytic enzymes, including an aminopeptidase and pepsin. The coagulation process has been shown to have diagnostic significance in that the semen from males with bilateral congenital absence of the vasa deferentia and seminal vesicles fails to coagulate because of the absence of the coagulation substrate (Amelar, 1962). Liquefaction should be complete within 30 minutes. It is important to distinguish persistent increased viscosity from delayed liquefaction.

Volume. The normal semen volume averages 3.5 ml with a usual range of 1.5 to 5.0 ml. Paradoxically males associated with infertile marriages tend to have an increased rather than a decreased semen volume, which is frequently associated with a significantly diminished sperm count. Postcoital studies suggest, however, that greatly decreased semen volumes may result in poor penetration of the cervical mucus by the sperm (MacLeod, 1965). Semen volume does not vary significantly with the period of continence (MacLeod, 1951).

MICROSCOPIC EXAMINATION

Sperm Counts. Following liquefaction of the semen, the spermatozoa may be counted in

---

*Milex Seminal Pouch, Milex Products, Chicago, Illinois.

a hemocytometer chamber following initial dilution in a white blood cell pipette. Mix the semen sample thoroughly and draw an aliquot to the 0.5 mark on the pipette. Dilute to the 11 mark with the following solution:

Sodium bicarbonate	5 g
Formalin (neutral)	1 ml
Distilled water	100 ml

After charging the hemocytometer chamber, 2 minutes are allowed for the immobilized sperm to settle. The spermatozoa in 2 sq mm (two large squares) are counted. This number multiplied by 100,000 gives the number of spermatozoa per milliliter. The entire counting procedure including the initial dilution should be repeated at least once and the results averaged.

Considerable difficulty may be encountered in diluting semen of greatly increased viscosity. Under these circumstances the counting will be facilitated if the semen is diluted 1:1 with the mucolytic agent Alevaire (Brean Laboratories, Inc.) prior to pipette dilution and the final count is multiplied by two (Amelar, 1977).

The hemocytometer method of counting sperm is relatively imprecise. Freund (1964) found that duplicate sperm counts by the same technologist varied by a mean difference of 20 per cent. For counts performed by three technicians, each of whom used duplicate pipettings on the same sample, the 95 per cent confidence limit was ±52 per cent. In the author's experience, however, these variations seem unduly high.

The sperm count of normal semen will usually fall in the range of 60 to 150 million per ml., with a mean of about 100 million per ml. Counts of less than 20 million per ml are usually considered to be distinctly abnormal, although successful impregnation may occur. MacLeod (1951), in studying the semen of 1000 fertile males and 800 males associated with infertile marriages, found that 5 per cent of the fertile group and 17 per cent of the "infertile" group had sperm counts in the range of 1 to 20 million per ml.

Motility. In order for the spermatozoa to penetrate the cervical mucus and subsequently migrate to fertilize the ovum in the fallopian tubes, active motility is necessary. To evaluate motility, a small drop of liquefied semen is placed on a microscope slide prewarmed approximately to body temperature and then covered with a coverslip which has been ringed with petrolatum. Motility can be evaluated by scanning several fields with the high dry objective until a total of at least 200 spermatozoa have been observed. It is essential to focus through the entire depth of a given field so as to include non-motile sperm which may have settled to the bottom of the medium. The percentage of sperm showing actual progressive motion should be recorded. It is also desirable to render a qualitative estimate of sperm motility. Watson (1966), for example, assigns sperm to one of three categories: progressive motility, non-progressive motility, and non-motility. He furthermore grades those showing progressive motility according to the following code: grade I, minimal forward progression; grade II, poor to fair activity; grade III, good activity with tail movements visualized; grade IV, full activity with tail movements difficult to visualize.

Although it is frequently stated that normal semen contains more than 70 per cent or even 80 per cent motile sperm, this criterion would seem entirely too rigid in view of several large studies. For example, MacLeod (1951) found a mean of only 58 per cent motile sperm with a standard deviation of ±16 per cent in 732 males of proven fertility. In contrast, he found a mean motility of 51 per cent ±19 in 869 males associated with infertile marriages. These results may be somewhat low in that some specimens were evaluated as late as 5½ hours after collection. Many feel that semen should be considered abnormal if fewer than 60 per cent of spermatozoa show progressive motion in specimens examined within 3 hours of collection.

Some investigators have previously recommended motility estimates at intervals during the 24 hours following collection, e.g., 3, 6, 12, and 24 hours. The motile forms will decrease by about 5 per cent per hour after the fourth hour following collection. Since sperm must penetrate the cervical mucus within a few minutes following ejaculation (or be inactivated by the relatively low pH of the vaginal secretions), the seminal plasma is not a physiologic medium for prolonged evaluation of sperm activity. Furthermore, the metabolic activity of the sperm as well as bacterial growth will significantly alter the pH of semen after a few hours.

Sperm Morphology. Sperm morphology is evaluated by performing differential counts of morphologically normal and abnormal spermatozoa types on stained smears. Smears are

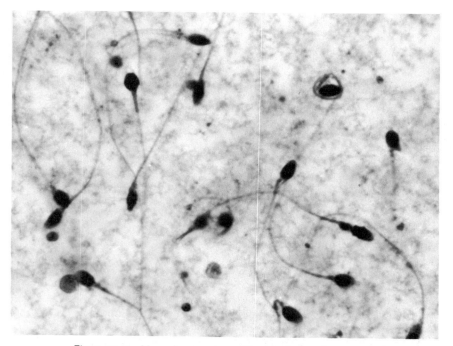

Figure 21-1. Normal spermatozoa. Papanicolaou stain; ×1580.

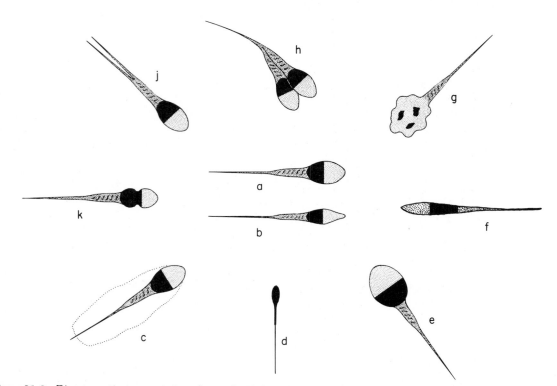

Figure 21-2. Diagrammatic representation of normal and abnormal spermatozoa. *a,* Normal, face view. *b,* Normal, lateral view. *c,* Immature spermatozoon (spermatid). *d–k,* Morphologically abnormal types: *d,* pin-head; *e,* giant head; *f,* acute tapering form; *g,* amorphous form; *h,* double head; *j,* double tail; *k,* constricted head. (Tails on all forms are disproportionately short.)

prepared on clean microscope slides in a manner identical to blood films. The best stain for morphologic detail is the Papanicolaou stain (Fig. 21-1). Although somewhat complicated and time consuming, the Papanicolaou technique is to be recommended, particularly in the laboratory that uses this stain routinely for exfoliative cytology. It is essential that the smear be placed immediately into fixative, either 95 per cent (v/v) ethanol or 50 per cent (v/v) ethanol ether, before drying has occurred.

A method which is also satisfactory but gives somewhat poorer differentiation of sperm detail is the hematoxylin method described by Amelar (1977). In this method the film is air dried and then treated as follows: (1) 10 per cent (v/v) formalin, 1 minute; (2) water rinse; (3) Meyer's (or Harris) hematoxylin, 2 minutes; (4) water rinse; (5) air dry. Other staining techniques which have been recommended include Giemsa, basic fuchsin, and crystal violet. The last two named require preliminary heat fixing, which has been demonstrated to cause some degree of artifactual distortion of the spermatozoa.

At least 200 spermatozoa should be examined under oil immersion and the percentage of abnormal forms recorded (Fig. 21-2). Normal semen has fewer than 30 per cent abnormal forms. In addition to sperm morphology, the presence of red blood cells, leukocytes, and epithelial cells should be noted. Immature cells of the germinal line may appear in the semen and must be differentiated from macrophages or leukocytes. Numerous granules and globules are normally present in semen. These presumably originate from the secretion of glandular cells or perhaps from autolysis of epithelial lining cells in the accessory reproductive structures.

OTHER TESTS OF SEMEN

Postcoital (Sims-Huhner) Test. This test consists of the examination of cervical mucus following coitus. It is intended as a measure both of the quality of cervical mucus and the ability of the spermatozoa to penetrate the mucus and maintain activity. The cervical mucus undergoes both quantitative and qualitative changes, which are correlated with the menstrual cycle. In the ovulatory phase at midcycle, the amount of mucus is maximum while the viscosity is significantly diminished, thus facilitating penetration of the mucus by the spermatozoa. Progesterone in the secretory phase causes increased viscosity of the mucus.

During the ovulatory phase, as determined by basal temperature records, the female is instructed to report to the physician within several hours of coitus. The results of the test are constant for about 8 hours after coitus (Danezis, 1962). The external cervical os is wiped clear of mucus. The endocervical mucus sample may be obtained by aspiration with a glass cannula attached by a rubber tube to a Luer syringe. The specimen may then be delivered to the laboratory in the syringe. The volume of mucus is measured. Following discharge into a Petri dish, its color and viscosity are noted. At midcycle the mucus should be clear and watery. One further property that is commonly evaluated is the spinnbarkeit, which refers to the tenacity of the mucus. This is tested by grasping a portion of the mucus with forceps and noting the distance which it can be drawn before breaking. A good spinnbarkeit, which should prevail at midcycle, is at least 10 cm. A drop of mucus is then placed on a microscope slide, covered with a coverslip, and examined for the presence of sperm. An estimate of the number of sperm per highpower field with percentage of motile forms should be reported. The material may also be examined for leukocytes, erythrocytes, and trichomonads.

The postcoital test typically shows better quality of mucus and better sperm penetration at the ovulatory phase than at other times in the ovulatory cycle. The degree of sperm penetration is correlated with the quality of semen as well as with the fertility of the mating, although the differences are usually not striking.

Antibodies to Spermatozoa. Recently considerable interest has focused on the occurrence of antibodies to spermatozoa, both in males with semen abnormalities and in females of infertile marriages. The extensive experimental and clinical work in this complex and as yet rather poorly understood field has recently been reviewed by Schulman (1971). Investigations thus far have established a firm immunologic basis for spermatozoal antibodies. There appear to be several antigens that are specific for the sperm cell line. Using immunofluorescence, antibodies have been found to react with four distinct regions of the spermatozoa: the front part of the acrosome, the post-nuclear cap, the equatorial segment of the acrosome, and the tail piece (Husted, 1975). Other techniques for detecting antibodies to spermatozoa include agglutination, immobilization, precipitation, complement fixation, passive hemagglutination, and cytotoxicity. Some of these techniques have not yet proved to be technically reliable, however, and widely variant results often occur among laboratories performing the same test.

A causal relationship between spermatozoal antibodies and disease has not been clearly established. The antibodies are found in some human males with testicular disease and also in association with autoimmune aspermatogenesis experimentally induced by immunization with spermatozoa, semen, or testicular homogenates and appropriate adjuvants. Sperm agglutinins appear in the sera of many men following vasectomy. In one study, sperm agglutinins occurred in 60 per cent of 52 men during the first year following vasectomy (van Lis, 1974).

There is by no means unanimity of opinion regarding the importance of spermatozoal antibodies in the serum of females, but available evidence strongly suggests a cause and effect relationship to otherwise unexplained infertility. One of the earliest and still controversial reports is that of Franklin (1964), who employed a straightforward agglutination reaction between serum and semen. Results were read microscopically after a four-hour incubation at 37°C. Using this method, they were able to detect antibodies in the serum of 31 out of a group of 43 female partners of infertile marriages in which there was no other demonstrable cause for infertility in either husband or wife. In contrast, such antibodies were present in the female in only two of 35 fertile marriages. Antibodies were variously individual specific, in that they agglutinated only the husband's spermatozoa, or species specific, in that they agglutinated the spermatozoa of all males tested. The clinical importance of this test was further demonstrated by the fact that the antibody levels diminished markedly in each of 13 infertile females who were persuaded to practice continence or to restrict coitus to the use of condoms over a period of two to six months. Nine of these patients eventually became pregnant upon resumption of unrestricted coitus.

EXAMINATION FOR THE PRESENCE OF SEMEN

The clinical pathology laboratory may be requested to investigate material from the vagina or stains from clothing, skin, or hair for the presence of semen. Such cases will usually involve alleged rape or suspected sexual assault in association with homicide. In all medicolegal cases special precautions are indicated to identify specimens properly and to maintain the chain of evidence.

Obtaining the Sample. Secretions from the vagina may be obtained by direct aspiration or saline lavage. A preliminary scan with ultraviolet light may prove helpful in selecting specific areas of clothing or other fabrics for further investigation. Semen stains frequently result in a greenish white fluorescence, although this may occur with stains from other body fluids as well. A 1 sq cm portion of the stained fabric should be cut out and soaked in 1 or 2 ml of physiologic saline for 1 hour. The fluid from this washing may be subjected to further tests for semen. It is desirable to include as a control, particularly for acid phosphatase determination and the detection of blood group substances, a piece of fabric remote from the stain.

Examination for Sperm. Prior to aspiration or lavage it is desirable to prepare direct smears from the vagina for Papanicolaou staining. Alternatively, such smears may be prepared from the aspirate or lavage. Contrary to some expressed opinions, well-preserved sperm may be recovered from the vagina many hours after coitus and even from exhumed bodies, if they have been properly embalmed. Smears should also be prepared from the washings of fabric stains. The wash fluid may be first concentrated by centrifugation and a smear prepared from the sediment. Such smears may be stained with hematoxylin and eosin. The fragile tails of the sperm are frequently broken off, thus making identification somewhat more difficult.

Acid Phosphatase Determination. Acid phosphatase should be determined on the vaginal aspirate or lavage or on the wash fluid from stains. High values of acid phosphatase will render positive identification of semen even if the male involved is aspermic. Determination of acid phosphatase is significantly more sensitive than a microscopic search for spermatozoa in detecting intravaginal semen (Schumann, 1976). Seminal fluid averages about 2500 King-Armstrong units per ml of acid phosphatase, while other body fluids and extraneous foreign materials will have well under 5 units per ml. Acid phosphatase can be reliably determined on the wash fluid from stains which are many months old. The acid phosphatase method selected should have a high degree of specificity for prostatic acid phosphatase. (See Chapter 12.)

Detection of Blood Group Substances. In the case of positive identification of fluid or a stain as semen, the presence of A, B, or H blood group substances may be investigated. Approximately 80 per cent of individuals, those having the dominant secretor gene in homozygous or heterozygous state, will secrete the water-soluble form of blood group substances in body fluids, including semen. The identification of the specific substance is based on the ability of the semen to partially or completely neutralize the agglutinating activity of the specific antiserum. With this determination, it may be possible on occasion to demonstrate that the seminal fluid of a suspect differs from that recovered from the victim.

Florence Test. This test is a preliminary screening method and has been largely replaced by the far more dependable acid phosphatase determination. It is usually performed on stains from clothing, other fabric, or hair and depends on the presence of choline, which is found in high concentration in seminal fluid. A portion of the stained sample is extracted with distilled water by using gentle heat. Several drops of the extract are placed on a microscope slide and treated with an equal volume of a reagent composed of the following: iodine, 2.54 g; potassium iodide, 1.65 g; distilled water, 30 ml. In a positive test, rhombic or needle-like crystals of periodide of choline will be noted. The test may yield false positive results because of the high choline content occasionally found in other tissue fluids of human or animal origin.

Other Tests. A precipitin test can be used to detect semen of human origin and is therefore helpful in rendering positive identification of semen stains on clothing. The test requires specific antiserum obtained by immunizing suitable animals with human semen and absorbing the non-specific antibodies with human serum. It is performed as a capillary tube precipitin reaction by overlaying the antiserum with washings from the stain.

Determination of the sperm-specific lactate dehydrogenase isoenzyme has been reported to provide a specific differentiation of human semen from other body fluids and from the semen of other animals (Mokashi, 1976).

REFERENCES

Amelar, R. D.: Coagulation, liquefaction and viscosity of human semen. J. Urol., *87*:187, 1962.

Amelar, R. D.: Male Infertility. Philadelphia, W. B. Saunders Company, 1977.

Danezis, J., Sujan, S., and Sabrero, A. J.: Evaluation of the postcoital test. Fertil. Steril., *13*:559, 1962.

Franklin, R. R., and Dukes, C. D.: Further studies on sperm-agglutinating antibody and unexplained infertility. J.A.M.A., *190*:682, 1964.

Freund, M., and Carol, B.: Factors affecting haemocytometer counts of sperm concentration in human semen. J. Reprod. Fertil., *8*:149, 1964.

Hustad, S.: Sperm antibodies in men from infertile couples. Analysis of sperm agglutinins and immunofluorescent antibodies in 657 men. Int. J. Fertil., *20*:113, 1975.

MacLeod, J.: Semen quality in one thousand men of known fertility and in eight hundred cases of infertile marriage. Fertil. Steril., *2*:115, 1951.

MacLeod, J.: The semen examination. Clin. Obstet. Gynecol., *8*:115, 1965.

MacLeod, J., and Gold, R. Z.: The male factor in fertility and sterility. III. An analysis of motile activity in the spermatozoa of 1,000 fertile men and 1,000 men in infertile marriage. Fertil. Steril., *2*:187, 1951.

Mann, T.: The Biochemistry of Semen and of the Male Reproductive Tract. London, Methuen and Co. Ltd., 1964.

Mokashi, R. H., and Madiwale, M. S.: The use of sperm-specific lactate dehydrogenase isoenzyme for the identification of semen in dried stains. Forensic Sci., *8*:269, 1976.

Raboch, J., and Skachova, J.: The pH of human ejaculate. Fertil. Steril., *16*:252, 1965.

Schulman, S.: Sperm antibodies as a cause of infertility. CRC Crit. Rev. Clin. Lab. Sci., *2*:393, 1971.

Schumann, G. B., Badawy, S., Peglow, A., and Henry, J. B.: Prostatic acid phosphatase. Current assessment in vaginal fluid of alleged rape victims. Am. J. Clin. Pathol., *66*:944, 1976.

van Lis, J. M. J., Wagenaar, J., and Soer, J. R.: Sperm-agglutinating activity in serum of vasectomized men. Andrologia, *6*:129, 1974.

Watson, A. A., and Robertson, C. M. G.: Male infertility: A reappraisal of semen analysis. J. Med. Lab. Tech., *23*:1, 1966.

22

SPUTUM

Daniel C. Niejadlik, M.D.

PHYSIOLOGY OF SPUTUM

Tracheobronchial secretions are an inconstant mixture of plasma, water, electrolytes, and mucin. As these secretions pass through the lower and upper respiratory tract, they become contaminated with cellular exfoliations, nasal and salivary gland secretions, and normal bacterial flora of the oral cavity. This mixture of secretions and particulate is collectively referred to as sputum.

The principal sources of tracheobronchial secretions are the mucous glands and the goblet cells. The surfaces of the trachea, bronchi, and bronchioles are lined by ciliated columnar cells and goblet cells, with the goblet cells being more numerous proximally in the upper respiratory tract. Between the surface epithelial cells and the cartilaginous plates are the submucous gland cells. The goblet cells produce a thick mucin type secretion which is diluted by a more serous mixture of acid glycoproteins, sialoproteins, and sulfoproteins secreted by the submucous glands. Both types of secretions are increased by vagal nerve stimulation and cholinergic drugs, although nerve impulses are not necessary for goblet cells to discharge their content.

Under appropriate immunologic or inflammatory stimulus, mast cells, eosinophils, and plasma cells may contribute to the secretions. An undetermined volume of the sputum occurs as a transudate from the serum in mucosal capillaries and under normal conditions appears to be quite small. With severe inflammation, though, the tracheal fluid may virtually all be a serum transudate.

The physical properties of sputum reveal the secretions to be viscoelastic, that is, some of the properties of a liquid and some of a solid. The consistency is dependent mainly on the molecular structure of the glycoproteins and on the degree of hydration. Clinicians have long recognized that patients with chronic obstructive airway disease have greater difficulty in evacuation of secretions and that rehydration by water mist aerosol is followed by easier clearing of the respiratory tract.

Throughout the normal respiratory tract there is a two-layered mucous blanket with a fairly constant depth of 7 μm. The inner 5 μm layer lies beneath a 2 μm higher shear gel of greater viscoelasticity. This gel layer is impermeable to water and contains immunoglobulins to protect the underlying cilia and epithelium from toxic damage (Newhouse, 1976).

Chemical composition of the sputum reveals it to be composed of approximately 95 per cent water and 5 per cent total solids. The solids are primarily carbohydrates, proteins, lipids, and deoxyribonucleic acid (DNA). These solids increase in amount with increasing inflammation. The DNA originates from disrupted leukocytes, macrophages, and bronchial epithelial cells, and in some diseases such as cystic fibrosis may increase to thirty times normal levels. Numerous enzymes have been identified and studied in pathologic and normal sputum; among them are alpha$_1$-antitrypsin, lactoferrin, complement lysozymes, and lactate dehydrogenase.

Although large numbers of viable microorganisms are inhaled, the lower respiratory tract is maintained virtually sterile. Two mechanisms are responsible: the alveolar macrophage system, and the mucociliary system. The alveolar macrophage system will be discussed later in this chapter.

The mucociliary system provides both a mechanical removal of inhaled organisms and an antimicrobial activity in the secretions within the mucus.

The mechanical removal of inhaled organisms depends on three mechanisms to maintain a continuous outward flow of sputum. The first mechanism is the tapering of the bronchial lumen to produce a vector force directed toward the larger diameter. When sputum impinges upon the wall, this force moves the sputum forward. The second mechanism is the continuous alteration in the diameter of the bronchial lumen produced by respiration. Again, a vector force is formed which leads to the expulsion of sputum. The final and most important mechanism is the effect of the ciliary border of the respiratory epithelium. The cilia move sequentially in metachronal waves and carry the sputum lining the bronchi outward to the oropharynx where it is imperceptibly swallowed. Expectoration of sputum then depends on cough. Excessive mucus can inhibit the action of the cilia. Increased "thickness" is noted in response to irritation or infection, as both gland cells and goblet cells increase in activity and number. Absent mucociliary function is not incompatible with a relatively

normal existence, as shown from data in patients with Kartagener's syndrome.

The antimicrobial activity of sputum is composed of many factors (Yeager, 1971). Lysozymes and secretory immunoglobulins are the principal secretions, with the latter the more important. Specific antibodies in the respiratory tract are predominantly dimeric IgA to which is attached an additional structure known as the secretory piece. This immunoglobulin is mostly produced locally by plasma cells in the mucosa, and the secretory piece is added by the epithelial cells in transport of the IgA across the mucosa and into the secretions. Small amounts of IgG and IgM are present, but without the secretory piece. IgE reagin is predominately synthesized locally in the mucous membranes. Currently, the only known function is to sensitize mast cells and basophiles involved in the inflammatory response. Deficiency in either IgA production or attachment of the secretory piece significantly reduces the amount of immunoglobulin present and may render the individual more susceptible to increased infections of the respiratory tract. Also, the high or low pH of the secretions contributes to antimicrobial properties. Finally, systemically administered antibiotics diffuse into tracheobronchial secretions fairly effectively and are of importance in the laboratory when interpreting the results of a sputum culture.

SPECIMEN COLLECTION

Specimens labeled "sputum" seldom contain only lower respiratory tract secretions. Saliva, nasopharyngeal secretions, and bacteria or food particles often contaminate these specimens. Prerinsing the mouth prior to collection will remove most of these contaminants and will not affect the result of the bacteriologic examination. Sputum collection should be supervised by professional personnel familiar with the methods discussed later if proper clinical correlations are to be obtained.

For most examinations, a first morning specimen is best, since it represents the pulmonary secretions accumulated overnight. However, most tracheobronchial secretions are not ejected from the mouth, but are swallowed during sleep.

Contamination of the first coughed specimen may occur in catarrhal inflammation of the nasopharynx, as mucous may accumulate in the bronchi at night. Also gastric contents may enter the bronchi in patients with hiatal hernias who have slept in the recumbent position.

To obtain a proper specimen, the most important step is gaining the patient's cooperation and understanding. Usually no problems are encountered in adults, but in children lack of comprehension and cooperation presents a problem. To circumvent this, three different methods are widely used and advocated: In the first method a nasopharyngeal swab is obtained in children with bronchial disease and is said to be representative of the bronchial pathogens. Advocates of this method believe that the viral or bacterial pathogens affect the ciliated columnar epithelium of the nasal passages as well as the respiratory tract. In the second method a cough plate is held before the child's mouth and the child is urged to cough. The third and recommended method, the cough swab technique, is an easy procedure to do and gives the most representative, non-contaminated sputum sample. In this technique the child's mouth is held open with the aid of a tongue blade. The tongue is depressed and the visualized epiglottis is touched with a swab to induce a cough. Material from the trachea expelled from the cough deposits on the swab, and the swab is plated onto the appropriate culture medium. Contamination is avoided if the swab does not touch the nasopharyngeal walls.

In patients who are either non-cooperative or unable to produce sputum spontaneously, sputum induction is becoming a popular means of obtaining specimens. Induction both promotes an increased flow of bronchial secretion and stimulates a cough.

Among the popular inductants are 10 per cent sodium chloride, acetylcysteine, and sterile or distilled water aerosols. Nebulizers are used to deliver these particles, which condense on the bronchial mucosa and increase the volume of mucus present. The fine particles also have an irritant effect, causing a cough that expectorates the diluted secretions.

Sodium chloride aerosols have an additional effect, as the increased hypertonicity causes a shift in fluid from the bronchial mucosa into the lumen to further increase the volume of secretions. Distilled water and sodium chloride concentrations greater than 10 per cent are very irritating, and in patients with asthma or chronic bronchitis, bronchospasm can be wor-

sened. Bronchodilators can be given by aerosol after the above are used. Also, propylene glycol in a 10 per cent concentration is usually added to the saline solvent to increase penetration and minimize evaporation of these particles. In concentrations greater than 20 per cent, propylene glycol has an inhibitory effect on *Mycobacterium tuberculosis* by destroying or preventing its growth on culture.

Acetylcysteine and other related drugs are thought to act by breaking disulfide bonds which aid in maintaining the gel structure of mucus. Acetylcysteine is delivered by aerosol in combination with a bronchodilator; it is one of the most widely used inductants today.

The specimen should be collected in a sterile, disposable, impermeable container with a screw cap or tightly fitting cap or cork. After the patient expectorates the sputum into the container, care should be taken to see that no sputum has been smeared by the patient on the outsides of the container. The sputum specimen should be delivered to the laboratory immediately and not be allowed to stand. If 24-hour specimens are being collected for identification of tubercle bacilli or for volume measurements, a large mouth container can be used. Culturing for bacterial organisms is not recommended or suitable from these 24-hour collections.

Finally, to obtain a specimen in problem cases such as severely debilitated patients, patients with a possible anaerobic pulmonary infection, or patients with equivocal sputum culture findings, a 15-gauge needle with an intracatheter can be inserted into the trachea below the cricoid cartilage. Secretions can be aspirated with a connecting syringe or, if secretions are scant, sterile saline can be injected and reaspirated. However, transtracheal aspiration has numerous complications: transient hemoptysis, subcutaneous emphysema, myocardial arrythmias, mediastinal emphysema, and aspiration of gastric contents during a coughing paroxysm.

SPUTUM EXAMINATION

The sputum specimen should be transferred to a sterile empty Petri dish placed against a dark background. Sterile disposable wooden applicator sticks are used to spread it thinly, and the specimen can be examined carefully with the naked eye or a hand lens.

MACROSCOPIC EXAMINATION

With gross examination of the sputum the following macroscopic findings are of importance and should be noted.

Volume. Occasionally 24-hour sputum collections may be performed on patients with chronic bronchitis, lung abscesses, or bronchial asthma. The volume is used as an index of prognosis, decreasing as the patient's condition improves or increasing as his disease progresses. The volume may decrease, however, as the patient's condition deteriorates and he is unable to cough up any sputum.

Consistency and Appearance. Sputum may be described as liquid (serous), mucoid, purulent, bloody, or combinations of these, i.e., seropurulent, mucopurulent. Usually specific diseases have characteristic consistencies and appearances; e.g., in pulmonary edema, the sputum is often described as serous, frothy, and blood-tinged. In most normal sputum specimens, the appearance is clear and watery, and any opaqueness results from cellular material suspended in it. Most opaque particles are masses of pus and epithelium. Other infrequent material seen in sputum can be Curshmann's spirals, lung stones, Dittrich's plugs, caseous material, bronchial casts, or food substances. Particular attention should be paid to the examination of these opaque materials, as their presence may be the initial laboratory clue in the diagnosis of the disease.

Color. The color of sputum is determined by the material contained, and often the color can indicate the pathologic process. Sputum color, though, is an unreliable indicator of the cellular composition. A yellow color indicates pus and epithelial cells are present and is commonly seen in pneumonic processes. When coupled with a green tint, Pseudomonas may be implicated as the etiologic agent. Variation of the color red in sputum can be used as an aid in the differential diagnosis, too. Rust-colored sputum is due to decomposed hemoglobin and is seen in such diseases as pneumococcal pneumonia or pulmonary gangrene, while a bright red is found in recent hemorrhage secondary to a variety of diseases such as acute cardiac failure, pulmonary infarction, or extension of a tuberculous caseous lesion or neoplasm invading and rupturing a blood vessel. Rarely a pigmented bacteria, *Serratia marcescens*, has contributed a red tinge to sputum.

Odor. Usually no odor is present in normal and pathologic sputums, but if bacterial decomposition has taken place within the body or after expectoration, a variety of odors will be present. Suppurative conditions such as lung abscesses, cavitary tuberculosis, or gangrene produce the most putrid odors. A ruptured subphrenic or liver abscess often imparts a fecal odor.

Miscellaneous Findings. Other macroscopic findings which may be observed in sputum in certain diseases are listed below:

CHEESY MASSES. These are fragments of necrotic pulmonary tissue primarily seen in such diseases as pulmonary gangrene or tuberculosis.

BRONCHIAL CASTS. These are branching treelike casts of bronchi whose size varies with that of the bronchi in which they are formed. They are frequently composed of fibrin and are white or gray in color. At one time bronchial casts were commonly seen during the consolidation stage of lobar pneumonia, but with the advent of drug therapy, they are rarely seen today. Their expulsion is similar to that of a foreign body, and when expelled they are so tangled that they cannot be recognized until they are floated on water against a black background.

BRONCHOLITHS (LUNG STONES). These are usually formed by calcification of necrotic or infected tissue within a larger bronchus or cavity. Chronic tuberculosis is the most common cause for the formation of broncholiths, but occasionally a foreign body or fungus growth may serve as a nidus for formation. Nevertheless, broncholiths are rarely present in sputum specimens.

DITTRICH'S PLUGS. These are most frequently observed in putrid bronchitis and bronchiectasis. They occasionally are coughed up alone and appear as yellowish or gray caseous bodies which vary in size from the head of a pin to a navy bean. When crushed they are found to be composed of cellular debris, fatty acid crystals, fat globules, and bacteria. They appear most commonly in chronic bronchitis, bronchiectasis, and bronchial asthma.

FOREIGN BODIES. Infrequently, foreign bodies may be expelled during a violent coughing spell. In children, foreign bodies can be any small object a child may place into his mouth and inhale. Among the more common objects are peanuts and buttons. In adults, foreign bodies are either food particles or gastric contents aspirated during convulsions, drug intoxication, or operative anesthesia. Since seeds are frequently part of the average diet, the diagnosis of aspiration is simplified by demonstrating these vegetable particles in the sputum either by gross examination or with a periodic acid–Schiff (PAS) stain on microscopic examination.

PARASITES. These are extremely rare in the United States and thus are infrequently seen in sputum. As worldwide travel increases, the laboratory is bound to see more in the future. Among the "common" ones in this country are *Ascaris lumbricoides, Echinococcus granulosus,* and *Toxocara canis.* In Japan *Paragonimus westermani,* the lung flukeworm, may be encountered, with ova found in sputum.

MICROSCOPIC EXAMINATION

After macroscopic examination is performed, all suspicious particles are transferred by a sterile instrument to a clear slide where they are examined unstained if necessary. The remaining portion of the specimen is cultured. Examination of the unstained specimen is universally neglected, yet valuable information not visualized well on a stained preparation is present. Among the more important structures to be seen are elastic fibers, Curschmann's spirals, crystals, fungi, and myelin globules. Forming the background are usually granular debris and mucus, which at times may interfere in structural visualization.

Examination of the stained specimen reveals best any bacteria and cells (Fig. 22–1). When making smears, it is best to air dry the smear first, then flame it to kill all infectious organisms before applying the Gram stain. Specialized stains for specific cells or organisms can also be made at this time, e.g., Wright's stain for blood cells, buffered crystal violet for bronchial epithelial cells, Ziehl-Neelsen stain for *M. tuberculosis,* Papanicolau stain for malignant cells, and so forth.

By observing the bronchial epithelial cells present it is possible to determine the adequacy of the sputum specimen. Chodosh (1970) strongly recommends that cellular morphology be the basis for a decision whether or not further tests are to be performed on the sputum. If cells characteristic of the bronchopulmonary tree are not present, then the sample should be regarded as contaminated for culture and discarded. The presence of squamous cells signifies the specimen as being more representative of the mouth or pharynx rather than the bronchopulmonary tree.

The presence of the alveolar macrophage is the best assurance that the material being examined arises from the lower respiratory tract, as macrophages have not been reported in the secretions of the upper respiratory tract. The nuclei of the alveolar macrophage are pyknotic, variable in size, and usually peripherally located. The cytoplasm often contains granules of carbonaceous material or has a foamy vacuolated appearance. Alveolar macrophages are derived from bone marrow and are activated during an infectious process. When activated, they possess a higher bacteriocidal activity, are more phagocytic, and have a higher lysosomal enzyme level.

Three types of cells from the bronchial epithelial layer may be noted. The basal bronchial epithelial cell is usually about the size of a lymphocyte and has the greatest nuclear to cytoplasmic ratio of the three forms. Columnar bronchial epithelial cells are seen in two forms. Both forms are rectangular, with one

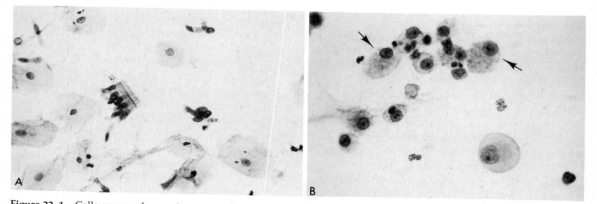

Figure 22–1. Cells commonly seen in sputum. Squamous and respiratory epithelial cells (*A*). Alveolar macrophages (arrows) and an alveolar cell (*B*). Appearance of macrophages indicates sample from lower respiratory tract. (Papanicolaou ×650.)

end tapered and containing a bulging nucleus. One form contains the ciliated border and is more common, while the other is the non-ciliated goblet type and is infrequently seen.

Blood cells are best identified with a Wright or Giemsa strain. Neutrophils may be present as partially disintegrated cells in almost every sputum specimen, and their presence most frequently indicates a pyogenic infection. Lymphocytes are the predominant cell seen in early cases of tuberculosis. Eosinophils are found in large numbers in the sputum of patients with bronchial asthma, but their presence is not pathognomonic of asthma. Erythrocytes are usually present as contaminants in all sputums, but in large numbers indicate an exudate or hemorrhage.

The various bacteria seen in sputum will be discussed later in relation to the disease with which they are associated.

SPUTUM CULTURE

When culturing sputum for a possible pathogen, two methods can be used: The first and most popular is the classic technique of streaking on an agar plate. In our laboratory, each specimen is routinely plated in sheep blood agar, chocolate agar, MacConkey's agar, and thioglycolate broth. The plates are incubated at 37°C. for 24 hours with the chocolate and blood agar plates in a 5 per cent carbon dioxide atmosphere. All known pathogens are identified and semiquantitated as to many, moderate, or few organisms present. Specific identification of all pathogens is performed by standard methods described elsewhere in this book. If no pathogens are present, the predominating organism or normal flora is reported.

The culture should be correlated with the previous Gram stain. If many organisms were seen on Gram stain, but only scant numbers or no growth on culture, then either the culture method was inadequate or the flora was suppressed by antibiotics. The hypothesis underlying the streak method is that the pathogenic organism will be present in greater numbers than any other superficial contaminating organism. However, even in sputum minimally contaminated with saliva it is possible to take the loopful of sample entirely from this contaminated area.

The second method is quantitative analysis of the organisms present. The sputum is homogenized and various dilutions of the sample are made. The method's hypothesis is that the organisms causing inflammation will be present in greater numbers than any other superficial contaminating organisms. Also, other problems such as overgrowth with *Proteus*, mixed infections, and even superinfections by a single organism are easier to identify.

The reluctance to adopt the method of quantitative analysis centers on the prolonged processing of the specimen required and the numerous agar plates needed.

A more extensive discussion of quantitative versus streak plate methods may be found in papers by Monroe (1969) and Pirtle (1969).

MYCOBACTERIA

According to the National Tuberculosis Association, any mycobacterial disease of the lungs other than that caused by *M. leprae* can be designated as tuberculosis. In this country the etiologic agent is *M. tuberculosis* in 97 to 99 per cent of the cases, with the remaining ones caused by the atypical mycobacteria. In sputum examination no differentiation by various staining techniques can be made between *M. tuberculosis* and the atypical mycobacteria. For this reason, a culture should always be performed in a previously undiagnosed case of tuberculosis. Treatment and public health procedures are different for these organisms.

In the classic or fulminant forms of the disease, large amounts of mucopurulent sputum are raised. Evidence of pulmonary hemorrhage and particles of caseous and necrotic material are present.

Within the necrotic tissue, elastic fibers are often present. These fibers are derived from blood vessels, alveoli, and bronchi. Their presence indicates destruction of pulmonary tissue, and thus they may appear in other diseases such as lung abscesses, bronchiectasis, or malignancy. Most often they are seen in advanced cases of tuberculosis. Careful selection of necrotic material will demonstrate the presence of fibers. Optimal demonstration is achieved by a concentration method— boiling with equal parts of 10 per cent sodium hydroxide and centrifuging. Upon examination these fibers appear as curled, slender, highly refractile, wavy fibrils of uniform diameter. Highly characteristic are the graceful curves without sharp bends.

Within the caseous material, large numbers

of bacilli are usually present. Staining procedures are best performed on this material for bacillus demonstration.

The problem confronting the laboratory centers on the recognition of the disease in its early stages. To aid in the early diagnosis, efforts have involved three parameters: (1) sputum induction and collection; (2) specimen concentration and decontamination procedures; and (3) organism demonstration by more sensitive staining techniques.

In the earliest stages of disease, sputum is present only in the morning in scant amounts and appears primarily mucoid with occasional yellow flakes. Compared with tuberculosis in later stages, the volume of sputum raised is not a criterion of the extent of pulmonary disease. To overcome this problem of small volumes, 24-hour pooled specimens and gastric lavage were collected in the past. Contamination with bacterial organisms was great. In 1966 Yue demonstrated that sputum induction by the newer inhalation methods gave a higher recovery rate of tubercle bacilli in a single morning specimen when compared with the older methods.

With the exception of the occasional stat requests for examination of acid-fast organisms, pretreatment of sputum by digestion procedures facilitates organism demonstration by: (1) liquefying the sputum for a more even distribution of organisms; (2) lowering the specific gravity for centrifugation of the organism; and (3) decontaminating the specimen of other organisms to allow the maximal survival of the acid-fast organism.

The methods currently in use employ either sodium hydroxide, N-acetyl-L-cysteine, Zepharin-trisodium phosphate (Z-TSP), or combinations thereof. Each method has its attributes, whether in preparation time, tubercle bacilli survival, or isolation rate. Compared with sodium hydroxide and N-acetyl-L-cysteine methods, a more dependable decontamination and greater mycobacterial survival appear to be present with the Zepharin-trisodium phosphate digestion procedure.

Procedure
REAGENTS

1. Zepharin-trisodium phosphate solution, one part Zepharin (benzalkonium chloride) to 3000 parts of 24 per cent trisodium phosphate.

2. M/15 phosphate buffer, pH, 6.6, prepared with two stock solutions, each M/15.

   a. KH_2PO_4 9.08 g/l 630 ml mixed with;

   b. Na_2HPO_4 9.48 g/l 370 ml for a final pH of 6.6.

METHOD

1. Place an appropriate volume of specimen in a sterile 50-ml screwcap tube and add an equal volume of Z-TSP solution.

2. Shake the specimen for 20 minutes and then leave at room temperature for an additional 30 minutes.

3. Centrifuge at 2000 rpm for 20 minutes.

4. Remove supernatant fluid by aspiration or decanting.

5. Resuspend sediment in 10 to 20 ml of M/15 sterile phosphate buffer, pH 6.6.

6. Allow to set for 15 minutes and recentrifuge for 20 minutes.

7. Remove supernatant fluid and prepare appropriate slides and media.

Preferably slides should be stained by the auramine-rhodamine (A-R) stain and a modification of the Ziehl-Neelsen (ZN) method.

The effectiveness of the acid-fast smear for detection of pulmonary tuberculosis has been well documented in many areas of the world. However, in the United States where the prevalence of tuberculosis is decreasing, acid-fast smear techniques alone for case finding have been recently shown to be less reliable. Boyd (1975) noted that for every true positive result, a false positive result was obtained; this suggests that the acid-fast smear is a poor screening technique in a population where the prevalence of tuberculosis is low.

At present the use of fluorescent microscopy is regarded as the most reliable method for the examination of acid-fast bacilli in smears. In 1962 Traunt described the auramine-rhodamine dye combination. Its superiority in comparison with the Ziehl-Neelsen staining procedure is due to more intensive binding of mycolic acid of the tubercle bacillus to carbol auramine than to carbol fuschin.

The auramine-rhodamine dye combination stains non-viable bacilli. Since bacilli viability is important in the evaluation of the drug effect, an acid-fast stain should be performed on all positive A-R stains. The acid-fast method stains only viable organisms.

With atypical mycobacteria, all strains of Runyon's Groups I, II, and III are auramine-rhodamine fast, while the majority of group IV do not stain by this dye technique.

Procedure (Traunt, 1962)
REAGENTS

1. Stain:

Auramine	1.5 g
Rhodamine	0.75 g
Phenol (liquefied at 50° C.)	10 ml
Glycerol	75 ml
Distilled H₂O	50 ml

2. Decolorizing solution: 0.5 per cent in 70 per cent ethanol.

3. Counterstain: 0.5 g potassium permanganate in 100 ml distilled water.

TECHNIQUE

1. Heat fix slides on a slide warmer.

2. Stain for at least 15 minutes at room temperature.

3. Rinse with distilled water.

4. Decolorize with acid alcohol for 2 to 3 minutes.

5. Counterstain with potassium permanganate solution for 2 to 4 minutes.

6. Rinse, dry, and examine under the fluorescent microscope using the filter combinations suggested by Traunt.

In summary, the superiority of the A-R staining technique to the acid-fast smear is attributed to the following factors: (1) the tubercle bacilli have a higher affinity for A-R dye; (2) the entire smear can be examined, since the low-power objective is used; and (3) the black background in fluorescent microscopy makes the bacilli stand out more sharply to allow more rapid and accurate slide screening.

MYCOTIC DISEASE

The identification of fungal organisms in sputum plays a vital role in diagnosis of pulmonary lesions of mycotic disease. Mycotic disease of the lungs often mimics either inflammatory or neoplastic disease in clinical symptoms or roentgenographic findings. If the presence of fungi in sputum is noted, valuable time is saved in the diagnosis for both the clinician and the mycologist. By recognizing characteristic morphology on sputum wet mount preparations, the mycologist can isolate and identify the organism more promptly by selecting appropriate media.

Poor communication between the clinician and mycologist often limits the effectiveness of rapid diagnosis. For example, the identification of *Actinomyces israelii* in sputum requires communication among the following: (1) clinician for the symptoms; (2) roentgenologist for evidence of pulmonary lesion; and (3) mycologist for significance of isolation.

Otherwise, a possible pathogenic organism might be considered a "usual" contaminant of sputum.

A first morning specimen is preferred, as it represents the overnight secretions of the tracheobronchial tree. A sterile container should be used to collect the specimen. In the laboratory the specimen should be placed in another sterile container and examined against a dark background. Fungi are usually present in tiny flecks or particles which appear yellow-gray in color and more dense than the surrounding sputum (Fig. 22-2).

A direct mount with 10 per cent sodium hydroxide should be made and examined under the low- and high-powered lens. If no fungi are found, the specimen can be concentrated by various techniques using either 4 per cent NaOH or the enzyme pancreatin. It is recommended that microscopic findings be confirmed by cultural methods. Sputum concentrate should never be cultured, as this procedure kills the fungi.

The primary isolation medium used by many laboratories is modified Sabouraud's dextrose agar. However, when utilizing this medium, bacteria and molds in sputum often overgrow and the yield of isolates is poor. If the degree of suspicion of mycotic infection is high, initial culture on selective isolation media such as modified Sabouraud's dextrose agar or heart brain infusion agar is recommended.

Pathologic Fungi

Actinomyces israelii. Although this is not a true fungus, most clinicians erroneously consider *Actinomyces israelii* and *Nocardia asteroides* to be fungi. *Actinomyces israelii* is a gram-positive organism that tends to grow slowly, with branching filaments. It can be cultured from most of the human tonsils removed at routine tonsillectomy and from scrapings of gum and teeth. Why the organism becomes invasive is not known, as it is a commensal organism. It is the only species of Actinomyces known to cause pulmonary actinomycosis. In sputum *A. israelii* appears macroscopically as yellow sulfur granules, usually less than 1 mm in diameter. Microscopically these granules appear as a mass of gram-positive mycelial filaments surrounded by a sheath of eosinophilic material, which gives a club-shaped appearance to the ends of these filaments.

Nocardia asteroides. In pulmonary nocardiosis caused by *N. asteroides* the pulmonary

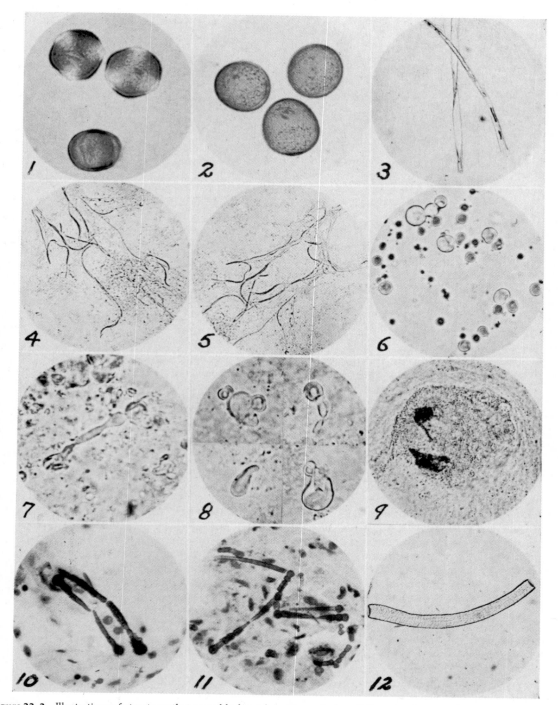

Figure 22–2. Illustrations of structures that resemble fungi found in sputum. *1*, Pollen, timothy grass (×800). *2*, Pollen, maple (×800). *3*, Cotton fibers (×100). *4* and *5*, Elastic tissue (×200). These are slender, highly refractile, wavy fibrils of uniform diameter and double contour. They may appear as single strands or in bundles and frequently show an alveolar arrangement. Their ends are often frayed or split. *6*, Fat cells (×800). *7* and *8*, Myelin globules (×800). Colorless globules occurring in a variety of sizes and bizarre forms. *9*, Bacterial colony (×400). Frequently found in sputum as small, gray or yellowish granules. They consist of a mass of either cocci or bacilli. *10* and *11*, Asbestos bodies (×800). They may occur as single structures or in small bundles and have a yellowish color. *12*, Wool fiber (×100). (From Kurung, J. M.: Am. Rev. Tuberc., *55*:387, 1947.)

lesions may resemble tuberculosis or histoplasmosis. Since treatment is radically different in all three diseases, sputum examination can play a vital role in early diagnosis. Nocardia morphology is similar to Actinomyces, but its granules, if present, lack the clubbing of peripheral filaments and are not so compact. The filaments are gram-positive, bacilliform in shape, and in some stains are partially acid fast.

Isolation from a solitary specimen is not presumptive of the diagnosis, since it may occasionally be a saprophyte in the upper respiratory tract. Its repeated presence is diagnostic of pulmonary nocardiosis.

Cryptococcus neoformans. The India ink technique is recommended for direct examination of sputum. India ink is mixed undiluted with the specimen; experience indicates the correct amount of ink to use. A negative India ink does not contraindicate performing a culture. (Most pulmonary lesions are clinically inapparent, while the disseminated lesions are more apparent and severe.)

The organism appears as a single budding blastospore, 5 to $20\,\mu$ in diameter, and is surrounded by a capsule from 3 to $5\,\mu$ in thickness.

Histoplasma capsulatum. The disease frequently starts as a flu-like syndrome; with healing, the pulmonary lesions become fibrotic and calcified, resembling healed primary tuberculosis. Occasionally the disease may become progressive and disseminated to all organs.

Direct microscopic examination of fresh preparations rarely results in identification of the organism. Staining of sputum with either Wright's or Giemsa's stain often reveals macrophages with characteristic intracellular small yeast cells in the cytoplasm. The specimen should be cultured upon receipt, as sputum contains enzymes fungicidal for the organism.

Coccidioides immitis. The primary pulmonary disease usually has minimal manifestations. Approximately 5 per cent of patients are left with residual lesions of the lung such as nodules, abscesses, and cavities. Locally destructive pulmonary lesions rarely progress to the disseminated form.

Sputum should be examined by wet direct mounts. The organism appears as a spherule, measuring 20 to $60\,\mu$ in diameter and being filled with endospores (2 to $5\,\mu$ in diameter). In the chronic cavitary form of the disease, hyphae may be seen.

Blastomyces dermatitidis. The initial infection begins in the lungs, with subsequent hematogenous spread to other organs of the body. In direct wet mounts, the organisms appear as 8 to $15\,\mu$ in diameter spherical cells with a thick, double, contoured refractile wall. Buds are attached to the mother cell by a broad base with a characteristic septum between them. The single bud distinguishes *B. dermatitidis* from its South American counterpart, *Paracoccidioides brasiliensis*, whose pathogenic phase is a multiple budding yeast. No mycelium occurs in sputum.

Candida albicans. *Candida albicans* is part of the normal throat flora. With widespread antibiotic and immunosuppressive therapy there is often an overgrowth of *C. albicans*. Its appearance on repeated examination indicates it as a possible pathogen. Close communication with the attending physician is needed for proper interpretation of the results.

Candida multiply readily at room temperature, and if the sputum sits at room temperature, the overgrowth may lead to erroneous interpretation. The report should include an evaluation of the number of organisms seen per field. On direct mount the organisms measure about $4\,\mu$ in diameter, are thin walled, and may appear singly, in pairs, or in small clusters. Budding forms and pseudomycelia may be formed. The organisms stain intensely positive with Gram stain.

Aspergillus fumigatus. Like *C. albicans*, the organisms appear often as a sputum contaminant, and if demonstrated repeatedly in a specimen, it can be implicated as the principal pathogen. Again, communication is essential between the mycologist and the clinician. Pulmonary disease caused by *Aspergillus* may present as either an allergic bronchitis or a localized "aspergilloma."

Phycomycosis. Mucor is the most common species of the genera disease. Mucormycosis is now referred to as phycomycosis and rarely causes pulmonary lesions. When it does, it is seen usually in patients on steroids, in diabetics, or in severely burned patients. Direct wet mounts may reveal broad, 6 to $50\,\mu$ nonseptate hyphae. Isolation on culture is needed for definite identification.

BRONCHIAL ASTHMA

Laboratory examination of sputum for evidence of bronchial asthma is often neglected, although characteristic patterns can be seen in

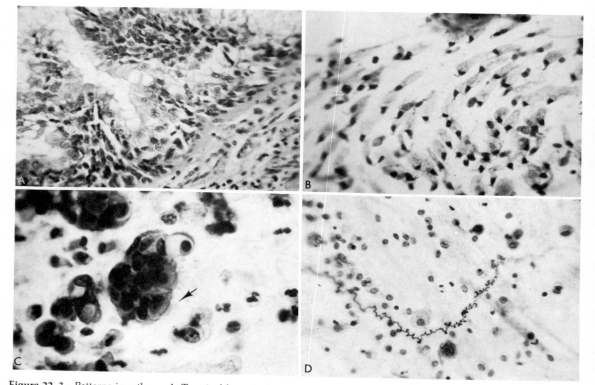

Figure 22–3. Patterns in asthma. *A,* Terminal bronchiole showing goblet cell hyperplasia (H & E stain ×650); *B,* Exfoliated goblet cells (Papanicolaou ×650); *C,* Creola body. Note presence of cilia (arrow) (Papanicolaou ×650); *D,* Curschmann's spiral. Note elongated wavy central thread (Gram stain ×250).

sputum (Fig. 22-3). The sputum is usually white and mucoid and contains no blood or pus unless an underlying bacterial infection is present. Approximately one third of all asthmatics will have sputum showing evidence of intercurrent respiratory infection. Some of the following findings are frequently observed in sputum. (Sanerkin, 1965).

Eosinophilia. The sputum has distinctive eosinophilic staining properties which have been attributed to an increased number of eosinophils and to the increased accumulation of serum proteins from the inflammation of the allergic reaction. This eosinophilic staining property has been used to differentiate asthma from chronic bronchitis. Also, sputum eosinophilia appears to be associated with a better response to prednisone.

Blood Cells. The cell seen in the greatest number is the eosinophil, both intact and degenerated. Unless there is an underlying infection, neutrophils are not present. Monocytes and histiocytes appear in significant numbers during the recovery phase.

Charcot-Leyden Crystals. They are rarely found in sputum except in cases of bronchial asthma. They may be absent in fresh sputum but make their appearance if the specimen is allowed to sit. The crystals are colorless, pointed hexagons and vary greatly in size. The average length is about three to four times the diameter of a red blood cell. Often they appear needle-like. They are derived from the disintegration of eosinophils; hence, they stain strongly with eosin.

Bronchial Epithelial Cells. The epithelial cells often occur singly and show hydropic degeneration, with poor definition of the original morphology. During acute exacerbations, these cells gather in larger clusters, display a vacuolated cytoplasm with ciliated borders, and are known as Creola bodies. Also present are well-preserved, hypersecretory goblet cells occurring singly or in clusters.

Creola Bodies. These are seen almost exclusively in the sputum of asthmatic patients and occur in approximately one half the cases. Their appearance in large or increasing numbers is a poor prognostic sign. They are large, compact clusters of ciliated columnar cells, occasionally having vacuoles in the cytoplasm.

Curschmann's Spirals. They are found most frequently in bronchial asthma and are fairly characteristic of the disease. Occasionally they may be observed in chronic bronchitis and other respiratory diseases, but in these cases there is nearly always an underlying asthmatic tendency. Macroscopically they can sometimes be recognized by the naked eye and appear as yellow-white, mucoid, wavy threads frequently coiled into little balls. Unraveled, their length rarely exceeds 1.5 cm. Microscopically a central thread is seen around which mucus is wrapped, supported by a fibril network. The central thread is formed by the shedding of the lining epithelium. Often embedded within the mucus are leukocytes and Charcot-Leyden crystals.

Future and promising studies center on chemical abnormalities of asthmatic sputum in the hope of improving pharmacologic approaches to asthma. Among the abnormalities identified are increased levels of sialomucins, histamine, antitrypsin, kallikrein, and IgE. Clinical and laboratory application of their measurements is still in the future.

BRONCHIECTASIS

Bronchial dilatation of the saccular or cylindrical form *per se* will not cause symptoms unless a superimposed infection is present. The production of a mucopurulent sputum is one of the cardinal symptoms of this disease, and the amount expectorated varies with the posture. In the morning, production of sputum is usually the greatest, as the contents of the dilated lung sacs empty into the larger bronchi.

Characteristically, sputum is putrid, gray-green in color, and varies in volume from 50 to 250 ml daily. Occasional blood streaking may be present. The source of this blood is usually the chronic granulation tissue of the chronically infected bronchial wall. If the sputum is allowed to sit, it separates into three layers: an upper frothy layer which later subsides, a middle turbid mucus layer, and a bottom layer composed primarily of pus cells and various organisms. Closer examination of the bottom layer reveals the presence of bronchial epithelial cells, fatty crystals, various bacteria, and, occasionally, Dittrich's plugs (see p. 723). Occasionally elongated fatty acid crystals appear to be elastic tissue but lack the characteristic wavy appearance. The presence of elastic fibers may be used to differentiate the sputum of bronchiectasis from that of gangrene or lung abscesses.

CHRONIC BRONCHITIS

In chronic bronchitis the bronchioles as well as the bronchi may be inflamed, and the inflammatory reaction may be either cellular or catarrhal. The mildest and most frequent form of the disease in the United States is smoker's cough. Of all the criteria required to establish the diagnosis of chronic bronchitis, sputum production is accepted as the necessary minimum.

Macroscopically the sputum is tenacious, white, and mucoid in appearance. During superimposed infections, the secretions increase in volume and become purulent yellow-green in color. The average volume expectorated is about 60 ml per day, but volumes as high as 600 ml per day have been produced. Some clinicians use increasing or decreasing volume as a parameter in assessing the activity of the disease.

Microscopically the presence of histiocytes and monocytes can help in assessing the activity of the disease. In early chronic bronchitis, large numbers of histiocytes and monocytes indicate a stable phase, but during exacerbation these cells disappear. When entering clinical remission again, these cells reappear. A similar pattern holds true for leukocytes and epithelial cells. In remission, a few cells are noted. The presence of necrotic tissue or elastic fibers is an ominous sign, as this indicates a superimposed severe process such as abscess formation or bronchiectasis.

Examination of the Gram stain and subsequent culture usually reveals the presence of mixed organisms without a predominant pathogenic organism. Indeed, there is little difference in the bacterial flora in the sputum of patients in remission or exacerbation. *Hemophilus influenzae* and pneumococci are frequently cultured, but their pathologic significance is difficult to assess, especially if they are present in small numbers. For example, *H. influenzae* is cultured in more than 50 per cent of patients clinically ill; however, in patients not ill, 10 to 20 per cent grow *H. influenzae* on culture.

Chemical analysis of sputum is a relatively new but promising procedure. Further clinical studies need to be performed before sound clinical applications can be construed.

The activity of the enzyme lactic dehydrogenase (LDH) can be measured in sputum. It originates from serum, the inflammatory cells, and the mucosal surface. Thus, with destructive inflammatory changes in the bronchial mucosa, increased LDH activity may be expected. During exacerbation of chronic bronchitis, total LDH activity increases, with the greatest increase occurring in the electrophoretically faster isoenzyme fractions. With improvement, the reverse is seen. When bacterial resistance to antibiotic therapy is developing, increased LDH activity may be observed before clinical deterioration. Hence, appropriate changes in antibiotics may be made sooner than waiting for culture or clinical changes (Levine, 1969).

DNA in sputum can be demonstrated either by fluorescent microscopy or by chemical determination. It originates from disintegrated inflammatory cells and the destruction of bronchial epithelial cells. Thus, in infected secretions, DNA levels are high as a result of extensive cellular damage. Levels fall as improvement is noted.

Finally, elevated neuraminic acid levels have been measured in the sputum of patients with chronic bronchitis.

LUNG ABSCESS

Unless the abscess ruptures into a bronchus, there is little or no sputum production. Most abscesses are initiated by bronchial occlusion, by virtue of either aspirations, tumor, or foreign body occlusion. Those originating from a bacterial pneumonia usually have as their etiologic agent *Klebsiella, Hemophilus, Staphylococcus aureus*, or *Streptococcus pyogenes* because these organisms may cause tissue necrosis.

When rupture occurs, a large amount of bloody, creamy, foul-smelling pus is suddenly and violently expectorated. Close examination reveals the presence of elastic fibers, cellular debris, and leukocytes. Usually more than one organism will be seen with Gram staining. A search for tubercle bacilli or malignant cells must also be made.

PNEUMONIA

In the early diagnosis of pneumonia a Gram stain of the sputum is perhaps the most essential examination. Proper interpretation leads to institution of appropriate therapy at least 24 hours before the results of the culture are available. However, certain hazards in the interpretation of the Gram stain are present. These include the following. Gram-negative organisms are often overlooked, as non-bacterial elements stain gram-negative. Conversely, gram-positive debris is often mistaken for organisms, especially by the novice. Smears are often stained improperly. The occurrence of more than a faint trace of positive stain in the cytoplasm of white blood cells indicates undercolorization. Finally, the description of the Gram stain is often inadequate. For example, "gram-positive cocci" does not distinguish between pneumococcus and staphylococcus, two pathogenic organisms whose antibiotic treatment is different.

Gram-positive Cocci

Of the gram-positive pneumonias, the principal pathogen is *Streptococcus pneumoniae;* rarely are staphylococci and other streptococci involved.

The *S. pneumoniae* organism is a gram-positive lancet-shaped diplococcus with the long axis in a straight line. Occasionally, a capsule may be seen on Gram stain. A Quelling reaction is used to differentiate pneumococci into 75 types. These types have different virulence with the type III organism being associated with the most virulent form of pneumococcal pneumonia.

Since pneumococci quickly autolyse, they should be cultured as soon as possible or immediately refrigerated. Thorsteinsson (1975) has shown that a sputum specimen is as accurate as either a transtracheal or bronchial aspirate in the diagnosis of acute pneumococcal pneumonia.

In pneumococcal pneumonia the character of the sputum varies with the stage of the disease. In the early stages of typical lobar pneumonia, the sputum is scanty and transparent, with occasional blood flecks. As the disease progresses to the red-hepatization stage, the sputum becomes rust red, very tenacious, and mucopurulent. Microscopic examination reveals the presence of many intra- and extracellular organisms, epithelial cells, leukocytes, and erythrocytes. During the stages of resolution, the sputum becomes more abundant and less tenacious and assumes the appearance of that seen in chronic bronchitis. The rusty character of the sputum is absent during this stage, and the reappearance of this characteristic should alert the clinician that the disease is progressing or has involved the opposite lung. Daily sputum Gram stains should be performed on these patients for two reasons; to follow the effect of treatment on the disease, and to rule out secondary infection.

In staphylococcal pneumonia, a yellow, purulent, voluminous sputum is present. On Gram stain, large numbers of staphylococci in grapelike clusters and neutrophils are present.

GRAM-NEGATIVE BACILLI

The gram-negative pneumonias are hard to diagnose initially on sputum examination. Gram stains of sputum may be confusing, since morphologically similar organisms are present in normal throat flora. Almost any of the gram-negative aerobic organisms have the potential to cause disease of the lower respiratory tract, but the more common ones are *Klebsiella, Hemophilus, Enterobacter, Pseudomonas,* and *Escherichia coli*. With the exception of the foul green sputum seen in *Pseudomonas* infections, no "classic" macroscopic findings are present in these sputums.

Hemophilus influenzae is often missed on Gram stain. The organism binds the safranine stain poorly and it is misinterpreted as background debris. *Hemophilus* is particularly important as a pathogen in adults with a diagnosis of chronic bronchitis or bronchiectasis. The methylene blue stain permits easier recognition of *H. influenzae* than does the Gram stain. If the organism suspected is *H. influenzae* and no methylene blue stain is available, 0.2 per cent fuchsin solution can be used as the counterstain instead of safranine.

Klebsiella, Enterobacter, Escherichia coli, and *Pseudomonas* are common gastrointestinal inhabitants which may cause pneumonia. Conditions leading to this disease are aspiration, host immunosuppression, and antibiotics. However, patients with chronic disease apparently unrelated to previous antibiotic therapy often have stable flora in the upper respiratory tract that are predominantly gram-negative bacilli. Therefore, a culture or Gram stain should never be the sole reason for patient treatment without clinical indications.

Various anaerobes such as Bacteroidaceae and anaerobic streptococci have been implicated in essentially all types of pulmonary infections (Bartlett, 1974). The sputum is characteristically putrid. Gram stain usually reveals primarily gram-negative organisms of mixed morphology. In pneumonia caused by the anaerobic streptococci, the sputum is not foul smelling and on Gram stain, tiny gram-positive cocci in chains are noted.

Percutaneous transtracheal aspiration is recommended for specimen collection for culture. Expectorated sputum is often heavily contaminated by the indigenous anaerobic flora of the mouth and oropharynx.

PNEUMOCONIOSIS

The term pneumoconiosis refers to a fibrosis of the lung secondary to inhalation of an organic or inorganic dust. The disease is primarily occupational and its severity differs according to the type of inhaled dust.

To reach the alveoli and initiate a reaction, the particles usually have to be less than $5\,\mu$ in diameter. In the alveoli the reaction to the dust particle depends upon its composition. In general, particles are engulfed by macrophages and deposited in peribronchial lymph channels or are carried onto the regional lymph nodes. By far the commonest and severest form of pneumoconiosis in the United States is silicosis. Other types of pneumoconiosis are asbestosis, anthracosilicosis, berylliosis, bagassosis, and byssinosis. The latter two are caused by cane sugar and cotton dust, respectively.

The character and production of sputum varies with the severity and stage of the disease. Macroscopically the sputum is tenacious and can sometimes display the color of the dust inhaled. Microscopically various diagnos-

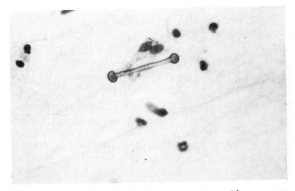

Figure 22–4. Asbestosis body from patient with pneumoconiosis; characteristics may occasionally be overlooked and considered artefact. (Papanicolaou ×650.)

tic features can differentiate the pneumoconiosis, but their presence is difficult to demonstrate (Fig. 22-4).

In anthracosilicosis angular black granules will be both intracellular and extracellular. Unfortunately the presence of these cells is not pathognomonic for anthracosilicosis, as similar cells with smaller carbon particles are abundant in heavy tobacco smokers and people living in highly polluted areas.

In asbestosis the presence of dumbbell-shaped asbestos needles in clusters is diagnostic. They stain yellow to dark brown and measure 10 to 80 μ in size. Numerous multi-nucleated giant cells and histiocytes may also be observed.

In silicosis the particles are detected with polarized light. The crystals appear sharp, elongated, and fragmented. Numerous neutrophils, macrophages, and multinucleated giant cells are present.

In byssinosis polarized light should also be used to demonstrate the crystals. They appear as rectangular, prism-shaped crystals that shine brightly with polarized light.

PULMONARY EMBOLISM

If pulmonary infarction is secondary to thromboembolus, sputum examination shortly afterward reveals the presence of bright red blood in a very tenacious, mucoid background. As the infarction resolves, the sputum becomes progressively darker in color. Microscopic examination reveals erythrocytes, altered hemoglobin, and macrophages with denatured hemoglobin products in the cytoplasm. Bacteria usually start to appear at this stage as infarcted lung is an excellent culture medium.

Sputum examination in fat embolism is non-definitive. Lipid-laden macrophages and fat droplets may be found in normal persons and especially in persons who are cigarette smokers. Endogenous fat and tobacco tar stain are positive by oil red O but can be differentiated in that the tar has fluorescent properties.

HEART DISEASE

Sputum examination has characteristic findings in some types of heart disease.

In acute edema, a condition in which large amounts of serous exudate pass from the cap-

illaries into the alveoli, the sputum is abundant, frothy, and pink. As much as 1 liter a day may be expectorated in severe conditions. Microscopically the sputum may be shown to contain numerous erythrocytes and large hyaline masses. These hyaline masses are the protein component of the serous exudate.

In mitral heart disease the sputum is tenacious and blood is present, either in streaks or in dark masses mixed with mucus.

In chronic congestive heart failure, the sputum is frothy and rust colored. Microscopic examination reveals the presence of erythrocytes and "heart failure cells." In fresh unstained sputum these cells appear as round colorless bodies filled with various-sized granules of yellow to brown pigment. This pigment may be demonstrated to be hemosiderin by staining with 10 per cent potassium ferrocyanide for a few minutes and then with 0.1 N HCl. Hemosiderin pigment stains a blue color.

PULMONARY ALVEOLAR PROTEINOSIS

In this disease, eosinophilic material which is positive for periodic acid–Schiff (PAS) stain is deposited in the alveoli without serious alteration of lung structure. The disease usually pursues a chronic course ending in death but may resolve spontaneously. Diagnosis is confirmed by lung biopsy but can be made by sputum examination. Microscopic examination reveals an increase of hypertrophic, hyperplastic alveolar cells, with a granular protein deposit in the background. If formalin-fixed sections are made, PAS-positive alveolar casts with laminated bodies and acicular spaces are present.

PNEUMOCYSTIS CARINII

Pneumocystis carinii is a protozoan parasite which can cause an interstitial pneumonia in the immunologically impaired host. Expectorated sputum is a poor source to demonstrate the presence of the organism. In a study of patients with known *Pneumocystis carinii* pneumonia, Lau (1976) found the organism present in sputum in approximately 1 per cent of the cases. The best yield for diagnosis is obtained in lung biopsy. Transtracheal or postbronchoscopy aspirations may also be successful. The Gomori silver stain best delineates the cysts of the organism. The cysts measure $4.5\,\mu$ in diameter and are round or cup-shaped, with a thin black wall enclosing a cylindrical or comma-shaped structure within the cyst. If one desires a more prompt interpretation, smears made from aspirated specimens and imprint preparations from lung biopsies may be stained by the Gram-Weigert procedure (Rosen, 1977) or by a variation of the Gomori method (Charukian, 1977).

GOODPASTURE'S SYNDROME

This syndrome or disease is characteristically seen in young males and usually terminates in death within two years secondary to kidney failure or pulmonary hemorrhage. Immunoglobulins are deposited on the basement membranes of both lung and kidney. Sputum examination reveals the presence of large numbers of hyperplastic alveolar cells mixed with an abundance of large hemosiderin-laden macrophages.

VIRAL INFECTIONS

Viruses have been estimated to cause between 70 and 90 per cent of all respiratory infections. Six large groups of viruses are capable of causing infections, and almost all the groups include a great number of serotypes. Since the prognosis of respiratory tract infections is usually excellent, little attention has been paid to identifying the specific etiologic viral agents.

Viruses are composed of a core of RNA or DNA covered by a protein coat. All viruses require living cells for growth. After penetration into a cell, the nucleic acid of the virus takes control of the enzymatic machinery of the infected cell, which results in multiplication of the virus and often leads to destruction of the cell. Infected cells show viral aggregates (inclusion bodies) in the nucleus (herpes simplex virus), in the cytoplasm (parainfluenza), or in both the nucleus and cytoplasm (cytomegalovirus).

Preparation of specimens for viral examination is similar to sputum cytology for malignancy. Instead of examining for malignant changes in cells, the presence of inclusion bodies is looked for.

The inclusion bodies of herpes simplex and adenovirus are intranuclear. Herpes simplex is the easier of the two to identify, and in the bronchial epithelium, the changes involve only

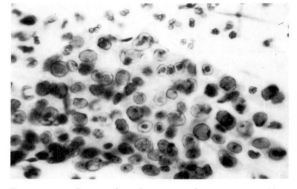

Figure 22-5. Sputum from herpes simplex pneumonia. Note presence of amphophilic intranuclear inclusion, margination of chromatin, and opaqueness of nuclei. (Papanicolaou ×650.)

the young columnar or squamous exfoliated cells (Fig. 22-5). These mononuclear cells, along with giant cells, develop intranuclear eosinophilic inclusion bodies surrounded by a halo. Decreased nuclear basophilia is also evident in these cells except in areas where the chromatin clump has adhered to the inner surface of the nuclear membrane. In contrast to herpes simplex and other viruses, the adenovirus infection is compatible with cellular life.

Eosinophilic intracytoplasmic inclusions are seen in parainfluenza and measle viral infections, while basophilic intracytoplasmic inclusions are present in respiratory syncytial and cytomegalic viral infections.

Of these viruses, the cytomegalic viral infection is associated with the highest morbidity, and recent evidence indicates that few individuals escape infection during life. The majority of generalized severe infections occur in the newborn period and presumably originate from intrauterine infections. Infants with this disease may harbor the virus in the nasopharynx and act as a reservoir similar to infants with congenital rubella. Since prompt identification of the disease is important, rapid diagnosis can sometimes be made by obtaining sputum by tracheal aspiration. The presence of large epithelial cells with both intranuclear and intracytoplasmic inclusion bodies is diagnostic.

CYTOLOGIC EXAMINATION IN MALIGNANCY

The cytologic examination of sputum is the single most reliable method for diagnosis of

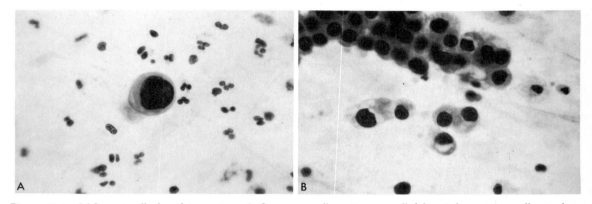

Figure 22–6. Malignant cells found in sputum. *A*, Squamous cell carcinoma, well-delineated squamous cell cytoplasm; *B*, alveolar cell carcinoma—can be confused with cells of sputum of patients with resolving pulmonary infarction. (Papanicolaou ✕650.)

early pulmonary carcinoma, having a positive yield of approximately 50 per cent as compared to 25 per cent when bronchoscopy and bronchial biopsy are performed. In combination with bronchoscopy and radiography, the number of early cases detected has significantly increased, although unfortunately the survival rate has not improved.

Since methods of specimen collection and preparation vary considerably, it is advisable to consult with the pathologist prior to specimen collection and to follow his instructions.

The most common specimen is the single, early morning, "deep cough" sputum. These specimens should be collected on a minimum of three and preferably five consecutive mornings and submitted to the laboratory fresh without prior fixation. The fresh specimen is examined, and bloody areas and tissue flecks are selected and smeared onto a slide. Other methods of preparing smears include blenderizing, enzymatic digestion, and concentration of the sediment. The accepted criterion for a satisfactory sputum sample is the presence of alveolar macrophages. Four slides are pre-

pared for examination and stained with the Papanicolaou stain.

If multiple sputum collections are impractical, the most reliable sputum sample is the postbronchoscopy specimen.

Central bronchogenic carcinoma gives the highest percentage positive results in sputum examination, although it is not uncommon for peripheral lesions and metastatic carcinomas to yield positive smears.

Interpretation of smears is difficult, as many diseases cause cellular changes mimicking carcinoma. Inflammatory pulmonary lesions, and especially tuberculosis, form atypical squamous cells which are difficult to distinguish from squamous cell carcinoma (Fig. 22-6). Pulmonary infarction, chronic bronchitis, and especially bronchial asthma may cause profound atypical terminal bronchiolar metaplasia and alveolar pneumocyte dysplasia which closely mimics pulmonary adenocarcinoma. Other diagnostic problems are caused by viral pneumonias, especially those due to herpes simplex and to cytotoxic drugs such as busulfan, cyclophosphamide, and azathioprine.

REFERENCES

Baldry, P. E., and Josse, S. E.: The measurement of sputum viscosity. Amer. Rev. Resp. Dis., *98*:392, 1968.

Bartlett, J. G., Gorback, S. L., and Finegold, S. M.: The bacteriology of aspiration pneumonia. Am. J. Pathol., *84*:372, 1976.

Boyd, J. C., and Marr, J. J.: Decreasing reliability of acid-fast smear techniques for detection of tuberculosis. Ann. Intern. Med., *82*:489, 1975.

Bürgi, H., Wiesmann, U., Richterich, R., Negli, K., and

Medici, T.: New objective criteria for inflammation in bronchial secretions. Br. Med. J., *2*:654, 1968.

Charukian, C. J., and Schenk, E. A.: Rapid Grocotts methenamine-silver nitrate method for fungi and Pneumocystis carinii. Am. J. Clin. Pathol., *68*:427, 1977.

Chodosh, S.: Examination of sputum cells. N. Engl. J. Med., *282*:854, 1970.

Epstein, R. L.: Sputum eosinophilia in obstructive lung disease. Ann. Intern. Med., *75*:317, 1971.

Heller, C.: Fluorostaining of tubercle bacilli. Am. Rev. Resp. Dis., *95*:1068, 1967.

Joseph, S. W., and Houk, V. N.: Evaluation and application of the fluorochrome stain for microscopic detection of mycobacteria in clinical specimens. Am. Rev. Resp. Dis., *98*:1044, 1968.

Kubica, G. P., Dye, W. E., Cohn, M. L., and Middlebrook, G.: Sputum digestion and decontamination with N-acetyl-L-cysteine sodium hydroxide for culture of mycobacteria. Am. Rev. Resp. Dis., *87*:775, 1963.

Kurung, J. M.: The isolation and identification of pathogenic fungi from sputum. Am. Rev. Tuberc., *55*:387, 1947.

Lau, W. K., Young, L. S., and Remington, J. S.: Pneumocystis carinii pneumonia. Diagnosis by examination of pulmonary secretions. J.A.M.A., *236*:2399, 1976.

Levine, I., Flief, A., Sansur, M., and Wroblewski, F.: Clinical implications of LDH activity in sputum. J.A.M.A., *207*:2436-2437, 1969.

Monroe, P. W., Muchmore, H. G., Felton, F. G., and Pirtle, J. K.: Quantitation of microorganisms in sputum. Appl. Microbiol., *18*:214, 1969.

Naib, Z. M., Stewart, J. A., Dowdle, W. R., Casey, H. L., Marine, W. M., and Nahmias, A. J.: Cytological features of viral respiratory tract infections. Acta Cytol., *12*:162, 1968.

Newhouse, M., Sanchis, J., and Bienenstock, J.: Lung defense mechanisms. N. Engl. J. Med., *295*:990, 1976.

Pirtle, J. K., Monroe, P. W., Smalley, T. K., Mohr, J. A., and Rhoades, E. R.: Diagnostic and therapeutic advantages of several quantitative cultures of fresh sputum in acute bacterial pneumonia. Am. Rev. Resp. Dis., *100*:831, 1969.

Rosen, P. R.: Frozen section management of a lung biopsy for suspected Pneumocystis pneumonia. Am. J. Surg. Pathol., *1*:79, 1977.

Sanerkin, N. G., and Evans, D. M.: The sputum in bronchial asthma: Pathognomonic patterns. J. Pathol. Bacteriol., *89*:535, 1965.

Thorsteinsson, S. B., Mosher, D. M., and Fagan, T.: The diagnostic value of sputum culture in acute pneumonia. J.A.M.A., *233*:894, 1975.

Traunt, J. P., Brett, W. A., and Thomas, W.: Fluorescence microscopy of tubercle bacilli stained with auramine and rhodamine. Henry Ford Hosp. Med. Bull., *10*:287, 1962.

Yeager, H., Jr.: Tracheobronchial secretions. Am. J. Med., *50*:493, 1971.

Yue, W. U., and Cohen, S. S.: Sputum induction in patients with pulmonary tuberculosis by newer inhalation methods. Am. Rev. Resp. Dis., *94*:502, 1966.

23

EXAMINATION OF EXOCRINE PANCREATIC FUNCTION

Wei T. Wu, Ph.D.,
Myrton F. Beeler, M.D.,
and Yuan S. Kao, M.D.

PHYSIOLOGY OF PANCREATIC SECRETION

The pancreas produces from 1000 to 2500 ml of juice in 24 hours. This fluid is slightly alkaline and, besides water, contains mainly enzymes, sodium, potassium, sodium bicarbonate, chloride, and phosphate. Secretin, an intestinal hormone produced under stimulation by hydrochloric acid, causes production of fluid high in bicarbonate level, low in enzyme activity; while cholecystokinin-pancreozymin, an intestinal hormone produced under stimulation by gastrin, causes production of fluid high in enzyme activity, low in bicarbonate level. Enzymes include amylase, lipase, trypsinogen, chymotrypsinogens A and B, procarboxypeptidases A and B, proelastase, and prophospholipase. Duodenal enterokinase catalyzes formation of trypsin from trypsinogen. Trypsin catalyzes conversion of the proteolytic proenzymes and prophospholipase to their active forms.

SCREENING FOR PANCREATIC DISORDERS

Determination of altered activity of amylase and lipase in body fluids has, for years, been the keystone of the laboratory approach to the diagnosis of acute and relapsing (chronic) pancreatitis, in which there is increased release of these substances into blood and urine, whereas, for the diagnosis of pancreatic carcinoma and chronic pancreatitis, examination of stimulated pancreatic fluid through duodenal aspiration has been, until recently, the only reliable means of assessing pancreatic secretory function. These tests are not suitable for detecting the pancreatic disease-prone individual or for screening for the predisease state. However, there are predisposing conditions which can be screened for. For example, alcoholism or gallstone disease is present in over 80 per cent of patients with pancreatitis, so biochemical tests sensitive to liver damage—such as serum aspartate aminotransferase or gamma glutamyl transpeptidase—may be useful. In alcoholics, hypertriglyceridemia may trigger the pancreatitis; therefore, serum triglyceride determinations may also be useful. Serum calcium level measurements may be indicated, since patients with hyperparathyroidism are at increased risk of developing pancreatitis. Hyperparathyroidism merits a screening procedure on its own. Steroids, thiazides, sulfonamides, azathioprine, and birth control pills have also been implicated as causes of pancreatitis, although not commonly. A family history can serve as a good screening test for cystic fibrosis of the pancreas. Unfortunately, because pancreatic carcinoma is the fourth leading cause of cancer deaths in the United States and because the five-year survival rate is only 1 to 2 per cent, there is no established effective screening test for early diagnosis of this form of cancer, although abdominal ultrasound has recently been recommended followed by a pancreatic function test using cholecystokinin-stimulated enzyme output (DiMagno, 1977). Specific pancreatic tumor-associated glycoproteins, recently described by researchers at Roswell Park Memorial Institute and at the University of Chicago, may provide leads toward development of such a screening test.

AMYLASE
(α-1, 4-glucan-4-glucanohydrolase)

BIOCHEMISTRY AND PHYSIOLOGY

Amylases are enzymes that catalyze the hydrolysis of polysaccharides such as amylose, amylopectin, glycogen, and their partially hydrolyzed products. α-Amylase (α-1, 4-glucan-4-glucanohydrolase, E.C. 3.2.1.1) occurs in animal tissues and fluids. It splits α-1, 4-glucosidic linkages in random fashion. Upon hydrolysis by α-amylase, amylose gives rise to a mixture of maltose and glucose, whereas amylopectin yields a mixture of branched and unbranched oligosaccharides. Since α-amylase is unable to attack α-1, 6-glucosidic linkages, the polysaccharides which remain after hydrolysis are dextrins. α-Amylase is an endo-enzyme and was so named because all the hydrolysis products have α configuration at C_1 of the reducing glucose unit. α-Amylase rapidly decreases the ability of amylose to stain blue with iodine and decreases the viscosity of starch solutions.

Other amylases include β-amylase, found in both animals and plants, an exo-enzyme (α-1, 4-glucanomaltohydrolase, E.C. 3.2.1.2), and γ-amylase (α-1, 4-glucanglucohydrolase, E.C. 3.2.1.3) found in numerous fungi.

Of these three amylases, only α-amylase is of clinical interest. α-Amylase is stable at room temperature for at least one week and at refrigeration temperature for at least two months. It may be kept in the frozen state much longer without appreciable loss of activity.

In humans, α-amylase is normally present in pancreas (approximately 200 mg/kg), salivary glands, liver, muscle, adipose tissue, saliva, blood, urine, feces, milk, semen, kidney, brain, lung, fallopian tube, intestine, spleen, and heart. The α-amylase present in blood and urine of normal individuals is predominately of pancreatic and salivary origin. α-Amylases of pancreatic and salivary origins we abbreviate to P-type and S-type amylase, respectively, whenever such distinction is needed. These two types of amylase are closely related enzymes but also exhibit organ-specific variation. They yield the same amino acid composition and similar, but not identical, peptide maps. Each appears to consist of a single polypeptide chain. Pancreatic amylase has a molecular weight of 54,000 daltons. Higher molecular weights have been reported for salivary amylase (CDC Survey, 1975). Both amylases contain sulfhydryl groups. Amylases are metallo-enzymes containing at least one atom of calcium per molecule and require this metal for their catalytic activities. The pH for optimal activity ranges from 6.9 to 7.0. The pH optimum for salivary amylase varies with the anion used as activator, of which chloride is most important. Optimal chloride concentration is 10 mmol/l and the activation is allosteric (Levitski, 1974). Bromide and iodide ions also activate amylase.

The optimal temperature for α-amylase assay is 50°C., but most determinations are carried out at 37°C. Several recently described automated amylase methods employ 40°C., 45°C., and 50°C. (Fridhandler, 1970; Wu, 1972; Matthews, 1973). The Q_{10} factors (p. 351) have been reported to be 1.2 between 40 and 50°C. (Proelss, 1975) and 1.4 between 30 and 50°C.

Like most other enzymes, there is no known function of α-amylase in serum. Wilding (1967) remarked that "it is possibly fair to say that the amylase of normal serum has no function, but is merely a waste product on its way to excretion in the urine. The amount of amylase circulating in the blood may then be considered as the net result of the amount entering the extracellular fluid from tissues and the amount being cleared by the kidneys. Under normal conditions, activity in any one patient is fairly constant."

Also, little is known about the normal mechanism of entrance of pancreatic enzymes, such as amylase, into blood, where normally the pancreatic enzyme appears to account for less than 50 per cent of serum amylase activity. Increased serum activity in acute pancreatitis presumably results from escape of enzymes into the interstitial tissue and peritoneal cavity, with increased absorption through the lymphatics and veins. The renal clearance of amylase has been estimated to be 1 to 3 ml/min, appearing to be constant over a wide range of urine flow; therefore, increased release into the blood is followed by increased excretion in the urine (Levitt, 1968).

Amylase is first detectable in serum of infants between the ages of one and two months, and by one year of age low normal adult levels are reached.

INTERPRETATION

Serum amylase activity rises within a few hours of onset in patients with acute pancreatitis, but not proportionally to severity of the disease. Values over five times the upper limit of normal are highly suggestive of the diagnosis. Activity usually returns to normal in two to five days in patients with the milder edematous forms of the disease. Elevated values persisting longer than this suggest continuing necrosis or possible pseudocyst formation. The urine amylase activity rises promptly, often within several hours of the rise in serum activity (Gambill, 1963). Urine activity may remain abnormal after the serum activity has returned to the normal range. Values over 1000 Somogyi units per hour are seen almost exclusively in patients with acute pancreatitis (Bockus, 1965).

As may be surmised from this, increased renal clearance of amylase accounts for the greater sensitivity of the urine amylase in acute and relapsing pancreatitis (Levitt, 1969; Warshaw, 1975), and the ratio of amylase clearance to the creatinine clearance expressed as a percentage has been used diagnostically. It can be calculated by the following formula:

Clearance ratio (%)
$$= \frac{\text{Urine amylase activity}}{\text{Serum amylase activity}}$$
$$\times \frac{\text{Serum creatinine concentration}}{\text{Urine creatinine concentration}} \times 100$$

The normal ratio averages from 2 to 3 per cent, while that for patients with pancreatitis averages about 10 per cent (Warshaw, 1975; Johnson, 1976). Unfortunately, about one third of pancreatitis patients have normal ratios, and elevated ratios may be found in patients with burns, ketoacidosis, renal insufficiency, and duodenal performations, and after thoracic surgery (Levine, 1975; Jacobson, 1975). Thus, the ratio adds little to the diagnostic armamentarium (Dürr, 1977).

The ratio is very low—less than 1 per cent—in patients with macroamylasemia (Levitt, 1968), a condition whose importance lies in the fact that the correspondingly high serum amylase may be misinterpreted as indicating a clinically serious condition. Macroamylase (Wilding, 1964; Berk, 1967) is a large amylolytic enzyme, presumably a complex of normal-size amylase bound to glycoprotein(s) (Take, 1970; Levitt, 1972). It has been found in patients with malabsorption and/or alcoholism (Berk, 1970) but does not directly correlate with any single disease state.

Serum amylase may be elevated in patients with pancreatic carcinoma, but too late to be useful. It is also elevated frequently (over 60 per cent of patients) in diabetic ketoacidosis. Polyacrylamide gel electrophoresis has demonstrated that in this condition it is usually salivary rather than pancreatic amylase that is elevated. Serum activity may also be elevated in patients with cholecystitis, peptic ulcer, and postoperatively following gastric resection. Fewer patients may be found to have intestinal obstruction, mesenteric thrombosis, and peritonitis. In some of these patients, pancreatic secretions find their way into the peritoneal cavity and are absorbed into the blood stream; in others there may be inflammation involving the pancreas.

Less-than-normal serum amylase activity may be found in patients with chronic pancreatitis and pancreatic carcinoma, and has also been reported in such diverse and unexpected conditions as congestive heart failure, gastro-intestinal cancer, bone fractures, and pleurisy (Casey, 1971).

ISOENZYMES

Isoenzyme fractionation is technically feasible but has not found wide clinical acceptance, perhaps because of lack of availability, perhaps because of limited usefulness. However, since the electrophoretic fractionation of human salivary and pancreatic α-amylase into different isoenzymes was accomplished in early 1960 by Norby (1964) and others (Aw, 1966), there have been numerous studies focused on this subject. Recent investigations have revealed that human pancreatic and salivary amylases appear to have the same amino acid composition and exhibit the same substrate specificity, although there are differences in molecular weight and carbohydrate content (Stiefel, 1973).

After electrophoresis of human serum on agar gel, Kamaryt (1965) observed two bands with amylolytic activity. They both appeared in the gamma globulin region. The mobility of the less anodic isoenzyme corresponded to that of the amylase band obtained from pancreas and the more anodic one corresponded to the band of amylase from salivary gland. A minimum of three and a maximum of five serum amylases were found by De la Lande (1969) using polyacrylamide gel electrophoresis. These isoenzymes were designated as Amy SE-1, -2, -3, -4, and -5, respectively, according to their mobilities (Amy = amylase and SE = serum electrophoresis). They concluded that Amy SE-1 and SE-2 were likely of pancreatic origin and SE-2 and SE-3 were the most active isoenzymes in normal human serum. In his study of 1000 blood donors, Vacikova (1969) reported the presence of four amylase monomers and five possible combinations of the isoenzymes designated as SP, sSP, SPp, sSpP, and P.

Fridhandler (1972) observed two components in human serum, urine, fallopian tube, and liver homogenates, with chromatographic characteristics resembling pancreatic and salivary amylases. Similar results were reported by Takeuchi (1974, 1975).

With refinement of separation techniques (Spiekerman, 1974), it was found that human amylase of pancreatic origin contained one or two major and one or more minor isoenzymes, whereas salivary amylase generally yielded one or two major and three to six minor amylolytic bands. In his attempt to establish the normal pattern of amylase isoenzymes and to evaluate the usefulness of the isoenzyme patterns in clinical diagnosis, Otsuki (1976) determined amylase iosenzymes in serum and urine of 3036 normal persons by electrophoresis on polyacrylamide gel as well as the isoenzymes in saliva, pancreatic juice, and homogenates of human pancreas, parotid glands, and liver. In addition, serum and urine samples from patients with mumps, pancreatitis, pancreatectomy, and chronic relapsing pancreatitis were analyzed. As many as seven amylase isoenzymes were separated from these specimens. His work suggested that essentially all the isoenzymes in human serum and urine were derived from the pancreas and salivary gland, and that the isoenzymes of more than 98 per cent of normal individuals consist of two major and two to three minor isoamylases. The patterns of amylase isoenzymes from pancreas and from serum obtained from patients with acute pancreatitis were the same, but differed from those from saliva and serum of patients with mumps or who had undergone total pancreatectomy.

Assigning "amylase-1" to the isoenzyme with the slowest mobility and "amylase-7" to the one with the fastest mobility toward the anode at pH 8.8, Otsuki (1976) reported that amylase isoenzymes-1, -2, -4, and -6 in serum and urine had electrophoretic mobilities identical with those of pancreatic isoamylase, and amylases-3, -5, and -7 had mobilities identical with those of salivary isoamylase. Among the first group, amylase-1 was the major fraction and among the second group, amylase-3 was the predominating isoenzyme. This is in agreement with the findings of Spiekerman (1974) that, as a group, the isoenzymes of human pancreatic origin migrated more slowly in the electrical field toward the anode than did those of human salivary amylases.

The numbering of amylase isoenzymes with respect to their electrophoretic mobilities from cathode to anode is contrary to the commonly accepted numbering practice and doubtless causes some confusion. Lactic dehydrogenase, for example, has five isoenzymes. The one which moves fastest in the electrical field toward the anode is the HHHH tetramer. This isoenzyme was numbered as LDH_1 originally by Europeans but LDH_5 by Americans.

After much confusion, this most anodic iso-enzyme is universally recognized as LDH_1. By this convention, "amylase-7," being the fastest migrating isoenzyme, should be assigned am-ylase-1, and "amylase-1" should be assigned amylase-7, since it is the slowest migrating isoenzyme.

The nomenclature of amylase isoenzymes is further complicated by the reports of Aw (1966) and Legaz (1976), in which the faster moving isoamylases of salivary origin were named S_3, S_2, and S_1 (S_3 being the most anodic among three S-type isoenzymes) and the slower moving isoamylases of pancreatic ori-gin were named P_3, P_2, and P_1. P_1, the least anodic isoenzyme, was found in fewer than 2 per cent of the 240 subjects studied. The major S-type isoenzyme was S_1, and that of the P-type was P_2, in normal serum and urine.

In their studies, Legaz (1976) used cellulose acetate electrophoresis, whereas Otsuki (1976) used polyacrylamide gel electrophoresis. The former technique separates isoenzymes based on their different electrical charges, but sepa-ration by the latter is based not only on the charges but also on the molecular shape and size of the component isoenzymes. It is not surprising that more fractions were obtained by Otsuki's study. By comparing the patterns of their separations, "amylase-1" probably is the counterpart of P_2; "amylase-2" the coun-terpart of P_3; "amylase-3" the counterpart of S_1; "amylase-4" the counterpart of S_2; "amy-lase-5" the counterpart of S_3; and "amylase-6" and "amylase-7" the counterparts of amylase isoenzymes O_1 and O_2 found in the beta-glob-ulin zone in Aw's (1967) report on human urine isoamylase study.

The relative proportions of the P and S type isoamylases in normal serum and urine have been intensively studied. After fractionation by physical methods such as electrophoresis, chromatography, or electrofocusing, each iso-enzyme was quantitated either by direct den-sitometry or by amyloclastic or saccharogenic techniques. A unique method, involving no electrophoresis or chromatography for differ-ential serum amylase determination, has also been reported by O'Donnell (1977).

In normal serum the P-type amylase was reported to comprise less than half of the total activity (28 to 49 per cent) by Fridhandler (1972), and in the corresponding urine, the percentage of pancreatic amylase was signif-icantly higher. There were no statistically sig-nificant differences between results for normal males and females. On the other hand, it was found by Otsuki that, for normal adult serum, the activity of the P-type amylases averaged 52.3 per cent of the total and the P-type activ-ity was higher than that of the S-type in al-most all normal adults. In serum and urine of newborn infants, pancreatic isoamylase activ-ity was quite low but increased gradually after four months of age. This may reflect the post-natal development of exocrine function in the pancreas.

The question of whether the isoenzyme de-termination of amylase is of diagnostic value has been controversial. It certainly adds little additional information to the differential di-agnosis of pancreatitis and parotitis, since the clinical symptoms are quite different and eas-ily differentiated. However, in the investiga-tion of clinically unexplained hyperamylase-mia, isoenzyme analysis may yield important information because it may be possible to dis-tinguish acute pancreatitis from other intra-abdominal catastrophes associated with ele-vated activities.

There have been a great number of reports supporting the finding that, in acute pancrea-titis, the P-type amylase is greatly elevated in both serum and urine (Otsuki, 1976; O'Donnell, 1977), whereas the S-type isoen-zyme is decreased to 0 to 15 per cent of the total activity of hyperamylasemic serum of patients with acute pancreatitis, 12 to 25 per cent in the case of chronic relapsing pancrea-titis, and 0 per cent in the case of carcinoma of the head of pancreas. S-type amylase was found to be increased in serum of patients with chronic pancreatitis, mumps, Sjögren's syndrome (Wolf, 1976), cholelithiasis, common duct narrowing, alcohol ingestion, acute gas-troenteritis, acute respiratory insufficiency, and chronic renal failure (Benjamin, 1974). Isoenzyme studies on serum, urine, and duo-denal fluid from 19 patients with cystic fibro-sis revealed that two thirds of the patients had no or little pancreatic amylase (Taussig, 1974).

At the present time, then, clinical useful-ness of isoamylase determination is still somewhat limited (Benjamin, 1974). The evi-dence available today indicates that most am-ylase isoenzymes are highly organ-specific, based on their different electrophoretic mobil-ities (Taussig, 1974). It is expected that amy-lase isoenzyme determination may become more common practice in the near future in many clinical laboratories, especially those which are performing other types of electrophoretic fractionations.

LIPASE
(triacylglycerol acyl hydrolase)

BIOCHEMISTRY AND PHYSIOLOGY

Lipases hydrolyze glycerol esters of long-chain fatty acids preferentially at the carbons' 1 and 3 ester bonds, producing two moles of fatty acids and one mole of β-monoglyceride per mole of triglyceride. After isomerization the third fatty acid can be split off.

Lipase acts only on emulsified fats at a rate proportional to surface area, and absence of bile salts in duodenal fluid with resultant lack of emulsification renders lipase ineffective.

Activators of lipase, in addition to bile salts, include albumin and ionized calcium; inhibitors include heavy metals and quinine. The optimal pH is 8.8. Pancreatic lipase is to be differentiated from lipoprotein lipase, aliesterase, and aryl-ester hydrolase, which are related but different enzymes. Lipase is also present in stomach, intestine, white blood cells, fat cells, and milk.

INTERPRETATION

Serum pancreatic lipase activity rises more slowly than serum amylase activity in patients with acute pancreatitis, sometimes as late as 24 to 48 hours after onset, often peaking on the fourth day. It may remain elevated longer than the serum amylase; however, the evidence is contradictory. Although it is a less sensitive test than the serum amylase, it provides confirmatory evidence for the diagnosis when positive (Beeler, 1970; Lifton, 1974). Serum lipase activity elevation in patients with mumps strongly suggests significant pancreatic as well as salivary gland involvement by the disease.

OTHER PANCREATIC ENZYMES

Proteolytic enzymes, such as trypsin, chymotrypsin, and carboxypeptidase, in pancreatic juices may, in acute pancreatitis, leak into the interstitial fluid and eventually reach the plasma. Attempts to assay trypsin in the blood of patients with acute pancreatitis have not generally been very successful, possibly because of inactivation of the enzyme by naturally occuring trypsin inhibition (Babson, 1962).

In the case of pancreatic insufficiency it has been shown that trypsin in duodenal fluid following stimulation of pancreas by secretin has to fall to 10 per cent or less of normal for creatorrhea to occur (Haverback, 1963) (as lipase must fall to a similarly low level to cause steatorrhea). Urinary excretion of chymotrypsin following pancreatic stimulation has also been shown to be lower than normal in about half of patients with chronic pancreatitis with insufficiency and in half of those with pancreatic carcinoma.

Trypsin and chymotrypsin are nearly always present in grossly measurable quantities in the stools of normal young children. There is frequently much less activity detectable, however, in the adult stool, except when there is rapid transit through the gastrointestinal tract. The enzymes are apparently partially destroyed by bacteria within the gastrointestinal tract, and activity is seldom detectable at all by the cruder tests when there is constipation. The simpler tests are therefore not very useful for adults. On the other hand, many bacteria produce proteolytic enzymes which may give positive tests in the absence of pancreatogenous enzymes. For this reason, results must be interpreted with caution in children also (Ammann, 1968). In spite of these drawbacks, the tests have gained wide popularity.

A number of methods have been devised for detecting and measuring proteolytic enzyme activity in stools and duodenal fluid. These include tests based on ability of stool solutions to digest such substrates as serum proteins, hemoglobin, casein, and gelatin. The methods lack specificity and precision. One has been widely used as a screening test for fibrocystic disease of the pancreas. It depends on the ability of stool suspension to digest the gelatin emulsion of x-ray film.

Serial dilutions are made of stool with barbital buffer, pH 8. Strips of x-ray film are partially immersed in them and are incubated for 1 hour at 37°C. Proteolytic activity is indicated by digestion and removal of the opaque emulsion from the film.

Table 23-1. PATTERNS OF SECRETION OBSERVED FOLLOWING
THE AUGMENTED SECRETIN TEST*

	VOLUME	HCO$_3^-$		AMYLASE
		Concentration	Output	
Normal	↑↑	↑	↑↑	↑↑
Chronic pancreatitis	↑	= or ↓	↑↑	↑
Pancreatic cancer	= or ↓	↑	↑	↑

*Modified from Bordalo, O., Noronha, M., Lamy, J., and Dreiling, D. A.: Standard and augmented secretin testing in chronic pancreatic disease. Am. J. Gastroenterol., *64*:125, 1975.

SECRETIN TEST

According to Wormsley (1970) the exocrine secretory capacity of the pancreas is best studied by intubating the duodenum and subjecting the pancreas to direct stimulation with secretin and pancreozymin, preferably in the form of continuous intravenous infusion. Bicarbonate secretory capacity is best expressed in terms of output (secretory rate). It appears that the distribution of bicarbonate output of normal subjects is very skewed, with a sharp cut-off at the lower end of the normal range. Subjects with normal pancreatic function generally secrete more than 15 mEq in 30 minutes. Wormsley has shown that the diagnostic discrimination between normal and chronic pancreatitis may be improved by considering bicarbonate concentration and volume together or by calculating bicarbonate output. He recommends that the bicarbonate concentration always be assessed in conjunction with the secretory rate (p. 774).

Dreiling (1970) has published the most extensive study of the secretin test. Using his criteria for the lower limit of normality for volume, bicarbonate concentration, and enzyme output, there were false positives in 5.1 per cent of 2723 patients without pancreatic disease and false negatives in 5.2 per cent of 1725 patients with proven pancreatic diseases.

AUGMENTED SECRETIN TEST
(Bordalo, 1975)

The standard test is adequate for the diagnosis of well-established pancreatic lesions causing gross destruction of the parenchyma. The augmented test (4.0 to 5.0 secretin U/kg) is of particular value if the response to 1.0 U/kg is equivocal, inasmuch as augmented stimulation enhances secretory deficiencies in inflammation and cancer. See Table 23-1 for abnormal patterns and Table 23-2 for normal values.

Until recently, attention has been directed largely toward the secretory deficiency pattern. Discordant secretion is a pattern of increased flow after secretin stimulation with lesser increases in bicarbonate secretion. This condition is demonstrated in cases of the Zollinger-Ellison syndrome, hemochromatosis, and alcoholic and non-alcoholic cirrhosis. A preliminary report of the secretory patterns in these patients is as follows: (1) biliary cirrhotics and non-alcoholic cirrhotics had elevated volumes and high normal bicarbonate secretion; (2) patients with the Zollinger-Ellison syndrome, hemochromatosis, and alcoholic cirrhosis had marked increase in volume and a lesser increase in bicarbonate secretion, above the upper limit of normal.

SERUM CHOLECYSTOKININ-PANCREOZYMIN

Harvey (1973) has shown that in patients with deficient pancreatic secretion, fasting serum levels of cholecystokinin-pancreozymin were 300 times those of healthy adults. Yet those results remain to be confirmed.

MISCELLANEOUS TESTS

There is usually leukocytosis in patients with acute pancreatitis, white blood cell counts sometimes reaching 30,000/mm^3. There may also be signs of hemoconcentration. A falling serum calcium points to the more serious form of pancreatitis, as does turbidity of the serum. The falling calcium presumably results from formation of calcium soaps of the fatty acids liberated by the action of pancreatic lipase. Hyperbilirubinemia occurs in many patients, not only those with gallstones but those in

Table 23-2. NORMAL RANGES FOR STANDARD AND AUGMENTED SECRETIN TEST*

	STANDARD	AUGMENTED
Volume (ml/kg)	2.0–4.4	4.5–8.1
HCO_3 (mEq/l)	90–130	93–141
HCO_3 (mEq)	12.2–31.0	22.5–58.9
Amylase (U/kg)	6.6–35.2	8.3–65.1

*From Dreiling, D. A.: The early diagnosis of pancreatic cancer. Scand. J. Gastroenterol., 5(Suppl. 6):115–122, 1970.

whom the pancreatitis appears to be related to alcoholism. The reason is not well understood. Results of other liver function tests may also be abnormal. Transient hyperglycemia may also occur.

Malabsorption is discussed in Chapter 25. Since it may be caused by inadequacy of pancreatic secretion, and may result from chronic pancreatitis or pancreatic carcinoma, various tests for malabsorption, such as the serum carotenoid level, the glucose tolerance test, the ^{131}I-labeled triolein absorption test, the starch tolerance test, and the three-day fecal fat determination, may be useful diagnostically, as may gross and microscopic examination of stools. Although these tests are discussed in greater detail elsewhere (Chap. 25), it should be stated that the ^{131}I-triolein test yields many false positive and false negative results, which has prompted most gastroenterologists to abandon it. Only about one third of patients with pancreatic carcinoma are reported to have abnormal starch tolerance test results. A similar percentage have abnormal ^{131}I-triolein test results. A larger percentage may have a "flat" glucose tolerance curve; but this is very non-specific diagnostically. The d-xylose test, discussed in Chapter 25, is a very useful test for distinguishing malabsorption caused by pancreatic disease from that caused by intestinal disorders.

Recent reports have suggested a possible association between α-1 antitrypsin deficiency and chronic pancreatitis (Mihas, 1976).

SWEAT TEST

PRINCIPLE

Pilocarpine is iontophoresed into the skin to stimulate locally increased sweat gland secretion (Gibson, 1959). The resulting sweat is absorbed by filter paper, weighed, diluted with distilled water, and analyzed for sodium and chloride content. The method is painless and reliable. Total body sweating in patients with cystic fibrosis is hazardous, and a number of deaths from the procedure have been recorded. Cellulose sponges have been used successfully in place of filter paper, although we have found that use of a syringe to express the sweat from the cellulose sponge is inefficient and necessitates use of ultra-micro techniques, whereas the method described is suitable to micro techniques. Potentiometric methods are also available.

INTERPRETATION

Fibrocystic disease (mucoviscidosis) is a familial, mendelian-recessive disease characterized by abnormal secretion by the various exocrine glands of the body, including pancreas; salivary glands; peritracheal, peribronchial, and peribronchiolar glands; lacrimal glands; sweat glands; mucosal glands of the small bowel; and even the bile ducts.

Involvement of the intestinal glands may result in presence of meconium ileus at birth. Chronic lung disease and malabsorption resulting from pancreatic involvement are the major clinical problems of those who survive beyond infancy. The histologic appearance of the pancreas is one of dilatation of ducts and acini, with plugging by acidophilic material and flattening of the lining epithelial cells. There may be an increased amount of fibrous tissue present.

Laboratory diagnosis depends largely on demonstration of increased sodium and chloride in the sweat, found in about 99 per cent of patients. Screening tests for sweat chloride have also been used and depend on hand imprints on silver nitrate–containing agar or paper. The sweat chloride precipitates with silver, and the intensity of the print is roughly proportional to the sweat chloride concentration. We believe that a careful history and physical are better screening procedures, and that the definitive sweat test should be applied only when indicated. In children, chloride concentrations over 60 mEq/l of sweat are diagnostic. Levels between 50 and 60 mEq/l are suggestive in the absence of adrenal insufficiency. Sodium concentrations are usually about 10 to 20 mEq/l higher than chloride.

Sweat electrolytes in about half of a group of premenopausal adult women have been shown to undergo cyclic fluctuation, reaching a peak chloride concentration most commonly 5 to 10 days prior to the onset of menses. Peak values were slightly under 65 mEq/l. Men showed random fluctuations up to just under 70 mEq/l. For this reason, interpretation of values in adults must be approached with caution.

NORMAL VALUES IN CHILDREN

CHLORIDE	SODIUM
Below 50 mEq/l: normal	Below 70 mEq/l: normal
50 to 60 mEq/l: equivocal	70 to 90 mEq/l: equivocal
Over 60 mEq/l: abnormal	Over 90 mEq/l: abnormal

METHODOLOGY

AMYLASE: GENERAL METHODOLOGY

OVERVIEW

Like any other enzyme determination in a clinical laboratory, the activity of amylase rather than the quantity is determined. The activity of amylase is expressed in some arbitrary unit that is calculated from the production of a certain amount of reaction product or from the disappearance of a certain amount of substrate under defined conditions, such as the concentration of the substrate and cofactors, pH, and temperature. In the case of amylase determinations in which starch or another type of polysaccharide is used as substrate, the concentration term is rather difficult to define. Polysaccharides possess many potential points of cleavage, and amylases "attack" a polysaccharide molecule in multiple fashion (Caraway, 1959; Robyt, 1967). During the course of hydrolysis, the number of polysaccharides of smaller sizes and oligosaccharides increases until the later stage of the reaction.

A great number of methods for amylase activity determination are available today, and the majority of these methods use starch as substrate, although recently, dye-coupled polysaccharides, such as Cibachron Blau F36GA dyed amylose, and some smaller molecules containing α-1,4-glucosidic linkages, such as maltopentose, have been used as substrates in place of the classic substrate, starch.

By principle, amylase methods can be categorized as follows:

Saccharogenic method

The reducing power resulting from the amylase reaction on substrate is measured. The products in the early stage of amylase action on amylose, the linear unbranched polysaccharide, are maltose, maltotriose, maltotetraose, and higher oligosaccharides. In the later stage of amylolysis, the main products are maltose and maltotriose in the ratio of 2.39:1. The final products are maltose and the hydrolysis products of maltotriose, glucose, and maltose. Maltose itself is not further hydrolyzed. With amylopectin, the branched polysaccharide with α-1,6-glucosidic linkages at the branching points (which are not attacked by α-amylase), the breakdown products in the first stage are maltose (42 per cent), maltotriose (28 per cent), and α-limit dextrins (30 per cent). α-Limit dextrins contain both α-1,4- and α-1,6-glucosidic linkages, and the smallest dextrin was found to be pentasaccharide, containing one single α-1,16 linkage. The larger α-limit dextrins contain two or more branching points per molecule. In the second stage, the smallest α-limit dextrin has been reported to be tetrasaccharide. Glucose is also formed from maltotriose. The amylolysis products of glycogen are the same as those of amylopectin.

In the saccharogenic method, the reducing substances of the reaction products are measured. Somogyi's saccharogenic method (Somogyi, 1960) is the best known procedure. In its original form, it employs no buffer for pH control and the color reagent does not always react stoichiometrically with liberated reducing compounds of different chain length. Also, it is difficult for inexperienced persons to perform reproducibly. It is not, therefore, an accurate method. However, modifications (Henry, 1960) of it serve as the reference methods for the iodometric procedure and the many modifications of it. Most clinicians are familiar with the normal range when expressed in Somogyi units (the amount of enzyme in 100 ml of serum which produces reducing substances equivalent to 1 mg of glucose from starch substrate in 30 minutes at 40°C. under the conditions specified in his test). Therefore, it is still considered the reference method by many in this country.

The reducing substances produced by the reaction may be quantitatively determined by copper reduction as described by Somogyi, or for example, by ferricyanide reduction, picric acid reduction, or dinitrosalicylic acid reduction.

Several automated saccharogenic methods have been developed and are routinely used by a number of large hospital and research laboratories (Fridhandler, 1970; Wu, 1972; Matthews, 1973). Except for a few newly published procedures (Proelss, 1975; James, 1977), in which quantitation of the reducing power is based on the amount of maltose produced by coupled enzymatic reactions, all saccharogenic methods require a blank for each specimen in order to compensate for endogenous glucose and other reducing substances present in the specimen.

Conversion of the Somogyi Unit to the International Unit

The Somogyi unit, as mentioned, is defined as the amount of enzyme in 100 ml of specimen which liberates reducing substances equivalent to 1 mg of glucose from starch in 30 minutes at 40°C. To convert Somogyi units/dl into International units/l, the following isothermal conversion factor (ICF) may be used (Sax, 1972):

$$ICF = \frac{1 \text{ mg glucose}}{30 \text{ min} \times 100 \text{ ml sample}}$$
$$\times \frac{1000 \text{ micromole} \times 1 \text{ (SF)}}{180 \text{ mg glucose}}$$
$$\times \frac{1000 \text{ ml}}{1 \text{ liter sample}} = 185$$

where SF = 1 (each enzymatic cleavage gives rise to one glucose equivalent of reducing power).

The validity of the definition of a Somogyi unit and of this conversion factor depends upon the following assumptions:

a. that the cleavage rate of undegraded and partially degraded substrate molecules are identical.

b. that the reducing powers of glucose, maltose, maltotriose, maltotetraose and higher oligosaccharides are the same on a molar basis.

Amyloclastic and iodometric methods

The coloration of starch by iodine has been widely used since 1908 for the measurement of amylase activity. Amylose, the linear polysaccharide which is more water soluble and less viscous in solution, is primarily responsible for the blue iodine reaction of starch. The iodine color produced by a given amount of amylose is approximately six times as intense as the iodine color produced by an equal amount of amylopectin, which is less water soluble and more viscous in solution. Two factors which influence the iodine color given by a particular starch are the length of the glucose chain involved and the degree of branching of the chain. Amylose takes up approximately one iodine molecule per six glucose units, which make up each turn of starch helix. Starches containing 45 glucose residues or more turn blue with iodine. Polysaccharides containing 36 to 48 glucose residues yield a purple color, those with 18 to 30 residues a red color, with 12 to 18 a brown color, and with less than 12 residues no color.

Amyloclastic methods involve measuring the time required to reach the achromic point (the point at which the blue color produced by iodine and starch is no longer visible), and *iodometric* methods involve measuring photometrically (Van Loon, 1952) the amount of blue color lost in a given interval of time. The Somogyi amyloclastic method, as modified by Dade Reagents (Miami, Florida, 1975), and an iodometric method, also modified by Dade Reagents (1975), are both in common use, and their results can be made to correlate with those of the Somogyi saccharogenic method. Many modifications of the Somogyi starch-iodine method have been developed and made available commercially (such as those manufactured by Harleco, Biomedix, Cordis, and Sigma). Unfortunately, they each employ different types of substrates and use different expressions for units, which makes interlaboratory comparison extremely difficult.

The amyloclastic procedure has been criticized in that the enzyme reaction does not proceed under optimal conditions (Searcy, 1967) because "substrate exhaustion" is used as the criterion for the end point. However, the method has worked well in our laboratory for many years as a quick screening test, and results compare closely with those obtained by Somogyi's saccharogenic procedure.

Use of starch iodine kits for routine amylase determinations probably warrants further evaluation. A recent Center for Disease Control survey (1975) showed that over three fourths of the 227 laboratories using starch-iodine methods reported elevated values on specimens containing normal amylase activities. It also showed that, among the various starch-iodine methods and kits, only the Dade and Sigma kits (and a few other miscellaneous procedures) generally yielded a normal amylase value for normal human serum and had a reasonably narrow range of distribution of intervals.

Chromolytic (dyed-starch) methods

In the past several years, many dyed-starch substrates (in which a dye is covalently coupled to an insoluble polysaccharide) have been introduced.

These include:

Remazol Brilliant Blue R-Amylopectin (Alpha-Amylase Fast Pack)

Reactone Red 2B-Amylopectin (DyAmyl)

Procion Brilliant Red M-2BS-Amylopectin

Cibachron Blau F36GA-Amylose (Amylochrome)

Cibachron Blau F3GA-d-crosslinked potato starch polymer

In all of the above methods, hydrolysis of substrate by amylase liberates water-soluble, colored starch fragments into the solution. After terminating the reaction, by either increasing or decreasing the pH, and subsequent separation of the insoluble residues, the absorbance of the solution is determined and the amylase activity read from a calibration curve constructed by using an empirical dye standard or a reference serum with known amylase activity as determined by a commonly accepted method.

The dyed-starch methods have received general approval and acceptance, since they offer simplicity and sensitivity. However, because different methods use different reaction conditions, enzyme units and normal ranges, it is virtually impossible to compare results from one method with those from another, although reasonably good correlations with a modified saccharogenic method (Klein, 1970) and an amyloclastic method (Dalal, 1971) have been reported. Some of the dyed-starch substrates have also been used in automated systems (Hathaway, 1970; Mazzuchin, 1973).

In the recent survey of amylase methodology (1975) by the Center for Disease Control, it has been shown that dyed-starch methods (209 laboratories) generally yielded more "accurate" results, both in normal human specimens and in those with elevated activity, than did starch-iodine procedures (227 laboratories).

Turbidimetric and nephelometric methods

When a starch solution, which is colloidal in nature, is hydrolyzed by amylase, the molecular size of polysaccharides decreases rapidly owing to the fragmentation by amylase action. This results in diminishing turbidity (absorbance) and light scatter of the original solution. The decrease in turbidity can be measured absorptiometrically and the decrease in light scatter can be measured nephelometrically and related to the amylase activity. A rapid procedure employing the turbidimetric principle was described in 1955 (Peralta), and a rapid nephelometric method has recently become available. Turbidimetric and nephelometric methods have the advantages of simplicity and rapidity. The major disadvantages of these procedures have been the lack of proper standards, poor substrate stability, and relatively poor precision at near normal levels of amylase activity, but a recently introduced commercial nephelometric method (Perkin-Elmer, Coleman 91) yields satisfactory results. Using these methods, decrease in turbidity or light scatter as a function of time is generally recorded continually (Shipe, 1972; Zinterhofer, 1973), and amylase activity is calculated from a calibration curve. Most turbidimetric and nephelometric methods use an amylopectin preparation as substrate, but corn starch, dextrin, and a special liquid laundry starch have been successfully used. Any spectrophotometer (turbidimetry) or nephelometer or fluorometer (nephelometry) of good quality with temperature-controlled cuvettes and a chart recorder may be used. Turbidimetric and nephelometric determinations of amylase have been found to correlate closely with Somogyi units when a conversion factor is applied. Nephelometric methods have an outstanding advantage over turbidimetric methods in that measurement of decreased light scatter is much more sensitive than measurement of decreased turbidity.

Nephelometric methods have been in very little use until recently, when Perkin-Elmer Corporation (Norwalk, Connecticut) introduced its Model 91 Amylase-Lipase Analyzer, which automatically monitors the activity of amylase (or lipase) in serum or urine. This method, which has been evaluated extensively by Yourno (1978), is an adaptation of the procedure introduced by Zinterhofer in 1973. Amylose-free amylopectin is used for substrate preparation. The same substrate has also been used on the Perkin-Elmer KA-150 kinetic analyzer with good results (Malkus, 1977). It is likely that more laboratories will adopt nephelometric methods in the future for their routine amylase determinations.

Viscosimetric methods

When the size of the swollen starch granules decreases as a result of amylase action, the viscosity of the starch solution decreases accordingly, because viscosity is a function of interference between granules. This can be made the basis of an amylase assay. However, this method has not been well accepted by clinical laboratories for routine use.

AMYLASE: RECOMMENDED METHODOLOGY

Four methods for determination of amylase activities are recommended for different types of laboratories. The recommendations are based on our own experience or evaluations published in literature and on other considerations as described under each method. The common feature of these methods is that their results are expressed in Somogyi units, or can be converted to Somogyi units by a rather simple factor (Koch, 1971).

Regardless of the method chosen for amylase determination, caution must be exercised to avoid contamination of specimens with saliva, since its amylase content is approximately 700 times that of serum. Red cells contain no amylase, so hemolysis generally presents no problem with most of the methods. Heparinized plasma and serum yield identical results. Oxalated or citrated plasma may give low results by up to 20 per cent. Fasting and postprandial venous blood samples yield similar results. For routine determinations, a timed, two-hour urine collection, with activity expressed on a per hour basis, is of greatest clinical value.

Serum and urine samples are stable at room temperature for at least one week; up to several months, if refrigerated. Samples diluted with an equal volume of glycerol are stable for up to two years at refrigerator temperatures.

Automated saccharogenic amylase determinations

For a laboratory where a large number of amylase determinations are performed, an automated method is necessary. The automated method of Wu (1972) or that of Matthews (1973) will serve this purpose well. The major features of these two methods are discussed subsequently.

Substrate. Wu's method uses Argo corn starch purified according to Somogyi. We have used this procedure for the past eight years, during which time over 100,000 serum, urine, or fluid amylase determinations have been

performed. There is virtually no batch-to-batch variation in the starch. The cost for starch substrate, including purification, is amazingly low. Matthews uses glycogen (Calbiochem No. 3615) as substrate, with no laboratory preparation necessary before the solution is constituted.

Quantitation of Reducing Substances. The total reducing capacity of the amylase reaction products, including glucose, maltose, and other oligosaccharides, is quantitated as milligrams of glucose equivalents per deciliter by an alkaline ferricyanide reduction procedure using the AutoAnalyzer I (Technicon Instrument Corporation, Tarrytown, N.Y.) in Wu's method. The incubation, however, is carried out separately in a 50°C. water bath, manually. In Matthews' method, the reducing power of the major reaction product, maltose, is quantitated by copper neocuproine method. Since maltose is a disaccharide and possesses only one reducing end per molecule, it has less than 50 per cent reducing power per unit weight when compared with that of glucose. This method uses a dual-channel AutoAnalyzer. No separate water bath for incubation is required.

Calibration and Calculation. Wu's method determines the endogenous glucose and other reducing substances in the specimen by a separate blank which may be assayed during the incubation period of the specimen with substrate. The instrument is calibrated against glucose standard solutions. Specimens containing higher than 300 mg/dl glucose equivalent of endogenous reducing power must be diluted and the assay repeated. After subtracting the blank value from the total reducing power of the test run, the amylase activity of the specimen is calculated using a factor derived from a reference standard serum with known activity. The method is linear up to 450 Somogyi units/dl. A coefficient of variation of less than 5 per cent for both the normal and elevated amylase levels is routinely obtained by different technologists. In Matthews' method, blank and test are run simultaneously, since a dual-channel analyzer is used. Glucose oxidase is incorporated into the reagent, so that endogenous glucose up to 800 mg/dl and the glucose produced by amylase action are eliminated from the calculation. The blank channel measures the reducing substances other than glucose, and this value is subtracted from the value measured by the test channel. The instrument is first checked and calibrated separately with glucose and maltose standard solutions, and a standard amylase activity curve is constructed using pooled serum with known amylase activity. It is convenient for the blank and test recordings to be "in phase," but it is not essential. The linearity of this procedure is up to 800 Somogyi units/dl, with inter- and intra-day coefficients of variation of 9 per cent and 3 to 5 per cent for normal and elevated amylase levels, respectively.

Choice of Method. Both methods are considered sufficiently efficient, accurate, and precise for routine amylase determinations. The choice of method should probably be made on the availability of experienced personnel and instrumentation.

Manual amyloclastic amylase determination (Somogyi, 1938)

Principle. Amylase present in serum is permitted to act on starch substrate of known concentration at 40°C. The reaction is followed by periodically transferring aliquots of the starch solution to an iodine solution and observing the color; first blue, then purple, then reddish brown. The end point is noted in the tube showing the last trace of purple in the developing red-brown of the erythrodextrin mixture.

Procedure

1. Remove starch solution from refrigerator and mix well.

2. Flame mouth of flask and pour out about 6 ml of starch solution.

3. Transfer 4 ml of starch solution (containing 3 mg starch) to a test tube and incubate in 40°C. water bath for 5 minutes.

4. While incubating, transfer 0.5 ml of dilute iodine solution to each of the nine test tubes (7 mm inside diameter).

5. Add 1 ml serum (or urine or diluted duodenal or peritoneal aspirate) to starch solution and start stopwatch. Mix well and return to water bath.

6. After 1 minute, transfer 0.5 ml of the starch-serum mixture to the first iodine tube, noting color immediately before a "daylight" lamp.

7. If the color is dark blue, wait 2 more minutes and try a second sample.

8. If the sample is blue, double the waiting period and continue in this manner until the first purple is obtained.

9. Judging from the time of appearance of the first purple, take subsequent samples until the end point is reached (a barely perceptible tint of purple in the red-brown). It may be helpful to go past the end point in order to be sure it has been reached. With experience, one learns to judge the shade of purple signaling the halfway point.

10. If the end point is reached before 8 minutes,

dilute serum appropriately with 0.5 per cent (w/v) sodium chloride and repeat the test, using 0.3 ml aliquots of iodine rather than the 0.5 ml aliquots called for with undiluted serum. (This balance is important.)

11. Occasional urine-starch incubates cause fading of the iodine solution when aliquots are added. The cause in most or all cases is the presence in urine of Telapaque, Aggrafin, or other radiopaque media. Color can be restored for a sufficient duration to read the end point by judicious addition of extra iodine to the urine-starch-iodine mixture. Alternatively, one can dilute out the interference and still have an end point, although this results in a rather lengthy test. The interference has not been encountered in serum determinations.

Calculation

$$\frac{1600}{\text{time in minutes}} = \text{Somogyi units/dl}$$

Somogyi arbitrarily defined these units to correspond to those of his saccharogenic method. The Somogyi unit may be defined in terms of the amount of reducing substance produced by incubation of serum with buffered starch substrate for 30 minutes at 40°C. It is expressed as milligrams of glucose equivalent per 100 ml of serum. It would be appropriate to check the factor for the brand of starch used, although Somogyi noted it to be relatively constant over many years when cornstarch was used.

Reagents

1. Iodine solution (stock). Dissolve 2.5 g potassium iodide and 1.27 g resublimed iodine in distilled water and dilute to 100 ml.

2. Iodine solution (working). Dilute 2 ml stock iodine solution to 100 ml with 2 per cent (w/v) potassium iodide.

3. Dry starch (can be purchased prepared from Dade Reagents, Inc., Miami, Fl.). Suspend 100 g Argo cornstarch in 1 liter of approximately 0.01 normal HCl and agitate frequently for 1 hour. Let stand (may take several hours to settle out) and decant HCl. Add 1 l of approximately 0.05 per cent (w/v) NaCl and let stand until starch settles out. Decant. Repeat wash with 0.05 per cent NaCl. Decant and spread starch on evaporating dishes. Blot surface with coarse filter paper to absorb moisture. Spread out on filter paper to dry in air overnight. When thoroughly dry, transfer to brown, stoppered bottle.

4. Starch solution. (A) Grind 10 g washed starch in mortar with 50 ml water; add to 400 ml boiling distilled water in beaker with constant stirring. Wash mortar with 50 ml distilled water and add to contents of beaker. Boil while stirring for 1 min. Add 5 ml 25 per cent NaCl and heat for 30 min in boiling water bath with inverted beaker over mouth of flask. Let settle in refrigerator overnight. Centrifuge at 3000 rpm for 30 min. Decant and save supernatant. (B) Dilute supernatant fluid to

proper volume (see below) with NaCl and buffer solution. Distribute in Erlenmeyer flasks stoppered with gauze-covered cotton. Autoclave. Keep in refrigerator, sterile.

DETERMINING PROPER FINAL DILUTION FOR STARCH (75 g STARCH PER 100 dl, 250 mg NaCl PER 100 dl)

1. Hydrolyze aliquot of starch solution: Into a 25×200 mm NPN tube, place 5 ml starch solution, 1 ml 3.6 N HCl. Stopper with one-hole rubber stopper fitted with two-foot glass tube to act as reflux condenser, and immerse in boiling water bath for $2\frac{1}{2}$ hours. (This converts the starch to glucose.) Neutralize with NaOH (phenol red indicator, red to yellow). This requires approximately 6 ml of 20 per cent NaOH.

2. Dilute to 25 ml with distilled water and determine the glucose content. We prefer the automated ferricyanide reduction method. To convert answer from glucose to starch, results must be multiplied by 0.9 to correct for equivalent weight of starch compared with that of glucose.

3. Calculate proper dilution of starch solution (75 mg starch and 250 mg NaCl per 100 ml) and potassium phosphate buffer 0.012 M pH 6.8.

This is easy once the principle is understood. If one dilutes 75 ml of the stock starch solution to the same number of milliliters as the numerical value of its concentration (in mg/dl) one will always end with a working solution containing 75 mg starch/dl. For example, if the stock starch solution contains 434 mg/dl, then:

$$\frac{75 \text{ ml stock starch solution}}{434 \text{ ml working starch solution}}$$

$$\times \frac{434 \text{ mg starch}}{100 \text{ ml stock starch solution}}$$

$$= \frac{75 \text{ mg starch}}{100 \text{ ml}}$$

Let C = starch content of stock starch solution (mg/100 ml). Then,

$$A = \frac{C}{2} - 75 = \text{ml } 0.25 \text{ per cent NaCl needed}$$

$$B = \frac{C}{2} \div 2 = \text{ml mixed buffer needed}$$

$$C = \frac{C}{2} \div 2 = \text{ml } 0.5 \text{ per cent NaCl needed}$$

$$D = 75 = \text{ml stock starch solution needed}$$

Example

Stock starch solution contains 434 mg/dl.

$$A = \frac{434}{2} - 75 = 142 \text{ ml } 0.25 \text{ per cent NaCl}$$

$$B = \frac{C}{2} \div 2 = 109 \text{ ml mixed buffer needed}$$

$$C = \frac{C}{2} \div 2 = 109 \text{ ml } 0.5 \text{ per cent NaCl needed}$$

$$D = 75 \text{ ml stock starch solution needed}$$

Reagents for preparation of starch solution:

1. HCl, 3.6 N
2. HCl, 0.01 N
3. NaCl, 25 per cent (w/v)
4. NaCl, 0.5 per cent (w/v)
5. NaCl, 0.25 per cent (w/v)
6. NaCl, 0.05 per cent (w/v)
7. NaOH, 20 per cent (w/v)
8. Phenol red indicator
9. 0.05 M phosphate buffer: KH_2PO_4, 3.6280 g/ 500 ml H_2O; K_2HPO_4, 3.6448 g/500 ml H_2O. Mix in equal proportions.
10. Reagents for glucose determination

Discussion. According to Somogyi, one should be able easily to reproduce the end point within 1 minute, and we have found this to be true in our laboratory. On serum diluted 1:1, the calculated amylase activities at end points of 12 and 13 minutes are 266 and 246 units, respectively, a difference of no clinical significance. For this reason we currently see no great advantage to the increased precision resulting from the many photometric adaptations of the procedure. In addition, they may yield artificially high results in some circumstances because of fading of color caused by albumin or radiographic contrast media.

Preparation of the starch substrate is tedious. In our laboratory Argo cornstarch has been consistently satisfactory. Reif (1962) has confirmed Somogyi's findings that cornstarch, not soluble starch, must be used to prepare a standard substrate. He proposed a simplified method for standardizing the starch but stated that the determination of glucose equivalence is preferable. The starch is stable for several months if kept sterile in the refrigerator. Commercially prepared starch substrate is available.

Determination of amylase by a dyed-starch method (Phadebas Procedure, Pharmacia, Piscataway, N.J.)

Principle. A reagent tablet of water-insoluble starch polymer containing cross-linked dye is used as substrate by the addition of water. Amylase hydrolyzes this polymer into water-soluble blue starch fragments. After stopping the reaction by raising the pH and subsequent separation of the soluble reaction products from the insoluble residue of the blue starch polymer, the absorbance of the blue-colored solution is determined. The amylase activity of the sample is read from a standard curve.

Procedure

1. Pipette 4.0 ml distilled or deionized water into a test tube. Mark the tube "Test."
2. Pipette 4.2 ml distilled or deionized water

into another tube. Mark the tube "Blank." For urine amylase, use 4.1 ml water.

3. Add one tablet to each tube and shake vigorously by hand or mixer.

4. Preincubate all tubes at 37°C. for 5 minutes.

5. Add 0.2 ml serum sample. For urine specimens, add 0.1 ml.

6. Incubate at 37°C. for exactly 15 minutes.

7. Add 1.0 ml 0.5 M NaOH to stop the reaction. Shake vigorously.

8. Filter or centrifuge at 1500 g for 5 minutes.

9. Measure the absorbance of the clear blue supernatant/filtrate at 620 nm against distilled water using a 1 cm cuvette. Any spectrophotometer with a band width less than 10 nm is satisfactory.

10. Subtract the blank value from unknowns.

11. Read amylase activity from a standard curve (see Discussion). For serum, the amylase is directly read. For urine samples, the activity is read from the standard curve first and then multiplied by 2 to correct for the smaller sample volume.

Discussion

1. Our recommendation of Phadebas is based on the following considerations:

a. The Phadebas method has been reported to be the simplest of four dyed-starch kits evaluated. It differentiates normal and abnormal levels of serum amylase exactly as does one of the modified saccharogenic procedures. It was rated as having the lowest coefficient of variation, better linearity as determined by dilution techniques, and lowest cost per test.

b. Using 15 minute incubation at 37°C., as recommended by the manufacturer, amylase activity up to at least 20 times normal for serum and 7.5 times normal for urine can be measured without requiring any dilutions.

c. Judging by results of a Hyland Regional Quality Control Program in which over 150 hospital laboratories took part, Phadebas gave an average for elevated/normal serum amylase ratio of 5.5. The same ratio determined by our automated saccharogenic method was 5.0. Other dyed-starch methods gave a much lower ratio, ranging from 3.0 to 4.4. This indicates that results from the Phadebas kit parallel more closely Somogyi's saccharogenic method than do those from other dyed-starch methods.

2. In constructing a calibration curve, Phadebas uses three-cycle logarithmic graph paper because the logarithm of absorbance is proportional to the logarithm of enzyme activity. Phadebas is the only dyed-starch kit with this property (Ceska, 1969).

3. For specimens with very high activities, the incubation time may be shortened to 5 minutes and results multiplied by a factor of 3 (15/5 = 3).

4. For routine and stat amylase determinations, incubation may be performed at 52°C. instead of at 37°C. as recommended by the manufacturer (Creno, 1976).

5. The Phadebas method has been reported to underestimate amylase activities on urine, saliva, and pancreatic and duodenal contents when compared with results by a saccharogenic procedure (O'Donnell, 1974; Wiener, 1977a). The incorporation of at least 3 μmol/l albumin, 5 mg/dl bovine albumin (Irie, 1972), or 50 mg/l PVP (polyvinylpyrrolidone) (Wiener, 1977a) is recommended to correct for this deficiency. It may be used in place of water for the preparation of the substrate.

6. The calibration of the Phadebas method is not an easy matter, and difficulties have been noticed (Hamlin, 1974). The manufacturer claimed that batch-to-batch variation of dye content has been less than 3 per cent and recommended that reagent from the same batch be purchased, if desired, for a one-year supply (Ali, 1974). It also recommended that laboratories prepare or purchase a supply of reference serum for calibration of the Phadebas kit. Hyland Multi-Enzyme Reference Serum (Hyland, Division Travenol Laboratories, Inc., Costa Mesa, Cal. 92626) lists amylase values by both the saccharogenic (Henry, 1960) and Phadebas methods. Pharmacia has recently made available its own Amylase Calibration Reference Serum, with approximately 1,100 U/l activity, and recommends that this be used for calibration of their procedure.

7. The normal range for serum is 70 to 300 U/l and that for urine is 100 to 2,000 U/l. Approximate conversion from U/l to Somogyi U/dl may be made by multiplying by 0.54.

Determination of amylase with the Perkin-Elmer Amylase-Lipase Analyzer

Principle. The instrument measures kinetically and automatically the reduction of light scattering by the substrate, amylopectin, as a result of the action of amylase. The reaction follows zero order kinetics up to 500 Somogyi U/dl. Between 500 and 1000 Somogyi U/dl the unit scale is progressively compressed to correct for slight non-linearity.

System Description. The Perkin-Elmer Analyzer is basically a nephelometer. A tungsten light is used as the light source. At right angles to the light beam are two selenium photodetectors located on opposite sides of the 12.5 mm square cuvette. The cuvette is maintained at 37°C. ± 1°C. There are 12 additional wells available for preincubation of the substrate. After adding 50 μl of sample into the substrate cuvette with mixing, the cuvette is inserted into the test compartment. The insertion starts the automatic sequence. In the first 15 seconds the electronic circuitry automatically counteracts the detected signals so that the meter stays at zero deflection. During the next two minutes, the meter starts to register as the light scattering decreases. A cycle indicator flashes to signal completion of the test. Results are expressed as Model 91 Amylase Units and the scale may be adjusted to Somogyi U/dl. A dilute indicator lights up in case the specimen contains very high amylase activity beyond the measurable range.

Discussion

1. For operation of the Model 91 Analyzer, please refer to Instruction Manual.

2. This method for amylase determination has the advantages of simplicity, speed, and good precision. Results are not affected by color of the specimen.

3. This instrument may be calibrated in Somogyi units by using a reference serum with known Somogyi amylase value. However, careful evaluation is necessary.

4. There are no means provided for checking the actual temperature of the sample well and incubator. Routine verification with a precalibrated thermometer is recommended.

5. All cuvettes must be kept meticulously clean or an error will be introduced. Disposable cuvettes are available and have been found to be satisfactory. To eliminate potential light-scattering error caused by dust particles in the reaction mixture, use of a strip-chart recorder to monitor the detector signals is strongly recommended. Without such a recorder, an average error of ±25 per cent may occur in 10 per cent of the assays (Grove, 1977).

6. Substrate may be prepared in the laboratory. Amylopectin is commercially available from Calbiochem (Los Angeles, Cal.).

LIPASE

General discussion

The classic method is that of Cherry (1932), in which olive oil is used as a substrate, avoiding inclusion of non-specific esterase activity in the assay result. Oleic acid released after a 16 to 18 hour incubation at 37°C. is titrated with standard alkali and results are expressed as ml 0.05 N NaOH (corrected for blank). Normal serum activity is up to 1.5 units/ml. The procedure is too slow to be useful. Many modifications of this procedure have been developed, largely aimed at speeding up the test and improving its sensitivity and reproducibility. One of the more successful is the Tietz-Fierech (1972) modification.

Vogel (1963) published the first method measuring decreased turbidity spectrophotometrically. Shihabi published a modification of the procedure in 1971. Shipe modified the procedure by using fluorometry to measure light scattering.

Despite drawbacks, such as the care required for preparation of substrate, its limited stability, and interference by jaundice (Zieve, 1966), we have used the turbidimetric method with reasonable success.

Lipase determination (serum, urine)
(Vogel, 1963)

Principle. Lipase activity of serum is determined by the decrease in absorbance of purified, buffered (pH 9.1) olive oil emulsion when incubated at room temperature (23°C.) for 20 minutes with diluted serum. Absorbance is measured at 650 nm. Units are equivalent to change in absorbance (O.D.) × 1000.

Procedure

1. To 0.8 ml of buffer diluent add 0.2 ml of serum and mix well.

2. Start timing clock. Add 0.2 ml of diluted serum to 4 ml of substrate. Mix five times by inversion. Transfer mixture immediately to a 1 cm cuvette and determine absorbance.

3. Let stand at room temperature (23°C.) for 20 minutes and again determine absorbance.

Reagents

1. Tris buffer (0.05 M, pH 9.1). Dissolve 6.057 g tris-(hydroxymethyl)-aminomethane in about 980 ml of water and adjust to pH 9.1 with 1 N HCl. Bring to a volume of 1 liter.

2. Buffer diluent. Dissolve 3.5 g sodium deoxycholate in above buffer and make up 1 liter with distilled water. Readjust to pH 9.1 if necessary.

3. Purified olive oil. Pass U.S.P. olive oil through alumina to remove free fatty acids. Collect nearly colorless effluent after a few hours. (Add reagent aluminum oxide to a 2 × 32 cm chromatographic tube fitted with a coarse disk. Pour in double this amount of olive oil. Let filter.)

4. Stock olive oil solution (10 per cent v/v). Dissolve 10 g of treated olive oil in reagent grade acetone to volume of 100 ml.

5. Olive oil solution (1 per cent, v/v). Dilute 10 ml of stock solution to 100 ml with acetone.

6. Triglyceride substrate (0.05 per cent, v/v) (available commercially). Set metal container from homogenizer containing 100 ml of buffer diluent in vigorously boiling steam bath. When temperature reaches 92°C., remove from bath and place on homogenizer base connected to Powerstat variable voltage transformer set at 35 volts. Add 4 ml of the 1 per cent olive oil solution at once, drop by drop, over a two-minute interval. Then run homogenizer uncovered at 110 volts for 10 minutes. Transfer substrate to a reagent bottle. Our reagent has had an absorbance of about 0.650 at 650 nm when measured against the buffer diluent. It has a pearly opalescence. At room temperature there is a tendency for a rim of olive oil to form on the bottle. The reagent should be shaken vigorously prior to use. It appears to be stable over a period of four to five days at room temperature. If absorbance is less than 0.600, it may be increased by reheating and remixing in the blender.

Calculation. Absorbance at time 0 minus absorbance at 20 minutes × 100 = units of lipase activity/ml (1000 × absorbance units per 0.04 ml serum per 20 minutes).

Discussion. Values up to 10 units/ml are normal; values above 15 units/ml are definitely abnormal; values from 11 to 15 units/ml are doubtful.

This method has the great advantages of speed and simplicity. The high pH is said to be optimum for lipase activity in the pancreatitis sera studied. It is above the optimum for lipase activity of normal serum. The reaction is non-linear and, therefore, the technique should be adhered to rigidly. Unfortunately, this procedure may give spuriously elevated results in the presence of jaundice. In 1966 Zieve published a procedure for eliminating effects of bilirubin on this lipase procedure. Although what some authorities consider the limited usefulness of the serum lipase measurement seems hardly to justify the extra trouble involved, others place great emphasis on lipase assays. Hence, for the purpose, clean commercial DEAE-cellulose with 0.5 sodium hydroxide, wash with distilled water, methanol, and chloroform (the last two alternately four times), and then air dry. Suspend 3 g in 75 ml ice-cold 0.1 molar Tris buffer (pH 8.8). Pipette 4 ml aliquots into centrifuge tube and spin in the cold at 3000 rpm for 10 minutes. Discard supernatant and wash residue three times with cold buffer, spinning each time. Loosen final compacted residue with a stirring rod. Add 0.5 ml serum and spin, then 1 ml cold buffer and spin. Combine washings with original supernatant and bring final volume to 5 ml. Final dilution is 1:10. Use 0.4 ml of final dilution for assay.

Determination of lipase with the Perkin-Elmer Amylase-Lipase Analyzer

Principle.   Automatic measurement of decrease in light scatter of the substrate, olive oil emulsified with deoxycholate. Kinetics are reasonably linear in the normal range and tend to greater non-linearity in the elevated range.

System Description.   See description of nephelometer above (nephelometric determination of amylase). The automatic sequence in this measurement requires 1 minute lag time and 5 minute measurement time. The Model 91 lipase scale may be adjusted to a convenient unitage, e.g., Sigma-Tietz units/ml.

Discussion

1. Operation: refer to Instruction Manual.
2. Like nephelometric amylase, this method has the advantage of simplicity, speed, good precision, and generally good accuracy.
3. Kinetics may be linear or slightly non-linear in the normal range. Kinetics tend to greater non-linearity in the elevated range, but may be linear in the slightly to moderately elevated range. With elevated lipase up to four times normal, non-linearity is seldom of clinical significance. Above this range specimens must be diluted to achieve an on-scale value (Yourno, 1978).
4. Calibration in Sigma-Tietz U/ml may be achieved with a reference serum with a known Sigma-Tietz value (Yourno, 1978).
5. Temperature checks: see above (nephelometric amylase).
6. Precautions against light scatter error should be followed as discussed above (nephelometric amylase).

7. A small fraction of specimens is encountered with normal amylase and titrimetric lipase, but transiently elevated nephelometric lipase. This probable false positive nephelometric lipase may be easily spotted by assay of serial dilutions of specimens. Pancreatitis lipase values (in U/ml) increase or remain constant, while false positive lipase values decline with increasing dilution (Yourno, 1978).

Fecal trypsin

Principle **(Wiggins, 1967).**   The rate at which hydrogen ions are liberated by the hydrolysis of the specific substrate N-benzoyl-L-arginine ethyl ester hydrochloride (B.A.E.E.) is measured. This is achieved by noting the time required to neutralize a known amount of alkali.

Reagents
1. 0.04N NaOH
2. 1% (w/v) sodium barbiturate
3. B.A.E.E.
4. 0.05 molar acetate buffer pH 5.8, containing 0.5 g $CaCl_2$ per liter.

Equipment
1. Stopwatch
2. pH meter with small electrodes, preferably with expanded scale
3. Vials, approximately 1 inch in diameter and 3 inches high
4. Magnetic stirrer

Procedure.   Dissolve 0.5 g of B.A.E.E. in 100 ml of a 1:10 dilution of 1% (w/v) sodium barbiturate. Adjust the pH to 9 and bring to 25°C. before use. (Sometimes the substrate solution becomes more acid on standing. If so, readjust pH before use.)

Mix 1 ml of intestinal contents with 9 ml of 0.05 M acetate buffer and bring to 25°C.

Mix 1 ml of the diluted intestinal contents with 5 ml of substrate in the reaction vial and place on the stirrer, with electrodes immersed.

The initial pH should be about 8.5, the reading falling continuously. When the pH reads 8, start the stopwatch and add 0.1 ml of 0.04 N NaOH to the reaction mixture. The pH will rise to about 8.4. Follow until it again decreases to 8, then stop the stopwatch.

The time elapsed is that during which 4 μEq of H^+ is released.

Calculation

$$\frac{\mu\text{Eq NaOH added}}{\text{time (minutes)}} \times \text{dilution of intestinal contents}$$

$$= \mu\text{Eq } H^+ \text{ released/min/ml intestinal contents}$$

Explanation of dilution factor:

$$\frac{1 \text{ ml intestinal contents}}{10 \text{ ml dilutional contents}}$$

$$\times \frac{1 \text{ ml diluted contents}}{6.1 \text{ ml final dilution}}$$

$$= \frac{1 \text{ ml intestinal contents}}{61 \text{ ml final dilution}}$$

Dilution factor, therefore, is 61.

Discussion. Samples with normal tryptic activity will take less than 4 minutes. If the time interval is greater than 10 minutes the reaction should be repeated with a 1:5 dilution of intestinal contents. If the reaction still takes more than 10 minutes, the results should be reported as $<2\,\mu Eq/ml/min$.

This method is easy to perform, has been found suitable for occasional use, requires only normal laboratory equipment, and yields results directly in International Units ($\mu Eq\ H^+$ released/ml/min).

Secretin test (Dreiling and Hollander, 1948)

Principle. A double-lumen tube, providing for separate aspiration of gastric and duodenal contents, is passed into the duodenum, using fluoroscopic guidance and maintaining constant aspiration of gastric contents. Duodenal contents are aspirated until clear. The patient is then given secretin ($1\,\mu/kg$) intravenously, and the pancreatic secretion entering the duodenum is collected for 80 minutes. The aspirate is examined for volume, bicarbonate content, and amylase activity.

Procedure

1. After a 12-hour fast, pass a radiopaque double-lumen tube under fluoroscopic guidance through the mouth to beyond the ampulla of Vater.

2. Maintain constant suction on both gastric and duodenal outlets with a negative pressure of 25 to 40 mm Hg. Gastric content must be completely and continuously removed to prevent contamination of duodenal aspirate.

3. When duodenal aspirate is clear and alkaline (determined by pHydrion paper), collect aspirate for a controlled period of 20 minutes.

4. Perform intradermal skin test with secretin for sensitivity. (Do not use in patients with atopic asthma.)

5. If no hypersensitivity is present, inject 1.0 clinical unit of secretin per kilogram of body weight intravenously.

6. Collect duodenal aspirate for 80 minutes, fractionally, at 20 minute intervals.

7. Clear tube between fractions by injecting air.

8. Place containers with duodenal aspirate in ice.

9. Transport to laboratory for analysis of volume, bicarbonate content, amylase activity, and pH. (Drop of pH below 7 indicates contamination by gastric juice and invalidates other results.) Microscopic examination may be performed to note presence or absence of cholesterol crystals, calcium bilirubinate pigment, and parasites. Cytologic study may also be performed.

10. Draw blood samples at 1, 4, and 24 hours following the injection of secretin for determination of serum amylase.

A number of technical problems may complicate the procedure. Incomplete gastric drainage may lead to inactivation of enzymes by contamination with gastric content. This may also alter bicarbonate content. Secretion can be lost by regurgitation into stomach (signaled by sudden increase in volume, pH, and appearance of bile in gastric aspirate) or by passage into jejunum, especially in uncooperative patients.

Results in health and disease states have been discussed previously (p. 744).

Method for augmented secretin test (Bordalo, 1975)

1. A standard secretin test, using 1.0 IU/kg secretin and collecting sequentially for 80 minutes, is routinely performed.

2. If the standard test shows an abnormal pattern of secretion or if pancreatic disease is strongly suspected, this is followed seriatim by the augmented test, employing 4.0 IU secretin/kg body weight.

3. The data of the augmented response are interpreted not only in accordance with classic patterns of secretion derived from the standard test, but, more importantly, by the response parameters of the standard test compared with the corresponding parameters for the augmented test.

Sweat electrolytes by pilocarpine iontophoresis (Gibson, 1959)

Principle. Pilocarpine iontophoresed into the skin stimulates locally increased sweat gland secretion. The resulting sweat is absorbed by filter paper, weighed, diluted with distilled water, and analyzed for sodium and chloride content.

Procedure

1. Transfer a salt-free filter paper disc, 2.5 cm in diameter, to a weighing bottle, using dry, clean forceps, and weigh on an analytical balance to the nearest 0.1 mg. (S and S No. 589 Green Ribbon is satisfactory.)

2. Tape a 2×2 inch gauze square to each of the two electrodes of the iontophoresis unit. The metal must not come in contact with the patient's skin, or pain and a burn may result.

3. Saturate the gauze covering the positive electrode with pilocarpine solution and apply to the patient's forearm, halfway between wrist and elbow.

4. Saturate the gauze covering the negative electrode with bicarbonate solution and apply to the extensor surface of the forearm directly opposite the other electrode.

5. Press electrode firmly, wiping the skin around the electrode thoroughly.

6. Place rubber strap around forearm to hold electrodes in place.

7. Turn iontophoretic unit on. (We have been satisfied with the Alloyd Iontophoresor. Other instruments are available.)

8. Adjust rheostat to 2.5 milliamps.

9. Allow to run for 10 to 12 minutes unless the patient complains of discomfort or pain, in which case double check to be sure that the gauze com-

pletely covers the electrodes and that the electrodes are in firm contact with the skin. Burns can be caused by incomplete saturation of the gauze with the solutions or by inadequate electrode contact caused by loose application as well as by direct contact of metal of electrode with skin.

10. Remove electrodes and thoroughly wash forearm area of positive electrode with distilled water, drying with 4 × 4 inch gauze squares previously determined to have a low NaCl content.

11. Using dry, clean forceps, remove filter paper discs from weighing jar and place over reddened area of patient's forearm where positive electrode had been.

12. Cover filter paper with Parafilm.

13. Tape each edge of Parafilm with waterproof adhesive tape, making sure that the seal is airtight.

14. Leave in place for 1 hour.

15. Remove tape and Parafilm carefully; transfer filter paper with dry, clean forceps to weighing jar without delay to avoid evaporation; and send to laboratory.

16. Reweigh jar to nearest 0.1 mg. Satisfactory collection requires at least a 100 mg increase in weight. Further procedure will depend on chloride and sodium method.

17. Add distilled water equivalent to 1:40 dilution and let stand with intermittent swirling for at least 5 minutes.

18. Determine chloride in 1 ml aliquot. Depending on result, add appropriate amount of lithium nitrate solution to remainder of sample (to make final concentration identical with that of standard) and determine sodium content by flame photometry.

Calculations. Calculate milliequivalents of chloride per liter of sweat. Using the Schales method, titrate 1 ml aliquot of diluted sweat and 1 ml aliquot of standard (10 mEq of chloride per liter) correcting for chloride dilution:

Chloride (mEq/liter of sweat)

$$= 400 \times \frac{\text{ml of unknown titration}}{\text{ml of standard titration}}$$

Reagents

1. Pilocarpine solution (1.5 per cent, w/v). Dissolve one-quarter grain (0.016 g) pilocarpine hydrochloride tablet in 3.2 ml of distilled water. Prepare fresh for each test.

2. Add bicarbonate solution.

REFERENCES

Ali, R.: Standardization of Phadebas alpha-amylase procedure. Clin. Chem., *20*:91, 1974.

Ammann, R. W., Tagwercher, E., Kashiwagi, H., and Rosenmund, H.: Diagnostic value of fecal chymotrypsin and trypsin assessment for detection of pancreatic disease. Am. J. Dig. Dis., *13*:123, 1968.

Aw, S. E., and Hobbs, J. R.: Human isoamylases. Biochem. J., *99*:16P, 1966.

Aw, S. E., Hobbs, J. R., and Wooton, I. D. P.: Urinary isoamylases in the diagnosis of chronic pancreatitis. Gut, *8*:402, 1967.

Babson, A. L., Read-Williams, P. A., and Phillips, G. E.: An evaluation of serum "trypsin" tests. Clin. Chem., *8*:62, 1962.

Beeler, M. F.: Amylase and lipase. Check Sample Program, Council on Clinical Chemistry, Commission on Continuing Education, American Society of Clinical Pathologists, 1970.

Benjamin, D. R., and Kenny, M.: Clinical value of amylase isoenzyme determinations. Am. J. Clin. Pathol., *62*:752, 1974.

Berk, J. E., Kizu, H., Take, S., and Fridhandler, L.: Macroamylasemia: Clinical and laboratory features. Am. J. Gastroenterol., *53*:211, 1970.

Berk, J. E., Kizu, H., Wilding, P., and Search, R. L.: Macroamylasemia: A newly recognized cause for elevated serum amylase activity. N. Engl. J. Med., *27*:941, 1967.

Bockus, H. L., Lopusniak, M. S., and Tachidjean, V.: *In* Bockus, H. L.: Gastroenterology, 2nd ed., Vol. III. Philadelphia, W. B. Saunders Company, 1965, pp. 892–931.

Bordalo, O., Noronha, M., Lamy, J., and Dreiling, D. A.: Standard and augmented secretin testing in chronic pancreatic disease. Am. J. Gastroenterol., *64*:125, 1975.

Caraway, W. T.: A stable starch substrate for the determination of amylase in serum and other body fluids. Am. J. Clin. Pathol., *32*:97, 1959.

Casey, A. E., Gilbert, F. E., Gravlee, J. F., and Downey, E. L.: Disease and chemical syndromes associated with serum levels of glucosyl transferases. Alabama J. Med. Sci., *8*:322, 1971.

Center for Disease Control, U.S. Department of Health, Education, and Welfare: Alpha-amylase methodology survey I, 1975.

Ceska, M., Birath, K., and Brown, B.: A new and rapid method for the clinical determination of alpha-amylase activities in human serum and urine. Optimal conditions. Clin. Chim. Acta, *26*:437, 1969.

Cherry, I. S., and Crandall, L. A., Jr.: The specificity of pancreatic lipase: Its appearance in the blood after pancreatic injury. Am. J. Physiol., *100*:266, 1932.

Creno, R. J., and Wenk, R. E.: A rapid, manual test for amylase at 52°C. Am. J. Med. Technol., September: 310, 1976.

Dalal, F. R., and Winsten, S.: Laboratory evaluation of a chromogenic amylase method. Clin. Chim. Acta, *32*:327, 1971.

De la Lande, F. A., and Boettcher, B.: Electrophoretic examination of human serum amylase isoenzymes. Enzymologia, *37*:335, 1969.

DiMagno, E. P., Malagelda, J. R., Taylor, W. F., et al.: A prospective comparison of current diagnostic tests for pancreatic cancer. N. Engl. J. Med., *297*:737, 1977.

Dreiling, D. A.: The early diagnosis of pancreatic cancer. Scand. J. Gastroenterol., *5*(Suppl. 6):115, 1970.

Dreiling, D. A., and Hollander, F.: Studies in pancreatic function. I. Preliminary series of clinical studies with the secretin test. Gastroenterology, *11*:714, 1948.

Dreiling, D. A., and Hollander, F.: Studies in pancreatic

function. II. A statistical study of pancreatic secretion following secretin in patients without pancreatic disease. Gastroenterology, 15:620, 1950.

Dürr, H. K., Bode, J. C., Lankisch, P. G., and Koop, H.: Amylase-creatinine clearance ratio in pancreatitis. N. Engl. J. Med., 296:635, 1977.

Fridhandler, L., Berk, J. E., and Ueda, M.: Isolation and measurement of pancreatic amylase in human serum and urine. Clin. Chem., 18:1493, 1972.

Fridhandler, L., and Berk, J. E.: Automated saccharogenic assay of alpha-amylase activity in serum. Clin. Chem., 16:911, 1970.

Gambill, E. E., and Mason, H. L.: One-hour value for urine amylase in 96 patients with pancreatitis. J.A.M.A., 186:24, 1963.

Gibson, L. E., and Cooke, R. E.: A test for concentration of electrolytes in sweat in cystic fibrosis of the pancreas utilizing pilocarpine by iontophoresis. Pediatrics, 23:545, 1959.

Grove, T. H., and Hohnadel, D. C.: Source of error in amylase estimation with the Perkin-Elmer Model 91 Amylase/Lipase Analyzer. Clin. Chem., 23:1512, 1977.

Hamlin, C. R., and Schwede, K.: Standardization of an alpha-amylase kit procedure. Clin. Chem., 20:96, 1974.

Harvey, R. F., Dowsett, L., Hartog, M., and Read, A. E.: A radioimmunoassay for cholecystokinin-pancreozymin. Lancet, 2:826, 1963.

Hathaway, J. A., Hunter, D. T., and Barrett, C. R.: An automated method for the determination of amylase. Clin. Biochem., 3:217, 1970.

Haverback, B. J., Dyce, B. J., Gutentag, P. J., and Montgomery, D. W.: Measurement of trypsin and chymotrypsin in stool: A diagnostic test for pancreatic insufficiency. Gastroenterology, 44:588, 1963.

Henry, R. J., and Chiamori, N.: Study of the saccharogenic method for the determination of serum and urine amylase. Clin. Chem., 6:434, 1960.

Hoffman, N. E., LaRusso, N. F., and Hoffman, A. F.: An improved method for fecal collection: A fecal field kit. Lancet, 1:1422, 1973.

Irie, A., Hunaki, M., Bando, K., and Kawai, K.: Determination of amylase activity in serum and urine using blue starch substrate. Clin. Chim. Acta, 42:63, 1972.

Jacobson, G.: Amylase-creatinine clearance ratio in pancreatitis. N. Engl. J. Med., 292:293, 1975.

James, G. P., Passey, R. B., Fuller, J. B., and Giles, M. L.: Evaluation of the DuPont aca alpha-amylase procedure. Clin. Chem., 23:546, 1977.

Johnson, S. G., Ellis, C. J., and Levitt, M. D.: Increased renal clearance of amylase: Creatinine in acute pancreatitis. N. Engl. J. Med., 295:1214, 1976.

Kamaryt, J., and Laxova, R.: Amylase heterogeneity, some genetic and clinical aspects. Humangenetik, 1:579, 1965.

Klein, B., Forman, J. A., and Searcy, R. L.: New chromogenic substrate for determination of serum amylase activity. Clin. Chem., 16:32, 1970.

Koch, P., and Tonks, D. B.: A comparison of various methods for assaying amylase activity. Presented at the Joint Meeting of the American Association of Clinical Chemists and the Canadian Society of Clinical Chemists, Seattle, Washington, 1971.

Legaz, M. E., and Kenny, M. A.: Electrophoretic amylase fractionation as an aid in diagnosis of pancreatic disease. Clin. Chem., 22:57, 1976.

Levine, R. I., Glauser, F. L., and Berk, J. E.: Enhancement of the amylase-creatinine clearance ratio in disorders other than acute pancreatitis. N. Engl. J. Med., 292:329, 1975.

Levitski, A., and Steer, M. L.: The allosteric activation of mammalian alpha-amylase by chloride. Eur. J. Biochem., 41:171, 1974.

Levitt, M. D., and Cooperband, S. R.: Hyperamylasemia from the binding of serum amylase by 11S IgA globulin. N. Engl. J. Med., 278:474, 1968.

Levitt, M. D., Duane, W., and Cooperband, S. R.: Study of macroamylase complexes. J. Lab. Clin. Med., 80:414, 1972.

Levitt, M. D., Rapoport, M., and Cooperband, S. R.: The renal clearance of amylase in renal insufficiency, acute pancreatitis and macroamylasemia. Ann. Intern. Med., 71:919, 1969.

Lifton, L. J., Slickers, K. A., Katz, L. A., and Pragay, D. A.: Amylase vs. lipase in the diagnosis of acute pancreatitis. Clin. Chem., 20:880, 1974.

Malkus, H., Ibanez, J., Castro, A., and DiCesare, J. L.: Automated turbidimetry of amylase activity by use of a discrete kinetic analyzer. Clin. Chem., 23:122, 1977.

Matthews, W. S., Sterling, R. E., Boyd, T., and Flores, O. R.: Modified automated saccharogenic determination of serum and urinary amylase activity. Clin. Chem., 19:1384, 1973.

Mazzuchin, A., Weggel, C., and Porter, C. J.: Automated method for determining amylase activity in serum and urine. Clin. Chem., 19:1187, 1973.

Mihas, A. A., and Hirschowitz, B. I.: Alpha-1-antitrypsin and chronic pancreatitis. Lancet, 2:1032, 1976.

Norby, S.: Electrophoretic non-identity of human salivary and pancreatic amylases. Exp. Cell Res., 36:633, 1964.

O'Donnell, M. D., Fitzgerald, O., and McGenney, K. F.: Differential serum amylase determination by use of an inhibitor, and design of a routine procedure. Clin. Chem., 23:560, 1977.

O'Donnell, M. D., and McGenney, K. F.: Comparison of saccharogenic and Phadebas methods for amylase assay in biological fluids. Enzyme, 18:348, 1974.

Otsuki, M., Saeki, S., Yuu, H., Maeda, M., and Baba, S.: Electrophoretic pattern of amylase isoenzymes in serum and urine of normal persons. Clin. Chem., 22:439, 1976.

Peralta, O., and Reinhold, J. G.: Rapid estimation of amylase activity of serum by turbidimetry. Clin. Chem., 1:157, 1955.

Proelss, H. F., and Wright, B. W.: New, simple maltogenic assay for mechanized determination of alpha-amylase activity in serum and urine. Clin. Chem., 21:694, 1975.

Reagent Insert, CH89-0138E. Amyloclastic amylase (Modified Somogyi's method). Miami, Fla., Dade Division, American Hospital Supply Corporation. March, 1975.

Reagent Insert, CH11-0139E. Iodometric amylase (modified Caraway's method). Miami, Fla., Dade Division, American Hospital Supply Corporation. March, 1975.

Reif, A. E., and Nabseth, D. C.: Serum amylase determination by Somogyi's amyloclastic method with use of a photometric end point. Clin. Chem., 8:113, 1962.

Robyt, J. F., and French, D.: Multiple attack hypothesis of alpha-amylase action: Action of porcine pancreatic, human salivary, and aspergillus oryzae alpha-amylase. Arch. Biochem., 122:8, 1967.

Sax, S. M.: Interconversion of enzyme units. Santa Monica, Cal., Clinton Laboratories, 1972.

Searcy, R. L., Wilding, P., and Berk, J. E.: An appraisal of methods for serum amylase determination. Clin. Chim. Acta, 15:189, 1967.

2

Shihabi, Z. K., and Bishop, C.: Simplified turbidimetric assay for lipase activity. Clin. Chem., *17*:1150, 1971.

Shipe, J. R., and Savory, J.: Kinetic nephelometric procedure for measurement of amylase activity in serum. Clin. Chem., *18*:1323, 1972.

Somogyi, M.: Micromethods for the estimation of diastase. J. Biol. Chem., *125*:399, 1938.

Somogyi, M.: Modification of two methods for the assay of amylase. Clin. Chem., *6*:23, 1960.

Spiekerman, A. M., Perry, P., Hightower, N. C., and Hall, F. F.: Chromogenic substrate method for demonstrating multiple forms of alpha-amylase after electrophoresis. Clin. Chem., *20*:324, 1974.

Stiefel, D. J., and Keller, P. J.: Preparation and some properties of human pancreatic amylase including a comparison with human parotid amylase. Biochim. Biophys. Acta, *302*:345, 1973.

Take, S., Fridhandler, L., and Berk, J. E.: Macroamylasemia: Possible role of polysaccharide in composition of macroamylase. Clin. Chim. Acta, *27*:369, 1970.

Takeuchi, T., Matsushima, T., and Sugimura, T.: Separation of human alpha amylase isoenzymes by electrofocusing and their immunological properties. Clin. Chim. Acta, *60*:207, 1975.

Takeuchi, T., Matsushima, T., Sugimura, T., Kozu, T., Takeuchi, T., and Takemoto, T.: A rapid new method for quantitative analysis of human amylase isoenzymes. Clin. Chim. Acta, *54*:137, 1974.

Taussig, L. M., Wolf, R. O., Woods, R. E., and Deckelbaum, R. J.: Use of serum amylase isoenzyme in evaluation of pancreatic function. Pediatrics, *54*:229, 1974.

Tietz, N. W., and Fiereck, E. A.: Measurement of lipase activity in serum. *In* Cooper, A. R. (ed.): Standard Methods of Clinical Chemistry, Vol. 7. New York, Academic Press, 1972, p. 19.

Vacikova, A., and Blochova, L.: Isoamylases in blood donors. Humangenetik, *8*:162, 1969.

Van Loon, E. J., Likins, M. R., and Seger, A. J.: Photometric method for blood amylase by use of a starch-iodine color. Am. J. Clin. Pathol., *22*:1134, 1952.

Vogel, W. C., and Zieve, L.: A rapid and sensitive turbidimetric method for serum lipase based upon differences between the lipases of normal and pancreatitis serum. Clin. Chem., *9*:168, 1963.

Warshaw, A. L., and Fuller, A. F.: Specificity of increased renal clearance of amylase in diagnosis of acute pancreatitis. N. Engl. J. Med., *292*:325, 1975.

Wiener, K., and Foot, C. H.: A study of some factors affecting the Phadebas amylase test. Clin. Chim. Acta, *75*:177, 1977a.

Wiener, K., and Foot, C. H.: Interlaboratory variability in amylase assay. Clin. Chem., *23*:1506, 1977b.

Wiggins, H. S.: Simple method of estimating trypsin. Gut, *8*:415, 1967.

Wilding, P., Cooke, W. T., and Nicholson, G. I.: Globulin-bound amylase. A cause of persistently elevated levels in serum. Ann. Intern. Med., *60*:1053, 1964.

Wilding, P., and Dawson, H. P.: Serum amylase. A brief biochemical evaluation. Clin. Biochem., *1*:101, 1967.

Wolf, R. O., Ross, M. E., and Tarply, T. M.: Changes in serum salivary isoamylases in Sjögren's syndrome. Am. J. Clin. Pathol., *65*:1022, 1976.

Wormsley, K. G.: Test of pancreatic function. Proc. R. Soc. Med., *63*:431, 1970.

Wu, W. T., and Beeler, M. F.: A simplified semi-automatic saccharogenic method for amylase assay. Am. J. Clin. Pathol., *57*:497, 1972.

Yourno, J., and Henry, J. B.: Rapid amylase and lipase determination by nephelometry. Am. J. Clin. Pathol., in press.

Yourno, J., and Henry, J. B.: Transiently elevated apparent lipase by nephelometry. Am. J. Clin. Pathol., in press.

Zieve, L., and Doizaki, W. M.: Influence of jaundice on turbidimetric measurement of serum lipolytic activity. J. Lab. Clin. Med., *67*:127, 1966.

Zinterhofer, L., Wardlaw, S., Jatlow, P., and Seligson, D.: Nephelometric determination of pancreatic enzymes. 1. Amylase. Clin. Chim. Acta, *43*:5, 1973.

24

EXAMINATION OF GASTRIC AND DUODENAL CONTENTS

Donald C. Cannon, M.D., Ph.D.

EXAMINATION OF GASTRIC CONTENTS

Although it is true that analysis of gastric secretion has not fulfilled some of the previous claims and expectations, this procedure maintains a useful role in clinical diagnosis and in the evaluation of therapy. As with most other laboratory examinations, information derived from gastric analysis is by itself seldom of pathognomonic significance but rather must be interpreted in light of the patient's history and with the results of other pertinent clinical, roentgenologic, and laboratory examinations. For example, anacidity does not invariably indicate pernicious anemia, although it is true that adult patients with pernicious anemia invariably have anacidity. Studies of peripheral blood and bone marrow, an investigation of intrinsic factor activity, or measurement of plasma gastrin may be necessary to substantiate or eliminate the diagnosis of pernicious anemia. Furthermore, in interpreting the results of gastric analysis, it must be kept in mind that there exists no sharply delineated normal range such as one is accustomed to use as a reference point for many laboratory measurements in chemistry, hematology, or serology. It is indeed only at the extremes of gastric secretion—anacidity or the marked hypersecretion such as is seen in the Zollinger-Ellison syndrome or in some cases of duodenal ulcer—that one can say with certainty that an underlying disease exists.

Considering both its limitations and its value, it is probable that a properly performed gastric analysis is done too infrequently at the present time. Among the factors that have contributed to this situation is the fact that many of the previously held beliefs regarding gastric secretion have been disproved by newer tests and better controlled surveys, thus adding a note of bewilderment and pessimism in the mind of the physician confronted with a patient having gastrointestinal complaints. For example, studies using the augmented histamine test have disproved the notion engendered by the older and now obsolete tests—standard histamine, alcohol stimulation, or various test meals—that anacidity is frequently a variant of normal. Anacidity, furthermore, is no longer considered to be a reliable screening test for gastric carcinoma, since most afflicted individuals do not have gastric anacidity; when anacidity occurs it is usually only in the more advanced cases. Gastroscopy, roentgenography, and gastric cytology are far more useful in establishing the diagnosis of probable gastric carcinoma than is gastric analysis. Even in the diagnosis of duodenal ulcer, the hypersecretory state that was once considered typical for the disease does not occur in most affected patients. An element of confusion has perhaps been added by the fact that the physicochemical basis for the older concept of "free," "combined," and "total" acid has now been found untenable.

The properly performed gastric analysis requires a relatively large investment of time by the physician who must perform the intubation and supervise the collection of samples. Although in itself a benign procedure, intubation is apt to be an unpleasant experience for the patient, not a few of whom submit to the procedure with reluctance. In view of these facts and the inherent limitations of the information to be gained, it is essential that there be a definite indication for performing routine gastric analysis. In general there are four clear-cut indications:

1. To determine whether or not the patient can secrete any gastric acid. The finding of anacidity is of major importance in three situations: the patient with macrocytic anemia, neurologic disorders, or other signs and symptoms of pernicious anemia; the patient suspected of having pernicious anemia who has been treated with vitamin B_{12} before the diagnosis was unequivocally established; and the exclusion of simple peptic ulceration in a patient with a suspicious ulcerating lesion of the stomach.

2. To measure the amount of acid produced by a patient with symptoms of peptic ulcer, particularly a patient with suspected duodenal or postoperative stomal ulcer who has no roentgenographically demonstrable lesion.

3. To reveal the hypersecretory state characteristic of the Zollinger-Ellison syndrome.

4. To determine the completeness of vagotomy by the insulin test.

In addition, gastric analysis is considered by some to be helpful for judging the efficacy of surgical, medical, or roentgen therapy for peptic ulcer and for determining the proper type of surgical procedure to be performed in the patient with peptic ulcer.

PHYSIOLOGY OF GASTRIC SECRETION

Gastric secretion has three major physiologic functions—the initiation of protein digestion, the physical and chemical preparation of ingested food resulting in an optimal mixture for subsequent digestion in the small intestine, and the secretion of intrinsic factor which promotes vitamin B_{12} absorption in the ileum. The first of these functions is not absolutely essential to the welfare of the human body, as shown by the fact that individuals with anacidity of long duration and therefore with failure of gastric protein digestion can exist free of gastrointestinal complaints and in good nutritional status.

Stimuli to gastric secretion are classically considered to occur in three phases, although present information demonstrates a relationship among these various phases. The cephalic or neurogenic phase consists of stimuli that are transmitted by the vagus nerves. This phase consists of anticipatory stimuli which arise from visual or olfactory perceptions associated with the ingestion of food and psychogenic stimuli which are derived from mental processes not related to the ingestion of food. Vagal impulses directly stimulate the parietal cells to secrete acid but also stimulate the antral mucosa to secrete gastrin into the blood. The polypeptide hormone, gastrin, is the most powerful known stimulus to gastric secretion, being many times as potent on a weight basis as histamine. Its elaboration and secretion are the paramount features of the second or gastric phase of secretion. In addition to vagal stimulation, gastrin is released by distention of the antrum with food or fluid and by contact of protein and protein breakdown products, the so-called secretagogues, with the antral mucosa. Secretagogues probably also act to stimulate the parietal and chief cells directly. The gastric phase is thus diminished but not abolished by vagotomy. The intestinal phase is quantitatively the least important phase of gastric secretion and is presumably mediated by humoral substances secreted into the blood by the duodenum in response to the entry of digestive products. It is probable that gastrin, formed by the duodenum, is the major humoral agent in this phase. Gastrin or a very similar substance has also been isolated from non–beta-cell adenomas of the pancreas associated with the hypersecretory state of the Zollinger-Ellison syndrome.

Various mechanisms serve to inhibit gastric secretion. Particularly important is the inhibition of gastrin secretion which occurs when the acidity of antral contents falls below a pH of about 1.5. An additional effect of high acidity of antral contents has been postulated to be the secretion of an inhibitory hormone by the antrum. A variety of inhibitory and neural reflex mechanisms have also been postulated to originate in the duodenum. It appears well established that an inhibitory hormone, enterogastrone, is liberated into the blood following contact of fatty acid breakdown products with the duodenal mucosa. Psychic mechanisms can inhibit gastric secretion as shown by the diminished secretion reported in patients suffering from chronic depression, and under other circumstances can stimulate gastric secretion.

COMPOSITION OF GASTRIC SECRETION

Gastric secretion is a complex solution the synthesis of which is not completely understood. Although the cells which secrete hydrochloric acid, pepsin, and mucus have been clearly identified, the varying concentration of inorganic ions in particular remains the object of speculation. The most widely popularized theory is the two-component hypothesis of Hollander (1952), which states that gastric secretion is composed of a parietal or acid component of fixed composition and a nonparietal or alkaline component consisting of a mixture of several secretions in varying proportions (Table 24-1). According to this theory, the variations in electrolyte concentrations are a reflection of the degree of dilution and neutralization of the parietal component by the alkaline component. Although it has served as a useful concept, the two-component hypothesis fails to explain some of the more important facts regarding the composition of gastric secretion. The following are components of gastric secretion:

Hydrochloric Acid. It is a remarkable biochemical feat that the stomach can secrete

Table 24-1. THE CONCENTRATION OF ELECTROLYTES IN GASTRIC SECRETION (mEq per liter)*

ION	COMPONENT	
	Parietal	Nonparietal
Hydrogen	160	—
Sodium	—	160
Potassium	10	10
Calcium	—	4
Chloride	170	125
Bicarbonate	—	45
Phosphate	—	6

*From the data of Hunt (1959) as interpreted by Sparberg, M., and Kirsner, J. B. (1964).

hydrogen ions at a concentration of more than one million times the plasma concentration—a concentration of about 160 mEq/l prior to dilution with the other secretory components. Hydrochloric acid is secreted by the parietal cells which are located in the isthmus and neck of the gastric glands of the fundus and body of the stomach but not those at either anatomic extreme—the narrow rim of cardia or the pylorus and antrum. The major importance of hydrochloric acid to digestion is to provide the high acidity necessary for the activation of pepsin from pepsinogen but also to a limited extent to hydrolyze polypeptides and disaccharides directly. As a result of the ease of measurement and relatively good correlation with disease states, the determination of gastric acidity is the most commonly used clinical index of gastric secretory activity.

Digestive Enzymes. The major digestive enzyme of gastric secretion is pepsin, which is elaborated by the chief or peptic cells located at the base of the gastric glands of the body and fundus. Pepsin is secreted as the zymogen, pepsinogen, which is activated by gastric acid at an optimal pH of 1.6 to 2.4. Pepsin catalyzes the degradation of proteins to proteoses and peptones but does not liberate free amino acids, this being the function of the more potent proteases in the secretions of the pancreas and small intestine. A small amount of pepsinogen enters the blood, presumably by direct absorption from the peptic cells, and is secreted in the urine as uropepsinogen. It has recently been shown that gastric proteolytic activity is shared by several enzymes. At least one of these, gastricsin, has a higher pH optimum (approximately 3.2) than pepsin. Gastricsin apparently arises from the same zymogen precursor as pepsin, and its concentration in gastric secretion is about one third that of pepsin. The significance of multiple gastric proteolytic enzymes is not yet known.

Other digestive enzymes include rennin and gastric lipase. Rennin has weak proteolytic activity and is best known for its ability to coagulate caseinogen in milk. Its high pH optimum (approximately 5 to 6) would seem to obviate any important contribution to gastric digestion. Gastric lipase, similarly, has a high pH optimum and appears to be of no importance to digestion.

Mucus. Gastric mucus is a chemically complex mixture of mucoproteins and mucopolysaccharides, the physiologic significance of which is poorly understood. Attempts have been made to correlate alterations or deficiencies in gastric mucus with the occurrence of peptic ulcer, but such studies are inconclusive. Mucus is secreted by specialized cells of the gland necks in the fundus and body of the stomach, by cells of the surface epithelium, and by the acinar cells of the cardia, antrum, and pylorus. Mucus secretion is probably stimulated largely by mechanical and chemical stimuli.

Electrolytes. Gastric secretion contains all the electrolytes found in other body fluids in a combined osmolar concentration equal to or slightly greater than plasma. The individual electrolytes vary widely in concentration, and with the exception of hydrogen ion, such variations have no known clinical significance. The concentration of electrolytes in the parietal and non-parietal components is shown in Table 24-1.

Nondigestive Enzymes. Using the technique of intragastric neutralization, various enzymes have been described in gastric secretion including lactic dehydrogenase, aspartate aminotransferase, isocitric dehydrogenase, leucine amino peptidase, alanine aminotransferase, beta-glucuronidase, alkaline phosphatase, and ribonuclease. These enzymes are doubtless the result of active gastric metabolism and have no function in digestion, particularly since all are inactivated by gastric acid except perhaps ribonuclease. Attempts have been made to correlate the levels of lactic dehydrogenase and beta-glucuronidase with gastric malignancy, but the results are equivocal (Piper, 1963).

Serum Proteins. Small amounts of serum albumin and gamma globulin are normally present in gastric secretion. Their presence can usually be detected only in the anacid stomach or by use of intragastric neutralization. Albumin may be increased in the gastric secretion in cases of giant hypertrophic gastritis or Menetrier's disease, in carcinoma, and in benign peptic ulcer.

Miscellaneous Substances. The most important component in this group and probably in the gastric secretion as a whole is intrinsic factor, which is elaborated and secreted by the gastric mucosa. It is a mucoprotein with molecular weight of about 17,000. The manner in which intrinsic factor promotes vitamin B_{12} absorption in the ileum is uncertain, but it has been convincingly shown to involve a complex between the two substances.

In approximately 80 per cent of individuals, those possessing the dominant secretor gene in homozygous or heterozygous state, the water-soluble blood group specific substances are present in the gastric secretion. This is of no particular significance to gastric secretion, since in these individuals the group specific substances are present in all body fluids.

NOMENCLATURE OF GASTRIC SECRETION

At present the nomenclature relating to the measurement of gastric secretion is in a state of transition. As previously mentioned, the concept underlying the older terminology has recently been justifiably challenged on the grounds that it lacks physicochemical validity. Nevertheless, such terms as "free acid," "combined acid," "total acid," and "clinical units" continue in common but hopefully diminishing usage. For this reason the intended meaning of these terms will be reviewed.

It was previously believed that the hydrochloric acid in gastric secretion existed in two distinct phases, the relative amounts of which depended on the pH of the secretion. At high pH values, generally taken to be greater than 3.0 or 3.5, the acid supposedly existed almost exclusively as a mixture of organic salts formed from combination of the acid with proteins and peptones in the gastric secretion. This phase, the "combined acid," was a direct reflection of the buffering capacity of the gastric secretion. Only when the buffering capacity was exceeded could the hydrochloric acid supposedly exist as ions in solution or as "free acid." Acidity was measured in "clinical units" or "degrees of acidity" which were equal to the number of milliliters of 0.1 N NaOH required to titrate 100 ml of gastric secretion to the endpoint of Topfer's reagent (pH 2.8 to 3.5) for "free acid" or to the endpoint of phenolphthalein (pH 8.2 to 10) for "total acid."

The older concept of gastric acidity was supported by titration curves obtained from the neutralization of gastric acid with sodium hydroxide. Such curves were similar to the titration curve of an aqueous solution of hydrochloric acid at pH values below about 2.8, but above this pH the curves resembled more closely those of a buffer mixture composed of a weak acid and its salt. As pointed out by Bock (1962), however, such studies failed to take into account the buffering effect of the various test meals then in use as gastric stimulants, an effect which could prove considerable. It has, in fact, now been shown that the titration curve of gastric secretion collected after histamine or Histalog stimulation rather closely resembles that of a solution of pure hydrochloric acid, although a slight buffering effect is evident at high pH values, generally above pH 4.0 (Moore, 1965). It is clearly apparent from such studies that a significant amount of "free" hydrochloric acid is present in gastric secretion at pH values greater than 3.5.

It is therefore recommended that the older terms of "free," "combined," and "total" acid be avoided entirely. Gastric secretion can best be described in terms of three measurements to be performed on each sample of gastric secretion:

1. *Volume* in milliliters.
2. *Titratable acidity* expressed in milliequivalents per liter. This is determined by titration of a suitable aliquot of gastric secretion with 0.1 N NaOH to neutrality (pH of 7.0 or 7.4 as preferred by some). The endpoint should be measured electrometrically with a suitable pH meter. If a pH meter is not available, the endpoint can be determined colorimetrically with phenol red (color change of yellow to red in the pH range of 6.8 to 8.4).
3. The *pH* measured electrometrically.

The *acid output* in milliequivalents for each sample can be calculated by multiplying its volume in milliliters by the titratable acidity and dividing by 1000. In addition to reporting the measured *volume*, *titratable acidity*, and *pH* and the calculated *acid output* for each individual sample, the *total volume* and *total acid output* will usually be reported for a given test by adding the individual sample values. Thus, for the study of basal secretion, a one-hour collection is generally employed consisting of four individually segregated 15-minute samples. The *basal acid output* in milliequivalents per hour is reported as the sum of the acid outputs for the four samples.

Nomenclature related to stimulated gastric secretion has developed in recent years largely in reference to histamine stimulation. The various terms can logically be applied to stimulation using pentagastrin, which is now the preferred gastric stimulant because the pattern of acid output following stimulation with pentagastrin is similar to that with histamine (Khodadoost, 1972).

The *maximal acid output* was originally defined as the milliequivalents of acid secreted in the hour following injection of histamine in the augmented or maximal histamine test. This is not to be confused with the *maximal histamine response*, which was defined by Kay (1953) as the output of acid in milliequivalents in the period from 15 to 45 minutes after histamine injection. Since these terms are easily confused, the term *maximal histamine response* is best avoided.

The *peak acid output* was originally defined as the greatest acid output in any two successive 15-minute periods in the augmented histamine test (Baron, 1963).

Various terms have been employed to describe qualitatively the results of gastric secretion tests. Most of these terms originated in relation to the older concepts of gastric acid and therefore must be redefined or discarded. Some useful terms have been given different definitions by different investigators. Only with the anticipation of vociferous objection can any definition of these terms be attempted.

Anacidity was previously defined as the absence of "free" acid, usually taken to mean a failure of the gastric secretory pH to fall below 3.5. Most investigators now define *anacidity* as a failure of the pH to fall below either 6.0 or 7.0 in the augmented histamine or Histalog tests. It is the most reasonable compromise between clinical usefulness and strict physicochemical definition to define *anacidity* as a failure of the pH to fall below 6.0 following augmented or maximal histamine or Histalog stimulation. The reason for choosing 6.0 is that *anacidity* so defined will apply to virtually all adult patients with pernicious anemia. Some of these patients, however, will secrete gastric juice with pH values a fraction of pH unit below strict neutrality, pH 7.0, at some time during the maximal histamine test (Callender, 1960).

Achlorhydria is used synonymously with

anacidity by some investigators but is defined differently by others. Some define *achlorhydria* as a gastric secretion with pH persistently above 3.5 and with failure of the pH to fall more than one unit with maximal histamine stimulation (Callender, 1960). *Hypochlorhydria*, on the other hand, has been used to refer to gastric juice with a pH persistently above 3.5 but falling more than one pH unit with maximal histamine stimulation. This fine distinction does not appear justified on clinical grounds. Furthermore, since pH 3.5 has been shown to have neither a unique physicochemical significance nor any particular clinical usefulness, the terms *achlorhydria* and *hypochlorhydria* should probably be avoided entirely.

Hyposecretion and hypersecretion are relative terms referring to the secretion of acid in amounts less than or greater than normal. Since the normal range for gastric secretion is not sharply delineated from that of pathologic states, these two terms, though admittedly useful clinically upon occasion, do not admit to strict definitions.

GASTRIC INTUBATION

The general procedure of intubation should be carefully explained to the patient in order to obtain the fullest possible cooperation and to avoid undue apprehension. The best recovery of gastric secretion will be obtained with the patient in a sitting position. Towels or a large apron should be provided to protect clothing. The bedfast patient should lie on his left side with his head elevated approximately 45 degrees. For intubation, a Levin tube, usually number 14F or 16F, may be passed through the nose, or a Rehfuss or similar tube may be passed through the mouth. Whether to use oral or nasal intubation depends largely on the preference of the individual examiner. It is likely that less difficulty will be encountered with nasal intubation if the patient has a hyperactive gag reflex. It is essential for the tube to have a radiopaque tip so that it can be adjusted fluoroscopically.

Many recommend preliminary chilling of the tube with ice in the belief that nausea during intubation is diminished. For oral intubation the patient is instructed to open his mouth and project his chin slightly forward and upward. The tip of the tube is placed on the superior aspect of the posterior portion of the tongue and pushed gently to the posterior pharynx, avoiding the uvula as much as possible. After the patient has closed his mouth gently on the tube he should be encouraged to alternate swallowing and deep oral breathing, the tube being pushed intermittently to its destination as he swallows. It is common for gastric tubes to be calibrated with several measurements, one of which is likely to be 55 cm, which corresponds to the approximate distance from the mouth to the antrum. It is imperative, however, for the position of the tube to be adjusted fluoroscopically so that the tip lies in the most dependent portion of the stomach, which will usually be the antrum if the patient is sitting and in the middle of the greater curvature if he is lying on his left side. Placement of the gastric tube on the basis of measurement, clinical judgment, or trial aspiration will be unsuitable for maximal aspiration in at least half of the intubation attempts. Following correct positioning, the tube should be directed lateral to the third molar tooth and can be maintained in position by taping to the patient's face. Value has been attributed to the water recovery test and fluoroscopic screening in positioning a nasogastric tube during gastric secretory studies (Findlay, 1972).

The principles of nasal intubation are similar to those of oral intubation. With the patient's chin elevated, the tube is directed slightly upward and then pushed gently posteriorly into the nasopharynx and esophagus. Some recommend preliminary spraying of the nasopharynx with a local anesthetic, although this should rarely be necessary.

If gastric secretion is to be collected over a period of time, as in the basal one-hour secretion test, continuous aspiration should be employed, since intermittent withdrawal of secretion has been shown to result in significantly lower recovery volumes (Kay, 1953). Continuous aspiration can be performed either with a syringe or by mechanical means. In one study in which isotopically (^{131}I) labeled human serum albumin was instilled into the esophagus during gastric intubation in order to simulate gastric secretion, significantly greater recovery was achieved with continuous aspiration with a glass syringe than with suction apparatus (Johnston, 1958). After brief instruction, the patient can usually be depended upon to operate the syringe successfully. It is important to caution the patient to expectorate all saliva and nasorespiratory secretions while aspiration is in progress.

Gastric intubation for secretory studies may be contraindicated for patients with esophageal varices, diverticula, stenosis, or malignant neoplasms of the esophagus, aortic aneurysm, recent severe gastric hemorrhage, congestive heart failure, or pregnancy.

PHYSICAL EXAMINATION OF GASTRIC CONTENTS

Secretion from the normal fasting stomach is a pale gray, translucent, slightly viscous fluid with a faintly pungent odor. The fasting volume varies up to about 50 ml. Following a 12-hour fast the presence of food particles is distinctly abnormal and indicates delayed gastric emptying, often the result of pyloric obstruction.

Bile.   Yellow to green coloration is the result of bile, which is occasionally regurgitated in the normal stomach and frequently accompanies excessive gagging during intubation. Large amounts of bile may be present with obstructing lesions of the small intestine distal to the ampulla of Vater.

Mucus.   The mucus normally present is largely responsible for the viscosity of gastric secretion. In addition to mucus of gastric origin, important contributions of mucus result from swallowed saliva and nasorespiratory secretions and to a minor degree from the reflux of duodenal contents. The latter is identified by its bile staining. Saliva is identified by its frothy flocculent nature, which causes it to float on the surface of the gastric secretion. Nasorespiratory mucus is highly tenacious and may contain dust particles.

Blood.   Flecks or streaks of blood are commonly seen as a result of minor trauma during intubation. Blood of greater amount and longer duration in the acid-secreting stomach will be brown and granular, the so-called "coffee-ground" appearance. Such quantities of blood may be from a gastric lesion such as gastritis, ulcer, or carcinoma or may be swallowed from the mouth, nasopharynx, or lungs. The presence of significant quantities of blood should be confirmed by the orthotolidine (Hematest) or guaiac tests.

pH.   pH should be measured electrometrically with a reliable pH meter. There may be occasions when a rapid bedside estimate is indicated, in which case the use of pH indicator paper is permissible if due regard is given to the inherent inaccuracies.

MICROSCOPIC EXAMINATION OF GASTRIC CONTENTS

A variety of structures may be recognized on microscopic examination. Components which may be present in the normal stomach include erythrocytes, leukocytes, epithelial cells, yeast, bacteria, and particles of mucus. Cellular elements are usually in various stages of autolysis, and their specific identity may be difficult.

As noted previously, small numbers of erythrocytes are of no consequence.

Leukocytes may be of gastric origin or may be from swallowed secretions. Small numbers of leukocytes are present in normal gastric secretion. Increased numbers may result from inflammation of the gastric mucosa, mouth, paranasal sinuses, or nasorespiratory tract, or, less commonly, from the pancreas, biliary tract, or duodenum.

Epithelial cells will be found in small numbers as a result of desquamation from various mucosal surfaces. Squamous cells may be dislodged from the mouth, nose, pharynx, or esophagus during intubation and may even appear in small clumps. Gastritis may result in a significant increase in columnar epithelial cells, but this is usually not a helpful criterion.

As a result of the high acid secretion and perhaps other secretory factors inimical to the survival of bacteria, the normal stomach does not have an established microbiologic flora. Although bacteria and yeasts can be regularly cultured from gastric secretion, these usually reflect the flora of the mouth and nasorespiratory tract from the swallowing of secretions. These same bacteria probably do exist as an established flora in the anacid stomach. Yeasts may be present in large numbers in retention of gastric contents, such as occurs with pyloric obstruction.

In the past, considerable interest has focused on the Boas-Oppler bacillus, a species of lactobacillus. These large, nonmotile, gram-positive bacilli commonly occur in chains or clumps. Although once attributed special significance in the diagnosis of gastric carcinoma, their proliferation is probably the result of a favorable fermentative environment created by retention of gastric contents and decreased or absent hydrochloric acid.

Protozoan and metazoan parasites occur rarely and then usually with reflux of duodenal content. *Giardia lamblia* trophozoites or cysts, strongyloides larvae, or ascaris or hookworm ova may be found.

TESTS OF GASTRIC FUNCTION

Basal Gastric Secretion. Basal gastric secretion represents the response of the stomach to endogenous stimuli which are continually present in the interdigestive or fasting state. These endogenous stimuli include psychoneurogenic influences mediated by the vagus nerves and hormonal stimuli, such as gastrin and perhaps adrenocorticosteroids. For clinical validity it is essential that basal physiologic and environmental conditions be maintained as much as possible during collection of the secretion. Minimum requirements include the following: (1) the patient must be in the fasting state and free from the sight or odor of food. (2) All medications influencing gastric secretion must be withheld for 24 hours. The most obvious medications in this regard include antacids and antisecretory (anticholinergic) drugs and also such secretory stimulants as reserpine, alcohol, adrenergic blocking agents, and adrenocorticosteroids. (3) The patient should be removed from environmental situations evoking untoward psychological reactions such as fear, anger, or depression.

The one-hour morning aspiration is now the standard method of measuring basal secretion, having replaced the cumbersome and inherently less precise 12-hour nocturnal aspiration.

TECHNIQUE

1. Following a 12-hour overnight fast, the patient is intubated. Water may be taken until 8 hours prior to intubation.

2. The residual volume of gastric secretion is measured and qualitatively examined.

3. Continuous aspiration is begun, preferably manually with a syringe. The aspirate should be segregated into 15-minute samples. Usually the first one or two samples are discarded to allow for adjustment of the patient to the intubation procedure. Subsequent to this adjustment period, four 15-minute samples are taken.

4. For each 15-minute sample, the volume, pH, and titratable acidity are measured and the acid output calculated. The sum of the acid outputs in the four samples, expressed in milliequivalents, represents the one-hour basal acid output.

CLINICAL EVALUATION. The mean basal acid output reported for normal males ranges from 1.3 to 4.0 mEq per hour in various series. This variation among series is a reflection, in part at least, of different collection techniques and methods of measuring titratable acid. Lower values occur in females and with aging. Somewhat lower than normal values are reported in most large series for gastric carcinoma and benign gastric ulcer and distinctly higher values for duodenal ulcer or jejunal ulcer following partial gastrectomy with gastrojejunostomy (Table 24-2). Extremely high acid output is present in patients with the Zollinger-Ellison syndrome. In 25 such patients reviewed by Ellison and Wilson (1964), the one-hour basal acid output varied from 11 to greater than 80 mEq. A high ratio of basal acid output to maximal acid output is of even greater significance, however, in the diagnosis of the Zollinger-Ellison syndrome.

It is important to emphasize that no pathognomonic range exists for any of the disease states listed, with the possible exception of the very high acid output found in patients with the Zollinger-Ellison syndrome. For example, in the series of 20 normal individuals reported by Marks (1962), the acid output in normal individuals ranged from 0 to 13.8 mEq per

Table 24-2. BASAL AND MAXIMAL ACID OUTPUT IN VARIOUS CONDITIONS*

CONDITION	SEX	NUMBER OF PATIENTS	ACID OUTPUT (mEq/hour)	
			Basal	Maximal
Controls	Male	35	4.2	22.6
	Female	26	1.8	15.2
Medical students	Male	145	5.3	26.7
	Female	16	3.3	21.4
Duodenal ulcer	Male	256	7.1	35.2
	Female	64	4.2	25.7
Gastric ulcer	Male	117	2.9	19.6
	Female	43	1.6	13.1
Gastric carcinoma	Male	74	1.5	6.7
	Female	32	0.7	3.0
Jejunal ulcer	Male†	10	7.9	25.1
	Female	4	5.5	16.4
	Male‡	4	9.1	36.1

* From Marks, I. N., et al.: S. Afr. J. Surg., 1:53, 1963.
† Following partial gastrectomy with gastrojejunostomy.
‡ Following gastroenterostomy alone.

hour. Nevertheless, a basal acid output greater than 10 mEq per hour is found in only about 4 per cent of normal individuals but about 13 to 19 per cent of duodenal ulcer patients (Marks, 1961).

The volume of gastric secretion in the basal hour, which ranges from about 50 to 100 ml, has by itself little diagnostic significance.

Augmented Histamine Test. Histamine is a powerful stimulant to gastric secretion and for several decades has been used clinically in gastric function tests. Earlier studies, including the "standard histamine test," utilized small doses of histamine and consequently resulted rather frequently in the incorrect diagnosis of anacidity. The augmented, or maximal, histamine test was introduced by Kay (1953), who showed that a dose of histamine acid phosphate of 0.04 mg/kg of body weight resulted in an acid output which did not increase further with larger doses of histamine. In order to avoid the undesirable side effects of histamine, however, the augmented histamine test has now largely been replaced by the pentagastrin test, which results in a similar magnitude of acid output with considerably fewer side effects.

The untoward systemic effects of histamine are largely prevented by a previous injection of antihistamine which does not interfere significantly with the stimulatory effect on gastric secretion. Side effects were recorded in one series of 166 patients and, although frequent, were for the most part relatively mild clinically (Callender, 1960). A decrease in blood pressure lasting from 30 to 45 minutes occurred in 61 per cent of the patients. The fall in blood pressure varied from 3 to 65 mm Hg systolic with a mean of 19 mm and from 3 to 40 mm diastolic with a mean of 13 mm. Hypotension necessitated discontinuation of the test in only one patient, however. In contrast, a slight rise in blood pressure occurred in 12 per cent. Other side effects of less significance were as follows: subjective feeling of warmth usually lasting approximately 30 minutes, 95 per cent; increased pulse rate (mean increase of 11 per minute with a maximum of 52 per minute), 70 per cent; drowsiness attributable to administration of antihistamine, 61 per cent; decreased pulse rate, 16 per cent; generalized patchy erythema, 12 per cent; headache, 7 per cent; lacrimation and nasal obstruction, 6 per cent.

A history of bronchial asthma or urticaria, the presence of severe cardiac, pulmonary, or renal disease, and paroxysmal hypertension or other possible signs and symptoms of pheochromocytoma are contraindications to the performance of this test.

TECHNIQUE

1. Following a 12-hour fast, basal secretion is collected for one hour as previously described.

2. Thirty minutes before completion of the basal secretion collection, a suitable dose of antihistamine is administered intramuscularly, e.g., 10 mg chlorpheniramine maleate (Chlor-Trimeton), 50 mg pyrilamine maleate (Neo-Antergan), or 50 mg diphenhydramine hydrochloride (Benadryl).

3. After the conclusion of the basal secretion study, histamine acid phosphate is administered subcutaneously in a dose of 0.04 mg/kg body weight.

4. Gastric contents are then collected in 15-minute samples for one hour.

5. The volume, pH, and titratable acidity are measured for each sample and the acid output is calculated. From these the one-hour or maximal acid output in milliequivalents is calculated.

CLINICAL EVALUATION. The maximum rate of acid secretion is characteristically attained within 15 minutes after histamine injection and is maintained for approximately 30 minutes. By 60 minutes after histamine injection acid secretion usually will have fallen to basal levels. The maximum acid output, representing the sum of the acid outputs for four consecutive 15-minute posthistamine samples (one hour), is the most generally accepted expression of gastric acid secretion. Values for various conditions are listed in Table 24-2.

As in the case of basal acid secretion, the extended range of the maximal acid output for normal individuals obviates strict diagnostic categorization. Thus, in the series of Marks (1962), the range for maximal acid output in normal males was 4.9 to 38.9 mEq per hour. Some generalizations are useful, however. A maximal acid output of greater than 40 mEq per hour is found in about 40 per cent of males with duodenal ulcer but only rarely in normal individuals (Marks, 1961). In addition to the marked hypersecretion, patients with the Zollinger-Ellison syndrome have a high ratio of basal to maximal acid output. Ratios greater than 60 per cent are strongly indicative of this disorder, while ratios between 40 to 60 per cent are suggestive. The maximal acid output is not of great help in distinguishing benign gastric ulcer from gastric carcinoma unless anacidity is found, in which case benign peptic ulceration can be excluded.

Anacidity in the augmented histamine test is most commonly found in adults with pernicious anemia or gastric carcinoma. Nevertheless, it has been reported in a variety of other conditions, including hypochromic anemia, rheumatoid arthritis, steatorrhea, aplastic anemia, myxedema, nutritional megaloblastic anemia, and the asymptomatic relatives of patients with pernicious anemia. Such cases are uncommon, as indicated by the series of Card (1955) in which, of 500 consecutive patients subjected to the maximal histamine test, all patients with anacidity proved to have pernicious anemia. Pernicious anemia in adults is virtually always accompanied by anacidity, but this does not hold true for the rare cases of juvenile pernicious anemia, in which normal acid secretion may be present. In a series of 30 patients with classic pernicious anemia reported by Callender (1960), the pH of the gastric contents remained above 6.0 in all samples during both the basal and augmented histamine studies. Furthermore, following histamine stimulation, the pH actually increased from basal levels in 25 of the 30 patients, failed to show any change in three, and fell slightly to acid levels in two. In neither of the two cases did the pH fall more than a fraction of one unit.

Anacidity with gastric carcinoma is the exception rather than the rule. In one series, 10 of 38 males and six of 14 females with gastric carcinoma had anacidity in the augmented histamine test (Marks, 1962).

Data from the basal and augmented histamine tests have been used by some physicians as an aid in determining which surgical procedure should be employed in the treatment of peptic ulcer. It has been suggested that an increased functioning parietal cell mass evidenced by an elevated maximal acid output indicates the need for gastric resection. On the other hand, elevated basal secretion with normal or only slightly elevated maximal secretion has been interpreted as an indication for vagotomy with drainage procedure. These are by no means universally accepted dictums.

Acid secretion is not expressed solely in terms of pH and maximal acid output by all workers. The *maximal histamine response,* which is the acid output in the interval from 15 to 45 minutes after histamine, was proposed on the basis of its high reproducibility (Kay, 1953). More recently, the similar concept

of peak acid output has been used to represent the greatest acid output in any two successive 15-minute posthistamine samples. In about one-half of the cases, the peak acid output will occur in the period from 15 to 45 minutes after histamine (Baron, 1963). The peak acid output does not occur at the same interval in repeated tests on the same patient, but its value is the most reproducible measurement of acid secretion in the augmented histamine test. Some confusion has been introduced by the fact that some investigators have reported the peak acid output as a rate of acid output, i.e., milliequivalents per hour, by doubling the peak half-hour value.

Pentagastrin Stimulation Test. Pentagastrin is a synthetic pentapeptide derivative which contains the four C-terminal amino acids of gastrin linked to substituted alanine. Pentagastrin retains a significant fraction of the biologic activity of gastrin and therefore is a potent stimulus to the secretion of acid, pepsin, and intrinsic factor by the stomach. It also stimulates secretion of both bicarbonate and enzymes by the pancreas, relaxation of the sphincter of Oddi, and contraction of the gallbladder.

Pentagastrin has been commonly used in Europe for gastric stimulation tests since 1966. It was not until 1975, however, that it was approved for routine clinical use in the United States. It is commercially available as Peptavlon (Ayerst).

Side effects following pentagastrin administration are relatively slight and include transitory dizziness, faintness, flushing, and numbness of the extremities.

A dose of 6 μg/kg of body weight is injected subcutaneously for maximal acid secretion. Otherwise, the test is conducted identically to the augmented histamine test except that prior injection of an antihistamine is not necessary.

Acid output following the recommended dose of pentagastrin is very similar to that following augmented histamine stimulation in the first hour and in the earlier peak (15 to 30 minutes) (Khodadoost, 1972). The duration of histamine stimulation is somewhat longer, as evidenced by its greater residual effect on acid output in the second post-stimulation hour. The interpretation of the two tests appears to be the same for all practical purposes.

Histalog Test. Histalog (3-B-aminoethyl pyrazole dihydrochloride, betazole), an analogue of histamine, is frequently used in place of histamine as a stimulus in gastric secretory studies. Histalog has the distinct advantage that side effects are minimal or absent; thus, premedication with antihistamines can be omitted. Results of Histalog stimulation are as reproducible as those of the augmented histamine test.

The dose of Histalog which gives maximal acid response, the augmented Histalog dosage, has been determined to be 1.7 mg/kg body weight injected intramuscularly (Zaterka, 1964). Somewhat smaller doses, e.g., 1.5 mg/kg body weight or a fixed dose of 100 mg, intramuscularly, are commonly used. The test is performed in the same manner as the augmented histamine test except that (1) prior administration of an antihistamine is omitted, and (2) eight instead of four 15-minute post-Histalog samples are collected.

The acid secretory response to Histalog is similar to that of histamine but has a distinctly greater latency period and longer duration of action. Whereas the peak secretion is regularly attained in the second or third 15-minute period in the augmented histamine test, it is not reached until some time in the second to fifth 15-minute period in the augmented Histalog test. The peak secretory rate may last for 45 to 90 minutes in the augmented Histalog test. The peak 30-minute acid output is comparable in the two tests, being approximately 12 to 14 mEq in normal subjects.

Insulin Hypoglycemia Test. Hypoglycemia resulting from the administration of insulin is a potent stimulus to gastric acid secretion. The major component of this stimulus is transmitted by the vagus nerves and can be abolished by vagotomy. The hypoglycemic response is complex, however, and probably consists of three phases. For about 30 minutes after insulin injection there is a slight depression of gastric secretion, the mechanism of which has not been explained. The predominant effect during the remainder of the first two hours consists of marked enhancement of gastric secretion. It is believed that this results from stimulation of the anterior hypothalamus by the hypoglycemia and subsequent transmission of this stimulus to the vagal centers of the brain. The final effect, which is manifested after two hours, also stimulates gastric secretion but presumably by a humoral mechanism. This late effect may result from initial stimulation of the posterior hypothalamus, with secondary neurohumoral stimulation of the anterior pituitary to release adrenocorticotropic hormone. The adrenocortical hormones which are thereby released probably act directly on the parietal cells, since this late effect of insulin hypoglycemia may be clearly manifested after complete vagotomy.

TECHNIQUE (Modified from Hollander, 1948)

1. After a 12-hour overnight fast the patient is intubated. A two-hour basal secretion is obtained in 15-minute samples.

2. Blood samples for glucose determinations are obtained upon completion of the basal secretion study and at 30, 60, and 90 minutes after insulin injection.

3. Insulin is administered intravenously either at a fixed dosage of 15 or 20 units or at a calculated dosage of 0.20 unit/kg body weight. It is essential that a 50-ml syringe filled with 50 per cent (w/v) glucose solution be readily available to counteract any serious hypoglycemic effects.

4. Gastric secretion is collected in 15-minute samples for two hours after insulin.

5. For each basal and postinsulin gastric sample, the volume and titratable acidity are determined, and the acid output is calculated.

CLINICAL EVALUATION. The insulin test is valid only if the blood glucose falls below 50 mg/100 ml at some point in the test, which will usually be 30 minutes after insulin administration. The test is furthermore valid only for the stomach that has been shown to be capable of secreting hydrochloric acid. Therefore, if no acid is present in either the basal or postinsulin periods, it is necessary to perform an augmented histamine test in an attempt to evoke acid secretion. If the stomach is truly anacid, no conclusion can be drawn regarding the completeness of vagotomy, but the question of simple peptic ulceration is then effectively excluded.

The assessment of gastric function following vagotomy has been recently reviewed (Read, 1974). There is no clear delineation of normal from abnormal results in the insulin test. Nevertheless, several generalizations can be made. The patient can be considered to be completely vagotomized if the acid output in the greater of the two postinsulin hours is less than the greater of the two basal hours. Incomplete vagotomy is likely if the acid output in the two-hour postinsulin period exceeds that of the two-hour basal period by more than 0.5 mEq (Stempien, 1962). Incomplete vagotomy is also suggested by an acid output of greater than 2 mEq in either basal hour.

The time of increased acid output in the insulin test appears to be of some prognostic significance in incompletely vagotomized patients. Bell (1965) reported the clinical course of 42 patients shown to be incompletely vagotomized by the insulin test. Of 28 patients giving an elevated acid output in the first postinsulin hour, 10 eventually developed recurrent peptic ulceration. In contrast, ulceration recurred in only one of the remaining 14 patients who showed an elevated acid output in the second postinsulin hour.

Twelve-hour Nocturnal Aspiration. This method of determining basal gastric secretion continues to be used, although the much less complicated one-hour morning basal collection has been shown to give qualitatively comparable results (Levin, 1951). The 12-hour collection has no proven superiority over the one-hour morning collection. It has been claimed to be more representative of basal gastric secretory activity by allowing freer expression of the normal fluctuations in gastric secretion, but this theoretical advantage is probably largely offset by the mechanical difficulties attendant upon the prolonged aspiration. Other disadvantages of the 12-hour nocturnal aspiration include the following: (1) Hospitalization is required, whereas the one-hour morning basal collection followed by the pentagastrin stimulation test may be performed on an outpatient basis. (2) The test requires continual attention to proper functioning of the suction pump, including intermittent flushing with air. (3) The swallowing of saliva and nasorespiratory secretions cannot be avoided. (4) The test unduly extends for the patient the discomfort which is attendant upon any intubation procedure.

TECHNIQUE (Levin, 1948)

1. For 24 hours prior to the start of aspiration, all medication influencing gastric secretion is withheld.

2. The usual diet is allowed until 12:30 P.M. on the day of the test, and normal activity is conducted until 5:30 P.M. At this time the patient is hospitalized and given a clear liquid meal. Food and water are subsequently withheld.

3. At 8:00 P.M., nasogastric intubation is performed and the stomach emptied completely. Continuous aspiration is begun.

4. At 8:30 P.M. and continuing for the next 12 hours the gastric secretion is collected by continuous aspiration. Hourly samples are segregated. Suction should be frequently interrupted and the tubing flushed with air.

5. For each hourly sample, the volume and titratable acidity are measured and the acid output is calculated. Samples contaminated with bile are discarded. The total acid output and volume are also reported.

CLINICAL EVALUATION. Levin (1948) studied 21 normal males and 12 normal females and found a mean 12-hour nocturnal volume of 643 ml and 460 ml respectively. In contrast, the mean volume was 1004 ml in 32 duodenal ulcer patients. The secretory volumes were not significantly different from normal in patients with gastric ulcer (623 ml) or gastric carcinoma (436 ml).

The total acid output for the 12 hours is about 15 to 30 mEq for normal individuals.

The 12-hour nocturnal aspiration has been thought to have special usefulness in the diagnosis of the Zollinger-Ellison syndrome, but the one-hour basal test combined with the pentagastrin stimulation test is probably superior in distinguishing this entity from other hypersecretory states such as duodenal ulcer. Overnight secretion was studied in 55 patients of the series collected by Ellison (1964). Total secretory volumes ranged from 250 ml to greater than 4000 ml. In 85 per cent of the patients, the volume exceeded 1 liter, 49 per cent exceeded 2 liters, 22 per cent exceeded 3 liters, and 14 per cent exceeded 4 liters. Data on acid output were available on 54 patients. In 74 per cent of these the acid output exceeded 100 mEq, and in 35 per cent it exceeded 300 mEq. In view of the normal range reported for the 12-hour nocturnal aspiration, it may be concluded that the Zollinger-Ellison syndrome is to be considered probable if the total volume exceeds 2 liters and the acid output exceeds 100 mEq.

Tubeless Gastric Analysis. The tubeless gastric analysis is an indirect method for detecting gastric acid secretion and has as its only significant advantage the elimination of gastric intubation. The method utilizes a carboxylic cation exchange resin, the hydrogen ions of which have been replaced by those of an indicator cation. After ingestion the indicator cations are in turn released from the resin by hydrogen ions if acid is present in the gastric secretion. The indicator cations which are released are subsequently absorbed in the small intestine and eventually excreted in the urine. The measurement of the quantity of indicator cations in the urine is thus an indication of gastric acidity.

Initially quininium was used as the indicator but was later replaced by the dye azure A.

Azure A has the advantage that its excretion can be estimated by direct visual inspection.

A variety of stimulants to gastric secretion have been recommended for use in this test, including oral caffeine sodium benzoate, Histalog, or alcohol and parenterally administered histamine or Histalog. Orally administered caffeine sodium benzoate and Histalog are the ones most commonly used.

The test reagents and comparator block are now commercially available as a complete kit (Diagnex Blue Test, Squibb).

TECHNIQUE (Segal, 1960)

1. Upon rising, the patient urinates and discards the urine. No food is ingested until completion of the test.

2. The gastric stimulant, either 500 mg caffeine sodium benzoate or 50 mg Histalog, is taken with a glass of water. Alternatively, histamine or Histalog can be administered subcutaneously.

3. One hour later the patient urinates and again discards the sample. Immediately thereafter, 2 g of azuresin (U.S.P. granules) are ingested with one half glass of water.

4. Two hours later the patient again urinates and saves the entire sample. The urine sample is diluted to 300 ml with water, and a 10-ml aliquot is placed in each of three test tubes.

5. Two of the tubes serve as color controls, and to each of these approximately 300 mg of L-ascorbic acid is added. This reduces the azure A to a colorless form.

6. The tubes are then placed in a comparator block containing azure A standards of 0.3 mg/300 ml and 0.6 mg/300 ml. If the color of the test urine is more intense than that of the 0.6-mg standard, the test is completed and the patient is presumed to secrete hydrochloric acid.

7. If the color of the test urine is less than that of the 0.6-mg standard, a drop of a solution containing 195 mg $CuSO_4 \cdot 5H_2O$ in 100 ml of 18 per cent HCl (Diagnex Blue reagent, Squibb) is added to each of the three urine tubes. All three tubes are placed in a boiling water bath for 10 minutes.

8. After cooling at room temperature for two hours, the color development is again compared to the standard solutions. The results are reported as less than 0.3 mg, 0.3 to 0.6 mg, or greater than 0.6 mg.

CLINICAL EVALUATION. The tubeless gastric analysis is strictly a qualitative test. An excretion of greater than 0.6 mg azure A in two hours is considered to be indicative of hydrochloric acid secretion, while values less than 0.3 mg are considered presumptive evidence of anacidity. Values between 0.3 and 0.6 mg represent borderline secretion.

Considerable difference of opinion exists regarding the reliability of the tubeless gastric analysis. Much of the reported variation in false positives and false negatives is the result of differences in the standard of comparison for the tubeless analysis, different methods of gastric stimulation, and problems in the definition of anacidity. Marks (1960) compared the results of the azure A tubeless gastric analysis following caffeine sodium benzoate with those of the augmented histamine test in 85 selected patients. Defining anacidity as a failure of the pH to fall below 6.0 in the augmented histamine test, they found one of the 85 patients to show a false positive tubeless analysis result and 14 to show a false negative result. Most of the false negative results occurred in patients with greatly diminished secretion.

Histalog given orally appears to be a more effective gastric stimulant than caffeine sodium benzoate. Segal (1959) administered the tubeless analysis following stimulation with 50 mg of oral Histalog in 149 patients who were anacid according to the results with 500 mg caffeine sodium benzoate stimulation. They found that 51 per cent of these patients secreted detectable acid with the Histalog stimulus.

The tubeless gastric analysis is considered unreliable in patients with previous subtotal gastrectomy, gastroenterostomy, or pyloroplasty. These conditions have been reported as causing both false positive and false negative results, both due to the rapid transit of the resin through the stomach. False positive results in this case are caused by release of the azure A by cations in the small intestinal secretion such as sodium, magnesium, potassium, and calcium. It is recommended that oral administration of salts containing barium, iron, calcium, magnesium, or aluminum be discontinued for 48 hours prior to testing. A single case of diverticulosis of the small intestine has been reported as causing false positive results, probably as a result of altered bacterial flora (Forster, 1961). Other conditions which make the tubeless analysis unreliable are malabsorption syndromes, severe diarrhea, pyloric obstruction, severe hepatic or renal disease, marked dehydration, and urinary retention.

Some recommend repeating the tubeless gastric analysis following apparent negative or borderline results. It is advisable that five days be allowed to elapse before repeating the test in order to allow for delayed excretion of the azure A.

Many gastroenterologists consider tubeless gastric analysis to be a discredited procedure, although it still attracts considerable attention.

MISCELLANEOUS STUDIES

Mycobacterial Culture. Aspiration of gastric contents for mycobacterial culture is indicated in patients who are suspected of having pulmonary tuberculosis but who are unable to produce adequate sputum samples. The procedure is particularly indicated for young children, since it is not until the age of about seven years that children can effectively expectorate pulmonary secretions. It is essential that the gastric content be collected in the early morning prior to eating or drinking and preferably immediately upon awakening before increased motor activity of the stomach has largely emptied its contents. Since gastric acidity is inimical to the survival of *Mycobacterium tuberculosis*, as well as to most other bacteria, it is important that specimens be submitted immediately for decontamination and culture. Acid-fast stains on gastric contents are unreliable because of the frequent presence of saprophytic acid-fast organisms originating in the mouth.

Exfoliative Cytology of the Stomach. Gastric cytology, gastroscopy, and roentgenography are at present the most useful procedures for investigating lesions of the stomach for possible malignancy. To a large extent the three procedures complement one another, but in the final analysis the most discriminating information is provided by exfoliative cytology. Multiple techniques for obtaining specimens have been reported, including simple aspiration of gastric content, the use of abrasive balloons or brushes, and gastric lavage with saline, buffered salt solutions, or solutions of papain or chymotrypsin. Chymotrypsin is believed to facilitate the exfoliation of cells by liquefying the mucous coating. Accuracies of greater than 90 per cent have been reported for exfoliative cytology in the diagnosis of gastric carcinoma.

OTHER PROCEDURES IN GASTRIC ANALYSIS

Determination of Hydrogen Ion Concentration from Electrode pH Measurements. Moore (1965) has recommended, on the basis of both practicality and accuracy, the determination of hydrogen ion concentration from electrode pH measurements. This method utilizes the interrelationships between pH, hydrogen ion activity (a_{H+}), the hydrogen ion activity coefficient (γ_{H+}), and hydrogen ion concentration (c_{H+}) represented by the two equations:

$$pH = -\log_{10} a_{H+}$$
$$\gamma_{H+}\, c_{H+} = a_{H+}$$

The activity coefficient is a function of both total ionic strength and pH. Since the ionic strength of gastric juice is largely determined by the concentration of major cations, sodium, potassium, and hydrogen, it has been possible to tabulate the activity coefficients and therefore the concentration of hydrogen ions for various concentrations of sodium and potassium at a given pH. This method thus requires precise measurement of pH with a glass electrode and determination of the sum of potassium and sodium. This approach has not been widely accepted and does not appear to provide any additional information which is of unique clinical value.

Electrophoresis of Gastric Secretion. Electrophoresis of gastric secretion reveals distinct bands of albumin and gamma globulin (Cohen, 1962), multiple bands composed largely of mucopolysaccharides, and perhaps a band of pepsin (Glass, 1961). Electrophoresis has proved helpful in detecting the marked loss of albumin into the gastric contents which occurs in Menetrier's disease (giant hypertrophic gastritis with hypoproteinemia). Losses of albumin have also been described in benign gastric ulcer and gastric carcinoma. This technique requires special attention to the collection of samples, intragastric neutralization usually being necessary to avoid autodigestion of proteins. Electrophoresis of gastric content requires further evaluation, but studies thus far do not indicate the likelihood of adoption of this technically involved, time-consuming procedure for routine clinical use.

Determinations of Intrinsic Factor. Until recently intrinsic factor activity could be determined only by *in vivo* methods, such as the Schilling test, which measure the absorption of cobalt-60–labeled vitamin B_{12}. Several *in vitro* methods for assaying intrinsic factor have now been reported which utilize various immunologic methods and such techniques as starch-gel or paper electrophoresis, column chromatography, or charcoal absorption. None of these methods has as yet received general acceptance, but it is anticipated that in the near future *in vitro* assays for intrinsic factor will become established as an important supplement to gastric analysis in selected cases.

Determination of Plasma Gastrin. Although not an integral part of gastric analysis *per se*, radioimmunoassay of plasma or serum gastrin is now available as a sensitive (5 pg/ml) and specific clinical laboratory determination. The assay is a valuable adjunct in diagnosis of the Zollinger-Ellison syndrome and pernicious anemia, both of which are associated with marked elevations of gastrin. The two diseases are readily distinguished on the basis of concomitant gastric acid secretion studies and by the fact that intragastric installation of dilute hydrochloric acid results in a precipitous decrease in plasma gastrin in pernicious anemia, whereas no appreciable change occurs in the Zollinger-Ellison syndrome (Yalow, 1970). In general in normal individuals, fasting plasma gastrin levels, which range up to approximately 300 pg/ml, are inversely related to the rate of gastric acid secretion. Fasting plasma gastrin concentrations in duodenal ulcer patients do not differ from those of normal individuals; however, after a meal there is a greater response of the plasma gastrin in duodenal ulcer patients (Levine, 1977). Small increases in plasma gastrin are associated with gastric ulcers and with aging (Trudeau, 1971).

TESTS OF GASTRIC FUNCTION NO LONGER RECOMMENDED FOR ROUTINE CLINICAL USE

Determination of Organic Acids. Small quantities of organic acids are occasionally present in the gastric content either as a result of ingestion with food or more importantly as a result of putrefaction. Putrefaction is apt to occur only in the stomach with the combination of retained contents and diminished acid secretion. Under these circumstances lactic acid is more commonly present, but acetic or butyric acid may be detected upon occasion. Lactic acid can be determined by several methods which have in common color development with ferric chloride. Lactic acid in increased amounts was formerly considered an important indication of gastric obstruction, particularly due to carcinoma, but this information can now be gained by far more discriminating clinical tests.

Determination of Peptic Activity. Pepsin is the most important digestive enzyme in gastric secretion. Detailed methods of analysis have been described based on the digestion of protein substrates such as egg albumin or hemoglobin and immunoassays (Samloff, 1974). The peptic activity of gastric juice closely parallels the level of acid secretion, and its measurement has not been shown to add significant additional clinical information. Although formerly a common procedure, this analysis is no longer indicated for routine clinical use.

Determination of Rennin. Rennin, which is derived from renninogen in the presence of hydrochloric acid, can be detected by incubation of an aliquot of gastric juice with fresh milk, which results in coagulation of the milk. The level of rennin activity has no special clinical significance. Deficiencies parallel those of pepsin and hydrochloric acid, and routine clinical determinations are therefore not indicated.

Determination of "Free," "Combined," and "Total" Acidity. As previously discussed, these older concepts of gastric acid are no longer tenable. Detailed methodology is given in previous editions of this book, to which the reader is referred for purposes of historical completeness.

Test Meals. A variety of substances have been used in the past to stimulate gastric secretion, including test meals ingested by the patient, ethyl alcohol (50 ml of a 7 per cent [v/v] solution) or caffeine (0.2 g in 200 ml of water) introduced through a gastric tube, or plain water. The most common test meal has been Ewald's test breakfast, which consists of two slices of bread without butter or eight arrowroot cookies and 350 ml of water or unsweetened tea. Among other test meals used on occasion was Riegal's test meal, consisting of 400 ml of bouillon, 200 g of broiled beefsteak, and 150 g of mashed potatoes.

Although test meals are physiologic gastric stimulants, they share with alcohol and caffeine the disadvantage that the stimulus is submaximal. A further disadvantage of the test meals is the fact that the acid output cannot be reliably quantitated because of the buffering effect of the test meal itself. In view of these facts and particularly the need for confirming the diagnosis of anacidity with a maximal stimulation test, the test meals and other submaximal stimulants are now largely considered to be obsolete.

Fractional Gastric Analysis. The fractional gastric analysis was designed to measure the free acid present at varying times after a test meal stimulus. Following an overnight fast the patient is intubated and then given a test meal such as the Ewald test breakfast. After ingestion of the test meal, 10-ml aliquots of gastric contents are removed at 15-minute intervals for a period of two hours. Each aliquot is grossly examined and its free acid determined by titration.

The fractional gastric analysis was originally intended only to be a qualitative test. Some feel that it gives useful information regarding the chymification and emptying functions of the stomach in addition to the acid concentration. The information to be gained, however, is not adequate justification for the continued clinical use of this test.

Tetracycline Fluorescence. It has recently been found that the gastric sediment from patients with carcinoma of the stomach shows strong autofluorescence following prolonged administration of tetracycline or one of its derivatives. The test has resulted in many false positive as well as false negative results and is distinctly inferior to good cytologic techniques.

EXAMINATION OF DUODENAL CONTENTS

The duodenal contents are composed of exocrine pancreatic secretion, bile, and the succus entericus or secretion of the intestine itself mixed with gastric secretion which may contain partially liquefied and digested food particles. Clinical examinations are usually performed in the fasting state, and samples are collected in such a manner that gastric secretion is effectively excluded.

PANCREATIC EXOCRINE SECRETION

Pancreatic exocrine secretion probably exceeds 1500 ml per day in the normal adult and is thus the major contributor to duodenal contents from the standpoint of volume. It is a colorless, clear, non-viscid, highly alkaline solution with a pH of approximately 8.0. The secretion consists of 1 to 2 per cent organic material, mostly enzymes or their precursors including trypsinogen, chymotrypsinogen, amylase, lipase, lecithinase, elastase, collagen-

ase, leucine aminopeptidase, and various esterases. The secretion contains about 1 per cent inorganic material, with sodium the major cation and bicarbonate the major anion. Compared with serum, sodium and potassium are present in about the same concentrations, while calcium and magnesium are present in lower concentrations. The bicarbonate concentration varies directly with the rate of pancreatic secretion from about 25 to 150 mEq/l, while chloride varies inversely with the rate of secretion, so that the sum of these two ions remains approximately constant (Table 23-1, p. 744).

Pancreatic exocrine secretion occurs in response to both vagal and hormonal stimuli. The vagal component is relatively slight and results in a small volume of secretion that is rich in enzymes. Two hormones, secretin and pancreozymin, which are elaborated in the duodenal mucosa, are potent stimuli to pancreatic secretion. They are released into the blood following the entry of peptones, amino acids, or fluid into the duodenum. Acid by itself can apparently stimulate the release of secretin. Secretin results in a copious flow of pancreatic secretion that is low in enzyme content and high in bicarbonate. Pancreozymin, on the other hand, stimulates the pancreas to secrete enzymes and consequently results in degranulation of the acinar cells. Investigations over the past several decades have established useful clinical tests using these two hormones (see Chap. 23, p. 744).

BILE

Approximately 500 to 1000 ml of bile enters the duodenum daily. Bile is yellow to brown or green and usually alkaline, with a pH of 7.0 to 8.5. In addition to the bile salts, chiefly sodium glycocholate and taurocholate, bile contains the bilirubin pigments, cholesterol, phospholipids, and various inorganic salts. The only enzyme present in a significant amount is alkaline phosphatase, which has no function in digestion. Bile flow is enhanced by two substances which have been termed choleretics and cholagogues. Choleretics are substances, such as bile salts and secretin, which increase the secretion of bile by the hepatic cells. Cholagogues, on the other hand, increase bile flow by causing contraction of the gallbladder and relaxation of the sphincter of the common bile duct. Magnesium sulfate and the hormone cholecystokinin are included in this category.

Cholecystokinin is secreted by the duodenum in response to the entry of acid, fats, or partially digested protein, and perhaps also in response to nervous reflex mechanisms. This hormone is of some importance in clinical laboratory tests for the collection of stimulated bile and also for the reason that it is commonly present as an impurity in preparations of pancreozymin.

SUCCUS ENTERICUS

The duodenal secretion, like the pancreatic secretion, contains a variety of digestive enzymes which are capable of breaking down fats, proteins, and carbohydrates. Unlike the pancreatic secretion, however, the enzymatic activity of the succus entericus is considered to be relatively weak. The daily volume of duodenal secretion is not known, but it is mildly alkaline with a pH of about 7.6. Various disease states of the small intestine are not reflected in abnormalities of the succus entericus.

DUODENAL INTUBATION

Duodenal intubation is usually performed in the fasting state by a double-lumen tube, such as the Diamond, Lagerlöf, or Dreiling tube. A simple new device described by Linscheer (1976) eliminates effectively the need for the uncomfortable and prolonged technique associated with use of a Dreiling or Diamond tube. Instruments that have been developed for the purpose of obtaining small bowel biopsies can achieve duodenal intubation in less than 10 minutes. This allows simultaneous collection of gastric and duodenal contents and largely eliminates entrance of gastric secretion into the duodenum. This same result has been achieved with a variety of other techniques, each of which has its advocates, such as the use of two separate tubes or a three-lumen tube, one lumen of which is used to inflate one or more balloons for sealing the duodenum from the stomach. It is essential for the tube to be equipped with a radiopaque tip so that its position may be verified fluoroscopically.

A rapid method of intubation has been described by Raskin (1958): Following an overnight fast, a sedative dose of pentobarbital is administered parenterally. A double-lumen Diamond tube is inserted into the mouth and passed a distance of 45 cm, which brings the tip approximately to the cardia. The patient is then placed in a left lateral decubitus position on a table, the cephalic end of which is elevated 16 inches. The tube is then slowly swallowed for another 15 cm, which results in its being positioned along the greater curvature. The patient then sits on the edge of the examining table with his body bent forward at the waist as far as possible. Several deep inspirations will assist entrance of the tube into the antrum. Peristalsis will move the tube into the duodenum if the patient lies in the right lateral decubitus position with his feet elevated for about 5 minutes. Finally the patient lies on his back for another 5 minutes while the tube is slowly advanced another 10 to 15 cm. The tube is adjusted with fluoroscopic visualization so that its tip is located in the middle of the third portion of the duodenum. Proper location of the tube can be maintained by taping it to the patient's face. This entire procedure can usually be completed in about 15 minutes in contrast to the one or two hours required for many other methods of intubation.

Secretions are collected with continuous suction by a vacuum pump or other suitable apparatus to obtain a pressure of at least 25 mm Hg. During aspiration the patient may lie either on his back or right side. The duodenal aspirate can be collected in suitable containers, such as centrifuge tubes, which can be placed as a trap in the suction line. This will facilitate the frequent changing of containers that is required. The character of the aspirate may be continuously monitored by placing a section of glass tubing in the duodenal tube just before the collection container. The gastric aspirate is discarded.

In addition to the conditions which are contraindications to gastric intubation, duodenal intubation should not be performed as a general rule in patients with acute cholecystitis or acute pancreatitis.

PHYSICAL EXAMINATION OF DUODENAL CONTENTS

In the fasting state the residual content of the duodenum varies up to 20 ml. The fluid may be slightly turbid as a result of mixture with gastric secretion; normal duodenal fluid from which gastric juice is excluded is transparent or slightly translucent, pearly gray, and moderately viscid. Bile staining is usually absent, but its presence is of no significance. Slight blood streaking may result from the intubation procedure. Larger amounts of blood suggest neoplasm involving usually the ampulla of Vater. The presence of food particles is distinctly abnormal and usually indicates either intestinal obstruction or a duodenal diverticulum. Sediment or flocculent debris may be seen in inflammation of the duodenal mucosa, pancreas, or biliary tract.

MICROSCOPIC EXAMINATION
OF DUODENAL CONTENTS

For maximum preservation of cellular elements, the duodenal secretion should be collected in containers chilled in an ice bath and should be examined as soon as possible. Following centrifugation, a drop of sediment may be examined unstained. A few leukocytes or epithelial cells are normal. Increased numbers of polymorphonuclear leukocytes and exfoliated epithelial cells, with or without masses of bacteria, enmeshed in mucus may be found in inflammation of the duodenum, bile ducts, or pancreas. The presence of bile staining may prove of some help in differentiating inflammatory conditions of the biliary tract. Rarely, parasites such as the larvae of *Strongyloides stercoralis*, cysts or trophozoites of *Giardia lamblia* or *Entamoeba histolytica*, or the ova of *Necator*, *Ancylostoma*, or *Ascaris* may be found.

BACTERIOLOGIC EXAMINATION
OF DUODENAL CONTENTS

Normally the duodenal content is nearly sterile, largely as a result of the bactericidal effect of gastric acid. Elaborate mechanisms have been devised for the collection of culture specimens from the duodenum, but these are not indicated for routine clinical use. One of these utilizes a gelatin cap to cover the sterilized duodenal tube, the cap being forced off after the tube is in place. Although seldom indicated, bacterial cultures can be removed from the aspirate of residual duodenal content or following stimulation of pancreatic or biliary secretion.

CHEMICAL EXAMINATION OF
DUODENAL CONTENTS

The most important electrolyte in the duodenal contents is bicarbonate, but its measurement is indicated only in tests of pancreatic function, such as the secretin test. Chloride is infrequently determined and provides no useful information.

The determination of amylase, lipase, or trypsin activity in the pancreatic secretion following secretin or pancreozymin stimulation is an important index of pancreatic exocrine function. Variations in the three enzyme levels usually parallel one another so that only one of the determinations is indicated. Amylase is the most commonly measured and has the advantage of greatest stability. Determination of lipase and trypsin, in addition to amylase, is occasionally helpful in infants with suspected cystic fibrosis or with diarrhea or steatorrhea of unknown etiology. Methods for determining either serum amylase or lipase may be easily adapted to duodenal content following an appropriate initial dilution. The Somogyi method for serum amylase, for example, may be adapted to duodenal content by eliminating the initial protein precipitation and substituting a 1:50 or 1:250 dilution of duodenal fluid for the sample (Dreiling, 1955). Trypsin activity may be determined by testing for digestion of the gelatin coating on x-ray film as is done for fecal trypsin. As in the case of fecal trypsin determination, false positive tests may occur as a result of bacterial gelatinase.

Determination of bilirubin and urobilinogen in duodenal contents yields no information that cannot be deduced from measurements of serum bilirubin, urine bilirubin or urobilinogen, or fecal urobilinogen.

PROVOCATIVE TESTS OF
PANCREATIC SECRETION

The most important of these are the secretin and pancreozymin tests, which are discussed in Chapter 23.

EXAMINATION OF
STIMULATED BILE

Since bile flow into the duodenum is intermittent in the fasting state, it is usually necessary to induce bile flow with a suitable stimulant if examination of bile is indicated. Although secretin is a potent choleretic agent, the increased volume of bile produced by the liver is stored in the gallbladder if the cystic duct is patent. In the presence of normal gallbladder function, secretin may result in a decrease or even disappearance of bile flow into the duodenum. Pancreozymin, on the other hand, will usually result in abundant bile flow as a result of its content of cholecystokinin. Magnesium sulfate, olive oil, and purified cholecystokinin have all been used to stimulate bile flow. Magnesium sulfate functions as an active cholagogue when applied topically to the duodenal mucosa but not when administered orally. Olive oil is probably an even more potent cholagogue but has the disadvantage that the oil interferes with subsequent microscopic examination of the bile. Commercial preparations of cholecystokinin have been used clinically but have no significant advantage over the other more readily available substances.

TECHNIQUE (Lyon, 1919)

1. Duodenal intubation is performed and the position of the tube confirmed fluoroscopically. The test may be performed following the secretin test for pancreatic function.

2. Following aspiration of the residual duodenal content, slowly introduce 50 to 100 ml of a sterile 25 per cent saturated solution of magnesium sulfate through the duodenal tube.

3. After a minute or so, aspirate the magnesium sulfate and duodenal content. The collections are pooled and discarded until yellow bile first appears in quantity; this usually requires about 2 to 10 minutes.

4. Three fractions of bile are subsequently collected in separate containers. The first of these to appear, the "A" bile, is light yellow and watery. After 1 to 3 minutes, it will normally give way abruptly to a viscid deep yellow-brown bile, the "B" bile. Eventually the bile again becomes pale yellow and watery, heralding the appearance of the "C" bile.

5. If no "B" bile appears after 15 to 20 minutes, stimulation with magnesium sulfate and the entire collection may be repeated one or two times.

CLINICAL EVALUATION. "A" bile will usually amount to 5 to 20 ml and originates in the common duct. "B" bile is the result of concentration and probably comes solely from the gallbladder under normal circumstances. Approximately 30 to 75 ml of "B" bile will normally be recovered. It may be absent in advanced cholecystitis, cholelithiasis with obstruction of the cystic duct, or recent cholecystectomy. Absence of "B" bile is not proof of gallbladder disease, and this finding should be confirmed with cholecystography and other examinations. On the other hand, it has been demonstrated that "B" bile can be obtained following cholecystectomy or in cases of congenital absence of the gallbladder. This is probably the result of other portions of the extrahepatic ducts assuming the function of bile concentration. This explanation is supported by the observation that usually a year or more is required for "B" bile to reappear following cholecystectomy. The hepatic ducts and intrahepatic radicles are presumed to be the source of "C" bile.

Inflammation of the biliary tract may be evidenced by the presence of flocculent debris, which will be found to consist of bile-stained epithelial cells, and leukocytes in a mucous network, often with clumps of bacteria. The finding of bile sand, often in deep red-brown bile, is highly suggestive of cholelithiasis or calculus elsewhere in the biliary tract.

The importance of microscopic examination of bile for crystals, particularly the transparent rectangular or rhomboidal crystals of cholesterol or the amorphous yellow to orange masses of calcium bilirubinate, is to be emphasized. Bockus (1931) found that the presence of either or both of these crystals was associated with calculi in approximately 90 per cent of patients. Indeed, examination for bile crystals has real clinical importance (Juniper, 1957) with emphasis given to cholesterol crystals (individual contents) in the absence of jaundice as a means of diagnosing biliary tract disorders.

Culture of stimulated bile is occasionally informative. As a consequence of the circumstances of the collection, interpretation is frequently difficult and depends on quantitative as well as qualitative evaluation of cultures. The coliform organisms (*Escherichia coli* and the *Klebsiella-Aerobacter* group), staphylococci, beta-hemolytic or anaerobic streptococci, enterococci, and various species of *Salmonella* may be found in cases of acute or chronic cholecystitis and cholangitis.

REFERENCES

Baron, J. H.: Studies of basal and peak acid output with an augmented histamine test. Gut, *4*:136, 1963.

Bell, P. R. F., Checketts, R. G., Johnston, D., and Duthie, H. L.: Augmented histamine response after incomplete vagotomy. Lancet, *2*:978, 1965.

Bock, O. A. A.: The concepts of "free acid" and "total acid" of the gastric juice. Lancet, *2*:1101, 1962.

Bockus, H. L., Shay, H., Willard, J. H., and Pessel, J. F.: Comparison of biliary drainage and cholecystography in gallstone diagnosis with especial reference to bile microscopy. J.A.M.A., *96*:311, 1931.

Callender, S. T., Retief, F. P., and Witts, L. J.: The augmented histamine test with special reference to achlorhydria. Gut, *1*:326, 1960.

Card, W. I., Marks, I. N., and Sircus, W.: Observations on achlorhydria. J. Physiol. (London), *130*:18, 1955.

Cohen, N., Horowitz, M. I., and Hollander, F.: Serum albumin and gammaglobulin in normal human gastric juice. Proc. Soc. Exp. Biol. Med., *109*:463, 1962.

Dreiling, D. A.: The technique of the secretin test: Normal ranges. J. Mount Sinai Hosp., *21*:363, 1955.

Ellison, E. H., and Wilson, S. D.: The Zollinger-Ellison

syndrome: Re-appraisal and evaluation of 260 registered cases. Ann. Surg., *160*:512, 1964.

Findlay, J. M., Prescott, R. J., and Circus, W.: Comparative evaluation of water recovery test and fluoroscopic screening in positioning a nasogastric tube during gastric secretory studies. Br. Med. J., *4*:458, 1972.

Forster, G. M.: An unusual false-positive response to the azuresin test. J.A.M.A., *176*:619, 1961.

Glass, G. B. J.: Paper electrophoresis of gastric juice in health and disease. Am. J. Dig. Dis., *6*:1131, 1961.

Hollander, F.: Laboratory procedures in the study of vagotomy (with particular reference to the insulin test). Gastroenterology, *11*:419, 1948.

Hollander, F.: Gastric secretion of electrolytes. Fed. Proc., *11*:706, 1952.

Hunt, J. N.: Gastric emptying and secretion in man. Physiol. Rev., *39*:491, 1959.

Johnston, D. H., and McCraw, B. H.: Gastric analysis—evaluation of collection techniques. Gastroenterology, *35*:512, 1958.

Juniper, K., and Burson, E. N.: Biliary tract studies. II. The significance of biliary crystals. Gastroenterology, *32*:175, 1957.

Kay, A. W.: Effect of large doses of histamine on gastric secretion of HCl, an augmented histamine test. Br. Med. J., *2*:77, 1953.

Khodadoost, J., Leitao, O., and Glass, G. B. J.: Comparison of pentagastrin and augmented histamine stimulation as tests of gastric acid secretion. Am. J. Gastroenterol., *57*:311, 1972.

Levin, E., Kirsner, J. B., and Palmer, W. L.: A simple measure of gastric secretion in man: Comparison of one hour basal secretion, histamine-secretion and twelve hour nocturnal gastric secretion. Gastroenterology, *19*:88, 1951.

Levin, E., Kirsner, J. B., Palmer, W. L., and Butler, C.: The variability and periodicity of the nocturnal gastric secretion in normal individuals. Gastroenterology, *10*:939, 1948.

Levine, R.: Personal communication, Dec. 21, 1977.

Linscheer, W. G., and Abele, J. E.: A new directable small bowel biopsy device. Gastroenterology, *71*:575, 1976.

Lyon, B. B. V.: Diagnosis and treatment of diseases of the gallbladder and biliary ducts, preliminary report on a new method. J.A.M.A., *73*:980, 1919.

Marks, I. N.: The augmented histamine test. Gastroenterology, *41*:599, 1961.

Marks, I. N., Bank, S., Louw, J. H., and van Embden, B. H.: The augmented histamine test, an analysis of 672 consecutive tests. S. Afr. Med. J., *36*:807, 1962.

Marks, I. N., Bank, S., Moshal, M. G., and Louw, J. H.: The augmented histamine test, a review of 615 cases of gastroduodenal disease. S. Afr. J. Surg., *1*:53, 1963.

Marks, I. N., and Shay, H.: Augmented histamine test, Ewald test meal, and Diagnex test, comparison of results. Am. J. Dig. Dis., *5*:1, 1960.

Moore, E. W., and Scarlata, R. W.: The determination of gastric acidity by the glass electrode. Gastroenterology, *49*:178, 1965.

Piper, D. W., Macoun, M. L., Broderick, F. L., Fenton, B. H., and Builder, J. E.: The diagnosis of gastric carcinoma by the estimation of enzyme activity in gastric juice. Gastroenterology, *45*:614, 1963.

Raskin, H. F., Wenger, J., Sklar, M., Pleticka, S., and Yarema, W.: The diagnosis of cancer of the pancreas, biliary tract, and duodenum by combined cytologic and secretory methods. 1. Exfoliative cytology and a description of a rapid method of duodenal intubation. Gastroenterology, *34*:996, 1958.

Read, R. C., and Hall, W. H.: Objective assessment of gastric function after vagotomy. Curr. Probl. Surg. 1, July, 1974.

Samloff, I. M., and Liebman, W. M.: Radioimmunoassay of Group I pepsinogens in serum. Gastroenterology, *66*:494, 1974.

Segal, H. L.: Clinical measurement of gastric secretion: Significance and limitations. Ann. Intern. Med., *53*:445, 1960.

Segal, H. L., Rumbold, J. C., Friedman, B. L., and Finigan, M. M.: Detection of achlorhydria by tubeless gastric analysis with betazole hydrochloride as the gastric stimulant. N. Engl. J. Med., *261*:544, 1959.

Sparberg, M., and Kirsner, J. B.: Gastric secretory activity with reference to HCl, clinical interpretations. Arch. Intern. Med. (Chicago), *114*:508, 1964.

Stempien, S. J.: Insulin gastric analysis: Technic and interpretations. Am. J. Dig. Dis., *7*:138, 1962.

Trudeau, W. L., and McGuigan, J. E.: Relations between serum gastrin levels and rates of gastric hydrochloric acid secretion. N. Engl. J. Med., *284*:408, 1971.

Yalow, R. S., and Berson, S. A.: Radioimmunoassay of gastrin. Gastroenterology, *58*:1, 1970.

Zaterka, S., and Neves, D. P.: Maximal gastric secretion in human subjects after Histalog stimulation. Comparison with augmented histamine test. Gastroenterology, *47*:251, 1964.

MALABSORPTION, DIARRHEA, AND EXAMINATION OF FECES

Myrton F. Beeler, M.D.,
Yuan S. Kao, M.D.,
and W. Douglas Scheer, Ph.D.

THE PHYSIOLOGY OF DIGESTION AND ABSORPTION

Mechanisms of transport of nutrients across the intestinal mucosa include (1) active transport, (2) passive diffusion, (3) facilitated diffusion, and (4) pinocytosis. A brief review of digestion and absorption of major categories of foodstuffs follows:

Amino Acids. Dietary proteins are initially degraded in the stomach by pepsin. The resulting peptides are further degraded by the action of pancreatic enzymes—trypsin, chymotrypsin, aminopeptidase, and carboxypeptidase—to dipeptides and tripeptides plus a small amount of amino acids. Dipeptides and tripeptides are further hydrolyzed by dipeptidase at the brush border of the intestinal epithelium. Only L-amino acids are actively transported.

Carbohydrates. Starch and glycogen are hydrolyzed by salivary and pancreatic amylases to disaccharides. These are split by disaccharidases located on the brush border or within microvilli of the intestinal epithelial cells. Thus, lactose is split into glucose and galactose, sucrose into glucose and fructose, and maltose into two molecules of glucose. The monosaccharides, such as glucose and galactose, are absorbed by active transport.

Fat. Ingested fat is digested mainly in the small intestine. The time interval for gastric emptying is longer following a fatty meal than following a meal containing less fat.

Dietary fat is digested and absorbed in the following sequence: (1) hydrolysis of triglycerides by pancreatic lipase to free fatty acids and 2-monoglycerides, (2) formation of micelles by aggregation of fatty acids and 2-monoglycerides with bile salts, (3) passage of the micelles into jejunal mucosal cells where esterification and chylomicron formation occur, and finally, (4) transport of chylomicrons from the mucosal cells into the intestinal lymphatics.

Water and Electrolytes. The small intestine absorbs water at an average minimal rate of 200 to 400 ml/hour. Water is absorbed throughout the small intestine, but the main site of absorption following a meal is in the upper part of the small intestine. Water and electrolytes can freely penetrate the membrane through aqueous channels, especially in the jejunum, where the effective pore radius is relatively large. In the ileum and colon the pore size is believed to be smaller; therefore sodium cannot pass freely but rather is absorbed actively. Potassium appears to be passively absorbed in the upper part of the small intestine, but it is secreted in the terminal ileum and colon.

INTESTINAL HORMONES

Secretin is produced in the duodenal mucosa by S-cells—one of the types of cells (along with those producing gastrin and cholecystokinin) which may give rise to apudomas, so called because of their amine precursor uptake and decarboxylation activities. Cholecystokinin-pancreozymin is produced in duodenal and jejunal mucosa. These are discussed in Chapter 23. Intestinal mucosal cells also produce enteroglucagon and VIP (a vasodilator and smooth muscle relaxant which inhibits acid secretion and stimulates pancreatic secretion and flow of bile).

COLONIC PHYSIOLOGY

Water and electrolytes, as mentioned, are absorbed from the colon, whose other function is to serve as a reservoir, allowing storage and evacuation of feces as orderly processes. Up to 1500 ml of water is delivered to the colon daily, depending on the tone of the ileocecal sphincter. Gastrin releases the sphincter as it stimulates propulsive motility of the ileum. The colon itself undergoes slow segmented contractions which impede the flow of contents, followed eventually by mass movements which propel the feces forward into the sigmoid colon. Resulting distention of the rectal walls initiates the defecation reflex, during which there are contraction of the abdominal muscles and relaxation of the anal sphincter.

The average healthy adult defecates at frequencies varying from three times a day to three times a week. The common pattern is once a day. The stool tends to be small and dry on a diet high in meat, soft and bulky on a diet high in vegetables and fiber. Two thirds of the weight of the average stool is attributable to bacteria, indigestible material such as cellulose, undigested or unabsorbed food, gastrointestinal secretions, and desquamated cells. The normal brown color is of still undetermined origin. The odor results largely from indole and skatole, produced by bacteria from tryptophan.

THE MALABSORPTION SYNDROMES

CLASSIFICATION

The malabsorption syndromes result from impaired digestion or assimilation of foodstuffs by the small bowel.

Maldigestion usually results from pancreatic disease (see Chap. 23), such as chronic pancreatitis, carcinoma of the pancreas, or fibrocystic disease of the pancreas, and subsequent lack of pancreatic digestive enzymes. Generally there are associated creatorrhea, evidenced by presence of undigested meat fibers in the feces, and steatorrhea, an increase in fat—largely triglycerides.

Hepatogenous maldigestion results from interference with bile flow. Loss of bile salts interferes with fat emulsification, diminishing the surface area available for lipolytic action. In addition, there is loss of bile salt activation of lipase activity. The diseases with which this syndrome is associated are discussed in Chapter 12. Patients are usually jaundiced, pass dark urine, and have other signs of liver disease. Hepatogenous steatorrhea may coexist with pancreatic steatorrhea, as when there is a neoplasm obstructing the ampulla of Vater.

Enterogenous malabsorption comprises a variety of conditions which have in common normal digestion but inadequate net assimilation of foodstuffs. This may result from competition by bacteria or altered bacterial flora, as in the blind loop syndrome or diverticulosis of the small bowel; from obstruction to the flow of lymph, as in Whipple's disease and lymphoma; from diseases affecting the small bowel mucosa, as in amyloidosis, inflammation following radiation, and other types of small bowel inflammation; from diminished mucosal surface area, as in gastroileostomy or small bowel resection; or from alterations in small bowel mucosal function, as in atrophy secondary to gliadin (a fraction of gluten) sensitivity in celiac disease or secondary to relative vitamin B_6 or B_{12} deficiency. Malassimilation may also occur in patients with vasculitis, diabetes mellitus, the carcinoid syndrome, hypoparathyroidism, hypothyroidism, and hypogammaglobulinemia. In some of these situations it may result from rapid transit of small bowel contents—as diarrheal syndromes may be associated with malabsorption.

The conditions listed above all cause general malabsorption, of which steatorrhea is a major sign. Steatorrhea may be defined as the presence of more than 5 g of lipid (measured as fatty acids) in feces per 24 hours. Normal individuals on a normal fat intake excrete up to 5 g of lipid daily (Frazer, 1955). While the source of fecal lipid is largely dietary, gastrointestinal excretions, cellular desquamation, and bacterial metabolism also contribute (Frazer, 1956). Lipids are normally present as soaps and triglycerides. In addition, lipoids are present, including higher alcohols, paraffins, and vegetable carotenoids. Although diet has some effect on it, the pattern of lipids excreted may be very different from that of the diet, and the quantity of fat ingested by the normal individual has a relatively small effect on the total output of fat. According to one study, the fecal lipid is equal to a constant (2.93 g) plus 2.1 per cent of the dietary fat intake. On a fat-free diet, the output of fat normally varies from 1 to 4 g/day (Wollaeger, 1947). In severe cases of steatorrhea, stools are generally fluid, semifluid, or soft and pasty, bulky, pale, and foul smelling. They may be foamy and may tend to float on water. Floating stools contain gas, which may also appear in stools from healthy people, so the sign is not specific.

Patients with malabsorption are liable to development of deficiencies of fat-soluble vitamins (A, D, E, and K). Primary and secondary alterations of bowel mucosa may also result in deficiency of water-soluble vitamins. In addition, these patients are liable to weight loss because of large caloric loss, and are likely to have other evidence of nutritional deficiencies, such as hypoprothrombinemia, glossitis, anemia, edema, ascites, and osteomalacia.

Malabsorption may also involve a single foodstuff or vitamin or only a small group of substances. For example, pernicious anemia results from failure to absorb vitamin B_{12} because of deficiency of intrinsic factor. Then, too, different foodstuffs are absorbed primarily in different locations, so that a lesion of regional enteritis localized to the distal ileum may affect only Vitamin B_{12} and bile salt absorption. Lactose intolerance caused by lactase deficiency is an example of a specific malabsorption syndrome.

SCREENING TESTS

Screening tests are available for detection of steatorrhea, such as determination of serum carotene, which tends, along with fat-soluble vitamin A, to be lower than normal; or microscopic examination of the stool for fat globules. Definitive diagnosis depends upon quantitative demonstration of increased fecal lipid (Frazer, 1955).

DIFFERENTIATING CAUSES

When the diagnosis of malabsorption has been established, differential diagnosis becomes important for determining treatment. The usual problem is differentiation of pancreatogenous from enterogenous malabsorption. In children the definitive test for mucoviscidosis, their main cause of pancreatic malabsorption, is the sweat electrolyte determination described in Chapter 23. This test should be used whenever clinical evidence warrants it, although screening tests based on absent stool trypsin and on semiquantitative demonstrations of increased sweat chloride have been applied. One of the most valuable of the differential diagnostic tests, for adults especially, has been the D-xylose absorption test (Santiago-Borrero, 1971). In this procedure, a 25 g dose of the pentose sugar in water is administered orally, and the amount excreted in the urine over a five-hour period is determined. If the amount excreted is less than 3 g, the diagnosis is most likely enterogenous malabsorption, as pancreatic enzymes are not required for absorption of D-xylose. Poor kidney function may also result in low excretion, and for this reason, the test is difficult to interpret in patients with renal disease. If the test is performed under these circumstances, blood levels should also be assayed. High blood values coupled with low urine values are expected in renal disease. Because reference values in this situation are not available, the test is better avoided in patients with renal disease.

There is no fully satisfactory alternative to the D-xylose test, although isotopic techniques and starch tolerance tests have been used by some workers for this purpose. In the latter, absorption of starch is followed by serial blood glucose determinations. The rise in blood glucose is compared with that following a glucose tolerance test. Theoretically, if a patient lacks pancreatic amylase, the glucose tolerance test will yield higher values than the starch tolerance test. Quantitative, specific stool trypsin and chymotrypsin assays may be helpful (Haverback, 1963), as may the Schilling test for vitamin B_{12} absorption, which tends to be abnormal in patients with enterogenous steatorrhea and is not correctable with intrinsic factor. Probably the best alternative laboratory diagnostic aid, although unpleasant for the patient, is duodenal intubation as described in Chapter 23.

DEFINITIVE TEST FOR STEATORRHEA

The definitive test for steatorrhea is the fecal fat determination. The amount of fat in feces may be determined and expressed as per cent by weight of wet stool, per cent by weight of dry stool, or per cent of ingested fat retained (absorbed), or as chemically determined amount of fat per 24-hour stool collection. Because of wide variation in water content of the stool, wet weight concentration is the least informative. Dry weight concentration is only slightly less variable because of the effect of diet on bulk. Total output of fat per 24 hours, based on chemical analysis of at least a three-day stool collection, is the most reliable measurement. For this purpose, the patient is placed on a standard diet containing 100 g of fat per day. In infants and children, for whom the standard 100 g diet cannot be used, "per cent coefficient of fat retention" is the more useful expression. This is the difference between fecal fat and ingested fat expressed as a percentage of the ingested fat $\left(\dfrac{\text{dietary fat} - \text{fecal fat}}{\text{dietary fat}} \times 100\% \right)$. The coefficient of fat retention of normal children and adults is 95 per cent or higher, although in

premature infants it may be much lower than this. A low value, otherwise, is indicative of steatorrhea.

DIARRHEA

GENERAL CONSIDERATIONS

The large intestine receives about 500 to 1500 ml of fluid from the ileum daily, but only about 150 ml is normally lost in the stool each day. The large intestine normally absorbs water, chloride, and sodium, but excretes bicarbonate and potassium. Under normal conditions the large intestine of an adult can absorb about double the amount of fluid coming from the ileum daily. If the amount of fluid either entering or secreted into the large intestine exceeds the capacity for absorption, diarrhea will result.

Table 25-1 is an outline of the stool patterns and types of pathophysiology associated with common clinical conditions causing diarrhea (Haubrich, 1976).

STOOL EXAMINATION

When working up a patient for the differential diagnosis of diarrhea, a history is most important. Additionally, establishing presence or absence of fecal polymorphonuclear or mononuclear leukocytes is very useful. Fecal leukocytes are usually present in bacterial infection of the intestines by such organisms as *Salmonella, Shigella, Yersinia,* and invasive *Escherichia coli,* as well as in non-bacterial inflammatory processes, such as ulcerative colitis, and occasionally in antibiotic-associated colitis. Fecal leukocytes are usually not present in the stools of diarrhea secondary to viruses, toxigenic bacteria (*Staphylococcus, E. coli, Clostridium perfringens, Vibrio cholera*) and parasites (*Giardia, Entamoeba*). A modified version of an algorithm for the differential laboratory diagnosis of diarrhea is shown in Figure 25-1.

INTESTINAL DISACCHARIDASE DEFICIENCY

Many of the previously listed conditions causing malabsorption may also be associated with intolerance to disaccharides; disaccharide absorption is diminished because of deficient disaccharidase activity in the small intestinal

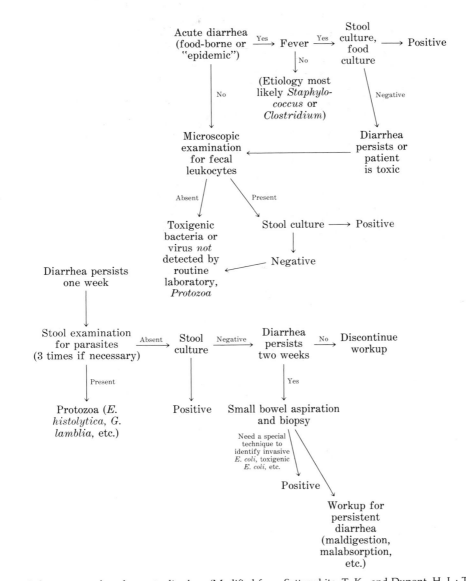

Figure 25–1.   Laboratory workup for acute diarrhea. (Modified from Satterwhite, T. K., and Dupont, H. L.: The patient with acute diarrhea: An algorithm for diagnosis. J.A.M.A., *236*:2663, 1976. Copyright 1976, American Medical Association.)

Table 25–1. CLASSIFICATION AND CAUSES OF DIARRHEA*

STOOL PATTERN	PATHOPHYSIOLOGY	COMMON CLINICAL CONDITIONS
Watery diarrhea	Secretory diarrhea	1. Specific enteric infection (*Salmonella, Shigella, Staphylococcus,* pathogenic *Escherichia coli,* cholera, clostridia, and *Protozoa*) 2. Non-specific enteric mucosal injury (idiopathic ulcerative colitis, regional enteritis, irradiation enteritis, drug injury (methotrexate, lincomycin, clindamycin, digitalis, alcohol, and reserpine) 3. Neoplasms (villous adenoma, abdominal lymphoma, carcinoid, pancreatic islet cell tumors, medullary carcinoma of the thyroid) 4. Hyperthyroidism 5. Post-vagotomy state
	Osmotic diarrhea	1. Post-surgical (pyloroplasty, gastroenterostomy, resection of jejunum and proximal ileum) 2. Primary disease of the intestine (celiac disease, tropical sprue, dermatitis herpetiformis, Whipple's disease, lymphoma, ulcerative colitis) 3. Infestation by parasites (giardiasis, strongyloidiasis) 4. Drug-induced osmotic cathartics (sorbital, lactulose, antacids, phenformin, tetracycline, lincomycin) 5. Mucosal digestive defects (specific disaccharidase deficiencies) 6. Mucosal transport defect (glucose-galactose malabsorption) 7. Immunoglobulin deficiencies (congenital or acquired) 8. Chloridorrhea
	Altered intestinal transit, hypermotility	1. Secretory and osmotic diarrhea 2. Carcinoid syndrome 3. Post-vagotomy state 4. Functional gastrointestinal disorders 5. Hypocalcemia 6. Hyperthyroidism 7. Hypoadrenalism 8. Hypopituitarism 9. Pancreatic cholera syndrome 10. Gastrin-secreting tumors
Steatorrhea	Maldigestion	1. Pancreatic exocrine insufficiency (chronic pancreatitis, cystic fibrosis) 2. Altered bile salt circulation (steatorrhea of newborn, disorders of liver, blind-loop syndrome, resection of ileum)
	Malabsorption	1. Primary intestinal malabsorption (celiac disease, tropical sprue, Whipple's disease, abetalipoproteinemia, blind-loop syndrome)
Small stool diarrhea	Rectocolic irritability	1. Functional bowel disorder, inflammatory disease of the colon and rectum (ulcerative proctocolitis, Crohn's disease, diverticulitis, irradiation proctocolitis, anorectal tumor)

*Modified from Haubrich, W. S.: Diarrhea and Constipation. *In* Bockus, H. L. (ed.): Gastroenterology, Vol. 2. Philadelphia, W. B. Saunders Company, 1976, pp. 921-922.

mucosa. These acquired (secondary) lactase deficiencies are usually transient. Permanent intolerance results from primary disaccharidase deficiency, possibly resulting from a genetically determined enzyme defect or from environmental factors, or both (Cook, 1966; Keusch, 1969). Lactose intolerance is by far the most common of these disorders. Unhydrolyzed disaccharides are fermented by intestinal bacteria, producing gas and lactic acid. The osmotic effect of the lactose and its metabolites and the irritation of the bowel by the lactic acid produced often result in diarrhea as well as complaints of bloating and flatulence. Primary sucrase and maltase intolerance, although rarely seen, have been reported (Anderson, 1963).

The stools are usually acid (pH 5.5 or below). The lactic acid content of the stools (in the case of lactase deficiency) is usually greater than 100 mg/24 hr. The most consistent test result is sugar content higher than 240 mg/100 ml of stool (lactose, glucose, and galactose) (Anderson, 1966). Stool can be analyzed for sugars by chromatography or by one of the semi-quantitative, non-specific tests for urinary sugars adapted for stool analysis. The Clinitest tablet (Ames Company, Elkhart, In-

Table 25–2. RISE IN BLOOD GLUCOSE OVER FASTING LEVEL

CARBOHYDRATE INGESTION	BLOOD GLUCOSE INCREASE (mg/dl)		
	Normal	Lactose Intolerance	Idiopathic Sprue
Lactose, 50 g	14–60 (35)*	2–11 (6)	0–19 (9)
Glucose, 25 g Galactose, 25 g	25–66 (49)	20–71 (40)	24–34 (28)
Maltose, 50 g	(28–80) (52)	57–92 (74.5)	19 (one case)

*Figures in parentheses are average values. (From Basford, R. L., and Henry, J. B.: Postgrad. Med., *41:*A70, 1967.)

Table 25–3. CLASSIFICATION OF TYPES OF SUGAR INTOLERANCE*

TYPES OF SUGAR	INTOLERANCE	
	Disaccharide	Monosaccharide
Primary	Sucrase-isomaltase deficiency	Glucose-galactose intolerance (fructose absorbed)
	Lactase deficiency a. congenital alactasia b. late onset hypolactasia (isolated lactase deficiency)	
Secondary	Mucosal damage Lactase deficiency	Monosaccharide intolerance (all sugars)
	Deficiency of all disaccharidases	

*Modified from Anderson, C. M., and Burke, V.: Disorders of Carbohydrate Digestion and Absorption. *In* Anderson, C. M., and Burke, V.: Pediatric Gastroenterology. Oxford, Blackwell Scientific Publications, Ltd., 1975.

diana) is suitable for the purpose (Kerry, 1964). Abnormally high results with this test are common, however, in normal infants between the ages of 3 and 7 days (Davison, 1970).

Definitive diagnosis depends on demonstrating low lactase activity in small bowel biopsy material; normal intestinal sucrase and maltase activity; intolerance to orally administered lactose; and a flat lactose tolerance test curve (Newcomer, 1967; Basford, 1967).

Krasilnikoff (1975) found the lactose tolerance test to have an incidence of 23 to 30 per cent false positives following oral administration of lactose, i.e., flat tolerance curve, <20 mg/dl (1.1 mmol/l) increase in blood sugar. Delayed gastric emptying appears to be the cause, since duodenal instillation of lactose eliminates the flat tolerance curve. The use of capillary blood glucose values can eliminate the flat tolerance curve in normal individuals, but lactase-deficient patients have shown normal tolerance curves with capillary blood glucose values.

GLUCOSE-GALACTOSE MALABSORPTION

Primary glucose-galactose malabsorption is a rare hereditary disorder of active absorption of glucose and galactose from the small intestine. Recent studies suggest an autosomal recessive mode of inheritance (Melin, 1969). Symptoms and signs are similar to those seen in patients with disaccharide malabsorption, diarrhea being the main problem. Stools are watery and always contain several grams per 100 ml of glucose and galactose. Fructose absorption is normal in this disorder (Linquist, 1963).

Laboratory Tests. Diagnostic laboratory tests for this disorder include identification of glucose and galactose in the stools, using glucose oxidase, galactose oxidase, or chromatography, and oral glucose tolerance tests and oral galactose tolerance tests, in which a flat curve is expected. Fructose tolerance tests should also be performed, results of which should be normal. A flat glucose tolerance curve alone does not, of course, indicate the presence of this disorder. Many variables affect blood glucose levels. Flat glucose tolerance curves are normal in newborn babies. Furthermore, blood glucose levels are affected by oral fructose loading (Meeuwisse, 1969; 1970). If oral sugar tolerance tests yield equivocal results, intubation and perfusion of a segment of the small intestine may be indicated to establish the diagnosis (Kaijser, 1970).

FECAL BLOOD

Bleeding into the gastrointestinal tract may be acute or chronic, massive or slight, obvious or occult, and may originate anywhere from the gingiva or nasal cavity to the rectum. It should never be ignored, although often it results from minor pathology, such as hemorrhoids and anal fissures. Of one group of patients with significant gastrointestinal bleeding, 18 per cent were found to have malignant tumors and 30 per cent benign peptic ulcer. Slightly over 50 per cent had their bleeding source in the esophagus, stomach, or duodenum; 45 per cent in the colon and rectum (Thompson, 1949). Bleeding from the jejunum and ileum was seen in very few of the patients.

Drugs, particularly salicylates, steroids, rauwolfia derivatives, indomethacin, and colchicine, have been shown to be associated with increased gastrointestinal blood loss in normal subjects and even more pronounced increase in blood loss in patients with gastrointestinal tract pathology (Bockus, 1964). This effect may follow even parenteral administration of the drugs (Grossman, 1961). Apparent fecal peroxidase activity has also been shown to increase with use of carmine as a stool marker (Kirschen, 1942) and occasionally with massive iron therapy. The latter, however, may result from actual bleeding secondary to gastrointestinal irritation produced by some iron compounds (Brayshaw, 1963).

Loss of more than 50 to 75 ml of blood from the upper gastrointestinal tract generally imparts a dark red to black color and a tarry consistency to the stool (Daniel, 1939). Persistence of a tarry appearance for two or three days suggests loss of at least 1000 ml of blood. Following this amount of bleeding, occult blood may persist for 5 to 12 days (Schiff, 1942). Somewhat smaller quantities entering the lower gastrointestinal tract may produce similar appearing stools, or may appear as bright red blood. Such stools should be considered grossly bloody only after verification with chemical tests to avoid confusion with coloring from dietary substances or medications. Smaller increases in blood content may not alter appearance of the stool. Such stools are said to contain "occult blood," detection of which can be most useful in uncovering or localizing disease. This is especially important because over half of all cancers (excluding skin) are those of the gastrointestinal tract, and early diagnosis and treatment of patients with colonic cancer results in a relatively good prognosis for survival (Greegor, 1971).

According to Winawer (1977), 139 cancers were detected with the Hemoccult test (Smith-Kline Diagnostics, Sunnyvale, Cal.), of which only 20 were within reach of the standard sigmoidoscope. Only one patient had a false negative result. Of 47 "silent" cases, 85 per cent were localized to the bowel wall. The authors noted that only one or two specimens examined out of six are usually positive.

COLLECTION OF FECES

Uninstructed patients sometimes exhibit considerable ingenuity in collecting stool specimens, but a few simple instructions are likely to produce more satisfactory specimens. A scoured, well-rinsed bedpan is a convenient collection container. If the patient does not own one, a carefully cleaned, rinsed, and boiled glass jar of suitable size is a satisfactory alternative. Patients should be warned against passing urine at the same time into the bedpan or container because, among other things, urine has a harmful effect on protozoa. Tongue depressors or pieces of cardboard are reasonably convenient instruments for transferring the stool from bedpan to transport vessel, for which plastic, cardboard, and glass containers are available. We prefer two-ounce ointment jars with screw caps for small stool samples because they are odor free, leak proof, and easy to transport. Patients should be instructed not to contaminate the outside of the container and not to overfill the container. Gas, which frequently accumulates, should be released gradually by careful loosening of the cap. Failure to observe this simple precaution, especially in the case of an overfilled container, can result in an explosive release of contents.

Fecal matter left on the physician's gloved finger at the time of a rectal examination may be transferred to a piece of filter paper for inspection and testing for occult blood.

Because of wide variation in bowel habits, intestinal transit time, and bulk of stool, special consideration must be given to methods of timed stool collection. For collection of timed urine specimens, the urinary bladder can be emptied before and at the end of the collection period; the gastrointestinal tract, however, cannot be emptied completely at will. Therefore, the amount of stool collected in a 24-hour period usually correlates very poorly with the amount of food ingested over a similar period of time. For determining the 24-hour fecal excretion of any substance, stools should be collected over a period of at least three days, and calculations should be based on the entire specimen divided by the number of days of collection. The accuracy of this method can be enhanced somewhat by having the patient ingest carmine dye (0.3 g) at the beginning and charcoal (1 g) at the end of a collecting period, collecting the stools from the beginning of the appearance of the dye to the beginning of the appearance of the charcoal. However, *Salmonella cubana* outbreaks in Massachusetts and California were traced to carmine dye (Lang, 1967). Another method of signaling the collection period involves use of inert, non-absorbable stool markers. These are taken in divided, uniform doses for several days prior to the beginning of the collection, continuing through the collection period. The concentration of the material found in the stool specimen is then used to determine the quantity of stool containing one day's ingestion of the material as an indication of the 24-hour output. For this purpose, chromium sesquioxide (Cr_2O_3) has been used and its concentration in the feces determined chemically (Rose, 1964). The substitution of radioactive chromium isotopes has made it possible to determine concentration by measurement of radioactivity of the stool (Spencer, 1969). Zirconium-95 oxide has been used in a similar manner (Weber, 1969). The latter methods as currently used are too time-consuming for routine determinations, but they may lead to future modifications, permitting analysis of random specimens instead of the three-day collections now generally required.

Hoffman (1973) has described a sample collection method which has the advantages of ease of transportation and storage, not requiring special equipment and being acceptable to patients and laboratory staff. They use a plastic bag cut halfway down each side seam, with double-sided adhesive tape attached on both sides to the upper outer lip. The bag is opened and placed in a toilet, its top sides attached by the adhesive tape, laterally, to an ordinary toilet seat. After collection it can be closed with a twist tie and placed in a bag with an air-tight closure, which, in turn, can be placed in a paint can. There are problems with this method of collection at home. For example, cultural conditions in rural and ghetto circumstances may make it very difficult for people to collect such samples; and one can not always be sure that the sample brought in actually corresponds to a particular member of the family.

A pediatric method described by Jelliffe (1974) includes using a thick-walled glass tube ($\frac{1}{4}$ inch I.D.), lubricated by dipping into water and then inserted into the young child's rectum. In about two thirds of the cases, a core of feces can be obtained, which can be poked out with an applicator into a container. During the procedure, the child can be held on the mother's lap, with the buttocks separated by the operator's left hand, while the tube is inserted with the right hand.

METHODS AND METHODOLOGY

INSPECTION OF FECES

Inspection of the feces is important, for it may lead to a diagnosis of parasitic infestation, obstructive jaundice, diarrhea, malabsorption, rectosigmoidal obstruction, dysentery, ulcerative colitis, or gastrointestinal tract bleeding.

The quantity, form, consistency, and color of the stool should be noted. Normally, 100 to 200 g of stool is passed per day. When there is diarrhea, the stool is watery. Passage of large amounts of mushy, foul-smelling, gray stool which floats on the water is characteristic of steatorrhea. Constipation may be associated with passage of small, firm, spherical masses of stool (scybala). Constipation most often results from the irritable colon syndrome of patients with anxiety or from overuse of laxatives. In such patients, repeated tests for occult (hidden) blood are called for to detect more serious organic problems such as carcinoma, which may also, of course, afflict those patients.

A narrow, ribbon-like stool suggests the possibility of spastic bowel or rectal narrowing or stricture. Clay color suggests diminution or absence of bile or presence of barium sulfate. Blood, especially when originating from the lower gut, may cause the stool to be red; beets in the diet may mimic this. Bleeding from the upper gastrointestinal tract is more likely to cause the stool to be black and of a tarry consistency. Bismuth, iron, and charcoal may also color the stool black. Standing in the air for a time may cause the stool to darken on the surface. Green stools may result from ingestion of spinach and other green vegetables or calomel, or may result from the presence of biliverdin, seen in patients taking antibiotics orally. It is not unusual to see seeds and vegetable skins. Parasites are considered in Chapter 51.

Mucus

Presence of recognizable mucus in a stool specimen is abnormal and should be reported. Translucent gelatinous mucus clinging to the surface of the formed stool suggests spastic constipation or mucous colitis. It is seen in stools of emotionally disturbed patients and may result from excessive straining. Bloody mucus clinging to the fecal mass suggests neoplasm or inflammatory processes of the rectal canal. Mucus associated with pus and blood is found in stools of patients with ulcerative colitis, bacillary dysentery, ulcerating diverticulitis, and intestinal tuberculosis. Patients with villous adenoma of the colon may pass copious quantities of mucus, aggregating up to 3 or 4 liters in 24 hours. They frequently develop severe dehydration and electrolyte disturbances, especially hypokalemia (Wells, 1962).

Pus

Patients with chronic ulcerative colitis and chronic bacillary dysentery frequently pass large quantities of pus with the stool, for the recognition of which microscopic examination is required. This also occurs in patients with localized abscesses or fistulas communicating with the sigmoid colon, rectum, or anus. Large amounts of pus seldom accompany the stools of patients with amoebic colitis. Therefore, its presence is evidence against this diagnosis. No inflammatory exudate is seen in the watery stools of patients with viral gastroenteritis.

MICROSCOPIC EXAMINATION OF FECES
(Pihl, 1953; Drummey, 1961)

Fat

The crudest technique is microscopic examination using Sudan III, Sudan IV, or oil red O stains. The procedure has been widely employed for screening because of its simplicity. In our experience, results have correlated well with quantitative measurements when aliquots of the same homogenized stool have been analyzed. For this purpose, a small aliquot of stool suspension is placed on a slide and mixed with 2 drops of 95 per cent ethanol, followed by addition of 2 drops of saturated ethanolic solution of Sudan III, with mixing. It is then coverslipped. Under these conditions fatty acids are present as lightly staining flakes or as needle-like crystals which do not stain and which, therefore, may be missed. Soaps also do not stain, but

appear as well-defined amorphous flakes or as rounded masses or coarse crystals. Neutral fats, however, appear as large orange or red droplets. When 60 or more stained droplets of neutral fats per high-power field are seen, one may be reasonably certain that the patient has steatorrhea. (Caution is advisable in interpretation, as mineral oil or castor oil may mimic neutral fat.) The procedure is then repeated, adding several drops of 36 per cent (v/v) acetic acid to the stool mixture and warming the slide several times over a flame until slight boiling occurs. This converts neutral fats and soaps to fatty acids and melts the fatty acids, causing them to form droplets which stain strongly with Sudan III. The slide is then examined while warm. After this procedure, presence of up to 100 stained droplets per high-power field is considered normal. Patients with pancreatogenous steatorrhea are likely to show greater increases in fatty acids and soaps. Use of oil red O has been advocated by some because it permits substitution of isopropanol for ethanol.

Meat fibers (Moore, 1971)

The technique for sampling is identical to that for Sudan preparations for fecal fat. The stool is mixed thoroughly on a slide with a 10 per cent alcohol solution of eosin, allowed to stain for 3 minutes, and examined for muscle fibers. The entire area under the coverslip is examined, and only rectangular fibers with clearly evident cross-striation are counted.

It appears that examination for meat fibers yields results that correlate well with chemical determination of fat excretion.

Leukocytes (Harris, 1972)

1. Place a small fleck of mucus or a drop of liquid stool on a glass microscopic slide with a wooden applicator stick.
2. Add 2 drops of Loeffler's methylene blue.
3. Mix thoroughly and carefully.
4. Place a coverslip on the mixture.
5. Let stand for 2 to 3 minutes for good nuclear staining.
6. With low-power scanning, make rough quantitative counts by approximating the average number of leukocytes and erythrocytes. All differential counts should be made under high power, counting 200 cells when possible. Only those cells clearly identified as either mononuclear or polymorphonuclear are included in the differential count. Macrophages and epithelial cells that can not be clearly identified are ignored. The initial cell counts should be performed at the time of presentation of the sample to the physician.

SERUM CAROTENOIDS

Carotenoids are a group of compounds which are the major precursors of vitamin A in man. They are synthesized by plants and some animals, excluding man. The absorption of carotenoids in the intestine is dependent on the presence of dietary fat and its normal absorption. Since carotenoids are not stored in the body to any appreciable degree, lack of carotenoids in the diet or disturbances in absorption of lipids from the intestine can result in decreasing levels of serum carotenoids. This is a simple and useful screening test for steatorrhea. In addition to steatorrhea and poor diet, low levels of serum carotenoid may also be caused by liver disease and high fever. Elevated serum carotenoid levels can be caused by hypothyroidism, diabetes, hyperlipidemia, and excessive intake of carotene (ingestion of carrots) (Wegner, 1957).

Principle (Kolmer, 1951). Carotenoids are normally transported as complexes with lipoproteins in serum. These carotenoid bonds are broken with ethanol and the pigments extracted with petroleum ether. After the absorbance is determined at 420 nm, the concentration is calculated by reference to a potassium dichromate standard. Alternatively, one may use a β-carotene standard.

Reagents

1. Ethanol—95 per cent
2. Petroleum ether, boiling point 35° to 60°C.
3. Artificial carotene standard. Add 200 mg of potassium dichromate to a 1 liter volumetric flask, add a small amount of distilled water to dissolve the crystals, and dilute to the mark with distilled water. The concentration of the standard equals 1.12 μg carotenoids/ml of petroleum ether extract.

Procedure (Kolmer, 1951)

1. Pipette 1 ml of serum into each of two 15 ml centrifuge tubes.
2. Add 1 ml of 95 per cent ethanol to each tube.
3. Add 2 ml of petroleum ether to each tube.
4. Stopper the centrifuge tubes with Parafilm-covered stoppers and shake vigorously for 5 minutes.
5. Remove stoppers, seal the tubes with Parafilm, and centrifuge for 5 minutes at 2000 to 2500 rpm.
6. Carefully remove the petroleum ether from the duplicate specimens and combine in one cuvette. Cover the cuvettes to prevent evaporation.
7. Read the absorbance of each specimen at 420 nm against a petroleum ether blank.
8. Determine the absorbance of the potassium dichromate standard at 420 nm against a water blank.

Calculation

$$\frac{1.12\,\mu\text{g/ml} \times 2 \times 100\text{ ml/dl}}{A_S} \times A_U$$

$$= \mu\text{g carotenoids/dl}$$

where

1.12 μg/ml = the equivalent carotenoid concentration of the potassium dichromate standard

2 = dilution factor owing to petroleum ether

100 = factor to convert to 100 ml of serum

A_S = absorbance reading of standard

A_U = absorbance reading of unknown

Normal values are 40 to 300 μg carotenoids/dl serum (0.74 to 5.58 mmol/l as β-carotene).

Comments

1. The serum for the determination of carotenoids should be free from hemolysis, protected from light, and collected when the patient is in the fasting state.

2. Carotene-loading tests in which serum carotenoids are measured before and after oral administration of carotene have been reported to provide greater diagnostic specificity and sensitivity than a single fasting serum carotenoid value (Finley, 1958; Onstad, 1972). However, the loading tests are not practical for screening purposes, because they require that blood be collected anywhere from 3 to 7 days after administration of the carotene in order to determine the peak serum value.

STARCH TOLERANCE TEST

The starch tolerance test has been used to differentiate pancreatogenous from enterogenous malabsorption. In the presence of pancreatic amylase, starch is hydrolyzed into dextrins, maltose, and glucose. Other enzymes are then able to hydrolyze the dextrins and maltose into their monosaccharide components, which can be absorbed in the intestine. After ingestion of 100 g of soluble starch, in the morning after an overnight (8 hr.) fast, hydrolysis and absorption of starch are followed by serial blood glucose determinations. The rise in blood glucose is compared with that following a glucose tolerance test. If the pancreas is unable to synthesize amylase or the ductal system is unable to deliver it to the intestine, the glucose tolerance test will result in significantly higher blood glucose values than those of the starch tolerance test.

Method (Althausen, 1954). One hundred grams of soluble starch (prepared according to the method of Lintner and marketed by Merck and Company, Inc.) are suspended in 150 ml of water by mixing with a spoon. Just before the test this suspension is poured into 300 ml of water which has just ceased boiling and is thoroughly stirred. The fasting patient should ingest the starch as soon as the temperature has cooled sufficiently. Blood specimens are drawn at 30 minutes, one hour, two hours, and three hours after administration of the starch, for glucose determinations. To arrive at the correct answer it is necessary to obtain, in addition, a standard three-hour glucose tolerance test following ingestion of 100 g of glucose. The two tolerance tests should be performed on two consecutive days.

Calculation. The extent to which the maximal rise in blood glucose exceeds that after starch is expressed as a percentage and is calculated as follows:

$$\text{percentage} = \frac{(P' - F') - (P - F)}{P - F} \times 100$$

where

percentage = the extent to which the maximal rise in blood glucose exceeds that after starch.

P′ = the peak blood glucose value after glucose ingestion.

F′ = the fasting blood glucose before glucose ingestion.

P = The peak blood glucose value after starch ingestion.

F = the fasting blood glucose value before starch ingestion.

Normal Values.   Althausen (1961) recommended that values below 70 per cent be considered normal. Results falling between 70 and 100 per cent should be considered borderline, while values above 100 per cent should be interpreted as definitely abnormal. A positive starch tolerance test (values above 100 per cent) is a reliable indicator of chronic pancreatic disease, but a negative result does not rule out pancreatic disease (Sun, 1961).

Comments

1. It is absolutely necessary to prepare the starch test meal properly. If the suspension of starch is allowed to boil, the starch may be partially hydrolyzed by heat into a less complex carbohydrate, thereby facilitating absorption in the gastrointestinal tract. Patients with severe pancreatic insufficiency may then exhibit normal responses to the starch tolerance test. If the starch is mixed with cold water and administered at this temperature, normal subjects may have a flat blood glucose curve.

2. The starch test meal must be ingested as soon as prepared and at a temperature of 50° to 55°C. The ingestion of the gel form of the starch meal may result in a flat blood glucose curve even in normal patients (Sun, 1961).

3. False negative results may be obtained in patients with achlorhydria. It is possible that the lack of hydrochloric acid allows the digestion of starch by salivary enzymes to continue in the stomach and small intestine (Althausen, 1961).

4. It is important to regulate the time of insulin administration on the days prior to the test for diabetic patients. If a single dose of insulin is being used it should be given at 1 P.M. on the day preceding each tolerance test.

D-XYLOSE TEST

The D-xylose absorption test is a valuable test for the differential diagnosis of malabsorption. In this procedure, a 25 g dose of the pentose sugar in water is administered orally, and the amount excreted over a five-hour period in the urine determined. If the amount excreted is less than 3 g, the diagnosis

is most likely enterogenous malabsorption, as pancreatic enzymes are not required for absorption of D-xylose. D-Xylose is passively absorbed in the small intestine and is not metabolized by the liver, though a portion of an orally or intravenously administered dose is destroyed. The accuracy of the method depends not only on the rate of absorption of D-xylose but also on the rate of excretion by the kidneys.

Method (Reiner, 1965)

Principle.   D-Xylose 25 g is administered orally. Blood level is determined two hours later; urine excretion over a five-hour postadministration period is also determined. Chemical determination depends on dehydration of pentose to furfural in the presence of acid, followed by condensation of furfural with *p*-bromoaniline to form a colored compound.

At 70°C. about 9 per cent of the available pentose is converted to furfural, but at this temperature very little furfural is formed from other precursors. *p*-Bromoaniline is used because it does not form any appreciable color with other substances; and thiourea, which is an antioxidant, also helps to prevent the formation of interfering colored compounds.

Sample Collection

1. Allow patient nothing by mouth after midnight on the day of the test.

2. Between 8:00 and 9:00 A.M., have patient void. Discard urine.

3. Immediately after patient has voided, give orally 25 g of D-xylose dissolved in 250 ml (8 oz.) of tap water. Follow immediately with an additional 250 ml of tap water. Note time. In the case of children, administer 0.5 g of xylose per pound of body weight up to 25 g, with the amount of water adjusted accordingly.

4. Exactly two hours following administration of D-xylose, draw 3 ml of anticoagulated venous blood. This should be sent to the laboratory immediately.

5. Allow patient no further fluid or food and keep on bed rest or in a chair until completion of the test. Patient may experience a mild diarrhea later in the day from the D-xylose.

6. Save all urine voided during the test. Five hours after the test was started have the patient void. Add this urine to the rest. Send pooled urine to the laboratory immediately.

Reagents

1. Stock D-xylose standard solution (2 mg/dl). Dissolve 0.02 g Pfanstiehl D-xylose (Pfanstiehl Laboratories, Waukegan, Il.) in 0.3 per cent (w/v) benzoic acid in a 100 ml volumetric flask and dilute to volume with 0.3 per cent (w/v) benzoic acid.

2. Working D-xylose standard (0.04 mg/ml). Dilute 2.0 ml of the stock D-xylose standard to volume in a 100 ml volumetric flask with 0.3 per cent (w/v) benzoic acid.

3. Working D-xylose standard (0.10 mg/ml). Di-

lute 5.0 ml of the stock D-xylose standard to volume in a 100 ml volumetric flask with 0.3 per cent (w/v) benzoic acid.

4. Working D-xylose standard (0.20 mg/ml). Dilute 10 ml of the D-xylose stock standard to volume in a 100 ml volumetric flask with 0.3 per cent (w/v) benzoic acid.

5. Somogyi deproteinizing reagents (same as those used in Somogyi-Nelson blood glucose):

    a. $ZnSO_4 \cdot 7H_2O$, 10.5 g; distilled water, 1000 ml.

    b. $Ba(OH)_2 \cdot 8H_2O$, 9.5 g; distilled water, 1000 ml.

To adjust the solutions, remove 100 ml from each. Using these solutions, titrate 10 ml of the $ZnSO_4$ solution with the $Ba(OH)_2$ solution. Use 1 drop of 1 per cent alcoholic phenolphthalein as the indicator and the first faint pink as the end point. Dilute the remaining 900 ml of the stronger solution so that 10 ml of the $ZnSO_4$ requires 10 ml (± 0.05 ml) of the $Ba(OH)_2$ solution to neutralize it. Supernates using these solutions should be crystal clear.

6. Glacial acetic acid saturated with thiourea (Matheson, Coleman, and Bell); use approximately 4 g thiourea per 100 ml glacial acetic acid. Keep 250 ml on hand. It is stable.

7. D-Xylose color reagent. Make fresh just before use. Add 4 g p-bromoaniline (Eastman No. 473) to 200 ml glacial acetic acid saturated with thiourea. This is enough for one complete set.

Procedure

1. Prepare appropriate quantity of D-xylose color reagent.

2. Prepare a protein-free supernate 1:10 as follows: Mix 1 ml whole blood, 4.5 ml $ZnSO_4$, and 4.5 ml $Ba(OH)_2$. Shake and centrifuge at 200 rpm for 10 minutes.

3. Measure the volume of urine and prepare 1:50, 1:100, and 1:250 dilutions with distilled water.

4. Pipet 1.0 ml of water, standards, blood filtrate, and urine dilutions in a series of duplicate tubes.

5. Add 5.0 ml of p-bromoaniline reagent to all tubes.

6. Incubate one of the duplicate tubes in a water bath at 70°C. ± 2°C. for 10 minutes. Cool tubes in running water to room temperature. Use the unheated set of tubes as blanks.

7. Place the heated and unheated tubes in a dark place for 70 minutes.

8. Read each set of tubes in a spectrophotometer at 520 nm. The unheated tube serves as a blank for each corresponding heated tube. Read within 30 minutes.

9. Construct a standard curve by plotting corrected absorbance vs. D-xylose concentration in mg/ml for the three xylose standards. The corrected absorbance for both standards and samples is absorbance (test) minus absorbance (blank). The standard curve should be linear and pass through the origin.

Calculations

BLOOD CONCENTRATION. Read the concentration of D-xylose in mg/ml corresponding to the cor-

rected absorbance for the blood supernatant from the standard curve.

URINE CONCENTRATION. Read the concentration of D-xylose in mg/ml corresponding to the corrected absorbance for the diluted urine from the standard curve.

for 1:50 dilution

    D-Xylose excreted in g/5 hr = (mg/ml D-xylose) $\times$ (50/1) $\times$ (urine volume in liters)

for 1:100 dilution

    D-Xylose excreted in g/5 hr = (mg/ml D-xylose) $\times$ (100/1) $\times$ (urine volume in liters)

for 1:250 dilution

    D-Xylose excreted in g/5 hr = (mg/ml D-xylose) $\times$ (250/1) $\times$ (urine volume in liters)

Normal Values. With a 25 g dose of D-xylose, adults should excrete at least 4 g of xylose in the five-hour urine specimen. The blood concentration should be 36 ± 16 mg/dl (2.4 ± 1.07 mmol/l). Children should normally excrete 16 to 33 per cent of the dose in the five-hour urine, and the blood concentration should be greater than 30 mg/dl (2.01 mmol/l).

FECAL FAT DETERMINATIONS

The normal fat content of feces consists primarily of fatty acids, fatty acid salts (soaps), and neutral fats, with higher alcohols, paraffins, sterols, and vegetable carotenoids present in significantly smaller amounts. Fractionation of the total lipids into free fatty acids and neutral fats was formerly thought to aid in the assessment of the exocrine functions of the pancreas. However, because of the presence of bacterial lipase and the spontaneous hydrolysis of neutral fats, fractionation of the total lipid provides no additional information about the cause of steatorrhea.

A number of methods are available for the measurement of fecal fat. Titrimetric and electrical capacitance methods quantitate various chemical forms of fatty acids, while gravimetric procedures quantitate total fecal lipids. Radioisotope techniques measure the ability of the gastrointestinal tract to assimilate free fatty acids and triglycerides rather than quantitating the fecal lipids.

Gravimetric Methods. A weighed aliquot of feces, either as homogenized wet specimen or as dried specimen, is extracted with an organic solvent, such as xylene or petroleum ether. The extract is evaporated to dryness and the residue is weighed. The weight is taken to represent the amount of fat present in the specimen. There have been many modifications of this general procedure (Webb, 1959), the chief differences among them being the spectrum of lipids and lipoids included in the measurement.

Electrical Capacitance Method (*Wolochow, 1965*). A rapid method for quantitative determination of fecal fat has been described in which electrical capacitance is used. For this purpose an aliquot of fecal suspension is extracted with solvent consisting chiefly of chlorinated benzenes. The extract is filtered, and its electrical capacitance is measured and compared with standards of triolein similarly treated.

Even though it is a relatively simple and rapid procedure it has not gained wide acceptance in the clinical laboratory.

Isotopic Techniques (*Rufin, 1961*).   Oleic acid or triglycerides are labeled with ^{131}I and given orally to the patient. Subsequently, the blood or stool is examined for ^{131}I by gamma spectrography. The difference between the absorption rate of ^{131}I-labeled triglyceride and that of similarly labeled oleic acid has been interpreted as a measure of enzyme activity in the gastrointestinal tract and has been applied in the differential diagnosis of pancreatogenous and enterogenous steatorrhea. Theoretically the test should be extremely useful, but in practice it has been found to be unreliable and has been largely abandoned as a diagnostic procedure (Tuna, 1963; Spencer, 1969).

Titrimetric Method of Van de Kamer

PRINCIPLE.   Fats and fatty acids are converted to soap by boiling with alcoholic potassium hydroxide. After cooling, excess hydrochloric acid is added to convert soaps to fatty acids. These are extracted with petroleum ether. An aliquot is evaporated, taken up in neutral alcohol, and titrated with sodium hydroxide. Fats are calculated as fatty acids.

PROCEDURE.   All refluxing, evaporating, blending, and transferring of fecal emulsion should be done in a motorized hood. Ground glass joints are used throughout.

1. Weigh container in which stool is to be homogenized (paint can, blender, etc.) before use.
2. Blend, adding water to bring the consistency to that of ice cream mix.*
3. Reweigh container and contents.
4. Weigh 125 ml flask with ground glass stopper.
5. Transfer (using open [broken]-tip, 10 ml serologic pipette, and rubber bulb) about 8 to 10 ml of emulsion to weighed flask.
6. Reweigh flask, stopper, and contents.
7. Repeat steps 4 to 6 with a second flask.
8. Add 10 ml 6 N KOH to each flask, using graduated cylinder.
9. Add 40 ml ethanol with 0.4 per cent isoamyl alcohol to each flask, using graduated cylinder.
10. Add five glass beads to each flask.
11. Remove stopper from first flask, place on hot plate, and couple to reflux condenser.
12. Reflux for 20 to 30 minutes.
13. Remove flask from condenser, replace stop-

per, place in ice bath. Place a strip of paper between the stopper and flask neck to prevent formation of a vacuum in the flask as it cools.
14. Connect second flask to condenser and reflux for 20 to 30 minutes.
15. When first flask has cooled to room temperature or below, add 17 ml 6.8 N HCl, using graduated cylinder, and restopper (without paper).
16. When flask is again cold, add 50 ml petroleum ether, using a rubber bulb and a 50 ml transfer pipette.
17. Stopper and shake vigorously for 90 to 120 seconds by the clock.
18. When the upper petroleum ether has separated, transfer 25 ml of this layer, using a rubber bulb and a 25 ml transfer pipette, to a 125 ml Erlenmeyer flask.
19. Connect flask (containing 25 ml aliquot of petroleum ether) to distilling apparatus. (Apparatus is a safety measure to minimize fire and explosion hazard from evaporated petroleum ether.) Place flask in 56°C. water bath. Evaporate almost to dryness.
20. Remove from bath, add 10 ml ethanol, using a serologic pipette, rinsing down the sides of the flask with the alcohol.
21. Add 3 drops of thymol blue indicator.
22. Titrate with standard NaOH until yellow color begins to change.
23. Repeat steps 13 and 15 to 22, inclusive, with second flask.

REAGENTS
1. KOH, aqueous 6 N (33 per cent w/v)
2. Ethanol 95 per cent (v/v) with 0.4 per cent (v/v) isoamyl alcohol
3. HCl 6.8 N (25% w/v)
4. Petroleum ether, B.P. 40° to 60°C. (approximately)
5. Ethanol 95 per cent (v/v) neutral
6. Thymol blue, 0.2 per cent (w/v) in 50 per cent ethanol
7. Standard aqueous NaOH, 0.1 N

EQUIPMENT
1. Hood
2. Electric hot plate (about 500 watts)
3. Two ring stands—one burette clamp and one condenser clamp
4. Ice bath
5. Waring blender, Osterizer, or equivalent
6. Two-kg platform balance and weights
7. Glass beads
8. Rubber bulb (or Propipette)
9. Two 125 ml flasks, ground glass neck 24/40 (A.H. Thomas No. 5343). Two stoppers, ground glass (A.H. Thomas No. 9314-J)
10. One 50 ml burette
11. Two 125 ml Erlenmeyer flasks
12. Two 25 ml volumetric pipettes and one 50 ml volumetric pipette
13. One 10 ml serologic pipette with tip broken off (to transfer the fecal emulsion of step 5)
14. Two 10 ml serologic pipettes

---

* It has been suggested that coarse silica be added to the specimen when using the paint can method to hasten homogenization and dispersion of the feces. Cellulose gum is also added to stabilize the mixture. Ethanol is also added before blending.

15. One 50 ml graduated cylinder and one 25 ml graduated cylinder

16. One distilling head (Claisen) with West condenser and ground glass joints 24/40 (Corning Cat. No. 3560)

17. One distilling tube with suction tube and ground glass joints 24/40 (Corning Cat. No. 9420)

CALCULATION

1. Calculate the total weight of the emulsion from steps 1 and 3.

2. Calculate the weights of aliquots in each flask from steps 4, 6, and 7.

3. Calculate ml standard NaOH used to titrate the fatty acids in flasks from step 22.

4. Using the formula below, calculate the $\dfrac{\text{g fatty acids}}{24 \text{ hr}}$ for each flask.

5. Average results and report as $\dfrac{\text{g total fat}}{24 \text{ hr}}$.

(In this method the g total fat is calculated as fatty acid.)

FORMULA

$$\frac{\text{g fatty acids}}{24 \text{ hr}}$$

$$= \frac{\begin{array}{c}\text{ml NaOH used} \times \text{normality NaOH used} \\ \times \text{ gm fecal emulsion} \times 0.5907\end{array}}{\begin{array}{c}\text{g of aliquot of emulsion taken} \\ \times \text{ number of days of collection}\end{array}}$$

where

$$0.5907 = \frac{50 \text{ ml petroleum ether extract}}{25 \text{ ml petroleum ether extract}}$$

$$\times \frac{1.04 \text{ g fatty acids (total)}}{1.00 \text{ g fatty acids (extract)}} \times \frac{284 \text{ g fatty acids}}{1000 \text{ ml NaOH}}$$

EXPLANATION. Assumed average molecular weight of fatty acids is 284. When 50 ml extract is made, 25 ml is evaporated. A further correction is made for the partition of fatty acids between the emulsion and petroleum ether.

Normal Adults:

FAT INTAKE (g/24 hr)	FATTY ACIDS EXCRETED (g/24 hr)	PER CENT OF INTAKE EXCRETED/24 hr
50	2–3	4–6
100	4–5	4–5

Children: 5 per cent or less of daily dietary intake.

COMMENT. In some cases of malabsorption, the coefficient of fat retention can be improved by substituting medium chain fatty acids for long chain fatty acids in the diet. The Van de Kamer method does not quantitatively recover medium chain fatty acids (Saunders, 1967). Braddock (1968) has improved the recovery of medium chain fatty acids from feces by slightly modifying the Van de Kamer procedure. He reduced the amount of water during saponification and distilled off the excess alcohol prior to extraction, resulting in complete recovery of medium chain and long chain fatty acids.

CLINITEST FOR REDUCING SUBSTANCES IN STOOL (Kerry, 1964)

Procedure. Add 1 volume of stool to 2 volumes of distilled water and mix thoroughly. Transfer 15 drops of this suspension to a clean test tube and add a Clinitest tablet. The reaction and interpretation of results are described in Chapter 17.

Interpretation. Presence of 0.25 g/dl reducing substance or less is considered normal; from 0.25 g/dl to 0.5 g/dl is regarded as suspicious; greater than 0.5 g/dl is interpreted as indicating abnormal amounts of sugar. Sucrose, of course, is not a reducing sugar and will not react in this test. However, in the case of sucrose intolerance, little sucrose but large amounts of glucose and fructose are found in the stool, presumably due to hydrolysis of sucrose by intestinal bacteria, so that the test is positive nonetheless.

ORAL LACTOSE TOLERANCE TEST (Basford, 1967; Gudmand-Hoyer, 1977)

Following an overnight fast, administer, orally, 50 g lactose dissolved in 400 ml of water. Draw fasting blood and blood samples at 30, 60, and 120 minutes after ingestion, as for a glucose tolerance test. Also collect a five-hour stool specimen, examining and recording appearance, consistency and pH.

Patients with lactase deficiency exhibit a peak rise of less than 20 mg/dl in reducing substances expressed as glucose. In all persons with flat tolerance curves, the test should be repeated within two days and the less abnormal of the two curves used for interpretation. A control test may be performed, using 25 g glucose and 25 g galactose if the lactose test indicates malabsorption. Some investigators use a 100 g dose, which has been reported by some to yield more definitive results. It may cause symptoms in cases of mild lactase deficiency. In children, the dosage of lactose or other sugars is 2 g/kg of body weight.

ASSAY OF INTESTINAL DISACCHARIDASES (Dalhquist, 1968)

Principle. Homogenized intestinal mucosa is incubated with disaccharide substrate; the enzyme is then inactivated, and the amount of liberated glucose is estimated photometrically by a second incubation step, using glucose oxidase, peroxidase, and chromogen.

Method (Dahlquist, 1968). Preparation of intestinal homogenate. Weigh and record specimen. Do not wash with water, as this may alter enzyme activity (Antonowicz, 1970). When a whole piece of intestine is available:

1. Scrape off the mucosa with a piece of glass.
2. Add four parts of distilled water.
3. Homogenize.
4. Chill the mucosa and water well with crushed ice for at least 5 minutes before and during homogenization.
5. Centrifuge at 2000 to 4000 rpm for 10 minutes in order to remove layer of cell debris.

When only a very small amount of mucosa is available:

1. For 10 to 20 mg of mucosa, add 0.5 ml water.
2. Chill the tube with its contents (including the pestle) with crushed ice for at least 5 minutes prior to homogenization and then during the whole homogenization procedure.
3. Homogenize in a glass pestle homogenizer (Potter and Elvehjem, or in some similar type) for 1 to 2 minutes, with motor speeds of 200 to 300 rpm.

Reagents

1. *Substrate.* Maltose, sucrose, trehalose, lactose, and isomaltose are available commercially. Impurity of substrate will be revealed by a high blank reading in the assay procedure.
2. *Buffer* (sodium maleate buffer (0.1 mol/l, pH 6.0)). Dissolve 1.16 g maleic acid in 15.3 ml 1 mol/l NaOH and dilute with distilled water to 100 ml. Measure the pH and adjust, if necessary, to 6.0.
3. *Substrate-buffer solution.* An 0.056 mol/l solution of the appropriate disaccharide in 0.1 mol/l sodium maleate buffer, pH 6.0. Substrate-buffer solutions are stored frozen in small aliquots.
4. *Glucose oxidase reagents:*

STOCK SOLUTION

a. Tris buffer (0.5 mol/l, pH 7.0). Dissolve 61 g Tris in 85 ml 5 mol/l HCl and dilute with water to 1000 ml. Measure the pH and adjust, if necessary, to 7.0.

b. Peroxidase solution. Dissolve 10 mg peroxi-dase (grade D, Worthington Biochemical Company, Freehold, N.J.) in water to 10 ml. Store frozen in small aliquots.

c. Detergent solution. Dissolve 20 g Triton X-100 (Rohm & Haas Company, Philadelphia, Pa.) in 80 g 95 per cent ethanol.

d. O-Dianisidine solution. Dissolve 100 mg o-dianisidine (technical, Eastman, Rochester, N.Y.) in ethanol to 10 ml. Store in dark; discard when it becomes brown by oxidation. Tris-glucose oxidase reagent (TGO-reagent). Dissolve 2 mg glucose oxidase 130,000 (Fermco Laboratories, Chicago, Ill. 60680) in 100 ml 0.5 mol/l Tris buffer. Add 1.0 ml o-dianisidine solution, 1.0 ml detergent solution, and 0.5 ml peroxidase solution. Mix well. This is stable for several days if stored in refrigerator. TGO reagent will interrupt disaccharidase activity.

STANDARD GLUCOSE SOLUTIONS

Prepare solutions of glucose in distilled water containing:

a. 100 μg/ml
b. 300 μg/ml
c. 500 μg/ml

Store frozen in small aliquots.

Method. The enzyme preparation should be diluted to contain a suitable activity of the disaccharidase to be assayed. If 1 molecule of glucose is formed per substrate molecule hydrolyzed, the diluted solution should contain somewhat less than 0.1 unit/ml; if 2 molecules of glucose are formed, it should contain a little less than 0.05 unit/ml. When homogenates of peroral biopsy specimens are analyzed and have been prepared as described above, suitable dilutions for the different activities usually are about the following:

Maltase	1:50
Isomaltase	1:20
Sucrase (invertase)	1:10
Trehalase	1:5
Lactase	1:5
Cellobiase	1:2

The readings obtained with the incubated sam-

Table 25–4. DISACCHARIDASE ACTIVITIES AT THE LIGAMENT OF TREITZ IN 100 HEALTHY SUBJECTS*

DISACCHARIDASE	NO. OF SUBJECTS	ACTIVITY (WET WT.)				ACTIVITY (PROTEIN)				
		Mean	SD (units/g)	SEM	Range	CV (%)	Mean	SD (units/g)	SEM	Range	CV (%)
Lactase	100	3.3	2.0	0.2	0–11.1	60.6	29.0	18.6	1.9	0–82.8	64.1
Normal	94	3.5	1.9	0.2	0.7–11.1	54.2	30.9	17.6	1.8	3.0–82.8	56.9
Deficient	6	0.2	0.2	0.07	0–0.5	100.0	1.3	1.4	0.6	0–4.1	108.0
Sucrase	100	5.9	2.3	0.2	1.2–14.0	39.0	51.3	22.9	2.3	4.6–121.0	44.6
Maltase	100	22.3	7.2	0.7	6.5–39.1	32.2	195.2	78.1	7.8	27.7–446.5	40.0
Isomaltase	14	7.2	2.6	0.7	3.0–12.1	36.1	67.3	19.4	5.2	28.5–103.0	28.8

*From Newcomer, A. D., and McGill, D. B.: Disaccharidase activity in the small intestine: Prevalence of lactase deficiency in 100 healthy subjects. Gastroenterology, *53*:884, 1967.

ples should not exceed the highest point of the standard curve. If they do, the enzyme must be further diluted and a new incubation performed.

1. Transfer to a conical test tube 100 µl diluted enzyme solution.

2. Incubate in a 37°C. water bath for a few minutes to bring to temperature.

3. Add 100 µl of substrate-buffer solution and mix. The reaction is started at this point.

4. Incubate for exactly 60 minutes.

5. Add 3 ml TGO reagent. Mix well. This will immediately interrupt the disaccharidase reaction.

6. Let stand in the water bath at 37°C. for 60 minutes for development of color.

BLANK

1. Transfer to a conical test tube, in order: 100 µl diluted enzyme solution, 3 ml TGO reagent, 100 µl substrate-buffer solution.

2. Mix.

3. Incubate in 37°C. water bath for 60 minutes.

REAGENT BLANK

1. To a conical test tube add: 200 µl distilled water, 3 ml TGO reagent.

2. Mix.

3. Incubate in 37°C. water bath for 60 minutes.

After the development of color, measure sample in a spectrophotometer at 420 nm against the reagent blank.

Standard Series. Mix in three test tubes 200 µl of standard solutions a, b, and c, respectively, with 3 ml of TGO reagent. These tubes will contain, in order, 20, 60, and 100 µg glucose.

Incubate the tubes in a water bath at 37°C. for 60 minutes for development of color.

Calculation

1 unit of enzyme hydrolyzes 1 µmol disaccharide per minute. The disaccharidase activity per milliliter enzyme preparation is then calculated by the following formula:

$$10 \times \frac{a}{180} \times \frac{1}{60} \times \frac{1}{n} \times d \quad \text{or} \quad \frac{a \times d}{n \times 1080} \text{ units/ml}$$

where:

a = µg glucose liberated in 60 minutes (sample-blank)

d = dilution factor for the enzyme solution of which 100 µl are used

n = number of glucose molecules per molecule of disaccharide (for maltose, isomaltose, trehalose, and cellobiose, n = 2; for sucrose and lactose, n = 1)

180 = molecular weight of glucose

10 = factor to convert 0.1 ml to 1.0 ml

Method for assay with a final volume of 320 microliters

When limited amounts of material are available, as in the analysis of peroral biopsy specimens, amounts are employed which give a final volume of 320 µl.

In this procedure, special ultramicro test tubes are used. The tubes of the standard series will contain 2, 6, and 10 µg glucose, respectively. All volumes in the procedure described above are reduced ten-fold. A spectrophotometer with an ultramicro cuvette is used for the readings. The disaccharidase activity is calculated in the following way (for symbols, see above):

$$100 \times \frac{a}{180} \times \frac{1}{60} \times \frac{1}{n} \times d \quad \text{or} \quad \frac{a \times d}{n \times 108} \text{ units/ml}$$

The disaccharidase unit is defined as the activity hydrolyzing 1 µmol of disaccharide per minute under the conditions used, i.e., temperature 37°C., substrate concentration 0.028 mol/l, pH 6.0.

The disaccharidase activity finally is expressed as units per gram (wet weight) or units per gram of protein. In the latter instance, protein content of the homogenate is measured.

Discussion. These assay methods are performed in two separate incubation steps. Although accurate and sensitive, they are somewhat laborious and time-consuming. The one-stage ultramicro method is convenient and can be used for tiny tissue specimens obtained from peroral biopsies. However, maltase activity with this method was found to be 40 per cent lower than when measured with the micro method (Messer, 1966).

Fecal Blood

Quantitative methods have been developed for study of gastrointestinal bleeding by use of radioactive chromium-51 (Fall, 1971). These methods have greater specificity than peroxidase tests. Furthermore, they can be combined with other techniques to determine the location of bleeding, when present. As they involve considerable time, effort, and expense, their use should be reserved for patients presenting special diagnostic problems.

The procedures are based on ability of radioactive chromium to be bound to red blood cells and on the fact that radioactive chromium is not reabsorbed from the gastrointestinal tract but is excreted in the feces, where it can be measured by gamma-ray spectrometry. For this purpose a sample of blood is withdrawn from the patient, mixed with citrate solution containing chromium-51 as sodium chromate, and then reinjected into the patient. Most of the sodium chromate is bound to the red blood cells and remains so bound until they are destroyed or lost through hemorrhage. Subsequently, stools contain quantities of chromium-51 quantitatively related to the blood content. Gamma ray activity of the stool specimen is determined and the blood loss is calculated from comparison with activity of patient's blood. Bleeding source may be localized by similarly examining for blood fluid removed from various levels of the gastrointestinal tract through a Miller-Abbot tube or by use of an umbilical tape attached to a small bag of mercury in a lead sinker, swallowed by the patient, located by fluoroscope, then withdrawn and examined for blood staining.

The commonly applied screening tests depend on the determination of the peroxidase activity of hemoglobin for the semiquantitation of blood in feces. Reagents used include guaiac, benzidine,* ortho-tolidine, and ortho-dianisidine. Peroxidases (including hemoglobin, which can act as either a catalase or peroxidase) catalyze oxidation of the test substance by hydrogen peroxide, causing development of various shades and intensities of blue, depending on reagent, concentration of hemoglobin or other peroxidases, presence of other coloring matter, and presence (or absence) of inhibitors. The reagents differ chiefly in sensitivity. Benzidine gives a positive result with blood in a 1:100,000 dilution with saline; ortho-tolidine is positive in a 1:20,000 dilution, and guaiac is positive in 1:100 to 1:5000 dilution, depending on the age and hemoglobin concentration of the blood (Hoerr, 1949). The more sensitive reagents can be adapted to provide a less sensitive test by manipulation of techniques. Hematest (Ames Company, Inc.) incorporates ortho-tolidine, while Hemoccult (SmithKline Corporation) employs guaiac-impregnated filter paper. These commercial tests have sensitivities intended to be consistent with the uses for which they are designed. The normal individual loses 2.0 to 2.5 ml of blood into the gastrointestinal tract daily (Ebaugh, 1958). Therefore, it is reasonable to use a test which begins to turn positive with a blood loss greater than 5 to 10 ml per day. This corresponds to 5 to 10 mg of hemoglobin per gram of stool, assuming a blood hemoglobin of 15 g/dl and an average 150 g stool. Morris (1976) found, in comparing three screening procedures (1:60 alcoholic solution of guaiac, Hematest, and Hemoccult) with the quantitative radioassay technique, that guaiac and Hematest detected 95 per cent of stools

with more than 5 mg hemoglobin/g stool. Hemoccult detected 37 per cent of stools in the 2.0 to 5.0 mg hemoglobin/g stool range, 60 per cent of stools containing 5.0 to 20.0 mg hemoglobin/g stool, and 95 per cent of stools with greater than 20.0 g hemoglobin/g stool. Earlier authors comparing either the volume of ingested blood or fecal quantitation of ingested ^{51}Cr-labeled red cells with different screening methods have, in some cases, confirmed the relative sensitivities of these reagents, while others have come to different conclusions. Ostrow (1973) found guaiac and Hematest consistently detected as little as 2.0 mg hemoglobin/g stool, while Hemoccult detected only 50 per cent of the stools with 5 to 10 mg hemoglobin/g stool and most of the stools with greater than 10 mg hemoglobin/g stool. However, Peranio (1951) found ortho-tolidine to be more sensitive than guaiac, requiring only 1 ml of ingested blood to yield a positive test, whereas guaiac required 20.0 ml. These differences in relative sensitivity illustrate how the same basic reagents used under different conditions can yield markedly different results.

Stroehlein (1976) found that the ratio of volume of blood loss to stool volume, as well as the amount of blood loss, was an important factor in obtaining a positive fecal occult blood result. Two thirds of the stools were positive for occult blood with Hemoccult when the calculated volume of fecal blood loss was 10 per cent of stool volume, and nearly all specimens were positive when the volume of blood loss was 30 per cent of the stool volume.

Numerous modifications have been developed based on the same fundamental processes in efforts to improve test precision and specificity and diagnostic accuracy. Of the commercially available screening tests, Hemoccult seems to have the lowest percentage of false positive results, approximately 1 to 12 per cent (Stroehlein, 1976; Morris, 1976). The range of false positives reported for other guaiac-based procedures is 6 to 76 per cent (Morgan, 1957; Morris, 1976). Hematest has been reported to have a 27 to 76 per cent false positive rate (Ostrow, 1973; Morris, 1976). The high rate of false positives is influenced by the lack of specificity of the reagents and the presence of peroxidase activity in other fecal constituents, as well as the sensitivity of the different chromogens to peroxidase activity. The myoglobin and hemoglobin of ingested meat and fish have peroxidase activity that

---

*The use and marketing of benzidine is restricted by federal regulations due to its carcinogenicity, and its use should be eliminated whenever possible. Some or all of the alternative chemicals may also be carcinogenic.

may falsely indicate the presence of occult blood. The necessity of eliminating meat from the diet before and during the test period is dependent on the sensitivity of the occult blood test used. In general, the less sensitive guaiac methods are the least affected by meat in the diet, although there are reports of a significant number of false positives caused by meat with the guaiac procedures (Greegor, 1971; Ostrow, 1973).

Bacteria in the bowel as well as ingested vegetables, such as horseradish and turnips, also have peroxidases and can falsely elevate fecal peroxidase activity. Modifications of tests intended to destroy plant and bacterial peroxidases by boiling or heating the fecal suspension may also denature some of the peroxidase activity of hemoglobin (*Lancet*, 1970) and are therefore not recommended.

The possibility of false positives owing to the presence of iron in the diet is widely recognized and has been reported for guaiac (Johnson, 1941), and for ortho-tolidine (Peranio, 1951). Later studies have failed to confirm these findings (Morgan, 1957; Morris, 1976). In fact, in the presence of iron, the percentage of false positives was decreased with Hemoccult and the false negatives tended to be lower with guaiac, Hematest, and Hemoccult (Morris, 1976). Morris also found that laxatives and barium did not interfere with the performance of the occult blood test. There has been some evidence that false negatives occur with guaiac, benzidine, ortho-tolidine, and ortho-dianisidine in the presence of large amounts of vitamin C (Jaffe, 1975).

As blood traverses the gut, it is broken down into its constituents, which may have decreased or no peroxidase activity. The actual form of hemoglobin most commonly found in the colon is hematin, which has much less peroxidase activity than heme. A source of hemorrhage in the upper gastrointestinal system or an increased transit time through the bowel will, therefore, decrease the peroxidase activity of hemoglobin.

One group found an 80- to 120-fold decrease in the peroxidase activity of blood passing through the gastrointestinal tract as compared to blood added directly to the feces (Ebaugh, 1958). Furthermore, because of inhibiting substances in the stool, similar loss of activity may be found by adding blood to feces, as compared with adding similar quantities of blood to water. Ebaugh and associates suggest that this inhibition results from masking of indicator color by added color from the feces. Another factor may be competition for nascent oxygen by reducing substances in the feces.

Finally, techniques for measuring peroxidase activity are subject to considerable experimental error, particularly when large numbers of stool specimens must be screened by mass production methods. Specimens show marked variability in consistency and in their tendency to disperse in suspensions. This leads to inconsistencies in amount of aliquot used and in the portion of the aliquot actually available to react in suspension. Filter paper techniques are also limited in reproducibility by the tendency for liquid stools to be absorbed into the substance of the paper.

Further errors result from inaccurate measurement of reagents, inaccurate timing of the reaction, and variable interpretation of the color developed. Inconsistencies may also arise from sampling because of incomplete mixing of blood with the stool. Blood arising in the upper gastrointestinal tract is relatively uniformly mixed throughout the specimen, but blood from the lower gastrointestinal tract is likely to be segmental in distribution within the stool, or it may only coat the surface. Anorectal blood frequently produces red streaking of the surface. The presence of such focally distributed blood should be reported after chemical verification. In routine testing for occult blood, an attempt is made to use an aliquot from the center of the formed stool.

In the patient with severe gastrointestinal hemorrhage, the diagnostic problems are not such as to need a very sensitive test to detect blood in feces. The real benefit of these tests is as a screening procedure for hemorrhage from colonic carcinoma and other occult sources of hemorrhage which may bleed intermittently. To be valid, the test employed must be repeated at least three and preferably six times with the patient on a diet free of the exogenous sources of peroxidase activity. In addition, the patient should be requested to include liberal amounts of high residue foods such as prunes, bran, raw vegetables, corn, and peanuts. This regimen is usually unacceptable to the patient, so that positive tests on a normal diet must be repeated following a three- or four-day period of abstinence from meats, fish, and vegetable sources of peroxidase activity. Only after this regimen can a positive series of tests be considered an indication for further evaluation of the patient.

Methodology

The guaiac method to be described represents a compromise suitable for routine screening. It will detect 0.5 to 1.0 mg of hemoglobin per ml of aqueous solution. If one substitutes 0.2 per cent ortho-tolidine for guaiac and 0.3 per cent hydrogen peroxide for 3 per cent hydrogen peroxide in the same procedure, one obtains approximately the same sensitivity. We have found the Hematest techniques to be capable of detecting as little as 0.1 mg blood in an aqueous solution. It has an unacceptable number of false positive reactions when patients are on a regular diet (Ostrow, 1973; Morris, 1976). Paradoxically, however, Hematest sometimes gives only a trace or 1+ reaction with tarry stools. We believe this results from improper mixing of hematin with reagent, probably because of the tarry consistency of the stool. Mixing (not recommended by the manufacturer) obviates the problem.

We advise use of a saturated solution of guaiac because of the tendency of weaker solutions to fade. Addition of extra powdered guaiac will restore the coloring in these cases. The problem may also be overcome by observing for maximal color development.

Hemoccult, employing guaiac-impregnated filter paper, is of lower sensitivity and begins to turn positive in the presence of about 5.0 mg of hemoglobin per gram of stool. This is the upper limit of normal peroxidase activity of stool and as this represents a significant improvement in methodology, false positives can be kept in the range of 1 to 12 per cent (Stroehlein, 1976; Morris, 1976). The Hemoccult test also has the advantage of being so simple and esthetically acceptable that specimens can be collected at home and mailed for evaluation. However, Morris (1976) and Winawer (1977) have found that some specimens may convert from positive to negative after storage for two days.

Guaiac test for occult blood
Reagents
1. 1:60 (w/v) solution of gum guaiac in 95 per cent (v/v) ethyl alcohol or, preferably, a saturated solution
2. Glacial acetic acid
3. 3 per cent (v/v) hydrogen peroxide

Procedure
1. Place about 0.5 g of feces in a 10 × 100 mm test tube.
2. Add about 2 ml of tap water and mix with applicator sticks.
3. Add 0.5 ml of glacial acetic acid and mix well.
4. Add about 2 ml of the gum guaiac solution and mix well.
5. Add about 2 ml of hydrogen peroxide and mix; start timer.
6. Observe for 2 minutes and record the maximal color development during that time as trace, 1+, 2+, 3+, or 4+, depending on the intensity of the blue color. Strongly positive reactions will fade rapidly and should be read according to maximal color development rather than the appearance at the end of the time period.
7. Reagents should be checked daily by testing a sample known to contain blood.

Hemoccult slide test for occult blood
(SmithKline Corp., Sunnyvale, Cal. 94806)
Procedure
1. Collect a very small stool specimen on tip of wooden applicator.
2. Apply thin smear of specimen inside the circle.
3. Close cover; dispose of applicator.
4. Allow specimen to dry (important that specimen dry completely).
5. Open perforated window in back of slide.
6. Apply two or three drops of developing solution to slide opposite specimen.
7. Read results after 30 seconds.
Positive: Trace of blue indicates test is positive for occult blood.
Negative: No detectable blue anywhere on slide indicates test is negative for occult blood.

REFERENCES

Althausen, T. L., and Uyeyama, K.: A new test of pancreatic function based on starch tolerance. Ann. Intern. Med., *41*:563, 1954.

Althausen, T. L., and Uyeyama, K.: Further experience with the starch tolerance test for pancreatic insufficiency. Gastroenterology, *40*:470, 1961.

Anderson, C. M., Messer, M., Townley, R. R. W., and Freeman, M.: Intestinal sucrase and isomaltase deficiency in two siblings. Pediatrics, *31*:1003, 1963.

Anderson, C. M., and Burke, V.: Disorders of carbohydrate digestion and absorption. *In* Anderson, C. M., and Burke, V. (eds.): Pediatric Gastroenterology. Oxford, Blackwell Scientific Publications, Ltd., 1975.

Anderson, C. M., Burke, V., Messer, M., and Kerry, K. R.: Sugar intolerance and celiac disease. Lancet, *1*:1322, 1966.

Antonowicz, I., Ishida, S., Khaw, K. T., et al.: Effect of tissue preparation on determinations of disaccharidase activities in intestinal mucosa. Pediatrics, *45*:104, 1970.

Basford, R. L., and Henry, J. B.: Lactose intolerance in the adult. Postgrad. Med., *41*:A70, 1967.

Bockus, H. L.: Gastroenterology, 2nd ed. Philadelphia, W. B. Saunders Company, 1964.

Braddock, L. I., Fleisher, D. R., and Barbero, G. J.: A physical chemical study of the Van de Kamer method for fecal fat analysis. Gastroenterology, *55*:165, 1968.

Brayshaw, J. R., Harris, F., McCurdy, P. R., et al.: The effect of oral iron therapy on stool guaiac and ortho-tolidine reactions. Ann. Intern. Med., *59*:172, 1963.

Cook, G. C., and Kajubi, S. K.: Tribal incidence of lactase deficiency in Uganda. Lancet, *1*:725, 1966.

Dahlquist, A.: Assay of intestinal disaccharidases. Anal. Biochem., *22*:99, 1968.

Daniel, S. A., Jr., and Egan, S.: The quantity of blood required to produce a tarry stool. J.A.M.A., *113*:2232, 1939.

Davison, A. G. F., and Mullinger, M.: Reducing substances in neonatal stool detected by Clinitest. Pediatrics, *46*:632, 1970.

Drummey, G. D., Benson, J. A., and Jones, G. M.: Micro-scopical examination of the stool for steatorrhea. N. Engl. J. Med., *264*:85, 1961.

Ebaugh, F. G., Jr., Clements, T., Jr., Rodan, G., et al.: Quantitative measurement of gastrointestinal blood loss. Am. J. Med., *25*:169, 1958.

Fall, D. J., Kupier, D. H., and Pollard, H. M.: Use of isotopes of various tests for occult blood in feces. Cancer, *28*:135, 1971.

Finley, P. R., Doe, R., and Doyle, R.: The use of standardized carotene loading test in the diagnosis of malabsorptive states. Clin. Res., *6*:275, 1958.

Frazer, A. C.: Steatorrhea. Br. Med. J., *2*:805, 1955.

Frazer, A. C., and Sammons, H. G.: Fat synthesis by intestinal bacteria. Clin. Chem., *2*:272, 1956.

Goldman, P., Paver, W. K., and Corbett, W. H.: The detection of occult blood in the feces. Med. J. Aust., *1*:755, 1964.

Greegor, D. H.: Detection of silent colon cancer in routine examination. CA, *19*:330, 1969.

Greegor, D. H.: Occult blood testing for detection of asymptomatic colon cancer. CA, *28*:131, 1971.

Grossman, M. I., Matsumoto, K. K., and Litcher, R. J.: Fecal blood loss produced by oral and intravenous administration of various salicylates. Gastroenterology, *40*:383, 1961.

Gudmand-Hoyer, E., and Simony, K. O.: Individual sensitivity to lactose in lactose malabsorption. Am. J. Dig. Dis., *22*:177-181, 1977.

Harris, J. C., Dupont, H. L., and Hornick, R. B.: Fecal leukocytes in diarrhea illness. Ann. Intern. Med., *76*:697-703, 1972.

Haubrich, W. S.: Diarrhea and constipation. *In* Bockus, H. L. (ed.): Gastroenterology, vol. I. Philadelphia, W. B. Saunders Company, 1976, pp. 921-922.

Haverback, B. J., Dyce, B. J., Gutentag, P. J., et al.: Measurement of trypsin and chymotrypsin in stool. Gastroenterology, *44*:588, 1963.

Hoerr, S. O., Bliss, W. R., and Kaufman, J.: Clinical evaluation of various tests for occult blood in the feces. J.A.M.A., *141*:1213, 1949.

Hoffman, N. E., LaRusso, N. F., and Hoffman, A. F.: An improved method for fecal collection: The fecal field-kit. Lancet, *1*:1422, 1973.

Jaffe, R. M.: False negative stool occult blood tests caused by ingestion of ascorbic acid (vitamin C). Ann. Intern. Med., *83*:842, 1975.

Jelliffe, D. B., and Jelliffe, E. F. P.: Collection of stool sample. Lancet, *2*:618, 1973.

Johnson, A. S.: Effect of ingested iron on tests for occult blood in stools. J. Lab. Clin. Med., *26*:727, 1941.

Kaijser, K., and Ockerman, P. A.: Diagnostic problems in glucose-galactose malabsorption. A case report. Acta Paediatr. Scand., *59*:214, 1970.

Kerry, K. R., and Anderson, C. M.: A ward test for sugar in faeces. Lancet, *1*:981, 1964.

Keusch, G., Troncale, T. J., Miller, L. H., et al.: Acquired lactose malabsorption in Thai children. Pediatrics, *43*:540, 1969.

Kirschen, M., Sorter, H., and Necheles, M.: Occult blood with note on the use of carmine for marking of stools. Am. J. Dig. Dis., *9*:154, 1942.

Kolmer, J. A., Spaulding, E. H., and Robinson, H. W.: Approved Laboratory Technique. 5th ed. New York, Appleton-Century Crofts, Inc., 1951, p. 1066.

Krasilnikoff, P. A., Gudmand-Hoyer, E., and Moltke, H. H.: Diagnostic value of disaccharide tolerance tests on children. Acta Paediatr. Scand., *64*:693, 1975.

Lancet: Occult blood tests. *Lancet*, *1*:819, 1970.

Lang, D. J., Kunz, L. J., Martin, A. R., et al.: Carmine as a source of nosocomial salmonellosis. N. Engl. J. Med., *276*:829, 1967.

Linquist, B., and Meeuwisse, G. W.: Intestinal transport of monosaccharides in generalized and selective malabsorption. Acta Paediatr. Scand., *146*(Suppl.):110, 1963.

Meeuwisse, G. W., and Melin, K.: Glucose-galactose malabsorption, a clinical study of 6 cases. Acta Paediatr. Scand., *188* (Suppl.): 3, 1969.

Meeuwisse, G. W., and Linquist, B.: Glucose-galactose malabsorption—studies on the intermediate carbohydrate metabolism. Acta Paediatr. Scand., *59*:74, 1970.

Melin, K., and Meeuwisse, G. W.: Glucose-galactose malabsorption. A genetic study. Acta Paediatr. Scand., *188* (Suppl.):19, 1969.

Messer, M., and Dahlquist, A.: A one-step ultramicro method for the assay of intestinal disaccharidases. Anal. Biochem., *14*:376, 1966.

Moore, J. G., Engler, E., Jr., Bigler, A. H., et al.: Simple fecal tests of absorption—a prospective study and critique. Am. J. Dig. Dis., *16*:97, 1971.

Morgan, E., et al.: Evaluation of tests for occult blood in the feces. J.A.M.A., *164*:1664, 1957.

Morris, D. W., Hansell, J. R., Ostrow, J. D., et al.: Reliability of chemical tests for fecal occult blood in hospitalized patients. Am. J. Dig. Dis., *21*:845, 1971.

Newcomer, A. D.: Disaccharidase deficiencies. Mayo Clin. Proc., *48*:648, 1973.

Newcomer, A. D., and McGill, D. B.: Disaccharidase activity in the small intestine: Prevalance of lactase deficiency in 100 healthy subjects. Gastroenterology, *53*:881, 1967.

Onstad, G. R., and Zieve, L.: Carotene absorption, a screening test for steatorrhea. J.A.M.A., *221*:677, 1972.

Ostrow, J. D., Mulvaney, C. A., and Hansell, J. R.: Sensitivity and reproducibility of guaiac, Hematest, and Hemoccult test for fecal occult blood. Ann. Intern. Med., *76*:860, 1972.

Ostrow, J. D., Mulvaney, J. R., Hansell, J. R., et al.: Sensitivity and reproducibility of chemical tests for fecal occult blood with an emphasis on false-positive reactions. Am. J. Dig. Dis., *18*:930, 1973.

Peranio, A., and Bruger, M.: The detection of occult blood in the feces including observation on the ingestion of iron and whole blood. J. Lab. Clin. Med., *38*:433, 1951.

Pihl, H. D., and Hepler, P. E.: Stains for fat in feces. Am. J. Clin. Pathol., *23*:1373, 1953.

Reiner, M., and Cheung, H. L.: Xylose. *In* Meites, S. (ed.): Standard Methods of Clinical Chemistry. New York, Academic Press, 1965, vol. 5, p. 257.

Rose, G. A.: Experiences with the use of interrupted carmine red and continuous chromium sesquioxide marking of human feces with reference to calcium, phosphorus, and magnesium. Gut, *5*:274, 1964.

Rufin, F., Blahd, W. H., Nordyke, R. A., et al.: Reliability of I^{131}-triolein test in the detection of steatorrhea. Gastroenterology, *41*:220, 1961.

Santiago-Borrero, P. J., Santini, R., Jr., and Moldonado,

N.: The xylose excretion test in normal children and in pediatric patients with tropical sprue. Pediatrics, *48*:59, 1971.

Satterwhite, T. K., and Dupont, H. L.: The patient with acute diarrhea: An algorithm for diagnosis. J.A.M.A., *236*(23):2662, 1976.

Saunders, D. R.: Medium chain triglycerides and the Van de Kamer method. Gastroenterology, *52*:135, 1967.

Schiff, L., Stevens, R. J., Shapiro, N., et al.: Observation on the oral administration of citrated blood in man: The effects on the stool. Am. J. Med. Sci., *203*:409, 1942.

Spencer, R. P.: Use of radioisotopes in evaluation of the gastrointestinal canal. *In* Behrens, C. F., King, E. R., and Carpender, J. W. J.: Atomic Medicine, 5th ed. Baltimore, The Williams & Wilkins Co., 1969, pp. 672.

Stroehlein, J. R., Farrbanks, U. F., McGill, D. B., et al.: Hemoccult detection of fecal occult blood quantitated by radioassay. Am. J. Dig. Dis., *21*:841, 1976.

Sun, D. C. H., and Shay, H.: An evaluation of the starch tolerance test in pancreatic insufficiency. Gastroenterology, *40*:379, 1961.

Thompson, H. L., and McGuffin, D. W.: Melena, a study of underlying causes. J.A.M.A., *141*:1208, 1949.

Tuna, N., Mangold, H. K., and Mosser, D. G.: Re-evaluation of the I[131]-triolein absorption test. J. Lab. Clin. Med., *61*:620, 1963.

Van de Kamer, J. H., ten Bokel Huinink, H., and Weyers, H. W.: Rapid method for the determination of fat in feces. J. Biol. Chem., *177*:347, 1949.

Watson, C. J., Schwartz, S., Sbarov, V., et al.: Studies of urobilinogen. V. A simple method for the quantitative recording of the Ehrlich reaction as carried out with urine and feces. Am. J. Clin. Pathol., *14*:605, 1944.

Weber, P. M., O'Reilley, S., Pollycover, M., et al.: Gastrointestinal absorption of copper. Studies with ^{64}Cu, ^{95}Zr. A whole-body counter and the scintillation camera. J. Nucl. Med., *10*:591, 1969.

Wegner, J., Kirsner, J. B., and Palmer, W. L.: Blood carotene and steatorrhea and the malabsorptive syndrome. Am. J. Med., *22*:373, 1957.

Wells, C. L., Moran, T. J., and Cooper, W. M.: Villous tumors of the rectosigmoid colon with severe electrolyte imbalance, a cause of unexplained morbidity and sudden mortality. Am. J. Clin. Pathol., *37*:507, 1962.

Wollaeger, E. E., Comfort, M. W., and Osterberg, A. E.: Total solids, fat and nitrogen in the feces. III. A study of normal person taking a test diet containing a moderate amount of fat, comparison with result obtained with normal person taking a diet containing a large amount of fat. Gastroenterology, *9*:272, 1947.

Wolochow, D. A.: A rapid method for quantitative determination of fecal fat based on the principle of electrical capacitance. J. Lab. Clin. Med., *65*:334, 1965.

Winawer, S. J., and Sherlock, P.: Detecting early colon cancer. Hosp. Prac., March, 49–56, 1977.

26

CYTOGENETICS

Jorge J. Yunis, M.D.,
and Mary E. Chandler, Ph.D.

Human cytogenetics evolved into a medical discipline after Tjio (1956) found the correct number of chromosomes in man and a simple technique for obtaining metaphase chromosomes by lymphocyte culture was introduced (Hungerford, 1959; Moorhead, 1960). Autosomal trisomies 21, 18, and 13 were soon described (Lejeune, 1959; Edwards, 1960; Patau, 1960); Turner's and Klinefelter's syndromes were confirmed as sex chromosome anomalies by karyotype analysis (Ford, 1959; Jacobs, 1959); and the consistent association of the Philadelphia chromosome with chronic myelogenous leukemia became established (Nowell, 1960b).

Autoradiographic techniques were found to be useful in identifying the X chromosome and the autosomes most frequently involved in chromosomal anomalies owing to their differential times of replication (Yunis, 1965). However, cytogeneticists were not yet able to identify most of the human chromosomes with certainty. Although many cases exhibiting abnormal chromosomes or chromosome segments were known, it was not possible to correlate clinical signs with specific chromosome abnormalities.

In 1968 Caspersson reported that plant chromosomes exhibit a distinctive fluorescence pattern after quinacrine mustard staining. The importance of this finding was not immediately realized until the same technique was applied to human chromosomes and a specific banding pattern was observed in each chromosome pair (Caspersson, 1970).

This development, as well as that of other staining techniques which also allow the visualization of differentially stained bands in chromosomes, proved to be the beginning of a series of explosive advances in human cytogenetics. Since then, at least eight tumors and myeloproliferative disorders have been found to exhibit a consistent chromosome defect; over 30 new congenital chromosomal syndromes have been defined; and a large number of isolated cases of partial trisomy or partial deletion have been described involving every chromosome (Lewandowski, 1975; Sanchez, 1977). In many instances, one of the parents of an individual with partial trisomy or deletion is found to be a carrier of a balanced chromosome translocation, making proper counseling and prenatal diagnosis particularly useful in preventing the recurrence of these disorders.

Recently developed techniques for the routine analysis of high resolution early mitotic chromosomes in man (Yunis, 1976; Yunis, 1978c and 1978d) can be used to uncover previously undetected chromosome defects, to localize the exact break points involved in numerous duplication-deficiencies, and to establish possible phenotype-genotype relationships at a refined level (Yunis, 1977b). It is likely that minute chromosome defects will be uncovered with this technology in a large number of patients previously diagnosed as having "idiopathic" mental retardation, "idiopathic" growth retardation, multiple miscarriages, or antisocial behavior, and in patients with neoplasia or multiple congenital defects previously diagnosed as having "normal" chromosomes by metaphase analysis.

INDICATIONS FOR CYTOGENETIC TESTING

Chromosome defects are relatively common in the human population. While some of them are acquired after birth, such as those found in neoplastic tissue, many are congenital, including those associated with the chromosomal syndromes. A list of clinical situations which benefit from chromosome or sex chromatin analysis is shown in Table 26-1. As discussed below, these conditions illustrate the propensity for certain types of phenotypic findings among the congenital chromosome defects, as well as the role of chromosomes in other genetically predisposed and acquired clinical entities.

It has been estimated that close to 0.7 per cent of liveborn infants have a chromosomal aberration (Hook, 1977). These patients can generally be recognized because they exhibit

Table 26-1. INDICATIONS FOR CYTOGENETIC ANALYSIS

Multiple congenital anomalies associated with mental retardation
Unexplained mental or growth retardation
Infertility
Cryptorchidism, small testes, and/or hypogonadism
Primary amenorrhea
Ambiguous genitalia
Multiple miscarriages
Neonatal death and stillbirths associated with congenital defects
Prenatal diagnosis for advanced maternal age or familial chromosome translocation
Malignancies
Myeloproliferative syndromes and refractory anemias
Bone marrow transplant
Chromosomal breakage syndromes

certain features characteristic of either an autosomal defect or a sex chromosome anomaly. Those with multiple congenital defects at birth and with associated delayed growth and neuromotor development in infancy should be suspected of having an autosomal abnormality. Persons exhibiting disturbance of gonadal function or of reproductive ability either at puberty or in adult life may have a sex chromosome defect. More specifically, cytogenetic evaluation (sex chromatin and/or chromosome analysis) should be considered in females with poor development of secondary sexual characteristics, primary amenorrhea, or sterility. In these cases it is not uncommon to find trisomy-X, Turner syndrome (XO), or the XO/XX or XO/XXX mosaicism forms of Turner syndrome. Male hypogonadism with small testicles and/or sterility should bring to mind the possibility of Klinefelter syndrome, since it has been detected in 10 per cent of males examined in infertility clinics (Williams, 1966). Infants born with ambiguous genitalia require sex chromatin or chromosome analysis to determine the true genetic sex so that proper corrective measures can be instituted. Often these patients have one of the various forms of adrenogenital syndrome and can be effectively treated with steroid therapy.

Prenatal diagnosis is indicated in mothers over the age of 35, since advanced maternal age is known to be associated with an increased frequency of autosomal trisomy (chromosomes 13, 18, or 21) and sex chromosome aneuploidy (XXX, XXY, XYY). Indeed, it has been determined that there is a 1 in 50 chance of having a chromosomally defective child by mothers between the ages of 35 and 39, and that the risk rises to 1 chance in 30 for mothers aged 40 to 44 years (Milunsky, 1977). Another group for whom prenatal diagnosis is recommended is that of couples in which one has been previously diagnosed as carrying a balanced reciprocal translocation. The parents may have been recognized because they had a child with a chromosome defect or are close relatives of an affected child. Known carriers have a theoretical risk of 50 per cent of having an abnormal child. However, the actual risk in each case depends upon the chromosomes involved, the specific type of chromosome translocation, selection against abnormal gametes, and lower viability of chromosome deletions. Also, in cases of Robertsonian translocation or centric fusion, as is usually the case in familial

Down's syndrome between chromosomes 21 and 14, or 21 and 22, carriers have a theoretical risk of 33 per cent of having an abnormal child. In practice, if the female is the carrier, there is a risk of approximately 8 per cent, while male carriers have a risk of only about 2 per cent of having an offspring with Down's syndrome.

Parents who carry a balanced chromosome translocation, as well as those who have an inversion of a chromosome segment, may be found among couples who experience three or more first trimester miscarriages. The analysis of late prophase or prometaphase chromosomes in these patients is of particular importance since these more finely banded chromosomes can reveal subtle types of structural rearrangements.

A specialized situation in which cytogenetic analysis is becoming of increasing importance is in following the progress of bone marrow transplants. When the donor and recipient are of opposite sex, the simple analysis of sex chromosomes in metaphase cells from marrow or blood is useful to determine the origin of the cells populating the marrow. When they are of the same sex, however, the study of polymorphic variations of centromeric regions, such as those seen with Q- or C-banding, is essential.

Another application of chromosome analysis is in the differential diagnosis of certain syndromes which exhibit an increased predisposition to chromosome breakage, such as Fanconi's anemia, Bloom's syndrome, and ataxia telangiectasia. For example, the presence of a high percentage of chromosome breaks in a patient suspected of having Fanconi's anemia and the presence of a large number of sister chromatid exchanges in a patient thought to have Bloom's syndrome become quite useful in the clinical assessment of these conditions (German, 1974).

As mentioned previously, neoplasias are well known to exhibit many different types of chromosomal changes. Recently it has become apparent that chromosome analysis of malignant tissues, particularly of bone marrow in leukemia, represents an important part of the management of such patients. This is due to the fact that specific defects have been consistently found in certain types of neoplasia and that the chromosomal findings have a prognostic and therapeutic value. For example, the 90 per cent of patients with chronic myelogenous leukemia (CML) who exhibit a 22/9 translocation have a longer mean survival time and respond better to treatment than CML patients without this specific defect.

CHROMOSOME BANDING, NOMENCLATURE, AND IDENTIFICATION

BANDED CHROMOSOMES

Four basic staining techniques were initially developed for chromosome banding, that is, Q-banding, C-banding, G-banding, and R-banding. Because these methods are still the most widely used, a brief description follows.

The *Q-banding* technique, the first banding procedure described (Caspersson, 1970), utilizes either quinacrine mustard or quinacrine dihydrochloride. After staining, each chromosome exhibits a characteristic sequence of bands, alternately brightly and faintly fluorescent, along the length of each arm (Fig. 26-1) such that all chromosomes can be readily identified (Caspersson, 1970). The distal half of the long arm of the Y chromosome fluoresces intensely, allowing easy recognition of this chromosome in interphase as well as in mitotic cells (see p. 829 on Sex Chromatin Tests) (Pearson, 1970; Mittwoch, 1974). In addition, pericentromeric regions exhibit polymorphic variations in size and staining intensity which are simply inherited (Fig. 26-2). Although the Q-bands were accepted as a main reference banding pattern and the technique remains one of the simplest of the banding methods, fluorescence microscopy is required, the preparations are not permanent, and the fluorescence of small minor bands or subbands is difficult to appreciate. This technique has been largely replaced by the G- and R-banding techniques in routine blood culture studies but continues to be utilized in some laboratories for staining bone marrow chromosomes, owing to difficulties in obtaining satisfactory G- or R-banding in cells from this tissue (Rowley, 1974). Also, because of the clear visualization of polymorphic pericentromeric variations, Q-banding is used in specialized situations, such as in following the progress of bone marrow transplants, in determining the parental origin of the extra or missing chromosome in aneuploid patients, and in paternity cases.

In 1971, Yunis and Arrighi described techniques which induce intensive staining with

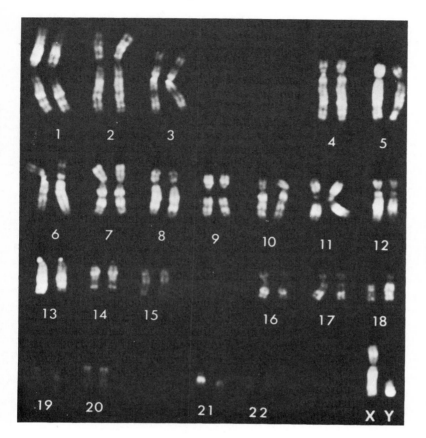

Figure 26–1. Flourescent banding pattern of chromosomes of a normal male. Note characteristic differential features of each chromosome pair. Bright fluorescence of the distal half of the long arm of the Y chromosome is equivalent to the Y body of interphase nuclei. (From Uchida, 1974.)

Giemsa of pericentromeric regions and the distal half of the long arm of the Y chromosome. Designated as *C-banding*, these methods make use of denaturation/renaturation of chromosomal DNA using heat or alkaline-heat treatment and are selective for constitutive heterochromatin. This small well-defined chromatin fraction remains condensed and darkly staining in interphase and is located around the centromeres on both the short and long arms of all chromosomes, except for the Y chromosome in which it is located in the distal end of the long arm. C-bands vary greatly in size between the various chromosomes, depending upon the amount of constitutive heterochromatin present, with chromosomes 1, 9, and 16 and the distal segment of the long arm of the Y chromosome exhibiting the largest amounts. Almost every individual with a normal phenotype has polymorphic size variations of one or several pericentromeric regions, similar to that observed with Q-banding (Fig. 26-3). These variants make C-banding useful in similar types of specialized situations, such

as transplant studies, determinations of the parental origin of extra or missing chromosomes, and in paternity studies.

Based on variations of the C-banding techniques, several investigators independently observed that it was possible to elicit a banding pattern throughout the chromosome arms with Giemsa and related Romanowsky stains, which was designated as *G-banding*. These G-banding techniques, as well as others subsequently developed, require a chromosomal pretreatment step using one of many diverse reagents, such as trypsin or a heated salt solution, to induce chromosome bands (Yunis, 1974a). Such pretreatments are difficult to control with precision and may destroy or affect the quality of minor fine bands, particularly on elongated chromosomes. This problem has been circumvented by the development of a simple and direct Wright's staining technique that produces excellent G-banding in two or three minutes (Fig. 26-4 and p. 824).

G-banding shows a similar banding pattern to that obtained with Q-banding except that

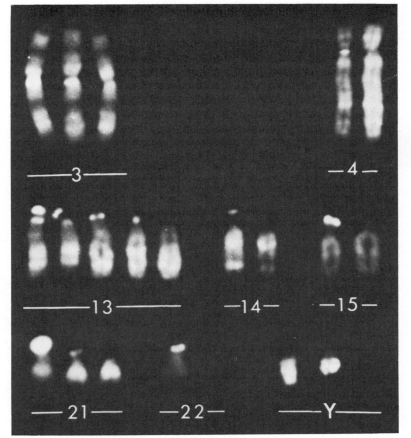

Figure 26–2. Some normal morphologic variants in fluorescent bands obtained from different subjects. The sizes and intensities of the bright bands are constant for a subject and for those among his relatives who have inherited the same chromosome. Chromosomes 3 and 4 have the variant bands adjacent to the centromere. The acrocentric chromosomes are characterized by satellites and short arms of different intensities and sizes. Note in particular the unusually large satellite on one chromosome No. 21. Three Y chromosomes are shown ranging in size from a large 13-like to a tiny and barely visible chromosome. Since these variants are inherited, they are useful as genetic markers. (From Uchida, 1974.)

Figure 26–3. Normal and polymorphic patterns of C-bands in autosomes 1, 9, and 16 and in the Y chromosome from human leukocytes. For autosomes 1, 9, and 16 the first pair shows the normal pattern of C-bands, while the other two are polymorphic. The Y chromosomes show a small amount of positive staining on the pericentromeric regions and varying amounts on the distal portion of the long arms. (From Yunis, 1972.)

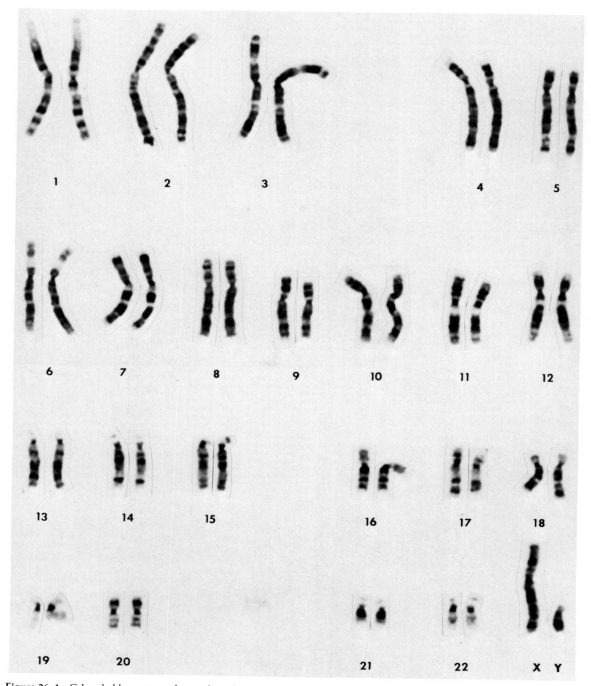

Figure 26–4. G-banded karyotype of metaphase from an amethopterin-synchronized lymphocyte of a normal male. Over 440 bands per haploid set are observed. (From Yunis, 1977b.)

most pericentromeric regions are negatively stained with quinacrine but darkly stained with the G-banding technique. In addition, the distal half of the long arm of the Y chromosome stains less intensely with Giemsa. One disadvantage of G-banding is that several telomeric bands stain lightly and are difficult to visualize with accuracy at mid-metaphase. G-banding is the most widely utilized banding method in the United States, since it is simple, produces permanent chromosome preparations, and requires only standard laboratory and microscopic equipment.

Based on minor modifications of the original technique for C-bands of Yunis (1971), Dutrillaux (1971) described a heat-Giemsa staining procedure that elicits banding patterns on chromosomes which are, in general, the reverse of those induced by Q- and G-banding methods. Known as *R-banding*, positively stained R-bands are Q- and G-negative and vice versa (Fig. 26–5). Recently, R-bands have also been obtained with the use of high concentrations of sodium phosphate and staining with acridine orange. As with the G-banding techniques, most of the R-banding methods described require aging of slides and a pretreatment step (Dutrillaux, 1977). One of the important features of this technique is that most of the telomeric and centromeric regions stain positively, permitting a more precise analysis of chromosome arm and total chro-

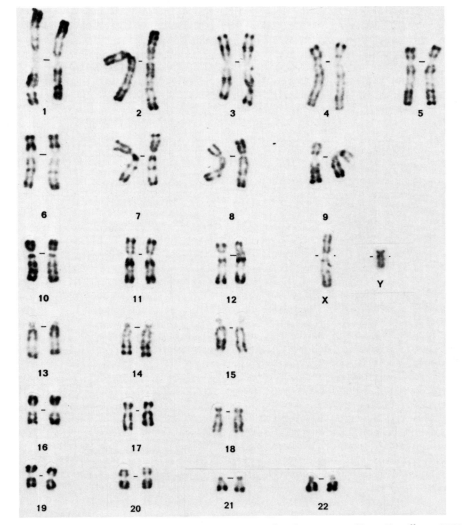

Figure 26–5. Karyotype of a male metaphase showing R-banding pattern. (From Dutrillaux, 1977.)

mosome length, as well as the detection of small abnormalities affecting telomeres.

Numerous new banding techniques have been developed since the four major methods (Q, C, G, and R) were originally described. Because most of them represent only staining or chromosome pretreatment variations that yield one of the already established banding patterns, they have been given the appropriate letter designation of Q-, C-, G-, or R-band techniques. Certain others represent new methods, such as those that preferentially stain telomeres (T-bands) or permit visualization of sister chromatid exchanges, and are useful in specialized situations (Dutrillaux, 1977; Sanchez, 1977).

NOMENCLATURE OF BANDED CHROMOSOMES

The advent of the chromosome banding techniques prompted an international conference in Paris in 1971 for agreement on a nomenclature system to describe the bands of mid-metaphase chromosomes (Paris Conference, 1971). To accomplish this, the specific banding patterns obtained in each chromosome pair with the use of Q- and G-banding were used to construct a banded ideogram of the human karyotype (Fig. 26-6). Constant and distinctive morphologic features, such as centromeres, telomeres, and well-defined bands, were selected as "landmarks." The chromosomal arms (p designating short arm and q long arm) were divided into "regions," a region being defined as "the area of a chromosome lying between two adjacent landmarks." The regions in each arm, as well as the bands contained within each region, were numbered consecutively from the centromere toward the telomere (Fig. 26-7A).

Using the recommendations set forth by the Paris Conference, each band is described by listing in order, without spacing or punctuation, the chromosome number, arm symbol, region number, and band number. For example, 6p23 indicates chromosome 6, short arm, region 2, band 3. To describe a subband, a decimal point is placed after the original band designation, followed by the number assigned to the subband. Subbands derived from a given band are also numbered sequentially from the centromere outward; the first subband proximal to the centromere of the above example would thus be written 6p23.1 (Fig. 26-7B).

The participants of the Paris Conference (1971) developed two systems for the designation of structural abnormalities: a "short system," which is a simple modification of the Chicago nomenclature (Chicago Conference, 1966), and a "detailed" system, which identifies precisely the type of arrangement and defines each abnormal chromosome by its band composition. Table 26-2 lists symbols commonly used in the descriptions; a more complete listing can be found in Sanchez, 1977. The short system is easier to understand, is much more commonly used, and is more appropriate for those who are clinically oriented. In this system, the total number of chromosomes is indicated first, followed by the sex chromosome constitution; next comes the symbol representing the chromosomal abnormality, followed in parentheses by the number(s) of the involved chromosome(s) and, in a second parentheses, the band number(s) where the breaks occurred. From this information the band composition of the abnormal chromosome(s) can be inferred. For example, 46,XY,t(2;6)(q34;p12) describes a male karyotype of 46 chromosomes in which a reciprocal translocation has occurred between chromosomes 2 and 6 with break points in the long arm of chromosome 2, region 3, band 4, and in the short arm of chromosome 6, region 1, band 2. Note that the first chromosome listed (number 2) corresponds to the first band indicated in the following parentheses (q34) and both are separated by semicolons from the

Table 26-2. COMMONLY USED SYMBOLS RECOMMENDED BY THE CHICAGO (1966) AND PARIS (1971) CONFERENCES

X, Y	the sex chromosomes
diagonal (/)	separates cell lines in describing mosaicism
cen	centromere
dic	dicentric
i	isochromosome
inv	inversion
mar	marker chromosome
mat	maternal origin
p	short arm of chromosome
pat	paternal origin
q	long arm of chromosome
r	ring chromosome
t	translocation
del	deletion
dup	duplication
ins	insertion
ter	terminal end (pter = end of short arm; qter = end of long arm
→	from-to

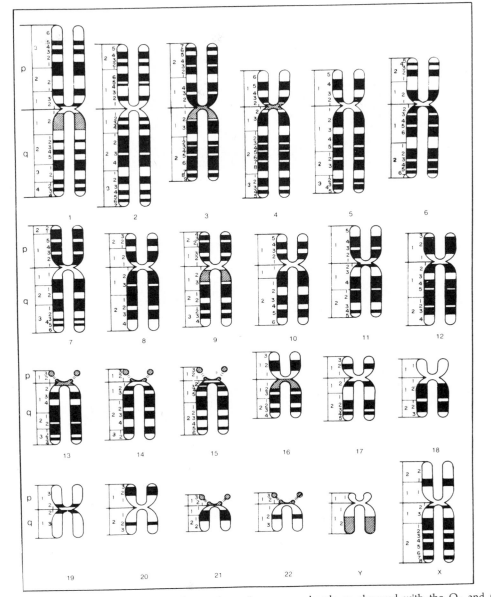

Figure 26–6. Diagrammatic representation of metaphase chromosome bands as observed with the Q- and G-banding methods; centromeres representative of Q-banding method only. (Reproduced from the report of the Paris Conference, 1971.)

other chromosome (number 6) and its corresponding band (p12). In this example, it can be inferred that the person carrying the translocation has two abnormal chromosomes, a number 2 having a segment of the short arm of chromosome 6 attached to its long arm, and a number 6 carrying a segment of the long arm of chromosome 2 attached to its short arm (Fig. 26–8).

The nomenclature of the Paris Conference also provides a way to designate an unbalanced karyotype, such as those possible in the offspring of a balanced translocation carrier. Referring back to the previous example in which the short system is used, if a son received from his carrier father the abnormal chromosome 2 and a normal chromosome 6 (all other paternal and maternal chromosomes assumed to be normal), his karyotype would be written as follows: 46,XY,der(2)t(2;6)(q34;p12)pat. This indicates that a male with 46 chromosomes has an abnormal chromosome 2 derived from a

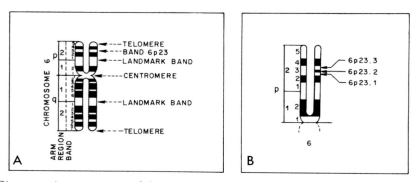

Figure 26-7. *A,* Diagrammatic representation of chromosome 6 in mid-metaphase according to the Paris Conference (1971). *B,* Diagrammatic representation of chromosome 6 in an earlier stage of mitosis, illustrating the denotation of subbands of band 6p23. (From Sanchez, 1977.)

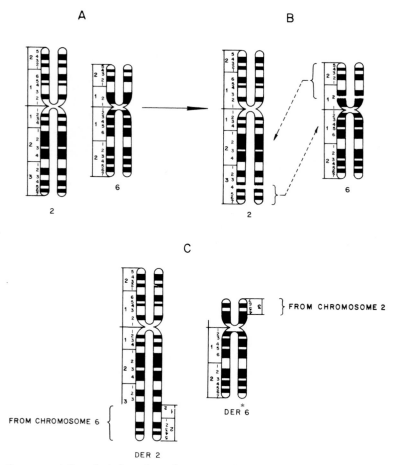

Figure 26–8. Schematic representation of a balanced translocation involving chromosomes 2 and 6.* Derivative chromosome. (From Sanchez, 1977.)

balanced translocation in the father involving chromosomes 2 and 6. This description also implies that the boy has a partial trisomy for a segment of the short arm of chromosome 6 (6p12 to 6pter, which is attached to the derivative chromosome 2) and a monosomy for part of the long arm of chromosome 2 (2q34 to 2qter, which is absent in the derivative chromosome 2). Additional examples and information can be found in Sanchez (1977) and the Paris Conference (1971).

Although the Paris Conference banding pattern ideogram has been widely accepted for the general identification of metaphase chromosomes, it has been found to be of limited value in defining chromosome segments because the representation of bands was constructed with the use of visual estimates. A revised ideogram, based on measurements of the actual placement, width, and number of bands and utilizing 6 different shades to describe various staining intensities of G-banded chromosomes, has been recently reported by Yunis (1978c) (Fig. 26-9). In comparing the mid-metaphase ideogram of Yunis with that of the Paris Conference (1971), 74 additional subbands, as well as differences in the size and position of many bands, are observed (Fig. 26-9). These discrepancies are due to improvements in the more recent study, which include minimal exposure of cells to colcemid to minimize chromosome condensation, increased resolution, and the more accurate method used to characterize bands. In addition, in a few areas only one band is seen instead of the two or three depicted in the Paris Conference ideogram. These generally occur in pericentromeric regions that stain positive with G-banding but negative with the Q-banding, which was used as the reference pattern in representing these regions at the Paris Conference.

With the introduction of high resolution chromosome techniques, cells in the various early stages of cell division, namely, late prophase, prometaphase, and early metaphase, as well as mid-metaphase, can now be routinely used (Yunis 1978c and d). Using a large number of representative chromosomes, it has been possible to draw a schematic representation of every chromosome at each of the four mitotic stages, based on their average length, width, and centromeric position, which illustrate the size, position, and staining intensity of every band. These schemes are shown in Figure 26-10. As seen in these figures, the G-positive and, to some extent, the G-negative bands of mid-metaphase result from a coalescence of finer subbands of earlier stages. Each band and its corresponding subbands maintain a constant position relative to its centromere-telomere length and usually, although not always, a similar staining intensity throughout cell division. Late prophase chromosomes were found to exhibit twice the length and slightly more than half the width of mid-metaphase chromosomes. Similarly, each segment of bands in late prophase corresponding to a major band in mid-metaphase was twice as long as its metaphasic counterpart. Chromosomes and chromosome bands in prometaphase and early metaphase were found to be intermediate in length.

In assigning band and subband numbers to the longer and finely banded chromosomes, the Paris Conference (1971) recommendation was followed which states that any subband, seen either in mid-metaphase or in an earlier stage, should be classified as a subband and assigned an arbitrary number (Fig. 26-10). This nomenclature is advantageous in that it is easy to use, subbands are readily related to the well-known bands of mid-metaphase, and even the highly banded chromosomes of late prophase can be reasonably described (Fig. 26-10). However, ambiguities may arise, such as in describing the precise location of a gene or a pathogenic segment, since the numbers assigned to certain subbands vary from stage to stage. It may be necessary, therefore, to develop a different international nomenclature for use with prophasic chromosomes based on the maximum number of bands observed rather than the minimum, as was done with mid-metaphases.

CHROMOSOME IDENTIFICATION

When human chromosomes are closely examined at various stages of chromosome condensation, it is apparent that the banding patterns are consistent at any given stage and that the general appearance of a particular chromosome usually remains similar from late prophase to mid-metaphase (Fig. 26-10). In addition, certain bands are quite conspicuous and serve as useful markers for identification of chromosomes and chromosome segments. The combined use of size, centromeric index, and distinctive bands makes possible a general description of characteristic features that facilitates the identification of G-banded chro-

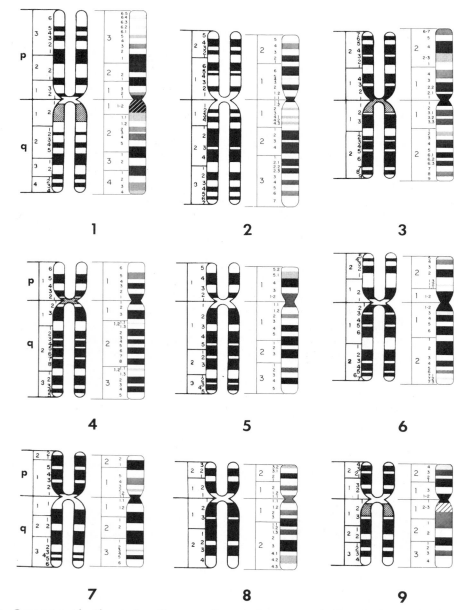

Figure 26–9. Comparison of mid-metaphase ideograms. For each chromosome, the Paris Conference (1971) representation is on the left and the pattern found by Yunis (1978d) on the right. In the latter schematic representation of chromosomes, shading illustrates the staining intensities of G-positive bands. Variable regions are indicated by diagonal stripes. Note differences in the size, position, and number of bands. (From Yunis, 1978d.) (*Illustration continued on opposite page*)

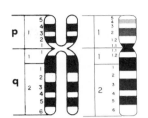

10

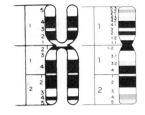

11

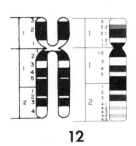

12

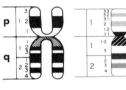

13

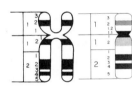

14

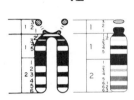

15

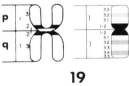

16

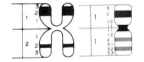

17

18

19

20

21

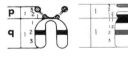

22

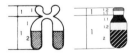

Y

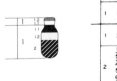
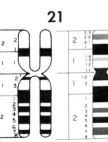

X

Figure 26–9 *continued.*

mosomes. Unless indicated, the following description of bands and subbands of the individual chromosomes will be based on patterns seen in mid-metaphase, but it is also applicable to the corresponding subbands present in early metaphase, prometaphase, and late prophase.

Chromosome 1. Chromosome 1 is the largest and most metacentric chromosome in the complement. It is readily identified by its size, its centromeric position, and its charac-

teristic banding pattern which is distinguished by the weakly staining distal third of the short arm and the darkly staining centromeric block of the long arm (q12). Inherited variations in size occur in this heterochromatic material, so that in some individuals, band q12 may be quite small and in others it may contain as much as twice the usual amount. The distal half of the long arm is characterized by three dark bands of similar size (q31, q41, q43), which are progressively less stained toward

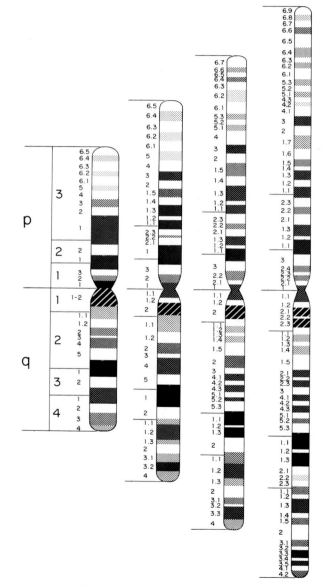

Figure 26–10. Schematic representation of G-banded human chromosomes at different stages of mitosis: from left to right, each chromosome is represented in mid-metaphase, early metaphase, prometaphase, and late prophase. (From Yunis, 1978c and d.)

the telomeric end. The very dark band in the middle of the long arm (q31) and the one in the proximal segment of the short arm (p21) remain conspicuous and basically undivided from late prophase to mid-metaphase.

Chromosome 2. Chromosome 2 is the largest submetacentric chromosome and its dark bands stain with a similar intensity. The short arm is somewhat evenly banded, with the first proximal dark band (p12) being prominent, particularly in prometaphase and early metaphase. The long arm has a more distinctive appearance, with the proximal region (q1) being the lightest staining segment of the chromosome. In this region, the two dark subbands of band q14 (q14.1 and q14.3) are especially prominent as a pair in late prophase and prometaphase. In addition, the two

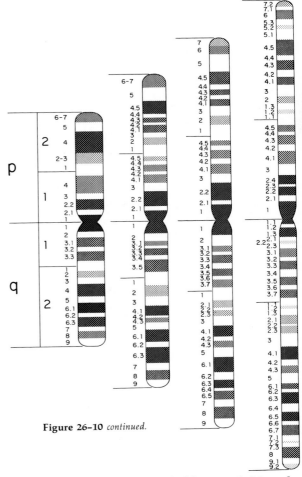

Figure 26–10 *continued.*

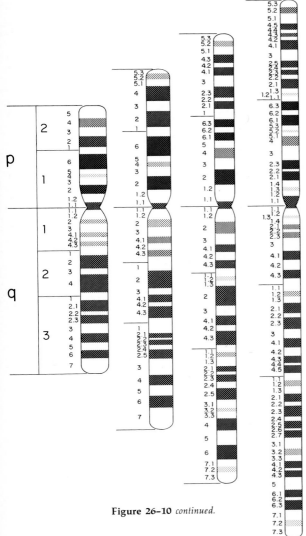

Figure 26–10 *continued.*

most distal dark bands of this arm (q34 and q36) remain distinctive features from prophase to metaphase.

Chromosome 3. Chromosome 3 is the second largest metacentric chromosome and the two arms give the impression of a symmetrical banding pattern. It usually appears very darkly stained throughout with a prominent light area midway in the short arm (p21) and slightly above midway in the long arm (q21). The short arm has a characteristically rounded and darkly staining end. The proximal regions of both the short (p1) and long (q1) arm are dark and exhibit a relatively non-distinct banding pattern. In the long arm, the most distal dark band (q28) is relatively thin but distinctive, followed by a lightly staining telomere.

Chromosome 4. Chromosome 4 is a darkly staining and large submetacentric chromosome. The short arm has a relatively large and faintly staining telomere and two prominent dark bands in its middle portion (p13 and p15). Of these two bands, the more proximal (p13) is more intensely stained and is subdivided in late prophase. The more distal dark band (p15) is subdivided in both late prophase and prometaphase. The long arm has a somewhat evenly banded appearance, with the proximal dark band (q13) being the largest and most conspicuous.

Chromosome 5. Chromosome 5 is a large submetacentric chromosome similar in size and centromeric position to chromosome 4. The short arm exhibits a prominent very dark band in the middle (p14), and the long arm is characterized by a dark block of bands located in the central one-third of the arm (q14-q23). Other important features are the two prominent dark bands of the distal third of the long arm (q32 and q34), which generally remain as single bands throughout mitosis. Together the above-mentioned characteristics make chromosome 5 rather easy to identify at all stages.

Chromosome 6. Chromosome 6 is the

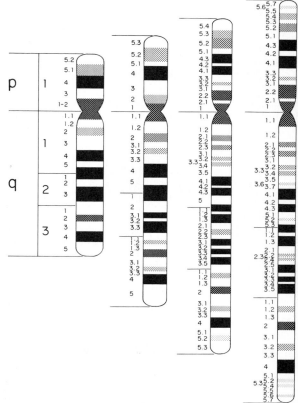

Figure 26-10 *continued.*

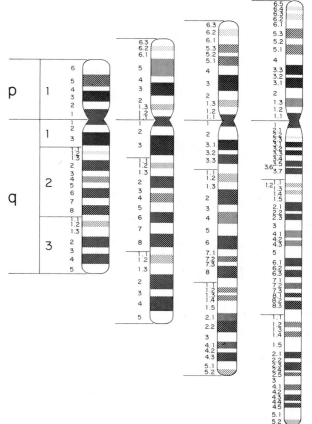

Figure 26-10 *continued.*

largest of the intermediate-sized submetacentric chromosomes (6-12 and X). The short arm is readily recognized by a very large light staining band (p21), which is usually subdivided in the middle by a minute weakly staining subband (p21.2). Except for an average-sized light band in its mid-portion (q21), the long arm features a predominance of darkly staining bands. Of these, the dark bands q16 and q22 appear more intensely stained in prometaphase and late prophase.

Chromosome 7. Chromosome 7 exhibits a distinctive large dark band in the distal end of the short arm (p21). It is followed by a very faintly staining telomere, often causing this band to appear terminal, particularly at mid-metaphase. The middle portion of the long arm shows two very large and very dark bands (q21 and q31), representing a coalescence of several closely apposed dark subbands of late prophase and prometaphase. Because of its overall characteristic appearance, this is one of the easiest chromosomes to identify.

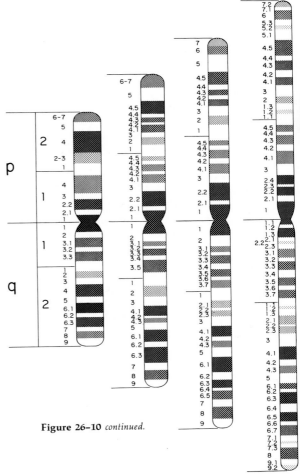

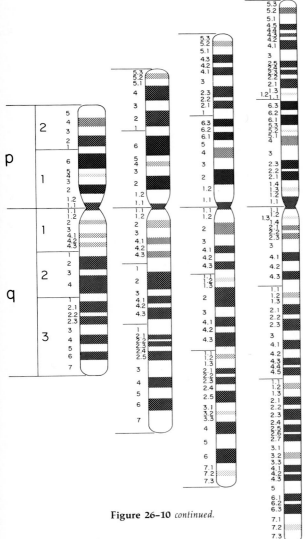

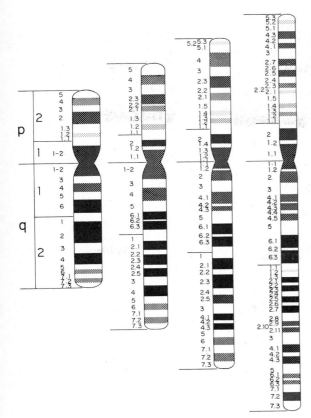

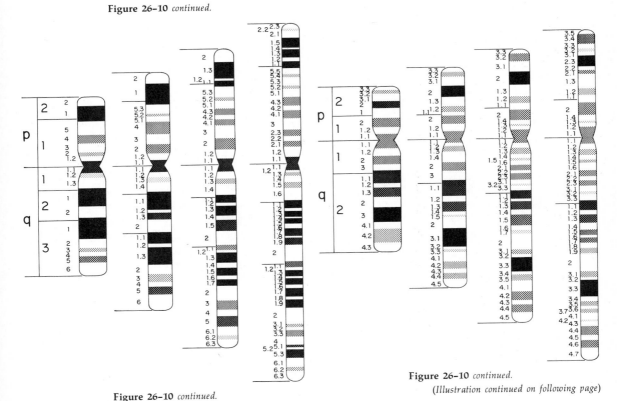

Chromosome 8. Chromosome 8 has a rather indistinct pattern except for the small but intensely staining band (p22) in the distal half of the short arm, which helps to identify this chromosome in all stages. In mid- and early metaphase, the long arm is identified by a prominent dark band (q23) in its distal third. This chromosome may at times be confused with chromosome 9, particularly in late prophase.

Chromosome 9. The short arm of chromosome 9 has a relatively large proximal light band (p13), followed by two dark bands (p21 and p23). This large light band (p13), as well as the central position of the more prominent dark band (p21), stands out as one of the major differential features between chromosomes 8 and 9. The long arm of chromosome 9 shows a pericentromeric band (q12) of variable size and staining intensity, followed by a large and moderately stained dark band (q21). In addition, in the middle of the long arm there is a large light band (q22) which maintains its obvious appearance in late prophase and prometaphase.

Chromosome 10. In this chromosome, the short arm is characterized by a dark band near the middle (p12) and a second, less prominent

Figure 26–10 *continued.*

Figure 26–10 *continued.*

Figure 26–10 *continued.*

(Illustration continued on following page)

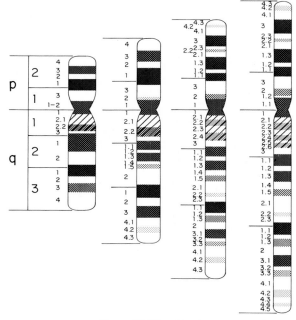

Figure 26–10 *continued.*

although they are more subtle in late prophase due to the delicate subbanding pattern. The most proximal band (q21) is typically the most intensely stained. The light bands that space the three dark bands are helpful in late prophase to distinguish chromosome 10 from 8 and 9.

Chromosome 11. Chromosome 11 is the least submetacentric chromosome of the 6-12 and X group. The short arm is larger than that of chromosome 12 and can be distinguished by two conspicuous dark bands (p12 and p14.1), the latter being the more prominent and located in the middle. The long arm is distinctive, with a very large, weakly staining band near the centromere (q13) and two large and very dark bands (q14 and q22) located in the middle portion of the arm.

Chromosome 12. Chromosome 12 is the most submetacentric of the 6-12 and X group with a central large dark band (p12) occupying most of its short arm. The long arm has a very noticeable proximal light band (q13), smaller than that found in chromosome 11. The central portion of this arm is dominated by a large dark block of bands (q14-q23), which is more subdivided and occupies a greater portion of the arm than the central dark block in chromosome 11. In late prophase and prometaphase the distal third of the long arm of chro-

dark band adjacent to the telomere (p14). The long arm is distinctive, showing three somewhat evenly spaced dark bands in metaphase. These three bands are apparent at all stages,

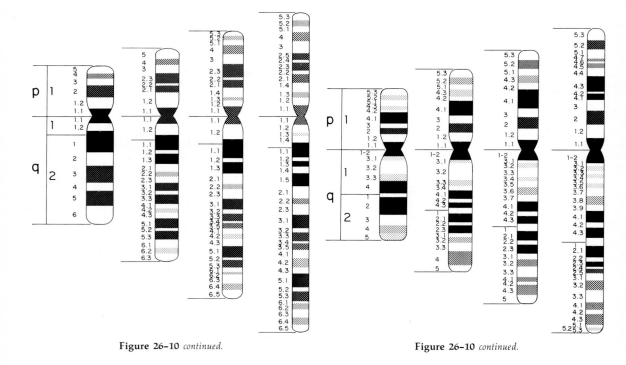

Figure 26–10 *continued.*   **Figure 26–10** *continued.*

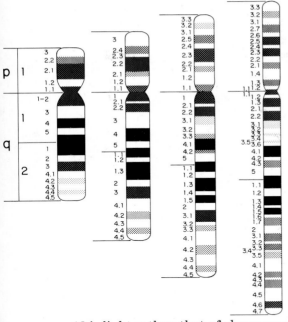

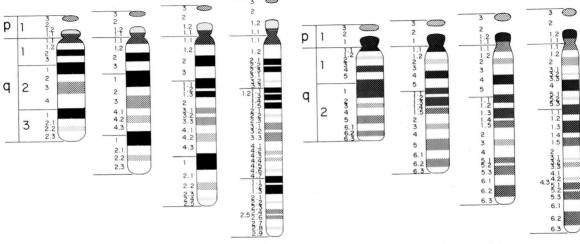

Figure 26–10 *continued.*

mosome 12 is lighter than that of chromosome 11 and can be used as an additional differential feature.

Chromosome 13. Chromosome 13 is the only one of the large acrocentric chromosomes (13-15 group) in which the distal portion of the long arm appears more darkly staining than the proximal segment. The middle third of the long arm has two rather large and very dark bands (q21 and q31), which are followed by another less intensely staining distal dark band (q33). The proximal segment of the long arm stains weakly except for band q13.

The short arm of chromosome 13, as well as that of the other large (14-15) and small (21-22) acrocentric chromosomes, is polymorphic in nature. Variations in size may occur in the heterochromatic satellite region (p13), the nucleolar organizer or secondary constriction (p12), and the short arm proper (p11).

Chromosome 14. The long arm of this acrocentric chromosome has two very dark bands in its proximal third (q12 and q21) and a conspicuous, very darkly staining band (q31) within an otherwise lightly staining distal portion. This dark band is usually undivided and serves as the main identifying characteristic at any stage.

Chromosome 15. Chromosome 15 is the most weakly staining of the larger acrocentric chromosomes. The distal half of the long

Figure 26–10 *continued.*

Figure 26–10 *continued.*

(Illustration continued on following page)

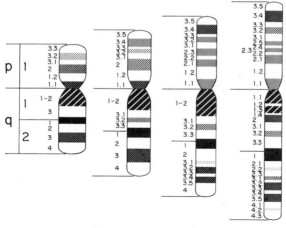

Figure 26–10 continued.

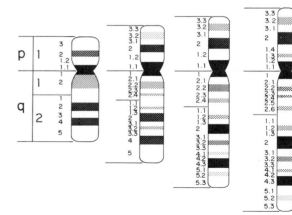

Figure 26–10 continued.

arm is light, while the proximal half is distinguished by two moderately staining bands, one small (q14) and the other large (q21). In prophase, the large dark band is subdivided and the two distal dark bands (q25 and q26.2) are more prominent, making the long arm appear evenly banded but with less staining intensity distal to the middle.

Chromosome 16. Chromosome 16 is the largest and most metacentric of the smaller 16-18 group chromosomes. The G-positive bands and subbands of the short arm are lightly to moderately stained and poorly differentiated, giving this chromosome arm a characteristic indistinct appearance. In the long arm the most prominent feature is the large darkly staining pericentromeric heterochromatic region (band q11), which may show variable length between individuals. In the middle of the long arm there is an intensely staining band (q21) and, more distally, a moderately staining band (q23), both of which remain as blocks from prophase to metaphase and are useful distinguishing features.

Chromosome 17. Chromosome 17 is a small lightly staining submetacentric chromosome with a medium staining dark band (p12) near the middle of the short arm and a pair of dark bands (q22 and q24) in the distal half of the long arm. In the space between the latter two bands, a distinct subband is clearly seen in late prophase and prometaphase. This third band also occurs in early metaphase but is less pronounced. The light staining band (q21) in the proximal portion of the long arm is useful in discerning chromosome 17 from chromosome 18.

Chromosome 18. Chromosome 18 is small, submetacentric, and one of the most darkly staining chromosomes. The short arm is small and has a G-positive telomere. The long arm is characteristically dark and evenly banded with a distinctive light band in the middle (q21), which is most pronounced in prometaphase and early metaphase. Its location is more distal than the similar appearing band in chromosome 17.

Chromosome 19. Both the short and long arms of this small metacentric chromosome are very weakly staining, the short arm being the lightest staining region in the entire chromosome complement. Only the relatively large pericentromeric area (p11-p12 and q11-q12) stains intensely. This segment often shows variation in the proportions of pericentromeric material located on the short and long

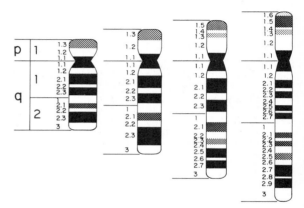

Figure 26–10 continued.

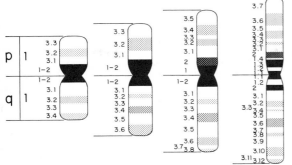

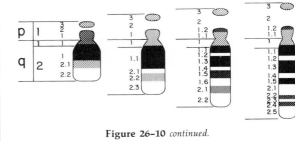

Figure 26–10 *continued.*

Figure 26–10 *continued.*

arms. The lightly staining subbands seen in both chromosome arms are more obvious in early stages, such as subbands p13.2 and q13.4, which also appear subdivided in late prophase.

Chromosome 20. Chromosome 20 is a small metacentric chromosome, appearing much like 19 except for a very characteristic dark band in the short arm (p12). It has a darkly staining pericentromeric region, which is smaller than that of chromosome 19, and two evenly spaced dark bands (q12 and q13.2) distinguishing the long arm. In late prophase these bands are rather diffuse, leading to some confusion between it and chromosome 19.

Chromosome 21. Chromosome 21 is a very small and easily identifiable acrocentric chromosome. It stains darkly except for the lightly staining distal half of the long arm. This band (q22) often shows a delicate darker staining subband (q22.1), which in turn is subdivided in late prophase.

Chromosome 22. Chromosome 22 is also acrocentric and, along with chromosome 19, is one of the lightest staining chromosomes in the complement. It characteristically has a

darkly staining centromeric region and a fine dark band slightly above the middle of the long arm (q12). In earlier stages, this band is subdivided, giving the chromosome a distinctive appearance.

Y chromosome. The Y chromosome is the smallest submetacentric chromosome of the complement and has a dark staining appearance. The distal portion of the long arm (q12) stains intensely, exhibits the most variation in size of any segment in the complement, and is subdivided into several subbands in prometaphase and late prophase.

X chromosome. The X chromosome is a medium-sized submetacentric chromosome having a relatively long short arm with a noticeable broad dark band (p21) in its mid-portion. The long arm has a large darkly staining proximal band (q21) followed distally by three smaller and moderately staining bands (q23, q25, and q27). These features are recognizable in prometaphase, early metaphase, and mid-metaphase. In late prophase, however, the long arm has a more evenly banded appearance, while the short arm maintains its broad, dark band in the middle of the short arm. Sometimes this chromosome is confused with the number 10, but by carefully noting the intensities of the bands it becomes apparent that chromosome 10 in late prophase is more intensely stained in the proximal portion of

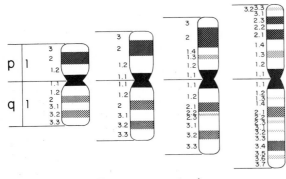

Figure 26–10 *continued.*

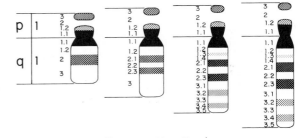

Figure 26–10 *continued.*
(*Illustration continued on following page*)

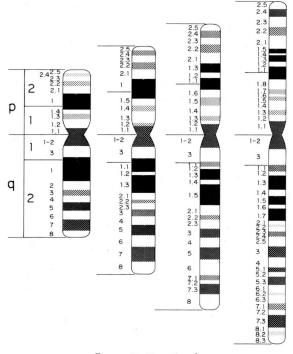

Figure 26–10 *continued.*

the long arm, while the X chromosome is darker in the distal portion of the long arm (bands q23, q25, and q27).

CHROMOSOME TECHNIQUES

Tissues which are utilized for chromosome analysis are composed of cells that either exhibit an inherently high mitotic rate or can be readily stimulated to divide in culture (Yunis, 1974). Those in which cells are actively dividing (bone marrow, tumors) can be treated briefly with colcemid, passed directly into hypotonic solution, and then fixed and stained. If

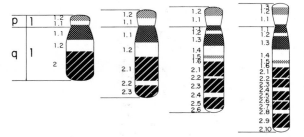

Figure 26–10 *continued.*

desired, the yield of mid-metaphases can be increased by incubating the tissue with colcemid for an extended period (one to four hours) before hypotonic treatment. Other types of tissue (blood, skin, amniotic fluid) are cultured until active cell division is initiated. Blood is the tissue of choice for routine chromosome analysis of birth defects owing to its accessibility, satisfactory response to stimulation, short culture (three to four days), and high quality of chromosomes obtained.

From blood, only lymphocytes undergo division in culture. Lymphocytes are very hardy cells and have been successfully cultured as long as two days post mortem. Their capability for survival under adverse conditions also makes it feasible to mail blood over long distances that may require one to two days for transit (Mellman, 1974). It should be noted, however, that blood samples yield few mitoses unless a mitogenic agent is added. Phytohemagglutinin (PHA) is by far the most efficient and widely used mitogen.

Bone marrow chromosome spreads may be examined within a few hours of sampling or after an overnight culture. This is due to the high mitotic activity of marrow, which virtually guarantees that metaphase figures will be obtained. Unfortunately, bone marrow is inconvenient to sample and not recommended for routine use except when hematopoietic disorders, such as leukemias and refractory anemias, are being investigated.

Fetal cells, obtained by drawing a small amount of amniotic fluid transabdominally during the fourteenth to sixteenth week of pregnancy, is the method of choice for prenatal diagnosis of chromosome defects. Fetal cells require a longer culture time than blood lymphocytes in order to obtain a sufficient number of dividing cells, generally 10 to 14 days.

Of several solid tissues used for chromosome analysis, the most common are skin and tumor tissue (Harnden, 1974). Skin samples are inconvenient to obtain and, once cultured, require several (two to four) weeks for adequate growth. During this time, they are susceptible to contamination, sensitive to alterations of pH and electrolyte content of the medium, and require frequent medium changes. Although skin tissue is not recommended for routine use, it becomes of value when searching for an elusive mosaic chromosome pattern. Tissue from solid tumor is usually directly harvested or cultured overnight. The technique is simple but has not become of practical importance in the diagnosis, prognosis, and treatment of solid neoplasms. Instead, direct analysis of pleural effusions or ascites fluid is used in some laboratories to rule out the possibility of metastatic processes (Dewald, 1976).

Occasionally, chromosome analyses of specialized tissues are undertaken in the routine laboratory. For example, postmortem tissue may be the only material accessible. In this case, cultures can be obtained from either skin, fascia, spleen, bone marrow, or lymph nodes. Placental tissue can be used in the study of habitual abortion, and testicular biopsies provide meiotic figures for the study of certain chromosome rearrangements.

BLOOD

As mentioned earlier, peripheral blood lymphocytes, stimulated to divide in culture and then arrested in mitosis, are the most widely used cell type for obtaining human chromosomes. This has been made possible by the recognition of the stimulatory property of phytohemagglutinin (Nowell, 1960) and the development of a simple peripheral blood culture method (Moorhead, 1960). Incorporated into a basic culturing technique, either whole blood or separated leukocytes are incubated in defined culture medium supplemented with serum and phytohemagglutinin at 37°C. for three to four days. The dividing cells are then arrested in mitosis with the use of colcemid, exposed to hypotonic treatment, "fixed" in an alcohol–acetic acid fixative, and air dried on slides (Mellman, 1974). The standard techniques yield almost exclusively midmetaphase chromosomes because a long exposure to colcemid is used (two to three hours) to obtain sufficient mitoses (1 to 5 per cent) for analysis.

A major advance in obtaining high numbers of mitotic cells at various stages of cell division was recently made with the recognition of the usefulness of synchronized cell cultures. In 1976, Yunis developed a lymphocyte culture technique which utilizes amethopterin (Methotrexate) as a cell synchronizing agent. Cells are prevented from replicating their DNA in the presence of this compound and accumulate at the G_1/S border. Upon release of the block with the addition of thymidine, cells complete DNA replication in synchrony and can be arrested as mitosis is reached. With this synchronization technique, the wave of mitotic cells may be collected early (5 hours and 5 minutes after release) with only a minimal

exposure to colcemid (0.06 $\mu g/ml$ for 10 min). This serves to inhibit spindle fiber formation while minimizing chromosomal condensation, and allows the attainment of a relatively large number of cells (8 to 13 per cent) in late prophase, prometaphase, early metaphase, and mid-metaphase.

Cell Culture and Synchronization. One ml of peripheral blood is drawn into a sterile syringe containing approximately 20 units of preservative-free heparin (Upjohn) and mixed well. Blood may also be obtained by a finger or toe prick. RPMI 1603 media (Gibco, special order) is supplemented with 20 per cent fetal calf serum (Gibco), 2.0 per cent penicillin-streptomycin (5000 units/ml penicillin and 5000 $\mu g/ml$ streptomycin; Microbiological Associates), and 0.25 per cent mycostatin (Squibb). Four drops of heparinized blood and 0.2 ml phytohemagglutinin M (Difco) are added to 5 ml of complete media in a 30-ml culture flask (Falcon), which is tightly capped and placed in an upright position in a water-jacketed incubator at 37°C. After 72 hours growth, amethopterin (Methotrexate; Lederle) is added at a final concentration of 10^{-7} M (e.g., 50 μl of 10^{-5} M solution to each 5-ml culture) to induce synchrony (Yunis, 1976). Following 17 hours of additional incubation at 37°C., cells are released from the amethopterin block. To this end, the contents of two flasks are combined into one sterile 16 by 125 mm tube (Falcon) and centrifuged at 200 g (1100 rpm in clinical centrifuge) for 8 minutes. The supernatant is aspirated off, leaving approximately 0.5 ml above the pellet. Ten ml of unsupplemented RPMI 1603 media at room temperature is then added and the pellet is resuspended by inversion and centrifuged. After completion of a second wash, the cells in each tube are resuspended in 10 ml of complete RPMI 1603 media containing 10^{-5} M thymidine (Sigma) (e.g., 1 ml of a 10^{-3} M solution per 100 ml media), which is then placed in a clean, sterile culture flask and returned to the incubator. The cells are allowed to grow at 37°C. for 5 to 5½ hours, followed by treatment with 0.05 to 0.12 $\mu g/ml$ colcemid (Gibco) for 10 to 120 minutes at 37°C. It has been our experience that a release period of 5 hours, 5 minutes or 5 hours, 10 minutes, followed by a 10 minute colcemid treatment of 0.06 $\mu g/ml$, usually results in the most elongated chromosomes as well as a high mitotic index (see below).

To harvest the cells, the contents of each flask are poured into a siliconized 15-ml centrifuge tube and centrifuged at 200 g for 8 minutes. The supernatant is aspirated off, leaving approximately 0.5 ml above the pellet, which is then gently resuspended by tapping the tube with a finger. Eight ml of 0.075 M KCl at 37°C. is gently added in 2 to 3 ml amounts and then mixed gently but thoroughly with a siliconized Pasteur pipette. Cells are placed in an incubator or water bath at 37°C. for 10 minutes. The tubes are then centrifuged at 200 g for 5 minutes, after which the supernatant is aspirated off except for 0.2 to 0.4 ml and the cells resuspended in fresh 3:1 methanol:acetic acid fixative exactly according to the following. The pellet is first partially resuspended by tapping the tube, and the fixative is then slowly added drop by drop with a Pasteur pipette, while gently shaking the tube to keep the cells in suspension during the process of fixation. Approximately 1 to 2 ml of fixative is added in this manner, followed by thorough mixing with the pipette; an additional 4 to 5 ml is added and mixed thoroughly. Each tube is then tightly sealed with Parafilm. After a period of 20 to 30 minutes, the tubes are centrifuged at 200 g for 5 minutes and the fixative changed. The fixative change should be repeated at least 4 to 6 times to eliminate cell debris and insure excellent spreading and staining of mitoses. If possible, chromosome preparations should be made the same day; otherwise, cells may be stored in the refrigerator overnight in 4 to 6 ml of fixative in tubes tightly covered with double Parafilm, but they must be allowed to come to room temperature and be rinsed 2 to 3 times with fresh fixative before spreading onto slides.

Slide Preparation and Spreading. Chromosome spreading is an important aspect of slide preparation with cells of any stage but becomes increasingly difficult with prometaphase and late prophase chromosomes owing to their increased length and tendency to overlap. Adequate separation of early mitotic chromosomes is possible if several essential steps are followed. Slides should be cleaned thoroughly with 70 per cent ethanol in distilled water. The cells, after fixation and rinsing with 3:1 methanol:acetic acid, are resuspended in freshly prepared 6:1 methanol:acetic acid at a dilute concentration. For example, a cell pellet of less than 0.1 ml is diluted with approximately 1 ml, followed by the addition of more diluent as needed. This is most easily determined by checking the first two slides of each pellet for cell concentration under phase microscopy or with brightfield microscopy using a lowered condenser. Preparations are made by dropping 2 to 3 drops of the cell suspension from a height of approximately $2\frac{1}{2}$ to 3 feet onto each slide set at a 30 to 45 degree angle. Both wet cold (4°C.) and dry room temperature slides should be tested, since one method may be more successful than the other with a particular pellet.

Relationship of Colcemid Treatment to Mitotic Stages Obtained. Colcemid, as well as its natural analog colchicine, is very effective in preventing formation of the spindle fiber, thereby arresting cells in mitosis. Unfortunately, it also causes condensation and contraction of the chromosomes directly. The number of cells arrested in mitosis and the degree of chromosome contraction, which determines the actual stages in which the cells are harvested, are directly correlated with colcemid concentration, exposure time, and temperature. By varying these parameters of colcemid

treatment on amethopterin-synchronized cells, it is possible to obtain selectively the types of cells desired. For example, 17 to 25 per cent of mid-metaphases can be harvested with 0.12 μg/ml (e.g., 120 μl of a 10 μg/ml solution/10 ml culture) colcemid for 2 hours at 37°C. To obtain approximately 8.0 to 12.5 per cent mitoses with a predominance of early metaphases and some prometaphases, 0.08 μg/ml colcemid for 30 minutes at 37°C. is suggested. For more refined studies, such as in cases where a minute chromosome defect is suspected, the use of 0.05 to 0.06 μg/ml colcemid for 10 minutes at room temperature (20 to 22°C.) or 37°C. will result in 6 to 8 per cent of cells in mitosis, with a majority in prometaphase or late prophase.

Staining of G-bands. The technique recommended is advantageous in that it requires no chromosome pretreatment yet elicits sharp and well contrasted G-bands with a minimum of time, reagents, and equipment. It is, however, important that the details given, such as source of stain, preparation of stock solution and buffer, and the actual staining procedure, are followed closely. Wright's stain (Manufacturing Chemists) is prepared at a concentration of 0.25 per cent in anhydrous acetone-free methanol in 1-liter quantities. After stirring in an airtight container with an electric stirrer for 30 to 60 minutes, the stain is filtered with double No. 1 filter paper into clean, dark 1-pint bottles and stored airtight for at least one month. Phosphate buffer for dilution consists of 490 ml solution A (0.06 M Na_2HPO_4) and 510 ml solution B (0.06 M KH_2PO_4), adjusted to pH 6.8 and stored airtight.

During the staining procedure exact timing is extremely important; therefore, a maximum of two slides should be stained at one time. Optimum time appears to be between $2\frac{1}{2}$ and 4 minutes, and the stock solution should be diluted with methanol, if necessary, to achieve this range. For each bottle of stock solution, several trials are necessary to determine the approximate staining time; the exact time will then vary by several seconds depending on the source of cells, age of slides, and room temperature (ideal temperature and relative humidity for banding appear to be 22 to 24°C. and 40 per cent respectively). It should also be noted that prophases require a few seconds longer than metaphases.

To stain, the Wright's stock solution is diluted 1:3 with phosphate buffer (4 ml total/slide) in a clean tube, mixed rapidly, and poured *immediately* onto the slide. After exact timing, the slide is rinsed quickly with tap water and dried with an air jet.

Inadequately stained slides can sometimes be improved by further rinsing and restaining. For example, a 5 to 30 second rinse in running tap water may be employed to minimize cytoplasmic background or improve overstained slides. Rinsing may even be as long as several minutes, followed by restaining for 30 to 60 seconds, and possibly another rinse. Understained slides may also be restained or rinsed and restained. Progress of staining is most easily monitored with the use of an Epiplan 80× microscope objective which does not require the application of oil to the slide.

Ideally, slides should be aged at least 10 and up to 60 days before staining to ensure excellent banding patterns. For more routine chromosome studies, however, it is often possible to forgo the aging requirement by destaining with a series of alcohol solutions and then restaining with Wright's stain. To destain, fresh slides which have already been stained are dipped into the following reagents in the given order for the stated time: 95 per cent ethanol—2 minutes; chloroform—15 seconds; 95 per cent ethanol containing 1 per cent concentrated HCl—30 seconds; methanol—2 minutes.

Slides are dried with an air jet between solutions, which are changed daily. A maximum of two slides should be destained at the same time. If a slide has previously been checked with the use of an oil immersion objective, the oil must be removed by rinsing in several changes of xylol and dried before destaining. Restaining is carried out in the same manner as the initial staining and for a similar time. For very freshly made preparations, two to three destain/restain series may be best, but more than three times usually affects the chromosome morphology. This procedure can also be used to improve slides that were initially over- or under-stained.

Scanning of Cells. Slides are most easily scanned using a low-power (for example, 10× or 16×) brightfield objective and 12.5× wide-angle oculars. Satisfactory mitotic figures should be moderately numerous (one or two per low-power field with low exposure to colcemid and three or four with more extensive colcemid treatment). When selecting cells for analysis, they should appear well-spread, rounded, and well-banded. Elongated or extensively stretched out spreads may actually be broken cells with artificially missing or sometimes extra chromosomes. Satisfactory mitoses are recorded by use of stage coordinates.

Chromosome Analysis. The number of chromosomes per mitosis is most easily counted directly using a 100× oil immersion objective. Although there are many different counting techniques, it is probably easiest to mentally divide each mitotic figure into imaginary geographic areas and count the chromosomes in each. Most laboratories determine the chromosome number in 20 to 30 well-spread and intact mitoses. Counts can be recorded in a tabular form, such as the following:

Chromosome	<45	45	46	47	>47
Number of cells	1	1	28	0	0

The modal number is the number of chromosomes present in the largest number of cells, which is 46 in the example above. Counts below the modal number are to be expected, since even in good preparations, 3 to 5 per cent of cells will be non-modal through chromosome loss (factitious hypoploidy). This percentage increases if excessive hypotonic treatment has been used. As stated earlier, this is most likely to be encountered in elliptical or strung out mitotic figures.

Mosaics exhibit two or more modal numbers owing to the presence of two or more cell lines with different chromosome constitutions. If there is the slightest suspicion that more than one cell line may be present—for example, if two or more cells have the same chromosome extra or missing—it is necessary to analyze an additional 50 to 70 mitoses to rule out mosaicism.

When screening for structural defects, selected mitoses should be analyzed under oil immersion, as with determinations of chromosome number. In fact, it is easiest to first count the chromosomes of a particular spread, and then to analyze each chromosome pair and its banding patterns carefully. An abnormality noted must be substantiated in at least 5 to 10 of the best quality spreads, since one of several morphologic artifacts may be present in a given cell. For example, homologous chromosomes in the same cell may appear not to exhibit the same banding pattern owing to slight differences in the degree of contraction and non-uniform staining. In addition, there can be a mosaic pattern for a given structural defect, making it difficult to conclude that an abnormality is present and emphasizing the need for thorough analysis of an adequate number of cells.

Photography. It is usually easier, better, and less expensive to analyze mitoses directly through the microscope. Photography, however, is important in certain difficult cases and is useful for confirmation and permanent recording of what was observed. Mitoses are selected for photography on the basis of (a) containing the modal number of chromosomes; (b) having sharply banded chromosomes; (c) having a clear background; (d) showing no artifacts (air bubbles, stain particles, coverglass imperfections, etc.); (e) being rounded or oval (elongated and elliptical mitoses often have lost chromosomes); and (f) showing little or no chromosome overlap.

Of critical importance for chromosome analysis and photography is the use of high quality microscopic equipment, as well as certain procedures which maximize resolution. Microscopes with excellent optical systems (Zeiss, Leitz), a planachromat or a planapochromat 100× oil objective (N.A. 1.3), and a planachromat condenser (N.A. 1.4), are highly recommended. A monochromatic light filter, such as Schott filter, type PIL, which blocks all but a narrow wavelength range of monochromatic light, and the placement of oil (Cargille oil R.I. 1.515) between slide and condenser are important in photography to increase detail.

Proper illumination is best provided by Kohler's illumination and brightfield optics. Built-in lamps can be easily adjusted for Kohler's illumination, and the technique should be reviewed and mastered before photography is attempted (Yunis, 1965).

The most commonly available photographic setup for routine photography of metaphases is the microscope-mounted 35 mm camera. Photographs are taken with black-and-white film. Kodak Plus-X Pan or Panatomic-X 35 mm film has been satisfactory in our laboratory for mid- and early metaphases.

When photographing more elongated chromosomes, such as those from late prophase and prometaphase cells, a 4 by 5 inch microscope-mounted camera should be used to record the very fine banding patterns observed. This attachment magnifies the image by a factor of 1.6, providing a $1600\times$ final magnification when used with a $100\times$ oil objective and a $10\times$ eyepiece. For adequate illumination, the 4 by 5 inch camera necessitates the utilization of a high-intensity xenon lamp instead of the more common tungsten light system. Film recommended is 4 by 5 inch Kodak Plus-X professional film 4147 because of its fine grain and good tone range. We have obtained excellent results with this film when it is slightly underexposed and overdeveloped (15 minutes at 20 to 22°C. with Kodak D-76 instead of the recommended 6 minutes) to improve contrast. Using a high-quality enlarger (Omega) with variable condenser and componon objectives, prints should be exposed on Kodabromide F-5 photographic paper such that development with Dektol requires $1\frac{1}{2}$ to 2 minutes. Careful attention to these details ensures excellent band contrast without loss of fine detail.

Interpretation of Analyses. Interpretation is facilitated if the clinical features of the patient are known. As a general rule, the larger the autosome or autosome segment affected, the worse the phenotypic defect produced. Gains of chromosomal material are better tolerated than losses. Extra autosomes larger than 13 have not been found (except in mosaic patterns, such as trisomy 8 or 9 mosaics) in living patients, nor have missing autosomes (except, rarely, a chromosome 21 or 22).

Deciding whether mosaicism is truly present is not easy if one cell line accounts for less than 10 per cent of the total cell population. Criteria for identifying true mosaicism include (1) the incidence of non-modal cells should be greater than chance expectation; (2) the non-modal cells must have the same karyotype; (3) the mosaic pattern persists on repeated examination of the same tissue and is demonstrable in different tissues.

AMNIOTIC FLUID

The use of transabdominal amniocentesis to obtain fetal cells for cytogenetic evaluation is now an integral part of prenatal diagnostic procedures. Amniocentesis should be performed as early as possible so that proper treatment can be initiated if desired and in case the cells do not grow and the procedure must be repeated. However, since the procedure is difficult and hazardous when performed before the fourteenth week of gestation, the recommended time is usually between the fourteenth and seventeenth weeks of gestation, with the optimum time at 16 weeks. (See Chapter 20.)

The amniotic fluid contains cells derived mainly from fetal skin, genitourinary, alimentary and respiratory tracts, vagina, conjunctiva, and amnion, which divide in culture. It is important to realize that both fibroblast-like cells and epithelium-like cells, which are morphologically distinguishable from each other, may proliferate. In every culture the proportion of each can be extremely variable and should be followed. This is because the fibroblast-like cells grow fast, readily undergo long-term culture, and usually present no problem in obtaining good cytogenetic preparations. On the other hand, epithelium-like cells grow slowly and senesce in two to four weeks. Chromosome preparations should be obtained as early as possible (within 10 to 20 days), although this will essentially depend upon the growth rate of cells in culture. To obtain a large number of mitotic cells for chromosome analysis, it is important to maintain an optimum density of amniotic cells in culture. Too sparse a population causes cells to undergo a lag phase of growth, whereas too dense a population causes contact inhibition.

Amniocentesis is now a routine procedure that may be performed as an office procedure by an obstetrician. The risk appears to be very low. In fact, a four-year Amniocentesis Registry Project study by the National Institutes of Child Health and Human Development Department, published in 1976, showed no increase in fetal loss in 1040 cases of mid-trimester amniocentesis as compared with 992 matched controls. In experienced laboratories where care is taken to maintain proper cell culture techniques, successful results can be obtained in 95 per cent of the cases.

Many variations in the method of culturing amniotic cells can be found. For instance, samples may be concentrated by gentle centrifugation (100 g for 10 minutes) and resuspended in a small amount of amniotic fluid or fetal calf serum (Nadler, 1974). The concentrated cells can then be suspended in growth medium or amniotic fluid and cultured in culture flasks (Coriell, 1973), Petri dishes (Milunsky, 1971), or tissue culture chambered slides (Lab Tech Laboratories). In some instances, a sterile coverslip can be used to immobilize the amniotic fluid cells (Nadler, 1974). The method described below is the one currently in use in our laboratory. Like others in the literature, it is primarily used for the analysis of mid- and early metaphases. In the future, it may be possible to adapt microculture cell synchronization techniques, such as that described by Singh, 1975, for the rapid analysis of earlier mitotic cells.

Method

Approximately 10 ml of amniotic fluid in a sterile tube is gently mixed and placed into two sterile 30-ml flasks (Falcon). Flasks are incubated lying flat with screw caps slightly loosened in 5 per cent carbon dioxide at 37°C. The culture flasks may be checked after two to three days of culture for signs of cell attachment and growth. Small isolated colonies of long, spindle-shaped fibroblasts can usually be observed after five to seven days. After this time, the original amniotic fluid is replaced with 5 ml of Dulbecco's Modified Eagle Medium (Gibco) containing 20 per cent fetal calf serum (Gibco), 2 per cent penicillin-streptomycin (5000 units/ml penicillin and 5000 μg/ml streptomycin; Microbiological Associates), and 0.25 per cent mycostatin (Squibb). The medium is then changed every two to three days by pipetting or pouring off the old medium and replacing it with fresh complete medium. When three to five large colonies (over 100 cells per colony) are observed in a flask with the aid of an inverted microscope, the cells are trypsinized to promote even growth. To this end, the medium is removed from the flask and the cells washed three to four times with 3 to 4 ml of Puck's saline A (Gibco) adjusted to a pH of 7.5 with 4.3 per cent sodium bicarbonate. 0.5 ml of 0.25 per cent trypsin EDTA (Difco) in Puck's saline is then added to the flask and the cells are watched with the use of an inverted microscope. When the cells are seen to detach from the surface (approximately 3 to 5 minutes), 2 ml of complete medium is added and the cells are drawn up into a pipette and blown out several times to break up the colonies. The medium is then added up to 5 ml per flask and the cultures are returned to the incubator. Subsequently, when flasks have an even and heavy, yet non-confluent growth, they are each subdivided into two to four flasks.

Usually the best time to harvest is 24 hours after trypsinization. To determine whether the cultures are suitable for harvesting, flasks can be scanned under the inverted microscope. "Rounded-up" cells are usually undergoing mitosis and if the number of these cells is sizable, the culture can be harvested. To harvest, colcemid is added to each flask at 0.06 μg/ml. After 30 to 60 minutes, the cells are trypsinized as described above and the cell suspensions from three or four flasks are pooled into one tube and centrifuged at 200 g for 10 minutes. The procedures for swelling, fixation, and spreading of the cells on slides are similar to those described for peripheral blood lymphocytes, except that amniotic cells appear to be more fragile. To minimize cell breakage during spreading, the suspension is dropped from a height of only two inches.

Special Precautions. Some of the problems that may be encountered in prenatal diagnosis of cytogenetic aberrations include maternal cell contamination, polyploidy, mosaicism, and bacterial or mycoplasmal contamination. Maternal cells grow rapidly in tissue culture by comparison with amniotic cells. Caution should be exercised, therefore, when cultures grow more rapidly than usual. To help prevent the problem of maternal cells, it has been suggested that the first 2 ml of amniotic fluid drawn be discarded (Nadler, 1974). Also, whenever possible, chromosome analysis should be performed separately on two or more different culture vessels.

Polyploidy, in particular tetraploidy, is observed in some amniotic cell cultures, particularly if harvested after three or four weeks growth. Since individuals with tetraploidy/diploidy mosaicism are very rare, and tetraploid cells in amniotic cultures may be found with relatively high frequency in some laboratories, it is best to assume that this phenomenon is generally a culture artifact and to explain this to parents seeking prenatal studies in case a true diploid/tetraploid mosaic is missed.

Other factors that should be considered with amniotic cell culture include contamination by bacteria or mycoplasma and pH variation of the culture medium. The medium for culturing amniotic cells should be kept between pH 6.8 and 7.2. Variation in pH can stop cell growth, and alkaline pH in particular may induce aneuploidy (Ford, 1973). Of critical importance is maintenance of sterile culture conditions. Contamination by mycoplasma, for instance, has been found to cause a significant increase in chromosome breakage (Scheider, 1974). Sterile disposable plasticware should be used whenever possible and airborne contamination can be effectively avoided by working in a laminar flow hood. For a detailed discussion of quality control measures in tissue culture, the reader is referred to Kruse, 1973.

Bone Marrow

Unlike peripheral blood lymphocytes, bone marrow cells exhibit a high mitotic activity and can be harvested directly and karyotyped. However, it is advisable to set up short-term cultures (16 to 20 hours) whenever enough material is obtained, since the number and quality of mitotic cells available for analysis is extremely variable from one patient to another. Bone marrow studies are routinely performed on persons suspected of possessing a hematopoietic disorder and especially on those with leukemias, myeloproliferative syndromes, refractory anemias, and tumor metastases.

A disadvantage of the study of marrow cells, particularly leukemic cells, is that the chromosomes often have a "fuzzy" appearance. Another problem relates to the difficulty in consistently obtaining a large number of well-spread and relatively elongated metaphases, since a brief exposure of cells to colcemid (15 to 20 minutes) results in fewer available mitoses, and longer colcemid exposure (1 to 2 hours) tends to produce an undesirable contraction of chromosomes.

A short-term culture of marrow (16 hours) followed by 5 hours exposure of cells to cold (4°C.) results in a relatively large number of elongated mitoses, since cold inhibits the formation of spindle fibers and cells accumulate in mitosis without the undesirable condensation effect of colcemid.

Direct Harvest. Two or three drops (0.1 to 0.2 ml) of well-mixed marrow are added within 5 minutes of aspiration to a siliconized tube containing 10 ml of 0.075 M KCl and 0.02 μg/ml of colcemid (Gibco). Contents in the tube are mixed by inversion and incubated in a 37°C. water bath for 20 minutes. At the end of the incubation, the mixture is centrifuged at 200 g for 8 minutes and the supernatant is aspirated, leaving approximately 0.5 ml above the pellet. The tube is gently tapped to resuspend the pellet and the cells are fixed, spread, and stained as described for peripheral blood lymphocyte preparations. It is important to process samples immediately after aspiration, since they generally yield a significantly higher number of mitoses than those processed 30 minutes to an hour later. Also, it should be noted that when colcemid is used in combination with the hypotonic treatment, it is much more effective and a lower dose (0.02 vs. 0.08 μg/ml) is needed.

Short-term Culture. 0.5 ml of heparinized bone marrow is added to a culture flask with 6 ml of Eagle's Minimal Essential Medium (Microbiological Associates) containing 20 per cent fetal calf serum (Gibco), 2 per cent penicillin-streptomycin (5000 units/ml penicillin and 5000 μg/ml streptomycin; Microbiological Associates), and 0.25 per cent mycostatin (Squibb) (Morse, 1977). After incubation at 37°C. for 16 hours, the cultures are chilled in an ice bath at 4°C. and exposed to the same temperature (in a cold room or refrigerator) for 5 to 5½ hrs. At the end of this period, the contents of the flask are poured into a siliconized centrifuge tube and centrifuged at 200 g for 8 minutes. The supernatant is aspirated and the cells are resuspended in 8 ml of 0.075 M KCl at 37°C. for 10 minutes. The mixture is then centrifuged at 200 g for 5 minutes and the supernatant is aspirated, leaving approximately 0.5 ml above the pellet. The cells are fixed, spread on slides, and stained as described for peripheral blood lymphocyte preparations.

Q-banding Technique. Some laboratories experience difficulties in eliciting satisfactory G-bands in mitotic spreads from bone marrow and prefer the Q-banding method for this tissue. The technique described can also be used on chromosome preparations from other tissues.

Q-bands are observed on mitotic chromosomes after staining with certain fluorochromes, generally quinacrine mustard (Caspersson, 1970) or quinacrine dihydrochloride (Uchida, 1974), and exposure to ultraviolet light. In order to obtain clear banding patterns, it is necessary to have well-spread chromosomes with chromatids positioned closely together. Preparations should be made without flame drying on high quality microscope slides (Clay-Adams Gold Seal) to avoid background. Freshly prepared slides produce the best results, although older slides also can be well banded, particularly if stored under refrigeration or below freezing.

Quinacrine dihydrochloride stain consists of 5 g quinacrine dihydrochloride (G. T. Gurr, Ltd., England), 45 ml glacial acetic acid, and 55 ml distilled water. This solution can be stored at room temperature for one to two months. Slides are immersed for 5 minutes, then rinsed in three changes of distilled water at pH 4.5, which should be lowered with increasing age of the slides. After air drying, coverslips are mounted with a drop of distilled water. To minimize the thickness of the water layer and prevent a hazy image due to light scattering, excess water should be removed by blotting. The edges of the coverslip are then sealed with paraffin wax, beeswax, or clear nail polish. Slides should be examined immediately under a fluorescent microscope, but may be refrigerated up to several hours if absolutely necessary (Uchida, 1974).

Quinacrine mustard (Sterling Winthrop Research Institute, Rensselaer, New York) stain is made by dissolving 0.5 mg of the powder per 10 ml of MacIlvaine's buffer. MacIlvaine's buffer consists of 86.3 ml of 0.1 M citric acid and 453.7 ml of 0.2 M disodium phosphate, diluted to 1 liter with distilled water and adjusted to pH 7.0. Slides are stained in a horizontal position for 20 minutes, washed in three changes of buffer or distilled water (pH 7.0) for a total of three minutes, and then mounted with buffer or distilled water as described for quinacrine dihydrochloride (Caspersson, 1970).

Fluorescence Microscopy and Photography. Any good microscope setup for fluorescence photography can be used. For example, the standard Zeiss GFL fluorescence microscope equipped with an HBO 200 W/Z DC exciter unit and an ultra-darkfield condenser for transmitted illumination is satisfactory. The use of the exciter unit allows a decrease in the film exposure time, since it has a more stable light source as well as a substantial increase in light intensity. A 16× or 40× objective is used to scan slides; for photography a 100× planapochromat oil objective equipped with an iris is necessary.

Since fluorescent preparations fade on exposure to light, only a rapid evaluation is possible directly under the microscope, and photographs are used to carry out a detailed evaluation. For photography it is important that the microscope be located in an area free of vibration. Highly sensitive black and white films (Kodak Tri-X; Illford HP 4) are recommended for routine use. Printing is done on Kodabromide F2 or F3 paper. Karyotypes are prepared by mounting the chromosomes on an exposed sheet of Kodabromide paper.

Following completion of the fluorescence photography, the coverslip should be removed immediately by freezing. The slide can then be stored for future restaining with quinacrine or conventional stains, if needed.

SOLID TUMORS

Karyotypic changes in tumors can be evaluated by the analysis of both direct preparations of tumor cells and of short-term cultures. Cytogenetic studies of tumor tissue may be of diagnostic value, particularly when clinical and cytologic criteria are equivocal.

For the successful analysis of a direct preparation, it is crucial that the tissue be as fresh as possible in order to obtain sufficient cells in mitosis. With some specimens, short-term cultures (16 to 24 hours) may provide more analyzable material than direct preparations (Kotler, 1967); therefore, the two techniques should be employed in parallel. Long-term culture of tumor tissue leads to the selective growth of normal cells. For this reason, the culture of tumor cells usually should not exceed 72 hours (Kotler, 1967; Harnden, 1974).

Direct Preparation of Tumor Tissue. Fresh tumor specimens are freed from fat tissue and blood. The tissue is minced with scissors or two scalpel blades into small pieces (approximately 0.1 to 0.2 mm) in Dulbecco's medium (Gibco) supplemented with 20 per cent fetal calf serum (Gibco) and 0.06 to 0.1 μg/ml colcemid (Gibco). To convert the solid tumor into a suspension of cells, two methods can be used. In the first, the minced tissue is suspended in 5 ml of unsupplemented Dulbecco's medium, which is then poured into a small beaker and stirred gently with a magnetic bar and stirrer. Alternatively, the tissue can be incubated at 37°C. for three hours and the cells loosened from the tissue by gently shaking the culture bottle at the end of the incubation period (Kotler, 1967). In either case, the mixture of cells and tissue is transferred to a siliconized centrifuge tube. Large fragments of tissue are allowed to sediment under gravity, and the cell suspension is decanted into a second centrifuge tube. In the case of lymph nodes, mincing is not necessary, since the capsule can be torn off with a pair of dissecting needles, releasing the cells into the medium.

The cell suspension is centrifuged, exposed to hypotonic treatment and fixation, and spread onto slides, as described on page 823.

Short-term Incubation. Tumor specimens (except lymph nodes) are minced with scissors in 5 ml of Dulbecco's medium (Gibco) supplemented with 20 per cent fetal calf serum (Gibco), 2 per cent penicillin-streptomycin (5000 units/ml penicillin and 5000 μg/ml streptomycin; Microbiological Associates), and 0.25 per cent mycostatin (Squibb) and incubated at 37°C. in air supplemented with 5 per cent CO_2 for 16 to 24 hours. Colcemid (Gibco) is added to the culture at a final concentration of 0.06 to 0.1 μg/ml 15 to 60 minutes before harvesting (Harnden, 1974). To obtain midmetaphases as well as mitotic cells in earlier stages, it is best to divide the sample into two parts. Half is exposed to a high concentration of colcemid for a long exposure (e.g., 0.1 μg/ml for 60 minutes) to obtain midmetaphases, and the other half to a minimal amount of colcemid (e.g., 0.06 μg/ml for 15 minutes) to obtain cells in midmetaphase as well as in earlier stages of mitosis. At the end of the incubation, the mixture is gently shaken to loosen cells from the minced tissue, and the cell suspension is decanted into a siliconized centrifuge tube. Hypotonic treatment, fixation, and preparation of chromosomes are the same as described for peripheral blood (p. 823).

SEX CHROMATIN TESTS

Methods for the detection of the Barr body or X chromatin body in interphase nuclei were the first cytogenetic techniques to find practical clinical application. The Barr body was fortuitously discovered in neuronal cells of cats by Barr (1949), who later extended his investigations to humans. Initially, biopsy material was used; later Moore (1955) developed the buccal smear technique which is still in general use.

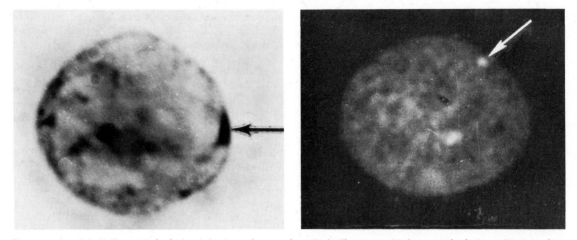

Figure 26-11. *Left,* X-chromatin body (arrow) in interphase nucleus. *Right,* Fluorescent Y-chromatin body (arrow) in interphase nucleus. The other fluorescent body (center) represents strongly fluorescent chromosomal material that may in some patients be mistaken for a Y body. (From Lewandowski, 1975.)

The Y body can also be detected in interphase nuclei by the use of quinacrine staining and fluorescence microscopy, due to its characteristic intense staining property (Pearson, 1970). Tests for the X and Y bodies are valuable screening procedures in cases where a sex chromosome anomaly is suspected and sometimes provide enough information so that karyotyping is not necessary.

Barr Body. The Barr body appears as a mass of chromatin attached to the nuclear membrane, usually with a planoconvex shape measuring about 1.2 by 0.7 μ (Fig. 26-11). Occasionally, it appears bipartite or as an inverted pyramid. The Barr body is easily seen in any nucleus with an open, vesicular chromatin pattern, e.g., the nuclei of basal layer epithelial cells.

ORIGIN OF THE BARR BODY. Soon after the discovery of the existence of the Barr body or chromatin body in normal mammalian females, it was determined that each is derived from one entire X chromosome (Ohno, 1959). Along the same line, Mary Lyon postulated in 1961 that the condensed X chromosome which appears as the Barr body is inactivated in somatic cells of females, leaving only one X chromosome active.

The inactivated X can be of either paternal or maternal origin. Inactivation occurs at the time of embryonic implantation in the uterus and is entirely random. Once the process of inactivation has occurred, however, all descendants of each particular cell will have the same X inactivated. The inactivation of the X chromosome is reflected morphologically by *heterochromatinization.* In interphase and in early prophase, it is shorter, more darkly staining, and more condensed than its active counterpart.

If more than one X chromosome is present in a cell, all but one will be inactivated. Thus, the number of X chromatin masses (m) expected can be predicted using the formula m = n − 1, where n is the number of X chromosomes in the cell (Table 26-3). Males having a single X chromosome do not exhibit an X chromatin mass (1 − 1 = 0). Normal females having two X chromosomes have a single chromatin mass (2 − 1 = 1). Trisomy X females (XXX) have two X chromatin masses in their nuclei (3 − 1 = 2).

In sex chromatin preparations from normal females, an X chromatin body is usually found in about 30 per cent of nuclei, with a range of 15 to 40 per cent, depending on the individual laboratory. Barr bodies are probably present in most somatic cells, but owing to the fact that they are adherent to the nuclear membrane and many fall behind or in front of the nucleoplasm in the preparation, they cannot be identified with certainty.

BARR BODY TECHNIQUE. The Barr body may be seen in any tissue in which the cells have large, open nuclei. Cells from buccal or vaginal smears, the epithelial cells of urinary sediment, and the cells of amniotic fluid can be used. In addition, in a normal female, sex chromatin can be identified in the nuclei of almost any tissue that has been paraffin sectioned. By far the source of cells most commonly used for the study of Barr bodies is the buccal mucosa.

Using a sterile metal spatula, the inner surface

Table 26-3. IDENTIFICATION OF SEX CHROMOSOME
DISORDERS USING THE SEX BODIES OF THE
INTERPHASE NUCLEUS

X OR BARR BODIES	Y BODIES	DISORDER
0	0	XO (Turner syndrome)
1	0	XX (Normal female)
2	0	XXX syndrome
3	0	XXXX
4	0	XXXXX
0	1	XY (Normal male)
1	1	XXY (Klinefelter syndrome)
2	1	XXXY (Klinefelter variant)
3	1	XXXXY
0	2	XYY syndrome
1	2	XXYY (Klinefelter variant)

of the cheek is firmly scraped and the cells are spread on a clean glass slide. It is important that firm pressure be used in order to dislodge deeper cells with the desired vesicular nuclei. It is a good practice to make two slides, scraping the same area of the cheek both times. The second scraping usually yields the more satisfactory deeper cells with no bacterial contamination. Smears should not be spread too thin on the slides, since this may make the cells difficult to examine. Slides are fixed immediately without air drying in 70 per cent ethanol for a minimum of 10 minutes and a maximum of 24 hours.

If needed, the slides can be treated with parlodion prior to spreading to minimize cell loss during staining. Slides are immersed in absolute ethanol for 3 minutes, followed by 2 minutes in a 0.2 per cent solution of parlodion in equal parts of absolute ethanol and ether. The slides are air dried and then immersed in 70 per cent ethanol for 5 minutes, followed by 5 minutes each in two changes of distilled water.

Any nuclear stain will stain the Barr body. These include hematoxylin-eosin and Papanicolaou stains, as well as special stains, such as orcein, cresylecht violet, thionine, Feulgen stain, the Guard stain, or carbolfuchsin (Mittwoch, 1974). Probably the most satisfactory routine stain for the X chromatin body is carbolfuchsin.

A carbolfuchsin stock solution is made by dissolving 3 g of basic fuchsin in 100 ml of 70 per cent ethanol. This stock solution is good for several months. To prepare the carbolfuchsin working solution, 10 ml of the stock solution is added to 90 ml of 5 per cent phenol in water. Ten ml of glacial acetic acid and 10 ml of 37 per cent formaldehyde are then added to the mixture. The solution is thoroughly mixed and allowed to stand for 24 hours before use. Working solutions should be prepared fresh every month.

Slides are stained for 5 to 10 minutes with the working solution followed by 1 minute in 95 per cent ethanol and 1 minute in absolute alcohol. They are cleared in xylol and mounted with Permount.

Stained smears are examined with oil immersion. One hundred suitable (open and vesicular) nuclei from several areas on the slides should be examined and the percentage of X chromatin-positive nuclei determined. As mentioned earlier, in normal women and girls the range of X chromatin-positive nuclei varies from 15 to 40 per cent. A normal range of values should be established for each individual laboratory. Smears from normal males are X chromatin negative.

Y Body. Pearson (1970) described the presence of the fluorescent Y body in nuclei of buccal mucosa cells, lymphocytes, and fibroblasts which had been stained with quinacrine dihydrochloride. The proportion of cells derived from male subjects in which this body was visible varied between 25 and 50 per cent. It usually had the form of a single fluorescent spot of about 0.25 μm in diameter and was seen midway between the center and periphery of the nucleus (Fig. 26-11B). In buccal smears from men with two Y chromosomes (47,XYY or 48,XXYY; Table 26-3), two Y bodies could be seen in about 30 per cent of nuclei and a single body in approximately 10 to 20 per cent of cells.

ORIGIN AND SIZE VARIATION OF THE Y BODY. The distal end of the long arm of the Y chromosome displays a brilliant fluorescence with quinacrine, allowing for its easy recognition in interphase and mitosis. This phenomenon has been found only in man and gorilla, and in man is due to the presence of human-specific nongenic, highly repetitive DNA sequences (Jones, 1977). The length of the long arm of the Y chromosome varies in different individuals, and it has been shown that this is closely correlated with the size of the highly fluorescent segment in both interphase and metaphase. The variation is so extreme that in a few individuals the brilliant segment may be twice the usual size or may be completely absent with no effect on the phenotype. These differences in size represent normal polymorphic variations that can be followed through many generations. The use of the Y body complements the use of the Barr body for the simple determination of sex chromosome numbers. Unlike the Barr body, however, which is present for each X chromosome in excess of one, each Y chromosome present forms a Y body (Table 26-3).

Y BODY TECHNIQUE. Buccal smears are fixed in 70 per cent ethanol for at least 10 minutes. The slides are then stained for 5 minutes in 0.5 per cent aqueous quinacrine hydrochloride. (This may be prepared from either pure quinacrine hydrochloride powder or from dissolved and filtered atabrine tablets). They are then rinsed for 3 minutes each in two changes of distilled water and 3 minutes each in phosphate-citrate buffer (0.01 M citric acid, pH 5.5) and phosphate buffer (0.01 M, pH 7.4). Coverslips are mounted and cleared with nail polish, and the slides are examined using fluorescent light microscopy. The use of quinacrine hydrochloride in conjunction with an alkaline buffer, such as the one described above, makes it possible to use the slides for a considerable time after staining (Hollander, 1971).

Reporting and Interpreting Sex Chromatin Bodies.

Buccal chromatin tests are properly reported as X and/or Y body positive or negative. If more than one X or Y body is present per nucleus, or if there is a lowered incidence of sex chromatin-positive nuclei, these findings should be reported.

Interpreting variations in the number of Barr bodies per cell is simple if the relationship $m = n - 1$ is kept in mind. Increases in the percentage of X chromatin-positive nuclei per smear are rarely of significance but should alert one to look for extra Barr bodies. Diminution in the percentage of X chromatin-positive nuclei is usually not significant unless the percentage falls to a low value for a given laboratory. In this case, sex chromosomal *mosaicism* (e.g., XO/XX) is a diagnostic possibility and chromosome analysis should be entertained.

Erroneous results in the number of Barr bodies present may arise from artifacts in the laboratory. Laboratory errors include false positives produced by bacteria, wrinkles in the nuclear membrane, or analysis of pyknotic nuclei. Careful microscopy will readily differentiate any of these from chromatin masses. False negatives may be produced by analysis of degenerating cells or the usage of outdated stain. Nuclei always display other small,

darkly staining clumps of chromatin representing pericentromeric heterochromatin, and these small masses can be used to monitor the quality of cells and stain used (Fig. 26-11).

The incidence of chromatin-positive nuclei has been reported to be sensitive to a variety of stimuli. The oral ingestion of antibiotics may sometimes reduce the percentage of chromatin-positive nuclei in buccal smears. Also, the frequency may fall to as low as 4 or 5 per cent in both the mother in the postpartum state and in the normal female newborn.

Actual alterations in the size of the X chromatin mass may reflect structural alterations of the X chromosome and are comparatively infrequent except in cases suspected of Turner's syndrome. More often, however, they may reflect differences in preparation, or tissue and type of stain used. For instance, Barr bodies appear smaller in hematoxylin-eosin than in carbolfuchsin-stained preparations. Variation in Barr body size may also be noted in smears from different body sites. The Barr bodies of vaginal cells are often larger than those seen in buccal smears from the same patient. In general, sex chromatin size is not a reliable indicator of the size of an X chromosome, and when there is doubt a chromosome analysis should be performed.

Analyses of the Y body present fewer technical difficulties because of its typical brilliance and the ease of discerning it. Cells do not have to be the basal ones to be detectable. Also, if the Y chromosome is larger than usual, the Y body is easier to detect. In cases in which the Y body is very small, there can be problems in analysis. However, the study of both the X and Y bodies in a phenotypic male is quite helpful in this unusual situation.

Often chromosome regions, such as the pericentromeric heterochromatin of chromosomes 3, 4, and 13 and the satellites of certain acrocentric chromosomes are fluorescent (see Fig. 26-1). Uptake of the stain varies considerably in these chromosomes between homologues and between one individual and another (see Fig. 26-2). Occasionally, one of these segments is notably fluorescent and, in interphase nuclei, can be confused with the Y chromosome (Fig. 26-11 *right*). This problem is compounded when there are several highly fluorescent polymorphic regions that coalesce in interphase (Dutrillaux, 1977). These possibilities render prenatal detection of sex by the study of sex bodies of limited value, unless cells from both parents are examined concomitantly.

Table 26-4. TYPES OF CHROMOSOME DEFECTS

NUMERICAL	STRUCTURAL	
Trisomy	Deletion	Partial duplication-deficiency
Monosomy	Interstitial	Isochromosome
Polysomy	Terminal	Ring chromosome
Aneuploid mosaicism	Inversion	Dicentric
Polyploidy	Pericentric	Translocation
Triploidy	Paracentric	Reciprocal
Tetraploidy	Partial trisomy	Robertsonian
		Insertion

TYPES AND ETIOLOGY OF CHROMOSOME DEFECTS

The human cell has a great propensity for chromosomal error. These errors can occur during gametogenesis or embryonic development, giving rise to the chromosomal syndromes, or can be acquired after birth, such as those which occur after irradiation or viral infections and those found in neoplasia.

Types of Chromosome Defects. There are many different types of chromosome defects, such as deletions, inversions, ring formations, trisomies, and polyploidy. They can all be grouped into two major types: those involving an abnormality in the number of chromosomes and those involving structural changes in one or more chromosomes. A summary of the types of defects most commonly observed in man is shown in Table 26-4.

Numerical abnormalities arise through errors in normal chromosome migration during meiotic or mitotic division. In the first meiotic division, homologous chromosomes, each with two chromatids, synapse and then move toward opposite poles, providing daughter cells with one chromosome of each pair or half the original number of chromosomes. During the second meiotic division, as well as in mitosis, each replicated chromosome splits longitudinally into two sister chromatids, which move to opposite poles (*disjunction*). As an end result, each of the daughter cells of meiosis, which form the gametes, contain a *haploid* number (n) of chromosomes, while somatic cells have a *diploid* number (2n).

Errors in normal chromosome distribution are primarily due to failure of paired chromosomes or sister chromatids to separate and move to opposite poles (*non-disjunction*). In the chromosomal syndromes, this can occur during either the first or the second meiotic division of maternal or paternal gametogenesis, as is the case in Down's syndrome (Uchida, 1977). The resulting gametes and the cells fertilized from them contain chromosome complements that are not exact multiples of n and are termed *aneuploid*. Aneuploid cells with three members of a particular chromosome are *trisomic* (2n + 1), such as in trisomy 21, and those with a missing chromosome (2n − 1) are said to be *monosomic* (e.g., X-monosomy) (Fig. 26-12). Non-disjunction for a given chromosome can occasionally occur successively in both meiotic divisions in a given individual or at one division in each of the two parents. This results in *polysomy*, which has been found in cases involving the X chromosome (e.g., XXXXX or XXXXY) or the Y chromosome (e.g., XYYY), or in double trisomy and/or monosomy, such as those involving two autosomes (e.g., +8, +21) or a sex chromosome and an autosome (e.g., XXX, +21).

An error originating during gametogenesis results in an individual who is aneuploid in all the body cells. Non-disjunction, however, can also occur in the zygote, usually giving rise to *mosaicism*. For example, it can produce both a trisomic and a monosomic daughter cell line (e.g., XXX/XO mosaicism) or a diploid and a monosomic cell line (e.g., XX/XO mosaicism). The latter phenomenon is due to anaphase lag and subsequent loss of an X chromosome in the cytoplasm.

In addition to aneuploidy, *polyploid* zygotes, either triploid (3n) or tetraploid (4n), arise either from mitotic anomalies in germ cell precursors, complete failure of a meiotic division to occur, or dispermy. Polyploidy is rarely compatible with life, and the few cases reported of either triploidy or tetraploidy exhibit many congenital anomalies and generally do not survive the first year of life.

Structural defects result from chromosome breakage, followed by reunion of the broken ends in an abnormal combination. The two most common types found in man are inter-

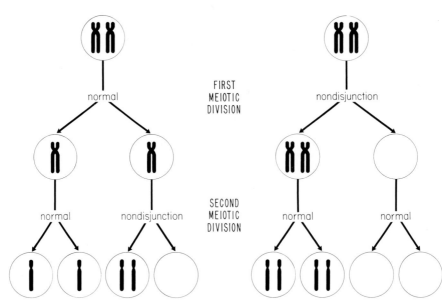

Figure 26–12. Nondisjunction at first and second meiotic divisions, producing gametes with an extra or missing chromosome. Only the chromosome pair involved in nondisjunction is shown.

stitial deletions and reciprocal translocations. *Interstitial deletions* arise following two breaks in the same chromosome and loss of the segment between the breaks. Interstitial or terminal deletions of a chromosome segment are not uncommon in man. One example is the cat cry syndrome, in which part of the short arm of chromosome 5 is deleted.

When breakage occurs in two chromosomes and each of the broken pieces reunites with the other chromosome, the result is a *reciprocal translocation*. An example involving chromosomes 2 and 6 is shown in Figure 26-8. In this case, the distal segment of the short arm of chromosome 6 is translocated to the distal end of the long arm of chromosome 2, and the telomere end of the long arm of chromosome 2 is translocated to the short arm of chromosome 6. A parent with this translocation has all the genetic material in each cell and is phenotypically normal. However, a child receiving only one of the two abnormal chromosomes has not only a partial trisomy or a partial deletion, but a combination of both (a partial duplication-deficiency). This technically produces a double chromosome defect in each instance that can be translated clinically into varying admixtures of two given syndromes or defects and may pose a diagnostic difficulty, since the patient may not present with a readily identifiable syndrome. Fortu-

nately, it is not uncommon for one chromosome to break at the most distal end of one of its arms, thus contributing little, if any, loss or gain of clinically significant material. In these cases, the patients are said to have a "pure" partial trisomy or deletion (Fig. 26-13).

A special type of translocation involving breakage near the centromeric regions of two acrocentric chromosomes and reunion of their long arms is known as *Robertsonian translocation*. As illustrated by a translocation involving chromosomes 14 and 21 in Figure 26-14, a break can occur in the short arm of chromosome 14 and another near the centromere in the long arm of chromosome 21, followed by fusion of the long arms and loss of the heterochromatic and genetically inactive short arm of the chromosome 21. Since the translocated chromosome has the centromere of the chromosome 14, it moves at random with respect to the other chromosome 21 in the first meiotic anaphase, leading to four possible types of gametes: one with a normal chromosome 14 and a normal chromosome 21; one with a balanced translocation 14/21; one containing the translocation 14/21 and an additional chromosome 21; and one gamete with only a chromosome 14 and no chromosome 21. Fertilization with normal gametes would produce one normal and one balanced translocation karyotype, both of which would result in a normal pheno-

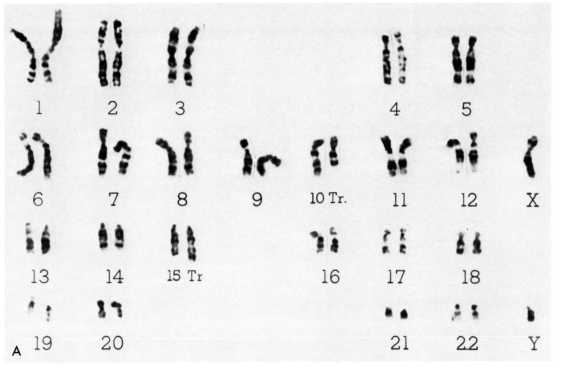

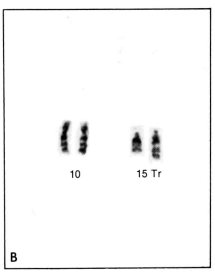

Figure 26–13. *A*, G-banded karyotype of a man with a balanced translocation involving chromosomes 10 and 15. *B*, Partial karyotype of son demonstrating abnormal chromosome 15, making the patient partially trisomic for the distal segment of the long arm of chromosome 10. (From Yunis, 1974b.)

type; one zygote with trisomy 21; and one zygote with monosomy 21 (which is inviable). Therefore, when one of the parents has a balanced karyotype with a 14/21 translocation, there is theoretically a one in three chance of having a viable abnormal child (trisomy 21). In practice, the observed risk is much lower, being approximately 8 per cent for female carriers and 2 per cent for male carriers (Hamerton, 1971).

Another relatively common structural de-

fect, in particular involving the X chromosome, is the formation of an *isochromosome*. This occurs when the centromere of a chromosome divides perpendicular to the long axis of the chromosome instead of parallel to it. As a result, each of the two daughter chromosomes carries identical arms on either side of the centromere, causing partial duplication and partial deletion. For instance, a person carrying an isochromosome for the long arm of an X chromosome is monosomic for the short arm

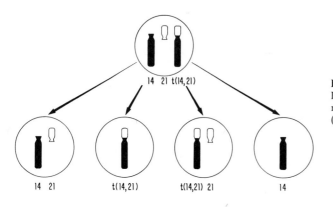

Figure 26–14.   Gametogenesis in a carrier of a Robertsonian translocation of the long arm of chromosome 21 (white) to the short arm of chromosome 14 (black). For details, see text.

and trisomic for the long arm. These patients usually present themselves clinically with Turner's syndrome, since the short arm of the X chromosome is the causative segment of this disorder and partial or complete trisomy X produces little or no phenotypic effect (see p. 846).

In addition to the anomalies described above, several types of rarer structural defects can also be found. For instance, a chromosome broken at two points may reunite with the interstitial piece inverted. Such a rearrangement is called an *inversion* and can involve the centromere (pericentric inversion) or a segment of a chromosome arm (paracentric inversion). Usually the change in gene order produced by an inversion does not lead to an abnormal phenotype, but problems arise during meiosis when pairing of homologues cannot occur normally. Unbalanced gametes often result, which may give rise to sterility in the carrier and/or offspring possessing partial duplications and deficiencies (Benirschke, 1974).

Sometimes *ring chromosomes* are formed when breakage occurs simultaneously at both ends of one chromosome and the two proximal ends join, the two distal acentric fragments being lost. Chromosome 18 and the X chromosome are the best known for their involvement in ring formation. In the case of chromosome 18, 46,18r patients have features of both 18p- and 18q- individuals. In the case of the X chromosome, the 46,Xr patient may have features of Turner's syndrome.

Another uncommon structural defect, which is more frequent among neoplasias and rarely congenital, is the formation of a dicentric chromosome. This occurs when two chromosome fragments, each with a centromere and usually of relatively long length, fuse. Only dicentric chromosomes with centromeres close together are reasonably stable, since they otherwise form bridges at anaphase, leading to breakage. The most common dicentric chromosome in man involves the Y chromosome: 46,X,dic(Y). It may arise after replication by breakage of the short arm and fusion of the proximal ends of the two chromatids. Individuals with this defect may express Turner's syndrome (Armendares, 1972; Cohen, 1973), since there appears to be homology between the short arms of the X and Y chromosomes.

Causes of Chromosomal Aberrations. Although we understand some of the mechanisms that produce aberrations of chromosome number and structure and we know that they can be produced in man both by genetic factors and by various clastogens (e.g., radiation, viruses, chemicals), we do not know much about the specific factors that predispose to the formation of these aberrations in certain situations. A number of factors which have been implicated as causative agents of chromosomal aberrations are listed in Table 26-5.

One very significant biologic factor in the predisposition to chromosomal trisomies is elevated maternal age. For example, it is known

Table 26-5.   ETIOLOGY OF CHROMOSOME DEFECTS

Intrinsic factors
    Age—especially maternal age
    Autoimmune disease
    Short arms of acrocentric chromosomes
    Structural chromosome abnormalities
    Gene defects
Extrinsic (environmental) factors
    Ionizing radiation
    Viral infections
    Drugs

that while the incidence of Down's syndrome is one in 2000 for mothers of age 20, it is one in 300 at age 35, one in 100 by age 40, and one in 50 in mothers over 45 years of age (Penrose, 1966; Stene, 1970). Furthermore, if all chromosome defects are considered, a woman between the ages of 35 and 39 years stands a one in 50 chance of having a child with a chromosome defect, and the risk increases to one in 30 if the woman is between 40 and 44 years of age (Milunsky, 1977). It is possible that if women over 35 would abstain from having children or would seek prenatal diagnosis, the incidence of trisomies could be decreased by one third.

Attempts have been made to explain this age-dependent phenomenon as a tendency to non-disjunction during oogenesis in older mothers, owing to known differences between oogenesis and spermatogenesis. Developing ova are arrested in the first meiotic prophase in embryogenesis and remain at this stage until ovulation, which, for a particular ovum, may not be until 35 or 45 years later. Spermatozoa, on the other hand, undergo a developmental period of no more than 48 days after meiosis begins. Recently, it has been suggested that non-disjunction may also occur in a sizable minority of older fathers, as evidenced by the finding of paternal origin of the extra chromosome 21 in a number of cases of Down's syndrome (Wagenbichler, 1976).

Radiation has also been postulated to be a cause of non-disjunction during meiotic division, since many parents of aneuploids, particularly mothers of Down's syndrome children, have significant radiation histories (Uchida, 1977). In addition, radiation is known to be a chromosome breaking agent and there is suggestive evidence that exposure to radiation in prospective mothers, such as that used for diagnostic purposes, may be an etiologic factor in the origin of *de novo* structural chromosome abnormalities (Patil, 1977).

A large number of viruses have been implicated as causative agents of chromosomal abnormalities, at least when tested with cells in culture. Furthermore, chromosomal changes have been described in patients suffering from viral infections, such as measles, mumps, chicken pox, and rubella (Ansari, 1977). The established relationship between DNA and RNA oncogenic viruses, chromosome aberrations, and mammalian tumors has given credence to the possibility that some human neoplasias may also show a similar relationship. Burkitt's lymphoma and its association with the Epstein-Barr virus, as well as a translocation involving chromosomes 8 and 14, is a potential example of such a relationship. While very little work has been done regarding the effect of viruses on gametogenesis, indirect evidence suggests that they may be of some importance. For example, Robinson (1969) showed a high incidence of elevated levels of IgM in the cord blood of newborns with aneuploidy, suggesting intrauterine infection in the mothers.

Autoimmune disease has been suggested to play a role in the pathogenesis of non-disjunction, in view of the correlation in some families between high thyroid autoantibody levels in parents and chromosomal anomalies in the offspring. Fialkow (1971) has shown a two- to threefold excess of seropositivity in mothers of Down's syndrome children, as well as an increased frequency of thyroid autoantibodies in the sisters and other first-degree relatives of the mothers. In addition, thyroid antibodies are elevated in Turner's syndrome, particularly in the X/isochromosome X form (Sparkes, 1967).

Some chromosomes appear to be more predisposed to involvement in aberrations of number and structure. For example, the sex chromosomes are most often involved in numerical defects, possibly due to the fact that they pass through the meiotic cycle slightly out of phase with the remainder of the chromosomes. Also, the 13-15 and 21-22 acrocentric chromosomes tend to lie in close association at their satellited ends in the formation of the nucleoli, and this may make them "sticky," promoting non-disjunction as seen in trisomies 13, 21, and 22. These same chromosomes, with their heterochromatic short arms and satellites, also appear to exhibit an increased propensity for breakage in these regions, as evidenced by the relatively high incidence of Robertsonian translocations in the normal adult population. Indeed, 1 to 3 of 1000 individuals have been found to carry a Robertsonian translocation, particularly between chromosomes 13 and 14 and between 14 and 21, leading in part to multiple miscarriages and trisomic offspring (Benirschke, 1974).

Balanced reciprocal translocations appear to be a very important factor in the causation of chromosomal syndromes, since of approximately 0.2 per cent of newborns with a partial duplication and/or deletion, probably half are the product of a familial translocation, while in the other half the defect occurs *de novo*. Another chromosomal rearrangement that may be a significant factor in reproductive failure, congenital defects, and early infant mortality is that of chromosomal inversion. However, the frequency and importance of this factor remains to be determined. Another possible factor is the presence of pericentric inversions involving the heterochromatic regions of various chromosomes, particularly of chromosome 9, which occurs in at least 1 per cent of the population (Sanchez, 1977). This may give rise to a high frequency of sterility or multiple miscarriages, owing to the production of unbalanced gametes.

Genes predisposing to non-disjunction have been suspected in humans, since such genes are known to exist in several organisms. The evidence in man so far relates to a few reports of pedigrees with clusters of aneuploids of the same or different chromosomes (Hamerton, 1971). In addition, there are several rare diseases due to gene defects (Fanconi's anemia, Bloom's syndrome, ataxia telangiectasia), which have a propensity for "spontaneous" chromosomal breakage and a tendency to malignancy (See Chromosome Defects in Neoplasia, p. 848).

CHROMOSOMAL SYNDROMES

Recent studies indicate that 0.7 to 0.8 per cent of all newborns possess a chromosome defect of sufficient size to be detected with current cytogenetic methods. Approximately one third of these (0.25 per cent) have a sex chromosome anomaly, in particular XXY, XYY, and XXX, and exhibit relatively mild or no phenotypic effects. Another one third are due to an extra or missing autosome, primarily an extra chromosome 21, 18, or 13, manifest multiple congenital defects and severe mental and growth retardation, and, like the sex chromosome anomalies, are generally sporadic in nature. The remaining one third are predominantly partial trisomies or partial monosomies, the majority of which have been characterized following the advent of the banding techniques. These patients usually exhibit severe phenotypic effects like the previous group, although some are closer to normalcy, depending upon the particular defect. A large number of these cases are familial, that is, occurring in progeny of balanced translocation carriers, and could be effectively prevented through counseling and prenatal diagnosis.

GENERAL PHENOTYPE AND VIABILITY

Before chromosome banding, it was known that the only autosomal trisomies that are viable at birth are trisomy 13, trisomy 18, trisomy 21, and rarely trisomy 22. Monosomies are not found in newborns, except for XO Turner's syndrome and a very few cases of monosomy involving the smallest autosomes (21 and 22). Other possible trisomies and monosomies were believed to be incompatible with life, and studies have confirmed that the great majority of fetuses which are monosomic or have a trisomy for a large autosome are lost early in embryogenesis (Carr, 1977). The finding that trisomies are more common than monosomies also indicates that the absence of an autosome is much less tolerated than the presence of an extra one. Although the effects of sex chromosome abnormalities are generally less severe than those of autosomal defects, the severity increases as the imbalance becomes more extensive. For example, XXX females may be normal or exhibit mild mental retardation and minor physical abnormalities, whereas those with an XXXX sex chromosome constitution usually have severe growth and mental deficiency, reduced fertility, and associated facial defects. On the other hand, females with an XXXXX sex complement show serious growth and mental deficiency, as well as multiple congenital defects.

With the advent of the banding techniques that allow individual chromosomes and chromosome segments to be identified with reasonable accuracy, more than thirty new chromosomal syndromes resulting from either a partial trisomy or monosomy have been characterized (Fig. 26-15). Partial trisomies are more common than partial monosomies, again supporting the idea that deletions of genetic material are less viable than duplications. In addition, it has been found that individuals with trisomies other than the classic ones, such as trisomy 8 or 9, survive if they are mosaics and possess a sufficient number of normal cells to help sustain life.

Diagnosis of an autosomal syndrome depends to a large extent on recognition of a particular constellation of phenotypic features, since many effects observed overlap among the various syndromes (Table 26-6). However, recent studies indicate that some of the phenotypic features, especially those seen in the new chromosomal syndromes, are relatively uncommon or discriminating (Table 26-7). Recognition and characterization of

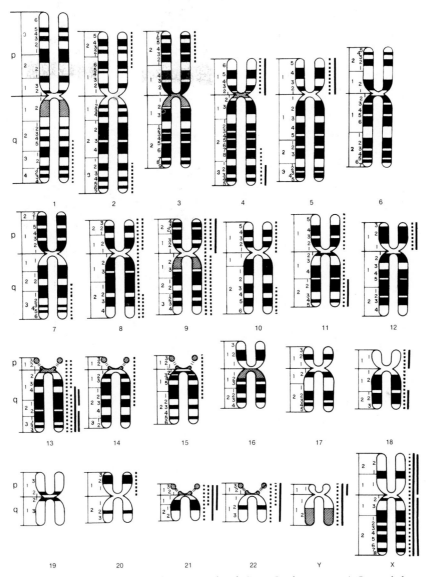

Figure 26–15. Representation of mid-metaphase chromosome bands (Paris Conference, 1971). Currently known chromosomal syndromes are each illustrated by a vertical line on the right corresponding to the chromosome or chromosomal segment involved. Dotted lines represent trisomic state. Solid lines represent monosomic state. (From Yunis, 1977b.)

these discriminating features are very helpful in diagnosis, as well as in attempts to understand the pathophysiology of the autosomal chromosome abnormalities. For example, deletion 13q syndrome, due to the loss of the distal three fifths of the long arm of chromosome 13, usually includes mental retardation; prominence of the forehead, root of the nose, maxilla, and superior incisors; large ears with deep sulci helici and small lobes; hypoplasia to aplasia of thumbs and first metacarpals; syn-

ostoses of fourth and fifth metacarpals; and predisposition to bilateral retinoblastoma. By comparing patients with smaller deletions of the long arm of chromosome 13, it has been possible tentatively to sublocalize predisposition to bilateral retinoblastoma to a portion of band 13q14; hypoplasia of thumbs and synostoses of fourth and fifth metacarpals to bands q31-32; and prominence of nose bridge, maxilla, and upper incisors, as well as large ears with deep sulci helici and small lobes, to band

Table 26–6. SELECTED OVERLAPPING PHENOTYPES OF CHROMOSOMAL SYNDROMES

	dup 1q	dup 2q	dup 3p	del 4p	dup 4p	dup 4q	del 5p	dup 5p	dup 7q	dup 8	dup 9	dup 9p	del 9p	dup 9q	dup 10p	dup 10q	dup 11p	dup 11q
Mental retardation	++	+	++	++	++	++	++	++	++	+	++	++	++	++	++	++	+++	++
Growth retardation	+		++	++	++	++	++	++	++		++	++	++	++	++		+++	+
Low birth weight		++		++		++	++		+									
Microcephaly		+	+	++	++		++				+	+				++	+	+
Downward slanting eyes					++		+									++		
Upward slanting eyes				+				++									+	
Hypertelorism		+	+	++	+		+	+	+			+	+					
Microphthalmia													+				+	
Small palpebral fissures						++										++		
Strabismus		++		++		++			++		+							
Broad nasal bridge		+		++	+		++		++	+			+		+++		++++	
Cleft upper lip				++						+								
Cleft palate				++						+								
Micrognathia	+	+	++	++	++	++	++		++	+++						++++		++++
Low-set ears					++	++	++		++		+			+				
Short neck			+							++		+	+		+			
Clinodactyly																		
Camptodactyly					+			+			+		+					
Congenital heart disease	+	++	+	++	+		+	+		++	+		+	++	+++	++	+	+
Cryptorchidism		+		++	+	+			+						+	+		
Elevated axial triradius							++											
Transverse palmar crease				+					+			+		+	+	+		

Table 26-6. SELECTED OVERLAPPING PHENOTYPES OF CHROMOSOMAL SYNDROMES (continued)

	del 11q	dup 12p	del 12p	dup 13	dup 13qp*	dup 13qd*	del 13q	dup 14q	dup 15q	dup 18	del 18p	del 18q	dup 20p	dup 21	del 21q	dup 22	del 22
Mental retardation	+ +	+ +	+ +	+ +	+ +	+ +	+ +	+ +	+ +	+ +	+ +	+ +	+	+ +	+ +	+ +	+ +
Growth retardation	+ +	+ +	+ +	+ +	+ +	+ +	+ +	+ +	+ +	+ +	+ +	+ +		+ +	+ +	+ +	+ +
Low birth weight	+	+		+ +							+	+			+ +	+ +	
Microcephaly	+			+		+	+	+	+						+	+	
Downward slanting eyes													+				
Upward slanting eyes			+								+		+	+			
Hypertelorism	+															+	
Microphthalmia				+	+												
Small palpebral fissures							+	+	+								
Strabismus						+	+	+	+	+		+	+	+			
Broad nasal bridge		+		+			+	+							+		
Cleft upper lip			+	+								+					
Cleft palate			+	+								+			+		
Micrognathia	+ +	+		+	+	+	+	+	+	+	+ +				+		
Low-set ears	+ +						+	+	+	+	+	+		+ +	+		+
Short neck				+				+	+	+				+ +		+	+
Clinodactyly			+	+				+		+				+		+	
Camptodactyly				+				+		+			+	+		+	
Congenital heart disease				+			+	+		+		+		+			
Cryptorchidism		+		+			+	+	+	+		+			+	+	+
Elevated axial triradius		+								+		+			+		
Transverse palmar crease	+				+		+			+							

*"p" refers to partial trisomy for the proximal one-third, and "d" to partial trisomy for the distal two-thirds of the long arm of chromosome 13. (From Lewandowski, 1977.)

Table 26-7. DISCRIMINATING PHENOTYPES OF CHROMOSOMAL SYNDROMES

PHENOTYPE	SYNDROME
Laryngomalacia, premature graying of hair	del 5p
Retinoblastoma	del 13q
Polydactyly	dup 13
Agenesis of thumb and first metacarpal	del 13q
Bony syndactyly of fourth and fifth metacarpals	del 13q
Hypoplasia of first metacarpal	del 18q
Delayed ossification carpus, tarsus, pelvis	del 4p
Persistence of fetal hemoglobin and neutrophils	dup 13
Thymic aplasia	dup 1q
Absent patella	dup 8
Anal stenosis	dup 22q, del 13q
Holoprosencephaly	dup 13, del 13q, del 18p
Orbital hypotelorism	dup 21, del 13q, del 18p

From Lewandowski, 1977.

q34 (Fig. 26-16). Relatively discriminating phenotypic findings of the trisomy 13 syndrome have been similarly sublocalized. For example, genetic material responsible for delayed disappearance of fetal neutrophils and for fetal hemoglobin is located in bands q12 and q14, respectively; tendency to arrhinencephaly in chromosome band q14; and polydactyly in chromosome segment q31-qter (Fig. 26-16).

ABNORMALITIES OF AUTOSOMES

Both numerical and structural defects involving the 22 pairs of homologous chromosomes are observed. While the variety of numerical defects is quite limited, some of them occur with a relatively high frequency. In contrast, the number of different duplication deficiencies is almost unlimited, with each occurring at a relatively low frequency. A few of the more significant autosomal disorders are discussed in this section; for a more complete review, see Yunis, 1977a.

Down's Syndrome. Down's syndrome, due to trisomy of chromosome 21, is the most common chromosomal syndrome, with a general incidence of 1 in 650 among newborns. This fact, as well as its severity, relatively long life span, frequency of recurrence, identifiable high-risk mothers, and possibility of prenatal diagnosis, makes Down's syndrome uniquely important.

The clinical diagnosis is almost always obvious at birth, owing to the distinctive facial appearance of upward slanting eyes, small and malformed ears, and large protruding tongue; poor muscle tone; short stubby hands with incurved fifth fingers (clinodactyly); and abnormal dermatoglyphics, including simian creases, distal axial triradii in the palms, and arch tibial patterns on the big toes. Major visceral anomalies of the heart, gastrointestinal tract, and urinary system are not uncommon, and the patient's longevity is usually less than normal, such that the mean survival age is about 20 years. The intelligence quotient ranges from 25 to 70, with an average of 50 to 59 in patients less than 3 years of age, and a lower average (25 to 49) with increasing age. Patients with Down's syndrome exhibit a twentyfold increased risk over that of the general population of developing acute leukemia.

Approximately 95 per cent of the cases each possess 47 chromosomes, including an extra 21 (Fig. 26-17). This is due to non-disjunction of a chromosome 21 during meiosis, the incidence of which increases with maternal age. A mother less than 20 years of age has a risk of

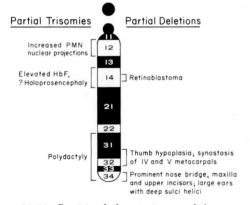

Figure 26-16. Provisional phenotypic map of chromosome 13. (From Yunis, 1977b.)

Figure 26–17. Selected chromosomes involved in trisomy 21 in three different patients. *A, Left,* Trisomy 21 due to non-disjunction. *B, Center,* Trisomy 21 resulting from a parental balanced translocation t(14;21). *C, Right,* Trisomy 21 resulting from a t(21;21) balanced translocation in one of the parents.

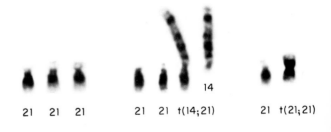

21   21   21   21   21   t(14;21)   21   t(21;21)

about 1 in 2500 of having a child with trisomy 21. This risk gradually increases and at 35 years of age is about 1 in 250; over 45 years of age the prospective mother has a 1 in 50 chance of having a child with Down's syndrome.

About 3 per cent of cases of Down's syndrome have 46 chromosomes, the extra chromosome 21 being attached to another chromosome. Translocation Down's syndrome, which cannot be differentiated from the trisomic form on the basis of clinical features, is not age-dependent. This form may be either sporadic or familial. In most cases of the familial form, one of the parents has 45 chromosomes instead of the normal 46, and one of the chromosomes 21 is involved in a Robertsonian translocation with another acrocentric chromosome, chromosome 14 in about half the cases (Fig. 26-17), and chromosome 22 in most other cases. This is thought to be due to the fact that the very small, short arms of acrocentric chromosomes, with their nucleolar organizers and heterochromatic regions, are more likely to break than other chromosome segments on other autosomes, producing a high frequency of structural aberrations in these chromosomes. The parent carrying the translocation chromosome is phenotypically normal, since no significant amount of genetic material has been lost in the translocation process. When the chromosome 21 is translocated to either a chromosome 14 or 22, the chance of having an abnormal offspring is relatively high if the mother is the carrier (about 10 per cent) and low if the father is the carrier (approximately 2.5 per cent). The reason for this difference is not known. In persons carrying a translocation between two 21 chromosomes, the risk is 100 per cent, since conceptuses are either trisomic 21 (Fig. 26-17) or monosomic 21 lethals.

The third or mosaic form constitutes about 2 per cent of all patients with Down's syndrome and is caused by having two different cell populations, one trisomic for chromosome 21 and the other normal. This form is usually suspected when the phenotypic expression of trisomy 21 is not fully expressed or when the intelligence of the patient is higher than expected, since individuals having trisomy 21 mosaicism may vary in phenotype from typical Down's syndrome to normal. In addition, they may have children with the typical Down's syndrome.

Trisomy 13. Trisomy 13 syndrome is a devastating disorder, resulting in severe growth and mental retardation, arrhinencephaly, and polydactyly, as well as other major and minor defects such as congenital heart disease and polycystic kidneys. There is a delayed disappearance of fetal hemoglobin and fetal neutrophils. In the absence of mosaicism, about 45 per cent of affected individuals die within the first month, 70 per cent by the sixth month, and more than 95 per cent by three years of age. This syndrome has an incidence of about 1 in 6000, is more commonly seen in female infants, and, like Down's syndrome, has more than one type of chromosomal basis.

About 75 per cent of cases have three chromosomes 13, as a result of primary non-disjunction in meiosis. The mean age for mothers of trisomy 13 infants of this type is 32.4 years, suggesting that the risk increases with advancing maternal age. About 20 per cent of the cases of trisomy 13 are caused by a translocation, most of them (85 per cent) of the Robertsonian type between a chromosome 13 and another of the 13-15 group. As with Down's syndrome, the other acrocentric is usually a number 14. In addition, there are numerous instances of the syndrome resulting from the extra presence of only part of chromosome 13. These patients vary in severity, depending upon the length of the segment involved, but usually exhibit a clinically milder phenotype. Partial trisomy 13 generally occurs in offspring of parents who carry a reciprocal translocation between a segment of the long arm of chromosome 13 and another chromosome segment.

The remaining 5 per cent of trisomy 13 cases are caused by mosaicism. About half of these patients have 2 cell populations, one of which possesses an extra chromosome 13. The other half result from a complex assortment of chromosomal abnormalities. As expected, the clinical findings are often less severe in mosaic infants than in those with classical trisomy 13.

Trisomy 18.   Trisomy 18 syndrome is similar to trisomy 13 in severity, preponderance of affected females, and dependence of incidence on maternal age (mean age is over 32 years). Recent surveys have varied in their reported incidence of trisomy 18 from 1 in 3500 to 1 in 7000 births. Thirty per cent fail to survive more than one month, 50 per cent die by two months, and over 90 per cent by one year. The average survival time for females is 134 days and for males 15 days (overall average 70 days).

The main features of trisomy 18 are microcephaly, prominent occiput, microphthalmia, abnormally shaped ears, prominent tip of the nose, small mouth, micrognathia, short sternum, congenital heart disease, hypoplastic labia in females, overriding clenched fingers, and rocker-bottom feet. The combination of micrognathia and prominent occiput result in a characteristic "pointed-face" appearance when the affected infant is viewed from the side. Even more distinctive is the hand deformity, in which the hand is clenched, the index finger overlaps the third, the fourth finger overlaps the fifth, and most fingertips show simple arches. The hand defect, present in most trisomy 18 infants, is sufficient indication for chromosome studies.

It is thought that about 10 per cent of trisomy 18 individuals are mosaics. As expected, they may exhibit a milder phenotype and may survive longer. There are also reported cases of partial trisomy 18 resulting from chromosomal translocations.

Trisomy 8 Syndrome.   Trisomy 8 syndrome is one of the new chromosomal syndromes described since the advent of the banding techniques. Most cases known are mosaics, having normal and trisomy 8 cell lines. Phenotypic features include mental retardation; normal height; long and slender trunk; anomalies of vertebrae and ribs; limited joint function; absent knee caps; bulging skin with deep furrows in palms and soles; de-formed skull; strabismus; low-set or dysplastic ears; and micrognathia. It is not uncommon for these patients to live to be 28 years of age. In suspected cases, such as an infant presenting with mental retardation, long and slender trunk, absent knee caps, restricted articular function, and deep furrows, blood chromosome analysis should be performed.

In addition to trisomy 21, 13, and 18 and trisomy 8 mosaicism, trisomy 9 mosaicism, trisomy 22, monosomy 21, and monosomy 22 have occasionally been found among liveborns (Table 26-6). All other clinically distinctive autosomal abnormalities are due to partial trisomies or partial deletions (Table 26-6 and Figure 26-15). Among the deletion disorders, the best known are the 5p- and 18q- syndromes. Of the partial trisomies, +9p syndrome is the most common and the +10q syndrome results in the most severely affected and characteristic phenotype. These disorders are reviewed below.

5p- or Cat-cry Syndrome.   Patients with the cat-cry syndrome usually show a deletion of one half to two thirds of the short arm of one of the chromosomes 5. The distinguishing feature is a weak, shrill cat-like cry in infancy caused by hypoplasia of the larynx. The cry, almost one octave higher than normal and monotone in quality, usually disappears with time, even within a few weeks of age. Other features include microcephaly, round face, hypertelorism, antimongoloid obliquity of palpebral fissures, epicanthus, bilateral alternating strabismus, severe mental retardation, and failure to thrive. Preauricular tags are occasionally noted. Life expectancy is fairly long and older patients develop premature graying of hair and overbite malocclusion, while the roundness of the face and the ocular hypertelorism disappear.

18q- Syndrome.   Long arm deletion of chromosome 18 can be recognized by characteristic facial changes, including midface hypoplasia, deep-set eyes, ophthalmologic defects, short nose, and carp-shaped mouth; unusual pinnae; and an excess of whorls in the fingertips. Mental retardation is severe.

Trisomy +9p.   Trisomy for the short arm of chromosome 9 is probably the most commonly occurring autosomal syndrome after Down's syndrome. Except for mental retardation, the phenotypic effects are relatively mild and include moderate microcephaly, brachycephaly, flat forehead, enophthalmos, prominent nose with inverted nostrils, a short upper lip with the corners of the mouth slanting downward, and protuberant ears. In addition, the hand shows a distinct morphology, including hypoplasia of phalanges, a transverse palmar flexion crease, decreased number of whorls on the fingers, and the absence of b or c triradius. Mortality from this syndrome appears low and patients are known to live at least to their teens. Cases in which 9p trisomy is limited to the distal half of the short arm of chromosome 9 exhibit a *form fruste* of the syndrome.

Trisomy +10q. Trisomy for the distal segment of the long arm of chromosome 10 has a low frequency of occurrence and results in a phenotype comparable in severity to that of the classic full trisomies. Because of characteristic facial features and unusual anomalies of the extremities, this syndrome is readily identifiable. Patients exhibit severe psychomotor and growth retardation, hypotrophy, microcephaly, a spacious forehead, flat and round face, arched or cleft palate, micrognathia, malformed or low-set ears or both, and short neck. In the hands and feet, findings frequently include syndactyly of the second and third toes, an excess of ulnar loops, a simian crease, proximally implanted thumbs or toes, overlapping fingers, webbing of fingers, camptodactyly, a space between the first and second toes, and deep plantar furrows. The chromosome segment which appears to be responsible for the phenotype is 10(q25 → qter), as illustrated by the case shown in Figure 26-13. The G-banded karyotype of the father shows a balanced translocation involving chromosomes 10 and 15 (Fig. 26-13*A*). The son, however, has an unbalanced karyotype, since he received the abnormal chromosome 15 and the normal chromosome 10, resulting in +10q (Fig. 26-13*B*). Prognosis is poor, with about half of the patients dying by one year of age.

SEX CHROMOSOME DEFECTS

The X and Y chromosomes are involved in numerical and structural defects more frequently than any other chromosome. Among the various abnormalities that may occur, the basic but not sole alteration is impairment of gonadal function, the degree depending upon the magnitude of the chromosome defect as well as the percentage of body cells affected. Other common features, which may be found either alone or in combination, include very tall or very short stature, skeletal anomalies, abnormal dermatoglyphic patterns, mental retardation, and abnormal behavior.

The relative mildness of the phenotypic effects observed in sex chromosome anomalies as compared with that of autosomal defects is related to the fact that in early embryogenesis any X chromosome exceeding one is inactivated in somatic cells and the Y chromosome contains only a small number of structural genes. Another feature of the sex chromosome anomalies is the relatively high frequency of mosaicism, especially in Turner's syndrome, which can reduce the severity of the particular defect.

Sex chromosome anomalies become evident at birth (such as in Turner's syndrome, in XO/XY mosaicism, and in individuals with an XXXX or XXXXY sex complement), at puberty (e.g., hermaphroditism), or adulthood (e.g., trisomy X, Klinefelter syndrome, and XYY syndrome).

At Birth. Intersexes can be detected in infancy by external genitalia that are either completely ambiguous or show marked impairment of normal differentiation. Some of them are due to XO/XY mosaicism, or they may be true hermaphrodites with an XX, XY, XX/XY, XX/XXY, or other types of mosaicism with a line containing a Y chromosome. More frequently, however, newborns or infants with ambiguous genitalia may represent cases of adrenogenital syndrome in females with signs of virilism. These can be detected with a urinary 17-ketosteroid assay; the presence of Barr bodies in the buccal smear is quite helpful for confirmation. If neither cytogenetic nor hormonal assays are diagnostic, surgical exploration and gonadal biopsy are usually necessary to resolve the ambiguity. In cases of possible true hermaphrodites or intersexes with normal urinary ketosteroids, chromosome studies are carried out to determine the true genetic sex so that appropriate corrective measures may be instituted. The more common sex chromosome defects are rarely symptomatic at birth, except for Turner's syndrome (45,XO), in which webbing of the neck or edema may be seen. Even in this syndrome, however, the infant's secondary sex characteristics are normal.

At Puberty. Children with the more common sex chromosome anomalies (e.g., 47,XXX; 47,XXY; and 47,XYY) usually develop more or less normally until puberty. XXX females may then exhibit amenorrhea, XXY males have small testes and cannot procreate, and XYY males may present with aggressive behavior and tallness. In cases of true hermaphrodites or XO/XY mosaics with a female phenotype, virilization at puberty may provide the first clue to these conditions.

In Adults. If gonadal function is not depressed to the degree that pubertal sexual development is impaired, otherwise "normal" adults with sex chromosome anomalies may exhibit sterility. Two examples in which this may occur are Trisomy X (47,XXX) and mosaic variants of Klinefelter syndrome.

Turner's Syndrome. Of the syndromes due to sex chromosome anomalies, Turner's syndrome shows the most severely affected phenotype. The frequency of occurrence is about 1 per 2500 female births. It may be caused by X monosomy, either complete or in a mosaic form (XO/XX, XO/XXX); or by deletion of the short arm of one X chromosome, which is present as a "pure" short arm deletion, a ring chromosome, or an isochromosome for the long arm of an X chromosome. Phenotypic features may vary, although certain characteristics are usually found. Among the most consistently noted are short height (adult height generally less than 57 inches) and streak ovaries (consisting of long strands of white wavy connective tissue without follicles), which result in primary amenorrhea and sterility. Breast development is usually absent and the nipples are widely spaced and hypoplastic. The external genitalia are infantile and pubic hair sparse. Other common features include webbing of the neck, shield chest, increased numbers of cutaneous nevi, cubitus valgus, short fourth metacarpals, hypoplastic and deep-set toenails, coarctation of the aorta, and horseshoe kidney. Facial features include triangular face with epicanthal folds, ptosis of upper eyelids, prominent ears, and micrognathia. The hairline is low at the nape, and the neck is often short. Mental retardation is not a feature of Turner's syndrome, although many patients exhibit a defect in space perception and orientation.

About 60 per cent of cases of Turner's syndrome have an XO sex complement and are, in general, the most severely affected. Diagnosis is readily made, since buccal cells are X-chromatin negative and karyotyping reveals a single population of cells with a modal number of 45 chromosomes, with one X and no Y chromosome.

Approximately 10 per cent of patients with Turner's syndrome are XO/XX mosaics, probably resulting from early loss of an X chromosome in a female embryo. Clinical features vary, depending on the time of loss and on the cell composition of the various tissues. Because the two cell population types may appear throughout the body or preferentially in certain tissues, the study of chromosomes or the X body in a single tissue does not necessarily give an accurate picture. In general, a low percentage (5 to 12 per cent) of Barr bodies is found, but the clinical spectrum is wide, ranging from cases with typical Turner's syndrome to cases with normal gonads and normal stature. About 20 per cent menstruate, but the great majority of patients are sterile.

About 5 per cent of the cases of Turner's syndrome are XO/XXX mosaics. Clinically they resemble the XO/XX mosaics, but they may exhibit mental retardation.

Approximately 20 per cent of patients with Turner's syndrome have an isochromosome for the long arm of the X chromosome (Xqi). These patients exhibit many of the features seen in those with XO Turner's syndrome, i.e., short stature, sexual infantilism, primary amenorrhea, and skeletal anomalies, but they are less likely to have webbed neck and aortic coarctation. Of the cases with an iso-X chromosome, less than one third have a true XXqi chromosome constitution; the remainder are mosaics (XO/XXqi). Turner's syndrome may also result when one of the X chromosomes has a short arm deletion or is in a ring configuration with substantial deletion of the short arm. This suggests that the short arm of the X-chromosome is the most important pathogenic segment and contains gene(s) involved in ovarian differentiation and determination of height.

XO/XY Mosaicism. The phenotype of these individuals is quite variable, depending upon when in embryogenesis a cell loses the Y chromosome and how the resulting two cell types populate the various tissues of the body. About 80 per cent have ambiguous genitalia, 15 per cent have a female phenotype with some features of Turner's syndrome, and 5 per cent have a male phenotype (with bilateral undescended testes). Patients with XO/XY mosaicism and a Turner's phenotype usually become hirsute and develop hypertrophy of the clitoris at puberty. Also, about 25 per cent of these patients, along with those exhibiting ambiguous genitalia, develop seminoma or gonadoblastoma in their teens or adulthood.

Since these patients are reared as females, develop virilism, and have a propensity for malignancy, it is a common practice to remove the gonads once the diagnosis is established.

Trisomy X. XXX females usually exhibit a mild but variable phenotype. Although the incidence in the population is only about 0.73 per 1000 liveborn females, approximately 4 to 5 per 1000 institutionalized females have been found to have trisomy X, supporting the finding of intellectual or emotional impairment in about 25 per cent of these patients. In addition, approximately 25 per cent have some type of congenital deformity, 25 per cent exhibit mild developmental lags, and 25 per cent are essentially normal. The effects on sexual development vary from none (75 per cent) to mild menstrual disorders to hypoplastic ovaries associated with poor breast development, amenorrhea, and sterility. Fertility is not uncommon, and the resulting offspring have a normal chromosome constitution, suggesting the occurrence of selection against ova possessing two X chromosomes. Maternal age is elevated, as in other human trisomies. Studies of somatic cells show a large number with two X chromatin bodies, as would be expected.

Tetrasomy and Pentasomy X. Females with more than three X chromosomes almost always exhibit mental retardation. XXXX females also frequently have ocular hypertelorism, epicanthal folds, mild mandibular prognathism, and reduced fertility. XXXXX females are more severely affected and show some resemblance to XXXXY males. These patients have severe mental deficiency; ocular hypertelorism with uncoordinated eye movements; broad flat nose; everted and furrowed lips; short neck; low hairline; abnormal development of sexual organs such as infantile breasts and uterus; scanty pubic hair; increased number of digital arches; and a variety of skeletal anomalies. In addition, pentasomy X females may exhibit hypoplastic frontal sinuses, microbrachycephaly, and malformed sacral vertebrae.

Buccal mucosa cells from XXXX and XXXXX females exhibit up to three and four X chromatin bodies, respectively. Of the cases studied with regard to parental origin, the extra X chromosomes have been found to be inherited from the mother.

Klinefelter's Syndrome. Klinefelter's syndrome, which occurs at a frequency of 1 in 700 live male births, is primarily due to an XXY constitution (80 per cent) or mosaicism (15 per cent). The remaining 5 per cent are XXYY, XXXY, or XXXXY Klinefelter variants and are generally more severely affected. This syndrome is also known as X chromatin-positive testicular dysgenesis and usually results in sterility.

XXY Klinefelter patients develop the characteristic clinical features at puberty, including long lower extremities, great arm span, and small, firm, insensitive testes with hyalinized seminiferous tubules and abnormal Leydig cells. Other abnormalities may include gynecomastia, sparse facial and axillary hair, a female pattern of pubic hair distribution, and decreased libido and potency. Klinefelter patients tend to be passive and poorly motivated, yet may display inappropriately aggressive behavior when confronted with stressful situations. Approximately 20 to 25 per cent of XXY males have reduced intelligence.

In Klinefelter's syndrome, maternal age is significantly advanced and non-disjunction occurs in the mother in about 60 per cent of the cases.

Klinefelter males with the less common XXYY, XXXY, and XXXXY chromosome constitutions exhibit the same symptoms with greater severity, often including severe mental retardation and aggressive behavior. In addition, they may have some somatic anomalies, such as hypoplastic penis in XXXY and XXXXY males, and hypertelorism, strabismus, epicanthus, mandibular prognathism, short neck, and skeletal anomalies in XXXXY males.

Klinefelter mosaics generally have an XXY, XXXY, or XXXXY sex chromosome constitution in one cell line and an XX or XY karyotype in the other. The actual phenotype depends upon the sex chromosome constitution of the predominant cell type present in critical tissues, such as the brain and gonads, at a given stage of development.

XYY Syndrome. XYY males appear to be either normal or minimally affected by the extra Y chromosome. The frequency in newborn male infants is about 1 per 700 births, and parental age is not elevated. Patients are usually above the ninetieth percentile in height by age 6 owing to increased leg and trunk length, but other features are less frequent and may be subtle, such as muscle weakness, poor coordination, mild facial asymmetry, mild pectus excavatum, mild scapular winging, long ears, and bony chin point. XYY men usually have normal testes, external genitalia, and fertility. The extra Y chromosome is not transmitted to progeny, suggesting a marked selection against the abnormal sperm.

Following studies which indicated a disproportionately high percentage (2 to 4 per cent) of XYY males to be in prisons or mental hospitals, extensive psychiatric investigations were carried out. It appears that cases with subnormal intelligence and criminality are few, while aggressive and explosive behavior, as well as a propensity to destroy property, may be a more common feature of XYY males.

CHROMOSOME DEFECTS IN NEOPLASIA

Cancer cells have been shown to exhibit an extremely wide range of chromosome defects that vary in both degree and number among different cells in the same tissue. These defects include aneuploidy, polyploidy, and numerous types of structural abnormalities. Until recently, most investigators considered chromosomal abnormalities in human cancer to be an epiphenomenon of neoplasia. This was due to the fact that, except for the association of the Philadelphia chromosome with chronic myelogenous leukemia, no specific chromosome abnormalities were consistently observed. Indeed, patients with the same type of neoplastic process, for example, acute myelogenous leukemia, were usually seen to exhibit quite different karyotypes. The development of chromosome banding techniques (for a review, see Yunis, 1974), however, helped to advance cytogenetic tumor research, resulting in the discovery of several constant associations between specific types of neoplasia and chromosomal changes (Table 26-8) (Mitelman, 1976; Rowley, 1976; Mark, 1977).

The first malignancy associated with a specific chromosome defect was chronic myelogenous leukemia (CML), in which approximately 90 per cent of cases were found to exhibit a small chromosome 22 (Philadelphia or Ph[1] chromosome). With the use of the banding methods, it has been possible to show that the distal half of the long arm of the chromosome 22 is actually translocated to another chromosome, usually onto the end of the long arm of a chromosome 9 (Fig. 26-18). This translocation has been shown to be acquired and limited to hematopoietic cells of the granulocytic, erythrocytic, and megakaryocytic types. In some

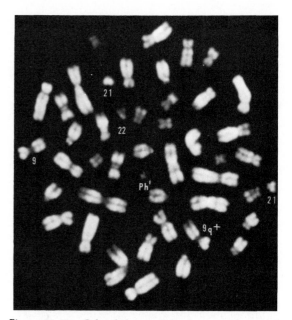

Figure 26–18.   Q-banded metaphase from a patient with CML. Note balanced 22(Ph[1]);9(9q+) translocation. (From Rowley, 1974.)

cases of CML, the overt clinical manifestations of leukemia may be preceded by a relatively long symptom-free period. In these cases, the finding of the Ph[1] chromosome allows for early diagnosis and treatment of this disorder.

The observation of the Philadelphia chromosome in CML is also of prognostic value. Ph[1]-positive patients respond better to chemotherapy than Ph[1]-negative patients and have a significantly longer mean survival time (42 months for Ph[1]-positive compared with 15 months for Ph[1]-negative patients). Later in the course of the disease, a change in the karyotype of a Ph[1]-positive patient is a strong indication of onset of the acute or blast phase. The additional chromosome defects usually seen include the presence of an extra copy of the Ph[1] chromosome, an isochromosome for the long arm of chromosome 17, and/or trisomy 8.

The Ph[1] chromosome has been found in several patients with acute lymphocytic leukemia (ALL) and acute non-lymphocytic leukemia (ANLL). A recent evaluation (Bloomfield, 1977) on the clinical significance of Ph[1]-positive ALL has indicated that these patients are older and have a higher frequency of lymphadenopathy and splenomegaly than Ph[1]-negative ALL patients. Remissions were obtained in all nine adults with Ph[1]-negative ALL, but

Table 26-8. CONSISTENT CHROMOSOME DEFECTS OBSERVED IN SPECIFIC NEOPLASMS AND MYELOPROLIFERATIVE DISORDERS

NEOPLASIA	CHROMOSOME(S) INVOLVED												
	1	5	7	8	9	13	14	15	17	18	20	21	22
CML					t(9,22)								t(9,22)
CML-Blast crisis				+8	t(9,22)				i(17q)				t(9,22) 22q−
ALL and ANLL (subtype)					t(9,22)								t(9,22)
AML			−7	t(8,21) +8								t(8,21)	
APL								t(15,17)	t(15,17)				
Polycythemia vera											20q−		
Refractory anemia (subtype)		5q−											
Burkitt's lymphoma				t(8,14)			t(8,14)						
Other lymphomas							14q+						
Ataxia telangiectasia							14q−						
Retinoblastoma						13q14−							
Meningioma				−8									−22
Colonic polyps				+8			14+						

in only three of six with Ph[1]-positive ALL. Similarly, adults with Ph[1]-positive ANLL all survived significantly shorter periods than adults with Ph[1]-negative ANLL.

Acute myelogenous leukemia (AML), in contrast to CML, is not characterized by a single chromosome defect. Approximately 40 per cent of these patients exhibit a normal karyotype, and 60 per cent show relatively non-specific, but not completely random, chromosomal changes. Indeed, 80 per cent of the defects discovered involve either an additional chromosome 8, a missing 7, and/or a translocation between chromosomes 8 and 21 (Levan, 1977) (Fig. 26-19). As in the case of CML, cytogenetic studies in these patients provide valuable information on the prognosis and response to therapy. For example, patients with AML and a normal karyotype have approximately an 87 per cent rate of remission and a mean survival of 8 months, whereas patients with an abnormal karyotype have only a 20 per cent remission rate and a 2-month mean survival time (Rowley, 1976). Subgroups of AML with specific defects are now beginning to be uncovered, such as those patients with the Philadelphia chromosome. A second possible subgroup is suggested by the finding in several unrelated patients with acute promyelocytic leukemia (APL) of a con-

sistent chromosome change involving an insertion of band 17q21 into the middle of the long arm of chromosome 15 (Rowley, 1977).

Burkitt's lymphoma is a type of neoplastic process associated with the Epstein-Barr virus which has been found to exhibit an abnormally long chromosome 14. This marker chromosome has been shown to represent part of a reciprocal translocation between the distal ends of the long arm of a chromosome 8 and the long arm of a chromosome 14 (Zech, 1976). It is also evident that certain other non-Hodgkin B cell lymphomas exhibit what appears to be a similar marker chromosome 14.

Retinoblastoma is a tumor appearing in childhood with a high frequency among two groups of genetically predisposed individuals: those who inherit a tumor predisposition in an autosomal dominant fashion, and those born with a partial deletion of the long arm of chromosome 13, who usually also exhibit mental retardation and congenital defects. The latter group is of particular importance because it is the only instance known in man in which a specific chromosome defect that occurs prezygotically can consistently predispose affected individuals to a certain tumor. Studies of 11 patients with retinoblastoma, as well as various associated congenital defects and mental retardation, showed the deletion

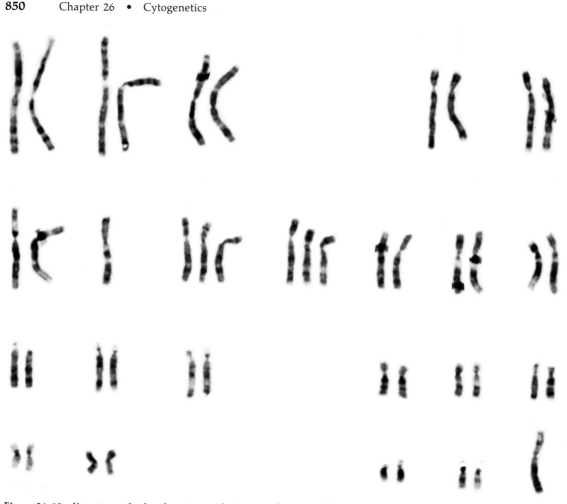

Figure 26-19. Karyotype of a female patient with acute myelogenous leukemia showing monosomy 7 and X and trisomy 8 and 9.

in common to be band 13q14. Recently, analysis of the fine subbanding pattern in late prophase chromosomes of a retinoblastoma patient revealed a deletion of the minute subband 13q14.2 and a portion of each of the adjacent subbands 13q14.1 and 13q14.3 (Yunis, 1978; Fig. 26-20).

Two additional and more unusual types of chromosomal aberrations found in malignant tumor cells, particularly those of neurogenic origin, include very long marker chromosomes and double minutes. The very long marker chromosomes have each been found to contain, with the use of chromosome banding, a lightly and homogeneously staining region (HSR). HSR-containing chromosomes in man have been observed thus far only in neuroblastomas and differ in each line studied. Double minutes are small, paired, acentric, and weakly staining chromatin bodies whose number and size vary from cell to cell. They are found most frequently in neuroblastomas and gliomas, although the abnormality has also been occasionally detected in other neoplasias such as acute leukemia. The origin and function of double minutes is unclear. Because of their association with tumors of neurogenic origin, especially neuroblastomas, and the propensity for this kind of tumor to regress spontaneously, it has been suggested that they serve a role in the neoplastic process (Balaban-Malenbaum, 1977).

Until recently, it was believed that only malignant tumors would show an abnormal karyotype. However, it is now evident that certain benign tumors, as well as some myeloproliferative syndromes and refractory anemias, have consistent chromosome defects. For example, meningiomas have been found to exhibit a partial or complete loss of chromosome 22 and/or monosomy 8 in over 90 per cent and over 50 per cent of the cases, respectively. Trisomy 8 and trisomy 14 have been discovered in a high percentage of colonic polyps. Polycythemia vera cases often possess a chromosome 20 which has about half of its long arm deleted. A specific subset of patients with refractory anemia exhibit a partial deletion of the long arm of a chromosome 5 (Sokal, 1975).

In addition to benign and malignant tumors known to exhibit specific chromosome defects, it has been observed that certain autosomal recessive disorders have a tendency to show "spontaneous" chromosome aberrations and to develop neoplasms at an increased frequency. These conditions include Fanconi's anemia, Bloom's syndrome, and ataxia telangiectasia. Patients with Fanconi's anemia, who often exhibit pancytopenia and congenital defects, have a propensity to develop malignancies, particularly leukemia. Approximately 10 per cent of metaphases from direct bone marrow preparations and a larger number from lymphocyte cultures are found to have chromatid gaps and breaks as well as chromosome rearrangements. The finding of a high incidence of chromatid breakage has been found useful in the diagnosis of this condition. Bloom's syndrome is characterized by stunted growth, sunlight sensitivity, facial telangiectasia, chromosome instability, and frequent development of leukemia or other neoplasias, particularly those of gastrointestinal origin. Besides increased breakage, quadriradial figures, i.e., four armed figures generally derived from the exchange of chromatid segments of two homologous chromosomes, are often seen (German, 1974). In addition, a large number of chromatid exchanges per chromosome is often observed using the sister chromatid exchange technique (Sanchez, 1977). Ataxia telangiectasia is characterized by progressive cerebellar ataxia, oculocutaneous telangiectasia, and immunodeficiency; approximately 10 per cent of these patients develop lymphoma. In addition to a relatively high frequency of chromosome breaks, chromosome 14 often shows a preferential break in the proximal portion of its long arm (q11-12), leading to 14q- cell lines (Wyandt, 1977).

HIGH RESOLUTION CHROMOSOMES IN CLINICAL MEDICINE

Many advances in human cytogenetics have been accomplished within the past several years with the study of banded midmetaphase chromosomes, in which some 320 bands per haploid set were observed. Improvements in methodology, such as the recently developed technique involving lymphocyte synchronization with amethopterin and minimal exposure to colcemid (see p. 823), allows for the analysis of chromosomes arrested earlier in mitosis. Of importance is the fact that late prophase chromosomes, exhibiting an average of 1035 bands per haploid set; prometaphase chromosomes with an average of 750 bands; early metaphase chromosomes, with an average of 543 bands; and midmetaphase chromosomes, with an average of 401 bands, can now be routinely studied. The increase in resolution should have a dramatic impact on basic and clinical disciplines, such as the study of gene mapping, neoplasia, and birth defects.

Before the advent of the banding techniques, chromosome aberrations observed in malignant tumors were thought to be an epiphenomenon of the neoplastic process. Since 1971, with the use of banded midmetaphases, approximately 12 specific types of malignant and benign tumors, as well as certain myeloproliferative disorders, have been found to exhibit a consistent chromosome defect (p. 848). With the recent use of prophase chromosomes it has been possible to localize with precision the chromosome band deletion in chromosome 13 (q14) responsible for predisposition to bilateral retinoblastoma. It is likely that further use of these finely banded chromosomes will result in a surge of new discoveries. For example, about half of patients with acute myelogenous leukemia (AML) have a "normal" karyotype, and it should be possible, with the high resolution technique, to uncover subtle defects in some of these patients. Furthermore, while chronic myelogenous leukemia (CML) and Burkitt's lymphoma cells have been found to have reciprocal translocations (9q; 22q and 8q; 14q, respectively), it remains

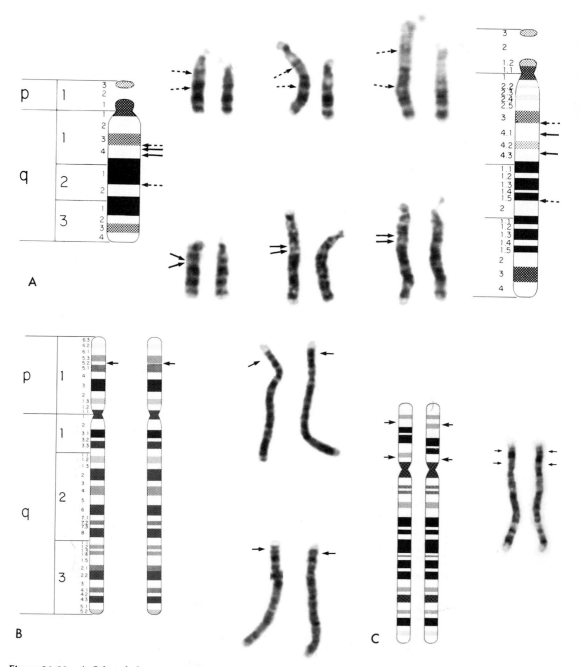

Figure 26–20. *A,* Selected chromosomes 13 in various stages of mitosis from two patients with retinoblastoma. Schematic representation of chromosome 13 at mid-metaphase (*left*) and prometaphase (*right*). Dotted and solid arrows indicate deleted segments in the two patients, respectively. *Upper center,* G-banded chromosomes from a patient showing deletion of subbands 13q14.1 to q21.5 (dotted arrows). *Lower center,* G-banded chromosomes from a second patient showing deletion of subband 13q14.2 and a portion of both subbands 13q14.1 and 13q14.3 (solid arrows). (Modified from Yunis, 1978a.)
B, Schematic representation (*left*) and selected G-banded prometaphase chromosomes (*right*) of a patient with the 4p − phenotype and deletion of subband 4p15.2. (From Yunis, 1977b.)
C, Schematic representation (*left*) and selected G-banded prometaphase chromosomes 5 (*right*) from a patient with a history of multiple miscarriages and paracentric inversion of a segment of the short arm of chromosome 5.

to be seen if these translocations are balanced or if there is a minute band deletion or genetic inactivation involved in the translocation process.

In the case of bilateral retinoblastoma and associated congenital defects, it was difficult to determine the band deletion in chromosome 13 responsible for tendency to the disease using midmetaphase chromosomes, since the major metaphase bands of chromosome 13 are not clearly distinguishable among themselves. However, in more elongated chromosomes, such as prometaphase and late prophase, the refined subbanding patterns allowed a critical analysis of break points, and a common deletion of a portion of band q14 was uncovered (Fig. 26-20A) (Yunis, 1978a). Retinoblastoma is one of about seven types of embryonic tumors with small, round cells that are often clinically associated with congenital defects (Anderson, 1976). It is possible that other neoplasms in this group also have specific chromosome defects involved. Indeed, in Wilms' tumor (nephroblastoma usually associated with aniridia and other congenital abnormalities), an interstitial deletion of the short arm of chromosome 11 has been recently found (Riccardi, 1978).

In studies of patients exhibiting multiple congenital defects and abnormal dermatoglyphics with or without growth and mental retardation, it is not uncommon to find "normal" metaphase chromosomes. This occurs even in some patients fulfilling all criteria for having a specific chromosome defect, such as the 4p- and 5p- syndromes. Following the introduction of prophasic chromosomes in our laboratory, we have uncovered minute chromosome defects in several patients, such as that illustrated in Figure 26-20B. In this patient, who presented with the typical 4p- syndrome, only a deletion of the minute light subband 4p15.2 was found.

It is also becoming evident that patients who exhibit variations of normalcy, such as "idiopathic" mental retardation, unexplained growth retardation, or short stature with only a few minor anomalies, should be scrutinized. This is in contrast to approaches in the past, when chromosome studies were indicated primarily in patients with sex anomalies or newborns with multiple congenital defects and associated developmental lag. In this regard, of the individuals with relatively mild phenotypic changes who are being studied in our

laboratory, several instances of a band or subband duplication have been found to be responsible for the phenotype. Since 3 per cent of the population have an IQ of < 70 and about 10 per cent have an IQ of < 90, and since a large number of retarded individuals are known to have a chromosome defect (Penrose, 1971), it is important to screen this population with the use of banded prophases.

As indicated above, a subgroup in which high resolution chromosome studies may be beneficial is that of individuals with short stature. It is known that about 15 to 20 per cent of patients with the clinical manifestations of Turner's syndrome are mosaics and that in those with an XO/XX or XO/XXX constitution, the syndrome can be mild. In fact, these individuals may be normal or present themselves with "idiopathic" shortness of stature (Leão, 1966). It is also known that the short arm of the X chromosome, perhaps the distal end, as well as the short arm of the Y, carry gene(s) important for determination of height. Since structural chromosome defects involving the sex chromosomes are relatively common, it is therefore likely that minute deletions may be found in patients with unexplained short stature.

Another subgroup for whom analysis of prophase chromosomes is indicated is that of infertile couples, which account for about 10 per cent of all marriages in the general population (Novak, 1975). Relatively large inversions and translocations have been found to be the cause in a few cases with the study of midmetaphase chromosomes (Benirschke, 1974). Recently, several patients who exhibit habitual abortions yet have "normal" chromosomes by metaphase analysis have been found with the use of prometaphases and prophases to carry chromosomal rearrangements (Fig. 26-20C).

The fine detail offered by prophasic chromosomes also allows the determination of the precise break points involved in chromosome defects, providing a more definitive characterization of the chromosome segments involved. This and the recognition of single subband defects, such as that found for bilateral retinoblastoma, should enable one to gain a better understanding of how genes affect morphogenesis to produce specific phenotypic anomalies. Indeed, recent work suggests that the light staining or G-negative chromosome bands contain the bulk of the structural genes and that in late prophase light subbands may only have 10 to 60 genes each (Yunis, 1977b). Thus, it is evident that we are finally bridging the gap between genes and chromosomes and we can now begin to visualize, at a refined level, how the human genome is organized.

REFERENCES

Anderson, W.A.D., and Scotti, T.: Synopsis of Pathology, 9th ed. St. Louis, The C. V. Mosby Co., 1976.

Ansari, B. M., and Mason, M. K.: Chromosomal abnormality in congenital rubella. Pediatrics, 59:13, 1977.

Armendares, S., Buentello, L., Salamanca, F., and Cantu-Garza, J.: A dicentric Y chromosome without evident sex chromosomal mosaicism, 46,XYq dic, in a patient with features of Turner's syndrome. J. Med. Genet., 9:6, 1972.

Arrighi, F. E., and Hsu, T. C.: Localization of heterochromatin in human chromosomes. Cytogenetics, 10:81, 1971.

Arrighi, F. E., and Hsu, T. C.: Staining constitutive heterochromatin and Giemsa crossbands of mammalian chromosomes. In Yunis, J. J. (ed.): Human Chromosome Methodology, 2nd ed., New York, Academic Press, Inc., 1974.

Balaban-Malenbaum, G., and Gilbert F.: Double minute chromosomes and the homogeneously staining regions in chromosomes of a human neuroblastoma cell line. Science, 198:739, 1977.

Barr, M. L., and Bertram, E. G.: A morphologic distinction between the neurones of the male and female, and the behavior of the nucleolar satellite during accelerated protein synthesis. Nature, 163:676, 1949.

Benirschke, K.: Chromosomal errors and reproductive failure. In Coutinho, E. M., and Fuchs, F. (eds.): Physiology and Genetics of Reproduction—Basic Life Sciences, Vol. 4A. New York, Plenum Press, 1974.

Bloomfield, C. D., Peterson, L. C., Yunis, J. J., and Brunning, R. D.: The Philadelphia chromosome (Ph¹) in adults presenting with acute leukaemia: A comparison of Ph¹+ and Ph¹− patients. Br. J. Haematol., 36:347, 1977.

Carr, D. H., and Gedeon, M.: Population cytogenetics of human abortuses. In Hook, E. B., and Porter, I. H. (eds.): Population Cytogenetics. New York, Academic Press, Inc., 1977.

Caspersson, T., Farber, S., Foley, G. E., Kudynowski, J., Modest, E. J., Simonsson, E., Wagh, E., and Zech, L.: Chemical differentiation along metaphase chromosomes. Exp. Cell Res., 49:219, 1968.

Caspersson, T., Zech, L., Johansson, C., and Modest, E. J.: Identification of human chromosomes by DNA-binding fluorescent agents. Chromosoma, 30:215, 1970.

Chicago Conference: Standardization in human cytogenetics. Birth Defects, Original Article Ser. 2, No. 2. New York, The National Foundation for Birth Defects, 1966.

Cohen, M. M., Macgillivray, M., Capraro, V., and Aceto, R.: Human dicentric Y chromosomes. J. Med. Genet., 10:74, 1973.

Dewald, G., Dines, D. E., Weiland, L. H., and Gordon, H.: Usefulness of chromosome examination in the diagnosis of malignant pleural effusions. N. Engl. J. Med., 295:1494, 1976.

Dutrillaux, B.: New chromosome techniques. In Yunis, J. J. (ed.): Molecular Structure of Human Chromosomes. New York, Academic Press, Inc., 1977.

Dutrillaux, B., and Lejeune, J.: Sur une nouvelle technique

d'analyse du caryotype humain. C. R. Acad. Sci. (Paris), 272:2638, 1971.

Edwards, J. H., Harnden, D., Cameron, A., Crosse, V., and Wolff, O.: A new trisomic syndrome. Lancet, 1:787, 1960.

Fialkow, P. J., Thuline, H. C., Hecht, F., and Bryant, J.: Familial predisposition to thyroid disease in Down's syndrome: Controlled immunoclinical studies. Am. J. Hum. Genet., 23:67, 1971.

Ford, C. E., Jones, K., Polani, P., de Almeida, J., and Briggs, J.: A sex chromosome anomaly in a case of gonadal dysgenesis (Turner's syndrome). Lancet, 1:711, 1959.

German, J. (ed.): Chromosomes and Cancer. New York, John Wiley & Sons, Inc., 1974.

Harnden, D. B.: Skin culture and solid tumor technique. In Yunis, J. J. (ed.): Human Chromosome Methodology, 2nd ed. New York, Academic Press, Inc., 1974.

Hollander, D. H., and Borgaonkar, D. S.: The quinacrine fluorescence method of Y chromosome identification. Acta. Cytol., 15:452, 1971.

Hook, E. B., and Porter, I. H. (eds.): Population Cytogenetics. New York, Academic Press, Inc., 1977.

Hungerford, D. A., Donnelly, A. J., Nowell, P. C., and Beck, S.: The chromosome constitution of a human phenotypic intersex. Am. J. Hum. Genet., 11:215, 1959.

Jacobs, P. A., and Strong, J. A.: A case of human intersexuality having a possible XXY sex-determining mechanism. Nature (London), 183:302, 1959.

Jones, K. W.: Repetitive DNA and primate evolution. In Yunis, J. J. (ed.): Molecular Structure of Human Chromosomes. New York, Academic Press, Inc., 1977.

Kotler, S., and Lubs, H. A.: Comparison of direct and short-term tissue culture technics in determining solid tumor karyotypes. Cancer Res., 27:1861, 1967.

Kruse, P. F., Jr., and Patterson, M. K. (eds.): Tissue Culture: Methods and Applications. New York, Academic Press, Inc., 1973.

Leão, J. C., Voorhess, M. L., Schlegel, R. J., and Gardner, L. I.: XX/XO mosaicism in nine preadolescent girls. Pediatrics, 38:972, 1966.

Lejeune, J., Turpin, R., and Gautier, M.: Le mongolisme. Premier exemple d'aberration autosomique humaine. Ann. Genet., 1:41, 1959.

Levan, A., Levan, G., and Mitelman, F.: Chromosomes and cancer. Hereditas, 86:15, 1977.

Lewandowski, R. C., and Yunis, J. J.: New chromosomal syndromes. Am. J. Dis. Child., 129:515, 1975.

Lewandowski, R. C., and Yunis, J. J.: Phenotypic mapping in man. In Yunis, J. J. (ed.): New Chromosomal Syndromes. New York, Academic Press, Inc., 1977.

Lyon, M. F.: Gene action in the X-chromosome of the mouse. (Mus musculus L.). Nature, 190:372, 1961.

Mark, J.: Chromosomal abnormalities and their specificity in human neoplasms: An assessment of recent observations by banding techniques. Adv. Cancer Res., 24:165, 1977.

Milunsky, A., and Atkins, L.: The frequency of chromosomal abnormalities diagnosed prenatally. *In* Hook, E. B., and Porter, I. H. (eds.): Population Cytogenetics. New York, Academic Press, Inc., 1977.

Mitelman, F., and Levan, G.: Clustering of aberrations to specific chromosomes in human neoplasms. II. A survey of 287 neoplasms. Hereditas, *82*:167, 1976.

Mittwoch, U.: Sex chromatin bodies. *In* Yunis, J. J. (ed.): Human Chromosome Methodology, 2nd ed. New York, Academic Press, Inc., 1974.

Moore, K. L., and Barr, M. L.: Smears from the oral mucosa in the detection of chromosomal sex. Lancet, *2*:57, 1955.

Moorhead, P. S., Nowell, P. C., Mellman, W. J., Battips, D. M., and Hungerford, D. A.: Chromosome preparations of leukocytes cultured from human peripheral blood. Exp. Cell Res., *20*:613, 1960.

Nadler, H. L., and Ryan, C. A.: Amniotic cell culture. *In* Yunis, J. J. (ed.): Human Chromosome Methodology, 2nd ed. New York, Academic Press, Inc., 1974.

NICHD National Registry for Amniocentesis Study Group: Midtrimester Amniocentesis for Prenatal Diagnosis. J.A.M.A., *236*:1471, 1976.

Novak, E. R., Seegar Jones, G., and Jones, H. W.: Textbook of Gynecology, 9th ed. Baltimore, Williams and Wilkins Co., 1975.

Nowell, P. C.: Phytohemagglutinin: An initiator of mitosis in cultures of normal human leukocytes. Cancer Res., *20*:462, 1960a.

Nowell, P. C., and Hungerford, D. A.: A minute chromosome in human chronic granulocytic leukemia. Science, *132*:1497, 1960b.

Ohno, S., Kaplan, W. D., and Kinosita, R.: Formation of the sex chromatin by a single X-chromosome in liver cells of *Rattus norvegicus*. Exp. Cell Res., *18*:415, 1959.

Paris Conference: Standardization in human cytogenetics. Birth Defects, Original Article Ser. 3, No. 7. New York, The National Foundation for Birth Defects, 1971.

Patau, K., Smith, D., Therman, E. M., Inhorn, S. L., and Wagner, H. P.: Multiple congenital anomaly caused by an extra autosome. Lancet, *1*:790, 1960.

Patil, S. R., Lubs, H. A., Kimberling, W. J., Brown, J., Cohen, M., Gerald, P., Hecht, F., Moorhead, P., Myrianthropoulos, N., and Summitt, R. L.: Chromosomal abnormalities ascertained in a collaborative survey of 4,342 seven and eight-year old children: Frequency, phenotype and epidemiology. *In* Hook, E. B., and Porter, I. H. (eds.): Population Cytogenetics. New York, Academic Press, Inc., 1977.

Pearson, P. L., Bobrow, M., and Vosa, C. G.: Technique for identifying Y chromosomes in human interphase nuclei. Nature (London), *226*:78, 1970.

Penrose, L. S., and Smith, G. F.: Down's Anomaly. London, J. & A. Churchill, 1966.

Riccardi, V. M., Sujansky, E., Smith, A. C., and Francke, V.: Chromosomal imbalance in the aniridia—Wilms' tumor association: 11p interstitial deletion. Pediatrics, *61*:604, 1978.

Robinson, A., Goad, W. B., Puck, T. T., and Harris, J. S.: Studies on chromosomal non-disjunction in man. III. Am. J. Hum. Genet., *21*:466, 1969.

Rowley, J. D.: Identification of human chromosomes. *In* Yunis, J. J. (ed.): Human Chromosome Methodology, 2nd ed. New York, Academic Press, Inc., 1974.

Rowley, J. D.: The role of cytogenetics in hematology. Blood, *48*:1, 1976.

Rowley, J. D., Golomb, H. M., and Dougherty, C.: 15/17

translocation, a consistent chromosomal change in acute promyelocytic leukemia. Lancet, *1*:549, 1977.

Sanchez, O., and Yunis, J. J.: New chromosome techniques and their medical applications. *In* Yunis, J. J. (ed.): New Chromosomal Syndromes. New York, Academic Press, Inc., 1977.

Sokal, G., Michaux, J. L., Van Den Berghe, H., Cordier, A., Rodhain, J., Ferrant, A., Moriau, M., De Bruyere, M., and Sonnet, J.: A new hematologic syndrome with a distinct karyotype: The 5q- chromosome. Blood, *46*:519, 1975.

Sparkes, R. S., and Motulsky, A. G.: The Turner syndrome with isochromosome X and Hashimoto's thyroiditis. Ann. Intern. Med., *67*:132, 1967.

Stene, J.: Detection of higher recurrence risk for age-dependent chromosome abnormalities with an application to trisomy G_1 (Down's syndrome). Hum. Hered., *20*:112, 1970.

Tjio, J. H., and Levan, A.: The chromosome number of man. Hereditas, *42*:1, 1956.

Uchida, I. A.: Maternal radiation and trisomy 21. *In* Hook, E. B., and Porter, I. H. (eds.): Population Cytogenetics. New York, Academic Press, Inc., 1977.

Uchida, I. A., and Lin, C. C.: Quinacrine fluorescent patterns. *In* Yunis, J. J. (ed.): Human Chromosome Methodology, 2nd ed. New York, Academic Press, Inc., 1974.

Wagenbichler, P., Killian, W., Rett, A., and Schnedl, W.: Origin of the extra chromosome No. 21 in Down's syndrome. Humangenetik, *32*:13, 1976.

Williams, D. L., and Runyan, J. W., Jr.: Sex chromatin and chromosome analysis in the diagnosis of sex anomalies. Ann. Intern. Med., *64*:422, 1966.

Wyandt, H. E., Magenis, R. E., and Hecht, F.: Abnormal chromosomes 14 and 15 in abortions, syndromes, and malignancy. *In* Yunis, J. J. (ed.): New Chromosomal Syndromes. New York, Academic Press, Inc., 1977.

Yunis, J. J. (ed.): Human Chromosome Methodology. New York, Academic Press, Inc., 1965.

Yunis, J. J. (ed.): Human Chromosome Methodology, 2nd ed. New York, Academic Press, Inc., 1974.

Yunis, J. J.: High resolution of human chromosomes. Science, *191*:1268, 1976.

Yunis, J. J. (ed.): New Chromosomal Syndromes. New York, Academic Press, Inc., 1977a.

Yunis, J. J., and Chandler, M. E.: The chromosomes of man—clinical and biologic significance. Am. J. Pathol., *88*:465, 1977b.

Yunis, J. J., and Ramsay, N.: Retinoblastoma and subband deletion of chromosome 13. Am. J. Dis. Child., *132*:161, 1978a.

Yunis, J. J., and Bahr, G.: Chromatin fiber organization of human interphase and prophase chromosomes. Exp. Cell Res. (in press, 1978b.)

Yunis, J. J., Kuo, M. T., and Saunders, G. F.: Localization of sequences specifying messenger RNA to light-staining G-bands of human chromosomes. Chromosoma, *61*:335, 1977c.

Yunis, J. J., Roldan, L., Yasmineh, W. G., and Lee, J. C.: Staining of satellite DNA in metaphase chromosomes. Nature (London), *231*:532, 1971.

Yunis, J. J., and Sanchez, O.: A new syndrome resulting from partial trisomy for the distal third of the long arm of chromosome 10. J. Pediatr., *84*:567, 1974.

Yunis, J. J., Sawyer, J. R., and Ball, D. W.: The characterization of high-resolution G-banded chromosomes of man. Chromosoma, *67*:293, 1978c.

Yunis, J. J., Sawyer, J. R., and Ball, D. W.: G-banding patterns of high resolution human chromosomes 6-22 and X, Y. Human Genetics, (in press, 1978d).

Yunis, J. J., and Yasmineh, W. G.: Model for mammalian constituitive heterochromatin. Adv. Cell Mol. Biol., *2*:1, 1972.

Zackai, E. H., and Mellman, W. J.: Human peripheral blood leukocyte cultures. *In* Yunis, J. J. (ed.): Human Chromosome Methodology, 2nd ed. New York, Academic Press, Inc., 1974.

Zech, L., Haglund, U., Nilsson, K., and Klein, G.: Characteristic chromosomal abnormalities in biopsies and lymphoid-cell lines from patients with Burkitt and non-Burkitt lymphomas. Int. J. Cancer, *17*:47, 1976.

Part 3

HEMATOLOGY AND COAGULATION

Edited by Douglas A. Nelson, M.D.,
and John Bernard Henry, M.D.

27

BASIC METHODOLOGY

Douglas A. Nelson, M.D.

The branch of laboratory medicine known as hematology focuses chiefly on the cellular elements of the blood and on coagulation.

Included in its concerns are:

1. The concentration of different types of cells in the blood.
2. The status and proliferative behavior of their precursor cells in the hematopoietic organs.
3. The structure, chemical content, and functional activity of blood cells.
4. Certain chemical constituents of plasma or serum which are intimately linked with blood cell structure and function.
5. The role of blood vessels, platelet function, and blood coagulation in maintaining vascular integrity.

Aberrations in these characteristics may produce hematologic disease or may be hema-tologic manifestations of disease processes initiated elsewhere in the body.

In this chapter we consider hematologic methods widely or "routinely" used in studying disease.

BLOOD COLLECTION

The two sources of blood for hematologic tests are capillary or peripheral blood and venous blood.

CAPILLARY OR PERIPHERAL BLOOD

Free flowing "capillary" or peripheral blood is more nearly arteriolar than capillary.

For hematologic examination, blood is best obtained from a vein. When this is not possible, many determinations may be performed on blood obtained from the lobe of an ear, the palmar surfaces of the tip of a finger, or, in the case of infants, the plantar surfaces of the great toe or the heel. In the case of the ear, the free margin of the lobe, not the side, should be punctured. Puncture can be made deliberately and slowly because there is almost no pain connected with it. The puncture should be about 3 mm deep. If the patient is bedridden, the finger will be found more convenient. An edematous or congested site should not be used. Free flow of blood is essential to obtain reproducible results comparable to those with venous blood. Cold, cyanotic skin is a source of errors. It is responsible for falsely high figures for hemoglobin and cell counts, but can be avoided by massage before the puncture until the skin is pink and warm. Vigorous squeezing after the puncture is another source of errors.

Equipment. Equipment consists of gauze pads, 70 per cent alcohol, and a lancet or scalpel blade. Disposable lancets or blades are recommended. Reusable blades must be sterilized by autoclaving before being used on different patients.

Technique. The site is first rubbed well with a gauze pad moistened with 70 percent alcohol to remove dirt and epithelial debris and to increase the amount of blood in the part. After the skin has dried and the circulation has returned, a puncture 2 to 3 mm deep is made with the blade or lancet. The puncture is practically painless if properly made with a sharp blade. It should be made expeditiously with a firm stab, which, however, must not be made so quickly or from so great a distance that its site and depth are uncertain. A deep puncture is no more painful than a superficial one and makes it unnecessary to repeat the procedure.

The first drop of blood that appears is wiped away because it contains tissue juices; the second is used for examination. If the skin at the site of the puncture is not dry, the blood will not form a rounded drop as it exudes. The blood must not be pressed out, since this dilutes it with fluid from the tissues, but moderate pressure some distance above the puncture is allowable. After the needed blood has been obtained, a pad of sterile gauze is applied to the puncture and the patient instructed to apply slight pressure until bleeding has ceased. When the heel is used, it must be made warm; this may be done by immersion in warm water or by use of a hot-water compress.

Otherwise, values significantly higher than in venous blood may be obtained, especially in the newborn.

Precision is poorer in capillary than in venous blood because of variation in flow. Initial capillary samples tend to give lower cell counts because of dilution with interstitial fluid; in freely flowing blood, results gradually approach those from venous samples. Even with freely flowing blood, the cell counts and hemoglobin are probably slightly lower in blood from a skin puncture. This is a mixture of capillary and arteriolar blood, and it is clear that the venous hematocrit is significantly greater than the whole body hematocrit by a factor of 1/0.9 (ICSH, 1973). It is undesirable to use capillary blood for platelet counts because of the rapidity with which platelets adhere to wound surfaces and aggregate, tending to lower the platelet count; here the need for free flow is especially great. Blood films made from capillary blood are preferable to those made from blood taken into an anticoagulant, but the blood must flow freely to avoid an altered distribution of leukocytes.

VENOUS BLOOD

Three factors are involved in a good venipuncture: the venipuncturist, the patient and his veins, and the equipment (see Chap. 3).

Venipuncturist. The venipuncture is in most instances a relatively simple procedure. The operator must be aware of the old phrase in ancient medicine that the doctor's main motto should be *primum non nocere*—"the first thing is not to inflict damage." The vein that one tries to enter should be preserved for innumerable future uses. Actually, the life of the patient may sometimes depend on vein patency.

The hematomas displaying all the colors of the rainbow in antecubital fossae, around wrists, and in various other places testify eloquently to the operator's lack of skill or judgment. As a rule, the damage is only temporary, but it may be long-lasting or even permanent. A venipuncture must be approached with due care and deliberation.

The Patient and His Veins. The patient should be reassured with a few words well chosen to fit the particular situation. Self-assurance and poise will do much to establish the proper rapport. The patient should be made comfortable, and the approach to his arm should be convenient for the operator.

There is no need to add to the difficulties by trying to do the puncture in an inconvenient position. Ambulatory patients should be seated comfortably, preferably in a chair provided with an armrest or at a table on which the arm can be placed comfortably.

The veins should be inspected and evaluated. When veins are deep and not felt distinctly, an attempt to enter them is bad practice because it amounts to blind probing. One can minimize this difficulty by using a tourniquet, which makes the veins more prominent and palpable for orientation. Such trial compression should be released and repeated again when one is ready for the actual puncture.

In patients who have had many punctures in the past and sequelae thereof, such a preliminary study of the veins is particularly important and may reveal more available veins than would seem apparent at first glance.

Equipment. The syringe should be of the proper size for the amount of blood to be drawn. Disposable plastic syringes are widely used. With reusable glass syringes, the fit of the plunger and barrel and the integrity of the syringe tip should be checked; following use, the syringe should be rinsed in cold water to remove the blood.

The gauge and length of the needle are chosen for the specific task. The gauge number expresses the diameter of the needle. The smaller the number, the larger the needle. The length of the needle used depends upon the depth of the vein. The tip should be inspected carefully. A blunt or bent tip will damage the patient's vein and often leads to failure.

Method of Obtaining Blood from a Vein. Whether the patient is lying down or sitting, his arm should be firmly supported. Never have the patient standing or seated on a high stool. Although few patients faint as a result of venipuncture, this danger must be kept in mind.

A rubber tourniquet is placed around the upper arm to increase venous pressure and to make the veins more prominent and easier to enter, but to prevent hemoconcentration the pressure should not be maintained longer than necessary.

The outer end of the tourniquet should be tucked under the last round in such a manner that a slight pull will release the bandage. The cuff of a blood pressure apparatus answers admirably; it has the advantage that it permits adjustment of the compression to a level

midway between systolic and diastolic pressures, which reduces the flow of venous blood without stopping arterial circulation. Also, reduction or release of pressure after the needle has entered the vein is facilitated. Occasionally it will be sufficient for an assistant or even the patient to grasp the upper arm firmly. If one uses a rubber tubing as tourniquet, he can apply the proper pressure by first compressing the arm so as to suppress the radial pulse and then releasing the pressure just enough to feel the radial pulse feebly. The patient is asked to open and close his fist several times. This causes the veins to become distended. Giving the patient an active role in the procedure helps to take his mind off the puncture. Even if not seen, veins can usually be felt beneath the skin. In fat persons, veins that show as blue streaks are usually too superficial and too small.

After all preliminary steps have been taken, the skin is cleansed with 70 per cent alcohol or another suitable disinfectant and allowed to dry. It is desirable to apply the tourniquet while the alcohol is drying. The next step is to fix the vein in position. This is done by supporting the patient's forearm with the operator's hand and compressing and pulling the soft tissues just below the intended puncture site with the operator's thumb. The syringe is held between the thumb and the last three fingers of the other hand. The back of these fingers are rested on the patient's arm. The free index finger rests against the hub of the needle and serves as a guide. A prominent vein may be entered with a single direct puncture of skin and vein. This one-step procedure is less painful.

When veins are difficult to find, a two-step procedure is used. First the skin is punctured in the vicinity of the vein and then the vein itself is punctured. Successful entrance into the vein is followed immediately by appearance of blood in the syringe. If that does not take place, the plunger is withdrawn slightly and in most instances blood appears. The tourniquet may be loosened if blood flows freely; otherwise, it may be left in place until the desired amount of blood is obtained. At this point the patient is asked to open his fist, the tourniquet is released, a small additional amount of blood is permitted to enter the syringe, the needle is withdrawn, gentle pressure is applied to the site of the puncture with a pad of dry gauze or cotton, and the patient is instructed to take over pressing the pad and to raise the outstretched arm for a few minutes. This usually stops the bleeding and prevents formation of a hematoma. A small dressing (Band-Aid) may be applied, mainly to prevent a stain on the rolled-down sleeve. The operator must see that the patient's condition is satisfactory before he is dismissed. If there is any sign of continued discomfort, anxiety, bleeding, or shock, the patient should be kept lying down and seen by a physician.

It is usually easy to secure 5 to 15 ml of blood, or even more, if required. If the needle is sharp and smooth, the procedure causes the patient surprisingly little inconvenience. There is rarely any difficulty in inserting a needle into a vein except in children and in patients in whom the arm is fat and the veins are small. If necessary, one of the veins about the ankle can be used. In infants, blood may be secured from the femoral or the external jugular vein.

When the blood has been expelled, the plunger should be separated from the barrel of reusable syringes, and both washed in cold water. Otherwise the syringe may become "frozen" when the blood clots or dries.

Instead of syringes, evacuated blood collection tubes may be employed (see Chap. 3, p. 53). Evacuated tubes, sealed with a stopper, are supplied with a measured amount of anticoagulant (or none) and sufficient vacuum to draw a predetermined volume of blood. A disposable needle screws into a holder and the evacuated tube is placed in the holder so that the tube stopper just reaches the guide line. The short needle is thereby embedded in the tube stopper but does not penetrate through it to break the vacuum. After the needle is inserted into the arm vein as described above, the tube is pushed all the way into the holder, vacuum is broken, and the blood flows into the tube. After the flow ceases, the tube may be removed and another tube inserted into the holder, or if only one tube is needed, the whole unit is withdrawn as described above for the syringe. This convenient system eliminates the need for syringes and uses disposable needles and tubes.

Hemolysis interferes with many examinations. It can be minimized by using clean glassware and clean and not too thin needles, by drawing the blood slowly, no faster than the vein is filling; by avoiding admixture of air with frothing; and, after the blood is drawn, by removing the needle and then emptying the blood again slowly and without force into the test tube.

Complications of Venipunctures and Suggestions for Their Prevention

IMMEDIATE LOCAL COMPLICATIONS. Hemoconcentration is the result of prolonged application of the tourniquet. Over 60 seconds will produce measurable increases in the concentration of the blood cells.

Failure of blood to enter the syringe is the result of several factors. Excessive pull on plunger may collapse a small vein. Piercing the outer coat of the vein without entering the lumen may also account for the failure of blood to enter the syringe. This may be remedied by withdrawing lightly and reentering the vein. This complication may occasionally be followed by hematoma formation. As soon as signs of beginning hematoma are noticed, the tourniquet should be released, the needle withdrawn, and local pressure applied. Venipuncture should then be attempted on the other arm. Transfixation of the vein also accounts for failure to obtain blood. This may be remedied by slight withdrawal followed by gentle aspiration to see whether blood appears. If this fails, the puncture may have to be repeated. This complication is frequently followed by formation of a hematoma, and the same remedy is followed as outlined above. Circulatory failure is another cause, and the situation is entirely beyond the control of the operator.

In the case of these or of any other complications, failure to draw blood after two attempts should be an indication to request another operator to try.

Another not infrequent immediate complication is syncope. This is best treated by having the patient lie down, if he is not already in this position. A physician should check the patient immediately.

Continued bleeding may occur in patients with a hemorrhagic tendency. Local pressure, as a rule, controls the bleeding.

LATE LOCAL COMPLICATIONS. Thrombosis of the vein is sometimes due to trauma, especially following many venipunctures at the same site. Rarely, infection results in thrombophlebitis. These complications are rare if the precautions and recommendations discussed in this chapter are observed.

LATE GENERAL COMPLICATIONS. Serum hepatitis may be caused by transmission of the virus by contaminated needle or syringe. The use of disposable needles has virtually eliminated this source of transmitted disease.

Venipuncture in Infants.

In infants and children venipuncture presents special problems because of the small size of the veins and the difficulty controlling the patient. However, even here much can be achieved by the same approach that was outlined for procedures in adults.

Restraining the infant to reduce mobility, use of sharp needles of appropriate size, careful inspection of the veins, and making certain that the pressure applied with the tourniquet is not excessive (best checked by feeling pulsation of the radial artery) will contribute to a successful venipuncture when others may have failed. External jugular puncture may be tried in difficult cases and is frequently successful. Occasionally the internal jugular vein may have to be used.

For hematologic examination, blood obtained by venipuncture is delivered without delay to tubes containing a suitable anticoagulant. Mixing with the anticoagulant is accomplished by thorough but gentle rotation of the container. A drop of blood from the needle or syringe tip is placed on two or more slides and films are made directly. As soon as the collection is completed, before leaving the patient, it is essential to label the tubes and slides with the patient's name and identification number.

To obtain serum, blood is kept at room temperature or in a 37°C. incubator until a clot has formed and begins to retract; then it is centrifuged and the serum pipetted off. To accelerate retraction the clot may be separated from the wall of the container with a platinum needle, a thin glass rod, or wooden applicator before it is incubated. To obtain serum more rapidly, the blood may be defibrinated with glass beads or a glass rod.

Anticoagulants. The four used in hematology are a mixture of ammonium and potassium oxalate, trisodium citrate, the dipotassium or disodium salts of ethylenediamine tetraacetic acid (EDTA), and heparin. The first three prevent coagulation by removing calcium from the blood plasma by precipitation or binding in un-ionized form. Heparin acts by forming a complex with plasma antithrombin III, which inhibits thrombin and other stages of clotting factor activation.

The mixture of ammonium oxalate (three parts) and potassium oxalate (two parts), 2 mg per 1 ml of blood, does not affect the mean corpuscular volume and may be used for hemoglobin, hematocrit, and red and white cell counts. Its usefulness for blood films is limited to the first few minutes because of the sever-

ity of leukocytic changes such as cytoplasm vacuoles, phagocytosis of oxalate crystals, and irregular nuclear lobulation. It is unsuitable for platelet counting because it allows platelet clumps.

Trisodium citrate is used in a mixture of one part of a 3.8 per cent aqueous solution and nine parts of blood for blood coagulation studies.

EDTA is used in a concentration of 1 to 2 mg per 1 ml of blood and is probably the most widely used anticoagulant for blood cell counts. It must be mixed thoroughly with the blood. It equals oxalate for hematocrit studies and is superior for morphologic studies because artifacts form slowly, only on prolonged standing. Acceptable blood films can be prepared after 2 to 3 hours and cell counts even up to 24 hours, if the blood is refrigerated. It prevents platelet clumping and is the anticoagulant of choice for platelet counting.

Heparin, 0.1 to 0.2 mg per 1 ml of blood, does not affect the corpuscular size and hematocrit. It is the best anticoagulant for prevention of hemolysis and for osmotic fragility tests. It is not satisfactory for leukocyte or platelet counts, because of cell clumping. It produces a troublesome blue background in Wright's-stained blood films.

SOURCES OF ERROR. Even with the use of the preferred anticoagulant for cell counting, EDTA, changes take place that may lead to errors unless suitable precautions are taken.

Blood films should be prepared immediately. If other determinations cannot be performed within 2 or 3 hours, the blood should be refrigerated at 4°C. If the blood is kept at room temperature, sometime between 6 and 24 hours swelling of erythrocytes raises the hematocrit and mean corpuscular volume (MCV) and lowers the mean corpuscular hemoglobin concentration (MCHC) and the erythrocyte sedimentation rate. At 24 hours, however, the white cell count (WBC), red cell count (RBC), hemoglobin, hematocrit, and the red cell indices are all unchanged if the blood has been anticoagulated with EDTA and stored at 4°C. (Brittin, 1969b); under these conditions this is true also for the reticulocyte count and the platelet count (Lampasso, 1968). The sedimentation rate should be performed within two hours (Morris, 1975).

Before taking a sample from a tube of venous blood for a hematologic determination, it is important to mix the blood thoroughly. This requires at least 60 inversions of the tube, which is easily accomplished in two minutes on a mechanical rotator; less than this leads to unacceptable deterioration in precision (Fairbanks, 1971).

HEMOGLOBIN (Hb)

Hemoglobin (Hb), the main component of the red blood cell, is a conjugated protein that serves as the vehicle for the transportation of oxygen and CO_2. When fully saturated, each gram of hemoglobin holds 1.34 ml of oxygen. The red cell mass of the adult contains approximately 600 g of hemoglobin, capable of carrying 800 ml of oxygen. The terminology and symbols employed in this discussion are given in Table 27-1.

A molecule of hemoglobin consists of two pairs of polypeptide chains ("globin") and four prosthetic heme groups, each containing one atom of ferrous iron. Each heme group is precisely located in a pocket or fold of one of the polypeptide chains. Located near the surface of the molecule, the heme reversibly combines with one molecule of oxygen or carbon dioxide.

The main function of hemoglobin is to transport oxygen from the lungs, where oxygen tension is high, to the tissues, where it is low. At an oxygen tension of 100 mm Hg in the pulmonary capillaries, 95 to 98 per cent of the hemoglobin is combined with oxygen. In the tissues, where the oxygen tension may be as low as 20 mm Hg, the oxygen readily dissociates from hemoglobin; in this instance, less than 30 per cent of the oxygen would remain combined with hemoglobin.

Reduced hemoglobin (Hb) is hemoglobin with iron unassociated with oxygen. When each heme group is associated with one molecule of oxygen, the hemoglobin is referred to

Table 27-1. NOMENCLATURE OF HEMOGLOBIN DERIVATIVES

TERM USED	SYMBOL	OTHER TERMS
Hemoglobin	Hb	
Oxyhemoglobin	HbO_2	
Carboxyhemoglobin	HbCO	
Sulfhemoglobin	SHb	
Carboxysulfhemoglobin	SHbCO	
Hemiglobin	Hi	Methemoglobin
Hemiglobincyanide	HiCN	Cyanmethemoglobin

(Modified from van Assendelft, O. W.: Spectrophotometry of Haemoglobin Derivatives. Assen, The Netherlands, Royal Van Gorcum Ltd., 1970.)

as oxyhemoglobin (HbO_2). In both Hb and HbO_2, iron remains in the ferrous state. With iron oxidized to the ferric state, methemoglobin (hemiglobin; Hi) is formed, and the molecule loses its capacity to carry oxygen or carbon dioxide.

Hemoglobinometry is the measurement of the concentration of hemoglobin in the blood. Anemia, a decrease below normal of the hemoglobin concentration, erythrocyte count, or hematocrit, is a very common condition and frequently a complication of other diseases. Clinical diagnosis of anemia based on estimation of the color of skin and of visible mucous membranes is highly unreliable. Anemia is frequently masked in many diseases by other manifestations. To a limited extent similar considerations apply to conditions with abnormally high hemoglobin. For all these reasons the correct estimation of hemoglobin is important and is one of the routine tests done on practically every patient.

DETERMINING THE CONCENTRATION OF HEMOGLOBIN

The concentration of hemoglobin is expressed in grams per 100 ml of blood, or grams per deciliter (g/dl). The custom of recording hemoglobin as a percentage of some arbitrary normal is ambiguous and should not be used.

When one evaluates the relative merits of clinical laboratory tests, at least four desiderata are considered: the accuracy of a single determination as compared with a known standard; the reproducibility of a series of determinations when done by the same technician, by a group of technicians in the same laboratory, and by different laboratories; the speed from the point of view of availability in case of emergency; and the simplicity of the procedure from the point of view of economy.

The methods used in hemoglobinometry can be grouped into four main classes, depending on the basic technique employed: colorimetric methods, gasometric methods, specific gravity methods, and chemical methods.

Colorimetric methods

Principle. Hemoglobin is measured as HbO_2 or is first converted into cyanmethemoglobin (hemiglobincyanide; HiCN). The measurement is done by comparing the optical density of the unknown sample with that of a standard, using a colorimeter or spectrophotometer.

Oxyhemoglobin (HbO₂) Method.   No longer
widely used, but still a satisfactory method is the
determination of hemoglobin as oxyhemoglobin.
The main disadvantage is the lack of a stable
standard for HbO_2. Because of the method's simplicity, it is often used to compare levels of hemoglobin when the absolute quantity is not needed, as
in the osmotic fragility or the HbA_2 determinations. The HbO_2 method does not measure carboxyhemoglobin (HbCO), methemoglobin (Hi), or sulfhemoglobin (SHb), all of which are inactive in
transporting oxygen.

In this procedure 0.02 ml of blood measured with
a Sahli-type hemoglobin pipette is washed into
5.0 ml of approximately 0.007 N ammonium hydroxide solution prepared by adding 4 ml of reagent grade NH_4OH to 1 liter of water and mixing.
Rinse the pipette three times with diluting fluid.
The water used in the preparation of ammonia
solution must be glass distilled, because minute
amounts of copper in distilled water or other diluents employed in HbO_2 determinations may cause
HbO_2 to be converted to Hi and lower the values.
Shake well to insure mixing and oxygenation of
hemoglobin. The solution is read in a photometer in
which are used a green filter (540 nm) and a 0.007 N
ammonium hydroxide solution as blank. The test
can be read within a few seconds or with a stoppered cuvette any time up to three days. The
standard curve can be set up with one of the procedures to be listed later.

Hemiglobincyanide (HiCN) Method.   This
method is the outcome of the long-felt need for
improvement of standardization of hemoglobin determinations; it is now the method of choice.

In 1964 the Subcommittee on Hemoglobinometry
of the International Committeee for Standardization in Hematology proposed that hemoglobinometry be standardized by international agreement.
The HiCN method was recommended, with HiCN
solution as a standard. Hemoglobin constants and
the standard were defined. In the United States,
the College of American Pathologists is entrusted
with the certification of standards. Among the
forms of hemoglobin well adapted to photometry,
HiCN has outstanding advantages. All forms of
hemoglobin likely to be found in blood—HbO_2, Hb,
HbCO, and Hi, but not SHb—are quantitatively
converted to HiCN upon the addition of a single
reagent.

Solutions of HiCN are the most stable of the
various hemoglobin pigments; they are stable for
at least six months when kept in the refrigerator.
Another advantage of HiCN solutions is that they
can be standardized accurately. The absorption
band of cyanmethemoglobin in the region of
540 nm is broad rather than sharp (Fig. 27-1), and
consequently its solutions can be used in filter-type
photometers and in narrow-band spectrophotometers. These instruments are discussed in Chapter 4.

It is advisable to have an independent "photometric" standard in addition to the HiCN standards. This will help to check both the instrument
and the HiCN standard if the photometric readings
of the standard used in the test show excessive
variations in duplicate readings.

Preparation of independent "photometric"
standards:

Copper sulfate · $5H_2O$	1.5 g
2 M ammonium hydroxide	500.0 ml

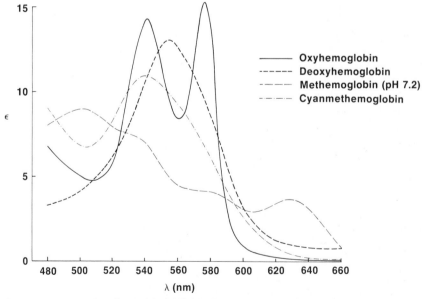

Figure 27-1.   Absorption spectra of oxyhemoglobin (HbO₂), deoxyhemoglobin (Hb), methemoglobin (hemiglobin, Hi), and
cyanmethemoglobin (hemiglobin-cyanide, HiCN). (From Bunn, H. F., Forget, B. G., and Ranney, H. M.: Human Hemoglobins.
Philadelphia, W. B. Saunders Company, 1977.)

Store in tightly stoppered Pyrex flasks. Keep for a year.

Preparation of 2 M ammonium hydroxide: Dilute 136 ml of concentrated reagent grade ammonium hydroxide to 1 liter with distilled water.

SELECTION AND MATCHING OF CUVETTES

Round Cuvettes

1. Clean and dry several dozen cuvettes inside and out.

2. Examine each cuvette and select only those free of scratches or other flaws.

3. Add 0.2 ml of whole blood to 50 ml of distilled water, mix well, and fill each cuvette with this solution.

4. Set the photometer at the 540 nm band or insert the appropriate green filter.

5. Set a water blank at 100 on the transmittance scale (T) or at zero on the density scale (D). This setting should be checked frequently.

6. Insert a filled cuvette in the well. Set the galvanometer beam near the middle of the scale. Rotate the tube slowly, watching the movement of the beam. At the midpoint of the beam's swing, mark the cuvette with a diamond point pencil in relation to a stable mark on the housing of the well.

7. Repeat the same procedure with each cuvette and rotate it until the reading of the galvanometer corresponds with the reading of the first cuvette, marking each in relation to the same stable mark of the colorimeter.

8. All precautions should be taken to avoid scratching the cuvettes. For that reason wooden or coated wire test tube racks are preferable.

Square Cuvettes. Steps 1 to 5 are identical.

6. Place each cuvette in the well. If inexpensive cuvettes are used, only those giving identical readings should be kept. If high-grade expensive cuvettes are used, a correction factor has to be determined for each and applied each time the cuvette is used.

PIPETTES. The 0.02 ml (20 μl) pipette (Sahli) that is used to measure the blood should be accurate to ± 1 per cent. Several supply houses offer 0.02 ml pipettes with a claimed accuracy of this order, both disposable pipettes and reusable glass pipettes. It would appear advisable to calibrate a few reusable pipettes in order to verify the degree of accuracy. (For technique of calibration see p. 867.) The pipettes should be acid cleaned and thoroughly washed with water at least once a week. They should be washed and thoroughly dried between each measurement.

The transfer pipettes used to measure the diluent solution should be of a good order of accuracy, preferably within ± 0.5 per cent. Some of the commercially available pipettes are well within these limits. (The Bureau of Standards tolerance on 5 ml pipettes is ± 0.2 per cent.) If a burette or automatic pipette is used for this purpose, it should be of the same order of accuracy. The task of matching cuvettes can be bypassed by using the flow-through cuvette with which most instruments are now sup-plied. After each reading, the solution is discarded by means of a valve in the bottom of the cuvette. Since all readings, both standards and unknowns, are taken through the same cuvette, errors due to imperfectly matched cuvettes are eliminated.

STANDARD

Principle. Potassium ferricyanide-cyanide solution is used. Ferricyanide converts hemoglobin iron from the ferrous to the ferric state to form Hi, which combines with potassium cyanide to produce the stable HiCN.

The stock standard, which has been certified by the College of American Pathologists, is available commercially from several firms. The exact concentration is within ± 2 per cent of the value stated on the label. It is about 60 mg of HiCN per 100 ml. The spectrophotometric characteristics of HiCN are such that optical density is directly proportional to the concentration. Three different concentrations of the reagent must be used for the preparation of a standard curve, the one purchased containing 60 mg and two more with 40 and 20 mg of HiCN per 100 ml. They are equivalent to 15, 10, and 5 g of hemoglobin per 100 ml when blood is diluted 1:251.

Dilution of Standard

1. Transfer 5 ml of the stock standard to each of three large clean test tubes, using a clean 5-ml volumetric pipette. Allow the pipette to drain. Do not blow it out. Add a second 5-ml volume of the standard to the second tube, using the same pipette.

2. Rinse pipette five times with Drabkin's diluent.

3. Add 5 ml of the diluent to tube 2 and 10 ml to tube 3.

4. Mix contents of tube 3 and of tube 2 in the order mentioned.

5. Beginning with tube 3 and continuing with tubes 2 and 1, transfer 5 ml of contents of each tube into each of three matched cuvettes.

6. The concentration of cyanmethemoglobin in tube 1 is the same as stated on the label of the standard solution. The concentration in tube 2 is two thirds and in tube 3, one third of the standard.

7. The procedure is different if one uses a photometer in which the dilution of blood must be 1:501. Therefore, 5 ml of the stock standard is added to each of the three test tubes, followed by 5 ml of the diluent to tube 1, 10 ml to tube 2, and 20 ml to tube 3. The resulting concentration of cyanmethemoglobin in tube 1 is one half of the stock solution, one third in tube 2, and one fifth in tube 3.

Drabkin's Diluent Solution

Sodium bicarbonate (NaHCO$_3$)	1.0 g
Potassium cyanide (KCN)	0.05 g
Potassium ferricyanide (K$_3$Fe(CN)$_6$)	0.20 g
Distilled water to make	1000.0 ml

This is a clear, pale yellow solution. It should be discarded if it turns turbid. It should be kept in a

3

brown bottle and not more than a month's supply should be prepared. Reagent grade quality chemicals should be used.

PRECAUTIONS IN THE USE OF CYANIDE. Salts and solutions of cyanide are poisonous, and care should be taken to avoid getting them into the mouth or inhaling their fumes.

The concentration of cyanide in the stock standard and the diluent is 50 mg per liter. The smallest dose of potassium cyanide that has been known to kill a human is 300 mg. Nonetheless, this is not a substance to be handled by irresponsible persons. Especially the salt itself must be handled with great circumspection. The following precautions have been recommended:

1. A suction bulb should be employed to fill pipettes.

2. Blood should be mixed with the cyanide solution by swirling.

If the standard or the diluent is prepared in the laboratory, special care must be taken in handling the chemical. If during weighing it is spilled accidentally on the bench or floor, the dry powder should be wiped up with a damp cloth. The cloth should be carefully discarded into a suitable closed container. The solution or powder should not be placed in a sink with acid. The solution may be discarded into a sink if the water is flowing freely. The solid potassium cyanide should be kept under lock and key.

The diluent is now available commercially, either as a solution or as premeasured chemical in a dry pack, so that handling of the salt is avoided.

The standard solution is bacteriostatic and will remain free of bacterial growth if not contaminated in handling. It is recommended that the standard be placed in clean matched cuvettes and sealed permanently. Stoppers are not recommended. It should be stored in a refrigerator in darkness together with the blank solution at about 5° C. but not frozen. Before use, the outside of the cuvettes should be wiped free of moisture, finger marks, and lint, and the standard should be permitted to reach room temperature to prevent condensation on the cuvettes and formation of bubbles when the cold solution is heated suddenly by the light source. Both events may be a source of error. The standard must be discarded every six months.

CALIBRATION OF INSTRUMENT WITH THE CYAN-METHEMOGLOBIN STANDARDS

1. The readings are taken at the 540 nm band. The filter appropriate for the instrument must be in place.

2. The current is turned on and the instrument allowed to warm up according to the instructions of the manufacturer.

3. Distilled water or the diluent solution is used as blank. The absorption of light by the diluent at 540 nm is negligible.

4. The blank is set at 100 on the per cent transmittance (T) scale or at zero on the optical density (OD) scale.

5. The three standard tubes are placed in the cuvette well and the readings recorded beginning with the tube with the lowest concentration and proceeding with next higher concentration tubes. This standardization procedure takes about 5 minutes. It should be done by the beginner before each determination. Later, as experience grows and the instrument performs well and reliably, checking with the standards may be done at intervals to be determined by the operator's and supervisor's judgment.

PREPARATION OF A STANDARD CURVE AND TABLE. The following formula is used:

$$\frac{S \times D}{1000} = g \text{ Hb per dl}$$

where S is concentration of HiCN standard and D is the dilution of the blood sample. For example, if the concentration of the HiCN standard is 60.4 mg per 100 ml and the dilution is 251, then

$$\frac{60.4 \times 251}{1000} = 15.16 \text{ g Hb per dl}$$

The procedure may be facilitated by preparing a curve from which the readings of the galvanometer can be readily translated into hemoglobin values.

If the galvanometer readings are in terms of per cent of transmission (T), the readings of the standards are entered on semilogarithmic graph paper. The abscissa (bottom axis) represents grams of hemoglobin, and the ordinate, the percentage of light transmittance. A line is drawn through the three points. It should pass through or very near T per cent = 100. This graph will show the value in grams of hemoglobin per deciliter corresponding to each reading. When many tests are done, it may be more convenient to construct a table of hemoglobin values for every possible per cent reading. Each photometer must be standardized individually against the standards and should be checked frequently.

If the meter readings are in terms of optical density (OD), the values are plotted on linear graph paper with the density values on the ordinate and the hemoglobin in g/dl on the abscissa. A line connecting the three points should pass through or very near zero. The readings for unknown can be translated into grams of hemoglobin.

PROCEDURE

1. Exactly 5 ml of Drabkin's solution is transferred into each of two matched cuvettes, using an accurate volumetric transfer pipette (meeting U.S. Bureau of Standards requirements of tolerance). A suction bulb, an automatic pipette, or a burette should be used, depending on the amount of work.

2. The blood sample may be taken from a freely bleeding capillary puncture or from a venous sample. The latter must be thoroughly mixed by gently tipping the tube at least 60 times before blood is taken from it. Exactly 0.02 ml of whole blood is transferred with an accurate standardized Sahli pipette into one of the two cuvettes. Great care

must be exerted to fill the pipette exactly to the mark. If the excess is minimal (not more than 2 mm), it may be removed by touching the point of the pipette with a cloth; otherwise the pipette has to be emptied, cleaned, and dried, and the procedure repeated.

3. The blood and solution are mixed by swirling the cuvette. They are left standing for 10 minutes to permit formation of cyanmethemoglobin.

4. The second cuvette serves as a blank. (Instead of Drabkin's solution, distilled water may be used.)

5. If a filter-type photometer is used, the filter appropriate for the make of the instrument is put in place. If the instrument is a spectrophotometer, the wavelength scale is adjusted to 540 nm. Then proceed for the blank and unknown as described previously (see p. 866). The hemoglobin values are read from the curve or table.

The details of procedure may vary with different instruments.

SOURCES OF ERROR—PIPETTE. In view of the fact that 0.02 ml Sahli pipettes may be less accurate than claimed, it is desirable to reserve several carefully calibrated pipettes for Hb measurements. Calibration of blood-diluting pipettes can be carried out by the following procedure recommended by Stevenson (1951).

Equipment. Redistilled mercury; tuberculin syringe; single-hole, size O rubber stopper; mineral oil or stopcock grease; apparatus support stand; 50-ml beaker; weighing bottles; thermometer; analytical balance.

Calibration

1. 0.02 ml pipettes are cleaned with concentrated nitric acid, washed, and dried.

2. The equipment is kept at room temperature. The mercury and pipettes are allowed to reach room temperature before calibration is started. The temperature of the mercury is recorded. Mercury is placed in the beaker. The weighing bottles are weighed and the weight recorded.

3. The plunger of the syringe is coated with mineral oil or grease and the syringe assembled. The tip of the syringe is inserted into the hole of the rubber stopper, which is then clamped vertically to a heavy apparatus support about 18 inches above the bench.

4. The proximal end of the pipette is inserted into the other end of the stopper.

5. The plunger of the syringe is slightly withdrawn. The tip of the pipette is immersed in the mercury. Slow withdrawal of the plunger fills the pipette with mercury. When the 0.02 mark is reached, the beaker is removed. If some mercury is lost in this procedure, the procedure must be repeated. The mercury is emptied into the weighing bottle. The determination should be done in duplicate. The weight of the mercury is established by subtracting the weight of the empty weighing bottle from the final weight with mercury.

6. The volume of the weighed mercury is established by dividing the weight by a temperature correction factor (the specific gravity of mercury in g/ml.):

TEMPERATURE (°C.)	CORRECTION FACTOR
20	13.547
21	13.545
22	13.543
23	13.541
24	13.539
25	13.537
26	13.534
27	13.532
28	13.530
29	13.528
30	13.526

7. The actual volume of the pipette expressed in milliliters divided by the number of milliliters supposed to be measured by the pipette (0.02) gives a correction factor for the pipette, which should be scratched on the pipette with a diamond pencil.

Example

(1) Weight of weighing
bottle = 39.8731 g
(2) Weight of weighing
bottle plus mercury = 40.1311 g
Weight of the mercury 0.2580 g
= (2) − (1)

Volume of mercury delivered by pipette

$$\frac{W}{TCF} = \frac{0.2580\ g}{13.528\ g/ml} \text{ at } 29°C. = 0.0191\ ml$$

where W is the weight of mercury and TCF is the correction factor for the temperature.

Correction factor for the pipette =

$$\frac{VM}{SVP} = \frac{0.0191}{0.0200} = 0.96,$$

where VM is the volume of mercury delivered at prevailing temperature and SVP is the supposed volume measured by the pipette.

OTHER SOURCES OF ERROR. Hyperlipemia, when due to chylomicrons, may falsely elevate the Hb concentration. This can be corrected by centrifuging the blood and replacing the plasma with saline (Gagné, 1977).

Occasionally hypochromic red cells or cells containing Hb S or Hb C will not be lysed by the Drabkin's solution, and the resulting dilution of unknown blood in diluent is turbid. In this case, exactly 5 ml of distilled water added to the turbid fluid will lyse the cells and make it clear. The value determined for the hemoglobin from the calibration curve must then be corrected for the additional dilution by multiplying by 2.

Since leukocytes are not lysed by Drabkin's diluent, high leukocyte counts (over $25 \times 10^9/l$) may falsely elevate the Hb concentration. Centrifugation of the hemolysate will remove the turbidity and the problem. According to Green (1959), falsely high hemoglobin values were seen in two patients with easily precipitable globulins, one with myeloma and the other with idiopathic macroglobulinemia. Adding 0.1 g of K_2CO_3, which increased the alkalinity of the reagent, corrected the problem;

the globulin remained in solution. Otherwise the composition of the reagent remained identical.

Omission of the sodium bicarbonate from Drabkin's reagent and addition of 140 mg of KH_2PO_4 and 0.5 ml of Sterox SE (Hartman-Leddon Co., Philadelphia), a nonionic detergent, will also minimize turbidity due to protein precipitation. In addition, time for full color development is shortened to 3 minutes with this reagent, compared to 20 minutes with Drabkin's (van Assendelft, 1970).

Gasometric method

Van Slyke's Oxygen Capacity Method. This is an indirect method, which estimates the amount of HbO_2 from the amount of oxygen it will bind and utilizes the Van Slyke apparatus. It serves as an accurate method for determining HbO_2 concentration in order to standardize instruments that measure absorbance, but is too complicated for clinical work (Henry, 1964a.) It will not measure Hi, SHb, or HbCO and therefore will underestimate the total hemoglobin, especially in smokers.

Specific gravity method

The specific gravity of the blood is the ratio of the weight of a volume of blood to the weight of the same volume of water at a temperature of 4° C. The normal specific gravity ranges from 1.048 to 1.066. The average for men is 1.057 and for women 1.053. Reflecting the normal diurnal variation in hemoglobin concentration of blood, there is a variation of about 0.003, the values in the afternoon and after meals being somewhat lower and those after exercise and at night, higher. The specific gravity of the serum is 1.026 to 1.031 and that of the erythrocytes, 1.092 to 1.095.

The copper sulfate method of measuring the specific gravity of the blood is a simple and rapid procedure requiring no precision equipment. Drops of blood are permitted to fall into a series of solutions of copper sulfate of known specific gravity, and one observes whether the drops sink or rise in the solutions. Upon immersion, the drops of blood become coated with a layer of copper proteinate, remain discrete for 15 to 20 seconds, and fall if their specific gravity is higher than that of the copper sulfate solution and vice versa. The accuracy of the method depends on the number of solutions used. If 16 are used with specific gravity intervals of 0.004, the gravities are accurate to 0.001. The solutions can be used repeatedly.

The procedure is given by Phillips, (1950). The method has found its main use in screening potential blood donors for anemia. The same method can be used for measuring plasma protein.

Chemical method

Iron Content. Hemoglobin may be measured by determining its iron content. Iron must first be separated from hemoglobin, usually by acid or by ashing. It is then either titrated with $TiCl_3$ or complexed with a reagent to develop color that can be measured photometrically. Satisfactory methods are described by van Assendelft (1970) and by Henry (1964b).

The value for the iron content may be transposed into grams of hemoglobin per deciliter of blood by dividing the amount of iron in milligrams per deciliter by 3.47. According to the recommendation of the Subcommittee on Hemoglobinometry of the International Committee for Standardization in Hematology, the iron content in hemoglobin is 0.347 per cent. Determination of the concentration of hemoglobin by measurement of iron content is too complex for routine work, but from it one can construct calibration curves for both the HbO_2 method and the HiCN method. It is used for standardization in hemoglobinometry if desired or if certified cyanmethemoglobin standards are not available. The iron method, of course, measures total hemoglobin; the HbO_2 method measures only Hb and HbO_2; and the HiCN method measures Hb, HbO_2, Hi, and HbCO.

Errors in hemoglobinometry

The sources of error may be those of the sample, the method, the equipment, or the operator. Some of these have been discussed under the descriptions of the different methods.

Errors Inherent in the Sample. Improper venipuncture technique may introduce hemoconcentration, which will make hemoglobin concentration and cell counts too high. Improper technique in finger-stick or capillary sampling can produce errors in either direction.

Errors Inherent in the Method. The oxyhemoglobin method measures Hb and HbO_2, but not Hi, HbCO, or SHb. It is therefore the method that most closely determines physiologically active hemoglobin. This may be important to recognize in some patients.

The HiCN method is now the method of choice. The use of HiCN standard for calibration of the instrument and for the test itself eliminates one major source of error and provides comparability among all laboratories employing it. The broad absorption band of HiCN in the region of 540 nm makes it convenient to use it both in filter-type photometers and in narrow-band spectrophotometers. With the exception of SHb, all other varieties of hemoglobin are converted to HiCN.

Errors Inherent in the Equipment. The accuracy of equipment is not uniform. A good grade of pipette with a guaranteed accuracy of less than 1 per cent is desirable. Calibration of pipettes will lessen errors inherent in the use of reusable glass pipettes. Significant error will be introduced by the use of unmatched cuvettes. Flow-through cuvettes are preferred because they eliminate the small error present even in the use of matched cuvettes.

The photometer must be calibrated in the laboratory before its initial use and must be rechecked frequently. The wavelength settings, the filters, and the meter readings require checking.

When used with a properly standardized and regularly checked photometer, the HiCN method's error can be reduced to ±2 per cent (expressed as ±C.V.).

Operator's Errors. Most of the human errors are the same in all technical procedures. They can be reduced by good training, meticulous understanding of the clinical significance of the test and of the necessity for a dependable method, adherence to oral and written instructions, and familiarity with the equipment and with the sources of error. The technologist should be well trained, familiar with the performance of his instrument, and able to identify its misbehavior. Errors have been shown to increase with fatigue and tend to be greater near the end of the day than at the beginning. The technologist who is patient and critical by nature and by training and who is interested not only in the *what* and *how* of his work, but also in the *why*, will be less prone to make errors than the one not so constituted.

The above discussion applies to manual techniques of hemoglobinometry. Semiautomated and automated equipment is widely used and has the virtue of eliminating components of the error in individual pipettes and cuvettes and much of the human error.

ABNORMAL HEMOGLOBIN PIGMENTS

The two physiologic hemoglobins, the oxyhemoglobin and the reduced hemoglobin, are readily converted into a series of compounds through the action of acids, alkalies, oxidizing and reducing substances, heat, and other agents. Their gross presence can be distinguished with the spectroscope. For small concentrations (less than 10 per cent) and for quantitative measurements, spectrophotometric, colorimetric, and gasometric methods have to be used.

Hemiglobin (Methemoglobin; Hi). Hi is a derivative of hemoglobin in which the ferrous iron is *oxidized* to the ferric state. The polypeptide chains are not altered.

Hi is part of the "inactive" hemoglobin; it is unable to combine reversibly with oxygen. Although oxygen affinity increases within the Hb tetramer if only partial oxidation of the heme occurs, the oxygen-hemoglobin dissociation curve does not usually shift to the left; this is probably because of the interaction of remaining ferrous hemes with 2,3-diphosphoglycerate tending to shift the curve to the right (Schwartz, 1978). Abnormal amounts of Hi will cause cyanosis and functional "anemia" if high enough, and cyanosis at lower concentrations. Cyanosis may occur at a concentration of 0.5 g of Hi per dl of blood. Comparable degrees of cyanosis will be caused by 5 g Hb/dl blood, 1.5 g Hi/dl blood, and 0.5 g SHb/dl blood. The degree of cyanosis, however, is not necessarily correlated with the concentration of Hi.

The normal individual may have up to 0.24 g Hi/dl blood. The average normal concentration is about 0.4 per cent of the total hemoglobin or about 0.06 g Hi/dl blood.

A small amount of Hi is always being formed but is reduced by enzyme systems within the erythrocyte. At least four pathways exist by which methemoglobin (Hi) may be reduced to hemoglobin (Schwartz, 1978). The most important is the NAD-methemoglobin reductase system. Others, which may function mainly as reserve systems, are ascorbic acid, reduced glutathione, and NADP-methemoglobin reductase. The latter requires a natural cofactor or an auto-oxidizable dye such as methylene blue for activity (Fig. 29-10).

Methemoglobinemia, an increased amount of Hi in the erythrocytes, results from either an increased production of Hi or a decreased NAD-reductase activity, and may be hereditary or acquired. The hereditary form is divided into two major categories. In the first, methemoglobinemia is due to a decrease in the capacity of the erythrocyte to reduce the Hi that is constantly being formed back to Hb.

This is most often due to deficiency in the activity of NAD-methemoglobin reductase, which is inherited as an autosomal recessive characteristic. Heterozygotes have normal levels of Hi but intermediate levels of NAD-methemoglobin reductase activity. The homozygote has methemoglobin levels of 10 to 50 per cent and is cyanotic. Only occasionally is polycythemia present as a compensating mechanism. Hemiglobin concentrations of 10 to 25 per cent may give no apparent symptoms; levels of 35 to 50 per cent result in mild symptoms, such as exertional dyspnea and headaches; and levels exceeding 70 per cent are probably lethal. Therapy with ascorbic acid or methylene blue in this form of hereditary methemoglobinemia will reduce the level of Hi, the latter apparently by activation of the NADP-methemoglobin reductase system.

Heterozygotes have intermediate levels of NAD-methemoglobin reductase activity and normal blood levels of Hi. They may become cyanotic because of methemoglobinemia after exposure to oxidizing chemicals or drugs in amounts that will not affect normal individuals.

In the second major category of hereditary methemoglobinemia, the reducing systems within the erythrocyte are intact, but the structure of the hemoglobin molecule itself is abnormal. A genetically determined alteration in the amino acid composition of two of the four polypeptide chains (either alpha or beta chains) gives rise to a hemoglobin molecule that has an enhanced tendency toward oxidation and a decreased susceptibility of the methemoglobin formed to reduction back to hemoglobin. Five abnormal hemoglobins have been identified whose principal consequence is asymptomatic cyanosis due to methemoglobinemia; they are designated as various forms of hemoglobin M (HbM). They are inherited as autosomal dominants (Bunn, 1977). Methylene blue therapy in these individuals is without effect.

Most cases of methemoglobinemia are classified as secondary or acquired methemoglobinemia. They are due mainly to poisoning with drugs and chemicals that cause increased formation of hemiglobin (Wintrobe, 1974). Chemicals or drugs that directly oxidize HbO_2 to Hi include nitrites, nitrates, chlorates, and quinones. Other substances, which are aromatic amino and nitro compounds, probably act indirectly through a metabolite, since they do not cause Hi formation *in vitro*. These include acetanilid, phenacetin, sulfonamides,

and aniline dyes. Ferrous sulfate has been reported to produce methemoglobinemia after ingestion of very large doses. Levels of drugs or chemicals that would not cause significant methemoglobinemia in a normal individual may do so in someone with a mild reduction in NAD-reductase activity who, under ordinary circumstances, is not cyanotic. Such individuals are newborn infants and persons heterozygous for NAD-reductase deficiency (Cohen, 1968).

Hemiglobin is reduced back to Hb by the erythrocyte enzyme systems. It can also be reduced (slowly) by the administration of reducing agents, such as ascorbic acid or sulfhydryl compounds (glutathione, cysteine, BAL); these, as well as methylene blue, are of value in cases of hereditary NAD-methemoglobin reductase deficiency. In cases of acquired or toxic methemoglobinemia, methylene blue is of great value; its rapid action is not based on its own reduction capacity but on its acceleration of the normally slow NADP-methemoglobin reductase pathway.

Hemiglobin can combine reversibly with various chemicals (e.g., cyanides, sulfides, peroxides, fluorides, and azides). Because of its strong affinity for cyanide, the therapy of cyanide poisoning is to administer nitrites to form hemiglobin, which then combines with the cyanide. Thus, the free cyanide (which is extremely poisonous to the cellular respiratory enzymes) becomes less toxic when changed to hemiglobincyanide.

Hemiglobin (methemoglobin) and sulfhemoglobin are quantitated by the method of Evelyn (1938). If Hi is elevated, the following causes should be considered. Drugs or toxic substances must first be eliminated as a cause. Congenital methemoglobinemia due to NADH-methemoglobin reductase deficiency is determined by assay of the enzyme (Hegesch, 1968). An abnormal hemoglobin (HbM; p. 870) may also be responsible for methemoglobinemia noted at birth or in the first few months of life.

Sulfhemoglobin. *In vitro* and in the presence of oxygen, hemoglobin reacts with hydrogen sulfide to form a greenish derivative of hemoglobin called sulfhemoglobin. Since oxygen is necessary for the formation, it is assumed that oxyhemoglobin reacts directly with the H_2S. The role of sulfur or compounds containing sulfur in the *in vivo* production of sulfhemoglobin is unclear. Sulfhemoglobin implies an irreversible change in the polypeptide chains of the molecule. It may form in

$$Hb \underset{\text{tissues}}{\overset{\text{lungs}}{\rightleftharpoons}} HbO_2 \underset{\text{NAD-reductase}}{\overset{\text{Oxidation}}{\rightleftharpoons}} Hi \longrightarrow SHb \longrightarrow \begin{array}{c} \text{Denatured} \\ \text{hemoglobin} \\ \text{(Heinz bodies)} \end{array}$$

Figure 27–2. Simplified concept of oxidation of hemoglobin (Hb) as proposed by Jandl (1960). Reversible binding and release of oxygen occurs in lungs and tissues; oxidation of ferrous ions and formation of hemiglobin is reversible in the red cell to a limited extent; continued oxidation leads to irreversible conformational changes and sulfhemoglobin; still further oxidation results in denaturation of the hemoglobin and precipitation within the erythrocyte as Heinz bodies.

response to an oxidant stress; further change can result in denaturation and precipitation of hemoglobin as Heinz bodies (Fig. 27-2).

Sulfhemoglobin cannot transport oxygen, but it can combine with CO to form carboxy-sulfhemoglobin. Unlike methemoglobin, sulf-hemoglobin cannot be reduced back to hemoglobin, and it remains in the cells until they break down (see Fig. 15-10, pp. 510 and 511).

Sulfhemoglobin has been reported in patients receiving treatment with sulfonamides, aromatic amine drugs (phenacetin, acetanilid), and sulfur as well as in those with severe constipation, and in cases of bacteremia due to *Clostridium welchii*, and in a condition known as enterogenous cyanosis. The concentration of sulfhemoglobin *in vivo* is within the range of a few percentage points, as a rule, and seldom exceeds 10 per cent. The reason some patients develop methemoglobinemia, some sulfhemoglobinemia, and others Heinz bodies and hemolysis is not well understood.

Carboxyhemoglobin, HbCO. Hemoglobin has the capacity to combine with carbon monoxide in the same proportion as with oxygen. However, the affinity of the hemoglobin molecule for carbon monoxide is 210 times greater. This means that carbon monoxide will bind with hemoglobin even if its concentration in the air is extremely low (e.g., 0.02 to 0.04 per cent). In those cases, HbCO will build up until typical symptoms of poisoning appear.

HbCO cannot bind oxygen and therefore is not available as an oxygen carrier. Furthermore, the HbO$_2$, in a mixture with HbCO, does not release oxygen so readily as in normal blood, thus adding to the anoxia. If a patient poisoned with carbon monoxide receives pure oxygen, the conversion of HbCO to HbO$_2$ is greatly enhanced. HbCO is light sensitive and has a typical, brilliant, cherry red color.

Acute carbon monoxide poisoning has long been well known. Chronic poisoning, due to prolonged exposure to small amounts of carbon monoxide, is less well known but is assuming increasing importance. The chief sources of the gas are gasoline motors, illumi-nating gas, gas heaters, defective stoves, and the smoking of tobacco. Exposure to carbon monoxide is thus one of the hazards of modern civilization. The gas has even been found in the air of busy streets of large cities in sufficient concentration to cause mild symptoms in persons such as traffic policemen who are exposed to it over long periods of time. The chronic exposure to CO through tobacco smoking may lead to chronic elevation of HbCO and an associated left shift in the oxygen dissociation curve; smokers tend to have higher hematocrits than non-smokers and may have polycythemia (Smith, 1978).

Healthy persons exposed to various concentrations of the gas for an hour do not experience definite symptoms (headache, dizziness, muscular weakness, and nausea) unless the concentration of the gas in the blood reaches 26 or 30 per cent of saturation; however, it appears that in chronic poisoning, especially in children, serious symptoms may occur with lower concentrations.

Tests for Abnormal Hemoglobin Pigments. Some information can be obtained by naked eye examination of the blood specimen. Normal appearance of the serum or plasma identifies the red cells as the site of the pigment. Shaking of normal whole blood in the air for 15 minutes imparts to it a bright red color as the Hb is converted to HbO$_2$. The blood is cherry red when the pigment is HbCO in carbon monoxide poisoning. The color is chocolate brown in methemoglobinemia and mauve-lavender in sulfhemoglobinemia.

The specimen must be obtained carefully to avoid hemolysis and promptly analyzed, because certain abnormal pigments disappear on institution of therapy. If carbon monoxide is suspected, dry sodium citrate in small well-stoppered tubes should be used. If methemoglobin is to be tested for, heparin is the anticoagulant of choice, because oxalate tends to elevate the pH and favors conversion of neutral to alkaline methemoglobin. For all other tests, dry oxalate anticoagulant is preferable. Plasma containing hemoglobin is pink or red; it is brown in the presence of methemoglobin or met-hemalbumin. The red cells and the plasma or serum must be examined.

IDENTIFICATION OF HEMOGLOBIN PIGMENTS WITH

THE HAND SPECTROSCOPE. Whole blood or washed red cells are added to distilled water in a ratio of 1 to 10 or 1 to 100, depending on the concentration of the abnormal pigment. A few milliliters of the hemolyzed blood are placed in each of two test tubes. In the case of methemoglobin and methemalbumin, a dark band is seen in the spectroscope between 620 and 630 nm in the red portion of the spectrum. Sulfhemoglobin produces a similar band at 618 nm. To distinguish the pigments, 2 to 3 drops of a 5 per cent solution of potassium cyanide are added (with a dropper, not a pipette) to the second tube with blood. The band will disappear if the pigment is methemoglobin, and the color of the specimen will change from brown or black to dark red, but not if it is sulfhemoglobin or methemalbumin. Three per cent hydrogen peroxide causes the bands of sulfhemoglobin and methemoglobin to disappear. Carboxyhemoglobin and oxyhemoglobin are difficult to distinguish with the spectroscope. Both produce bands at approximately the same location (570 nm.) (see Fig. 15–11, p. 511).

OTHER TESTS. Naked eye examination of diluted blood (one drop in 5 ml of water) shows a yellow-red color of oxyhemoglobin and pink or red-blue color of carboxyhemoglobin.

Alkali Test. Two drops each of normal blood and of the patient's blood are placed on a spot plate. Two drops of 25 per cent sodium hydroxide are added to each. Carboxyhemoglobin remains unchanged. The normal control turns brown.

A simple qualitative test may be useful in an emergency and will be described.

Katayama's Test (1888). This simple test for HbCO will detect as little as 10 per cent of saturation. Place about 10 ml of water in each of two test tubes. To one tube, add 5 drops of the suspected blood and to the other add 5 drops of normal blood to serve as a control. To each tube, add 5 drops of fresh orange-colored ammonium sulfide. Mix gently and make faintly acid with acetic acid. The color of blood containing HbCO becomes more or less rose red, depending on the concentration of the gas; normal blood becomes a dirty green brown.

Spectrophotometric Identification of Hemoglobins. The various hemoglobins have characteristic absorption spectra, which can be determined easily with a spectrophotometer. The useful absorbance maxima are given in Table 27–2. The maxima for Hi vary considerably with pH. The maxima given in the two right hand columns are useful for distinguishing among these forms of hemoglobin. The absorbance between 405 and 435 nm (the Soret band) is considerably greater and may be used when small concentrations of hemoglobin are to be measured.

The identification of different forms of hemoglobins by determining absorption spectra can be carried out in a very simple way. Approximately one half of a drop of blood is put into a test tube and diluted with approximately 20 ml of de-ionized or double-distilled water. The actual dilution of the hemoglobin depends on the concentration of the

Table 27–2. ABSORPTION MAXIMA OF HEMOGLOBINS

	λ	ε	λ	ε	λ	ε
Hb	431	(140)	555	(13.04)		
HbO$_2$	415	(131)	542	(14.37)	577	(15.37)
HbCO	420	(192)	539	(14.36)	568.5	(14.31)
Hi (pH 7 to 7.4)	406	(162)	500	(9.04)	630	(3.70)
HiCN	421	(122.5)	540	(10.99)		

The Wavelength (λ) in nanometers for each maximum is followed by the extinction coefficient (ε) placed in parentheses.

Data are from van Assendelft, 1970.

hemoglobin. For maximal accuracy, the peak of absorption should be somewhere between 60 and 40 per cent transmittance. After the blood has been diluted with water, samples are read in a spectrophotometer with water as the blank. A recording spectrophotometer is especially convenient for this determination. Otherwise, the absorption is read at intervals of 5 nm (see Fig. 27–1).

HEMATOCRIT (PACKED CELL VOLUME)

Definition. The hematocrit of a sample of blood is the ratio of the volume of erythrocytes to that of the whole blood. It is expressed as a percentage or, preferably, as a decimal fraction. The units (l/l) are implied. The venous hematocrit agrees closely with the hematocrit obtained from a skin puncture; both are greater than the total body hematocrit. Dried heparin, balanced oxalate, or EDTA is satisfactory as an anticoagulant.

Macromethod of Wintrobe

Equipment. The Wintrobe hematocrit tube is a thick-walled glass tube with a uniform internal bore and a flattened bottom. It is graduated in millimeters from 0 to 105 and has a rubber cap to prevent evaporation during the long period of centrifugation. A disposable capillary (Pasteur) pipette with a rubber bulb is used to fill the tube.

The essential requirement of a centrifuge is that it generate a centrifugal field of not less than 2500 g at the bottom of the cup.

Procedure. After adequate mixing of the sample to ensure even distribution and oxygenation of red cells, the hematocrit tube is filled. The tip of the pipette is introduced to the bottom of the tube. As filling proceeds, the tip of the pipette is raised, but it remains under the rising blood meniscus in order to avoid foaming. The level of the blood should be noted and the tubes capped to avoid evaporation during the required centrifugation for 30 minutes at 2500 g.

Reading is done without disturbing the specimen. The result is calculated from the formula:

$$\text{Hematocrit} = \frac{L_1}{L_2}$$

where L_1 is the height of the red cell column in mm and L_2 is the height of the whole blood specimen (red cells and plasma). The gray-white layer of leukocytes and platelets above the erythrocytes is not included in L_1.

Micromethod

Equipment. A capillary hematocrit tube about 7 cm long with a uniform bore of about 1 mm is recommended. For blood collection directly from a skin puncture, capillaries are filled with a 1 to 1000 dilution of heparin, dried at 56 or 37°C., and stored. Special centrifuges are available, producing centrifugal fields ranging from 5000 to over 10,000 g. This permits shortening of centrifugation to 5 minutes for the latter and 10 minutes for the former.

Procedure. The microhematocrit (capillary) tube is filled by capillary attraction, either from a free-flowing puncture wound or a well-mixed venous sample. The capillary tube should be at least half full. The empty end is sealed in a small flame of a microburner or plugged with modeling clay. The filled tube is placed in the radial grooves of the microhematocrit centrifuge head with the sealed end away from the center.

The air at the outermost end of the capillary will be displaced in the course of centrifugation and the air gap will disappear. Leakage, especially if modeling clay was used for sealing, can be prevented by using a rubber gasket at the periphery of the hematocrit head to act as a cushion. Place the bottom of the tube against the rubber gasket to prevent breakage. Centrifugation for 5 minutes at 10,000 to 12,000 g is satisfactory unless the hematocrit exceeds 50 per cent; in this case an additional 5 minutes' centrifugation should be employed in order to ensure that plasma trapping has been minimized.

The capillary tubes are not graduated. The length of the whole column, including the plasma, and of the red cell column alone must be measured in each case with a millimeter rule and a magnifying lens or with one of several commercially available measuring devices. The instructions of the manufacturer must be followed.

Interpretation of Results. The normal hematocrit for adult males is 0.40 to 0.54, for females 0.37 to 0.47. A value below an individual's normal or below the reference interval for age and sex indicates anemia, and a higher value, polycythemia. The hematocrit reflects the concentration of red cells, not the total red cell mass. The hematocrit is low in hydremia of pregnancy, but the total number of circulating red cells is not reduced. The hematocrit may be normal or even high in shock accompanied by hemoconcentration, though the total red cell mass may be considerably decreased owing to blood loss.

Sources of Error

Centrifugation. Adequate duration and speed of centrifugation are essential for a correct hematocrit. The red cells must be packed so that additional centrifugation does not further reduce the packed cell volume. In general, the higher the hematocrit, the greater the centrifugal force required.

In the course of centrifugation, a small proportion of the leukocytes, platelets, and plasma are trapped between the red cells. The error resulting from the former is, as a rule, quite insignificant. The increment of the hematocrit due to trapped plasma is somewhat greater than that due to leukocytes and platelets, but this too is of little practical consequence. The lower the relative centrifugal force, the larger the amount of trapped plasma; therefore, the amount of trapped plasma is larger in high hematocrits than in low hematocrits, and is larger with the macromethod than the micromethod. With the micromethod, trapped plasma accounts for about 3 per cent of the red cell column in normal blood (about 0.014 in a hematocrit of 0.47), slightly more in macrocytic anemias, and up to 5 or 6 per cent in hypochromic anemias (England, 1972). Even greater amounts of trapped plasma occur in the hematocrits of patients with sickle cell anemia and vary depending upon the degree of sickling and consequent rigidity of the cells. Because less time is necessary for centrifugation, and because there is less error due to trapping of plasma, the micromethod is preferred over the macromethod.

Sample. Posture can cause the same order of changes in hematocrit and cell concentrations as it does for non-filterable soluble constituents (Chapter 1, p. 7). The hematocrit is lower after a period of recumbency than in ambulatory subjects; the difference may be 0.04 or about 9 per cent (Mollison, 1967). Vigorous exercise may increase the hematocrit by 0.02 to 0.05. After a meal, the hematocrit tends to fall slightly, about 0.015, in two to four hours (Chanarin, 1975). Prolonged stasis caused by constriction with a tourniquet for one or two minutes may result in a falsely high hematocrit of 0.005 to 0.03 (2 to 6 per cent) (Mollison, 1967). This error will also apply to hemoglobin and cell counts. Unique to the hematocrit is the error due to excess EDTA (inadequate blood for a fixed amount of EDTA): the hematocrit will be falsely low due to cell shrinkage, but the hemoglobin and cell counts will not be affected (Lampasso, 1967). The hematocrit of deoxygenated blood is about 2 per cent lower than fully oxygenated blood (Dacie, 1975).

A free flow of blood from a skin puncture for microhematocrit is essential. The hematocrit is unreliable as an estimate of anemia immediately after a loss of blood, even if moderate, and immediately following transfusions.

Other Errors. Technical errors include failure to mix the blood adequately before sampling, improper reading of the level of cells and plasma, and inclusion of the buffy coat as part of the erythrocyte volume. Irregularity of the inside diameter of the tubes will also lead to inaccurate hematocrits.

With good technique the precision of the hematocrit, expressed as ±2 C.V. (coefficient of variation), is ±1 per cent. With low hematocrit values, the C.V. is greater, especially with the microhematocrit method, owing to reading error.

Macroscopic Examination. When the hematocrit is performed by centrifugation, inspection of the specimen after spinning may furnish valuable information. The relative heights of the red cell column, buffy coat, and plasma column should be noted.

The buffy coat is the red-gray layer between the red cells and plasma; it includes platelets and leukocytes. In the centrifuged hematocrit tube each 1 per cent buffy coat is roughly equivalent to 10×10^9 leukocytes per liter, if the platelet count is normal. For example, a buffy coat of 1 per cent of the total volume in the tube indicates a leukocyte count in the range of 10×10^9/l. If the leukocyte count is over 12×10^9/l, a buffy coat of 1 per cent of the total volume represents a leukocyte count closer to 20×10^9/l because of greater packing. (Wintrobe, 1974). The size of the cells will alter the estimate if they are much different from normal. These estimates apply best to the macrohematocrit; in the microhematocrit they underestimate the leukocyte count because of the greater packing. The estimates give only a crude idea of the count, but they are sometimes useful.

An orange or green color of the plasma suggests increased bilirubin, and pink or red suggests hemoglobinemia. It should be kept in mind that poor technique in collecting the blood specimen is the most frequent cause of hemolysis. If the specimens are not obtained within an hour or two after a fat-rich meal, cloudy plasma may point to nephrosis or certain abnormal hyperglobulinemias, especially cryoglobulinemia.

BLOOD CELL COUNTING

Quantitative studies of the formed elements of the blood—red cells, white cells, and platelets—are concerned with the concentration of each in a given volume of blood. The unit of volume for cell counts traditionally has been expressed as cubic millimeters (mm^3) because of the linear dimensions of the hemacytometer (cell counting) chamber. The International Committee for Standardization in Hematology has now recommended that all units of volume be expressed in liters. Since $1\ mm^3 = 1.00003\ \mu l.$, the preferred mode of expressing blood cell counts for the examples below is on the right:

Erythrocytes
$$5 \times 10^6/mm^3 = 5 \times 10^6\ \mu l = 5 \times 10^{12}/l$$

Leukocytes
$$7 \times 10^3/mm^3 = 7 \times 10^3/\mu l = 7 \times 10^9/l$$
Platelets
$$300 \times 10^3/mm^3 = 300 \times 10^3/\mu l = 300 \times 10^9/l$$

Except for platelet counts, the hemacytometer is no longer used for routine blood cell counting in any but the smallest of laboratories. Yet it is still necessary for the technologist to be able to use this method effectively and to know its limitations.

Any cell counting procedure includes three steps: dilution of the blood, sampling the diluted suspension into a measured volume, and counting the cells in that volume.

ERYTHROCYTE COUNTS

Hemacytometer method

Counting Chamber. The type of hemacytometer or counting chamber most widely used consists of a heavy, colorless glass slide, on the middle third of which are fixed three parallel platforms extending across the slide. In the "double counting chamber," the central platform is subdivided by a transverse groove into two halves, each wider than the two lateral platforms and separated from them and from each other by moats. The central platforms or "floor pieces" are exactly 0.1 mm lower than the lateral platforms. Each of the central platforms has a so-called improved Neubauer ruling (Fig. 27-3), which consists of a square measuring 3 by 3 mm (9 sq mm) subdivided into nine secondary squares, each 1 by 1 mm (1 sq mm). The four corner squares, labeled A, B, C, D in this figure, are used for the white cell count and are subdivided into 16 tertiary squares.

The central square millimeter is divided into 25 tertiary squares, each of which measures 0.2 by 0.2 mm. Each of these is further subdivided into 16 smaller squares. The total number of the smallest squares in the central square is 400. As a rule, five of the tertiary squares, amounting to 80 of the smallest squares, are used for red cell counts.

A thick coverglass, ground to a perfect plane, accompanies the counting chamber. Ordinary coverglasses have uneven surfaces and should not be used. When the coverglass is in place on the platform of the counting chamber (Fig. 27-3), there is a space exactly 0.1 mm thick between it and the ruled platform; therefore, each square millimeter of the ruling forms the base of a space holding exactly 0.1 cu mm.

Counting chambers and coverglasses should be rinsed immediately after use in lukewarm water, wiped with a clean lint-free cloth, and allowed to dry in the air. The surfaces must not be touched with gauze or linen, because they may scratch the ruled areas. A scratch across the chamber or coverglass ruins it. The chamber and coverglass should not be touched because fingerprints are difficult to

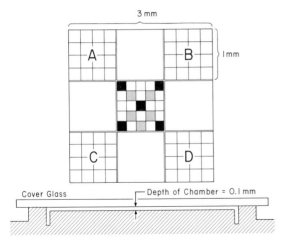

Figure 27-3. The upper figure is a diagram of the improved Neubauer ruling; this is etched on the surface of each side of the hemacytometer. The large corner squares, A, B, C, and D, are used for leukocyte counts. The five black squares in the center are used for red cell counts or for platelet counts, and the 10 black plus shaded squares for platelet counts. Actually, each of the 25 squares within the central sq mm has within it 16 smaller squares for convenience in counting.

The lower figure is a side view of the chamber with the coverglass in place.

remove and may be responsible for errors. Before use, the surfaces must be absolutely clean, dry, and free from lint and water marks. After they have been cleaned they must not be touched except at the edges.

Pipette. The Thoma glass pipettes (Fig. 27-4) consist of a graduated capillary tube, divided into 10 parts and marked 0.5 at the fifth mark and 1.0 at the tenth, a mixing bulb above it containing a glass bead, and above the bulb, another short capillary tube with an engraved mark 11 on the white and 101 on the red cell pipette. The red cell pipette has a red bead in the mixing bulb and the white cell pipette a white bead. The graduations on the pipettes are arbitrary. The volume of the red cell pipette is made up of one half part at the level of the 0.5 mark, one part at the level of the 1.0 mark, and 100 parts in the bulb. When the blood is drawn to the 0.5 mark and the diluting fluid to the 101

mark, all the blood cells are washed into the bulb and the resulting dilution in the bulb is 1 to 200. The capillary portion of the pipette contains no blood but only diluting fluid; therefore, it is not included in the total volume, and its contents must be expelled before the cell suspension is introduced into the chamber.

Pipettes should have a guaranteed error of no more than ± 1.0 per cent. Inferior pipettes should not be used. Alternatively it is perfectly acceptable to make the 1:200 dilution of blood with a 20 μl pipette into an ordinary test tube containing exactly 4 ml of red cell diluting fluid.

The rubber tubing that is attached to the pipette should be sufficiently heavy-walled to resist collapse during suction and should be long enough (at least 10 inches) to permit easy reading of the graduation marks.

After use, pipettes should be rinsed with tap water and then three times with distilled water, filling the bulb through the capillary end, shaking, and emptying through the large-bore end. This is followed by similar treatment with acetone or 95 per cent alcohol and finally with ether, using a water suction pump. The interior of the pipettes should then be dried with a current of dry air. The bulb is dry if the bead rolls freely. If the lumen of the capillary pipette contains coagulated blood or other debris, it can be cleaned with a special, delicate, commercially available wire. Washing devices are available that permit cleansing and drying many pipettes simultaneously. Care must be exerted to prevent damage to the delicate point of the pipette, for even the slightest damage that affects the bore makes the pipette useless because it leads to inaccuracy in the dilution.

Diluting Fluid. The diluting fluid must be isotonic to prevent lysis and crenation of red cells. It may contain a fixative to preserve the shape of the cells and to prevent agglutination and autolysis if the count cannot be performed within an hour. Gower's solution (sodium sulfate, 12.5 g; glacial acetic acid, 33.3 ml; distilled water, 200 ml) meets these requirements; it should be filtered before use. It is even simpler to use Isoton* or its equivalent,

---

*Coulter Diagnostics, Hialeah, Fla.

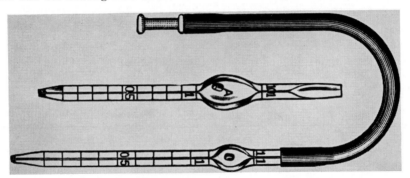

Figure 27-4. Thoma red and white cell diluting pipettes.

which is likely to be readily available if an electronic flow-through counter is in the laboratory.

Procedure

1. Venous blood in EDTA as anticoagulant is suitable. Before diluting, it must be thoroughly mixed by inversion at least 60 times.

2. The tip of the pipette is placed beneath the surface of the blood, which is then quickly aspirated just to the 0.5 mark on the red cell pipette. No air bubbles can be in the column of blood. If the blood rises slightly above the mark, it can be drawn back to the mark by touching the tip of the pipette to the finger. If a large excess of blood has been drawn up, the pipette should be cleaned and the procedure repeated, because even though it is withdrawn, enough will remain adhering to the inside of the pipette to introduce a significant error. Painstakingly accurate technique in this part of the procedure is important, because any error is magnified by the subsequent dilution.

3. The blood adhering to the tip is wiped off quickly, the tip is placed into the diluting fluid, and the fluid is drawn up to the mark 101, while rotating the pipette. It is best to hold the pipette nearly horizontally in order to avoid aspiration of air bubbles in the bulb, but when the bulb is almost full the pipette should be raised to the vertical position. At this stage the blood sample has been diluted 1 to 200.

4. The ends of the pipette are now closed with the thumb and middle finger, and the pipette is shaken for about 30 seconds to facilitate the initial mixing. The bead contained in the bulb should move freely. The shaking should be done at a 90 degree angle to the long axis of the pipette.

When it is not convenient to count the erythrocytes at once, a heavy rubber band is placed around the pipette to close both ends.

5. The coverglass is adjusted in place on the hemacytometer. The pipette is held between the thumb and middle finger or in a special shaking machine and shaken for 2 to 3 minutes at right angles to the long axis of the pipette.

6. The first 3 to 4 drops are discarded to eliminate the cell-free fluid from the capillary tube. The pipette is held at an angle of about 35 degrees while the tip is touched to the angle between the edge of the coverglass and one of the projecting ends of the floor piece. The fluid will run under the coverglass by capillary attraction. The fluid is allowed to enter in a controlled manner by pressure from the index finger on the open end of the pipette or from the pressure of the tongue on the mouthpiece of the pipette. Care must be exercised to permit just enough fluid to fill the space beneath the coverglass.

The characteristics of a properly filled counting chamber are that the fluid fills the space beneath the coverglass entirely or almost entirely, none of the fluid has run over into the moat, and there are no bubbles. If any of these conditions are not met, the count will not be reliable and the chamber has to be cleaned, dried, and recharged.

7. The cells in the chamber are permitted to settle for several minutes. Then the ruled area is surveyed with the low-power objective to see whether they are evenly distributed. If they are not, the procedure has to be repeated. If the chamber is filled and the cells not counted promptly, the fluid should be protected against evaporation by placing the chamber under a Petri dish containing a moistened piece of filter paper, which is applied to the top inner surface.

8. Counting. The square millimeter with the 400 small squares in the center of the ruled area lies under a volume of $1/10 \, \mu l$. In this volume, one usually counts the red cells in 80 small squares (5 of the 25 tertiary squares, see Fig. 27-3); in other words, the cells in one fifth of this volume of $1/10 \, \mu l$ of the diluted cell suspension. Since the dilution is 1 to 200, one is counting the number of red cells in $1/5 \times 1/10 \times 1/200 = 1/10,000 \, \mu l$ of blood. This means that the red cell count in $1 \, \mu l$ of blood is the number of cells counted $\times 10,000$.

9. In counting the 5 tertiary squares, each with 16 small squares, the following rule is suggested to avoid confusion in counting cells that lie on borderlines: Erythrocytes that touch any one of the three lines or the single line on the left and the top borders of the small square should be counted as though they were within the squares, but those that touch any of the lines on the right and the bottom borders of the small squares should not be counted. In this way no cell is counted twice. The cells are counted in each small square, first from left to right, beginning with the top of four small squares, and then from right to left for the next row, and so on. The number of cells for each of the five groups of 16 squares is recorded separately and the results are added.

Sources of Error. Numerous possibilities for error exist in all cell counts using the hemacytometer. Errors may be due to the nature of the sample, to the operator's technique, and to inaccurate equipment. Errors that are inherent in the distribution of cells in the counting volume are called "field" errors and can be minimized only by counting more cells.

ERRORS DUE TO THE NATURE OF THE SAMPLE. Partial coagulation of the venous blood introduces errors by changes in the distribution of the cells or decrease of their number.

The influence of prolonged application of the tourniquet, the patient's posture, and the time relationship to exercise and meals have been discussed (p. 873) and influence all cell counts as well as hematocrit. Failure to mix the blood thoroughly and immediately before drawing the sample into the pipette introduces an error, which depends upon the degree of sedimentation during the interval since the blood was mixed.

OPERATOR'S ERRORS. Errors due to faulty technique may occur when blood and the diluting fluid are drawn into the pipette, when the chamber is loaded, and when the cells are counted. A frequent source of trouble is faulty application of the coverglass, especially when it is raised by introduction of an excess of diluted blood, or movement of the coverglass after the counting chamber has been filled. Overflowing of the suspension into the moat is another example.

ERRORS DUE TO EQUIPMENT. Inaccuracies in the graduations of the pipettes and of the ruled areas and depth of the counting chambers are frequent sources of error. They can be diminished by using pipettes and hemacytometers certified by the U.S. Bureau of Standards.

INHERENT OR FIELD ERROR. Even in a perfectly mixed sample, variation occurs in the number of suspended cells that are distributed in a given volume (i.e., come to rest over a given square).

According to Poisson's law of distribution, the variation among the different squares in the chamber is given by the formula S.D. = $\sqrt{m}$, where m is the mean number of cells per unit area and S.D. is the standard deviation of the counts in these areas. *Example:* The mean count per 80 squares is 500 (as for a count of 5,000,000 per μl). The S.D. of counts of different sets of 80 squares in the chamber will be $\sqrt{500}$ or 22.4. Expressed relatively as a per cent, this is $\frac{22.4}{500} \times 100 = 4.5$ per cent. This expression of the standard deviation as a percentage of the mean $\left(\frac{\text{S.D.}}{\text{mean}} \times 100 \right)$ is known as the coefficient of variation (C.V.), which, for the Poisson distribution $100 \frac{\sqrt{m}}{m} = \frac{100}{\sqrt{m}}$.

This "error of the field" is the minimal error. Another error is the "error of the chamber," which includes variations in separate fillings of a given chamber, and in sizes of different chambers. Still another is the "error of the pipette," which includes variations in filling a given pipette, and in the sizes of different pipettes.

Berkson (1940) experimentally determined for hemocytometer red cell counts the following coefficients of variation, expressed as a percentage: the field error = $\frac{0.92 \times 100}{\sqrt{n_b}}$; the error of the chamber $= \frac{4.6}{\sqrt{n_c}}$; the error of the pipette $= \frac{4.7}{\sqrt{n_p}}$, where n_b = number of blood cells counted, n_c = number of chambers examined, and n_p = number of pipettes used. Experimentally, the field error for the red cell count (but not for the white cell count) was slightly lower than that given by the Poisson distribution $\left(\frac{100}{\sqrt{n_b}} \right)$. The total

$$\text{C.V.} = \sqrt{\frac{(0.92 \times 100)^2}{n_b} + \frac{4.6^2}{n_c} + \frac{4.7^2}{n_p}}.$$

If, for example, 500 cells are counted in doing the red cell count, the C.V. = 7.7 per cent if one chamber and one pipette are used. This corresponds to an experimental error of ± 15.4 per cent (twice the C.V.).

Using two pipettes and two chambers and counting twice as many cells reduces the experimental error to ± 11 per cent.

Dilutors

The method previously described for diluting the blood for hemoglobin or for cell counts can be performed more rapidly and accurately both manually and semiautomatically (Bull, 1971).

Semiautomated Methods. Several instruments are now available for precise and convenient diluting, which both aspirate the sample and wash it out with the diluent. In some instruments the volumes are adjustable; in others, one or both volumes are fixed. In either case the dilutor should perform a 1:250 or 1:500 dilution with a coefficient of variation of less than 1 per cent.

A semiautomatic dilutor, the Hem-Aliquanter (Bull, 1968), dispenses the diluent and the sample separately. The sample is dispensed simultaneously for several tests with errors of less than 1 per cent. This dilutor should be considered for the laboratory without a multichannel instrument.

Manual. For capillary sampling, manual methods are still necessary. Accurate disposable pipettes are now available; some are similar to the classic Sahli pipette. More convenient and reliable are microcapillary pipettes that fill by capillarity and cannot overfill;[*] when added to the diluent in an appropriate-sized test tube they empty satisfactorily, with sufficient washout of sample by diluent. These pipettes are available with an accuracy of ± 0.25 per cent, which is suitable for calibration. Less expensive pipettes with an accuracy of ± 1 per cent are usually used for routine work.

Combining a microcapillary tube with a plastic vial containing a premeasured volume of diluent, the Unopette[†] is a valuable system for manual dilutions. After the capillary is filled, it is pushed into the container and the sample is washed out by squeezing the soft plastic vial. This system is especially convenient for finger-puncture sampling. Unopettes are available with diluents for red cell counts, white cell counts, platelet counts, eosinophil counts, and hemoglobin determinations.

---

[*]Drummond Hemocaps, Drummond Scientific Company, Broomall, Pa.
[†]Becton-Dickinson, Rutherford, N.J.

Electronic counting method

(Brittin and Brecher, 1971; Ackermann, 1972)

The most widely used methods of cell counting today are electronic, employing one of two principles:

1. Cells passing through an aperture cause changes in electrical resistance which are counted as voltage pulses. This principle is used in the Coulter Counter* and in the Celloscope.†

2. Cells passing through a flow cell cause deflections in a beam of light which are converted to electric pulses by a photomultiplier tube. This principle is used in the Technicon Autoanalyzers‡ and the Fisher Autocytometer.§

Counting Voltage Pulses

Principle. Cells passing through an aperture through which a current is flowing cause changes in electrical resistance which are counted as voltage pulses. This principle, used in the Coulter Counter and in the Celloscope, is illustrated in Figure 27-5. An accurately diluted suspension of blood (CS) is made in 0.85 per cent saline or, preferably, in an isotonic conductive solution (such as Isoton*) which preserves the cell shape. The instrument has a glass cylinder (GC) that can be filled with

---

*Coulter Diagnostics, Hialeah, Fla.
†Lars Ljungberg & Co., Stockholm, Sweden.
‡Technicon Co., Ardsley, N.Y.
§Fisher Scientific Co., Pittsburgh, Pa.

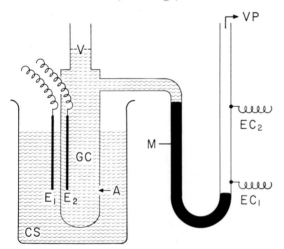

Figure 27–5. Schematic diagram of particle counter in which changes in electrical resistance are counted as voltage pulses. CS = cell suspension, GC = glass cylinder, A = aperture, E_1 and E_2 = platinum electrodes, V = valve, M = mercury column, EC_1 and EC_2 = electrical contacts, VP = vacuum pump. (Diagram adapted from Ackermann, 1972.)

the conducting fluid and has within it an electrode (E_2) and an aperture (A) of 100 μm diameter in its wall. Just outside the glass cylinder is another electrode (E_1). The cylinder is connected to a U-shaped glass tube which is partly filled with mercury (M) and which has two electrical contacts (EC_1 and EC_2). The glass cylinder is immersed in the suspension of cells to be counted (CS) and is filled with conductive solution and closed by a valve (V). A current now flows through the aperture between E_1 and E_2. Then, as a vacuum pump (VP) draws the mercury up the tube, the cell suspension flows through the aperture into the cylinder. Each cell that passes through the aperture displaces an equal volume of conductive fluid, increasing the electrical resistance and creating a voltage pulse, because its resistance is much greater than that of the conductive solution. The pulses, which are proportional in height to the volume of the cells, are counted.

The counting mechanism is started when the mercury contacts EC_1 and stopped when it contacts EC_2; during this time the cells are counted in a volume of suspension exactly equal to the volume of the glass tubing between contact wires EC_1 and EC_2.

If two or more cells enter the aperture simultaneously, they will be counted as one pulse; this produces a coincidence error for which a correction must be made. The size of the coincidence error can be diminished by decreasing the concentration of cells and decreasing the size of the aperture. However, decreasing the cell concentration increases the effect of errors in dilution, increases the inherent counting error, and makes more critical the error due to the background "noise" of contaminating particles. With decreased aperture size, partial or complete plugging of the aperture with debris becomes a problem. Therefore, a balance is struck, and for a given count above a critical number, a coincidence correction is made by referring to a chart supplied by the manufacturer.

A threshold setting or pulse discriminator allows the exclusion of pulses below fixed heights for red cell and white cell counts on the Coulter Counter Model D, and below an adjustable height on the Models ZF and ZBI. On the Model ZBI, a second threshold also excludes the counting of pulses *above* a certain height. One therefore counts only the cells in the "window" between the two settings. By systematically changing each threshold by given increments, one can determine a frequency distribution of relative cell volumes. Such cell size distributions can now be automatically plotted by attachments available for the Coulter Counter Model ZBI (Channelyzer) and may be valuable in the study of red cells or platelets when two or more changing populations of cells are present.

Instruments that handle the data from the changes in electrical resistance digitally (e.g., the Coulter Counter) are stable and infrequently require calibration. Therefore, they can be relied upon as primary reference machines to give a correct red cell count if the specimens are properly mixed and diluted (Brittin, 1971; Bull, 1971).

Before counting, the adjustment of the threshold is checked by counting the diluted suspension of red cells at successively increasing increments. To ensure that smaller particles (background "noise") are excluded from the count, the adjustment should be in the middle of the plateau. Larger foreign particles in the diluent are quantitated in a background or blank count which may be subtracted from the cell count. However, if the blank count is too high, the accuracy of the cell count will be impaired. The final cell dilution should allow a particle count of at least 5000, which should be at least 20 times the blank count. Specific directions for operation of the instruments are given by the manufacturer.

In the Coulter Counter, the dilution for the red cell count is $1:50,000$, usually made in two steps: first, 20 μl of blood in 10 ml ($1:500$), followed by 100 μl of the first dilution in 10 ml of diluent ($1:100$). Since 0.5 ml of the cell suspension is counted, 50,000 cells (after correction for coincidence) will be counted for a normal red cell count of $5 \times 10^{12}/l$.

For a normal red cell count, therefore, the Poisson error will be about 0.5 per cent

$\left(\text{C.V.} = \dfrac{\sqrt{n}}{n}\right)$ and for a very low count, closer to 1 per cent. The actual precision of red cell counting is about twice this, or 1 to 2 per cent (C.V.), and errors of dilution bring the precision achieved in practice to 2 to 4 per cent (Brittin, 1971).

The Celloscope 401 operates on the same principle as the Coulter Counter, but deals with the problem of coincidence in a different way. Instead of counting all the pulses and correcting for coincidence, the Celloscope 401 counts every 64th pulse and no coincidence correction is necessary. The precision of red cell counting is comparable to that of the Coulter Counter; Lappin (1972) found the mean coefficient of variation to be 1.2 per cent.

Counting Light-Scattering Events. In electron-optical counters (Fig. 27–6) a photomultiplier tube detects light scattering either from external reflections from the surface of cells, from transmitted and refracted light passing through the cells, or from diffracted light which has passed tangential to cell surfaces (Mansberg, 1970). In the Technicon cell counter, the intensity of the diffraction events provides the highest signal-to-noise ratio (about $100:1$) in the small scattering angle that is necessary for adequate depth of focus. Because of a uniform pulse amplitude, the high signal-to-noise ratio, and the forward-angle scattering character of the system, there is a broad threshold curve that is the same for leukocytes and erythrocytes. A small sensing volume (44×10^3 fl) is defined by illumination in the flow cell and allows a lesser dilution ($1:10,000$) than the voltage pulse counter, resulting in minimal coincidence. The characteristics described yield an accuracy and precision in cell counting that is limited only by the qualities of the pumping system.

The Technicon cell counter consists basically

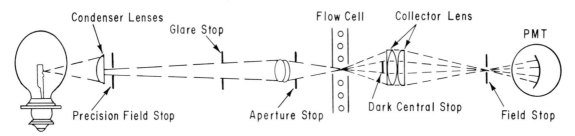

Figure 27–6. Schematic diagram of the electron-optical cell counter. Light is focused on the flow cell. Only light scattered by a cell reaches the photomultiplier tube (PMT), which converts it to an electrical pulse. (From Mansberg, H. P.: Advanc. Automated Anal. *1*:213, 1970.)

of the following modules: sampler, proportioning pump with manifolds having plastic tubing, glass helical mixing and phasing coils, a cell counter, and a single pen recorder. Anticoagulated blood in a tube or sample cup is mixed by two paddles (one minute each) before being sampled during a third minute. The capacity is 60 samples/hour.) The continuous flow system incorporates dilution with diluent and mixing before the diluted cell suspension reaches the flow cell for counting. The output of the photomultiplier tube is recorded by the pen on moving preprinted paper. The instrument must be calibrated with a known blood or particle suspension at the beginning of each series of counts; since this takes a relatively large volume of known or reference standard blood, it is not practical to run small numbers of samples.

The Technicon red cell counter is now almost always used as part of a multichannel instrument, the Hemalog 8/60 or 8/90. The coefficient of variation of the red cell count on these instruments is between 1 and 1.5 per cent (Thom, 1977).

Erythrocyte Indices

Wintrobe introduced calculations for determining the size, the content, and Hb concentration of red cells; these erythrocyte indices have been useful in the morphologic characterization of anemias. They may be calculated from the red cell count, hemoglobin concentration, and hematocrit.

Mean Cell Volume (MCV). The MCV is the average volume of red cells and is calculated from the hematocrit (Hct; packed cell volume) and the red cell count (RBC). MCV = Hct × 1000/RBC (in millions per μl), expressed in femtoliters or cubic micrometers. If the hematocrit = 0.45 and the red cell count = 5×10^{12}/l, one liter will contain 5×10^{12} red cells, which occupy a volume of 0.45 l. The MCV $= \dfrac{0.45\,\text{l}}{5 \times 10^{12}} = 90 \times 10^{-15}$ liters (fl). One femtoliter (fl) $= 10^{-15}$ liters $= 1$ cubic micrometer (μm^3).

Mean Cell Hemoglobin (MCH). The MCH is the content (weight) of Hb of the average red cell; it is calculated from the Hb concentration and the red cell count.

$$MCH = \frac{\text{Hb (in g per liter)}}{\text{RBC (in millions per } \mu l)}$$

expressed in picograms. If the Hb = 15 g/dl and the red cell count is 5×10^{12}/l, one liter contains 150 g of Hb distributed in 5×10^{12} cells.

$$MCH = \frac{150\,\text{g}}{5 \times 10^{12}} = 30 \times 10^{-12}\,\text{g (pg)}$$

One picogram (pg) $= 10^{-12}\,\text{g}$
$\qquad\qquad\qquad = 1$ micromicrogram ($\mu\mu g$)

Mean Cell Hemoglobin Concentration (MCHC). The MCHC is the average concentration of Hb in a given volume of packed red cells. It is calculated from the Hb concentration and the hematocrit.

$$MCHC = \frac{\text{Hb (in g/dl)}}{\text{Hct}}, \text{ expressed in g/dl}$$

If the Hb = 15 g/dl and the Hct = 0.45, the MCHC $= \dfrac{15\,\text{g/dl}}{0.45} = 33.3$ g/dl.

Discussion. Indices are determined in the Coulter Counter Model S (p. 885) somewhat differently. The MCV is derived from the mean height of the voltage pulses formed during the red cell count, and the Hb is measured by optical density of HiCN. The other three values are calculated: Hct = MCV × RBC; $MCH = \dfrac{\text{Hb}}{\text{RBC}}$; $MCHC = \dfrac{\text{Hb}}{\text{Hct}}$.

The reference values for the indices will depend on whether they are determined from the centrifuged hematocrit or the Coulter Model S. The values in normal individuals will be similar if both are corrected for trapped plasma. Because of increased trapped plasma in hypochromic anemias and sickle cell anemia, however, the MCHC calculated from the microhematocrit will be significantly lower than the MCHC derived from the Coulter Model S.

With the Coulter Model S, calibrated with correction for trapped plasma, our 95 per cent reference intervals for normal adults are: MCV = 80 to 96 fl; MCH = 27 to 33 pg; and MCHC = 32 to 36 g/dl. In a healthy person there is very little variation, no more than ±1 unit in any of the indices. Deviations from the reference value for an individual or outside the reference intervals for normal persons are useful particularly in characterizing morphologic types of anemia.

In *microcytic anemias*, the indices may be as low as an MCV of 50 fl, an MCH of 15 pg, and an MCHC of 22 g/l; rarely do any become lower.

In *macrocytic anemias*, the values may be as high as an MCV of 150 fl, an MCH of 50 pg, but the MCHC is normal or decreased (Dacie, 1975). The MCHC increases only in spherocytosis, and rarely is over 38 g/dl.

LEUKOCYTE COUNTS

In the total leukocyte count, no distinction is made among the five normal cell types (neutrophils, lymphocytes, monocytes, eosinophils, and basophils). Each cell type has its own particular function in defending the body against foreign threats. How they are distinguished from one another is considered later; here we are concerned with the total leukocyte concentration in the blood. The reference interval for adults is 4.5 to $11.0 \times 10^9/l$.

Sample. Heparin is unsatisfactory as an anticoagulant; EDTA or double oxalate should be used.

Hemacytometer Method. Though this method is rarely used in routine leukocyte counting any longer, the technologist should be able to perform it (1) as a check on the validity of electronic methods for calibration purposes; (2) as a check on the validity of electronic counts in cases with profound leukopenia or with leukemia; and (3) as a back-up method.

Equipment. The white cell pipette has a stem and a mixing chamber (Fig. 27-4). The stem has 10 gradations, marked at 0.5 and 1.0. The mixing chamber extends from the mark 1.0 to 11.0. It contains a white bead, which aids in the mixing. When blood is drawn to the 0.5 mark (1 volume) and the diluting fluid to the 11.0 mark (11 volumes), the dilution of the blood sample is 1 to 20 and the dilution factor is 20. When blood is drawn to the 1.0 mark and the diluting fluid to 11.0, the dilution factor is 10.

The counting chamber with the improved Neubauer ruling is used.

Diluting fluid. The diluting fluid lyses the erythrocytes so that they will not obscure the leukocytes. The simplest diluting fluid is a 2 per cent solution of acetic acid. More satisfactory is the following:

Glacial acetic acid	2 ml
1 per cent aqueous solution of gentian violet	1 ml
Distilled water	100 ml

The fluid must be filtered frequently to remove yeasts and molds.

Technique. Refer to the general recommendations made for the red cell count (p. 874).

1. The blood is drawn carefully to the 0.5 mark and the level adjusted to the mark by touching the tip of the pipette.
2. The outside of the tip of the pipette is wiped with gauze and the diluting fluid is drawn to fill the mixing chamber to the mark 11.
3. Mixing the pipette for 3 minutes, discharging the first few drops of diluting fluid from the stem, and loading the two counting chambers are performed as described for the red cell count.
4. The condenser diaphragm of the microscope is partially closed to make the leukocytes stand out clearly under a low-power ($10\times$) objective lens. The diluting fluid lyses the red cells but not the leukocytes. If the distribution of the latter in the four corner squares is uneven, the procedure thus far must be repeated with clean hemacytometer and pipette.
5. The leukocytes are counted in each of the four large (1 sq mm) corner squares (A, B, C and D in Fig. 27-3), each of which is divided into 16 smaller squares for convenience. Eight large squares in two chambers are counted.
6. Each large square encloses a volume of $1/10$ mm^3 and the dilution is 1 to 20. Therefore, in the volume in the chamber over one large square, one is counting the number of leukocytes in $1/10 \times 1/20 = 1/200$ mm^3 of blood. This means that the leukocyte count is the average number of cells in each large square (N) multiplied by 200. A general formula is:

$$\text{leukocyte count (cells/mm}^3) = \frac{cc}{lsc} \times d \times 10$$

where cc is the total number of cells counted, d is the dilution factor, 10 is the factor transforming volume over one large square ($1/10$ mm^3) to the volume in mm^3, and lsc is the number of large squares counted.

In leukopenia, with a total count below 2500, the blood is drawn to the 1.0 mark and the dilution factor is 10.

Example. 120 cells counted in eight squares; dilution factor = 10.

$$\text{Leukocyte count} = \frac{120}{8} \times 10 \times 10$$

$$1500/\text{mm}^3 \ (= 1.5 \times 10^9/l).$$

In leukocytosis, red cell pipettes are used, and the dilution may be 1 to 100 or even 1 to 200.

Sources of Error. The errors are caused by the same factors as in counting red cells (q.v.). The largest element is the small number of cells counted and the field error contributed by the Poisson distribution. According to Berkson (1940), the

$$CV \ (\%) = \sqrt{\frac{100^2}{n_b} + \frac{4.6^2}{n_c} + \frac{4.7^2}{n_p}}$$ where the first

term is the field error, with n_b = the number of blood cells counted; the second term is the error of the chamber, with n_c = the number of chambers; and the third term is the error of the pipette, with n_p = the number of pipettes used.

If 200 cells are counted using two chambers and one pipette, the C.V. = 9.1 per cent, corresponding to 95 per cent confidence limits of ±18.2 per cent (twice the C.V.). Using four chambers and two pipettes and counting twice as many cells reduces the 95 per cent confidence limits to ±12.8 per cent. Though this is a larger percentage error than the hemacytometer red cell counts, it is of less practical consequence because of the greater physiologic variation of the leukocyte count.

Nucleated red cells will be counted and cannot be

distinguished from leukocytes with the magnification used. If their number is high as seen on the stained smear, a correction should be made according to the following formula:

$$\text{True leukocyte count} = \frac{\text{total count} \times 100}{100 + \text{No. of NRBC}}$$

where the No. of NRBC = the number of nucleated red cells which are counted during the enumeration of 100 leukocytes in the differential count of 100 leukocytes.

Example. The blood smear shows 25 nucleated red cells per 100 leukocytes. The total white cell count is 10,000.

$$\text{True leukocyte count} = \frac{10,000 \times 100}{125}$$

$$= 8000/\mu l \ (8.0 \times 10^9/l)$$

Electronic Counting of Leukocytes. (Gagon, 1966; Brittin, 1971). The principle is the same as that of red cells, except that in either electro-optical or voltage pulse counting, the red cells are lysed before counting. Discussion here will be confined to voltage pulse counting, since this is the more widely used of the methods.

Diluent Solution

1. Physiologic saline, Isoton,* or one of the other commercially available diluting fluids is used, 10 ml for 20 μl of blood.

   a. To this are added two drops of a 3 per cent saponin solution (or one of the commercially available reagents, e.g. Zaponin*) for lysis of the red cells. Five minutes are required to ensure complete stromatolysis.

   b. Alternatively, one can use a commercially available reagent that both lyses red cells and converts Hb to HiCN (e.g., Zapoglobin*); this allows the hemoglobin concentration and the leukocyte count to be determined from the same dilution.

2. Cetrimide-citrate-saline has advantages over saponin in that stromatolysis and dilution occur with one procedure and the leukocytes are stable for several hours (Cartwright, 1968). A 1:500 dilution is made by diluting 20 μl of blood directly in 10 ml of cetrimide-citrate-saline.

Threshold (Pulse Discriminator) Setting. Prior to counting with any new instrument, diluent, or lysing agent, it is necessary to construct a threshold curve. This is done by performing multiple leukocyte counts on a normal blood sample at threshold settings differing by small increments from zero to a point at which the cells are no longer being counted. They may have to be done at different aperture current settings in order to select one that yields a good plateau. The threshold setting is selected so that baseline noise and small particles are not included in the count. The height of the

plateau should be checked by several replicate hemacytometer leukocyte counts.

Technique. Details of operation and coincidence correction charts are supplied by the instrument manufacturer. Background counts greater than 100 should be corrected for coincidence and subtracted from the corrected leukocyte count; if less than 100, background counts can be ignored.

Sources of Error. With the Coulter counter, 0.5 ml of the 1 to 500 dilution of blood is counted, so that 10,000 cells are actually counted for a white cell count of 10,000 per μl. If two counts are made from one dilution and averaged, the error (±2 C.V.) is approximately ±10 per cent in the normal range. If two dilutions of blood are made with an automatic dilutor and triplicate counts are done on each and averaged, the error (±2 C.V.) is ±4.6 per cent in the normal range. Gagon (1966) showed that the leukocyte concentration in blood anticoagulated with EDTA is stable for 24 hours at 8°C. or 25°C. Counts with heparinized blood were often higher than those with other anticoagulants and were not reproducible.

The speed of performance, the elimination of visual fatigue of the technician, and the improved precision are decisive advantages of the electronic cell counter over the hemacytometer.

PLATELET COUNTS

Normally 2 to 4 μm in diameter on stained films and 4 to 7 fl in volume, the platelets are the smallest formed elements in the blood. They function in hemostasis and in maintaining vascular integrity in addition to participating in the process of blood coagulation. The normal range is 140 to 440 × 10^9/l.

Platelets are difficult to count, because they are small and must be distinguished from debris. Another source of difficulty is their tendency to adhere to glass, to any foreign body, and particularly to each other. It is often possible to recognize a significant decrease in the number of platelets by a careful inspection of stained films. With capillary blood, films must be made evenly and very quickly after the blood is obtained in order to avoid clumping and to minimize the decrease due to adhesion of platelets to the margins of the injured vessels. A better estimate is possible by examining stained films made from venous blood with EDTA as an anticoagulant (EDTA-blood), in which platelets are evenly distributed and where clumping does not occur. Their morphology on films is described on page 910.

The visual method of choice employs the phase contrast microscope. This is the reference method. Laboratories performing over 20 platelet counts per day can justify electronic

---

*Coulter Diagnostics, Hialeah, Fla.

platelet counting; both the voltage pulse counting and the electro-optical counting systems are satisfactory.

Hemacytometer method

Phase Contrast Microscope (Brecher, 1964).

Specimen. Venous blood should be collected in a siliconized glass tube with EDTA as an anticoagulant. Plastic tubes may be satisfactory but should be checked against siliconized glass tubes in a trial before use. Several types of plastic tubes have been found to give significantly lower platelet counts than siliconized glass tubes (Lewis, 1971).

Equipment. Flat bottom counting chamber and a No. 1 or $1\frac{1}{2}$ coverslip. "Long-working distance" phase condenser with $43 \times$ annulus and matching $43 \times$ phase objective and $10 \times$ eyepiece. For American Optical Company equipment, "medium dark contrast" should be specified.

Diluent Solution. One per cent ammonium oxalate in distilled water. Stock bottle is kept in refrigerator. The amount needed for the day is filtered before use and the unused portion discarded at end of day.

Procedure

1. Though blood collected in plastic or siliconized syringes and test tubes is theoretically preferable, glass tubes in the Vacutainer system have proved satisfactory. Platelet clumping must be avoided by a good venipuncture and prompt anticoagulation. EDTA is the anticoagulant of choice. Although less desirable, blood from a skin puncture wound may be used if only the first few drops are used and the blood is flowing freely.

2. Two red cell pipettes (Fig. 27–4) are used. Each is filled rapidly with blood exactly to the 1 mark, carefully wiped, then filled with ammonium oxalate to the 101 mark, and rotated in a mechanical pipette rotor. The Bryant-Garrey rotors have been found satisfactory. Rotation for as long as 8 hours does not affect the counts.

3. The hemacytometer is filled in the usual fashion, using a separate pipette for each side.

4. The chamber is covered by a Petri dish for 15 minutes to allow settling of the platelets in one optical plane. A piece of wet cotton or filter paper is left beneath the dish to prevent evaporation.

5. The platelets appear round or oval and frequently have one or more dendritic processes. Their internal granular structure and a purple sheen allow the platelets to be distinguished from debris, which is often refractile. Ghosts of the red cells which have been lysed by the ammonium oxalate are seen in the background.

6. Platelets are counted in 10 small squares (as for red cell counts, the black squares in Figure 27–3), 5 on each side of the chamber. If the total number of platelets counted is less than 100, more small squares are counted until at least 100 platelets have been recorded; 10 squares per side (black plus checked squares, Figure 27–3) or all 25 squares

in the large central square on each side of the hemacytometer, if necessary. If the total number of platelets in all 50 of these small squares is less than 50, the count should be repeated with 1:20 dilutions of blood in white cell pipettes.

Calculation. Since each of the 25 small squares defines a volume of $1/250 \, \mu l$ $(1/25 \, mm^2$ area $\times 1/10 \, mm$ depth), the platelet count (per μl.)

$$= \frac{\text{No. cells counted}}{\text{No. squares counted}} \times \text{dilution} \times 250.$$

By adjusting the number of squares so that at least 100 platelets are counted, the field error (the statistical error due to counting a limited number of platelets in the chamber) can be kept in the same range for low platelet counts as for high platelet counts. It has been shown that the coefficient of variation (C.V.) due to combined field, pipette, and chamber errors is about 11 per cent when at least 100 platelets are counted, 15 per cent when 40 platelets are counted, and 30 per cent when only 10 platelets are counted. With this method the range of values in 95 per cent of healthy controls is from 140 to $440 \times 10^9/l$.

Sources of Error. Most of the sources of error are the same as those discussed previously for the red cell and white cell counts. Blood in EDTA is satisfactory for 5 hours after collection at 20°C. and 24 hours at 4°C., provided no difficulty was encountered in collection. Platelet clumps present in the chamber imply a maldistribution and negate the reliability of the count; a new sample of blood must be collected. The causes of platelet clumping are likely to be initiation of platelet aggregation and clotting before the blood reaches the anticoagulant, imperfect venipuncture, delay in the anticoagulant contacting the blood, or, in skin puncture technique, delay in sampling. Capillary blood gives similar mean values, but errors are about twice those with venous blood, probably because the platelet level varies in successive drops of blood from the skin puncture wound.

Electronic counting

Voltage Pulse Counting

Sample. In order to use the Coulter Counter or Celloscope for platelet counts, the red cells must first be removed from the blood sample by one of three methods:

1. Bull (1965) devised a sedimentation method in which a short length of plastic tubing (sealed at one end) is filled with blood and placed at an angle in a rack to speed sedimentation, which provides sufficient separation of red cells from platelet-rich plasma in 10 to 50 minutes.

2. Fry (1969) showed that closely controlled centrifugal force (300 g for 5 minutes) can provide reproducible separation of red cells without significant loss of platelets from the plasma.

3. Vertically held test tubes in a modified table top centrifuge (Serufuge, Clay-Adams, New York) can be spun at 40 g for 25 seconds to produce rouleaux, which then rapidly sediment to yield platelet-rich plasma in 2 minutes (Bull, 1970).

Equipment. The Coulter Counter model ZBI is more convenient than the Model ZF because it has two thresholds; the lower one excludes particles smaller than platelets, and the upper one excludes red cells or white cells larger than platelets. With the Coulter Counter Model ZF or the Celloscope 401, two counts must be taken at different thresholds and the platelets determined by subtraction. A 70-μm aperture is used with the Coulter Counters. The procedure for setting the amplification and aperture current controls and thresholds is given by Bull (1965).

Procedure. A 1:3000 dilution of platelet-rich plasma is made in Isoton* or saline using a 3-μl capillary pipette in 9 ml of diluent or 3.33 μl in 10 ml. The background count should not exceed 300; if over 150, it should be corrected for coincidence and subtracted from the corrected platelet count before calculation. Two or three counts are made and the results averaged. For platelet counts of less than 25×10^9/l, a 1:300 dilution is made by adding 20 μl of plasma to 6 ml of diluent.

Calculation. Since the number of platelets is expressed per liter of whole blood, a correction must be made for the hematocrit. In addition, platelet-free plasma is trapped by red cells during sedimentation, giving an excess of platelets in the supernatant plasma. For this, an experimentally derived correction also dependent on the hematocrit is applied and is available in a table (Bull, 1965). These corrections have been combined with that for coincidence into a circular slide rule (commercially available); from the uncorrected plasma platelet count and the hematocrit one can read the whole blood platelet count (Bull, 1970).

The coefficient of variation of this method is about 4 per cent, which compares favorably with the hemacytometer-phase contrast method of 11 to 16 per cent. The reference intervals are the same.

Sources of Error. Careful technique is especially important at all steps in platelet counting: collection of blood, having a particle-free diluent, obtaining platelet-rich plasma without losing platelets or having too many red cells remain, microtechnique in diluting, and cleanliness in glassware and in the aperture of the counter.

Excessive numbers of red cells in the plasma will give falsely low counts, because platelets entering the aperture at the same time as red cells will not be detected. High leukocyte counts will also produce a falsely low platelet count, because white cells erratically filter out platelets when aspirating into the microcapillary tube. Platelets as large as red cells will be screened out by the upper threshold, also giving a falsely low count. On the other hand, if the sample is hemolyzed, or if red cell fragments are present in the blood, the platelet count is apt to be falsely high.

Always in platelet counting the blood film must be examined before reporting the count, both for concordance of the apparent numbers on the film with that from the machine, and to detect abnormalities such as those just mentioned that are prone to produce erroneous counts.

Electro-optical Counting (Brittin, 1971; Simmons, 1971). A semiautomatic instrument for counting platelets, the Autocounter* utilizes the darkfield optical microscope system (Fig. 27-6) described previously for red cell counts. Whole blood is sampled automatically from test tubes or plastic cups, diluted approximately 1:1500 in 2 M urea which lyses the red cells. Platelets and leukocytes are counted. For a platelet count of 350×10^9/l, about 10,000 light-scattering events are counted in a small optically determined sensing volume (44,000 fl) in the flow cell; this gives a linear response with no significant coincidence. The results are recorded on a moving pen recorder. The instrument is calibrated with fresh normal EDTA-blood, using the average of multiple phase contrast hemacytometer counts. A stable Platelet Reference N (normal)* suspension is available; this should be used as a control or secondary standard rather than to calibrate the instrument. For each sample, the leukocyte count is separately determined and subtracted from the total count.

This instrument counts platelets with a greater precision than the voltage pulse counters in most hands (C. V. = 1 to 3 per cent versus 4 to 6 per cent for the Coulter method).

The Autocounter has the advantage of using whole blood and automatic mixing, diluting, and counting. Consequently it is easier to use and more reliable, since it is less prone to technical errors in handling samples. In addition, it is readily used for skin-puncture sampling using prediluted whole blood taken with the Unopette system.†

Sources of Error. No matter which method is used for platelet counting, the blood film (prepared from EDTA-blood) must be checked to corroborate the height of the count and to detect abnormalities in platelets or other blood elements that may give a false value. If Howell-Jolly bodies or other red cell inclusions are present, they will falsely elevate the count. So too will fragments of leukocyte cytoplasm that are sometimes numerous in leukemias. The

---

*Coulter Diagnostics, Hialeah, Fla.

*Technicon Corporation, Tarrytown, N.Y.
†Becton-Dickinson, Rutherford, N.J.

phase contrast hemocytometer method must be employed in these cases. Falsely low counts occur if platelets adhere to neutrophils (platelet satellitism) or if there is platelet clumping due to agglutinins, spontaneous aggregation, or incipient clotting. The first two of these phenomena appear to depend upon EDTA (Dacie, 1975).

Platelet counts tend to be the least reproducible of the blood cell counts, and the technologist must use constant vigilance to ensure their accuracy. This also includes the readiness to confirm suspicious or abnormal results with a freshly drawn sample.

Multichannel Instruments

Coulter Counter Model S

Description. The Coulter Counter Model S produces seven simultaneous measurements (leukocyte count, red cell count, hemoglobin, hematocrit, and the red cell indices) in 40 seconds' time, employing the principles of voltage pulse counting and size analysis together with a photosensitive device for measuring hemoglobin concentration. A power supply provides a vacuum and pressure to aspirate the blood and moves the diluting fluids and dilutions through the system. The instrument can accept a new sample every 20 seconds, as it counts one sample while diluting the next. The analysis may be performed on whole blood, of which the machine aspirates about 1.3 ml; most is used for flushing, then 44.7 μl is diluted 1:224 with Isoton* (Fig. 27-7). From this (Dilutor I) a second dilution of 1:224 is made, and from the resulting 1:50,000 dilution the red cell count and the MCV are determined by each of three Coulter counters (C). From Dilutor I, also, the original dilution is brought to a mixing chamber where a lysing agent is added to lyse the red cells and convert the hemoglobin to hemiglobincyanide, and the dilution from 1:224 to 1:250. After the hemoglobin concentration is measured, the suspension of white cells (in dilute HiCN solution) is brought to three counters (C). The red cells and white cells are counted simultaneously, in triplicate, and each group is averaged. This result is printed out unless one result disagrees with the other two by more than 3 standard deviations from the mean, in which case the discordant result is discarded and the mean of the other two is printed out. If all

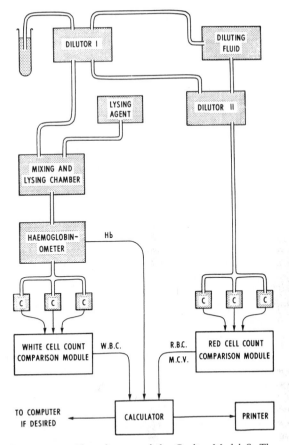

Figure 27-7. Flow diagram of the Coulter Model S. The blood sample is presented manually to the instrument as indicated by the tube, upper left. (From Pinkerton, P. H., et al.: J. Clin. Pathol. 23:68, 1970.)

three results disagree by more than 3 standard deviations, none is accepted and the print-out reads zero. After each sample the hemoglobinometer is automatically zeroed. The MCV is determined directly from voltage pulse heights, and the hematocrit is calculated from the MCV and the red cell count. The other indices are calculated and the seven results appear in digital print-out form on a special card that has been inserted in the printer to receive the data. Simultaneously, the results can pass to a computer.

Capillary blood from skin-puncture sampling can be easily handled by diluting 44.7 μl of blood in 10 ml of Isoton. This prediluted sample can then bypass the first dilution step by means of a separate aspirator. The instrument is not fully automatic, in that the technologist must hold the tube of blood up to the aspirator. This is not entirely disadvantageous in that it allows interruption for the rapid

*Coulter Diagnostics, Hialeah, Fla.

processing of urgent specimens with minimal trouble. Also, the operator is continually watching the oscilloscope screen, the diluting chambers and other working parts, which helps in early detection of malfunction.

The Coulter Model S has been thoroughly evaluated and found to correlate well with the results from the routine laboratory methods (Brittin, 1969a; Pinkerton, 1970). It is currently the most widely used multichannel instrument in hematology. The precision in all the red cell measurements, actual and calculated, has proved to be in the vicinity of 1 per cent (C.V.); the white count slightly higher, 2 to 3 per cent. These values for the coefficient of variation are superior to the routine methods discussed, even when automatic pipettes are used. The reason for this appears to lie in the automatic diluting system which itself has excellent precision.

Calibration. No certified standard cell suspensions are available, though several stabilized suspensions are commercially available. These stabilized cell suspensions, however, should not be used for calibration. Fresh normal blood should be used for calibration, as recently emphasized by Gilmer (1977) and earlier described by Brittin (1969a). Our method follows the latter. We prefer to calibrate the instrument with normal fresh blood in EDTA, which is analyzed by conventional methods as described by Brittin (1969a). Hemoglobin is determined by the HiCN method, using a certified standard and the Coleman Jr. spectrophotometer. Hematocrit is measured by the microhematocrit technique. Red cell counts and white cell counts are performed with the Coulter Counter Model F. For the former, the 1:50,000 dilution is made in a single step to reduce error. A 2 μl ±0.25 per cent Microcap[*] pipette is used to deliver the blood into 100 ml (±0.08) of Isoton[†] in a volumetric flask. The blood for white cell count is diluted 1:500, again with a Microcap, 20 μl ±0.25 per cent. Each of the above is performed on the normal blood in 5 to 10 replicate determinations, except that only two separate dilutions are made for the red cell count. The values are averaged and the hematocrit is corrected for trapped plasma by subtracting 3 per cent of its value, e.g., $0.44 - 0.013 = 0.427$ (England, 1972). Then the red cell indices are calculated. The white cell count is checked by performing du-

plicate hemacytometer counts. Using this normal blood, the Model S is primed several times and the average values set in. Now that the initial calibration is made, it is desirable to carry out final calibration over a period of several days to get the benefit of a larger number of determinations and to minimize any day-to-day variation in the less precise conventional methods. It is important that this calibration not be changed until a "drift" away from these values has been demonstrated on a statistical basis by quality control procedures. At that time, after any necessary maintenance work has been done, the instrument is recalibrated in the same fashion. The calibration settings must not be changed on the basis of a single determination of a control suspension of cells. The Model S has been found to be quite stable; recalibration is usually unnecessary oftener than every two or three weeks.

The method of calibration described gives values for red cell indices from the Model S comparable to those calculated from the individual methods except that the reference values reflect the slight difference due to correction of the hematocrit for trapped plasma. It is clear that in disorders in which trapped plasma is considerably increased (in the microhematocrit) owing to rigidity or shape of red cells, such as iron deficiency anemia and sickle-cell disease, the hematocrit and MCV are lower and the MCHC slightly higher with the Model S than with conventional methods. It appears quite likely that the Model S gives the more correct values.

Quality Control. A commercially available cell control blood may be used and charted every morning and at intervals during the day, but this is quite expensive and not entirely satisfactory. Brittin (1971) has discussed this problem in his excellent review of instrumentation, and Brittin (1969b) presented a useful method for using patient blood samples in quality control. He demonstrated that all seven values are stable in blood collected in EDTA for at least 24 hours at 4°C. At least five and preferably 10 specimens with hematologic values in the normal range are selected on Day 1, kept in the refrigerator, and re-analyzed on Day 2. A significant change in any channel between the two days can be detected statistically using the Student-t test for paired samples:

$$t_n = \frac{\overline{d}}{S_d} \sqrt{n}, \text{ with } n - 1 \text{ degrees of freedom}$$

---

[*] Drummond Scientific Co., Broomall, Pa.
[†] Coulter Diagnostics, Hialeah, Fla.

n = number of pairs of observations

$\bar{d}$ = mean of the differences (from day to day)

S_d = standard deviation of the differences

$$= \sqrt{\frac{\sum(d^2) - \frac{(\sum d)^2}{n}}{n - 1}}$$

The t value is calculated for each channel. If the calculated t value exceeds that critical value for the 95 per cent limits found in a statistical table of t-values, the difference is significant at the 5 per cent level. For n = 5, the critical t value is 2.78. For example, if the t score calculated from the five pairs of white cell counts exceeds 2.78, we can be 95 per cent confident that there is a significant difference between the two days, and we must look for trouble in the white cell channel. Often it is possible to ascertain from simple inspection of the values whether the mean difference from one day to the next differs significantly from zero. The calculations can be easily programmed for a desk top computer, and it is helpful to chart the t values for each channel.

The tendency for drift throughout the day can be monitored by repeating this procedure twice a day, or more simply by running two or three specimens from the first morning batch at intervals throughout the day.

This method will detect a developing loss of calibration, such as may be due to electronic drift. It is likely, however, to miss a significant loss of calibration that occurs more abruptly, due to mechanical or electronic breakdown. Bull (1974) has shown that calculation of a moving average for the MCV, MCH, and MCHC of each successive 20 samples run on the Coulter S throughout the day provides an effective, rapidly available indicator of loss of calibration. It is based on the demonstrated constancy of the mean values for these indices in medium- to large-sized hospitals from day to day and week to week. If the moving average changes by 3 per cent, the calibration must be checked at once. Variations of this method, of increasing complexity, may be performed on a hand calculator or a programmable calculator or be programmed into the laboratory computer system. The more complex variations are slightly more effective; of course, somewhat less of the technologist's time is required if the computer is available for this function.

Sources of Error. Carry-over is a problem with the Coulter Model S,[*] especially on low white cell counts, since it amounts to about 2 to 3 per cent. If the ratio of successive counts exceeds 3.3 : 1, the second count will be in error by 5 per cent (Brittin, 1971). It is therefore necessary to repeat any low white count (following a normal or high one) and to use the second value; this should also be done with very low red cell counts.

Increased white cell counts, over $25 \times 10^9/l$, usually produce a slight but significant false elevation of the hemoglobin as a result of turbidity. A very high white count can also elevate the hematocrit and the MCV because the white cells are counted and sized with the red cells.

Errors that influence the MCV determined by voltage pulse analysis have been reviewed by England (1976). From his studies it appears that if the MCV is calibrated in the normal range only, microcytic MCV's will be overestimated when compared with those determined by microhematocrits corrected for plasma trapping. They suggest that the MCV be calibrated with both small cells and normal-sized cells.

Cold agglutinins in high titer tend to give spurious macrocytosis and low red cell counts with impossibly high MCHCs (Hattersley, 1971). Warming the blood or the diluent eliminates this problem.

In some patients with leukemia the white cells appear to be fragile and escape being counted, giving a falsely low count. Erroneously low white counts may also be found in uremia or in some patients receiving immunosuppressive drugs (Luke, 1971). Hemacytometer counts should be used to check the white counts of such patients.

The following instruments have been discussed by Brittin (1971), to which the reader should turn for a critical analysis.

Technicon Hemalog 8

The successor to the Technicon SMA 4A/7A is the Hemalog 8, a continuous-flow system for automation of routine methods in hematology. This instrument uses the electro-optical principle (described on p. 879) to count red cells, white cells, and platelets; it measures hemoglobin by the HiCN method; it incorporates a

---

[*]But not with the succeeding model, the Coulter Model S-Senior.

unique centrifuge method for the microhematocrit, which is read automatically without stopping the centrifuge head. From the three red cell measurements, the MCV, MCH, and MCHC are calculated and the eight results are printed out (Saunders, 1974). This system operates without the need for the constant presence of a technologist, at the rate of 60 or 90 samples per hour. It does, however, require calibration for each batch of test samples. Evaluations have shown good correlation with other methods. The recent models can incorporate an optional automatic identification system and can be linked to a differential white cell counter (the Hemalog D, p. 909), so that all results are obtained from one sampling event at 60 or 90 patient specimens per hour.

Ortho Hemac*

This automated system counts light impulses that are scattered and diffracted from cells flowing through a laser beam. The impulses are detected by a silicon photovoltaic cell that counts them and generates pulses proportional to the cell size; the sum of their amplitudes determines the hematocrit. White cells are counted as a second, hemolyzed sample flows through the optical chamber. Hemoglobin is determined by the HiCN method, and the red cell indices are calculated. The instrument requires an operator to present each specimen; the results are available in 60 seconds. The instrument must be calibrated daily.

The precision is satisfactory, within a C.V. of 2 per cent for each measurement (Miale, 1977). According to Lewis (1977), the MCV appears to correlate better with the MCV calculated from a microhematocrit (corrected for plasma trapping) than does the Coulter Model S, which overestimates the MCV of microcytic blood. This difference is not likely to have clinical significance.

Fisher Hem-Alyzer†

A multichannel version of the Fisher Autocytometer, the Hem-Alyzer counts red cells and white cells by the electro-optical principle and measures hemoglobin as oxyhemoglobin. It does not have a hematocrit mode, and

therefore does not provide the MCV or the MCHC.

Reticulocyte Count

Principle. During erythropoiesis, after cell division is finished and cytoplasmic maturation is nearly complete, the orthochromatic normoblast loses its nucleus. A variable amount of ribonucleic acid (RNA) remains in the young red cell, and hemoglobin synthesis continues at a slow rate. When blood is mixed with a solution of brilliant cresyl blue or new methylene blue, the dye enters the young red cells and precipitates the RNA into a dark-blue network (reticulum) or as granules. Red cells that contain precipitated dye-ribonucleoprotein complex in any amount are known as reticulocytes.

Reagent. Dissolve 1.0 g new methylene blue (CI 52030) in 100 ml citrate-saline (one part 30 g/l sodium citrate plus four parts 9 g/l sodium chloride).

Procedure. Place three drops of dye solution in a small test tube, add three drops of blood, and mix. Incubate for 15 minutes at 20°C. Mix the suspension well, make two films on glass slides, and allow them to dry in air.

Viewed with the oil-immersion lens without further staining, reticulocytes have the appearance shown in Figure 27-8. The precipitated RNA is reticular or granular and stains deep blue; the red cells themselves stain paler blue or blue-green.

Examine at least 1000 erythrocytes (preferably 3000) for precipitated dye on several different portions of the slide. To obviate the difficulty of examining large fields that contain a confusing number of erythrocytes, the field of vision may be made smaller by placing a metal or paper diaphragm in the oculars to show about 25 cells per field.

The Miller ocular is a convenient device which aids in the rapid counting of large numbers of red cells and, hence, the reticulocytes among them (Brecher, 1950). It is a glass insert that fits into the eyepiece of the microscope and imposes a large square onto the field of view. In one corner of the large square is a smaller square equal to one ninth the area of the large square. Traversing the slide, count the reticulocytes in the large square and the red cells in the small square in successive fields. Count at least 300 red cells in the small square; this provides an estimate of reticulocytes among 300 × 9 red cells, providing an estimate of reticulocytes among 2700 red cells. The calculation is:

$$\text{Reticulocytes (\%)} = \frac{\text{No. reticulocytes in large square}}{\text{No. red cells in small square} \times 9} \times 100$$

After the reticulocyte percentage has been calculated, determine the absolute reticulocyte count

---

*Ortho Instruments, Westwood, Mass.
†Fisher Scientific Co., Pittsburgh, Pa.

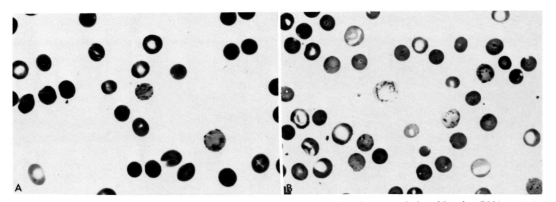

Figure 27–8. Reticulocytes; on air-dried film made after vital staining of blood with new methylene blue dye. RNA precipitates with the dye and appears as blue granules, which are sometimes connected into a network or reticulum.

by multiplying the percentage by the red cell count.

Normal Values. Normal adults have a reticulocyte count of 0.5 to 1.5 per cent or 24 to 84 $\times$ 10⁹/l. In newborn infants the percentage is 2.5 to 6.5 per cent; this falls to the adult range by the end of the second week of life.

Interpretation. Because reticulocytes are immature red cells that lose their RNA in a day or so after reaching the blood from the marrow, a reticulocyte count provides an estimate of the rate of red cell production. An absolute reticulocyte count or reticulocyte production index is more helpful than the percentage (p. 933).

Sources of Variation. Because such a small number of actual reticulocytes are counted, the sampling error in the reticulocyte count is relatively large. The 95 per cent confidence

limits may be expressed as $R \pm 2 \sqrt{\dfrac{R\,(100 - R)}{N}}$

where R is the reticulocyte count in per cent and N is the number of erythrocytes examined. This means that if 1000 erythrocytes are evaluated, the error expressed as ±2 C.V. for a 1 per cent reticulocyte count is 60 per cent and, for a 10 per cent count, 19 per cent. In practical terms, this is less disturbing than it seems, since the 95 per cent confidence limits for a 1 per cent count are 0.4 to 1.6 per cent; for a 5 per cent count, 3.6 to 6.4 per cent; and for a 10 per cent count, 8.1 to 11.9 per cent. It is important that this unavoidable sampling variation be kept in mind when one evaluates the significance of day-to-day changes in the reticulocyte count.

The films may be counterstained with Wright's stain which produces beautiful preparations.

BLOOD FILM EXAMINATION

MAKING AND STAINING BLOOD FILMS

The information gathered from the examination of the blood smear is extremely impor-

tant. It may furnish the diagnosis as does a histologic section; it may serve as a guide to therapy or as an indicator of harmful effects of chemotherapy and radiotherapy. The reliability of the information obtained depends to a considerable extent on the quality of the smears. Properly spread films are essential to accurate work. They more than compensate for the time spent in learning to make them.

The slides and coverglasses must be *perfectly clean* and free of grease. Commercially available precleaned slides are usually quite satisfactory. Otherwise the following procedures may be used.

Wash the slides with soap and water, then with abundant clean hot water (the water should not be permitted to cool before all the soap has been removed), followed by distilled water, and then dry and polish with a clean, lint-free cloth. From then on they must be handled by touching only their edges. Washed slides and coverglasses may be stored in 95 per cent alcohol. Dry coverglasses may also be stored in a clean, dry Petri dish.

The drop of blood must *not be too large.* The work must be done *quickly*, before coagulation begins. The blood is obtained from the fingertip or the lobe of the ear, as for a blood count. Only a very small drop is required, usually about twice the size of a pinhead. The size of the drop largely determines the thickness of the film. The proper thickness depends on the purpose for which the film is made. For a study of the structure of blood cells and examination for malarial parasites, it should be so thin that, throughout a considerable part of the film, the erythrocytes lie in a single layer, close together but not overlapping. In some cases of severe anemia, it is very difficult to make good films because of the large proportion of plasma, which leads to slow drying with consequent distortion of the erythrocytes and the appearance of artifacts. To overcome this, the films should be thin and dried quickly.

Three methods of making films are described: the

two-slide or wedge method, the coverglass method, and the spinner method.

The Two-Slide or Wedge Method.   Place a drop of blood 2 to 3 mm in diameter about 1 cm from the end of a clean, dust-free slide. Place the slide on a table or flat surface. With the thumb and forefinger of the right hand hold the end of a second (spreader) slide against the surface of the first at an angle of 30 to 45 degrees (the free edge of the spreader slide will then be about 5 cm above the table) and draw it back against the drop of blood until contact is established. Allow the blood to run completely across the end, filling the angle between the two slides. Push the "spreader slide" at a moderate speed forward so that the blood spreads evenly on the other side behind the edge of the spreader, keeping contact between the two until all the blood has been spread into a moderately thin film. The spreader slide should be slightly narrower than the first slide so that the edges can be easily examined with the microscope. A "margin-free" spreader slide can be prepared by cutting off the corners of a regular slide.

The slides are rapidly air dried; rapid drying is aided by waving the slide in the air or by using an electric fan. If the drop of blood was of appropriate size, the thin portion of the film is about 3 cm long. The thickness of the film can be regulated by changing the angle at which the spreader slide is held, by varying the pressure and the speed of spreading, and by using a smaller or larger drop of blood. At a given speed, increasing the angle at which the spreader slide is held will increase the thickness of the film. At a given angle, increasing the speed with which the spreader slide is pushed will increase the thickness of the film. The film should not cover the entire surface of the slide. In a good film there is a thick portion and a thin portion and a gradual transition from one to the other. The film should have a smooth, even appearance and be free from ridges, waves, or holes. The edge of the spreader must be absolutely smooth. If it is rough, the film has ragged tails containing many leukocytes.

In films of optimum thickness there is some overlap of red cells in much of the film but even distribution and separation of red cells toward the thin tail. The faster the film is air dried, the better the spreading of the individual cells on the slide. Slow drying (in humid weather, for example) results in contraction artifacts of the cells.

It is very easy by this method to make large numbers of thin, even films.

The slide may be labeled by writing the identification with a lead pencil directly on the thicker end of the blood film.

Portable instruments that automatically produce consistent wedge films of good quality are commercially available.*

Two-coverglass Method.   This method is recommended, but considerable practice is required to get good results. No. 0 or No. 1 coverglasses 22 mm square are recommended. No. 2 coverglasses are too thick for oil immersion.

Touch a coverglass to the top of a small drop of blood (about 2 to 3 mm in diameter) without touching the skin and place it, blood side down, crosswise on another coverglass so that the corners appear as an eight-pointed star. If the drop is not too large and if the coverglasses are perfectly clean, the blood will spread out evenly and quickly in a thin layer between the two surfaces. Just as it stops spreading and before it begins to coagulate, pull the coverglasses quickly but firmly apart on a plane parallel to their surfaces. They should not be separated by lifting. They should be placed film side up on clean paper and allowed to dry in the air, or they may be inserted back to back in slits made in a cardboard box.

Films from venous blood may be prepared similarly by touching the tip of the needle or syringe to a coverslip, placing on it a drop and proceeding as described. Venous blood with an anticoagulant is less suitable for the study of white cells. EDTA is perhaps the most satisfactory anticoagulant for examining the morphology of blood cells because vacuoles and other degenerative changes appear more slowly than with other anticoagulants; only minimal changes occur within 2 or 3 hours of collection. Blood with other anticoagulants and defibrinated blood are less satisfactory for the study of leukocytes.

Separation of the coverglasses must be done just at the right moment to get good results. If it is done too soon, the smear will be too thick. If it is done too late, the blood will clot and it may be difficult to pull the coverglasses apart. The blood usually is much more evenly spread on one of the coverglasses than it is on the other.

Spinner Method.   Blood films that combine the advantages of easy handling of the wedge slide and uniform distribution of cells of the coverglass preparation may be made with special types of centrifuges known as spinners* (Rogers, 1973). In such a device, a platen holds the slide in a horizontal plane perpendicular to the rotor. A low inertia, high torque motor spins the rotor, rapidly accelerates to about 5000 rpm, and quickly stops after a spinning time of a few seconds. To operate, the technologist places about 0.2 ml of EDTA blood in the center of the slide (on the platen) and closes the cover of the centrifuge, which activates the motor. In order to produce uniform slides, the duration of spinning must be proportional to the red cell concentration. An adjustment must be made, therefore, for the hematocrit; this is done by setting a knob on the instrument.

---

*Hemaprep, Geometric Data Corp., Wayne, Pa.

*LARC Spinner, Corning Medical, Medfield, Mass.

The spinner slide is covered by a uniform blood film, in which all cells are separated and do not overlap (a uniform monolayer). White cells can be easily identified at any spot in the film, which is ideal for differential counting and is used in at least one of the automatic white cell differential systems available. The distribution of the different types of white cells in spinner slides is indistinguishable from that in cover glass films and is presumably random. This contrasts with the wedge slide, in which there is a disproportion of monocytes at the tip of the feather edge, of neutrophils just in from the feather edge, and of both at the lateral edges of the film (Rogers, 1973). This is of little practical significance, but it does result in slightly higher monocyte counts in cover glass or spinner films (Table 27-3). A minor disadvantage of the spinner slide is the tendency of the red cells to have eccentric central pallor, mimicking the appearance of spheroidocytes.

Of the three, the coverglass film and the spinner slide have the advantage of an even distribution of white cells. The spinner slide and the wedge film have the advantages of ease of handling and of labeling. The spinner slide requires 0.2 ml of blood (which usually must contain an anticoagulant), requires a special centrifuge, and cannot easily be made at the bedside.

Fixation. In general, films must be "fixed" before they are stained. Stains that are dissolved in methyl alcohol, e.g., Wright's stain, combine fixation with the staining process. Fixation takes place during the first minute when the undiluted stain is applied. With aqueous stains, chemicals or heat must be used prior to application of the stain.

CHEMICAL FIXATION. Soak the film 1 to 2 minutes in pure methyl alcohol or absolute ethyl alcohol, or 15 minutes or longer in equal parts of absolute alcohol and ether. One minute in a 1 per cent solution of mercuric chloride or in a 1 per cent solution of formalin in alcohol is preferred by some workers. The film must be well washed in water after fixation with mercuric chloride. Chemical fixation may precede staining with hematoxylin and eosin and with other simple stains.

FIXATION WITH HEAT. This may precede any of the methods that do not combine fixation with a staining process. The best method is to place the film in an oven, raise the temperature to 150°C., and allow to cool slowly. Without an oven, the proper degree of fixation is difficult to attain.

Blood stains

The aniline dyes, which are extensively used in blood work, are of two general classes: basic dyes, such as methylene blue, and acid dyes, such as eosin. Nuclei and certain other structures in the blood are stained by the basic dyes and, hence, are called basophilic. Certain structures take up only acid dyes and are called acidophilic, oxyphilic, or eosinophilic. Certain other structures are stained by a combination of the two and are called neutrophilic. Recognition of these staining properties marked the beginning of modern hematology.

Polychrome Methylene Blue and Eosin Stains. These stains, which are the outgrowth of the original time-consuming

Table 27-3. ABSOLUTE LEUKOCYTE COUNTS, 95 PER CENT REFERENCE INTERVALS, ADULTS

	(1)	(2)	(3)
Total leukocytes	4.5 –10.1 Wh 3.6 –10.2 Bl	4.5 –11.0 Wh 3.8 –10.0 Bl	4.5–11.0
Neutrophil bands	0.2 – 2.1 Wh 0.06– 1.6 Bl	0 – 0.96 Wh 0 – 0.6 Bl	0– 0.7
Neutrophils	1.5 – 6.0 Wh 1.1 – 6.7 Bl	1.6 – 6.9 Wh 1.2 – 6.0 Bl	1.8– 7.0
Eosinophils	0 – 0.7	0 – 0.6	0– 0.45
Basophils	0 – 0.15	0 – 0.19	0– 0.2
Lymphocytes	1.5 – 4.0	1.2 – 3.9	1.0– 4.8
Monocytes	0.2 – 0.95	0.12– 1.2 (Sp) 0.1 – 0.8 (We)	0– 0.8

Data from three studies giving absolute leukocyte counts (cells $\times$ 10^9/l):
(1) Orfanakis, et al., 1970: Based on 200 cell differential counts on coverslip preparations, electronic total leukocyte counts; 226 whites (Wh), 65 blacks (Bl); Salt Lake City, Utah.
(2) Our data: Based on 100 cell differential counts on wedge films (We) and spinner films (Sp) which are similar except for monocytes, electronic total leukocyte counts; 300 white young adults (Wh), 56 black adolescents (Bl); Syracuse, New York.
(3) Altman and Dittmer, 1961: Data compiled from the literature, for 21-year-old individuals.

Romanowsky method, have largely displaced other blood stains for routine laboratory use. They are polychromatic stains; that is, they stain differentially most normal and abnormal structures in the blood.

The basic components of the Romanowsky-type stains are thiazines, and the acidic components are eosins; this class of stains is known, therefore, as thiazine eosinates (Lillie, 1977). The thiazines present consist of methylene blue (tetramethylthionine) and in varying proportions its analogues produced by oxidative demethylation: azure B (trimethylthionine); azure A (asymmetrical dimethylthionine); symmetrical dimethylthionine; and azure C (monomethylthionine). The acidic component, eosin, is derived from a xanthene skeleton (Baker, 1958).

Most of them are dissolved in methyl alcohol and combine the fixing with the staining process. Numerous methods of preparing and applying these stains have been devised, among the best known being Giemsa's and Wright's.

WRIGHT'S STAIN. This is a methyl alcoholic solution of eosin and a complex mixture of thiazines, including methylene blue (usually 50 to 75 per cent), azure B (10 to 25 per cent), and other derivatives (Lubrano, 1977). It is one of the best and is the most widely used stain. Wright's stain certified by the Biological Stain Commission is commercially available as a solution ready for use or as a powder.[*]

Reagents. The staining solution is prepared by dissolving 0.1 g of powder per 60 ml of chemically pure absolute methyl alcohol (C.P., acetone-free). The powder (0.1 g) is ground in a mortar, adding a few milliliters of the alcohol at a time until 60 ml have been added and the entire stain has gone into solution. This requires 20 to 30 minutes. The stain should then be left standing for a day or two and filtered before use. The stock dye is filtered when prepared and each time when samples are taken from the stock. The dye is sensitive to contamination with water in reagents or glassware. The reagent bottle must be tightly stoppered at all times to prevent entry of water vapor. Exposure to acid or alkaline fumes must also be avoided.

The Buffer solution (pH 6.4) contains: primary (monobasic) potassium phosphate (KH_2PO_4), anhydrous 6.63 g; secondary (dibasic) sodium phosphate (Na_2HPO_4), anhydrous 2.56 g; and distilled water to make 1 liter. A more alkaline buffer (pH 6.7) may be prepared by using 5.13 g of the potassium salt and 4.12 g of the sodium salt.

Procedure

1. For best results stain the films as soon as they have been dried in the air or within a few hours. If they must be kept longer without staining, they should be fixed. In smears left unfixed for a day or more, the dried plasma may stain and produce a background of pale blue.

2. Place the slide with the air-dried film side up on a stain rack over a pan; the coverslip is placed best on a support, i.e., a cork attached to the bottom of a pan with paraffin.

3. Without previous fixation, cover the film with the staining solution with a medicine dropper. There must be plenty of stain in order to avoid evaporation that leads to precipitates on the film. This step fixes the film.

4. After 2 minutes, add to the staining fluid on the film an equal quantity of the buffer solution with a second medicine dropper. To mix the stain with the diluent, blow gently on the diluted stain on several portions of the slide to set up gentle currents and to make an even distribution. The quantity of the fluid on the preparation must not be so large that some of it runs off; yet if too little fluid covers the slide, precipitates floating in the mixture will settle on the surface of the blood film. Look for a green metallic scum to appear. The margins should show a reddish tint. The time for optimal staining has to be established for each batch. Eosinophilic granules are best brought out by a short period of staining. The optimal time for the most effective combination of stain and diluent may vary from batch to batch.

5. Float off the stain with a stream of water (preferably distilled), first slowly and then more vigorously, preferably from an overhead water bottle, until all traces of excessive stain have disappeared. During the entire procedure the slide must remain horizontal. The washing takes 5 to 30 seconds until the thinner portions of the film become pink in color. If the stain is poured off before rinsing, the scum tends to settle on the blood film, where it clings in spite of subsequent washing. If the color is too dark, the excessive blue can be removed by further washing. The stain remaining on the back of the dried slide is removed with gauze moistened in alcohol.

6. The washing completed, drain the excessive water by tilting the slide and touching a blotter with the lower edge.

7. The slide may be dried by evaporation by leaving it in the tilted position, or by blotting gently with filter paper.

8. The coverglass, film side down, is mounted on a slide with neutral Canada balsam. Coverglass films may be mounted temporarily by placing them, blood slide down, on a glass slide on which a drop of immersion oil has been placed. Using a drop of isobutyl methacrylate dissolved in xylol or toluol at an approximately neutral pH will give permanent mounts.

---

[*]H. J. Conn and M. S. Darrow: Staining Procedures Used by the Biological Stain Commission, 2nd ed. Baltimore, The Williams & Wilkins Co., 1960.

Films stained well with Wright's stain have a pink color when viewed with the naked eye. When inspected under low power magnification of the microscope, the cells should be evenly distributed and separated from each other. The red cells are pink, not lemon yellow or red; they are lying flat without overlapping or forming rouleaux. At least eight satisfactory low power fields on a slide are present in a good preparation. There should be only a minimum of precipitate. The areas between the cells are clear. The color of the film should be uniform without pale or dark green areas indicative of excessive staining of thick portions of film. The blood cells should be free from artifacts, such as vacuoles. The nuclei of leukocytes are blue to purple, the basi- and oxychromatin (chromatin and parachromatin) clearly differentiated, and the cytoplasmic neutrophilic granules tan in color. The eosinophilic granules are red-orange and each distinctly discernible, so that one may count the individual granules.

The basophil has dark blue to purple granules. Platelets have dark lilac granules. Bacteria (if present) are blue. The cytoplasm of lymphocytes is generally robin's-egg blue; that of the monocytes has a faint bluish tinge. Malarial parasites stain characteristically: the cytoplasm, sky blue; the chromatin, red-purple. These colors are not invariable; two films stained from the same bottle sometimes differ greatly. In general, a preparation is satisfactory when both the nuclei and the neutrophilic granules are distinct, regardless of their color, and when the film is free from precipitated dye. The colors are prone to fade if the preparation is mounted in a poor quality of balsam or if it is exposed to the light.

Staining Problems

Excessively Blue Stain. Thick films, prolonged staining time, inadequate washing, or too high an alkalinity of stain or diluent tends to cause excessive basophilia. In such smears the erythrocytes appear blue or green, the nuclear chromatin is deep blue to black, and the granules of the neutrophils are deeply overstained and appear large and prominent. The granules of the eosinophils are blue or gray. Such stain may be corrected by staining for a shorter time or by using less stain and more diluent. If these steps are ineffective, the buffer may be too alkaline and a new one with a lower pH should be prepared.

Excessively Pink Stain. Insufficient staining; prolonged washing time; mounting the coverslips before they are dry; or too high an acidity of the stain or buffer may cause excessive acidophilia. In such films the erythrocytes are bright red or orange and not pink, the nuclear chromatin is pale blue, and the granules of the eosinophils are sparkling brilliant red. One of the causes of the increased acidity is exposure of the stain or buffer to acid fumes. The problem may be in a low pH of the buffer, or it may be in the methyl alcohol, which is prone to develop formic acid as a result of oxidation

on standing. A given powder may afford perfect results when dissolved in fresh methanol, but poor results when dissolved in the same lot of methanol after some months of exposure to air. After these steps have been checked, one might suspect that the dye does not have the proper polychrome components and try another lot.

Inadequately Stained Red Cells, Nuclei, or Eosinophilic Granules may be due to understaining or excessive washing. Prolonging the staining or reducing the washing may solve the problem.

Precipitate on the Film may be due to unclean slides, drying during the period of staining, inadequate washing of the slide at the end of the staining period, especially failure to hold the slide horizontally during initial washing, inadequate filtration of the stain, or permitting dust to settle on the slide or smear.

OTHER STAINS. Besides Wright's stain, Romanowsky-type stains include a number of others: Giemsa, Leishman, Jenner, May-Grünewald, MacNeal, and various combinations. Some have been particularly recommended for certain purposes, such as Giemsa's stain for excellence in staining malarial parasites and protozoa.

These Romanowsky-type stains (thiazine eosinates) generally vary in the proportions of methylene blue and its demethylated polychrome intermediates (azure B, azure A, etc.). The latter may be developed by "aging" the stain or by adding various oxidizing agents; or they may be more or less purified elsewhere and added. A combination of these thiazine dyes seems to be necessary to produce the subtle varieties of color in well-stained blood cells.

Slight variations in staining quality that are common in most laboratories can be accommodated by the trained observer's eye without difficulty. The recent advent of automated leukocyte differential counting systems, however, has demanded a much more consistent stain. This demand has stimulated several studies in an attempt to achieve a better understanding and control of the process.

Marshall (1975), using thin layer chromatography, and Lubrano (1977), using high performance liquid chromatography, have analyzed the composition of a large number of commercially available Romanowsky dyes. They have shown that the composition of the dyes in the same stain often varies among different suppliers, and even may vary considerably from batch to batch from the same supplier. In addition, during storage at 25°C. (but not at 4°C.) degradation products that are not polychrome dyes form in methanol; these impair staining intensity but not color (Dean, 1977).

Marshall (1975a) correlated the staining performance of a number of commercial stains with their chemical composition on thin-layer chromatography. Although the results did not show a precise relationship, he was able to determine that: methylene blue, azure B, and eosin when used alone produced consistent and satisfactory staining; poor results were correlated with the presence of methylene violet Bernthsen and methyl thionoline/thionoline; and that the stain must not be contaminated with metal salts. On the basis of these studies they have produced a standardized Romanowsky stain from purified dyes (Marshall, 1975b). Unfortunately, purified, metal-free dyes are not yet available as such commercially. It seems likely, however, that the impetus for more consistent performance will improve the consistency of dye formulation, as well as improve our understanding of the polychromatic staining process.

ERYTHROCYTES

The stained films furnish the best means of studying the morphology of the blood and blood parasites, and, to an experienced person, they give a fair idea of the amount of hemoglobin and of the number of erythrocytes, leukocytes, and platelets. An oil-immersion objective is required.

In a healthy person the erythrocytes, when not crowded together, appear as circular, homogeneous discs of nearly uniform size, ranging from 6 to 8 μm in diameter (Fig. 27-9). However, even in normal blood there may be individual cells as small as 5.5 μm and as large as 9.5 μm. The center of each is somewhat paler than the periphery. Erythrocytes are liable to be crenated when the film has dried too slowly. In disease, erythrocytes vary in their hemoglobin content, size, shape, staining properties, and structure.

Variation in Color

HEMOGLOBIN CONTENT. The depth of staining furnishes a rough guide to the amount of hemoglobin in red cells, and the terms normochromic, hypochromic, and hyperchromic are used to describe this feature of red cells. *Normochromic* refers to normal intensity of

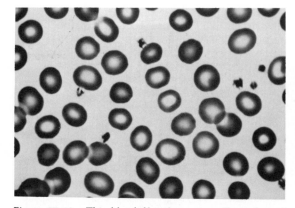

Figure 27-10. This blood film shows a small number of slightly hypochromic red cells; most are normochromic. Cell diameters are normal. MCV and MCHC were normal. The irregular bodies 2 to 3 μm in diameter are normal blood platelets (×875).

staining (Figs. 27-9 and 27-10). When the amount of hemoglobin is diminished, the central pale area becomes larger and paler. This is known as *hypochromia*. The MCH and MCHC are usually decreased (Fig. 27-11). In megaloblastic anemia, because the red cells are larger and hence thicker, many stain deeply and have less central pallor (Figs. 27-12 and 27-14). These cells are *hyperchromic* because they have an increased hemoglobin content (MCH), but the hemoglobin concentration (MCHC) is normal. In hereditary spherocytosis the cells are also hyperchromic (Fig. 27-13); though the hemoglobin content (MCH) is normal, the hemoglobin concentration (MCHC) is usually increased because of a reduced surface/volume ratio.

The presence of hypochromic cells and normochromic cells in the same film is called

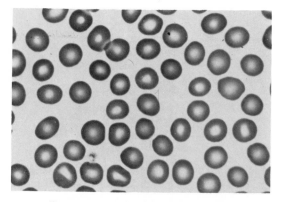

Figure 27-9. Normal blood film (×875).

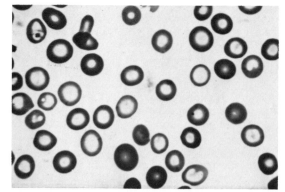

Figure 27-11. Iron deficiency anemia. Most of the cells are hypochromic and microcytic. Note elliptical cells. Anisocytosis is slight in degree (×875).

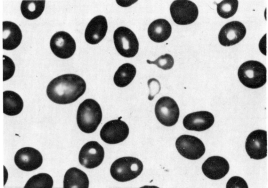

Figure 27-12. Megaloblastic anemia. Macrocytosis. Marked anisocytosis. Note elliptical cells and teardrop-shaped cells (×875).

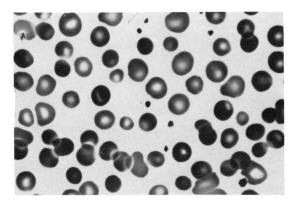

3

Figure 27-13. Hereditary spherocytosis. The denser cells are more spherocytic. Note that they have minimal and eccentric pallor, moderate anisocytosis. Though the cell diameter is reduced, the MCV is within the normal range (×875).

Figure 27-14. Megaloblastic anemia, macrocytosis, marked anisocytosis (×875).

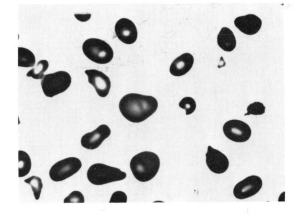

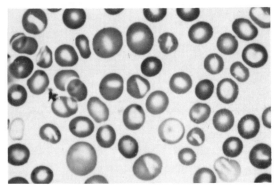

Figure 27-15. Sideroblastic anemia. Dimorphic populations of hypochromic cells and normochromic cells, some of which are macrocytic. Moderate anisocytosis (×875).

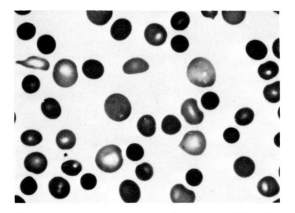

Figure 27-16. Autoimmune hemolytic anemia. The paler, large cells are polychromatic macrocytes (i.e., young reticulocytes.) The small, dense cells are spherocytes. Moderate anisocytosis (×875).

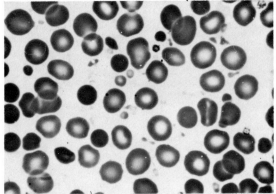

Figure 27-17. Blood film from a patient who has just suffered extensive body burns. Note the many tiny red cell fragments that have budded off the red cells as a result of the heat, leaving spherocytes. Marked anisocytosis (×875).

anisochromia or, sometimes, a dimorphic anemia (Fig. 27-15). This is characteristic of sideroblastic anemias, but also is found some weeks after iron therapy for iron deficiency anemia or in a hypochromic anemia after transfusion with normal cells.

POLYCHROMATOPHILIA. A blue-gray tint to the red cells (polychromatophilia or polychromasia) is a combination of the affinity of hemoglobin for acid stains and the affinity of RNA for basic stains. The presence of residual RNA in the red cell indicates that it is a young red cell which has been in the blood one to two days. These polychromatic red cells are larger than the mature red cells and may lack the central pallor (Fig. 27-16). Young cells with residual RNA are polychromatophilic red cells on air-dried films stained with Wright's stain, but are reticulocytes when stained supravitally with brilliant cresyl blue. Therefore, increased polychromasia implies reticulocytosis; it is most marked in hemolysis and in acute blood loss.

Variation in Size. The red cells may be abnormally small or *microcytes* (Figs. 27-11, 27-14, and 27-17), abnormally large or *macrocytes* (Figs. 27-12, 27-14, and 27-15), or show abnormal variation in size (*anisocytosis*) (Figs. 27-11 through 27-17). Anisocytosis of varying degree is a feature of most anemias; when it is marked in degree, both macrocytes and microcytes are usually present (Figs. 27-12 and 27-14). In analyzing causes of anemia, the terms *microcytic* and *macrocytic* have most meaning when considered as cell volume rather than cell diameter. The mean cell volume, of course,

is measured directly on the Coulter Counter Model S, or is calculated from the spun hematocrit and the red cell count. The diameter we perceive directly from the blood film, and infer from it (and the hemoglobin content) the volume. Thus, the red cells in Figure 27-11 are microcytic; since they are hypochromic they are thinner than normal and the diameter is not decreased proportionately to the volume. Also, the mean cell volume in the blood of the patient with spherocytosis (Fig. 27-13) is in the normal range; though many of the cells have a small diameter, their volume is not decreased because they are thicker than normal.

Variation in Shape. Variation in shape is called *poikilocytosis*. Any abnormally shaped cell is a poikilocyte. Oval, pear-shaped, tear drop-shaped, saddle-shaped, helmet-shaped, and irregularly shaped cells may be seen in a

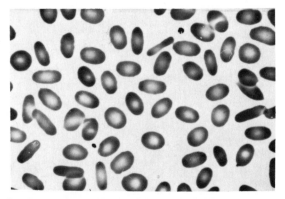

Figure 27-18. Hereditary elliptocytosis. Incidental finding, no anemia (×875).

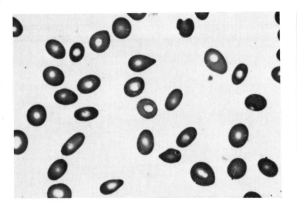

Figure 27-19. Blood film from patient with myelofibrosis with myeloid metaplasia. Numerous elliptocytes. Teardrop-shaped cells (×875).

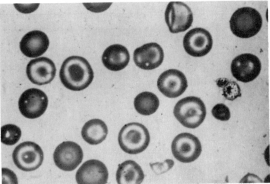

Figure 27-21. Target cells that have an increased cell diameter. Blood film from a patient with obstructive jaundice (×875).

3

single case of anemia such as megaloblastic anemia (Figs. 27-12 and 27-14).

Elliptocytes are most abundant in hereditary elliptocytosis (Fig. 27-18), in which the majority of the cells are elliptical; this is a dominant condition that is only occasionally associated with hemolytic anemia. Elliptocytes are seen in normal persons' blood, but number less than 10 per cent of the cells. They are more common, however, in iron deficiency anemia, myelofibrosis with myeloid metaplasia (Figs. 27-19 and 27-20), megaloblastic anemias (Figs. 27-12 and 27-14), and sickle cell anemia.

Spherocytes are nearly spherical erythrocytes in contradistinction to normal biconcave discs. Their diameter is smaller than normal. They lack the central pale area or have a smaller, often eccentric, pale area (because the cell is thicker and can come to rest somewhat tilted instead of perfectly flattened on the

slide). They show increased fragility in hypotonic salt solutions and are found in hereditary spherocytosis (HS, Fig. 27-13), in some cases of acquired hemolytic anemia (AHA, Fig. 27-16), and in some conditions in which there has been a direct physical or chemical injury to the cells, such as heat (Fig. 27-17). In each of these three instances tiny bits of membrane (in excess of hemoglobin) are removed from the adult red cells, leaving the cell with a decreased surface/volume ratio. In HS and AHA this occurs in the reticuloendothelial system; in other instances (e.g., the patient with body burns), this may occur intravascularly.

Target cells are erythrocytes that are thinner than normal (leptocytes) and when stained show a peripheral rim of hemoglobin with a dark, central, hemoglobin-containing area. The two are separated by a pale unstained ring, which contains less hemoglobin. These cells, as well as other hypochromic cells, seem to be more resistant to hypotonic salt solution than are normal erythrocytes. They are found in obstructive jaundice (e.g., Fig. 27-21), in which there appears to be an augmentation of the cell surface membrane; in the postsplenectomy state, in which there is a lack of normal reduction of surface membrane as the cell ages; in any hypochromic anemia, especially thalassemia; and in hemoglobin C disease.

Schistocytes (cell fragments) indicate the presence of hemolysis, whether in megaloblastic anemia (Fig. 27-14), severe burns (Fig. 27-17), or microangiopathic hemolytic anemia (Fig. 27-22). The latter process is associated with either small blood vessel disease or fibrin in small blood vessels and results in intravas-

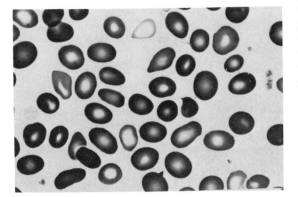

Figure 27-20. Same as Figure 27-19. A few hypochromic microcytic cells are present also (×875).

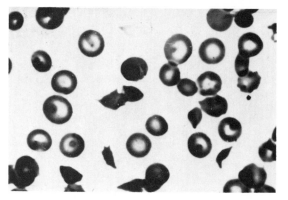

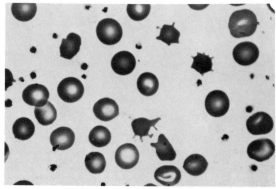

Figure 27-22. Microangiopathic hemolytic anemia; hemolytic-uremic syndrome. Note irregularly contracted cells, schistocytes, a few crenated cells. One nucleated red cell (×875).

Figure 27-23. Acanthocytes. Note the long spicules, which tend to have bulbous ends (×875).

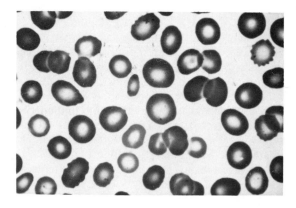

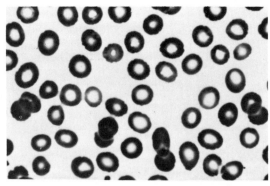

Figure 27-24. Megaloblastic anemia. A few crenated cells are present (×875).

Figure 27-25. Artifact due to water in the methyl alcohol fixative. If bubbles are small in size (as here) they cause an indented appearance which may be confused with crenation (×875).

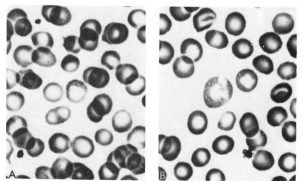

Figure 27-26. Basophilic stippling. One stippled red cell in the center of each field. *A*, thalassemia minor; *B*, lead poisoning (×875).

cular fragmentation; particularly characteristic are helmet cells and triangularly shaped cells. Burr cells are irregularly contracted red cells with prominent spicules and are seen in the same process; however, this term is used differently by different hematologists, and therefore leads to confusion.

Acanthocytes are spiculated red cells in which the ends of the spicules are bulbous and rounded (Fig. 27-23); they are seen in abetalipoproteinemia, hereditary or acquired, and certain cases of liver disease. *Crenated cells* or echinocytes (Fig. 27-24) are regularly contracted cells which may commonly occur as an artifact during preparation of films, or may be due to hyperosmolarity, or to the discocyte-echinocyte transformation. *In vivo* the latter may be associated with decreased red cell ATP due to any of several causes (Brecher, 1972).

Artifacts resembling crenated cells consisting of tiny pits or bubbles indenting the red cells (Fig. 27-25) may be caused by a small amount of water contaminating the Wright's stain (or absolute methanol, if this is used first as a fixative).

Variations in Structure

BASOPHILIC STIPPLING (PUNCTATE BASOPHILIA). This is characterized by the presence, within the erythrocyte, of irregular basophilic granules, which vary in size from scarcely visible dots to granules nearly as large as azurophil granules of promyelocytes (Fig. 27-26). The number of these granules present in an erythrocyte commonly varies in inverse ratio to their size. They stain deep blue with carbolthionin blue or Wright's stain. The erythrocyte containing them may stain normally in other respects or it may exhibit polychromatophilia. Fine stippling is commonly seen when there is increased polychromatophilia, and, therefore, with increased production of red cells. Coarse stippling may be seen in lead poisoning or other diseases with impaired hemoglobin synthesis, in megaloblastic anemia, and in other forms of severe anemia; it is attributed to an abnormal instability of the RNA in the young cell.

Red cells with inorganic iron-containing granules (as demonstrated by stains for iron) are called *siderocytes*. Sometimes these granules stain with Wright's stain; if so, they are called *Pappenheimer bodies*. In contrast to basophilic stippling, Pappenheimer bodies are few in number in a given red cell and are rarely seen in the peripheral blood except after splenectomy.

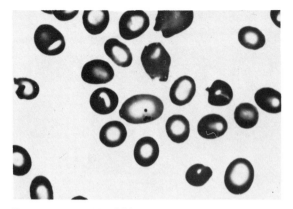

Figure 27-27. Megaloblastic anemia. The central oval macrocyte has four Howell-Jolly bodies; the lower three are touching one another ($\times$875).

HOWELL-JOLLY BODIES. These particles are smooth, round remnants of nuclear chromatin. Single Howell-Jolly bodies may be seen in megaloblastic anemia, hemolytic anemia, and after splenectomy. Multiple Howell-Jolly bodies in a single cell (Fig. 27-27) usually indicate megaloblastic anemia or some other form of abnormal erythropoiesis.

CABOT RINGS. These are ring-shaped, figure-of-eight, or loop-shaped structures. Occasionally they are formed by double or several concentric lines. They have been observed rarely in erythrocytes in pernicious anemia, lead poisoning, and certain other disorders of erythropoiesis. They stain red or reddish purple with Wright's stain and have no internal structure (on close examination they are seen to consist of fine granules). In addition to Cabot's rings, erythrocytes may occasionally contain basophilic granules, nuclear fragments, or even complete nuclei. The rings have been thought to be the remains of a nuclear membrane or microtubules remaining from a mitotic spindle, but no convincing evidence exists for either hypothesis. They are interpreted as evidence of abnormal erythropoiesis.

MALARIAL STIPPLING. This term has been applied to the finely granular appearance of erythrocytes that harbor the parasites of tertian malaria. It was formerly classed with basophilic stippling but is undoubtedly different. Not all stains show it. With Wright's stain it can be brought out by staining longer and washing less than when ordinary blood is examined. The minute granules, "Schüffner's granules," stain purplish red. They are sometimes so numerous that they almost hide the

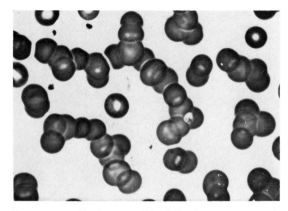

Figure 27–28. Rouleaux in a blood film from a patient with multiple myeloma (×875).

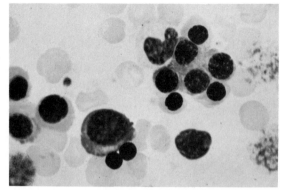

Figure 27–30. Normoblasts in the marrow from a patient with hemolytic anemia. Largest cell is a basophilic normoblast (×875).

parasites. These red cells are, as a rule, larger than normal.

ROULEAU FORMATION. This is the alignment of red cells one upon another so that they resemble stacks of coins in wet preparations. On air-dried films, rouleaux appear as in Figure 27-28; the red cells are not evenly distributed. Elevated plasma fibrinogen or globulins cause rouleaux to form and, because of this, also promote an increase in the erythrocyte sedimentation rate. Rouleau formation is especially marked in paraproteinemia (monoclonal gammopathy). *Agglutination* or clumping of red cells is more surely separated from rouleaux in wet preparations, but on air-dried films (Fig. 27-29) tends to show more irregular and round clumps than the linear rouleaux. Cold agglutinins are responsible for this appearance.

Nucleated Red Cells. In contrast to eryth-rocytes of lower vertebrates and to other cells of the body, a unique characteristic of the mammalian erythrocyte is the absence of a nucleus.

Nucleated red cells (*normoblasts*) are precursors of the non-nucleated mature red cells in the blood. In the human, normoblasts are normally present only in the bone marrow (Fig. 27-30). The stages in their production (described on p. 922) from the earliest to the latest are the pronormoblast, basophilic normoblast, polychromatophilic normoblast, and orthochromatic normoblast.

In general, nucleated red cells that might appear in the blood in disease are polychromatic normoblasts. In some, however, the cytoplasm is so basophilic that it is difficult to recognize the cell as erythroid except by the character of the nucleus: intensely staining chromatin; sharp separation of chromatin from parachromatin. Such erythroid cells are often mistaken for lymphocytes, an error that usually can be prevented by careful observation of the nucleus. The *megaloblast* (Fig. 27-31) is a distinct, nucleated erythroid cell, not merely a larger normoblast. It is characterized by large size and abnormal "open" nuclear chromatin pattern. Cells of this series are not found in normal marrow, but are characteristically present in the marrow and sometimes the blood of patients with pernicious anemia or other megaloblastic anemias. They are described on page 925.

SIGNIFICANCE OF NUCLEATED ERYTHROCYTES. Normoblasts are present normally only in the blood of the fetus and of very young infants. In the healthy adult they are confined to the bone marrow and appear in the circulating blood only in disease, in which their presence

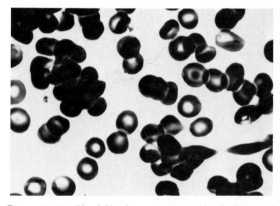

Figure 27–29. Blood film from a patient with a high titer of cold agglutinins. Red cells aggregate in clumps. Separation of cells during making the film may distort the cells (lower right) (×875).

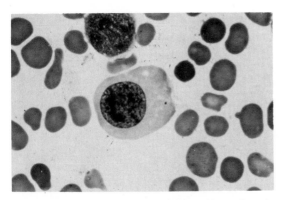

Figure 27-31. Polychromatic megaloblast. Above: "smudge cell" (damaged nucleus; no cytoplasm) (×875).

Table 27-4. CONDITIONS ASSOCIATED WITH LEUKOERYTHROBLASTOSIS

0.63	0.26	Solid tumors and lymphomas
	0.24	Myeloproliferative disorders including CML
	0.13	Acute leukemias
0.37	0.03	Benign hematologic conditions
	0.08	Hemolysis
	0.26	Miscellaneous, including blood loss

Data are from Weick, J. K., Hagedorn, A. B., and Linman, J. W.: Leukoerythroblastosis: Diagnostic and prognostic significance. Mayo Clin. Proc., *49*:110, 1974.

Proportions are based on a series of 215 cases discovered in a prospective study of 50,277 blood film examinations in a six-month period, a proportion of 0.004.

CML = Chronic myelogenous leukemia

usually denotes an extreme demand made on the blood-forming organs to regenerate erythrocytes. Such increased red cell production occurs in response to acute blood loss or to hemolytic anemia, which includes a group of conditions characterized by increased red cell destruction. Large numbers of circulating nucleated red cells are particularly found in hemolytic disease of the newborn (erythroblastosis fetalis, p. 1010) and thalassemia major (p. 999). In the latter, circulating normoblasts may be extremely numerous, an observation that led to an older name for the condition, "erythroblastic anemia."

Leukoerythroblastotic Reaction. The presence of normoblasts and immature cells of the neutrophilic series in the blood is known as a "*leukoerythroblastotic reaction.*" This may be found in the conditions just mentioned (infancy, blood loss, and malignancy). In addition, it often indicates space-occupying disturbances of the marrow, such as myelofibrosis with myeloid metaplasia, metastatic carcinoma, leukemias, multiple myeloma, Gaucher's disease, and others. Nonetheless, in the study of Weick (1974), over a third of the patients with a leukoerythroblastotic reaction did not have malignant or potentially malignant disease (Table 27-4). In patients with metastatic malignancy, a leukoerythroblastotic reaction is good evidence for marrow involvement by tumor.

The presence of megaloblasts indicates a change in the type of blood formation. This is seen most characteristically in pernicious anemia and other megaloblastic anemias. It indicates the presence of megaloblasts in the marrow and is therefore important in the diagnosis of this disease.

LEUKOCYTES

Differential leukocyte count

Before evaluating leukocytes on the Romanowsky-stained blood film, one should first determine that the film is well made, the distribution of the cells is uniform, and the staining of cells is satisfactory. Learning to identify normal cells with low power (100× magnification) as well as with the oil immersion lens (1000×) will enable one to find abnormal cells readily when they are present.

One first scans the counting area of the slide and in wedge films, the lateral and feather edges where monocytes, neutrophils, and large abnormal cells (if present) tend to be disproportionately represented. Suspicious cells are detected at 100× magnification, but of course are identified with the oil immersion lens. Since nucleated red cells, macrophages, immature granulocytes, immature lymphoid cells, megakaryocytes, and abnormal cells are not normally found in blood, they should be noted if present.

While scanning under low power, it is advisable to estimate the leukocyte count from the film. Even though it is a crude approximation, it sometimes enables one to detect errors in total count. One then proceeds to determine the percentage distribution of the different types of leukocytes, which is known as the differential leukocyte count. In the crenellation technique of counting, the field of view is moved from side to side across the width of the slide in the "counting area," just behind the feather edge, where the red cells are separated from one another and are free of artifacts. As each leukocyte is encountered, it is

Table 27-5. NINETY-FIVE PER CENT CONFIDENCE LIMITS FOR THE PERCENTAGE OF CELLS WITH A PARTICULAR CHARACTERISTIC, GIVEN THAT *a* PER CENT OF CELLS WITH THIS CHARACTERISTIC ARE FOUND IN A STUDY OF *n* CELLS*

					n			
a		100		200		500		1000
0	0	4	0	2	0	1	0	1
1	0	6	0	4	0	3	0	2
2	0	8	0	6	0	4	1	4
3	0	9	1	7	1	5	2	5
4	1	10	1	8	2	7	2	6
5	1	12	2	10	3	8	3	7
6	2	13	3	11	4	9	4	8
7	2	14	3	12	4	10	5	9
8	3	16	4	13	5	11	6	10
9	4	17	5	14	6	12	7	11
10	4	18	6	16	7	13	8	13
15	8	24	10	21	12	19	12	18
20	12	30	14	27	16	24	17	23
25	16	35	19	32	21	30	22	28
30	21	40	23	37	26	35	27	33
35	25	46	28	43	30	40	32	39
40	30	51	33	48	35	45	36	44
45	35	56	38	53	40	50	41	49
50	39	61	42	58	45	55	46	54

*For $n = 100$, the confidence limits were calculated exactly; for *n* over 100, with $a \times n$ over 2000, the normal approximation was applied; and for *n* over 100 with $a \times n$ under 2000, Poisson's approximation was used.

For *x* over 50, obtain confidence limits by reading limits for $100 - x$ in the table and subtracting them from 100. For example, the confidence limits for 75 per cent in a sample of $n = 100$ are 65 and 84.

From C. L. Rümke: Variability of results in differential counts on blood smears. Triangle, the Sandoz Journal of Medical Science, *4*:156, 1960.

classified, until 100, 200, 500, or 1000 leukocytes have been counted. The greater the number of cells counted, the greater the precision (Table 27-5), but for practical reasons 100 or 200 cell counts are usually made. Another technique is to count all the cells as the field of view is moved longitudinally from the thick end to the feather end, encompassing the cells from one part of the original drop of blood. The disadvantage of this latter method is the difficulty in identifying contracted, heavily stained cells in the thicker part of the film.

A record of the count may be kept by placing a mark for each leukocyte in its appropriate column, ruled on paper. It is more convenient to use one of several commercially available recording tabulators. They have a separate key for each type of cell, and the

percentages can be read directly as the instrument automatically indicates when 100 corpuscles have been counted. Leukocytes that cannot be classified should be placed together in an unidentified group. In some conditions, notably leukemia, there may be many of these unidentified leukocytes. During the differential leukocyte counting procedure the morphology of erythrocytes and platelets is examined and the number of platelets is estimated.

The absolute number of each variety of leukocyte in a microliter (or liter) is easily calculated from these percentages and the total leukocyte count. It should form part of the record if this is to be complete. An increase in absolute concentration is an *absolute increase;* an increase in percentage only is a *relative increase.* With a low total leukocyte count, for example, the neutrophil count may be relatively normal (normal percentage) but absolutely decreased. Reference intervals are more useful if given as absolute concentrations rather than percentages (see Table 27-3, p. 891).

Leukocytes normally present in blood

Neutrophil (Polymorphonuclear Neutrophilic Leukocyte; Segmented Neutrophilic Granulocyte). Neutrophils average $12\,\mu m$ in diameter; they are smaller than monocytes and eosinophils and slightly larger than basophils. The nucleus stains deeply; it is irregular and often assumes shapes comparable to such letters as E, Z, and S. What appear to be separate nuclei normally are segments of nuclear material connected by delicate filaments.

A filament has length but no breadth as one focuses up and down. A *segmented neutrophil* has at least two of its lobes separated by such a filament. A *band neutrophil* has either a strand of nuclear material thicker than a filament (as described above) connecting the lobes, or a U-shaped nucleus of uniform thickness. The nucleus in both types of neutrophil has coarse blocks of chromatin and rather sharply defined parachromatin spaces. If, because of overlapping of nuclear material, it is not possible to be certain whether or not a filament is present, the cell should be placed in the segmented category (Mathy, 1974). The number of lobes in normal neutrophils ranges from two to five, with a median of three.

The cytoplasm, itself colorless, is packed full of tiny granules (0.2 to $0.3\,\mu m$) that stain tan to pink with Wright's stain (Figs. 27-32*A* and

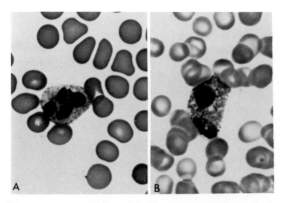

A B

Figure 27-32. *A*, Neutrophil. The cytoplasm is filled with tiny granules, some of which stain more deeply than others (toxic granulation). Note that most of the red cells lack central pallor, an artifact seen near the feather edge of the film. *B*, Eosinophil. Typically this cell has fewer nuclear lobes and larger cytoplasmic granules than the neutrophil (×875).

Plate 27-1). About two thirds of these are specific granules and one third azurophil granules. The intensity of the red-blue or purple staining of the azurophil granules in the more immature neutrophils (p. 935) has diminished; with light microscopy the two types of granules often can not be distinguished in the mature cell.

Segmented neutrophils average 56 per cent of leukocytes; reference intervals are 1.5 to 7.0 × 10^9/l in white adults; but have a lower limit of about 1.1 × 10^9/l in blacks. Band neutrophils average 3 per cent of leukocytes; the upper reference value is about 1.0 × 10^9/l in whites and slightly lower in blacks (using the above definition and counting 100 cells in the differential, Table 27-3).

Normally about 35 per cent of the segmented neutrophils have two lobes, 41 per cent have three lobes, 17 per cent four, and no more than 3 per cent have five lobes. A "shift to the left" occurs when there are increased bands and less mature neutrophils in the blood, as well as a lower average number of lobes in segmented cells.

Neutrophil production and physiology are discussed on page 937. Neutrophilia or neutrophilic leukocytosis is an increase in the absolute count, and neutropenia is a decrease; they are discussed in Chapter 30.

Eosinophil (Eosinophilic Granulocyte). Eosinophils average 13 μm in diameter. The structure of these cells is similar to that of the polymorphonuclear neutrophils, with the striking difference that, instead of the neutrophilic granules, their cytoplasm contains larger round or oval granules having a strong

affinity for acid stains (Figs. 27-32*B* and Plate 27-1*F* and *G*). They are easily recognized by the size and color of the granules, which stain bright red with stains containing eosin. In well-stained preparations a distinct highlight can be seen on each granule. Their cytoplasm is colorless or has a faint sky-blue tinge. The nucleus stains somewhat less deeply than that of the polymorphonuclear neutrophils and usually has two connected segments, rarely more than three.

Eosinophils average 3 per cent of the leukocytes in adults and the upper reference value is 0.6 × 10^9/l when calculated from the differential count. If allergic individuals are excluded, and if direct hemacytometer counts of eosinophils are performed, the upper limit is probably 0.35 × 10^9/l or 350/μl (Beeson, 1977). The lower reference value is probably 40/μl; a decrease in eosinophils (eosinopenia) can be detected only by counting large numbers of cells as in direct hemacytometer counts (Dacie, 1975) or with a flow-through automated differential counter (p. 908).

Eosinophilia, an increase in eosinophils, and eosinopenia are discussed on page 908.

Basophil (Basophilic Granulocyte). In general, basophilic granulocytes resemble polymorphonuclear neutrophils, except that the nucleus is less segmented (usually merely indented or partially lobulated) and granules are larger and have a strong affinity for basic stains (Figs. 27-33 and Plate 27-1*H* and *I*). They are easily recognized. In some basophils, most of the granules may be missing because they are readily soluble in water, leaving clean-cut openings in the cytoplasm. The granules then are a mauve color. In a well-

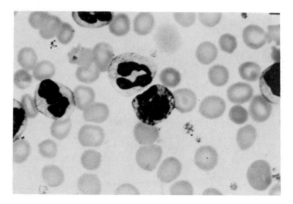

Figure 27-33. Neutrophil (below) and basophil (above). The basophil is smaller, has large deeply basophilic granules which often can be partially washed out, leaving vacuoles (×875).

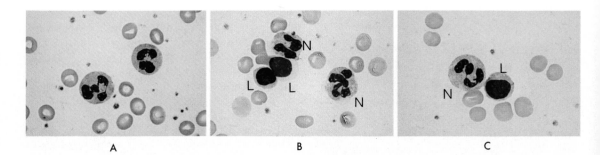

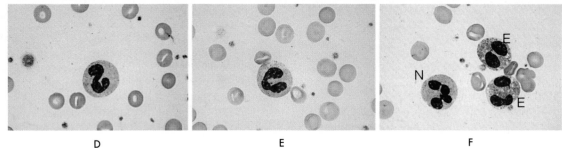

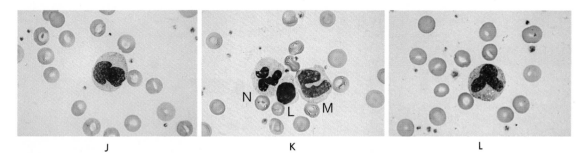

Plate 27–1. These photomicrographs are from buffy coat preparations of blood from a normal individual. The number of leukocytes and platelets per field, therefore, is greater than in blood films made directly. *A,* Neutrophils. The cell on the right has a few nuclear spicules or extensions. These rather pointed spicules are directed toward the centrosomal region of the cell. Such nuclear extensions may be found in normal individuals but are more frequent in those with chronic illnesses (Bessis, 1977). They should be distinguished from the sex chromatin appendages, which have a drumstick appearance. *B,* Lymphocytes (L) of slightly different size and chromatin condensation, and neutrophils (N). *C,* Neutrophil (N) and lymphocyte (L). *D and E,* Band neutrophils. In *E,* note the incomplete segmentation. *F,* Neutrophil (N) and eosinophils (E). Eosinophils have larger granules and, on the average, fewer lobes than do neutrophils. *G,* Eosinophil. *H,* Basophil. *I,* Basophil (B); neutrophil (N). *J,* Monocyte. *K,* Neutrophil (N); lymphocyte (L); monocyte (M). The monocyte has more delicately staining chromatin than the other cells; this usually can be appreciated at low magnification. *L,* Monocyte.

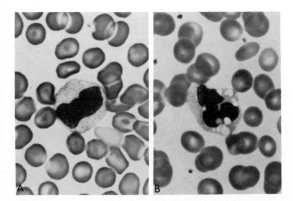

Figure 27-34. *A* and *B,* Monocytes. Of the normal blood cells, the monocyte is the largest and has the most delicate chromatin pattern; it has a propensity to form cytoplasmic vacuoles (*B*) which usually indicate phagocytosis (×875).

prepared smear stained with Wright's stain, the granules are deep purple, while the nucleus is somewhat paler and is often nearly hidden by the granules so that its form is difficult to distinguish.

Unevenly stained granules of basophils may be ring shaped and resemble *Histoplasma capsulatum* or protozoa.

Basophils are the least numerous of the leukocytes in normal blood and average 0.5 per cent of the total leukocytes. The 95 per cent reference values for adults are 0 to $0.2 \times 10^9/l$ when derived from the differential count. Direct hemacytometer counts employing Alcian blue (Gilbert, 1975) or the Hemalog D (p. 909) allow a narrower reference interval of 10 to 80 per microliter (0.01 to $0.08 \times 10^9/l$).

Basophilia (basophilic leukocytosis) and basopenia (decreased absolute basophil count) are discussed on page 941.

Monocyte. The monocyte is the largest cell of normal blood (Figs. 27-34 and Plate 27-1*J,* *K,* and *L*). It generally is about two to three times the diameter of an erythrocyte (14 to 20 μm), although smaller monocytes sometimes are encountered. It contains a single nucleus, which is partially lobulated, deeply indented, or horseshoe-shaped. Occasionally the nucleus of a monocyte may appear round or oval. Viewing the nucleus at different focal planes with the oil immersion lens often reveals that even in those cases there is an indentation of the nucleus, which is obscured by the position of the cell.

The cytoplasm is abundant. With Wright's stain the characteristic feature of the nucleus is for the chromatin to be in strands. There is also a relatively sharp distinction between the chromatin and the parachromatin, which results in a less densely stained nucleus than that seen in the lymphocyte. The cytoplasm is blue-gray and has a ground glass appearance and often contains fine red to purple granules that are less distinct and smaller than the granules of neutrophilic leukocytes. Occasionally blue granules may be seen.

When the monocyte transforms into a macrophage, it becomes larger (20 to 40 μm); the nucleus may become oval and the chromatin more reticular or dispersed so that nucleoli may be visible (Plate 27-2*I*). A perinuclear clear zone (Golgi) may be evident. The fine red or azurophil granules are variable in number or may have disappeared. The more abundant cytoplasm tends to be irregular at the cell margins and to contain vacuoles. These are phagocytic vacuoles, which may contain ingested red cells, debris, pigment, or bacteria. Evidence of phagocytosis in monocytes or the presence of macrophages in directly made films of capillary blood is pathologic and often indicates the presence of active infection.

The size of the cell, the width of the zone of cytoplasm, the blue-gray color, evidences of phagocytosis, and the depth of color and the folds and indentations of the nucleus, usually with the absence of peripheral condensation of nuclear chromatin, are the points to be considered in distinguishing monocytes that have a round nucleus from lymphocytes. For comparison, condensation of nuclear chromatin in clumps and at the nuclear margin, a perinuclear clear zone in the cytoplasm, and a homogeneous agranular cytoplasm are characteristic for lymphocytes. It must be borne in mind that the thickness of the film has a great influence on the apparent size of all leukocytes. They are larger and paler when flattened out in the thin part of the film where they are most easily identified.

The monocytes average 4 per cent of leukocytes and the reference interval for adults is approximately 0.15 to $1.0 \times 10^9/l$, depending on the method of performing the differential count (Table 27-3, p. 891).

Monocyte production is discussed on page 943. An increase in monocytes (monocytosis) and a decrease (monocytopenia) are discussed beginning on page 944.

Lymphocyte. Lymphocytes are mononuclear cells without specific cytoplasmic granules. Small lymphocytes are about the size of an erythrocyte or slightly larger (6 to 10 μm), although their diameter is influenced by the

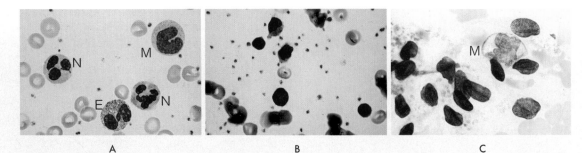

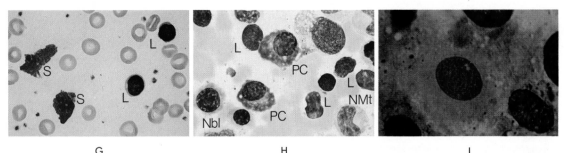

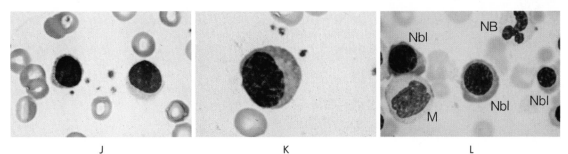

Plate 27–2. Photomicrographs A, B, F, G, J, and K are from buffy coat preparations from a normal individual. As in Plate 27–1, the number of leukocytes and platelets per field is greater than in blood films made directly. *A*, Neutrophils (N), eosinophil (E), and monocyte (M) are easily identifiable in this thin, well-spread area of the film. *B*, Thick area of same film as Plate 27–2*A*, same magnification. Slow drying and shrinkage has made cell identification much less certain. *C*, Endothelial cells and a monocyte (M) at the feather edge of a normal blood film. Endothelial cells have an oval nucleus that is folded or "creased" and abundant, ill-defined cytoplasm. *D*, Two neutrophil myelocytes and the nucleus of a broken or smudged cell (S). Normal marrow. *E*, Neutrophil myelocytes (NMy), neutrophil metamyelocytes (NMt), and neutrophil band forms (NB). Normal marrow. *F*, Monocyte (M) and neutrophil (N). *G*, Lymphocytes (L) and broken, smudged nuclei (S). *H*, Plasma cells (PC), normoblasts (Nbl), lymphocytes (L), neutrophil metamyelocyte (NMt); normal marrow. *I*, Macrophage. These cells have reticular nuclei and abundant cytoplasm containing scattered pigment granules. Bone marrow. *J*, Lymphocytes. *K*, Atypical lymphocyte. Increased cytoplasmic basophilia and more distinct separation of chromatin from parachromatin distinguish this "activated lymphocyte" from resting normal lymphocytes (Plate 27–2*J*). *L*, Normoblasts (Nbl), monocyte (M), and neutrophil band (NB). Normal marrow.

thickness of the film, being greatest in very thin films in which the leukocytes are much flattened (Plates 27-1 and 27-2). The typical lymphocyte has a single, sharply defined nucleus containing heavy blocks of chromatin. The chromatin stains dark blue with Wright's stain, while the parachromatin stands out as lighter stained streaks; at the periphery of the nucleus, the chromatin is condensed. The characteristic feature of the nucleus is that there is a gradual transition between the chromatin and the parachromatin so that it is practically impossible to tell where chromatin ends and parachromatin begins. The nucleus is generally round but is sometimes indented at one side. The cytoplasm stains pale blue except for a clear perinuclear zone.

Larger lymphocytes, 12 to 15 μm in diameter, with less densely staining nuclei and more abundant cytoplasm, are frequently found, especially in the blood of children, and may be difficult to distinguish from monocytes. The misshapen, indented cytoplasmic margins of lymphocytes are due to pressure of neighboring cells. In the cytoplasm of about one third of the large lymphocytes, a few round, red-purple granules are present. They are larger than the granules of neutrophilic leukocytes (Fig. 27-35). It appears that there is a continuous spectrum of sizes between small and large lymphocytes, and, indeed, there can be a transition from small to large to blast forms as well as the reverse (Plate 28-3J and K). It does not appear to be meaningful to classify small lymphocytes and large lymphocytes separately in differential counting. The presence of a significant proportion of atypical lymphocytes and the presence of blast forms (non-leukemic lymphoblasts; reticular lymphocytes) must be noted; these findings indicate transformation of lymphoid cells as a response to antigenic stimulation (p. 951).

Plasma cells have abundant blue cytoplasm, often with light streaks or vacuoles, an eccentric round nucleus, and a well-defined clear (Golgi) zone adjacent to the nucleus (Plate 27-2H). The nucleus of the plasma cell has heavily clumped chromatin, which is sharply defined from the parachromatin, and often arranged in a radial or "wheel-like" pattern. Plasma cells are not present normally in blood.

Lymphocytes average 34 per cent of all leukocytes, and range from 1.5 to 4 $\times$ 10^9/l in adults.

The lymphocytes and their derivatives, the plasma cells, operate in the immune defenses of the body. Lymphocytosis is discussed beginning on page 949, plasmacytosis on page 951.

Artifacts

Broken Cells. Damaged or broken leukocytes constitute a small proportion of the nucleated cells in normal blood. Bare nuclei from ruptured cells vary from fairly well preserved nuclei without cytoplasm to smudged nuclear material (Plate 27-2G), sometimes with strands arranged in a coarse network, the so-called basket cells (Fig. 27-36). They probably represent fragile cells, usually lymphocytes, that have been broken in preparing the film. They are apt to be numerous when there is an atypical lymphocytosis (p. 949), in chronic lymphocytic leukemia, and in acute leukemias.

Degenerative Changes. As EDTA-blood stands in the test tube, changes in leukocyte morphology begin to take place (Sacker, 1975). The degree of change varies among cells and

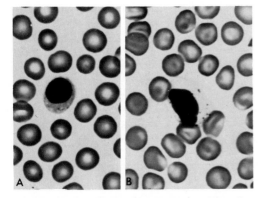

Figure 27-35. *A*, Small lymphocyte. *B*, Larger lymphocyte with granules; note that many of the red cells are target cells ($\times$875).

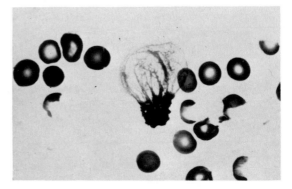

Figure 27-36. Basket cell. This is a nuclear remnant from a damaged or broken cell ($\times$875).

in different individuals. Within a half hour the nuclei of neutrophils may begin to swell, with some loss of chromatin structure. Cytoplasmic vacuoles appear especially in monocytes and neutrophils. Nuclear lobulation appears in mononuclear cells; deep clefts may cause the nucleus to resemble a clover leaf (radial segmentation of the nuclei; Rieder cells). Finally, loss of the cytoplasm and a smudged nucleus may be all that remains to be seen of the cell.

Degenerative changes occur more rapidly in oxalated blood than in EDTA-blood. They arise more rapidly with increasing concentrations of EDTA, such as occur when evacuated blood collection tubes (with a given amount of EDTA) are incompletely filled.

Contracted Cells.   In the thicker part of wedge films, drying is slow. The obvious changes in the film are rouleaux of the erythrocytes and shrinkage of the leukocytes. Since the leukocytes are contracted and heavily stained, mononuclear cells are difficult to distinguish from one another. Optimal cell identification is usually impossible in these areas (Plate 27-2*B*).

Endothelial Cells.   Endothelial cells from the lining of the blood vessel may appear in the first drop of blood from a fingerstick specimen, or, rarely, in venous blood (Plate 27-2*C*). They have an immature reticular chromatin pattern and may be mistaken for histiocytes or for tumor cells.

Sources of error in the differential leukocyte count

Even in the most perfectly made blood films, the differential count is subject to the same errors of random distribution as are other cell counts. For interpretation of day-to-day or slide-to-slide differences in the same patient, it is helpful to see how much of the variation is ascribable to chance alone. Table 27-5 gives 95 per cent confidence limits for different percentages of cells in differential counts performed, classifying a total of 100 to 1000 leukocytes. In comparing the percentages from two separate counts, if one number lies outside the confidence limits of the other, it is probable that the difference is significant (i.e., not due to chance). Thus, on the basis of a 100-cell differential count, if the monocytes were 5 per cent one day and 10 per cent the next, it is quite probable that the difference is due solely to sampling error. Although the difference *could be* real, one cannot be confident that it *is* real, because of the small number of cells counted. If, on the other hand, the differential count totaled 500 cells, the difference between 5 per cent and 10 per cent is significant; one can be reasonably certain (with a 5 per cent chance of being wrong) that the difference is a real one and not due to chance alone. Of course, this is a minimal estimate of the error involved in differential counts, since it does not include mechanical errors (due to variations in collecting the blood samples, inadequate mixing, irregularities in distribution depending on the type and quality of the blood films, and poor staining) or errors in cell identification, which depend upon the judgement and experience of the observer. Meticulous technique and accurate and consistent cell classification are therefore demanded of the technician. The physician who interprets the results must be aware of the possible sources of error, especially the minimal error due to chance in the distribution of cells. The latter is a major source of variation in the absolute leukocyte counts when they are computed from electronically derived total leukocyte counts.

Table 27-3 shows the distribution of the various types of leukocytes in the blood of normal persons. Absolute concentrations are given, as these have considerably greater significance than percentages alone.

Automated differential leukocyte counting

A brief, useful appraisal of automated systems for differential leukocyte counting is that of Bentley (1977). Ideally, the requirements should include the following: (1) the distribution of cells analyzed should be identical with that in the blood; (2) all leukocytes usually found in blood diseases should be accurately identified, or detected and "marked" in some way; (3) the speed of the process should enable a large number of cells to be counted in order to minimize statistical error; and (4) the instrument should be cost effective.

Two general principles have been employed in the systems available to date: digital image processing systems, which use computer identification of cells on stained blood films; and flow-through systems, which analyze cells suspended in a liquid.

Digital Image Processing.   A uniformly made and stained blood film is placed on a microscope stage, which is driven by a motor. A computer controls the movement, scans the slide, stopping it when leukocyte(s) are in the field. The optical images, e.g., nuclear size, shape, and color; and cytoplasmic size and color are recorded by a television camera, analyzed by the computer, and converted to digital form; these characteristics are then compared with a memory bank of such characteristics for the different cell types. If the pattern "fits" that of a normal cell type, it is identified as such; otherwise it is classed as unknown. The coordinates of the unknown cells are kept by the instrument and can be relocated at the end of the count so that the technologist can classify them.

Two instrumental systems have been available commercially and have undergone clinical evaluations, the LARC* (Leukocyte Automatic Recognition Computer) and the Hematrak†; a third, the "diff-3 system,"‡ is newly available.

The LARC (Megla, 1973) uses slides made with a spinner (p. 890) and stained in a carefully controlled manner, and classifies 100 cells in about 50 seconds, during which time the operator can evaluate red cell morphology and estimate the number of platelets. These observations can be entered on a console. After reviewing and identifying the unclassified cells, which the instrument has relocated on demand, the results are printed out and, if desired, sent to a computer. The results have shown reasonable agreement with "manual" differential counts, including band neutrophil counts and the detection of abnormal cells (unclassified, for review) (Cotter, 1976; Arkin, 1977). A reticulocyte program has been added as an optional program, but not yet evaluated.

The Hemtrak (Dutcher, 1974) uses Romanowsky-stained wedge films and classifies 100 cells in about 25 seconds. Red cell morphology and platelet estimate are made after or before the count and entered on the console. Programs are available for automated reticulocytes, automated platelet estimate, and automated red cell measurements. The utility of these optional systems has not been established by clinical trial. The identification of leukocytes, including band neutrophil counts, and the detection of abnormal cells have been reported to be satisfactory (Benzel, 1974; Egan, 1974).

The "diff-3 system," which also uses the

stained blood film, has recently become available but has not been clinically evaluated. It has the capacity to perform the leukocyte differential count, evaluate red cell morphology, and estimate platelet number and size, and has available a reticulocyte program.

Having Romanowsky-stained blood films for verifying cell identification is an advantage in these digital image processing systems. They are somewhat more consistent than a group of technologists. At the present time, however, their operating speed is too slow to count the large number of leukocytes which would be necessary to significantly improve the random statistical error that has afflicted differential counting. Also, they are marginally cost effective.

Flow-through Systems. The *Hemalog D** automatically samples blood from cups on a turntable sampler at the rate of 60 or 90 per hour. Red cells are lysed, leukocytes are separated into three channels and fixed, and reagents are introduced for cytochemical reactions (Mansberg, 1974). In a photo-optical system, measurements of light scattering and of light absorption are made while the cells are being counted. In the *peroxidase channel* immature neutrophils, neutrophils, and eosinophils (which all contain peroxidase) absorb light. A pH of 3.2 is used; eosinophils stain more deeply than neutrophils and are discriminated from them by greater absorption and less scatter. Immature neutrophils have greater peroxidase activity than mature neutrophils and are designated "high peroxidase cells"; they, too, are separated by greater absorption and equal or greater scatter. Lymphocytes are discriminated by low scatter and low absorption. "Large unstained cells" have high scatter and low absorption and include atypical lymphocytes and blasts. The cells are counted and instantaneously plotted (scatter versus absorption) on a scattergram, which is electronically displayed and may be photographed. Platelets and red cell stroma are excluded by a lower threshold. In the *lipase channel*, monocytes are stained by alpha naphthyl butyrate esterase activity and counted; they are separable from other cells by high scatter and high absorption. In the *third channel*, basophils are counted by their staining reaction with Alcian blue.

Ten thousand leukocytes are counted in each

*Corning Medical Instruments, Medfield, Mass.
†Geometric Data, Wayne, Pa.
‡Coulter Electronics, Inc., Hialeah, Florida (Manufactured by Perkin Elmer).

*Technicon Instruments Corp., Tarrytown, N.Y.

channel; the results are expressed in both per cent and absolute concentrations. An optional addition is an automatic slide maker that makes and stains blood films on a roll of plastic tape and identifies them by accession number for reference or examination if needed.

The reference intervals achieved with the Hemalog D are similar to those with manual technique (Simmons, 1974).

Flow cell cytofluorometry (Adams, 1977) using the Cytofluorograf* can differentiate six classes of cells that appear to represent lymphocytes, monocytes, basophils, eosinophils, neutrophils, and immature neutrophils. The cells are stained supravitally in a hypotonic solution of acridine orange and are identified on a scatter plot of green nuclear fluorescence against red cytoplasmic fluorescence. This system has not been clinically evaluated.

Flow-through systems have the advantage of rapidly analyzing larger numbers of cells, significantly reducing the statistical error of counting. They can be more fully automated than the digital image processors. The disadvantage is that the categories of cells are not completely consonant with those with which we are familiar on Romanowsky-stained films. An "unclassified" category is difficult to analyze. When an abnormal result occurs, a film must be made and examined. Yet this kind of precision in differential leukocyte counting has not previously been available. Analytic variation in the Hemalog D is sufficiently small that physiologic variations previously undetected become apparent, and an individual's own baseline reference values become meaningful (Statland, 1978). For example, the significance of changes in basophil counts in disease appears to become more useful (Gilbert, 1975). As clinical significance of the results of the Hemalog D are determined, it is likely that our knowledge of leukocytic changes in disease will increase and the differential leukocyte count will become more useful in diagnostic work.

PLATELETS

In films made from EDTA-blood and stained with Romanowsky stains, platelets are round or oval, 2 to 4 μm in diameter, and well separated from one another (Plate 27-1). The platelet count may be estimated from such films when the distribution is uniform. On the average, if the platelet count is normal, about one platelet is found per 10 to 30 red cells. Using the A-O Microstar* microscope at 1000 × magnification, this is equivalent to about 5 to 20 platelets per oil immersion field in the areas where red cell morphology is optimal.

Platelets contain fine purple granules which usually fill the cytoplasm. Occasionally granules are concentrated in the center (the "granulomere") and surrounded by a pale cytoplasm (the "hyalomere"); these are probably activated platelets, the appearance resulting from contraction of the microtubular band (p. 1110). A few platelets may have a decreased concentration of granules (hypogranular platelets).

In EDTA-blood from normal individuals, the fraction of platelets that exceed 3 μm in diameter and the fraction of platelets that are hypogranular are both less than 5 per cent if the films are made at 10 minutes or 60 minutes after the blood is drawn. If films are made immediately or at 3 hours after blood drawing, the fraction of large platelets and the fraction of hypogranular or activated platelets are increased (Zeigler, 1978). These artifacts make it necessary to standardize time of film preparation when evaluating platelet size from films.

In patients with immune thrombocytopenia large platelets are increased in number. They are also increased in patients with the rare Bernard-Soulier syndrome (p. 1119) and in patients with infiltrated bone marrows or myeloproliferative syndromes; in the latter, the platelets are frequently hypogranular or are "activated", i.e., have a distinct granulomere and hyalomere.

In blood films made from skin puncture wounds, platelets assume irregular shapes with sharp projections and tend to clump together in proportion to the time after the wound is made.

PHYSIOLOGIC VARIATION

PHYSIOLOGIC VARIATION IN ERYTHROCYTES

Changes in red cell values are greatest during the first few weeks of life (Fig. 27-37). At the time of birth, as much as 100 to 125 ml of

---

*Biophysics Systems, Division of Ortho Instruments, Westwood, Mass. 02090

*American Optical Co., Buffalo, N.Y.

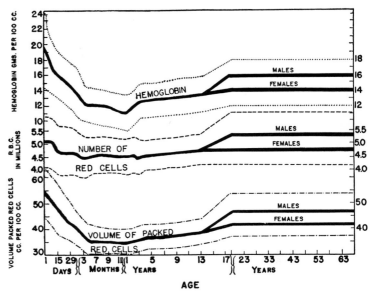

Figure 27–37. Values for hemoglobin, hematocrit (volume of packed red cells), and red cell counts from birth or old age. Mean values are heavy lines. Reference interval for hemoglobin is indicated by dotted lines, for red cell counts by interrupted lines, and for hematocrit by dotted interrupted lines. The scales on the ordinate are similar so that relative changes in hemoglobin, red cell count, and hematocrit are apparent on inspection. The scale for age, however, is progressively altered. (From Wintrobe, M. M.: Clinical Hematology, 6th ed. Philadelphia, Lea & Febiger, 1967.)

placental blood may be added to the newborn if tying the cord is postponed until its pulsation ceases. In a study of newborns whose cords had been clamped late, the average capillary red cell counts were $0.4 \times 10^{12}/l$ higher 1 hour after and $0.8 \times 10^{12}/l$ higher 24 hours after birth compared with newborns whose cords had been clamped early.

Capillary blood (obtained by skin prick) gives higher RBC and Hb values than venous blood (cord). The differences may amount to about 0.5×10^{12} RBC/l and 3 g Hb/dl. The slowing of capillary circulation and the resulting loss of fluid may be the responsible factor. Examination of venous blood furnishes more consistent results than examination of capillary blood.

In the full-term infant, *nucleated red cells* are most numerous at birth with about $500/\mu l$. The normoblast count declines to about $200/\mu l$ at 24 hr., $25/\mu l$ at 48 hr., and less than $5/\mu l$ at 72 hr. By four days it is rare to find circulating normoblasts (Oski, 1972).

The normal *reticulocyte count* at birth ranges from 3 to 7 per cent during the first 48 hours, during which time it rises slightly. After the second day it falls rather rapidly to 1 to 3 per cent by the seventh day of life.

Hemoglobin concentration in capillary blood during the first day of life averages 19.0 g/dl, with 95 per cent of normal values falling between 14.6 and 23.4 g/dl. In cord blood the average is 16.8 g/dl., with 95 per cent of normals between 13.5 and 20.1 g/dl (Oski, 1972).

There is frequently an initial increase in the hemoglobin level of venous blood at the end of 24 hours compared with that of cord blood. At the end of the first week, the level is about the same as in cord blood and it does not begin to fall until after the second week. During the first two weeks the lower limit of normal is 14.5 g/dl for capillary blood and 13.0 g/dl for venous blood.

The hematocrit in capillary blood on the first day of life averages 61 per cent, with 95 per cent of normal values between 0.46 and 0.76. In cord blood, the average is 0.53. The changes during the first few weeks parallel the hemoglobin concentration.

The Hb and Hct are highest at birth but fall rather steeply in the first days and weeks of life to a minimum average Hb of 10.7 g/dl and Hct of 0.31 at about two months of age. Though the lower limit of the 95 per cent reference values in some studies is as low as 9 g Hb/dl and 0.26 Hct, these probably include children with nutritional deficiencies. The level to define anemia probably should be no lower than 10.5 g Hb/dl or 0.33 Hct (Williams, 1977).

The normal MCV at birth ranges from 104 to 118 fl, compared with the adult reference interval of 80 to 96 fl. Since the RBC does not fall to the degree the Hb and Hct do, the MCV decreases abruptly, then gradually, during the first few months of life. The lowest value is reached at about one year. In a study using the Coulter Model S in which iron deficiency and

Table 27–6. ERYTHROCYTE AND LEUKOCYTE VALUES IN NORMAL ADULTS, 95 PER CENT REFERENCE INTERVALS

	1 DACIE AND LEWIS (1975)		2 WILLIAMS AND SCHNEIDER (1977)		3 UPSTATE MEDICAL CENTER
Leukocyte count	4.0 –11.0		M	3.9 – 10.6	4.5 –11.0
(× 10⁹/l)			F	3.5 – 11.0	
Erythrocyte	M	4.5 – 6.5		4.4 – 5.9	4.5 – 6.0
count (× 10¹²/l)	F	3.8 – 5.8		3.8 – 5.2	4.2 – 5.4
Hemoglobin	M	13.0 –18.0		13.3 – 17.7	13.5 –17.5
(g/dl)	F	11.5 –16.5		11.7 – 15.7	11.5 –15.5
Hematocrit	M	0.40– 0.54		0.40– 0.52	0.43– 0.51
(l/l)	F	0.37– 0.47		0.35– 0.47	0.36– 0.45
MCV		77–93	M	80.5 – 99.7	80–96
(fl)			F	80.8 –100.0	
MCH		27–32	M	26.6 – 33.8	27–33
(pg)			F	26.4 – 34.0	
MCHC		31–35	M	31.5 – 36.3	32–36
(g/dl)			F	31.4 – 35.8	

Data from Williams, W. J., et al.: Hematology, 2nd ed. New York, McGraw-Hill Book Company, 1977.

thalassemia were excluded, Koerper (1976) found the following MCVs (average; 95 per cent reference intervals):

age 10 to 17 months   = 77 fl; 70 to 84 fl
age 18 months to 4 years = 80 fl; 74 to 86 fl
age 4 years to 7 years   = 81 fl; 76 to 86 fl

The MCV very gradually rises until after puberty, when adult levels are reached.

Reference intervals for red cell values in sexually mature adults are given in Table 27–6. The indices are similar in males and females, but the Hb is 1 to 2 g/dl higher in males, with commensurate increments in Hct and RBC. This is believed to be mainly the effects of androgen in stimulating erythropoietic production and its effect on the marrow. Estrogen probably has a slight suppressing effect on red cell production (Erslev, 1977).

In older men the Hb tends to fall and in older women the Hb tends to fall to a lesser degree (in some studies) or even rise slightly (in other studies). In older individuals, therefore, the sex difference is less than 1 g Hb/dl (Dacie, 1975).

Posture and muscular activity change the concentration of the formed elements. The Hb, Hct, and RBC increase by several per cent when the change from recumbency to standing is made (Mollison, 1967; p. 873) and strenuous muscular activity causes a further increase, presumably due primarily to loss of plasma water.

Diurnal variation that is not related to exercise or to analytical variation also occurs (Statland, 1978). The Hb is highest in the morning, falls during the day, and is lowest in the evening, with a mean difference of 8 to 9 per cent (Dacie, 1975).

In persons living at a higher altitude, the Hb, Hct, and RBC are elevated over what they would be at sea-level. The difference is about 1 g Hb/dl at 2 kilometers altitude and 2 g Hb/dl at 3 km. Increased erythropoiesis is secondary to anoxic stimulation of erythropoietin production. People who are smokers also tend to have a mild erythrocytosis (p. 1012).

PHYSIOLOGIC VARIATION IN LEUKOCYTES

The total white cell count at birth and during the first 24 hours varies within wide limits. Neutrophils are the predominant cell, varying from 6 to 28 × 10⁹/l; about 15 per cent of these are band forms (Altman, 1974), and a few myelocytes are present. Neutrophils drop to about 5 × 10⁹/l and remain at about the same level thereafter. Lymphocytes are about 5.5 × 10⁹/l at birth, and change little during the first week. They become the predominant cell, on the average, after the first week of life and remain so until about age seven, when neutrophils again predominate. The upper limit of the 95 per cent reference interval for lymphocytes at age 6 months is 13.5; at 1 year, 10.5; at 2 years, 9.5; at 6 years, 7.0; and 12 years, 6.0 × 10⁹/l; for neutrophils at the same ages the values are 8.5, 8.5, 8.5, 8.0, and 8.0 × 10⁹/l, all somewhat higher than those for adults (Table 27–3, p. 891).

Some studies suggest a slightly higher neutrophil level in adult women, but this has not been found in all studies (England, 1976).

Diurnal variation has been recognized in the

neutrophil count, with highest levels in the afternoon and lowest levels in the morning at rest. Statland (1978) has shown, however, using precise methods (Hemalog D), that diurnal variation in neutrophils and in total WBC varies from subject to subject; in some there is very little diurnal variation, but the pattern is quite consistent for the individual.

Exercise produces leukocytosis, which includes an increased neutrophil concentration due to a shift of cells from marginal to circulating granulocyte pool (p. 937); increased lymphocyte drainage into blood also appears to contribute to the total increase.

Both the average and the lower reference value for neutrophil concentration in the black population is lower than in the white (Table 27–3); this difference must be taken into account in assessing neutropenia.

Cigarette smokers have higher average leukocyte counts than non-smokers. The increase is greatest (about 30 per cent) in heavy smokers who inhale, and affects neutrophils, lymphocytes, and monocytes (Corre, 1971).

There appear to be mild changes during the menstrual cycle (England, 1976). Neutrophils and monocytes fall and eosinophils tend to rise during menstruation. Basophils have been reported to fall during ovulation (Mettler, 1974).

The availability of precise automated leukocyte analyzers (p. 909) provides the potential for investigating physiologic sources of variation that have been obscured by the statistical error in traditional microscopic differential counts (Statland, 1978). Reference intervals for each type of leukocyte could be established for an individual. This potential appears promising; its value is beginning to be established in some areas (Gilbert, 1975) and needs to be investigated further.

PHYSIOLOGIC VARIATION IN PLATELETS

The average platelet count is slightly lower at birth than in older children and adults, and may vary from $84 \times 10^9/l$ to $478 \times 10^9/l$ (Oski, 1972). After the first week of life the reference intervals are those of the adult. No sex difference is clearly established. In women, the platelet count may fall at the time of menstruation.

ERYTHROCYTE SEDIMENTATION RATE

Principle. After placing well-mixed venous blood in a vertical tube, erythrocytes will tend to fall toward the bottom. An increase in this tendency of erythrocytes to "sediment" is found in certain pathologic conditions, especially in inflammatory disorders. The length of fall of the top of the column of erythrocytes in a given interval of time is the erythrocyte sedimentation rate (ESR). Several factors are involved.

Plasma Factors. An accelerated ESR (erythrocyte sedimentation rate) is favored by elevated levels of fibrinogen and, to a lesser extent, of globulin. These asymmetric protein molecules have a greater effect than other proteins in decreasing the negative charge of erythrocytes (zeta potential) that tends to keep them apart. The decreased zeta potential promotes the formation of rouleaux, which sediment more rapidly than single cells. Removal of fibrinogen by defibrination lowers the ESR, except when plasma globulin is markedly elevated.

The effect of globulin on acceleration of the ESR is less pronounced than that of fibrinogen, except in liver disease, in which close correlation between the two has been noted in the presence of low fibrinogen levels. There is no absolute correlation between the ESR and any of the plasma protein fraction. Alpha and beta globulins are more effective than gamma globulin. Albumin retards sedimentation. Cholesterol accelerates and lecithin retards the ESR.

Red Cell Factors. Anemia is responsible for an accelerated ESR. The change in the erythrocyte-plasma ratio favors rouleaux formation. These changes are independent of changes in the concentration of the plasma proteins. By any method of measurement, the ESR is most sensitive to altered plasma proteins in the hematocrit range of 0.30 to 0.40 (Bull, 1975).

Microcytes sediment significantly more slowly and macrocytes somewhat more rapidly than normocytes. The larger the cells, the smaller the surface in relation to the volume. The sedimentation rate is directly proportional to the weight of the cell aggregate and inversely proportional to the surface area. Rouleaux have decreased surface area in relation to the volume of the aggregates than do individual cells. The result is acceleration of the ESR. If the red cells have an abnormal or irregular shape which does not allow rouleaux formation, the ESR will be low; sickle cell disease and spherocytosis are cases in point.

Stages in the ESR. Three stages can be

observed: (1) The initial period of aggregation. During this phase the rouleaux are formed and the sedimentation is relatively slow. It lasts about 10 minutes of the 1-hour observation period. (2) The period of fast settling. During this period the settling rate is constant. It lasts about 40 minutes. (3) The final period of packing continues for the balance of the hour and for a longer time afterwards.

Methods

Westergren Method. Because of its simplicity the Westergren method is widely used. The National Committee for Clinical Laboratory Standards has recommended it as the basis for an acceptable standard method.

Equipment. The Westergren tube is a straight pipette 30 cm long and 2.5 mm in internal diameter. It is calibrated in millimeters from 0 to 200. It holds about 1 ml. The Westergren rack is also used.

Reagent

A 0.105 molar solution of sodium citrate is used as the anticoagulant-diluent solution (31 gm of $Na_3C_6H_5O_7 \cdot H_2O$ added to 1 liter of distilled water in a sterile glass bottle). This is filtered and kept without preservatives.

Technique

1. Exactly 1.0 ml of the sodium citrate is transferred with a graduated pipette to a tube with a mark at the 5-ml level.

2. Five milliliters of venous blood are withdrawn in a dry syringe, and 4 ml of it are placed in the tube containing the anticoagulant. The tube, now filled to the 5-ml mark, is inverted two or three times to mix thoroughly the anticoagulant with the blood. This blood-citrate mixture should be used within 2 hours if kept at 20°C. or within 12 hours if kept at 4°C.

3. A Westergren pipette is filled exactly to the 0 mark and placed in the rack. The bottom of the tube must be pressed firmly against the rubber stopper in the base of the rack before removing the finger from the top of the tube. The tube must be held firmly by the clip at the top of the rack in an *exactly vertical* position. The rack is constructed to hold 12 or more tubes.

4. The room temperature must be constant and the tube cannot be exposed to direct sunlight. The tube must not be disturbed, either by moving it or by vibrations of the bench.

After exactly 60 minutes, the distance from the bottom of the surface meniscus to the top of the column of red cells is recorded in millimeters as the ESR value. If the demarcation between plasma and red cell column is hazy, the level is taken where the full density is first apparent.

MODIFIED WESTERGREN METHOD. A modification of the Westergren method employs blood anticoagulated with EDTA rather than citrate. This is more convenient, since it allows the ESR to be performed

from the same tube of blood as is used for other hematologic studies. Two milliliters of well-mixed EDTA-blood is diluted either with 0.5 ml of 3.8 per cent sodium citrate (Dawson, 1960) or with 0.5 ml of 0.85 per cent sodium chloride (Gambino, 1965), which yields the same degree of dilution as is used in the classic Westergren method. Results are reproducible and are almost identical with those obtained by the classic Westergren method. The blood must be diluted, since undiluted blood anticoagulated with EDTA or double oxalate gives poorly reproducible results. Blood anticoagulated with EDTA may be kept for 12 hours at 4°C. without affecting the ESR.

The ESR is higher in women than in men and gradually increases with age. Westergren's original upper limits of normal (10 mm per hour for men and 20 mm per hour for women) appear to be too low. After studying a large number of healthy working people, Böttiger (1967) recommended that the upper limit of normal should be 15 mm per hour for men and 20 mm per hour for women below the age of 50 and 20 mm per hour for men and 30 mm per hour for women over the age of 50.

SOURCES OF ERROR

1. If the concentration of the anticoagulant is higher than recommended, the ESR may be slowed. Sodium citrate or EDTA does not affect the rate of sedimentation if used in the proper concentration. Heparin, however, alters the membrane zeta potential, and cannot be used as an anticoagulant.

2. Hemolysis may modify the sedimentation.

3. The cleanliness of the tube is important, and all traces of alcohol and ether must be removed.

4. Tilting the tube accelerates the ESR. The red cells aggregate along the lower side while the plasma rises along the upper side. Consequently, the retarding influence of the rising plasma is less effective. An angle of even 3 degrees from the vertical may accelerate the ESR by as much as 30 per cent.

5. Bubbles left in the tube when it is filled will affect the ESR.

6. Temperature should be within the range of 20 to 25°C. Lower or higher temperatures in some cases alter the ESR. If the blood has been kept refrigerated, it should be permitted to reach room temperature before the test is performed.

7. The test should be set up within 2 hours after the blood sample is obtained (or 12 hours if EDTA is used as the anticoagulant and the blood is kept at 4°C.); otherwise, some samples with elevated ESR's will be falsely low. On standing, erythrocytes tend to become spherical and less inclined to form rouleaux.

8. A decrease in the number of erythrocytes, i.e., anemia, accelerates the ESR; an increase as in polycythemia retards it. These changes are independent of any changes in the plasma proteins. There is no effective method for correcting for anemia in the Westergren method.

9. Anisocytosis may interfere with rouleaux for-

mation. Pronounced poikilocytosis, for example, sickling, may inhibit sedimentation.

10. Factors that tend to decrease the ESR are defibrination, partial clotting with resulting defibrination, low temperature, excess of dry anticoagulant, and diameter of tube less than 2 mm.

Zeta Sedimentation Ratio. A centrifugal device (the Zetafuge*) spins capillary tubes in a vertical position in four 45-second cycles (Bull, 1972). This results in controlled compaction and dispersion of erythrocytes, allowing rouleaux to form and sediment in this 3-minute period of time. The capillary tube is then read as if it were a standard hematocrit tube, giving a value referred to as a zetacrit. The true hematocrit is divided by the zetacrit, and the result, expressed as a percentage, is the zeta sedimentation ratio (ZSR). It is not affected by anemia, which should make it easier to interpret. Its sensitivity to elevation of the ESR by fibrinogen is the same as the Westergren method. This ZSR requires only a 100-μl sample and is considerably faster. The reference interval is 41 to 54 for both sexes. If the hematocrit is elevated, some of the red cells must be removed and the procedure repeated.

Interpretation

The ESR is higher in women than in men. In pregnancy, the ESR increases moderately, beginning in the tenth to twelfth week. Nor-

---

*Coulter Diagnostics, Hialeah, Fla.

mal rates return about one month post partum.

The ESR tends to be markedly elevated in monoclonal blood protein disorders such as multiple myeloma or macroglobulinemia, in severe polyclonal hyperglobulinemias due to inflammatory disease, and in hyperfibrinogenemias.

Moderate elevations are common in active inflammatory disease such as rheumatoid arthritis, chronic infections, collagen disease, and in neoplastic disease. The major use at present is as an indication of the presence of active disease of these sorts. It is a simpler test than protein electrophoresis, which has tended to replace it, and it has few false negative results.

The ZSR has been shown to be a satisfactory alternative to the ESR in a few clinical trials (e.g., Morris, 1977).

The Westergren method is somewhat less useful in the presence of anemia. If the Wintrobe method (Wintrobe, 1974) is used, it probably should be corrected for anemia using the method of Hynes and Whitby, for there is evidence (once again) that this is useful (Bull, 1974). It must be remembered, however, that the sensitivity of the ESR in detecting plasma protein abnormalities is best in the non-anemic state (Bull, 1975).

REFERENCES

Ackerman, P. G.: Electronic Instrumentation in the Clinical Laboratory. Boston, Little, Brown and Company, 1972.

Adams, L. R.: Staining for the Cytograf and Cytofluorograf. J. Histochem. *25*:965, 1977.

Altman, P. L., and Dittmer, D. S. (eds.): Blood and Other Body Fluids. Washington, Federation of American Societies for Experimental Biology, 1961, p. 125.

Altman, P. L., and Dittmer, D. S.: Biology Data Book, 2nd ed., Vol. III. Bethesda, Federation of American Societies for Experimental Biology, 1974, p. 1856.

Arkin, C. F., Sherry, M. A., Gough, A. G., and Copeland, B. E.: An automatic leukocyte analyzer. Validity of its results. Am. J. Clin. Pathol., *67*:159, 1977.

Baker, J. T.: Principles of Biological Microtechnique. New York, John Wiley & Sons, Inc., 1958.

Beeson, P. B., and Bass, D. A.: The Eosinophil. Vol. XIV in the series Major Problems in Internal Medicine, Smith, L. H., Jr., (ed.). Philadelphia, W. B. Saunders Company, 1977.

Bentley, S. A., and Lewis, S. M.: Automated differential leukocyte counting: The present state of the art. Br. J. Haematol., *35*:481, 1977.

Benzel, J. E., Egan, J. J., Hart, D. J., and Christopher, E. A.: Evaluation of an automated differential leukocyte counting system. II. Normal cell identification. Am. J. Clin. Pathol., *62*:530, 1974.

Berkson, J., Magath, T. B., and Hurn, M.: The error of estimate of the blood cell count as made with the hemocytometer. Am. J. Physiol., *128*:309, 1940.

Bessis, M.: Blood Smears Reinterpreted, trans. G. Brecher. New York, Springer-Verlag, 1977.

Böttiger, L. E., and Svedberg, C. A.: Normal erythrocyte sedimentation rate and age. Br. Med. J., *2*:85, 1967.

Brecher, G., and Bessis, M.: Present status of spiculated red cells and their relationship to the discocyte-echinocyte transformation: A critical review. Blood, *40*:333, 1972.

Brecher, G., and Cronkite, E. P.: Estimation of the number of platelets by phase microscopy. *In* Tocantins, L. M., and Kazal, L. A.: Blood Coagulation, Hemorrhage and Thrombosis. New York, Grune & Stratton, Inc., 1964.

Brecher, G., and Schneiderman, M.: A time-saving device for the counting of reticulocytes. Am. J. Clin. Pathol., *20*:1079, 1950.

Brittin, G. M., and Brecher, G.: Instrumentation and automation in clinical hematology. Prog. Hematol., *7*:299, 1971.

Brittin, G. M., Brecher, G., and Johnson, C. A.: Evaluation of the Coulter Counter Model S. Am. J. Clin. Pathol., *52*:679, 1969a.

Brittin, G. M., Brecher, G., Johnson, C. A., and Elashoff, R. M.: Stability of blood in commonly used anticoagulants. Use of refrigerated blood for quality control of the Coulter Counter Model S. Am. J. Clin. Pathol., *52*:690, 1969b.

Brittin, G. M., Dew, S. A., and Fewell, E. K.: Automated optical counting of blood platelets. Blood, *38*:422, 1971.

Bull, B. S.: Aids to electronic platelet counting. Am. J. Clin. Pathol., *54*:707, 1970.

Bull, B. S.: Automation in haematology. *In* Goldberg, A., and Brain, M. C. (eds.): Recent Advances in Haematology. Edinburgh, Churchill-Livingstone, 1971, p. 357.

Bull, B. S.: Is a standard ESR possible? Lab. Med., *6*:31, 1975.

Bull, B. S., and Brailsford, J. D.: The zeta sedimentation ratio. Blood, *40*:550, 1972.

Bull, B. S., and Brecher, G.: An evaluation of the relative merits of the Wintrobe and Westergren sedimentation methods, including hematocrit correction. Am. J. Clin. Pathol., *62*:502, 1974.

Bull, B. S., Dutcher, T. F., and Siggard-Andersen, O.: The Hem-Aliquanter: A dispenser-dilutor for hematology. Am. J. Clin. Pathol., *49*:295, 1968.

Bull, B. S., Elashoff, R. M., Heilbron, D. C., and Couperus, J.: A study of various estimators for the derivation of quality control procedures from patient erythrocyte indices. Am. J. Clin. Pathol., *61*:473, 1974.

Bull, B. S., Schneiderman, M. A., and Brecher, G.: Platelet counts with the Coulter Counter. Am. J. Clin. Pathol., *44*:678, 1965.

Bunn, H. F., Forget, B. G., and Ranney, H. M.: Human Hemoglobins. Philadelphia, W. B. Saunders Company, 1977.

Cartwright, G. E.: Diagnostic Laboratory Hematology, 4th ed. New York, Grune & Stratton, Inc., 1968.

Chanarin, I.: Critical appraisal of the PCV. *In* Lewis, S. M., and Coster, J. F. (eds.): Quality Control in Haematology. London, Academic Press, 1975, p. 103.

Corre, F., Lellouch, J., and Schwarz, D.: Smoking and leukocyte counts. Results of an epidemiological survey. Lancet, *2*:632, 1971.

Cotter, D. A., and Sage, B. H.: Performance of the LARC classifier in clinical laboratories. J. Histochem. Cytochem., *24*:202, 1976.

Dacie, J. V., and Lewis, S. L.: Practical Haematology, 5th ed. Edinburgh, Churchill-Livingstone, 1975.

Dawson, J. B.: The E.S.R. in a new dress. Br. Med. J., *1*:1697, 1960.

Dean, W. W., Stastny, M., and Lubrano, G. J.: The degradation of Romanowsky-type blood stains in methanol. Stain Technol., *52*:35, 1977.

Dutcher, T. F., Benzel, J. E., Egan, J. J., Hart, D. J., and Christopher, E. A.: Evaluation of an automated differential leukocyte counting system. I. Instrument description and reproducibility studies. Am. J. Clin. Pathol., *62*:525, 1974.

Egan, J. J., Benzel, J. F., Hart, D. J., and Christopher, E. A.: Evaluation of an automated differential leukocyte counting system. III. Detection of abnormal cells. Am. J. Clin. Pathol., *62*:537, 1974.

England, J. M., and Bain, B. J.: Total and differential leucocyte count. Br. J. Haematol., *33*:1, 1976.

England, J. M., Bashford, C. C., Hewer, M. G., Hughes-Jones, N. C., and Down, M. C.: Simple method for automating the differential leukocyte count. Lancet, *1*:492, 1975.

England, J. M., and Down, M. C.: Measurement of the mean cell volume using electronic particle counters. Br. J. Haematol., *32*:403, 1976.

England, J. M., Walford, D. M., and Waters, D. A. W.: Reassessment of the reliability of the haematocrit. Br. J. Haematol., *23*:247, 1972.

Erslev, A. J.: Anemia of endocrine disorders. *In* Williams, W. J., Beutler, E., Erslev, A. J., and Rundles, R. W.: Hematology, 2nd ed. New York, McGraw-Hill, 1977.

Evelyn, K. A., and Malloy, H. T.: Microdetermination of oxyhemoglobin, methemoglobin, and sulfhemoglobin in a single sample of blood. J. Biol. Chem., *126*:655, 1938.

Fairbanks, V. F., Fahey, J. L., and Beutler, E.: Clinical Disorders of Iron Metabolism, 2nd ed. New York, Grune & Stratton, Inc., 1971.

Fry, G. L., and Hoak, J. C.: Improved method for electronic counting of platelets. J. Lab. Clin. Med., *74*:536, 1969.

Gagné, C., Auger, P. L., Moorjani, S., Brun, D., and Lupien, P. J.: Effect of hyperchylomicronemia on the measurement of hemoglobin. Am. J. Clin. Pathol., *68*:584, 1977.

Gagon, T. E., Athens, J. W., Boggs, D. R., and Cartwright, G. E.: An evaluation of the variance of leukocyte counts as performed with the hemocytometer, Coulter, and Fisher instruments. Am. J. Clin. Pathol., *46*:684, 1966.

Gambino, S. R., DiRe, J. J., Monteleone, M., and Budd, D. C.: The Westergren sedimentation rate, using K_3EDTA. Am. J. Clin. Pathol., *43*:173, 1965.

Gilbert, H. S.: The clinical application of automated cytochemical techniques in patient management. *In* Advances in Automated Analysis. Technicon International Congress. Mediad, Inc., Tarrytown, N.Y., 1973, p. 51.

Gilbert, H. S., and Ornstein, L.: Basophil counting with a new staining method using Alcian blue. Blood, *46*:279, 1975.

Gilmer, P. R., Jr., Williams, L. J., Koepke, J. A., and Bull, B. S.: Calibration methods for automated hematology instruments. Am. J. Clin. Pathol., *68*:185, 1977.

Green, P., and Teal, C. F. J.: Modification of hemoglobin in order to avoid precipitation of globulins. Am. J. Clin. Pathol., *32*:216, 1959.

Hattersley, P. G., Gerard, P. W., Caggiano, V., and Nash, D. R.: Erroneous values on the Model S Coulter due to high titer cold agglutinins. Am. J. Clin. Pathol., *55*:442, 1971.

Hegesh, E., Calmanovici, N., and Avron, M.: New method for determining ferrihemoglobin reductase (NADH-methemoglobin reductase) in erythrocytes. J. Lab. Clin. Med., *72*:339, 1968.

Henry, R. J.: Clinical Chemistry: Principles and Technics. New York, Harper & Row, 1964.

ICSH: Standard techniques for the measurement of red cell and plasma volume. A report by the International Committee for Standardization in Hematology (ICSH): Panel on diagnostic applications of radioisotopes in haematology. Br. J. Haematol., *25*:801, 1973.

Jandl, J. H., Engle, L. K., and Allen, D. W.: Oxidative hemolysis and precipitation of hemoglobin. I. Heinz body anemias as an acceleration of red cell aging. J. Clin. Invest., *39*:1818, 1960.

Karayalcin, G., Rosner, F., and Sawitsky, A.: Pseudo-neutropenia in Negroes. N.Y. State J. Med., *72*:1815, 1972.

Koerper, M. A., Mentzer, W. C., Brecher, G., and Dallman, P. R.: Developmental change in red cell volume: Implication in screening infants and children for iron deficiency and thalassemia trait. J. Pediatr., *89*:580, 1976.

Lampasso, J. A.: Changes in hematologic values induced by storage of ethylene diaminetetraacetate human blood for varying periods of time. Am. J. Clin. Pathol., *49*:443, 1968.

Lampasso, J. A.: Error in hematocrit value produced by excessive ethylenediamine-tetraacetate. Am. J. Clin. Pathol., *44*:109, 1965.

Lappin, T. R. J., Lamont, A., and Nelson, M. G.: An evaluation of the Celloscope 401 electronic blood cell counter. J. Clin. Pathol., *25*:539, 1972.

Lewis, S. M., and Bentley, S. A.: Haemocytometry by laser-beam optics: Evaluation of the Hemac 630L. J. Clin. Pathol., *30*:54, 1977.

Lewis, S. M., and Stoddart, C. T. H.: Effects of anticoagulants and containers (glass and plastic) on the blood count. Lab. Pract., *20*:787, 1971.

Lillie, R. D. (ed.): H. J. Conn's Biological Stains, 9th ed. Baltimore, The Williams & Wilkins Company, 1977.

Lubrano, G. J., Dean, W. W., Heinsohn, H. G., and Stastny, M.: The analysis of some commercial dyes and Romanowsky stains by high-performance liquid chromatography. Stain Technol., *52*:13, 1977.

Luke, R. G., Koepke, J. A., and Siegel, R. R.: The effects of immunosuppressive drugs and uremia on automated leukocyte counts. Am. J. Clin. Pathol., *56*:503, 1971.

Mansberg, H. P., Saunders, A. M., and Groner, W.: The Hemalog D white cell differential system. J. Histochem. Cytochem., *22*:711, 1974.

Mansberg, H. P.: Optical techniques of particle counting. Technicon International Congress, 1969. Advances in Automated Analysis, *1*:213, 1970.

Marshall, P. N., Bentley, S. A., and Lewis, S. M.: An evaluation of some commercial Romanowsky stains. J. Clin. Pathol., *28*:680, 1975a.

Marshall, P. N., Bentley, S. A., and Lewis, S. M.: A standardized Romanowsky stain prepared from purified dyes. J. Clin. Pathol., *28*:920, 1975b.

Mathy, K. A., and Koepke, J. A.: The clinical usefulness of segmented vs. stab neutrophil criteria for differential leukocyte counts. Am. J. Clin. Pathol., *61*:947, 1974.

Megla, G. K.: The LARC automatic white blood cell analyzer. Acta Cytol., *17*:3, 1973.

Mettler, L., and Shirwani, D.: Direct basophil count for timing ovulation. Fertil. Steril., *25*:718, 1974.

Miale, J. B.: Laboratory Medicine: Hematology, 5th ed. St. Louis, The C. V. Mosby Co., 1977.

Morris, M. W., Pinals, R. S., and Nelson, D. A.: The zeta sedimentation ratio (ZSR) and activity of disease in rheumatoid arthritis. Am. J. Clin. Pathol., *68*:760, 1977.

Morris, M. W., Skrodzki, Z., and Nelson, D. A.: Zeta sedimentation ratio (ZSR), a replacement for the erythrocyte sedimentation rate (ESR). Am. J. Clin. Pathol., *64*:254, 1975.

Oski, F. A., and Naiman, J. L.: Hematologic Problems in the Newborn, 2nd ed. Philadelphia, W. B. Saunders Company, 1972.

Phillips, R. A., VanSlyke, D. D., Hamilton, P. B., Dole, V. P., Emmerson, K., and Archibald, R. M.: Measurement of specific gravities of whole blood and plasma by standard copper sulfate solutions. J. Biol. Chem., *183*:305, 1950.

Pinkerton, P. H., Spence, I., Ogilvie, J. C., Ronald, W. A., Marchant, P., and Ray, P. K.: An assessment of the Coulter Counter Model S. J. Clin. Pathol., *23*:68, 1970.

Rogers, C. H.: Blood sample preparation for automated differential systems. Am. J. Med. Technol., *39*:435, 1973.

Rutten, W. P. F., Scholtis, R. J. H., Schmidt, N. A., and van Oers, R. J. M.: A systematic investigation on the Hemalog. Z. Klin. Chem. Klin. Biochem., *13*:387, 1975.

Sacker, L. S.: Specimen collection. *In* Lewis, S. M., and Coster, J. F. (eds.): Quality Control in Haematology. New York, Academic Press, 1975, p. 211.

Saunders, A. M., and Scott, F.: Hematologic automation by continuous flow systems. J. Histochem. Cytochem., *22*:707, 1974.

Schwartz, J. M., and Jaffé, E. R.: Hereditary methemoglobinemia with deficiency of NADH-dehydrogenase. *In* Stanbury, J. B., Wyngaarden, J. B., and Fredrickson, D. S.: The Metabolic Basis of Inherited Disease, 4th ed. New York, McGraw-Hill Book Co., 1978, p. 1452.

Simmons, A., Leaverton, P., and Elbert, G.: Normal laboratory values for differential white cell counts established by manual and automated cytochemical methods (Hemalog D). J. Clin. Pathol., *27*:55, 1974.

Simmons, A., Schwabbauer, M. L., and Earhart, C. A.: Automated platelet counting with the Autoanalyzers. J. Lab. Clin. Med., *77*:656, 1971.

Smith, J. R., and Landaw, S. A.: Smokers' polycythemia. N. Engl. J. Med., *298*:6, 1978.

Statland, B. E., Winkel, P., Harris, S. C., Burdsall, M. J., and Saunders A. M.: Evaluation of biologic sources of variation of leukocyte counts and other hematologic quantities using very precise automated analyzers. Am. J. Clin. Pathol., *69*:48, 1978.

Stevenson, G. F., Smetters, G. W., and Cooper, J. A. D.: A gravimetric method for the calibration of hemoglobin micropipets. Am. J. Clin. Pathol., *21*:489, 1951.

Thom, R.: Evaluation of the new model Hemalog 8, which operates at 90 samples per hour, using 400 microliters of blood. *In* Advances in Automated Analysis, Technicon International Congress. Mediad, Inc., Tarrytown, N.Y., 1977.

van Assendelft, O. W.: Spectrophotometry of haemoglobin derivatives. Assen, The Netherlands, Royal Van Gorcum Ltd., 1970.

Weick, J. K., Hagedorn, A. B., and Linman, J. W.: Leukoerythroblastosis: Diagnostic and prognostic significance. Mayo Clin. Proc., *49*:110, 1974.

Wintrobe, M. M.: Clinical Hematology, 7th ed. Philadelphia, Lea & Febiger, 1974, p. 125.

Zeigler, Z., Murphy, S., and Gardner, F. H.: Microscopic platelet size and morphology in various hematologic disorders. Blood, *51*:479, 1978.

28

HEMATOPOIESIS

Douglas A. Nelson, M.D.

WITH A SECTION ON LYMPHOCYTES BY
Frederick R. Davey, M.D.

STEM CELLS

In postnatal life in man, erythrocytes, granulocytes, monocytes, and platelets are produced only in the bone marrow. Lymphocytes are produced in the secondary lymphoid organs, as well as in the bone marrow and thymus gland.

Most bone marrow cells are morphologically recognizable precursors of granulocytes, erythroid cells, or platelets. Small numbers of monocytes, macrophages, endothelial cells, and

918

plasma cells are noted, and a small fraction of cells in adults is identifiable only as lymphocytes.

Stem cells are cells that can both reproduce themselves and give rise to more differentiated cells; they are not morphologically identifiable as stem cells.

HEMATOPOIETIC STEM CELLS

A pluripotential or multipotential stem cell is present in the marrow and is a common precursor cell for granulocytes and monocytes, erythrocytes, and megakaryocytes. Evidence for this in animal models was demonstrated experimentally by Till (1961), who injected isologous bone marrow cells into irradiated mice. Seven to ten days later spleen colonies formed which contained erythroid cells, granulocytes, megakaryocytes, or a mixture of cell types. It could be shown that all the differentiating cells in a single colony were derivatives of a single stem cell (Becker, 1963), and by retransplanting cells from a single colony with only one differentiated cell type present, multipotential stem cells were still present in the individual colonies (Lewis, 1964). These multipotential stem cells have been operationally designated colony-forming units—spleen (CFU-S).

Evidence in the human for a multipotential hematopoietic stem cell derives from myeloproliferatve disorders (polycythemia vera, myelofibrosis with myeloid metaplasia, chronic myelogenous leukemia) in which it has been shown that one precursor cell gives rise to the abnormal erythrocytes, granulocytes, and megakaryocytes, but not to lymphocytes, marrow fibroblasts, or other cell lines (Fialkow, 1977).

These multipotential hematopoietic stem cells (HSC's) are present in small numbers in blood and marrow and have a very slow turnover—they comprise a dormant reserve. The mechanism by which HSC's are induced to become committed stem cells for the various cell lines is not known, but there is evidence that it is under the control of environmental factors. Proliferating hematopoietic cells are therefore confined to certain locations in the body (Metcalf, 1977).

COMMITTED PROGENITOR CELLS

Committed progenitor cells (committed stem cells) are characterized by their ability to form colonies *in vitro* in response to a soluble factor. Bradley (1966) and Izikawa (1966) described *in vitro* culture systems in which granulocytic differentiation occurred from normal mouse hemopoietic cells; the technique was later adapted for human cells by Pike (1970). The status of this exciting field, the growth of hematopoietic cells in semisolid media, has been reviewed by Metcalf (1977). The cultures consist of two layers of cells in agar: an upper layer of blood or bone marrow contains "target" stem cells (colony-forming cells, CFC; or colony-forming units in culture, CFU-C); a lower layer of blood cells (feeder layer) contains a diffusable substance (colony-stimulating factor, CSF) necessary to stimulate the CFC to proliferate and differentiate into colonies. After a period of 7 to 14 days, colonies become visible in the upper layer; these are composed of neutrophils, monocytes (macrophages), or a mixture of the two. The CSF necessary in the feeder layer is produced by monocytes or activated lymphocytes. It was shown that each colony was derived from a single progenitor (stem) cell. Since both neutrophils and monocytes were found in the same colony, it became obvious that neutrophils (granulocytes) and monocytes were both derived from a single committed progenitor cell (GM-CFC) in response to a soluble substance (GM-CFS).

Modifications in culture systems have permitted *in vitro* colony growth and differentiation of erythroid precursors from erythropoietic progenitor cells (E-CFC) in response to erythropoietin, and eosinophils from eosinophil progenitor cells (EO-CFC) in response to EO-CSF produced by activated lymphocytes. Megakaryocytes have been grown from MEG-CFC in response to MEG-CSF from activated lymphocytes. All have been demonstrated with both human and mouse cells, except for the megakaryocyte, which has been grown from mouse cells only (Metcalf, 1977).

The various CFC's are regarded as committed progenitor cells that have receptors for the appropriate humoral factor (e.g., erythropoietin, CSF) and that respond by proliferation and differentiation (Fig. 28-1). These committed progenitor cells are self-sustaining for long periods of time and are signaled to proliferate by the humoral messenger in response to need.

Neither the multipotential hematopoietic stem cells nor the committed stem cells are

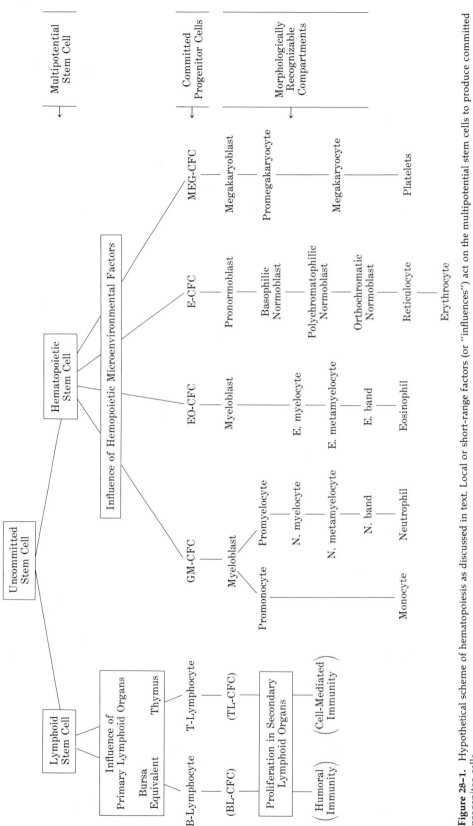

Figure 28–1. Hypothetical scheme of hematopoiesis as discussed in text. Local or short-range factors (or "influences") act on the multipotential stem cells to produce committed progenitor cells.

GM-CFC = granulocyte-monocyte colony forming cell
EO-CFC = eosinophil colony forming cell
E-CFC   = erythrocyte colony forming cell
MEG-CFC = megakaryocyte colony forming cell
BL-CFC = B-lymphocyte colony forming cell
TL-CFC = T-lymphocyte colony forming cell

Though lymphocytes can be induced to grow in colonies, these CFC's are not analogous to the committed progenitor cells of the myeloid lines. The latter respond to specific hormones (e.g., erythropoietin for E-CFC, GM-CSF for GM-CFC) by proliferation and differentiation into mature cells of the particular series.

morphologically identifiable. They have no differentiation characteristics by which they can be recognized. Evidence exists that they have the appearance of small to medium-sized lymphocytes; by immunologic criteria they are neither T-lymphocytes nor B-lymphocytes but are null cells.

There is more recent evidence that T-lymphocytes (from mouse or human) and B-lymphocytes (from mouse) can proliferate in agar culture under appropriate conditions (TL-CFC and BL-CFC; Metcalf, 1977). At least in the case of the BL-CFC, these lymphocytes that proliferate in culture do not appear to be progenitor cells but more differentiated B-lymphocytes.

HEMATOPOIETIC TISSUES
(Weiss, 1977)

Organs or tissues in which blood cell production occurs are known as hematopoietic tissues.

EMBRYONIC AND FETAL HEMATOPOIESIS

Beginning in the first month of prenatal life, the first blood cells arise outside the embryo in the mesenchyme of the yolk sac, as *blood islands*. The cells are predominantly *primitive erythroblasts*, which are large and megaloblastic, are formed intravascularly, and retain their nuclei. At the sixth week, hematopoiesis begins in the liver, and this becomes the major hematopoietic organ of early and mid fetal life. *Definitive erythroblasts*, which become non-nucleated red cells, are formed extravascularly in the liver; granulopoiesis and megakaryocytes are present to a lesser degree. In the middle part of fetal life, the spleen and to a lesser extent lymph nodes have a minor role in hematopoiesis, but the liver continues to dominate. In the later half of fetal life, the bone marrow becomes progressively more important as a site of blood cell production; as this occurs, the liver's role diminishes.

POSTNATAL HEMATOPOIESIS

Shortly after birth, hematopoiesis in the liver ceases and the marrow is the only site for the production of erythrocytes, granulocytes, and platelets. Hematopoietic stem cells and committed progenitor cells are maintained in the marrow. Lymphocytes (of the B cell type) continue to be produced in the marrow, as well as in the secondary lymphoid organs, whereas T-lymphocytes are produced in the thymus and also in the secondary lymphoid organs (p. 949).

At birth, the total marrow space is occupied by active hematopoietic (red) marrow. As body growth progresses and marrow space increases during infancy, only part of that space is needed for hematopoiesis; the remaining space is occupied by fat cells. Later in childhood, only the flat bones (the skull, vertebrae, thoracic cage, shoulder, and pelvis) and the proximal parts of the long bones (femora and humeri) are sites of blood formation. The remaining marrow space is fatty or yellow marrow; this can be replaced by hematopoietic cells if continuous, intensive stimulation exists.

The marrow circulation is closed, that is, arterioles deriving from central longitudinal arteries (i.e., in long bones) connect directly with broad venous sinuses which anastomose and eventually empty into central longitudinal veins. The flattened endothelium of the sinuses is partially covered by adventitial reticular cells, a form of fibroblast that elaborates argentophilic reticulin fibers. These reticular cells and fibers form the supporting meshwork of the marrow stroma, where the hematopoietic cells reside. The reticular cells are but minimally phagocytic; they may swell and take up water, may become fat cells, and possibly may induce hematopoietic stem cells to become committed progenitor cells (Weiss, 1977). After proliferation and maturation has occurred in the marrow stroma, blood cells gain entrance to the blood through or between the endothelial cells of the sinus wall. This requires displacement of adventitial cells. Little is known about this process of "release"; in the case of red cells (reticulocytes), erythropoietin appears to play a role.

ERYTHROCYTE PRODUCTION*

The erythrocyte is a vehicle for the transport of hemoglobin, which is produced in precursor cells of the erythrocytes, the normoblasts. The function of hemoglobin is

---

*See Hillman, 1974; and Izak, 1977.

the transport of oxygen and carbon dioxide. The erythrocyte is also metabolically capable of keeping hemoglobin in a functional state.

It is believed that the pluripotential hematopoietic stem cell (HSC) is induced by certain microenvironmental influences to become the committed erythroid progenitor cell (E-CFC), which is sensitive to erythropoietic stimulation (Fig. 28-1). These cell types are not morphologically identifiable and probably have the appearance of small lymphocytes.

In response to a hormone, erythropoietin (p. 927), the committed progenitor cells (E-CFC) in the marrow undergo mitosis and one or both daughter cells enter the erythroid maturation sequence.

The committed progenitor cell compartment for erythropoiesis (E-CFC) in both the mouse and the human probably consists of two components (Metcalf, 1977). These are defined operationally by their behavior in *in vitro* culture systems as burst-forming units (BFU-E) and colony-forming units (CFU-E). The BFU-E is probably the earlier form, responding to erythropoietin by forming CFU-E's, and the latter responding to lower amounts of erythropoietin by forming morphologically recognizable pronormoblasts. BFU-E are present in small numbers in peripheral blood, as well as in marrow.

NORMOBLASTIC MATURATION
(PLATE 28-1)

The earliest recognizable erythroid precursor is the *pronormoblast* (Fig. 28-1 and Plate 28-1A and I). At about 20 μm diameter, it is the largest of the erythroid precursors. The nucleus has a fine, uniform chromatin pattern which is somewhat more distinct and more intensely staining than that of the myeloblast. The nuclear membrane appears prominent. One or more prominent nucleoli are present. The cytoplasm has a heterogeneous rather than smooth quality and is moderate in amount and moderately basophilic; no granules are present. The pronormoblast undergoes mitosis and forms two basophilic normoblasts.

The *basophilic normoblast* (Plate 28-1B, C, J, and K) is somewhat smaller and has slightly coarser chromatin which stains intensely; the chromatin may be partially clumped and the pattern may suggest a wheel with broad spokes. The parachromatin (the non-chromatin part of the nucleus) is distinct and stains

pink. Nucleoli are present but not often visible. The nuclear/cytoplasmic ratio (i.e., the ratio of the area occupied by the nucleus to that of the cytoplasm) is moderate; about one fourth of the total cell area appears to be cytoplasm. The cytoplasm is deeply basophilic owing to the abundance of ribonucleic acid (RNA); much of this is evident as polyribosomes in electron micrographs (Fig. 28-2A). The cell borders of both this and the preceding stage frequently are made irregular by pseudopodia.

After mitosis of the basophilic normoblast, continuing hemoglobin production becomes visible in the cytoplasm of the two daughter cells as polychromasia, i.e., mixtures of the red-staining of hemoglobin with the blue of RNA in varying shades of grey. This cell is the *polychromatophilic normoblast* (see Fig. 27-30 and Plate 28-1C, J, K, L, and M), which is slightly smaller than the basophilic normoblast. The nucleus occupies about half of the area of the cell; it stains intensely and has moderately condensed chromatin which is sharply distinct from the pink parachromatin. In electron micrographs (Fig. 28-2) the chromatin clumps are larger than in the basophilic normoblast, and fewer polyribosomes and more hemoglobin are present in the cytoplasm. The polychromatophilic normoblast undergoes one or two mitotic divisions.

After the last mitosis, the nucleus becomes small and dense (pyknotic) and the *orthochromatic normoblast* stage is reached (see Fig. 27-30 and Plate 28-1D). Mitosis is no longer possible. The cell is smaller than the polychromatophilic normoblast and has a lower N/C ratio. The cytoplasm contains more abundant hemoglobin and fewer polyribosomes (Fig. 28-2) and remains polychromatophilic.

Finally, accompanied by cytoplasmic contractions and undulations, the nucleus and a small rim of cytoplasm are ejected from the orthochromatic normoblast (Fig. 28-2; see also Lessin, 1977) forming the *reticulocyte* (Fig. 28-3A). On air-dried films with Romanowsky stains, the reticulocyte is polychromatophilic due to the retention of RNA.

In the marrow, developing erythroid cells are usually in contact with macrophages in what are termed "erythroblastic islands" (Fig. 28-3C and Plate 28-1M). It is likely that ferritin and possibly other substances move directly from one cell to the other, but the extent of this and the direction of movement are not clearly understood. These erythroblastic

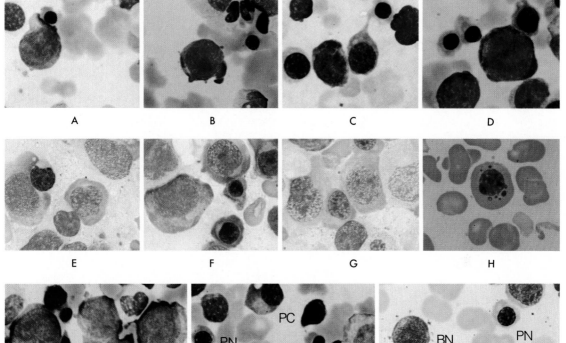

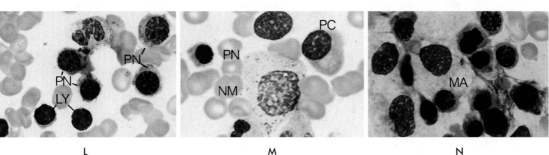

Plate 28–1. Normoblastic series, *A* to *D*; megaloblastic series, *E* to *H*; same magnification. *A*, Pronormoblast, normal marrow. A small orthochromatic normoblast is in contact with the pronormoblast. A broken nucleus of an unidentifiable cell is partly in the field. *B*, Basophilic normoblast, normal marrow. Note the intense cytoplasmic basophilia and irregular cytoplasmic protrusions, which are common. *C*, Basophilic normoblast, center; polychromatophilic normoblasts (PN) on either side. The PN on the right is more mature, having more condensed nuclear chromatin and more cytoplasmic hemoglobin than the PN on the right. *D*, Orthochromatic normoblasts; *left*, normal marrow. Note the pyknotic nuclei. Cytoplasm retains RNA and is polychromatophilic. A basophilic normoblast and a polychromatophilic normoblast are in the field. *E*, Promegaloblast, *left*. Overlying its edge is a small cell with intensely staining nuclear chromatin, probably part of a late polychromatophilic megaloblast. In the center, an earlier polychromatophilic megaloblast is in contact with a lymphocyte. *F*, Basophilic megaloblast, *left*; polychromatophilic megaloblasts, *center*. *G*, Polychromatophilic megaloblasts. Note, in addition to the large size (compared with *C*), the prominent parachromatin; this is an "open" nuclear chromatin pattern. *H*, Orthochromatic megaloblast with karyorrhexis and multiple Howell-Jolly bodies. *I*, A group of four pronormoblasts, one basophilic normoblast, and a few later forms, from a marrow aspirate showing normoblastic hyperplasia. *J*, Contrast the basophilic normoblast (BN) and the polychromatophilic normoblasts (PN) with the plasma cell (PC); these cells are sometimes confused. *K*, Basophilic normoblast (BN) with several "pseudopods," four polychromatophilic normoblasts (PN), and a neutrophil band form (NB). *L*, Contrast the lymphocytes (Ly) with smudged nuclear chromatin, and the polychromatophilic normoblasts (PN) which are sometimes confused. Here, the PN have delayed cytoplasmic maturation (less hemoglobin than expected for the degree of nuclear development). The normoblasts have sharper separation of nuclear chromatin and parachromatin than the lymphocytes. *M*, Small polychromatophilic normoblast (PN), damaged early neutrophil myelocyte (NM), and plasma cell (PC). *N*, Erythroblastic island. The macrophage in the center (MA) has abundant partially vacuolated cytoplasm which is in contact with several normoblasts; one of the latter is in mitosis.

923

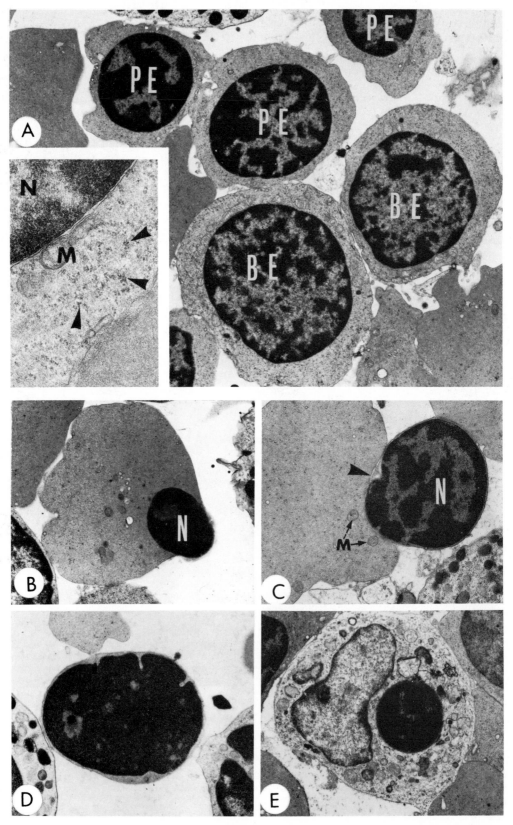

Figure 28–2. *See opposite page for legend.*

islands are usually broken up when aspirated marrow is spread on slides, but fragments of macrophage cytoplasm may sometimes be seen attached to the separated normoblasts, especially on Prussian blue-stained films.

During proliferation and maturation, most of the iron is transferred from the plasma transferrin into the cells in the pronormoblast and basophilic normoblast stages. These cells have the highest content of RNA, which begins to decline in the polychromatophilic normoblasts as hemoglobin increases in amount. Synthesis of RNA gradually decreases in each stage through the orthochromatic normoblasts. Of course, when the nucleus is no longer present (in the reticulocyte), RNA synthesis ceases, yet the RNA already present remains for a few days, and protein and heme synthesis continue in the reticulocyte until the cell loses its mitochondria and RNA.

During this maturation process, three or four mitotic divisions occur in a period of three days, resulting in the potential production of 16 reticulocytes from each pronormoblast. The reticulocytes are larger than mature red cells and are sticky. They remain in the marrow stroma for one to two days before they are released into the blood.

The reticulocytes in the marrow are about equal in number to the nucleated erythrocytes in the marrow and slightly greater in number than the reticulocytes in the circulating blood. If sufficiently severe hypoxia is present, this marrow pool of reticulocytes can be released. This approximately doubles the number of circulating reticulocytes. Normally, reticulocytes remain as such, slowly synthesizing hemoglobin, for one day in the marrow and one day in the blood. Residual ribosomes, mitochondria, and other organelles are then removed, probably by a process called autophagy by which they are ejected from the cell into the surrounding medium (Bessis, 1973).

The mature erythrocytes circulate for about 120 days. During this time they gradually age, certain enzymatic activities diminish, and they are finally destroyed within phagocytic cells of the reticuloendothelial system.

MEGALOBLASTIC MATURATION
(PLATE 28-1)

Abnormal maturation of erythroid precursors that occurs in vitamin B_{12} deficiency or folic acid deficiency (p. 969) is known as megaloblastic maturation, and the abnormal erythroid cells are called *megaloblasts*. Because of impaired ability of the cells to synthesize deoxyribonucleic acid (DNA), the intermitotic phase as well as the mitotic phase is prolonged. This results in enlarged cells, with nuclear maturation lagging behind cytoplasmic maturation (cytonuclear dissociation). The nuclear chromatin pattern is more delicate and more "open," with prominent parachromatin. Karyorrhexis, or breaking-up of the nucleus, and Howell-Jolly bodies, are frequently noted. Megaloblastic development parallels normoblastic maturation; the stages of promegaloblast, basophilic megaloblast, polychromatophilic megaloblast, and ortho-

---

Figure 28-2. Five normoblasts from a bone marrow spicule are seen in A ($\times 6600$). They are at various stages of maturation. The younger cells, basophilic normoblasts (BE), are larger, and their nuclei have coarse, partially clumped or condensed chromatin; nucleoli, which are present at this stage, are not included in this plane of section. The basophilia of the cytoplasm as seen by light microscopy is due to the presence of numerous clusters of five or six ribosomes, grouped because they are joined together by a thread of mRNA. These polyribosomes (arrows), better seen at higher magnification in the inset ($\times 34,000$) are the site for synthesis of the polypeptide chains of hemoglobin. Mitochondria (M) play an important role in the formation of hemoglobin by providing the enzymatic machinery for the synthesis of the heme ring.

The more mature cells, the polychromatophilic normoblasts (PE), are smaller and have denser chromatin clumping; they have a decreased number of polyribosomes and mitochondria. The cytoplasm appears darker as a result of the accumulation of electron-dense hemoglobin. This corresponds to decreased basophilia and increased eosinophilia in Romanowsky-stained material visualized by light microscopy.

In the orthochromatic normoblast (B—$\times 7700$) fewer ribosomes and mitochondria remain. The small pyknotic nucleus (N) becomes eccentric and bulges out on one side of the cell.

In the process of extrusion (C—$\times 8800$), the nucleus (N) is surrounded by a very narrow, barely visible rim of cytoplasm. The plasma membrane (arrow) constricts about the neck formed between the nucleus and the main portion of the cytoplasm. Mitochondria (M) aggregate in the region of the constriction, presumably providing energy for the synthesis of the new plasma membrane and for the eventual complete separation of the nucleus from the young reticulocyte. The expelled nucleus, with its thin rim of hemoglobin-rich cytoplasm (D—$\times 10,500$), is soon phagocytized by a macrophage and digested (E—$\times 8000$). The hemoglobin which is lost with the nucleus comprises much of the ineffective hemoglobin production (or ineffective erythropoiesis) in normal people, i.e., the 10 to 15 per cent of hemoglobin produced that never reaches the circulating blood. (From Fresco, R.: Ultrastructure of the blood cells and their precursors. *In* Davidsohn, I., and Henry, J. B.: Clinical Diagnosis by Laboratory Methods, 15th ed. Philadelphia, W. B. Saunders Company, 1974.)

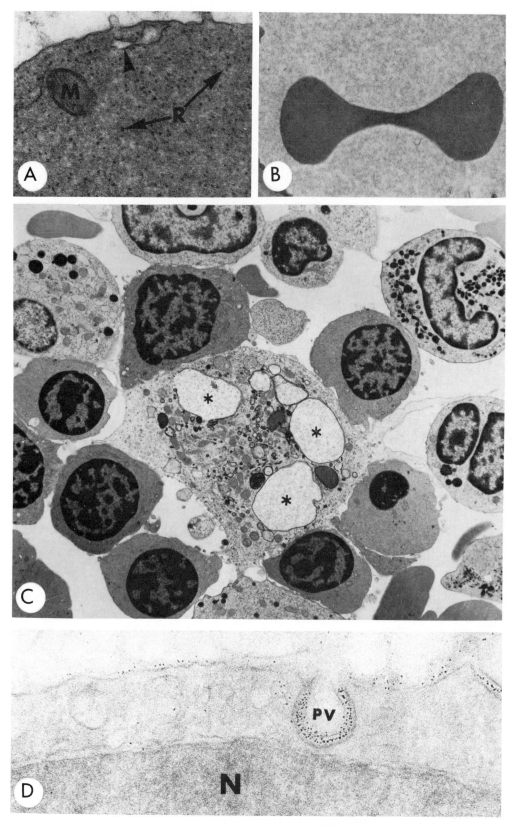

Figure 28–3. *See opposite page for legend.*

chromatic megaloblast may be recognized (Plate 28-1*E* to *H*).

REGULATION OF ERYTHROCYTE PRODUCTION

The number of erythrocytes in the blood may be regulated by changing the rate of production. The rate of erythrocyte destruction does not vary appreciably in normal individuals. The evidence indicates that increased production of erythrocytes occurs when oxygen transport to the tissues is impaired, as in anemia, in cardiovascular disorders, and low oxygen tension, such as occurs at high altitudes. On the other hand, production of erythrocytes is decreased when an individual is hypertransfused or exposed to high oxygen tension.

In general, the hemoglobin level is adjusted according to the delivery of oxygen to the tissues, but this is modified by the oxygen affinity of hemoglobin, which is modulated by the concentration of certain phosphates in the red cell. Intracellular phosphates, in particular 2,3-diphosphoglycerate (2,3-DPG), combine with reduced hemoglobin and diminish its affinity for oxygen (Fig. 28-4). In areas of tissue hypoxia, as oxygen moves from hemoglobin into the tissues, the amount of reduced hemoglobin in the red cells increases, binding more 2,3-DPG, depleting free 2,3-DPG in the cell, leading to increased glycolysis with the production of more 2,3-DPG. In turn, the latter is bound by hemoglobin, further reducing its oxygen affinity so that more oxygen can be delivered to the tissues (Erslev, 1971).

Tissue hypoxia induces formation of a factor or hormone that travels in the plasma to the marrow, where it effects the production of more red cells. This erythropoietic factor is known as *erythropoietin*. It is found in the mucoglycoprotein fraction of the plasma and migrates electrophoretically in the alpha-2-globulin range. It is relatively heat stable and is inactivated by proteolytic enzymes. Erythropoietin is produced mainly in the kidney. Erythropoietin appears to act by inducing committed progenitor cells of the marrow to differentiate into erythropoietic cells. The rate of cell division is also increased, and the release of reticulocytes from the marrow is promoted. When we sample a marrow which is producing more erythrocytes than normal, we see increased numbers of normoblasts but in a normal ratio of cell types, a condition known as normoblastic hyperplasia.

Measurement of erythropoietin requires a bioassay procedure (Erslev, 1977). The patient's plasma or urine is injected into the polycythemic mouse. The mouse is made polycythemic by transfusions or hypoxia in order to depress its own erythropoietin production and to make it more sensitive to any injected activity. The response of the mouse is measured by the incorporation of radioactive iron into circulating erythrocytes. Increased amounts of erythropoietin can be detected in the plasma of patients with certain types of anemia, but in plasma, normal or decreased levels cannot be detected. Methods for concentrating the urine have been devised, and well-defined levels of erythropoietic activity can be measured in normal urine (Adamson,

---

Figure 28-3.   The young reticulocyte (A—×52,000) still often shows portions of plasma membrane clefts (arrow) at the site of nuclear expulsion as well as a few mitochondria (M) and ribosomes (R), which continue to synthesize small amounts of hemoglobin for about one to two days, at which time the cytoplasmic organelles have disappeared. The mature erythrocyte can be seen as the familiar biconcave disk bound by a plasma membrane and rich in electron-dense hemoglobin (B—×8800).

After from 80 to 120 days, the aged erythrocytes are phagocytized in turn by the reticulum cells of the bone marrow (C—×4000), and some appear within the cytoplasm as whole cells, fragments, or "ghosts" (*). The hemoglobin is broken down and its iron is released and stored in the form of ferritin. The plasma membranes of normoblasts are in contact with that of the macrophage, forming an erythroblastic island.

At higher magnification (D—×100,000—unstained) dense ferritin molecules can be seen on the surface of these cells and in pinocytotic vesicles (PV). It was originally suggested by Bessis and Breton-Gorius (1957) that, in a process they called "rheopeocytosis," ferritin is taken up by maturing erythroblasts surrounding the reticulum cell (erythroblastic island) to be resynthesized into new hemoglobin, but others have questioned the validity of this interpretation and have suggested a movement of ferritin in the opposite direction, namely, that iron not required for hemoglobin synthesis in red cell precursors is incorporated into ferritin and returned to the macrophage. In either case, an intimate relationship between normoblasts and macrophages in the marrow exists and is recognized morphologically as "the erythroblastic island." To some extent normally, and to a greater extent in some abnormal circumstances, the spleen and liver are also involved in destroying erythrocytes. (From Fresco, R.: Ultrastructure of the blood cells and their precursors. *In* Davidsohn, I., and Henry, J. B.: Clinical Diagnosis by Laboratory Methods, 15th ed. Philadelphia, W. B. Saunders Company, 1974.)

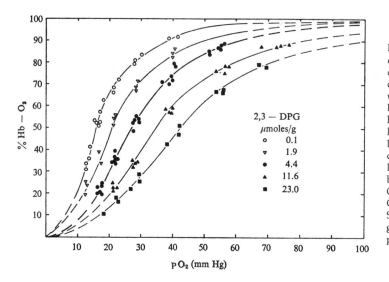

Figure 28-4. Oxygen dissociation curves of hemoglobin at different concentrations of 2,3-diphosphoglycerate (DPG). The curve is sigmoidal and shifts to the right with increasing concentrations of 2,3-DPG; this results in decreased affinity of hemoglobin for oxygen and increased delivery of oxygen to the tissues. (From Duhm, J.: The effect of 2,3-DPG and other organic phosphates on the Donnan equilibrium and the oxygen affinity of human blood. *In* Rørth, M., and Astrup, P. (eds.): Oxygen Affinity of Hemoglobin and Red Cell Acid Base Status. (Alfred Benzon Symposium IV). Copenhagen, Munksgaard International Publishers, 1972, p. 583.)

1966). Elevated levels are detected in patients with erythroid hyperplasia and in aplastic anemia. Decreased levels below the normal range are found in normal individuals after transfusion and in polycythemia vera.

Synthesis of Hemoglobin

HEME SYNTHESIS. Heme synthesis occurs in most cells of the body, except the mature erythrocytes, but most abundantly in the erythroid precursors. Succinyl-coenzyme A condenses with glycine to form the unstable intermediate alpha-amino beta-keto-adipic acid, which is readily decarboxylated to delta-amino-levulinic acid (ALA) (Fig. 28-5). This

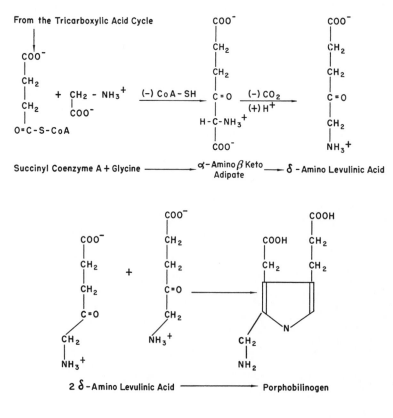

Figure 28-5. Formation of porphobilinogen from succinyl-coenzyme A and glycine. (From Leavell, B. S.: Fundamentals of Clinical Hematology, 4th ed. Philadelphia, W. B. Saunders Company, 1976.)

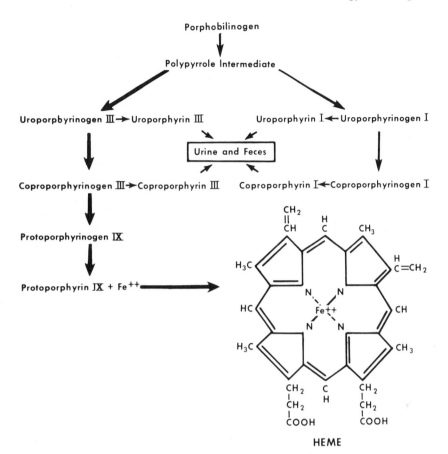

Porphobilinogen

Polypyrrole Intermediate

Uroporpbyrinogen Ⅲ → Uroporphyrin Ⅲ   Uroporphyrin Ⅰ ← Uroporphyrinogen Ⅰ

Urine and Feces

Coproporphyrinogen Ⅲ → Coproporphyrin Ⅲ   Coproporphyrin Ⅰ ← Coproporphyrinogen Ⅰ

Protoporphyrinogen Ⅸ

Protoporphyrin Ⅸ + Fe^{++} ⟶

HEME

Figure 28–6. Formation of heme from porphobilinogen. (From Leavell, B. S.: Fundamentals of Clinical Hematology, 4th ed. Philadelphia, W. B. Saunders Company, 1976.)

condensation requires pyridoxal phosphate (vitamin B_6) and must take place in intact mitochondria.

ALA is excreted normally in small amounts in the urine; in certain abnormalities of heme synthesis (for example, lead poisoning) excretion is increased. Two molecules of ALA condense to form the monopyrrole, porphobilinogen, catalyzed by the enzyme ALA-dehydrase. Porphobilinogen is also normally excreted in small amounts in the urine. Markedly elevated amounts appear in the urine in acute intermittent porphyria, easily detected by a color reaction with Ehrlich's aldehyde reagent.

Four molecules of porphobilinogen react to form uroporphyrinogen III or I (Fig. 28-6). It is the type III isomer that is converted, by way of coproporphyrinogen III and protoporphyrinogen, to protoporphyrin. In certain diseases when this pathway is partially blocked, the type I isomers of uroporphyrinogen and coproporphyrinogen are formed and their oxi-

dized excretion products, uroporphyrin I and coproporphyrin I, are increased in amount.

Protoporphyrin is normally found in mature erythrocytes. In abnormalities of heme synthesis, levels of free erythrocyte protoporphyrin may be increased.

Iron is inserted into protoporphyrin by the mitochondrial enzyme ferrochetalase to form the finished heme moiety.

GLOBIN SYNTHESIS. Globin synthesis occurs in the cytoplasm of the normoblast and reticulocyte. According to the prevailing doctrine of protein synthesis, the polypeptide chains (which constitute the protein part of hemoglobin) are manufactured on the ribosomes, which are located mainly in the cytoplasm of the young erythroid cell. Specific small sRNA (soluble RNA) molecules attach to each amino acid and determine the placement of that amino acid according to the code in the mRNA (messenger RNA). Progressive growth of the polypeptide chain begins at the amino end.

This process of protein synthesis occurs on ribosomes clustered into polyribosomes or polysomes, which are probably held together by the messenger RNA strand. Since the reticulocyte can synthesize hemoglobin for at least two days after loss of its nucleus, it appears that the messenger RNA for hemoglobin is quite stable. It is probable that the globin polypeptide chains formed on the polysome are folded into their three-dimensional configurations spontaneously.

Control of hemoglobin synthesis is not entirely elucidated, but it has been shown that hemin inhibits heme synthesis (probably at the ALA-synthetase step) and either hemin or iron increases globin synthesis.

STRUCTURE AND FUNCTION OF HEMOGLOBIN. (See Bunn, 1977.) In each hemoglobin molecule, one heme group is inserted into a hydrophobic pocket of one folded polypeptide chain. Normal adult hemoglobin A consists of four heme groups and four polypeptide chains (two alpha chains and two beta chains) which form a roughly globular hemoglobin molecule (Fig. 28-7). The ferrous iron atoms have six coordination bonds, four to the pyrrole nitrogens of heme, one to the imidazole nitrogen of histidine of the globin chain (87 alpha or 92 beta), and one that is reversibly bound to oxygen. As the oxygen partial pressure increases, the four heme groups sequentially bind one molecule of oxygen each. In the process, a change in the overall configuration of the hemoglobin molecule occurs, and this altered configuration appears to favor the heme-heme interaction in the binding of oxygen.

The sigmoid-shaped oxygen dissociation curve of hemoglobin reflects this affinity for oxygen with increasing partial pressure of oxygen, such as occurs in the lungs (Fig. 28-4). With the conditions prevailing in the tissues of decreasing pH, conversion of $HbO_2 \rightarrow Hb$,

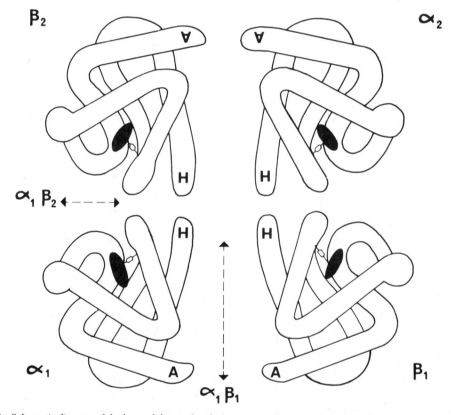

Figure 28-7. Schematic diagram of the hemoglobin molecule (tetramer, molecular weight 64,500 daltons). The heme group for each monomeric polypeptide chain is depicted as a black disc, connected to an imidazole group of histidine, and located near the surface of the molecule in a "pocket" formed by the polypeptide chain. Letters A and H designate alphahelical segments of each polypeptide chain; A is the N-terminal segment and H is the C-terminal segment. The four monomers are separated in this drawing, but actually make contact along a relatively large area ($\alpha_1 \beta_1$), which is thought to be the relatively fixed or stabilizing contact area, and a smaller ($\alpha_1 \beta_1$) area thought to be the functional contact area, where movement occurs during oxygenation and deoxygenation, changing the molecular configuration. (From White, J. M., and Dacie, J. V.: The unstable hemoglobins. Prog. Hematol., 7:69–109, 1971. Grune & Stratton, Inc., New York, by permission.)

binding of more 2,3-DPG to Hb (p. 927), and increasing temperature produced by metabolic events, the curve shifts downward and to the right, favoring the release of oxygen. Rapidly metabolizing tissue will extract more oxygen from hemoglobin than will metabolically inactive tissue.

Carbon dioxide (CO_2) is also transported in erythrocytes as well as in plasma. A small part of red cell CO_2 is dissolved, a small part is bound to amino groups of hemoglobin as carbamino-CO_2, but most is in the bicarbonate form (Henry, 1964). The enzyme carbonic anhydrase catalyzes the transformation of carbon dioxide to bicarbonate in the red cell while in the tissue capillary bed and catalyzes the reverse reaction (the release of carbon dioxide from bicarbonate) in the erythrocyte when it is in the capillary bed of the lungs.

ERYTHROCYTE DESTRUCTION

From the time an erythrocyte enters the circulation and loses its RNA, it gradually undergoes metabolic changes over the course of its 120-day life span. At this time, the less viable senescent cell is removed from the circulation. We know that certain glycolytic enzymes diminish in activity as the cell ages. Older red cells have a smaller surface area and an increased MCHC compared with younger cells (Ganzoni, 1971). It is probable that changes in the cell surface, possibly indirectly related, render the cell more liable to phagocytosis. Fragmentation of the red cell, without hemolysis, can occur with the formation of schistocytes or cell fragments. These particles are then readily removed by the reticuloendothelial system. Some have held that this process of fragmentation prior to removal by phagocytosis plays an important role in eliminating senescent erythrocytes from the circulation. This explanation has been used to account for the lack of morphologic evidence of erythrophagocytosis in the reticuloendothelial system of the normal individual, despite the removal from the blood of three million erythrocytes every second. The other possibility is phagocytosis of the intact aged erythrocytes and rapid breakdown within the phagocytes.

Whether one process predominates or both coexist, it seems clear that the cells are removed by the macrophages of the reticuloendothelial system.

Under normal conditions in man, the major part of erythrophagocytosis appears to occur in the bone marrow (Bessis, 1973). In pathological states when the erythrocyte is damaged and the red cell survival is shortened, the site of destruction depends upon the extent to which the erythrocyte is damaged. If the damage is small, the erythrocytes are removed primarily by the spleen. If the damage is great, the cells are removed mainly by the liver.

DEGRADATION OF HEMOGLOBIN

After removal of the red cell from the circulation, hemoglobin is broken down within the macrophages of the reticuloendothelial system into its three constituents—iron, protoporphyrin, and globin. The iron goes into storage and may be completely reutilized. The polypeptide chains of globin are probably degraded and returned to the amino acid pool of the body. In contrast, the protoporphyrin ring is split, converted to bilirubin, and excreted from the body.

In the macrophage, the protoporphyrin ring is cleaved by a heme oxidase enzyme at the alpha-methene bridge, yielding one mole of carbon monoxide (CO) and one mole of biliverdin (see Fig. 11-2). The CO appears in the blood as HbCO and is eventually exhaled. Biliverdin is reduced to bilirubin in the macrophage, and bilirubin is transported to the liver by plasma albumin (p. 309). It is removed from the plasma by the liver cell, conjugated mainly with glucuronide and excreted in the bile. In the intestine, reduction by bacteria occurs, and bilirubin is transformed into urobilinogen, mesobilirubinogen, and stercobilinogen, compounds which are collectively designated urobilinogens (see Fig. 11-1).

Estimation of exhaled CO, HbCO, or fecal urobilinogen can be used as measures of hemoglobin breakdown. When production of red cells is diminished and the level of circulating hemoglobin is low, as in aplastic anemia, urobilinogen excretion is reduced. When destruction of erythrocytes is increased, as in hemolytic anemia, all three are increased in amount.

In normal man about 80 to 90 per cent of the excreted bile pigment measured as fecal urobilinogen is derived from breakdown of senescent erythrocytes which have lived 100 to 120 days. However, about 10 to 20 per cent of the pigment is excreted within the first few days. This early labeled bile pigment could not be derived from erythrocytes destroyed at the end of their normal life span. Although a small amount of this comes from non-hemoglobin heme formed in the liver, most of this early labeled pigment comes from the breakdown of newly formed hemoglobin in the bone marrow. Much of it may represent hemoglobin from the nucleus and pieces of cytoplasm of the orthochromatic normoblast that are lost during the process of nuclear extrusion.

In certain hematologic diseases, notably thalassemia, pernicious anemia, refractory normoblastic anemia, and erythropoietic porphyria, this early labeled bile pigment fraction may be markedly increased. This excessive intramedullary destruction of hemoglobin, which never appears in circulating erythrocytes, is known as ineffective erythropoiesis.

ERYTHROKINETICS

The balance between delivery of erythrocytes to the blood and removal of erythrocytes from the blood is maintained tenaciously and results in a relatively constant hemoglobin mass in the circulation. Anemia results when the removal of erythrocytes from the blood is increased and cannot be compensated for by increased production or when the delivery of erythrocytes or hemoglobin to the blood is decreased or when both processes exist together.

When anemia develops, the resultant tissue hypoxia leads to elevated levels of erythropoietin in the plasma. Resultant normoblastic hyperplasia produces more erythrocytes for delivery to the circulation. The marrow in a normal individual is capable of six to eight times the normal output of erythrocytes with extreme stimulation. This capacity must be compared with the output actually attained when one is evaluating the marrow response of a given patient.

Measurements that assess effective erythropoiesis (production and delivery of erythrocytes to the circulation), ineffective erythropoiesis, and destruction of erythrocytes are often necessary to determine the mechanism and the cause of anemia (Harris, 1970).

Measurements of Total Production of Erythrocytes or Hemoglobin. The *total mass of erythropoietic cells* in the body cannot be easily measured. An estimate is made by examining a sample of bone marrow from a normally active site and determining the cel-

lularity (ratio of the volume of hematopoietic cells to the volume of fat plus hematopoietic cells compared with the normal) and the percentage of total nucleated cells that are erythropoietic (see section on bone marrow, p. 957). When marrow activity increases, usually the additional hematopoietic cells replace the fat in the red marrow sites before extension occurs into the yellow marrow of the long bones. One assumes that the sample is representative of the marrow as a whole, an assumption that usually holds, but one sometimes finds exceptions.

The *plasma iron turnover* is calculated from the serum iron level and the rate of removal of injected radioactive iron from the plasma. About 25 to 30 per cent of the iron is not used in erythropoiesis and is probably taken up by the liver. The remaining 70 to 75 per cent is taken up by erythropoietic cells and is therefore a measure of total erythropoiesis, both effective and ineffective.

Measurement of Total Destruction of Erythrocytes or Hemoglobin. Determination of *fecal urobilinogen* is an estimate of the total excretion of bile pigments—the breakdown products of heme. This measurement includes pigment derived from hemoglobin formed and destroyed in the marrow without ever reaching the circulation, as well as that from the destruction of circulating erythrocytes. Limitations include diminished conversion of bilirubin to urobilinogen because of oral administration of broad-spectrum antibiotics and failure of pigment to reach the intestine in obstructive jaundice. In severe liver disease less reabsorbed urobilinogen is excreted in the bile and more is excreted in the urine. The urine urobilinogen is not so good a measure of urobilinogen excretion for two reasons: Removal by the kidney is usually a minor component of the total excretion, and with a normally functioning liver, clearance of reabsorbed urobilinogen in the plasma is so effective that considerable increases in the circulating blood may result in little or no elevation of the urine urobilinogen.

Measurement of Effective Production of Erythrocytes

RETICULOCYTE COUNT. Since the RNA of the reticulocyte disappears about a day after its entry into the blood, enumeration of reticulocytes will be a measure of the number of cells being delivered by the marrow to the blood, that is, a measure of effective erythropoiesis. The normal absolute reticulocyte count is approximately $50 \times 10^9/l$ or 1 per cent of the circulating erythrocytes. If the erythrocyte count is determined, one can calculate the absolute reticulocyte count by multiplying the reticulocyte percentage by the erythrocyte count. To give a meaningful expression of erythropoiesis, the absolute reticulocyte count, or some estimate of it, and not simply the percentage must be used (Hillman, 1967, 1974).

A second consideration is an increased maturation time of reticulocytes in the blood due to accelerated release from the marrow, an effect of erythropoietin. The need for this is recognized by the presence of large, polychromatic cells or nucleated red cells in the blood film, indicating a shift of excessively immature reticulocytes from the marrow into the blood. An approximate correction is to assume that the reticulocyte life span has doubled.

If a patient has a Hct = 0.26, red count = $2.89 \times 10^{12}/l$, and a reticulocyte count = 7 per cent, he will have an absolute reticulocyte count = $202 \times 10^9/l$. Since the average normal absolute reticulocyte count is $50 \times 10^9/l$, he has $\dfrac{202 \times 10^9/l}{50 \times 10^9/l}$, or four times as many reticulocytes as normal. However, this must be corrected for the increased maturation time (shift): $4 \times \frac{1}{2} = 2$. Therefore, two times as many reticulocytes are entering his blood per day as in a normal individual; that is, his red cell production is two times normal.

If only the hematocrit is available, this same correction can be made as follows:

Correction for hematocrit:

"absolute percentage" = reticulocyte
$$\text{count (7\%)} \times \frac{\text{Patient's Hct. (0.26)}}{\text{Normal Hct. (0.45)}} = 4\%$$

Correction for shift:

Corrected reticulocyte count
$$= \frac{\substack{\text{Absolute reticulocyte} \\ \text{percentage (4\%)}}}{\text{Maturation time (2 days)}} = 2$$

Corrections are necessary in order to assess the degree of red cell production in response to anemia.

A normal individual with a normal supply of iron can increase red cell production by two times normal within a week if the hematocrit drops to 0.35, or to three times normal if the hematocrit drops to 0.25. Only if there is a parenteral supply of iron (such as in hemolysis) can the maximal red cell production of six to eight times normal be achieved (Hillman, 1969).

If an appropriate marrow response to anemia has not been reached in one to two weeks, we can infer that some impairment of red cell production exists.

The *erythrocyte utilization of iron* is a measure of the amount of an injected dose of iron which appears in the hemoglobin of circulating erythrocytes. It is derived from the plasma iron turnover and the percentage of radioactive iron which has been injected and which appears in the circulating erythrocytes after two weeks, assuming that none of the newly formed cells have been destroyed in that time interval. This, too, is a measure of effective erythropoiesis.

Measurement of Effective Survival of Erythrocytes in the Blood. The *erythrocyte survival* can be determined by removing a sample of blood, labeling the erythrocytes with ^{51}Cr, inactivating the excess ^{51}Cr remaining in the plasma, and reinjecting the labeled erythrocytes into the patient. The ^{51}Cr is bound to the beta chain of the hemoglobin molecule and for the most part is not released until the red cell is removed from the circulation and the hemoglobin is degraded. Measurements of radioactivity in the red cells are made at 2 hours or 24 hours (the zero time, or 100 per cent level) and at 1- to 3-day intervals until over 50 per cent of the activity has disappeared. The results are usually expressed as the ^{51}Cr half survival time. The normal range is 28 to 38 days. (The reason it is not 60 days is that ^{51}Cr is eluted from the hemoglobin at the rate of about 1 per cent per day.) If the production of erythrocytes equals destruction (i.e., if a steady state exists), the erythrocyte survival is also a measure of effective production of erythrocytes.

Summary. Total erythropoiesis refers to the total production of hemoglobin or red cells; effective erythropoiesis refers to production of hemoglobin or red cells that reach the circulation; and ineffective erythropoiesis refers to production of hemoglobin or red cells that never reach the circulating blood. These concepts of the *erythrokinetic* approach to the study of anemia are useful, especially in situations that defy easy classification.

Neutrophils (Plate 28-2)

It is likely that the common progenitor cell for neutrophils and monocytes (GM-CFC) divides and gives rise to the myeloblast, the earliest recognizable granulocyte-monocyte

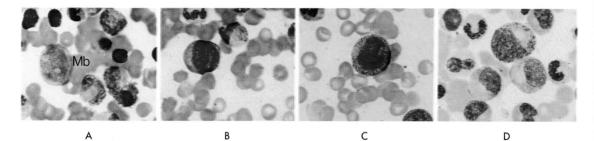

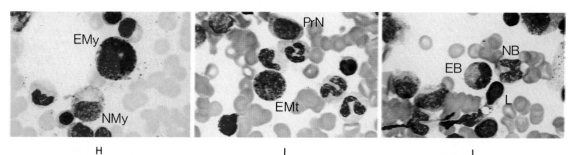

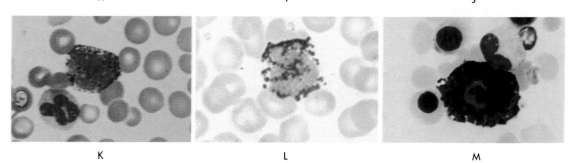

Plate 28-2. *A*, Myeloblast (Mb). *B*, Early promyelocyte has more basophilic cytoplasm than the myeloblast. A few azurophilic granules are in the vicinity of the Golgi zone. *C*, Promyelocyte. Later stage has more numerous azurophilic granules. *D*, Neutrophil myelocytes. Newly formed specific granules have appeared in the Golgi zone adjacent to the nucleus. The azurophilic granules, which were formed in the promyelocyte stage, are best seen in the upper cell. As maturation proceeds, the azurophilic staining quality is lost. *E*, Neutrophil myelocytes (NMy), a late polychromatophilic normoblast, and three neutrophils. In the NM on the left, opaque granules overlying the nucleus give it a pale or "moth-eaten" appearance. *F*, N. myelocyte (NMy), N. metamyelocytes (NMt), and N. band form (NB). NMt and monocytes are frequently confused with one another. *G*, N. myelocyte (NMy), N. metamyelocytes (NMt), N. band forms (NB), and a broken or smudged cell. *H*, Eosinophil myelocyte (EMy), contrasted with a neutrophil myelocyte (NMy), is larger and has larger granules. The eosinophil granules that appear early in development have a basophilic staining reaction; as the cell matures they become olive-green, then eosinophil in their staining characteristics. *I*, Eosinophil metamyelocyte (EMt). Neutrophils and a pronormoblast (PrN) are present. *J*, Eosinophil band form (EB), neutrophil band form (NB), and lymphocyte (Ly). The granules in the EB have the staining reaction characteristic of the mature cell. *K*, Basophil and neutrophil. *L*, Mature basophil. The nuclei in basophils do not normally segment. Immature basophils have cytoplasmic basophilia (outside of the granules) which this cell lacks. *M*, Tissue mast cell; *center*, bone marrow. Mast cell granules are smaller, rounder, less water soluble, and more abundant than basophil granules; they usually obscure the nucleus.

precursor, under stimulation by a hormone, colony-stimulating factor for granulocytes and monocytes (GM-CSF).

MORPHOLOGY OF NEUTROPHIL PRECURSORS

Air-dried films

The *myeloblast* (Plate 28-2A) is a cell about 15 µm in diameter with a moderately high N/C ratio, a large oval to quadrangular nucleus, very fine, uniform chromatin pattern, delicate nuclear membrane, and 2 to 5 nucleoli. The cytoplasm is pale, clear blue, and without granules. The appearance of azurophil granules (~0.5 µm diameter) heralds the earliest promyelocyte (Plate 28-2B) and indicates that the cell is to be a neutrophil. The *promyelocyte* stage encompasses the entire period of production of azurophil granules. The promyelocyte is slightly larger than the myeloblast. The nuclear chromatin begins to condense a bit, and the nucleoli are less obvious. The cytoplasm is basophilic and is filled by more and more azurophil granules (Plate 28-2C). The *neutrophil myelocyte* stage begins with the appearance of specific neutrophil granules, at first only in the Golgi region; as more specific granules develop they spread throughout the cytoplasm (Plate 28-2D to H). With successive mitoses the number of azurophil granules (which have ceased production at the end of the promyelocyte stage) are diminished. The early neutrophil myelocyte, therefore, has a rather fine, dispersed nuclear chromatin pattern, many azurophil granules, and few specific granules. The late neutrophil myelocyte has a somewhat more condensed chromatin pattern, a cytoplasm well filled with specific granules, and rather few azurophil granules. The myelocyte is the latest stage capable of cell division. No cytoplasmic granules are formed, and no cell division occurs in later stages. Next is the *neutrophil metamyelocyte*, distinguished by an indented, kidney-shaped nucleus with more condensed chromatin (Plate 28-2F and G). From this stage on, changes in the cytoplasm are insignificant. In the *band neutrophil* (stab form) the nucleus has more

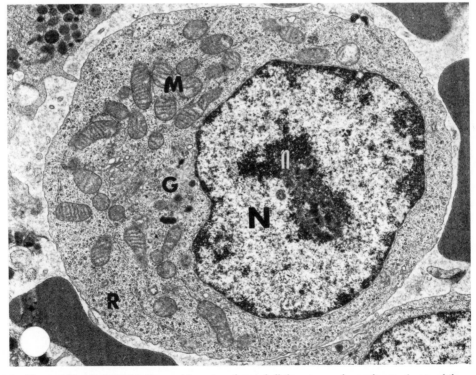

Figure 28–8.   The *myeloblast* (×13,200) is the most immature form of all three types of granulocytes (neutrophils, eosinophils, and basophils). The nucleus (N) is spherical to slightly angular, with finely granular evenly distributed chromatin, except for some clumps adjacent to the nuclear envelope. One or more nucleoli (n) are present near the center of the nucleus. The cytoplasm is relatively abundant, with numerous large mitochondria (M), a well-developed Golgi complex (G) often showing a few small dense granules associated with it, polyribosomes (R) which are responsible for the cytoplasmic basophilia seen by light microscopy, and a few profiles of rough-surfaced endoplasmic reticulum. (From Fresco, R.: Ultrastructure of the blood cells and their precursors. *In* Davidsohn, I., and Henry, J. B.: Clinical Diagnosis by Laboratory Methods, 15th ed. Philadelphia, W. B. Saunders Company, 1974.)

condensed chromatin and a rather uniform elongated shape. Partial constriction of the nucleus occurs in the band stage, until a fine filament (length but no breadth) is formed between two of the lobes, at which point the cell is classified as a *segmented neutrophil*.

Electron microscopy

The ultrastructural characteristics of the neutrophil series are illustrated in Figures 28-8 through 28-11. The myeloblast has few or no granules yet visible (Fig. 28-8). It is probable that during the myeloblast stage, enzymes destined to be localized in granules are synthesized and carried in the rough-surfaced endoplasmic reticulum to the Golgi area. There they are packaged into the granules

that begin to spread out from the Golgi area in the promyelocyte stage (Fig. 28-9). The azurophil granules that are formed in the promyelocyte arise from the concave aspect of the Golgi apparatus (Bainton, 1966). During the myelocyte stage (Fig. 28-10), only specific granules are being formed, arising from the opposite or convex surface of the Golgi apparatus. These are morphologically different granules when viewed with the electron microscope; this is best seen in Figure 28-11A and B. The mature human neutrophil has twice as many specific granules as azurophil granules. The azurophil granules (formed in the promyelocyte stage) contain lysosomal enzymes (acid hydrolases: acid phosphatase, β-glucuronidase, etc.), acid mucosubstance, per-

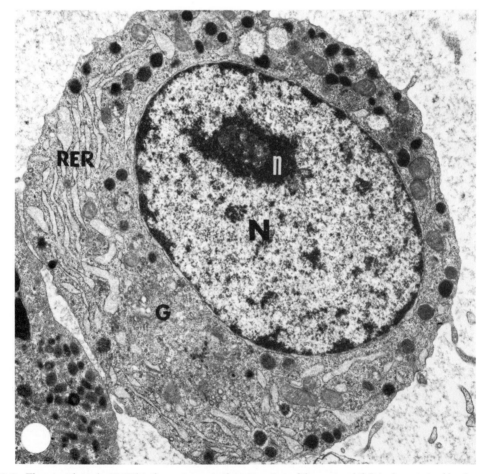

Figure 28–9.   The *promyelocyte* (× 13,200) is the next stage in the maturation of the neutrophil. It is characterized by the presence of numerous profiles of rough-surfaced endoplasmic reticulum (RER) and numerous round or elongated primary (azurophil) granules scattered throughout the cytoplasm. The Golgi complex (G) is prominent, and a moderate number of mitochondria and free ribosomes are seen. The nucleus (N) is usually oval and shows increased condensation of its chromatin. A nucleolus (n) is still present at this stage. (From Fresco, R.: Ultrastructure of the blood cells and their precursors. *In* Davidsohn, I., and Henry, J. B.: Clinical Diagnosis by Laboratory Methods, 15th ed. Philadelphia, W. B. Saunders Company, 1974.)

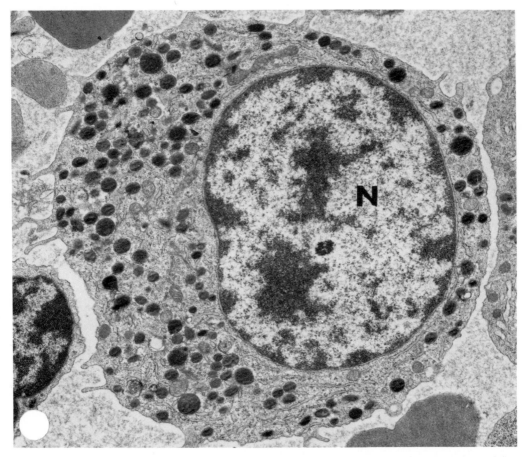

Figure 28-10. A *neutrophil myelocyte* is illustrated here ($\times$ 13,200). At this stage of development the primary (azurophil) granule formation has ceased and has been replaced by the production of secondary (specific) granules. The specific neutrophil granules are smaller and less dense than the azurophil granules and arise from the distal or convex face of the Golgi complexes by pinching-off and confluence of vesicles which have a finely granular content (Bainton, 1966).

The Golgi complex in the myelocyte continues to diminish in size and complexity. There is a depletion of rough endoplasmic reticulum and a decrease in the number of polysomes, free ribosomes, and mitochondria. The cytoplasmic matrix becomes denser and contains increasing amounts of particulate glycogen. The nucleus (N) begins to show an indentation. The nuclear chromatin is more condensed and the nucleoli disappear. (From Fresco, R.: Ultrastructure of the blood cells and their precursors. *In* Davidsohn, I., and Henry, J. B.: Clinical Diagnosis by Laboratory Methods, 15th ed. Philadelphia, W. B. Saunders Company, 1974.)

oxidase, one third of the cell's muramidase, and cationic antibacterial proteins. The specific granules (formed in the myelocyte stage) contain lactoferrin, most of the muramidase, and collagenase (Bainton, 1976). Biochemical studies of mature human neutrophils have shown that alkaline phosphatase is not in either of the granule fractions, but is in a lighter membrane fraction (West, 1974).

DISTRIBUTION AND KINETICS

The distribution of this cell series in the body is depicted in Figure 28-12. For each neutrophil in the blood vessels, about 16 precursors are present in the marrow. From the time of differentiation into a myeloblast, through about five mitotic divisions (three of which occur at the myelocyte stage), it takes about 14 days until the progeny of that cell reach the blood. The last eight days are spent in the maturation and storage pool. When a neutrophil enters the blood, it moves readily between a circulating granulocyte pool (CGP), which is sampled in the leukocyte count, and a marginal granulocyte pool (MGP), which is not, but is either marginated along vessel walls or sequestered in capillary beds. In less

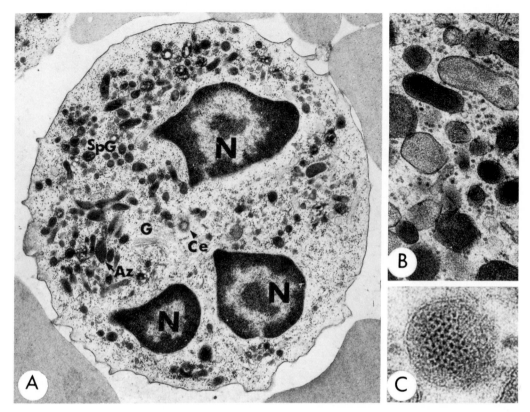

Figure 28–11. This mature *neutrophil* ($\times 12,400$) has three nuclear lobes (N) connected by thin filamentous strands not seen in this plane of section. The nuclear chromatin is condensed, particularly close to the nuclear membrane. A centriole (Ce) is situated close to the center of the cell, and the lamellae and cisternae of the Golgi complex (G) lie below and to the left of it. There are relatively few mitochondria. Ribosomes and glycogen granules are evenly distributed throughout the cytoplasm, as are numerous round or elongated specific granules (Sp G) and denser azurophil granules (Az). The heterogeneous appearance of the specific granules is better seen at higher magnification in B ($\times 52,000$), which reveals a variety of sizes, shapes, and densities. Occasionally the granules (C— $\times 170,000$) have an internal crystalloid organization, in the form of regularly arranged electron-dense particles. (From Fresco, R.: Ultrastructure of the blood cells and their precursors. *In* Davidsohn, I., and Henry, J. B.: Clinical Diagnosis by Laboratory Methods, 15th ed. Philadelphia, W. B. Saunders Company, 1974.)

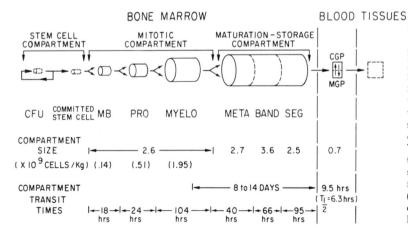

Figure 28–12. Neutrophil production, distribution, and kinetics. CFU = Multipotential stem cell; MB = myeloblast; PRO = promyelocyte; MYELO = myelocyte; META = metamyelocytes; SEG = segmented neutrophil; CGP = circulating granulocyte pool; MGP = marginal granulocyte pool. The cylinders representing the various compartments are drawn proportional to their sizes. The compartment transit times on the next to last line are from DF^{32}P studies; those on the last line are from tritiated thymidine studies. (From Wintrobe, M. M., et al: Clinical Hematology, 7th ed. Philadelphia, Lea & Febiger, 1974.)

than a day after it arrives, the neutrophil emigrates from the circulation in a random manner and enters the tissues. From there, if not utilized in an inflammatory exudate, neutrophils leave the body within a few days via secretions in bronchi, saliva, gastrointestinal tract, and urine, or they are destroyed by the reticuloendothelial system.

FUNCTION

Neutrophils are able to move in a zigzag manner, but their motion changes to a straight line path if a chemotactic attractant (e.g., a bacterium coated with certain components of complement) is within a certain distance. Neutrophils have receptors for the Fc portion of IgG as well as for complement (C3) and bind and phagocytize the coated particle. Phagocytosis occurs, with the formation of a phagocytic vacuole that contains the ingested particle; accompanying this process is an increase in metabolic activity and energy production. Specific granules, followed shortly by azurophil granules, empty their contents into the phagocytic vacuoles, a process known as degranulation. Bactericidal activity occurs within the vacuole, mediated by H_2O_2, peroxidase, and a halide ion generating the free halogen, or by other enzymatic activity.

Neutrophils thus are important in defense against infectious disease (see Chap. 40). If their enzymes are activated and released outside the cell, neutrophils can cause tissue necrosis, as occurs in the Arthus or Shwartzman reaction. Neutrophils, which are active in inflammation, release an endogenous pyrogen that produces fever by acting on the hypothalamus to set the body's thermostat at a higher level.

For a more detailed consideration of neutrophils consult Murphy (1976) or Cline (1975).

EOSINOPHILS

Eosinophils are produced in the bone marrow. It seems likely from *in vitro* culture studies that there is a separate eosinophilic committed progenitor cell (colony forming cell, EOS-CFC) in marrow that is distinct from the GM-CFC. The colony-stimulating factor that induces the EOS-CFC to proliferate and differentiate into eosinophil colonies (EO-CSF) is produced by lymphocytes when stimulated by pokeweed mitogen or mercaptoethanol (Metcalf, 1977).

MORPHOLOGY OF EOSINOPHIL PRECURSORS

Air-dried films

The cell that is the precursor for the earliest recognizable eosinophil, the eosinophil myelocyte, is presumably a distinctive myeloblast. However, it is morphologically indistinguishable from that which gives rise to neutrophils and monocytes or to basophils (Fig. 28-1 and Plate 28-2). In the early eosinophil myelocyte the granules are large and take the basophilic stain (Plate 28-2*H*). As the cell matures, the granules appear olive-green (Plate 28-2*I*) and finally the characteristic red-orange color (Plates 28-2*I* and 27-1*F* and *G*). Nuclear maturation is similar to that of the neutrophil. Eosinophils are slightly larger than neutrophils and have fewer nuclear lobes.

Electron microscopy

Electron micrographs of eosinophils show characteristic granules that have a dense crystalloid core in a less dense matrix (Figure 28-13). Immature granules, appearing in the myelocyte, at first have no crystalloid but develop them as maturation proceeds. Mature granules are of two types: the larger granule (0.5 to 1.5 μm in largest diameter) which contains a dense crystalloid; and a smaller granule (0.1 to 0.5 μm diameter) which contains no crystalloid. The smaller granules appear later during maturation, after the myelocyte stage.

Eosinophil granules contain peroxidase, acid hydrolase, phospholipase, and cathepsin. The small granules contain arylsulfatase; both granule types contain peroxidase and acid phosphatase. In the larger granules, the enzymes are localized in the matrix, not the crystalloid. Eosinophil granules have a different form of peroxidase than do neutrophils; also, eosinophils contain no alkaline phosphatase, muramidase, or phagocytin (Beeson, 1977).

DISTRIBUTION AND KINETICS

The kinetics of eosinophils are less well understood than those of neutrophils, but they are probably similar. They spend about the same half-time in the blood (less than eight hours) as neutrophils, and probably do not re-enter the circulation once they leave it. Eosinophils are considerably less numerous in blood and marrow than are neutrophils. Eosinophils in the tissues, however, are at least

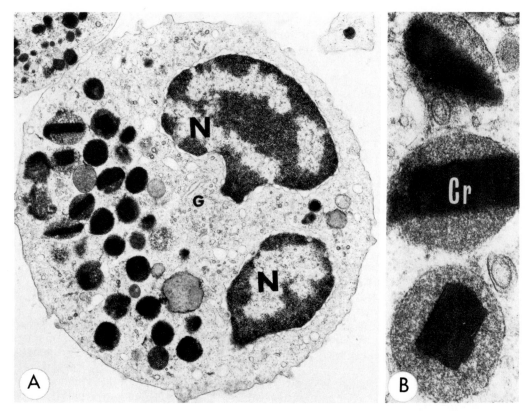

Figure 28-13. This *eosinophil* (×12,400) has a bilobed nucleus (N) showing chromatin condensation. A Golgi complex (G) occupies the center of the cell. The distinctive ultrastructural feature of the eosinophil is the presence of large round or oval membrane-bound specific granules with dense internal crystalloid structures (Cr) of various shapes. These structures are best seen at higher magnification (B—×52,000) (Miller, 1966). The smaller granules do not contain crystals.
  Like the azurophil granules of the neutrophil, the eosinophil granules are lysosomes, containing several acid hydrolases, including acid phosphatases, and also peroxidase (see text). (From Fresco, R.: Ultrastructure of the blood cells and their precursors. *In* Davidsohn, I., and Henry, J. B.: Clinical Diagnosis by Laboratory Methods, 15th ed. Philadelphia, W. B. Saunders Company, 1974.)

100 times as numerous as the total eosinophils in the blood; they are located primarily in skin, lung, and gastrointestinal tract, i.e., the epithelial barriers to the outside world.

FUNCTION (BEESON, 1977)

The function of eosinophils is not completely understood. Eosinophils leave the blood when adrenal cortical hormone increases. Eosinophils proliferate in response to immunologic stimuli; this proliferative response is mediated, at least with some antigens, by T-lymphocytes. Although eosinophils phagocytose foreign particles and antigen-antibody complexes, this may not be their main function. There is evidence that eosinophils modulate reactions that occur when tissue mast cells and basophils degranulate. Among the chemotactic factors that attract eosinophils, ECF-A

(eosinophil chemotactic factor of anaphylaxis) is present in basophils and mast cells; also, eosinophils contain substances that inactivate factors released by mast cells and basophils, such as histamine, slow-reacting substances of anaphylaxis, and platelet-activating factor. According to Beeson (1977), except for providing some defense against helminthic parasites, the primary functions of eosinophils seem to be in their reactions with endogenous substances: products from mast cells and from lymphocytes, coagulation factors, complement, hormones, and kinins.

BASOPHILS AND MAST CELLS

Because there is no evidence for basophil development in *in vitro* colonies containing neutrophils and monocytes or eosinophils, it is possible that basophils develop from a separate committed precursor cell; there is, however, no evidence for this.

MORPHOLOGY

Air-dried films

Basophils probably develop from a cell resembling a myeloblast. The first recognizable stage is a *basophil myelocyte*, with the appearance of the specific basophil granules. These granules (about 0.2 to 1 μm in diameter) are larger than the azurophil granules of promyelocyte and often are irregular in shape. As the cell matures, the granules become more metachromatic (red-purple) because of increasing acid mucopolysaccharide (heparin) content. During maturation, cytoplasmic RNA decreases, and the nucleus partially segments. Because of incomplete nuclear segmentation, stages analogous to the neutrophil are not readily identified. In mature basophils the nucleus has condensed but smudged chromatin and the background cytoplasm lacks basophilia (residual RNA) (Plate 28-2*K* and *L*).

In contrast, *tissue mast cells* are connective tissue cells of mesenchymal origin that contain metachromatic cytoplasmic granules. They are widely distributed throughout the organism, including bone marrow, thymus, and spleen, but they do not normally appear in blood. On Romanowsky-stained films (Plate 28-2*M*) they are usually larger than basophils and have a low N/C ratio and a round or oval reticular nucleus which is usually obscured by abundant red-purple granules. The granules are smaller, more round and regular, and less soluble than basophil granules. The cytoplasmic granules are often spindle-shaped rather than round.

Electron microscopy (Fig. 28-14)

The basophil granules are difficult to fix satisfactorily and show differing appearances, probably on this basis; these include fine gran-

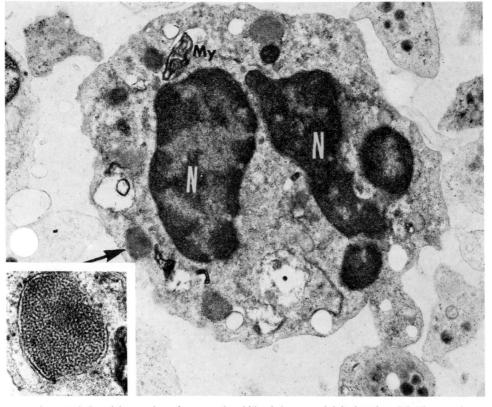

Figure 28-14. (×13,200). *Basophilic granulocyte* from peripheral blood showing a bilobed nucleus (N). The cytoplasm contains rare small mitochondria, a few profiles of rough endoplasmic reticulum, some free ribosomes and glycogen particles, and several specific granules. Some of these have lost their contents, leaving clear vacuoles lying close to the periphery of the cell. Myelin figures (My) are present in close association with the ruptured granules. One of the intact specific granules (arrow) is shown at higher magnification in the inset at the lower left-hand corner. It is bound by a "unit membrane" and is filled with uniform-sized particles, some of which are arranged in rows along and concentric with the unit membrane (×52,000) (Zucker-Franklin, 1967). (From Fresco, R.: Ultrastructure of the blood cells and their precursors. *In* Davidsohn, I., and Henry, J. B.: Clinical Diagnosis by Laboratory Methods, 15th ed. Philadelphia, W. B. Saunders Company, 1974.)

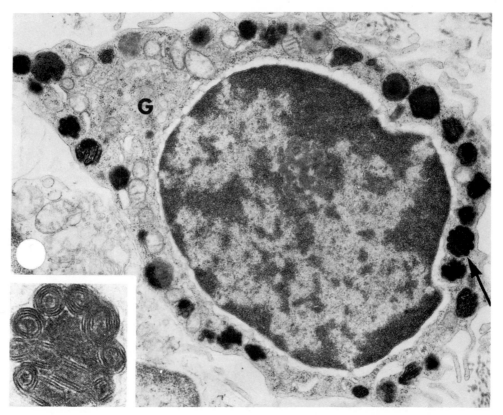

Figure 28–15 (×18,000). Though they bear a close functional relationship to the blood basophils and show similarities in the chemical composition and tinctorial qualities of their granules, the *tissue mast cells* (×18,000) show distinctive ultrastructural features. There is a single, rounded or oval nucleus. Several mitochondria are present in the cytoplasm, as well as a few profiles of rough endoplasmic reticulum and ribosomal clusters. A Golgi complex (G) is found in the upper left, close to the nucleus. Most of the cytoplasm is filled with large electron-dense granules showing a complex internal organization. This is demonstrated by the granule indicated by the arrow, which is seen at higher magnification in the inset at the lower left-hand corner. Bound by a unit membrane, it contains structures which, when cut longitudinally, appear as parallel lines, and when seen in cross-section have a spiral configuration. These have been called scroll forms but could also be described as resembling locks of hair in curlers(!) (×75,000). The fine structure and cytochemical composition of mast cell granules vary considerably in different species. The scroll-like lamellae appear to be characteristic of human mast cells (Kobayasi, 1968) but their composition is as yet unknown. Like basophils, mast cell granules are rich in heparin and histamine, and in some species, but not in man, also contain serotonin. (From Fresco, R.: Ultrastructure of the blood cells and their precursors. *In* Davidsohn, I., and Henry, J. B.: Clinical Diagnosis by Laboratory Methods, 15th ed. Philadelphia, W. B. Saunders Company, 1974.)

ules, crystals, and myelin figures (Parwaresch, 1976). It is probable that only one type of basophil granule exists; there is no convincing evidence to the contrary (Cawley, 1973).

Mast cell granules have a different ultrastructural appearance (Fig. 28-15).

KINETICS

Because the basophil is relatively the least numerous of the leukocytes, the kinetics have been difficult to discover and information is sparse. Production is believed to be similar to that of the neutrophil and eosinophil. Its time in the marrow is probably somewhat shorter than that of the neutrophil, and its half-time in the blood is about the same. Its fate in the tissues is not well understood.

FUNCTION

With regard to circulating numbers, basophils respond to adrenal cortex hormones in similar fashion to eosinophils.

Basophil granules contain histamine, heparin, and peroxidase (Dvorak, 1975). Basophils synthesize and store histamine and eosinophil chemotactic factor of anaphylaxis (ECF-A). They synthesize and release slow-reacting substance of anaphylaxis (SRS-A) and probably platelet activating factor (PAF) at the time of stimulation, but do not store them. Basophils lack hydrolytic enzymes such as alkaline and acid phosphatase, at least in significant amounts. Glycogen is abundant outside the granules. Though ultrastructurally different, mast cells have similar cytochemical characteristics except for the presence of proteolytic enzymes and serotonin, which basophils lack. In tissues the two cell types appear to function in a similar manner.

Basophils (as well as mast cells) appear to be involved in immediate hypersensitivity reactions, such as allergic asthma (Dvorak, 1975). Immunoglobulin E (reagin) binds readily to basophil and mast cell membranes. When specific antigen reacts with the membrane-bound IgE, degranulation occurs with the release of mediators of immediate hypersensitivity, e.g., histamine, SRS-A, PAF, heparin, and ECF-A. The latter leads to the accumulation of eosinophils, which contain substances that tend to counteract these mediators (Beeson, 1977). Basophils are also involved in some delayed hypersensitivity reactions, "cutaneous basophil hypersensitivity," such as contact allergies, in which they appear to undergo a different type of degranulation response (Dvorak, 1975).

MONOCYTES AND MACROPHAGES

Monocytes share the same committed progenitor cell as neutrophils, the GM-CFC (Figure 28-1).

MORPHOLOGY

Air-dried films

In normal marrow it is not possible to distinguish the "monoblast" from the myeloblast. The earliest recognizable cell in this series is the *promonocyte*, which is 15 to 20 μm in diameter, somewhat larger than the myeloblast. The N/C ratio is moderate, and the nucleus may be oval or indented with a fine uniform or slightly streaked chromatin pattern and two to five nucleoli. The cytoplasm is basophilic with a ground-glass appearance and a variable number of fine azurophilic granules (Plate 28-3A). The *monocyte*, which is present in both blood and marrow, is only slightly smaller, has a moderate to low N/C ratio, and an indented or lobed nucleus with a finely streaked, only slightly condensed, delicate chromatin pattern. Nucleoli are indistinct or obscured. The cytoplasm is opaque, more grey than blue, and contains an abundance of fine azurophilic granules (Plate 28-3B).

Electron microscopy

The granules in *promonocytes* have a characteristic peripheral clear zone not seen in later stages. The Golgi zone is well developed, there is moderately abundant rough-surfaced endoplasmic reticulum (RER), and small bundles of microfibrils are frequently seen (Cawley, 1973). The mature monocyte is depicted in Figure 28-16. As the monocyte transforms into a macrophage, in its tissue phase, the cytoplasm increases in extent, the azurophilic granules disappear as they are used in the digestive processes, and large numbers of digestive vacuoles are present. Rough surfaced endoplasmic reticulin, mitochondria, and Golgi apparatus all increase in amount, and a large number of small, coated vesicles appear (Nichols, 1971).

In the promonocyte stage the granules contain acid hydrolase, arylsulfatase, and peroxidase; they represent primary lysosomes. There may be more than one type of granule (Cawley, 1973). As the cell matures, peroxidase activity diminishes and acid phosphatase and arylsulfatase activity increases. The enzyme activity is in the RER, Golgi zone, coated vesicles, and digestive vacuoles, suggesting that in the macrophage the coated vesicles are a second form of primary lysosome that shuttles hydrolytic enzymes from the Golgi to the digestive vacuoles (Bainton, 1976).

KINETICS

After promonocytes are formed, they undergo two mitotic divisions in a period of about 50 to 60 hours before being released into the blood (Meuret, 1974). Under conditions of increased demand, the cycle time can shorten, with earlier release of more immature cells into the blood. Blood monocytes are distributed in a circulating monocyte pool and a marginal monocyte pool, in a ratio of 1 to 3.5 (Meuret, 1973). Once monocytes enter the blood, they leave randomly with a half-time of 8.4 hours; this time period is shortened in splenomegaly or acute infection, and may be prolonged in monocytosis. After monocytes leave the blood, they spend several months, perhaps longer, in the tissue phase.

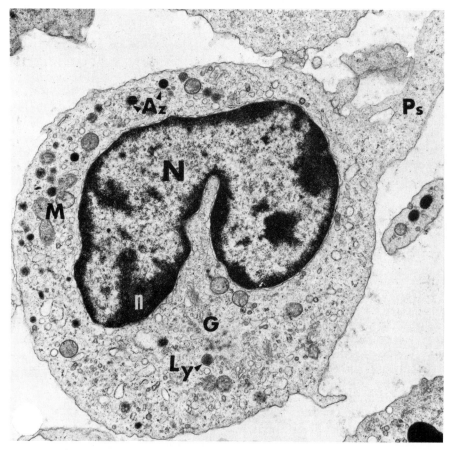

Figure 28–16 ($\times$ 12,400).   The *monocyte* has a horseshoe-shaped nucleus (N), with clumped chromatin occurring predominantly adjacent to the nuclear membrane. A nucleolus (n) is present. The cytoplasm is more abundant than in the lymphocyte, shows a better developed Golgi complex (G), several mitochondria (M), scattered free ribosomes, numerous vesicles of various sizes, as well as lysosomal (Ly) and denser azurophilic (Az) granules. The abundance of these various organelles is responsible for the "ground glass" appearance of the cytoplasm as seen by the light microscope. A large pseudopod (Ps) extends in the right upper corner. (From Fresco, R.: Ultrastructure of the blood cells and their precursors. *In* Davidsohn, I., and Henry, J. B.: Clinical Diagnosis by Laboratory Methods, 15th ed. Philadelphia, W. B. Saunders Company, 1974.)

FUNCTION (CLINE, 1975; 1977)

The monocyte is formed in the marrow, transported by the blood, and migrates into the tissues where it transforms into a histiocyte or macrophage (p. 905; Plate 27-2*I*) to spend the majority of its life span. The blood monocytes and tissue macrophages make up a mononuclear phagocyte system (reticuloendothelial system).

The mononuclear phagocyte system has an important role in defense against microorganisms, including mycobacteria, fungi, bacteria, protozoa, and viruses. The cells are motile and respond to chemotactic factors (complement components and factors from activated lymphocytes); they become immobilized by migration-inhibition factor (MIF) from activated lymphocytes. They engage in phagocytosis, a process that is enhanced if the particle is coated by IgG or complement for which the macrophages have membrane receptors. After phagocytosis, they kill ingested microorganisms.

These mononuclear phagocytes are an integral part of both humoral and cell mediated immunity. They handle or process antigens, providing contact of the antigen (or antigenic information) with lymphocytes. They also respond to various lymphokines and act as effector (e.g., cytotoxic) cells in the cell-mediated immune response.

Macrophages remove and process senescent cells and debris through phagocytosis and digestion: for example, erythrocytes, leukocytes, megakaryocyte nuclei by macrophages in the marrow; inhaled particulate material by alveolar macrophages in the lungs.

Macrophages may be "activated" by either specific factors (e.g., cytophilic antibody) or non-specific factors (e.g., in response to phag-ocytized material). Activation results in en-largement of the cell and enhanced me-tabolism, phagocytosis, microbicidal activity, cytotoxicity, etc.

Macrophages also synthesize and secrete several biologically active molecules such as certain complement components, transferrin, muramidase, and interferon. An important role in regulation of hematopoietic activity may be played by GM-CSF, the colony-stimu-lating factor for neutrophils and macrophages (p. 919; Metcalf, 1977). Although GM-CSF may be found in serum and urine, it is likely that its biologic activity is at shorter range, as it is secreted by macrophages in the marrow. It has been shown *in vitro* that when GM-CSF in-creases beyond a critical concentration, mac-rophages then produce prostaglandin E (PGE), which inhibits the response of the GM-CFC, opposing the effect of GM-CSF (Kurland, 1978). Thus, the net myeloproliferative activ-ity of monocyte and neutrophil may be deter-mined by the balance between GM-CSF and PGE, both produced by the mononuclear phagocyte.

This system, therefore, appears to have multiple functions which include host defense, some control of hematopoiesis, and policing of the environment within the body (Cline, 1977).

MEGAKARYOCYTES

Platelets originate in the marrow from megakaryocytes, which are the largest of all hematopoietic cells and number less than 1 per cent of the total nucleated marrow cells. They arise from the multipotential hematopoietic stem cell, probably directly from a committed progenitor cell (Fig. 28-1). It is likely that megakaryocyte proliferation is regulated by the action of a humoral substance (analogous to erythropoietin) called *thrombopoietin*. The evidence for this, however, is incomplete (Ebbe, 1976).

MORPHOLOGY

Air-dried films

The *megakaryoblast* is the earliest cell in this series. By the time it is recognizable, it is 20 to 30 μm in diameter and has basophilic cytoplasm and an oval to irregularly lobulated nucleus (Plate 28-3*D*). The chromatin pattern is reticular and somewhat densely staining; nucleoli are small. Megakaryoblasts engage in DNA synthesis and division of the nucleus several times, without cytoplasmic division, a process known as endomitosis. The ploidy var-ies from 4N to 64N; about two thirds are 16N; 8N and 32N each account for about one sixth of the total. DNA synthesis is virtually com-plete before the nucleus enlarges or begins to form lobules.

In the *promegakaryocyte*, nuclear segmen-tation has become visible, and the cytoplasm has a basophilic granularity. Near the nucleus, fine red-pink granules begin to appear (in the Golgi region) and spread throughout the cyto-plasm. A peripheral hyaline (clear) basophilic zone may be evident.

In the *megakaryocyte*, cytoplasmic baso-philia has disappeared and red-pink granules fill the cytoplasm. At first the granules are diffusely distributed; later they cluster in small aggregates (Plate 28-3*E*, lower and upper cells, respectively). The nucleus is irreg-ularly lobulated; the number of lobes does not correlate precisely with ploidy. The nuclear chromatin, though intensely staining, is rather dispersed early, but later becomes more compact and dense. Small nucleoli may be vis-ible. (*Note:* Nucleoli are *small* at all stages of megakaryocyte development.) Platelets are shed as cytoplasmic fragments (Plate 28-3*F*) by fusion of demarcation membranes (Fig. 28-18). In the marrow, the megakaryocyte is adjacent to the sinus wall, and platelets are released into the lumen.

Electron microscopy
(Figs. 28-17, 28-18, and 28-19)

Granules are formed from the Golgi com-plexes; they are electron dense, about 0.2 μm in diameter, and encompassed by a unit mem-brane. Demarcation membranes, which form from the confluence of cytoplasmic mem-branes and vesicles, are the walls of channels which are in contact with the outside of the cell. When they fuse with one another, frag-ments of megakaryocyte cytoplasm (the platelets) are released. The ultrastructure of platelets is considered in Chapter 32.

MEGAKARYOCYTES IN BLOOD

Whole megakaryocytes or fragments may occasionally be found in normal blood films. If buffy coat films are examined, they are con-

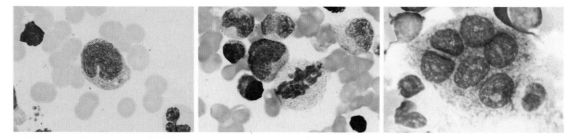

A   B   C

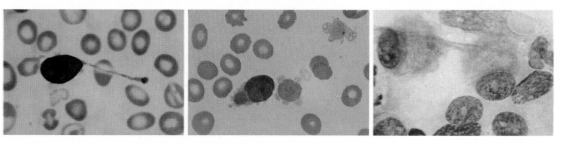

D   E   F

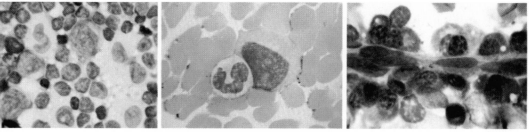

G   H   I

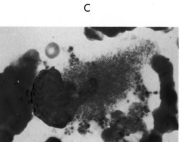

J   K   L

Plate 28-3. *A,* Promonocyte. Multiple fine granules and a deeply indented nucleus help identify this cell as a monocyte. That this is an immature monocyte is evident from the delicate nuclear chromatin, obvious nucleoli, and blue-tinted cytoplasm. *B,* Three neutrophil metamyelocytes at the top, a monocyte in the center of the group of cells, a small plasma cell, and a neutrophil myelocyte in mitosis. *C,* Osteoclast. Separate nuclei with relatively large nucleoli are the major features that distinguish this cell from a megakaryocyte. *D,* Megakaryoblast. *E,* Early megakaryocyte (bottom); the later megakaryocyte at the top has more compact nuclear material and clustering of granules. *F,* Megakaryocyte, releasing platelets. *G,* Megakaryocyte nuclear fragment with long strand of cytoplasmic material. *H,* Dwarf megakaryocyte and two atypical platelets from the blood of a patient with myelofibrosis with myeloid metaplasia. The atypical platelets are large, lack the normal number of granules, and have pseudopods. *I,* Osteoblasts. The eccentric nucleus, reticular chromatin pattern, large nucleolus, basophilic cytoplasm, and large pale Golgi zone separated from the nucleus are characteristic. *J,* Lymph node imprint from a patient with reactive lymph node hyperplasia. Note four or five histiocytes with abundant cytoplasm; numerous small lymphocytes; and stages in blast transformation, including three large reticular lymphocytes (non-leukemic lymphoblasts). *K,* Reticular lymphocyte (non-leukemic lymphoblast) in the blood of a patient with atypical pneumonitis and increased cold agglutinins. Note the large nucleoli, reticular nuclear chromatin, and moderately abundant, opaque, basophilic cytoplasm. *L,* Plasma cells lining sinusoidal endothelium in a marrow film from a patient with rheumatoid arthritis. In reactive plasmacytosis in marrow, plasma cells are frequently oriented in this manner. The chromatin in coarse blocks and the pale Golgi zone immediately adjacent to the nucleus are in contrast to the appearance of osteoblasts (Plate 28–3*I*).

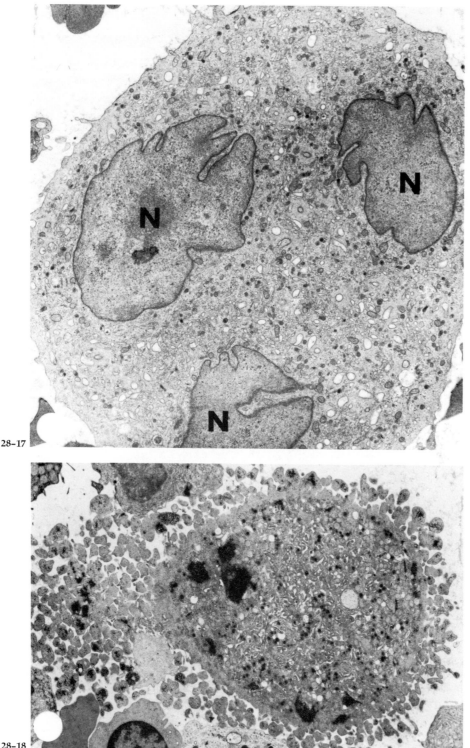

28–17

28–18

Figures 28–17 and 28–18. The *megakaryocytes* are the largest cells found in the normal bone marrow, sometimes measuring up to 150 μm in diameter. They have large multilobed nuclei. Figure 28–17 (×6000) is an electron micrograph of a developing megakaryocyte showing three nuclear lobes (N) with irregular borders, the lobe on the left showing a nucleolus. The abundant cytoplasm contains numerous electron-dense granules, small Golgi complexes, and small round mitochondria, as well as numerous vesicles. These vesicles elongate, coalesce, and become continuous with the cell surface; these *demarcation membranes* "mark off" segments of cytoplasm (containing organelles) that will become platelets when the membranes fuse (Fig. 28–18—×4400). Channels enclosed by the demarcation membranes are continuous with the interstitial fluid outside the cell. (From Fresco, R.: Ultrastructure of the blood cells and their precursors. *In* Davidsohn, I., and Henry, J. B.: Clinical Diagnosis by Laboratory Methods, 15th ed. Philadelphia, W. B. Saunders Company, 1974.)

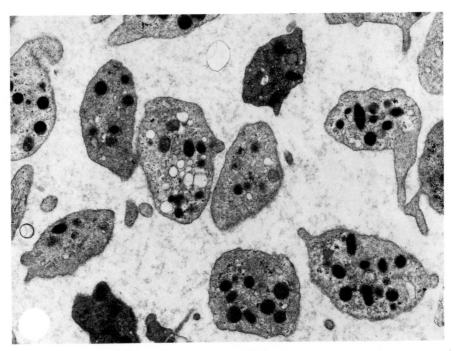

Figure 28–19 (× 13,200). *Platelets.* As seen in Figure 28–18, the *platelets* are fragments of the megakaryocyte cytoplasm and, as such, have no nucleus and rarely show structures such as Golgi complexes and endoplasmic reticulum, but retain organelles or inclusions such as vesicles, mitochondria, electron-dense granules, and glycogen particles from the megakaryocyte (Fig. 28–17). The circulating human platelets are disc-shaped structures with an average diameter of 2 μm but can easily acquire irregular shapes during processing for electron microscopy through the action of anticoagulants, centrifugation, cold fixatives, and, in fact, almost any stimulus. (From Fresco, R.: Ultrastructure of the blood cells and their precursors. *In* Davidsohn, I., and Henry, J. B.: Clinical Diagnosis by Laboratory Methods, 15th ed. Philadelphia, W. B. Saunders Company, 1974.)

sistently present. Efrati (1960) found mega-karyocytes in all of 55 normal individuals studied, an average of 22 per ml of venous blood. Megakaryocytes are frequently found in the capillaries of the lungs. Kaufman (1965a) presented experimental data suggesting that pulmonary megakaryocytes do not originate in the lungs but are carried there in venous blood; they calculated that 7 to 17 per cent of the body's platelets may be released from pulmonary capillaries (Kaufman, 1965b).

Megakaryocyte fragments in blood films may be as small as lymphocytes and are recognized by the deeply stained chromatin (which has sharper chromatin-parachromatin separation than do lymphocytes) and by fragments of attached megakaryocyte cytoplasm (Plate 28–3G). They are found more frequently than normal in myelophthisic processes, myeloproliferative disorders, or after stress or injury to the marrow.

Dwarf megakaryocytes (Plate 28–3H), on the other hand, show evidence of abnormal megakaryopoiesis: agranular cytoplasm with hyaloplasmic zones or pseudopods; and association with large atypical platelets having sim-ilar cytoplasmic characteristics. These abnormal dwarf megakaryocytes are rarely found in any condition except myeloproliferative disorders, and they are especially apt to be found in myelofibrosis with myeloid metaplasia (p. 1074).

KINETICS

The maturation time for megakaryocytes in the marrow is about five days in man. Platelets are released into the marrow sinuses over a period of several hours, and the megakaryocyte nuclei are phagocytosed by macrophages. Newly released platelets appear larger, more active metabolically, and more effective hemostatically (Fig. 32–11). Platelets circulate at a stable concentration that averages $250 \times 10^9/l$. At any one time, about two thirds of the total platelets are in the circulation, and about one third are present in the spleen. In asplenic individuals, 100 per cent of platelets are circulating; on the other hand, in diseases characterized by splenic enlargement 80 to 90 per cent of platelets are sequestered in the spleen, resulting in a decreased concentration of circulating platelets (thrombocytopenia) on the basis of this altered distribution (Aster, 1977).

Platelets survive 8 to 11 days in the circulation. Some platelets are probably utilized in maintaining vascular integrity and in plugging small vascular injuries (random loss), and others are probably removed by the mononuclear phagocytic system when they become senescent.

FUNCTION

Platelets normally function in (1) maintaining the integrity (leak-free state) of blood vessels; and (2) forming hemostatic plugs to stop blood loss from injured vessels, and, in the process, promoting coagulation of plasma factors. These matters are considered in Chapters 32 and 33.

LYMPHOCYTES

PRIMARY LYMPHOID TISSUE

According to current concepts (Craddock, 1971), during fetal life lymphocyte precursors originate in the bone marrow and are influenced or programmed to perform a certain function by one of the primary lymphoid organs, either the thymus gland for T-lymphocytes or the "bursal equivalent" for B-lymphocytes. A distinct organ, the bursa of Fabricius, is present in birds and serves as the primary site of B-lymphocyte development. In man and other mammals a bursal equivalent is postulated to exist; evidence in mice suggests that the fetal liver may be a primary site of B lymphocyte development (Owen, 1974). Lymphopoiesis within primary lymphoid organs is vigorous and antigen independent.

Thymus

The human thymus has two parts. The cortex is populated predominantly by small lymphocytes with a few scattered epithelial cells. In contrast, the medulla is composed mostly of epithelial cells with a small component of lymphocytes. The cortex is subdivided by several fibrous septa extending from the capsule to the medullary region. In the medulla, Hassall's corpuscles are present. Hassall's corpuscles are small islands of partially hyalinized epithelial cells of no known functional significance (Douglas, 1977). The thymus reaches a maximum size (approximately 40 g) during adolescence and then gradually undergoes involutional changes. Some functional activity may be present throughout life.

SECONDARY LYMPHOID TISSUE

In late fetal and postnatal life, lymphocytes are produced in the secondary lymphoid tissue: spleen, lymph nodes, and intestine-associated lymphoid tissue. Lymphocytes of the secondary lymphoid organs are progeny from stem cells which have been influenced by primary lymphoid organs. The secondary lymphoid organs are thus composed of a mixture of B cells and T cells. Lymphopoiesis in secondary lymphoid organs depends solely on antigenic stimulation (Miller, 1977). B cells and T cells tend to localize in anatomically distinct parts of the lymphoid tissue where proliferation can take place.

Lymph nodes

Lymph nodes are surrounded by a fibrous capsule which is penetrated by afferent lymphatic vessels. These afferent lymphatic vessels carry lymph and lymphoid cells into the subcapsular sinus. The intermediate and radial sinuses bring the lymph from the subcapsular sinus to the efferent lymphatics in the medullary portion of the node. The outer layer of the lymph node (cortex) contains nodules of lymphocytes (primary and secondary follicles). Some of these nodules contain a center (germinal center) composed of macrophages and lymphoid cells of various stages of maturation. When a germinal center is present, the nodule is referred to as a secondary follicle. A strip of loosely packed lymphoid cells is present between follicles (paracortical areas) and as cords extending into the medullary areas (medullary cords). Macrophages capable of phagocytizing antigen line the sinuses. Dendritic macrophages, located in the germinal center, localize and retain antigen. B cells are located predominantly in the germinal centers and in the medullary cords. Although a few T cells are located in germinal centers, T cells are principally found in the paracortical areas.

Spleen

The spleen is divisible grossly into *white pulp* (lymphoid area) and red pulp (vascular sinuses and blood). The white pulp is composed of lymphocytes forming a sheath (periarteriolar lymphocyte sheath) around central arteries and its tributaries. T cells are located within the periarteriolar lymphocytic sheath. B cells are present in the primary and secondary follicles, which are in and around the sheath. Surrounding the germinal center is a mantle of small lymphocytes.

The *red pulp* is a network of branching sinuses separated from each other by the splenic cords, which are filled with a variety of cellular blood elements.

The sinuses and cords receive blood from tributaries of the central artery (arteries of the red pulp or penicilliary arteries). Blood cells that have entered the cords must regain the circulation through narrow (3 μm diameter) apertures in the sinusoidal wall. Cells that are inflexible or otherwise abnormal may be trapped and destroyed in the cords. The contents of the venous sinuses, in turn, flow into the pulp veins, trabecular veins, capsular veins, and finally the splenic vein (Weiss, 1977).

The marginal zone represents the junction between the periarterial lymphatic sheath and the red pulp. In the marginal zone small recirculating lymphocytes may leave the venous sinuses and enter the lymphatic sheath.

LYMPHOCYTE FUNCTION AND PHYSIOLOGY (Craddock, 1971)

Those lymphocytes influenced by the thymus (thymus-dependent lymphocytes or T cells) and their progeny function in cell-mediated immunity, which includes delayed hypersensitivity, graft rejection, graft-versus-host reactions, defense against intracellular organisms (such as tubercle bacillus and brucella), and probably defense against neoplasms. The lymphocytes influenced by the bursal equivalent (bursa-dependent lymphocytes or B cells) and their progeny perform in humoral immunity, or the production of antibodies, either as a lymphocyte or after transformation into a plasma cell.

The majority of the circulating lymphocytes are T cells, which have a life span of months to years. The B cells are a minor population (10 to

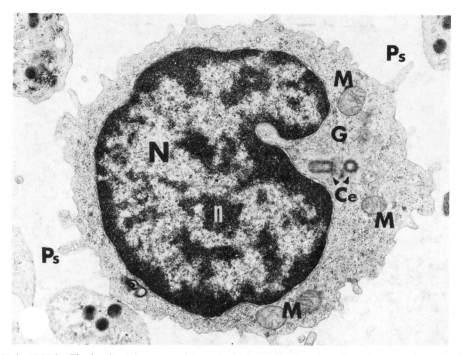

Figure 28-20 (×15,000).   The *lymphocyte* has a round, or as in this case slightly indented, nucleus (N) with highly condensed chromatin. It is this dense chromatin which obscures the nucleolus (n) in conventionally stained blood smears, but which is often seen in thin sections and in electron micrographs. Thus, the mere presence of a nucleolus does not denote cell immaturity. A relatively scanty cytoplasm surrounds the nucleus. A poorly developed Golgi complex (G) and a pair of centrioles (Ce) arranged at right angles to one another are seen close to the nuclear indentation. Free ribosomes are distributed throughout the cytoplasm, and a few mitochondria (M) are present. Several small pseudopods (Ps) project from the surface. (From Fresco, R.: Ultrastructure of the blood cells and their precursors. *In* Davidsohn, I., and Henry, J. B.: Clinical Diagnosis by Laboratory Methods, 15th ed. Philadelphia, W. B. Saunders Company, 1974.)

20 per cent of the lymphocytes), probably have a short life span measured in days, and are distinguished by the presence of considerable immunoglobulin on their surface membrane.

Lymphocytes, especially T cells, recirculate from blood to lymph; in the postcapillary venule in lymphoid tissue the lymphocyte travels from the blood through the endothelium and into the lymphoid tissue, where it may stay or percolate through and return to the blood via the thoracic duct lymph. Small lymphocytes (Plate 28-3*J*) have little cytoplasm and, in electron micrographs, few organelles and relatively little RNA (Fig. 28-20). After antigenic stimulation, small lymphocytes (B cells or T cells, depending on the nature of the antigen) become activated, increase their RNA synthesis, and undergo blast transformation. On Wright's stained films, these blasts are large cells (15 to 25 μm) with abundant rather deep blue cytoplasm, a large reticular nucleus with uniform chromatin, and prominent nucleoli (Plate 28-3*J* and *K*). This is the cell which is called the *reticular lymphocyte* (non-leukemic lymphoblast; "immunoblast"). If the blasts are derived from B cells, the new lymphocytes function in the production of antibodies (B cells, plasma cells); or, if the blasts are derived from T cells, the progeny act in the cellular immune response. The latter is mediated by several soluble factors produced by the activated T cell, including transfer factor, which can transfer the capacity for delayed hypersensitivity to another cell; lymphotoxin, which is directly toxic to cells; and migratory inhibition factor, which promotes adherence of macrophages and keeps them at the site.

Plasma cells have abundant blue cytoplasm, often with light streaks or vacuoles, an eccentric round nucleus, and a well-defined clear (Golgi) zone adjacent to the nucleus. The nucleus of the plasma cell has heavily clumped chromatin, which is sharply defined from the parachromatin, and often arranged in a radial or "wheel-like" pattern (Plate 27-2*H* and 28-3*L*).

In electron micrographs (Fig. 28-21) the large, relatively central Golgi area appears to displace the nucleus to the side. The abundant rough-surfaced endoplasmic reticulum and large Golgi area are characteristic of cells which are producing protein for secretion outside of the cell (e.g., immunoglobulins). This is in contrast to the abundance of non-membrane-bound polyribosomes in cells synthesizing protein for use within the cell; an example

is the basophilic normoblast, synthesizing hemoglobin (see Fig. 28-2). Both cell types are intensely basophilic with Wright's stain, because of the high RNA content.

BONE MARROW EXAMINATION

Marrow aspiration biopsy, introduced by Arinkin in 1929, was considered at first a formidable and highly specialized procedure. It is now widely used in the diagnosis of hematologic diseases and many conditions not primarily affecting the blood system. A number of techniques have been devised by which a suitable specimen of marrow can be obtained with little discomfort to the patient. The simple aspiration type of biopsy can be carried out as an office procedure on ambulatory patients. The risks involved are minimal. They compare favorably with ordinary venipuncture and are less traumatizing than a lumbar puncture. As for any other special procedure, however, the indications for marrow examination should be clear. In each instance the physician should have in mind some reasonable prediction of its result and consequent benefit to the patient. Without exception, the peripheral blood should be examined carefully first. It is a relatively uncommon circumstance to find hematologic disease in the bone marrow either earlier or more certainly than evidence of it can be discovered in the peripheral blood. If an examiner is not able to find at least suggestive evidence of abnormality referable to the marrow from the clinical data or the study of the peripheral blood, he is not likely to do better with the marrow.

It is estimated that the weight of the marrow in the adult is 1300 to 1500 g. A unique feature of this organ is its lability. It can undergo complete transformation in a few days and occasionally even in a few hours. As a rule, this rapid transformation involves the whole organ, as evidenced by the fact that a small sample represented by a biopsy or aspiration is usually fairly representative of the whole marrow. This conclusion is in accord with results of studies of biopsy samples simultaneously removed from several sites. According to these observations, the various sites chosen for removal of marrow for studies are in most instances equally good. Consequently, the difficulty of access, the risks involved, the ease of obtaining a good biopsy, and the discomfort of the patient are the main reasons

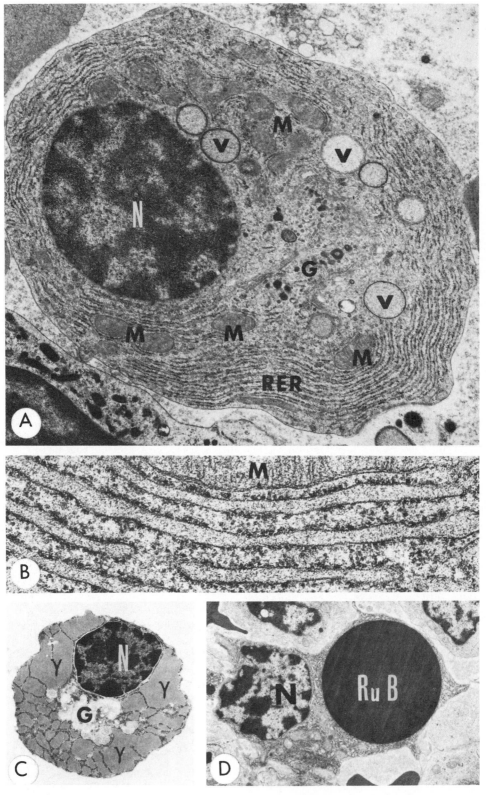

Figure 28–21. *See legend on opposite page.*

for selection of a site in the particular patient. Occasionally the failure to obtain quantitatively or qualitatively adequate material in one site may be followed by success in another location. Also, the need for repeated aspirations or biopsies may indicate the use of several different sites. We regard the posterior iliac crest as the preferred site. The large marrow space allows both aspiration and biopsy to be performed with ease at one time.

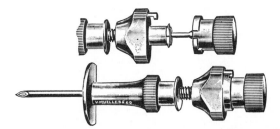

Figure 28–22. University of Illinois sternal needle with adjustable guard, special locking device for the stylet, and Luer-Lok hub set into the needle. (Courtesy of V. Mueller and Co., Chicago.)

TECHNIQUE OF MARROW ASPIRATION BIOPSY

In the adult patient, the sternum, the spinous processes of the vertebrae, and the anterior or posterior iliac crest are readily accessible areas from which bone marrow material can be obtained. In infants the upper end of the tibia may be conveniently used to obtain marrow. The various methods of obtaining and handling material are essentially identical in principle so that comparable results are achieved by workers of equal skill and experience.

Surgical biopsy has been largely replaced by aspiration and needle biopsy techniques which have the advantages of simplicity and less discomfort to the patient. Stained sections are not as suitable for accurate differentiation of cell types as the smeared preparations. In addition to aspiration, needle biopsy should be used when it is important to see the cells in their anatomic relation to one another and to the inactive fat or connective tissue stroma (as in aplastic anemia and myelofibrosis) or in diseases that produce focal rather than diffuse changes (Hodgkin's disease, multiple myeloma, malignant lymphoma, metastatic tumors, granulomatous diseases, and so forth). Histologic examination may also be performed with aspirated marrow particles (fragments of marrow tissue) which are clotted together with thrombin and plasma, placed in fixative, and processed for tissue sectioning. Histologic sections of needle biopsy and of aspirated particles will usually yield sufficient information in the situations mentioned above so that surgical biopsy will be unnecessary.

The technique for handling aspirated marrow outlined here is known to yield good films and to show reasonably smooth distribution of cells, and it can be carried out with a minimum of technical complexity.

Equipment. The needle must be of stout construction, properly molded for a firm grasp, with a short bevel and well-fitted stylet. The lumen needs to be rather large, not less than about 14 gauge. Several varieties of needles are available. A widely used needle is the University of Illinois sternal needle* (Fig. 28–22). It has an adjustable guard, which, when properly set, will prevent perforation of the inner plate of the sternum. With each complete turn the guard moves 1 mm. The stylet can be fixed firmly. A small needle of same construction is available for infants and children.

The Jamshidi bone marrow biopsy needle† (Fig. 28–23) is preferred for biopsies of adequate size and free of crushing artifact (Jamshidi, 1971). The tapered distal end of the biopsy needle makes loss of the sample less probable. Biopsies 1 to 3 cm long and 2 mm in diameter are easily obtained.

Other biopsy needles, such as the Westerman-Jensen and the stout Vim-Silverman needles, are also satisfactory.

Clean glass slides, coverslips, test tubes, and watch glasses should be available.

Ten- or 20-ml syringes are preferred over smaller sizes because they allow a stronger pull. Syringes

---

*V. Mueller & Co., Chicago, Ill.

† Kor Med Corporation, Minneapolis, Minn.

Figure 28–21. *A* ($\times 132,000$), The mature plasma cell from the bone marrow has a round eccentric nucleus (N) with clumped chromatin occurring mostly at the periphery, a distribution responsible for the wheel-like appearance seen by light microscopy. The salient ultrastructural feature of the plasma cell is the presence of abundant arrays of well-packed rough-surfaced endoplasmic reticulum (RER) throughout most of the cytoplasm. The cell also displays a prominent Golgi complex (G) composed of stacks of flattened sacs and vesicles, lined by smooth membranes. Several of the peripheral vesicles (V) are dilated, some containing a fluffy material. Several mitochondria (M) are present, mostly at the periphery of the Golgi complex. The RER is responsible for the basophilia of the cytoplasm seen in the light microscope, and the paranuclear clear zone or "Hof" of the German authors is due to the Golgi and adjacent mitochondria.

The RER is seen at higher magnification (B— $\times 68,000$) to consist of flattened membranous sacs containing finely granular material and lined on the outer surfaces by electron-dense ribosomes. These ribosomes are the sites of antibody formation. The newly synthesized immunoglobulins accumulate in the cisternae. Sometimes the cisternae become distended by the globulin (γ) as is seen in C ($\times 6600$), forming what has been called a "flame cell." The lack of demonstrable membranes in this cell is due to aldehyde fixation without postosmication. Occasionally plasma cells show localized, dense, rounded accumulations of protein, known as Russell bodies (Ru B) (D— $\times 5500$). (From Fresco, R.: Ultrastructure of the blood cells and their precursors. *In* Davidsohn, I., and Henry, J. B.: Clinical Diagnosis by Laboratory Methods, 15th ed. Philadelphia, W. B. Saunders Company, 1974.)

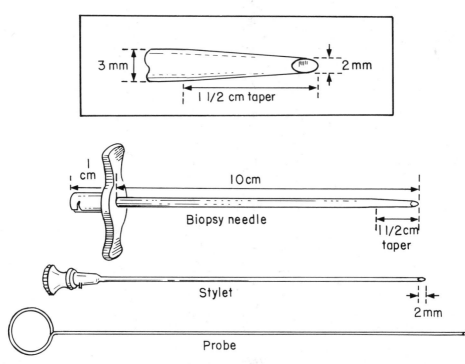

Figure 28–23. Jamshidi biopsy needle. The device has a uniform, external cylindrical configuration with a core of substantially constant internal diameter except for the tapered distal portion. The distal tip is beveled and has a sharp cutting edge. The interior diameter of the distal portion is tapered radially toward the cutting tip. This provides space within the interior of the instrument which has a larger diameter than the cutting tip, avoids compression of the tissue, and allows one to obtain specimens without plugging the lumen of the needle. The proximal end is calibrated for syringe attachment and has finger grips. The stylet is designed to interlock, to fit the tapered internal core, and projects 1 to 2 mm beyond the tip in order to protect the cutting edge and provide a means of entering the marrow. (From Jamshidi, K., and Swaim, W. R.: Bone marrow biopsy with unaltered architecture. J. Lab. Clin. Med., 77:335, 1971.)

with metal tips are preferable. An extra syringe and a *separate* small syringe for the anesthetic should be available.

Sterile equipment to be used by the operator should be ready on a marrow puncture tray. It should contain the following: towels, emesis basin, cotton sponges, hemostat, two 10-ml syringes preferably with metal tips, one 5-ml syringe, one 24-gauge hypodermic needle, one 22-gauge needle, a surgical blade (No. 11 Bard-Parker), and a marrow needle (University of Illinois type) wrapped and sterilized. In addition: several pairs of sterile rubber gloves, procaine, alcohol, iodine, or another local antiseptic (e.g., 4 per cent chlorhexidine solution), clean and preferably new glass slides, Band-Aids, and collodion.

If buffy coat films of aspirated marrow are to be made, EDTA is the preferred anticoagulant for preservation of cellular detail.

Iliac Crest Aspiration and Biopsy. Occasionally a mild, rapidly acting sedative may be useful, though for most patients it will be unnecessary.

The patient should be informed and reassured concerning the nature of the procedure to put him in the proper frame of mind. The next step is to put him at ease physically by having him lie comfortably on his side with his back flexed and knees drawn toward his chest.

The site for the puncture is selected. The posterior superior iliac spine is located and marked. With the use of sterile technique, the skin is prepared with an antiseptic solution over the entire posterior iliac crest and several centimeters around it. The field surrounding the puncture site is protected with a sterile drape or sterile towels. Sterile gloves are worn. Aseptic technique should be used during the operation.

Using a solution of 1 per cent procaine or lidocaine (Xylocaine), raise a skin wheal just over the posterior iliac spine. Change to the 22-gauge needle and infiltrate the subcutaneous tissue and the periosteum over a few square centimeter area of the iliac crest.

One must make sure that the patient is not sensitive to the particular anesthetic; if sensitivity is known or demonstrated, another should be chosen. Another recommended precaution is to withdraw the needle slightly at the start of the injection to make certain that the local anesthetic is not being injected intravenously.

A 3 mm skin incision avoids the possibility of pushing a plug of skin into the marrow cavity.

With its stylet in place and locked in position, the University of Illinois needle is grasped firmly and introduced vertically through the anesthetized area until its point impinges upon the outer table of the bone. The guard is screwed down until it touches the skin. It is then screwed back about four turns. Now, with steady pressure and a slight clockwise-counterclockwise rotation of the needle, push the needle firmly into the bone. A sudden loss of resistance may be felt as the needle enters the marrow cavity.

When the point of the needle is in the marrow, the stylet is removed and a 10- or 20-ml syringe is attached. Using sharp, firm aspiration, quickly withdraw not more than 0.2 to 0.3 ml of material. The small amount is more suitable for cytologic studies. When greater volumes are aspirated, sinusoidal blood predominates, and differential cell counts may be completely vitiated by dilution. A slightly larger amount may be drawn if the specimen is to be concentrated by centrifugation. Many patients experience pain or distress when marrow is being aspirated. Prepare the patient for the pain by warning him or her just before aspirating; it does not come as a surprise and is tolerated better. If material is not obtained at once, the stylet can be replaced and the needle advanced further after rotating back the guard.

The syringe and needle are removed and handed to an assistant who proceeds to make the slides. If a biopsy is not to be done, the operator places a sterile compress over the wound and holds it firmly in place for a few minutes. Then a sterile gauze or cotton bandage is taped over the wound, after making certain that its edges are approximated.

A biopsy can easily be performed through the same incision used for the aspiration. With the stylet in place, the operator now takes the Jamshidi biopsy needle and advances it through the skin incision to a point on the periosteum a centimeter or two superior to the previous site on the iliac crest. The needle is pointed toward the anterior iliac spine (in a slight superior and lateral direction) as it is firmly pushed through the bony cortex. When decreased resistance indicates that the marrow cavity has been entered, the stylet is removed and the biopsy needle is slowly and smoothly advanced while rotating it in a clockwise-counterclockwise manner. After 2 to 3 cm of further advance, the biopsy needle is rotated completely several times and then slowly removed while continuing a slight rotational motion. The wound is treated as described above. The probe is inserted through the distal cutting end to push the marrow core out of the biopsy needle.

The biopsy specimen, if handled gently, can be used for smears or imprints before being fixed in Zenker's acetic solution for 18 to 24 hours.

Sternal Aspiration. The same basic technique for preparation, anesthesia, and aspiration is used; of course, biopsy must not be performed in the sternum because of the danger of penetrating the inner cortex and piercing the heart or great vessels beneath.

The patient lies on his back with arms at his sides. Find the sternomanubrial prominence (angle of Louis) and, using a skin pencil, mark this with a horizontal line. Locate the jugular notch of the manubrium and mark the midline of the sternum in its long axis. The site of puncture in the body of the sternum will lie in the midline or slightly to one side of the midline, 1 to 2 cm below the angle of Louis, opposite the second interspace. This location is recommended because it contains marrow and is rarely deformed. The outer table in that region varies from 0.2 to 3 mm in thickness and the marrow cavity from 5 to 15 mm in depth. The area between the costal insertions should not be used; it may be cartilaginous. The manubrium itself should be avoided because it is often more fatty than the rest of the sternum.

The University of Illinois needle is especially recommended for sternal puncture. With the stylet in place, the needle is advanced vertically, at right angles to the sternum in the midline opposite the second interspace and placed firmly on the periosteum. The guard is rotated down until it is tightly flush with the skin, then rotated back three turns. Firm pushing with only slight rotation of the needle will advance the needle into the marrow cavity; the guard will prevent its going through the inner cortex (because it allows only a 3 mm advance from the outside of the outer cortex) (Fig. 28–22).

Aspiration is performed as described previously. Sternal aspiration should not be used in children before adolescence.

Anterior Iliac Crest Aspiration. The patient lies on his back. The puncture site is about 1 cm below the crest posterior to the anterior iliac spine. The needle is directed slightly cephalad.

Vertebral Spinous Process Aspiration. This site has the psychologic advantage that the patient cannot see the operation. The patient sits leaning forward or lies on his side or with his face down. The lower thoracic or lumbar vertebral spinous process is punctured. More pressure is needed than for sternal puncture. The needle should be inserted slightly to the side of the middle at a right angle to the skin surface.

Obtaining Marrow from Infants and Children

TIBIA. This site is frequently used in infants and may be used in children up to about two years of age. The preferable site for the puncture is the superior medial surface of the tibia, inferior to the medial condyle and medial to the tibial tuberosity.

POSTERIOR ILIAC CREST. The procedure is essentially the same as for the adult, except that a smaller needle is used. This is the most useful site for children after infancy as well as for adults.

Complications of Marrow Aspiration and Biopsy. Hematoma formation may occur if the patient has a bleeding tendency. Local pressure for several minutes will forestall this complication in most individuals.

Death has been reported from puncture of the heart and tamponade after an overaggressive sternal puncture. Caution is essential. Indications for the procedure should be observed. Neophytes should be carefully trained and closely supervised, especially with sternal marrow puncture.

PREPARATION OF THE ASPIRATE FOR EXAMINATION

Many procedures are in use and each has its advocates. The three most frequently used are marrow films, gross quantitative study, and histologic sections.

Marrow Films. Delay, no matter how brief, is undesirable. To avoid delay in handling aspirated bone marrow, it is well to have an assistant on hand to prepare the smears. When small amounts of material are taken as suggested previously, films can be made in a similar manner as for ordinary blood counts. Grey particles of marrow are usually seen with the naked eye. They are the best material for the preparation of good films and serve as landmarks for the microscopic examination of stained smears.

DIRECT FILMS. A drop of marrow is placed on a slide a short distance away from one end. A film 3 to 5 cm long is made with a spreader, not wider than 2 cm, dragging the particles behind but not *squashing* them. A trail of cells is left behind each particle.

IMPRINTS. Marrow particles can also be used for preparation of imprints. One or more visible particles are picked up with a capillary pipette, the broken end of a wooden applicator, or a toothpick and transferred immediately to a slide and made to stick to it by a gentle smearing motion. The slide is air dried rapidly by waving and then is stained.

CRUSH PREPARATIONS. Marrow particles in a small drop of aspirate may be placed on a slide near one end. Another slide is carefully placed over the first. Slight pressure is exerted to crush the particles, and the slides are separated by pulling them apart in a direction parallel to their surfaces.

All films should be dried rapidly by whipping them through the air or by exposing them to a fan.

As the aspirated material is being spread, the appearance of fat as irregular holes in the films gives assurance that marrow and not just blood has been obtained.

Gross Quantitative Study. The aspirate is added to EDTA (1.5 mg/ml), mixed, and transferred to a Wintrobe hematocrit tube with a capillary pipette. Some or all of the visible particles are included, depending on their use for preparation of direct smears. The tube is centrifuged at 2500 rpm for 10 minutes. Four layers can be distinguished in the centrifugate: fat, plasma, myeloid-erythroid (M : E) portion, and erythrocytes. Their height is recorded in percentages by reading on the scale of the tube. Normally the fat layer is 1 to 3 per cent of the total volume and the M : E layer, 5 to 8 per cent. The

volumes of the plasma and erythrocyte layers vary considerably depending upon the degree of dilution with sinusoidal blood. Smears of the M : E layer may be made by aspirating this complete layer with an equal volume of plasma, mixing in a watch glass, and preparing films.

High myeloid-erythroid and low fat values, in the absence of a significant peripheral leukocytosis, suggest marrow hyperplasia. Low myeloid-erythroid and high fat values suggest hypoplasia, at least of the aspirated sample. If the myeloid-erythroid layer is less than 2 per cent and fat is absent, the sample is mainly sinusoidal blood. Examination of histologic sections is an essential check on the quantitative data. This type of preparation allows an optimal cell density and freedom from erythrocytes and fat cells on the films, and many such slides may be easily prepared.

Histologic Sections. The needle biopsy and the clotted marrow particles (fragments) are fixed in Zenker's acetic acid solution (5 per cent glacial acetic acid; 95 per cent Zenker's) for 6 to 24 hours. The longer time interval promotes adequate decalcification of most biopsies; excessive time in fixative makes the tissue brittle. The tissue is processed routinely for embedding in paraffin. Embedding the tissue in plastic materials allows thinner sections of 1 to 4 μm (Dancey, 1976); though this has some advantages it is not yet a routine procedure.

Sections provide the best estimate of cellularity and a picture of marrow architecture but are somewhat inferior for the study of cytologic details. Another disadvantage is that particles adequate for histologic sections are not always obtained, especially in conditions in which the diagnosis depends on marrow evidence, e.g., myelofibrosis or metastatic cancer.

Berman (1953) recommended the following technique for marrow particles. The aspirated marrow is deposited in a paraffin-coated vial. A small amount of powdered topical thrombin is placed on a clean glass slide, dissolved in a drop of water, and allowed to dry. The marrow particles in the aspirate tend to stick to the paraffin coating. They are transferred with the broken end of a wooden applicator and placed close to each other on the thrombin-coated area on the slide. A few drops of plasma from the centrifuged aspirate are added. The plasma clots by action of thrombin. The marrow particles are included in the clot, which is transferred to a suitable fixative. The latter is changed repeatedly until it remains water clear and then the tissue is processed.

Staining marrow preparations

Romanowsky Stain. Marrow films should be stained with a Romanowsky stain (e.g., Wright-Giemsa) in a similar manner to blood films (p. 891). A longer staining time may be necessary for marrows with greater cellularity.

Prussian Blue Reaction for Iron. Two films should also be stained for iron using the Prussian blue reaction. Marrow particles must be on the films because they contain numerous macrophages, the site of storage iron. Normoblasts are also examined for the presence of particulate iron.

Reagents

1. Potassium ferrocyanide, 2 per cent
2. Hydrochloric acid, 1 per cent
3. Nuclear Fast Red

Prepare 5 per cent solution of aluminum sulfate (anhydrous), using heat to dissolve. Allow solution to cool. Filter and add a crystal of thymol as preservative. Dissolve 0.1 g Nuclear Fast Red* in 100 ml of the 5 per cent aluminum sulfate solution. This solution keeps indefinitely.

Procedure

1. Use only marrow films which contain particles. A slide known to contain iron should be included as a positive control.
2. Fix slides for 10 minutes in a Coplin jar containing a filter paper moistened with two drops of 10 per cent formalin.
3. Prepare staining solution just before use by mixing 12 ml of 2 per cent potassium ferrocyanide with 36 ml of 1 per cent hydrochloric acid (HCl).
4. Remove filter paper and add staining solution to Coplin jar.
5. Stain for 10 minutes.
6. Rinse slides with distilled water and allow to dry.
7. Counterstain one slide with Nuclear Fast Red for 10 minutes.
8. Rinse counterstained slide with tap water and allow to dry.
9. Coverslip.

Result. The slide without the counterstain is most easily read for storage iron, and the slide counterstained with Nuclear Fast Red for sideroblasts (see below).

Hemosiderin and ferritin are blue; iron in hemoglobin is not stained. Report as negative or 1+ to 5+. Storage iron, which is contained in macrophages, can be evaluated only in the marrow particles on the smear. In adults, 2+ is normal, 3+ slightly increased, 4+ moderately increased, and 5+ markedly increased. Marrow hemosiderin is comparable to hemosiderin in the rest of the body.

Interpretation. Storage iron in the marrow is located in macrophages. Normally a small number of blue granules are seen. In iron deficiency, blue-staining granules are absent or extremely rare. Storage iron is increased in infections, pernicious anemia, hemolytic anemia, hemochromatosis, hemosiderosis, hepatic cirrhosis, uremia, and cancer, and after repeated transfusions (Plate 29-1*D* and *E*).

---

*Kernechtrot; Chroma-Gesellschaft, Schmidt and Co. Distributed by Roboz Surgical Instrument Co., 810 18th St. N.W., Washington, D.C. 20006

Sideroblasts are normoblasts which contain one or more particles of stainable iron. Normally, from 20 to 60 per cent of the late normoblasts are sideroblasts; in the remainder, no blue granules can be detected. The percentage of sideroblasts is decreased in iron deficiency anemia (where storage iron is decreased) and also in the common anemias associated with infection, rheumatoid arthritis, and neoplastic disease (where storage iron is normal or increased). The number of sideroblasts is increased when erythropoiesis is impaired for other reasons; it is roughly proportional to the degree of saturation of transferrin (Bainton, 1964). The Prussian blue reaction can also be performed on slides previously stained with a Romanowsky stain (Sundberg, 1955) to identify sideroblasts or to determine whether iron is present in other cells of interest.

Sections. Routine hematoxylin and eosin stains are satisfactory for most purposes. Romanowsky stains can be used to good advantage with Zenker-fixed material. Block (1976) successfully relies on the study of routine Romanowsky-stained marrow biopsy preparations almost to the exclusion of marrow films; most people, however, find the combination of marrow films and biopsy specimen to be preferable.

Iron stains may be performed on sections but are less sensitive than films because some iron is lost in the processing of sections (more lost in Zenker's than in formalin-fixed tissue) and much thicker pieces of marrow tissue (whole particles) are visualized on the films.

EXAMINATION OF MARROW

It is desirable to establish a routine procedure in order to obtain the maximum information from examination of the marrow.

Peripheral Blood. The complete blood cell count, including platelet count and reticulocyte count, should be performed on the day of the marrow study and the results incorporated in the report. The pathologist or hematologist who examines the marrow should also carefully examine the blood film as previously described (p. 889) and incorporate the observations in the marrow report.

Cellularity of the Marrow. The marrow cellularity is expressed as the ratio of the volume of hematopoietic cells to the total volume of the marrow space (cells plus fat and other stromal elements). Cellularity varies with the age of the subject and the site. For example, at age 50 years, the average cellularity in the vertebrae is 75 per cent; sternum, 60 per cent; iliac crest, 50 per cent; and rib, 30 per cent (Custer, 1974). Normal cellularity of the iliac bone at different ages has been well defined by Hartsock (1965), as summarized in Figure 28–

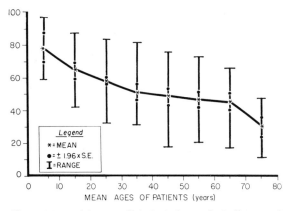

Figure 28–24. Marrow cellularity in hematologically normal individuals. Percent cellularity on the ordinate, versus age, grouped by decade, on the abscissa. (From Hartsock, et al.: Am. J. Clin. Pathol. *43*:326, 1965.)

24. If the percentage is increased for the patient's age, the marrow is hypercellular, or hyperplastic; if decreased, the marrow is hypocellular, or hypoplastic.

Marrow cellularity is best judged by histologic sections of biopsy or aspirated particles (see Fig. 28–26) but should be also estimated from the particles that are present in marrow films. This is done by comparing the areas occupied by fat spaces and by nucleated cells in the particles as well as the density of nucleated cells in the "tail" or fallout of the parti-

cles. Comparison of films and sections on each marrow will enable the observer to estimate cellularity reasonably well from films, a skill that is useful in the instances when sectioned material is unavailable.

Distribution of Cells. The distribution of the various cell types can be ascertained in two ways. First, by scanning several slides under low, then high dry, and finally under oil-immersion magnification; and on the basis of previous experience, one can arrive at impressions concerning the number and distribution of cells in very much the same manner as the pathologist reads his sections of tissue. Second, one can actually make a differential count of 300 to 1000 cells and calculate the percentage of each type of cell. A combination of both methods is preferred.

The second of these methods, careful differential counting, is an essential part of training in this work without which accuracy in the first method may be difficult to achieve. The differential count also affords an objective record from which future changes may be measured.

One first scans the marrow films under low power (100 × or 200 × magnification), looking for irregularities in cell distribution, the number of megakaryocytes, and the presence of abnormal cells. Then one selects areas on the

Table 28–1. DIFFERENTIAL CELL COUNTS OF BONE MARROW IN PER CENT OF TOTAL NUCLEATED CELLS

| | ROSSE (1977) Birth | | 1 Month | | MAUER (1969) over 4 months | WINTROBE (1974) Adult |
	Mean S.D.		Mean S.D.		Mean Range	Mean Range
Normoblasts, total	14.5 ± 7.2		8.0 ± 5.0		23.1	25.6 (18.4–33.8)
Pronormoblasts	0.02 ± 0.06		0.10 ± 0.14		0.5 (0 – 1.5)	(0.2– 1.3)
Basophilic N.	0.24 ± 0.24		0.34 ± 0.33		1.7 (0.2– 4.8)	(0.5– 2.4)
Polychromatophilic N.	13.1 ± 6.8		6.9 ± 4.4		18.2 (4.8–34.0)	(17.9–29.2)
Orthochromatic N.	0.69 ± 0.73		0.54 ± 1.88		2.7 (0 – 7.8)	(0.4– 4.6)
Neutrophils, total	60.4 ± 8.7		32.4 ± 7.7		57.1	53.6 (49.2–65.0)
Myeloblasts	0.31 ± 0.31		0.62 ± 0.50		1.2 (0 – 3.2)	(0.2– 1.5)
Promyelocytes	0.79 ± 0.91		0.76 ± 0.65		1.4 (0 – 4.0)	(2.1– 4.1)
Myelocytes	3.9 ± 2.9		2.5 ± 1.5		18.3 (8.5–29.7)	(8.2–15.7)
Metamyelocytes	19.4 ± 4.8		11.3 ± 3.6		23.3 (14.0–34.2)	(9.6–24.6)
Bands	28.4 ± 7.6		14.1 ± 4.6			(9.5–15.3)
Segmented	7.4 ± 4.6		3.6 ± 3.0		12.9 (4.5–29.0)	(6.0–12.0)
Eosinophils	2.7 ± 1.3		2.6 ± 1.4		3.6 (1.0– 9.0)	3.1 (1.2– 5.3)
Basophils	0.12 ± 0.20		0.07 ± 0.16		0.06 (0 – 0.8)	0.1 (0 – 0.2)
Lymphocytes, total	15.6		49.0		16.0 (4.8–35.8)	16.2 (11.1–23.2)
Transitional	1.2 ± 1.1		2.0 ± 0.9			
Small (mature)	14.4 ± 5.5		47.0 ± 9.2			
Plasma cells	0.00 ± 0.02		0.02 ± 0.06		0.4 (0.2– 0.6)	1.3 (0.4– 3.9)
Monocytes	0.88 ± 0.85		1.01 ± 0.89			0.3 (0 – 0.8)
Megakaryocytes	0.06 ± 0.15		0.05 ± 0.09			0.1 (0 – 0.4)
Reticulum cells						0.3 (0 – 0.9)
M : E Ratio	4.4		4.4		2.9 (1.2– 5.2)	2.3 (1.5– 2.3)

Data from Mauer, A. M.: Pediatric Hematology. New York, McGraw-Hill Book Company, 1969; and Wintrobe, M. M., et al.: Clinical Hematology, 7th ed. Philadelphia, Lea & Febiger, 1974.

films where marrow cells are both undiluted with blood cells and separated and spread out sufficiently to allow optimal identification. These areas are usually just behind marrow particles on the direct film, or near the particles on the crushed films. The differential count is performed at 400 × or 1000 × magnification.

Examples of reference intervals for differential counts of the marrow at selected different ages are given in Table 28-1.

Changes in the marrow cell distribution are most dramatic in the first month of life (Fig. 28-25), during which a predominance of granulocytic cells at birth changes to a predominance of lymphocytes. This predominance of lymphocytes characterizes the bone marrow during infancy. A small proportion of "immature" or transitional lymphocytes (fine nuclear chromatin, high N/C ratio, intermediate cell size) is normally present; it may be that included in these are stem cells and progenitor cells, but this has not been demonstrated in human marrow (Rosse, 1977). Normoblasts fall after birth, rise to a maximum at two months, then fall to a stable, relatively low level by four months and remain there during most of infancy.

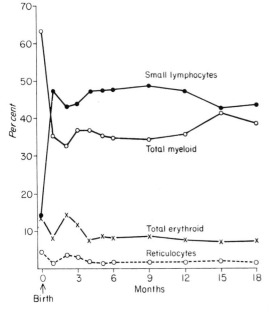

Figure 28-25. Mean percentages of three classes of marrow cells and blood reticulocytes in bone marrow of normal infants. Infants were clinically healthy and had normal leukocyte counts, serum proteins, and transferrin saturations. The values for birth (month 0) were collected during the first four days of life. (From Rosse, C., et al.: Bone marrow cell populations of normal infants: The predominance of lymphocytes. J. Lab. Clin. Med., *89*:1225–1240, 1977.)

The myeloid:erythroid (M:E) ratio is the ratio of total granulocytes:total normoblasts. In newborns and infancy it is somewhat higher than in later childhood or adult life (Table 28-1). In adults the range is broad, varying from 2:1 to 4:1.

Both the differential count and the M:E ratio are relative values and must be interpreted with respect to the cellularity or with respect to other evidence that one of the systems is normal.

An *increased* M:E ratio, e.g., 6 to 1, may be found in infection, chronic myelogenous leukemia, or erythroid hypoplasia. A *decreased* M:E ratio, i.e., less than 2 to 1, may mean a depression of leukopoiesis or a normoblastic hyperplasia, depending upon the marrow cellularity.

The number of megakaryocytes is estimated more reliably in sections than in marrow films. In scanning areas of films with good cellularity under low power (100 ×), an average of one to three megakaryocytes should be found in each field in a normal marrow.

Maturation. While examining the cells during the differential count, one should evaluate whether maturation is normal, that is, whether nuclear and cytoplasmic development is in balance. Impaired cytoplasmic maturation in normoblasts, for example, occurs when hemoglobin synthesis is impaired; impaired nuclear maturation occurs in megaloblastic anemias. Bizarre or dysplastic maturation occurs as a result of certain drugs, in some leukemias, and in dysmyelopoietic syndromes.

Presence of Rare Cell Types or Abnormal Cells. In scanning the marrow, one looks for the presence of rare or unexpected cell types.

Tissue mast cells (Plate 28-2*M*) are normally very infrequent. They are increased in number in aplastic or refractory anemias, and in macroglobulinemia.

Osteoblasts (Plate 28-3*I*) are cells which synthesize the collagen matrix of bone. *Osteoclasts* (Plate 28-3*C*) are cells that resorb bone and are thought to result from the fusion of histiocytes. Both cell types are normally present in small numbers in the aspirates of infants and children. They are uncommonly seen in adult marrow, except when bone destruction or repair is occurring, as in hyperparathyroidism, Paget's disease, metastatic tumor, or a recent biopsy at the same site.

Osteoblasts are large cells with a single eccentric nucleus which has reticular chromatin and a prominent nucleolus. The cytoplasm is moderately basophilic; a large pale Golgi zone is separated from the nucleus, rather than abutting it as in plasma cells. Osteoblasts are often present in clusters and may be confused with immature plasma cells or myeloma cells.

Osteoclasts are large, multinucleated cells up to 100 μm diameter that may be mistaken for megakaryocytes. They have multiple nuclei which are separate (not joined as in megakaryocytes). The chromatin is reticular, and a prominent nucleolus is usually present. The cytoplasm may be basophilic but usually has pink-purple granules that resemble megakaryocyte granules. Coarse fragments of purple-staining material are often present.

Clusters of *metastatic neoplastic cells* may be found in one or more marrow films of patients with metastatic tumor in the bone sampled; they may be found in biopsy sections and not films, in both, or, less commonly, in one or more films and not the biopsy. Some metastatic neoplastic cells resemble myeloblasts or other primitive blasts. The clue to recognizing them is that they almost always appear in clusters or clumps of cells; this is not true of hematopoietic blast cells.

Evaluation of the Biopsy. Histologic sections allow better estimates of the marrow cellularity and the number of megakaryocytes than do marrow films (Fig. 28-26). In good histologic preparations, the cell distribution and maturation abnormalities can be quite reliably determined. In addition to more reliable detection of the presence of lymphomas or metastatic tumor, the histologic pattern can often be diagnostic of the type of neoplasm. Other focal lesions not found in films include granulomas, abscesses, and vascular lesions.

In some conditions, such as myelofibrosis and leukemic reticuloendotheliosis (hairy cell leukemia), the bone marrow cannot be aspirated, and biopsy is necessary to establish a diagnosis.

Trabeculae should always be examined in order to detect bony abnormalities. Osteosclerosis with thickened bone trabeculae may accompany myelofibrosis or be congenital. In osteoporosis the bone trabeculae are thin. Osteomalacia is characterized by a recognizable osteoid seam. Osteitis fibrosa occurs in hyperparathyroidism and is characterized by irregular osteoclastic bony resorption, endosteal fibrosis, and some osteoblastic activity in areas of bone regeneration. Irregularly widened

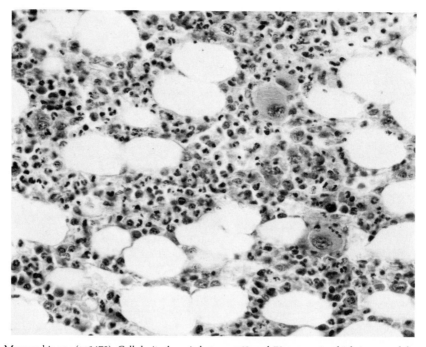

Figure 28-26. Marrow biopsy ($\times$1470). Cellularity here is between 60 and 70 per cent, which is normal for an adult. Three megakaryocytes are present, which is normal for this size field. Granulocytic maturation appears normal with all stages present. Very few normoblasts are noted. (Normoblasts have intensely staining nuclei and tend to occur in clusters.) The M:E ratio is higher than 4:1, indicating erythroid hypoplasia. No other abnormalities are noted.

trabeculae with a "mosaic" pattern are typical findings in Paget's disease of bone (Rywlin, 1976).

Interpretation. The *summary* of the marrow report should include an estimate of cellularity, an estimate of the number of megakaryocytes, the M:E ratio, statements about any cytologic or maturation abnormalities, an estimate of the storage iron and proportion of sideroblasts, and statements about any other abnormal findings present. A summary of the abnormalities in the blood cell counts and morphology is also made.

Then an *interpretation* of the observed findings should be made, which would of course include a diagnosis if this is possible. In making such an interpretation, one should include an integration of the marrow and blood observations with clinical findings and other laboratory data.

Alterations in blood and marrow cells are discussed with reference to the disease and disorders considered in subsequent chapters.

Indications for marrow study (Wintrobe, 1974)

In the differential diagnosis of macrocytic anemia, there are some cases in which the changes in the blood are minimal, yet the marrow is megaloblastic.

In microcytic anemias, evaluation of the iron stores and sideroblasts allow categorization of the anemia, i.e., iron deficiency, anemia of chronic disease, sideroblastic.

In normocytic anemias, marrow examination is less often useful. Comparing the level of marrow erythroid precursors with the reticulocyte count allows an estimation of the degree of ineffective erythropoiesis, or lack of erythropoiesis, as in pure red cell aplasia.

In neutropenia, thrombocytopenia, or pancytopenia, marrow study is helpful in assessing the presence and normality of the precursor cells in each series. This enables one to assess the probabilities of decreased production, impaired maturation, or increased destruction as the mechanism of the disorder.

In immunoglobulin abnormalities, the diagnosis of plasma cell myeloma or macroglobulinemia may be confirmed if infiltrations of abnormal plasma cells or lymphocytes are present.

If the marrow cannot be aspirated ("dry tap"), biopsy is essential. Marrow biopsy should also be performed if there are blood changes suggesting myelofibrosis with myeloid metaplasia, or if granulomatous disease or metastatic tumor is suspected.

CELL CULTURE SYSTEMS

Although *in vitro* semisolid cell culture systems are not yet established as essential clinical laboratory procedures, their potential importance merits comment.

As noted in this chapter, most of the major hematopoietic cell lines can now be studied with these techniques in man, as well as in animals. Development of these methods is allowing intensive investigation of the regulation of hematopoiesis: stimulators, inhibitors, cell-cell interaction. It is likely that our understanding of the biology of hematopoiesis will be measurably enhanced as a result; it is also likely that some of these techniques will demand a place in the next edition of this book as necessary tools in the clinical hematology laboratory. Metcalf (1977) discusses the principles and the technical details of these systems as currently used.

REFERENCES

Adamson, J. W., Alexanian, R., Martinez, C., and Finch, C. A.: Erythropoietin excretion in normal man. Blood, *28*:354, 1966.

Bainton, D. F., and Farquhar, M. G.: Origin of granules in polymorphonuclear leukocytes. J. Cell. Biol., *28*:277, 1966.

Bainton, D. F., and Finch, C. A.: The diagnosis of iron deficiency anemia. Am. J. Med., *37*:62, 1964.

Bainton, D. F., Nichols, B. A., and Farquhar, M. G.: Primary lysosomes of blood leukocytes. *In* Dingle, J. T., and Dean, R. T. (eds.): Lysosomes in Biology and Pathology 5. Amsterdam, North Holland Publishing Company, 1976, p. 3.

Bainton, D. F., Ullyot, J. L., and Farquhar, M. G.: The development of neutrophilic polymorphonuclear leukocytes in human bone marrow. J. Exp. Med., *134*:907, 1971.

Becker, A. J., McCulloch, E. A., and Till, J. E.: Cytological demonstration of the clonal nature of spleen colonies derived from transplanted mouse marrow cells. Nature, *197*:452, 1963.

Beeson, P. B., and Bass, D. A.: The Eosinophil. Volume XIV in Major Problems in Internal Medicine. Philadelphia, W. B. Saunders Company, 1977.

Berman, L.: A review of methods for aspiration and biopsy of bone marrow. Am. J. Clin. Pathol., *23*:385, 1953.

Bessis, M.: Living Blood Cells and Their Ultrastructure. Trans. by R. I. Weed. New York, Springer-Verlag, 1973.

Bessis, M. C., and Breton-Gorius, J.: Iron particles in normal erythroblasts and normal and pathological erythrocytes. J. Biophys. Biochem. Cytol., 3:503, 1957.

Block, M. H.: Text—Atlas of Hematology. Philadelphia, Lea & Febiger, 1976.

Bradley, T. R., and Metcalf, D.: The growth of mouse bone marrow cells in vitro. Aust. J. Exp. Biol. Med. Sci., 44:287, 1966.

Bunn, H. F., Forget, B. G., and Ranney, H. M.: Human Hemoglobins. Philadelphia, W. B. Saunders Company, 1977.

Cawley, J. C., and Hayhoe, F. G. J.: Ultrastructure of Haemic Cells. Philadelphia, W. B. Saunders Company, 1973.

Cline, M. J.: The White Cell. Cambridge, Harvard University Press, 1975.

Cline, M. J., and Golde, D. W.: Granulocytes and monocytes: Function and functional disorders. In Hoffbrand, A. V., Brain, M. C., and Hirsh, J. (eds.): Recent Advances in Haematology 2. Edinburgh, Churchill Livingstone, 1977.

Craddock, C. G., Longimire, R., and McMillian, R.: Lymphocytes and the immune response. N. Engl. J. Med., 285:324 and 378, 1971.

Custer, R. P.: An Atlas of the Blood and Bone Marrow, 2nd ed. Philadelphia, W. B. Saunders Company, 1974.

Dancey, J. T., Deubelbeiss, K. A., and Harker, L. A.: Section preparation of human marrow for light microscopy. J. Clin. Pathol., 29:704, 1976.

Douglas, S. D., and Ackerman, S. K.: Anatomy of the immune system. Clin. Haematol., 6:299, 1977.

Duhm, J.: The effect of 2,3-DPG and other organic phosphates on the Donnan equilibrium and the oxygen affinity of human blood. In Rorth, M., and Astrup, P. (eds.): Oxygen Affinity of Hemoglobin and Red Cell Acid Base Status. New York, Academic Press, Inc., 1972, p. 583.

Dvorak, H. F., and Dvorak, A.: Basophilic leukocytes: structure, function and role in disease. Clin. Haematol., 4:651, 1975.

Efrati, P., and Rozenszajn, L.: The morphology of buffy coat in normal human adults. Blood, 16:1012, 1960.

Erslev, A. J.: Anemia of chronic renal failure. In Williams, W. J., Beutler, E., Erslev, A. J., and Rundles, R. W. (eds.): Hematology. New York, McGraw-Hill Book Co., Inc., 1972, p. 237.

Erslev, A. J.: Erythropoietin assay. In Williams, W. J., Beutler, E., Erslev, A. J., and Rundles, R. W. (eds.): Hematology, 2nd ed. New York, McGraw-Hill Book Co., 1977, p. 1616.

Fialkow, P. J., Jacobson, R. J., and Papayannopoulou, T.: Chronic myelocytic leukemia: Clonal origin in a stem cell common to the granulocyte, erythrocyte, platelet, and monocyte/macrophage. Am. J. Med., 63:125, 1977.

Ganzoni, A. M., Oakes, R., and Hillman, R. S.: Red cell aging in vivo. J. Clin. Invest., 50:1373, 1971.

Harris, J. W., and Kellermeyer, R. W.: The Red Cell: Production, Metabolism, Destruction: Normal and Abnormal, rev. ed. Cambridge, Harvard University Press, 1970.

Hartsock, R. J., Smith, E. B., and Petty, C. S.: Normal variations with aging of the amount of hematopoietic tissue in bone marrow from the anterior iliac crest. Am. J. Clin. Pathol., 43:326, 1965.

Henry, R. J.: Clinical Chemistry: Principles and Technics. New York, Harper & Row, Publishers, Inc., 1964, p. 435.

Hillman, R. S., and Finch, C. A.: Erythropoiesis: Normal and abnormal. Semin. Hematol., 4:327, 1967.

Hillman, R. S., and Finch, C. A.: Red Cell Manual, 4th ed. Philadelphia, F. A. Davis Co., 1974.

Ichikawa, Y., Pluznik, D. H., and Sachs, L.: In vitro control of the development of macrophage and granulocyte colonies. Proc. Natl. Acad. Sci. U.S.A., 56:488, 1966.

Izak, G.: Erythroid cell differentiation and maturation. Prog. Hematol., 10:1, 1977.

Jamshidi, K., and Swaim, W. R.: Bone marrow biopsy with unaltered architecture: A new biopsy device. J. Lab. Clin. Med., 77:335, 1971.

Kaufman, R. M., Airo, R., Pollack, S., Crosby, W. H., and Doberneck, R.: Origin of pulmonary megakaryocytes. Blood, 25:767, 1965a.

Kaufman, R. M., Airo, R., Pollack, S., and Crosby, W. H.: Circulating megakaryocytes and platelet release in the lung. Blood, 26:720, 1965b.

Kobayasi, T., Midtgard, K., and Asboe-Hansen, G.: Ultrastructure of human mast cell granules. J. Ultrastruct. Res., 23:153, 1968.

Kurland, J. I., Bockman, R. S., Broxmeyer, H. E., and Moore, M. A. S.: Limitation of excessive myelopoiesis by the intrinsic modulation of macrophage-derived prostaglandin E. Science, 199:552, 1978.

Lessin, L. S., and Bessis, M.: Morphology of the erythron. In Williams, W. J., Beutler, E., Erslev, A. J., and Rundles, R. W. (eds.): Hematology, 2nd ed. New York, McGraw-Hill Book Co., 1977, p. 103.

Lewis, J. P., and Trobaugh, F. E., Jr.: Haematopoietic stem cells. Nature, 204:589, 1964.

Mauer, A. M.: Pediatric Hematology. New York, McGraw-Hill Book Co., 1969.

Metcalf, D.: Hemopoietic Colonies. In vitro cloning of normal and leukemic cells. Recent Results in Cancer Research, vol. 61. New York, Springer-Verlag, 1977.

Meuret, G., and Hoffmann, G.: Monocyte kinetic studies in normal and disease states. Br. J. Haematol., 24:275, 1973.

Meuret, G., Bammert, J., and Hoffmann, G.: Kinetics of human monocytopoiesis. Blood, 44:801, 1974.

Miller, F., de Harven, E., and Palade, G. E.: The structure of eosinophil leukocyte granules in rodents and in man. J. Cell Biol., 31:349, 1966.

Miller, J. F. A. P.: The cellular basis of immune responsiveness. Clin. Haematol., 6:277, 1977.

Murphy, P.: The neutrophil. New York, Plenum Medical Book Co., 1976.

Nichols, B. A., Bainton, D. F., and Farquhar, M. G.: Differentiation of monocytes. Origin, nature and fate of their azurophil granules. J. Cell Biol., 50:498, 1971.

Owen, J. J. T., Cooper, M. D., and Raff, M. C.: In vitro generation of B lymphocytes in mouse foetal liver, a mammalian bursa equivalent. Nature, 249:361, 1974.

Parwaresch, M. R.: The Human Blood Basophil. Morphology, origin, kinetics, function and pathology. New York, Springer-Verlag, 1976.

Pike, B. L., and Robinson, W. A.: Human bone marrow colony growth in agar-gel. J. Cell. Physiol., 76:77, 1970.

Rosse, C., Kraemer, M. J., Dillon, T. L., McFarland, R., and Smith, N. J.: Bone marrow cell populations of normal infants: The predominance of lymphocytes. J. Lab. Clin. Med., 89:1225, 1977.

Rywlin, A. M.: Histopathology of the bone marrow. Boston, Little, Brown and Co., 1976.

Sundberg, R. D.: Myeloid metaplasia. In Klein, H. (ed.):

Polycythemia. Theory and Management. Springfield, Ill., Charles C Thomas, Publisher, 1973, p. 112.

Sundberg, R. D., and Broman, H.: The application of the Prussian blue stain to previously stained films of blood and marrow. Blood, *10*:160, 1955.

Till, J. E., and McCulloch, E. A.: A direct measurement of the radiation sensitivity of normal mouse bone marrow cells. Rad. Res., *14*:213, 1961.

Weiss, L.: The Blood Cells and Hematopoietic Tissues. *In* Weiss, L., and Greep, R. O. (eds.): Histology, 4th ed. New York, McGraw-Hill Book Co., 1977.

West, B. C., Rosenthal, A. S., Gelb, N. A., and Kimball, H. R.: Separation and characterization of human neutrophil granules. Am. J. Pathol., *77*:41, 1974.

White, J. M., and Dacie, J. V.: The unstable hemoglobins—molecular and clinical features. Progr. Hematol., *7*:69, 1971.

Wintrobe, M. M., Lee, G. R., Boggs, D. R., Bithell, T. C., Athens, J. W., and Foerster, J.: Clinical Hematology, 7th ed. Philadelphia, Lea and Febiger, 1974.

Zucker-Franklin, D.: Electron microscopic study of human blood basophils. Blood, *29*:878, 1967.

3

29

ERYTHROCYTIC DISORDERS

Douglas A. Nelson, M.D.

WITH SECTIONS ON ACQUIRED HEMOLYSIS, ERYTHROCYTE SURVIVAL, AND ERYTHROCYTE AND PLASMA VOLUME BY

Frederick R. Davey, M.D.

ANEMIAS

GENERAL MANIFESTATIONS

Anemia is considered to be present if the hemoglobin concentration or the hematocrit is below the lower limit of the 95 per cent reference interval for the individual's age, sex, and geographic location (altitude) (see Fig. 27-37, p. 910, Table 29-1). This is not an absolute definition of anemia, however. An individual's hemoglobin may fall within the reference interval for his age and sex yet be below his own normal reference value; he then should be considered anemic. Conversely, an individual may have a physiologically normal hemoglobin concentration which happens to be below the reference interval.

Causes of anemia fall into three major pathophysiologic categories: impaired red cell production; blood loss; or accelerated red cell destruction (hemolysis) in excess of the ability of the marrow to replace these losses. The presence of anemia is not a disease in itself but a sign of an underlying disorder whose cause should be identified, since correction may be very important to the individual.

Anemia may be classified by red cell morphology as macrocytic, normocytic, or microcytic, an approach that is especially useful in differential diagnosis (p. 1028). Or anemia may be classified by the pathophysiologic mechanism involved, which is useful in understanding the disease process. Neither satisfies completely; both should be understood. Some

Table 29-1. REFERENCE VALUES BELOW
WHICH ANEMIA IS CONSIDERED TO
EXIST AT SEA LEVEL

AGE (YEARS)	Hb (g/dl)	Hct (Liter/liter)
0.6 to 4	11	0.33
5 to 9	11.5	0.345
10 to 14	12	0.36
Adults—men	14	0.42
Adults—women	12	0.36
Pregnant women	11	0.33

From Committee on Iron Deficiency: Iron deficiency in
the United States. J.A.M.A., *203:*407, 1968. Copyright 1968,
American Medical Association.

anemias have more than one pathogenetic
mechanism and go through more than one
morphologic stage, e.g., blood loss anemia.

Clinical signs of anemia

Certain clinical signs and symptoms result
from the diminished delivery of oxygen to the
tissues and, therefore, are roughly proportional to the hemoglobin concentration. It is
not possible to state a critical level beyond
which vital processes are deranged, since there
are always a number of factors operating at
one time. Consideration must be given to the
underlying disease process and its complications other than anemia, the metabolic requirements of the tissues as conditioned by
the illness, the capacity of the cardiovascular
and pulmonary systems to compensate, and
the rate at which the anemia develops. When
anemia develops slowly in a patient who is not
otherwise severely ill, erythrocyte counts
below $2 \times 10^{12}/l$, or hemoglobin concentrations as low as 6 g/dl, may develop without
producing any discomfort or physical signs as
long as the patient is at rest.

In general, the anemic patient complains of
easy fatigability and dyspnea on exertion. He
may complain also of faintness, vertigo, and
palpitation. Headache is a common symptom.
Tinnitus is occasionally mentioned. The more
common physical findings are pallor, a rapid
bounding pulse, low blood pressure, slight
fever, some dependent edema, and systolic
murmurs. In addition to these general signs
and symptoms certain clinical findings are
characteristic of the specific type of anemia. It
is not our present purpose to discuss these in
full, but the point to be emphasized is that the
anemias are not laboratory diseases but are

conditions in which the clinical findings have
both specific and differential diagnostic value.

BLOOD LOSS ANEMIA

Acute posthemorrhagic anemia (Wintrobe, 1974)

Blood may be lost from the circulation ex-
ternally, into the gastrointestinal tract, or into
a tissue space or body cavity. If blood is lost
over a short period of time in amounts sufficient to cause anemia in the face of adequate
iron stores, *acute posthemorrhagic anemia*
occurs.

After a single episode of bleeding which is
short in duration, there follows a characteristic sequence of events. For the first one to
three days, the major manifestations are those
due to depletion of blood volume (hypovolemia). The clinical features depend upon the
rate and amount of blood loss. When blood
volume is returned to previous levels by movement of fluid into the circulation, anemia and
signs of increased red cell production become
evident.

The earliest hematologic changes are a
transient fall in the platelet count and the
whole blood coagulation time. Within an hour,
however, the platelet count may rise to elevated levels. The next development is a moderate neutrophilic leukocytosis with a shift to
the left; a maximum leukocyte count of 10 to
$35 \times 10^9/l$ is reached in two to five hours. The
hemoglobin concentration and hematocrit do
not fall immediately, but only slowly over the
course of the first 24 hours. Tissue fluids move
into the circulation to compensate for the lost
blood volume; this is responsible for the progressive fall in Hb and Hct, which may not
reveal the full extent of the red cell loss until
two or three days after the hemorrhage.

The anemia that develops at first is normochromic and normocytic, with a normal MCV
and MCHC and only minimal anisocytosis and
poikilocytosis. Increased erythropoietin secretion stimulates erythroid proliferation in the
marrow, and reticulocytes begin to reach the
circulation in three to five days, reaching a
maximum by 10 days or so. During this period
transient macrocytosis (increased MCV), increased polychromasia, and normoblasts may
appear in the blood. It takes about two weeks
after the blood loss for the morphologic
changes to disappear, and two to four days for

the leukocyte count to return to normal. Return of red cell values is slower. Red cell count becomes normal in about four to six weeks; the hemoglobin may take slightly longer.

Chronic posthemorrhagic anemia

If blood is lost in small amounts over an extended period of time, both the clinical and hematologic features that characterize acute posthemorrhagic anemia are lacking. Regeneration of red cells occurs at a slower rate, and significant anemia may not develop until after storage iron is depleted.

The reticulocyte count may be within the normal reference interval or slightly increased. Significant anemia does not usually develop until after storage iron is depleted; the anemia, therefore, is one of iron deficiency (q.v.). The anemia is at first normochromic and normocytic, and gradually the newly formed red cells become microcytic, then hypochromic. The leukocyte count is normal or slightly decreased owing to neutropenia. Platelets are commonly increased, and only later, in severe iron deficiency, are they likely to be decreased.

The source and cause of blood loss must be identified, for it is toward these that definitive treatment must be directed.

IMPAIRED PRODUCTION— IRON DEFICIENCY

Iron metabolism (Hillman, 1974; Worwood, 1977)

The physiologic chemistry of iron and clinicopathological correlations are reviewed in Chapter 9.

Iron is an essential component of hemoglobin, of myoglobin (in muscle cells), and of certain enzymes (in most body cells). The major "pools" of iron in the body are illustrated in Figure 29-1. Two thirds or more of the body's total iron is in the erythron (normoblasts and erythrocytes); each milliliter of red cells contains about 1 mg of iron. Storage iron is present in macrophages of the reticuloendothelial system as ferritin (iron bound to the protein, apoferritin, molecular weight 460,000) and as hemosiderin, a more complex storage form with a lesser proportion of protein than ferritin (Wintrobe, 1974). Most of the iron utilized in hemoglobin synthesis is that recently released from degraded Hb in macrophages and transported to the normoblasts by plasma transferrin (a beta globulin, molecular weight 80,000).

Very little iron is lost from the body, and this mainly from loss of cells in the gastrointestinal tract and to a lesser extent from the skin and in the urine. The iron excreted in women averages more than that in men because of menstrual blood loss. Iron balance is maintained by control of absorption. In the United States, dietary iron in men averages 15 mg/day with 6 per cent absorption, and 11 mg/day in women with 12 per cent absorption (Hillman, 1974). Absorption can be increased in iron deficiency, but only to about 20 per cent of ingested iron in meat-containing diets, and less in vegetarian diets. Absorption takes place largely in the small intestine, most efficiently in the duodenum.

In the plasma, the total iron averages 110 μg/dl (1.1 mg/l or 19.7 μmol/l). The great majority of this is bound to the transferrin, which has a capacity to bind 330 μg of iron/dl (or 59.1 μmol/l) and therefore is about one third saturated. A very small amount of iron in plasma is bound to ferritin. Plasma (or serum) ferritin averages about 100 μg/l in men (less in women, about 50 μg/l). If serum ferritin contains the same proportion of iron as tissue ferritin (20 to 25 per cent), plasma ferritin would normally contain about 20 μg of iron per liter (Siimes, 1974b).

Iron deficiency anemia

When iron loss exceeds iron intake for a time long enough to deplete the body's iron stores, insufficient iron is available for normal hemoglobin production. When well developed, iron deficiency anemia is characterized by a decrease of hemoglobin and, to a lesser degree, of the hematocrit, both more marked than the decrease in the number of red cells: a hypochromic microcytic anemia.

Iron deficiency results only when there is an increased need for iron (e.g., during rapid growth in infancy and childhood or during pregnancy) or when excessive loss of blood has reduced the body's reserves of iron (e.g., following repeated hemorrhages, excessive menstruation, or multiple pregnancies).

In infancy and childhood, iron deficiency is probably the most common cause of anemia, especially between the ages of six and 24 months. It is caused by an amount of dietary iron insufficient to meet the needs of rapid growth. After the first four to six months of life, the iron stores of the normal infant present from birth have been exhausted, and he depends on his diet for iron. If the infant is maintained on milk and carbohydrates without supplements of iron-containing foods, he is likely to develop an iron deficiency anemia, The so-called milk anemia of infancy. Defective absorption of iron and eventual iron deficiency anemia occur in most patients after total gastrectomy and in nearly half the patients after subtotal gastrectomy (Fairbanks, 1971). Except for the sprue syndrome, other causes of malabsorption of iron are extremely rare.

The adult male has no increased physiologic demands for iron. If he had absolutely no iron intake or absorption (which would be extremely rare), his body iron stores of 1000 mg would last for three to four years before he would even begin to become iron deficient. Therefore, almost all cases of iron deficiency

anemia in adult males are due to chronic blood loss.

An understanding of the sequence of events or stages in the development of iron deficiency anemia is helpful (Harris, 1970; Hillman, 1974). When blood loss exceeds absorption, a negative iron balance exists. Iron is mobilized from stores, storage iron decreases, plasma ferritin decreases, iron absorption increases, and plasma iron-binding capacity (transferrin) increases. This stage is known as *iron depletion*. After iron stores are depleted, the plasma iron concentration falls, saturation of transferrin falls below 15 per cent, and the percentage of sideroblasts decreases in the marrow. As a result of lack of iron for heme synthesis, red cell protoporphyrin increases. This second

3

IRON METABOLISM

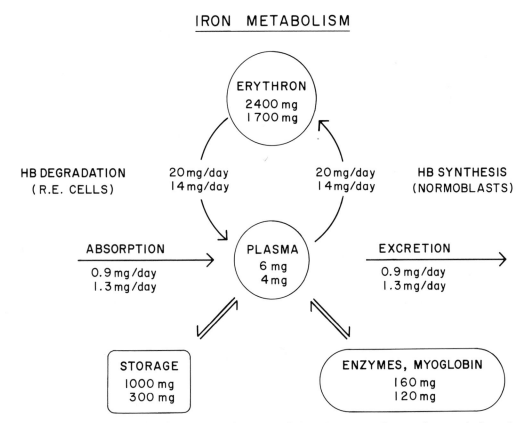

Figure 29–1. Scheme of iron metabolism. The upper figure in each position is average for an 80 kg man; the lower figure is for a 65 kg woman. (Data from Hillman, 1974.) The plasma iron, bound largely to transferrin, is central in one scheme. It completely turns over several times a day in supplying iron for heme synthesis.

Each day, about $\frac{1}{120}$ of the total circulating red cells are destroyed and the same number of new red cells are delivered to the blood. That proportion of the total erythron iron enters the plasma from the site of Hb degradation, the macrophages of the RE system, and travels (bound to transferrin) to the normoblasts in the marrow. Storage iron largely resides also in the macrophages of the RE system. Absorbed iron enters the plasma pool, bound to transferrin. Excreted iron is largely from loss of cells.

stage is *iron deficient erythropoiesis;* anemia may not yet be present. The third stage is *iron deficiency anemia;* in addition to the above abnormalities, anemia is detectable. The anemia is at first normochromic and normocytic, gradually becomes microcytic, and finally microcytic and hypochromic.

Clinical Findings. Clinical findings may be due to the underlying cause of the blood loss itself, to the general manifestations of anemia (p. 964), or to iron deficiency. Those which are probably attributable to lack of tissue iron include: paresthesias, such as numbness and tingling; atrophy of epithelium of the tongue with burning or soreness; fissures or ulcers at the corners of the mouth (angular stomatitis); chronic gastritis, which leads to decreased gastric secretions but few symptoms; "pica," which is the craving to eat unusual substances such as dirt or ice; concave or spoon-shaped nails (koilonychia); difficulty swallowing due to "webs" of tissue or partial strictures at the junction of the esophagus and hypopharynx (Wintrobe, 1974). The latter two findings are relatively uncommon. Splenomegaly may occur but is quite uncommon.

Laboratory Findings

BLOOD. In early iron deficiency anemia, the stained blood film often shows normochromic normocytic erythrocytes (Fairbanks, 1971). In later stages the picture is one of microcytosis, anisocytosis, poikilocytosis (including elliptical and elongated cells), and varying degrees of hypochromia (see p. 894). Reticulocytes are usually decreased in absolute numbers except following iron therapy. The number of red cells is rarely as low as in pernicious anemia. The hemoglobin and hematocrit may be extremely low. Osmotic fragility may be decreased because the red cells are thinner than normal (Fig. 27-11; Plate 29-1J).

The white blood cell count is normal or slightly lowered. Granulocytopenia, relative lymphocytosis, and a small number of hypersegmented neutrophils may be present. Platelets may be increased, whether the iron lack is due to blood loss or dietary deficiency, but tend to be decreased in severe anemia.

MARROW. Normoblastic hyperplasia occurs early, but in later stages the limiting effect of severe iron deficiency restricts erythropoiesis to the basal level. The normoblasts are smaller than normal, deficient in the amount of hemoglobin in the cytoplasm, and irregular in shape with frayed margins (Plate 29-1G). Giant neutrophil bands or metamyelocytes, if present, are rarely due to iron deficiency per se; usually they indicate an associated vitamin

B_{12} or folate deficiency (p. 971). Iron stains should be performed routinely (p. 957, Plate 29-1D and E). *Storage iron* is absent, unless iron has recently been administered in some form. The proportion of normoblasts that are *sideroblasts* is decreased (less than 20 per cent); this proportion is usually about the same as the per cent saturation of transferrin (or TIBC) and is a measure of iron delivery to the normoblasts.

SERUM IRON. The reference interval is 65 to 175 $\mu g/dl$ (11 to 31 $\mu mol/l$) in adults. The level is lower in iron deficiency but also in infections and the anemia of chronic disease.

SERUM IRON-BINDING CAPACITY. The reference interval for adults is 300 to 360 $\mu g/dl$ (54 to 64 $\mu mol/l$). In iron deficiency anemia, the serum total iron-binding capacity (TIBC) is increased. It is normal or decreased in the anemia of chronic disease. If chronic infection coexists with chronic blood loss, the TIBC may not be increased, even though the patient is iron deficient.

PER CENT SATURATION OF TIBC. The ratio of serum iron to TIBC is the per cent saturation of the TIBC. Normally this is 20 to 55 per cent; values below 15 per cent indicate iron deficient erythropoiesis.

There is normally a marked diurnal variation in serum iron, with highest values in the morning and lowest values late in the day. Consequently, fasting morning blood specimens are preferred for the diagnosis of iron deficiency.

Somewhat lower reference intervals for serum iron are normal in iron sufficient infants from the second month through the twelfth month. Saarinen (1977) studied infants in whom iron deficiency was excluded by normal hemoglobin, MCV, and serum ferritin values. The TIBC gradually rose during the first year of life. After the first four months of life, through the first year, the lower reference value for per cent saturation in normal infants was 10 per cent rather than 20 per cent as in adults. Thereafter, values slowly rise to adult levels at about the age of two years (Jacobs, 1974).

SERUM FERRITIN. In adults, the reference values are 12 to 300 $\mu g/l$, with higher values in men than women. Although the precise role of serum ferritin in iron metabolism is not worked out in man, it appears to be in equilibrium with tissue ferritin and is a good reflection of storage iron in normal subjects and in most disorders (Jacobs, 1975). The equivalence of 1 $\mu g/l$ of serum ferritin with 8 mg storage iron has been suggested. In patients with tissue injury, especially liver necrosis, abnormal release of tissue ferritin may destroy this relationship. Also, leukemic cells appear to synthesize ferritin at a high rate, so that these patients have higher levels of serum ferritin disproportionate to their stores. A *low* value, however, below 12 µg/l, indicates low iron stores; falsely low values mimicking iron deficiency have not been found.

In infancy and childhood, between the ages of 6 months and 15 years, the reference interval for serum ferritin is 7 to 142 µg/l (Siimes, 1974a) somewhat lower than early infancy or adult life. In men, serum ferritin gradually rises between the ages of 18 and 30 years, whereas in women it does not (Finch, 1977); representative geometric mean values of the skewed distribution of reference values were 127 µg/l for men, 46 µg/l for women.

ERYTHROCYTE PORPHYRINS. Since heme is formed by insertion of iron into protoporphyrin IX, the latter is increased in iron deficient erythropoiesis, whether due to iron deficiency or anemia of chronic disease. It is also increased in lead poisoning and in the idiopathic form of sideroblastic anemia (Wintrobe, 1974) but is normal in thalassemia. A relatively simple micromethod measuring "free erythrocyte porphyrins" (FEP) in whole blood (Piomelli, 1973) has been shown to be useful in distinguishing microcytosis due to iron deficiency from that due to beta thalassemia minor (Stockman, 1975). The normal reference interval was 10 to 90 µg/dl of erythrocytes; in iron deficiency, the erythrocyte porphyrins became elevated when the saturation of the TIBC was less than 15 per cent.

Differential diagnosis

The utility of serum iron, TIBC, and per cent saturation may be seen in Table 10–10, p. 296, and in Table 29–12, p. 1031.

Anemia due to iron deficiency usually must be distinguished from other microcytic or hypochromic anemias. These include the thalassemia traits (p. 998), long-standing anemia of chronic disease (p. 977), and the sideroblastic anemias (p. 983). Bone marrow storage iron and serum ferritin will be decreased in iron deficiency and normal or elevated in all others. In addition, in *thalassemia trait*, the FEP is normal, serum iron is normal, the Hb A_2 and, occasionally, Hb F are increased (in beta-thalassemia trait), and the condition is present in family members; indeed, the Hb A_2 is often decreased in iron deficiency. In *anemia of chronic disorders* (chronic infection, rheumatoid arthritis, or neoplastic disease),

although the serum iron is low, as in iron deficiency, the TIBC is low or normal. In the *sideroblastic anemias*, which include chronic lead poisoning, the serum iron and per cent TIBC saturation are increased, and pathologic "ring" sideroblasts are present in the marrow.

Management. The first principle in therapy is that the underlying cause be identified and corrected. Ferrous iron is given orally, about 200 mg per day, in three doses between meals. This will provide 20 to 40 mg of absorbed iron per day, which, with the iron produced by turnover of senescent red cells, will be sufficient to increase production to two or three times normal (Hillman, 1974). The reticulocyte count will reach a maximum at 5 to 10 days, then gradually decrease toward normal. Monitoring the hemoglobin is best; Hb should increase by 0.2 g/dl per day after the fifth day and by 3 g/dl in three weeks. After the hemoglobin has returned to normal, iron therapy should be continued for at least two months in order to replenish storage iron.

IMPAIRED PRODUCTION— MEGALOBLASTIC ANEMIA

Macrocytosis with normoblastic marrow

Macrocytic anemias which are not megaloblastic may be due to early release of erythrocytes from the marrow, as in response to acute blood loss or hemolysis; this is a "shift" macrocytosis, since it results from a premature release of reticulocytes from the marrow (Hillman, 1974). Macrocytosis not due to reticulocytosis is found commonly in hypothyroidism and in individuals with an excessive alcohol intake, and in some cases of aplastic or refractory anemias and of non-alcoholic liver disease (Chanarin, 1976).

Megaloblastosis

Macrocytic anemias associated with megaloblastic changes in the bone marrow have certain morphologic differences from non-megaloblastic macrocytic anemias in the peripheral blood (Chanarin, 1969). The finding of macro-ovalocytes and giant hypersegmented neutrophils is distinctive of megaloblastic anemia.

Megaloblastic anemia is characterized by enlargement of all rapidly proliferating cells of the body. Both nucleus and cytoplasm are enlarged, but the increase is more pronounced in the cytoplasm. The major cellular abnormality appears to be the diminished capacity of the cells to synthesize DNA.

The cells have both a prolonged intermitotic resting phase and a block early in mitosis. The number of mitotic figures is increased. RNA synthesis is less impeded than is DNA synthesis; hence, cytoplasmic maturation and growth continue, accounting for enlargement of the cells. In the bone marrow, hemoglobin appears at an unusually early stage in the erythroid cells, as judged by nuclear maturation. The delicate, finely reticulated chromatin and the prominent parachromatin result in a distinctly more "open" chromatin pattern than is seen in the normoblastic series (Plate 28-1*E* to *H*; Plate 29-1*H*). The nuclei undergo karyorrhexis readily, and multiple Howell-Jolly bodies may be present. Basophilic stippling is frequently seen. There are relatively more cells analogous to the pronormoblast and basophilic normoblast (i.e., the promegaloblast and basophilic megaloblast) than are seen in normal erythropoiesis. This has sometimes been termed "maturation arrest," or nuclear cytoplasmic asynchrony. Giant polychromatic megaloblasts are especially distinctive. The same general features are seen in the other cell lines. In the granulocytic series, the cells are larger, with retarded nuclear maturation and large cytoplasmic mass; often the specific granules themselves are distinctly larger. The chromatin pattern is less condensed (more "open") and, as a result, the nucleus appears to stain poorly. Abnormally contorted nuclear configurations are common. The giant metamyelocyte is the most characteristic of the abnormal granulocytes. Megakaryocytes, too, are large and have abnormally pronounced nuclear segmentation and often fragmentation.

All these features characterize the *morphologic entity* of megaloblastic anemia.

The *etiology* of megaloblastic anemia is almost always vitamin B_{12} or folic acid deficiency.

Vitamin B_{12} metabolism

Vitamin B_{12} (cyanocobalamin) has a molecular weight of 1355. The molecule's two major parts are (1) a "planar group" (the corrin nucleus), a ring structure surrounding a cobalt atom, and (2) a "nucleotide" group, which consists of the base, 5,6-dimethylbenzimidazole, and a phosphorylated ribose esterified with 1-amino, 2-propanol. A cyanide group is in coordinate linkage with the trivalent cobalt. Different forms of vitamin B_{12} result from replacement of the cyanide by hydroxy, aquo, or nitro groups.

Vitamin B_{12} is unique in that it is the only vitamin exclusively synthesized by microorganisms. It is found in practically all animal tissues. It is stored primarily in the liver. The human liver contains approximately 1 μg per gram of liver. Vitamin B_{12}, in its coenzyme form, is released by digestion of proteins of animal origin and then is bound by gastric intrinsic factor (I.F.), which is essential for absorption. This vitamin B_{12}-I.F. complex then adheres to specific receptor sites on the epithelial cells of the ileum, at which site the vitamin B_{12} is absorbed. Several hours are required for absorption.

Once absorbed, vitamin B_{12} is transported in the plasma bound to a group of proteins, called transcobalamin I (TC I), transcobalamin II (TC II), and transcobalamin III (TC III) (Allen, 1976). Ninety per cent of newly absorbed vitamin B_{12} is bound to TC II, which serves as the chief transport protein, rapidly delivering the vitamin to the liver, hematopoietic cells, and other dividing cells. Some vitamin B_{12} attaches to TC I; this appears to be a passive reservoir which is in equilibrium with body stores in the liver. The reference interval for plasma vitamin B_{12}, which varies with different methods of assay, commonly is 200 to 900 mg/l (150 to 670 pmol/l). One third of the vitamin B_{12} binding sites on transcobalamins are normally occupied. TC I is 70 to 90 per cent saturated and binds most of the plasma vitamin B_{12}; this is very slowly cleared from the plasma. TC II is only about 5 per cent saturated; much of newly absorbed vitamin B_{12} bound to TC II is removed from the plasma during the first few hours, but a small fraction remains bound for several weeks (Hall, 1975).

The relative importance of the transcobalamins is illustrated by the effects of congenital absence (Hall, 1973). Lack of TC II results in severe megaloblastic anemia in infancy; yet the serum vitamin B_{12} level is normal. Lack of TC I is not accompanied by anemia or megaloblastosis; yet the serum vitamin B_{12} level is decreased.

TC I and III are R-type proteins, appear to differ only in their carbohydrate proportions, and have been called cobalophilin (Stenman, 1976). Much of the serum TC III is released from granulocytes during blood clotting *in vitro;* TC III does not appear to bind significant amounts of plasma B_{12} under normal conditions. TC I may arise from granulocytes as well as other tissues. Elevation of TC I and III accounts for the elevation of total vitamin B_{12} binding proteins in myeloproliferative diseases. TC II is probably produced in the liver.

The daily requirement of vitamin B_{12} is in the range of 2 to 5 μg per day. The body's stores of 2 to 5 mg will last for several years if intake is cut off, as is the case if total gastrectomy is performed (Beck, 1977).

Vitamin B_{12} deficiency

Vitamin B_{12} deficiency is produced by any of several mechanisms.

Inadequate Intake. A dietary deficiency is an *extremely rare* cause of megaloblastic anemia and is seen only in persons who completely abstain from animal food, including milk and eggs. For example, strict vegetarians are known to develop this form of vitamin B_{12} deficiency.

Defective Production of Intrinsic Factor. This is the most common cause of vitamin B_{12} deficiency.

PERNICIOUS ANEMIA (PA). Pernicious anemia is a "conditioned" nutritional deficiency of vitamin B_{12} which is caused by a failure of the gastric mucosa to secrete intrinsic factor. This abnormality is genetically determined but usually is not manifested until late in life.

Clinical Features. The disorder is equally common in males and females. Anorexia, malaise, weakness, shortness of breath, and the combination of skin pallor and jaundice giving a lemon-yellow appearance of the skin are often present. The tongue may be sore, smooth, and pale (atrophic glossitis) or red and raw (acute glossitis). Three systems are commonly involved: *Gastrointestinal symptoms* may be prominent and include episodic abdominal pain, constipation, and diarrhea. Diffuse and irregular degeneration of the white matter of the *central nervous system* characteristically involves the posterior and lateral columns of the spinal cord (subacute combined degeneration) and sometimes other sites. Symmetrical sensations of "pins and needles" of the distal extremities, numbness and tingling, loss of position sensation (difficulty with balance and gait), and loss of vibratory sensation (perhaps the most constant sign) are indicative of posterior column lesions. Lateral column involvement gives rise to weakness, spasticity, and increased deep tendon reflexes. Sometimes, in advanced cases, the brain may be affected, and the patient shows irritability, emotional instability, or a change in personality; the term "megaloblastic madness" has sometimes been applied to the latter.

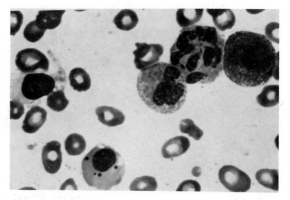

Figure 29–2. Megaloblastic anemia. Below, orthochromatic megaloblast with four Howell-Jolly bodies. Above, right, two giant neutrophils (one of which has nine nuclear lobes and could be called a macropolycyte) and an eosinophil with poor nuclear maturation. ($\times$875.)

Peripheral Blood (Figs. 27-12, 27-14, 27-24, 27-27, 27-31, 29-2; Plate 29-1K). The *hematopoietic* is the third system involved. Pancytopenia (a decrease in all the formed elements of the blood) is the rule. The anemia is macrocytic with an elevated MCV and is characterized by macro-ovalocytes and often extreme degrees of anisocytosis and poikilocytosis. Microcytes and teardrop forms are common. Basophilic stippling, multiple Howell-Jolly bodies, nucleated red cells with karyorrhexis, and even megaloblasts may be seen. Leukopenia is present. Granulocytes have increased numbers of lobes, presumably a result of abnormal nuclear maturation. Five or more lobes in more than 5 per cent of the neutrophils constitute hypersegmentation (Herbert, 1976), as do any neutrophils with six or more lobes. Thrombocytopenia is usually encountered and on rare occasions is sufficiently severe to be responsible for bleeding. It is worth noting that significant morphologic changes may occur in the blood in the absence of anemia and also that neurologic symptoms may be present in the absence of anemia.

Bone Marrow (Plate 28-1E to H; Plate 29-1B and H). The bone marrow is hyperplastic. The fat is replaced, and red marrow extends into the long bones. The number of erythroid precursors (megaloblasts) is increased. Instead of the normal myeloid-erythroid ratio of 3 to 1, the ratio is more likely to approach 1 to 1. The cytologic changes have been described. If the megaloblastic process is incompletely developed, or if the patient has been inadequately treated, the findings may be only partial. Since they persist longer, the granulocytic alterations are especially helpful in assessing partially treated megaloblas-

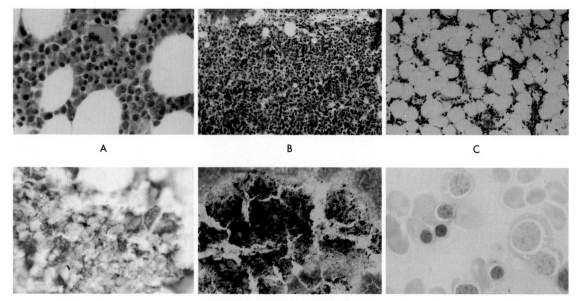

A

B

C

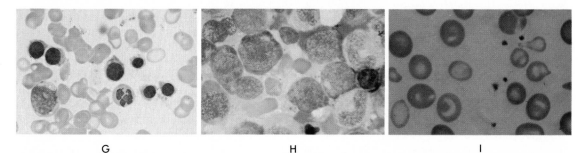

D

E

F

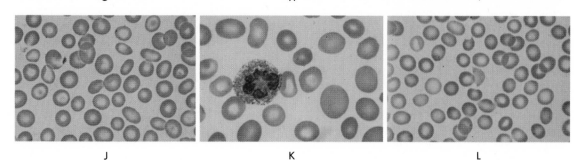

G

H

I

J

K

L

Plate 29-1. *A*, Section of normal marrow. The cellularity (i.e., the ratio of the space occupied by cells to the total) is about 0.5 to 0.6. The E/G ratio is normal, about $\frac{1}{3}$. A megakaryocyte is in the upper center. *B*, Section of hyperplastic marrow, megaloblastic anemia. The cellularity is over 0.95. *C*, Section of hypocellular marrow, aplastic anemia. The cellularity is about 0.10 or less. Though not discernible at this magnification, most of the cells are lymphocytes and plasma cells. *D*, Marrow film, Prussian blue reaction, no counterstain, normal marrow. Storage iron stains blue-green and is within macrophages. On a scale of 0 to 5+, the amount of storage iron here is judged as 1+, which is in the normal range for a woman, probably somewhat low for a man. In iron deficiency anemia, no blue-green staining iron is visible. *E*, Marrow film, Prussian blue reaction, no counterstain; sideroblastic anemia. On a scale of 0 to 5+, the amount of storage iron is judged at 5+, which is markedly increased. *F*, Marrow film, Prussian blue reaction, counterstained with nuclear fast red, sideroblastic anemia. The normoblasts in the field contain multiple siderotic granules. Two ring sideroblasts are left of the center. The wide perinuclear space in some cells is an artifact. *G*, Marrow film, iron deficiency anemia. The six normoblasts have irregular margins and irregular clear spaces, reflecting lack of hemoglobin synthesis, i.e., defective cytoplasmic maturation. Also in the field are a neutrophil and an immature monocyte. *H*, Marrow film, megaloblastic anemia. Basophilic and polychromatophilic megaloblasts predominate in this field; two giant-band neutrophils are present. The "open," non-condensed chromatin pattern and large cell size are characteristic of defective nuclear maturation. *I*, Blood film, primary acquired sideroblastic anemia. Dimorphic red cell

(legend continued on the following page)

tic anemia. The marrow findings are due to the effects of the vitamin B_{12} deficiency on nucleic acid synthesis (DNA synthesis impeded more than RNA synthesis) and to hypoxic stress, giving rise to increased numbers of erythroid cells. If the patient is transfused with packed red cells, the number of erythroid precursors diminishes but the cytologic abnormalities persist.

Stomach. In man both intrinsic factor and HCl are secreted by parietal cells. Gastric atrophy involving all coats of the wall is found in approximately 40 per cent of cases; the remainder show varying degrees of atrophic gastritis. It is generally held that these are successive stages of the same process. Except for the few patients with juvenile pernicious anemia who have free acid secretion but no intrinsic factor, adult patients with pernicious anemia have histamine-refractory achylia and achlorhydria—a decreased volume of gastric juice and a total lack of acid secretion. It must be remembered that a small proportion of hematologically normal persons over the age of 60 have histamine-fast achlorhydria but usually not achylia.

Historical Observations. Addison's name has been linked with pernicious anemia because of his clinical description of the disease in 1855. The term pernicious anemia reflected the inevitable fatal outcome. Gastric atrophy was later noted on autopsy of these patients.

Whipple's observations that liver was a particularly effective food to induce hemoglobin production in dogs led Minot and Murphy to feed raw liver in huge amounts to patients with pernicious anemia. Their success and their recognition of the importance of the gastric lesion won them a Nobel prize and led Castle to his classic experiments, which defined the extrinsic factor and the intrinsic factor.

Castle used the daily reticulocyte count to assess the effectiveness of his therapeutic efforts. For 10 days he gave beef and normal human gastric juice, 12 hours apart; the result was no reticulocytosis. Then, for a succeeding 10-day period, he gave the beef and normal human gastric juice together and achieved a reticulocyte response. He reasoned that for effective erythropoietic activity the interaction of an extrinsic factor (beef) and an intrinsic factor (in normal gastric juice) was essential.

Later, vitamin B_{12} was crystallized (1948), and after enormous effort its structure was determined (1955). Vitamin B_{12} experimentally was shown to be identical to Castle's extrinsic factor. Intrinsic factor is a mucoprotein secreted by the parietal cells of the stomach. It binds vitamin B_{12} and facilitates its absorption in the ileum.

Erythrokinetics in Pernicious Anemia. As previously noted, the mass of erythroid tissue in the marrow is increased. The plasma iron turnover is very rapid, with uptake in the marrow. From the marrow the iron does not move into the circulating red cells but to the liver instead. Fecal urobilinogen is usually increased. Thus, measures of total erythropoiesis indicate an *increase* of up to three times normal.

In untreated pernicious anemia, in addition to poor RBC utilization of iron, the reticulocyte count is low and the survival of circulating erythrocytes is shortened. Effective erythropoiesis is below normal. Since total erythropoiesis is increased, this implies that a great deal of the erythropoietic activity is *ineffective.* This has also been directly shown with glycine-^{15}N studies.

Diagnosis of Pernicious Anemia. The symptoms are non-specific, except that evidence of neurologic involvement is highly suggestive of the diagnosis.

Laboratory Findings

1. Blood and marrow evidence of megaloblastosis.

2. Histamine-fast achlorhydria and achylia (gastric juice, p. 768).

3. Evidence of vitamin B_{12} deficiency.

Microbiological assay of serum vitamin B_{12} employs the organism *Euglena gracilis*, which requires vitamin B_{12} for growth (Anderson, 1964).

Plate 29–1 (Continued.)
populations: normocytic to macrocytic and normochromic, microcytic, and hypochromic, *J*, Blood film, iron deficiency anemia, same patient as in *G* above. The red cells are microcytic; some are also hypochromic; a few target cells and an increased proportion of elliptocytes are present. *K*, Blood film, megaloblastic anemia. The oval macrocytes and hypersegmented neutrophil are presumptive evidence of megaloblastosis. Note the prominent large neutrophil granules. *L*, Blood film, lead poisoning. The red cells are slightly microcytic with some hypochromic cells. The poikilocyte in the center contains basophilic stippling.

A radioisotope dilution assay gives more rapid results, which are comparable to the Euglena assay. One uses $^{57}CoB_{12}$, a standardized intrinsic factor preparation, and albumin-coated charcoal (Lau, 1965). Mollin (1976) discusses the problems that have been encountered with B_{12} radioassays; he believes radioassays should be used as a screening test with results checked by an established micro-biological assay. By either method, the normal serum B_{12} level is 200 to 900 pg/ml.

Measurement of urinary methylmalonic acid: Since a vitamin B_{12} coenzyme is essential for the isomerization of methylmalonate, excretion of in-creased amounts of methylmalonate in the urine is found in vitamin B_{12} deficiency. This is a sensitive test, provided the inborn error of metabolism, methylmalonic aciduria, is not present. Thin-layer chromatography, gas chromatography, or colori-metric methods are available (Hoffbrand, 1971). This measurement is not usually necessary for di-agnosis of vitamin B_{12} deficiency.

Demonstration of a typical reticulocyte response and clinical response with administration of physi-ologic doses of vitamin B_{12} (parenteral, 2 μg per day): The reticulocytes begin to rise on about the fourth day and reach a peak somewhere between the seventh and tenth days, at which time the hemoglobin and number of red blood cells have begun to rise on their way back to normal levels. This shows that vitamin B_{12} deficiency was respon-sible for the anemia.

4. Demonstration that the patient lacks in-trinsic factor.

Several methods have been used for the *in vitro* assay of intrinsic factor activity in the gastric juice (Yamaguchi, 1967). These remain research proce-dures and are not available in most laboratories.

In vivo determination of the ability of the pa-tient to absorb an oral dose of radioactive vitamin B_{12} has become standard practice in the diagnosis of pernicious anemia. This can be done in several ways—measuring fecal excretion, hepatic uptake, urinary excretion, plasma uptake, or even whole body counting. The most convenient is the Schilling test, the measurement of radioactivity in a 24-hour sample of urine. Two hours after oral administra-tion of 0.5 to 2.0 μg of radioactive vitamin B_{12}, a large "flushing" dose of non-labeled vitamin B_{12} is given parenterally. Normal individuals will excrete over 7 per cent of a 1 μg dose of ingested vitamin B_{12} in the urine in 24 hours, whereas patients lack-ing intrinsic factor excrete less. If the excretion is low, the test must be repeated using the same procedure except that hog intrinsic factor is given orally along with the labeled vitamin B_{12}. If the 24-hour excretion is normal, the low value in the first part was due to intrinsic factor deficiency. If the excretion remains abnormal in the second part of the procedure, another explanation for malab-sorption of vitamin B_{12} must be sought (Beck, 1977). The validity of the results depends upon good renal function and an accurate urine collection. The determination of whether the patient has intrinsic factor activity in his gastric juice is the one finding that is demonstrable in both remission and relapse.

5. Serum antibody studies (Hoffbrand, 1971; Taylor, 1976). (See Chap. 38, p. 1280.)

Two types of autoantibodies have been found in the serum of patients with pernicious anemia. One reacts with gastric parietal cells and is present in 85 to 90 per cent of patients who have been tested. This parietal cell antibody is also present in pa-tients with chronic gastritis, such as that associ-ated with iron deficiency, and in some patients with thyroiditis and myxedema; it may be present in healthy controls, especially in older age groups. This is a non-specific finding that probably indi-cates the presence of gastritis. The other autoanti-bodies are directed against intrinsic factor. Almost 75 per cent of patients with pernicious anemia have in their serum anti-intrinsic factor antibodies of the "blocking" type (which block the binding of intrin-sic factor to B_{12}) with or without the "binding" type (which inhibit the binding of intrinsic factor to the ileal mucosa and are present in up to 48 per cent of patients). Intrinsic factor antibodies in the absence of PA have not been found, except in hyperthyroidism (Graves' disease), where the inci-dence is 3 to 6 per cent, and in a similar percentage of insulin-dependent diabetics. There appears to be an immunologic relationship of some kind between stomach and thyroid.

Family studies in patients with pernicious anemia have shown an increased incidence of the disease in relatives, and many relatives have achlorhydria and partial defects of vitamin B_{12} absorption. Relatives of patients with pernicious anemia also have a higher incidence of gastric parietal cell antibodies and of thyroid antibodies than normal.

These and other studies reviewed by Taylor (1976) have led to the suggestion that adult perni-cious anemia may be a genetically determined au-toimmune gastritis. It must be stated, however, that the etiology of the gastric lesion of pernicious anemia remains unknown.

Therapy of Pernicious Anemia. Parenteral injection of hydroxycobalamin at regular in-tervals is the therapy of choice. The maximal reticulocyte response occurs in seven to 10 days. Within 4 to 6 hours after the initial injection, the bone marrow shows a decrease in the number of early megaloblasts and the appearance of normal pronormoblasts. Pro-gressive change toward normal occurs so that by two to four days the marrow is predomi-nantly normoblastic. Of help to the hematolo-gist in partially treated patients is the fact that the cytologic abnormalities in the granu-locytes return to normal more slowly than do those in the erythroid cells. Patients with per-nicious anemia can be kept in complete remission with parenteral injections of hydroxy-cobalamin every one to three months in sufficient amounts to supply about 5 μg/day (Chanarin, 1976). Since up to eight per cent of patients with pernicious anemia have been reported to develop carcinoma of the stomach, annual physical examination, CBC, and erythrocyte sedimentation rate should be performed.

It is important to recognize that treatment with large doses of folic acid (pharmacologic doses of 5 to 15 mg per day) will provide a hematologic response in patients with vitamin B_{12} deficiency while failing to effect any improvement in the neurologic lesions. Failure to recognize that a patient has pernicious anemia may be due to masking of the diagnosis by folic acid therapy; this allows the neurologic complications to progress to an irreversible stage.

Let us return to our classification of vitamin B_{12} deficiency.

GASTRECTOMY. Surgical removal of the stomach (total or even subtotal occasionally) will remove the source of intrinsic factor. This will lead to clinical and laboratory findings almost identical with those of PA after the body's stores of vitamin B_{12} have been exhausted, in three to six years.

Defective Absorption of Vitamin B_{12}

MALABSORPTION SYNDROMES. Celiac disease, tropical sprue, resection of small bowel, or inflammatory disease of the small bowel may be associated with multiple defects of absorption, including other vitamins. Folic acid deficiency (absorbed principally in the upper small bowel) is more commonly seen than vitamin B_{12} deficiency (absorbed principally in the lower small bowel) in diseases leading to malabsorption. The reason for this is probably the lesser time necessary for depletion of body stores of folic acid.

Cases have been reported in which there is specific intestinal failure of absorption of vitamin B_{12} in the presence of normal intrinsic factor, the Immerslund-Gräsbeck syndrome (Cooper, 1976).

LACK OF AVAILABILITY OF VITAMIN B_{12}. In certain countries infestation with the fish tapeworm (*Diphyllobothrium latum*) is common enough so that vitamin B_{12} deficiency may occur occasionally when it is present. The worm successfully competes with the host for the ingested vitamin B_{12}. Most common in Finland, it is rarely seen in the United States.

Bacteria in a blind-loop of intestine may also preferentially utilize ingested vitamin B_{12} to the detriment of the host.

In all these latter conditions, due to malabsorption or lack of availability of vitamin B_{12}, the Schilling test will show lack of absorption of vitamin B_{12} which is not corrected by intrinsic factor.

Folic acid metabolism (Beck, 1977)

Folic acid or pteroyl monoglutamic acid contains three parts: a pteridine derivative; a para-aminobenzoic acid residue; and an L-glutamic acid residue. In nature, folic acid occurs mainly as less soluble polyglutamates, with multiple glutamic acid residues attached to one another. Folic acid is present in a wide variety of foods, such as eggs, milk, leafy vegetables, yeast, liver, and fruits, and also is formed by intestinal bacteria.

Conjugase enzymes in bile and intestine hydrolyze the folylpolyglutamates prior to absorption, which is rapid and occurs in the proximal jejunum. Folate is rapidly removed from plasma to cells and tissues for utilization. The principal form of folate in serum, erythrocytes, and liver is 5-methyl tetrahydrofolate (5-methyl-FH_4); the liver is the chief storage site. The minimal daily requirement is about 50 μg of pteroyl monoglutamate or 400 μg of total folate; the reference interval for serum folate is 5 to 21 μg/l (11 to 48 nmol/l) and for red cell folate 150 to 600 μg/l (340 to 1360 nmol/l) of red blood cells.

Folic acid deficiency (Hoffbrand, 1971; Streif, 1970)

Inadequate Intake of Folic Acid

EVOLUTION OF LABORATORY ABNORMALITIES. Experimental dietary folic acid deficiency in normal man (Herbert, 1962) has elucidated the sequence of events in the onset of folate-deficient megaloblastic anemia. After the folate-deficient diet was initiated, the various abnormalities were established as follows: 3 weeks, low serum folate; 11 weeks, hypersegmentation of neutrophils; 13 weeks, high excretion of formiminoglutamic acid (FIGLU) in urine; 17 weeks, low erythrocyte folate; 18 weeks, macro-ovalocytosis of erythrocytes; 19 weeks, megaloblastic bone marrow; 19 to 20 weeks, anemia.

At this time, changes in the intestinal epithelium had not yet appeared. Therefore, in man, with no dietary intake of folic acid, anemia will appear in three to six months. The peripheral blood and bone marrow features of megaloblastic anemia due to folic acid deficiency are similar to those of vitamin B_{12} deficiency; however, leukopenia and thrombocytopenia are less constant. Folic acid deficiency has usually been found in association with some complicating factor.

NUTRITIONAL FOLATE DEFICIENCY. On a worldwide basis, megaloblastic anemia due to lack of folate is most commonly associated with insufficient dietary intake. The usual diet does not contain much above the minimal requirements, and body stores (in the adult) are sufficient for only about three months' needs. Dietary folate deficiency is especially common in the tropics and in India, and even there it is usually associated with increased demand for folate in pregnancy, rapid growth in infancy, infection, or hemolytic anemia.

Folate deficiency in infancy is uncommon in the United States. Human milk or fresh cow's milk contains sufficient folate, but heated milk, powdered milk, and goat's milk do not. If the infant's milk lacks folate, if the diet is low in ascorbic acid, or if infections or diarrhea are a problem, then megaloblastic anemia may occur (Mauer, 1969).

Megaloblastic anemia in pregnancy is not uncommon, because of the fetal requirements for folate. The mother's plasma folate level gradually falls during pregnancy, and at birth the plasma level in the newborn averages five times that of the mother. Megaloblastic anemia is more frequent in multiparae, may be precipitated by infection, and is usually due to folate deficiency rather than B_{12} deficiency. Pregnant women should receive, in addition to iron, folic acid supplements of about 500 μg per day (WHO Report, 1972).

Elderly persons on inadequate diets in this country may develop folate-deficient megaloblastic anemia, a fact increasingly recognized in recent years.

LIVER DISEASE. Liver disease associated with alcoholism may lead to folate-deficient megaloblastic anemia because of the grossly inadequate diet of the alcoholic. With an adequate dietary folic acid intake, however, the anemia that is found with liver disease is macrocytic and normoblastic, not megaloblastic.

Defective Absorption of Folic Acid. Defective absorption of folic acid occurs in association with malabsorption syndromes discussed above and in the blind-loop syndrome, in which bacteria preferentially utilize folate.

Non-tropical sprue, or adult celiac disease, is an important cause of malabsorption in adults or children that, in some unknown way, is related to dietary gluten (wheat protein) (Sleisenger, 1975). Included among the signs of malabsorption may be megaloblastic anemia due to folic acid deficiency (Beck, 1977). Jeju-

nal biopsy shows villous atrophy. The folate deficiency as well as the malabsorption responds to a gluten-free diet. Folic acid therapy (parenteral) corrects the folate deficiency but not the general malabsorption.

Tropical sprue is common in the Caribbean, India, and Southeast Asia, and is generally similar to non-tropical sprue. It may in part be due to folate deficiency, but bacterial contamination of the small intestine also appears to play a causative role (Sleisenger, 1975). Evidence of malabsorption (p. 780) includes megaloblastic anemia due to folate deficiency. Treatment with folic acid brings considerable improvement in the general malabsorption as well as the anemia, but antimicrobial treatment is recommended in addition.

Megaloblastic anemia or decreased serum and red cell folate without anemia has been associated with the long-term use of anticoagulant drugs, phenytoin, phenobarbital, and primidone. There is considerable evidence that absorption of folate is impaired in the presence of the drug, but the mechanism is not completely understood. Oral contraceptives may adversely affect folate metabolism in a small proportion of women, probably those who have an underlying defect in absorption, utilization, or storage (Stebbins, 1976).

Increased Requirements for Folic Acid. The increased need in pregnancy and in infants (multiple birth) has been mentioned. The increased cell turnover that occurs in neoplasia or in the markedly stimulated hematopoiesis of hemolytic anemias may result in megaloblastic erythropoiesis. The basis for this is increased need for a marginal supply of folate.

Inadequate Utilization of Folic Acid. Inadequate utilization of folic acid is relatively rare but applies in certain cases.

Folic acid antagonists, such as methotrexate, block folic acid metabolism and because of this are used in therapy of some malignant neoplasms. In addition to inhibiting the growth of the tumor, they will also induce megaloblastic erythropoiesis.

In addition to the previously mentioned nutritional problem in alcoholics, *alcohol* may exert a direct effect in suppressing hematopoiesis by blocking metabolism of folate.

DIAGNOSIS OF FOLIC ACID DEFICIENCY. Folic acid deficiency or vitamin B_{12} deficiency is suspected when the blood and bone marrow show findings characteristic of megaloblastic anemia; usually serum folate and B_{12} levels are then determined.

Serum and Red Cell Folate. A microbiologic assay for folic acid activity employing *Lactobacillus casei* has been widely used, and remains the most reliable method for the definitive diagnosis (Beck, 1977a). Radioisotopic methods employing different folate binders are increasingly used because of rapidity and greater convenience. Although the correlation with the microbiologic assay is generally good, discrepancies seem to be frequent and, on the basis of other data, tend to be resolved in favor of the microbiologic assay (Rudzki, 1976).

The serum folate is decreased ($< 3\,\mu g/l$) in megaloblastic anemia due to folate deficiency but is usually normal in vitamin B_{12} deficiency. A low serum folate level precedes decrease of red cell or tissue folate; it indicates a negative folate balance but does not by itself indicate tissue folate deficiency. A low red cell folate level ($< 150\,\mu g/l$) is definite evidence of folic acid deficiency.

Urinary Formiminoglutamic Acid (FIGLU). Folic acid coenzymes are required for the conversion of FIGLU to glutamic acid in the catabolism of histidine. When oral histidine is given, FIGLU will appear in increased amounts in the urine if folate deficiency is present. However, its value in discriminating between vitamin B_{12} and folate deficiency is lessened by the fact that many patients (50 per cent) with pernicious anemia who are not deficient in folic acid have increased FIGLU excretion.

Therapeutic Trial. The therapeutic trial remains an excellent way to discriminate between folic acid and vitamin B_{12} deficiency. Physiologic doses of folic acid (parenteral, 50 to 200 μg/day) will allow an adequate reticulocyte response in patients with folic acid deficiency, but not in vitamin B_{12} deficiency. Physiologic daily doses of vitamin B_{12} (parenteral, 1 to 5 μg/day) will lead to hematologic response in patients with vitamin B_{12} deficiency and not folic acid deficiency.

On the other hand, the usual therapeutic doses of folic acid (5 to 15 mg/day) or larger doses of vitamin B_{12} (500 to 1000 μg) may induce a partial response in a patient with megaloblastic anemia due to the other deficiency.

The therapy of pernicious anemia with folic acid sufficient to lead to a hematologic response (5 to 15 mg/day) must be condemned because of the danger of allowing the neurologic manifestation of PA (subacute combined degeneration of the spinal cord) to progress and become irreversible.

Other Defects of Nucleoprotein Synthe- ***sis.*** Other defects of nucleoprotein synthesis may lead to megaloblastic anemias which do not respond to vitamin B_{12} or folic acid.

CONGENITAL DEFECTS. Oroticaciduria is a very rare autosomal recessive condition in which certain enzymes required for pyrimidine synthesis are absent. The findings are excessive urinary excretion of orotic acid, failure of normal growth and development, and megaloblastic anemia which is refractory to vitamin B_{12} and folate but which responds to uridine.

SYNTHETIC INHIBITORS. Synthetic inhibitors of purine synthesis (6-mercaptopurine, thioguanine, azathioprine), of pyrimidine synthesis (5-fluorouracil), or of deoxyribonucleotide synthesis (cytosine arabinoside or hydroxyurea) are used in chemotherapy for neoplasia and may concomitantly produce megaloblastosis.

REFRACTORY ANEMIAS. Anemias that are megaloblastic and that fail to respond to vitamin B_{12} or folic acid are considered with the refractory anemias (p. 982). Usually the megaloblastic changes are not typical and do not include the characteristic granulocytic changes.

IMPAIRED PRODUCTION—OTHER

Anemia of chronic disorders

The anemia most commonly seen in chronic infections, rheumatoid arthritis, and neoplastic disease is usually mild and is overshadowed by the basic disease. Occasionally the basic disease may be obscured by the anemia. Usually, the anemia does not progress in severity and has characteristic morphologic, biochemical, and kinetic disturbances (Cartwright, 1966; 1971).

Blood. The erythrocytes are usually normocytic and normochromic, but they are often normocytic and hypochromic and occasionally microcytic and hypochromic. As the anemia develops, hypochromia usually precedes the development of microcytosis; this is in contrast to iron deficiency anemia, in which the reverse is usual. Anisocytosis and poikilocytosis are slight. The reticulocyte count is usually not elevated. Leukocytes and platelets are not distinctively altered, except by the causative disease.

Marrow. The marrow is normocellular or minimally hypocellular or hypercellular, and the cell distribution is not greatly disturbed. The normoblasts may have frayed hypochromic cytoplasm and the appearance of hemoglobin in the cells may be delayed (as in iron deficiency anemia). Sideroblasts are decreased, but storage iron is normal or increased.

Biochemical Features. The serum iron is characteristically decreased, the total iron-binding capacity (TIBC) is decreased or normal (in contrast to iron deficiency anemia, in which the TIBC is elevated), and the per cent saturation is somewhat decreased. Erythrocyte protoporphyrin and serum ferritin are elevated.

Erythrokinetics. Red cell production, though normal or even slightly increased, is insufficient to compensate for a moderately decreased red cell survival. In these patients, the marrow is capable of responding to erythropoietin; but for unknown reasons, erythropoietin production is inappropriately low. Erythropoietin can be produced in response to other types of stimulation, for example, cobalt.

The defect in iron metabolism is principally a block in the movement of iron from the storage sites in the reticuloendothelial cells to the erythroid marrow; this results in the low serum iron and in an iron-deficient type of erythropoiesis, despite the presence of adequate storage iron. The anemia usually fails to respond to therapy with iron or other measures; spontaneous improvement will occur when the underlying disorder is corrected.

The abnormalities are characteristic of a large number of anemias secondary to systemic disease. Cartwright (1966) has proposed the term "sideropenic anemia with reticuloendothelial siderosis" as more descriptive than "simple chronic anemia" for a condition that is not simple and that is not always chronic.

Anemia of renal insufficiency

The correlation between the severity of the anemia and the degree of elevation of the blood urea nitrogen is positive but not strictly linear. When the blood urea nitrogen (BUN) exceeds 100 mg/dl (36 mmol/l), the hematocrit is usually below 0.30 (Erslev, 1977).

Several factors are often involved in the anemia of chronic renal failure. Decreased production of erythropoietin by the damaged kidney is probably the important factor in most cases in which the blood urea nitrogen exceeds 100 mg/dl. Even with complete loss of kidney function (e.g., bilateral nephrectomy) there is a basal level of erythropoiesis; it is not known whether this is the result of extrarenal erythropoietin production. Both ineffective erythropoiesis and impaired ability of the marrow to respond to erythropoietin appear to be present in some degree.

Hemolysis is a significant feature in many cases of chronic renal failure. There appears to be an extracorpuscular factor in uremic plasma which has a detrimental effect on red cell metabolism and results in morphologically deformed cells (irregularly contracted and spiculated red cells). Numerous irregularly contracted and fragmented cells are seen in the hemolytic uremic syndrome and in malignant hypertension as a result of traumatic damage incurred by the red cells in traversing the damaged small blood vessels (Brain, 1962).

In addition, bleeding is a common problem in chronic renal disease, probably due either to thrombocytopenia, in some patients, or to platelet functional defects, which are present in most patients. Anemia due to iron deficiency from blood loss should always be suspected. Folic acid deficiency may be a problem in patients in a dialysis program, since folic acid is readily moved into the dialysis bath.

Anemia of liver disease

Chronic posthemorrhagic anemia, folate-deficient megaloblastic anemia due to poor nutrition in alcoholic cirrhosis, and acquired hemolytic anemias associated with either Coombs' positive red cells, congestive splenomegaly, or lipid disturbances may occur in liver disease.

In addition to these, there is an anemia associated with liver disease which is characterized by shortened red cell survival and relatively inadequate red cell production. It is exaggerated by an increased blood volume which appears to correlate with the degree of portal hypertension (Wintrobe, 1974). The red cells are normocytic or macrocytic (thin macrocytes). Frequently target cells are present, especially in obstructive jaundice (see Fig. 27-21); these have increased surface membrane with increased cholesterol and lecithin content. Their survival is decreased if there is splenomegaly due to cirrhosis (Cooper, 1977a). Reticulocytes may be slightly increased, and platelets may be normal or decreased. The bone marrow may be slightly hypercellular and erythropoiesis is macronormoblastic rather than megaloblastic. Changes in leukocytes, such as are present in megaloblastic anemias, are not seen, and this type of anemia does not respond to vitamin B_{12} or folic acid. The anemia is of unknown origin.

A small proportion of patients with severe cirrhosis have a hemolytic anemia associated with "spur cells," which are red cells with thorny projections similar to acanthocytes. As with target cells, the spur cells are secondary to lipid abnormalities in the plasma; they have increased surface membrane with increased cholesterol but normal phospholipid content in the membrane. These irregular cells have decreased deformability and tend to be trapped in the spleen and destroyed (Cooper, 1977b).

Anemia in endocrine disease

Uncomplicated anemia in hypothyroidism is mild to moderate; it is normochromic and normocytic without reticulocytosis and with normal red cell survival. It reflects a decreased marrow production due to a smaller tissue oxygen requirement. Hypothyroidism may, of course, be complicated by iron deficiency or folic acid or vitamin B_{12} deficiency. The pathogenesis of a similar anemia in adrenal cortical hormone deficiency is less clear; it is corrected by hormone replacement.

Deficient testosterone secretion in the man results in a decrease in red cell production of 1 to 2 g Hb/dl (to a value comparable to that of the woman); this appears to be due to the effect of androgens on erythropoietin secretion.

Pituitary deficiency tends to result in a greater depression of hemoglobin concentration because of the effect on multiple endocrine glands and possibly the loss of growth hormone effect (Erslev, 1977).

Anemia associated with bone marrow infiltration (myelophthisic anemia)

This anemia is associated with marrow replacement by (or involvement with) metastatic carcinoma, multiple myeloma, leukemia, lymphoma, lipidoses or storage disease, and certain other conditions.

The characteristic finding in the blood is the presence of varying numbers of normoblasts and immature neutrophils; these are responsible for the descriptive terms *leukoerythroblastotic reaction, leukoerythroblastic anemia,* and *leukoerythroblastosis* (see Table 27-4, p. 901).

Normochromic and normocytic (occasionally macrocytic) anemia of varying severity is present. Reticulocytes are often increased, and the number of normoblasts is usually out of proportion to the severity of the anemia. The leukocyte count is normal or reduced (occasionally elevated), and immature neutrophils and even myeloblasts may be found. Platelets are normal or decreased, and bizarre, atypical platelets can sometimes be seen.

Examination of the marrow will usually reveal the condition responsible for this reac-

tion. Mechanical crowding out of the hematopoietic tissue by the pathologic process has been assumed but not proved and probably is not the usual cause. Often the amount of erythropoietic tissue in the marrow as determined by morphologic and kinetic studies is normal or increased. The mechanism described in the section on anemia of chronic disorders (p. 977) may often play a role, but the reason for the outpouring of immature cells into the blood is not clear.

In addition to myelophthisic anemias, circulating normoblasts and immature neutrophils can also be seen in severe anemias due to other causes, severe infections, and congestive heart failure, but usually the normoblasts are not so numerous.

The *leukoerythroblastotic reaction* associated with myelophthisic anemias cannot always be distinguished from the blood picture of myelosclerosis with myeloid metaplasia (MMM), which is usually regarded as one of the myeloproliferative disorders. In MMM, enlargement of the spleen and liver is almost always found. In the blood film, more severe red cell abnormalities, leukocytosis, myeloblasts and immature granulocytes of all varieties (not just neutrophils), increased basophils, more atypical platelets, more numerous megakaryocyte fragments, and dwarf megakaryocytes are all findings more characteristic of MMM than of a leukoerythroblastotic reaction of some other cause. Examination of the bone marrow by a needle biopsy or surgical biopsy is necessary to differentiate MMM from other myelophthisic anemias (see p. 951).

Aplastic anemia

The term aplastic anemia usually refers to pancytopenia associated with hypocellularity of the bone marrow—that is, a severe reduction in the amount of hematopoietic tissue which results in deficient production of blood cells. The marrow, though hypocellular, may have patchy areas of normocellularity or even hypercellularity.

The clinical course may be acute and fulminating, with profound pancytopenia and a rapid progression to death, or the disorder may have an insidious onset and a chronic course. The symptoms and signs are related to the degree of the deficiencies: bleeding may be caused by thrombocytopenia; infection may be the result of neutropenia; and other signs and symptoms are those of anemia. As a rule, splenomegaly and lymphadenopathy are absent.

3

Aplastic anemias are of diverse etiology. In approximately half the cases, the marrow has apparently been injured by ionizing radiation, drugs, or chemicals; and in the remainder, no antecedent cause of exposure to an injurious agent can be found (Lewis, 1965).

Aplastic Anemia Associated with Chemical or Physical Agents

TOXIC APLASTIC ANEMIAS.   Toxic aplastic anemias are caused by a number of physical and chemical agents that produce marrow damage in all humans and animals exposed to a sufficient dose. Here belong ionizing radiation, mustard compounds, benzene, and antineoplastic agents, such as busulfan, urethane, and antimetabolites.

Benzene Poisoning.   The changes in the blood frequently include anemia, either alone or in combination with leukopenia and thrombocytopenia. Occasional changes are eosinophilia, leukocytosis, and leukemoid reactions. The marrow may vary from acellular to hypocellular to hypercellular. Occasionally extramedullary hematopoiesis and splenomegaly may be present.

Ionizing Radiation.   The effects on blood cells depend on the radiosensitivity of the cells, the capacity of the cells to regenerate, and the survival rate of the cells in the peripheral blood. The erythroid cells are most sensitive, granulocytes have intermediate sensitivity, and the megakaryocytes are the least sensitive of the three. Reticulum cells and connective tissue cells are relatively insensitive.

After acute exposure to radiation, the reticulocyte count falls, but the red cells decline very slowly because of their long survival. Within the first few hours there is a neutrophilic leukocytosis due to a shift from marginal and probably marrow storage pools. A fall in lymphocytes occurs after the first day and is responsible for the early leukopenia. After five days or so, granulocytes begin to fall. The last cells to decrease are usually the platelets; these are often the last to return to normal in the recovery phase.

The effects of massive exposure depend on the dose and sensitivity. In the acute radiation syndrome, systemic effects (prostration, fever), leukopenia, and infection may lead rapidly to death. Or thrombocytopenia and purpura may develop. This form may lead to diarrhea, dehydration, infection, aplastic anemia, hemorrhage, and death in weeks. The effect of radioactive isotopes is more gradual, more persistent, and longer lasting. Late effects of ionizing radiation include increased susceptibility to leukemia.

Blood counts at regular intervals for persons exposed occupationally to ionizing radiation have been recommended, but this practice is ineffective in detecting dangerous doses of radiation before the damage is done. The use of film badges is more practical.

HYPERSENSITIVE APLASTIC ANEMIAS.   A large number of drugs produce marrow damage in some individuals after single or repeated exposures. These drugs are not capable of damaging the marrow of animals, as are the chemicals in the first group. They include antimicrobial drugs (salvarsan, chloramphenicol, sulfonamides, chlortetracycline, streptomycin), anticonvulsants (Mesantoin, Tridione), analgesics (phenylbutazone), antithyroid drugs (carbimazole), antihistaminics (Pyribenzamine), insecticides (DDT), and other chemicals—some known (gold compounds, Atabrine, chlorpromazine, hair dyes, bismuth, mercury) and others to come.

Chloramphenicol is a drug in this category that appears important in the causation of aplastic anemia. Reactions of the marrow to chloramphenicol are of two types which are possibly unrelated (Yunis, 1964; Wintrobe, 1974).

In about half the patients who receive chloramphenicol, a reversible increase in serum iron, reticulocytopenia with anemia, neutropenia, and thrombocytopenia occur. The marrow may show decreased erythroid cells and vacuolization of primitive erythroid and granulocyte precursors. These changes are dose- and time-dependent and reversible.

In a very small proportion of persons receiving chloramphenicol, an irreversible aplastic anemia develops which may be fatal. No relationship has been established between the reversible erythropoietic lesion and the development of aplastic anemia; it may be that individual susceptibility is responsible for the latter. For this reason it is essential that restraint be employed in using the drug, because monitoring its administration with blood cell counts is unlikely to be an effective preventive measure (Wintrobe, 1974).

Aplastic Anemia Associated with Other Disease

INFECTION.   Marrow aplasia has been described as an infrequent sequel to infectious hepatitis, occurring a few months after onset when the hepatitis is resolving. These patients are usually males and under age 20; the prognosis is usually grave (Hagler, 1975). Other viral infections can cause hematopoietic depression and rarely are followed by aplastic anemia.

PAROXYSMAL NOCTURNAL HEMOGLOBINURIA (PNH). This rare hemolytic process (p. 987) may be followed by aplastic anemia. Usually in PNH a variable degree of marrow hypofunction coexists. Curiously, in some patients who present with aplastic anemia, the red cell defect of PNH may be present or may appear during the course of the disease. According to Lewis (1967), about 15 per cent of patients with aplastic anemia have a demonstrable PNH red cell defect, with or without clinical hemolysis.

Idiopathic Aplastic Anemia. In patients with pancytopenia and a hypocellular bone marrow, search should be made for evidence of significant exposure to radiation, drugs, and chemicals of known or possible propensity to injure the marrow so that further exposure can be eliminated. Nevertheless, in approximately half the cases of aplastic anemia, no suspected causal relationship to toxic agents can be found, and it is these that are designated as idiopathic.

The symptoms and signs do not differ, but the onset is commonly more insidious than in toxic or hypersensitive aplastic anemias.

BLOOD. The red cells are usually normal in size and shape, though in some cases there may be varying degrees of anisocytosis and poikilocytosis or macrocytosis. Polychromasia, stippling, and normoblasts are most often conspicuously absent. Leukopenia with marked decrease in granulocytes and a relative lymphocytosis are observed. In severe leukopenia there is often also an absolute lymphocytopenia. Neutrophil granules may be larger than normal and may stain dark red (unlike the "toxic" granules found in infections), and the leukocyte alkaline phosphatase may be elevated (Lewis, 1962). Thrombocytopenia is part of the picture. The serum iron is usually increased.

BONE MARROW. In most cases the aspirate consists of red cells, lymphocytes, some plasma cells, and fatty particles. Marrow sections will show fatty tissue with inconspicuous fibrosis and islands of lymphocytes and plasma cells (Plate 29-1*C*). Though focal areas of normocellularity or hypercellularity may sometimes be present, the overall cellularity is decreased. Storage iron is increased.

ERYTHROKINETIC STUDIES. The increased serum iron is a valuable early sign of erythroid hypoplasia and reflects the decreased plasma iron turnover. In addition, the erythrocyte utilization of iron is decreased. Both effective and total erythropoiesis, therefore, are decreased in aplastic anemia.

Constitutional Aplastic Anemia (Fanconi's Anemia; Congenital Pancytopenia). Pancytopenia becomes obvious after infancy and usually by the eighth year of life. Often more than one member of a family is affected. The anemia is usually normochromic and may be macrocytic; the marrow is generally hypocellular. Developmental anomalies are present and may include short stature, hypogonadism, malformations of the extremities (e.g., aplasia of the radius and abnormalities of the thumbs), and malformations of other organs (e.g., heart and kidneys). Chromosomal defects have been described (Fanconi, 1967).

PATHOGENESIS OF APLASTIC ANEMIA. Some kind of damage to the hematopoietic stem cell appears to be likely in most cases of aplastic anemia, by a known or unknown agent that in some way alters the ability of the cell to proliferate or differentiate (L.A., 1977). Although hematopoietic stem cells cannot be assayed in humans, the committed granulocyte-monocyte precursor cells (GM-CFC) are decreased in blood and marrow in most patients with aplastic anemia (Kern, 1977). In a small proportion of cases, it may be that the defect is in the hematopoietic microenvironment which fails to support stem-cell growth; this may be the case when bone marrow transplants repeatedly will not "take." Also, evidence is accumulating that inhibition of stem-cell growth may be mediated by peripheral blood or bone marrow lymphocytes in some cases of aplastic anemia (Good, 1977).

MANAGEMENT. Treatment in aplastic anemia is aimed at blood replacement, stimulation of any residual marrow (androgens, adrenal corticoids), combating infection (antibiotics, isolation), and controlling bleeding problems. Bone marrow transplantation, when a suitable donor is available, is successful in selected patients but as yet requires a vast array of support services and fails in a fair proportion of trials because of marrow graft rejection, graft-versus-host disease, or infections (Storb, 1976).

PROGNOSIS. Complications are related to infection, bleeding, and problems of iron overload from repeated transfusion. The prognosis appears to depend upon the severity of marrow damage. In the series from Utah analyzed by Williams (1973), 25 per cent of patients died within four months of the onset of symptoms, 50 per cent died within 12 months, and 71 per cent within five years. There was no prognostic influence of age of the patient or the etiology of the aplasia. Those who died within four months had significantly lower reticulocyte, neutrophil, and platelet counts; lower per cent of myeloid cells in the marrow; and a shorter interval between onset of symptoms and visit to the physician (Lynch, 1975). In the survivors, partial recovery is common. A small proportion of survivors eventually have been found to develop leukemia or paroxysmal nocturnal hemoglobinuria.

Aplastic anemia has a high mortality rate. It may be important to identify early those who have a particularly grim prognosis for potential marrow transplantation.

Pure Red Cell Aplasia

TRANSITORY ARREST OF ERYTHROPOIESIS. This may occur during the course of a hemolytic anemia (often preceded by an infection), and the combination of aplasia and hemolysis becomes a threatening situation (Bauman, 1967). Red cell production may occasionally cease during rather minor infections in normal children or adults, at which time the marrow will show absence of all but a few of the most immature erythroid precursors. Since a temporary arrest in production, e.g., a week or two, may not result in enough fall in hemoglobin to become symptomatic, it is quite possible that such events are considerably more common than we realize. If the arrest in erythropoiesis persists, anemia will result (Chanarin, 1964).

CONGENITAL HYPOPLASTIC ANEMIA (ERYTHRO-GENESIS IMPERFECTA; THE ANEMIA OF BLACKFAN AND DIAMOND). This is a rare pure red cell aplasia which usually becomes obvious during the first few months of life. The severe anemia is normochromic and slightly macrocytic; reticulocyte level is low; leukocytes and platelets are normal; and the marrow shows a marked reduction in all developing erythroid cells except pronormoblasts, but normal granulocytic and megakaryocytic cell lines. Fetal hemoglobin (Hb F) is elevated (5 to 25 per cent) to a degree not expected for the patient's age and the antigen "i" (little i) is often present (Diamond, 1976). These findings contrast with those of transient arrest of erythropoiesis (transient erythroblastopenia of childhood). In the latter, the red cells are normocytic, the Hb F is normal, the antigen "i" is absent, and red cell enzymes are at a lower level (characteristic of an older cell population) (Wang, 1976).

Conflicting evidence has been presented regarding the nature of the defect. Hoffman (1976) demonstrated that lymphocytes from six patients suppressed growth of normal erythroid cells *in vitro*, suggesting a cellular immune phenomenon. Nathan (1978) on the other hand could not demonstrate such a phenomenon in their 11 patients; they showed that the committed erythroid precursor cells were qualitatively or quantitatively unresponsive to erythropoietin.

Most patients respond at least partially to corticosteroids, but only 25 per cent or so achieve long-term remissions without the drug (Diamond, 1976).

ACQUIRED PURE RED CELL APLASIA. In adults, selective failure of production of red cells is also rare. Reticulocytopenia and a cellular marrow devoid of all but the most primitive erythroid precursors are characteristic. Leukocyte and platelet production are normal. About half the cases are associated with a thymoma, a relationship that must be more than accidental (Havard, 1965). Remission of the anemia occurs in about one fourth of patients when the thymoma is removed. Autoimmune phenomena are present in some patients. Krantz (1974) has presented evidence for cytotoxic antibody against erythroid precursors and a plasma inhibitor of heme synthesis in the majority of patients he has studied; this kind of humoral activity has not been found in the anemia of Blackfan and Diamond.

Refractory Anemia with Hypercellular Bone Marrow.
Anemia or pancytopenia of unknown cause is sometimes associated with a hypercellular bone marrow showing erythroid hyperplasia and low or inadequate levels of reticulocytes in the blood. Red cell life span may be somewhat shortened, but hemolysis is not a major problem. Plasma iron turnover is increased, but the erythrocyte utilization of

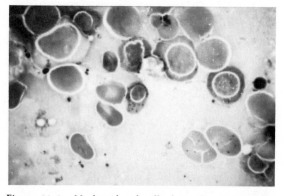

Figure 29-3. Nucleated red cells from the marrow of a patient with sideroblastic anemia. The Prussian blue reaction stains non-hemoglobin iron as blue granules (here shown as dark granules) in the cytoplasm. The perinuclear space is artifactually widened. In the center is a late normoblast with multiple granules of iron, hence, a sideroblast; it is a ring sideroblast, since the granules almost completely surround the nucleus. In the lower right are two siderocytes, i.e., non-nucleated red cells containing stainable iron granules. (×875.)

iron is decreased. Characteristically, therefore, ineffective erythropoiesis is increased. These anemias have been reviewed by Vilter and his associates (1967).

Sideroblastic Anemia. This is characterized by hypochromic, often microcytic, red cells in the blood, with or without leukopenia and thrombocytopenia. The serum iron is increased, and the per cent saturation of the iron-binding protein is greatly elevated. The marrow shows markedly increased storage iron, erythroid hyperplasia with evidence of defective hemoglobinization, and increased numbers of sideroblasts. In addition to increased numbers of sideroblasts, there are increased numbers of granules per cell, and granules surround the nucleus (at least three fourths of the circumference) forming "ring sideroblasts" (Dacie, 1966) (Fig. 29–3; Plate 29–1*E* and *F*). In the latter, iron loading of mitochondria is seen by electron microscopy (Fig. 29–4). In the hereditary form and in primary acquired sideroblastic anemia usually over half of the normoblasts are ring sideroblasts, whereas in the other forms ring sidero-

blasts are fewer. These findings probably reflect defective synthesis of protoporphyrin, which may be due to any of several possible enzyme defects (Hoffbrand, 1977). Occasionally, megaloblast-like changes are seen in the erythroid cells, but changes typical of vitamin B$_{12}$ or folate deficiency are not seen in granulocytes unless folate deficiency coexists. The following classification is that of Hines (1970):

HEREDITARY SEX-LINKED SIDEROBLASTIC ANEMIA. This occurs in males and may not appear until adolescence. It is rare, but a few well-documented family studies exist.

ACQUIRED REFRACTORY SIDEROBLASTIC ANEMIA. *Primary acquired sideroblastic anemia* is more common and has its onset in later adult life and in either sex. This is usually a dimorphic anemia with both normochromic and hypochromic red cells. In addition to the marrow findings described previously, tissue mast cells are usually increased in number. The marrow is megalobastic in over half the cases, and usually remains so after therapy with vitamin B$_{12}$ and folic acid. A small pro-

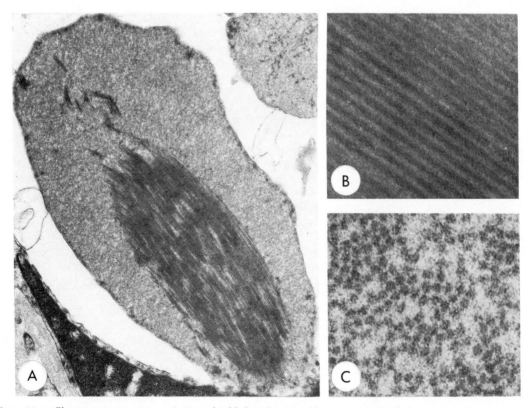

Figure 29–4. Electron microscopic examination of sickled erythrocytes (A— × 11,000) reveals the presence of numerous long, slender, parallel rods, representing polymerized reduced hemoglobin S, along the long axis of the deformed erythrocyte. At higher magnification (B— × 150,000), as described by Stetson (1966), the rods can be seen to have a diameter of about 15 nm, and on cross-section (C— × 150,000) show a tubular configuration with electron-dense borders. As discussed by Bunn (1977), each "rod" probably represents an eight-stranded helix, with each strand composed of a chain of interconnected tetramers of reduced Hb S. (From Fresco, R.: Ultrastructure of the blood cells and their precursors. *In* Davidsohn, I., and Henry, J. B.: Clinical Diagnosis by Laboratory Methods, 15th ed. Philadelphia, W. B. Saunders Company, 1974.)

portion of patients has either folic acid deficiency or an abnormality in pyridoxine metabolism, or both, and show partial improvement when treated with these agents. A likely explanation for the combination of impaired heme synthesis and megaloblastosis is a somatic mutation. If leukocyte and platelet abnormalities are present, this may be at the hematopoietic stem cell level; if not, it presumably is at the erythroid-committed progenitor cell level (Hoffbrand, 1977). A small proportion, perhaps 10 per cent, of these patients eventually develop acute leukemia (Gralnick, 1977).

Secondary acquired sideroblastic anemia is associated with another disease (which may or may not be hematologic) and usually shows fewer ring sideroblasts than the primary form. Hines (1970) states that about half the patients in this group show a hematologic response to folic acid, or pyridoxine, or both.

Reversible Sideroblastic Anemia. This is due to some agent which interferes with heme synthesis; recognition is important because hematologic improvement occurs if the agent is removed.

The *antituberculosis drugs* isoniazid, cycloserine, and pyrazinamide cause sideroblastic abnormalities in some patients on long-term therapy.

Lead poisoning is an important member of this group because environmental exposure to lead is usually unrecognized and needs to be detected. Lead interferes with heme synthesis by blocking the enzymes ALA synthetase, ALA dehydrase, and heme synthetase. These blocks are only partial and of different degree; aminolevulinic acid and coproporphyrin are increased in the urine. *Chloramphenicol* also results in ring sideroblast formation, probably by inhibiting mitochondrial protein synthesis.

Alcoholism is perhaps the most common of the reversible sideroblastic anemias. Folate deficiency, hypomagnesemia, and hypokalemia are concomitant findings. After withdrawal of alcohol intake, the abnormal sideroblasts usually disappear within a few days.

Pyridoxine-responsive Anemia. Individuals who partially respond to pyridoxine have been included in other categories above. Those in whom anemia is completely corrected form a smaller group. They are young or middleaged males with a severe microcytic and hypochromic anemia and are dependent upon extraordinary amounts of dietary pyridoxine to maintain a normal hemoglobin level.

Refractory Anemia with Excess of Blasts (Dysmyelopoiesis). Included here is a group of ill-defined refractory anemias with hypercellular marrow, macrocytic or normocytic anemia, usually with neutropenia and thrombocytopenia. The marrow shows bizarre megaloblastoid erythropoiesis but is without all the characteristic morphologic alterations seen in typical megaloblastic anemia of vitamin B_{12} and folate deficiency, and the process does not respond to these agents. Sideroblasts may or may not be prominent here, and the erythroblasts may have PAS-positive cytoplasm. Abnormalities in the granulocytes may be present, and the leukocyte alkaline phosphatase is sometimes very high or very low. Abnormalities in megakaryocytes are common and include bizarre giant forms, complete separation of nuclear lobes, or small fragmented forms with one or two small nuclei. Myeloblasts may be increased up to about 20 per cent for long periods of time, accounting for the name. Among the refractory anemias with a hypercellular marrow, this group may be particularly likely to eventuate in acute myelogenous leukemia or erythroleukemia; this has occurred in about 28 per cent of patients (Gralnick, 1977). It is classified among the dysmyelopoietic syndromes (p. 1075).

Anemia in Alcoholism. An excessive alcoholic intake leads to macrocytosis, at first without anemia (Chanarin, 1976). Eichner and Hillman (1971) have provided evidence suggesting stages in the evolution of anemia of alcoholism. *First,* negative vitamin balance is associated with regular alcohol ingestion and decreased food intake; the serum folic acid is low and the marrow shows cytoplasmic vacuoles in the erythroid precursors. *Second,* the erythroid marrow becomes megaloblastic, and the anemia (usually but not always present) is characteristic of folate deficiency. *Third,* sideroblastic anemia (characterized by ring sideroblasts) develops, but only in certain patients who have either pyridoxine deficiency or some ethanol-induced interference with pyridoxine metabolism. *Fourth,* early resolution occurs when alcohol ingestion is stopped or normal diet is started. The marrow becomes normoblastic, reticulocytosis occurs, but some ring sideroblasts persist. *Finally,* 10 days or so after the onset of stage four, the ring sideroblasts have disappeared and the marrow and blood picture resembles hemolytic anemia. Different hematologic patterns, therefore, may depend upon the time of the evaluation.

In the presence of cirrhosis with splenomegaly other changes complicate these findings (p. 978).

CONGENITAL DYSERYTHROPOIETIC ANEMIA (CDA). Several forms of apparently hereditary anemias characterized by abnormal erythropoiesis with ineffective erythropoiesis and splenomegaly have recently been identified. They appear to have an autosomal recessive mode of inheritance. In general, they tend to be more benign than β thalassemia major, which forms another group of hereditary anemias with ineffective erythropoiesis.

At least three types have thus far been separated on the basis of marrow and serologic findings (Lewis, 1973). CDA-I has megaloblastic changes with some binuclearity, internuclear chromatin bridges, and a macrocytic anemia. CDA-II shows binuclearity and multinuclearity of erythroid precursors with pluripolar mitoses and karyorrhexis. The anemia is normocytic. CDA-II is distinguished from the others because it has a positive acidified serum test (with some, but not all normal sera) and a negative sucrose hemolysis test. It is known as Hereditary Erythroblastic Multinuclearity with Positive Acidified Serum test (HEMPAS). The red cells have an antigen not present on normal or PNH cells and about one third of normal sera contain the corresponding antibody. CDA-III, described first by Björkman in 1965, has more pronounced multinuclearity, with giant erythroid precursors and a macrocytic anemia.

HEMOLYSIS—GENERAL

Definitions

Anemias which are due primarily to increased red cell destruction are *hemolytic anemias*. A shortened red cell survival, therefore, proves that hemolysis is present; this measurement is usually unnecessary in practice.

Hemolytic anemias may be due to a defect of the red cell itself, an *intrinsic hemolytic anemia:* these are usually hereditary, and are commonly grouped as *membrane, metabolic,* or *hemoglobin* defects. Or the hemolysis may be due to a factor outside the red cell and acting upon it, an *extrinsic hemolytic anemia:* these are almost always acquired. The terms *intravascular hemolysis* and *extravascular hemolysis* refer to the *site* of the destruction of the red cell: within the circulating blood, or outside it, respectively.

Hemoglobin Destruction. Laboratory findings differ, depending on the site of blood destruction, the amount of destroyed blood, and the rate of destruction. If the destruction is *intravascular* and the quantity of destroyed blood is large, free hemoglobin and methemalbumin will be present in the plasma (hemoglobinemia and methemalbuminemia). The urine may contain free hemoglobin and may also show hemosiderin.

Free hemoglobin readily dissociates into αβ dimers ($\alpha_2\beta_2 \rightarrow 2\alpha\beta$). These are bound to haptoglobin, an α_2-globulin, and the hemoglobin-haptoglobin complex is rapidly removed from the circulation and catabolized by the liver parenchymal cells. This process prevents hemoglobin from appearing in the urine. However, when the plasma hemoglobin level exceeds 50 to 200 mg/dl (8 to 31 µmol/l), which is the capacity of haptoglobin to bind hemoglobin, the free αβ dimers of hemoglobin readily pass through the glomerulus of the kidney. Part of the hemoglobin is then absorbed by the proximal tubular cells where the hemoglobin iron is converted to hemosiderin. When these tubular cells are later shed into the urine, *hemosiderinuria* results. If the amount of hemoglobin in the tubular lumen exceeds the capacity of the tubular cell to absorb it, it reaches the urine (*hemoglobinuria*). In the process, it may be oxidized to methemoglobin. Plasma hemoglobin not bound to haptoglobin nor removed by the kidney is oxidized to hemiglobin (methemoglobin). The oxidized heme groups (hemin) are bound to *hemopexin*, a beta globulin, and the complex is rapidly cleared by the hepatic parenchymal cells. If hemopexin is depleted, hemin groups bind to albumin, forming methemalbumin. Once hemopexin again becomes available, it removes the hemin groups from albumin for hepatic clearance (Hillman, 1974).

Lactate dehydrogenase (LD) is released from red cells and is increased in serum in hemolysis, especially in intravascular hemolysis; it is cleared more slowly than is hemoglobin. If the upper reference value is 207 IU/l, the LD in hemolytic anemia may be increased as much as 800 IU/l. In megaloblastic anemia, for reasons that are unclear, the LD is greatly increased to several thousand units (Chap. 12). Serum LD is also increased in other forms of cellular injury (p. 368 and Chapter 12).

The normal plasma hemoglobin level is 0.5 to 5 mg/dl (0.08 to 0.78 µmol/l). A rise to 10 mg/dl imparts to the plasma a yellow to orange color. With further increase the color becomes pink. Levels up to 25 to 30 mg/dl are common in hemolytic anemia. Higher levels usually indicate intravascular hemolysis and are seen in hemolytic transfusion reactions and in paroxysmal cold and nocturnal hemo-globinurias.

If hemolysis is primarily *extravascular,* no hemoglobinemia, hemoglobinuria, or hemosid-erinuria is present. Hemolysis is detected by measuring an increase in one of the products of heme catabolism (see also p. 931):

1. An increase in CO expired (a research technique), or in the blood carboxyhemoglobin level.

2. An increase in indirect-reacting serum bilirubin; since this is bound to albumin, it will not appear in the urine.

3. An increase in urine urobilinogen or, more consistently, in fecal urobilinogen.

The normal urobilinogen in a 24-hour speci-men is 0.05 to 2.5 mg (0.08 to 4.23 μmol) in urine and 40 to 200 mg (0.068 to 0.340 mmol) in the stool. Following excessive hemolysis it may increase to 5 to 200 mg in the urine and to 300 to 400 mg in the stool. The examination of feces is more dependable than examination of the urine because it may show an increase when the urine shows none. It may show an increase even when the serum bilirubin is not raised. This is explained by the fact that the normal liver has the capacity to remove large amounts of (indirectly reacting) bilirubin and of reabsorbed urobilinogen from the blood.

Hemolytic anemia is characterized also by increased red cell production. Because of the availability of maximal amounts of iron for hemoglobin formation, red cell production reaches the maximal degree possible (about eight times normal) in severe chronic hemo-lytic anemia, if complicating factors such as folate deficiency do not intervene. If the red cell destruction exceeds the capacity of the marrow to replace red cells at the same rate, hemolytic anemia occurs. With less severe he-molysis, the marrow may be able to produce enough red cells so that anemia does not occur; this is called compensated hemolysis.

Blood Film. The anemia is normocytic or macrocytic. Macrocytosis is an expression of the presence of immature red cells, which are larger than normocytes. Polychromasia is usu-ally prominent; it may be excessively baso-philic and normoblasts may be present, both of which indicate a "shift" of marrow reticulo-cytes into the blood.

Other red cell abnormalities may give a clue to the nature of the hemolytic process. Sphero-cytes suggest hereditary spherocytosis or au-toimmune hemolysis (see Figs. 27-13 and 27-16); schistocytes suggest traumatic hemolytic anemia (see Fig. 27-22); sickle cells, target cells, or crystals suggest a hemoglobinopathy

(Figs. 29-8 and 29-9; Plate 29-2). When hemo-lytic anemia is acute, numbers and younger forms of leukocytes and platelets are often released from the marrow together with erythrocytes. The result is leukocytosis with a "shift to the left" and thrombocytosis with both normal and giant platelets.

Bone Marrow. Normoblastic hyperplasia is the rule and may be striking in degree. Storage iron is usually increased and sidero-blasts are normal or increased in number, re-flecting the abundance of available iron for hemoglobin synthesis.

Sudden worsening of the degree of anemia may occur in chronic hemolytic anemias and be due to either of two basic mechanisms. Occasionally episodes of bone marrow failure (transient arrest of erythropoiesis, p. 982) characterized by erythroid hypoplasia and re-ticulocytopenia may upset the equilibrium be-tween production and destruction of red cells. In most instances these "aplastic crises" are thought to be precipitated by infection (Bauman, 1967). On the other hand, a sudden increase in the rate of red cell destruction may occur accompanied by an increased reticulocy-tosis in an insufficient attempt to compensate. This is called a "hemolytic crisis."

HEMOLYSIS—MEMBRANE DISORDERS

Hereditary Spherocytosis. Hereditary spherocytosis is characterized by spherocytic red cells which are intrinsically defective, splenomegaly, and familial occurrence (most often autosomal dominant). The hemolytic process is variable in severity and is corrected by splenectomy, though the spherocytosis re-mains.

The laboratory findings are those of a chronic extravascular hemolytic process: evi-dence of increased pigment catabolism, eryth-roid hyperplasia, and reticulocytosis. The Coombs' test is negative, spherocytes are present, and osmotic fragility is increased. Spherocytes have a smaller diameter and are more intensely stained than normal cells. They have decreased or absent central pallor; if present, the pallor may be eccentric (Fig. 27-13; Plate 29-2J). The MCHC is often in-creased, reflecting a decrease in cell surface.

The osmotic fragility of freshly drawn blood is usually increased but may be normal in mildly affected patients; that of blood incu-bated at 37°C. for 24 hours is uniformly in-creased (p. 1017). The increased osmotic fragil-ity of freshly drawn blood is characteristic, but not specific; it may occur in some acquired hemolytic anemias. The autohemolysis test (p. 1024) shows increased lysis at 48 hours; with added glucose, lysis is diminished except in the more severe cases.

Since the diagnosis is established by familial occurrence, siblings and the parents should be studied. In a few families, neither parent may be affected.

The erythrocytes are abnormally permeable to sodium, and there is no defect in energy metabolism, which is, in fact, increased. The increased metabolic activity has been explained as an attempt to compensate for a membrane defect which leaks cations, with degenerative changes and the loss of cell surface accelerated by the metabolic and physical stress of passage through the spleen (Jandl, 1968). The primary defect appears to be in the erythrocyte membrane, probably an abnormal structural protein (Jacob, 1971). Attention has been directed to a decreased phosphorylation of membrane protein by ATP that is present in HS, but the molecular abnormality is not yet defined (Valentine, 1977).

Hereditary Elliptocytosis. This autosomal dominant condition probably includes more than one genetic variant. Non-hypochromic ovalocytes (elongated erythrocytes) are abundant in the blood film, numbering over 25 per cent (see Fig. 27-18), whereas in normal individuals less than 15 per cent of the red cells are elliptical. The deformity is increased in sealed, moist preparations. Most persons with this cellular abnormality are asymptomatic. About 10 to 15 per cent develop a mild to moderate hemolytic anemia; in these patients the osmotic fragility and autohemolysis tests may show similar abnormalities to hereditary spherocytosis, whereas in the trait the tests are normal (Dacie, 1960).

Hereditary Stomatocytosis. Stomatocytes are cells which on air-dried films have a slit-shaped rather than circular pallor; in wet preparations their shape is that of a bowl rather than a biconcave disc. Rh null red cells are stomatocytes and have a shortened survival. A syndrome of hereditary hemolytic anemia with stomatocytes includes cases with considerable variability of hemolysis both within and between families. In some cases, the cells appear as target cells on air-dried films. In common there is increased sodium permeability and flux, but there is variability in ion content and water content (Wiley, 1975).

Paroxysmal Nocturnal Hemoglobinuria (PNH) (Dacie, 1972; Rosse, 1977). PNH is an acquired intrinsic defect of red cells which renders them unusually sensitive to complement. The nature of the defect is unknown, but PNH cells bind more C3 than do normal cells whether complement is activated by the classic or the alternate pathway. Two or three populations of cells of different complement sensitivity are present, and one is almost always normal (Rosse, 1977). Hemolysis *in vivo* probably occurs primarily via activation of the alternate pathway (Götze, 1972). Platelets and neutrophils also appear to be sensitive to complement.

Clinically, PNH usually occurs in young adults and is characterized by chronic intravascular hemolysis with or without obvious hemoglobinuria. Hemosiderinuria is, however, almost constantly present. Typical nocturnal or sleep-related hemoglobinuria is present in less than 25 per cent of patients.

The blood usually shows a normocytic anemia with a reticulocytosis that is often less than expected for the degree of anemia. Hypochromic microcytic anemia is not uncommon, however, and is due to loss of iron in the urine. Neutropenia occurs in three fifths and thrombocytopenia in two thirds of patients at some time during the course of disease, so that pancytopenia is common. The direct antiglobulin test is usually negative. Red cell acetylcholinesterase and neutrophil alkaline phosphatase are usually decreased. Osmotic fragility is not increased. The autohemolysis test shows increased lysis at 48 hours; with added glucose the degree of lysis is not diminished but may be accentuated.

The marrow is usually hypercellular with normoblastic hyperplasia, but it may be hypocellular. In some patients marrow failure may occur during the course of PNH; in others, aplastic anemia is the initial diagnosis, with signs of PNH later manifesting themselves. An abnormal line of cells probably develops in an aplastic or regenerating marrow (Lewis, 1967).

Thrombotic complications are common. The disease may undergo partial remissions and exacerbations. In over half of patients, both the proportion of abnormal cells and the clinical severity decrease with time.

A sucrose hemolysis test (p. 1027) should be performed whenever the diagnosis of PNH is considered, also in hypoplastic anemias, and in any hemolytic anemia of obscure origin. The confirmatory sucrose hemolysis test is rarely positive except in PNH. The definitive diagnosis of PNH requires a positive acidified serum test (Ham's test). Both tests depend

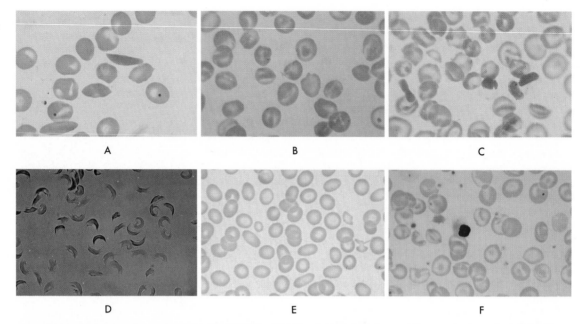

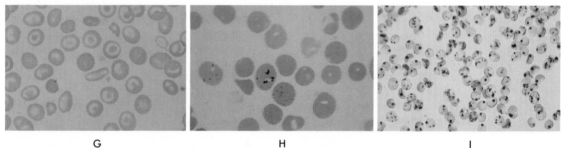

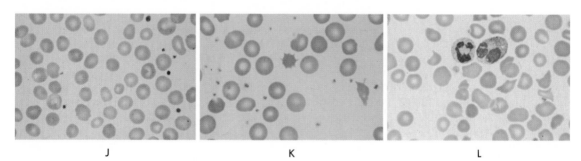

Plate 29-2. *A*, Blood film, sickle cell anemia, adult. In contrast to elliptocytes, sickled cells have a densely staining center and pointed ends; three are shown here. Two Howell-Jolly bodies are present, suggesting asplenia. *B*, Blood film, hemoglobin C disease. The numerous target cells and cells with an elongated central density are characteristic. *C*, Blood film, hemoglobin C disease, same patient as in *B* after splenectomy. Four of the red cells here contain densely staining aggregations of Hb C, which tend to become crystals and assume an elongated hexagonal shape. *D*, Sickle cell preparation, in sodium metabisulfite, sickle cell anemia; all the cells are sickled. *E*, Blood film, beta-thalassemia trait. Microcytosis; increased number of elliptocytes. Note that target cells may not be prominent. *F*, Blood film, homozygous beta thalassemia. This patient, a black woman, had a relatively mild hemolytic process, a previous splenectomy, and had not been recently transfused. This is in contrast to the greater severity of the usual homozygous beta thalassemia in Mediterranean peoples. The localized dense hemoglobin in the normoblast suggests precipitation of alpha chains; note the Howell-Jolly body. *G*, Blood film, hemoglobin H disease. A form of alpha-thalassemia, this has the combination of microcytic hypochromic red cells and hemolysis. Target cells are numerous. *H*, Film made after incubation of blood with brilliant cresyl blue, hemoglobin H disease, same patient as in *G*. Two reticulocytes have dark blue precipitates of RNA. Several red cells contain multiple smaller pale blue precipitates of Hb H (*G* and *H*: Courtesy of Dr. McDonald K. Horne). *I*, Heinz bodies. Normal red cells incubated with an oxidant drug, acetyl-phenylhydrazine, and stained while in suspension by methyl violet; finally, an air-dried film was made and stained with Wright's stain.

(*legend continued on opposite page*)

upon the increased susceptibility of PNH red cells to lysis by complement.

HEMOLYSIS—HEMOGLOBIN DISORDERS

In 1949 Pauling and his associates described specific properties of a hemoglobin type in patients with sickle cell anemia. Their studies initiated the concept of molecular disease; that is, a molecular variation in a single protein can be responsible for the entire spectrum of clinical, laboratory, and pathologic manifestations that characterize a disease. The subsequent finding that the abnormality was due to the substitution of a single amino acid in a polypeptide chain of hemoglobin inaugurated the exciting field of biochemical genetics.

At present, over 250 different hemoglobins have been described. The great majority of these have been characterized as a single amino acid substitution in one of the polypeptide chains (α, β, γ, or δ), which can be explained by a single base substitution in the corresponding triplet codon of the gene. In a small number of abnormal hemoglobins, the polypeptide chain is abnormally long or short due to termination errors, frame-shift mutations, crossover in phase, deletion of codons, or fused or hybrid chains (Bunn, 1977).

Normal hemoglobins

The heme group is identical in all variants of human hemoglobin. The protein part of the molecule (globin) consists of four polypeptide chains. At least three distinct hemoglobin types are found postnatally in normal individuals, and the structure of each has been determined.

Hb A ($\alpha_2\beta_2$). Hemoglobin A is the major normal adult hemoglobin. The polypeptide chains of the globin part of the molecules are of two types: two identical alpha chains, each with 141 amino acids, and two identical beta chains, with 146 amino acids each. Each chain is linked with one heme group. The molecule is ellipsoidal, with the four heme groups at the surface of the molecule, where they function by combining reversibly with oxygen or carbon dioxide (see Figs. 28–7 and 29–5).

Hb F ($\alpha_2\gamma_2$). Hemoglobin F is the major hemoglobin of the fetus and the newborn infant. The increased affinity for oxygen of fetal blood over adult blood is not due to the hemoglobin itself, but probably to the environment in the red cell. The two alpha chains are identical to those of Hb A, and two gamma chains, with 146 amino acid residues, differ from beta chains. During fetal life, Hb F predominates, as alpha chain production and gamma chain production are high (Fig. 29–6). Beta chain production begins before the twentieth week of prenatal life, so that Hb A is 10 per cent of the total between 20 and 35 weeks and 15 to 40 per cent at the time of birth. After birth, smaller amounts of Hb F are produced; by 6 months Hb F is usually 1 per cent of the total Hb or less. In some normal children, however, Hb F may be as high as 5 per cent for 12 to 24 months (Chernoff, 1952). Only traces of Hb F (<0.5 per cent) are found in adults. The mechanism of "switching" from gamma to beta chain production is unknown. If for some reason beta chain production is impaired during this time of switching, gamma chain production may continue in considerable degree into adult life, so that high levels of Hb F often indicate an anemia of early onset (e.g., thalassemia major).

Hb A$_2$ ($\alpha_2\delta_2$). Hemoglobin A$_2$ accounts for 1.5 to 3.5 per cent of normal adult hemoglobin. Its two alpha chains are the same as in Hb A and Hb F; its two delta chains differ from beta chains in only eight of their 146 amino acids.

Delta chain synthesis begins late in fetal life and occurs only in normoblasts (not reticulocytes). The level of Hb A$_2$ gradually increases during the first year of life at which time the adult level is reached. Quantitation has become important, for Hb A$_2$ is increased

---

Plate 29–2 (Continued.)
Purple-staining Heinz bodies are precipitates of denatured hemoglobin which tend to be attached to the cell membrane. *J*, Blood film, hereditary spherocytosis. In milder cases, the morphologic clues are a decreased red cell diameter and a decreased amount of central pallor which tends often to be eccentric. *K*, Blood film, pyruvate kinase deficiency, post-splenectomy. The contracted, deformed cells were not present prior to splenectomy; they probably represent the most ATP-depleted cells. *L*, Blood film, hemolytic-uremic syndrome. Note the irregularly shaped schistocytes, including helmet cells.

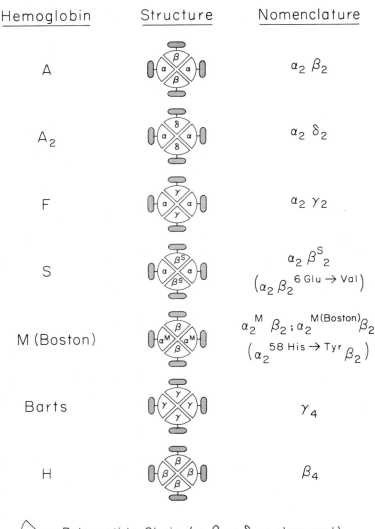

Hemoglobin	Structure	Nomenclature

A — $\alpha_2 \beta_2$

A_2 — $\alpha_2 \delta_2$

F — $\alpha_2 \gamma_2$

S — $\alpha_2 \beta^S{}_2$

$$\left(\alpha_2 \beta_2{}^{6\,Glu \rightarrow Val}\right)$$

M (Boston) — $\alpha_2{}^M \beta_2 \,;\, \alpha_2{}^{M(Boston)} \beta_2$

$$\left(\alpha_2{}^{58\,His \rightarrow Tyr}\beta_2\right)$$

Barts — γ_4

H — β_4

$\Diamond$ = Polypeptide Chain (α, β, γ, δ or abnormal)

⬮ = Heme Group (attached to polypeptide chain)

Figure 29–5. Configuration and nomenclature of normal and abnormal hemoglobins. Each triangle represents one folded polypeptide chain; the bar attached to its external surface represents a heme group. The drawing is schematic. Each heme group is near the surface of the molecule, located in a pocket formed by folds of its polypeptide chain and attached to that chain by an imidazole group. In most hemoglobinopathies (e.g., Hb S, Hb G$_{Philadelphia}$), the affected polypeptide chain differs from normal in only one amino acid. In Hb S, the designation could also be written $\alpha_2\beta_2{}^{6\,Val}$, and in Hb G$_{Philadelphia}$, $\alpha_2{}^{68\,Lys}\beta_2$, indicating the site of the substitution and the amino acid which replaces the one usually present (After Krieg, 1967).

in some beta-thalassemias. Iron deficiency causes decreased Hb A_2 synthesis.

Embryonic Hemoglobins. Hb Gower-1 (ϵ_4 or $\zeta_2\epsilon_2$) and Hb Gower-2 ($\alpha_2\epsilon_2$) are embryonic hemoglobins; they have been found in normal human fetuses with a gestational age of less than three months (Fig. 29-6). The epsilon (ϵ) polypeptide chain is distinct from the α, β, γ, and δ chains. The zeta (ζ) chain is similar to the α chain; combined with the γ chain it forms Hb Portland-1 ($\zeta_2\gamma_2$). Hb Portland-1 is normally present in the embryo and in trace amounts in cord blood (Bunn, 1977).

Investigations of hemoglobin structure and inheritance of abnormal hemoglobins have re-

sulted in the concept of genetic loci on chromosomes, which govern the structure of the polypeptide chains. Available evidence indicates that the alpha locus is duplicated in some, but not necessarily all, human population groups. Also, at least two structural genes exist for gamma chains, because normal individuals have two types of Hb F: one has glycine in position 136 ($^G\gamma$); the other has alanine in position 136 ($^A\gamma$). The ratio of $^G\gamma$ to $^A\gamma$ chains changes from 3:1 at birth to 2:3 by age 12 months (Weatherall, 1974). The beta and delta loci appear to be single and are closely linked. The alpha locus is either farther removed from the others or is on a different chromosome.

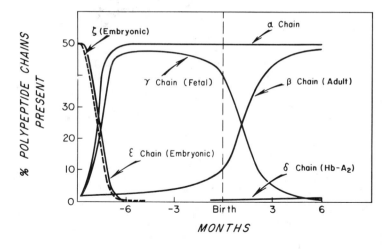

Figure 29-6. Relative proportions of polypeptide chains of hemoglobin present during fetal and neonatal life. (From Bunn, H. F., Forget, B. G., and Ranney, H. M.: Human Hemoglobins. Philadelphia, W. B. Saunders Company, 1977.)

Abnormal hemoglobins and nomenclature

Normal adult hemoglobin was designated Hb A; fetal hemoglobin, Hb F; and that found in sickle cell anemia, Hb S. Thereafter, as hemoglobin variants were discovered, they were given sequential letters of the alphabet. When more than one hemoglobin was found with the same electrophoretic mobility, it was designated with the subscript indicating the geographical location in which it was found; there are several variants of Hb D, G, J, and M, for example. After the letter Q was used, it became obvious that the alphabet would not supply sufficient letters to designate newly found hemoglobins. The investigator describing a new hemoglobin thereafter gave it a specific name, usually geographic. The polypeptide chain on which the abnormality is present can be indicated as a superscript; e.g., $HbS = \alpha_2^A$ β_2^S; $HbI = \alpha_2^I \beta_2^A$. The common designation now is the number of the amino acid residue in the superscript along with the substituted amino acid; e.g., $HbS = \alpha_2\beta_2^{6Val}$; $HbI = \alpha_2^{16Asp}\beta_2$ (Fig. 29-5). Amino acid substitutions in some of the known hemoglobin variants are listed and classified by functional characteristics in Table 29-2.

Abnormal hemoglobin syndromes

In *hemoglobinopathies* the structure of one of the four types of polypeptide chains formed is abnormal; this is usually due to substitution of a single amino acid. A larger number of hemoglobin variants which do not cause disease have been discovered in surveys. In clinically significant disease, either the beta chain or the alpha chain is affected. Involvement of the gamma chain and delta chain occurs, but because of the small amount of hemoglobin involved they are less often detected and rarely of any clinical significance. Depending on the type of amino acid and the site involved, the hemoglobin may be functionally abnormal and have altered chemical and physical properties.

In *thalassemias*, globin chains of normal structure are formed, but the rate of production of one type of polypeptide chain is diminished. Beta thalassemia refers to decreased production of beta chains; therefore HbF $(\alpha_2\gamma_2)$ or HbA$_2$ $(\alpha_2\delta_2)$ would be expected to be relatively increased with respect to Hb A $(\alpha_2\beta_2)$. Alpha thalassemia refers to decreased production of alpha chains: Hb A $(\alpha_2\beta_2)$, Hb A$_2$ $(\alpha_2\delta_2)$ and Hb F $(\alpha_2\gamma_2)$ are proportionally decreased.

In *homozygous beta hemoglobinopathies*, both allelic genes for the abnormal beta chains are present, so that no normal beta chains (hence, no Hb A) are produced. Examples are sickle cell disease (Hb SS) and hemoglobin C disease (Hb CC). Since alpha, gamma, and delta genes (and chain production) are normal, the Hb F and Hb A$_2$ formed are structurally normal, though they may be increased in amount.

Homozygous alpha hemoglobinopathies have not been described.

In *heterozygous beta hemoglobinopathies*, the abnormal hemoglobin is present in addition to Hb A; Hb F and Hb A$_2$ again are structurally normal, since only a portion of the beta chains are abnormal. Examples are sickle cell trait (Hb AS) and hemoglobin C trait (Hb AC). The normal Hb A quantitatively exceeds the abnormal hemoglobin present because of either slower production of abnormal beta chains than of normal beta chains or selective early destruction of the red cells with higher concentrations of the abnormal hemoglobin or selective removal of the abnormal hemoglobin from the cell.

In *heterozygous alpha hemoglobinopathies,* the abnormality in the alpha chain will affect all three hemoglobin types. Therefore, six different hemoglobin types are found—the three normal hemoglobins and the three abnormal forms. Examples are Hb D$_{Baltimore}$, Hb Ann Arbor, and Hb M$_{Boston}$.

Combinations of abnormalities exist. *Double heterozygotes for two beta chain abnormalities* produce two different abnormal beta chains; therefore, there are two abnormal hemoglobins and no hemoglobin A. An example of this is Hb S-C disease. Double heterozygotes for beta and delta chain abnormalities and for alpha and beta chain abnormalities are rare but have provided important information. The latter will have four major hemoglobin types on electrophoresis: $\alpha_2^A\beta_2^A$; $\alpha_2^X\beta_2^A$; $\alpha_2^A\beta_2^Y$; and $\alpha_2^X\beta_2^Y$.

Double heterozygotes for beta hemoglobinopathy and beta thalassemia are well known. Here, the quantity of abnormal hemoglobin exceeds the normal hemoglobin, in contrast to the heterozygous beta hemoglobinopathies, in which the reverse is true. Examples are Hb S thalassemias and Hb E thalassemia.

Beta hemoglobinopathies

Hemoglobins S, C, D, and E are believed to be polymorphisms because their frequency is greater than can be explained by mutation alone (Lehmann, 1977). They occur in homozygous as well as heterozygous form and involve the beta chain.

Sickle Cell Disease.   Homozygous Hb S disease is a serious chronic hemolytic anemia, first manifest in early childhood and often fatal before the age of 30 years. With modern medical care, however, many patients live longer. Hemoglobin S is found almost exclusively in the black population; 0.1 to 0.2 per cent of the blacks born in the United States have sickle cell anemia (Schneider, 1976).

In hemoglobin S the glutamic acid in the sixth position on the beta chain is replaced by valine. This substitution is on the surface of the molecule and changes its charge and, hence, its electrophoretic mobility. Hemoglobin S is freely soluble when fully oxygenated; when oxygen is removed from Hb S, polymerization of the abnormal hemoglobin occurs, forming tactoids (fluid crystals) which are

rigid and deform the cell into the shape which gave the cell its name (Fig. 29–7). In homozygous Hb S disease, sickling occurs at physiologic oxygen tensions and the rigidity of the red cells is responsible for the hemolysis as well as for most of the complications. The rigid cells are more vulnerable to trauma and are readily trapped by the reticuloendothelial system, especially the spleen, accounting for the hemolysis. As a result of the hemolysis, severe continued marrow hyperplasia during childhood produces bone changes: expansion of the marrow space, thinning of the cortex, and radial striations seen in the skull on x-ray. Leg ulcers are common.

COMPLICATIONS.   In early childhood, bilateral painful swelling of the dorsa of the hands or feet occurs as a result of sickling and capillary stasis; this is known as the *hand-foot syndrome* or sickle cell dactylitis. It lasts about two weeks, is accompanied by changes of periostitis as observed by x-ray, and does not occur after the age of four.

The spleen is central to three complications: A *sequestration crisis* refers to sudden pooling of blood and rapid enlargement of the spleen, resulting in hypovolemic shock. This may occur in early childhood when splenomegaly is present. *Functional asplenia* (Pearson, 1969) consists of inadequate antibody responses under some conditions and an impaired ability of the reticuloendothelial system to clear bacteria and particulate material from the blood, probably due to reticuloendothelial blockade. This may partly explain the increased risk of infection in children with the disease. Salmonella and pneumococcal infections are unusually prevalent in children with sickle cell anemia. *Autosplenectomy* is the result of vaso-occlusive episodes, resulting in progressive infarction, fibrosis, and contraction of the spleen. Though splenomegaly is present in childhood, a small fibrotic remnant is the rule in the adult.

From early childhood, patients cannot produce a concentrated urine, apparently as a result of anoxic damage to the vasa recta in the medullae of the kidneys. Hematuria as a result of papillary necrosis is common.

Vaso-occlusive crises are debilitating episodes of abdominal and bone or joint pain, accompanied by fever, which are probably due to plugging of small blood vessels by masses of sickled cells. Bone necrosis occurs and may be a focus for salmonella osteomyelitis. Aseptic necrosis of the femoral head is occasionally a complication. The various complications as a

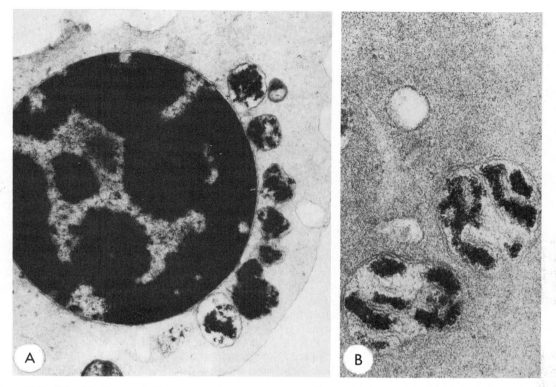

Figure 29-7. Sideroblastic anemia. Heme synthesis occurs within mitochondria, at least in part. In sideroblastic anemias, there appears to be a defect in mitochondrial enzymes involved in heme synthesis, and iron-laden mitochondria can be seen in erythroid precursors. In *A* ($\times 11,000$) note numerous iron-laden mitochondria surrounding the nucleus of a normoblast, the so-called ringed sideroblast. At higher magnifications the electron-dense iron is seen to accumulate in the matrix between the mitochondrial cristae (*B*—$\times 76,500$). (From Fresco, R.: Ultrastructure of the blood cells and their precursors. *In* Davidsohn, I., and Henry, J. B.: Clinical Diagnosis by Laboratory Methods, 15th ed. Philadelphia, W. B. Saunders Company, 1974.)

result of recurring vaso-occlusive crises involve many systems (Diggs, 1965).

Aplastic crises can occasionally afflict any patient with chronic hemolytic anemia. A temporary failure of red cell production which would not be noticed in a person with a normal red cell life span will cause a serious fall in hemoglobin concentration in hemolytic anemia. This may be a result of infection, exposure to toxic drugs, or folic acid deficiency; sometimes no cause can be found. *Hemolytic crises* are less common, and cannot be diagnosed without evidence of increased red cell or hemoglobin destruction.

BLOOD. The anemia is normochromic and normocytic; polychromasia is increased; normoblasts are present. Target cells are numerous (up to 30 per cent), and Howell-Jolly bodies are regularly seen in older children and adults, as a result of asplenia. Sickle cells are often found in the stained smear (Fig. 29-8; Plate 29-2*A*). The microhematocrit as an estimate

of degree of anemia is unreliable because of excessive plasma trapping. Osmotic fragility is usually decreased, and mechanical fragility is increased. Neutrophilia and thrombocytosis are usual. Sickle cell preparation and solubility test are positive. The marrow shows normoblastic hyperplasia and increased storage iron.

Hb ELECTROPHORESIS, pH 8.4. If the patient has not been recently transfused, no Hb A, over 80 per cent Hb S, 1 to 20 per cent Hb F, and 2 to 4.5 per cent Hb A_2 may be found (Wrightstone, 1974). The fetal hemoglobin is distributed unevenly among the red cells. Hb S, Hb D, and Hb G (Philadelphia) have the same electrophoretic mobility but, of these, only Hb S gives a positive sickle cell test. Hb D and Hb G also migrate differently from Hb S in agar gel electrophoresis at an acid pH (Fig. 29-16; p. 1022).

Sickle Cell Trait (Hb AS). Sickle cell trait is probably the most common hemoglobinopathy in the United States. This heterozygous

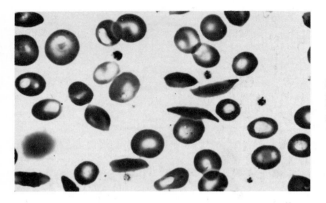

Figure 29–8. Sickle cell anemia. Note that the elongated, pointed cells have greater density in the center than near the edges, in contrast to elliptocytes. Linked molecules of reduced Hb S, forming tactoids, distort the cells. (× 875.)

condition (Hb A + Hb S) is present in about 9 per cent of American blacks (Schneider, 1976). Under normal circumstances no clinical signs of disease or hematologic abnormalities are present. However, acidosis or hypoxia due to aircraft flight, respiratory infection, anesthesia, or congestive heart failure may cause sickling and vascular complications with visceral infarcts, including hematuria. Impaired ability to concentrate urine is found in adults with the trait. Sickle cell trait confers protection on the individual from the lethal effects of falciparum malaria, which may account for the major distribution of Hb S in central Africa.

The stained blood film appears normal, except perhaps for a few target cells. Blood cell counts are normal. The sickle cell preparation is positive, and almost all the red cells eventually sickle. The solubility test is positive.

ELECTROPHORESIS. Hb A, 50 to 70 per cent; Hb S, 30 to 45 per cent; Hb F, normal; Hb A_2, normal to slightly increased, up to 4.5 per cent.

Hemoglobin C Disease. Homozygous hemoglobin C disease in a mild hemolytic anemia with splenomegaly which is often asymptomatic but occasionally results in jaundice and abdominal discomfort. In the United States, 0.02 per cent of blacks have Hb C disease (Schneider, 1976).

BLOOD.   Slight normochromic normocytic anemia with an admixture of microcytes and spherocytes, minimal increase in reticulocytes, and numerous target cells (40 to 90 per cent) are seen in the blood. Osmotic fragility is biphasic, with both increased and decreased fragility. Hexagonal or rod-shaped crystals may be seen in erythrocytes in the stained smear, especially after splenectomy or after slow drying of the smear (Fig. 29-9; Plate 29-2*B* and *C*). If red cells are incubated in 3 per cent saline, crystal-like inclusions appear in almost every cell. This tendency of the hemoglobin to form rod-shaped inclusions apparently increases the rigidity of the cells and increases their likelihood of being trapped and destroyed in the spleen (Conley, 1967).

ELECTROPHORESIS.   No Hb A; over 90 per cent Hb C; less than 7 per cent Hb F. Hb E and

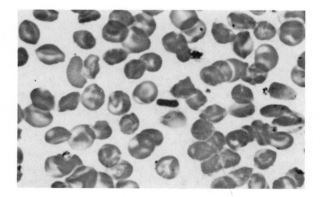

Figure 29–9. Hemoglobin C disease, postsplenectomy. Prior to splenectomy the only morphologic abnormality was the presence of target cells. After splenectomy Howell-Jolly bodies and hemoglobin crystals, such as that in the center, were present. Note that almost all the hemoglobin in this particular cell is in the dark bar, and the membrane is still visible. Some such crystals are distinctly hexagonal. (× 875.)

Hb O-Arab have the same migration as Hb C on alkaline electrophoresis. They can be separated on agar gel at an acid pH (Fig. 29-16; p. 1022).

Hemoglobin C Trait. Hemoglobin C is prevalent in West Africans and in about 2 to 3 per cent of American blacks. The heterozygous state is asymptomatic, without anemia, and mild hypochromia and target cells (up to 40 per cent) may be present.

ELECTROPHORESIS.   Hb C, 30 to 40 per cent; Hb A, 50 to 70 per cent.

Hemoglobin D Disease and Trait. Hemoglobin D is found in India. Hb D-Punjab and Hb D-Los Angeles are the same ($\alpha_2\beta_2^{121\ Gln}$) and constitute the most common D-variant in American blacks (<0.02 per cent). The trait is asymptomatic, with no anemia and a normal blood smear. Homozygous Hb D disease is very rare, with virtually no symptoms and no hemolytic anemia. In some individuals, target cells and decreased osmotic fragility are found.

ELECTROPHORESIS.   Hb D and Hb G Philadelphia ($\alpha_2^{68\ Lys}\beta_2$) have a mobility on alkaline electrophoresis identical to that of Hb S but have negative solubility and sickling tests. Hb D and Hb G migrate differently from Hb S on agar gel at an acid pH. Because alpha chains are affected, Hb G will show a double Hb A_2 band on alkaline electrophoresis. Hb G is probably somewhat more frequent than Hb D in American blacks (Schneider, 1976).

In Hb D disease, Hb D is about 95 per cent, and Hb A_2 is normal. In this trait, Hb D accounts for less than half of the total hemoglobin.

Hemoglobin E Disease and Trait. Hb E is found in Southeast Asia, primarily in orientals, but does occur in blacks. Hb AE (the trait) is asymptomatic and has no hematologic abnormalities. Individuals homozygous for Hb E have a mild anemia with microcytosis and target cells and a slightly decreased red cell survival. Osmotic fragility is decreased. In Southeast Asia, iron deficiency and thalassemias are prevalent. Hb E-beta thalassemia tends to be a severe disease resembling homozygous β thalassemia; Hb A is reduced or absent. In combination with α thalassemia, the proportion of Hb E is lower than in the trait (Hb AE) (Bunn, 1977).

ELECTROPHORESIS.   Hb E migrates similarly to Hb A_2, Hb C, and Hb O-Arab on alkaline electrophoresis. On agar gel at acid pH, Hb E migrates with Hb A, Hb O-Arab tends to separate from A, and Hb C is distinct. In the trait, Hb E is 30 to 45 per cent (Lehmann, 1977).

Doubly heterozygous states (beta hemoglobin)

A different abnormal beta chain inherited from each parent may result in interaction of Hb C, D, or E with Hb S to produce hemolytic anemia of variable severity.

Sickle Cell–Hemoglobin C Disease (SC Disease). The frequency of Hb SC disease is about the same as that of Hb SS disease in American blacks. The severity is intermediate between sickle cell trait and sickle cell disease, with almost all the manifestations of sickle cell anemia appearing but with less frequency. The onset is usually early in childhood, but real difficulties do not occur until the teens or later. Fatigue, dyspnea on effort, frequent upper respiratory infections, attacks of mild jaundice, and arthralgias are seen. Crises are usually rare and mild. Painful crisis occurs more often in joints and muscles than in the abdomen. Constant hip and low back pain may be present with aseptic necrosis of the head of the femur on x-ray. Hematuria and splenic infarcts have been described. Leg ulcers occur only occasionally. In pregnancy there is a tendency toward increased frequency of crises—both clinical and hematologic. Painful crises are related to infarction, and sudden death may occur following childbirth. In contrast to sickle cell anemia, splenomegaly is usually present. The body habitus is normal or stocky in contrast to the asthenic features in sickle cell anemia.

BLOOD.   Anemia varies from moderate to very mild and is normochromic normocytic. Anisocytosis and poikilocytosis are mild to severe, and target cells are numerous—up to 85 per cent of the erythrocytes. Plump and angulated sickled cells may be present on the film. The sickle cell test is positive.

ELECTROPHORESIS.   Hb C and Hb S occur in about equal amounts. Hb F ranges from normal to 7 per cent. Because no normal beta chains can be produced, Hb A is absent.

Sickle Cell–Hemoglobin D Disease (SD Disease). SD disease simulates but is less severe than sickle cell anemia, and thus may also resemble SC disease. The sickle cell test is positive.

ELECTROPHORESIS.   The pattern is indistinguishable from sickle cell anemia because

Hb S and Hb D cannot be separated on routine (alkaline) electrophoresis. Agar gel electrophoresis at pH 6.2 will separate Hb S and Hb D; solubility studies (Hb D is more soluble than Hb S) and family studies will help to reveal the true nature of the condition. One parent is likely to have a negative sickle cell test and an abnormal hemoglobin with the mobility of Hb S.

Other doubly heterozygous beta hemoglobinopathies are known but are even less common.

Heterozygous hemoglobinopathies

A number of amino acid substitutions occur in the heme pocket where they either increase the stability of the methemoglobin form (Hb M) or alter the affinity of the heme for oxygen; the latter usually alters the stability of the molecule as well.

Other substitutions affect the $\alpha\beta$ contact sites; these also can change stability and oxygen affinity of the molecule (Perutz, 1968).

These functionally significant hemoglobinopathies are heterozygous; usually the concentration of the abnormal hemoglobin is less than 50 per cent. Generally, the hemoglobins with abnormal alpha chains form a smaller proportion of the total (10 to 25 per cent) than do those with abnormal beta chains (35 to 50 per cent) (Bunn, 1977).

Hemoglobins Associated with Methemoglobinemia and Cyanosis

HEMOGLOBIN M. Five abnormal hemoglobins are associated with clinical methemoglobinemia and cyanosis which do not respond to methylene blue (Table 29-2). The common feature is that all have an amino acid substitution at or near the heme group so that a stable complex is formed with heme in the oxidized state; reduction to ferrous heme and hence reversible binding of oxygen are prevented.

Cyanosis from birth is seen in hemoglobin M disease with alpha chain abnormalities, but does not appear for two to four months if the abnormality is in the beta chain—that is, until beta chain production approaches adult levels. The cyanosis is, of course, not associated with enzyme abnormalities in the red cell, toxic drugs, or cyanotic heart disease, conditions which must be considered in the differential diagnosis.

All Hb M disorders thus far discovered are heterozygotes. Some types of Hb M will not separate from Hb A on alkaline electrophoresis. If the hemolysate is first converted to methemoglobin, the Hb M will migrate differently from normal methemoglobin at pH 7.1. Then absorption spectra of the eluted Hb M, which may be distinctive, can be compared with that of normal methemoglobin (Bunn, 1977). Amino acid analysis of peptide maps of tryptic digests of the abnormal hemoglobin will enable identification of the Hb M. This may be performed at a reference laboratory.

Hemoglobins Associated with Altered Oxygen Affinity

INCREASED AFFINITY AND POLYCYTHEMIA. Over 20 alpha and beta chain abnormalities have been described (Lehmann, 1977; Bunn, 1977). Some are listed in Table 29-2. The oxygen dissociation curve is shifted to the left. The P_{50}, the partial pressure of oxygen at which the hemoglobin is 50 per cent saturated, is decreased. Under physiologic conditions, the normal P_{50} of whole blood is 26 mm Hg; in this disorder it has ranged from 12 to 18 mm Hg. Since the hemoglobin has high affinity for oxygen, the tissues are relatively hypoxic at any given P_{O_2}, resulting in increased erythropoietin production and polycythemia. Since the amino acid substitution is inside the molecule, usually the abnormal hemoglobin is indistinguishable from Hb A on electrophoresis (Stamatoyannopoulos, 1971).

Hemoglobin Chesapeake. An alpha chain abnormality associated with mild asymptomatic polycythemia in a Caucasian family was the first described (Charache, 1966). The features were similar to those of benign familial polycythemia. The abnormal hemoglobin, accounting for about 30 per cent of the total, had an increased affinity for oxygen which resulted in significantly elevated hematocrit levels. The abnormal hemoglobin could be detected by starch block or starch gel electrophoresis.

These disorders are autosomal dominant; only heterozygotes have been described. The hemoglobin concentration has ranged from 15 to 23.8 g/dl. Only about half of these abnormal hemoglobins can be separated from Hb A by starch gel or cellulose acetate electrophoresis at pH 8.6. Measurement of oxygen affinity is required to establish the diagnosis (Bunn, 1977).

DECREASED AFFINITY AND CYANOSIS. Six abnormal hemoglobins are stable and have decreased oxygen affinity (Table 29-2, Bunn, et. al., 1977). The oxygen dissociation curve is

Table 29-2. FUNCTIONAL CLASSIFICATION OF HEMOGLOBIN VARIANTS

I. Homozygous: Hemoglobin polymorphisms; the variants that are most common.

Hb S	$\alpha_2\beta_2^{6Val}$	Severe hemolytic anemia; sickling
Hb C	$\alpha_2\beta_2^{6Lys}$	Mild hemolytic anemia
Hb D Punjab	$\alpha_2\beta_2^{121Gln}$	No anemia
Hb E	$\alpha_2\beta_2^{26Lys}$	Mild microcytic anemia

II. Heterozygous: Hemoglobin variants causing functional aberrations or hemolytic anemia in the heterozygous state.

  A. Hemoglobins associated with methemoglobinemia and cyanosis.

    1. Hb M Boston $\alpha_2^{58Tyr}\beta_2$ 3. Hb M Saskatoon $\alpha_2\beta_2^{63Tyr}$

    2. Hb M Iwate $\alpha_2^{87Tyr}\beta_2$ 4. Hb M Milwaukee $\alpha_2\beta_2^{67Glu}$

                                    5. Hb M Hyde Park $\alpha_2\beta_2^{92Tyr}$

  B. Hemoglobins associated with altered oxygen affinity.

    1. Increased affinity and polycythemia.

a.	Hb Chesapeake	$\alpha_2^{92Leu}\beta_2$
b.	Hb J Capetown	$\alpha_2^{92Gln}\beta_2$
c.	Hb Malmo	$\alpha_2\beta_2^{97Gln}$
d.	Hb Yakima	$\alpha_2\beta_2^{99His}$
e.	Hb Kemp	$\alpha_2\beta_2^{99Asn}$
f.	Hb Ypsi (Ypsilanti)	$\alpha_2\beta_2^{99Tyrl}$
g.	Hb Hiroshima	$\alpha_2\beta_2^{143Asp}$
h.	Hb Rainier	$\alpha_2\beta_2^{145Cys}$
i.	Hb Bethesda	$\alpha_2\beta_2^{145His}$

    2. Decreased affinity—may have mild anemia or cyanosis.

a.	Hb Kansas	$\alpha_2^{102Thr}\beta_2$
b.	Hb Titusville	$\alpha_2^{94Asn}\beta_2$
c.	Hb Providence	$\alpha_2\beta_2^{82Asn,Asp}$
d.	Hb Agenogi	$\alpha_2\beta_2^{90Lys}$
e.	Hb Beth Israel	$\alpha_2\beta_2^{102Ser}$
f.	Hb Yoshizuka	$\alpha_2\beta_2^{108Asp}$

  C. Unstable hemoglobins

    1. Hemoglobins which may precipitate as Heinz bodies after splenectomy: "Congenital Heinz body hemolytic anemia."

      a. α-chain abnormalities

Hb Torino	$\alpha_2^{42Val}\beta_2$
Hb L-Ferrara	$\alpha_2^{47Gly}\beta_2$
Hb Hasharon	$\alpha_2^{47His}\beta_2$
Hb Ann Arbor	$\alpha_2^{80Arg}\beta_2$
Hb Etobicoke	$\alpha_2^{84Arg}\beta_2$
Hb Dakar	$\alpha_2^{112Glu}\beta_2$
Hb Bibba	$\alpha_2^{136Pro}\beta_2$

      b. β-chain abnormalities

Hb Leiden	$\alpha_2\beta_2^{6or7}$	(Glu deleted)
Hb Sogn	$\alpha_2\beta_2^{14Arg}$	
Hb Freiburg	$\alpha_2\beta_2^{23}$	(Val deleted)
Hb Riverdale Bronx	$\alpha_2\beta_2^{24Arg}$	
Hb Genova	$\alpha_2\beta_2^{28Pro}$	
Hb Tacoma	$\alpha_2\beta_2^{30Ser}$	
Hb Philly	$\alpha_2\beta_2^{35Phe}$	
Hb Louisville	$\alpha_2\beta_2^{42Leu}$	
Hb Hammersmith	$\alpha_2\beta_2^{42Ser}$	
Hb Zurich	$\alpha_2\beta_2^{63Arg}$	
Hb Toulouse	$\alpha_2\beta_2^{66Glu}$	
Hb Bristol	$\alpha_2\beta_2^{67Asp}$	
Hb Sydney	$\alpha_2\beta_2^{67Ala}$	
Hb Shepherd's Bush	$\alpha_2\beta_2^{74Asp}$	
Hb Seattle	$\alpha_2\beta_2^{76Glu}$	
Hb Boras	$\alpha_2\beta_2^{88Arg}$	
Hb Santa Ana	$\alpha_2\beta_2^{88Pro}$	
Hb Gun Hill	$\alpha_2\beta_2^{91-97}$	(5 a.a. deleted)
Hb Sabine	$\alpha_2\beta_2^{91Pro}$	
Hb Köln	$\alpha_2\beta_2^{98Met}$	
Hb Kansas	$\alpha_2\beta_2^{102Thr}$	
Hb Wein	$\alpha_2\beta_2^{130Asp}$	
Hb Olmsted	$\alpha_2\beta_2^{141Arg}$	

    2. Tetramers of normal chains; appear in thalassemias.

Hb Bart's	γ_4
Hb H	β_4
Hb α_4^A	α_4

shifted to the right, and the P_{50} is increased. Two of these are associated with cyanosis. The hemoglobin level may be somewhat low on the basis of the high P_{50}.

Hemoglobin Kansas. This hemoglobin, described in a Caucasian boy, had just the opposite property from Hb Chesapeake, an abnormally low affinity for oxygen. The clinical features were cyanosis since infancy, normal arterial oxygen tension, and reduced oxygen saturation. Electrophoresis after conversion to methemoglobin allowed separation from Hb A (Reissman, 1961).

Unstable Hemoglobins
(White, 1971; Lehmann, 1977)

Over 60 variants have been described in which the hemoglobin precipitates within the red cell as Heinz bodies. Some are listed in Table 29-2. Most of the abnormalities are beta chain; some are alpha. Amino acid substitution or deletion renders the Hb molecule unstable through molecular mechanisms discussed in the references cited. Precipitated Hb attaches to the cell membrane and shortens its survival; the cells are inflexible; Heinz bodies are removed by the spleen; the further damaged cells have a shortened survival. The oxygen affinity is usually abnormal and may be increased or decreased. Some of these unstable hemoglobins have been defined as the cause of what were originally called "congenital Heinz body hemolytic anemias."

All patients have been heterozygous. The clinical features have shown considerable variation, from severe hemolytic anemia in the first year of life (e.g., Hb Hammersmith, Hb Bristol) to a very mild chronic hemolytic anemia (e.g., Hb Louisville, Hb Hasharon) which may be exacerbated by drugs (e.g., Hb Zurich). A few unstable hemoglobins have been discovered incidentally in clinically normal individuals (e.g., Hb Toulouse, Hb Sogn).

Jaundice and splenomegaly are common, as in other hemolytic anemias. More distinctive in some cases is the excretion of darkly pigmented urine (only during hemolytic crises in mild variants). The urine pigment appears to be a dipyrrole, probably a breakdown product of denatured hemoglobin. Cyanosis is present in some patients and is due to met- and sulfhemoglobinemia or to low oxygen affinity.

The anemia is normocytic and normochromic to hypochromic, the latter because of the loss of hemoglobin from the cells (in the form of Heinz bodies) in the reticuloendothelial organs. Patients with relatively high hemoglobin concentrations in the steady state usually have hemoglobin variants with a high oxygen affinity and an unexpectedly high reticulocyte count (e.g., Hb Köln, Hb Gun Hill). On the other hand, patients with rather low hemoglobin concentrations may be relatively asymptomatic if their hemoglobin has a low oxygen affinity; their reticulocyte counts are unexpectedly low for the hemoglobin concentration (e.g., Hb Hammersmith). Heinz bodies are rarely seen in circulating red cells before splenectomy, though sometimes they may be generated by incubating the red cells with brilliant cresyl blue or new methylene blue. After splenectomy, Heinz bodies are readily demonstrable in a large proportion of cells; blood film shows irregularly contracted cells and basophilic stippling which may be pronounced.

In splenectomized patients, the Heinz bodies interfere with hemoglobin determinations and with electronic platelet and white cell counts. Before reading the O.D. of the hemolysate it should be centrifuged to remove the Heinz bodies. Platelet and leukocyte counts should be performed by visual methods.

The key laboratory estimations are the heat stability and isopropanol precipitation tests (p. 1021). The hemoglobin electrophoresis may be either normal or abnormal. Hb A_2 may be elevated in β-chain variants because of the loss of the abnormal hemoglobin from the cells. Hb F may be increased to a level of 10 to 15 per cent.

THALASSEMIAS

Thalassemias comprise a heterogeneous group of hereditary diseases of hemoglobin synthesis in persons of Mediterranean, African, and Asian ancestry.

The common characteristic of this group of diseases is impaired production of one of the polypeptide chains of hemoglobin; that is, the *rate* of synthesis is diminished in varying degree, but the chain formed is, in most cases, structurally normal. In beta thalassemias, beta chain production is decreased. Alpha thalassemia and delta-beta thalassemia have decreased synthesis of the respective polypeptide chains. These various conditions constitute the "thalassemia syndromes" (Weatherall, 1972). Orkin (1976) and Weatherall (1977) have summarized evidence for the genetic defects in these syndromes, which, in the great majority of cases, result in a quantitative deficiency of messenger RNA (mRNA).

Beta thalassemia

Studies have shown that in most β thalassemias, the structural genes are present but the mRNA either is not produced efficiently or is degraded rapidly. The clinical, genetic, and hemoglobin findings in the β-thalassemias are summarized in Table 29–3.

Thalassemia Major (Homozygous Beta Thalassemia; Cooley's Anemia). With an absence (β°) or a marked decrease (β^+) in β-chain production, γ-chain production remains high (Hb F is elevated), and there is an excess of α-chains. Aggregates of the latter are unstable and precipitate in the normoblast or red cell and damage the cells. Precipitates and cells are removed, causing a severe hemolytic anemia.

Clinical findings include jaundice and splenomegaly, which become evident early in childhood. Prominent frontal bones, cheek bones, and jaws impart a mongoloid appearance. These changes and the roentgenographic findings of thinned cortex of the long and flat bones and thickening of the skull with osteoporosis ("hair-on-end" appearance) reflect the extreme bone marrow hyperplasia in response to the hemolytic process. Growth is stunted and puberty is delayed. Most patients require regular transfusions, and develop problems due to iron loading. Hemochromatosis commonly develops, and the major cause of death is cardiac failure due to myocardial siderosis by the end of the third decade.

BLOOD. Unlike most hemolytic diseases, the anemia is hypochromic and microcytic. This is probably due to the defect in hemoglobin synthesis. Extreme poikilocytosis with bizarre shapes, target cells, ovalocytosis, Cabot rings,

Table 29–3.   BETA THALASSEMIAS

CONDITION	PARENTAL GENOTYPES	RISK	HEMOGLOBIN PATTERN	SEVERITY	β MRNA	GENES
Homozygous states:						
β^+ thalassemia	Both β^+/β	$\frac{1}{4}$	↓Hb A, ↑Hb F, variable Hb A_2	Variable; usually Cooley's anemia	Marked deficiency of β mRNA	β genes present
β^0 thalassemia	Both β^0/β	$\frac{1}{4}$	0 Hb A, variable Hb A_2, residual Hb F	Cooley's anemia	(i) absent β mRNA (ii) mutant, non-functional β mRNA present in rare Oriental cases	β genes present
$\delta\beta^0$ thalassemia	Both $\delta\beta^0/\delta\beta$	$\frac{1}{4}$	0 Hb A, Hb A_2, 100% Hb F	Thalassemia intermedia	δ and β mRNA's absent	β genes deleted; probable δ-gene deletion.
Hb Lepore	Both Hb Lepore/β	$\frac{1}{4}$	0 Hb A, Hb A_2; 75% Hb F, 25% Hb Lepore	Cooley's anemia	β-like mRNA present in reduced amount	β-δ fusion genes present; no normal β & δ genes.
Heterozygous states:						
β^+ thalassemia	β^+/β, normal	$\frac{1}{2}$	↑Hb A_2, slight ↑Hb F	Thalassemia minor	Deficient β mRNA	β genes present
β^0 thalassemia	β^0/β, normal	$\frac{1}{2}$	↑Hb A_2, slight ↑Hb F	Thalassemia minor	Deficient β mRNA, or rarely non-functional β mRNA present	β genes present
$\delta\beta^0$ thalassemia	$\delta\beta^0/\delta\beta$, normal	$\frac{1}{2}$	5-20% Hb F	Thalassemia minor	Presumed deficiency of β & δ mRNA's	β & probable δ gene deletion on 1 homologous chromosome
Hb Lepore	Hb Lepore/β, normal	$\frac{1}{2}$	↑HbF, ↓Hb A_2, 5-15% Hb Lepore	Thalassemia minor	β-like mRNA present	Hb Lepore gene replaces normal β & δ genes on 1 chromosome

Reprinted by permission from Orkin, S. H., and Nathan, D. G.: The thalassemias. N. Engl. J. Med., *295*:710, 1976.

Howell-Jolly bodies, nuclear fragments, siderocytes, anisochromia, anisocytosis, and often extreme normoblastosis are present. Poikilocytosis is more striking in patients with intact spleens; normoblastosis is more severe after splenectomy. Normoblasts have hypochromic cytoplasm and, especially after splenectomy, an aggregate of densely staining hemoglobin (Plate 29-2*F*), which probably represents precipitated alpha chains (with heme attached). Incubation of the blood with methyl violet (as for Heinz bodies, p. 1024) stains these precipitates of alpha chains in both red cells and normoblasts. The reticulocyte count is less elevated than expected for the degree of anemia because of destruction of erythroid precursors in the marrow. Osmotic resistance of the red cells, serum iron, and indirect-reacting bilirubin are increased.

MARROW.   Marked normoblastic hyperplasia is present. Many late normoblasts show inclusion bodies as in the blood. Intramedullary destruction of hemoglobin (ineffective erythropoiesis) is markedly increased in thalassemia major. Storage iron and sideroblasts are increased.

HEMOGLOBIN STUDIES.   Almost all cases of thalassemia major fall into the group of the homozygous *high A₂ beta thalassemias* (true β thalassemia). Hb F is increased, usually 40 to 60 per cent, and may be as high as 90 per cent. Hb A is undetectable in some individuals. Hb A_2 is low, normal, or elevated, but the ratio of A_2 to A is always increased. In the very rare homozygous delta-beta thalassemia, no Hb A or Hb A_2 is formed; Hb F is 100 per cent. This form is of intermediate clinical severity ("thalassemia intermedia"). Blacks with homozygous thalassemia also usually have a milder clinical course, without need for transfusion. Thalassemia intermedia is a clinical, not a genetic, designation.

Thalassemia Minor (Heterozygous Thalassemia Minima; Cooley's Trait).   Clinical findings are as follows: The features in heterozygous beta thalassemia vary from moderately severe anemia (thalassemia intermedia) to completely normal clinical findings. The severe intermediate forms of heterozygous thalassemia are rare and are found in Mediterranean individuals but not in blacks; in the latter, heterozygous thalassemia is uniformly mild. In many persons, there is a mild hypochromic, microcytic anemia with slight hemolytic jaundice and splenomegaly. Most individuals with thalassemia minor, however, have no symptoms or abnormal physical signs.

BLOOD.   Usually there is no anemia. Most characteristically, the red cell count is elevated and the hemoglobin and hematocrit are reduced. The MCH is low, usually less than 22 pg; and the MCV is low, between 50 and 70 fl. The MCHC is sometimes low but often normal. On stained films, the cells have a moderate degree of microcytosis and poikilocytosis; target cells and basophilic stippling are often present. Osmotic fragility is decreased. The serum iron is normal or high and the serum ferritin is normal.

MARROW.   Normoblastic hyperplasia and elevated storage iron may be found.

HEMOGLOBIN STUDIES.   Most common is heterozygous *high A₂ beta thalassemia* (true beta thalassemia). Hb F is slightly elevated in 50 per cent of cases in the 2 to 6 per cent range. Hb A_2 is elevated in the 3.5 to 7 per cent range. The remainder is Hb A.

In heterozygous delta-beta thalassemia (high Hb F-beta thalassemia), the Hb F is elevated in the range of 5 to 20 per cent; Hb A_2 is normal or slightly decreased. This variant is much less common than beta thalassemia. Heterozygotes for delta-beta thalassemia may be distinguished from those for a non-thalassemic condition, *hereditary persistence of Hb F*, by the fact that in the latter the Hb F is uniformly distributed among the red cells. In thalassemias, Hb F is unevenly distributed in the red cell population, as shown by the acid elution staining technique (p. 1021). Other forms of beta thalassemia exist but are less common, and description in some is incomplete. It is evident that no single finding is diagnostic and that family studies are of great importance.

Hemoglobin Lepore Syndromes.   Hb Lepore is an abnormal hemoglobin that has a normal α-chain combined with a composite $\delta\beta$-chain (Weatherall, 1972). It probably occurred due to chromosome misalignment with crossing-over and fusion of genetic material at the $\delta\beta$-gene complex. Different Hb Lepores have been described, depending on the point of fusion. Because the composite $\delta\beta$-chain is synthesized at a slow rate, it results in a hypochromic microcytic red cell picture resembling the thalassemias (Table 29-3). Lepore migrates similarly to Hb S on alkaline electrophoresis.

Double heterozygosity for beta thalassemia and beta hemoglobinopathy

The beta thalassemia gene selectively depresses synthesis of the normal beta chains of

Hb A. For example, patients doubly heterozygous for beta thalassemia and Hb S have levels of Hb A which are *less* than the level of Hb S. In the simple sickle cell trait, the level of Hb A always exceeds that of Hb S.

Sickle Cell–Beta Thalassemia (S/β Thalassemia). S/β^0 thalassemia is more severe than S/β^+ thalassemia. The anemia and clinical findings vary from slight to severe, with manifestations similar to those in sickle cell anemia (SS). In contrast to SS, the spleen in S/β thalassemia remains enlarged after childhood and into adult life.

BLOOD.   Pronounced microcytosis, variable hypochromia, and many target cells are present. Sickled cells are uncommon. The MCV and MCH are low.

HEMOGLOBIN STUDIES.   The solubility test and sickling test are of course positive. In S/β^+ thalassemia, Hb A = 15 to 30 per cent, Hb S = over 50 per cent, Hb F = 1 to 20 per cent, and Hb A_2 is increased, usually over 4.5 per cent. Though these individuals clinically may resemble sickle trait (Hb AS), in S/β^+ thalassemia the amount of Hb S always exceeds Hb A; in Hb AS, Hb A always exceeds Hb S.

In S/β^0 thalassemia, Hb A is absent, Hb S is 75 to 90 per cent, Hb F is 5 to 20 per cent, and Hb A_2 is usually increased, over 4.5 per cent. This disorder clinically and hematologically resembles sickle cell disease (SS). The main difference is that in S/β^0 thalassemia, the MCV and MCH are lower and the Hb A_2 is increased. Family study is often necessary for a clear distinction (Lehmann, 1977; Wrightstone, 1974).

Hemoglobin C–Beta Thalassemia.   This occurs mainly in blacks, in whom it tends to result in little disability. Patients of Mediterranean extraction usually have moderately severe hemolytic anemia.

BLOOD.   The MCH and MCV are reduced. On the blood film are hypochromic target cells, fragmented red cells, and microspherocytes, many of which have a folded appearance.

HEMOGLOBIN STUDIES.   Hb C, 65 to 95 per cent; Hb F, variable; Hb A, about 20 per cent. Hb A_2 levels cannot be studied when Hb C is present, as there are no satisfactory methods for separating the two.

Hemoglobin E Thalassemia.   In this Southeast Asian disorder, a clinical and hematologic picture similar to thalassemia major is usual.

HEMOGLOBIN STUDIES.   Hb E, 15 to 95 per cent; Hb F, 5 to 85 per cent. It is of interest that Hb A is nearly always absent. This emphasizes the fact that absence of Hb A cannot be taken as proof of homozygosity; it must be supported by family studies.

Alpha thalassemias

Whereas there are two β-globin genes per diploid cell, evidence now indicates the presence of four α-globin genes per cell in Orientals and Caucasians, and two to four in blacks (Orkin, 1976). Also in contrast to β thalassemia, the defect in α thalassemia is usually *deletion* of genetic material, with consequent quantitative decrease of mRNA (Table 29-4).

Homozygous Alpha Thalassemia (Hydrops Fetalis with Hb Bart's).   Complete absence of α-chains is incompatible with life. Infants are stillborn with severe edema, marked anemia, and marked hepatosplenomegaly. The blood shows marked anisocytosis, poikilocytosis, microcytosis, and erythroblastosis. ABO or Rh incompatibility is absent. Because of the absence of α-chains, no Hb A $(\alpha_2\beta_2)$ or Hb F $(\alpha_2\gamma_2)$ is present. Large quantities of Hb Bart's (γ_4) and some Hb H (β_4) are present; both of these migrate faster than Hb A on alkaline electrophoresis.

Hemoglobin H Disease.   Three of the four α-genes are absent. A chronic anemia with the clinical picture of thalassemia intermedia is usual, though the severity varies. Hb H disease has been described in almost all racial groups, especially in Southeast Asia, Greece, and parts of the Middle East.

BLOOD.   The MCV and MCH are decreased. The blood film shows hypochromia, target cells, and anisopoikilocytosis (Plate 29-2G). Reticulocytes are usually 4 to 5 per cent. Vital staining of the blood with an oxidizing dye such as brilliant cresyl blue induces pale blue inclusion bodies (Hb H precipitates) in many of the red cells, which contrast with the deep blue precipitates of RNA in reticulocytes (Plate 29-2H, p. 1024). After splenectomy, single large Heinz bodies are seen.

HEMOGLOBIN STUDIES.   Hemoglobin electrophoresis shows a rapidly migrating band of Hb H (β_4) accounting for 4 to 30 per cent of the hemoglobin, and traces of the slightly less rapidly migrating Hb Bart's (γ_4). The percentage of Hb Bart's is about 25 per cent at birth; it gradually falls thereafter, but the level in adults is quite variable.

Heterozygous α Thalassemia (α Thalas-

Table 29-4 ALPHA THALASSEMIAS

CONDITION	PARENTAL GENOTYPES	RISK	HEMOGLOBIN PATTERN	SEVERITY	α mRNA	GENES
Homozygous α-thalassemia (hydrops fetalis with Hb Bart's)	Both α-thalassemia trait	$\frac{1}{4}$	80% Hb Bart's; remainder, Hb H & Portland.	Lethal	Absent	All α genes deleted
Hb H disease	(i) α-thalassemia trait, silent carrier	$\frac{1}{4}$	4-30% Hb H in adults: approximately 25% Hb Bart's in cord blood; when Hb CS gene present, 2-3% Hb CS.	Variable, usually thalassemia intermedia	Marked deficiency	(i) 3 of 4 α genes deleted
	(ii) α-thalassemia trait, Hb CS heterozygote	$\frac{1}{4}$				(ii) 2 of 4 deleted; 1 normal; 1 Hb CS gene
Heterozygous α thalassemia (α-thal trait)	α-thalassemia trait, normal	$\frac{1}{2}$	Approximately 5% Hb Bart's in cord blood	Mild; very mild in blacks	Presumed deficiency	2 of 4 α genes deleted; ? 1 of 3 deleted in blacks
Silent carrier	Silent carrier, normal	$\frac{1}{2}$	Approximately 1-2% Hb Bart's in cord blood	0	Presumed slight deficiency	1 of 4 α genes deleted
Heterozygous Hb Constant Spring (CS)	Hb CS heterozygote, normal	$\frac{1}{2}$	Approximately 1% Hb CS	0	Presumed deficiency	3 of 4 α genes present; 1 Hb CS gene

Reprinted by permission from Orkin, S. H., and Nathan, D. G.: The thalassemias. N. Engl. J. Med., *295*:710, 1976.

semia-1 Trait, α^0 Thalassemia Trait). Absence of two α-genes results in a clinical picture similar to β-thalassemia trait with very mild anemia, microcytosis, a normal serum iron, normal serum ferritin, and normal red cell protoporphyrin.

HEMOGLOBIN STUDIES. Diagnosis is best made by finding 5 to 6 percent Hb Bart's in cord blood; normally, only trace amounts (<0.5 per cent) are found. In adults Hb H inclusion bodies can be found in a very small percentage of red cells (perhaps 1 in 10^5), if *exhaustively sought after* (Wasi, 1974). Otherwise no evidence of hemoglobin imbalance is detectable by standard techniques, and the diagnosis is one of excluding iron deficiency and beta thalassemia or demonstrating a decreased α-chain/β-chain synthesis ratio (~0.6).

Silent Carrier of α Thalassemia (α Thalassemia-2 Trait; α^+ Thalassemia Trait). One of four α-globin genes is absent. No hematologic abnormality is detectable in adults; MCV, blood film, and hemoglobin studies are normal. In infants, Hb Bart's accounts for 1 to 2 per cent of the cord blood hemoglobin. The diagnosis cannot be reliably made in the adult.

Hemoglobin Constant Spring. Hb Constant Spring (Hb $\overline{CS}$) is an α-chain variant with 31 extra amino acids. It is synthesized slowly and therefore tends to result in a thalassemia-like picture (Table 29-4). The homozygous state appears as a mild thalassemia with microcytosis and 5 to 6 per cent Hb $\overline{CS}$, normal Hb A_2, trace amounts of Hb Bart's, and the rest Hb A (Weatherall, 1977b). The heterozygous state shows no hematologic abnormality: normal Hb A and A_2 and about 1 per cent Hb $\overline{CS}$. The abnormal Hb migrates more slowly than Hb A_2 at alkaline pH and is easily missed. The gene behaves similarly to that in a silent carrier (α^+ thalassemia trait) and is found in about 40 per cent of cases of Hb H disease in Southeast Asia (see Table 29-4).

Hereditary persistence of fetal hemoglobin F (HPFH)

A group of conditions with Hb F production persisting beyond infancy without significant hematologic abnormalities is known as HPFH. It is found in about 0.1 per cent of American blacks; there are also a Greek form and other variants.

In the blacks, the homozygote has slightly microcytic, hypochromic red cells without anemia. Hb F = 100 per cent; no Hb A or Hb A_2 is present. This lack of β- and δ-chain synthesis has been shown to be due to deletion of the $\delta\beta$-gene complex (Weatherall, 1977a).

In the heterozygote, Hb F = 20 to 30 per cent, Hb A_2 = 1 to 2.1 per cent, with the remainder Hb A. With the acid elution technique, the Hb F is homogeneously distributed among the red cells in contrast to β thalassemia, in which the distribution is heterogeneous (p. 1021). No hematologic abnormalities are found.

HEMOLYSIS—METABOLIC DISORDERS

Deficient enzyme activity in the erythrocyte may result in abnormalities that lead to premature destruction and hemolytic anemia; these disorders are usually inherited. Interference with or oxidative stress on erythrocyte metabolism, however, can sometimes result in hemolysis in individuals who have normal erythrocytes (see Table 12-19, p. 380).

Erythrocyte Metabolism. The mature red cell lacks mitochondria and therefore oxidative phosphorylation and Krebs' cycle activity. Energy production is mainly glycolytic, 90 per cent of which occurs through the Embden-Meyerhof pathway, as glucose goes to lactic acid with the net production of two moles of ATP (Fig. 29-10). ATP is needed for the en-

ergy-requiring reactions in the cell: for active cation transport across the membrane; for maintaining membrane deformability; and for preserving the cell's biconcave shape. Most of the hemiglobin (methemoglobin) produced in the normal cell (about 3 per cent of the total per day) is reduced by NAD-linked Met Hb reductase. The pentose phosphate pathway (hexose monophosphate shunt) generates NADPH in the first two steps, through the enzymes glucose-6-phosphate dehydrogenase (G6PD) and 6-phosphogluconate. NADPH production is linked to glutathione reduction and, through this mechanism, to preservation of vital enzymes and hemoglobin from oxidation. Small amounts of oxidized hemoglobin (methemoglobin) are reduced by GSH (glutathione). Activity of the pentose phosphate pathway increases when the cell is exposed to an oxidant drug, probably as a result of increased NADP production. If an enzyme in this pathway is lacking in activity, GSH cannot be produced and hemoglobin will be oxidized by the oxidant stress. Oxidation in the

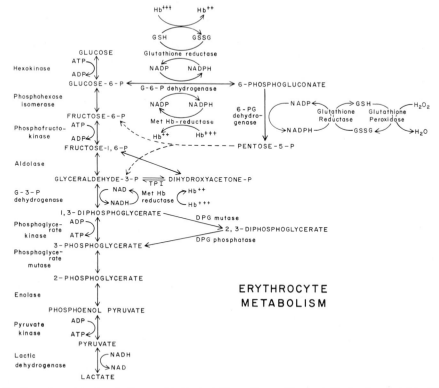

Figure 29–10. Erythrocyte metabolism is discussed in the text. Normally most hemoglobin (methemoglobin, Hb^{+++}) is reduced to hemoglobin (Hb^{++}) by nicotinamide adenine dinucleotide-linked methemoglobin reductase (NAD, Met Hb reductase). NADP-linked methemoglobin reductase requires methylene blue for activation and is more effective in drug-induced methemoglobinemia than the normal cell mechanism. GSH = reduced glutathione; GSSG = oxidized glutathione.

red cell is mediated by high energy derivatives of oxygen referred to collectively as activated oxygen (Carrell, 1975). Oxidized Hb denatures and precipitates as Heinz bodies which adhere to the membrane, inducing rigidity and a tendency to lysis. Moderate enzyme deficiencies in this pathway (e.g., G6PD) may not be associated with anemia; however, if the cells are challenged by an oxidizing drug an acute hemolytic episode occurs.

Deficiencies in the Embden-Meyerhof pathway result in impaired ATP generation and a chronic hemolytic anemia. The mechanism of the red cell destruction here is less clear. Heinz bodies are not formed. It appears that lack of cell deformability and impaired cation pumping may be important in the hemolytic process (LaCelle, 1971).

Another shunt, the Rapoport-Luebering shunt, provides for the conversion of 1,3-diphosphoglycerate (1,3-DPG) to 2,3-diphosphoglycerate (2,3-DPG) instead of directly to 3-phosphoglycerate (3-PG) (Fig. 29-10). If this shunt is operating, generation of two moles of ATP (per mole of glucose) is bypassed; the result is no net energy production in glycolysis. However, 2,3-DPG combines with the β-chain of hemoglobin and decreases the affinity of hemoglobin for oxygen. At a given partial pressure of oxygen, therefore, increased 2,3-DPG allows more oxygen to leave hemoglobin and go to the tissues; the oxygen dissociation curve is shifted to the right (p. 928, Fig. 28-4). Increased activity of this shunt is apparently stimulated by hypoxia.

Glucose-6-phosphate Dehydrogenase (G6PD) Deficiency

(Beutler, 1977; Carson, 1966). About 10 per cent of male American blacks who were given the anti-malarial drug primaquine during the Korean War developed a self-limited, acute hemolytic anemia. Only the older red cells were destroyed, and it was found that the deficiency in the susceptible red cells was in G6PD.

It has since been found that G6PD deficiency is widespread throughout the world. Among Caucasians, the highest incidence is in Kurdish Jews; the deficiency is also found in blacks and in Orientals.

Since G6PD is determined by a gene on the X-chromosome, full expression of the deficiency is found in the male hemizygote. Partial expression may be found in the heterozygous female who has two populations of red cells, one normal and one deficient. The deficiency of G6PD results in a limitation of the

regeneration of NADPH, which renders the cell vulnerable to oxidative denaturation of hemoglobin. Since, normally, G6PD is highest in young cells and decreases as the cell ages, in persons with G6PD deficiency the older cells are preferentially destroyed.

Hemolytic susceptibility in affected persons can increase greatly during intercurrent illness or upon exposure to various drugs (e.g., primaquine, sulfonamides, nitrofurans, and aminoquinolones) which have oxidant properties (Table 29-5).

The genetic heterogeneity is great and is expressed as variation in the stability and the electrophoretic and catalytic properties of the enzymes, in the degree of deficiency, in the types of cells in the body affected, in the types of drugs which will produce hemolysis, and in the susceptibility to chronic hemolysis or to neonatal jaundice (Oski, 1972). The most common ("normal") G6PD isozyme in all population groups is designated as B. In blacks, an electrophoretically more rapid variant, A, is prevalent and has almost the same activity; 30 per cent of black males have this variant. Eleven per cent of black males have the A- type of G6PD, which has only 5 to 15 per cent of the normal enzyme activity; it is these individuals who are susceptible to hemolysis after ingesting oxidant drugs or during infection. The most common variant in Caucasians is G6PD-Mediterranean, found in Mediterranean populations; the level of enzyme activity in affected males is low, often less than 1 per cent. These individuals usually are not anemic, but may have somewhat more severe and non-self-limited hemolytic anemia with infections, and with a wider variety of drugs than the black variant (Beutler, 1978). Severe hemolysis may occur within hours after eating fava beans ("favism"). Although the vast majority of G6PD-deficient patients worldwide are not anemic, a small proportion of persons with G6PD-Mediterranean (and persons with some rarer variants) have a chronic non-spherocytic hemolytic anemia.

The laboratory findings during active hemolysis are those of hemolytic anemia in general. In the blood film, poikilocytes, irregularly contracted cells, and occasional spherocytes may be found. After supravital staining with methyl violet, Heinz bodies may be present early in an acute hemolytic episode (p. 1024). G6PD deficiency may be detected by one of the screening tests: the incubated Heinz body test, the dye reduction test, the ascorbate cyanide test, or a fluorescence spot test. Confirmation may be made with a quantitative assay. These are discussed on page 1025.

Pyruvate Kinase (PK) Deficiency (Tanaka, 1962; 1971). Though G6PD deficiency is the most common red cell enzyme abnormality, it does not usually produce a chronic hemolytic anemia. Deficiency of the glycolytic enzyme *pyruvate kinase* is probably the most common cause of hereditary non-spherocytic hemolytic anemia. The type II pattern of autohemolysis is usually seen (p. 1024), although it is not established that all type II patterns are due to PK deficiency. It is inherited as an autosomal recessive characteristic. Heterozygotes are asymptomatic and have normal hemograms, but most can be detected by enzyme assay. The disease may appear in infancy. Irregularly contracted erythrocytes and crenated cells may be prominent on the blood film in some cases, especially after splenectomy (Plate 29-2*K*). Reticulocyte counts are often very high.

Heinz bodies are not found. The diagnosis is established by a specific screening test or by enzyme assay (p. 1026).

Splenectomy is usually advisable if transfusions are necessary to avoid symptoms of anemia. It is frequently helpful despite some continued hemolysis.

Deficiency of Other Enzymes. Hemolytic anemia has been described in deficiencies of several other enzymes of the Embden-Meyerhof pathway, the hexose monophosphate shunt, glutathione metabolism, and nucleotide metabolism. These are rare entities (Valentine, 1977b). Mild to moderate deficiency of glutathione reductase may be found in many disorders on the basis of flavin deficiency; it does not appear to play a measurable role in red cell destruction (Beutler, 1975).

In general, the deficiencies of the glutathione system that result in hemolytic anemia are rare; patients with these deficiencies show autosomal recessive inheritance, have increased susceptibility to oxidant drugs, and may be expected to show Heinz bodies during episodes of acute hemolysis (p. 1024).

After membrane defects, hemoglobin defects, G6PD deficiency, and pyruvate kinase deficiency have been excluded as causes of an intrinsic hemolytic anemia, consideration of the rare other enzyme defects is warranted. Consultation with a laboratory experienced in these assays is advisable (see Beutler, 1975).

HEMOLYSIS—ACQUIRED; EXTRINSIC

Chemical agents

Agents Hemolytic to Normal Cells. The action of chemical agents depends on the dose and on other factors, many of which are known only vaguely. They range from simple substances, such as water, to some that are highly complex.

When used as irrigating fluid, distilled water was found responsible for acute hemolytic anemia as a result of entry into venous channels during transurethral resection. In addition to anemia some of these chemicals produce methemoglobinemia, and some are responsible for cyanosis (toluene, trinitrotoluene, nitrobenzene, acetanilid, and phenacetin). Some may lead to aplastic anemia (toluene and trinitrotoluene). Promin, a sulfone derivative, makes blood turn chocolate brown. Lead administered therapeutically may produce progressive anemia, with basophilic stippling, reticulocytosis, normoblastemia, Cabot's rings, Howell-Jolly bodies, and leukocytosis. Lead not only causes damage to the red cell and hemolysis, but also produces defects in the heme synthetic pathway. In cases of chronic exposure to lead, basophilic stippling, more in the marrow than in the peripheral blood, and coproporphyrinuria are the characteristic findings. These changes produce defective erythrocytes, which are removed by the spleen.

Agents Hemolytic to Abnormal Cells. Certain drugs and chemicals which have oxidizing activity (Table 29-5) may produce hemolytic anemia in only a few of the many persons who are exposed to them. These biochemical defects have been mentioned in the section on metabolic defects of the cell (p. 1003) and include glucose-6-phosphate dehydrogenase (G6PD) deficiency, glutathione deficiency, and glutathione reductase deficiency. In addition, unstable hemoglobins such as Hb Zürich have a propensity for drug-induced hemolytic anemia. Premature infants, although they have high levels of G6PD, have glutathione instability and low levels of glutathione and may develop hemolytic anemia when given large doses of synthetic water-soluble analogues of vitamin K.

It must be remembered that, if the exposure to these oxidant substances is great enough, acute hemolytic anemia may be produced in

Table 29–5. COMPOUNDS RESPONSIBLE FOR CLINICALLY SIGNIFICANT HEMOLYSIS OF G6PD-DEFICIENT ERYTHROCYTES

Analgesics	*Non-sulfonamide Antibacterial Agents*
Acetanilid	Furazolidone
Acetylsalicylic acid[1]	Furmethanol
Acetophenetidin (phenacetin)[1]	Nitrofurantoin
Sulfonamides and Sulfones	Nitrofurazone
Sulfanilamide	Chloramphenicol[2]
Sulfapyridine	*Miscellaneous*
Diphenylsulfone	Naphthalene
N-Acetylsulfanilamide	Trinitrotoluene
Sulfacetamide	Methylene blue
Thiazolsulfone	Nalidixic acid
Salicylazosulfapyridine	Phenylhydrazine
Sulfamethoxypyridazine	Quinine[2]
Antimalarial	Quinidine[2]
Primaquine	Ascorbic acid[3]
Pamaquine	Niridazole
Pentaquine	
Quinocide	
Quinacrine	

From Beutler, E.: Glucose-6-phosphate dehydrogenase deficiency. *In* Stanbury, J. B., Wyngaarden, J. B., and Frederickson, D. A.: The Metabolic Basis of Inherited Disease, 4th ed. New York, McGraw-Hill Book Co., 1978, p. 1431.
[1] Only slightly hemolytic in G6PD A-, in large doses.
[2] Hemolytic in G6PD Mediterranean but not in G6PD A-.
[3] In massive doses.

normal individuals; persons with biochemical abnormalities are sensitive to lower doses.

During the acute hemolytic episode, Heinz bodies can frequently be demonstrated by direct vital staining of blood with methyl violet (p. 1024). Red cells with Heinz bodies are removed from the circulation by the spleen, or the Heinz bodies are extracted from the red cells by splenic action. Therefore, Heinz bodies may not be found in the blood if the spleen is effectively removing them or after the acute hemolytic process has abated.

Tests for G6PD deficiency, the most common underlying cause of drug-sensitive hemolytic anemia, are described on page 1025.

Physical agents

Heat. Extensive third-degree burns produce hemolytic anemia, probably because of direct damage to red cells. The blood film may show remarkable morphologic abnormalities of the red cells, including numerous schistocytes (fragments) and irregularly contracted cells. The most severe abnormalities are often found immediately after extensive burns before a reticulocyte response has had time to develop (Fig. 27-17). The badly damaged cells are rapidly removed from the circulation.

Traumatic Hemolysis. Hemolytic anemia characterized by striking morphologic abnormalities of the red cells and occurring in certain other conditions has been attributed to physical trauma to the red cells. The red cell abnormalities are present in varying degree and include fragments (schistocytes) and irregularly contracted cells (burr cells, triangular cells, helmet cells) (Fig. 27-22; Plate 29-2L). The basis of the hemolytic process has been thought to be physical damage to the red cells in their contact with loose fibrin meshworks (intravascular coagulation) or with pathologic vascular lesions. Fragmentation of the cells results with or without intravascular lysis. Two general categories are recognized in this group of disorders, aptly termed the "red cell fragmentation syndrome."

CARDIAC VALVULAR DISEASE AND PROSTHESES. Chronic intravascular hemolysis associated with low serum haptoglobin, hemosiderinuria, reticulocytosis, and red cell abnormalities (e.g., schistocytes and irregularly contracted cells) may occur after surgical replacement of a diseased heart valve with a prosthesis or after surgical repair of a septal defect with a plastic patch (Marsh, 1969). This has been attributed to mechanical damage of red cells in the turbulent environment of a leaky valve or of a roughened surface uncovered by endothelial cells. Repair of the valve or coverage of the patch by endothelium has improved the hemolytic process. Other studies have shown that some patients with cardiac valvular disease have a hemolytic process which may be altered by surgery.

MICROANGIOPATHIC HEMOLYTIC ANEMIA. Hemolytic anemia with red cell fragmentation (e.g., schistocytes and irregularly contracted cells) has been described in malignant hypertension, thrombotic thrombocytopenic purpura, and disseminated carcinoma, in which a common factor was the presence of pathologic lesions involving small blood vessels. The hypothesis was advanced that the hemolytic anemia in these conditions may be an expression of mechanical or perhaps chemical effects of the vascular lesions on the red cells, and the process was designated "microangiopathic" (Brain, 1962).The role of disseminated or local intravascular coagulation has been recognized as an important factor (though not necessarily the inciting factor) in the pathogenesis of microangiopathy and the resultant hemolysis (Brain, 1970; 1972).

A rather distinct clinical state that probably belongs in the latter group as far as the hemolytic mechanism is concerned is the hemolytic-uremic syndrome (Piel, 1966). It occurs most commonly in infants less than two years of age and is often preceded by a viral infection. Hemolytic anemia with bizarre red cells, variable thrombocytopenia, and uremia are the cardinal features. Death has occurred in almost half the cases; the renal pathology has included acute glomerulonephritis and thrombotic and necrotic vascular lesions associated with patchy, bilateral renal cortical necrosis. The disorder appears in some way to be related to thrombotic thrombocytopenic purpura. In some cases, laboratory findings suggestive of disseminated intravascular coagulation have been observed. In previous years, death occurred in over half the cases. More recently, an increasing number of children have recovered; some, however, have persistent impairment of renal function (Brain, 1974).

Vegetable and animal poisons

Inhalation of pollens of the fava bean plant or ingestion of the bean itself may be followed by a fulminant hemolytic anemia in sensitive persons, mainly of Mediterranean origin. Glucose-6-phosphate dehydrogenase (G6PD) deficiency of the red cells plus a serum factor makes the individual sensitive to the fava bean.

G6PD-deficient persons without the serum factor may be found in the same family and are not subject to favism. So-called Baghdad spring anemia is similar to the anemia caused by the fava bean. Some snake venoms and ricin contained in the castor bean are strongly hemolytic.

Infectious agents

Destruction of erythrocytes by plasmodia is responsible for the anemia in malaria. This is supported by the observation that the osmotic and mechanical fragility of parasitized erythrocytes is increased. Inhibition of marrow activity may be an additional factor. Fulminant hemoglobinuria (blackwater fever) is a complication of *P. falciparum* malaria. Its frequency after quinine therapy suggests an autoimmune mechanism mediated by the drug.

Oroya fever, a frequently fatal disease that occurs in Peru, is characterized by a hemolytic anemia and leukocytosis. *Bartonella bacilliformis* is the responsible agent.

Hemolytic anemia with cold agglutinins may complicate mycoplasma pneumonia and infectious mononucleosis. This is due to the effect of antibody on the cells (p. 1009).

Hemolytic anemia of varying severity is frequent in some bacterial infections. A notable example of the latter is *Clostridium welchii* septicemia following septic abortion or biliary tract surgery, which may be accompanied by a dramatic and life-threatening hemolytic crisis.

Immune hemolytic anemias

Immune hemolytic anemias are disorders in which erythrocyte survival is reduced because of the deposition of immunoglobulin and/or complement on the red cell membrane. The immune hemolytic anemias can be grouped according to the presence of autoantibodies, isoantibodies, or drug-related antibodies (Table 29-6).

Autoimmune Hemolytic Anemic (AIHA). The autoimmune hemolytic anemias are due to an altered immune response resulting in the production of antibody against the host's own erythrocytes, with subsequent hemolysis. The AIHA's can be classified according to serologic or clinical characteristics (Table 29-7). Dacie (1951) was the first to show that some AIHA's are mediated by antibodies with maximum binding affinity at 37°C. and other AIHA's are mediated by antibodies with their

Table 29-6. CLASSIFICATION OF IMMUNE HEMOLYTIC ANEMIAS

Autoimmune Hemolytic Anemias
    Associated with Warm Antibodies
    Associated with Cold Antibodies
Isoimmune Hemolytic Anemia
    Hemolytic Disease of Newborn
        Rh Incompatibility
        ABO Incompatibility
Drug-induced Hemolytic Anemia
    Adsorption of Immune Complexes to Red Cell Membrane
    Adsorption of Drug to Red Cell Membrane
    Induction of Autoantibody by Drugs
    Non-immunologic Adsorption of Immunoglobulin to Red Cell Membrane

maximum binding affinity at 4°C. In addition, AIHA's could be viewed according to their association with other disorders. Approximately 50 to 80 per cent of the cases of AIHA are associated with some underlying disorder and the remainder are idiopathic (Pirofsky, 1975; Dacie, 1969).

ETIOLOGY AND PATHOPHYSIOLOGY. The cause of the production of autoantibody in patients with AIHA is not yet known. However, several mechanisms have been suggested. Autoimmune antibodies are sometimes produced following an infection. This is typically seen with the elaboration of anti-I in patients with *Mycoplasma pneumoniae* infections. It has been hypothesized that the autoantibody may be a response to sensitization from a breakdown component of the *Mycoplasma pneumoniae* organism (Weens, 1974). In infectious mononucleosis, anti-i antibody is present in the serum of patients and it occasionally results in AIHA. Since the i-antigen is normally on the lymphocyte membrane, perhaps in this disorder the production of anti-i is part of an effort to remove host-infected B cells.

The development of AIHA in patients with lymphoproliferative disorders or with autoimmune disorders may relate to some abnormality with B cells, T cells, macrophages, or the interaction among these cells. Perhaps loss of T cell suppressor function could result in unrestrained production of red cell antibody by B cells (Weens, 1974).

In AIHA associated with warm type antibody, there is IgG coating of erythrocytes with or without complement fixation. Clearance of red cells occurs mostly in the spleen. In the absence of complement fixation, it appears that the Fc portion of the red cell–bound IgG immunoglobulin interacts with the Fc receptor present on the membrane of splenic macrophages located along the cords of Bilroth. Thus sensitized erythrocytes are either retained, phagocytosed, or fragmented by splenic macrophages during their passage through the spleen (Frank, 1977).

In AIHA associated with the production of cold type autoantibody, the erythrocytes are usually coated with IgM immunoglobulin. Under these circumstances, the fixation of complement frequently occurs. In paroxysmal cold hemoglobinuria, the offending antibody is an IgG immunoglobulin which fixes complement. If the entire complement sequence is activated, there may be intravascular hemolysis. This phenomenon may occur in cases of cold hemagglutinin disease as well as paroxysmal cold hemoglobinuria. If complement activation fails to proceed to completion but is halted at an intermediate stage, intravascular lysis of the erythrocytes may not occur. However, extravascular hemolysis can still continue. In this situation, sensitized cells with

Table 29-7. AUTOIMMUNE HEMOLYTIC ANEMIA

ASSOCIATED WITH WARM ANTIBODIES		ASSOCIATED WITH COLD ANTIBODIES	
Associated Disorder	Percentage of Patients	Associated Disorder	Percentage of Patients
Idiopathic	41	Idiopathic cold hemagglutinin disease	13
Lymphomas	13	*Mycoplasma pneumoniae*	8
Systemic lupus erythematosus	5	Infectious mononucleosis	1
Other autoimmune disorders	7	Lymphomas	2
Miscellaneous	5	Paroxysmal cold hemoglobinuria	5
Total	71		29

Modified from Dacie, J. V., and Worlledge, S. M.: Autoimmune-hemolytic anemias. Prog. Hematol., *6*:82, 1969.

C3b on the membrane are bound in the liver by the interaction of C3b and its receptors on Kupffer cells (Frank, 1977). Erythrocytes may be phagocytosed entirely or portions of the cells may be removed, resulting in fragmentation and spherocyte formation.

AIHA Associated with Warm Antibody. The warm antibody type of AIHA is slightly more frequent in females than males and most likely to occur in individuals 40 years or older. The clinical signs and symptoms frequently relate to the nature of an underlying disorder. However, in individuals with idiopathic AIHA, the patient may have noted the presence of a mild upper respiratory tract infection just prior to the onset of hemolysis. As the disorder progresses, there may be weakness, dizziness, and fever. Jaundice can be a presenting complaint.

Laboratory findings include the presence of a moderate to severe anemia. The neutrophil count may be increased. In a small proportion of cases thrombocytopenia can exist. The peripheral film frequently shows spherocytosis, red cell fragmentation, polychromasia, and a few normoblasts (see Fig. 27-16). Reticulocyte percentage is high in approximately 50 per cent of patients. The lack of reticulocytosis should not keep one from making a diagnosis of autoimmune hemolytic anemia (Pirofsky, 1976). The bone marrow exhibits normoblastic erythroid hyperplasia, sometimes with mild megaloblastic changes.

There is usually a decrease in serum haptoglobins and an increase in unconjugated bilirubin. The osmotic fragility and autohemolysis test can be either normal or abnormal.

The direct and indirect antiglobulin tests indicate the presence of erythrocyte antibodies. The specificity of the autoantibody is usually directed against antigens of the Rh system. However, activity against U, LW, Kell, jk^a, and Fy^a antigens may also occur. The warm antibody is most likely an IgG immunoglobulin with subclass IgG1; IgG2 and IgG3 are considerably less frequent, the IgG4 rare (Dacie, 1975). Occasionally the antibody may be an IgA immunoglobulin and rarely an IgM immunoglobulin. Complement may be detected on the erythrocyte membrane in slightly over half of the cases.

In some cases sensitized red cells contain less immunoglobulin than can be detected using commercially prepared antiglobulins, which are normally sensitive to 250 to 500

molecules of IgG/red cell (Gilliland, 1976). Under these circumstances the autoantibody can at times be detected with an antiglobulin consumption test (Rosse, 1974).

The clinical course of AIHA associated with warm antibody is characterized by periods of remissions and relapse. In secondary AIHA, the course and prognosis is related to the nature of the underlying disorder. In idiopathic AIHA, the complications of the hemolytic disorder may be severe and lead to the demise of the patient. The overall prognosis of this disorder is not good; the mortality rate is approximately 40 per cent (Pirofsky, 1975).

AIHA Associated with Cold Antibody. AIHA associated with cold antibody can be mediated by an IgM immunoglobulin and less frequently by an IgG immunoglobulin. The IgM autoantibody is associated with a syndrome known as cold hemagglutinin disease whereas the IgG autoantibody is seen with paroxysmal cold hemoglobinuria (Brown, 1977).

Cold Hemagglutinin Disease. Cold hemagglutinin disease occurs in individuals usually over the age of 50 years and in females more often than in males. In some cases cold hemagglutinin disease is associated with a lymphoreticular malignancy or autoimmune disorder. Other cases appear as a complication of infection (especially *Mycoplasma pneumoniae*). Cases unassociated with an underlying disorder are listed as idiopathic.

Symptoms and signs vary widely. Some individuals may complain of acrocyanosis or Raynaud's phenomenon. Others will have episodes of hemolysis following exposure to cold (Swisher, 1977).

The laboratory findings usually indicate an anemia. Spherocytes and polychromatophilic erythrocytes are present to a variable degree in the blood film. There may be marked red cell agglutination which should be differentiated from rouleaux formation (see Figs. 27-28 and 27-29). A mild leukocytosis can exist.

The cold antibody is usually an IgM immunoglobulin with anti-I specificity. Rarely do other specificities exist. In the chronic idiopathic form of cold hemagglutinin disease, the antibody tends to be monoclonal IgM, k. The autoantibody is also capable of fixing complement. When the titer of cold antibody is very high, the thermal range of antibody activity may extend up to 37°C. The direct antiglobulin test is positive only if the reagents contain anti-complement activity. Thus one usually observes a positive antiglobulin reaction with the broad spectrum and non-gamma reagents but no agglutination with only the gamma reagent.

Paroxysmal Cold Hemoglobinuria. Paroxysmal cold hemoglobinuria is a very rare disorder that can occur in an individual of any age. Females are as frequently involved as males. Patients present with symptoms of acute hemolysis following exposure to the cold. There are chills, fever, pain in the back and legs, and hemoglobinuria. The acute form may follow an acute viral illness, but the chronic form is associated with congenital syphilis.

The laboratory features consist of anemia, elevated reticulocyte count, increased concentration of conjugated bilirubin, and the presence of hemoglobin in the urine.

Serum from afflicted patients contains a cold hemolysin with biphasic activity. This antibody, first described by Donath and Landsteiner (1904), is an IgG immunoglobulin which fixes the first components of complement (C1-C4) in the cold (4°C.). As the temperature rises to 25 to 37°C., the remainder of the complement proteins are activated and erythrocyte lysis results. The specificity of the antibody is directed against the P antigen. In general, the prognosis of patients with paroxysmal cold hemaglobinuria is good.

Isoimmune Hemolytic Anemia. Isoimmune hemolytic anemia usually occurs in newborns following the transplacental passage of maternal anti-fetal red cell antibody. Isoimmune hemolytic disease of the newborn most frequently results from incompatibility in Rh and ABO erythrocyte antigens between mother and fetus. In rare cases some other red cell antigen may be responsible for this disorder. (See Chapter 43.)

In isoimmune hemolytic disease of the newborn due to Rh incompatibility, prior sensitization is necessary to initiate the disease process. This sensitization usually occurs during pregnancy when Rh(D) fetal red cells cross the placenta and enter the circulation of a mother with Rh negative cells. Maternal sensitization can also occur by a previous incompatible transfusion. Under either of these circumstances, maternal IgG antibodies are produced against the fetal cells. If a subsequent pregnancy occurs in a sensitized mother, fetal erythrocytes regain access to the maternal circulation. They restimulate an antibody response resulting in transfer of anti-Rh(D) antibody across the placenta and reduced red cell survival.

In the ABO system anti-A or anti-B antibodies of the IgG class may arise spontaneously in the mother, and thus their presence does not require prior transfusion or pregnancy. As a result, first-born children may suffer from isoimmune hemolytic disease when ABO incompatibility exists.

The clinical features of isoimmune hemolytic disease of the newborn due to Rh incompatibility vary greatly among affected infants. Some newborns experience only mild jaundice. Other infants may initially appear markedly pale and then develop jaundice. They can have prominent hepatosplenomegaly. The disease may be complicated by a bleeding diathesis, marked acid-base abnormalities, and kernicterus. In very severe cases, patients can present with hydrops fetalis (Zipursky, 1974).

Early examination of the blood usually reveals an increase of nucleated erythrocytes, which may include forms as immature as pronormoblasts. Although this finding gave the disease its name, *erythroblastosis fetalis,* erythroblastosis is not always present, especially if the examination is not done immediately after birth.

Up to 2.0×10^9 nucleated red cells per liter in term infants and up to $5.0 \times 10^9/l$ in premature infants are commonly seen in this disorder. Normally, nucleated red cells average $0.5 \times 10^9/l$ in term infants and 1.0 to $1.5 \times 10^9/l$ in premature infants. Blood from the umbilical vein for early examination is more reliable than peripheral (capillary) blood because the erythrocyte count and the hemoglobin may be significantly altered between birth and ligation of the cord.

Generally there are a macrocytic anemia of varying severity and an increase in reticulocytes. Occasionally anemia may appear suddenly on the second or third day. The leukocyte count is frequently elevated, with immature leukocytes. There is pronounced normoblastic hyperplasia of the marrow.

In severely affected infants, there may be thrombocytopenia, depression of the prothrombin complex procoagulants, or diffuse intravascular coagulation.

A direct antiglobulin test on fetal erythrocytes indicates the presence of an IgG antibody. When the maternal serum and an eluate from the fetal erythrocytes are incubated separately with a panel of O cells, one can usually demonstrate the presence of antibody with Rh(D) specificity. In Rh negative pregnant women known to be sensitized to Rh(D), the titer of antiRh(D) antibody is measured periodically during pregnancy to serve as a guide for performing amniocentesis (see p. 1495).

Isoimmune hemolytic disease of the newborn associated with ABO incompatibility is less severe than that observed with Rh incompatibility. Occasionally the diagnosis is suggested by the presence of unexplained hyperbilirubinemia in a group A or B newborn infant from a group O mother.

Laboratory findings usually show a mild anemia and modest reticulocytosis. In contrast to Rh isoimmune disease, spherocytosis in ABO isoimmune disease may be prominent. However, there may be no anemia. The fetal cells are usually weakly positive with the antiglobulin reagents. Eluates from the newborn's cells and serum from the newborn should demonstrate the presence of anti-A or anti-B antibody. In addition, the maternal serum should contain high titers of anti-A or anti-B antibodies of the IgG subclass.

Drug-Induced Immune Hemolytic Anemia. Immune hemolytic anemia may occur following the administration of drugs. Four mechanisms appear to mediate the immune hemolysis (Petz, 1975).

ADSORPTION OF IMMUNE COMPLEXES TO THE RED CELL MEMBRANE. Numerous drugs are known to provoke an antibody response with subsequent adsorption of immune complexes to the erythrocyte membrane (Table 29–8). The drug-induced antibody is usually of the IgM class and tends to fix complement, resulting in lysis of cells.

Table 29–8. DRUGS ACCEPTED AS CAUSING IMMUNE HEMOLYTIC ANEMIA BY THE ADSORPTION OF IMMUNE COMPLEXES TO RED CELLS

Stibophen
Quinidine
Para-aminosalicylic acid
Quinine
Phenacetin
Chlorinated hydrocarbon-containing insecticides
Antihistamines
Sulfonamides
Isonicotinic acid hydrazine
Chlorpromazine
Aminopyrine
Dipyrone
Melphalan
Mefanamic acid
Sulfonylureas
Insulin
Rifampicin

Modified from Petz, L. D., and Garratty, G.: Drug-induced haemolytic anemia. Clin. Haematol., *4*:181, 1975.

Patients present with acute intravascular hemolysis, hemoglobinemia, and hemoglobinuria. The direct antiglobulin reaction is positive if the reagents contain anti-complement activity. The reaction with the gamma reagent is usually negative because it contains little anti-IgM or complement specificity.

The diagnosis can be determined by incubating the patient's serum with the offending drug in the presence of target erythrocytes, and observing agglutination, lysis, or sensitization of the erythrocytes to antiglobulin era.

ADSORPTION OF DRUG TO RED CELL MEMBRANE. Penicillin and cephalosporin combine with protein normally present on the erythrocyte membrane. These drugs, once bound to the red cell membrane, form haptenic groups and provoke an immune response. Both IgM and IgG antibodies are made, but only the IgG antibodies are associated with the immune hemolysis. Complement is not involved. The erythrocytes, coated with IgG antibody, are presumably removed via the Fc receptors on macrophages in the spleen.

The direct antiglobulin test is strongly positive. Antibody eluted from patient's erythrocytes will react only with red cells previously treated with penicillin or cephalosporins.

INDUCTION OF AUTOANTIBODY BY DRUGS. In approximately 15 per cent of patients using the antihypertensive drug alpha-methyldopa, a positive direct antiglobulin reaction is present. The antibody is of the IgG class and in some studies appears to have Rh specificity (Croft, 1968). However, other studies indicate that there may be non-specific erythrocyte adsorption of γ-globulin following red cell exposure to alpha-methyldopa (Gottlieb, 1974).

The development of the positive antiglobulin reaction is dose-dependent. Thirty-six per cent of patients have a positive antiglobulin reaction when consuming 2 g or more of alpha-methyldopa per day, and 11 per cent have a positive reaction when taking only 1 g daily. An immune hemolytic anemia occurs in less than 1 per cent of patients (Petz, 1975).

NON-IMMUNOLOGIC ADSORPTION OF IMMUNOGLOBULIN TO RED CELL MEMBRANE. Cephalosporins and perhaps alpha-methyldopa appear to alter the erythrocyte membrane, resulting in the non-specific adsorption of plasma proteins to its surface. As a result, IgG and IgM immunoglobulin may be loosely bound to red cell membrane. This phenomenon can then cause a positive direct antiglobulin reaction (Petz, 1975).

POLYCYTHEMIA

Polycythemia is an increased concentration of erythrocytes in the blood that is above the normal for age and sex. Usually, but not always, the hematocrit and hemoglobin are also elevated.

Absolute polycythemia refers to an increase in the total red cell mass in the body; in *relative polycythemia*, the total red cell mass is normal, but the hematocrit is elevated because the plasma volume is decreased. Polycythemia may be classified as in Table 29-9.

Relative polycythemia

Relative polycythemia refers to an increase in hematocrit or red cell count due to decreased plasma volume; total red cell mass is not increased. This occurs in acute dehydration, e.g., in severe diarrhea or burns.

In cases of burns there is marked hemoconcentration as the fluid portion of the blood leaks into the tissues. The concentration of hemoglobin has been found to be reduced after hemorrhage and increased during shock. In shock there is reduction in the plasma volume, which results in hemoconcentration. Hemoconcentration may occur several hours before blood pressure sinks to critical levels. Studies of blood concentration made early may show a rising curve that acts as a warning signal of the more serious circulatory failure

that will follow unless active treatment is immediately carried out.

In spurious polycythemia (Gaisböck's syndrome), the red cell mass is often high normal and the plasma volume is low normal; these patients have been regarded as an extreme of the normal physiologic state. Almost all are men, have a high incidence of tobacco smoking, and tend to be obese and to have hypertension. Weinreb (1975) compared a group of these patients with a second group, similar except that the elevated hematocrit was due primarily to decreased plasma volume. The latter group had a greater tendency to hypertension and hypercholesterolemia, and had a poorer survival. Smoking as a cause of polycythemia has been recently stressed (Smith, 1978); it is likely that smoking is an important factor in some cases of "spurious polycythemia."

Absolute polycythemia

Secondary to Hypoxia

ARTERIAL OXYGEN UNSATURATION. Lack of oxygen reaching the blood for one reason or another results in arterial unsaturation, impaired oxygen delivery to the tissues, increased production of erythropoietin, erythroid hyperplasia in the marrow, and resultant erythrocytosis (Balcerzak, 1975). The red cell mass is increased. As a response to the hypoxia, the red cell 2,3-DPG and the P_{50} are increased. In contrast to polycythemia vera, there is usually no leukocytosis or thrombocytosis, and the neutrophil alkaline phosphatase is normal. Arterial oxygen unsaturation may be the cause of polycythemia in persons living at high altitudes; in patients with chronic pulmonary disease and a block in diffusion of oxygen into the blood; in cyanotic heart disease in which there is right to left shunt; in cigarette smokers (Smith, 1978); and in methemoglobinemia whether due to enzyme deficiency (p. 869), chronic drug effect, or a structurally abnormal hemoglobin (Hb M) (p. 996).

HIGH OXYGEN AFFINITY HEMOGLOBINOPATHY. Another cause of tissue hypoxia is the presence of a structurally abnormal hemoglobin which has a high affinity for oxygen (p. 996; Adamson, 1975). As in other functional hemoglobinopathies, the disorder occurs in the heterozygote. The abnormal hemoglobin releases less oxygen to the tissues than does normal hemoglobin at the same Po_2; the oxygen dissociation curve is shifted to the left and

---

Table 29-9. CLASSIFICATION OF POLYCYTHEMIA

Relative Polycythemia
1. Diminished plasma volume: dehydration; shock
2. Spurious polycythemia (stress polycythemia; Gaisböck's syndrome)

Absolute Polycythemia
1. Secondary polycythemia (increased erythropoietin)
   a. Hypoxia
      1. Arterial oxygen unsaturation: high altitude; pulmonary disease; cyanotic heart disease; smoker's polycythemia; methemoglobinemia; Hb M
      2. High oxygen affinity hemoglobinopathy
   b. Inappropriate erythropoietin production
      1. Neoplasms: renal carcinoma; cerebellar hemangioma; hepatoma; uterine fibroids; adrenal cortical neoplasms
      2. Renal pathology: cysts; hydronephrosis; transplantation
2. Recessive familial polycythemia
3. Polycythemia vera

Modified from Berlin, N. I.: Diagnosis and classification of the polycythemias. Semin. Hematol., *12*:339, 1975.

the P_{50} is decreased. The red cell 2,3-DPG is not increased. As in arterial oxygen unsaturation, there are increased erythropoietin production and erythrocytosis. It must be emphasized that routine hemoglobin electrophoresis usually does not detect these hemoglobin variants because the amino acid substitution is at one of the $\alpha\beta$ contact sites or near the heme pocket. A low P_{50} therefore is presumptive evidence for a hemoglobinopathy. The heat lability test for unstable hemoglobin should be done, since some hemoglobins with high affinity and polycythemia are unstable.

Secondary to Inappropriate Erythropoietin Production

Neoplasms, either benign or malignant, have been associated with polycythemia (Balcerzak, 1975). Renal neoplasms account for the majority. In almost all cases, erythrocytosis has disappeared after resection of the tumor. The mechanism is not clear. Some of these neoplasms have been shown to contain, and presumably produce, erythropoietin (e.g., cerebellar hemangioma, hypernephroma, some hepatomas). In other neoplasms or growths (e.g., renal cysts, hydronephrosis, ovarian carcinoma, some hepatomas) it appears that the mass impinging on the kidney induces increased renal production of ESF due to increased pressure or local hypoxia within the kidney. Renal ischemia (and hypoxia) due to arterial occlusion also is the probable mechanism for erythrocytosis in patients with renal transplants; narrowing of small arteries occurs during the rejection reaction. (See Balcerzak, 1975.)

Recessive Familial Polycythemia

In certain families erythrocytosis occurs in siblings but not in parents, and analysis has supported an autosomal recessive inheritance (Adamson, 1975). These individuals have no abnormalities in hemoglobin function nor do they have detectable renovascular or cardiopulmonary defects. Studies have shown increased erythropoietin production unrelated to hemoglobin concentration, and have suggested that the defect was in the regulation of erythropoietin production. Individuals with this disorder are involved earlier in life, have higher Hb and Hct levels, and more often have splenomegaly than do persons with autosomal dominant polycythemia (high-oxygen affinity hemoglobinopathy) (Adamson, 1975).

Benign Familial Polycythemia

Also known as primary erythrocytosis of childhood, benign familial erythrocytosis is a rare disorder. Originally this was described as a pure erythrocytosis without splenomegaly, and with normal leukocyte and platelet counts, occurring in one or more siblings and sometimes a parent (Abildgard, 1963). It now seems clear that at least some of the patients in families with autosomal dominant hereditary patterns in this group have high oxygen affinity hemoglobinopathies, and at least some with autosomal recessive hereditary patterns have autonomous ESF production (see above). What is not clear at the present time is whether different pathophysiologic mechanisms may be operative in other patients with "benign familial erythrocytosis," since most of the patients reported have not been studied with currently available techniques.

Polycythemia Vera (PV)

Polycythemia vera is a panmyelosis, that is, a condition in which excessive proliferation occurs in megakaryocytes and granulocytes as well as in erythrocytes. It is manifested by erythrocytosis, leukocytosis, and thrombocytosis of varying degree. The etiology is unknown. PV is discussed with the myeloproliferative disorders (p. 1072).

LABORATORY STUDIES

ERYTHROCYTE SURVIVAL STUDIES

Hemolytic anemias are caused by excessive destruction of red cells manifested by a shortening of the red cell survival. A shortened red cell survival constitutes the definition of hemolysis. If the hemolytic process is severe, other laboratory measurements will suffice to demonstrate that the hemolysis is in fact present. If the hemolytic process is mild or obscure, it may be necessary to perform red cell survival studies.

Differential agglutination method of Ashby (1919)

Compatible blood possessing a blood group factor that the recipient does not possess is transferred to the recipient, e.g., group O cells to group A, B, or AB recipient; and group ON cells to group M or MN recipients. After the transfusion, sera with potent agglutinins for the red cells of the recipient are added to samples of the recipient's blood and the unagglutinated red cells are counted. Using this technique, the life span of normal erythrocytes is determined to be between 110 and 120 days. Although accurate results can be obtained by this method, it is rarely used.

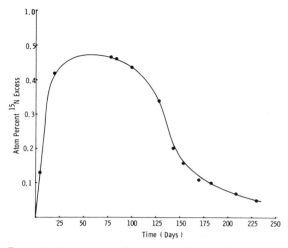

Figure 29–11. An example of cohort labeling of erythrocytes utilizing ^{15}N-glycine technique. Reutilization of the label accounts for the long persistence of activity. (From Bentley, S. A.: Red cell survival studies reinterpreted. Clin. Haematol., 6:601, 1977.)

The major disadvantages of this technique are that one is limited to suitably matched donors and recipients; the survival of the patient's cells in his own circulation cannot be studied; and it is necessary to transfuse large volumes of donor blood (Bentley, 1977).

Isotopic Tracer Techniques. The most convenient method of determining red cell survival is with the use of isotopic tracers. Radioisotopic techniques for measuring erythrocyte life span can be divided into two groups: cohort labeling and random labeling.

In *cohort labeling*, the isotope (^{15}N-glycine or ^{14}C-glycine) is incorporated into the cells during their formation. The labeled cells are followed as they appear in the circulation and subsequently as they are removed from the blood (Fig. 29–11). The curve shows a rising phase, a plateau, and finally a descending phase. The last phase represents the removal of erythrocytes from the circulation.

In *random labeling* techniques, a blood sample, consisting of erythrocytes of all ages, is labeled and reinjected into the subject. Beginning at time 0, therefore, senescent labeled cells begin to be removed. Random labeling is more practical, less time-consuming, and less expensive than the cohort labeling. Either radioactive chromium (^{51}Cr) or radioactive phosphorus (^{32}P) is used. Chromium-51 is used as sodium chromate ($Na_2{}^{51}CrO_4$) and ^{32}P is used as di-isopropyl-phosphofluoridate ($DF^{32}P$). Chromium-51 is the most widely used method (Dacie, 1975).

For specific details in measuring erythrocyte survival using ^{51}Cr and $DF^{32}P$ tracer techniques, consult the report by the International Committee for Standardization in Hematology (1971). The following is a general discussion.

RADIOACTIVE CHROMIUM METHOD. Chromium-51

binds to the β-chain of hemoglobin. Thus, chromated erythrocytes can be injected intravenously and the disappearance of the tracer can be measured by sampling and counting blood at intervals. The residual activity is an index of intravascular life span of the labeled erythrocytes. Since ^{51}Cr is a gamma ray emitter, external scanning for the presence of the tracer can detect sites of erythrocyte destruction.

Under sterile conditions, venous blood is withdrawn into a tube containing either acid-citrate-dextrose or citrate-phosphate-dextrose solution. In some methods the blood sample is centrifuged, the plasma is removed, and erythrocytes are washed prior to incubation with ^{51}Cr. If the leukocyte count is less than $25 \times 10^9/l$, ^{51}Cr can be added directly to the blood sample. Following a period of incubation, ascorbic acid is added to reduce the chromate to chromic ions, which cannot penetrate erythrocyte membrane and therefore cannot label the cell. A sample of labeled erythrocytes is injected intravenously, and, after 10 to 15 minutes a blood sample is collected from the opposite arm. This sample is used as the Day 0, or 100 per cent, sample. Samples of blood are withdrawn every 1 to 2 days for 10 to 14 days. With each sample, a part of the Day 0 specimen is counted. In this way, the activity of each sample is compared with a single standard and no decay corrections are required. The radioactivity is expressed as counts per minute (cpm) per gram hemoglobin or cpm/ml of whole blood or cpm/ml red cells. The ratio of this radioactivity on Day t/Day 0 $\times$ 100 is the per cent ^{51}Cr survival on Day t. This value is plotted against days on either linear or semilogarithmic graph paper, depending on accuracy of fit. The erythrocyte life span is usually expressed as the period during which one half of the radioactivity remains in the blood (the T $^{1}/_{2}$ ^{51}Cr; see Fig. 29–12).

Chromium normally elutes from the red cells at a rate of 1 per cent per day. Thus, the half-life of the ^{51}Cr-labeled erythrocytes in normal individuals is 25 to 32 days instead of 60 days.

$DF^{32}P$ METHOD. Approximately 90 per cent of $DF^{32}P$ binds intracellularly. The remainder binds to acetylcholinesterase confined to erythrocyte membrane (Bentley, 1977). The labeling of red cells with $DF^{32}P$ may be performed *in vivo* or *in vitro*. For labeling *in vivo*, intravenous or intramuscular injections of tracer are given. The *in vitro* labeling requires the removal of a large volume of blood and thus is less commonly performed. A blood sample is collected 60 minutes after injection of tracer, a second blood sample is collected at 24 hours, three samples are collected in the following five days, and then one sample is obtained each week until the termination of the study. Results are plotted on graph paper as above.

Since very little $DF^{32}P$ elutes from the erythrocytes, this technique affords more accuracy in judging life span of red cells. Cohen (1954) found in two normal individuals that red cell tracer activity was

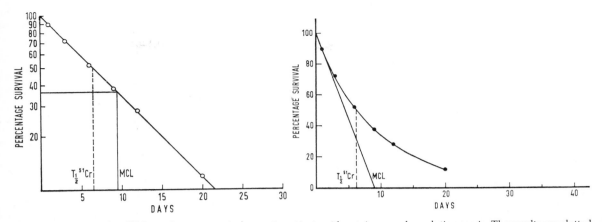

Figure 29-12. Results of ^{51}Cr erythrocyte survival curve in patients with autoimmune hemolytic anemia. The results are plotted on semilogarithmic graph paper. The mean cell life span (MCL) was 9 to 10 days and is recorded at a period when 37 per cent of cells are still circulating. The time of 50 per cent survival ($T_{1/2}$Cr) was 6 to 7 days. (From Dacie, J. V., and Lewis, S. M.: Practical Hematology, 5th ed. Edinburgh, Churchill Livingstone, 1975.)

a linear function of time and that erythrocyte life span could be calculated at approximately 120 days. These findings have been supported by other observers (Mayer, 1956). However, a high degree of accuracy is rarely needed in clinical studies. DF^{32}P, a beta emitter, does not permit external scanning, and thus this method is a less popular method of measuring red cell survival.

Interpretation. A steady state must exist for one to obtain accurate results. Blood loss, change in hematocrit, and recent blood transfusions can significantly complicate the interpretation of erythrocyte survival data.

In autoimmune hemolytic anemias the slope of erythrocyte survival produces a straight line when plotted on semi-logarithmic paper (Fig. 29–12).

However, in other hemolytic anemias, two cell populations may exist. In these situations the survival curve may be composed of an initial steep slope followed by flatter component (Fig. 29–13). This type of curve has been seen in hereditary enzyme-deficiency hemolytic anemias, sickle cell anemia, and paroxysmal nocturnal hemoglobinuria (Dacie, 1975).

ERYTHROCYTE AND PLASMA VOLUME

Principle. The erythrocyte and plasma volumes are measured by the use of radioactive isotopic tracers and the dilution principle. Many isotopic labels have been utilized, but the most commonly employed tracers are ^{51}Cr in the form of sodium chromate bound to erythrocytes for measurement of erythrocyte volume. Iodine-125 or iodine-131 is bound to albumin and can be used to measure plasma volume.

Method. For detailed description of measurement of red cell and plasma volume, see the report of the International Committee for Standardization in Hematology (1973).

Erythrocyte Volume. In brief, blood is collected from the patient and the erythrocytes are labeled with ^{51}Cr. The chromated erythrocytes are washed in saline. An aliquot of the ^{51}Cr erythrocytes diluted in saline is injected intravenously into the patient. After a period for equilibration, usually 10 to 20 minutes, a sample of blood is withdrawn from the opposite arm. In cases where the equilibration time is likely to be prolonged (as in splenomegaly, heart failure, or shock) another sample should be withdrawn 60 minutes after injection.

Radioactivity of each sample is recorded by a

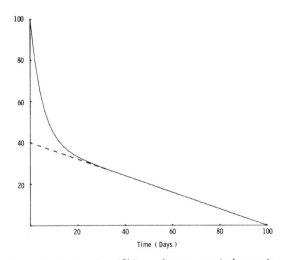

Figure 29-13. Results of ^{51}Cr erythrocyte survival curve in a patient with hemolytic anemia containing two cell populations. The per cent survival is on the ordinate. By extrapolating the flatter curve to time 0, it can be estimated that 40 per cent of the cells have a mean cell life span of 100 days. Sixty per cent of cells have a mean cell life span of five days. (From Bentley, S. A.: Red cell survival studies reinterpreted. Clin. Haematol., 6:601, 1977.)

scintillation counter. The erythrocyte volume (EV) is calculated using the formula:

$$EV \ (ml) = \frac{I(cpm)}{C(cpm/ml)}$$

where I = total injected radioactivity (counts per minute)

C = radioactivity in erythrocytes after mixing is complete (counts per minute per milliliter of erythrocytes).

Plasma Volume. Approximately 20 ml of blood is withdrawn from a patient. After centrifugation, the plasma is removed and radioiodine-labeled albumin is added. After mixing, the labeled plasma is injected intravenously into the patient. At 10, 20, and 30 minutes following the injection, 5 ml of blood is removed and the radioactivity is counted in a well-type scintillation counter. The radioactivity at zero time (P_o) is determined by plotting the three points on semilogarithmic graph paper and extrapolating to zero time. A standard is prepared by diluting an aliquot of the radioiodine-labeled albumin with saline containing a small amount of detergent.

The plasma volume (PV) is calculated using the formula

$$PV \ (ml) = \frac{S(cpm/ml) \times D \times V(ml)}{P_o \ (cpm/ml)}$$

where S = counting rate of standard (counts per minute/ml)

D = dilution of diluted standard solution

V = volume of radioiodine-labeled albumin solution injected

P_o = counting rate of plasma sample corrected to zero time (counts/minute/ml).

Interpretation. The normal red cell volume for men is 28.2 ± 4.0 ml/kg and for women it is 25.3 ± 3.0 ml/kg. The plasma volume for men is 34.2 ± 4.5 ml/kg and for women is 36.6 ± 4.3 ml/kg. In newborns and premature infants the red cell volume and plasma volume in ml/kg are higher than in adults.

Patients with polycythemia have red cell volumes exceeding 36 ml/kg for men and 32 ml/kg for women. Changes in erythrocyte volume and plasma volume in a variety of conditions are recorded in Table 29-10.

Table 29-10. CLINICAL EFFECT OF VARIABLE RELATIONSHIP BETWEEN RED-CELL VOLUME AND PLASMA VOLUME

RED-CELL VOLUME	PLASMA VOLUME	CAUSE	EFFECT
Normal	High	Pregnancy Cirrhosis Nephritis Congestive cardiac failure	Pseudo-anemia
Normal	Low	Stress Peripheral circulatory failure Dehydration Edema Prolonged bed rest	Pseudo-polycythemia
Low	Normal	Anemia	Accurate reflection of degree of anemia
Low	High	Anemia	Anemia less severe than indicated by blood count
Low	Low	Hemorrhage Severe anemia (when PCV below 0.2)	Anemia more severe than indicated by blood count
High	Normal to low	Polycythemia	Accurate reflection of polycythemia or polycythemia less severe than apparent
High	High	Polycythemia (when PCV > 0.5)	Polycythemia more severe than apparent
Normal or even high	High	Marked splenomegaly	Pseudo-anemia

From Dacie, J. V., and Lewis, S. M.: Practical Haematology, 5th ed. Edinburgh, Churchill Livingstone, 1975.

Tests for the Presence of Hemolysis

Plasma hemoglobin

Hemoglobin circulating in the plasma in amounts in excess of 5 mg/dl (0.05 g/l) is evidence for intravascular hemolysis *if* the lysis did not occur during or after venipuncture. Careful technique is therefore essential. In the small amounts to be measured, the method of Crosby (1956) is usually used. The principle is that heme catalyzes the oxidation of benzidine (or orthotolidine) by hydrogen peroxide. The color developed in the plasma-benzidine-H_2O_2 mixture is compared with that developed in an appropriately dilute standard Hb solution in a spectrophotometer or colorimeter at 515 nm.

The pathophysiology of intravascular hemolysis has been discussed (p. 985). At plasma hemoglobin levels in excess of 50 mg/dl, the plasma is red and intravascular hemolysis is present. Paroxysmal nocturnal hemoglobinuria, paroxysmal cold hemoglobinuria, traumatic hemolytic anemia, falciparum malaria, cold hemagglutinins, and septicemia due to a hemolytic organism are among the possible causes. Usually in extravascular hemolysis, the level of plasma Hb is only slightly to moderately increased. Violent exercise may also result in moderate hemoglobinemia (see Dacie, 1975).

Methemalbumin

The Schumm test is a qualitative test for methemalbumin. Nine volumes of plasma or serum are overlaid with a layer of ether in a large test tube. One volume of saturated solution of ammonium sulfide is added with a pipette. After thorough mixing, the contents is poured into a hand spectroscope. An absorption band at 558 nm indicates a positive test for methemalbumin. An ammonium hemochromogen formed from methemalbumin gives a more intense color at this wavelength than methemalbumin itself. (See Figure 15-10, p. 511.)

Methemalbumin can also be detected by its mobility in the electrophoretic determination of haptoglobin.

In intravascular hemolysis, when haptoglobin is depleted, hemoglobin in plasma is oxidized. The hemin (oxidized heme) groups, in excess of those that form a complex with hemopexin for removal, are bound to plasma albumin. The presence of methemalbumin, therefore, indicates that intravascular hemolysis has been occurring (see p. 985).

Serum haptoglobin

A semiquantitative method is based on simple serum electrophoresis. The haptoglobin-hemoglobin complex migrates faster than free hemoglobin and slower than methemalbumin. Known amounts of hemoglobin are added to the patient's (and a control's) serum. If hemoglobin is added in an amount less than the binding capacity of the haptoglobin present, only one band of hemoglobin will be seen on the unstained electrophoretic strip; this is the haptoglobin-hemoglobin complex which migrates as an α_2-globulin. If more hemoglobin is added than can be bound by haptoglobin, a second band of hemoglobin is seen, that of free hemoglobin which migrates with the β-globulins. Thus, if increasing amounts of hemoglobin are added to several samples of the patient's serum, the quantity of haptoglobin can be estimated. Absence of hemoglobin in the α_2-globulin region indicates absent haptoglobin. Hemoglobin migrating in the albumin band is methemalbumin; this is present in the absence of hemoglobin added *in vitro*. The presence of methemalbumin indicates intravascular hemolysis; usually in this case the haptoglobin band is missing. Details of the method may be found in Brus (1959) or Dacie (1975).

Another type of haptoglobin measurement is made by combining the available haptoglobin in plasma with methemoglobin and measuring the peroxidase activity, which is much greater than that of free methemoglobin (Owen, 1960). The measurement is spectrophotometric and is more convenient than the electrophoretic method when large numbers of samples must be investigated.

Decreased or absent haptoglobin, as mentioned above, indicates hemolysis, either intravascular or extravascular, but also may occur in infectious mononucleosis, severe liver disease, and congenital ahaptoglobinemia.

Increased serum haptoglobin may occur in any inflammatory disease or during steroid therapy; in such situations the presence of hemolysis cannot be ruled out if the haptoglobin concentration is normal.

Erythrocyte Osmotic Fragility Test

The osmotic fragility test provides an indication of the change of shape (surface/volume ratio) of the red cell from the normal biconcave disc. Its chief value is in establishing a diagnosis of hereditary spherocytosis.

Principle

Red cells suspended in hypotonic solution of sodium chloride take up water, swell, become spheroidal and, after reaching the critical volume, eventually burst. The cell that is thicker than normal (spheroidal as in hereditary spherocytosis) has a decreased surface/volume ratio, and its capacity to expand is limited. Consequently, it bursts upon intake of small amounts of water in relatively high concentrations of the salt. Its osmotic fragility is increased and its osmotic resistance is decreased. On the other hand, the thin or flat cell in hypochromic anemia can take up considerable amounts of water and reaches the critical volume for lysis at lower concentrations of sodium chloride than does the normal red cell. Its osmotic fragility is decreased; its resistance is increased.

The osmotic fragility test measures how nearly

spherical red cells are, but it does not measure the fragility of the red cells. Increased osmotic fragility or decreased resistance indicates spherocytosis.

Increased fragility is found in hereditary spherocytosis and in those idiopathic and symptomatic acquired hemolytic anemias in which a tendency to spherocytosis is present. In contrast, diminished osmotic fragility or increased resistance means excessive flatness of red cells; it is seen in the presence of obstructive jaundice, in iron deficiency anemias, in thalassemia, in sickle cell anemia, after splenectomy, and in a variety of anemias in which target cells are found. In thalassemia a portion of red cells may remain unlysed in 0.03 per cent saline and even in distilled water. In tests for osmotic fragility, identical amounts of blood are added to decreasing concentrations of sodium chloride solution. After a period of incubation, the highest concentration of sodium chloride with minimum hemolysis determines beginning hemolysis; the highest concentration in which hemolysis is complete expresses the complete hemolysis.

Osmotic fragility of red cells is increased if hemolysis occurs in concentrations greater than 0.5 per cent sodium chloride. On the other hand, osmotic fragility is decreased if hemolysis is incomplete in 0.3 per cent sodium chloride.

Two tests of osmotic fragility of varying degrees of simplicity will be described.

Screening test

REAGENTS

1. Stock solution of sodium chloride. A 1 per cent solution of sodium chloride is prepared by dissolving 1.0 g of C.P. sodium chloride in 100 ml of distilled water. The salt must be first dried in a desiccator.

2. Dilute solutions. The 0.85 per cent solution is prepared by placing 8.5 ml of the stock solution in a test tube and adding 1.5 ml of distilled water. Similarly, the 0.5 per cent solution is prepared by mixing 5.0 ml amounts of the stock solution and of distilled water.

PROCEDURE.   One milliliter of each of the two solutions is placed in one of two tubes. One-tenth milliliter of venous blood is added. To a similar set of two tubes, blood of a normal person is added and serves as a control. The control blood must be obtained approximately at the same time as the patient's. The tubes are shaken gently, and if the tube with the 0.5 per cent sodium chloride solution shows hemolysis and the one with 0.85 per cent is not hemolyzed, the osmotic fragility of the red cells is probably increased and a quantitative test is indicated.

Quantitative method—unincubated

EQUIPMENT

1. Test tube rack containing two rows of 13 matched, chemically clean, and dry colorimeter tubes.

2. Ten-milliliter serologic pipettes.

3. Pipettes calibrated to contain or deliver 0.05 ml.

Sahli pipettes delivering 20 μl are recommended for transfer of blood.

REAGENTS

1. Stock solution of 10 per cent NaCl (pH 7.4).

NaCl	180.00 g
Na$_2$HPO$_4$	27.31 g
NaH$_2$PO$_4 \cdot$ 2H$_2$O	4.86 g

Dissolve in distilled H$_2$O and dilute to 2 liters. Keeps well at room temperature in a tightly stoppered bottle.

2. Starting with a 1 per cent solution prepared from the 10 per cent solution, 50 ml of the following solutions are made: 0.85, 0.75, 0.65, 0.60, 0.55, 0.50, 0.45, 0.40, 0.35, 0.30, 0.20, 0.10, and 0.00 per cent NaCl.

The solutions can be prepared in 50 ml volumetric flasks as follows: To each flask the following volumes of the 1 per cent solution are added: 42.5, 37.5, 32.5, 30.0, 27.5, 25.0, 22.5, 20.0, 17.5, 15.0, 10.0, and 5.0 ml. The solutions are made up to volume (50 ml) with distilled water. A 1.2 per cent solution of sodium chloride is prepared by diluting 6 ml of the 10 per cent solution to 50 ml. The solutions keep well at 4°C. for weeks. They should be discarded if molds develop.

3. Freshly obtained heparinized or defibrinated blood is preferable to oxalated or citrated blood. To defibrinate, 10 to 15 ml of aseptically drawn venous blood is placed in a sterile flask containing one glass bead (3 to 4 mm in diameter) for each milliliter of blood. The flask should be rotated gently until the beads become coated with fibrin. The control blood should be obtained at approximately the same time.

PROCEDURE.   Five milliliters of each of the dilutions of sodium chloride are added to the 13 test tubes of each row. The second row of tubes is set up as a control. Five one-hundredths ml of the patient's blood is added to each tube of the first row, and the same amount of the normal control blood is added to the second row. After each transfer of blood, the pipettes should be rinsed thoroughly with saline and blown out vigorously. The tubes are immediately mixed well. They are allowed to stand at room temperature for 20 minutes, remixed, and centrifuged at 2000 rpm for 5 minutes. In a photoelectric colorimeter provided with a 540 nm filter, the degree of hemolysis in the supernatant (diluted 1 to 2 or 1 to 5) is measured by comparing with 100 per cent hemolysis in the tube with no saline and using the supernatant of the 0.85 per cent sodium chloride as a blank. The dilutions are made so that the optical density readings fall between 0.2 and 0.8. The per cent hemolysis in each of the tubes is calculated by dividing the hemoglobin value by the value in the tube containing no saline. A good colorimeter permits recognition of as little as 1 per cent hemolysis.

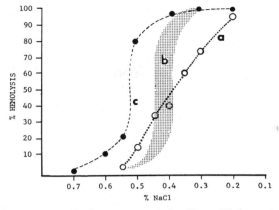

Figure 29–14. Erythrocyte osmotic fragility. *a*, Thalassemia, showing a small fraction of cells with increased fragility (lower left), and a larger fraction of cells with decreased fragility (upper right). *b*, Normal curves fall in shaded area. *c*, Hereditary spherocytosis, showing increased osmotic fragility.

The percentage of hemolysis in each tube is plotted against the corresponding concentration of sodium chloride (Fig. 29-14).

NORMAL REFERENCE VALUES

Values of osmotic fragility in normal blood:

Per Cent NaCl	Per Cent Hemolysis
0.30	97–100
0.40	50–90
0.45	5–45
0.50	0–5
0.55	0

Each laboratory should determine its own normal values.

Results may also be expressed as the median corpuscular fragility (MCF), which is the concentration of NaCl at which 50 per cent of the cells have lysed. Before incubation, the normal range for the MCF is 0.40 to 0.445 per cent NaCl.

INTERPRETATION. Although osmotic fragility is essentially a measure of spherocytosis, it provides a more objective measurement than inspection of a blood film. A difference of more than one tube between the patient and the control is significant.

SOURCES OF ERROR

1. Chemical purity of sodium chloride is essential. Even minute impurities may act as hemolytic agents.

2. Accuracy of the sodium chloride solution.

3. The relative volumes of blood and saline. A 1 to 100 dilution is recommended, because the degree of hemolysis can be read directly in most colorimeters without further dilution, and the minimal amount of plasma does not affect the tonicity of the solution. Because of differences between arterial and venous blood, the latter should be mixed until bright red.

4. A change of pH by 0.1 equals the change of tonicity by 0.01 per cent; a lowering of pH increases fragility.

5. A temperature rise increases fragility; a rise of 5°C. is equivalent to a change of tonicity of about 0.01 per cent. Room temperature is generally sufficiently constant.

Quantitative method after incubation

PROCEDURE. Duplicate 2-ml volumes of sterile, defibrinated blood from both patient and control in stoppered test tubes are incubated at 37°C. for 24 hours. The second test tube is included to have a spare in case of contamination. The test is set up similarly to the way described for the quantitative fragility test, but with the addition of a tube containing a 1.2 per cent solution of sodium chloride to serve as a blank in case of increased hemolysis.

As above, the per cent hemolysis is plotted against sodium chloride concentration on graph paper for both patient and control.

INTERPRETATION. The normal reference values for the MCF after incubation are 0.465 to 0.590 per cent NaCl. Incubation at 37°C. for 24 hours increases the fragility of normal erythrocytes (Fig. 29-15 [1A]). The increase is even more marked for red cells of hereditary spherocytosis and of congenital hemolytic anemia due to pyruvate kinase deficiency; hemolysis may begin between 0.70 and 0.65 per cent sodium chloride and may be complete at about 0.40 per cent (Fig. 29-15 [2A]). The test permits recognition of low-grade hereditary spherocytosis in which the unincubated osmotic fragility may be normal.

SOURCES OF ERROR. In addition to those sources mentioned for the unincubated test, bacterial contamination may occur and increase the degree of hemolysis.

INDICATIONS. Only when hereditary spherocytosis is suspected, e.g., unexplained hemolytic anemia

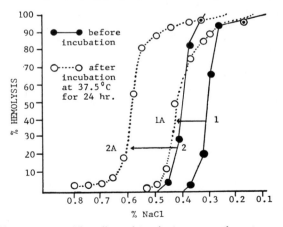

Figure 29–15. The effect of incubation on erythrocyte osmotic fragility. The change in the osmotic fragility curve from "before incubation" to "after incubation" is illustrated for normal blood (1 → 1A), and blood from a patient with hereditary spherocytosis (2 → 2A). Blood in hereditary spherocytosis characteristically shows a greater increase in fragility with incubation than does normal blood or even blood of acquired spherocytosis (e.g., autoimmune hemolytic anemia).

with splenomegaly or a family member of a known case, is the incubated osmotic fragility test indicated. Since the unincubated osmotic fragility test may be normal in mild hereditary spherocytosis, an abnormal incubated test may be decisive in establishing the diagnosis.

LABORATORY STUDIES IN HEMOGLOBINOPATHIES AND THALASSEMIAS

Careful history, with emphasis on anemic disorders, jaundice in the family, and ethnic background, and physical examination are necessary.

Routine hematologic studies will include red cell indices, reticulocyte count, and examination of a well-made blood smear.

If the red cells are hypochromic, iron deficiency anemia is first considered because of its frequency. Serum iron and iron-binding capacity, serum ferritin, or Prussian blue reaction of the marrow for sideroblasts and storage iron will effectively determine whether the patient has iron deficiency.

Demonstration that the patient is hemolyzing may require serum bilirubin, urine or fecal urobilinogen, serum haptoglobin, or red cell survival studies.

Osmotic fragility (see p. 1017) may be helpful. Unless some cells show increased resistance to hypotonic saline, a hemoglobinopathy is unlikely. If osmotic fragility is increased, the hemolytic process is not likely to be due to a hemoglobinopathy.

Sickling—Metabisulfite Microscopic Test

PRINCIPLE. Deoxygenated cells containing Hb S sickle. The process of deoxygenation is enhanced by adding a reducing substance to the preparation.

PROCEDURE. One drop of blood is added to 2 drops of freshly prepared 2 per cent sodium metabisulfite (conveniently available as 200-mg capsules ready to add to 10 ml of distilled water). A coverslip is placed on the slide and may be sealed with petrolatum, or the slide may be kept in a moist chamber, preferably at 37°C. A similar preparation, but with saline instead of the reducing agent, is set up as a control. The slides are examined under the microscope with the high dry objective at 30 minutes, at 2 hours, and at 24 hours before concluding that the test is negative. Sickling is best seen near the edge of the coverslip. Partially sickled cells have a "holly-leaf" shape (Plate 29-2D).

INTERPRETATION. The test does not differentiate sickle cell anemia from sickle cell trait or other Hb S syndromes; all the cells will sickle, since the Hb S is distributed homogeneously among the cells. Certain other abnormal hemoglobins (e.g., Hb C$_{Harlem}$, Hb I) will also sickle.

SOURCES OF ERROR. Deterioration of the reducing agent will give false negative results. False negative tests may also occur when the amount of Hb S is too small for detection (in a few patients with sickle trait), from admixture with alcohol (from skin preparation), from trapped air under

the coverslip, or from inadequate sealing. Distortion of cells caused by ovalocytosis, extreme poikilocytosis, and crenation may be distinguished from sickle cells by comparison with the saline control.

Sickling—Microscopic Test Without Reducing Agent

If a reducing solution is not available, a drop of blood may be placed on a slide, and a coverslip applied over it and sealed. Sickling will occur after several hours in sickle cell anemia; it will take longer in sickle cell trait. Placing a rubber band around the finger to deoxygenate the blood *in vivo* before sampling by finger puncture will shorten the times involved.

Solubility Test—Dithionite

PRINCIPLE. Hb S is reduced by dithionite and is insoluble in concentrated inorganic buffers. The polymers of reduced Hb S obstruct light rays from passing through the solution. This test is particularly useful for screening large numbers of people for Hb S. Positive results must be confirmed.

REAGENTS. Sickledex (Ortho Diagnostics, Raritan, N.J.) is a commercially available kit which provides all the reagents. Alternatively, these may be made up as follows at a considerable saving in cost per test (Greenberg, 1972):

1. Phosphate buffer, 2.36 M. Dissolve 236.7 g of potassium hydrophosphate and 135.9 g of potassium dihydrophosphate in distilled water and adjust the final volume to one liter. The pH should be about 7.0.
2. Precipitating reagent: Add 2 ml of 5 per cent saponin and 2 ml of 20 per cent sodium dithionite ($Na_2S_2O_4$) to 100 ml of the phosphate buffer. Fresh dithionite must be used each day, as it deteriorates readily.
3. Blood may be fresh or anticoagulated. Hemolysates may be used.

PROCEDURE. Patients and normal control blood are tested.

Place 0.02 ml of blood in a test tube 12 mm in diameter. Add 2 ml of the precipitating reagent. Invert the tube three times to mix. After three minutes' incubation at room temperature, examine the tube for opacity or transparency. Opacity is present when black newsprint cannot be seen through the solution in good light at a distance of 2.5 cm from the tube.

INTERPRETATION. Opacity indicates an insoluble hemoglobin which is almost always hemoglobin S (or a non-Hb S sickling hemoglobin), whether in homozygous, or heterozygous, or mixed heterozygous state. Normal blood or other abnormal hemoglobins result in transparency. Positive or doubtful tests are confirmed with the metabisulfite test and electrophoresis.

SOURCES OF ERROR

False positive reactions may occur:

1. In unstable hemoglobin disorders after splenectomy, when large numbers of Heinz bodies are present.

2. In blood protein disorders, such as multiple myeloma, due to precipitation of plasma proteins.

3. If the tube is held too far from the newsprint.

4. If there is too much blood for the quantity of reagent.

False negative reactions may occur if:

1. The patient is severely anemic. It is advisable to double the quantity of blood if the hematocrit is less than 30 per cent.

2. The dithionite has deteriorated, in which case the characteristic color (purple to red) may have changed to orange.

3. The saponin has deteriorated.

4. The tube is held too close to the newsprint.

5. The percentage of Hb S present is too small, for example, at birth or after transfusion.

Alkali Denaturation Test for Hb F (Singer, 1951). Fetal hemoglobin resists alkali denaturation; adult hemoglobin does not. A hemolysate is alkalinized and then neutralized, and the denatured adult hemoglobin is precipitated by ammonium sulfate. A filtrate will then contain only alkali-resistant hemoglobin, which is measured and expressed as a percentage of the total.

REAGENTS. N/12 KOH or NaOH, kept in refrigerator in plastic- or paraffin-lined containers (alkaline reagent). Fifty per cent saturated $(NH_4)_2SO_4$ is prepared by adding 500 ml saturated $(NH_4)_2SO_4$ to 500 ml distilled water; to this, 2.5 ml concentrated (11 N) HCl is added (precipitating solution).

PROCEDURE. A hemolysate is prepared by washing blood once with 0.85 per cent saline, centrifuging, discarding the supernatant, and adding 1.5 volumes of distilled water to the volume of cells plus 0.4 volume of toluene. Shake vigorously for 5 minutes. Centrifuge at 3000 rpm for 10 minutes. Discard the upper two layers. Adjust the concentration of hemoglobin in the hemolysate to about 10 g/dl with distilled water. Determine the hemoglobin concentration (H_1). Add 0.1 ml of the H_1 hemolysate to 1.6 ml of the alkaline reagent. To mix, rinse the pipette five to six times while shaking the tube.

After exactly 1 minute, add 3.4 ml precipitating reagent to stop the reaction and precipitate the non-resistant hemoglobin. Invert the tube three to four times and filter immediately. The filtrate (H_2) is a 1 to 50 dilution of the original hemoglobin solution (H_1). Measure the optical density of H_2 directly. Measure the optical density of a dilution of 0.02 ml of H_1 in 4 ml of distilled water (H_3) at 540 nm. The percentage of alkali-resistant hemoglobin is:

$$\frac{\frac{1}{4} \text{ optical density of } H_2}{\text{optical density of } H_3} \times 100$$

INTERPRETATION. The filtrate (H_2) from normal adult blood is colorless and is less than 2 per cent of the total hemoglobin. Filtrates from blood with over 2 per cent Hb F are brown to red. The alkali denaturation method is insensitive to less than 2 per cent Hb F, so all figures below that level are considered to be normal.

The modification of Betke (1959) gives slightly lower normal reference intervals, 0.2 to 1.0 per cent for adults.

At birth the predominant Hb is Hb F. In most infants Hb F is less than 2 per cent by the age of 6 months, but in a small proportion Hb F does not fall to adult levels for two or three years.

Elevated Hb F is found in some hemoglobinopathies, in beta thalassemias, and in hereditary persistence of fetal hemoglobin (HPFH). In heterozygous beta thalassemia, Hb F is normal in over half the cases, is less than 5 per cent in most of the rest, but may be as high as 12 per cent in *hemozygous beta thalassemia*, the Hb F is consistently elevated, usually comprising 10 to 90 per cent of the total hemoglobin, only occasionally less than 10 per cent. Only a few cases of homozygous HPFH, in blacks, have been reported; all have had Hb F = 100 per cent. *Heterozygous HPFH*, in blacks, has Hb F levels between 20 and 35 per cent. In double heterozygosity of Hb S and HPFH (S-HPHF), the Hb F levels are usually between 20 and 36 per cent. *Sickle cell anemia* and *sickle beta thalassemia* patients have similar levels of Hb F, 1 to 20 per cent. In sickle trait the level of Hb F is normal.

In certain *acquired hematopoietic disorders*, the Hb F level may be elevated. These include megaloblastic anemia, myelofibrosis, aplastic anemia, leukemias, erythroleukemia, refractory anemias, pregnancy, and paroxysmal nocturnal hemoglobinuria.

Acid Elution Slide Test for Hb F. If the alkali-resistant hemoglobin is in the range of 10 to 30 per cent in a person with clinical features of thalassemia minor, the distribution of Hb F in stained blood films should be examined. The modification of the original method of Kleihauer and Betke by Shepard (1962) is useful.

PRINCIPLE. Hemoglobins other than Hb F are eluted from the red cells on an air-dried blood film by a citric acid-phosphate buffer (pH 3.3). Only Hb F remains in the fixed red cells, and the distribution can be determined after staining.

INTERPRETATION. If the high Hb F is caused by the high F gene for hereditary persistence of Hb F, all the red cells will contain the same amount of Hb F. If the cause is thalassemia or a hemoglobinopathy, some red cells will contain little Hb F or none (ghosts), and others will contain considerable amounts.

Heat Instability Test. Most unstable hemoglobins will precipitate more rapidly than normal hemoglobins if incubated at 50°C. (Dacie, 1975). The choice of buffers makes a difference. Both normal and unstable hemoglobins precipitate more rapidly in Tris-buffer than in phosphate buffers.

REAGENTS

Buffer a. Tris-(hydroxymethyl) aminomethane (Tris), 0.1 M, pH = 7.4,

or b. Sodium barbital, 0.1 M, pH = 7.4.

PROCEDURE. Wash 1 ml of fresh blood from patient and from a normal individual (in any anticoagulant) twice in 0.9 per cent NaCl. Lyse the packed red cells by adding 5 ml distilled water and mixing gently. Add 5 ml of buffer and centrifuge at 1500 g for 10 minutes. Place 2 ml of the clear supernatant in a clean test tube and incubate at 50°C. in a waterbath. Examine the solution periodically during a period of 60 minutes for a precipitate.

If there is a precipitate, determine the amount of unstable hemoglobin present. Centrifuge the solution at 1200 g for 10 minutes. Dilute both the clear supernatant and the original hemolysate 1:20 with Drabkin's reagent. Read the optical density at 540 nm.

$$\% \text{ Unstable hemoglobin} =$$

$$\frac{(\text{OD unheated sample} - \text{OD heated sample}) \times 100}{\text{OD unheated sample}}$$

INTERPRETATION. An easily visible precipitate forms within an hour if a heat-precipitable, unstable hemoglobin is present. The control sample should show no precipitate or a slight cloudiness. Slight precipitation is equivocal; the test should be repeated and the isopropanol precipitation test performed as well.

Precipitates accounting for 10 to 40 per cent of the total Hb present are found in hemoglobinopathies owing to unstable hemoglobins.

Isopropanol Precipitation Test (Carrell, 1972)
PRINCIPLE. The internal bonding forces of hemoglobin are weakened by a relatively non-polar solvent, decreasing its stability. If a hemoglobin is unstable, it will precipitate more rapidly in a non-polar solvent than will normal hemoglobin.

REAGENTS

1. Isopropanol buffer: Isopropanol, 17 per cent (v/v) in 0.1 M Tris/HCl buffer, pH 7.4. Keep the solution stoppered.

2. Hemolysate. From both patient's and normal control blood, prepare a hemolysate as in the method for the heat instability test, and adjust to about 10 g Hb/dl.

PROCEDURE. Place two stoppered test tubes containing 2 ml isopropanol buffer each in a 37°C. waterbath and allow equilibration to occur. Add 0.2 ml of fresh control hemolysate to one tube, and 0.2 ml of test hemolysate to the other. Restopper the tubes, mix by inversion, and replace in the 37°C. waterbath. Observe for precipitates at 10-minute intervals for an hour.

INTERPRETATION. Normal hemoglobin remains clear in the isopropanol buffer for 30 to 40 minutes. Most unstable hemoglobins will form a flocculant precipitate within 20 minutes.

A false positive may occur if high levels of hemoglobin or of Hb F are present (Lehmann, 1977). The method has the advantage of being particularly suitable for separating an unstable hemoglobin from a normal hemoglobin under mild conditions for further study.

SOURCES OF ERROR. The concentration of isopropanol and the temperature should be exact. The pH should not be below pH 7.2. Although the

red cells may be several days old before the hemolysate is made, the hemolysate should be freshly prepared, since hemoglobin deteriorates in solution.

Hemoglobin Electrophoresis.
Hemoglobin molecules in an alkaline solution have a net negative charge and move toward the anode in an electrophoretic system at a speed proportional to the strength of their charge. Those with an electrophoretic mobility greater than that of Hb A at pH 8.6 in barbital buffer are known as the "fast hemoglobins"; these include Hb Bart's and the two fastest, Hb H and Hb I. Hb C is the slowest of the common hemoglobins. A few in order of increasing mobility are Hbs A_2, E=O=C, G=D=S, F, A, Bart's, N, and H (Fig. 29-16).

Different types of apparatus are commercially available or can be devised for Hb electrophoresis. The hemolysate is applied to a suspending medium (e.g., filter paper, cellulose acetate, starch gel, agar gel, or starch block) between chambers containing buffer solution, and a constant voltage is applied. Different media and different buffers vary in efficiency of separation. None is both practical and adequate for *all* separations and for screening purposes (Lehmann, 1966).

Filter paper electrophoresis with barbital buffer is simple and satisfactory for routine use and gives separations indicated above but will not show Hb A_2. Tris buffer will allow the demonstration of small Hb fractions, including Hb A_2, but is less satisfactory for separating S and C or S and E.

Starch-gel and starch-block electrophoresis provide more distinct separations and are particularly valuable for the best quantitation of Hb A_2 (the bands can be cut out, eluted, and the optical density measured), but they are more troublesome to employ. Agar gel appears to be best for electrophoretic separation of Hb F.

A practical method to employ for routine hemoglobin electrophoresis is cellulose acetate at alkaline pH (Briere, 1965). It is rapid and reproducible and separates hemoglobins S, F, C, A, and A_2. Quantification of the major bands is easily accomplished. If an S band is present, a solubility test or sickling test must be performed. Citrate agar electrophoresis at an acid pH (Milner, 1975) provides ready separation of hemoglobins that migrate together on cellulose acetate: S from D and G, and C from E and O (Fig. 29-16) (Schmidt, 1973).

Final characterization of abnormal hemoglobins is beyond the scope of the usual routine laboratory. It consists of purification of the abnormal hemoglobin with starch-block electrophoresis, hybridization experiments to determine whether the abnormality lies in the alpha or beta chain, and "fingerprinting." In the latter procedure, the polypeptide chains are split by enzymatic digestion into peptides that are separated by performing horizontal paper electrophoresis and vertical chromatography in sequence. This peptide map, or "fingerprint," is compared with that prepared from normal hemoglobin, and the peptide in which the

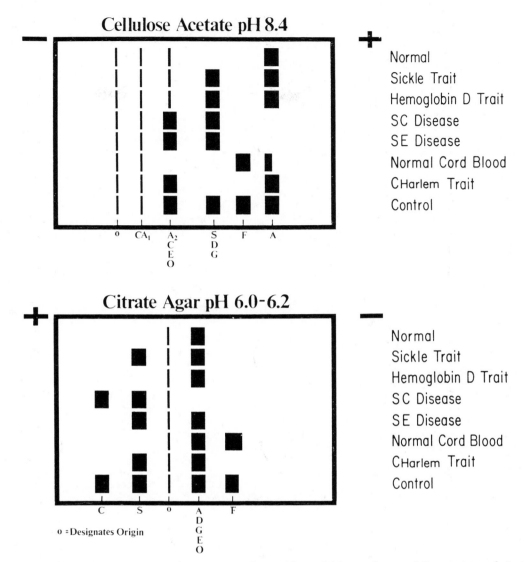

Figure 29-16. Hemoglobin electrophoresis. Comparison of various hemoglobin samples on cellulose acetate and citrate agar, showing relative mobilities. The control is a composite sample. The relative amounts of hemoglobin are not necessarily proportional to the size of the band; for example, in sickle trait (Hb AS), Hb A always exceeds Hb S in amount. (From Schmidt, 1976.)

abnormality occurs can be located. The abnormal peptide is then eluted and its amino acid content determined. Discussion of current techniques for identification of hemoglobins is provided by Huismann (1977).

   Hb A$_2$ Quantitation. For quantitation of Hb A$_2$, the starch block method of Kunkel (1957) is probably most consistently reliable; it is not practical for routine use.

   Estimating Hb A$_2$ visually or by densitometry from cellulose acetate membranes is unreliable (Schmidt, 1975). Satisfactory methods that can be

readily performed in a clinical laboratory are cellulose acetate electrophoresis followed by elution of the Hb A$_2$ band and measuring this spectrophotometrically as a percentage of the total (Marengo-Rowe, 1965). Somewhat more convenient for large numbers of samples is microchromatography using DEAE-cellulose and inexpensive glassware (Efremov, 1974). This method has been modified to minimize its sensitivity to pH changes of the developer and the ion exchanger (Huisman, 1975; Schleider, 1977).

   Reference intervals for Hb A$_2$ are 1.6 to 3.2 per

cent of the total hemoglobin. The intervals should be established on normal individuals by each laboratory for the method used.

Hb A_2 estimation is useful in identifying individuals with β thalassemia trait, in whom it is elevated, 3.5 to 7 per cent (see p. 000). It is also occasionally increased in megaloblastic anemia, but this causes no differential diagnostic problem. In an individual with iron deficiency, Hb A_2 may be somewhat decreased from his usual value. If an individual with β thalassemia trait has concomitant severe iron deficiency, the usually elevated Hb A_2 may be in the normal range; in this instance, retesting should be performed after the iron deficiency is corrected.

Hemoglobin H.   Hemoglobin H is an unstable hemoglobin composed of four beta chains (β_4). It is found in alpha-thalassemia trait in very small amounts and in hemoglobin H disease in larger amounts (Weatherall, 1972).

REAGENTS.   Brilliant cresyl blue, 1.0 g, in 100 ml of citrate-saline. Citrate-saline: 0.4 g sodium citrate in 100 ml of 0.9 per cent saline.

PROCEDURE.   Equal volumes of the dye solution and whole blood are placed in a small test tube, mixed, and incubated at 37°C. Films are made and air dried at 10 min., 1 hour, and 4 hours; they are examined without counterstaining.

RESULT.   Hemoglobin H inclusions are multiple, small, pale blue, round bodies. They must be distinguished from: (1) the granules and reticular networks in reticulocytes, which are darker blue in color; and (2) Heinz bodies, which are darker blue (with this stain), larger, and often attached to the membrane (Plate 29-2 *H* and *I*).

The 10-minute sample is the control by which to gauge the number of reticulocytes. Hemoglobin H inclusions should be present at 1 hour in over half the cells in hemoglobin H disease and in a very rare cell in alpha-thalassemia trait. Heinz bodies due to unstable hemoglobins are likely to appear only later (Atwater, 1977).

HEINZ BODIES

PRINCIPLE.   Heinz bodies are precipitates of denatured hemoglobin which characteristically attach themselves to the red cell membrane. Normally red blood cells do not contain Heinz bodies.

Heinz bodies cannot usually be detected in Wright's stained films but can be seen with phase microscopy or with the brightfield microscope following vital staining.

REAGENT.   Methyl violet, 0.5 g, or crystal violet, 2.0 g, is dissolved in 100 ml of 0.9 per cent saline and filtered.

PROCEDURE.   One volume of whole blood plus four volumes of the dye solution are incubated for 10 minutes in a small test tube. Films are then made, air dried, and examined without further staining. Alternatively, the incubation may be car-

ried out between a slide and coverslip and examined as a wet preparation.

INTERPRETATION.   Heinz bodies stain deep purple and vary from 1 to 4 μm in diameter. They tend to be attached to the red cell membrane (Plate 29-2 *I*). Reticulocytes do not stain with this dye. The presence of Heinz bodies in freshly drawn blood means that one of the following three situations exists: (1) A drug such as phenylhydrazine, chlorate, or an aromatic nitro or amino compound has been administered in an appropriate dose to the subject (or to the red cells *in vitro*), resulting in the oxidative denaturation of hemoglobin and the formation of Heinz bodies. (2) A drug such as primaquine or one of the above drugs in a lower dosage (insufficient to affect normal red cells) has been administered to a subject who has glucose-6-phosphate dehydrogenase deficiency (or some other red cell defect resulting in a deficiency of reduced glutathione) so that the hemoglobin cannot be protected from oxidative denaturation. (3) The subject has a hereditary defect, a hemolytic anemia associated with an unstable hemoglobin.

AUTOHEMOLYSIS TEST (Dacie, 1975)

PRINCIPLE.   When sterile defibrinated blood is incubated at 37°C., normal red cells undergo a complex series of changes with slow hemolysis. Cells with membrane or metabolic defects hemolyze to a greater extent than normal.

TEST.   Sterile defibrinated blood is used. The patient's blood and a normal control blood are tested in parallel. One-milliliter samples are delivered into four sterile screw-capped test tubes, and 0.05 ml of sterile 10 per cent glucose is added to two of the tubes. The tubes are incubated at 37°C. for 24 hours, then gently mixed by inversion and incubated for another 24 hours.

After the 48-hour incubation, the blood in each pair of tubes is pooled and well mixed (10 minutes on a rotary mixer at 15 revolutions/min.). A small sample is removed for microhematocrit and another for hemoglobin concentration (1:200 dilution) in Drabkin's solution. The remainder of each sample is centrifuged and the serum is placed in a clean test tube. A 1:10 dilution of the incubated serum is made in Drabkin's solution (a higher dilution is made if hemolysis is severe); the blank for the hemoglobin determination is a preincubation serum sample.

Calculation

$$\text{Lysis (\%)} = \frac{R_T \times (1\text{-Hct}) \times 100}{R_o} \times \frac{D_o}{D_T}$$

R_o = optical density of diluted whole blood
R_T = optical density of diluted serum at 48 h.
Hct = hematocrit at 48 hours (expressed as decimal)
D_o = dilution of whole blood (e.g., 1 in 200 = 0.005)

D_T = dilution of serum (e.g., 1 in 10 = 0.1)

NORMAL RANGE
Without added glucose 0.2 to 2.0 per cent
With added glucose 0 to 0.9 per cent

INTERPRETATION. In hereditary spherocytosis, lysis is almost always increased; with glucose, the lysis is diminished to a variable extent. In hereditary non-spherocytic anemias, Selwyn and Dacie found two patterns: Type I cases had slightly to moderately increased lysis without glucose; when glucose was added, some reduction in lysis occurred, but less than with normal blood. Type II cases had increased lysis but no improvement with added glucose.

It later was shown that glucose-6-phosphate dehydrogenase (G6PD) deficiency gave a Type I pattern and pyruvate kinase deficiency gave a Type II pattern of autohemolysis.

The autohemolysis test is usually used, at present, to study hemolytic anemias when other measurements have failed to give a definite answer.

TESTS FOR G6PD DEFICIENCY

Several methods may be used; they vary in their specificity, sensitivity to the heterozygous state, and the amount and freshness of blood required. For positive results in non-specific screening tests or for equivocal results in specific tests, the diagnosis must be confirmed by a quantitative assay.

Heinz Body Test for G6PD-Deficient Cells
(Beutler, 1955)

PRINCIPLE. Acetylphenylhydrazine, an oxidant drug, is added to the patient's and to control blood. After 2- and 4-hour incubation at 37°C., samples from each are examined for Heinz bodies.

REAGENTS
1. Acetylphenylhydrazine, 100 mg, is dissolved in 100 ml of 0.066 M phosphate buffer at pH = 7.6. To this is added 200 mg glucose. This solution must be freshly prepared.
2. Methyl violet, 0.5 g/dl saline, or crystal violet, 2 g/dl saline.
3. Blood sample: EDTA, double oxalate, or heparin may be used as anticoagulant, or defibrinated blood may be used.

PROCEDURE. To 2 ml of acetylphenylhydrazine solution in a test tube add 0.1 ml blood, mix well, and place in a 37°C. water bath. At 2 hours place a small drop of the mixture on a coverslip which is then inverted over a large drop of methyl violet or crystal violet on a slide. After 10 minutes examine slides from patient and control for Heinz bodies. This is repeated at 4 hours, if necessary.

RESULT. The percentage of cells with five or more Heinz bodies is determined for control and patient. Control values should be 0 to 30 per cent. Values for persons with G6PD deficiency (or defects in the glutathione system or unstable hemoglobins) will be greater, usually over 45 per cent.

Dye Reduction Test of Motulsky (Dacie and Lewis, 1968).

This test is conveniently performed using commercially available kits* which include detailed instructions. In principle, a mixture of glucose-6-phosphate, NADP, and brilliant cresyl blue dye in tris buffer is incubated with hemolysate. If G6PD is present, the NADP will be reduced to NADPH (Fig. 29-10), which, in turn, will reduce the blue dye to its colorless form. The time needed for this reduction to take place is noted for the patient's blood and for that of a normal control with an identical hemoglobin concentration (adjusted if necessary). This time is inversely proportional to the amount of G6PD present and is prolonged in G6PD-deficient subjects.

The dye reduction test is quite specific and can be performed on stored blood. It has the advantage that it can be performed on microsamples, but is likely to give false negative results in heterozygotes and black males with G6PD deficiency during a hemolytic episode (Fairbanks, 1969).

Ascorbate Cyanide Test (Jacob, 1966)

PRINCIPLE. Blood is incubated with a solution of sodium cyanide and sodium ascorbate. Hydrogen peroxide is generated from the coupled oxidation of ascorbate and hemoglobin. Since cyanide inhibits catalase, hydrogen peroxide is available to oxidize hemoglobin and the brown color of methemoglobin is discernible. This occurs more rapidly in G6PD-deficient cells than in normal cells.

REAGENTS
1. Sodium ascorbate, 10 mg, and glucose, 5 mg, are added to test tubes which are stoppered and may be stored indefinitely at −20°C.
2. Sodium cyanide, 500 mg, dissolved in 50 ml distilled water plus 20 ml of isotonic phosphate buffer, pH 7.4. The solution is neutralized to pH 7.0 with HCl, and the volume is made up to 100 ml with distilled water. This solution is stable indefinitely at room temperature.
3. Blood: EDTA, ACD, or heparin but not oxalate may be used as anticoagulant (hexose monophosphate shunt activity is inhibited by oxalate). Storage of blood at 4°C. for 14 days in ACD does not alter the results of the test.

PROCEDURE. Aerate the blood to a bright red color before adding 2 ml to the ascorbate and glucose mixture. Add 2 drops of the sodium cyanide solution and incubate the unstoppered blood suspension in a water bath at 37°C., preferably with agitation. Again mix the suspensions at 2 hours and at 3 or 4 hours, noting the color each time.

RESULT. G6PD-deficient blood appears brown after thorough mixing at a time normal blood remains red. For either hemizygote or heterozygote, this occurs at 1 to 2 hours when EDTA is the anticoagulant and at 2 to 4 hours when heparin or ACD is used. Normal blood changes color slowly over a period of several hours.

---

*G6PD kit, Dade, Miami, Fla.

INTERPRETATION. The ascorbate cyanide test is not specific, in that pyruvate kinase deficiency, paroxysmal nocturnal hemoglobinuria, and unstable hemoglobins will give a positive result. It is the most sensitive of the screening tests, in that it uses intact cells and will detect the deficiency in black males during hemolytic episodes and in heterozygotes (Fairbanks, 1969).

Fluorescence of NADPH (Beutler, 1975)

PRINCIPLE. Whole blood is added to a mixture of glucose-6-phosphate (G6P), NADP, saponin, and buffer, and a spot of this mixture is placed on filter paper and observed for fluorescence with ultraviolet light. If G6PD is present, NADP is converted to NADPH. Since phosphogluconate dehydrogenase is present in most hemolysates, further NADP is converted to NADPH (Fig. 29-10). NADPH fluoresces but NADP does not; therefore, lack of fluorescence indicates G6PD deficiency. By reoxidizing any small amounts of NADPH formed, oxidized glutathione (GSSG) enhances the ability of the test to detect mild G6PD deficiency.

REAGENTS

1. A screening mixture is made up with the following composition: G6P, 0.01 M, 1 part; NADP, 7.5 mmol, 1 part; saponin (Sigma) 1 per cent, 2 parts; tris-HCl buffer, 750 mmol, pH 7.8, 3 parts; GSSG, 8 mmol, 1 part; and water, 2 parts. This mixture is stable in the frozen state for several months. It is available in lyophilized form from Hyland Laboratories, Costa Mesa, California.

2. Whatman No. 1 filter paper (non-fluorescing).

3. Blood in heparin, ACD, or EDTA, which may be several weeks old. Spots of dried blood on filter paper are also satisfactory.

PROCEDURE. Add 10 μl of blood to 100 μl of the screening mixture and make a spot on the filter paper. After incubating the mixture at room temperature for 5 to 10 minutes, make a second spot. Examine spots under long-wave ultraviolet light.

INTERPRETATION. With the normal control sample, the first spot may fluoresce slightly and the second spot will fluoresce brightly. In G6PD deficiency, neither spot will show fluorescence.

Quantitative Assay of G6PD (and Other Red Cell Enzymes).

Methods are presented by Beutler (1975). For G6PD, most assays are based on the rate of reduction of NADP to NADPH, measured spectrometrically at 340 nm, when a hemolysate is incubated with G6P. Often an assay for G6PD activity is done simultaneously, using appropriate steps, because NADPH is formed in the first two reactions of the hexose monophosphate shunt.

In heterozygotes or in acute hemolysis in black subjects with G6PD deficiency, the diagnosis may be obscured even with the assay because of the increased level of G6PD in reticulocytes and younger erythrocytes. Usually, however, the ascorbate cyanide screening test will be positive in these instances.

TESTS FOR PYRUVATE KINASE (PK) DEFICIENCY (BEUTLER, 1975)

Screening Test for PK Deficiency

PRINCIPLE. Pyruvate kinase catalyzes the phosphorylation of ADP to ATP by phosphoenolypyruvate (PEP) with the formation of pyruvate. Pyruvate then reduces any NADH present to NAD with the formation of lactate (see Fig. 29-10). Loss of fluorescence of NADH under ultraviolet light is observed as evidence of the presence of PK.

Leukocytes must be removed from the sample because normally they contain about 300 times as much PK as do red cells, and in PK deficiency the red cells but not the leukocytes are deficient. Removing the buffy coat removes most of the leukocytes; lysing the red cells by hypotonicity allows the rest to remain intact, keeping the PK from the leukocytes out of the reaction.

REAGENTS

1. Mixture No. 1: In each milliliter are the following: phosphoenolypyruvate (PEP) cyclohexyl ammonium salt, 0.15 M (neut.), 30 μl; ADP, 30 mmol (neut.), 100 μl; MgCl$_2$, 80 mmol, 100 μl; KPO$_4$ buffer, 0.25 M, pH 7.4, 50 μl;* water, 720 μl. This mixture is stable indefinitely when frozen.

2. Dry NADH vial, 0.5 mg (Sigma).

3. Mixture No. 2: Add 0.5 ml of mixture No. 1 to a 0.5-mg NADH vial just before using.

4. Whatman No. 1 filter paper (non-fluorescing).

5. Blood may be collected in EDTA, ACD, or heparin.

PROCEDURE. After centrifuging the blood, carefully remove the buffy coat and plasma with a capillary pipette, and add 0.9 per cent NaCl to the red cells to make a 20 per cent suspension. Add 10 μl of the red cell suspension to 100 μl of mixture No. 2 screening mixture. Make one spot of this mixture on filter paper immediately and a second spot after 30 minutes' incubation at 37°C. After the spots are dry, examine them under long-wave ultraviolet light.

INTERPRETATION. With a normal control blood, the first spot should fluoresce brightly, but the second should have no fluorescence. Blood from a pyruvate kinase-deficient patient will show fluorescence in both spots.

Quantitative Assay of PK.

The same principle is employed as in the screening test, but the rate of decrease of O.D. at 340 nm is measured. A negative screening test or a normal PK assay (using the standard high substrate [PEP] concentrations) does not rule out PK-deficient hemolytic anemia. It has been clearly shown that hemolytic anemia may be associated with mutant PK enzymes which have

---

*KPO$_4$ buffer, 0.25 M, pH 7.4, is made up by mixing 8.25 ml of a stock solution of 1 M K$_2$HPO$_4$ with 1.75 ml of 1 M KH$_2$PO$_4$ and 30 ml of distilled water (Beutler, 1975, p. 22).

normal activity at high substrate concentration but decreased activity at a lower substrate concentration which prevails in the cell. Performing the PK assay at different substrate concentrations is therefore recommended (Beutler, 1975).

TESTS FOR PAROXYSMAL NOCTURNAL HEMOGLOBINURIA

Sucrose hemolysis tests (Hartmann, 1970)

Introduction. These tests should be performed whenever there is a suspicion of paroxysmal nocturnal hemoglobinuria (PNH). Since less than one fourth of patients have a history of sleep-related or nocturnal hemoglobinuria, the tests should also be performed in patients with hemolytic anemia of uncertain etiology. Patients with bone marrow hypoplasia and with myeloproliferative disorders frequently have a positive test.

Principle. In both the whole blood screening test and the confirmatory test, isotonic sucrose provides a medium of low ionic strength which promotes binding of complement components to the red cells. In paroxysmal nocturnal hemoglobinuria (PNH), a proportion of the red cells is abnormally sensitive to complement-mediated lysis.

Whole Blood Screening Test

SPECIMEN. Whole blood from patient collected in citrate or oxalate as anticoagulant.

REAGENTS. "Sugar water." Dissolve 10 g reagent grade sucrose in distilled water to make final volume of 100 ml. Prepare freshly each day.

PROCEDURE. Add one part blood to nine parts sugar water. Mix at once and incubate for 30 minutes at room temperature. Centrifuge and note any hemolysis in the supernate.

INTERPRETATION. Lack of hemolysis is evidence against PNH. Presence of hemolysis means that the confirmatory sucrose hemolysis test must be performed. A normal control blood sample must give a negative result.

SOURCES OF ERROR. False positive results are likely to occur (1) if defibrinated blood is used; (2) in anemic, non-PNH hematologic patients; or (3) if the sugar water is not freshly prepared. False negative results may occur if heparin or EDTA is used as an anticoagulant.

Confirmatory Sucrose Hemolysis Test

SPECIMEN. Wash red cells from patient and from a normal person, two times, and prepare 50 per cent suspensions in 0.15 M NaCl solution.

Use fresh ABO type compatible serum from a normal individual. Serum stored at $-70°C$. or below is satisfactory for at least a year.

REAGENTS. 1. Isotonic sucrose solution: Dissolve 92.4 g reagent grade sucrose in 91 ml of 50 mM NaH_2PO_4 and 9 ml of 50 mM Na_2HPO_4 and adjust the pH to 6.1 with HCl or NaOH. Add distilled water to a volume of 1000 ml. This solution may be kept for two weeks at 4°C. Fresh sugar water solution (above) can be used as an alternative.

2. Ammonium hydroxide (NH_4OH), 0.01 M.

PROCEDURE. In each of two tubes add 0.05 ml of serum to 0.85 ml sucrose solution and mix. Add 0.1 ml of patient's red cell suspension to one tube and 0.1 ml of normal red cell suspension to the other and mix promptly. Incubate the tubes at room temperature for 30 minutes. Centrifuge. If hemolysis is present in the supernate, determine percentage. Use as a blank the serum-sucrose mixture and as a standard 0.1 ml of the suspension of patient's red cells plus 0.9 ml of 0.01 M NH_4OH; read at 540 nm.

INTERPRETATION. Five per cent hemolysis or less is a negative result. A number of other hematologic diseases may cause this degree of hemolysis. Five to 10 per cent is doubtful and over 10 per cent is positive and virtually diagnostic for PNH.

SOURCES OF ERROR. False positive results may occur (1) rarely, in cases of autoimmune hemolysis or megaloblastic anemia (Rosse, 1977); (2) if sucrose solution is stored for a long period of time before use.

False negative results occur if the serum lacks complement activity, e.g., has been stored improperly.

Acidified Serum Test (Ham's Test) (Ham, 1939; Dacie, 1975)

INTRODUCTION. When the sucrose hemolysis test is positive, the acidified serum test is performed to confirm the diagnosis of paroxysmal nocturnal hemoglobinuria (PNH).

PRINCIPLE. Red cells in PNH are sensitive to lysis by complement, which is activated by the alternate pathway and bound to red cells in acidified serum. Individuals with PNH have a population of red cells that is unusually sensitive to lysis by complement.

SPECIMEN. 1. Wash red cells from patient and from an ABO-compatible normal person two times, and prepare 50 per cent suspensions in 0.15 M NaCl solution.

2. Use fresh serum (or properly stored at $-70°C$. or below) from patient and ABO-compatible normal control. To avoid hemolysed serum, the patient's serum should be obtained by defibrination.

3. Prepare heat-inactivated normal serum by heating at 56°C. for 30 minutes.

4. HCl, 0.2 N

5. NH_4OH, 0.01 M

PROCEDURE. Set up seven tubes. Add 0.5 ml normal serum to the four tubes indicated in Table 29-11, then add the other sera and acid as indicated and mix. After adding the red cell suspensions to the tubes, mix and incubate in a waterbath at 37°C. After one hour, centrifuge and examine supernatant serum for lysis.

The hemolysis is measured by pipetting 0.3 ml of the supernatant serum into 5.0 ml of 0.01 M NH_4OH and measuring the O.D. at 540 nm. As a blank use serum, and as a 100 per cent standard use 0.05 ml red cell suspension plus 0.55 ml water for the corre-

Table 29–11. ACIDIFIED-SERUM TEST*

	1	2	3	4	5	6	7
Fresh normal serum	0.5	0.5			0.5	0.5	
Patient's serum			0.5				
Heat-inactivated normal serum				0.5			0.5
0.2 N HCL		0.05	0.05	0.05		0.05	0.05
50% Patient's red cells	0.05	0.05	0.05	0.05			
50% Normal red cells					0.05	0.05	0.05
Pattern of lysis in positive test	Trace	+ + +	+	−	−	−	−

* Modified from Dacie, J. V., and Lewis, S. M.: Practical Haematology, 4th ed. New York, Grune & Stratton, Inc., 1968.

sponding test components; these are diluted in the same manner as the supernatant serum.

INTERPRETATION. Lysis of PNH cells occurs with acidified normal serum and acidified patient serum (often to a lesser degree). If lysis also occurs with heat-inactivated normal acidified serum, the test is not positive, as markedly spherocytic cells will react in this way. Normal cells should not lyse in any of the three tubes. Lysis of PNH cells is always partial, usually between 10 and 50 per cent.

A positive acidified serum test defines the PNH abnormality, whether in typical PNH or in aplastic anemia. A positive acidified serum test has also been found in a rare condition, congenital dyserythropoietic anemia, type II (CDA type II), or HEMPAS (p. 985). In CDA type II, however, lysis never occurs with the patient's own serum, and only with about 30 per cent of normal sera. In addition, the sucrose hemolysis test is negative in CDA type II; the hemolysis is believed to be due to an antibody present in some normal sera reacting to an unusual antigen (Dacie, 1975).

LABORATORY DIAGNOSIS OF ANEMIA

This section is based on the useful approach given by Wheby (1966). The diagnosis and study of anemia require the proper use and interpretation of laboratory measurements. Prerequisite for the efficient use of the laboratory are a careful history and physical examination, both of which lead to the initial laboratory measurements and provide important guidance in determining the nature of the anemia.

The first question to be answered is whether the patient is anemic (or polycythemic) and can be ascertained by determining whether his hemoglobin, hematocrit, or erythrocyte count lies outside the reference intervals for his age and sex. The second task is to define the underlying cause or mechanism for the anemia.

Usually the CBC (WBC, RBC, Hb, Hct, MCV, MCH, MCHC) and examination of a Wright's stained film are parts of the routine examination of the blood. It is possible that all these values could be normal in the presence of a mild macrocytic anemia, in which the RBC does not fall below the normal range, and the macrocytes present (and detectable on the blood film) do not elevate the MCV above the normal range.

Once anemia is discovered, the basic examination of the blood should include the following: (1) hemoglobin, hematocrit, and RBC count, for calculation of *indices* (if not already available with multichannel instrument); (2) blood film examination; (3) leukocyte count; (4) platelet count (if apparently abnormal on examination of the film or if suspected to be abnormal on clinical grounds); and (5) reticulocyte count.

With the Coulter Counter Model S, all red cell values and the indices have comparable precision. It must be remembered that indices are *mean* values, and will not detect different populations of cells which balance each other. For example, combined deficiencies of folate and iron may give rise to populations of macrocytic and hypochromic microcytic cells, which could yield normal indices. This emphasizes the need for careful examination of the blood film. Determination of erythrocyte indices and examination of the blood film are not substitutes for one another but are complementary.

Examination of the blood film will determine the *morphologic type* of anemia. In addition, certain changes or combinations of findings will suggest the mechanism involved.

Increased numbers of *polychromatic* macrocytes, with or without normoblasts, suggest increased erythropoiesis, and in the untreated patient this is usually due to hemorrhage or hemolysis. Here, the history (of blood loss) or physical examination (jaundice or splenomegaly) may help.

Findings suggestive of hemolysis are *poiki-*

locytes (abnormally shaped cells), *sickle cells, irregularly contracted forms* (including red cell fragments or schistocytes), and *spherocytes*. Sometimes it is difficult to detect spherocytes in hereditary spherocytosis because of minimal anisocytosis. The two findings in the red cells that are helpful here are the presence of a low MCD (mean cell diameter) between 6.0 and 6.5 μm (normal = 7.0 to 7.4) and spheroidocytes. Spheroidocytes are cup-shaped forms, spheroids, or flattened spheres as seen on the blood film or in a wet preparation.

Target cells may be found in hemoglobinopathies, especially in homozygous states for Hb C, Hb D, and Hb E, and in thalassemia. They may be present in any *hypochromic* anemia, though usually in smaller numbers. Target cells without microcytosis are also found in liver disease and in the absence of a spleen.

Fine *basophilic stippling* (which is due to precipitation of RNA) can be found in polychromatic red cells associated with a significant increase in the generation of erythrocytes, as in response to hemorrhage or hemolysis. Coarse basophilic stippling suggests an abnormality in hemoglobin synthesis. It is found in megaloblastic anemias, thalassemias, refractory anemias, and lead poisoning. In particular, hypochromasia or microcytosis with stippling is against the diagnosis of iron deficiency anemia and more suggestive of thalassemia or lead poisoning.

The combination of *oval macrocytes* and *hypersegmented neutrophils* indicates the very likely existence of megaloblastic anemia. In some laboratories the *lobe average* is used. This is computed on the basis of counting and averaging the number of nuclear lobes in 100 neutrophils. In the normal individual this is about three. The presence of megaloblastic anemia is strongly suggested by oval macrocytes, an increased lobe average (especially with giant PA neutrophils), and pancytopenia.

Finally, examination of the blood film allows the evaluation of *qualitative abnormalities in leukocytes and platelets* as well as an estimate of their numbers. Blood diseases that may be first suspected or detected in this manner are many and include chronic lymphocytic leukemia, compensated hemolytic anemia, early megaloblastic anemia, and anomalies of red cells, such as hereditary elliptocytosis, or of leukocytes, such as the Pelger-Huët anomaly.

After the routine studies just mentioned the choice of further procedures depends upon the morphologic type of the anemia as determined by the indices and the blood film.

Macrocytic anemia (MCV greater than 96 fl)

These anemias are normochromic, as determined by appearance on the film and by the MCHC. The first step is to ascertain whether the anemia is megaloblastic. The clues from the film have been mentioned. A *bone marrow aspiration* should be done to confirm the presence of megaloblastosis.

Megaloblastic Marrow. If the marrow is *megaloblastic*, with characteristic changes in both red cell and white cell precursors, the anemia in all likelihood is due to folate or vitamin B_{12} deficiency. We now have two questions: "Which type is it?" and "What is the *cause* of the deficiency?"

DIRECT METHODS OF DETERMINING DEFICIENCY OF VITAMIN B_{12} OR FOLATE. Serum and red cell assay for folic acid are low in folate deficiency and normal in vitamin B_{12} deficiency.

Serum assay for vitamin B_{12} is low in vitamin B_{12} deficiency and normal in folate deficiency.

INDIRECT METHOD OF DETECTING DEFICIENCY OF VITAMIN B_{12}. Urinary MMA (methylmalonic acid) is increased in vitamin B_{12} deficiency and normal in folate deficiency.

If the above measurements indicate a deficiency, the cause of the deficiency must still be found, and in vitamin B_{12} deficiency, this will include an assessment of gastric function, as indicated below. If the measurements described above are not available, a perfectly satisfactory alternative exists in the following.

GASTRIC ANALYSIS. The presence of free HCl provides valuable information, since it virtually excludes pernicious anemia in adults. The character and volume of the gastric juice should also be noted. In pernicious anemia the volume of gastric juice is small and the fluid is viscid, whereas with normal juice or with lack of free acid seen in many older people, the fluid is watery and of nearly normal volume.

Intrinsic factor assay, if possible, is helpful, for the gastric juice in pernicious anemia lacks intrinsic factor. This assay is not widely available.

TESTS OF VITAMIN B_{12} ABSORPTION. The Schilling test is most widely used and is discussed elsewhere (p. 974). It should be considered in two stages. If the initial absorption of vitamin B_{12}-^{60}Co is low, it indicates impaired absorption but does not distinguish between lack of intrinsic factor or defective absorption due to intestinal disease; therefore, the second stage must be performed—giving B_{12}-^{60}Co + intrinsic factor, which will correct impaired absorption caused by lack of intrinsic factor.

It is imperative that the Schilling test be delayed until bone marrow examination has been completed.

THERAPEUTIC TRIAL. If free acid is present in the gastric analysis, or if folic acid deficiency appears more likely than pernicious anemia, a therapeutic trial with 50 to 200 μg of folic acid (intramuscularly) per day would be a logical approach. Reticulocyte count and hematocrit are performed daily. A good response indicates folate deficiency. If there is no response, either a Schilling test or a similar therapeutic trial with 2 μg of vitamin B_{12} per day (intramuscularly) can then be performed.

Once the actual deficiency is established, the *cause* of it is ascertained by considering the various disorders discussed earlier (see pp. 971 and 975).

Non-megaloblastic Marrow. If the marrow is *not megaloblastic*, conditions which can be associated with macrocytosis should be investigated. These include liver disease, hemolytic anemias, hypothyroidism, alcoholism, and refractory or hypoplastic anemia. But anemias associated with these disorders, though they *may* be macrocytic, are more usually normocytic and thus are considered with the normocytic anemias.

Microcytic and hypochromic anemias (MCV < 80 fl; MCHC < 32 per cent)

If the counts are performed on a Coulter Counter Model S, the MCHC is likely to still be in the normal range, with slight to moderate degrees of hypochromia. Consequently the MCV has assumed the leading role in the detection of microcytic hypochromic anemias.

These anemias reflect a quantitative defect in hemoglobin synthesis.

1. *Iron deficiency anemias* are due to increased requirement or blood loss not balanced by intake.

2. *Anemia of chronic disorders,* otherwise known as sideropenic anemia associated with reticuloendothelial siderosis, or simple chronic anemia, is associated with infection, neoplasia, or collagen disease. This anemia may be normochromic and normocytic or hypochromic and normocytic but is sometimes hypochromic and microcytic.

3. *Thalassemia* is a genetically determined impairment in the rate of globin synthesis.

4. *Sideroblastic anemia* is that group of refractory anemias with erythroid hyperplasia of the marrow in which a defect in hemoglobin synthesis predominates. A few of these respond to pyridoxine and are called pyridoxine-responsive anemias.

Since *iron deficiency* is the most common, the first step is to determine whether the body lacks iron.

When blood loss cannot be documented, serum ferritin, serum iron and iron-binding capacity, or bone marrow study for iron should be performed. These will usually discriminate between the two most common anemias in this category, iron deficiency and simple chronic anemia associated with some other disease—frequently chronic infection or cancer. In both, the serum iron is low, but in iron deficiency the total iron-binding capacity is elevated, whereas in simple chronic anemia it is normal or decreased. Storage iron in the marrow is depleted in iron deficiency but is normal or elevated in simple chronic anemia. Iron deficiency anemia in an adult male almost always means chronic blood loss; the source must be found and corrected, if necessary.

Hypochromic anemias with basophilic stippling and increased serum iron are most likely *thalassemias,* and the next examinations to perform are hemoglobin electrophoresis and determination of Hb A_2 and Hb F. Investigation of other members of the patient's family is often essential in order to establish a diagnosis of thalassemia.

Least common in this group are the *sideroblastic anemias.* In addition to refractory sideroblastic anemia already discussed, a very similar picture may occur after therapy with certain drugs (e.g., isoniazid) and in chronic lead poisoning. Basophilic stippling is common in this group of anemias.

Table 29-12 summarizes the laboratory distinctions in hypochromic anemias.

Normocytic and normochromic anemias (MCV 80–96 fl)

This large group of anemias has many causes. A useful approach is evaluation of the erythrokinetics in a given patient (p. 932). Often a reticulocyte production index (RPI) or

Table 29–12. LABORATORY FEATURES IN MICROCYTIC HYPOCHROMIC ANEMIAS

	SERUM IRON	SERUM TIBC	% SATURATION	MARROW % Sideroblasts	Iron Stores	SERUM FERRITIN	FEP	Hb A₂	Hb F
Iron deficiency	↓	↑	↓	↓	↓	↓	↑	N-↓	N
β-Thalassemia trait	N (↑)	N	N	N	N-↑	N-↑	N	↑	N-↑
Anemia of chronic disease	↓	N-↓	↓	↓	N-↑	N-↑	↑	N	N
Sideroblastic anemia	↑	↓	↑	↑	↑	↑	↑(↓)	N	N-↑

TIBC = total iron binding capacity; FEP = Free erythrocyte porphyrins; ↓ = decreased; N = normal; ↑ = increased.

absolute reticulocyte count and evaluation of a bone marrow aspirate will suffice. The reticulocyte count is the simplest measure of effective erythropoiesis.

Optimal Marrow Response: Reticulocyte Production Index over Two Times Normal. If the output of reticulocytes has reached between three and six times normal, as determined by the absolute reticulocyte count or RPI, it can be assumed that the marrow has reached an optimal response. The cause for the anemia is then either *acute blood loss* or *hemolysis*. If blood loss cannot be proved, evidence that hemolysis is in fact present must be sought.

Erythroid hyperplasia of the marrow, serum bilirubin, urine or fecal urobilinogen will indicate whether erythropoietic activity and destruction are increased. Red cell survival determination may be needed to prove hemolysis in some cases. Low serum haptoglobin points to hemolysis, but a normal level does not exclude it. None of these measurements will specify whether hemolysis is intravascular or extravascular, but elevated plasma hemoglobin, hemoglobinuria, and hemosiderinuria indicate intravascular hemolysis.

Once it is determined that excessive hemolysis is occurring, the type of hemolytic mechanism must be ascertained.

The *direct antiglobulin (Coombs') test* is a useful guide to further study.

If the direct antiglobulin (Coombs') test is *positive*, tests to determine the type and specificity of the antibody should be undertaken. If the antibody is non-specific, tests such as cold agglutinins, the Donath-Landsteiner test, and serum protein electrophoresis may help to define the process.

If the direct antiglobulin (Coombs') test is *negative*, what examinations are performed next will depend upon the clinical findings and the results of the measurements already made.

If hereditary spherocytosis is suspected, osmotic fragility before and after 24-hour incubation at 37°C. and family studies will be necessary.

If a non-spherocytic congenital hemolytic anemia is suspected, an autohemolysis test, screening for glucose-6-phosphate dehydrogenase deficiency, hemoglobin electrophoresis, and a sickle cell test will be helpful.

If thalassemia seems likely, determinations of Hb A₂ and Hb F are appropriate. Thalassemia is unique in that it is both hypochromic and hemolytic. Again, family studies are often helpful.

If drug-induced hemolysis is suspected, a test for Heinz bodies, screening test for glucose-6-phosphate dehydrogenase and, if possible, tests for a drug-dependent autoantibody are indicated.

If the nature of the hemolytic anemia is obscure, a sugar-water test for paroxysmal nocturnal hemoglobinuria should be performed.

Inadequate Marrow Response: Reticulocyte Production Index under Two Times Normal. The mechanism of the anemia may be ineffective erythropoiesis. Conditions with the greatest degree of ineffective erythropoiesis appear in other categories (e.g., megaloblastic anemia and thalassemia), but some idiopathic refractory anemias have a hyperplastic bone marrow and impaired delivery of the cells to the blood. In some of these, abnormalities in erythroid precursors suggestive of megaloblastic change may be present, but the granulocytic and megakaryocytic changes usually seen in megaloblastic anemia are lacking.

A low reticulocyte count may indicate decreased production caused by inadequate stimulation of the marrow. Chronic renal disease may result in impaired production of erythropoietin. Certain endocrinopathies, such as hypopituitarism or hypothyroidism, may result in regulation of hemoglobin production at a lower level due to decreased tissue need for oxygen.

A large group of normochromic anemias associated with various chronic diseases form a heterogeneous group characterized by failure of the marrow to meet the need of a slightly decreased red cell survival. Some of these are anemia of chronic disorders associated with infection, cancer, or rheumatoid arthritis and have the defect in iron metabolism noted above under the hypochromic microcytic anemias. The reasons for inadequate stimulation or response of the marrow are not well understood.

Inability of the marrow to respond to erythropoietin may be due to damage to the marrow by drugs or toxic chemicals, to unknown causes, or to infiltration of the marrow by neoplastic cells or fibrous tissue.

In these conditions with low reticulocyte counts in which the marrow is not effectively producing erythrocytes, it is usually helpful to examine the bone marrow. Other studies to determine the underlying disease process can then proceed according to the marrow picture, the assessment of erythrokinetics, and the clinical findings.

REFERENCES

Adamson, J. W.: Familial polycythemia. Semin. Hematol., *12*:383, 1975.

Abildgard, C. F., Cornet, J. A., and Schulman, I.: Primary erythrocytosis. J. Pediatr., *63*:1072, 1963.

Allen, R. H.: The plasma transport of vitamin B$_{12}$. Br. J. Haematol., *33*:161, 1976.

Anderson, B. B.: Investigations into the *Euglena* method for the assay of the vitamin B$_{12}$ in serum. J. Clin. Pathol., *17*:14, 1964.

Atwater, J., and Schwartz, E.: Tests for hemoglobin H and other unstable hemoglobins. *In* Williams, W. J., Beutler, E., Erslev, A. J., and Rundles, R. W. (eds.): Hematology, 2nd ed. New York, McGraw-Hill Book Co., Inc., 1977, p. 1591.

Balcerzak, S. P., and Bromberg, P. A.: Secondary polycythemia. Semin. Hematol., *12*:353, 1975.

Bauman, A. W., and Swisher, S. N.: Hyporegenerative processes in hemolytic anemia. Semin. Hematol., *4*:265, 1967.

Beck, W. S.: Folic acid deficiency. *In* Williams, W. J., Beutler, E., Erslev, A. J., and Rundles, R. W.: Hematology, 2nd ed. New York, McGraw-Hill Book Co., 1977a, p. 334.

Beck, W.: Megaloblastic anemias. I. Vitamin B$_{12}$ deficiency. II. Folic acid deficiency. *In* Beck, W. (ed.): Hematology, 2nd ed. Cambridge, Mass.: The M.I.T. Press, 1977.

Bentley, S. A.: Red cell survival studies reinterpreted. Clin. Haematol., *6*:601, 1977.

Berlin, N. I.: Diagnosis and classification of the polycythemias. Semin. Hematol., *12*:339, 1975.

Betke, K., Marti, H. R., and Schlict, I.: Estimation of small percentages of foetal haemoglobin. Nature, *184*:1877, 1959.

Beutler, E.: Red Cell Metabolism. A Manual of Biochemical Methods, 2nd ed. New York, Grune & Stratton, Inc., 1975.

Beutler, E.: Glucose 6-phosphate dehydrogenase deficiency. *In* Williams, W. J., Beutler, E., Erslev, A. J., and Rundles, R. W.: Hematology, 2nd ed. New York, McGraw-Hill Book Co., 1977, p. 466.

Beutler, E.: Glucose-6-phosphate dehydrogenase deficiency. *In* Stanbury, J. B., Wyngaarden, J. B., and Fredrickson, D. A.: The Metabolic Basis of Inherited Disease, 4th ed. New York, McGraw-Hill Book Co., 1978, p. 1430.

Beutler, E., Dern, R. J., and Alving, A. S.: The hemolytic effect of primaquine: VI. An *in vitro* test for sensitivity of erythrocytes to primaquine. J. Lab. Clin. Med., *45*:40, 1955.

Brain, M. C.: Destruction of red cells by the vasculature and the reticuloendothelial system. *In* Nathan, D. G., and Oski, F. A. (eds.): Hematology of Infancy and Childhood. Philadelphia, W. B. Saunders Company, 1974, p. 241.

Brain, M. C.: Microangiopathic haemolytic anaemia (MHA). Br. J. Haematol., *23* (Suppl.):45, 1972.

Brain, M. C., Dacie, J. V., and Hourihane, D. O'B.: Microangiopathic haemolytic anaemia; the possible role of vascular lesions in pathogenesis. Br. J. Haematol., *8*:358, 1962.

Briere, R., Golias, T., and Batsakis, J. G.: Rapid qualitative and quantitative hemoglobin fractionation, cellulose acetate electrophoresis. Am. J. Clin. Pathol., *44*:695, 1965.

Brown, D. L.: Haematological disorders. *In* Holborow, E. J., and Reeves, W. G. (eds.): Immunology in Medicine. New York, Grune & Stratton, Inc., 1977, p. 911.

Brus, I., and Lewis, S. M.: The haptoglobin content of serum in haemolytic anaemia. Br. J. Haematol., *5*:348, 1959.

Bunn, H. F., Forget, B. G., and Ranney, H. M.: Human hemoglobins. Philadelphia, W. B. Saunders Company, 1977.

Carrell, R. W., and Kay, R.: A simple method for the detection of unstable hemoglobins. Br. J. Haematol., *23*:615, 1972.

Carrell, R. W., Winterbourn, C. C., and Rachmilewitz,

E. A.: Activated oxygen and hemolysis. Br. J. Haematol., *30*:259, 1975.

Carson, P. E., and Frischer, H.: Glucose-6-phosphate dehydrogenase deficiency and related disorders of the pentose phosphate pathway. Am. J. Med., *41*:744, 1966.

Cartwright, G. E.: The anemia of chronic disorders. Semin. Hematol., *3*:351, 1966.

Cartwright, G. E., and Lee, G. R.: The anemia of chronic disorders. Br. J. Haematol., *21*:147, 1971.

Chanarin, I.: Investigation and management of megaloblastic anaemia. Clin. Haematol., *5*:747, 1976.

Chanarin, I.: The Megaloblastic Anaemias. Oxford, Blackwell Scientific Publications, 1969.

Chanarin, I., Barkhan, P., Peacock, M., and Stamp, T. C. B.: Acute arrest of haemopoiesis. Br. J. Haematol., *10*:43, 1964.

Charache, S., Weatherall, D. J., and Clegg, J. B.: Polycythemia associated with a hemoglobinopathy. J. Clin. Invest., *45*:813, 1966.

Chernoff, A. I., and Singer, K.: Studies on abnormal hemoglobins. IV. Persistence of fetal hemoglobin in the erythrocytes of normal children. Pediatrics, *9*:469, 1952.

Clarke, C. A.: Prevention of rhesus iso-immunization. Lancet, *2*:1, 1968.

Cohen, J. A., and Warringa, M. G. P. J.: The fate of P[32] labelled diisopropylfluorophosphonate in the human body and its use as a labelling agent in the study of the turnover of blood plasma and red cells. J. Clin. Invest., *33*:459, 1954.

Conley, C. L., and Charache, S.: Mechanisms by which some abnormal hemoglobins produce clinical manifestations. Semin. Hematol., *4*:53, 1967.

Cooper, B. A.: Megaloblastic anaemia and disorders affecting utilization of vitamin B_{12} and folate in childhood. Clin. Haematol., *5*:631, 1976.

Cooper, R. A.: Destruction of erythrocytes. *In* Williams, W. J., Beutler, E., Erslev, A. J., and Rundles, R. W. (eds.): Hematology, 2nd ed. New York, McGraw-Hill Book Co., 1977a, p. 216.

Cooper, R. A., and Jandl, J. H.: Acanthocytosis. *In* Williams, W. J., Beutler, E., Erslev, A. J., and Rundles, R. W. (eds.): Hematology, 2nd ed. New York, McGraw-Hill Book Co., 1977b, p. 461.

Croft, J. D., Jr., Swisher, S. N., Gilliland, B. C., Bakermeier, R. F., Leddy, J. P., and Weed, R. I.: Coombs' test positivity induced by drugs: Mechanisms of immunologic reactions and red cell destruction. Ann. Intern. Med., *68*:176, 1968.

Crosby, W. H., and Furth, F. W.: A modification of the benzidine method for measurement of hemoglobin in plasma and urine. Blood, *11*:380, 1956.

Dacie, J. V.: Autoimmune hemolytic anemia. Arch. Intern. Med., *135*:1293, 1975.

Dacie, J. V.: Differences in the behavior of sensitized red cells to agglutination by antiglobulin sera. Lancet, *2*:954, 1951.

Dacie, J. V.: Paroxysmal nocturnal haemoglobinuria. The Scientific Basis of Medicine: Annual Reviews. London, The Athlone Press, 1972.

Dacie, J. V.: The Haemolytic Anaemias. Congenital and Acquired. Part I—The Congenital Anaemias. New York, Grune & Stratton, Inc., 1960.

Dacie, J. V., and Lewis, S. M.: Practical Haematology, 5th ed. Edinburgh, Churchill Livingstone, 1975.

Dacie, J. V., and Worlledge, S. M.: Auto-immune hemolytic anemias. Prog. Hematol., *6*:82, 1969.

Diamond, L. K., Wang, W. C., and Alter, B. P.: Congenital hypoplastic anemia. Adv. Pediatr., *22*:349, 1976.

Diggs, L. W.: Sickle cell crises. Am. J. Clin. Pathol., *44*:1, 1965.

Donath, J., and Landsteiner, K.: Über paroxysmale hämoglobinurie. Munchen. Med. Wochenschr., *51*:1590, 1904.

Efremov, C. D., Huisman, T. H. J., Bowman, K., Wrightstone, R. N., and Schroeder, W. A.: Microchromatography of hemoglobins. II. A rapid method for determination of hemoglobin A_2. J. Lab. Clin. Med., *83*:657, 1974.

Eichner, E. R., and Hillman, R. S.: The evolution of anemia in alcoholic patients. Am. J. Med., *50*:218, 1971.

Erslev, A. J.: Anemia of chronic renal failure. *In* Williams, W. J., Beutler, E., Erslev, A. J., and Rundles, R. W. (eds.): Hematology, 2nd ed. New York, McGraw-Hill Book Co., 1977, p. 288.

Erslev, A. J.: Anemia of endocrine disorders. *In* Williams, W. J., Beutler, E., Erslev, A. J., and Rundles, R. W. (eds.): Hematology, 2nd ed. New York, McGraw-Hill Book Co., 1977, p. 295.

Fanconi, G.: Familial constitutional panmyelocytopathy, Fanconi's anemia (F.A.). I. Clinical aspects. Semin. Hematol., *4*:233, 1967.

Finch, C. A., Cook, J. D., Labbe, R. F., and Culala, M.: Effect of blood donation on iron stores as evaluated by serum ferritin. Blood, *50*:441, 1977.

Frank, M. M., Schreiber, A. D., Atkinson, J. P., and Jaffe, C. L.: Pathophysiology of immune hemolytic anemia. Ann. Intern. Med., *87*:210, 1977.

Gilliland, B. C.: Coombs-negative immune hemolytic anemia. Semin. Hematol., *13*:267, 1976.

Good, R. A.: Aplastic anemia—suppressor lymphocytes and hematopoiesis. N. Engl. J. Med., *296*:41, 1977.

Gottlieb, A. J., and Wurzel, H. A.: Protein-quinone interaction: *In vitro* induction of indirect antiglobulin reactions with methyl-dopa. Blood, *43*:85, 1974.

Götze, O., and Müller-Eberhard, H. J.: Paroxysmal nocturnal haemoglobinuria: Hemolysis initiated by the C3 activator system. N. Engl. J. Med., *286*:180, 1972.

Gralnick, H. R., Galton, D. A. G., Catovsky, D., Sultan, C., and Bennett, J. M.: Classification of acute leukemia (N.I.H. conference). Ann. Intern. Med., *87*:740, 1977.

Greenberg, M. S., Harvey, H. A., and Morgan, C.: A simple and inexpensive screening test for sickle hemoglobin. N. Engl. J. Med., *286*:1143, 1972.

Hagler, L., Pastore, R. E., and Bergin, J. J.: Aplastic anemia following viral hepatitis: Report of two fatal cases and literature review. Medicine (Baltimore), *54*:139, 1975.

Hall, C. A.: Congenital disorders of vitamin B_{12} transport and their contribution to concepts. Gastroenterology, *65*:684, 1973.

Hall, C. A.: Transcobalamins I and II as natural transport proteins of vitamin B_{12}. J. Clin. Invest., *56*:1125, 1975.

Harris, J. W., and Kellermeyer, R. W.: The Red Cell: Production, Metabolism, Destruction: Normal and Abnormal, rev. ed. Cambridge, Harvard University Press, 1970.

Havard, C. W. H.: Thymic tumours and refractory anemia. Ser. Haematol., *5*:18, 1965.

Herbert, V.: Megaloblastic anemias. *In* Beeson, P., and McDermott, W. (eds.): Textbook of Medicine, 14th ed. Philadelphia, W. B. Saunders Company, 1975.

Hillman, R. S., and Finch, C. A.: Red Cell Manual, 4th ed. Philadelphia, F. A. Davis Co., 1974.

Hines, J. D., and Grasso, J. A.: The sideroblastic anemias. Semin. Hematol., *7*:86, 1970.

Hoffbrand, A. V.: The megaloblastic anaemias. *In* Goldberg, A., and Brain, M. C. (eds.): Recent Advances in

Haematology. Edinburgh, Churchill-Livingstone, 1971, p. 357.

Hoffbrand, A. V.: Sideroblastic anaemia. *In* Lewis, S. M., and Verwilghen, R. L.: Dyserythropoiesis. London, Academic Press, 1977, p. 139.

Hoffman, R., Zanjani, E. D., Vila, J., Zalusky, R., Lutton, J. D., and Wasserman, L. R.: Diamond-Blackfan syndrome: Lymphocyte-mediated suppression of erythropoiesis. Science, *193*:899, 1976.

Huisman, T. H. J., and Jonxis, J. H. P.: The Hemoglobinopathies. Techniques of Identification. New York, Marcel Dekker, Inc., 1977.

Huisman, T. H. J., Schroeder, W. A., Brodie, A. N., Mayson, S. M., and Jakway, J.: Microchromatography of hemoglobins. III. A simplified procedure for the determination of hemoglobin A_2. J. Lab. Clin. Med., *86*:700, 1975.

International Committee for Standardization in Hematology: Recommended Methods for Radioisotope Red-Cell Survival Studies. Br. J. Haematol., *21*:241, 1971.

International Committee for Standardization in Hematology: Standard Techniques for the Measurements of Red-Cell and Plasma Volume. Br. J. Haematol., *25*:801, 1973.

Jacob, H. S., and Jandl, J. H.: A simple visual screening test for glucose-6-phosphate dehydrogenase deficiency employing ascorbate and cyanide. N. Engl. J. Med., *274*:1162, 1966.

Jacob, H. S., Ruby, A., Overland, E. S., and Mazia, D.: Abnormal membrane protein of red blood cells in hereditary spherocytosis. J. Clin. Invest., *50*:1800, 1971.

Jacobs, A.: Erythropoiesis and iron deficiency anemia. *In* Jacobs, A., and Worwood, M.: Iron in Biochemistry and Medicine. New York, Academic Press, 1974, p. 405.

Jacobs, A., and Worwood, M.: The biochemistry of ferritin and its clinical implications. Prog. Hematol., *9*:1, 1975.

Jandl, J. H.: Hereditary spherocytosis. *In* Beutler, E. (ed.): Hereditary Disorders of Erythrocyte Metabolism. New York, Grune & Stratton, Inc., 1968.

Kern, P., Heimpel, H., Heit, W., and Kubanek, B.: Granulocytic progenitor cells in aplastic anaemia. Br. J. Haematol., *35*:613, 1977.

Koerper, M. A., and Dallman, P. R.: Serum iron concentration and transferrin saturation in the diagnosis of iron deficiency in children: Normal developmental changes. J. Pediatr., *91*:870, 1977.

Krantz, S. B.: Pure red-cell aplasia. N. Engl. J. Med., *291*:345, 1974.

Kreig, A. F., and Henry, J. B.: Hemoglobin electrophoresis. Clinical pathology correlations of hemoglobinopathies and thalassemias. N.Y. State J. Med., *67*:1275, 1967.

Kunkel, H. G., Ceppellini, R., Müller-Eberhard, U., and Wolf, J.: Observations on the minor basic hemoglobin component in blood of normal individuals and patients with thalassemia. J. Clin. Invest., *36*:1615, 1957.

L. A.: Aplastic anaemia: Seed or soil? Lancet, *2*:748, 1977.

LaCelle, P. L., and Weed, R. I.: The contribution of normal and pathologic erythrocytes to blood rheology. Prog. Hematol., *7*:1, 1971.

Lau, K. S., Gottlieb, C., Wasserman, L. R., and Herbert, V.: Measurement of serum vitamin B_{12} level using radioisotope dilution and coated charcoal. Blood, *26*:202, 1965.

Lehmann, H., and Huntsman, R. G.: Man's Haemoglobins. Philadelphia, J. B. Lippincott Co., 1966.

Lehmann, H., Huntsman, R. G., Casey, R., et al.: Erythrocyte disorders—anemias related to abnormal globin. *In*

Williams, W. J., Beutler, E., Erslev, A. J., and Rundles, R. W. (eds.): Hematology, 2nd ed. New York, McGraw-Hill Book Co., 1977, p. 495 ff.

Lewis, S. M.: Course and prognosis in aplastic anaemia. Br. Med. J., *1*:1027, 1965.

Lewis, S. M., and Verwilghen, R. L.: Dyserythropoiesis and dyserythropoietic anemias. Prog. Hematol., *8*:99, 1973.

Lynch, R. E., Williams, D. M., Reading, J. C., and Cartwright, G. E. The prognosis in aplastic anemia. Blood, *45*:517, 1975.

Marengo-Rowe, A. J.: Rapid electrophoresis and quantitation of haemoglobins on cellulose acetate. J. Clin. Pathol., *18*:790, 1965.

Marsh, G. W., and Lewis, S. M.: Cardiac haemolytic anaemia. Semin. Hematol., *6*:133, 1969.

Mauer, A. M.: Pediatric Hematology. New York, McGraw-Hill Book Co., 1969.

Meyer, K., and Ley, A. B.: The measurement of erythrocyte survival with P^{32}-tagged diisopropylfluorophosphate (DFP^{32}). Clin. Res., *4*:80, 1956.

Milner, P. F., and Gooden, H.: Rapid citrate-agar electrophoresis in routine screening for hemoglobinopathies using a simple hemolysate. Am. J. Clin. Pathol., *64*:58, 1975.

Mollin, D. L., Anderson, B. B., and Burman, J. F.: The serum vitamin B_{12} level: Its assay and significance. Clin. Haematol., *5*:521, 1976.

Nathan, D. G., Clarke, B. J., Hillman, D. G., Alter, B. P., and Housman, D. E.: Erythroid precursors in congenital hypoplastic (Diamond-Blackfan) anemia. J. Clin. Invest., *61*:489, 1978.

Orkin, S. H., and Nathan, D. G.: The thalassemias. N. Engl. J. Med., *295*:710, 1976.

Oski, F. A., and Naiman, J. L.: Hematologic Problems in the Newborn, 2nd ed. Philadelphia, W. B. Saunders Company, 1972.

Pearson, H. A., Spencer, R. P., and Cornelius, E. A.: Functional asplenia in sickle cell anemia. N. Engl. J. Med., *281*:923, 1969.

Perutz, M. F., and Lehmann, H.: Molecular pathology of human hemoglobin. Nature (London), *219*:902, 1968.

Petz, L. D., and Garratty, G.: Drug-induced haemolytic anemia. Clin. Haematol., *4*:181, 1975.

Piomelli, S.: A micromethod for free erythrocyte porphyrins: The FEP test. J. Lab. Clin. Med., *81*:932, 1973.

Pirofsky, B.: Immune hemolytic disease: The autoimmune hemolytic anaemias. Clin. Haematol., *4*:167, 1975.

Pirofsky, B.: Clinical aspects of autoimmune hemolytic anemia. Semin. Hematol., *13*:251, 1976.

Reissman, K. R., Ruth, W. E., and Nomura, T. A.: A human hemoglobin with lowered oxygen affinity and impaired heme-heme interactions. J. Clin. Invest., *40*:1826, 1961.

Rosse, W. F.: The detection of small amounts of antibody on the red cell in autoimmune hemolytic anaemia. Ser. Haematol., *7*:358, 1974.

Rosse, W. F.: Paroxysmal nocturnal hemoglobinuria. *In* Williams, W. J., Beutler, E., Erslev, A. J., and Rundles, R. W. (eds.): Hematology, 2nd ed. New York, McGraw-Hill Book Co., 1977, p. 560.

Rudzki, Z., Nazaruk, M., and Kimber, R. J.: The clinical value of the radioassay of serum folate. J. Lab. Clin. Med., *87*:859, 1976.

Saarinen, U. M., and Siimes, M. A.: Developmental changes in serum iron, total iron-binding capacity, and transferrin saturation in infancy. J. Pediatr., *91*:875, 1977.

Schleider, C. T. H., Mayson, S. M., and Huisman, T. H. J.: Further modification of the microchromatographic determination of hemoglobin A$_2$. Hemoglobin, *1*:503, 1977.

Schmidt, R. M.: Laboratory diagnosis of hemoglobinopathies. J.A.M.A., *224*:1276, 1973.

Schmidt, R. M., and Brosious, E. F.: Basic Laboratory Methods of Hemoglobinopathy Detection, 6th ed. Atlanta, U.S. Dept. Health, Education and Welfare, Center for Disease Control, 1976. [HEW Publ. No. (CDC) 77-8266]

Schmidt, R. M., Rucknagel, D. L., and Necheles, T. F.: Comparison of methodologies for thalassemia screening by Hb A$_2$ quantitation. J. Lab. Clin. Med., *86*:873, 1975.

Schneider, R. G., Hightower, B., Hosty, T. S., Ryder, H., Tomlin, G., Atkins, R., Brimhall, B., and Jones, R. T.: Abnormal hemoglobins in a quarter million people. Blood, *48*:629, 1976.

Shepard, M. K., Weatherall, D. J., and Conley, C. L.: Semiquantitative estimation of the distribution of fetal hemoglobin in red cell populations. Bull. Johns Hopkins Hosp., *110*:293, 1962.

Siimes, M. A., Addiego, J. E., and Dallman, P. R.: Ferritin in serum: diagnosis of iron deficiency and iron overload in infants and children. Blood, *43*:581, 1974a.

Siimes, M. A., and Dallman, P. R.: New kinetic role for serum ferritin in iron metabolism. Br. J. Haematol., *28*:7, 1974b.

Simmons, A., Schwabbauer, M. L., and Earhart, C. A.: Automated platelet counting with the autoanalyzers. J. Lab. Clin. Med., *77*:656, 1971.

Sleisenger, M. H.: Diseases of malabsorption. *In* Beeson, P. B., and McDermott, W. (eds.): Textbook of Medicine, 14th ed. Philadelphia, W. B. Saunders Company, 1975, p. 1217 ff.

Smith, J. R., and Landaw, S. A.: Smoker's polycythemia. N. Engl. J. Med., *298*:6, 1978.

Stamatoyannopoulos, G., Bellingham, A. J., Lenfant, C., and Finch, C. A.: Abnormal hemoglobins with high and low oxygen affinity. Ann. Rev. Med., *22*:221, 1971.

Stebbins, R., and Bertino, J. R.: Megaloblastic anaemia produced by drugs. Clin. Haematol., *5*:619, 1976.

Stenman, U-H: Intrinsic factor and the vitamin B$_{12}$ binding proteins. Clin. Haematol., *5*:473, 1976.

Stetson, C. A., Jr.: The state of hemoglobin in sickled erythrocytes. J. Exp. Med., *123*:341, 1966.

Stockman, J. A., Weiner, L. S., Simon, G. E., Stuart, M. J., and Oski, F. A.: The measurement of free erythrocyte porphyrin (FEP) as a simple means of distinguishing iron deficiency from beta-thalassemia trait in subjects with microcytosis. J. Lab. Clin. Med., *85*:113, 1975.

Storb, R., Thomas, E. D., Weiden, P. L., Buckner, C. D., Clift, R. A., Fefer, A., Fernando, L. P., Giblett, E. R., Goodell, B. W., Johnson, F. L., Lerner, K. G., Neiman, R. E., and Sanders, J. E.: Aplastic anemia treated by allogenic bone marrow transplantation: A report on 49 new cases from Seattle. Blood, *48*:817, 1976.

Swisher, S. N., and Burka, E. R.: Cryopathic hemolytic syndrome. *In* Williams, W. J., Beutler, E., Erslev, A. J., Rundles, R. W. (eds.): Hematology, 2nd ed. New York, McGraw-Hill Book Co., 1977, p. 596.

Taylor, K. B.: Immune aspects of pernicious anaemia and atrophic gastritis. Clin. Haematol., *5*:497, 1976.

Valentine, W. N.: The molecular lesion of hereditary spherocytosis: A continuing enigma. Blood, *49*:241, 1977a.

Valentine, W. N.: Deficiency of other enzymes leading to anemia. *In* Williams, W. J., Beutler, E., Erslev, A. J., and Rundles, R. W. (eds.): Hematology, 2nd ed. New York, McGraw-Hill Book Co., 1977b, p. 483.

Vilter, R. W., et al.: Refractory anemia with hyperplastic bone marrow. Blood, *15*:1, 1960; Semin. Hematol., *4*:175, 1967.

Wang, W. C., and Mentzer, W. C.: Differentiation of transient erythroblastopenia of childhood from congenital hypoplastic anemia. J. Pediatr., *88*:784, 1976.

Wasi, P., Na-Nakorn, S., and Pootrakul, S-N.: The alpha-thalassemias. Clin. Haematol., *3*:383, 1974.

Weatherall, D. J.: Abnormal haemoglobins and thalassaemia. *In* Hoffbrand, A. V., Brain, M. C., and Hirsh, J. (eds.): Recent Advances in Haematology, 2. Edinburgh, Churchill-Livingstone, 1977a, p. 43.

Weatherall, D. J.: The thalassemias. *In* Williams, W. J., Beutler, E., Erslev, A. J., and Rundles, R. W. (eds.): Hematology, 2nd ed. New York, McGraw-Hill Book Co., 1977b, p. 391.

Weatherall, D. J., and Clegg, J. B.: The Thalassaemia Syndromes, 2nd ed. Oxford, Blackwell Scientific Publications, 1972.

Weatherall, D. J., Pembrey, M. E., and Pritchard, J.: Fetal haemoglobin. Clin. Haematol., *3*:467, 1974.

Weens, J. H., and Schwartz, R. S.: Etiologic factors in autoimmune hemolytic anemia. Ser. Hematol., *7*:303, 1974.

Weinreb, N. J., and Shih, C-F.: Spurious polycythemia. Semin. Hematol., *12*:397, 1975.

Wheby, M. S.: Using a clinical laboratory in the diagnosis of anemia. Med. Clin. North Am., *50*:1689, 1966.

White, J. M., and Dacie, J. V.: The unstable hemoglobins—molecular and clinical features. Prog. Hematol., *7*:69, 1971.

W.H.O. Tech. Rep. Ser. 503, 1972. Nutritional Anemias: Report of a WHO group of experts.

Wiley, J. S., Ellory, J. C., Shuman, M. A., Shaller, C. C., and Cooper, R. A.: Characteristics of the membrane defect in the hereditary stomatocytosis syndrome. Blood, *46*:337, 1975.

Williams, D. M., Lynch, R. E., and Cartwright, G. E.: Drug-induced aplastic anemia. Semin. Hematol., *10*:195, 1973.

Wintrobe, M. M., Lee, G. R., Boggs, D. R., Bithell, T. C., Athens, J. W., and Foerster, J. (eds.): Clinical Hematology, 7th ed. Philadelphia, Lea & Febiger, 1974.

Wrightstone, R. N., and Huisman, T. H. J.: On the levels of hemoglobins F and A$_2$ in sickle-cell anemia and related disorders. Am. J. Clin. Pathol., *61*:375, 1974.

Yamaguchi, N., and Glass, G. B. J.: The determination of intrinsic factor in gastric secretory analysis. Ann. N.Y. Acad. Sci., *140*:924, 1967.

Yunis, A. A., and Bloomberg, G. R.: Chloramphenicol toxicity: Clinical features and pathogenesis. Prog. Hematol., *4*:138, 1964.

Zipursky, A.: Hemolytic disease of the newborn. *In* Nathan, D. G., and Oski, F. A. (eds.): Hematology of Infancy and Childhood. Philadelphia, W. B. Saunders Company, 1974, p. 280.

3

30

LEUKOCYTIC DISORDERS

Douglas A. Nelson, M.D.

With Sections on Lymphocytes, Chronic Lymphocytic Leukemia, Leukemic Reticuloendotheliosis, Malignant Lymphoma, and Blood Protein Disorders

by Frederick R. Davey, M.D.

NON-NEOPLASTIC DISORDERS

The examination of leukocytes includes two technical phases. In the quantitative phase, one determines the concentration of all the white cells, the total leukocyte count (white blood cell count; WBC) and the relative and absolute numbers of the various forms of white cells. The term *leukocytosis* refers to an increase in the total WBC above the upper limit of normal for age and sex. *Leukopenia* is a total WBC below normal. Although all leukocytes act in defending the body in one way or another, their functions are somewhat different and it is best to regard them as separate systems. An increase or decrease in the absolute number of cells in each series is termed: *neutrophilia* (neutrophilic leukocytosis) and *neutropenia; eosinophilia* (eosinophilic leukocytosis) and *eosinopenia; basophilia* (basophilic leukocytosis) and *basopenia; lymphocytosis* and *lymphocytopenia; monocytosis* and *monocytopenia*. In the qualitative phase, one determines structural abnormalities in cytoplasm and nucleus and, to an increasing extent, functional abnormalities as well (p. 1045). Examination also includes two anatomic phases: examination of peripheral blood (capillary or venous) and examination of marrow (obtained from sternum, tibia, ilium, or spinous process).

The purpose of the study of leukocytes is, first, to help in establishing a diagnosis. Occasionally the examination alone may furnish a positive specific diagnosis, for example, in leukemia. More frequently it may be diagnostically helpful together with other clinical or laboratory data, for example, in acute appendicitis or infectious mononucleosis. Another purpose is to help in establishing a prognosis. For example, a low white blood count in acute appendicitis or pneumonia is considered prognostically unfavorable.

Finally, study of the leukocytes is helpful in following the course of disease. For example, toxic effects of radiotherapy and chemotherapy may be recognized, and recovery monitored, by examination of leukocytes.

Examination of leukocytes may also reveal the existence of an entirely unsuspected disease. For example, leukemia may be found in a patient with the clinical picture of an acute infection, or infectious mononucleosis may be found in patients whose disease clinically resembles leukemia.

For these reasons the leukocyte count is one of the routine examinations which is performed on the blood of almost every patient admitted to the hospital regardless of disease.

In contrast to the red cells and platelets which function within the blood, the different white blood cells use the blood stream primarily for transportation; they perform their tasks in the tissues after leaving the blood. We have discussed the morphology, production, distribution within the body, life span, and function for each of the white cells in an earlier section, beginning on page 933. This background is assumed in the following sections, dealing with changes in number or function of the different cell types.

NEUTROPHILIA

Neutrophilic leukocytosis or neutrophilia refers to an absolute concentration of neutrophils in the blood above normal for age. Reference intervals are given in Table 27-3; age variations are discussed on page 912.

Mechanisms (Boggs, 1975; Finch, 1977). The primary factors influencing the neutrophil count are (1) the rate of inflow of cells from the bone marrow; (2) the proportion of neutrophils in the marginal granulocyte pool (MGP) and the circulating granulocyte pool (CGP); and (3) the rate of outflow of neutrophils from the blood (see p. 937).

Physiologic leukocytosis is produced by factors or situations that do not involve tissue damage. Severe exercise, hypoxia, stress, or the injection of epinephrine will result in a decrease in the MGP and a corresponding increase in the CGP, resulting in a pseudoneutrophilia. This is a simple redistribution of cells between the CGP and MGP.

Stress of greater severity or injection of endotoxin, corticosteroids, or etiocholanolone results in an increased inflow of cells to the blood from the marrow storage pool. As a result, the maturation and storage pool in the marrow is diminished, and both MGP and CGP are enlarged. A greater neutrophilia is possible here because of the much larger size of the storage pool than the CGP and MGP. Band neutrophils and metamyelocytes are likely to be present.

In both of the above an acute neutrophilia occurs as a result of redistribution of cells, without input from increased production. Chronic neutrophilia may be produced by corticosteroids, which decrease the egress of neutrophils from the blood and result in increased CGP and MGP without necessarily increasing the production of neutrophils.

In contrast to the above, *pathologic leukocytosis* is an increased WBC which occurs as a result of disease, and usually is a response to tissue damage (Table 30-1). This leukocytosis is most often a neutrophilia.

In addition to the random loss of neutrophils from the circulation in various body secretions, neutrophils leave the blood by ameboid movement when attracted to a focus of inflammation in tissues, presumably by chemotactic substances. It is from the marginal granulocyte pool (MGP) that the neutrophils leave the blood, pass between capillary endothelial cells, and reach the tissues.

In acute infection, increased margination of neutrophils and outflow from blood to tissues would lead to neutropenia were there not a flow of neutrophils from the marrow storage

Table 30–1. PATHOLOGIC LEUKOCYTOSIS

CAUSE	CELL TYPE
Allergy	Eosinophil
Brucellosis	Lymphocyte, monocyte
Convulsions	Neutrophil or lymphocyte
Drugs and poisons	
ACTH	Neutrophil
Adrenalin	
Camphor	Neutrophil and eosinophil
Copper sulfate, phosphorus, carpine	Eosinophil
Tetrachlorethane, Adrenalin	Monocyte, neutrophil, and lymphocyte
Other (acetanilid, arsenicals, benzene, CO, digitalis, lead, phenacetin, turpentine, venoms)	Neutrophil
Hemolysis	Neutrophil
Hemorrhage	Neutrophil
Hodgkin's disease	Neutrophil, eosinophil, and monocyte
Infectious lymphocytosis	Lymphocyte
Infectious mononucleosis	Lymphocyte, atypical changes
Leukemia	Granulocyte, lymphocyte, or monocyte
Loeffler's syndrome, periarteritis nodosa, pernicious anemia	Eosinophil
Polycythemia vera	Neutrophil, eosinophil, basophil
Toxemias:	
diabetic acidosis, eclampsia, gout, uremia	Neutrophil
Tuberculosis	Neutrophil, eosinophil, lymphocyte, monocyte
Tumors involving	
marrow and serous cavities	Neutrophil and eosinophil
ovary	Eosinophil
GI tract and liver	Neutrophil
Typhoid fever	Lymphocyte

compartment into the blood. Since the latter overcompensates, the result is a neutrophilia. Usually production and storage compartments then increase in the marrow and are able to sustain the increased CGP (i.e., neutrophilia) and MGP in the face of the increased flow of neutrophils from the blood into the inflammatory site. In these instances, the marrow will show granulocytic hyperplasia (decreased E/G ratio and increased cellularity), with maturation intact.

If the demand for neutrophils is extremely great, as in severe infection, there may be depletion of the marrow storage pool and a decreased CGP (i.e., neutropenia) and MGP, because the supply of cells is insufficient for the demand. In these instances, the marrow will show increased numbers of early neutrophil precursors, through the myelocyte stage, but decreased numbers of metamyelocytes, bands, and neutrophils.

Causes

INFECTION. Systemic infections due to various bacteria, fungi, spirochetes, and viruses may cause neutrophilia. In some, this may be preceded by a transient neutropenia, especially if the infection is severe. Some bacterial infections result in persistent neutropenia, such as typhoid fever, paratyphoid fever, and brucellosis. Whether this is due to the mechanism cited above for severe infection, or to a toxic depression of the marrow, or to a combination, is not clear.

Appendicitis, salpingitis, otitis media, and other localized infections caused by pyogenic organisms usually result in neutrophilia.

A characteristic pattern of response to infection includes progressive neutrophilic leukocytosis, increase of young forms (shift to the left), and fall in eosinophils. When the infection begins to subside and the fever drops, a gradual transformation in the blood picture occurs: the total number of leukocytes goes down, and the number of monocytes increases. This monocytic phase is gradually replaced by a relative or slight absolute lymphocytosis and eosinophilia as recovery proceeds.

Other disorders associated with neutrophilia

are listed below. In some of them, one or more of the mechanisms described above are operating; in others, the mechanism is unclear.

TOXIC

Metabolic. Uremia, eclampsia, gout, diabetic acidosis.

Drugs and Chemicals. Lead, mercury, potassium chlorate, digitalis, epinephrine, corticosteroids, turpentine, ethylene glycol, benzene.

PHYSICAL AND EMOTIONAL STIMULI. Heat, cold, muscular activity, anoxia, pain, fear, anger.

TISSUE DESTRUCTION OR NECROSIS. Myocardial infarction, burns, surgical operations, crush injuries, fractures, neoplastic disease (especially with extensive necrosis).

HEMORRHAGE. Especially if bleeding has occurred within a serous cavity (peritoneal, pleural, joint, subdural).

HEMOLYSIS. Especially with rapid hemolysis, as in hemolytic crises or hemolytic transfusion reactions.

HEMATOLOGIC DISORDERS. Myeloproliferative disorders, myelogenous leukemia, postsplenectomy state.

Determinants. Certain host factors modify the degree of neutrophilic response. Children respond more intensely than adults. The degree of neutrophilia produced may be impaired by the same factors that impair erythrocyte production (iron lack, folate or vitamin B_{12} deficiency) or by marrow failure due to other causes. Imperfectly defined factors which enable the body to localize an infection may play a role: the more localized the process, the more pronounced the neutrophilia.

Other factors modifying the neutrophilic response are due more to the microorganism than to the host. Pyogenic bacteria, especially, induce neutrophilia. Within limits the more virulent the agent, the higher the neutrophil count. When the infection is overwhelming, however, there is apt to be a neutropenia and greater shift to the left due to the mechanism described above.

It is claimed that the height of leukocytosis is an indicator of the resistance of the individual and that the degree of the shift to the left is an indicator of the severity of the infection. In keeping with this conception, a simultaneous fall of the former and a rise of the latter are prognostically unfavorable.

The following are hematologic signs of recovery from infectious diseases:

1. Drop of the total leukocyte count and of the number of neutrophils.

2. Disappearance of shift to the left.

3. Transient increase in number of monocytes.

4. Increase of eosinophils when they were decreased or absent during the height of the disease.

5. Increase in number of lymphocytes.

6. Disappearance of toxic granulation.

Therefore, the following are unfavorable hematologic signs:

1. A moderate or slight rise in the total number of leukocytes associated with a marked shift to the left during the height of the disease.

2. Failure of eosinophils to reappear in the end stages of an infectious disease when they were absent before.

3. Absolute reduction of lymphocytes.

4. Excessive number of cells with toxic granulation.

Therapy of infections with antibiotic agents may modify the leukocytic response to infection. Steroid therapy, though causing neutrophilia, tends to impair the host response to infection, probably because of diminished movement of neutrophils into the tissues and increased lysosomal stability.

NEUTROPENIA

Neutropenia is a reduction of the absolute neutrophil count below 2000 per μl for whites and below 1300 per μl for blacks. The term *agranulocytosis* has been used for severe neutropenia; this is almost always associated with depletion of eosinophils and basophils as well. If the neutrophil count is less than $1 \times 10^9/l$, the risk of infection is considerably increased over normal, and if there are less than 0.5×10^9 neutrophils per liter, the risk of infection is great.

Agranulocytic angina and malignant neutropenia are older terms that describe the common symptoms and rapidly fatal course that may be associated with infection and very severe neutropenia. Following a period of malaise comes the sudden onset of high fever and ulcerative lesions of the mouth, throat, and other mucous membranes. Death from sepsis occurs in a few days if effective antibiotic therapy cannot be achieved.

The mechanisms by which neutropenia occur include: (1) decreased flow of neutrophils from marrow into blood due to either lack of production or ineffective production; (2) increased removal of neutrophils from the blood; (3) altered distribution between circulating granulocyte pool (CGP) and marginal granulocyte pool (MGP); or (4) combinations of these. Neutropenias are not so neatly classified as anemias. In recent years, however, a sound approach has been made, using data from radioisotopic measurements of proliferative activity, maturation time, survival in the circulation, and measurement of MGP and CGP in addition to the usual bone marrow and peripheral blood studies (Cline, 1975; Finch, 1977). A classification is given in Table 30-2. It should be noted that drugs induce neutropenia through several mechanisms and are a very important consideration in any differential diagnosis of leukopenia.

Myeloid Hypoplasia. Kostman's infantile genetic agranulocytosis is a rare, autosomal recessive condition appearing in early infancy. The marrow usually shows increased early granulocytes but few maturing forms, and the neutrophil survival is normal. A soluble factor necessary for granulocyte maturation appears to be lacking (Barak, 1971).

Chronic familial neutropenia and cyclic neutropenia appear to be autosomal dominant conditions. The latter usually has a period of about 21 days, and appears to be due to periodic stem cell failure. Neutrophil precursors disappear prior to the fall in circulating neutrophils and reappear during the neutropenic phase. Other congenital and familial neutropenias have been described.

Isolated neutropenia or agranulocytosis is

Table 30-2. CLASSIFICATION OF NEUTROPENIA*

I. *Myeloid hypoplasia*
  A. Infantile genetic agranulocytosis (Kostman); familial neutropenia; cyclic neutropenia; chronic (hypoplastic) neutropenia; myelophthisic neutropenia.
  B. Drug induced:
    1. Cytolytic:
      a. Alkylating agents (nitrogen mustard, cyclophosphamide, chlorambucil, busulfan).
      b. Ionizing radiation.
      c. Mitosis inhibitors (colchicine, vinblastine, vincristine).
      d. DNA depolymerization (procarbazine).
    2. Metabolic interference with DNA synthesis:
      a. Purine and pyrimidine antagonists (cytosine arabinoside,† methotrexate,† 6-mercaptopurine, azathioprine, hydroxyurea).
      b. Phenothiazine type (phenothiazines, dibenzazepine compounds, antithyroid compounds,† sulfonamides,† antibiotics, anticonvulsants).
      c. Others (chloramphenicol,† benzene†).
    3. Idiosyncratic:
      a. Acute, days to weeks (quinine, quinidine, indomethacin, procainamide, thiazides, sulfonamides,† phenylbutazone,† antithyroids†).
      b. Chronic, months to years (chloramphenicol,† phenylbutazone,† benzene,† gold salts†).
II. *Marrow hyperplasia with ineffective granulocytopoiesis*
  A. Chediak-Higashi syndrome; megaloblastic anemia; myeloproliferative disorders (these may belong in IV).
  B. Drug induced:
    1. Impaired nucleic acid synthesis (cytosine arabinoside,† methotrexate,† phenytoin).
    2. Others (alcohol, chloramphenicol†).
III. *Decreased survival in circulation* due to increased utilization or increased destruction.
  A. Bacterial infections; viral infections; protozoal infections; chronic benign neutropenia of childhood; chronic idiopathic neutropenia in adults; splenic neutropenia; neonatal isoimmunization neutropenia; acquired immunoneutropenia.
  B. Drug induced (immunologic mechanism):
    Aminopyrine, amidopyrine, phenylbutazone,† sulfapyridine.†
IV. Combination of impaired production (I or II) and decreased survival (III).
  A. Megaloblastic anemia; severe bacterial infections; mycobacterial infections; chronic idiopathic myelokathexis.
  B. Drug induced (very likely):
    Alcohol, purine and pyrimidine inhibitors, aminopyrine.
V. Pseudoneutropenia (shift from CGP to MGP).
  A. Endotoxin.
  B. Drug induced: (?) anesthetic agents, ether, pentobarbital.

---

*Adapted from Finch, S. C.: *In* Williams, W. J., Beutler, E., Erslev, A. J., and Rundles, R. W. (eds.): Hematology. New York, McGraw-Hill Book Co., Inc., 1972.
†Drugs cited for more than one mechanism.

uncommon in adults. When the marrow is damaged, by a myelophthisic process such as metastatic carcinoma or Gaucher's disease replacing the marrow, or by drugs, usually the damage is not limited to granulopoiesis but affects normoblasts and megakaryocytes as well. Because of the short life span of granulocytes, however, neutropenia is the earliest recognizable effect in the blood. It takes weeks before damage to the erythropoietic tissue becomes manifest because of the long life span of erythrocytes. Platelets have a rather short life span but, on the other hand, megakaryocytes are more resistant to damage.

Drugs are an important cause of neutropenia, and, as outlined in Table 30-2, may act in different ways. Drugs that have the effect of destroying or interfering with mitosis of the proliferating cells are frequently used in the therapy of malignant disease. Important and limiting side effects of such chemotherapy are the results of marrow hypoplasia: severe neutropenia with its risk of infection, and severe thrombocytopenia with risk of bleeding; anemia is more readily controlled with transfusion. Of drugs used for therapy of other diseases, the phenothiazine group is responsible for most of the drug-related neutropenias at the present time.

Idiosyncratic drug effects refer to those in which host susceptibility factors predominate; that is, there is little relationship with dose and duration of drug therapy.

Ineffective Granulocytopoiesis. Neutropenia due to increased ineffective granulocytopoiesis occurs in megaloblastic anemias as a result of drugs that have an antifolate effect. Of course, anemia is usually present if therapy is prolonged, and often thrombocytopenia as well. The marrow is usually hyperplastic. In addition to increased destruction of cells in the marrow there is some evidence that circulating neutrophils have a shortened survival. Indirect evidence for increased granulocyte turnover in this group of neutropenias with hypercellular marrow is an increased serum muramidase (lysozyme) (Catovsky, 1971a).

Decreased Survival in Circulation. Transient neutropenia may occur early in some infections, followed by leukocytosis once the marrow production catches up with the demand. As previously noted, in severe, extensive bacterial infection, neutropenia with a shift to the left may be due to inability of marrow production to keep up with the peripheral utilization. Some bacterial infections, notably brucellosis and Salmonella infections, are prone to be associated with neutropenia; they may have some depressing effect on the marrow as well. Viral infections such as measles and rubella have neutropenia for several days after appearance of the rash; this is probably due in part to increased utilization. Lymphocytosis is present and persists after the neutropenia subsides.

The neutropenia of hypersplenism has been attributed to selective removal of neutrophils by the spleen. Described by Wiseman and Doan, it is associated with neutrophilic hyperplasia of the marrow and is corrected by splenectomy. Splenomegaly due to many causes may have shortened neutrophil survival and neutropenia; these include congestive splenomegaly, Felty's syndrome, Gaucher's disease, and lymphoma. In some cases of Felty's syndrome (neutropenia and splenomegaly in rheumatoid arthritis), there may be a neutrophil-specific antibody involved.

Evidence has been accumulating that there are antibodies capable of clumping leukocytes of all varieties under proper experimental conditions (leukoagglutinins). Leukopenia in the newborn may be produced by leukoagglutinins coming from the mother. Studies have demonstrated that autoantibodies also may be responsible for immune neutropenia or immune panleukopenia. Lalezari (1975) identified an antibody with agglutinating activity against a specific neutrophil antigen (NA2) that was responsible for neutropenia. An autoantibody with cytotoxic activity against mature granulocytes, monocytes, and lymphocytes as well as primitive myeloid cells has been shown to result in episodic autoimmune panleukopenia (Cline, 1976).

Drug-induced neutropenia due to immune mechanisms has been well described for aminopyrine since the first report in 1934 by Madison and Squier. In about 1 per cent of persons, seven to 10 days after first taking the drug, chills, headache, fever, and neutropenia with a shift to the left occur. Slight granulocytic hyperplasia is noted in the marrow. If the drug is continued, mucosal ulceration and sepsis may occur, and granulocytic precursors may disappear from the marrow. If, on the other hand, the drug is discontinued, the neutrophil count returns to normal levels in a week. An antibody develops in these patients which, in the presence of the drug, causes enhanced destruction of neutrophils. Of the possible mechanisms involved, a drug-plasma protein complex is probably the antigen; the antigen-antibody complex non-specifically adsorbs on the cells and leads to their destruction (Finch, 1977).

Combinations. As indicated, some of the conditions discussed above are probably combinations of increased destruction and impaired effective production. As more detailed studies are done, some of the entries in this classification will be clarified and probably changed.

Pseudoneutropenia. Small doses of endotoxin will cause a shift of neutrophils into the MGP from the CGP, giving an apparent neutropenia, prior to causing a leukocytosis. In animals, anesthetic agents such as ether will cause the same kind of pseudoneutropenia (Boggs, 1975).

MORPHOLOGIC ALTERATIONS IN NEUTROPHILS

In addition to quantitative changes, qualitative morphologic alterations also occur in neutrophils. Some of these, such as toxic granules or cytoplasmic vacuoles, are acquired and disappear after the stimulus which provoked them is gone. Others are hereditary and persist through life, with or without functional impairment. These are well illustrated and reviewed by Brunning (1970).

It should be noted that disorders of leukocyte function may exist without any structural abnormality detectable with the usual modes of morphologic examination. These are discussed on page 1044 and in Chapter 40.

Toxic Granulation. Toxic granules are dark blue to purple cytoplasmic granules in the metamyelocyte, band, or neutrophil stage. They are peroxidase positive and may be numerous or few in number; there may be less peroxidase activity in toxic than in normal neutrophils. Toxic granulation is found in severe infections or other toxic conditions (Plate 30-1A).

Normally neutrophil granules are tan to pink in color in neutrophil metamyelocytes, bands, and mature forms. Even the non-specific or azurophil granules which are dark blue on the promyelocyte stage normally lose their basophilia in the mature neutrophil, where they comprise about one third of the granules in the human. Toxic granules are azurophil granules that have retained their basophilic staining reaction by lack of maturation, or that have developed increased basophilia in the mature neutrophil. In addition, perhaps skipped divisions during the development of the neutrophil may result in a greater proportion of the granules being of the azurophil type. Increased basophilia of azurophil granules simulating toxic granules may occur in normal cells with prolonged staining time or decreased pH of the staining reaction (McCall, 1969; Bessis, 1973).

Irregular basophilia of the cytoplasm is also common in toxic conditions and appears to reflect impaired cytoplasmic maturation. If discrete, this focal basophilia is known as a Döhle inclusion body (v.i.).

Cytoplasmic vacuoles are also signs of toxic change if the possibility of degeneration artefacts can be eliminated by making films from fresh blood free of anticoagulant. Vacuoles imply that phagocytosis has occurred. One may also see irregular depletion of granules (Plate 30-1B).

Another toxic change in the neutrophil is

Plate 30-1. *A*, Toxic neutrophil, *left*, with cytoplasmic vacuoles and heavy azurophilic granules. Normal neutrophil, *center*. Lymphocyte, *right*. *B*, Toxic neutrophil. Partial degranulation, fusion of granules, vacuoles, and phagocytized diplococcus. Blood film from a patient with meningococcemia. *C*, May-Hegglin anomaly. Note the large pale blue inclusions at the outer margins of each neutrophil. *D*, Alder-Reilly anomaly, Hurler's syndrome. Deeply staining azurophilic granules almost obscure the nucleus of the neutrophil. The Alder-Reilly anomaly may be found in some cases of mucopolysaccharidosis (in which case the granules are usually metachromatic), or it may be found as a hereditary anomaly in apparently healthy persons. These cells resemble neutrophils with intense toxic granulation. *E*, Lymphocyte with basophilic inclusions surrounded by halos, characteristic of mucopolysaccharidosis. These inclusions are metachromatic. Peripheral blood film, Hurler's syndrome. *F*, Histiocyte or macrophage with numerous basophilic inclusions which are surrounded by clear spaces or halos. These granules are metachromatic and characteristic of mucopolysaccharidosis. Bone marrow film, Hurler's syndrome. *G*, Pelger-Huët anomaly, neutrophil. *H*, Chédiak-Higashi anomaly, band neutrophil. Neutrophil granules have fused into irregular masses which stain gray rather than tan. *I*, Chédiak-Higashi anomaly, lymphocyte. Azurophilic inclusions are much larger than azurophilic granules in lymphocytes of normal persons. *J*, Acute myelogenous leukemia. Several myeloblasts and one abnormal neutrophil myelocyte. *K*, Acute myelomonocytic leukemia. Blast, *left*; immature monocytes, *center* and *right*. *L*, Acute lymphocytic leukemia. The lymphoblasts have more nuclear irregularity and a higher nuclear to cytoplasmic ratio than myeloblasts.

3

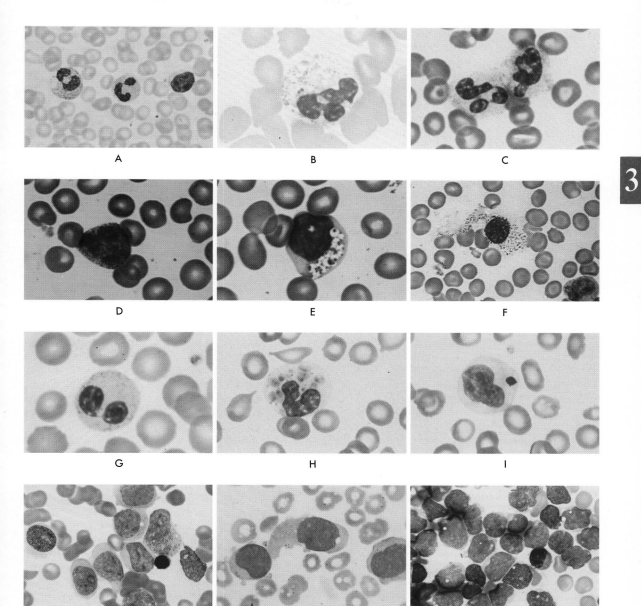

Plate 30–1. *See opposite page for legend.*

the occasional appearance of several sharp or blunt spicules extending out from the nucleus (see Plate 27-1*A*).

Döhle Inclusion Bodies. These are inclusions in the cytoplasm of polymorphonuclear neutrophils, which stain pale blue with Wright's stain. They are remnants of free ribosomes or rough surfaced endoplasmic reticulum persisting from an earlier stage of development (Bessis, 1973). The typical inclusion bodies are about the size of micrococci or a little larger; some of them are pear shaped; others appear as short rods or cocci lying in pairs. Smaller, discrete, punctiform granules are sometimes seen but do not have the same significance. Originally Döhle bodies were described as being especially prominent in scarlet fever, but they are seen in many other infectious diseases, in burns, in aplastic anemia, and following administration of toxic agents. Therefore, they frequently accompany toxic granulation in the neutrophil. With the light microscope, Döhle bodies resemble the inclusions seen in the May-Hegglin anomaly (Plate 30-1*C*).

May-Hegglin Anomaly. This is a rare autosomal dominant condition characterized by the presence of pale blue inclusions resembling Döhle bodies in neutrophils, giant platelets, and, in some persons, thrombocytopenia (Oski et al., 1962). The inclusions are larger and more prominent than the Döhle bodies found in infections (Plate 30-1*C*). They have been described in eosinophils, basophils, and monocytes as well as in neutrophils (Brunning, 1970). The blue staining of the inclusions can be abolished by prior treatment of the cells with ribonuclease. With electron microscopy, the appearance of the inclusions differs from that of Döhle bodies, suggesting structural alterations in RNA (Jenis, 1971).

Alder-Reilly Anomaly. Dense azurophilic granulation in all white blood cells was described by Alder in 1939 (Plate 30-1*D*). In neutrophils it may resemble toxic granulation but is unrelated to infection and is not transient. In 1940, Reilly described similar granulocytes in some but not all patients with gargoylism (the Hurler syndrome or, more generally, the genetic mucopolysaccharidoses). Other observations have shown that the heavy granulation in neutrophils can occur either as a feature of the genetic mucopolysaccharidoses or independently in otherwise healthy persons (Brunning, 1970).

Occurring more often than the Alder-Reilly anomaly in the genetic mucopolysaccharidoses is a metachromatic inclusion in the lymphocytes surrounded by a clear space (Plate 30-1*E*). Macrophages in the marrow frequently contain similar granulation (Plate 30-1*F*). This group of disorders is inherited and is characterized by deficiencies or derangement in various lysosomal enzymes required for degrading mucopolysaccharides. The result is abnormal deposition and storage of mucopolysaccharides in multiple organs. Skeletal abnormalities are prominent (Groover, 1972; McKusick, 1978).

Pelger-Huët Anomaly. This hereditary, autosomal dominant condition involves failure of normal segmentation of granulocytic nuclei. Most nuclei are band shaped or have two segments but no more (Plate 30-1*G*). The chromatin is quite coarse, and these are not normal young band forms. When a large number of band neutrophils appear in the differential count in a patient without infection or other cause, careful analysis of the smear of the patient and of family members will occasionally establish the presence of the Pelger-Huët anomaly.

A similar appearing, acquired disorder of nuclear segmentation in granulocytes may occasionally be found in cases of granulocytic leukemia, myeloproliferative disorders, some infections, and after exposure to certain drugs (Brunning, 1970); this is sometimes called the pseudo-Pelger anomaly. In addition to the band forms and neutrophils with only two segments, mature cells with round non-segmented nuclei and coarse chromatin are common, in contrast to the congenital Pelger-Huët anomaly.

Chediak-Higashi Syndrome. This rare, autosomal recessive disorder is characterized by partial albinism, photophobia, abnormally large granules in leukocytes and other granule-containing cells, and frequent pyogenic infections. An accelerated lymphoma-like phase occurs, with lymphadenopathy, hepatosplenomegaly, and pancytopenia; lymphoid infiltrates are widespread and death ensues at an early age (Blume, 1972). Granulocytes, monocytes, and lymphocytes contain giant granules (Plate 30-1*H* and *I*) which appear to be abnormal lysosomes (White, 1967). Leukocyte functional abnormalities exist (Stossel, 1977).

FUNCTIONAL DISORDERS OF NEUTROPHILS

Inherited and acquired disorders affecting leukocytes may result in abnormal function and consequent susceptibility to infections

(Stossel, 1977). Often, the leukocytes are normal in number and in morphologic appearance.

Deficiencies of humoral factors (antibodies; components of complement) may result in defective chemotaxis or opsonization. Cellular abnormalities (contractile protein dysfunction; enzyme deficiencies) may result in defects in chemotaxis, phagocytosis, or microbial killing.

These disorders are discussed in Chapter 40.

EOSINOPHILIA

Eosinophilia exists if blood eosinophils exceed 0.35×10^9/l when direct chamber counts are used, or 0.5×10^9/l when the count is calculated from the 100 or 200 cell differential and the total leukocyte count. The eosinophils in the blood come from the marrow; those in the tissues come from the blood.

Allergic Diseases. Allergic and atopic conditions such as bronchial asthma and seasonal rhinitis (hay fever) are characterized by eosinophilia. These immune reactions are mediated by IgE, which results in mast cell and basophil degranulation with the release of a chemotactic factor for eosinophils. Eosinophils are found in the blood, marrow, sputum (in bronchial asthma), and in nasal and conjunctival discharges (in hay fever). Blood eosinophilia is usually only mild or moderate (0.4 to 1.0×10^9/l).

In asthma, absolute eosinophil counts have been useful in management because the level of eosinophils positively correlates with pulmonary performance, indicates the adequacy of steroid therapy, and may indicate the presence of complicating infections (Beeson, 1977).

Skin Disorders. Atopic dermatitis and eczema are often accompanied by blood eosinophilia, especially in children. In pemphigus, eosinophilia is characteristic. Eosinophilia is frequently associated with acute urticarial reactions but is uncommon in chronic urticaria.

Parasitic Infestations. Eosinophilia is more pronounced if tissues are invaded (for example, trichinosis) than when parasites are inhabiting the lumen of a viscus (for example, tapeworm). The role of free exchange of tissue fluids (metabolic continuity) is evident by disappearance of eosinophilia in some forms of infestation when encystment occurs (for example, cysticerosis).

In trichinosis eosinophils begin to rise in the blood within days after infection. The peak of the eosinophilia, from 40 to 60 per cent, is during the third or fourth weeks.

Leukocytosis and eosinophilia extending over months are seen in visceral larva migrans (dog and cat round worm) infestation. In this condition pulmonary lesions (Loeffler's syndrome) may be present.

Another parasitic infestation with eosinophilia is creeping eruption caused by larvae of the dog or cat hookworm.

Eosinophilia may be absent in severe infestations with trichinae. The prognosis in such cases seems aggravated.

Infectious Diseases. Eosinophilia of various degrees is seen in some infectious diseases. Scarlet fever is one. It has a cutaneous rash, probably of allergic nature, and eosinophilia is common. Chorea may be associated with eosinophilia, but other forms of rheumatic fever are not.

In conditions characterized by neutrophilia, eosinophilia is uncommon; often this may be on the basis of increased adrenal corticosteroid secretion in disease. This is well shown in the disappearance of eosinophilia when a lesion that is responsible for eosinophilia (for example, echinococcus cyst) becomes infected, suppurates, and is followed by neutrophilia. The same phenomenon is also observed in acute infections (for example, pneumococcus pneumonia).

It is in infectious diseases that the depression of eosinophilia is particularly noticeable.

Pulmonary Eosinophilias

Loeffler's syndrome is characterized by repeated, transient pulmonary exudates accompanied by cough, often producing sputum which contains eosinophils. The syndrome resolves in a few weeks. It may be caused by certain drugs, inhaled antigens, or helminth (round worm) infestation during periods of dissemination when the parasites pass from the blood into the alveoli of the lung.

The *P.I.E.* syndrome (pulmonary infiltration with eosinophilia) refers to a more severe disorder characterized by fever, cough, dyspnea, and other symptoms. Etiology may be bacterial, viral, or fungal infection, allergic reaction to drugs, or parasitic infestations. The difference from Loeffler's syndrome appears to be one of severity (Wintrobe, 1974).

Tropical pulmonary eosinophilia is a syndrome of paroxysmal cough and bronchospasm associated with marked eosinophilia. It is found mainly in India, Southeast Asia, and the South Pacific. There is a predilection for males and for Indians, among racial groups living in an endemic area. Serum IgE levels are very high. Interestingly, epinephrine induces a rise instead of a fall in blood eosinophils (Beeson, 1977). The disease is caused by microfilariae, which may be found occasionally in lung or lymph node biopsies, but not in blood. The patients have a high titer of filarial complement-fixing antibodies in the blood. Response to the antifilarial drug diethylcarbamazine is curative (Marsden, 1975).

Hypereosinophilic Syndrome. Persistent high levels of eosinophils for long periods of time, no evidence of known causes of eosinophilia, and signs and symptoms of organ involvement are criteria for inclusion of patients in this syndrome (Chusid, 1975). The organ most consistently affected is the heart, with mural thrombi and endocardial and myocardial fibrosis. Hepatosplenomegaly is common. Poor prognostic signs are leukocytosis over $100 \times 10^9/l$, circulating myeloblasts, and leukemic markers such as elevated serum vitamin B_{12}, basophilia, low neutrophil alkaline phosphatase, and chromosomal abnormalities. Chusid, (1975) believes that most patients have a hypersensitivity reaction of some type; it is an open question whether some patients have a form of eosinophilic leukemia (p. 1070). Regardless of cause, large numbers of circulating eosinophils appear to damage the heart by some unknown mechanism.

Blood Diseases. In chronic myelogenous leukemia and, to a lesser extent, in other myeloproliferative disorders eosinophilia is common. Mild eosinophilia may be found in marrow and blood in pernicious anemia.

Other Conditions. Splenectomy is frequently followed by eosinophilia and lymphocytosis. Neutrophilia, if previously present, recedes. This may last for several months.

There is no satisfactory explanation for occasional instances of moderate and even severe eosinophilia, general or local, in patients with various neoplasms and a variety of other conditions (for example, ovarian cysts.). Eosinophilia is seen more frequently in neoplasms involving serous surfaces and bone and in those with necrosis. In Hodgkin's disease, the majority of patients do not have blood eosinophilia, though when present it is sometimes marked in degree (Beeson, 1977).

Various drugs have been reported to be responsible for eosinophilia: pilocarpine, physostigmine, digitalis, para-aminosalicylic acid, sulfonamides, and others. On the other hand, atropine is supposed to depress the eosinophils.

Hereditary eosinophilia occurs rarely in the absence of other recognized causes of eosinophilia (Naiman, 1964).

EOSINOPENIA

Eosinopenia is a decreased level of circulating eosinophils, below the lowest reference value of $0.04 \times 10^9/l$. In order to be detected, large numbers of cells must be counted, using direct hemacytometer counts (p. 875) or automated counts with an instrument such as the Hemalog D (p. 909).

Eosinopenia occurs in any situation that results in acute stress, due to adrenal glucocorticoid and epinephrine secretion (either causes eosinopenia), and also in acute inflammatory states. A rapid decrease in circulating eosinophils occurs due to margination or migration into inflammatory sites. Release of eosinophils from the marrow is temporarily inhibited, and later eosinophil production is inhibited. Once the acute process subsides, immune stimulation of eosinophil production may occur; this is mediated by T lymphocytes (Beeson, 1977). Eosinopenia of 0 to $0.03 \times 10^9/l$ also may occur in Cushing's syndrome, which is a chronic overproduction of adrenal glucocorticoids.

Following parenteral administration of adrenocorticotropic hormone (ACTH), an increased output of adrenal glucocorticoids results in eosinopenia. This is the basis of a test for adrenocortical function (Thorn, 1948). Absence of a significant drop in eosinophils after ACTH administration is interpreted as evidence of adrenocortical insufficiency. This test has been replaced by direct measurements of hormones (Chap. 14).

BASOPHILIA

Basophilia is an increase of basophils in the blood to a level above $0.2 \times 10^9/l$ if calculated from the differential count and the total leukocyte count, and above $0.08 \times 10^9/l$ if counted directly in a hemacytometer chamber or with the Hemalog D (Gilbert, 1975).

Basophilia is seen most frequently in allergic reactions, chronic granulocytic leukemia, myeloid metaplasia (extramedullary myelopoiesis), and polycythemia vera. Relative basophilia may be transient following irradiation. Basophilia may be present in hypothyroidism and chronic hemolytic anemia and following splenectomy.

BASOPENIA

A decreased basophil count (less than $0.01 \times 10^9/l$) can be detected only when large numbers of basophils are counted directly. With direct basophil counting, it has been determined that basophils, like eosinophils, show diurnal variation. The level is lowest in the morning and highest during the night. Sustained treatment with adrenal glucocorticoids induces a basopenia. Acute infection or stress results in a fall in basophils. About half of patients with hyperthyroidism have a basopenia (Gilbert, 1975).

MONOCYTOSIS

Monocytosis is an increase of monocytes above the upper reference value, usually $1.0 \times 10^9/l$ (Table 27–3).

Monocytosis is present during the recovery stage from acute infections and from agranulocytosis, where it is considered a favorable sign. In contrast, an increase of monocytes in tuberculosis is a poor prognostic sign.

Monocytosis may be present in subacute bacterial endocarditis. In this condition monocytes may show phagocytosis of other blood cells, red blood cells, and leukocytes. It may be present in mycotic, rickettsial, protozoal, and viral infections.

Infectious disease, however, is an uncommon cause of monocytosis. Maldonado and Hanlon (1965) reviewed 160 successive cases of absolute monocytosis at the Mayo Clinic. Over half (85) were associated with *hematologic disease:* 20 had monocytic or granulocytic leukemia; 20 had lymphoma (Hodgkin's disease was most frequent); 7 had multiple myeloma; 6 had myeloproliferative disorders; and, in 18, the cause was indeterminate. *Malignant disease* accounted for 13 cases; *connective tissue disorders*, 16; *infectious disease*, 9; *fever of unknown origin*, 7; *ulcerative colitis*, 4; *regional enteritis*, 4; *non-tropical sprue*, 2; and *cirrhosis*, 3 cases. *Miscellaneous and indeterminate causes* made up the remaining 17 cases. Among hematopoietic dysplasias, an unexplained monocytosis occasionally seems to precede the development of leukemia by months or years (p. 1075).

MONOCYTOPENIA

A decrease in circulating monocytes below the lower reference value of $0.2 \times 10^9/l$ is a monocytopenia. Few studies have dealt with monocytopenia, because of (1) the large number of cells that must be counted in a differential in order to obtain reliable counts; (2) the distributional bias of wedge blood film for monocytes compared with the spinner-made blood film (p. 891); and (3) the unavailability, until recently, of automation allowing large numbers of cells to be counted routinely (Hemalog D, p. 909).

During therapy with prednisone, monocytes fall during the first few hours after the first dose, but return to above original levels by 12 hours (Rinehart, 1975). Profound monocytopenia (0 to $0.017 \times 10^9/l$) has been observed in one study of five cases of leukemic reticuloendotheliosis or hairy cell leukemia (Seshadri, 1976). Appearance of monocytes in inflammatory exudates ("skin windows") was absent or reduced. These findings could be related to the increased susceptibility to infection in hairy cell leukemia.

LYMPHOCYTOSIS

Lymphocytes in normal individuals (see also Chapters 36, 38, and 39).

In normal individuals the absolute numbers of lymphocytes and T cells are highest at birth (Fig. 30–1). At this time, lymphocytes represent approximately 90 per cent of all leukocytes (Andersen, 1974). During the first three to seven days of life there is a slight decrease in the number of lymphocytes. However, during the second week of life, the lymphocyte count returns to the level observed at birth. Cellular immune function in the newborn is comparable to that in normal adults (Carr, 1974; Ceppellini, 1971).

During the first decade of life, the absolute lymphocyte count and the absolute number of T cells decrease but remain higher than observed in the adult. By the time of adolescence, the absolute lymphocyte count and the absolute number of T cells have leveled off at values observed throughout adulthood. The absolute number of B-lymphocytes remains stable during all stages of life (Davey, 1977). In adolescence and adulthood, lymphocytes constitute about 20 to 40 per cent of all leukocytes or 1.5 to 4.0×10^9 cells per liter (p. 891).

There is some disagreement regarding the

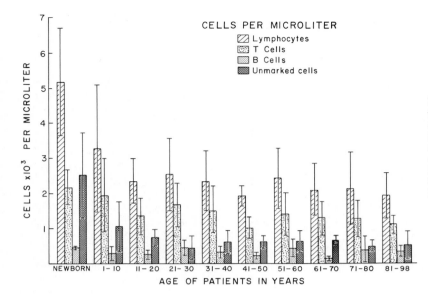

Figure 30–1. Absolute counts of total lymphocytes, T cells, B cells, and unmarked cells (non-T, non-B) in normal individuals at different ages, by decade. (From Davey, F. R., and Huntington, S.: Age-related variation in lymphocyte subpopulations. Gerontology, 23:381, 1977. Basel, S. Karger AG. Used by permission.)

absolute number of lymphocytes and number of T cells in aged individuals. Although some studies (Diaz-Jouanen, 1975; Smith, 1974) indicate that there is a decrease in total lymphocyte count and T cell numbers, other investigators find no significant change in total lymphocytes or T cells in aged individuals (Davey, 1977; Weksler, 1974). Elderly individuals have depressed delayed skin reactivity (Waldorf, 1968). In addition, lymphocytes from elderly individuals respond poorly to mitogens (Hallgren, 1974) and to allogenic lymphocytes (Weksler, 1974). Serum immunoglobulins, an index of B cell activity, are not reduced in the elderly (p. 1229). In fact, aged individuals have a higher frequency of anti–smooth muscle, antimitochondrial, antiparietal cell, antinuclear, rheumatoid, and lymphocytotoxic antibodies (p. 1263) (Ooi, 1974; Waldorf, 1968).

Lymphocytosis

Lymphocytosis is an increase in the number of lymphocytes in the peripheral blood; the reference intervals are 1.5 to 4.0 $\times$ 10^9/l in the adult and 1.5 to 8.8 $\times$ 10^9/l in the child. Relative lymphocytosis (an increase in the percentage of lymphocytes) is present in various conditions and is especially prominent in disorders with neutropenia.

Infectious lymphocytosis

This infectious and contagious disease, described by C. H. Smith (1941), is characterized by lymphocytosis and occurs mainly in children. The incubation period is 12 to 21 days.

Antibody and viral studies have indicated a relationship between infectious lymphocytosis and Coxsackie A virus (Horowitz, 1968), Coxsackie B6 virus (Nkrumah, 1973), ECHO viruses (Mandal, 1973) and adenovirus type 12 (Olson, 1964). No association has been noted with Epstein-Barr virus, cytomegalovirus, or herpes virus (Blacklow, 1970). Although the disease usually has no systemic manifestations, sometimes vomiting, fever, abdominal discomfort, signs suggesting involvement of the nervous system, cutaneous rashes, upper respiratory infections, and diarrhea occur. Leukocytosis (20 to 50 $\times$ 10^9/l, sometimes over 100 $\times$ 10^9/l) usually precedes the clinical manifestations. From 60 to 95 per cent of blood leukocytes are mature, small lymphocytes. In contrast to infectious mononucleosis, atypical lymphocytes (p. 1051) are uncommon. There is usually an eosinophilia. The lymphocytosis usually lasts three to five weeks, sometimes longer. Other blood changes are unusual. The marrow has no characteristic changes; an increased percentage of lymphocytes has been observed but is probably an artifact due to admixture of peripheral blood. Lymph node enlargement is rare and minimal when present. The spleen and liver are rarely if ever enlarged. Lymph node biopsy may show reactive follicular hyperplasia but no characteristic changes.

The tests for infectious mononucleosis (p.

1052) are negative. In some cases there has been an increase of white cells in the cerebrospinal fluid, with about 40 per cent lymphocytes. The course is benign.

Another form of infectious lymphocytosis in children has a chronic course. The leukocyte count is 10 to 25 × 10⁹/l with 60 to 80 per cent lymphocytes of normal appearance. Slight eosinophilia, monocytosis, and plasmacytosis are also present. As a rule, the children have enlargement of tonsils, lymph nodes, and spleen and a history of recurrent upper respiratory infections. The marrow shows no abnormalities.

Pertussis

Whooping cough (pertussis) occurs during childhood, especially in unimmunized children. The etiologic agent is *Bordetella pertussis* (hemophilus pertussis) which produces an inflammatory reaction of the entire respiratory tract.

The incubation period is approximately two weeks, and the first symptoms are those of a head cold. Later the patient develops paroxysms of coughing productive of thick sputum. There is frequently pain over trachea and bronchi (Brooksaler, 1967).

Patients frequently develop significant lymphocytosis. Counts higher than 30 × 10⁹/l have been recorded. The lymphocytes are small and mature. The lymphocyte count is highest during the first three weeks of the illness, then decreases during the fourth and subsequent weeks (Lagergren, 1963). The lymphocytosis is due to the release of lymphocytosis-promoting factor (LPF) from the organism. LPF causes a transient increased mobilization of lymphocytes from lymphoid organs followed by inhibition of recirculation of lymphocytes from blood into the lymph flow. Thus, the lymphocytosis is due to a redistribution of lymphocytes into the peripheral circulation without increased lymphopoiesis (Rai, 1971; Morse, 1970).

The diagnosis depends on identification of *B. pertussis*, cultured on Bordet-Gengou agar (p. 1625).

Infectious mononucleosis

Infectious mononucleosis is usually a self-limited infectious disease of the reticuloendothelial tissue produced by an infection with Epstein-Barr virus, a member of the herpes group. The disorder most frequently involves adolescent children and young adults. It has characteristic clinical, hematologic, and pathologic features and specific serologic alterations.

Etiology. Strong serologic and epidemiologic evidence now implicates the Epstein-Barr virus (EBV) as the cause of infectious mononucleosis (IM) (Henle, 1974). The EBV was originally found in cell culture of Burkitt's lymphoma. High titers of antibody to EBV are found in the serum of patients with Burkitt's lymphoma and carcinoma of the postnasal space.

Antibodies to EBV are consistently present in heterophil-positive IM. The EBV antibody is absent from serum prior to the development of IM. In several prospective studies only individuals without EBV antibody developed typical IM (Evans, 1977). All of these individuals later developed antibody to EBV in their sera during the course of the disease. IM does not occur in individuals with a low titer of antibody to EBV. About 10 per cent of adults and an even greater proportion of pediatric patients with IM have no heterophil antibody, but most have antibody to EBV (Henle, 1973). EBV has been isolated from the throats of patients with IM (Golden, 1971; Miller, 1973). Virus excretion may persist for prolonged periods of time. In addition, blood transfusions have resulted in the development of EBV-positive IM in individuals previously known not to have EBV antibodies (Carter, 1969).

Finally, heterophil and EBV antibodies have been produced in squirrel monkeys previously inoculated with EB virus-transformed autologous leukocytes (Shope, 1973).

The EBV is apparently spread to susceptible individuals through oral contact. When EBV gets into the mouth of a previously unexposed individual, it infects B-lymphocytes in the lymphoid tissue of the oral pharynx. Generalized disease occurs either as a result of a viremia with EBV traveling to B cell sites in other lymphoid tissues or as a result of EBV-infected B cells from the oral pharynx traveling to other lymphoid tissues (Epstein, 1977). During the acute phase of the disease, afflicted individuals develop antibodies to the viral capsid antigen, membrane antigen, and EBV-determined nuclear antigen. Some antibodies appear only transiently, whereas other antibodies remain for life.

Within the first week of the illness the patient develops a lymphocytosis. The atypical lymphocytes are due to changes in both B and

T cells. B-lymphocytes are transformed early in the disease owing to the direct effects of the EBV (Mangi, 1974). It appears that B cells bear receptors for EBV (Jondal, 1973). Later on, T cells form atypical lymphocytes as a response to neoantigen on the surface of B cells (Evans, 1974). The EBV induces the formation of a lymphocyte-detected membrane antigen which appears to be recognized by killer T cells (Rickinson, 1977). Thus, the B cell, infected with EBV, is responsible for the generation of activated T cells in the blood and in all the lymphoreticular system, resulting in a lymphocytosis, lymphadenopathy, and splenomegaly. Resolution of the illness is due in part to the elimination of infected B cells by the killer T cells. In addition, virus-neutralizing antibodies and T-lymphocytes reduce the number of productively infected cells in the oropharynx.

Clinical Features. The disease has been observed in patients from three months to 70 years of age but is most common in adolescents and young adults. The onset is vague, indefinite, and similar to the onset of other infectious diseases. Patients usually have fever, sore throat, and lymphadenopathy. They may also experience chills, sweats, headache, dizziness, malaise, retro-orbital aching, irritation, and prostration (Table 30-3).

The lymph node enlargement is usually moderate in degree. Cervical lymph nodes are most often the first to be enlarged; other regions, including mediastinal and inguinal, are then affected. The lymphadenopathy usually has regressed by three weeks. Splenomegaly is common. The spleen is usually tender to palpation, and the enlargement persists for a long time. The liver is less frequently enlarged. A rash may be observed in 3 to 6 per cent of patients. If ampicillin is administered, 69 to 100 per cent of patients may develop a rash (Karzon, 1976).

Relapses are not uncommon. Occasionally there may be several, and some may be more severe than the original attack.

Complications. Severe inflammatory and ulcerative lesions of the pharynx and laryngeal edema may occur and produce extreme dyspnea. Tracheostomy may be needed as a lifesaving operation.

Of the rare anemias associated with infectious mononucleosis, hemolytic anemia is the most common, occurring in 1 to 3 per cent of cases. The cause now appears to be related to the anti-i antibody produced frequently in this disease (Worlledge, 1969).

Mild thrombocytopenia occurs in about half the cases, but the platelet count is not often less than $100 \times 10^9/l$. Thrombocytopenic purpura with hemorrhagic complications is exceedingly rare (Sharp, 1969).

Rupture of the spleen may occur in the acute stage of the disease. Prompt recognition and immediate surgical intervention may be lifesaving.

Involvement of the liver demonstrable by biopsy is common in infectious mononucleosis. Abnormal liver function tests indicative of hepatitis occur in 85 to 100 per cent of patients. Usually there is a rise in the serum alkaline phosphatase, lactate dehydrogenase, alanine aminotransferase (ALT), and aspartate aminotransferase (AST). Mild hyperbilirubinemia up to $51\mu mol/l$ (3 mg/dl) has been noted in 30 to 50 per cent of patients (Finch, 1969). Clinical jaundice is rare, but cases have been reported in which jaundice and acute

Table 30-3. CLINICAL FINDINGS IN 106 CASES OF INFECTIOUS MONONUCLEOSIS

	NO. CASES	PER CENT		NO. CASES	PER CENT
Lymphadenopathy	101	95.3	Skin rash	5	4.7
Fever	93	87.7	Epistaxis	3	2.8
Pharyngitis	64	60.4	Icterus	3	2.8
without membrane	50	47.2	Loss of weight	2	1.9
with membrane	14	13.2	Diarrhea	2	1.9
Splenomegaly	51	48.1	Arthritic pains	2	1.9
Headache	26	24.5	Purpura	2	1.9
Hepatomegaly	24	22.6	Gingivitis	2	1.9
Prostration	11	10.4	Convulsions	1	0.9
Emesis	10	9.4	Toothache	1	0.9
Pain in abdomen	8	7.6	Albuminuria	14	13.2
upper abdomen	6	5.7	Positive test for syphilis	3	2.8
lower abdomen	2	1.9	Relapses (17 days to 2 months)	7	6.5
Stiffness or pain in neck	6	5.7	Recurrence (1 year)	1	0.9

pharyngitis were the only clinical manifestations of infectious mononucleosis, with positive hematologic and serologic findings. The jaundice is, as a rule, hepatocellular, with elevation of both conjugated and non-conjugated serum bilirubin, bilirubinuria, and elevated urine urobilinogen.

Other complications include superimposed infection with pyogenic bacteria and development of sinusitis, otitis, and bronchopneumonia. Approximately one third of patients with IM carry beta-hemolytic streptococci in the pharynx. Thus one should give attention to strict clinical, hematologic, and serologic criteria in distinguishing IM from streptococcal pharyngitis.

Hematologic Features. Leukocytes are increased, usually ranging from 12 to $25 \times 10^9/l$. Rarely, counts as high as $80 \times 10^9/l$ have been recorded. The leukocytosis is usually due to lymphocytosis (60 to 90 per cent) composed of a variety of atypical lymphocytes (Wood, 1967). The total leukocyte count, as a rule, returns to normal within three weeks. The atypical lymphocytes are the result of an increase in the amount and basophilia of cytoplasm and nuclear alterations.

Nuclear changes are characterized by an increased density of the chromatin and by changes in shape. They show deep indentations and many are lobated ("leukocytoid lymphocytes", Downey type I; Plate 30-2*E*). The cytoplasm shows basophilia, an increase of azurophilic granules, and frequently marked vacuolar degeneration. Some cells resemble plasma cells; some have nucleoli. Some cells resemble monocytes (monocytoid deviation). Cells which have a relatively smooth but still mature nucleus and abundant smooth cytoplasm with patchy peripheral and radial basophilia have been called "stress" lymphocytes or Downey type II (Plate 30-2*A* to *D*). They are often the most numerous. Occasionally lymphocytes have transformed into blast-like cells, presumably in response to the viral stimulation. These immature lymphocytes, usually representing only a small percentage of the total lymphocyte count, are large reticular lymphocytes (non-leukemic lymphoblasts) with a coarsely reticular nucleus and abundant deeply basophilic cytoplasm (Downey type III; Plate 30-2*C* and *G*; Plate 28-3*J* and *K*). In contrast, lymphoblasts of acute lymphocytic leukemia are usually smaller, with a very fine chromatin pattern and very little cytoplasm (Plate 30-1*L*, 30-2*H*, 30-3*G*) (Downey, 1923).

Not infrequently the number of monocytes rises transiently. The term mononucleosis refers to an increase of lymphocytes and not monocytes.

The cytologic alterations are not pathognomonic of IM. Similar cells are found in a variety of disorders including cytomegalovirus mononucleosis, toxoplasmosis, infectious hepatitis, and usually to a lesser extent in viral pneumonia, varicella, mumps, and viral exanthemas of children.

Neutrophils are relatively and absolutely decreased in most cases during the first week of illness. During this time there may be a shift to the left, with an increase of band cells and metamyelocytes. Toxic granules and Döhle bodies may be seen. The eosinophils are within normal limits.

The bone marrow from patients with IM usually shows an increased cellularity (Boyd, 1968). There is an increased number of lymphocytes, macrophages, plasma cells, megakaryocytes, and erythroid cells. The neutrophilic series appears decreased. About half of the cases may have collections of mononuclear cells forming loose granulomas (Hovde, 1950).

Early in the illness, the histopathology of lymph node cells usually shows a follicular hyperplasia with prominent germinal centers. In addition, there is intense hyperplasia of the interfollicular area. Throughout the follicle and especially at the margin of the germinal centers are large stimulated lymphocytes. Mitoses are frequent. Peripheral sinuses are filled with collections of histiocytes, mononuclear cells, and large stimulated lymphocytes. There may be lymphocytic infiltration of the capsule. The medullary cords are obscured and plasma cell elements do not appear increased. Blood vessels are prominent and endothelial cells are swollen and assume an epithelium-like appearance (Gall, 1940). Reed-Sternberg-like cells may also be present (Lukes, 1969). During later stages, hyperplasia of the follicles and paracortical areas is less pronounced and sinuses are less crowded. Medullary cords appear within normal limits (Carter, 1969).

In the spleen the capsule and trabeculae are edematous and are infiltrated with lymphocytes. The follicles are slightly increased in number and germinal centers are not prominent. Large stimulated lymphocytes, mononuclear cells, and small lymphocytes infiltrate the sinuses and cords. In addition, there are marked congestion and sometimes hemor-

Table 30–4. HIGH SHEEP CELL AGGLUTININ TITERS REPORTED IN CONDITIONS OTHER THAN INFECTIOUS MONONUCLEOSIS*

TITERS	CONDITIONS
56	Upper limit of normal.
112	Aplastic anemia, polycythemia, agranulocytosis, splenic thrombocytopenia, thyrotoxicosis, chronic nephritis.
224	Hodgkin's disease, myelogenous leukemia, staphylococcal infections.
448	Sarcoma, infectious hepatitis, tuberculosis.
896	Acute leukemia, injection of liver extract or blood group substance A.
3584	Monocytic leukemia, serum sickness.

*From Davidsohn, I., and Lee, C. L.: The clinical serology of infectious mononucleosis. *In* Carter, R. L., and Penman, H. G. (eds.): Infectious Mononucleosis. Oxford, Blackwell Scientific Publications, 1969. Used by permission.

rhages in the red pulp. Lymphoid infiltrates are present within trabecular vessels (Carter, 1969).

The prominent findings in the liver include an infiltrate of lymphoid and mononuclear cells in the portal areas and to a lesser extent in the lobular sinusoids. Kupffer cells are swollen. Hepatic cells usually show insignificant pathologic alterations (Finkel, 1964).

Serological Findings

HETEROPHIL ANTIBODY. Paul (1932) first described the presence of sheep cell agglutinins in the sera of patients with IM. Unfortunately, the presence of sheep cell agglutinins is not a specific finding for IM and can be present in other disorders (Table 30–4). Davidsohn (1937) demonstrated that the heterophil antibody in patients with IM differed from those seen in other illnesses by being absorbed with beef erythrocytes. In addition, heterophil antibodies present in conditions listed in Table 30–4 can be absorbed by Forssman antigen such as found in guinea pig kidney. The differential (Paul-Bunnell-Davidsohn) test is highly specific for IM. Only rare false positives have been reported. Less than 10 per cent of typical cases of IM are heterophil negative; in these, the diagnosis must be substantiated by the presence of antibody to EBV. Heterophil antibodies are considered IgM immunoglobulins (Davidsohn, 1969). The spot test for heterophil antibodies is a rapid differential test (p. 1087).

EPSTEIN-BARR VIRUS ANTIBODIES. Several antibodies are produced by the host in response to a variety of EBV antigens (Karzon, 1976) (Table 30–5). Antibody to the viral capsid antigen arises within the first two weeks of the onset. This antibody is measured by an immunofluorescent method and is probably the most widely used assay for determining exposure to EBV. Assaying for the presence of EBV antibody is usually limited to the few cases of heterophil negative IM.

OTHER SEROLOGIC REACTIONS. In addition to heterophil and EBV antibodies, patients with IM frequently produce antibodies to a wide variety of antigens. Antibodies against human erythrocytes, leukocytes, and platelets have been described. Patients with IM have an increased frequency of cold agglutinins. Positive tests to rheumatoid factor and antinuclear factor have been reported. There are elevated titers against a variety of organisms including *Proteus, Salmonella, Streptococcus* MG, *Listeria monocytogenes*, and Newcastle disease virus (Davidsohn, 1969).

Plate 30–2. *A,* Infectious mononucleosis. All the photographs of the lymphocytes of infectious mononucleosis are from patients with characteristic clinical findings and with positive differential tests. The lymphocyte is larger than any normal so-called large lymphocyte. The cytoplasm is abundant, clear, and moderately basophilic, especially close to the edges of the cell; red azure granules are accumulated along the upper periphery. The cytoplasm is delicate, and the surrounding red cells leave an indentation in the cytoplasm, giving it a scalloped appearance. The nucleus is oval, and the chromatin is delicate and less dense than in normal large lymphocytes. Three nucleoli are seen clearly. The two red cells adjacent on the right made indentations, even in the nucleus, suggesting that it is plastic. There is a light perinuclear zone. The characteristic lymphocytes in infectious mononucleosis are called atypical lymphocytes. *B,* Atypical lymphocyte, infectious mononucleosis. Notice sharp separation of nuclear chromatin and parachromatin, and basophilic cytoplasm. *C,* Reticular lymphocyte, (non-leukemic lymphoblast), *left;* atypical lymphocyte with greater nuclear maturity, *right.* Infectious mononucleosis. *D,* Atypical lymphocyte, *center;* normal lymphocyte, *right.* Infectious mononucleosis. *E,* Atypical lymphocyte with "leukocytoid" nucleus. Infectious mononucleosis. *F,* Normal monocyte. *G,* Reticular lymphocyte (non-leukemic lymphoblast); infectious mononucleosis. The nuclear chromatin is uniform and granular (or reticular). Nucleoli are conspicuous. The cytoplasm is deeply basophilic. Note the difference between this cell and the lymphoblast of acute leukemia (*H*). *H,* Lymphoblast, acute lymphocytic leukemia.

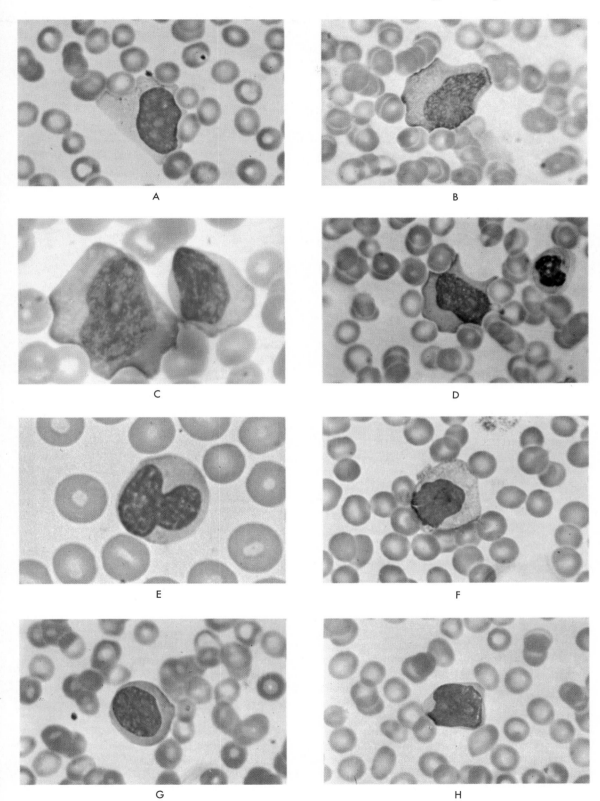

Plate 30–2. *See legend on opposite page.*

Table 30–5. MEASUREMENT OF ANTIBODIES TO EBV*

ANTIGEN	DETECTION SYSTEM†	TIME OF APPEARANCE	PERSISTENCE
Viral capsid antigens (VCA)	IF	Early	IgM—temporary IgG—life
Early antigen (EA): Diffuse (D)	IF	Early (80–85%)	Temporary
Restricted (R)	IF	Late (rare)	Temporary
Cell membrane antigen (MA)	IF	Intermediate	Life
Nuclear antigen (EBNA)	IF (anti-C')	Delayed	Life
Neutralizing	Neut.	Intermediate	Life
CF (Soluble or S)	CF	Delayed	Life
(Viral or V)	CF	? Early	? Life

*From Karzon, D. T.: Infectious mononucleosis. *In* Schulman, I., et al. (eds.): Advances in Pediatrics, vol. 22. Copyright © 1976 by Year Book Medical Publishers, Inc., Chicago. Used by permission.

†IF = immunofluorescence
CF = complement fixation

Differential Diagnosis. The clinical, hematologic, and serologic features of IM permit an accurate diagnosis to be made in over 90 per cent of the cases. When the spot test is negative, the test tube differential test may be done (Davidsohn, 1974). When this test is negative, one must consider several possibilities. The patient could still have EBV antibody-positive but heterophil-negative IM. However, cytomegalovirus infection is the most common cause of heterophil-negative mononucleosis. Other possibilities include toxoplasmosis, infectious hepatitis, and ingestion of drugs (*p*-aminosalicylic acid, phenytoin (Dilantin), and diaminodiphenylsulfone).

Course. IM is a benign disorder and complications occur in less than 5 per cent of patients (Finch, 1969). Fatalities are extremely rare. The disorder usually resolves in three to four weeks.

Cytomegalovirus infection

Cytomegalovirus infection may produce a variety of clinical syndromes (Weller, 1971). In the newborn infant cytomegalovirus infection is associated with microcephaly, jaundice, hepatosplenomegaly, and sometimes bleeding. The virus can also produce a pneumonitis in immunosuppressed patients.

Some individuals infected with cytomegalovirus develop a syndrome identical to infectious mononucleosis. This disorder can occur following massive blood transfusions (posttransfusion mononucleosis) or spontaneously in previously healthy individuals (cytomegalovirus mononucleosis) (Foster, 1969; Klemola, 1969). The patient has fever, chills, profound malaise, and myalgia. There may be a sore throat (but not exudative pharyngitis) and lymphadenopathy. Occasionally splenomegaly is found, but hepatomegaly does not occur.

Leukocytosis is characteristic with absolute lymphocytosis. Usually 20 per cent or more of the leukocytes are atypical lymphocytes. Bone marrow aspirates have shown an increased number of normal lymphocytes and atypical lymphocytes. Hepatic enzymes are frequently abnormal. In a small percentage of afflicted patients, there may be an increased titer of cold agglutinins, rheumatoid factor, and antinuclear antibodies. There is no rise in heterophil, Epstein-Barr virus, or toxoplasma antibodies. The diagnosis is usually made by isolating the cytomegalovirus from urine or demonstrating a rise in antibody by the complement fixation or indirect hemagglutination techniques (Jordan, 1973).

Toxoplasmosis

Toxoplasmosis can also produce several clinical syndromes. In the infant toxoplasmosis is responsible for hydrocephalus or microcephaly, brain damage with cerebral calcification, and chorioretinitis.

In children and adults, toxoplasmosis can produce a disorder similar to infectious mononucleosis (Beverley, 1958). Patients present with fever, lymphadenopathy, and an increased number of atypical lymphocytes in the peripheral blood (Siim, 1951). Rarely is there splenomegaly. Pharyngitis and upper respiratory tract infection are usually absent.

The histopathology of lymph nodes is usually distinctive and correlates closely with elevated toxoplasma antibody titers (Dorfman, 1973). Biopsies of lymph nodes usually show

Table 30-6.   CAUSES OF LYMPHOCYTOSIS*

LYMPHOCYTOSIS ASSOCIATED WITH ATYPICAL LYMPHOCYTES			LYMPHOCYTOSIS ASSOCIATED WITH SMALL MATURE LYMPHOCYTES
Per Cent of White Cells Which Are Atypical Lymphocytes		Uncommon Causes	
> 20	< 20		
Infectious mononucleosis Infectious hepatitis "Post-transfusion" syndrome Cytomegalovirus infection *p*-aminosalicylic acid (PAS) hypersensitivity Phenytoin (Dilantin) and mephenytoin (Mesantoin) hypersensitivity	(a) Infections Mumps,† varicella,† rubeola, rubella, atypical pneumonia, herpes simplex, herpes zoster, roseola infantum, influenza,† other viral illnesses, tuberculosis,† rickettsialpox, brucellosis,† toxoplasmosis† (b) Radiation (c) Other Letterer-Siwe disease Agranulocytosis Lead intoxication Stress Leukemia and lymphoma†	Tertiary syphilis† Congenital syphilis† Smallpox Tetrachlorethane poisoning TNT poisoning Organic arsenical hypersensitivity Severe dermatitis herpetiformis	Infectious lymphocytosis Pertussis

*Modified from Wood, T.A., and Frenkel, E.P.: The atypical lymphocyte. Am. J. Med., *42*:923, 1967.
†Higher counts of atypical lymphocytes occasionally found.

reactive follicular hyperplasia; clusters of epithelioid histiocytes and germinal centers, cortical and paracortical areas; and distension of sinuses by monocytoid cells (Saxen, 1959). Bone marrow biopsies usually have no specific pathologic lesion.

The diagnosis is established by demonstrating an elevation of toxoplasma antibodies by the Sabin-Feldman dye test, fluorescent-antibody, or hemagglutination techniques (Feldman, 1968).

Miscellaneous causes of lymphocytosis

Numerous disorders have been associated with lymphocytosis. A partial listing of illnesses associated with relative or absolute lymphocytosis is provided in Table 30-6.

LYMPHOCYTOPENIA

Lymphocytopenia is an absolute lymphocyte count below $1.5 \times 10^9/l$ in adults and below $3.0 \times 10^9/l$ in children. A number of immunologic deficiency disorders which are genetically determined have lymphocytopenia along with various other immunologic defects of either humoral or cell-mediated immunity (Hoyer, 1968). Lymphocytopenia in these disorders is due to impaired lymphopoiesis. In-

creased levels of adrenocortical hormones, the administration of chemotherapeutic drugs, or irradiation will result in lymphocytopenia. Impaired drainage of the intestinal lymphatics with loss of lymphocytes into the intestines due to a number of causes has been implicated as a mechanism for lymphocytopenia. Though decreased cell-mediated immunity may be evident early in the course of Hodgkin's disease, lymphocytopenia occurs late, in advanced disease (Cassileth, 1972; Zacharski, 1971).

PLASMACYTOSIS

Plasma cells are not normally present in circulating blood. They are increased in a variety of chronic infections, in allergic states, in the presence of neoplasms, and in other conditions in which the serum gamma globulin is elevated. Plasma cells have also been recorded in the blood of patients with viral disorders, including rubella, measles, chicken pox, and mumps. They are moderately increased in cutaneous exanthemas, infectious mononucleosis, syphilis, subacute bacterial endocarditis, sarcoidosis, and collagen diseases. Their increase is usually linked with an increase in lymphocytes, monocytes, and eosinophils.

In the marrow, an average of 1 per cent of

plasma cells is present in adults. An increase beyond 4 per cent is significant; lower values are found in children (see Table 28-1). Increases up to 20 per cent of plasma cells may be found in a variety of conditions other than multiple myeloma, including metastatic carcinoma, chronic granulomatous infections, conditions linked with hypersensitivity, and following administration of cytotoxic drugs. They are often increased in aplastic anemia, but this is probably just a relative increase. On the other hand, they are decreased or absent in agammaglobulinemia.

FUNCTIONAL DISORDERS OF LYMPHOCYTES

Functional disorders of lymphocytes can be inherited or acquired. The immune deficiency may be due to a disorder in B cells, T cells, stem cells, suppressor cells, or a combination. The inherited functional disorders are discussed on page 1398.

Acquired functional abnormalities of lymphocytes are most frequently observed in lymphoid malignancies. Decreased B cell function is observed in chronic lymphocytic leukemia in which two thirds of the patients have hypogammaglobulinemia. In multiple myeloma there is a diminished synthesis of normal immunoglobulin in the presence of high levels of paraprotein.

Diminished T cell activity has been described in patients with Hodgkin's disease, sarcoidosis, and leprosy. In autoimmune diseases, a loss of suppressor T cells has been observed.

In severe malnutrition and in patients with terminal malignancies there is diminished humoral and cell-mediated immunity.

The diagnosis of functional disorders of lymphocytes requires the use of skin tests, enumeration of B and T cells, measurement of serum immunoglobulin and antibodies, and a variety of *in vitro* lymphocyte assays which record their response to mitogens and antigens (p. 1325).

NEOPLASTIC AND RELATED DISORDERS PRIMARILY INVOLVING LEUKOCYTES

LEUKEMIA

Leukemia is a generalized neoplastic proliferation or accumulation of leukopoietic cells with or without involvement of the peripheral blood. Leukocytosis, abnormal circulating cells, and infiltration of non-hematopoietic tissues are frequently but not invariably present.

If no abnormal cells are present in the blood the leukemia is described as *aleukemic;* if abnormal cells are present but the total leukocyte count is not elevated, the term *subleukemic* leukemia is used.

The *acute leukemias,* if no remission is induced, usually are fatal within three months. The bone marrow is usually packed with primitive cells of the series involved with very little evidence of differentiation.

Subacute leukemias are often categorized with the acute leukemias, but when the term is used it implies a longer natural history of three to 12 months and cells of intermediate differentiation. Patients with *chronic leukemias* usually survive more than one year after the onset of symptoms if no remission occurs. The cell type is more differentiated.

Classification

1. *Chronologic* (based on natural history)
   a. Acute.
   b. Subacute.
   c. Chronic.
2. *Cytologic* (based on predominant cell type)
   a. Myelogenous leukemia: acute (myeloblast); chronic (myelocyte).
   b. Lymphocytic leukemia: acute (lymphoblast); chronic (lymphocyte).
   c. Monocytic leukemia: acute (monoblast), chronic (monocyte).
   d. Plasma cell leukemia.
   e. "Lymphosarcoma cell" leukemia.
3. *Functional capacity of release mechanism*
   a. Leukemic.
   b. Subleukemic.
   c. Aleukemic.
4. *Localized proliferation of cells of same type*
   a. Chloroma (myeloblast).
   b. Myeloma (plasma cell).
   c. Lymphoma (lymphoblast or lymphocyte).

Etiologic factors

The etiology of human leukemias remains unclear. Leukemia is an abnormal, uncontrolled proliferation or accumulation of one cell type at some level of maturation. It is probable that the initial event in the development of leukemia is a mutation in one cell, and that this event occurs as a result of one or more environmental determinants acting at a particular moment in a susceptible individual. It is also likely that more than one factor is involved.

Marrow Damage. Irradiation may result in an increased incidence of leukemia. In physicians the incidence is 1.7 times that in the general population, and in radiologists it is eight to 10 times that in other physicians. Following the dropping of the atomic bomb in 1945, an increased incidence of leukemia appeared in those of the Japanese population who were exposed to radiation. Treatment of ankylosing spondylitis with radiation has also been followed by an increased occurrence of leukemia. Generally, following radiation, when leukemia occurs it is acute or chronic myelogenous or acute lymphocytic.

Marrow damage due to *chemical agents* such as chloramphenicol, phenylbutazone, or benzene has been followed by a slightly increased frequency of acute myelogenous leukemia. *Aplastic anemia* of unknown cause and *paroxysmal nocturnal hemoglobinuria* are other examples of marrow injuries that are associated with a small but increased incidence of leukemia.

Immunologic Function. In patients with hereditary defects of the immune system, an increased frequency of lymphocytic leukemia and lymphoma has been noted. It may be that survival of malignant cells requires some defect in immune surveillance. Also, persons with a long-term proliferation of the lymphoid system, as in autoimmune hemolytic anemia, may eventually develop a lymphoma.

Genetic Factors. Multiple ocurrences of leukemia have been described in the same family, more in chronic lymphocytic than in chronic granulocytic leukemia. Monozygotic twins are much more likely to both have leukemia then are dizygotic twins.

Chromosome number 22 has shown an apparent deletion (and translocation) of one of the long arms in the myeloid cells of about 90 per cent of patients with chronic myelogenous leukemia. This abnormal chromosome is called the Philadelphia chromosome (Ph^1). Also, in children with an extra chromosome number 21 and Down's syndrome there is an increased incidence of both acute myelogenous leukemia and an unusual myeloid dysplasia that resembles leukemia but may be transient.

Viruses. In some animal leukemias, viruses have been proved to be the etiologic agent, and they are suspected to be so in human leukemia. It appears likely that the virus would be incorporated into the genome of cells with acquired or hereditary instability of DNA, increasing the risk of establishing a neoplastic clone of cells.

Incidence

Expected deaths from leukemia in the United States in 1978 are estimated to be 15,000, or 6.9 per 100,000 population; new cases in 1978 are expected to number 21,500. The age-adjusted death rate for leukemia in males in the United States increased from 3.4 per 100,000 in 1935 to 7.5 per 100,000 in 1960 and 1965; since then it has fallen slightly to 6.5 per 100,000 in 1975. The age-adjusted death rate for females in the United States is about 0.6 to 0.7 that of males (Silverberg, 1978).

Acute leukemias account for about 60 per cent of all leukemias; chronic myelogenous leukemia and chronic lymphocytic leukemia are each about 20 per cent of the total. Overall, males with leukemia outnumber females about 1.3 to 1; this ratio is larger in chronic lymphocytic leukemia.

Peaks in the age distribution for acute leukemia are at 3 to 4 years of age, and at 15 to 20 years of age. Acute lymphocytic leukemia accounts for most of the former and acute myelogenous leukemia for most of the latter. Most cases of chronic myelogenous leukemia occur between the ages of 20 and 50 years, and chronic lymphocytic leukemia, above 50. Monocytic leukemia, which is usually acute, favors middle age and is rare before age 30.

Acute leukemias

Clinical Features. The onset of the disease is sudden and differs strikingly from the insidious onset of chronic leukemia. The disease resembles an acute infectious or even a septic condition. Other changes include fever, rapidly developing anemia, and signs of granulocytic insufficiency, with ulcerations of mucous membranes, especially of the mouth and throat, and purpura. Enlargement of lymph nodes, spleen, and liver is not very pronounced. Rheumatoid pains, sometimes resembling acute rheumatic fever, are frequent. Marked prostration and general malaise may be present. The course is rapidly progressive. Acute leukemia may imitate a variety of diseases.

Lymph node enlargement is conspicuous only in acute monocytic leukemia, especially

3

cervical. Moderate generalized lymph node enlargement is more frequent in acute lymphocytic leukemia. In monocytic leukemia cervical lymph nodes are also tender.

The spleen in only slightly enlarged, except in acute lymphocytic leukemia, in which it may be moderately or even greatly enlarged.

Lesions in the mouth, with swelling, ulceration, and hemorrhages in the gums, are especially frequent in monocytic leukemia but may also occur in other forms. Mucosal ulcerations may also be present in other parts of the gastrointestinal tract. Also, these lesions are more frequent in monocytic leukemia.

In addition to rheumatoid pains previously referred to, there may also be tenderness of bones and swelling and tenderness of joints. The responsible pathologic lesion is the presence of subperiosteal leukemic infiltrations.

Signs of central nervous system (CNS) involvement are seen primarily in acute lymphocytic leukemia (ALL). CNS symptoms appear in about one third of children with ALL who live longer than one year. Usually due to meningeal infiltration with leukemic cells, the symptoms are related to increased pressure or to focal lesions. Other CNS problems are the result of high circulating blast counts leading to leukostatic thrombi and intracerebral hemorrhage, or to severe thrombocytopenia, which may result in subarachnoid hemorrhage.

Blood Findings. Anemia is present almost without exception in any case with fully developed clinical manifestations. It is usually normocytic. Frequently young nucleated red cells are present. Thrombocytopenia of moderate to marked degree is the rule. Prolonged bleeding time, poor clot retraction, and positive tourniquet test are present. The leukocyte count is occasionally very high (over $100 \times 10^9/l$), often is slightly elevated, but is perhaps most frequently normal or decreased. A combination of anemia, thrombocytopenia, and leukopenia is a common finding in acute leukemia.

The predominant cell is an immature blast cell, most frequently a myeloblast in the adult and a lymphoblast in the child (Plates 30–1*J* and *K* and 30–3).

Marrow Findings. By the time the patient is symptomatic, the hematopoietic cells and fat are usually replaced by diffuse infiltration of blasts. The bony trabeculae and cortex may be thin.

Chromosomal Abnormalities in Blood-Forming Cells. In almost half of patients with acute leukemia, the karyotype is normal. In the remainder, no consistent abnormality of the karyotype is found in any one form of acute leukemia. Most patients apparently have a normal (diploid) mode, but some have abnormal karyotypes, which are usually consistent for the individual but not for the type of leu-

---

Plate 30–3. *A*, Acute myelogenous leukemia (AML), Wright-Giemsa stain. No maturation is evident. This corresponds to the M_1 category of the French-American-British (FAB) classification (Table 30–8). *B*, AML, Sudan black B reaction. Same case as *A*. Though granules are not visible with the Wright-Giemsa stain, all of the blasts contain sudanophilic material (brown granules). The peroxidase reaction was similarly positive. *C*, Acute myelogenous leukemia with partial maturation (M_2). Naphthol AS-D chloroacetate esterase reaction. All stages of developing neutrophils have a positive reaction. *D*, Acute myelomonocytic leukemia (AMML), Wright-Giemsa stain. No cytoplasmic maturation is evident. This stain alone does not allow a definitive diagnosis. *E*, AMML, Sudan black B reaction. Same case as *D*. A moderate proportion of the blasts contains sudanophilic material. *F*, AMML, alpha naphthyl acetate esterase reaction. Same case as *D*. Most of the blasts contain non-specific esterase (which is fluoride-sensitive). Cytochemical reactions, therefore, lead to the diagnosis of myelomonocytic leukemia. *G*, Acute lymphocytic leukemia (ALL), Wright-Giemsa stain. Most of the blasts are small and the cytoplasm is scanty. This corresponds to the L_1 category of the FAB classification (Table 30–7). *H*, ALL, periodic acid–Schiff (PAS) reaction. Same case as *G*. A moderate proportion of the blasts contains one or more large granules or "blocks" of PAS-positive material. *I*, Acute promyelocytic leukemia, Wright-Giemsa stain. The majority of cells have abundant azurophil granules, often large. Usually, some cells contain multiple Auer rods, as in the cell at the right. The nuclei are irregularly shaped or indented (Rieder forms). This is the hypergranular promyelocytic category (M_3) of the FAB classification. *J*, Erythroleukemia, Wright-Giemsa stain. One primitive blast (*lower center*), one abnormal monocyte (*upper right*), one neutrophil, and five nucleated erythroid cells are present. Most of the latter are abnormal. *K*, Erythroleukemia, PAS reaction. Same case as *J*. Of the six nucleated erythroid cells in this field, five are PAS-positive: in the most immature the reactive material is granular (*lower center*); in the others it is diffuse. A monocyte and a blast are PAS-negative; a neutrophil is PAS-positive. *L*, Erythroleukemia, alpha-naphthyl butyrate reaction. Same case as *J*. Monocytes are strongly positive for this non-specific esterase reaction; they were increased in number and morphologically abnormal and part of the leukemic process. Erythroid, granulocytic, and monocytic cell lines are demonstrably involved in this case.

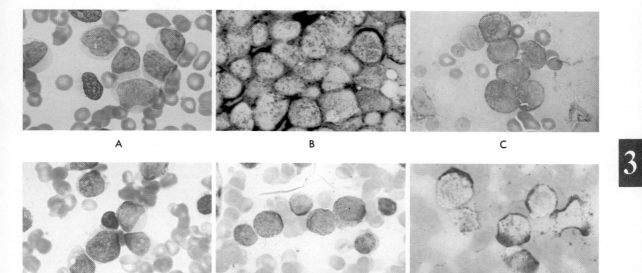

A   B   C

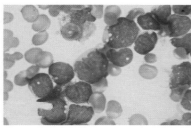

D   E   F

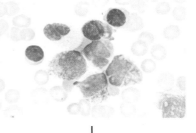

G   H   I

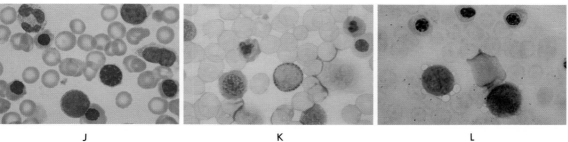

J   K   L

Plate 30-3. *See legend on opposite page.*

Table 30-7. FRENCH-AMERICAN-BRITISH (FAB)
CLASSIFICATION OF THE ACUTE LYMPHOBLASTIC
LEUKEMIAS (L)*

CYTOLOGY	L_1	L_2	L_3
Size	Small	Large	Large and Homogeneous
Chromatin	Homogeneous	Variable	Finely Stippled
Shape	Regular	Irregular	Oval to Round
Nucleoli	Rare	Present	1–3
Cytoplasm	Scanty	Moderate	Moderate
Basophilia	Moderate	Variable	Intense

*From Bennett, et al.: Proposals for the classification of the acute leukae-
mias. French-American-British (FAB) Co-operative group. Br. J. Haematol.,
*33:*451, 1976. Blackwell Scientific Publications, Ltd., Oxford.

kemia. Sandberg (1964) found that in the patients with acute myelogenous leukemia who
had an abnormal karyotype, the aneuploidy
was hypodiploid except for those with a bimo-
dal, unstable cell population. In acute lymphocytic leukemia, the aneuploidy in the patients
with abnormal karyotypes was hyperdiploid.

Cytochemistry. Hayhoe (1964) analyzed
140 cases of acute leukemia using standard
Romanowsky staining characteristics and four
cytochemical reactions: Sudan black B, peroxidase, neutrophil alkaline phosphatase, and per-
riodic acid-Schiff (PAS). Virtually all cases
could be classified into one of four groups:
lymphoblastic, myeloblastic, myelomonocytic,
and erythremic myelosis. Lymphoblastic was
quite clearly separable, but there was some

overlap among the other three groups. Later,
Hayhoe (1972) included data from cytochemical esterase reactions which have added some
discriminatory power. The usefulness of these
cytochemical characteristics is described in the
following sections, the methods are given beginning on page 1087, and some of the reactions are illustrated in Plate 30-3.

FAB Classification. A French-American-
British (FAB) cooperative group has published
proposals for the classification of acute leukemias (Bennett, 1976). The classification is
based on morphology of cells in Romanowsky-
stained blood and marrow films and certain
supplemental cytochemical reactions (Tables
30-7 and 30-8). They emphasized the need for
excellent technical preparations of blood and

Table 30-8. FRENCH-AMERICAN-BRITISH (FAB) CLASSIFICATION OF THE ACUTE
MYELOID LEUKEMIAS (M)*

A. Granulocytic Component Predominant

   M_1: Myeloblastic without Maturation
   ($>$ 3% blasts peroxidase positive, or azure granules $\pm$ Auer rods)

   M_2: Myeloblastic with Maturation
   ($>$ 50% cells = myeloblasts + promyelocytes; maturation beyond promyelocytes present)

   M_3: Hypergranular Promyelocytic
   (Majority of cells abnormal promyelocytes; Auer rods usual)

B. Monocytic Component Predominant

   M_4: Myelomonocytic
   ($>$ 20% monocytic; $>$ 20% myeloblasts + promyelocytes)

   M_5: Monocytic
   (Poorly differentiated or differentiated; $<$ 20% granulocytes)

C. Erythropoietic Component Predominant

   M_6: Erythroleukemia
   ($>$ 50% cells = erythroid, abnormal; or $>$ 30% cells erythroid + 10% bizarre erythroid cells + $>$ 30% myeloblasts
   and promyelocytes; $\pm$ Auer rods $\pm$ abnormal megakaryocytes)

*Modified from Bennett, et al.: Br. J. Haematol., *33:*451, 1976.

marrow films, and the need for caution before diagnosing leukemia from hypocellular specimens.

ACUTE LYMPHOCYTIC LEUKEMIA (ALL)

Morphology. The cell type is the lymphoblast. In the L_1 type according to the FAB classification (Table 30-7), the nuclear-cytoplasmic ratio is high. The nuclei may have deep clefts (known as Rieder cells) but are not indented or twisted. The chromatin pattern is fine and uniform. Usually only one or two nucleoli are present. The cytoplasm is scanty in amount, pale blue, and homogeneous, usually without granules (Plates 30-1L and 30-3G). The L_1 type is homogeneous in these characteristics and is the type of leukemia that is common in children. In L_2 a larger cell type prevails (Plate 30-2H), and usually there is more variation in cytologic features within and between cases. It is less common in children and is the usual adult type of ALL. L_3 represents the Burkitt type of ALL (see Plate

30-4H). The cells are large and uniform; they have a round or oval nucleus with prominent nucleoli and moderately abundant deeply basophilic cytoplasm.

Normoblasts are not usually found in the blood in ALL, nor are they predominant in the marrow. Auer rods, agranular neutrophils, or the acquired pseudo-Pelger anomaly are not found.

Cytochemistry (Table 30-9). The blasts are negative for Sudan black B, peroxidase, and naphthol AS-D chloroacetate esterase; Hayhoe (1972) states that no more than 5 per cent of the cells can be positive and the FAB classification puts 3 per cent as the upper limit for these staining reactions in the blasts. The diagnosis of ALL cannot be made with certainty until the Sudan black B or peroxidase reaction has been performed to show that the blasts are negative. In a few cases of L_2, azurophilic granules may be present, but they are Sudan black B and peroxidase negative. The acid phosphatase reaction is moderately or strongly positive in the blasts in about 20 per

Table 30-9. CYTOCHEMICAL REACTIONS IN NORMAL CELLS AND IN BLASTS AND IMMATURE CELLS OF ACUTE LEUKEMIAS*

	Sudan Black B Peroxidase	Chloroacetate Esterase	Non-specific Esterase	PAS
Cells				
Promyelocyte	+	+ (a)	−	±
Neutrophil	+ +	+ + (a)	−	+ + +
Monocyte	±	−	+ + +	±
Lymphocyte	−	−	− /± (b)	− /+
Normoblast	−	−	− (c)	− (d)
Megakaryocyte	−	−	+ +	+ + +
Leukemias				
ALL	−	−	± (e)	+ + (f)
AML	+ +	+ + (a)	−	±
APL	+ + +	+ + +	−	±
AMML	±	±	+ + +	+
AUL	−	−	−	−

Key: − negative
± weakly positive or few positive cells
+ moderately positive
+ + moderately to strongly positive
+ + + strongly positive (most cells)

ALL = acute lymphocytic leukemia
AML = acute myelogenous leukemia
APL = acute promyelocytic leukemia
AMML = acute myelomonocytic leukemia
AUL = acute unclassified leukemia

Comments: (a) Chloroacetate esterase is less consistently positive than SBB or PX.
(b) Some normal lymphocytes have *focal* positivity.
(c) Strong non-specific esterase activity is present in some cases of erythroleukemia and dyserythropoiesis.
(d) Positive in erythroleukemia, to a lesser degree in some cases of iron deficiency and thalassemia.
(e) Some cases of ALL have *focal* positivity.
(f) Some cases of ALL; coarse granules ± blocks.

*Modified from Nelson, D. A., and Davey, F. R.: Leukocyte esterases, *In* Williams, W. J., Beutler, E., Erslev, A. J., and Rundles, R. W. (eds.): Hematology, 2nd ed. New York, McGraw-Hill Book Co., 1977, p. 1633.

Table 30–10. MONONUCLEAR CELL MARKER CHARACTERISTICS

	T LYMPHOCYTES	B LYMPHOCYTES	MACROPHAGE OR MONOCYTE
E Rosette	+	–	–
EA Rosette	–	–	+
EAC Rosette	–	+	+
SMIg	–	+	–
Fc	–	+	+
Anti-T lymphocyte antisera	+	–	–
Anti-B lymphocyte antisera	–	+	–
Phagocytosis	–	–	+

E Rosette = Spontaneous sheep erythrocyte binding.
EA Rosette = Sheep erythrocyte-IgG antibody binding.
EAC Rosette = Sheep erythrocyte antibody complement complex binding.
SMIg = Surface membrane immunoglobulin.
Fc = Binding aggregated IgG via Fc receptors.
+ = Cell binds to reagents or cell can perform appropriate function.
– = Cell does not bind to reagent or perform appropriate function.

cent of cases of ALL. Most of these appear to be T-cell lymphomas (Catovsky, 1978). The PAS stain usually shows coarse blocks of material in at least some lymphoblasts (Plate 30-3*H*). The neutrophil alkaline phosphatase score is normal or high.

Immunologic Surface Markers. Surface markers which have been used in categorizing mononuclear cells as T cells and as B cells (Table 30-10) are being used to subclassify the blasts in ALL (Chessells, 1977; Kersey, 1978; Davey, 1974).

T-cell leukemias account for 15 to 25 per cent of ALL. They occur predominantly in boys who tend to be slightly older than children with the common ALL. T-cell ALL usually has a high leukocyte count and mediastinal widening by x-ray; the mediastinal involvement may be discovered and diagnosed as a poorly differentiated lymphocytic lymphoma before the process becomes leukemic. Frequently, these cells have deep nuclear indentations—the "convoluted lymphocyte" (Lukes, 1974). The prognosis in T-cell ALL is worse than in non B-, non T-cell ALLs.

The B-cell type of ALL has monoclonal surface membrane immunoglobulin and may correspond to either L_3 or L_2 of the FAB classification. It is the rarest of the subgroups of ALL and has the poorest prognosis. The L_3 or Burkitt's type may represent an advanced phase of non-African Burkitt's lymphoma and is more common in children. The L_2 type is usually seen in adults and probably represents

the leukemic phase of poorly differentiated lymphocytic lymphomas (Gralnick, 1977).

The non B-, non T-cell type is the commonest, accounting for about 75 per cent of ALL. In children, non B-, non T-cell leukemias have a better prognosis than the other subtypes.

ACUTE MYELOID LEUKEMIA

Acute Myelogenous Leukemia (AML). Acute myelogenous leukemia, myelomonocytic leukemia, and erythroleukemia share certain features. The latter two are usually considered variants of the former. This commonality suggests a common stem cell for granulocytes, monocytes, erythroid cells, and probably also megakaryocytes, since the latter are frequently abnormal when erythroid cells are involved (Hayhoe, 1972).

MORPHOLOGY. The cell type is the myeloblast, which is usually slightly larger than the lymphoblast (Plates 30-1*J* and 30-3*A*). The nuclear-cytoplasmic ratio is not high. The nucleus is round to oval. The chromatin is very fine, delicate, and uniform, without condensation. The nuclear membrane is indistinct. Three to five nucleoli are usually evident. The cytoplasm is homogeneous, without granules or with a very few azurophilic granules.

Less than 1 per cent of blood leukocytes are monocytes, and normoblasts do not predominate in the marrow. Promyelocytes are usually present, but intermediate cells between the blasts and mature neutrophils are not numerous. This lack of maturing cells is known as a *leukemic hiatus* and is characteristic of the M_1 type of AML according to the FAB classification (myeloblastic leukemia without maturation—Table 30-8). If maturation past the promyelocytic stage is present, the M_2 type is the appropriate category. If many myelocytes and metamyelocytes and increased basophils are present, it suggests that the picture may be one of a blast transformation of chronic granulocytic leukemia rather than *de novo* acute myelogenous leukemia.

Deficient granulation in mature neutrophils or hyposegmentation of the nuclei (pseudo-Pelger anomaly) may be present.

With Wright's stain, *Auer rods* are characteristic rod-shaped red to purple staining inclusions in the cytoplasm of myeloblasts or promyelocytes in AML (Plates 30-1*J* and 30-3*I*). Less commonly they may be seen in more mature neutrophils. Auer rods are derivatives of azurophilic granules and stain positively for Sudan black B, peroxidase, and naphthol AS-D chloroacetate esterase. Auer rods are found in the majority of cases of AML and almost never in any other condition except for myelomonocytic leukemia and erythroleukemia.

Acute promyelocytic leukemia or hypergranular promyelocytic leukemia (M_3) (Table 30-8) is a variant of AML in which promyelocytes predominate instead of myeloblasts. The azurophil granules tend to be abundant and darkly staining. This disorder usually has a fulminant course, punctuated by bleeding which is more severe than would be expected from the degree of thrombocytopenia. This is due to intravascular coagulation that in some way apparently is initiated by the procoagulant material from the granules of the abnormal cells.

CYTOCHEMISTRY. According to the defining criteria of Hayhoe (1972), over 5 per cent of the cells (and usually more than 85 per cent) have strong positive staining of granules with Sudan black B (Plate 30-3*B*). More than 5 per cent of the cells are also peroxidase positive. Staining of the late myeloblasts or early promyelocytes is the important criterion; occasionally the blasts fail to show these reactions if they have failed to show any development of azurophilic granules; on the other hand, sometimes no granules can be seen with Wright's stain, and yet the blasts are peroxidase and Sudan black B positive. Almost always these two stains react in parallel. Auer rods are positive with these staining reactions. Naph-

thol AS-D chloroacetate esterase is positive in developing granulocytes also, but alpha-naphthyl acetate esterase is negative. The PAS stain shows faint diffuse or granular staining in some blasts or early promyelocytes.

The neutrophil alkaline phosphatase score is usually low, suggesting that these neutrophils are derived from the leukemic blasts.

Acute Myelomonocytic Leukemia (AMML). In the past, two forms of monocytic leukemia were recognized. In the *Naegeli type*, myeloblasts are numerous and abnormal proliferation is evident in developing granulocytes as well as monocytes; this has been considered a variant of acute myeloid leukemia, with monocytes being derived from myeloblasts. The *Schilling type* of monocytic leukemia was considered a "pure" monocytic leukemia, with monocytes derived from the reticuloendothelial system, and with no evidence of abnormality in granulocyte development.

It seems now, however, improbable that monocytes have a dual origin and the terms Naegeli and Schilling should not be used in the classification of AMML. It now appears that monocytes originate in the bone marrow from a stem cell common to granulocytes, erythroid cells, and megakaryocytes. In the monocytic leukemias there is a spectrum, from cases with slight monocytic and strong myeloblastic components to those that are almost purely monocytic (Hayhoe, 1964; Hayhoe, 1972). When both components are present, the FAB category is myelomonocytic (M_4); pure or relatively pure monocytic leukemia is designated M_5 (Table 30-8). Cytochemistry is necessary, frequently, for these distinctions, and for distinguishing AMML from AML.

MORPHOLOGY. The nucleus has delicate reticular chromatin and several (three to five) nucleoli. The nucleus is folded, indented, and frequently twisted or even coarsely segmented. There is usually abundant cytoplasm (the nuclear-cytoplasmic ratio is not high) and often many fine azurophilic granules. Phagocytosis of red cells or cell debris may be seen. Auer rods may be present in the abnormal monocytes as well as in the blasts; neutrophils may have diminished granules; the pseudo-Pelger anomaly may be present; and eosinophils may be abnormal.

Monocytes comprise over 1 per cent of the circulating leukocytes. Normoblasts are not usually found in the blood, nor do they predominate in the marrow. Megakaryocytes are less likely to be depleted in the marrow in this form of acute leukemia, and thrombocytopenia is less frequent.

CYTOCHEMISTRY (Table 30-9). Sudan black B positivity is often present in the monocytes and is finer than that seen in granulocyte precursors. The peroxidase reaction also tends to be less strong, and usually is negative in the younger cells. The alpha-naphthyl acetate esterase reaction is positive in the monocytes (Plate 30-3*F*), and the naphthol AS-D chloroacetate esterase is negative, the reverse of the findings in the granulocyte precursors in acute myelogenous leukemia. This makes these esterase reactions particularly valuable in the diagnosis of myelomonocytic leukemia. The PAS reaction may be negative or show diffuse cytoplasmic staining of fine granules.

MURAMIDASE. Patients with myelomonocytic leukemia characteristically have markedly increased levels of muramidase (lysozyme) in the serum and urine (Osserman, 1966). Muramidase is an enzyme capable of lysing bacteria; it is present in normal neutrophils and monocytes. The source of the normal serum lysozyme is probably the neutrophil, and its concentration appears to correlate with neutrophil turnover. In myeloproliferative disorders the serum muramidase is also increased, and this correlation appears to hold (Catovsky, 1971a and b). The highest levels, however, occur in myelomonocytic leukemia, and here the muramidase level reflects the proliferation of monocytes. It appears probable that the muramidase is produced and secreted from the monocyte during its life, but that the muramidase is not released from the neutrophil until its death. If the cells are poorly differentiated or significantly abnormal morphologically they may not produce muramidase (Catovsky, 1971b).

Di Guglielmo Syndrome. Another variant of myeloid leukemias is erythroleukemia, which refers to an abnormal proliferation of both erythroid precursors and granulocytic precursors (M_6, Table 30-8). Morphologic abnormalities are usually pronounced.

Very rarely there is virtually no granulocytic involvement in the neoplastic process, in which case the condition is called *erythremic myelosis*. This disease has a rapid course resembling that of acute leukemia.

Usually there is a mixture of variable proportions of erythroid precursors and myeloblasts, *erythroleukemia*, which may include megakaryocytic and monocytic abnormal proliferations in addition. This also usually has a rapid course, but is more variable and sometimes may be subacute or even chronic.

When the abnormal erythroid proliferation is minimal and the myeloblastic proliferation predominates, the picture of *acute myelogenous leukemia* is seen.

Although each disorder may be seen *de novo*, occasionally one sees progression from an initial erythremic myelosis to erythroleukemia to a final termination in acute myelogenous leukemia in a single patient. This group of disorders has been designated the *Di Guglielmo syndrome* (Gunz, 1974).

MORPHOLOGY (Plate 30-3*J*). Erythroid precursors, though abnormal, usually are easily recognized. They predominate in the hyperplastic marrow and are usually present in the blood. They are irregular in outline, often with pseudopods. The nuclear:cytoplasmic ratio is not high. Nuclear shape is often bizarre, with atypical megaloblastic features. Nucleoli tend to be large. Mitoses and multinucleated giant forms are numerous. Vacuolation of cytoplasm in pro- and basophilic erythroblasts is often present. In erythremic myelosis and the more acute forms of erythroleukemia, there is an apparent arrest of maturation and fewer polychromatic and orthochromatic forms are present. In chronic forms of erythroleukemia, later normoblasts are present in larger numbers. Myeloblasts are increased in erythroleukemia, and Auer rods may be found in them or in promyelocytes. Abnormalities in neutrophils and eosinophils may be seen. Monocytic proliferation may be a part of the process. Abnormal megakaryocytes are often prominent and include giant forms with bizarre nuclear fragmentation and small fragmented megakaryocytes with one or two apparently diploid nuclei. Atypical platelets may be found in the blood (Plate 30-6*F* and *G*).

CYTOCHEMISTRY (Table 30-9). Some of the erythroid precursors at all stages of maturation show strong cytoplasmic PAS positivity. This is granular in early erythroid precursors and diffuse in later stages (Plate 30-3*K*). Erythroid precursors are normally PAS negative, and they are negative in most diseases, including nutritional megaloblastic anemia. They are sometimes positive, however, in iron deficiency anemia and thalassemia and in refractory sideroblastic anemia or refractory anemia with dyshematopoiesis (Hayhoe, 1964). The latter disorders are part of a heterogeneous group which have been regarded as chronic forms of the Di Guglielmo syndrome (Dame-shek, 1964).

In erythroleukemia increased numbers of primitive cells showing Sudan black and peroxidase positivity are found. A monocytic component is often evident (Plate 30–3L). Abnormal neoplastic erythroid precursors are also sometimes positive for the alpha-naphthyl acetate esterase reaction (Hayhoe, 1972).

CHRONIC LYMPHOCYTIC LEUKEMIA (CLL)

Clinical Findings. CLL is rare under the age of 40; most cases occur over the age of 60. It is more than twice as common in men as in women. The onset is insidious and the disease is commonly discovered by chance during the investigation of another problem. Lymphadenopathy, asymptomatic or associated with symptoms such as weakness, fatigue, anorexia, and weight loss, may cause the patient to come to the physician. Enlarged lymph nodes are usually evident, and frequently hepatosplenomegaly is also found, though splenomegaly is of lesser degree than that seen in CML or myelofibrosis with myeloid metaplasia (MMM). Skin lesions, gastrointestinal infiltration and symptoms, and bone pain or tenderness are rather common.

Blood. The leukocyte count is usually between 30 and $200 \times 10^9/l$, and 80 to 90 per cent of these are small lymphocytes. Damaged or smudged cells are common on the film, probably indicating fragile cells. Occasionally the leukocyte count by electronic counter will be significantly lower than a hemacytometer count because of the more fragile cells. It is advisable to check the electronic count by hemacytometer on new cases, and thereafter to check the appearance of the blood film with the count from the machine, keeping this problem in mind.

The lymphocytes are monotonously similar in appearance and usually look normal. Nuclear chromatin may be coarsely condensed and more sharply separated by parachromatin than in normal lymphocytes or, in some cases, the chromatin is less condensed than normal. Sometimes nucleoli are evident in many of the lymphocytes. Size variation is minimal. Cytoplasm is of small to moderate amount. In a minority of patients a small proportion of the lymphocytes is immature. Usually these are prolymphocytes or reticular lymphocytes (transformed lymphocytes).

Often there is neither anemia nor thrombocytopenia at the time of diagnosis. Anemia due to impaired production does develop as the marrow is replaced by leukemic cells. In addition, erythrocyte life span in some patients with CLL may be reduced. This is especially true when there is marked splenomegaly. Autoimmune hemolytic anemia develops in about 10 per cent of patients with advanced disease; among the leukemias, it has the greatest frequency in CLL. The Coombs' antiglobulin test is usually positive and the offending antibody is an IgG class immunoglobulin. Thrombocytopenia is often slight and occasionally becomes severe as the disease progresses, so that hemorrhagic manifestations appear. Thrombocytopenia is usually due to hypoproliferation but may also be secondary to an immune process or splenic sequestration.

Marrow. Very early in the disease marrow involvement may be lacking. The usual early finding, however, is the presence of slight to moderate lymphocytosis. Since the lymphocytes are morphologically normal, examination of marrow smears may be equivocal. Histologic sections of aspirated particles or biopsy material may then be very helpful. Small to medium-sized areas of lymphocytes are present and have indistinct margins; lymphocytes are infiltrating into adjacent hematopoietic tissue. If an autoimmune hemolytic anemia is present, erythropoiesis becomes prominent. Later in the disease, lymphocytes overrun the marrow, largely replacing hematopoietic tissue.

Differential Diagnosis. Persistent lymphocytosis in excess of $15 \times 10^9/l$ over a period of several weeks or months in an adult over 40 years of age is good evidence for CLL. Marrow examination, especially histologic sections, should confirm this diagnosis. In children lymphocyte counts in excess of $100 \times 10^9/l$, morphologically mimicking CLL, may be found transiently in infectious lymphocytosis or pertussis.

In contrast to CLL with normal-appearing lymphocytes is a somewhat less common variety, *lymphosarcoma cell leukemia*. In the latter the cells have variably condensed chromatin, usually less than in CLL, and notched nuclei. Deep clefts in the nuclei are characteristic. This type of lymphocytic leukemia is associated with poorly differentiated lymphocytic lymphoma, which is almost always nodular in its histologic pattern. In CLL, on the other hand, the histologic pattern of the in-

Table 30–11. RAI'S STAGING SYSTEM FOR CHRONIC LYMPHOCYTIC LEUKEMIA*

Stage 0	Absolute lymphocytosis of $>15 \times 10^9$ l
Stage I	Absolute lymphocytosis plus enlarged lymph nodes
Stage II[a]	Absolute lymphocytosis plus enlarged liver and/or spleen
Stage III[b]	Absolute lymphocytosis plus anemia (Hb < 11 g/dl)
Stage IV[b]	Absolute lymphocytosis plus thrombocytopenia (platelet ct. $< 100 \times 10^9$/l)

*From Phillips, E. A., Kempin, S., Passe, S., Miké, V., and Clarkson, B.: Prognostic factors in chronic lymphocytic leukemia and their implications for therapy. Clin. Hematol., 6:203, 1977.
[a]Stage II patients may or may not have adenopathy.
[b]Stage III and IV patients may or may not have adenopathy and/or organomegaly.

volved lymph node is a well-differentiated lymphocytic lymphoma that is diffuse.

Prolymphocytic leukemia is another variant of CLL (Galton, 1974). The disorder is characterized by a very marked lymphocytosis (mean 355×10^9/l), massive splenomegaly, moderate hepatomegaly, and inconspicuous lymphadenopathy. The malignant lymphoid cells have a large vesicular nucleolus, condensed nuclear chromatin, and moderate amount of cytoplasm.

Other Findings. Most patients with CLL have no detectable chromosomal abnormalities.

Hypogammaglobulinemia develops in 50 to 70 per cent of patients with CLL. Although all classes of immunoglobulin may be affected, IgM is usually most severely reduced. Along with neutropenia, this defect in humoral immunity accounts for an increased likelihood of infectious complications. In about 5 per cent of patients there is a monoclonal immunoglobulin elevation; usually this is IgM.

In studies thus far, virtually all patients with CLL have had surface immunoglobulins on most of the leukemic cells, indicating that they are probably B-lymphocytes (Aisenberg,

1972). It appears that the surface immunoglobulin is usually restricted to IgM and to a single light chain, supporting the clonal origin of the leukemic cells. The fact that most of the lymphocytes are B cells would explain their lack of responsiveness to phytohemagglutinin, which is considered to be a T cell characteristic. Lymphosarcoma cells (cells from poorly differentiated lymphocytic lymphoma) have been found to have greater concentrations of immunoglobulin, again mainly IgM, on their surfaces.

Course. Rai (1975) has devised a staging system for CLL (Table 30–11) based on degree of lymphocytosis, hemoglobin level, number of platelets in blood, lymphadenopathy, and presence of hepatosplenomegaly. A significant relationship exists between stage and survival (Table 30–12). For all patients regardless of stage, the median survival is about four years, but many patients live much longer than the median (Phillips, 1977). Very rarely (in contrast to CML) does a blastic phase supervene in CLL; in those rare cases the blasts morphologically resemble reticular lymphocytes ("transformed" lymphocytes).

Table 30–12. MEDIAN DURATION OF SURVIVAL FOR EACH STAGE OF DIAGNOSIS AS DETERMINED IN VARIOUS SERIES (CLL)*

Stage of Diagnosis	RAI'S SERIES		BOGGS'S SERIES		HANSEN'S SERIES		PRESENT SERIES	
	No. of Patients	Median Survival (months)	No. of Patients	Median Survival (months)	No. of Patients	Median Survival (months)	No. of Patients	Median Survival (months)
0	22	>150	3	–	6	180	11	150
I	29	101	7	130	52	60	25	84
II	39	71	41	108	23	47	60	48
III	21	19	13	9	32	26	29	24
IV	14	19	20	42	39	20	32	24

*From Philips, E. A., Kempin, S., Passe, S., Miké, V., and Clarkson, B.: Prognostic factors in chronic lymphocytic leukemia and their implication for therapy. Clin. Hematol., 6:203, 1977.

CHRONIC MYELOGENOUS LEUKEMIA (CML)

Clinical Findings. CML occurs primarily in young and middle-aged adults. The onset is insidious and the disorder may be discovered accidentally on a routine blood test. The patient may have symptoms of anemia and weight loss or he simply may complain of malaise. The spleen enlarges progressively, and the patient begins to lose weight and have fever and night sweats associated with the increased metabolism due to increased granulocyte turnover. The discomfort associated with an enlarged spleen may bring the patient to the doctor. Infarcts in the spleen may produce left upper quadrant pain. Excessive bleeding or bruising may occur in the later stages of the disease. Lymphadenopathy, though often present, is rarely prominent.

Laboratory Findings

BLOOD. The leukocyte count is usually over $50 \times 10^9/l$ and may exceed $300 \times 10^9/l$. The differential count is characteristic. There is a complete spectrum of granulocytic cells, from a few myeloblasts down to mature neutrophils. Myeloblasts are less than 10 per cent of the cells. Two peaks are present: myelocytes and neutrophils both exceed the other cell types. This is a feature that helps to exclude other myeloproliferative disorders and reactive leukocytoses (Spiers, 1977). The relative percentage of neutrophil myelocytes increases as the total leukocyte count increases. Basophilia is consistently present. Eosinophilia is almost always noted, along with the presence of eosinophil myelocytes. Monocytes are also absolutely increased in most patients.

Anemia is present in the majority of patients at the time of diagnosis. In others it appears during the course of the disease as a result of decreased RBC production. Erythrocytes are normochromic and normocytic. A few normoblasts can usually be found.

Thrombocytosis is present at the time of diagnosis in over half of patients. Less than 15 per cent of patients have a thrombocytopenia.

MARROW. The marrow is markedly hypercellular due primarily to granulocytic proliferation, with all stages represented. Eosinophil and basophil precursors are often increased. Normoblasts tend to be decreased. Frequently the marrow cannot be aspirated because of the density of cells packed together or (especially later in the disease) because of increased reticulin, which can be demonstrated on marrow biopsy. In a minority of patients are found macrophages laden with blue pigment (sea-blue histiocytes) or macrophages indistinguishable from Gaucher cells.

It is well to remember that even a typical bone marrow is not diagnostic of CML. On the other hand, the diagnosis can be made from the peripheral blood film alone in most cases.

NEUTROPHIL ALKALINE PHOSPHATASE (p. 1087). The neutrophil alkaline phosphatase (NAP) is greatly reduced or absent in over 90 per cent of patients with chronic myelogenous leukemia. It is greatly elevated in polycythemia vera; elevated, normal, or low in myelofibrosis with myeloid metaplasia; and normal or elevated in leukemoid reactions (Gunz, 1974). Although a low NAP is characteristic of chronic granulocytic leukemia, it is not specific, for low values may be found in paroxysmal nocturnal hemoglobinuria and in some cases of pernicious anemia, infectious mononucleosis, and aplastic anemia; these conditions do not, however, lead to diagnostic confusion. During remission of chronic myelogenous leukemia with a normal appearing blood picture, in most cases, the NAP continues to be low; in about one third of patients it returns to normal (Rosner, 1972). The NAP may increase in response to infection as it does in normal individuals.

CYTOGENETIC ABNORMALITIES. In direct bone marrow preparations and in metaphases of cultured peripheral blood, 90 to 95 per cent of patients with hematologically typical CML have an abnormally small acrocentric chromosome. With banding techniques this has been shown to be chromosome 22; part of the long arm has been translocated to another chromosome, usually chromosome 9. This was first described in 1960 by Nowell and Hungerford and is called the Philadelphia (Ph[1]) chromosome. The Ph[1] chromosome is present in blood and marrow cells during relapse and is demonstrable in the marrow also during remission. It appears that the Ph[1] chromosome is present in precursors of granulocytes, in normoblasts and megakaryocytes, but not in lymphocytes or skin cells.

Good evidence for a clonal origin of CML has been found in females who happen to be heterozygous for two isoenzymes of glucose 6-phosphate dehydrogenase (G6-PD) and who also have developed CML. Only one isoenzyme type is found in erythrocytes, granulocytes, monocytes, and platelets, but two types are found in skin cells (Fialkow, 1977).

The small proportion of patients with CML

3

who lack the Ph[1] chromosome are characteristic in most other respects: average age, spleen size, marrow and blood picture, and NAP values. On the average, however, the patients in this Ph[1]-negative group have less elevated white blood cell counts, have lower platelet counts, include a larger proportion of children, respond less well to therapy, and have a shorter survival (Tjio, 1966). Children with Ph[1]-negative CML ("juvenile CML") are usually one to two years old; their erythrocytes contain 30 to 70 per cent Hb F and also show other fetal characteristics (Mauer, 1974).

OTHER FINDINGS. Serum vitamin B_{12} and vitamin B_{12}-binding proteins are usually increased considerably, as a result of increased transcobalamin I, and are thought to reflect the size of the total blood granulocyte pool. The serum muramidase is also increased.

COURSE. Treatment with busulfan usually controls the disease in the chronic phase. After a median period of about three years, the disease changes into a more aggressive or accelerated phase. This is characterized by one or more features of progressive myeloproliferation: basophilia, thrombocytosis, leukocytosis, increasing splenomegaly, anemia, and reticulin myelofibrosis. These features become refractory to chemotherapy (Canellos, 1976). Preceding these changes, new clones of cells with cytogenetic abnormalities may be demonstrated, and, frequently, a change occurs in the *in vitro* growth characteristics of the committed progenitor cells in soft agar cultures (Metcalf, 1977).

In about one third of cases, the accelerated phase is characterized by a progressive increase in blasts and promyelocytes; when they exceed 30 per cent of cells in blood or marrow, it is regarded as the "acute blastic crisis" or blastic phase of the disease. In the majority of cases, the blastic phase follows the accelerated phase by a few months; in a small proportion of cases, the blastic phase may be the first presentation of the disease (Peterson, 1976). These patients usually have the Ph[1] chromosome, with or without morphologic evidence of CML, such as basophilia. The NAP becomes normal or high in most patients in the blastic phase.

The morphologic patterns in the blastic phase of CML resemble acute myeloblastic leukemia in the majority of cases, although Auer rods are found but rarely. In a substantial minority of cases, however, the appearance is that of acute lymphoblastic leukemia

(ALL) (Rosenthal, 1977). The distinction is useful because the latter (ALL) may respond to ALL-oriented therapy but the former (AML) do not (Peterson, 1976).

Median survival after onset of the blastic phase of CML is about 2 months overall and about 10 months in patients who respond by going into remission (Canellos, 1976).

LEUKEMIC RETICULOENDOTHELIOSIS ("HAIRY CELL" LEUKEMIA)

Bouroncle (1958) described this rare disorder which is clinically variable in its manifestations. It occurs more frequently in males than in females. The mean age of afflicted patients is 50 years. It has an insidious onset and is characterized by proliferation of the abnormal cells in the reticuloendothelial organs and blood. Splenomegaly is the predominant physical finding.

Pancytopenia or depression of only two cell lines is the usual finding, with variable numbers of RE cells. In the majority of cases bone marrow aspiration is difficult. Marrow biopsy shows a marrow that varies in cellularity, often having both hypocellular and hypercellular areas. RE cells are considerably increased in number.

Morphologically the cells are medium sized (10 to 20 μm diameter), with round to oval nuclei, though many are notched or dumbbell shaped. The chromatin pattern is usually uniformly reticular, and nucleoli are small and inconspicuous. In some cells chromatin is more condensed, resembling that of a lymphocyte. The cytoplasm is moderate in amount, often has numerous hair-like projections and frayed borders, and stains gray with Wright's stain (Plate 30-4L).

Cytochemically these cells contain acid phosphatase, which is resistant to inhibition by tartrate; this is in contrast to the isozymes of acid phosphatase present in other hemic cells (Yam, 1971a). The lineage of the reticuloendothelial cells is not yet known with certainty. The cells could be subtypes of B-lymphocytes, since in some cases the cells appear to synthesize surface immunoglobulin (Catovsky, 1977). However, other studies show that the cells have both phagocytic and B cell properties (Fu, 1974). The clinical course is usually chronic, but may be acute or subacute. The median survival is between two and four years. Splenectomy appears to be of significant benefit to many patients.

OTHER FORMS OF LEUKEMIA

Acute Undifferentiated (Stem Cell) Leukemia. This is a variety of acute leukemia in which the predominant cells are blast forms that cannot be classified as one of the types already discussed. Using cytochemical methods in classifying acute leukemia, Hayhoe (1964) was able to classify all cases of acute leukemia in other previously described categories, virtually eliminating the category of stem cell leukemia. We believe that it occurs, that it is very rare, and that it might better be designated "unclassifiable leukemia."

Plasma Cell Leukemia. Often in multiple myeloma a few plasma cells are found in the peripheral blood. Only in the rare instances of myeloma in which large numbers of plasma cells circulate is the term plasma cell leukemia used.

Chloroma. Rarely in AML there is formation of tumors originating from periosteum, especially of skull, orbits, nasal sinuses, ribs, and vertebrae. Exophthalmus with disturbances of vision may occur. The sectioned surface of the tumor shows a green color, and the tumor contains large amounts of verdoperoxidase and protoporphyrin. The color fades on exposure and can be restored with hydrogen peroxide and preserved by glycerin. There are aleukemic and leukemic forms, the latter with myeloblasts in the blood. Clinically the latter cases are identical with AML.

Myeloblastoma (*Granulocytic Sarcoma*). This localized tumor of myeloblasts differs from chloroma only by absence of pigment. Like chloroma it is rare, since the tissue involvement in AML is a diffuse infiltrative process.

Myeloblastoma may also occur preceding or at the time of the blastic phase of chronic myelogenous leukemia (CML) in skin, lymph nodes, and extradural masses or in localized, lytic bone lesions (Rosenthal, 1977). Diagnosis depends upon recognizing the nature of the primitive cells. This is facilitated by making touch imprint preparations of cut sections of the tumor and staining them with Romanowsky stains and cytochemical reactions. In formalin-fixed, embedded tissue, the naphthol AS-D chloroacetate esterase reaction may be helpful, since this enzyme resists destruction during tissue processing (p. 1090; Leder, 1964).

Eosinophilic Leukemia. This occurs but is extremely rare. Acute and chronic forms have been described; the cells infiltrating the tissues are immature eosinophils. It is generally regarded to be a variant of acute or chronic myelogenous leukemia, as the case may be, since other myeloid elements are usually involved, but to a lesser degree. It may be difficult or impossible to differentiate this lesion from the hypereosinophilic syndrome. Leukocytosis and eosinophilia, no matter how high, are not sufficient to establish the diagnosis of leukemia; both can be seen in parasitic infestation. But the diagnosis can be made when there are, in addition: persistent eosinophilia associated with immature forms in the blood as well as marrow; significantly increased blasts in the marrow (>5 per cent); tissue infiltration by immature eosinophils; and an acute course associated with anemia, thrombocytopenia, or increased susceptibility to infection (Rickles, 1972).

Basophilic Leukemia. Extremely high basophil counts overshadowing other myeloid involvement are seen occasionally in myelogenous leukemia, especially CML. A basophilic phase of CML is sometimes seen as part of the accelerated phase of the disease. It should be kept in mind that mast cells that resemble basophilic granulocytes are present in large numbers in the skin and marrow in urticaria pigmentosa.

Neutrophilic Leukemia. This is similar to eosinophilic and basophilic leukemia, but the cell type is the segmented granulocyte with very few immature forms. It is extremely rare.

Lymphosarcoma Cell Leukemia. See pages 1067 and 1078.

LEUKEMOID REACTIONS

A leukemoid reaction is an excessive leukocytic response to a stimulus that normally results in a lesser degree of leukocytosis or lesser immaturity in the circulating cells. It includes leukocytosis of $50 \times 10^9/l$ or higher with a shift to the left; lower counts, even below normal, with considerable numbers of immature granulocytes; and, similar quantitative or qualitative changes in lymphocytes or monocytes. Depending on the predominant cell, leukemoid reactions may be neutrophilic, eosinophilic, lymphocytic, or monocytic. No explanation for these apparent temporary aberrations in normal regulatory control mecha-

Tables 30–13. CONDITIONS WHICH MAY BE ASSOCIATED
WITH NEUTROPHILIC LEUKEMOID REACTIONS

CONDITION	COMMENTS
Hemolysis	Circulating normoblasts[a]
Hemorrhage	Circulating normoblasts[a]
Hodgkin's disease	Eosinophilia[b]
Infections	
Tuberculosis	Lymphocytic leukemoid reaction[c]
Congenital syphilis	Lymphocytic leukemoid reaction[c]
Pneumococcal infections	
Meningococcal infections	
Streptococcal infections	
Gas gangrene	
Diphtheria	
Leptospirosis	
Malaria	
Burns	
Eclampsia	
Vascular thrombosis	
Myelophthisic processes	Circulating normoblasts[a]
(e.g., myeloma, metastatic	Lymphocytic leukemoid reaction[c]
tumors)	Eosinophilic leukemoid reaction[c]

[a] Also present.
[b] May also be present.
[c] Another possibility in this condition.

nisms is yet available. The reactions are irregular in degree, even when associated with the same inciting agent.

Neutrophilic Leukemoid Reactions.
Leukemoid reactions involving neutrophils may occur in many situations. A list is provided in Table 30–13.

Examination of the blood is usually more helpful than marrow examination. Leukemoid reactions lack the characteristic differential count that is seen in CML, including the myelocyte "peak," eosinophilia, and basophilia (p. 1068). Also, the leukemic hiatus so characteristic of acute leukemia is absent.

Neutrophil alkaline phosphatase is decreased usually in AML and nearly always in CML, whereas it is elevated in leukemoid reactions, polycythemia vera, and sometimes in myelofibrosis with myeloid metaplasia (p. 1087).

Eosinophilic Leukemoid Reactions. Cells as immature as eosinophilic myelocytes rarely appear in the blood in reactive eosinophilia, in which the leukocyte count may excede $50 \times 10^9/l$. Eosinophilic leukemoid reactions usually occur in children and usually are caused by parasitic infections. The hypereosinophilic syndrome in adults is leukemoid (p. 1046).

Erythroblastosis. In patients with or without anemia, circulating normoblasts frequently are accompanied by a neutrophilic leukemoid reaction; this, then, is a *leuko-erythroblastotic reaction* (p. 901). A moderate anemia with normoblasts in the peripheral blood is fairly common in metastatic carcinoma involving bone marrow.

Lymphocytic Leukemoid Reactions. Extremely high counts of normal-appearing lymphocytes may occur in infectious lymphocytosis and in pertussis (p. 1048). When atypical lymphocytes are strikingly increased or immature (which may occur in conditions such as infectious mononucleosis), the distinction from leukemia may be difficult (p. 1051).

Examination of the marrow often is useful, since lymphocytes are minimally increased, if at all, in most leukemoid reactions in contrast to leukemia.

MYELOPROLIFERATIVE DISORDERS

The myeloproliferative disorders comprise a group of closely related syndromes characterized by self-perpetuating proliferation of bone marrow cells: erythroid precursors; granulocytes and monocytes; and megakaryocytes. The proliferation is abnormal, and the cause is unknown (Gunz, 1974). Marrow, spleen, liver, and lymph nodes may be involved; these are the organs that normally participate in fetal hematopoiesis. All cell lines may in involved in the proliferative process (panmyelosis) or a single cell line may predominate.

The acute myeloproliferative disorders include the Di Guglielmo syndrome (erythremic myelosis and erythroleukemia) (p. 1065), acute myelogenous leukemia (p. 1064), and acute myelomonocytic leukemia (p. 1064).

The chronic myeloproliferative disorders include polycythemia vera (PV), myelofibrosis with myeloid metaplasia (MMM), thrombocythemia, and chronic myelogenous leukemia (CML) (p. 1068). In addition, somewhat similar conditions, frequently called atypical myeloproliferative disorders or dysmyelopoietic syndromes, are probably related and will be discussed briefly.

It is known that erythroid, granulocytic-monocytic, and megakaryocytic cell lines are derived from a common hematopoietic stem cell (p. 919; see Figure 28-1). Studies in individuals with a myeloproliferative disorder who were heterozygous for glucose 6-phosphate dehydrogenase (G6-PD) isoenzymes have shown that only one isoenzyme was present in erythrocytes, granulocytes (and monocytes), and platelets, whereas both isoenzymes were found in other tissues of these patients. This has been demonstrated in CML (Fialkow, 1977), in PV (Adamson, 1976), and in MMM (Jacobson, 1978). Such evidence strongly supports the concept that myeloproliferative disorders are clonal in nature (and, by implication, neoplastic), having arisen from a single pluripotential hematopoietic stem cell. The fibrosis that may occur in the marrow in all of these conditions is not monoclonal and hence is likely to be reactive (Adamson, 1978).

The new clone appears to have a proliferative advantage over normal cells which it gradually replaces. Also, it has a variable degree of genetic instability and is predisposed to generate additional clones leading to an enhanced probability for acute leukemia to develop (Galton, 1977; Nowell, 1977). This increased probability of acute leukemia is greatest in CML, but is present in most of the myeloproliferative disorders.

Self-limited proliferative reactions of the marrow to known stimuli are not considered here to be among the myeloproliferative disorders.

Polycythemia Vera
(Erythremia, Vaquez-Osler Disease, Osler's Disease, Primary Polycythemia)

Polycythemia vera is characterized by panmyelosis (excessive proliferation of erythroid, granulocytic, and megakaryocytic elements in the marrow and also in extramedullary sites)

and reflected in the blood predominantly in an absolute increase in the red cell mass but also by leukocytosis and thrombocytosis. Erythropoietin excretion in the urine is decreased. The production of erythrocytes appears to be autonomous, but it does respond to erythropoietin when the patient has become anemic through blood loss. The cause of this panmyelosis and pancytosis in unknown.

Clinical Findings. The disease is more frequent in men than in women. It usually begins in middle age. Affected patients exhibit a peculiar and striking ruddy cyanosis. Splenomegaly is present in two thirds of patients. Thrombotic or hemorrhagic phenomena occur in about half of patients. Myocardial infarction, cerebral thrombosis, splenic infarction, pulmonary infarcts, and thrombophlebitis account for the most frequent thrombotic episodes; upper gastrointestinal bleeding, often from peptic ulcer, is the most common bleeding problem (Wasserman, 1966). Pruritus, especially after bathing, is common.

Blood. The erythrocytes number 6 to $12 \times 10^{12}/l$, and the hemoglobin is 18 to 24 g/dl. The MCV, MCH, and MCHC are normal or low. The erythrocytes are hypochromic and microcytic if chronic blood loss has occurred. Macrocytes, polychromatic cells, and normoblasts may be found but are not a prominent feature of the disease. Red cell production is increased. Red cell destruction is normal during the period of erythrocytosis; later in the disease, as splenomegaly develops, the red cell survival diminishes. The total blood volume is increased, primarily because of the increased red cell mass, though the plasma volume may also be elevated to a lesser degree. Blood viscosity is high, and it may be difficult to prepare good blood films. The ESR is reduced. The platelet count is increased in about two thirds of patients, often to levels exceeding $1000 \times 10^9/l$.

In 80 per cent of untreated patients, functional platelet abnormalities can be detected by platelet aggregation studies (Gilbert, 1975). Decreased aggregation in response to epinephrine is most common, but may be found in response to other reagents as well. No consistent clotting defect has been found in polycythemia vera. Clotting and clot retraction occur rapidly. Frequently, large numbers of erythrocytes remain outside the clot after clot retraction; this phenomenon of increased erythrocyte "fall out" is believed to be due to defective platelet aggregation (Gilbert, 1975). This may result in a false assumption of fibrinolysis, but the whole blood clot lysis and euglobulin clot lysis times are usually normal (Wasserman, 1964). Moderate neutrophilic leukocytosis in the range of 10 to $30 \times 10^9/l$ is common. Immature granulocytes are seen in about one half of cases and basophils are often absolutely increased. The neutrophil alkaline phosphatase is markedly elevated in 80 per cent of patients. Serum vitamin B_{12} binding capacity and serum muramidase are usually elevated.

The arterial oxygen saturation is normal. Hyperuricemia appears in many patients with polycythemia vera due to the increased nucleic acid metabolism, and in some patients, secondary gout or renal uric acid stones occur.

Soft agar culture of blood cells reveals normal to increased numbers of colonies (GM-CFC; p. 919). The colony stimulating activity (GM-CSF) in the blood is usually increased (Metcalf, 1977).

Marrow. The marrow is characteristically hypercellular, with all the elements (erythroid, granulocytic, and megakaryocytic) sharing the hyperplasia; fat is decreased (Plate 30-6*A*). In a study of patients of the Polycythemia Vera Study Group (PVSG) 90 per cent had moderate or marked hypercellularity; only 6 per cent were normocellular and none hypocellular (Ellis, 1975). Increased reticulin is often present and correlates positively with the cellularity. Storage iron is decreased or absent in 95 per cent of cases.

In vitro culture of marrow cells results in the growth of substantial numbers of erythroid colonies without added erythropoietin (EP); this suggests that the clone is EP independent or abnormally sensitive to EP (Prchal, 1974).

Diagnosis. Criteria for the diagnosis of PV established by the PVSG are as follows (Berlin, 1975):

1. Increased total erythrocyte volume (males, ≥ 36 ml/kg; females ≥ 32 ml/kg).
2. Normal arterial oxygen saturation (≥ 92 per cent).
3. Either splenomegaly, or two of the following:
   a. thrombocytosis ($> 400 \times 10^9/l$).
   b. leukocytosis ($> 12 \times 10^9/l$).
   c. increased neutrophil alkaline phosphatase.
   d. increased serum vitamin B_{12} (> 900 $\mu g/l$) or unsaturated B_{12} binding capacity (> 2200 $\mu g/l$).

If doubt remains about the diagnosis of polycythemia vera, a search for other causes of polycythemia should be made.

Course. Polycythemia vera is a chronic disease; patients usually live 10 to 20 years under good control. Phlebotomy, busulfan, and ^{32}P have been used to control the manifestations of the disease. Because of the high incidence of complications in untreated cases, surgery should not be undertaken unless the hematocrit has been reduced to normal levels (Wasserman, 1964).

In about 10 to 20 per cent of patients, progressive anemia, gradual splenic enlargement, and further elevation of the leukocyte count, with more immature granulocytes and more circulating nucleated red cells, may occur. Many erythrocytes become oval; tear drop-shaped cells (dacrocytes) become prominent; and poikilocytic red cells increase in number (see Figs. 27-19 and 27-20). Bone marrow aspiration becomes impossible because of myelofibrosis, and splenomegaly increases owing to extramedullary hematopoiesis. The manifestations at this stage of the disease are indistinguishable from myelofibrosis with myeloid metaplasia (Plate 30-6*B* to *D*). The latter, therefore, is not uncommonly a sequel of polycythemia vera (Gunz, 1974).

Another late complication of polycythemia vera is acute leukemia (Landaw, 1975). An increased risk of developing acute leukemia is associated with PV itself (phlebotomy treatment alone). To this is added the leukemogenic potential contributed by any of the effective myelosuppresive agents. It does appear, however, that treatment with phlebotomy alone results in shorter survival than treatment with myelosuppressive agents. The long-term prospective studies of the PVSG are likely to determine more clearly the risks associated with the different modes of therapy (Landaw, 1975).

MYELOFIBROSIS WITH MYELOID METAPLASIA

Synonyms for what is probably the same basic disease process include myelosclerosis with myeloid metaplasia, myeloid megakaryocytic hepatosplenomegaly, aleukemic myelosis, agnogenic myeloid metaplasia, and many others.

Definition. This is a chronic, progressive panmyelosis characterized by a triad of findings: varying degrees of fibrosis of the marrow, massive splenomegaly due to extramedullary hematopoiesis, and a leukoerythroblastic anemia with marked red cell abnormalities, circulating normoblasts, immature granulocytes, and atypical platelets (Gunz, 1974; Ward, 1971).

Clinical Findings. The disorder occurs typically in persons over the age of 50 and has an insidious onset, with weight loss, signs and symptoms of anemia, and abdominal discomfort due to the large spleen. Often the liver is enlarged as well, and the patient may be slightly jaundiced. On x-ray, diffuse or patchy osteosclerosis may appear in one third to one half of patients; osteoporosis may be seen also.

Blood. A moderate normochromic, normocytic anemia (frequently with some hypochromic cells and basophilic stippling), moderate anisocytosis, and marked poikilocytosis, including prominent teardrop forms (dacrocytes) and elliptocytes, are characteristic (see Figs. 27-19 and 27-20). Normoblasts are often present in numbers out of proportion to the degree of anemia, and a slight reticulocytosis is frequently found. The anemia may have a complicated origin, with components of marrow failure, ineffective erythropoiesis, and hemolysis. The leukocyte count is normal or, more commonly, moderately increased; immature neutrophils and occasionally even myeloblasts are present. The neutrophil alkaline phosphatase is most often elevated, but occasionally may be normal or decreased (Takácsi-Nagy, 1975). Chromosomal studies have not shown the presence of the Philadelphia (Ph[1]) chromosome, which is so characteristic of chronic granulocytic leukemia. Basophils are often increased in number. Platelets are normal or decreased in number (rarely increased) and often are atypical, with distinct "zones": a clear hyaloplasm and a central pale chromomere which lacks the usual concentration of azurophilic granules (Plate 30-6*E* to *G*). Small megakaryocytic fragments the size of lymphocytes with both nucleus and cytoplasm (dwarf megakaryocytes) or small megakaryoblasts may usually be found if searched for; on rare occasions, they are present in considerable numbers (Plate 30-6*E* to *G*; see also Plate 28-3*H*).

In vitro culture studies of blood cells have generally shown considerably increased colonies (GM-CFC) and clusters, which are similar to the pattern in CML. The serum colony stimulating activity (GM-CSF) appears to be very high (Metcalf, 1977).

Serum uric acid is frequently increased.

Serum vitamin B_{12} and unsaturated B_{12} binding globulin are normal or elevated.

Marrow. It is usually impossible to aspirate marrow, and a needle biopsy or a surgical biopsy is necessary for adequate study of the marrow; this is especially true later in the course of the disease. If examined early in the disease, the marrow may be hypercellular, with panmyelosis and prominently increased megakaryocytes which are frequently abnormal. On histologic sections there is a diffuse increase in reticulin fibers which is demonstrable with silver stains (Rappaport, 1966); patchy fibrosis may be present.

Later the marrow becomes more fibrotic, with residual islands of atypical megakaryocytes, erythroid, and granulocytic precursors. The fibrosis is of loose connective tissue with scanty collagen, but reticulin fibers are abundant. Foci of osteoid may be found, and the bony trabeculae are sometimes irregularly thickened (myelosclerosis). The marrow may show a mixture of hyperplasia and fibrosis in one sample or may differ in different sites of the body (Plate 30-6*A* to *E*).

Course. A significant proportion of cases of myelofibrosis with myeloid metaplasia represent a late stage, after many years' progression, of typical polycythemia vera. The usual course of MMM is one of progressive anemia and enlargement of the spleen; hemolysis frequently becomes an increasing element in the anemia. Infections may be a serious problem. Portal hypertension occurs in 10 to 20 per cent of cases and may result in bleeding esophageal varices. It may be due to portal vein thrombosis or intrahepatic obstruction due to myeloid metaplasia coupled with increased portal blood flow (Laszlo, 1975).

The median survival is about 5 years, slightly longer than that of chronic granulocytic leukemia, but considerably less than that of polycythemia vera; however, patients may occasionally live as long as 10 to 15 years. In patients with longer survival, frequently the terminal event is an acute leukemia.

THROMBOCYTHEMIA

As distinguished from *thrombocytosis*, the term *thrombocythemia* should probably be confined to situations in which the platelet count is persistently elevated to levels at least three times normal (Gunz, 1974). It will be evident that thrombocythemia, thus defined, will usually be part of the general picture of other myeloproliferative disorders: polycythemia vera, chronic myelogenous leukemia, and, rarely, myelofibrosis with myeloid metaplasia.

Occasionally, however, thrombocythemia may be the predominant feature of the hematologic picture, and in these cases it is commonly associated with bleeding problems. After reviewing most of the reported cases, Gunz (1960) regarded them as constituting a clinical syndrome of *hemorrhagic thrombocythemia.*

Clinical Findings. Characteristic are recurrent, spontaneous hemorrhages, which are most commonly gastrointestinal. Hemorrhages are occasionally preceded or accompanied by thrombosis in superficial or deep veins. Purpura has not been described. Slight splenomegaly is the rule.

Blood. The most striking feature is the marked increase in platelets (maximum values: 0.9 to 14.0 $\times$ 10^{12}/l, often with abnormal and giant forms and usually accompanied by fragments of megakaryocytes. Neutrophilic leukocytosis is almost always present, and the neutrophil alkaline phosphatase has been elevated in most cases in which it has been examined. Hypochromic microcytic anemia due to chronic blood loss is present in many cases; at other times, erythrocytosis may be evident. Platelet function defects in myeloproliferative diseases, especially thrombocythemia, are frequently demonstrable. The most typical finding is decreased aggregation in response to epinephrine (Spaet, 1969; Laszlo, 1975).

Marrow. The marrow shows a panmyelosis with increased megakaryocytes. Splenic extramedullary hematopoiesis may be present.

Gunz (1960) regards hemorrhagic thrombocythemia as a clinical syndrome; the pathologic features cannot be separated from those of the other myeloproliferative disorders. It is probably most closely related to polycythemia vera.

Dysmyelopoietic Syndromes

Certain hematopoietic proliferative disorders have a significantly increased risk of the subsequent development of acute leukemia; these have been designated by some as "preleukemia" (Saarni, 1973). Nowell (1977) recognizes three groups of disorders with such a risk: (1) Myeloproliferative disorders such as PV, MMM, and thrombocythemia, in which a small proportion of patients develop acute leu-

kemia; (2) Congenital and childhood disorders with chromosomal abnormalities (e.g., Fanconi's anemia) and some cases of aplastic and hypoplastic anemias; and (3) a spectrum of disorders characterized by a cellular marrow with disturbed maturation and often with increased blasts, and reduction of one or more blood elements, usually pancytopenia. A high proportion of this latter group develops acute leukemia. This is the "preleukemia" group reviewed by Saarni (1973).

The FAB Cooperative Group (Bennett, 1976) classifies these into two broad types: refractory anemia with excess of blasts (RAEB) and chronic myelomonocytic leukemia (CMML). These are distinguished mainly by a predominance of the erythroid component in the former and of the granulocytic and monocytic components in the latter.

Refractory Anemia with Excess of Blasts (RAEB). This is probably the most frequent of the dysmyelopoietic syndromes. It occurs in patients over age 50 as an anemia refractory to iron, vitamin B$_{12}$, folic acid, and pyridoxine therapy.

Blood. The anemia with reticulocytopenia is usually accompanied by neutropenia and often by thrombocytopenia. Neutrophil abnormalities such as hypogranularity or pseudo Pelger-Huët changes may be present. Monocytes are less than 1 $\times$ 10^9/l. A few blasts may be found in some patients.

Marrow. In the hypercellular marrow, erythroid cells usually predominate and dyserythropoietic changes are present, sometimes including ring sideroblasts. Abnormal granulocytic maturation is present, especially impaired nuclear maturation, and blasts and promyelocytes usually range from 10 to 30 per cent of the differential cell count. Megakaryocytes usually show morphologic changes: small binucleated or single nucleated (dwarf) megakaryocytes are frequently found, if sought (see Plate 28-3*H* and 30-6*E* to *G*).

Chronic Myelomonocytic Leukemia (CMML) (Miescher, 1974). CMML occurs after age 50 with a slight male predominance. Clinical findings are those of anemia; infections and hemorrhagic manifestations are common. One third of patients have slight splenomegaly.

Blood. Anemia is usually present, but less consistently than in RAEB. The absolute neutrophil count varies, but there is always an absolute monocytosis (>1 $\times$ 10^9/l). Neutrophil abnormalities as in RAEB may be found. Blasts are rarely present. Serum (and urinary) muramidase levels are consistently elevated. The neutrophil alkaline phosphatase may be low, normal, or elevated.

MARROW. The hypercellular marrow is similar to that in RAEB, though the E/G ratio tends to be lower. The principal cell type resembles a neutrophil myelocyte with impaired nuclear maturation. Blasts and promyelocytes number 10 to 30 per cent. Monocytosis is always present, but the morphologic distinction from myelocytes is often difficult; non-specific esterase stains (p. 1090) are helpful in demonstrating the monocytosis. A mild plasmacytosis is usually noted.

Cell Culture Studies. *In vitro* cultures using semisolid agar provide a means of studying disorders of myelopoiesis (p. 919; Metcalf, 1977). In RAEB, the number of colony forming cells (GM-CFC) formed by marrow cells is reduced, and the peripheral blood leukocytes fail to demonstrate colony stimulating factor (GM-CSF) activity. In contrast, marrow cells from CMML yield normal or increased numbers of GM-CFC's; and blood leukocytes produce GM-CSF (Sultan, 1977).

Although myeloproliferative disorders have yet to be thoroughly studied using *in vitro* culture techniques, abnormalities in GM-CFC growth have been noted in patients with several of these disorders (Metcalf, 1977). The presence of certain findings, such as low GM-CFC values in marrow, an increasing cluster/colony ratio,* or increased GM-CSF (or the change to such patterns) appears to precede or accompany the onset of acute leukemia in many patients (Greenberg, 1976).

MALIGNANT LYMPHOMA

Malignant lymphoma is a neoplastic proliferation of one of the cell types of the lymphopoietic-reticular tissue. Lymphocytes or histiocytes are the cells involved. If a mixture of more than one cell type appears to be present, it probably represents a variation in the size, configuration, or degree of differentiation of one cell type, rather than separate cell lines (Lukes, 1971).

Usually lymphoma begins in and involves

Colonies are aggregates of cells that contain more than 40 cells formed by proliferation *in vitro; clusters* are smaller aggregates containing 3 to 40 cells.

lymph nodes predominantly, although other sites such as the spleen and the gastrointestinal tract are frequent areas of origin as well. As the disease progresses, proliferation spreads to lymphoid tissue beyond the site of origin. In advanced disease, infiltrations of neoplastic cells are found in many organs throughout the body. When lymphoma originates in extranodal tissue, e.g., the stomach or lung, the course is likely to be more benign than otherwise.

NON-HODGKIN'S LYMPHOMAS

Classification

During the past 60 years numerous morphologic classifications of the non-Hodgkin's lymphomas have been presented. The classification offered by Rappaport (1966) has gained wide usage in the United States (Table 30-14). Studies have shown that this classification gives a good correlation between histopathology and clinical presentation, survival and response to therapy (Fig. 30-2; Table 30-15) (Jones, 1973). However, problems with the classification exist. Studies utilizing immunologic and cytochemical cell markers to determine the lineage of neoplastic lymphoreticular cells have shown that some of the terminology is inaccurate (Davey, 1976). In general, nodular lymphomas originate from follicular B-lymphocytes. Histiocytic lymphomas are rarely histiocytic; rather, the majority of these tumors are either B or null cell malignancies.

Undifferentiated lymphomas (Burkitt's lymphoma) are not truly undifferentiated but are B cell neoplasms. As a result of the problem with terminology, classifications by other investigators have been offered (Dorfman, 1974; Lukes, 1974). None of these classifications, however, has yet been shown in prospective studies to correlate well with survival. Until these data are available, we continue to use the Rappaport classification because of its popularity, simplicity, and clinical usefulness.

The Rappaport classification first divides the non-Hodgkin's lymphomas into two major categories, nodular and diffuse. In the former, neoplastic cells are arranged throughout the lymph node in a nodular pattern (Plate 30-4F). The normal architecture of the lymph node is lost (including normal germinal centers) in the proliferation, neoplastic cells infiltrate the capsule, and there is cellular atypia. In the diffuse lymphomas, no nodularity is

Table 30-14. CLASSIFICATION OF NON-HODGKIN'S LYMPHOMA

RAPPAPORT (1966)	DORFMAN (1974)	LUKES AND COLLINS (1974)
Nodular Lymphomas	Follicular Lymphomas	I. U cell (undefined cell) type

Lymphocytic, well differentiated
Lymphocytic, poorly differentiated
Mixed, lymphocytic-histiocytic
Histiocytic
	Small lymphoid
	Mixed small and large lymphoid
	Large lymphoid
		II. T cell types
		    Mycosis fungoides and Sézary's syndrome
		    Convoluted lymphocyte
		    ? Immunoblastic sarcoma (of T cells)
		    ? Hodgkin's disease

Diffuse Lymphomas	Diffuse Lymphomas	

Lymphocytic, well differentiated
Lymphocytic, poorly differentiated
Mixed, lymphocytic-histiocytic
Histiocytic
Undifferentiated
	Small lymphocytic
	Small lymphocytic with plasma-cytoid differentiation
	Atypical small lymphocytic
	Large lymphoid (pyroninophilic)
	Mixed small and large lymphoid
	Histiocytic
	Burkitt's lymphoma
	Mycosis fungoides
	Undefined
		III. B cell types
		    Small lymphocyte (CLL)
		    Plasmacytoid lymphocyte
		    Follicular center cell (FCC) types
		    (follicular, diffuse, follicular and diffuse, and sclerotic)
		      small cleaved
		      large cleaved
		      small non-cleaved
		      large non-cleaved
		    Immunoblastic sarcoma (of B cells)

		IV. Histiocytic type
		V. Unclassifiable

apparent in the specimen. Instead, the involved lymph node is composed of neoplastic lymphoid cells infiltrating the tissue in an even distribution (Plate 30-4C). The second requirement of the Rappaport classification is proper identification of the neoplastic cells according to five cytologic types. These include well-differentiated lymphocytic, poorly differentiated lymphocytic, mixed histiocytic-lymphocytic, histiocytic, and undifferentiated.

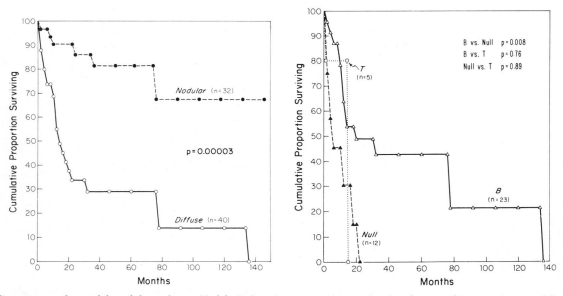

Figure 30-2. Survival for adults with non-Hodgkin's lymphoma according to the classification of Rappaport. *Left*, Diffuse versus nodular; *Right*, diffuse lymphoma according to subtype B, T, or null. (From Bloomfield, C. D., Kersey, J. H., Brunning, R. D., and Gajl-Peczalska, K. J.: Prognostic significance of lymphocyte surface markers in adult non-Hodgkin's malignant lymphoma. Lancet, 2:1330, 1976. Used by permission.)

Table 30–15.   CORRELATION OF MEDIAN SURVIVAL ACCORDING TO RAPPAPORT
CLASSIFICATION. STANFORD SERIES (1960–1971)*

| | NODULAR | | DIFFUSE | |
CYTOLOGIC TYPE	No. Cases	Med. Surv. (yrs)	No. Cases	Med. Surv. (yrs)
Lymphocytic, well differentiated	6	all alive > 5 yrs	10	1 Pt. dead at 3·5 yrs
Lymphocytic, poorly differentiated	69	7·5	44	1·8
Mixed lymphocytic-histiocytic	74	7·0	43	1·6
Histiocytic	29	2·9	116	1·1
Undifferentiated	0	—	14	0·5

*From Berard, C.W., and Dorfman, R.F.: Histopathology of malignant lymphomas. Clin. Hematol., *3*:39, 1974.

Well-differentiated lymphocytic lymphoma (Plate 30-4*A* and *B*)

The cell type is the small lymphocyte, with clumped chromatin indistinguishable from the normal lymphocyte. Mitoses are rarely seen. The pattern of node and marrow involvement is characteristically diffuse. Though it may begin in lymph nodes, the accumulative process involves the bone marrow quite early in its course, and the blood lymphocyte count is then elevated. The usual diagnosis, therefore, is chronic lymphatic leukemia rather than well-differentiated lymphocytic lymphoma. It is essentially the same disease.

This is a disorder of late adult life. Hypogammaglobulinemia is frequent, and autoimmune hemolytic anemia occurs in 10 to 20 per cent of patients.

Poorly differentiated lymphocytic lymphoma (Plate 30-4*D* and *E*)

The proliferating cell is a lymphocyte with a nucleus which has less condensation of chromatin than the normal circulating lymphocyte; irregular, cleft, or indented nuclear shape; and small inconspicuous nucleoli. The cytoplasm is scant in amount. It is similar to the cells in the germinal centers of normal lymph nodes. The pattern of node involvement is usually nodular, especially in adults. Spread to the marrow and other organs tends to be in nodular or discrete masses rather than diffuse. A few poorly differentiated lymphocytes occasionally enter the circulation. Late in the course of the disease in about 20 per cent of patients the marrow becomes more heavily involved, and larger numbers of these cleft or notched immature lymphocytes are found in the blood. The terms "lymphosarcoma cell leukemia" and "leukosarcoma" have been used to designate

Plate 30-4. *A*, Well-differentiated lymphocytic lymphoma. The lymph node is infiltrated by small lymphocytes. Hematoxylin and eosin (H & E), × 400. *B*, Touch preparation of well-differentiated lymphocytic lymphoma. The majority of lymphocytes are small lymphocytes; however, occasional stimulated lymphocytes are present. Wright-Giemsa, × 900. *C*, Non-Hodgkin's lymphoma with diffuse pattern. Compare with *F*. H & E, × 100. *D*, Poorly differentiated lymphocytic lymphoma. Note the presence of lymphoid cells with angulated and clefted nuclei, occasional nucleoli, and scant cytoplasm. Mitotic figures are more frequent than in *A*. H & E, × 400. *E*, Touch preparation of poorly differentiated lymphocytic lymphoma. The majority of cells are stimulated lymphocytes with occasional mature lymphocytes. Wright-Giemsa, × 900. *F*, Non-Hodgkin's lymphoma with follicular pattern. Compare with *C*. H & E, × 100. *G*, Burkitt's lymphoma. Large primitive lymphoid cells are positioned around tissue macrophages (H & E, × 400). *H*, Touch preparation of Burkitt's lymphoma. Neoplastic cells contain fine reticular chromatin. Cytoplasm is intensely basophilic and frequently contains multiple vacuoles. Wright-Giemsa, × 900. *I*, Sézary cells, blood film, from a patient with mycosis fungoides. Wright-Giemsa stain, × 400. These are mononuclear cells with scanty cytoplasm and a deeply indented or convoluted nucleus. The cell on the left has more chromatin condensation than the cell adjacent to the neutrophil on the right. *J*, Histiocytic lymphoma. Large lymphoid cells with prominent nuclei, thickened nuclear membrane, conspicuous nucleoli, and more abundant cytoplasm. H & E, × 400. *K*, Touch preparation of histiocytic lymphoma. Neoplastic cells are large, measuring approximately 20 μm in diameter. The nuclear chromatin is fine and reticular; nucleoli are prominent. Wright-Giemsa, × 900. *L*, Leukemic reticuloendotheliosis (hairy cell leukemia), blood film, Wright-Giemsa stain, × 400. The two left-most cells are "hairy cells." They have less condensed but more intensely staining chromatin and more irregular cytoplasmic margins than normal lymphocytes (cell at farthest right).

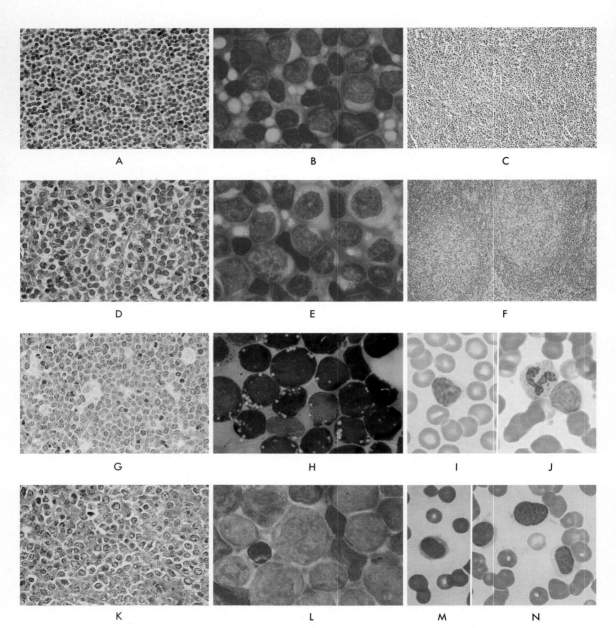

Plate 30-4. *See legend on opposite page.*

Table 30–17. CLASSIFICATIONS OF HODGKIN'S DISEASE*

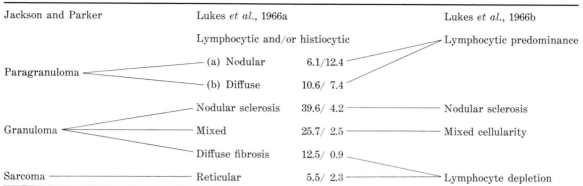

Jackson and Parker	Lukes *et al.*, 1966a	Lukes *et al.*, 1966b
	Lymphocytic and/or histiocytic	Lymphocytic predominance
Paragranuloma	(a) Nodular 6.1/12.4	
	(b) Diffuse 10.6/ 7.4	
Granuloma	Nodular sclerosis 39.6/ 4.2	Nodular sclerosis
	Mixed 25.7/ 2.5	Mixed cellularity
	Diffuse fibrosis 12.5/ 0.9	
Sarcoma	Reticular 5.5/ 2.3	Lymphocyte depletion

*The figures in the left column represent the per cent of cases of that type and the figures in the right column represent the median survival in years for all clinical stages of that type from the series reported by Lukes, R. J., Butler, J. J., and Hicks, E. B.: Cancer *19*:317, 1966.

The *mixed type* has a variety of cell types: lymphocytes, plasma cells, eosinophils, histiocytes, and Sternberg-Reed cells, which are often quite numerous. Necrosis and disorderly fibrosis may be present (Plate 30-5*D*).

The rare *lymphocyte depletion* type (Plate 30-5*E*) is more often diffuse fibrosis than reticular and is an acute febrile illness without lymphadenopathy associated with pancytopenia and lymphocytopenia. The lack of leukocytosis and thrombocytosis and more frequent involvement of the bone marrow contrast with other forms of Hodgkin's disease (Neiman, 1973).

Blood Findings. Normocytic, sometimes severe, anemia is seen in about 50 per cent of cases.

The leukocyte count may be elevated, normal, or reduced (leukopenic). The differential count shows neutrophilia, lymphocytopenia, monocytosis, and eosinophilia. Either all or any combination of these may be present.

Neutrophilic leukocytosis is seen, especially when lymph nodes are involved, and neutropenia, when bone marrow is involved. The blood changes seem to depend on the stage of the disease and on some individual, as yet unknown, factors. The neutrophil alkaline phosphatase is elevated during activity of the disease; it returns to normal during remissions.

The most frequent finding is a moderate leukocytosis, with white cell counts ranging from 12 to 25 × 10⁹/l and a relative and even absolute lymphopenia. In the differential count the lymphocytes may decrease below 10 per cent. A slight shift to the left may be present in the neutrophils. As a rule, lymphopenia is prognostically a poor omen.

Monocytosis is frequent, with values of 10 per cent or higher. Eosinophilia has been described in about 20 per cent of patients and may be extreme. The platelet count may be increased, normal, or decreased, the latter especially with marrow involvement.

Both the histologic changes noted above and the blood and marrow findings appear to be manifestations of different host responses to the disease.

Marrow Findings. Frequently there is a granulocytic hyperplasia with a shift to the left, slight monocytosis, and eosinophilia. As a rule, findings are not characteristic. Amyloid infiltration of various grades is sometimes present in various organs and with it plasma cell hyperplasia in the marrow.

If marrow biopsy is performed in patients with systemic symptoms or with clinical Stage III or Stage IV disease, it will be positive in about 10 per cent of patients (Rosenberg, 1971). Positive biopsy is interpreted as: (1) the presence of Reed-Sternberg cells in an appropriate pleomorphic cellular stroma; or, less commonly (2) abnormal infiltration of lymphocytes, histiocytes, and fibrosis without classic Reed-Sternberg cells, but with documented Hodgkin's disease in other sites.

In the rare lymphocyte depletion type of Hodgkin's disease, dissemination is widespread and bone marrow is involved in most cases.

Clinical Staging. Clinical staging is currently employed to determine the extent of the disease at the time of diagnosis. Besides history and physical examination, extensive radiographic studies, radioisotope scans, CBC, platelet count, erythrocyte sedimentation rate, neutrophil alkaline phosphatase, bone marrow biopsy, liver function studies, urinalysis, and skin tests for delayed hypersensitivity are performed. Stage I disease is limited to lymph nodes in one anatomic region or two contiguous regions on one side of the diaphragm. Stage II disease involves more than two contiguous regions or two non-contiguous regions on one side of the diaphragm. Stage III disease is present on both sides of the diaphragm but is confined to lymphoid tissue. Stage IV disease involves bone marrow or any other organ, in addition to lymphoid tissue. All stages are additionally classified as A if systemic symptoms are absent, B if they are present. This extensive diagnostic approach is to define areas of involvement and facilitate radiation therapy, which is combined with chemotherapy. It is part of the current aggressive approach to the management of Hodgkin's disease, which is resulting in longer survival and even apparent cure in some patients.

Immunologic studies in Hodgkin's disease have shown that cell-mediated immunity is defective when extensive disease is present.

MYCOSIS FUNGOIDES

Mycosis fungoides is a lymphoreticular neoplasm primarily involving the skin. As the disorder evolves, neoplastic cells infiltrate the lymph nodes and other visceral organs.

Mycosis fungoides occurs twice as frequently in men as in women. It usually affects individuals in their middle to late years.

The disorder first appears as an eczematoid, psoriaform, or generalized erythematous rash. The lesions tend to form plaques and then tumors which sometimes ulcerate.

Biopsies of the skin reveal lymphocytic and mononuclear cell infiltrates in the dermis. Neoplastic cells and normal-appearing lymphocytes infiltrate the epidermis and form clusters known as Pautrier abscesses. The nuclei of the neoplastic cells frequently have a cerebriform appearance.

In advanced stages of the disease, neoplastic cells infiltrate the lymph nodes, liver, spleen, and other organs (Rappaport, 1974).

Occasionally atypical mononuclear cells with cerebriform nuclei are present in the peripheral blood (Plate 30-4*I*). In addition, when lymphocytosis exists (especially in the erythremic patient) the disorder is called the *Sézary syndrome*. The cells with cerebriform nuclei (Sézary cells) have been demonstrated to be T-lymphocytes (Flandrin, 1974); mycosis

---

Plate 30-5. *A*, Hodgkin's disease, lymphocyte predominance type. The mature lymphocyte is the most common cell. Histiocytes are frequently present. Reed-Sternberg cells are rare. Eosinophils and plasma cells are infrequent. Hematoxylin and eosin (H & E), ×250. *B*, Hodgkin's disease, nodular sclerosis type. Broad bands of collagen course through the lymph node, forming nodules of lymphoid tissue. H & E, ×100. *C*, Hodgkin's disease, nodular sclerosis type. Note presence of "lacunar" Reed-Sternberg cells with multinuclei and pale cytoplasm. H & E, ×400. *D*, Hodgkin's disease, mixed type. There are numerous Reed-Sternberg cells and histiocytes. Eosinophils and plasma cells are characteristically present. H & E, ×400. *E*, Hodgkin's disease, lymphocyte depletion type. There are several multinucleated Reed-Sternberg cells and many abnormal mononuclear cells. Lymphocytes are less prominent. There is a background of proteinaceous material and disorderly fibrosis. H & E ×400. *F*, Reed-Sternberg cell, in Hodgkin's disease, mixed type. *G*, Poorly differentiated lymphocytic lymphoma, leukemic phase. Blasts, such as this cell, and cells with more chromatin condensation and notched nuclei (as in Plate 30-4*E*) are found in the blood in a minority of patients with PDLL, usually late in the disease. *H*, Lymphocytic reaction. This reticular lymphocyte in the blood of a patient with a viral infection resembles the malignant blast in *G*. This type of reactive blast form ("non-leukemic lymphoblast") usually has more deeply basophilic cytoplasm and is associated with numerous characteristic atypical lymphocytes, as in *I*. *I*, Atypical lymphocyte, blood film. *J*, Plasma cells adjacent to the endothelial cells lining a blood vessel in bone marrow film from a patient with rheumatoid arthritis. In mature plasma cells the nuclear chromatin is coarsely clumped and the cytoplasm is deeply basophilic. *K*, Multiple myeloma, bone marrow film. The abnormal plasma cells have abundant cytoplasm and eccentric nuclei. In contrast to normal plasma cells, however, the cytoplasm is less deeply basophilic, the chromatin is not coarsely clumped, and nucleoli are prominent. *L*, Multiple myeloma, bone marrow film. The dissociation between advanced cytoplasmic maturation (abundant, usually basophilic cytoplasm with a prominent Golgi zone) and delayed nuclear maturation (prominent nucleolus, less chromatin condensation) is the most useful feature in distinguishing the abnormal plasma cells in myeloma from normal plasma cells.

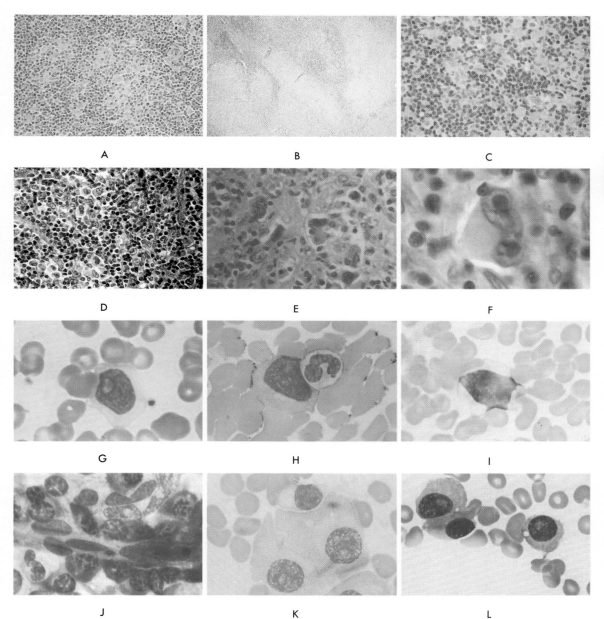

Plate 30–5. *See legend on opposite page.*

fungoides is now classified as a T-cell lymphoreticular neoplasm (see Tables 30-14 and 30-16).

The disorder may follow a prolonged chronic course. However, following lymph node infiltration, the disease becomes more progressive and death, usually due to infection, occurs within two years (Van Scott, 1977).

BLOOD PROTEIN DISORDERS

Immunoglobulins are discussed in Chapter 36 and 42.

Polyclonal gammopathy refers to an increase in the serum of several different immunoglobulins which are the products of many different clones of plasma cells. This is usually a response to antigenic stimulation.

Monoclonal gammopathy refers to an increase in the serum of one specific class, subclass, and type of immunoglobulin molecule (or fragment thereof); this is the product of plasma cells or lymphocytes which originated from a single cell or clone. Monoclonal gammopathy is found in multiple myeloma, some lymphomas (including Waldenström's macroglobulinemia and heavy chain diseases), some patients with primary amyloidosis, a few patients with carcinoma, and some individuals with no known underlying disease. The latter group may comprise up to one third of all monoclonal gammopathies (Ritzmann, 1972); it includes primarily elderly individuals who have a lower concentration of the homogeneous immunoglobulin (less than 2 g/dl) which does not change for long periods of time.

MULTIPLE MYELOMA

This is a neoplastic proliferation of plasma cells or morphologically abnormal plasma cells (myeloma cells), primarily occurring in the bone marrow either in nodules or diffusely. Though plasma cells also proliferate in lymph nodes and spleen, these organs are rarely enlarged.

Clinical. Multiple myeloma is rare under age 40. The mean age at the time of diagnosis is 62 years. The incidence of this disease is equal in men and women. Bone pain is the commonest symptom, and pathologic fractures are frequent. Neurologic symptoms may be prominent from encroachment of tumor which has broken through the bony cortex on spinal nerves or spinal cord. Bone destruction leads to calcium mobilization, with increase of calcium in the serum and metastatic calcification.

The growth of myeloma cells in the marrow produces multiple tumors, which appear on x-ray as multiple punched-out osteoporotic lesions; occasionally the growth is diffuse and appears as diffuse osteoporosis. An unusual propensity to infection is common because of impaired production of antibodies.

Blood. There is usually a normochromic normocytic anemia; normoblasts may be present in the blood. The leukocyte count is slightly decreased, normal, or slightly increased. Occasionally young neutrophils or even myeloblasts may be found. Usually myeloma cells can be located if careful search of the blood films or buffy coat films is made; on occasion, myeloma cells may be extremely numerous (plasma cell leukemia). The platelet count is usually normal, but may be decreased. The most striking feature of the blood smear is the marked degree of rouleaux formation, which may make cell counting difficult (see Fig. 27-28).

Marrow. The bone marrow shows the presence of plasma cells or myeloma cells, varying from less than 1 per cent to over 90 per cent, depending upon the degree of involvement in the site of marrow aspirated. Cytologically the cells may be indistinguishable from normal plasma cells, but they usually show abnormalities, such as less clumping of nuclear chromatin, large nucleoli, lack of a perinuclear clear zone, lighter blue cytoplasm, or varying degrees of anaplasia (Plate 30-5*K* and *L*). The dissociation of nuclear and cytoplasmic maturation is a distinctive feature of the myeloma cells (Bernier, 1976).

Immunoglobulins (see also p. 1217). Serum globulin is usually increased, often strikingly so. This increase is responsible for the tendency toward rouleaux formation and an elevated erythrocyte sedimentation rate (ESR). Serum protein electrophoresis usually shows an M-spot, a homogeneous band in the gamma or beta region; less commonly there is hypogammaglobulinemia (when only light chains are produced by the neoplastic plasma cells). Immunoelectrophoresis indicates that the monoclonal protein is IgG in over half the cases of multiple myeloma, IgA in about one fifth, IgD in less than 1 per cent, and IgE very rarely. In each of these groups of myeloma, some patients secrete Bence Jones protein (light chains, kappa *or* lambda) in addition to the whole immunoglobulin molecule. In about one quarter of patients with multiple myeloma, only light chains (Bence Jones protein) are produced by the abnormal plasma cells.

Hypogammaglobulinemia is found in the latter group because light chains are filtered through the renal glomerulus, leaving little or none in the serum, in addition to the fact that immunoglobulin production by the non-malignant plasma cells is greatly reduced in all patients with multiple myeloma.

Roughly 5 per cent of myeloma proteins are cryoglobulins, that is, proteins which precipitate from cooled serum and redissolve on warming.

Proteinuria is frequently present in multiple myeloma. In somewhat over 50 per cent of patients Bence Jones protein is present. This may be detected by its property of precipitating from acidified urine heated to 50°C. and redissolving when the urine is boiled, or by electrophoresis of a concentrate of urine on which it migrates as a narrow band in the gamma globulin region. If renal damage has occurred, albumin and whole immunoglobulin molecules are also found in the urine. Excretion of Bence Jones protein often results in obstruction and elimination of nephrons, and the so-called myeloma kidney. Renal insufficiency is common and is the presenting feature of multiple myeloma in some cases.

Amyloidosis, which is present in about 10 to 15 per cent of cases of multiple myeloma, may be a factor in the renal failure. Amyloid fibrils in cases of myeloma appear to have as the major protein component of their fibrils the light chains of immunoglobulin molecules (Glenner, 1973).

The diagnosis of multiple myeloma is secure if the marrow contains large numbers of morphologically bizarre, malignant-appearing plasma cells. If large numbers of normal-appearing plasma cells and plasma-cell precursors are present in the marrow, the diagnosis is not established unless punched-out, lytic bone lesions are demonstrated by x-ray, or Bence Jones proteinuria or a monoclonal gammopathy is also present (Rapaport, 1971).

Median survival after diagnosis is approximately three years. In almost 5 per cent of patients, acute leukemia develops (usually myelomonocytic) (Rosner, 1974). This may be preceded by sideroblastic anemia (Khaleeli, 1973).

WALDENSTRÖM'S MACROGLOBULINEMIA

Macroglobulins (IgM immunoglobulins) comprise 3 to 10 per cent of serum proteins. They have a high molecular weight (1,000,000), a sedimentation constant of 18 to 20 Svedberg units, and a high carbohydrate content and are characterized by a mu heavy chain and either kappa or lambda light chains. Increases of serum macroglobulins which are polyclonal may be seen in chronic infections or in collagen diseases. Monoclonal macroglobulinemia is found in a few individuals without detectable disease; in some cases of malignant lymphoma, chronic lymphocytic leukemia, and carcinoma; and in a syndrome known as Waldenström's macroglobulinemia. Though many have regarded the latter as primary macroglobulinemia and the others as secondary, MacKenzie (1972) states that this distinction cannot be maintained. They view monoclonal macroglobulinemia as a spectrum of disorders.

Clinical. Waldenström's macroglobulinemia is found in individuals over the age of 40, with a peak incidence between ages 60 and 70. It is characterized by a general proliferation of lymphocytes (and plasma cells) and the presence of at least 1 g/dl of monoclonal IgM in the serum, amounting to at least 15 per cent of the total serum protein.

The clinical features of the disease are effects of the increased serum macroglobulins, which commonly cause symptoms due to increased viscosity, and the cell proliferation itself, which accounts for hepatosplenomegaly and some degree of lymphadenopathy. In contrast to multiple myeloma, bone pain and osteolytic lesions on x-ray are rare. Hyperviscosity and sludging of blood may lead to visual disturbances, neurologic symptoms, impaired kidney function, and right-sided congestive heart failure. Hemorrhagic phenomena may be caused by the macroglobulins adhering to platelets, which interferes with their function, and forming complexes with plasma clotting factors, which impairs their activity. Cryoglobulinemia occurs somewhat more frequently than with myeloma and may be responsible for sensitivity to cold and Raynaud's phenomenon.

Blood. Normochromic, normocytic anemia is sometimes associated with thrombocytopenia or pancytopenia. Relative or slight absolute lymphocytosis is usually found. Marked rouleaux formation is present on the blood smear, and the sedimentation rate is usually extremely rapid, although it may be low if macrocryoglobulins are present and the test is carried out at a lower temperature. The anemia is occasionally hemolytic with a positive Coombs' test.

Marrow. Often the marrow cannot be aspirated readily. Lymphoid cells are increased in number. These usually resemble normal small lymphocytes, but sometimes plasmacytoid cells are present and plasma cells may be increased in number. PAS-positive inclusions are often seen in the cytoplasm and nucleus of the lymphoid cells. Tissue mast cells are increased in number.

Immunoglobulins (see also p. 1219). Serum globulin is usually markedly increased.

The *relative serum viscosity* may be simply measured using an Ostwald viscometer. The average time for descent of the serum at room temperature is expressed as a ratio to that of distilled water. The normal range is 1.4 to 1.8. It is considerably elevated in most patients with macroglobulinemia. Symptoms of hyperviscosity appear in most patients when the relative serum viscosity is between 6 and 8, though the threshold varies among patients (MacKenzie, 1972; see p. 1093).

The *Sia water test* is performed by allowing a drop of serum to fall into a tube of distilled water. Normally the drop disappears, leaving a faint haze. In macroglobulinemia a distinct precipitate forms, does not disappear, and falls to the bottom of the tube. The test is mentioned only because of its simplicity. It has the disadvantage of giving many false negative results, and it may be positive in polyclonal increases of IgM, such as rheumatoid arthritis and in a small proportion of patients with IgG myeloma, especially those with hyperviscosity (Pruzanski, 1972).

Zone electrophoresis of serum proteins on paper or cellulose acetate reveals a homogeneous band between the beta and gamma areas, which suggests a monoclonal gammopathy. If a disulfide reducing agent which splits the IgM into its component subunits (such as mercaptoethanol) is added to serum before electrophoresis, the single band will separate into two or more bands; this does not occur with non-aggregating immunoglobulins such as IgG.

Ultracentrifugal study shows the molecular size to be large, with a sedimentation constant of 19S.

Final identification is achieved by *immunoelectrophoresis*, which is required for definitive characterization of the protein; together with the mu heavy chains, only one type of light chain is found. The total monoclonal IgM exceeds 10 mg/ml (1 g/dl).

Bence Jones proteinuria occurs in about 10 per cent of patients.

Several studies have shown that in almost all cases of chronic lymphocytic leukemia (CLL), the lymphocytes are B cells; the surface immunoglobulin is monoclonal and, in most cases, is IgM. In about a third of cases of CLL, there is also a small amount of monoclonal serum immunoglobulin as well. In Waldenström's macroglobulinemia, lymphoid cells and plasma cells of the marrow and many of the circulating lymphocytes have a surface IgM with the same light chain type as the serum IgM. It appears that Waldenström's macroglobulinemia is a variant of CLL (or well-differentiated lymphocytic lymphoma) in which there is a greater degree of maturation of the B-lymphocytes into plasma cells (Preud'homme, 1972).

HEAVY CHAIN DISEASE

A small number of patients produce and excrete heavy chain fragments without associated light chains (see also p. 1218). Some of these proteins show structural mutations (Frangione, 1973).

Gamma Heavy Chain Disease (γ-HCD). This disorder clinically resembles malignant lymphoma rather than myeloma, with lymphadenopathy, hepatosplenomegaly, fever, and propensity to infections. Anemia is constantly present, often with leukopenia and thrombocytopenia. Atypical lymphocytes or plasma cells are frequently present in the blood, and two cases have terminated in plasma cell leukemia. The marrow is usually abnormal, with increased plasma cells and lymphocytes and eosinophils, but is not diagnostic. Usually, but not always, the histology of lymphoid tissue indicates a malignant lymphoproliferative disease. A rather broad serum protein "spike" has been found in the beta-gamma region in most patients, accompanied by hypogammaglobulinemia. The diagnosis is made by showing that the protein reacts on immunoelectrophoresis with antisera to γ-chains but not to light chains. The protein is also found in the urine in varying amounts, though concentration techniques may be necessary to demonstrate it.

Alpha Heavy Chain Disease (α-HCD). This disorder appears to be more common than γ-HCD, and involves a younger age group. The uniform clinical pattern in most patients is malabsorption and diarrhea accompanying a massive lymphoplasmacytic infiltration of intestinal mucosa, or a histiocytic lymphoma of the intestine. In a few patients, the respiratory tract has been involved instead. Bone marrow and other lymphoid organs have not been involved. Usually routine protein electrophoresis is negative, but small amounts of alpha chain may be detected in the serum and sometimes in the urine with immunoelectrophoresis. The abnormal protein does not contain light chains (Seligmann, 1975).

Mu Heavy Chain Disease (μ-HCD). The few patients who have been described have had chronic lymphocytic leukemia with vacuolated plasma cells in the marrow. Routine serum electrophoresis showed only hypogammaglobulinemia. The μ heavy chain was detected by serum immunoelectrophoresis; it was not found in the urine. In most patients, however, the urine contained light chains (κ) in large amounts (Franklin, 1975).

LABORATORY METHODS

The Spot Test for Infectious Mononucleosis (I.M.)

Principle. Agglutinins (heterophil antibodies) for red cells of sheep or horses may occur in normal sera and in conditions other than infectious mononucleosis (IM); these agglutinins are absorbed by the Forssman antigen (in guinea pig kidney) but not by beef red cells. The agglutinins for sheep or horse red cells that appear in IM are not absorbed by guinea pig kidney but are absorbed by beef red cells.

The spot test of Lee (1968) is based on the principle that (1) horse red cells are more sensitive than sheep red cells in the test for IM; (2) horse blood kept in sodium citrate is usable for three months and gives stronger and more rapid agglutination than formalinized horse red cells; (3) since some non-IM sera have high horse agglutinin titers, serologic diagnosis cannot depend upon titers alone; and (4) fine suspensions of guinea pig kidney and of beef red cell stroma result in rapid absorption of antibodies and a clear-cut differentiation between IM and non-IM sera.

Reagents. Reagents are available in kit form from Ortho Diagnostics, Raritan, New Jersey.

Method. The test is performed on a slide. Serum is mixed throughly with guinea pig kidney suspension on one part of the slide and with beef red cell stroma on another. Unwashed horse erythrocytes are added immediately to each spot, and mixed. The spots are observed for two minutes, and the occurrence and time of agglutination is noted (Fig. 30–3).

Interpretation. In a series of 200 samples of infectious mononucleosis sera, all showed agglutination within 2 minutes when absorbed with guinea pig kidney suspension, 76 per cent of them within 5 seconds, and 98 per cent within 1 minute. When absorbed with beef red cell stroma, only 30 per cent of the sera showed agglutination, which appeared later or was weaker than in the corresponding sera absorbed with guinea pig kidney suspension.

Ninety per cent of 300 samples of noninfectious mononucleosis sera showed no agglutination on both spots within 2 minutes. Of the remaining sera, 7 per cent showed earlier and/or stronger agglutination after absorption with beef red cell stroma than with guinea pig kidney suspension, and 3 per cent showed agglutination only after absorption with beef red cell stroma (Fig. 30–3).

Forty-five sera with sheep agglutinin titers of 56 or lower were examined with the spot test. The results were in complete agreement with the original diagnosis established by clinical, hematologic, and serologic findings, the latter with the differential test (Table 30–18).

In our laboratory, the spot test has proved to be simple, rapid, highly specific, and sensitive.

Neutrophil Alkaline Phosphatase (Kaplow, 1963)

Principle. The enzyme, located in the neutrophil-specific granules, is exposed to the substrate (a naphthol phosphate) in the presence of a diazonium salt (fast blue or fast violet) at an alkaline pH, 9.5. The substrate is hydrolyzed by the enzyme, releasing a phosphate and an arylnaphtholamide. The latter is immediately coupled to the diazonium salt, forming an insoluble azo dye.

Reagents
1. Fixative: 10 per cent formalin in absolute methanol. (To 10 ml 37 per cent formaldehyde add 90 ml absolute methanol. Store at −10 to −20°C.)

ABSORPTION WITH	AGGLUTINATION PATTERNS				
	POSITIVE		NEGATIVE		
	A	B	C	D	E
GUINEA PIG KIDNEY	5	3	NA	90	NA
BEEF RBC STROMATA	NA	20	NA	60	90

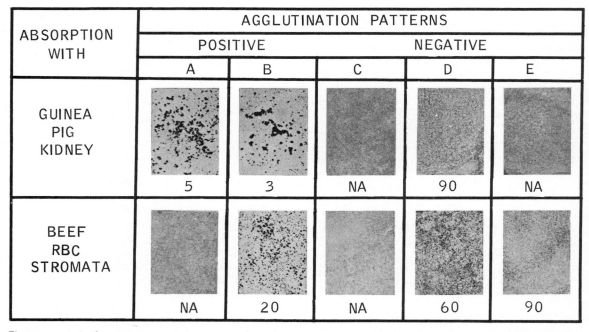

Figure 30–3. Agglutination patterns in spot test for infectious mononucleosis. (Numbers indicate time in seconds when aggregates appeared; NA indicates no agglutination within 2 minutes.)

2. Buffer: *Stock:* 0.2 M propanediol.* Dissolve 21 g of 2-amino-2-methyl-1,3-propanediol in distilled water and dilute to 1000 ml. Store at 4°C.

    Working: 0.05 M propanediol pH 9.4-9.6. Add 70 ml 0.1 N HCl to 250 ml of stock buffer and dilute to 1000 ml with distilled water. Store at 4°C, but warm to room temperature before using.

3. Substrate mixture: Dissolve 5 mg of naphthol AS-BI phosphate (or naphthol AS-MX phosphate or naphthol AS phosphate) in 0.2 to 0.3 ml dimethyl formamide* in a dry flask and add 60 ml of 0.05 M propanediol buffer and

*Eastman Organic, Rochester, N.Y.

40 mg of Fast Blue Salt RR, BB, or BBN* (or Fast Red Violet Salt LB). Shake well, filter through a Seitz filter into a Coplin jar, and use immediately.

4. Counterstain: Nuclear Fast Red. Prepare 5 per cent solution of aluminum sulfate (anhydrous), using heat to dissolve. Allow solution to cool. Filter and add a crystal of thymol as preservative.

    Dissolve 0.1 g Nuclear Fast Red† in 100 ml

*Sigma Chemical Co., St. Louis, Mo.

†Nuclear Fast Red (Kernechtrot); Chroma-Gesellschaft, Schmidt and Co. Distributed by Roboz Surgical Instrument Co., 810 18th St. N.W. Washington, D.C. 20006.

Table 30–18 SPOT TEST FOR INFECTIOUS MONONUCLEOSIS ON 45 LOW-TITER SERA‡

SHEEP-CELL AGGLUTININ TITER	NUMBER OF SERA	SPOT TEST OF IM		ORIGINAL DIAGNOSIS OF IM	
		Positive	Negative	Positive	Negative
56	18	15	3	15	3
28	14	7	7	7	7
14	12	4	8	4	8
<7	1	1		1	
Total	45	27	18	27	18

‡From Davidsohn, I., and Lee, C. L.: The clinical serology of infectious mononucleosis. *In* Carter, R. L., and Penman, H. G. (eds.): Infectious Mononucleosis. Oxford, Blackwell Scientific Publications, 1969. Used by permission.

of the 5 per cent aluminum sulfate solution. This solution keeps indefinitely.

Procedure. Use freshly made blood films. If venous blood is used, heparin should be the anticoagulant, as the enzyme activity diminishes rapidly in EDTA.

Fix air-dried blood films in 10 per cent formolmethanol for exactly 30 seconds at 0 to $-10°C$.

Wash in gently running tap water for 30 to 60 seconds.

Air dry slides, then place them in substrate mixture for exactly 10 min. Wash in gently running tap water again for 30 to 60 seconds.

Counterstain for 10 minutes in Nuclear Fast Red. Wash in running tap water briefly, and air dry.

Positive controls are run with each batch of slides. Women in the last trimester of pregnancy are good controls, because their scores are high normal or somewhat increased.

SCORING PROCEDURE. Examine 100 mature neutrophils in the thin part of the film, where red cells barely touch one another, and score each as follows:

Unstained cells	0
Cells stained faintly, diffusely, or a few discrete granules	1
Cells with moderate number of granules	2
Cells with granules filling the cell	3
Cells staining deeply, almost obscuring the nucleus	4

Adding the scores for the 100 neutrophils will give a total score with a possible range of 0 to 400.

REFERENCE VALUES. Each laboratory must establish its own reference values. Only a portion (up to 60 per cent) of the neutrophils normally stain under these conditions. With this method the reference values are about 20 to 100.

Interpretation. Increased activity is seen in infections with leukocytosis, polycythemia vera, some cases of myelofibrosis with myeloid metaplasia, and in Hodgkin's disease. Decreased activity is seen in chronic myelogenous leukemia, acute myelogenous leukemia, paroxysmal nocturnal hemoglobinuria, hereditary hypophosphatasia, and in some viral infections.

Sources of Variation. It is preferable to perform the reaction immediately or to fix the films and store in the freezer, in which case they will lose only 10 per cent activity in two to three weeks. At room temperature, unfixed air-dried films tend to have a small decrease in activity in the first 2 hours, then increasing to an average of 9 per cent above the original value at 4 to 6 hours, then declining gradually to 20 per cent below the original value at 24 hours and 35 per cent below at 48 hours (Kaplow, 1963).

The stained granules will fade if exposed to organic solvents. Avoid mounting media containing them. Avoid prolonged exposure to xylene or immersion oil.

SUDAN BLACK B STAIN
(SHEEHAN, 1947)

Principle. Sudan black B stains phospholipids and other lipids. It appears to stain both azurophilic and specific granules in neutrophils, whereas the peroxidase is found only in azurophilic granules. In early forms, late myeloblasts, and early promyelocytes, the Sudan black B reaction is therefore parallel to the peroxidase in its utility in separating acute lymphocytic from acute myelogenous leukemia.

Reagents

STOCK STAIN SOLUTION. Dissolve 0.3 g of Sudan black B powder in 100 ml ethyl alcohol.

BUFFER SOLUTION. Dissolve 16 g crystalline phenol in 30 ml ethyl alcohol. Add this to a solution of 0.3 g hydrated disodium hydrogen phosphate ($Na_2HPO_4 \cdot 12H_2O$) dissolved in 100 ml distilled water.

WORKING STAIN SOLUTION. Add 40 ml buffer solution to 60 ml stock stain solution. Filter, using Seitz filter. This solution is stable for approximately two months.

Procedure

1. Fix air-dried films in formalin vapor for 10 minutes. Slides need not be freshly made.

2. Wash slides in running tap water for 10 minutes.

3. Place slides in working stain solution (in Coplin jar) for 30 to 60 minutes.

4. Wash slides with 70 per cent ethyl alcohol for 2 to 3 minutes to remove excess dye.

5. Wash slides in tap water for 2 minutes.

6. Allow slides to dry. Counterstain slides with Wright's stain or hematoxylin.

Interpretation. Cytoplasmic granules stain faintly in neutrophil precursors and strongly in mature neutrophils with a brownblack color. Eosinophilic granules are brown, but often show a central pallor. Monocytes have scattered fine brown-black granules. Lymphocytes and lymphoblasts are negative, but at least some myeloblasts contain Sudan black-positive granules (Plate 30-3*B* and *E*).

The peroxidase and Sudan black B reactions show roughly similar patterns in the various cell types (see Table 30-9) (Hayhoe, 1964). The Sudan black B, however, is somewhat more sensitive than the peroxidase reaction in our experience. These techniques are most useful in distinguishing myeloblasts from lymphoblasts when large numbers of primitive blast forms are present in acute leukemias.

PEROXIDASE (MYELOPEROXIDASE)
(KAPLOW, 1965)

Principle. In the presence of hydrogen peroxide, peroxidase in leukocyte granules oxidizes benzidine from a colorless form to a blue or brown derivative which is localized at the site of the enzyme.

Reagents

Fixative: Mix 10 ml of 37 per cent formaldehyde with 90 ml of absolute ethanol.

Incubation mixture:

Ethanol, 30 per cent (v/v) in water	100 ml
Benzidine dihydrochloride	0.3 g
$ZnSO_4 \cdot 7 H_2O$, 0.132 M (3.8 per cent, w/v)	1.0 ml
Sodium acetate ($NaC_2H_3O_2 \cdot 3 H_2O$)	1.0 g
Hydrogen peroxide, 3 per cent	0.7 ml
Sodium hydroxide, 1.0 N	1.5 ml
Safranin O*	0.2 g

Reagents are mixed in the stated order. A precipitate forms after adding the zinc sulfate, but dissolves after other reagents are added. The pH is not critical between 5.8 and 6.5. The mixture is filtered and may be kept in a closed container and reused for a period of several months. Benzidine may not be available in the United States. Federal regulations require strict safety precautions (Federal Register, 1974).

If benzidine is not available, a method employing 3-amino-9-ethylcarbazole appears to be a satisfactory alternative (Kaplow, 1975).

Procedure

1. Freshly made films or imprints are used. Peroxidase is unstable in the light, but unfixed films are satisfactory for as long as 3 weeks if kept in the dark. Heparin, oxalate, or EDTA does not interfere with the reaction.

2. Place slides in fixative for 60 seconds at room temperature. Wash in gently running tap water.

3. Place slide in incubation mixture for 30 seconds at room temperature. Wash slides again in running tap water for 30 to 60 seconds.

4. Allow slides to dry, and examine under the microscope.

5. The slides may be counterstained with the Giemsa stain or with 1 per cent aqueous cresyl violet if greater nuclear detail is desired.

Interpretation. Peroxidase activity is indicated by blue granules in the cytoplasm. The nucleus and background cytoplasm stain red.

---

*Sigma Chemicals Co., St. Louis, Mo.

In the neutrophil series the peroxidase occurs in the azurophilic (nonspecific) granules in promyelocytes and is demonstrable in some myeloblasts before azurophilic granules are formed. Peroxidase positive granules increase in number in the promyelocytic stage; and with subsequent cell division one would expect them to become fewer in number in the mature neutrophils. However, there appears to be increased activity in the mature cell, probably because the activity as demonstrated in this reaction does not correlate with the number of granules. In eosinophils the specific granules contain peroxidase. Basophils, lymphocytes, and erythroid cells do not stain. Monocytes stain less intensely than do neutrophils, and the granules are smaller; some monocytes may be negative.

This peroxidase reaction finds its greatest usefulness in distinguishing between acute myelogenous and acute lymphocytic leukemia (see Table 30-9). It parallels the Sudan black B reaction; Auer rods are positive with both. Peroxidase appears earlier in cell development than the naphthol AS-D chloroacetate esterase activity.

Peroxidase activity may be absent in some toxic neutrophils in infection, in some neutrophils in acute myelogenous or myelomonocytic leukemia, and in the rare congenital myeloperoxidase deficiency.

ESTERASES

The cytochemical reactions for esterases are positive in many cell types. The *chloroacetate esterase* reaction, using napthol-AS-D-chloroacetate as a substrate, is positive in neutrophils and precursors and weak or negative in monocytes and precursors. The *non-specific esterases*, using α-naphthyl acetate or α-naphthyl butyrate as substrates are strongly positive in monocytes, but weak or negative in granulocytes. The more specific esterases that react in monocytes are inhibited by the presence of sodium fluoride in the incubation mixture. The two reactions presented here are useful in distinguishing neutrophil precursors from monocytes and precursors in the acute leukemias (see Tables 30-9) (Nelson, 1977).

NAPHTHOL AS-D CHLOROACETATE
ESTERASE (DANIEL, 1971)

Reagents

1. Fixative: Mix 10 ml of 37 per cent formaldehyde with 90 ml of absolute methanol.

2. Buffer: Michaelis veronal acetate buffer, pH 7.4.

Stock Solution A: Sodium acetate, anhydrous, 11.704 g. Sodium diethylbarbiturate (Barbital) 29.428 g. Distilled water, CO_2-free, to make 1000 ml.

Stock Solution B: HCl, concentrated, 8.4 ml. Distilled water, to make 1000 ml.

Mix 5.0 ml of Stock Solution A, 5.0 ml of Stock Solution B, and 13.0 ml of CO_2-free distilled water.

3. Incubation mixture: Add in the following order:

Distilled water	20 ml
Buffer	20 ml
Propylene glycol	1 ml
Naphthol AS-D chloroacetate,* (20 mg dissolved in 1.6 ml acetone)	20 mg
Fast Garnet GBC†	40 mg

Filter mixture through Seitz filter.

4. Harris hematoxylin

Procedure

1. Place air-dried blood or marrow films in fixative for 30 seconds at 4°C. The films can be stored unfixed at room temperature for 2 weeks without significant loss of activity. Wash in running tap water.

2. Place in incubation mixture for 30 minutes. Wash in running tap water.

3. Counterstain with hematoxylin for 10 minutes.

Interpretation. In neutrophils the naphthol AS-D chloroacetate esterase reaction parallels the peroxidase activity and is found in azurophilic granules (Plate 30-3*C*). In some cases blasts may be peroxidase positive and naphthol AS-D chloroacetate esterase negative, indicating that peroxidase reaction is either more sensitive or appears earlier in development. The chloroacetate esterase activity is weak or negative in monocytes and negative in lymphocytes.

ALPHA NAPHTHYL ACETATE ESTERASE
(YAM, 1971b)

Reagents

1. Fixative: Buffered formalin and acetone (pH 6.6): Formaldehyde, 37 per cent, 25 ml; Na_2HPO_4, 20 mg; KH_2PO_4, 100 mg; distilled water, 30 ml; acetone, 45 ml.

2. Buffer: Sorenson's phosphate buffer (M/15, pH = 7.6).

3. Incubation mixture: Add in the following order:

Buffer	44.5 ml
Hexazotized pararosaniline (1.5 ml pararosaniline* hydrochloride plus 1.5 ml fresh 4 per cent sodium nitrite)	3.0 ml
Alpha naphthyl acetate,† 50 mg dissolved in 2.5 ml ethylene glycol monomethyl ether	

Filter mixture through Seitz filter.

4. Harris hematoxylin

Procedure

1. Place air-dried blood or marrow films in fixative for 30 seconds at 4°C. Wash in running tap water.

2. Place slides in incubation mixture for 45 minutes. Wash in running water.

3. Counterstain with Harris hematoxylin for 10 minutes.

Interpretation. Red-brown precipitates are diffusely scattered through the cytoplasm of monocytes and of macrophages, but usually not in neutrophils or neutrophil precursors (Plate 30-3*F* and *L*). Megakaryoctyes are strongly positive. Plasma cells and many lymphocytes show one or two focal precipitates. Sodium fluoride inhibits the reaction in monocytes, megakaryocytes, platelets, and plasma cells but not that in neutrophils or lymphocytes (Li, 1973). Usually, however, fluoride inhibition studies are not necessary because neutrophils so rarely react positively with the alpha-napthyl acetate substrate.

PERIODIC ACID-SCHIFF
(PAS) REACTION (HAYHOE, 1964)

Principle. Periodic acid (HIO_4) is an oxidizing agent that converts hydroxy groups on adjacent carbon atoms to aldehydes. The resulting dialdehydes are combined with Schiff's reagent to give a red-colored product. A positive reaction is therefore seen with polysaccharides, mucopolysaccharides, and glycoproteins.

Reagents

1. Fixative: Mix 10 ml of 37 per cent formaldehyde with 90 ml of absolute ethanol.

2. Periodic acid, 5 g, is dissolved in 500 ml of distilled water. Stored in a dark bottle, the solution is good for three months.

3. Schiff's reagent: Dissolve 5 g of basic fuchsin in 500 ml of hot distilled water, and filter after it has cooked. Saturate with sulfur dioxide gas by

---

bubbling for 1 hour. Extract the solution with 2 g of activated charcoal for a few seconds in a hood and immediately filter through Whatman No. 1 filter paper into a dark bottle. The solution keeps for 2 to 3 months.

4. Harris hematoxylin

Procedure

1. Place air-dried blood and marrow films or imprints in fixative for 10 minutes. Wash briefly with tap water.

2. Control slides are exposed to digestion with saliva (salivary amylase) for 30 minutes. Place slides in periodic acid for 10 minutes. Wash briefly with tap water and blot dry.

3. Immerse slides in Schiff's reagent for 30 minutes.

4. Rinse slides in several changes of sulfur dioxide water for 20 to 30 minutes.

5. Wash for 5 to 10 minutes in tap water and counterstain with Harris hematoxylin for 10 minutes.

Interpretation. In blood cells a positive PAS reaction usually indicates the presence of glycogen. This is demonstrated by digestion with amylase and consequent loss of staining. Neutrophils react at all stages of development, the most strongly in the mature stage. The same is true of eosinophils. The glycogen is not in the granules, but in background cytoplasm. Myeloblasts contain a few small PAS-positive granules. Monocytes have a faint staining reaction in the form of fine granules. Lymphocytes may contain a few small or large granules. Normoblasts are normally PAS negative.

In erythroleukemia (Plate 30–3*K*) and in thalassemia some of the erythroid precursors are PAS positive. This is true to a lesser extent in iron-deficiency anemia and sideroblastic anemias. In acute lymphocytic leukemia the lymphoblasts often contain large coarse clumps of PAS-positive material (Plate 30–3*H*). In chronic lymphocytic leukemia and lymphomas as well as in infectious mononucleosis the lymphocytes may have increased numbers of PAS-positive granules.

ACID PHOSPHATASE
(KATAYAMA, 1977)

Principle

Acid phosphatase in the cells hydrolyzes the substrate, naphthol AS-BI phosphoric acid. The naphthol released is insoluble and couples with "hexazotized" pararosanilin. The colored precipitate in the cytoplasm of the cells indicates acid phosphatase activity. If L(+) tartaric acid is in the solution, it inhibits the isoenzymes of acid phosphatase that are present in most cells, but not that of the cells of hairy cell leukemia (leukemic reticuloendotheliosis).

Reagents

1. *Fixative:* Buffered formalin acetone mixture at pH 6.6 (20 mg Na_2HPO_4, 100 mg KH_2PO_4, 30 ml H_2O, 45 ml acetone, and 25 ml formalin). Store at 4 to 10°C.

2. *Acetate Buffer* (0.1M, pH 5)
a. 20 ml 0.1 M sodium acetate (2.051 g sodium acetate in 250 ml H_2O; refrigerate)
b. 5 ml 0.1 N HCl
c. 75 ml H_2O; adjust pH to 5.0 with 0.1 N HCl
If making more than 100 ml at a time, do not increase the 0.1 N HCl, just make up the difference with H_2O.

3. *Pararosanilin* (1 g pararosaniline* hydrochloride, 20 ml distilled H_2O, and 5 ml concentrated HCl, stored in dark at room temperature)

4. *Sodium Nitrite:* 4 per cent aqueous solution ($NaNO_2$). Hexazotization is performed by mixing equal volumes of pararosanilin and 4 per cent $NaNO_2$ one minute before use.

5. Naphthol AS-BI phosphoric acid†

6. N-N-dimethyl formamide

7. L(+) tartaric acid (for tartrate resistant acid phosphatase reaction).

8. One per cent aqueous methyl green buffered with 0.1 N sodium acetate to pH 4.2. Extract with chloroform until the solvent is clear.

Procedure

1. Fix the air dried films from the patient and from a normal individual in the buffered acetone fixative for 30 seconds at 4 to 10°C., wash with distilled water, air dry, and store at room temperature.

2. Mix 71.2 ml 0.1 M acetate buffer (pH 5.0) with 40 mg naphthol AS-BI phosphoric acid dissolved in 4 ml of N-N-dimethyl formamide.

3. To this solution (step No. 2) add 4.8 ml of hexazotized pararosanilin (2.4 ml 4 per cent $NaNO_2$ and 2.4 ml of pararosanilin) Total volume 80 ml.

4. For the tartrate-resistant acid phosphatase reaction add 300 mg L(+) tartaric acid to 40 ml of the mixture in step No. 3.

5. Adjust the pH of both mixtures to 5.1 with a saturated solution of sodium hydroxide.

6. Filter each into separate Coplin jars.

7. Incubate slides in solutions at 36°C. for one hour.

8. Wash slides with distilled water.

9. Counterstain with 1 per cent methyl green for two minutes.

10. Rinse in H_2O.

11. Dehydrate in ethanol.

12. Clear in xylene and mount with Permount.

---

*Fisher Scientific Co., Fair Lawn, N.J.
†Sigma Chemical Co., St. Louis, Mo.

Interpretation. Red granules in the cytoplasm indicate acid phosphatase activity. The reaction is positive to varying degrees in most normal (and abnormal) leukocytes. Monocytes stain more intensely than neutrophils and precursors. Lymphocytes normally contain little activity; T cells appear to react positively; B cells are usually negative (Tamaoki, 1969).

The acid phosphatase reaction is useful in two areas. First, one of the elements in confirming a diagnosis of *hairy cell leukemia* (p. 1069) is the presence of tartrate-resistant acid phosphatase in the abnormal cells. It must be realized, however, that a small fraction of cases of hairy cell leukemia do not show this reaction (Katayama, 1977). Second, in the subclassification of *acute lymphocytic leukemia,* definite positivity for acid phosphatase in the blasts is evidence in favor of T cell origin (Catovsky, 1978).

SERUM VISCOSITY

Principle. The viscosity of a fluid is the property that resists the force which causes it to flow. Serum viscosity depends on the concentration and physical properties of proteins.

The *relative serum viscosity* is determined by comparing the time needed for 5 ml of serum to flow between two measuring lines of the glass tubing of an Ostwald viscometer with the time needed for 5 ml of water to do the same. The ratio is the relative serum viscosity, which is useful in managing patients with the hyperviscosity syndrome.

Reagents and Equipment
1. Waterbath, 37°C.; laboratory stand with clamp; stopwatch; rubber tubing.
2. Ostwald viscometer: A U-shaped glass tubing with a reservoir arm and a measuring arm; the latter has a bulb separating two measuring lines. This simple apparatus is available through commercial supply houses.
3. 0.145 M sodium chloride (physiologic saline).
Procedure
1. Rinse the Ostwald viscometer with saline and suspend it in the waterbath by means of a laboratory stand.
2. Pipette 5 ml of the patient's serum into the reservoir arm, and allow it to reach 37°C.
3. Using suction, draw the serum up into the measuring arm to a level above the upper line.
4. Allow serum to fall and measure the time required for the upper meniscus of the serum to flow from the upper line to the lower line. Repeat twice, and average the times.

5. Rinse out the viscometer twice with saline and twice with distilled water.
6. Repeat steps 2 to 4 with distilled water and calculate.

$$\text{Relative serum viscosity} = \frac{\text{flow time of serum}}{\text{flow time of water}}$$

7. Normal reference values are 1.4 and 1.8.
8. If an Ostwald viscometer is not available, a red blood cell pipette or a 1 ml volumetric pipette may be used, supported vertically, at room temperature (Wright, 1970).

Interpretation. In normal individuals and in most patients with blood protein disorders, the relative serum viscosity (RSV) is similar at room temperature and at 37°C. If the RSV is increased at room temperature, the test should be repeated at 37°C.; if no difference is noted, serial studies may be performed at room temperature. Increased viscosity at room temperature compared to 37°C. suggests the presence of a cryoglobulin (Wright, 1970).

In patients with multiple myeloma and macroglobulinemia, high serum viscosity may give rise to symptoms of the *hyperviscosity syndrome:* bleeding not due to thrombocytopenia; retinopathy; variable neurologic symptoms and, more rarely, congestive heart failure. Symptoms do not occur unless the RSV exceeds 4.0; most patients have symptoms if the RSV is over 7.0 (Fahey, 1965). The hyperviscosity syndrome is more common in macroglobulinemia than in multiple myeloma, and probably more common in IgA than in IgG myeloma (Preston, 1978). Serum viscosity appears to depend on the aggregating tendency of the immunoglobulin as well as on the concentration.

THE LE (LUPUS ERYTHEMATOSUS CELL TEST

Hargraves described the LE cell in 1948; an interesting account of this discovery has been given (Hargraves, 1969).

Principle. A substance present in the gamma globulin fraction of the plasma or serum of patients with disseminated lupus erythematosus, the *LE factor*, reacts with the nucleoprotein of white cell nuclei. The LE factor appears to be an antinucleoprotein antibody. The transformed nucleoprotein acquires chemotactic properties and attracts phagocytes, usually segmented neutrophilic granulocytes and occasionally monocytes. Rarely other leukocytes may act as phagocytes. The phagocytes with the ingested nuclear material are the LE cells. The phenomenon of LE cell formation requires the presence in the serum of the LE factor, damaged leukocytes, complement, and normal active leukocytes.

Morphology. The LE cell contains two nuclei. The nucleus of the phagocyte is flattened out at the periphery of the cell. Its chromatin structure is well preserved. The bulk of the cytoplasmic portion of the cell is occupied by the ingested transformed nuclear mass. In the fully developed LE cell, the normal chromatin structure of the ingested nucleus is absent and is replaced by a lilac-colored, homogeneous, amorphous, round mass, which varies in size but is usually larger than the erythrocytes in the same preparation (Plate 30-6*J* and *K*). A phagocyte may engulf more than one nucleus. The transformation of the nucleus is a progressive process. The stages can be followed step by step. The early chemotactic action of the transforming or transformed nucleus may attract several neutrophilic granulocytes, which surround it and form a so-called "rosette." This finding is not diagnostic.

Nucleophagocytosis is a fairly common finding and is fundamentally different from the LE cell phenomenon. In such cases, the phagocyte is more frequently a monocyte but may be a granulocyte. The phagocytized nucleus retains the intact chromatin pattern. It may show degenerative changes, mainly pyknosis that is diffuse or appears along the margins, and nuclear vacuoles. The inclusion is frequently smaller than in a true LE cell. These are the so-called "tart cells" (Fig. 30-4).

Several tests and modifications are recommended.

Test No. 1. LE Clot Test (Magath, 1952)

1. About 8 ml of venous blood is collected in a sterile, dry, chemically clean test tube, allowed to clot, and left at room temperature for about 2 hours or at 37°C. for 30 minutes.

2. The clot is removed and passed through a copper wire screen of 30-mesh per inch, by use of the bottom of a test tube or a pestle. A special sieve and pestle are commercially available (Scientific Products Company). The effect of this procedure is twofold: the fibrin remains on the sieve, and some of the leukocytes are damaged.

3. The filtrate is transferred to several Wintrobe hematocrit tubes.

4. The tubes are centrifuged for 5 minutes at 1500 to 2000 rpm or until three distinct layers (serum, buffy coat, and red cells) have formed.

Plate 30–6. The stain is Wright's or Wright-Giemsa unless otherwise noted. *A,* Polycythemia vera, bone marrow biopsy. Hematoxylin and eosin. Solidly cellular marrow with panmyelosis, i.e., the hypercellularity is due to increased erythroid, granulocytic, and megakaryocytic proliferation. *B,* Myelofibrosis with myeloid metaplasia (MMM), bone marrow biopsy, H & E. Reticulin and collagen fibrosis accounts for the increased intercellular material; note the distortion of the megakaryocytes (*right center*). This marrow is considerably less cellular than *A. C,* MMM, bone marrow biopsy, reticulin stain. Reticulin fibers are coated with silver in this reaction and appear dark. They are the major component of the myelofibrosis in the early phases of MMM; only later does the collagen staining reaction appear. Note the large vascular space; these are often present in the marrow in MMM. *D,* MMM with osteosclerosis, bone marrow biopsy, H & E stain. Note the irregular new bone formation and the apparent continuity of fibers from the marrow with those in the bone (*upper center*). *E,* MMM, touch preparation of marrow biopsy. A mass of abnormal platelets, most with diminished granules, and many separate, small megakaryocytic nuclei (each the size of a small lymphocyte). These abnormal "dwarf" megakaryocytes and masses of atypical platelets can often be found on touch preparations of marrow biopsies in MMM. Usually aspiration of marrow tissue is impossible. *F,* MMM, blood film. Above the neutrophil myelocyte in the center is a dwarf megakaryocyte; note the intensely staining nuclear chromatin and the fine azure granules in the cytoplasm. These small megakaryocytes are often mistaken for lymphocytes. Also present are three large atypical platelets; two have a few azure granules and the third is rather basophilic. *G,* MMM, blood film. From the top and moving down, note two neutrophils, a neutrophil myelocyte, a dwarf megakaryocyte, and a large immature cell (probably an abnormal myeloblast). Note also several large atypical platelets. *H,* Thrombocythemia, bone marrow film, low power. An abundance of megakaryocytes dominates the marrow films from most aspirations in thrombocythemia. *I,* Thrombocythemia, blood film. Individual platelets usually appear normal, except that they are frequently large. The features of the blood film are considerably increased numbers of platelets, neutrophilia, and often-times hypochromic microcytic red cells as a result of chronic blood loss. *J,* Lupus erythematosus (LE) preparation, low power. Aggregates consisting of neutrophils and masses of extracellular altered nuclear material are usually the clue that the test will be positive. Here the aggregates of neutrophils include typical LE cells (see *K*). *K,* LE preparation, higher power. In a typical LE cell, the neutrophil's nucleus is displaced to the periphery by a large, homogeneous, lilac-colored mass of altered nuclear material. Three LE cells and several vacuolated neutrophils are present here. *L,* A "pseudo-LE cell," in a patient with cryoglobulinemia. Phagocytosis of masses of aggregated cold-precipitated proteins may simulate an LE cell. Distinction can be made using a specific DNA stain, such as the Feulgen reaction; the phagocytized body would be positive in the LE cell and negative in this type of cell.

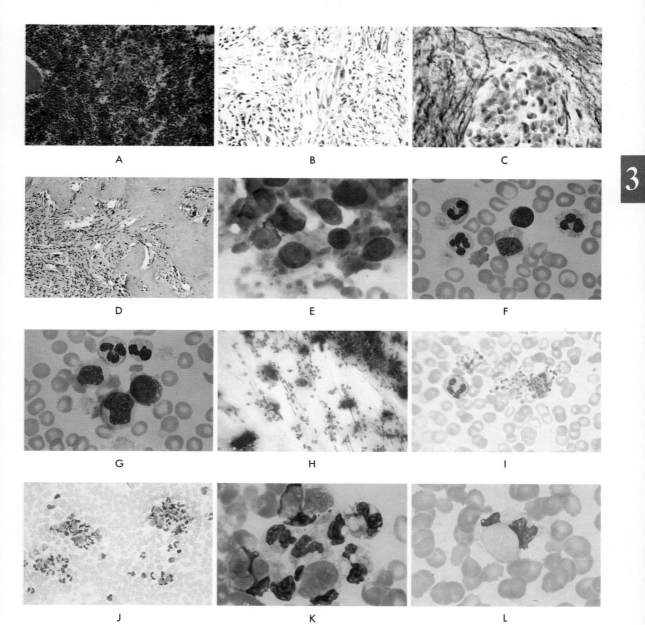

A

B

C

D

E

F

G

H

I

J

K

L

3

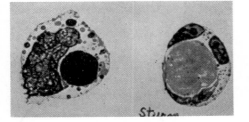

Figure 30–4. On the left is a monocyte with a phagocytized pyknotic nucleus (to be differentiated from lupus erythematosus cells). On the right is a neutrophil with a felt-like, purple staining mass in the cytoplasm; this is quite typical of an LE cell. (Permission for reproduction from *The Morphology of Blood Cells*, by L. W. Diggs, was obtained from Abbott Laboratories.)

5. The serum is discarded carefully with a pipette, leaving a layer of 1 or 2 mm above the buffy coat and the buffy coat layer. The latter is transferred drop by drop to slides on which it is mixed. Smears are made and stained with Wright's stain.

6. The slide is scanned with the low and high power of the microscope to locate areas suggestive of the presence of LE cells. These areas are then examined with the oil-immersion objective.

Test No. 2. Glass Bead, Heparin method (Zinkham, 1956)

1. Ten milliliters of venous blood is placed in a tube containing 3 drops of a 1 per cent aqueous solution of heparin (delivered with a 21-gauge needle) and 10 glass beads, 4 mm in diameter. It has been shown that excess heparin will decrease the number of positive tests (Dubois, 1957).

2. Let stand at room temperature for 90 minutes.

3. Rotate in a Shen type rotator set at 30 rpm for 30 minutes. Transfer to one or more Wintrobe hematocrit tubes. Continue as in Test No. 1.

Test No. 3. Defibrination and Rotation Method

1. Place 10 milliliters of venous blood in an Erlenmeyer flask containing 10 glass beads, and rotate and swirl the flask on a flat surface until defibrination has occurred.

2. Remove the clot, pour the defibrinated blood into a test tube containing 5 clean glass beads, and rotate at 30 rpm for 30 minutes.

3. Incubate the tube at 37°C. for 15 minutes.

4. Transfer to Wintrobe hematocrit tubes and continue as in Test No. 1.

Report. At least 1000 neutrophils should be examined, or a 20 minute search performed. A *positive* test is reported when four or more typical LE cells are found. If fewer than four typical LE cells or incompletely transformed inclusions are found, the test is designated as *suspicious.* Tart cells are of no significance (Fig. 30–4). Phagocytized non-nuclear material, such as cryoglobulins, may sometimes lead to erroneously positive tests (Plate 30–6L).

The LE Battery. If the LE test employed is suspicious but not definitely positive, or if the diagnosis of SLE is strongly suspected, a group or battery of three types of LE cell tests may be performed. Dubois (1957) showed that a battery produced more positives than any one single test. The rotary method (Test No. 2) was superior to the sieved clot method (Test No. 1). We prefer the defibrination and rotation method.

Interpretation. The LE cell phenomenon is positive in only 50 per cent of patients with SLE at the time of the first visit and in 70 or at most 80 per cent of patients at any time during the course of disease (Fries, 1975). It is not essential for the diagnosis of SLE and because of its insensitivity has been largely superseded by serologic tests for nuclear antigens (p. 1265).

REFERENCES

Adamson, J. W., and Fialkow, P. J.: The pathogenesis of myeloproliferative syndromes. Br. J. Haematol., *38*:299, 1978.

Adamson, J. W., Fialkow, P. J., Murphy, S., Prchal, J. F., and Steinman, L.: Polycythemia vera: Stem-cell and probable clonal origin of the disease. N. Engl. J. Med., *295*:913, 1976.

Aisenberg, A. C., and Bloch, K. J.: Immunoglobulins on the surface of neoplastic lymphocytes. N. Engl. J. Med., *287*:272, 1972.

Andersen, V., and Andersen, E.: Changes in blood lymphocytes during the neonatal period. Acta Paediatr. Scand., *63*:266, 1974.

Barak, Y., Paran, M., Levin, S., and Sachs, L.: *In vitro* induction of myeloid proliferation and maturation in infantile genetic agranulocytosis. Blood, *38*:74, 1971.

Beeson, P. B., and Bass, D. A.: The Eosinophil. Vol. XIV in the series Major Problems in Internal Medicine, Smith, L. H., Jr. (ed). Philadelphia, W. B. Saunders Company, 1977.

Bennett, J. M., Catovsky, D., Daniel, M-Th., Flandrin, G., Galton, D. A. G., Gralnick, H. R., and Sultan, C.: Proposals for the classification of the acute leukaemias. French-American-British (FAB) Co-operative Group. Br. J. Haematol., *33*:451, 1976.

Berard, C. W., and Dorfman, R. F.: Histopathology of malignant lymphomas. Clin. Haematol., *3*:39, 1974.

Bernier, G. M., and Graham, R. C., Jr.: Plasma cell asynchrony in myeloma: Correlation of light and electron microscopy. Semin. Hematol., *13*:239, 1976.

Beverley, J. K. A., and Beattie, C. P.: Glandular toxoplasmosis. A survey of 30 cases. Lancet, *2*:379, 1958.

Blacklow, N. R., and Kapikian, A. Z.: Serological studies with E B virus in infectious lymphocytosis. Nature, *226*:647, 1970.

Bloomfield, C. D., Kersey, J. H., Brunning, R. D., and Gajl-Peczalska, K. J.: Prognostic significance of lymphocyte surface markers in adult non-Hodgkin's malignant lymphoma. Lancet, *2*:1330, 1976.

Bloomfield, C. D., Kersey, J. H., Brunning, R. D., and Gajl-Peczalska, K. J.: Prognostic significance of lymphocytic surface markers and histology in adult non-Hodgkin's lymphoma. Cancer Treat. Rep., *61*:963, 1977.

Blume, R. S., and Wolff, S. M.: The Chediak-Higashi syndrome: Studies in four patients and a review of the literature. Medicine (Baltimore), *51*:247, 1972.

Boggs, D. R., and Winkelstein, A.: White Cell Manual, 3rd ed. Philadelphia, F. A. Davis Co., 1975.

Bouroncle, B. A., Wiseman, B. K., and Doan, C. A.: Leukemic reticuloendotheliosis. Blood, *13*:609, 1958.

Boyd, J. F., and Reid, D.: Bone marrow in nine cases of clinical glandular fever and a review of the literature. J. Clin. Pathol., *21*:638, 1968.

Brooksaler, F., and Nelson, J. D.: Pertussis. A reappraisal and report of 190 confirmed cases. Am. J. Dis. Child., *114*:389, 1967.

Brunning, R. D.: Morphologic alterations in nucleated blood and marrow cells in genetic disorders. Hum. Pathol., *1*:99,1970.

Canellos, G. P.: Chronic granulocytic leukemia. Med. Clin. North Am., *60*:1001, 1976.

Carr, M. C., Stites, D. P., and Fudenberg, H. H.: Cellular immune aspects of the human fetal-maternal relationship. III. Mixed lymphocyte reactivity between related maternal and cord blood lymphocyes. Cell. Immunol., *11*:332, 1974.

Carter, R. L., and Penman, H. G.: Histopathology of infectious mononucleosis. *In* Carter, R. L., and Penman, H. G. (eds.): Infectious Mononucleosis. Oxford, Blackwell Scientific Publications, 1969.

Cassileth, P.: Lymphocytopenia. *In* Williams, W. J., Beutler, E., Erslev, A. J., and Rundles, R. W. (eds.): Hematology. New York, McGraw-Hill Book Co., Inc., 1972.

Catovsky, D.: Hairy-cell leukaemia and prolymphocytic leukaemia. Clin. Haematol., *6*:245, 1977.

Catovsky, D., Cherchi, M., Greaves, M. F., Janossy, G., Pain, C., and Kay, H. E. M.: Acid-phosphatase reaction in acute lymphoblastic leukaemia. Lancet, *1*:749, 1978.

Catovsky, D., Galton, D. A. G., Griffin, C., Hoffbrand, A. V., and Szur, L.: Serum lysozyme and vitamin B_{12} binding capacity in myeloproliferative disorders. Br. J. Haematol., *21*:661, 1971a.

Catovsky, D., Galton, D. A. G., and Griffin, C.: Significance of lysozyme estimations in acute myeloid and chronic monocytic leukaemia. Br. J. Haematol., *21*:565, 1971b.

Ceppellini, R., Bonnard, G. D., Coppo, F., Miggiano, C., Pospisil, M., Curtoni, E. S., and Pellegrino, M.: Mixed leukocyte cultures and HL-A antigens. I. Reactivity of young fetuses, newborns, mothers at delivery. Transplant. Proc., *3*:58, 1971.

Chessells, J. M., Hardisty, R. M., Rapson, N. T., and Greaves, M. F.: Acute lymphoblastic leukaemia in children: Classification and prognosis. Lancet, *2*:1307, 1977.

Chusid, M. J., Dale, D. C., West, B. C., and Wolff, S. M.: The hypereosinophilic syndrome. Medicine (Baltimore), *54*:1, 1975.

Cline, M. J., Opelz, G., Saxon, A., Fahey, J. L., and Golde, D. W.: Autoimmune panleukopenia. N. Engl. J. Med., *295*:1489, 1976.

Coccia, P. F., Kersey, J. H., Gajl-Peczalska, K. J., Krivit, W., and Nesbit, M. E.: Prognostic significance of surface marker analysis in childhood non-Hodgkin's lymphoproliferative malignancies. Am. J. Hematol., *1*:405, 1976.

Daniel, M-Th., Flandrin, G., Lejeuene, F., Liso, P., and Lortholary, P.: Les estérases spécifiques monocytaires. Utilisation dans la classification des leucémies aiguës. Nouv. Rev. Fr. Hematol., *11*:233, 1971.

Davey, F. R., Goldberg, J., Stockman, J., and Gottlieb, A. J.: Immunologic and cytochemical cell markers in non-Hodgkin's lymphomas. Lab. Invest., *35*:430, 1976.

Davey, F. R., and Gottlieb, A. J.: Lymphocyte surface markers in acute lymphocytic leukemia. Am. J. Clin. Pathol., *62*:818, 1974.

Davey, F. R., and Huntington, S.: Age-related variation in lymphocyte subpopulations. Gerontology, *23*:381, 1977.

Davidsohn, I.: Serologic diagnosis of infectious mononucleosis. J.A.M.A., *108*:289, 1937.

Davidsohn, I., and Lee, C. L.: The clinical serology of infectious mononucleosis. *In* Carter, R. L., and Penman, H. G. (eds.): Infectious Mononucleosis. Oxford, Blackwell Scientific Publications, 1969.

Davidsohn, I., and Nelson, D. A.: The Blood. *In* Davidsohn, I., and Henry, J. B. (eds.): Clinical Diagnosis by Laboratory Methods, 15th ed. Phildelphia, W. B. Saunders Company, 1974, p. 262.

Diaz-Jouanen, E., Strickland, R. G., and Williams, R. C.: Studies of human lymphocytes in the newborn and the aged. Am. J. Med., *58*:620, 1975.

Dorfman, R. F.: Classification of non-Hodgkin's lymphomas. Lancet, *1*:1295, 1974.

Dorfman, R. F., and Remington, J. S.: Value of lymph-node biopsy in the diagnosis of acute acquired toxoplasmosis. N. Engl. J. Med., *289*:878, 1973.

Downey, H., and McKinlay, C. A.: Acute lymphadenosis compared with acute lymphatic leukemia. Arch. Intern. Med., *32*:82, 1923.

Dubois, E. L., and Freeman, V.: A comparative evaluation of the sensitivity of the L. E. cell test performed simultaneously by different methods. Blood, *12*:656, 1957.

Ellis, J. T., Silver, R. T., Coleman, M., and Geller, S. A.: The bone marrow in polycythemia vera. Semin. Hematol., *12*:433, 1975.

Epstein, M. A., and Achong, B. G.: Pathogenesis of infectious mononucleosis. Lancet, *2*:1270, 1977.

Evans, A. S.: Commentary: E B Virus, infectious mononucleosis, and cancer: The closing of the web. Yale J. Biol. Med., *47*:113, 1974.

Evans, A. S.: Infectious mononucleosis. *In* Williams, W. J., Beutler, E., Erslev, A. J., and Rundles, R. W. (eds.): Hematology, 2nd ed. New York, McGraw-Hill Book Co., 1977.

Fahey, J. L., Barth, W. F., and Solomon, A.: Serum hyperviscosity syndrome. J.A.M.A., *192*:464, 1965.

Federal Register 39, #20, p. 3756, Jan. 29, 1974.

Feldman, H. A.: Toxoplasmosis. N. Engl. J. Med., *279*:1370, 1431, 1968.

Fialkow, P. J., Jacobson, R. J., and Papayannopoulou, T.: Chronic myelocytic leukemia: Clonal origin in a stem cell common to the granulocyte, erythrocyte, platelet and monocyte/macrophage. Am. J. Med., *63*:125, 1977.

Finch, S. C.: Granulocytopenia (Chapter 83) and Granulocytosis (Chapter 84). *In* Williams, W. J., Beutler, E., Erslev, A. J., and Rundles, R. W. (eds.): Hematology, 2nd ed. New York, McGraw-Hill Book Co., Inc., 1977.

Finch, S. C.: Laboratory findings in infectious mononucleosis. *In* Carter, R. L., and Penman, H. G. (eds.): Infectious Mononucleosis. Oxford, Blackwell Scientific Publications, 1969.

Finkel, M., Parker, G. W., and Fanselau, H. A.: The hepatitis of infectious mononucleosis: Experience with 235 cases. Military Med., *129*:533, 1964.

Flandrin, G., and Brouet, J-C.: The Sézary cell: Cytologic, cytochemical and immunologic studies. Mayo Clin. Proc., *49*:575, 1974.

Foster, K. M., and Jack, I.: A prospective study of the role of cytomegalovirus in post-transfusion mononucleosis. N. Engl. J. Med., *280*:1311, 1969.

Frangione, B., and Franklin, E. C.: Heavy chain diseases: Clinical features and molecular significance of the disordered immunoglobulin structure. Semin. Hematol., *10*:53, 1973.

Franklin, E. C.: μ-chain disease. Arch. Intern. Med., *135*:71, 1975.

Fries, J. F., and Holman, H. R.: Systemic Lupus Erythematosus. A Clinical Analysis. Vol. VI in the series Major Problems in Internal Medicine. Philadelphia, W. B. Saunders Company, 1975.

Fu, S. M., Winchester, R. J., Rai, K. R., and Kunkel, H. G.: Hairy cell leukemia: Proliferation of a cell with phagocytic and B-lymphocyte properties. Scand. J. Immunol., *3*:847, 1974.

Gall, E. A., and Stout, H. A.: The histological lesion in lymph nodes in infectious mononucleosis. Am. J. Pathol., *16*:433, 1940.

Galton, D. A. G.: The chronic leukaemias. *In* Hoffbrand, A. V., Brain, M. C., and Hirsh, J.: (eds.): Recent Advances in Haematology, 2nd ed. Edinburgh, Churchill Livingstone, 1977.

Galton, D. A. G., Goldman, J. M., Wiltshaw, E., Catovsky, D., Henry, K., and Goldenberg, G. J.: Prolymphocytic leukaemia. Br. J. Haematol., *27*:7, 1974.

Gerber, P., Walsh, J. H., Rosenblum, E. N., and Purcell, R. H.: Association of EB-virus infection with the postperfusion syndrome. Lancet, *1*:593, 1969.

Gilbert, H. S.: Definition, clinical features and diagnosis of polycythaemia vera. Clin. Haematol., *4*:263, 1975.

Gilbert, H. S., and Ornstein, L.: Basophil counting with a new staining method using Alcian blue. Blood, *46*:279, 1975.

Glenner, G. G., Terry, W. D., and Isersky, C.: Amyloidosis: Its nature and pathogenesis. Semin. Hematol., *10*:65, 1973.

Golden, H. D., Chang, R. S., Lou, J. J., and Cooper, T. Y.: A filterable agent in throat washings of patients with infectious mononucleosis. J. Inf. Dis., *124*:422, 1971.

Gralnick, H. R., Galton, D. A. G., Catovsky, D., Sultan, C., and Bennett, J. W.: Classification of acute leukemia. Ann. Intern. Med., *87*:740, 1977.

Greaves, M. F.: Clinical applications of cell surface markers. Prog. Hematol., *9*:255, 1975.

Greenberg, P., Mara, B., Bax, I., Brossel, R., and Schrier, S.: The myeloproliferative disorders: Correlation between clinical evolution and alterations of granulopoiesis. Am. J. Med., *61*:878, 1976.

Groover, R. V., Burke, E. C., Gordon, H., and Berdon, W. E.: The genetic mucopolysaccharidoses. Semin. Hematol., *9*:371, 1972.

Gunz, F. W.: Hemorrhagic thrombocythemia: A critical review. Blood, *15*:706, 1960.

Gunz, F., and Baikie, A. G.: Leukemia, 3rd ed. New York, Grune & Stratton, Inc., 1974.

Hallgren, H. M., Kersey, J. H., Gajl-Peczalska, K. J., Greenberg, L. J., and Yunis, E. J.: T and B cells in aging humans. Fed. Proc., *33*:646, 1974.

Hargraves, M. M., Richmond, H., and Morton, R.: Presentation of two bone marrow elements: The "tart" cell and the "L.E." cell. Proc. Staff Meet. Mayo Clin., *23*:25, 1948.

Hayhoe, F. G. J., and Cawley, J. C.: Acute leukaemia: Cellular morphology, cytochemistry and fine structure. Clin. Haematol., *1*:49, 1972.

Hayhoe, F. G. J., Quaglino, D., and Doll, R.: The Cytology and Cytochemistry of Acute Leukaemias. London, Her Majesty's Stationery Office, 1964.

Henle, W., and Henle, G.: Epstein-Barr virus and infectious mononucleosis. N. Engl. J. Med., *288*:263, 1973.

Henle, W., Henle, G. E., and Horwitz, C. A.: Epstein-Barr virus specific diagnostic tests in infectious mononucleosis. Hum. Pathol., *5*:551, 1974.

Horowitz, M. S., and Moore, G. T.: Acute infectious lymphocytosis. An etiologic and epidemologic study of an outbreak. N. Engl. J. Med., *279*:399, 1968.

Hovde, R. F., and Sundberg, R. D.: Granulomatous lesions in the bone marrow in infectious mononucleosis. Blood, *5*:209, 1950.

Hoyer, J. R., Cooper, M. D., Gabrielsen, A. E., and Good, R. A.: Lymphopenic forms of congenital immunologic deficiency diseases. Medicine (Baltimore), *47*:201, 1968.

Jacobson, R. J., Salo, A., and Fialkow, P. J.: Agnogenic myeloid metaplasia: A clonal proliferation of hematopoietic stem cells with secondary myelofibrosis. Blood, *51*:189, 1978.

Jenis, E. H., Takeuchi, A., Dillon, D. E., Ruymann, F. B., and Rivkin, S.: The May-Hegglin anomaly: Ultrastructure of the granulocytic inclusion. Am. J. Clin. Pathol., *55*:187, 1971.

Jondal, M., and Klein, G.: Surface markers on human B and T lymphocytes. II. Presence of Epstein-Barr virus receptors on B lymphocytes. J. Exp. Med., *138*:1365, 1973.

Jones, S. E.: Clinical features and course of the non-Hodgkin's lymphomas. Clin. Haematol., *3*:131, 1974.

Jones, S. E., Fuks, Z., Bull, M., Kadin, M. E., Dorfman, R. F., Kaplan, H. S., Rosenberg, S. A., and Kim, H.: Non-Hodgkin's lymphomas. IV. Clinicopathologic correlation in 405 cases. Cancer, *31*:806, 1973.

Jordan, M. C., Rousseau, W. E., Stewart, J. A., Noble, G. R., and Chin, T. D. Y.: Spontaneous cytomegalovirus mononucleosis: Clinical and laboratory observations in nine cases. Ann. Intern. Med., *79*:153, 1973.

Kaplow, L. S.: Cytochemistry of leukocyte alkaline phosphatase. Am. J. Clin. Pathol., *39*:439, 1963.

Kaplow, L. S.: Simplified myeloperoxidase stain using benzidine dihydrochloride. Blood, *26*:215, 1965.

Kaplow, L. S.: Substitute for benzidine in myeloperoxidase stains. Am. J. Clin. Pathol., *63*:451, 1975.

Karzon, D. T.: Infectious mononucleosis. Adv. Pediatr., *22*:231, 1976.

Katayama, I., and Yang, J. P. S.: Reassessment of a cytochemical test for differential diagnosis of leukemic reticuloendotheliosis. Am. J. Clin. Pathol., *68*:268, 1977.

Kersey, J. H., Gajl-Peczalska, K. J., Coccia, P. F., and Nesbit, M. E.: The nature of childhood leukemia and lymphoma. Am. J. Pathol., *90*:487, 1978.

Khaleeli, M., Keane, W. M., and Lee, G. R.: Sideroblastic anemia in multiple myeloma: A preleukemic change. Blood, *41*:17, 1973.

Klemola, E., von Essen, R., Wager, O., Haltia, K., Koivuniemi, A., and Salmi, I.: Cytomegalovirus mononucleosis in previously healthy individuals. Ann. Intern. Med., *71*:11, 1969.

Lagergren, J.: The white blood cell count and the erythrocyte sedimentation rate in pertussis. Acta Paediatr., *52*:405, 1963.

Lalezari, P., Jiang, A-F., Yegen, L., and Santorineou, M.: Chronic autoimmune neutropenia due to anti-NA2 antibody. N. Engl. J. Med., *293*:744, 1975.

Landaw, S. A.: Acute leukemia in polycythemia vera. Semin. Hematol., *13*:33, 1975.

Laszlo, J.: Myeloproliferative disorders (MPD): Myelofibrosis, myelosclerosis, extramedullary hematopoiesis, undifferentiated MPD, and hemorrhagic thrombocythemia. Semin. Hematol., *12*:409, 1975.

Leder, L. D.: The selective enzymochemical demonstration of neutrophilic myeloid cells and tissue mast cells in paraffin sections. Klin. Wochenschr., *42*:533, 1964.

Lee, C. L., Davidsohn, I., and Panczyszyn, O.: Horse agglutinins in infectious mononucleosis. II. The spot test. Am. J. Clin. Pathol., *49*:12, 1968.

Li, C. Y., Lam, K. W., and Yam, L. T.: Esterases in human leukocytes. J. Histochem. Cytochem., *21*:1, 1973.

Lukes, R. J.: Malignant lymphoma: Histologic considerations. *In* Ultmann, J. E., Griem, M. L., Kirsten, W. H., and Wissler, R. W. (eds.): Current Concepts in the Management of Lymphoma and Leukemia. New York. Springer-Verlag, Inc., 1971, p. 6.

Lukes, R. J., Butler, J. J., and Hicks, E. B.: The natural history of Hodgkin's disease as related to its pathologic picture. Cancer, *19*:317, 1966a.

Lukes, R. J., and Collins, R. D.: Immunologic characterization of human malignant lymphomas. Cancer, *34*:1488, 1974.

Lukes, R. J., Craver, L. L., Hall, T. C., Rappaport, H., and Rubin, P.: Hodgkin's disease, report of Nomenclature Committee. Cancer Res., *26*:1311, 1966.

Lukes, R. J., Tindle, B. H., and Parker, J. W.: Reed-Sternberg-like cells in infectious mononucleosis. Lancet, *2*:1003, 1969.

MacKenzie, M. R., and Fudenberg, H. H.: Macroglobulinemia: An analysis of forty patients. Blood, *39*:874, 1972.

McCall, C. E., Katayama, I., Cotran, R. S., and Finland, M.: Lysosomal and ultrastructural changes in human "toxic" neutrophils during bacterial infection. J. Exp. Med., *129*:267, 1969.

McKusick, V. A., Neufeld, E. F., and Kelly, T. E.: The mucopolysaccharide storage diseases. *In* Stanbury, J. B., Wyngaarden, J. B., Fredrickson, D. S. (eds.): The Metabolic Basis of Inherited Disease. New York, McGraw-Hill Book Co., 1978, p. 1282.

Magath, T. B., and Winkle, V.: Technic for demonstrating "L.E." (lupus erythematosus) cells in blood. Am. J. Clin. Pathol., *22*:586, 1952.

Maldonado, J. E., and Hanlon, D. G.: Monocytosis: A current appraisal. Mayo Clin. Proc., *40*:248, 1965.

Mandal, B. K., and Stokes, K. J.: Acute infectious lymphocytosis and enteroviruses. Lancet, *2*:1392, 1973.

Mangi, R. J., Niederman, J. C., Keleher, J. E., Dwyer, J. M., Evans, A. S., and Kantor, F. S.: Depression of cell-mediated immunity during acute infectious mononucleosis. N. Engl. J. Med., *291*:1149, 1974.

Marsden, P.: The nematodes (Roundworms). *In* Beeson, P. B., and McDermott, W.: Textbook of Medicine, 14th ed. Philadelphia, W. B. Saunders Company, 1975, p. 522.

Mauer, A. M., Lampkin, B. C., and McWilliams, N. B.: The leukemias and reticuloendothelioses. *In* Nathan, D. G., and Oski, F. A. (eds.): Hematology of Infancy and Childhood. Philadelphia, W. B. Saunders Company, 1974, p. 665.

Metcalf, D.: Hemopoietic Colonies. *In vitro* cloning of normal and leukemic cells. Recent Results in Cancer Research, Vol. 61. New York, Springer-Verlag, Inc., 1977.

Miescher, P. A., and Farquet, J. J.: Chronic myelomonocytic leukemia in adults. Semin. Hematol., *11*:129, 1974.

Miller, G., Niederman, J. C., and Andrews, L. L.: Prolonged oropharyngeal excretion of Epstein-Barr virus after infectious mononucleosis. N. Engl. J. Med., *288*:229, 1973.

Morse, S. I., and Barron, B. A.: Studies on the leukocytosis

and lymphocytosis induced by Bordetella pertussis. III. The distribution of transfused lymphocytes in pertussis-treated and normal mice. J. Exp. Med., *132*:663, 1970.

Naiman, J. L., Oski, F. A., Allen, F. H., and Diamond, L. K.: Hereditary eosinophilia: Report of a family and review of the literature. Am. J. Hum. Genet., *16*:195, 1964.

Neiman, R. S., Rosen, P. J., and Lukes, R. J.: Lymphocyte-depletion Hodgkin's disease. N. Engl. J. Med., *288*:751, 1973.

Nelson, D. A., and Davey, F. R.: Leukocyte esterases. *In* Williams, W. J., Beutler, E., Erslev, A. J. and Rundles, R. W. (eds.): Hematology, 2nd ed. New York, McGraw-Hill Book Co., 1977, p. 1633.

Nkrumah, F. K., and Addy, P. A. K.: Acute infectious lymphocytosis. Lancet, *1*:1257, 1973.

Nowell, P. C.: Preleukemia: Cytogenetic clues in some confusing disorders. Am. J. Pathol., *89*:459, 1977.

Olson, L. C., Miller, G., and Hanshaw, J. B.: Acute infectious lymphocytosis presenting as a pertussis-like illness: Its association with adenovirus type 12. Lancet, *1*:200, 1964.

Ooi, B. S., Orlina, A. R., Masaitis, L., First, M. R., and Pollak, V. E.: Lymphocytotoxins in aging. Transplantation, *18*:190, 1974.

Osserman, E. F., and Lawlor, D. P.: Serum and urinary lysozyme (muramidase) in monocytic and monomyelocytic leukemia. J. Exp. Med., *124*:921, 1966.

Paul, J. R., and Bunnell, W. W.: The presence of heterophile antibodies in infectious mononucleosis. Am. J. Med. Sci., *183*:90, 1932.

Peterson, L. C., Bloomfield, C. D., and Brunning, R. D.: Blast crisis as an initial or terminal manifestation of chronic myeloid leukemia. A study of 28 patients. Am. J. Med., *60*:209, 1976.

Phillips, E. A., Kempin, S., Passe, S., Miké, V., and Clarkson, B.: Prognostic factors in chronic lymphocytic leukaemia and their implications for therapy. Clin. Haematol., *6*:203, 1977.

Pierre, R. V.: Preleukemic states. Semin. Hematol., *11*:73, 1974.

Prchal, J. F., and Axelrod, A. A.: Bone marrow responses in polycythemia vera. N. Engl. J. Med., *290*:1382, 1974.

Preston, F. E., Cooke, K. B., Foster, M. E., Winfield, D. A., and Lee, D.: Myelomatosis and the hyperviscosity syndrome. Br. J. Haematol., *38*:517, 1978.

Preud'homme, J. L., and Seligmann, M.: Surface bound immunoglobulins as a cell marker in human lymphoproliferative diseases. Blood, *40*:777, 1972.

Pruzanski, W., and Watt, J. G.: Serum viscosity and hyperviscosity syndrome in IgG multiple myeloma. Ann. Intern. Med., *77*:853, 1972.

Rai, K. R., Chanana, A. W., Cronkite, E. P., Joel, D. D., and Stevens, J. B.: Studies on lymphocytes. XVIII. Mechanisms of lymphocytosis induced by supernatant fluids of *Bordetella pertussis* cultures. Blood, *38*:49, 1971.

Rai, K. R., Sawitsky, A., Cronkite, E. P., Chanana, A. D., Levy, R. N., and Pasternack, B. S.: Clinical staging of chronic lymphocytic leukemia. Blood, *46*:219, 1975.

Rapaport, S. I.: Introduction to Hematology. New York, Harper & Row, Publishers, Inc., 1971.

Rappaport, H.: Tumors of the hematopoietic system. *In* Atlas of Tumor Pathology. Washington, D.C., Armed Forces Institute of Pathology, Section III, Fascicle 88, 1966.

Rappaport, H., and Thomas, L. B.: Mycosis fungoides: The pathology of extracutaneous involvement. Cancer, *34*:1198, 1974.

Rickinson, A. B., Crawford, D., and Epstein, M. A.: Inhibition of the *in vitro* outgrowth of Epstein-Barr virus-

3

transformed lymphocytes by thymus-dependent lymphocytes from infectious mononucleosis patients. Clin. Exp. Immunol., *28*:72, 1977.

Rickles, F. R., and Miller, D. R.: Eosinophilic leukemoid reaction J. Pediatr., *80*:418, 1972.

Ritzmann, S. E., Daniels, J. C., Lawrence, M. C., Beathard, G. A., and Levin, W. C.: Monoclonal gammopathies, present status. Texas Med., *68*:91, 1972.

Rinehart, J. J., Sagone, A. L., Balcerzak, S. P., Ackerman, G. A., and LoBuglio, A. F.: Effects of corticosteroid therapy on human monocyte function. N. Engl. J. Med., *292*:236, 1975.

Rosenberg, S. A.: Hodgkin's disease of the bone marrow. Cancer Res., *31*:1733, 1971.

Rosenthal, S., Canellos, G. P., DeVita, V. T., Jr., and Gralnick, H. R.: Characteristics of blast crisis in chronic granulocytic leukemia. Blood, *49*:705, 1977.

Rosner, F., and Grunwald, H.: Multiple myeloma terminating in acute leukemia. Report of 12 cases and review of the literature. Am. J. Med., *57*:927, 1974.

Rosner, F., Schreiber, Z. R., and Parise, F.: Leukocyte alkaline phosphatase. Fluctuations with disease status in chronic granulocytic leukemia. Arch. Intern. Med., *130*:892, 1972.

Saarni, M. I., and Linman, J. W.: Preleukemia. The hematologic syndrome preceding acute leukemia. Am. J. Med., *55*:38, 1973.

Sandberg, A. A., Ishihara, T., Kikuchi, Y., and Crosswhite, L. H.: Chromosomal differences among the acute leukemias. Ann. N.Y. Acad. Sci., *113*:663, 1964.

Saxén, E., and Saxén, L.: The histological diagnosis of glandular toxoplasmosis. Lab. Invest., *8*:386, 1959.

Seligmann, M.: Immunochemical, clinical and pathological features of α-chain disease. Arch. Intern. Med., *135*:78, 1975.

Sharp, A. A.: Platelets, bleeding and haemostasis in infectious mononucleosis. *In* Carter, R. L., and Penman, H. G. (eds.): Infectious Mononucleosis. Oxford, Blackwell Scientific Publications, 1969.

Sheehan, W. W.: The relationship between lymphocytic leukemias and lymphomas. *In* Ultman, J. E., Griem, M. L., Kirsten, W. H., and Wissler, R. D. (eds.): Current Concepts in the Management of Lymphoma and Leukemia. New York, Springer-Verlag, Inc., 1971.

Shope, T., and Miller, G.: Epstein-Barr virus. Heterophile responses in squirrel monkeys inoculated with virus-transformed autologous leukocytes. J. Exp. Med., *137*:140, 1973.

Siim, J. C.: Acquired toxoplasmosis. Report of seven cases with strongly positive reactions. J.A.M.A., *147*:1641, 1951.

Silverberg, E.: Cancer Statistics, 1978. CA-A Cancer Journal for Clinicians. New York, American Cancer Society, 1978. Vol. 28, p. 17.

Smith, C. H.: Infectious lymphocytosis. Am. J. Dis. Child., *62*:231, 1941.

Smith, E., Kochwa, S., and Wasserman, L. R.: Aggregation of IgG globulin *in vivo*. Am. J. Med., *39*:35, 1965.

Smith, M. A., Evans, J., and Steel, C. M.: Age-related variation in proportion of circulating T cells. Lancet, *2*:922, 1974.

Spaet, T. H., Lejnieks, I., Gaynor, E., and Goldstein, M. L.: Defective platelets in essential thrombocythemia. Arch. Intern. Med., *124*:135, 1969.

Spiers, A. S. D., Bain, B. J., and Turner, J. E.: The peripheral blood in chronic granulocytic leukemia. Study of 50 untreated Philadelphia-positive cases. Scand. J. Haematol., *18*:25, 1977.

Stossel, T. P., and Boxer, L. A.: Qualitative abnormalities of granulocytes. *In* Williams, W. J., Beutler, E., Erslev, A. J., and Rundles, R. W. (eds.): Hematology, 2nd ed. New York, McGraw-Hill Book Co., 1977, p. 756.

Sultan, C., Imbert, M., Riard, M. F., and Marquet, M.: Myelodysplastic syndromes. *In* Lewis, S. M., and Verwilghen, R. L. (eds.): Dyserythropoiesis. London, Academic Press, 1977.

Takácsi-Nagy, L., and Graf, F.: Definition, clinical features and diagnosis of myelofibrosis. Clin. Haematol., *4*:291, 1975.

Tamaoki, N., and Essner, E.: Distribution of acid phosphatase, β-glucuronidase, and N-acetyl-β-glucuronidase activities in lymphocytes of lymphatic tissues of man and rodents. J. Histochem. Cytochem., *17*:238, 1969.

Thorn, G. W., Forsham, P. H., Prunty, F. T. G., and Hills, A. G.: The response to pituitary adrenocorticotropic hormone as a test for adrenal cortical insufficiency. J.A.M.A., *137*:1005, 1948.

Tjio, J. H., Carbone, P. P., Whang, J., and Frei, E.: The Philadelphia chromosome and chronic myelogenous leukemia. J. Natl. Cancer Inst., *36*:567, 1966.

Van Scott, E. J., and Vonderheid, E. C.: Mycosis fungoides and Sezary syndrome. *In* Williams, W. J., Beutler, E., Erslev, A. J., and Rundles, R. D. (eds.): Hematology, 2nd ed. New York, McGraw-Hill Book Co., 1977.

Waldorf, D. S., Willkens, R. I., and Decker, J. L.: Impaired delayed hypersensitivity in an aging population. Association with antinuclear reactivity and rheumatoid factor. J.A.M.A., *203*:831, 1968.

Ward, H. P., and Block, M. H.: The natural history of agnogenic myeloid metaplasia (AMM) and a critical evaluation of its relationship with the myeloproliferative syndrome. Medicine (Baltimore), *50*:357, 1971.

Wasserman, L. R., and Gilbert, H. S.: Surgical bleeding in polycythemia vera. Ann. N.Y. Acad. Sci., *115*:122, 1964.

Wasserman, L. R., and Gilbert, H. S.: Complications of polycythemia vera. Semin. Hematol., *3*:199, 1966.

Weksler, M. E., and Hütteroth, T. H.: Impaired lymphocyte function in aged humans. J. Clin. Invest., *53*:99, 1974.

Weller, T. H.: The cytomegaloviruses: Ubiquitous agents with protean clinical manifestations. N. Engl. J. Med., *285*:203, 1971.

Williams, W. J.: Serum viscosity, *In* Williams, W. J., Beutler, E., Erslev, A. J., and Rundles, R. W.: Hematology, 2nd ed. New York, McGraw-Hill Book Co., 1977, p. 1639.

Wintrobe, M. M., Lee, G. R., Boggs, D. R., Bithell, T. C., Athens, J. W., and Foerster, J.: Clinical Hematology, 7th ed. Philadelphia, Lea & Febiger, 1974.

Wood, T. A., and Frenkel, E. P.: The atypical lymphocyte. Am. J. Med., *42*:923, 1967.

Worlledge, S. M., and Dacie, J. V.: Hemolytic and other anaemias in infectious mononucleosis. *In* Carter, R. L., and Penman, H. G. (eds.): Infectious Mononucleosis. Oxford, Blackwell Scientific Publications, 1969.

Wright, D. J., and Jenkins, D. E., Jr.: Simplified method for estimation of serum and plasma viscosity in multiple myeloma and related disorders. Blood, *36*:516, 1970.

Yam, L. T., Li, C. Y., and Lam, K. W.: Tartrate-resistant acid phosphatase isoenzyme in the reticulum cells of leukemic reticuloendotheliosis. N. Engl. J. Med., *284*:357, 1971a.

Yam, L. T., Li, C. Y., and Crosby, W. H.: Cytochemical identification of monocytes and granulocytes. Am. J. Clin. Pathol., *55*:283, 1971b.

Zacharski, L. R., and Linman, J. W.: Lymphocytopenia: Its causes and significance. Mayo Clin. Proc., *46*:168, 1971.

Zimmer, F. E., and Hargraves, M. M.: The effect of blood coagulation on lupus erythematosus cell phenomenon. Proc. Staff Meet. Mayo Clin., *27*:424, 1952.

Zinkham, W. H., and Conley, C. L.: Some factors influencing the formation of L.E. cells. Bull. Johns Hopkins Hosp., *98*:102, 1956.

31

BLOOD VESSELS AND HEMOSTASIS

Frederick R. Davey, M.D.

3

HEMOSTASIS

The hemostatic system provides for prompt repair of breaks in the circulation without compromising the free flow of the blood. Normal hemostasis depends on the integrity of blood vessels, function of platelets, interaction of circulating procoagulants with platelets, and activation of fibrinolysins.

ROLE OF BLOOD VESSELS IN HEMOSTASIS

Blood vessels are an important component in the hemostatic system. They are an appropriate conduit for the blood and nutrients to be circulated throughout the entire body. Under normal circumstances, the endothelium provides an inert surface over which blood passes without activation of coagulation. The tunica media (q.v.) provides sufficient strength to convey blood at optimal hydrostatic pressure. Under varied conditions, the blood vessels can constrict or dilate to change the rate of blood flow. In addition, constituents of blood vessels under certain circumstances initiate coagulation or activate fibrinolysins.

Anatomy of blood vessels

Capillaries, the smallest blood vessels, have an inner diameter of 5 to 10 μm. The lumen of the most common type of capillary is lined by a continuous endothelial layer, which is composed of flattened endothelial cells and supported by a thin continuous basal lamina or subendothelium (Stemerman, 1974) (Fig. 31-1). When a pericyte is present, the basal lamina splits to completely enclose it. The pericyte affords some contractile capability to the capillary.

The subendothelium has a widely diverse morphologic structure. The capillary basal lamina is approximately 50 to 70 nm thick and is a trilaminar structure in electron micrographs. The innermost layer has fine filaments of 5 nm diameter, and the outer margin contains filaments of 10 nm diameter with a periodicity of 20 nm. Fibers with a periodicity of 64 nm, typical of collagen, are present only peripheral to the outermost region of the basal

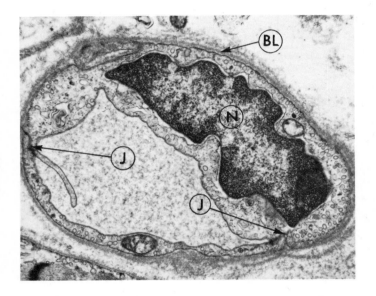

Figure 31–1. A blood capillary characterized by continuous endothelium and basement membrane (basal lamina, BL). In this section the endothelial lining is formed by parts of two cells separated by two intercellular junctions (J); the section passes through the nucleus (N) of only one of the cells. The narrow cytoplasmic projection into the lumen (at the left) is a common feature of capillaries. Prominent in the cytoplasm are numerous plasmalemmal vesicles (60 to 70 nm diameter) which act in the transfer of large molecules (> 10 nm diameter) across the endothelium.

The apparent thickening of the basement membrane at the bottom may be just a tangential section or may represent collagen. Typical cross-banded collagen strands are not included in this section.

Human muscle; ×16,500. (Courtesy of David B. Jones, M.D.)

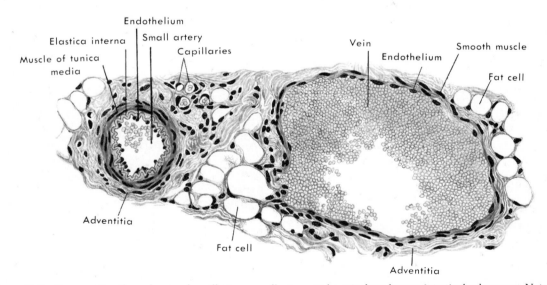

Figure 31–2. Cross-section through several capillaries, a small artery, and a vein from human intestinal submucosa. Note the relative diameters of the three types of vessel and the thickness of their walls. Smooth muscle in the tunica media and the elastica interna (internal elastic lamella) are prominent features of the artery. (From Bloom, W., and Fawcett, D. W.: A Textbook of Histology, 10th ed. Philadelphia, W. B. Saunders Company, 1975.)

lamina. A similar subendothelium is present in small veins.

Larger vessels, arteries and veins, have a more complex structure, consisting of a tunica intima (endothelium and subendothelium), tunica media (smooth muscle, collagen, and rare fibroblasts), and tunica adventitia (collagen, elastic fibers, and fibroblasts). An internal elastic lamella separates the tunica intima from the tunica media and the external elastic lamella separates the tunica media from the tunica adventitia (Fig. 31-2).

The subendothelium of larger vessels is approximately 100 nm wide and consists of a vestigal basal lamina, elastin, and microfibrils (Stemerman, 1974). In addition, larger vessels have vasa vasorum, small vessels which supply blood to the tunica media and tunica adventitia.

Veins differ from arteries in that the muscular and elastic tissues are not well developed; the tunica media in veins is thinner and the tunica adventitia is several times thicker than in arteries.

Vasoconstriction

Following vascular damage, vessels constrict transiently. The degree of vasoconstric-tion is in part a reflex response mediated by the autonomic nervous system (Bloom, 1975). Vasoconstriction is also due to local stimulation of smooth muscle fibers in the wall of vessels (Fig. 31-3). Smooth muscles may contract owing to the effects of epinephrine, serotonin (Zucker, 1955), and thromboxane A_2 (Moncada, 1976) released by the action of platelets. A small peptide from the amino-terminal end of the beta-chain of fibrinogen, fibrinopeptide B, may also play a role in vascular contraction (Colman, 1967). In addition, the pressure of extravasated blood on vessel walls (especially capillaries) may be sufficient to cause some degree of vascular collapse and cessation of hemorrhage.

Platelet adherence to subendothelial connective tissue

When vessels are damaged, platelets may be exposed to collagen located beneath the subendothelium. Through their interaction with the ϵ-amino groups of lysine in collagen, platelets may adhere to the subendothelial connective tissue after minor vascular injury (Wilner, 1968b). The active component is probably not native collagen, since the latter's 64 nm periodicity has not been identified in

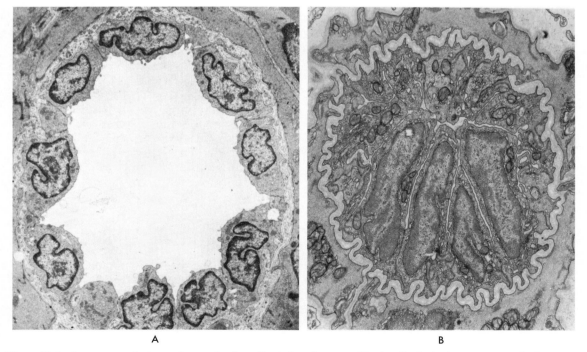

A   B

Figure 31-3. Low power electron micrograph of small arteries of comparable size. In *A,* the lumen is open. In *B* extreme vasoconstriction has occurred. The endothelial cells have increased in height and become narrower at their bases. It is evident that such vasoconstriction would markedly reduce blood flow and, in turn, reduce hemorrhage in tissue supplied by this artery. (From Bloom, W., and Fawcett, D. W.: A Textbook of Histology, 10th ed. Philadelphia, W. B. Saunders Company, 1975.)

the subendothelium by electron microscopy (Stemerman, 1974). Platelets interact with subendothelial microfibrils following the digestion of the subendothelium by collagenase on rabbit artery (Baumgartner, 1971).

Activation of circulating procoagulants by blood vessel components

Vascular components may activate circulating procoagulants through either the intrinsic or the extrinsic system. The free carboxyl groups of the glutamic and aspartic acids found in collagen and the triple helical structure of collagen have been shown to be critical in the activation of Hageman factor (Wilner, 1968a).

Substances rich in thromboplastic activity have been demonstrated in the endothelium of blood vessels. Indeed, abundant tissue factor antigen has been found in the intima, presumably the endothelial plasma membrane (Nemerson, 1972), but the tunica media contained very little tissue factor and the tunica adventitia almost none. Tissue factor reacts with plasma coagulation factor VII in the presence of calcium. This complex interacts with other procoagulants to activate thrombin which, in turn, interacts with platelets and fibrinogen to generate a clot.

Endothelial cells synthesize and secrete molecules that contain both factor VIII antigen and von Willebrand factor (Hoyer, 1973; Jaffe, 1973). Endothelial cells from patients with von Willebrand's disease lack both factor VIII antigen and the von Willebrand factor (Jaffe, 1973); these molecules appear to circulate free in plasma as well as bound to platelets (Jaffe, 1977). The von Willebrand factor, when bound to the platelet surface, enables the platelet to function normally by supporting platelet adhesion to exposed endothelial tissue. The circulating von Willebrand's factor may form a complex with the antihemophilic factor or be converted to a molecule with intrinsic clot-promoting activity (p. 1120).

Interaction of vascular factors with fibrinolysins

Plasminogen activators exist in abundant quantities in blood vessel walls (Warren, 1964). Some investigators claim that the fibrinolytic activity is slight in the intima and abundant in the adventitia (Baumgartner, 1971). In contrast, others claim that the endothelium contains significant quantities of plasminogen activator and that the high concentration in the adventitia is derived from the presence of plasminogen activator in the endothelium of the vasa vasorum (Astrup, 1966). The presence of fibrinolytic factors in the vascular walls permits removal of thrombi and restoration of the vascular lumens after healing. Fibrinolysis is discussed in Chapter 33, p. 1137.

Vascular factors influencing fluidity of blood

Recently it has been shown that microsomes from pig or rabbit aortas transform prostaglandin endoperoxides to an unstable principle, prostaglandin I_2 (PGI_2), which relaxes blood vessels and prevents platelet aggregation (Moncada, 1976b; Marx, 1977). Thus, the generation of PGI_2 by the vessel walls could be a mechanism which operates to keep blood fluid. In addition, the prostaglandin endoperoxides—prostaglandin G_2 (PGG_2) and prostaglandin H_2 (PGH_2)—in platelets may be converted to a non-prostaglandin compound thromboxane A_2 (TXA_2), which has platelet aggregating activity. Therefore, a balance between the amount of TXA_2 formed by platelets and PGI_2 formed by vessels might be critically important in maintaining normal hemostasis.

Factors influencing vascular integrity

Normal vascular integrity depends on several known factors. Thrombocytopenia results in increased capillary fragility (Aursness, 1974; Gimbrone, 1969); platelets, therefore, appear to play some role in maintaining normal vascular function. Therapy with adrenocortical steroids often reduces capillary fragility in thrombocytopenic patients (Faloon, 1952). In addition, ascorbic acid is necessary for the normal generation and maintenance of vascular connective tissue (Stolman, 1961).

VASCULAR DISORDERS

Hemorrhagic disorders may result in bleeding into deep tissues, into the gastrointestinal tract, or into the skin and mucous membranes. *Petechiae* are round hemorrhagic discolorations in skin and mucous membranes which vary in size from 1 to 3 mm, usually result from capillary bleeding, and tend to occur especially in the lower extremities or other areas

Table 31-1. BLEEDING ATTRIBUTED
TO VASCULAR DISORDERS

Purpura simplex
Stasis-induced purpura
Steroid purpura
Purpura due to inherited connective tissue disorders
Senile purpura
Scurvy
Purpura associated with dysproteinemia and cryoglobu-
   linemia
Purpura in benign hyperglobulinemia
Amyloidosis
Infectious purpura
Allergic purpura
Purpura associated with autoerythrocyte sensitization
Hereditary telangiectasis
Kaposi's sarcoma

of high venous pressure. *Ecchymoses* are
larger hemorrhagic discolorations which are
red, purple, yellow, green, or brown, depending upon the age of the lesion. *Purpura* refers
to a hemorrhagic state characterized by skin
and mucous membrane bleeding, i.e., petechiae and ecchymoses.

Bleeding into deep tissues and joints is usually the result of defects in coagulation factors
(Chap. 33). Petechiae and ecchymoses generally occur because of platelet disorders (Chap.
32) or vascular disorders. Usually, bleeding is
attributed to a vascular disorder only when no
other platelet or coagulation factor defect can
be identified (Table 31-1).

Purpura simplex is a mild disorder which is
common in women; it is characterized by
petechiae and small ecchymoses in the skin
(Davis, 1943). A similar disorder, *hereditary
familial purpura simplex,* has been described
in several families (Davis, 1941). The exact
etiology of the purpura is in many cases unknown and is probably due to a variety of
abnormalities. Some may be mild von Willebrand's disease or thrombocytopathies which
have not been detected. Others, however, may
be due to increased capillary pressure, since
they sometimes occur on the face following
coughing, vomiting, or crying (Zieve, 1976).

Stasis purpura, found in the legs of elderly
people, is due to extravasation of blood from
capillaries and small venules after prolonged
standing. A defect in the vascular supporting
framework may be an important contributing
factor.

Abnormalities in vascular connective tissue
may be a cause of bleeding in *senile purpura*
and *steroid purpura* (Scarborough, 1960), and
in several inherited connective tissue disorders (Gottlieb, 1977), such as pseudoxan-

thoma elasticum (Zieve, 1976), *Ehlers-Danlos
syndrome* (Day, 1961), *osteogenesis imperfecta,*
and *Marfan's syndrome* (Estes, 1965). Abnormalities in platelet function and blood coagulation, however, have also been described in
some of these disorders (Kashiwagi, 1965; Siegal, 1957).

Scurvy, a disorder due to vitamin C deficiency, is associated with a bleeding tendency.
This takes the form of perifollicular hemorrhages, bleeding gums, and a tendency to
bruise easily, particularly over the arms and
legs (Hodges, 1971). Frank hemorrhages into
the muscle may also be seen. Hyperkeratotic
hair follicles and short broken coiled hairs
occur in the skin. In animals, ascorbic acid
depletion is associated with degenerative
changes in connective tissue of blood vessel
walls and perivascular tissue (Stolman, 1961).
In addition, platelet functional abnormalities
have been described in some cases of scurvy in
man (Cetingil, 1958). The diagnosis should rest
on determination of the plasma ascorbic acid
level and satisfactory response to the administration of vitamin C.

Purpura and hemorrhage in the absence of
thrombocytopenia has been described in patients with *dysproteinemia* secondary to multiple myeloma and macroglobulinemia (Perkins, 1970). The paraprotein has been shown to
interfere with platelet function (Lackner, 1973),
to inhibit the conversion of fibrinogen to fibrin
(Coleman, 1972; Davey, 1976; Perkins, 1970),
and perhaps to have some inhibitory effects on
circulating procoagulants (Lackner, 1973).
Hemorrhage in these disorders is probably due
to several factors. Anoxic damage to blood
vessels resulting from increased blood viscosity has been postulated (Zieve, 1976). Also, a
correlation between overt hemorrhage and
platelet function has been observed (Perkins,
1970). Clinically significant hemorrhage is an
unusual complication of paraproteinemic
states. In general, plasmapheresis seems effective in maintaining normal hemostasis.

Purpura has been described in patients with
cryoglobulinemia unassociated with a malignant hematologic disorder (Firkin, 1958; Grey,
1973). In these circumstances, the bleeding has
been attributed to vascular anoxia secondary
to hyperviscosity.

In *amyloidosis,* purpura arises from the increased fragility of blood vessels involved with
amyloid deposits (Kyle, 1975). In some cases of
amyloidosis, there is a decreased plasma level
of factor X, probably due to its increased peripheral consumption (Furie, 1976).

Hemorrhage caused by an immunologic vascular injury appears to be one of the most common causes of non-thrombocytopenic purpura. *Hypergammaglobulinemic purpura* is a rare condition, frequently involving women with purpura primarily on the lower extremities. The disorder is characterized by a polyclonal gammopathy. Biopsies have shown vasculitis of the dermis and subcutaneous tissue. In 50 per cent of the cases, the disease was associated with collagen vascular disorders; in the remainder, the disease was considered primary, since no other abnormality was discovered (Kyle, 1971).

Allergic purpura (Henoch-Schönlein purpura) is attributed to vasculitis of arterioles arising from an immune response to foreign antigens. The disorder, usually found in children, may occur following bacterial infections, drug ingestion, and insect bites. Vascular lesions are found in skin, kidney, bowel, heart, liver, and lung. Polyarthralgias develop in about two thirds of patients. In a study of adults with allergic purpura, raised levels of serum cryoglobulins were observed in slightly less than 30 per cent of the patients; the cryoglobulin was usually an immune complex (Cream, 1970). Although the disease is usually of short duration, chronic cases have been observed.

Autoerythrocyte sensitization is a disorder found in women and is characterized by painful ecchymoses. In some patients, the lesions have been reproduced by the intradermal injection of autologous erythrocytes and erythrocyte stroma (Gardner, 1955; Ratnoff, 1968). The syndrome is confined to adult women who have multiple systemic and psychiatric complaints. This disorder may be similar to a syndrome known as deoxyribonucleic acid (DNA) sensitivity in which ecchymoses are produced by intracutaneous injections of DNA.

Infectious purpura appears in some cases to be the result of a vascular injury (Harker, 1974). In rickettsial disease, the organism produces a direct vascular lesion. However, in some bacterial infections, endotoxins may induce endothelial injury. Occasionally, there is a superimposed coagulation defect as in diffuse intravascular coagulation (DIC), which is described on page 1147.

Hereditary hemorrhagic telangiectasia is an autosomal dominant trait characterized by the presence of abnormally thin-walled capillaries and venules (Hodgson, 1959). The vascular abnormalities appear as flat, round, red lesions that blanch on pressure. Although they may be present anywhere on the body, they are commonly seen in the mouth, nasal mucosa, ears, and distal extremities. Bleeding from a gastrointestinal lesion may be massive and frequently is the problem that leads to the diagnosis. Platelet and coagulation studies are normal. Diagnosis depends on a family history and demonstration of telangiectases.

Kaposi's sarcoma is a neoplastic proliferation of vascular elements in tumor nodules, associated with localized hemorrhage and hemosiderin deposition (Reynolds, 1965). Involvement usually includes lower extremities. Tumor growth is usually slow. Visceral metastases exist in approximately 10 per cent of patients. The typical cutaneous lesions are ecchymotic nodules or plaques, but purpura and diffuse macular discoloration of the skin are also frequent.

MEASUREMENTS OF VASCULAR INTEGRITY

The *tourniquet test* (capillary fragility test) and the bleeding time have been used to measure vascular integrity. Neither is specific for vascular activity, however, since each also depends on platelet number and function.

Numerous variations of the tourniquet test have been used and no standard method exists (Kramar, 1962). All employ restricting venous return by compression around the upper arm; petechiae are counted distal to that site after removing the compression. A blood pressure cuff is applied to the upper arm and inflated to a pressure of 80 to 90 mm Hg. In different procedures, the length of stasis varies from 3 to 15 minutes and the length of time for recirculation before examining the arm for petechiae ranges from 0 to 5 minutes. In a standardized study of the tourniquet test, the number of petechiae on the dorsum of the hand was significantly greater in healthy elderly individuals than in the younger adults (Stavem, 1965). In addition, the number of petechiae in thrombocytopenic patients was similar to that observed in healthy elderly individuals. Others have recorded poor correlation between platelet count and number of petechiae elicited by the tourniquet test. As a result, the tourniquet test is rarely used as a screening test for hemostasis (Wintrobe, 1974).

Biopsy of vascular lesions may under certain circumstances be useful in the diagnosis of vascular tumors or vasculitis. It is of little use in defining the nature of other bleeding disorders.

The *bleeding time* is the elapsed time between making a cut of specified size in the skin and cessation of bleeding from the cut. It is discussed in Chapter 32 (p. 1122).

DIAGNOSIS OF DISORDERS OF VASCULAR INTEGRITY

The diagnosis of a vascular disorder as a cause of bleeding depends to a large extent on the clinical history and physical examination. With the exception of the tourniquet test and bleeding time, all other coagulation assays are usually normal. The tourniquet test and the bleeding time are not specific for vascular disorders, since they also measure platelet function. In addition, the tourniquet test and bleeding time are not invariably abnormal in the presence of a known vascular disorder. As a result, bleeding is attributed to vascular abnormalities when all other platelet and coagulation disorders appear unlikely and the appropriate clinical setting is present.

REFERENCES

Astrup, T.: Tissue activators of plasminogen. Fed. Proc., 25:42, 1966.

Aursnes, I.: Blood platelet production and red cell leakage to lymph during thrombocytopenia. Scand. J. Hematol., 13:184, 1974.

Baumgartner, H. R., Stemerman, M. B., and Spaet, T. H.: Adhesion of blood platelets to subendothelial surface: Distinct from adhesion to collagen. Experientia, 27:283, 1971.

Bloom, W., and Fawcett, D. W.: A Textbook of Histology. Philadelphia, W. B. Saunders Company, 1975.

Cetingil, A. I., Ulutin, O. N., and Karaca, M.: A platelet defect in a case of scurvy. Br. J. Haematol., 4:350, 1958.

Coleman, M., Vigliano, E. M., Weksler, M. E., and Nachman, R. L.: Inhibition of fibrin monomer polymerization by lambda myeloma globulins. Blood, 39:210, 1972.

Colman, R. W., Morris, R. E., and Osbahr, A. J.: New vasoconstrictor, Bovine Peptide B, released during blood coagulation. Nature, 215:292, 1967.

Cream, J. J.: Clinical and immunological aspects of cutaneous vasculitis. Q. J. Med., 45:255, 1976.

Cream, J. J., Gumpel, J. M., and Peadry, R. D. G.: Schönlein-Henoch purpura in the adult. A study of 77 adults with Schönlein-Henoch purpura. Am. J. Med., 39:461, 1970.

Davey, F. R., Gordon, G. B., Boral, L. I., and Gottlieb, A. J.: Gamma globulin inhibition of fibrin clot formation. Ann. Clin. Lab. Sci., 6:72, 1976.

Davis, E., and Manc, M. D.: Hereditary familial purpura simplex. Review of 27 families. Lancet, 1:145, 1941.

Davis, E.: Purpura of the skin. A review of 500 cases. Lancet, 2:16, 1943.

Day, J. H., and Zarafonetis, C. J. D.: Coagulation studies in four patients with Ehler-Danlos Syndrome. Am. J. Med. Sci., 242:565, 1961.

Estes, J. W., Carey, R. J., and Desai, R. G.: Marfan's syndrome. Hematological abnormalities in a family. Arch. Intern. Med., 116:889, 1965.

Faloon, W. W., Greene, R. W. and Lozner, E. L.: The hemostatic defect in thrombocytopenia as studied by the use of ACTH and cortisone. Am. J. Med., 13:12, 1952.

Firkin, B. G.: Essential cryoglobulinemia. Am. J. Med., 24:974, 1958.

Furie, B., Greene, E., and Furie, B. C.: Syndrome of acquired factor X deficiency and systemic amyloidosis. In vivo studies of the metabolic fate of factor X. N. Engl. J. Med., 297:81, 1977.

Gardner, F. H., and Diamond, I. K.: Autoerythrocyte sensitization. A form of purpura producing painful bruising following autosensitization to red blood cells in certain women. Blood, 10:675, 1955.

Gimbrone, M. A., Aster, R. H., Cotran, R. S., et al.: Preservation of vascular integrity in organs perfused in vitro with a platelet-rich medium. Nature, 222:33, 1969.

Gottlieb, A. J.: Disorders of hemostasis—non-thrombocytopenic purpuras. In Williams, W. J., Beutler, E., Erslev, A. J., and Rundles, R. W. (eds.): Hematology, 2nd ed. New York, McGraw-Hill Book Co., 1977, p. 1385.

Grey, H. M., and Kohler, P. F.: Cryoimmunoglobulins. Semin. Hematol., 10:87, 1973.

Harker, L. A.: Hemostasis manual. Philadelphia, F. A. Davis Co., 1974, p. 4.

Hodges, R. E., Hood, J., Canham, J. E., Sauberlich, H. E., and Baker, E. M.: Clinical manifestations of ascorbic acid deficiency in man. Am. J. Clin. Nutr., 24:432, 1971.

Hodgson, C. H., Barchell, H. B., Good, C. A., and Clagett, O. T.: Hereditary hemorrhagic telangiectasia and pulmonary arteriovenous fistula. N. Engl. J. Med., 261:625, 1959.

Hoyer, L. W., DeLosSantos, R. P., and Hoyer, J. R.: Antihemophilic factor antigen localization in endothelial cells by immunofluorescent microscopy. J. Clin. Invest., 52:2737, 1973.

Jaffe, E. A.: Endothelial cells and the biology of factor VIII. N. Engl. J. Med., 296:377, 1977.

Jaffe, E. A., Hoyer, L. W., and Nachman, R. L.: Synthesis of antihemophilic factor antigen by cultured human endothelial cells. J. Clin. Invest., 52:2757, 1973.

Kashiwagi, H., Riddle, J. M., Abraham, J. R., and Frame, B.: Functional and ultrastructural abnormalities of platelets in Ehlers-Danlos syndrome. Ann. Intern. Med., 63:249, 1965.

Kramár, J.: The determination and evaluation of capillary resistance—A review of methodology. Blood, 20:83, 1962.

Kyle, R. A., and Bayrd, E. D.: Amyloidosis: Review of 236 cases. Medicine (Baltimore), 54:271, 1975.

Kyle, R. A., Gleich, G. J., and Bayrd, E. D.: Benign hypergammaglobulinemic purpura of Waldenström. Medicine (Baltimore), 50:113, 1971.

Lackner, H.: Hemostatic abnormalities associated with dysproteinemias. Semin. Hematol., 10:125, 1973.

Marx, J. L.: Blood clotting: The role of prostaglandins. Science, 196:1072, 1977.

Moncada, S., Gryglewski, R. J., Bunting, S., and Vane, J. R.: A lipid peroxide inhibits the enzyme in blood vessel microsomes that generates from prostaglandin endoperoxides the substance (Prostaglandin X) which prevents platelet aggregation. Prostaglandins, *12*:715, 1976a.

Moncada, S., Gryglewski, R., Bunting, S., and Vane, J. R.: An enzyme isolated from arteries transforms prostaglandin endoperoxides to an unstable substance that inhibits platelet aggregation. Nature, *263*:663, 1976b.

Nemerson, Y., and Pitlick, F. A.: The tissue factor pathway of blood coagulation. Prog. Hemostasis Thromb., *1*:1, 1972.

Nossel, H. L.: The contact system. *In* Biggs, R. (ed.): Human Blood Coagulation, Haemostasis and Thrombosis. Oxford, Blackwell Scientific Publications, 1976.

Perkins, H. A., MacKenzie, M. R., and Fudenberg, H. H.: Hemostatic defects in dysproteinemias. Blood, *55*:695, 1970.

Ratnoff, O. D., and Agle, D. P.: Psychogenic purpura: A re-evaluation of the syndrome of autoerythrocyte sensitization. Medicine (Baltimore), *47*:475, 1968.

Reynolds, W. A., Winkelmann, R. K., and Soule, E. H.: Kaposi's sarcoma: A clinico-pathologic study with particular reference to its relationship to the reticuloendothelial system. Medicine (Baltimore), *44*:419, 1965.

Scarborough, H., and Shuster, S.: Corticosteroid purpura. Lancet, *1*:93, 1960.

Siegal, B. M., Friedman, I. A., and Schwartz, S. O.: Hemorrhagic disease in osteogenesis imperfecta, study of platelet functional defect. Am. J. Med., *22*:315, 1957.

Stavem, P.: The tourniquet test. The influence of age or hemorrhagic disorders on the distribution and size of petechiae. Scand. J. Clin. Lab. Invest., *17*:607, 1965.

Stemerman, M. B.: Vascular intimal components: Precursors of thrombosis. Prog. Hemostasis Thromb., *2*:1, 1974.

Stolman, J. M., Goldman, H. M., and Gould, B. S.: Ascorbic acid and blood vessels. Arch. Pathol., *72*:535, 1961.

Warren, B. A.: Fibrinolytic activity of vascular endothelium. Br. Med. Bull., *20*:213, 1964.

Wilner, G. D., Nossel, H. L., and LeRoy, E. C.: Activation of Hageman factor by collagen. J. Clin. Invest., *47*:2608, 1968a.

Wilner, G. D., Nossel, H. L., and LeRoy, E. C.: Aggregation of platelets by collagen. J. Clin. Invest., *47*:2616, 1968b.

Wintrobe, M. M., Lee, G. R., Boggs, D. R., Bithell, T. C., Athens, J. W., and Foerster, J.: Clinical Hematology, 7th ed. Philadelphia, Lea and Febiger, 1974, p. 1138.

Zieve, P. D., and Levin, J.: Disorders of Hemostasis. Philadelphia, W. B. Saunders Company, 1976, p. 16.

Zucker, M. B., and Borrelli, J.: Quantity assay and release of serotonin in human platelets. J. Appl. Physiol., *7*:425, 1955.

PLATELETS AND PLATELET DISORDERS

Frederick R. Davey, M.D.

3

PLATELET MORPHOLOGY

LIGHT MICROSCOPY

On air-dried, Romanowsky-stained blood films, platelets are round to oval cytoplasmic fragments which measure 2 to 4 μm in diameter. Characteristically, they contain multiple red-purple granules. The granules may be grouped in a central *granulomere* and surrounded by a peripheral homogeneous or slightly basophilic clear *hyalomere*. More commonly, the granules appear uniformly dispersed throughout the platelet.

In normal individuals, only 5 per cent of platelets measure greater than 2.5 μm in diameter on air-dried blood films (Howard, 1973). Platelet volume distribution for normal subjects is 5.17 ± 0.46 cu μm (SD) utilizing a computerized electronic particle counter (Corash, 1977). As platelets age, they decrease in size and density (Murphy, 1972). An increased number of large platelets usually is associated with increased platelet turnover. The large-sized platelets described in immune thrombocytopenic purpura are young platelets released from the marrow as a result of increased peripheral destruction of platelets. Yet the presence of large platelets in the peripheral blood does not always indicate young platelets. Large platelets are found in myelofibrosis, May-Hegglin anomaly, familial thrombopathic thrombocytopenia, macrothrombocytopathic nephritis and deafness, giant platelet syndrome, Bernard-Soulier syndrome, and other macrothrombopathic states. Small platelets are found in iron deficiency anemia and in the Wiskott-Aldrich syndrome (Stuart, 1975).

Although platelets usually contain multiple granules, certain disorders are characterized by the presence of hypogranular platelets. These include the Hermansky-Pudlak syndrome, myeloproliferative disorders (Weinfeld, 1975), and familial thrombocytopathic thrombocytopenia (Vossen, 1968).

In films made from blood collected in ethylenediaminetetraacetate as an anticoagulant (EDTA-blood), platelets appear randomly distributed, but in films made directly from a finger puncture, platelets tend to adhere to each other in clumps. In Glanzmann's thrombasthenia, platelets fail to form aggregates.

Some platelets enlarge and stain less intensely in films made from EDTA-blood which has been allowed to stand at room temperature longer than one hour. In a few individuals, the platelet count in EDTA-blood may be falsely low (Dacie, 1975): certain plasma factors may cause platelets to clump (platelet agglutinins) or to adhere to neutrophils in a rosette or satellite fashion (platelet satellite phenomenon).

ULTRASTRUCTURE OF PLATELETS

Several detailed reviews correlating platelet physiology with ultrastructural alterations are available (White, 1971; Rodman, 1971).

The ultrastructural features of platelets (glutaraldehyde-osmium fixation, transmission electron microscopy) are described in three zones: (a) peripheral zone, (b) sol-gel zone, and (c) organelle zone (Figs. 32-1 and 32-2).

The peripheral zone consists of the exterior coat (EC), cell membrane (CM), submembrane filaments (SMF), and the open canalicular system (CS). The exterior coat (10 to 20 nm in thickness) covers the trilaminar cell membrane. It contains a variety of proteins (i.e., fibrinogen, factor V, factor VIII, factor XI, and immunoglobulin IgM) that adsorb to the platelet surface. Actomyosin, adenyl cyclase, and glycosyl transferase also exist on the platelet surface. It is postulated that the exterior coat plays an important role in adhesion and aggregation (Weiss, 1975).

The platelet membrane, rich in phospholipoprotein, is similar to the trilaminar cell membrane present in other cells. Within the inner surface of the membrane is a system of submembrane filaments measuring 5 nm in diameter. The submembrane filaments may interact with the microtubules (MT) in maintaining the normal shape of platelets. They can also play a role in pseudopod formation and in the movement observed in clot retraction.

The open canalicular system consists of invaginated portions of cell membrane derived from the demarcation membrane system of megakaryocytes. The open canalicular system acts as a conduit for the release of endogenous substances during the platelet activation (Holme, 1973). The open canalicular system also functions in phagocytosis (Hovig, 1968). In addition, phospholipid (platelet factor 3) from the cell membrane and the open canalicular system functions in the activation of certain circulating procoagulants.

The *sol-gel zone* consists of submembrane filaments, microtubules, and microfilaments. The platelet microtubules are an annular band of tubules each 25 nm in diameter. Each tubule is composed of 12 to 15 subfilaments approximately 3.5 nm in diameter. The microtubules together with the submembrane filaments form a protein structure which serves as a skeleton for the platelet. Following the incubation of aggregating agents with platelets, pseudopod formation occurs and the band of microtubules moves toward the center of the platelets encircling the organelles (Fig. 32-3). If platelet release fails to occur, the band of microtubules and the mass of organelles will assume their original position and the platelet will return to a discoid shape.

The microfilaments represent the third system of filamentous protein structures in the platelets. The microfilaments, submembrane filaments, and the subfilaments of the microtubules are structurally similar and resemble actin filaments observed in muscle. It is postulated that the microfilaments are the actin components of the actomyosin contractile mechanism (Caen, 1977).

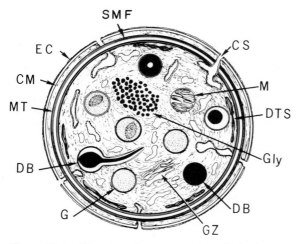

Figure 32–1. Diagrammatic representation of platelet sectioned along equatorial plane. *Peripheral zone:* exterior coat (EC); cell membrane (CM); canalicular system (CS); submembrane filaments (SMF). *Sol-gel zone:* microtubules (MT); canalicular system (CS); glycogen (Gly). *Organelle zone:* mitochondria (M); alpha granules (G); dense bodies (DB); Golgi zone (GZ); dense tubule system (DTS). (From White, J. C.: Platelet morphology. *In* Johnson, S. A. (ed.): The Circulating Platelet. New York, Academic Press, 1971, p. 45.)

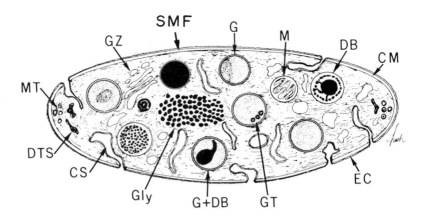

Figure 32–2. Diagrammatic representation of longitudinal section of platelet. Tubular structures (GT) resembling microtubules in granules. Other symbols as in Figure 32–1. (From White, J. C.: Platelet morphology. *In* Johnson, S. A. (ed.): The Circulating Platelet. New York, Academic Press, 1971, p. 45.)

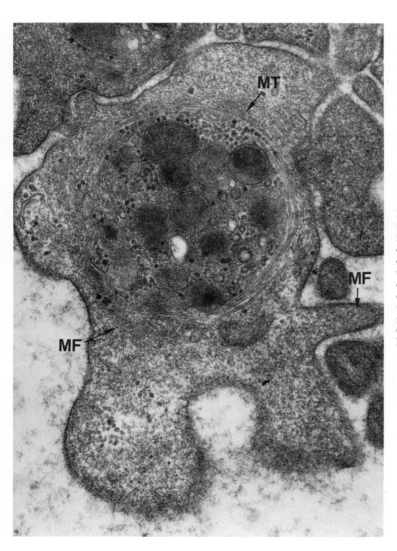

Figure 32–3. Platelet during ADP-induced aggregation. Internal changes include reduced circumference of microtubular band which brings the organelles closer together; organelles clumped together; swollen pseudopods with obvious microfilaments. These changes precede or coincide with the platelet release reaction (53,900×). (From White, J. C.: Platelet morphology. *In* Johnson, S. A. (ed.): The Circulating Platelet. New York, Academic Press, 1971, p. 45.)

The *organelle zone* contains granules, mitochondria, Golgi apparatus, and the dense tubular system. The alpha granules (G) measure 0.2 to 0.3 μm in diameter, are enclosed by a unit membrane, and are the most abundant platelet organelle. The alpha granules are lysosomes and contain acid hydrolases and cathepsins (Weiss, 1975).

A second type of granule appears as a dense body (DB). These granules contain ATP, ADP, serotonin, and calcium. The ADP stored in granules (*storage-pool ADP*) is released when platelets are incubated with ADP, epinephrine, serotonin, thrombin, or collagen. The *metabolic pool of ADP* which actively participates in platelet metabolism is not stored in granules.

Another type of platelet granule, not morphologically identifiable or separable from the others, contains platelet factor 4, β-thromboglobulin, and fibrinogen. The contents of this class of granules appear to be more easily released than those of the others.

Mitochondria (M) are relatively few in number. They function as a center for oxidative phosphorylation and can provide significant levels of ATP for cell metabolism. Electron-dense particles of glycogen (G) are the storage form of glucose needed for cell metabolism.

A Golgi zone (GZ), probably derived from the megakaryocyte, is present in approximately 10 per cent of platelets.

The dense tubular system (DTS) is closely associated with the annular band of microtubules but also wanders throughout the platelet substance. The dense tubular system contains filaments similar to those present as microfilaments, submembrane filaments, and subfilaments. It has been postulated that the dense tubular system may be involved in the manufacture of the filaments.

PLATELET FUNCTION

PLATELET ADHESION

Platelets adhere to collagen and microfibrils present in vascular basement membrane. Platelet adhesion to collagen is dependent on the degree of polymerization of collagen and presence of free epsilon-amino groups on collagen (Wilner, 1968). It has been suggested that an enzyme-substrate complex is formed between glucosyl transferase (located on platelet membranes) and galactosyl hydroxylysine groups on collagen (Jamieson, 1975),

though objection to this hypothesis has been made (Weiss, 1975). When platelets come in contact with collagen they lose their disc shape and pseudopods form. Release of platelet granules may occur following platelet adhesion.

Platelets also adhere to other foreign surfaces. Requirements for platelet adherence to glass beads include the presence of calcium ions, fibrinogen, plasma factors, and a moderate rate of blood flow (Bowie, 1969).

PLATELET AGGREGATION

Platelet aggregation indicates platelet-to-platelet adhesion. The formation of platelet clumps occurs normally *in vivo* following vascular injury. *In vitro*, platelet clumps can be demonstrated by placing platelet-rich plasma in a nephelometer at 37°C. while agitating continuously with a small magnetic stirrer (Born, 1962; O'Brien, 1962). Following the addition of an aggregating agent, platelets clump together, causing the turbidity of the platelet-rich plasma to decrease. The rate of platelet aggregation is dependent on the number of platelets, temperature, concentration of aggregating agents, calcium, and fibrinogen. Commonly employed aggregating agents include ADP, thrombin, epinephrine, serotonin, collagen, and ristocetin.

A curve plotting the change in per cent transmission against time is recorded on paper tape in a recorder linked to the nephelometer (Fig. 32-4). A reversible one-phase aggregation curve results from adding low concentrations of thrombin, ADP, or epinephrine to the platelet-rich plasma. At higher concentrations, a two-phase response occurs. The second-phase curve is due to release of endogenous ADP during the initial phase of aggregation.

Concentrations of ADP less than 0.5 μM usually elicit a reversible one-phase aggregation response. Higher concentrations of ADP result in a release of endogeneous ADP, which induces a second wave of aggregation (Hardisty, 1970). At higher concentrations of ADP, the aggregation response is irreversible (Fig. 32-4). The critical concentration for a two-phase platelet response is in the range of 0.1 to 1.0 μM for epinephrine. Thrombin causes a two-phase response at approximately 0.15 unit/ml. Serotonin infrequently causes a two-phase response, and collagen induces a one-phase response after a delay. Ristocetin can also elicit a two-phase response.

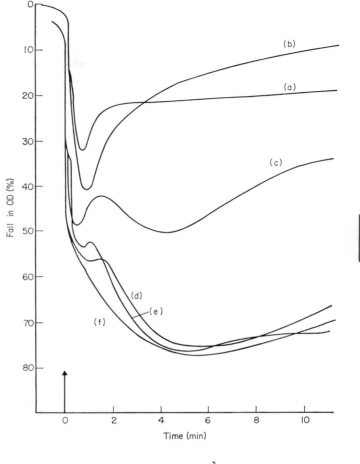

Figure 32–4. Changes in absorbance or optical density (O.D.) with time in platelet-rich plasma after the addition of ADP at zero time. Final concentrations are (a) 0.3 μM; (b) 0.4 μM; (c) 0.5 μM; (d) 0.6 μM; (e) 0.7 μM; (f) 0.8 μM. (From Hardisty, R. M., Hutton, R. A., Montgomery, D., Rickard, S., and Trebilcock, H.: Secondary platelet aggregation: A quantitative study. Br. J. Haematol., *19*:307, 1970.)

RELEASE REACTION

In the release reaction, platelets empty their granule contents into the external milieu. Release can be induced by ADP, serotonin, thrombin, collagen, and other materials. *Release I* refers to the emptying of dense bodies, a process which occurs in approximately 10 seconds (Day, 1971). In contrast, *release II* refers to alpha granules discharging their contents, which occurs in 40 to 60 seconds (Holmson, 1972). Epinephrine, ADP, and low concentrations of collagen induce a release I response. However, thrombin and high concentrations of collagen bring about both release I and II. Since aspirin inhibits release I, it is proposed that release I and II are mediated by different mechanisms.

The role of calcium in the release reaction is unclear. It has been suggested that calcium acts as the intracellular transmitter of the release reactions. Interaction of actin and myosin in the presence of ATP and calcium could provide the wave of contraction necessary for release (Holmson, 1976).

Prostaglandins play a major role in the induction of release I (Fig. 32–5). When platelets are incubated with a variety of aggregating agents, arachidonic acid is released from the platelet phospholipid pool, probably by the action of phospholipase A. Arachidonic acid is converted to cyclic endoperoxides (prostaglandins G_2 and H_2) by the action of cyclooxygenase (Hamberg, 1974). This reaction can be inhibited by aspirin. The endoperoxides are transformed by thromboxane synthetase (an enzyme present in platelets) to an unstable substance, thromboxane A_2, which is a potent platelet aggregating agent (Marx, 1977). Endoperoxides and their derivative, thromboxane A_2, induce release I and subsequently a second phase of aggregation. The mechanism by which the endoperoxides and thromboxane A_2 mediate the release I response is unknown. Thromboxane A_2 can also stimulate smooth muscle of rabbit aorta to contract.

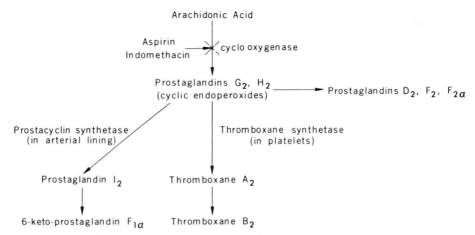

Figure 32–5. Sequence of reactions in the conversion of arachidonic acid to prostaglandins and thromboxanes. An enzyme in blood vessel walls forms prostaglandin I_2, which inhibits both platelet aggregation and vasoconstriction. An enzyme in platelets forms thromboxane A_2, which promotes platelet aggregation and vasoconstriction. 6-keto-prostaglandin $F_{1\alpha}$ and thromboxane B_2 are degradation products without significant activity. (From Marx, J. L.: Blood clotting. The role of the prostaglandins. Science, *196*:1072, 1977. Copyright 1977 by the American Association for the Advancement of Science.)

In the microsomes of blood vessels, endoperoxides are converted to prostaglandin I_2 by the action of prostacyclin synthetase (Marx, 1977). Prostaglandin I_2 prevents or reverses platelet aggregation and relaxes several kinds of blood vessels. The production of prostaglandins with opposite effects thus can serve as a controlling mechanism in normal coagulation. Presumably, platelets fail to adhere to normal blood vessels because the endoperoxides released by platelets are converted to prostaglandin I_2 by the blood vessel. However, in damaged blood vessels, prostaglandin I_2 may not be synthesized owing to the lack of prostacyclin synthetase. Thromboxane A_2 generated in platelets causes them to aggregate and vessel walls to constrict (Fig. 32–5).

ACTION OF PLATELETS ON FIBRIN FORMATION

Platelet membranes provide a phospholipid, platelet factor 3, which catalyzes the activity of certain calcium-dependent procoagulant interactions. Platelet factor 3 (PF3) accelerates the interaction of coagulation factors IXa, VIII, and calcium in the activation of factor X; PF3 also aids in the interaction of Xa, V, and calcium in the activation of prothrombin (Marcus, 1969).

Platelet factor 4 (PF4) has an anti-heparin-like activity and is liberated during release (Niewiarowski, 1968). PF4, therefore, prevents inhibition of coagulation in and around a platelet clot.

Platelets also contain plasminogen and antiplasmin (Caen, 1977). The role these platelet factors play in clinical fibrinolysis, however, is unclear.

CLOT RETRACTION

Clot retraction is due to the action of actomyosin (thrombosthenin), the platelet contractile protein. Antithrombosthenins appear to inhibit clot retraction. Platelet actomyosin represents approximately 15 to 20 per cent of platelet protein and is present at the platelet surface and within granules (Booyse and Rafelson, 1971; Nachman, 1967). It functions not only in clot retraction but also in pseudopod formation and platelet aggregation and release.

FORMATION OF HEMOSTATIC PLUG

In summary, platelets act by adhering to collagen or subendothelial connective tissue following vascular injury. Contact with collagen results in the release of ADP and other constituents from platelet granules. The endogenous ADP released from adherent platelets causes platelet aggregation and formation of a platelet plug within and outside the lumen of the vessel. Actomyosin causes the platelet plug to contract, decreasing its permeability.

Platelet factor 3, released during platelet aggregation, accelerates the activity of the

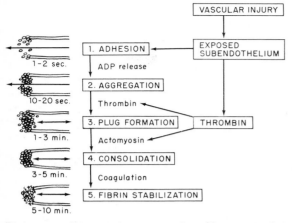

Figure 32-6. Diagramatic representation of hemostatic plug formation. (From Harker, L. A.: Hemostasis Manual. Philadelphia, F. A. Davis Co., 1974.)

intrinsic coagulation mechanism. Tissue thromboplastins and circulating procoagulants also interact to produce thrombin, which converts fibrinogen to fibrin. Thrombin also acts to aggregate more platelets and induce release of ADP and other biogenic amines, including serotonin and epinephrine. The latter agents may affect vascular tone to further maintain hemostasis (Fig. 32-6).

PLATELET METABOLISM

Adenine nucleotides (ATP and ADP) are present in two pools inside the platelet. The

metabolic pool is located in the cytosol, mitochondria, and membrane; it participates in normal metabolism of the cell. The storage pool, located in dense granules, is expelled in the release reaction and participates in promoting further platelet aggregation.

Platelets lack the ability to synthesize *de novo* adenine nucleotides. However, adenine and adenosine can be taken up by platelets and converted to adenine nucleotides by the action of adenine phosphoribosyl transferase and adenosine kinase (Weiss, 1975).

Most ATP production is the result of glycolysis (Embden-Myerhof pathway) and oxidative phosphorylation (Krebs cycle). The Embden-Myerhof glycolytic pathway provides 46 per cent of the total ATP, the Krebs cycle generates 41 per cent, and the hexose monophosphate shunt contributes 13 per cent (Hirsh, 1972).

Following activation of platelets by aggregating agents, there is an increase in glycolysis, glycogenolysis, and oxidative phosphorylation. This serves to restore the diminished ATP levels. ATP is necessary for clot retraction, platelet aggregation, release reaction, phagocytosis, and membrane transport. The ATP metabolized in the release reaction is not rephosphorylated but is degraded to inosine monophosphate and hypoxanthine (Fig. 32-7).

Platelets contain appropriate enzymes to synthesize glycogen from citrate. In addition, enzymes are present in platelets to store glycogen with α 1-4 and α 1-6 glycosyl linkages.

The level of cyclic AMP (cAMP) in resting

Figure 32-7. Diagram of platelet energy metabolism. About equal amounts of energy are derived from glycolysis and the tricarboxylic acid (TCA) cycle; as the initial fuel, however, fatty acids contribute less than glucose. Energy utilized for maintenance of structure and function is taken from the metabolic nucleotide pool, which is an energy reserve that is continually being used and renewed. The storage nucleotide pool in dense granules is expelled from the platelet during the release reaction. Abbreviations: ADP—adenosine diphosphate; ATP—adenosine triphosphate; AMP—adenosine monophosphate; IMP—inosine monophosphate. (Modified by Wintrobe (1974) from Hirsh, J., and Doery, J. C. G.: Platelet function in health and disease. Prog. Hematol., 7:185, 1971.)

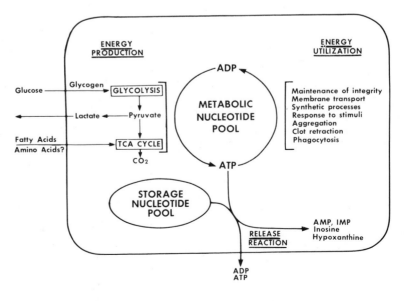

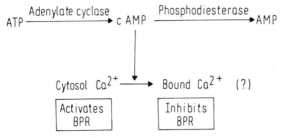

Figure 32–8. Postulated action of cyclic AMP system in regulating platelet function. Decreased cAMP promotes liberation of Ca++ from membrane, making it available for activity of contractile proteins and onset of platelet function. Abbreviation: BPR—Basic platelet reaction. (From Holmsen, H.: Classification and possible mechanism of action of some drugs that inhibit platelet aggregation. Ser. Haematol., 8:50, 1976. Copyright 1976, Munksgaard International Publishers, Ltd. Copenhagen, Denmark.)

platelets is $140 \, pm/10^9$ platelets. This level is maintained by the action of adenyl cyclase which catalyzes the synthesis of cAMP from ATP, and phosphodiesterase, which converts cAMP to AMP (Fig. 32-8). It has been postulated that cAMP activates a calcium pump that transports calcium ions from the cytosol into the platelet membrane and thus relaxes the platelet contractile protein (Holmsen, 1976). Therefore, substances which activate adenyl cyclase or inhibit phosphodiesterase will increase the level of cAMP and inhibit the activity of the platelet to aggregate and release. Adenosine, 2-chloroadenosine, isoprenaline, and prostaglandin E_1 and D_2 tend to enhance the activity of adenyl cyclase. Drugs which enhance the levels of cAMP by inhibiting phosphodiesterase in platelets include papaverine, dipyridamole, theophylline, caffeine, and aminophilline (Holmsen, 1976).

Platelets adsorb numerous plasma proteins on their surfaces. Most plasma coagulation factors have been found on the platelets. Immunoglobulins and fibrinogen are also present on platelets. In addition, young platelets are able to synthesize amino acids and proteins (Booyse, 1971). Platelet proteins include fibrinogen, actin, myosin, membrane proteins, and a variety of enzymes.

Platelets synthesize numerous lipids, and they can also take up lipids from the plasma (Lewis, 1969). Most of the platelet lipids are present within membranes and can be released or made "available" during platelet activation. These lipid moieties aid in the activation of certain procoagulants.

QUANTITATIVE PLATELET DISORDERS

THROMBOCYTOPENIAS

HYPOPROLIFERATIVE THROMBOCYTOPENIAS

In the hypoproliferative thrombocytopenias, platelet survival is normal and platelet production is decreased. There is a diminished number of megakaryocytes. However, the size of the megakaryocytes is slightly enlarged because of the increased thrombopoietic stress (Harker, 1969).

Decreased production of platelets is usually associated with marrow aplasia or hypoplasia (Table 32-1). The bone marrow may become hypoplastic following injury by drugs, chemicals, irradiation, or infections. Some hypoplastic marrows are related to genetic factors (Fanconi syndrome), but others have no known etiologic cause (idiopathic). Infiltration of bone marrow by neoplastic cells (such as in leukemia and carcinoma) may result in thrombocytopenia owing to deficient thrombocytopoiesis; the latter may also occur during a severe inflammatory reaction.

Congenital megakaryocytic hypoplasia is a rare disorder occurring in infants (Hall, 1969). Ecchymoses occur at birth and intracranial hemorrhage occurs frequently. Patients show thrombocytopenia, decreased numbers of megakaryocytes, and skeletal abnormalities.

Table 32–1. CAUSES OF THROMBOCYTOPENIA

Hypoproliferative thrombocytopenia
    Aplastic or hypoplastic marrow
    Infiltrative disease of marrow: carcinoma, leukemia, disseminated infection
    Specific megakaryocytic hypoplasia

Ineffective thrombopoiesis
    Folate deficiency
    Vitamin B_{12} deficiency

Platelet sequestration
    Pooling of platelets in enlarged spleen

Increased platelet destruction
    Immune thrombocytopenia
        Autoimmune
        Isoimmune
        Drug associated
    Disseminated intravascular coagulation
    Mechanical injury of platelets

Combination of several mechanisms

Chlorothiazides, estrogenic hormones, and corticosteroids have been reported to cause thrombocytopenia on rare occasions, owing to a specific suppression of platelet production (Wintrobe, 1974).

INEFFECTIVE THROMBOCYTOPOIESIS

Ineffective thrombopoiesis is associated with an increase in the megakaryocytic mass and a decrease in platelet production (Harker, 1974). The defect may be due to abnormal platelet production, abnormal release, or intramedullary destruction of platelets. Moderate shortening of platelet survival may contribute to the peripheral thrombocytopenia. Ineffective thrombopoiesis is a feature of megaloblastic anemias, owing to either vitamin B_{12} or folic acid deficiency. Ineffective thrombopoiesis has also been described in DiGuglielmo's syndrome, paroxysmal nocturnal hemoglobinemia, hereditary thrombocytopenias, and some forms of preleukemia.

PLATELET SEQUESTRATION

The spleen normally contains one third of the total platelet mass. In splenomegaly, up to 90 per cent of platelets can reside in the spleen. Platelet sequestration occurs, at times, in lymphomas, Felty's syndrome, Gaucher's disease, sarcoidosis, and splenomegaly associated with hepatic cirrhosis. Increased platelet sequestration can occur in any enlarged spleen regardless of etiology.

Since peripheral thrombocytopenia provides a thrombopoietic stress on the marrow, some increased platelet production results. Therefore, the level of peripheral thrombocytopenia results from the splenic platelet sequestration and the compensatory increase in platelet production by the marrow.

INCREASED PLATELET DESTRUCTION

Increased platelet destruction is usually due to (1) the removal of platelets by the reticuloendothelial system as a result of an immunologic reaction, (2) the removal of the platelets from the circulation in a consumptive process involving the coagulation system, or (3) destruction of platelets via contact with abnormal arterial surfaces. Thrombocytopenia caused by increased platelet destruction is usually associated with an increase in bone marrow megakaryocytic mass and an increase in platelet production.

Immune-mediated thrombocytopenia may be observed in a variety of clinical disorders. In idiopathic thrombocytopenic purpura, it is postulated that antigen-antibody complexes bind to platelets. Platelets are removed by macrophages in the liver or spleen. A similar mechanism may cause the thrombocytopenia observed in systemic lupus erythematosus, lymphoreticular disorders, and infectious mononucleosis. The antigenic specificity of the responsible antibody or antibodies is not known.

Isoimmune antibodies may arise in a mother immunized by fetal platelets and may cause neonatal thrombocytopenia. Immunization to four isoantigens has been described. They include PL^{A1} (ZW^a), PL^{E2}, $PlGrLy^{B1}$, and $PlGrLy^{C1}$ (Shulman, 1964). Compatible platelet transfusion can be performed using the mother as a donor (pp. 1475 and 1499).

Occasionally, drug-induced antibodies may result in thrombocytopenia. Numerous drugs, including quinidine, quinine, and sulfonamides, have been implicated in the formation of platelet antibodies. It has been hypothesized that the drug (hapten) binds with a plasma protein and together they stimulate an antibody response. A drug-antibody complex adsorbs to the platelet membrane; the platelets are then removed by macrophages of the reticuloendothelial system (Wintrobe, 1974).

Consumption of platelets is frequently observed in disseminated intravascular coagulation. This disorder frequently complicates septic and malignant diseases and is characterized by activation of the coagulation and fibrinolytic systems (Harker and Slichter, 1972b). In severe cases, there is consumption of factors V, VIII, XIII, prothrombin, fibrinogen, and platelets. In mild to moderate cases, the levels of these factors are sometimes not reduced from normal because of the compensatory increased production of circulating procoagulants and platelets.

Peripheral destruction of platelets can be due to platelet injury sustained by their passage over an abnormal arterial surface (Harker and Slichter, 1972b). Peripheral destruction of platelets owing to mechanical injury has been described in patients with prosthetic heart valves, prosthetic arteriovenous cannulas, prosthetic grafts, hemolytic uremic syndrome, thrombotic thrombocytopenic purpura, vasculitis, and arterial thrombosis.

In general, clinically significant bleeding rarely occurs in patients with a platelet count of greater than $40 \times 10^9/l$ unless there is a coexistent platelet functional disorder. Patients with immune thrombocytopenia may not experience hemorrhages at platelet counts as low as $10 \times 10^9/l$ because more of the circulating platelets are younger and more active hemostatically.

THROMBOCYTOSIS

Thrombocytosis occurs when the platelet count is greater than $440 \times 10^9/l$. Thrombocytosis can be reactive (secondary to some other process) or autonomous (primary or idiopathic thrombocythemia, Table 32-2).

In reactive thrombocytosis, the platelet count ranges from 400 to $1500 \times 10^9/l$. Total megakaryocytic mass and platelet production are increased and platelet survival is normal. Megakaryocytes and platelets are morphologically normal. Reactive thrombocytosis occurs in infectious and inflammatory disorders, malignancies, iron deficient states, following surgical procedures, and after splenectomy. In reactive thrombocytosis, the platelet count returns to normal when the primary disorder resolves.

In autonomous thrombocytosis, platelet production is unresponsive to normal regulatory processes. The platelet count is frequently greater than $1500 \times 10^9/l$. The total megakaryocyte mass and platelet production are increased. Platelet survival is normal to slightly decreased. In primary thrombocythemia, the platelets may appear abnormal

Table 32-2. CAUSES OF THROMBOCYTOSIS

Reactive thrombocytosis
  Infectious disorders
  Malignancies
  Iron deficiency anemia
  Following surgical procedures
  Post-splenectomy
  Inflammatory disorders (collagen vascular disease)
  Following hemorrhage
Autonomous thrombocytosis
  Idiopathic thrombocythemia (primary thrombocytosis)
  Myelofibrosis with myeloid metaplasia
  Polycythemia vera
  Chronic myelogenous leukemia

with marked anisocytosis (Lewis, 1972). There may be giant and bizarre shaped platelets. They may also show little granulation or be heavily granulated. Megakaryocyte fragments or dwarf megakaryocytes may be present in the peripheral blood. The bone marrow has increased numbers of large hyperlobulated megakaryocytes that tend to clump together. Masses of clumped platelets are numerous in marrow films. The erythroid to granulocytic ratio is normal. Silver staining of the marrow biopsy sometimes demonstrates increased reticulum, although not to the extent noted in myelosclerosis. Autonomous thrombocytosis is also found, at times, in other myeloproliferative disorders: polycythemia vera, myelofibrosis, and chronic myelogenous leukemia.

Patients with autonomous thrombocytosis may experience hemorrhagic or thrombotic episodes. Bleeding may include ecchymoses, epistaxis, and gastrointestinal hemorrhage. Qualitative platelet function defects are often present, especially reduced epinephrine-induced platelet aggregation. In contrast, somewhat less frequently, patients can develop thrombotic complications, e.g., deep vein thromboses and pulmonary embolism. The relationship of the platelet functional abnormalities to the thrombotic or hemorrhagic complications is not clear. Abnormal platelet function is uncommon in reactive thrombocytosis (Zucker, 1972).

FUNCTIONAL PLATELET DISORDERS

The incidence of platelet functional disorders is unknown. The diagnosis should be considered when a patient gives a significant bleeding history and has a prolonged bleeding time and a normal platelet count. Qualitative platelet disorders may be inherited or acquired.

INHERITED QUALITATIVE PLATELET DISORDERS

THROMBASTHENIA (GLANZMANN'S THROMBASTHENIA)

Thrombasthenia is a rare autosomal recessive disorder characterized by epistaxis, menorrhagia, gingival bleeding, and numerous ecchymoses (Caen, 1972). The platelet count and platelet morphology are normal

Table 32–3. LABORATORY FINDINGS IN DISORDERS OF PLATELET FUNCTION

TEST	THROMBASTHENIA	"STORAGE POOL DISEASE"	ABNORMAL RELEASE MECHANISM	BERNARD-SOULIER SYNDROME
Platelet count	U normal	U normal	U normal	Mild to moderate thrombocytopenia
Platelet morphology	Normal[1]	Normal; "microcytic" in some cases	U normal	Characteristic "giant" platelets
Bleeding time	M prolonged	V abnormality	U prolonged	U prolonged
Clot retraction	Deficient	Normal	Normal	Normal
PF-3 activity*	Abnormal[2]	V abnormality[3]	V abnormality	V abnormality
Platelet retention in glass bead columns	Reduced[2]	Reduced[3]	Reduced	—
Platelet aggregation by 5 µM ADP	Deficient	Normal	Normal	Normal[5]
Platelet aggregation by "threshold" concentrations of ADP (0.2-1.5 µM)	Deficient	V deficiency with subsequent disaggregation	V deficiency with subsequent disaggregation	Normal[5]
Platelet aggregation by dilute collagen suspensions and 5 µM epinephrine	Deficient	Deficient[4]	Deficient	Normal[5]
Storage nucleotide pool	Normal	Diminished	Normal	Normal[6]
Ancillary laboratory features	[1]Platelets appear discrete and rounded in stained smears. [2]Not corrected by ADP. Platelet fibrinogen commonly decreased.	[3]Corrected by ADP. [4]Second wave of epinephrine-induced aggregation absent or markedly reduced. Platelet dense bodies reduced in number.	In vitro effects of aspirin are additive.	Initial shape change lacking. [5]Aggregation may be abnormally rapid. [6]Corrected for increased platelet volume. Ristocetin-induced platelet aggregation deficient.

*Results vary depending on exact technique employed. Key: U—usually; M—markedly; V—variable. (From Wintrobe, M. M., Lee, G. R., Boggs, D. R., Bithell, T. C., Athens, J. W., and Foerster, J.: Clinical Hematology. Philadelphia, Lea & Febiger, 1974.)

(Table 32–3). The bleeding time is markedly prolonged, clot retraction is deficient, platelet adhesion to glass beads is reduced, and platelet aggregation by ADP, epinephrine, thrombin, or collagen is decreased, but aggregation by ristocetin is less impaired or even normal. The cause of the defect is unknown. Platelets from patients with Glanzmann's disease can release ADP, platelet factor 4, and prostaglandins when incubated with collagen and thrombin. However, thrombasthenic platelets have reduced actomyosin, glycoproteins, fibrinogen, and certain enzymes involved in glycolysis and the hexose monophosphate shunt pathway (Caen, 1977). The decrease in platelet fibrinogen and actomyosin may impair the platelet's ability to retract and aggregate. Malmsten (1977) has reported the loss of a glycoprotein (135,000 MW) which is postulated to serve as a receptor for ADP-induced liberation of arachidonic acid.

BERNARD-SOULIER SYNDROME

This rare disorder is inherited in an autosomal recessive manner. Patients have a moderate to marked degree of mucocutaneous hemorrhages. This purpuric bleeding may include epistaxis, menorrhagia, and gastrointestinal hemorrhage. There is usually a moderate thrombocytopenia associated with enlarged bizarre platelets which exceed 4 µm in diameter. The bleeding time is prolonged and clot retraction is normal. Platelets aggregate normally with ADP, epinephrine, thrombin, and collagen, but fail to aggregate with ristocetin. In addition, ristocetin-induced aggregation is not induced in the patient's platelets by adding normal plasma or purified factor VIII. Patients with Bernard-Soulier syndrome have normal concentrations of factor VIII and ristocetin co-factor.

The nature of this platelet dysfunction is

not entirely clear. However, Gröttum (1969) reported reduced sialic acid in platelet membrane and decreased electrophoretic mobility of the giant platelets. Nurden (1974) has demonstrated a reduction in a glycoprotein of 155,000 MW from platelet membranes. In addition, it has been reported that glycoproteins may play a functional role in ristocetin-induced aggregation (Jenkins, 1976).

**DEFICIENT RELEASE
REACTION**

Defects in release reaction may be due to a reduction in storage pool ADP or an inability to release ADP. Platelets with either type of defect do not aggregate normally to subendothelium. The inability of platelets to aggregate at sites of vascular injury may explain the bleeding diathesis observed in these patients.

The incidence of *storage pool disease* is unknown. In several kindreds, the defect appeared to be inherited as an autosomal dominant trait. In general, patients complain of mild to moderate mucocutaneous hemorrhages and occasionally of easy bruising. Patients usually have a prolonged bleeding time, normal platelet counts, diminished glass bead retention, and normal clot retraction (Holmsen and Weiss, 1972). There is a loss of second-phase aggregation when platelets are incubated with ADP or epinephrine, and an impairment in collagen-induced aggregation. The number of dense bodies is also diminished.

The decrease in storage pool ADP was documented by showing decreased platelet ATP and ADP, especially the latter; increased ATP/ADP ratio; and increased specific activity of ATP and ADP after incubation of platelets with ^{3}H-adenosine. Patients with storage pool disease show diminished release of platelet ATP and a greater reduction in ADP release (Holmsen and Weiss, 1972). Deficiency in storage pool ADP has been described in patients with Hermansky-Pudlak syndrome, Wiskott-Aldrich syndrome, and thrombocytopenia-absent radii syndrome.

Platelet dysfunction owing to *release defects* is a heterogeneous group of disorders. Patients may have a mild bleeding diathesis. The bleeding time is usually prolonged, platelet count is normal, clot retraction is normal, and the glass bead retention is reduced (Weiss, 1972). Collagen-induced aggregation is abnor-

mal, and secondary wave of aggregation by ADP or epinephrine is abnormal despite the presence of normal storage pool ADP documented by radioisotopic studies. In some patients, platelet factor 3 is diminished; in other individuals, platelet factor 4 is reduced. In addition, a release defect has been demonstrated in patients with glycogen storage disease (type I) (Czapek, 1973).

VON WILLEBRAND'S DISEASE

Von Willebrand's disease is inherited as an incompletely dominant autosomal trait. Bleeding problems most often begin in early childhood. The bleeding manifestations, though usually mild, may be severe. Mucocutaneous hemorrhages, epistaxis, and easy bruising are common. Some patients may be asymptomatic unless they have a major challenge to their hemostatic system; others may have serious bleeding problems with significant gastrointestinal hemorrhages. The severity of bleeding problems in von Willebrand's disease often lessens as the patient becomes older. The clinical bleeding tendency, as well as the characteristic laboratory abnormalities, may fluctuate widely in a given individual at different times. Repeated testing is often necessary for detection of the abnormalities and confirmation of the diagnosis.

The classic disease is characterized by prolonged bleeding time, reduction in platelet glass bead retention, decreased level of factor VIII procoagulant activity, diminished factor VIII antigen and abnormal ristocetin-induced aggregation (Hoyer, 1976). Following the infusion of factor VIII concentrates into a patient with the disease, coagulant activity of factor VIII remains for 24 to 48 hours, but antigenic factor VIII disappears more rapidly (Fig. 32-9). In addition to the classic form, several variants of von Willebrand's disease have been described. The plasma levels of procoagulant factor VIII, immunologic factor VIII, and the ristocetin co-factor are not always similar (Gralnick, 1977a). Although the exact relationship among the procoagulant factor VIII, antigenic factor VIII, and the von Willebrand co-factor is not yet understood, the data available support certain hypotheses. The current working hypothesis suggests that factor VIII antigen and von Willebrand co-factor are synthesized by endothelial cells under the direction of genes located on an autosome. The synthesis of procoagulant factor VIII is gov-

Figure 32–9. Transfusion response in von Willebrand's disease. Sequential measurements of factor VIII procoagulant (VIII AHF) and factor VIII antigen (VIII AGN) for two patients. *A* represents the results of a patient with moderately severe disease in whom there was a rapid fall of VIII AGN and a delayed rise in VIII AHF after infusion of 10 bags of cryoprecipitate prepared from normal donors. *B* represents a patient with moderately severe disease in whom there was a prolonged increase in both VIII AGN and VIII AHF levels after infusion of 12 bags of normal cryoprecipitate. (From Hoyer, L. W.: von Willebrand's disease. Prog. Hemostas. Thromb., *3*:231–287, 1976.)

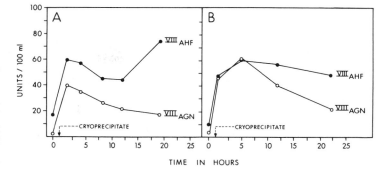

erned by a gene on the X chromosome; the site of its synthesis is unknown. The procoagulant factor VIII (low molecular weight) and the antigenic factor VIII and von Willebrand's co-factor (high molecular weight) circulate together as a complex, a single high molecular weight glycoprotein (see Fig. 33–8, p. 1144).

ACQUIRED QUALITATIVE DISORDERS OF PLATELETS

Acquired disorders of platelet function have been described in myeloproliferative disorders, including myelofibrosis with myeloid metaplasia, thrombocythemia, polycythemia vera, various leukemias, and preleukemic syndromes (Cowan, 1975). Guanidinosuccinic acid and phenolic acid are increased in the serum of patients with uremia and inhibit platelet function (Rabiner, 1972). Paraproteins in patients with plasma cell dyscrasias may coat platelet membranes to inhibit platelet adhesion and produce a prolonged bleeding time (Lackner, 1973). Patients with elevated fibrinogen-fibrin degradation products, liver disease, congenital heart disease, and scurvy may exhibit features of platelet dysfunction (Caen, 1977).

Inhibition of platelet function has been associated with ingestion of numerous drugs. Aspirin inhibits the synthesis of cyclic endoperoxides which can directly induce release I. Thus, aspirin ingestion is usually associated with a prolongation of bleeding time, inhibition of second phase of aggregation with ADP and epinephrine, and reduced collagen aggregation. The aspirin-induced injury lasts the life of the platelet.

Indomethacin and phenylbutazone also inhibit platelet release and aggregation. Other drugs that inhibit platelet function include antihistamines, sulfinpurazone, phenothia-

zines, and antibiotics. Several reviews have been published describing the inhibition of platelet function (Holmsen, 1976; Packham, 1977).

LABORATORY EVALUATION OF PLATELET DISORDERS

ESTIMATION OF PLATELET COUNT, BLOOD FILM

Platelets appear as purple granulated ovoid bodies of 2 to 4 μm in diameter when films are observed with Wright-Giemsa stain. Platelets are individually separated in EDTA-blood. In contrast, films made from a finger stick blood specimen frequently show platelets in clumps.

A rough estimate of the platelet count can be gauged from the examination of the peripheral blood film. On the average, one platelet is observed per 20 erythrocytes in the normal individual. The ratio of platelets among red cells in normal individuals can vary from 1 in 9 to 1 in 34. Thus, it is possible to judge only if platelets are absent, moderately reduced, normal, or significantly increased. Minor decreases or increases in platelet levels can be determined only by platelet counts, which are discussed in Chapter 27 (p. 882).

CLOT RETRACTION

Principle

Clot retraction is a commonly used but relatively insensitive test of platelet function. After blood coagulates, the platelet and fibrinogen network starts to contract, expressing serum and forming a firm, semigelatinous clot. This retraction is probably due to the action of platelet actomyosin in the presence of divalent cations.

Qualitative method (Owen, 1975)

One ml of blood is placed into each of three glass test tubes and the samples are maintained at 37°C. After two hours, the sample is judged normal if retraction is present in any tube.

Semiquantitative method (Owen, 1969)

Five ml of blood is allowed to clot for 1 hour in a 10 ml glass centrifuge tube at 37°C. The serum is removed from the blood and measured. The plasma volume is calculated by multiplying the plasmacrit by the volume of whole blood (5 ml). Clot retraction is the ratio of serum removed/plasma volume expressed as a percentage. The normal range is 40 to 94 per cent.

Interpretation

In the qualitative method, clot retraction is increased in anemia and decreased in polycythemia.

This variable is eliminated in the semiquantitative method. Clot retraction is usually decreased in thrombocytopenia but correlates poorly with platelet count. On rare occasions, it has been reported normal with platelet counts as low as $20 \times 10^9/l$. Clot retraction is significantly decreased in Glanzmann's thrombasthenia, afibrinogenemia, and some cases of hyperfibrinogenemia.

BLEEDING TIME

Principle

The bleeding time test is the duration of bleeding from a standardized skin wound. The test measures the *in vivo* function of the platelets' capacity to respond to injury. No attempt will be made to review all the numerous published methods and modifications of the bleeding time. The reader is referred to the excellent review by Bowie (1974).

Duke method (1910)

A small cut is made in the ear lobe with a disposable lancet. The drops of blood are blotted with filter paper at half-minute intervals until bleeding stops, normally within one to three minutes.

Ivy method (1935)

A blood pressure cuff is placed over the upper arm and inflated to 40 mm Hg to increase capillary and arteriolar pressure. The technique determines bleeding at the site of small punctures in the skin of the forearm. Normal time is from one to six minutes.

Standardized template bleeding time (Mielke, 1969)

A blood pressure cuff is placed around the upper arm and inflated to 40 mm Hg. Two accurate incisions 9 mm long and 1 mm deep are made on the forearm using a polystyrene template with a No. 11 Bard-Parker blade. The blood is blotted every 30 seconds with filter paper, taking care not to touch the wound itself. The average of the two determinations is recorded as the bleeding time. Normal bleeding time is 4.5 ± 1.5 minutes (1SD). A small linear scar may result. However, this can be minimized by applying a sterile tape across the wound to maintain the edges of the incision in apposition for 24 to 48 hours.

Interpretation

The Duke and Ivy methods are less sensitive than the standardized template bleeding time. Harker and Slichter (1972) found that patients with thrombocytopenia owing to impaired platelet production exhibited an inverse linear relationship between length of bleeding time and platelet count when the latter is between $10 \times 10^9/l$ and $100 \times 10^9/l$ (Fig. 32-10). They also noted prolonged bleeding times and normal platelet counts in patients with uremia or von Willebrand's disease and in individuals

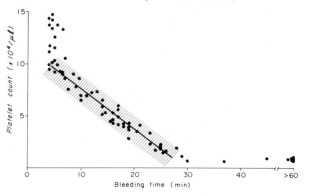

Figure 32-10. The platelet count (in the normal range and in thrombocytopenia due to impaired production) and the bleeding time are inversely related when the platelet count is below $100 \times 10^9/l$ ($10 \times 10^4/\mu l$) down to a level of about $10 \times 10^9/l$. The solid line is the regression line; the shaded area represents the 95 per cent confidence limits. (From Harker, L. A., and Slichter, S. J.: The bleeding time as a screening test for evaluation of platelet function. N. Engl. J. Med., *287*:155, 1972. Reprinted by permission.)

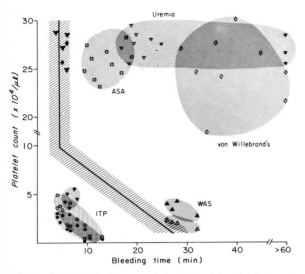

Figure 32–11. The inverse relationship of the platelet count and the bleeding time, as in Figure 32–10, is depicted by the solid line and shaded area. When the platelet population is young, as in immune thrombocytopenic purpura (ITP) or recovery from chemotherapy, the bleeding time is shorter than would have been predicted from the platelet count. When platelet function is impaired, as in von Willebrand's disease, uremia, acetylsalicylic acid (ASA) ingestion, or the Wiscott-Aldrich syndrome (WAS), the bleeding time is longer than predicted from the platelet count. (From Harker, L. A., and Slichter, S. J.: The bleeding time as a screening test for evaluation of platelet function. N. Engl. J. Med., *287*:155, 1972. Reprinted by permission.)

who had ingested aspirin (Fig. 32–11). In general, a prolonged bleeding time associated with a normal platelet count suggests platelet dysfunction. Bleeding times shorter than predicted, according to Harker and Slichter, indicate increased hemostatic function which is associated with young platelets. This phenomenon may be observed in immune thrombocytopenia (Fig. 32–11). In disorders attributed to vascular abnormalities, prolongation of the bleeding time is unusual.

GLASS BEAD RETENTION (ADHESION) ASSAY

Principle

The adhesion of platelets to the walls of an injured blood vessel is one of the events which occurs in hemostasis and thrombosis. The property of platelets to adhere to foreign surfaces varies in some disease states. In von Willebrand's disease, platelet adhesiveness or glass bead retention is usually diminished

(Strauss, 1965). In contrast, some investigators have reported enhanced platelet retention in thrombotic disorders (Owen, 1975).

Platelet retention has been measured by a variety of methods. Wright (1941) was the first to demonstrate that platelets adhere to glass when anticoagulated blood samples are rotated in a glass flask. Hellem (1960) was first to standardize a method of pumping citrated whole blood or platelet-rich plasma through a column of glass beads by means of an infusion pump. He expressed platelet adhesiveness as the per cent of platelets detained by the beads. Because blood flows slowly through the beads, the Hellem method does not clearly distinguish von Willebrand's disease from normal individuals. In addition, its complexity reduces its usefulness as a routine laboratory procedure.

Methods

In the Salzman (1963) method, a control sample of venous blood is collected from the arm into a vacuum tube containing EDTA. A second sample from the other arm is collected with a siliconized 20 gauge needle and is received through a glass bead filter column (1.0 g sodium-lime-silica glass beads) into a second vacuum tube containing EDTA. Platelet counts are performed on the two samples, and the difference is expressed as percentage of platelets retained by the glass beads (the difference between the counts divided by the control count). Under these conditions, Salzman found that normal platelet retention ranges from 26 to 60 per cent.

In the infusion pump technique, Bowie (1969) modified the Hellem and Salzman tests so that 10 ml of blood is collected in a plastic syringe containing 40 units of sodium heparin. The tube is gently inverted four times to ensure complete mixing, and 1 ml of blood is placed into a tube containing dried EDTA (0.1 ml of a 2 per cent solution) for the initial control platelet count. The remainder of the blood specimen is drawn into a 20 ml plastic syringe which is clipped into an infusion pump. A glass bead column containing 2.6 g of glass beads is attached to the end of the syringe by 1 cm lengths of polyvinyl tubing. The blood is pushed through the column by the pump at a flow rate of 5.1 ml/min. The first 3 ml are discarded and the last 2 ml of blood are collected separately into tubes containing EDTA. The final platelet count is calculated by averaging the values obtained in the last two tubes. The result is expressed as a percentage of platelet retention.

Platelet retention (%) =

$$\frac{\text{initial platelet} - \text{final platelet}}{\text{count} \qquad\qquad \text{count}} \times 100$$
$$\overline{\text{initial platelet count}}$$

3

Normal platelet retention is listed as 89.9 per cent $\pm$ 8.8.

Interpretation

Most workers agree that the Hellem method gives normal results in von Willebrand's disease. The Salzman method has been reported to show reduced platelet retention in von Willebrand's disease by some workers but not all. In a cooperative study, 15 per cent of patients with von Willebrand's disease had normal platelet retention and 20 per cent of normals had decreased platelet retention (Salzman, 1970). In the Salzman assay, the flow rate varies as the Vacutainer fills. O'Brien (1967) showed that the rate of flow is crucial in demonstrating a difference between platelet adhesiveness in patients with von Willebrand's disease and in normals. The infusion pump technique tends to circumvent this defect by providing constant flow rate of blood over glass beads.

Numerous sources of error exist in this procedure. One must be cautious to use polyvinyl plastic for the glass column, pack the glass beads with a vibrator before use, perform careful venipunctures, and handle the heparinized blood gently (Bowie, 1973). A decrease in platelet retention can be demonstrated in von Willebrand's disease as well as in many of the cases of familial and acquired platelet functional disorders (Bowie, 1969). An abnormal result, therefore, is not diagnostic of any single disorder.

PLATELET AGGREGATION

Principle

After an aggregating agent is added, platelets clump together, causing a decrease in the turbidity of platelet-rich plasma. The change in light transmission can be measured in a nephelometer with a graphic record.

Method

Born (1962) and O'Brien (1962) independently showed that under appropriate conditions a nephelometer can record platelet aggregation. Most aggregometers (nephelometers) measure a combination of light scatter and transmittance (Chap. 4, p. 93). The instrument maintains platelet-rich plasma at 37°C. by means of a small magnetic stirrer. The recorder is first adjusted to a light transmission of 10 per cent for platelet-rich plasma and 90 per cent for platelet-poor plasma. Four-

tenths ml of test sample platelet-rich plasma is placed in the cuvette of the aggregometer, followed by 0.02 ml of an aggregating agent. A control sample of platelet-rich plasma is analyzed simultaneously on dual channel aggregometers. The rate of aggregation depends on the number of platelets, temperature, rate of stirring, and concentration of the aggregating agents. The platelet count of the test sample should be between $200 \times 10^9/l$ and $400 \times 10^9/l$, and stirring rate between 900 and 1200 rpm. A reversible one-phase aggregation curve results from adding low concentrations of thrombin, ADP, or epinephrine to the platelet-rich plasma. At certain critical concentrations of the aggregating agents, a two-phase response occurs (see Fig. 32-4C to E). The second-phase curve is due to the release of endogenous ADP during the initial phase of aggregation. Tests are usually performed with two or three dilutions of ADP, epinephrine, and ristocetin. The light transmission curve is observed for at least three minutes. Useful final concentrations of aggregating agents are: ADP and epinephrine 6.4, 3.2, and 1.5 μM; ristocetin 1.5, 1.2, and 1.0 mg/ml.

ADP, epinephrine, ristocetin, and collagen can be obtained from commercial sources. Collagen also can be prepared by homogenizing 4 g fresh cadaver tendon in 50 ml 0.15 M NaCl in a blender. This is followed by centrifuging at 1800 g and discarding the pellet and the upper third. The remainder is kept at full strength and used at the highest dilution that still produces maximal aggregation with normal platelet-rich plasma. A method for preparing collagen from cadaver skin is given by Wilner (1968).

Interpretation

Since many drugs interfere with platelet aggregation, it should be performed after the patient has refrained from taking drugs for 7 to 10 days. In addition, some observers require the patient to be in a fasting state. Lipemic samples should be avoided. In general, a two-phase response is observed at 3.2 and 1.5 μM ADP and epinephrine. Collagen induces a one-phase response after a delay. Ristocetin usually evokes a rapid single-phase aggregation at 1.2 and 1.5 mg/ml in normal platelet-rich plasma.

In Glanzmann's thrombasthenia, platelets fail to aggregate with ADP, epinephrine, and collagen, but many aggregate with ristocetin. In storage pool disease and abnormal release disorders, no second-wave response occurs with epinephrine or threshold levels of ADP, and a reduced response to collagen is observed (Fig. 32–12). Ristocetin aggregation is abnormal in von Willebrand's disease and in Bernard-Soulier syndrome. In von Willebrand's

Figure 32–12. Typical platelet aggregation tracings in normal individuals and in patients with von Willebrand's disease (VWD), Bernard-Soulier syndrome (BSS), storage pool disease (SPD), acetylsalicylic acid–like disorders (ASA), and Glanzmann's thrombasthenia (TSA). The ASA and SPD defects lack a second wave of ADP aggregation and have impaired collagen aggregation because of impaired release of ADP. Cryoprecipitate corrects the abnormal ristocetin aggregation in VWD, but not in the BSS. (From Weiss, H. J.: Platelet physiology and abnormalities of platelet function. N. Engl. J. Med. *293*:531, 1975. Reprinted by permission.)

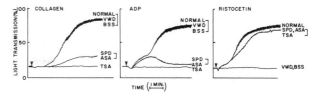

disease, but not in Bernard-Soulier syndrome, the ristocetin aggregation often becomes normal by the addition of pooled normal plasma (Jenkins, 1976). Platelet aggregation is abnormal in a variety of other illnesses, including Wiskott-Aldrich syndrome, uremia, leukemia, and myeloproliferative disorders.

Aspirin inhibits platelet aggregation with collagen and the second wave induced by ADP and epinephrine. Other commonly used drugs that interfere with the test include phenylbutazone, sulfenpyrazone, anti-inflammatory drugs, psychotropic agents of the phenothiazine and dibenzazepine classes, dipyridamole, and some antihistaminics.

PLATELET FACTOR 3 AVAILABILITY TEST

Principle

Platelet-rich plasma is incubated with kaolin, causing the release of phospholipid (platelet factor 3) and activating the plasma contact factors. At appropriate intervals, samples of platelet-rich plasma are removed and added to a second tube containing kaolin-activated normal platelet-poor plasma. A recalcification time is determined (p. 1155). Since the second tube will have a maximum contact activation of the plasma factors, the length of the recalcification time is inversely related to the amount of phospholipid released (or made "available") in the incubation mixture in the first tube. In normal individuals, there is a progressive shortening of the recalcification time (Fig. 32–13).

Method (Weiss, 1967)

One ml of platelet-rich plasma ($300 \times 10^9/l$) is incubated at 37°C. with 0.5 ml 8 per cent kaolin in 0.05 M imidazole buffered normal saline solution, pH 7.3 (tube 1). Immediately after preparing this incubation mixture (tube 1) the substrate is prepared by mixing 0.3 ml of normal platelet-poor plasma (kept on ice until needed) with 0.15 ml 2 per cent kaolin (tube 2) at 37°C. for four minutes. At two-minute intervals, 0.05 ml of the incubation mixture in tube 1 is added, with 0.4 ml of 0.025 M calcium chloride, to tube 2. The clotting time is determined.

Interpretation

In normal individuals, the clotting time shortens with increased incubation time of the mixture in tube 1 (Fig. 32–13). The most striking differences between normal subjects and patients with platelet factor 3 defects are seen after six minutes of incubation. In patients with von Willebrand's disease, the platelet factor 3 assay is normal. In patients with Glanzmann's thrombasthenia, the platelet factor 3 assay is abnormal and the addition of ADP to the incubation mixture in tube 1 has no effect. In some patients with ADP release defects, the platelet factor 3 assay is abnormal but is corrected with the addition of ADP to

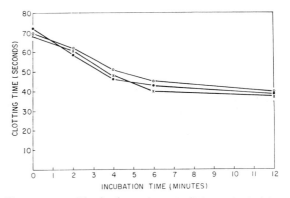

Figure 32–13. Platelet factor 3 assay. At two-minute intervals, samples are removed from an incubation mixture of platelet-rich plasma with kaolin and added with $CaCl_2$ to a substrate platelet-poor plasma with kaolin. Shortening of the clotting time of the substrate indicates platelet factor 3 availability or release. (From Weiss, H. J.: Platelet aggregation, adhesion and adenosine diphosphate release in thrombopathia (platelet factor 3 deficiency). A comparison with Glanzmann's thrombasthenia and von Willebrand's disease. Am. J. Med., *43*:570, 1967.)

the incubation mixture. In addition, platelet factor 3 activity increases after the addition of ADP, serotonin, and collagen to normal platelet-rich plasma. Thus, it appears that the liberation of platelet factor 3 requires the release of ADP. Decreased platelet factor 3 availability has been reported in some patients with uremia, myeloproliferative disorders, and macroglobulinemia, but an isolated deficiency of platelet factor 3 is extremely rare (ten Cate, 1972).

VON WILLEBRAND'S FACTOR (RISTOCETIN CO-FACTOR)

Principle

Formalin-fixed platelets (MacFarlane, 1975) or washed fresh platelets (Weiss, 1973) from normal individuals aggregate in response to ristocetin in the presence of normal platelet-poor plasma but not platelet-poor plasma in von Willebrand's disease. The time required for aggregation of platelets to occur is a function of the amount of von Willebrand's co-factor. Thus, a standard curve can be established relating percentage of von Willebrand's co-

factor to time of aggregation. This is performed by adding ristocetin to incubation mixtures of fixed platelet-rich plasma with various dilutions of pooled normal plasma in buffer and then measuring time for aggregation to occur. The end point of platelet clumping can be determined by a macroscopic tilt tube technique (Allain, 1975). An aggregometer can also be used to measure rate of aggregation (slope) or change in optical density (MacFarlane, 1975).

Method (Hoyer, 1977)

Preparation of Platelets. Whole blood is collected in siliconized centrifuge tubes containing $\frac{1}{6}$ volume of acid citrate dextrose anticoagulant. Platelet concentrates obtained from the Blood Bank can be used as a source of platelets. Platelet-rich plasma is obtained by centrifugation of blood at 460 g for eight minutes at room temperature. The platelet-rich plasma is incubated at 37°C. for one hour. An equal volume of phosphate-buffered 1.5 per cent formalin (pH 6.9) is added to platelet-rich plasma and incubated at room temperature for two hours. The mixture is diluted by the addition of an equal volume of phosphate buffer at pH 6.4 (made by mixing equal volumes of 0.15 M phosphate buffer at pH 6.4 and 0.15 M NaCl). This mix-

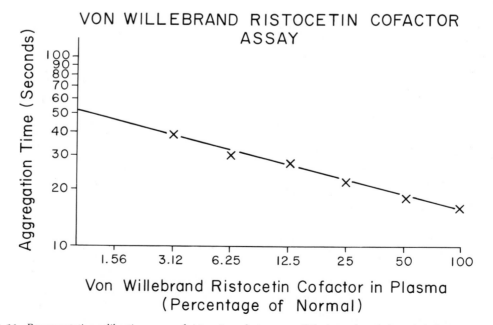

Figure 32–14. Representative calibration curve of ristocetin cofactor assay. Dilutions of pooled normal plasma are mixed with fixed normal platelet suspensions and ristocetin. Using log-log paper, the time to aggregation is plotted against the dilution, expressed here as "percentage of normal."

ture is centrifuged at 900 g for 10 minutes, and the supernate discarded. The platelet button is washed three times with 50 ml of 0.02 M imidazole buffered saline (pH 7.4) to which 40 g/l bovine serum albumin has been added. The platelets are adjusted to a count of $600 \times 10^9/l$ and kept at 4°C.

Assay. A suspension of the fixed platelets is well mixed and adjusted to a concentration of $300 \times 10^9/l$. A standard curve is made by incubating 0.1 ml of dilutions of pooled normal plasma (undiluted, $\frac{1}{2}$, $\frac{1}{4}$, $\frac{1}{8}$, $\frac{1}{16}$, $\frac{1}{32}$ with imidazole buffer containing 40 g/l of bovine serum albumin), 0.2 ml of fixed platelets and 0.1 ml ristocetin (4.0 mg/ml in 0.15 M NaCl). The tube is mixed and the time to aggregation is recorded using a tilt-tube method. One-tenth ml of test plasma is substituted for the pooled normal plasma, mixed with platelets and ristocetin, and the time to aggregation repeated. The plasma level of von Willebrand's factor in test plasma is obtained from the calibration curve (Fig. 32-14). Practice is necessary to determine the end point with reproducible results. Normal range is between 40 and 200 per cent.

Interpretation

Most patients with von Willebrand's disease have a level of von Willebrand's factor that is less than normal. In contrast, hemophiliac patients have normal levels of von Willebrand's factor. In general, the levels of factor VIII antigen and von Willebrand's factor parallel one another. In a few cases of von Willebrand's disease, the results of von Willebrand's factor have been much lower than the factor VIII antigen levels, suggesting a qualitative as well as quantitative defect in factor VIII molecule (Gralnick, 1977b).

PLATELET ANTIBODIES

Principle

An antiglobulin absorption assay measures the quantity of antibody bound to platelets. An optimal concentration of rabbit anti-human IgG is incubated with known numbers of washed platelets. Residual anti-IgG is then determined by measuring lysis of IgG-coated sheep red cells in the presence of complement. The degree of inhibition of this lysis is proportional to the amount of IgG on the surface of the platelet, which can be quantitated by constructing an appropriate calibration curve using purified IgG.

Free antiplatelet antibody in the serum can be determined by incubating washed, pooled normal platelets with the test serum. The platelets are again washed and then the bound IgG is determined as before.

Method

The method of Dixon (1975) and the modification of this by Hedge (1977) should be consulted for details.

Interpretation

Individuals may have platelet alloantibodies or autoantibodies. Platelet alloantibodies occur following transfusion or during pregnancy and have specificities against certain platelet antigens or against HLA antigens (Williams, 1972). Platelet autoantibodies (elevated levels of surface IgG) can be detected in most patients with idiopathic thrombocytopenic purpura (ITP) and systemic lupus erythematosus, and in some patients with lymphoproliferative disorders. Normal values of surface IgG on platelets were obtained in autoimmune hemolytic anemia (Hedge, 1977). In ITP the amount of platelet-bound IgG is inversely related to the platelet count and has been found helpful in predicting the clinical course of the disease (Dixon, 1975).

DRUG-MEDIATED PLATELET ANTIBODIES

Principle

Immune-mediated thrombocytopenia has been described following the ingestion of sedormid, anatazoline, imidazoline, quinine, carbromal, and quinadine (Ackroyd, 1962). The presence of this antibody can be demonstrated by incubating the test plasma with a saturated solution of the drug and freshly drawn blood and observing for inhibition of clot retraction.

Method (Dacie, 1975)

A saturated solution of the drug is made in 0.15 M NaCl. Two ml of fresh Group O blood is added directly to 0.2 ml of patient's serum and 0.2 ml of saturated drug solution in a glass tube. The mixture is incubated at 37°C. and inspected at 2 and 12 hours for clot retraction. Control samples are composed of (1) normal serum, drug solution, and blood and (2) patient's serum, saline solution without drug, and blood.

Interpretation

In the presence of drug-dependent anti-body, clot retraction occurs in the control samples but not in the test mixture.

DIAGNOSIS OF PLATELET DISORDERS

In the diagnosis of platelet disorders, knowledge of the clinical history and physical findings provides the proper data base to make an appropriate interpretation of the laboratory assays.

Platelet disorders (thrombocytopenia or platelet function defects) are characterized by petechiae and ecchymoses of skin and mucous membranes, in contrast to the deep tissue and joint bleeding that is more typical of coagulation disorders.

The bleeding time and the platelet count are the two most significant screening tests for platelet function. A prolonged bleeding time and a platelet count less than $50 \times 10^9/l$ indicate that thrombocytopenia is the likely cause of bleeding. Bone marrow examination should then be performed to evaluate the number of megakaryocytes. An increased number of megakaryocytes, which tend to be large, points to increased destruction or sequestration. Decreased numbers of megakaryocytes imply a hypoproliferative state. A normal or increased number of megakaryocytes in a megaloblastic marrow sometimes accompanies thrombocytopenia owing to ineffective thrombopoiesis. Platelet survival studies employing autologous platelets labeled with a radioisotope are sometimes useful when the etiology of thrombocytopenia remains in doubt; these studies are beyond the scope of most clinical laboratories.

A prolonged bleeding time and a normal, increased, or only slightly decreased platelet count indicate a qualitative platelet disorder. Measurements of platelet glass bead retention, platelet aggregation, clot retraction, and platelet factor 3 availability are then usually needed. Glanzmann's disease, von Willebrand's disease, Bernard-Soulier syndrome, and platelet release abnormalities can be characterized using these assays. The differentiation of storage pool defect from release reaction defects usually requires assays provided in research laboratories.

REFERENCES

Ackroyd, J. F.: The immunological basis of purpura due to drug hypersensitivity. Proc. R. Soc. Med., 55:30, 1962.

Allain, J. P., Cooper, H. A., Wagner, R. H., and Brinkhous, K. M.: Platelets fixed with paraformaldehyde: A new reagent for assay of von Willebrand factor and platelet aggregating factor. J. Lab. Clin. Med., 85:318, 1975.

Booyse, F. M., Zschocke, D., Hoveke, T. P., and Rafelson, M. E., Jr.: Studies on human platelets. IV. Protein synthesis in maturing human platelets. Thromb. Diath. Haemorrh., 26:167, 1971.

Booyse, F. M., and Rafelson, M. E., Jr.: Human platelet contractile proteins: Location, properties, and function. Ser. Haematol., 4:152, 1971.

Born, G. V. R.: Aggregation of blood platelets by adenosine diphosphate and its reversal. Nature, 194:927, 1962.

Bowie, E. J. W., Owen, C. A., Jr., Thompson, J. H., and Didisheim, P.: Platelet adhesiveness in von Willebrand's disease. Am. J. Clin. Pathol., 52:69, 1969.

Bowie, E. J. W., and Owen, C. A., Jr.: The value of measuring platelet "adhesiveness" in the diagnosis of bleeding diseases. Am. J. Clin. Pathol., 60:302, 1973.

Bowie, E. J. W., and Owen, C. A., Jr.: The bleeding time. Prog. Hemostasis Thromb., 2:249, 1974.

Caen, J.: Glanzmann's thrombasthenia. Clin. Haematol., 1:383, 1972.

Caen, J., Cronberg, S., and Kubisz, P.: Platelets: Physiology and Pathology. New York, Stratton Intercontinental Medical Book Corp., 1977.

Corash, L., Tan, H., and Gralnick, H. R.: Heterogenity of human whole blood platelet subpopulations. I. Relationship between buoyant density, cell volume and ultrastructure. Blood, 49:71, 1977.

Cowan, D. H., and Graham, R. C., Jr.: Structural-functional relationships in platelets in acute leukemia and related disorders. Ser. Haematol., 8:68, 1975.

Czapek, E. E., Deykin, D., and Salzman, E. W.: Platelet dysfunction in glycogen storage disease, Type I. Blood, 41:235, 1973.

Dacie, J. V., and Lewis, S. M.: Practical Hematology, 5th ed. Edinburgh, Churchill Livingstone, 1975.

Day, H. J., and Holmsen, H.: Concepts of the blood platelet release reaction. Ser. Haematol., 4:3, 1971.

Dixon, R., Rosse, W., and Ebbert, L.: Quantitative determinations of antibody in idiopathic thrombocytopenic purpura. N. Engl. J. Med., 292:230, 1975.

Duke, W. W.: The relation of blood platelets to hemorrhagic disease: Description of a method for determining the bleeding time and coagulation time and report of three cases of hemorrhagic disease relieved by transfusion. J.A.M.A., 55:1185, 1910.

Gralnick, H. R., Sultan, Y., and Coller, B. S.: Von Willebrand's disease: Combined qualitative and quantitative abnormalities. N. Engl. J. Med., 296:1024, 1977a.

Gralnick, H. R., Coller, B. S., Shulman, N. R., Andersen, J. C., and Hilgartner, M.: Factor VIII, NIH Conference. Ann. Intern. Med., 86:598, 1977b.

Gröttum, K. A., and Solum, N. O.: Congenital thrombocytopenia with giant platelets: A defect in platelet membrane, Br. J. Haematol., 16:277, 1969.

Hall, J. G., Levin, J., Kuhn, J. P., Ottenheimer, E. J., van

Berkum, K. A. P., and McKusick, V. A.: Thrombocytopenia with absent radius (TAR). Medicine (Baltimore), 48:411, 1969.

Hamberg, M., Svensson, J., and Samuelson, B.: Prostaglandin endoperoxides. A new concept concerning the mode of action and release of prostaglandins. Proc. Natl. Acad. Sci. U.S.A., 71:3824, 1974.

Hardisty, R. M., Hutton, R. A., Montgomery, D., Rickard, S., and Trebilcock, H.: Secondary platelet aggregation: A quantitative study. Br. J. Haematol., 19:307, 1970.

Harker, L. A.: Hemostasis Manual, 2nd ed. Philadelphia, F. A. Davis Co., 1974, p. 15.

Harker, L. A., and Finch, C. A.: Thrombokinetics in man. J. Clin. Invest., 48:963, 1969.

Harker, L. A., and Slichter, S. J.: The bleeding time as a screening test for evaluation of platelet function. N. Engl. J. Med., 287:155, 1972a.

Harker, L. A., and Slichter, S. J.: Platelet and fibrinogen consumption in man. N. Engl. J. Med., 287:999, 1972b.

Hedge, U. M., Gordon-Smith, E. C., and Worlledge, S.: Platelet antibodies in thrombocytopenic patients. Br. J. Haematol., 35:113, 1977.

Hellem, A. J.: The adhesiveness of human blood platelets in vitro. Scand. J. Clin. Lab. Invest., 12 (Suppl. 51):1, 1960.

Hirsh, J., and Doery, J. C. G.: Platelet function in health and disease. Prog. Hematol., 7:185, 1971.

Holme, R., Sixura, J. J., Mürer, E., and Hovig, T.: Demonstration of platelet fibrinogen secretion via surface connecting system. Thromb. Res., 3:347, 1973.

Holmsen, H.: The platelet: Its membrane, physiology and biochemistry. Clin. Haematol., 1:235, 1972.

Holmsen, H.: Classification and possible mechanism of action of some drugs that inhibit platelet aggregation. Ser. Haematol., 8:50, 1976.

Holmsen, H., and Weiss, H. J.: Further evidence for a deficient storage pool of adenine nucleotides in platelets from some patients with thrombocytopathias—"Storage Pool Disease." Blood, 39:197, 1972.

Hovig, T.: The ultrastructure of blood platelets in normal and abnormal states. Ser. Haematol., 1:3, 1968.

Howard, M. A., Hutton, R. A., and Hardisty, R. M.: Hereditary giant platelet syndrome: A disorder of a new aspect of platelet function. Br. Med. J., 2:586, 1973.

Hoyer, L. W.: von Willebrand's disease. Prog. Hemostasis Thromb., 3:231, 1976.

Hoyer, L. W.: Personal communication, 1977.

Ivy, A. C., Shapiro, P. F., and Melnick, P.: The bleeding tendency in jaundice. Surg. Gynecol. Obstet., 60:781, 1935.

Jamieson, G. A., Smith, D. F., and Kosow, D. P.: Possible role of collagen: Glucosyl transferase in platelet adhesion. Thromb. Diath. Haemorrh., 33:668, 1975.

Jenkins, C. S. P., Phillips, D. R., Clemetson, J. K., Meyer, D., Larrieu, M. J., and Lüscher, E. F.: Platelet membrane glycoproteins implicated in ristocetin-induced aggregation. J. Clin. Invest., 57:112, 1976.

Lackner, H.: Hemostatic abnormalities associated with dysproteinemias. Semin. Hematol., 10:125, 1973.

Lewis, N., and Majerus, P. W.: Lipid metabolism in human platelets. II. De novo phospholipid synthesis and the effect of thrombin on the pattern of synthesis. J. Clin. Invest., 48:2114, 1969.

Lewis, S. M., Szur, L., and Hoffbrand, A. V.: Thrombocythemia. Clin. Hematol., 1:339, 1972.

MacFarlane, D. E., and Zucker, M. B.: A method for assaying von Willebrand's factor (ristocetin cofactor). Thromb. Diath. Haemorrh., 34:306, 1975.

Maldonado, J. E.: The ultrastructure of the platelets in refractory anemia (preleukemia) and myelomonocytic leukemia. Ser. Haematol., 8:101, 1975.

Malmstein, C., Kindahl, H., Samuelsson, B., Levy-Toledano, S., Tobelem, G., and Caen, J. P.: Thromboxane synthesis and the platelet release reaction in Bernard-Soulier syndrome, thrombasthenia Glanzmann and Hermansky-Pudlak syndrome. Br. J. Haematol., 35:511, 1977.

Marcus, A. J.: Platelet function. N. Engl. J. Med., 280:1213, 1278, 1330; 1969.

Marx, J. L.: Blood clotting: The role of the prostaglandins. Science, 196:1072, 1977.

Mielke, C. H., Jr., Kanishiro, M. M., Maher, I. A., Weiner, J. M., and Rapaport, S. I.: The standardized normal Ivy bleeding time and its prolongation by aspirin. Blood, 34:204, 1969.

Murphy, S., Oski, F. A., Naiman, J. L., Lusch, C. S., Goldberg, S., and Gardner, F. H.: Platelet size and kinetics in hereditary and acquired thrombocytopenia. N. Engl. J. Med., 286:499, 1972.

Nachman, R. L., Marcus, A. J., and Safier, L. B.: Platelet thrombosthenin: Subcellular localization and function. J. Clin. Invest., 46:1380, 1967.

Niewiarowski, S., Lipinski, B., Farbiszewski, R., and Poplawski, A.: The release of platelet factor 4 during platelet aggregation and the possible significance of this reaction in haemostasis. Experientia, 24:343, 1968.

Nurden, A. T., and Caen, J. P.: An abnormal platelet glycoprotein pattern in three cases of Glanzmann's thrombasthenia. Br. J. Haematol., 28:253, 1974.

O'Brien, J. R.: Platelet aggregation. 1. Some effects of adenosine phosphates, thrombin, and cocaine upon platelet adhesiveness. J. Clin. Pathol., 15:446, 1962.

O'Brien, J. R., and Heywood, J. B.: Some interactions between human platelets and glass: Von Willebrand's disease compared with normal. J. Clin. Pathol., 20:56, 1967.

Owen, C. A., Bowie, E. J., Didisheim, P., et al.: The Diagnosis of Bleeding Disorders. Boston, Little, Brown and Company, 1969.

Owen, C. A., Bowie, E. J., and Thompson, J. H.: The Diagnosis of Bleeding Disorders, 2nd ed. Boston, Little, Brown and Company, 1975.

Packham, M. A., and Mustard, J. F.: Clinical pharmacology of platelets. Blood, 50:555, 1977.

Rabiner, S. F.: Uremic bleeding. Progr. Hemostasis Thromb., 1:233, 1972.

Rodman, N. F.: The morphologic basis of platelet function. In Brinkhous, K. M., Shermer, R. W., and Mostofi, F. K. (eds.): The Platelet. Baltimore, The Williams & Wilkins Co., 1971, p. 55.

Salzman, E. W.: Measurement of platelet adhesiveness. A simple in vitro technique demonstrating an abnormality in von Willebrand's disease. J. Lab. Clin. Med., 62:724, 1963.

Salzman, E. W.: Platelet adhesiveness in von Willebrand's disease: A cooperative study. In Brinkhous, K. M. (ed.): Hemophilia and New Hemorrhagic States. Chapel Hill, University of North Carolina Press, 1970, p. 205.

Shulman, N. R., Marder, J. J., Hiller, M. C., and Collier, E. M.: Platelet and leukocyte isoantigens and their antibodies: Serologic, physiologic and clinical studies. Prog. Hematol., 3:222, 1964.

Strauss, H. S., and Bloom, G. E.: Von Willebrand's disease. Use of a platelet adhesiveness test in diagnosis and family investigation. N. Engl. J. Med., 273:171, 1965.

Stuart, M. J.: Inherited defects of platelet function. Semin. Hematol., 12:233, 1975.

ten Cate, J. W.: Platelet function tests. Clin. Haematol., *1*:283, 1972.

Vossen, M. E. M. H., Stadouders, A. M., Kurstjens, R., and Haanen, C.: Observations on platelet ultrastructure in familial thrombocytopathic thrombocytopenia. Am. J. Pathol., *53*:1021, 1968.

Weinfeld, A., Branehög, I., and Kutti, J.: Platelets in the myeloproliferative syndrome. Clin. Haematol., *4*:373, 1975.

Weiss, H. J.: Platelet aggregation, adhesion and adenosine diphosphate release in thrombopathia (platelet factor 3 deficiency). A comparison with Glanzmann's thrombasthenia and von Willebrand's disease. Am. J. Med., *43*:570, 1967.

Weiss, H. J., and Rogers, J.: Thrombocytopathia due to abnormalities in platelet release reaction—studies on six unrelated patients. Blood, *39*:187, 1972.

Weiss, H. J., Hoyer, L. W., Ricklers, F. R., Varma, A., and Rogers, J.: Quantitative assay of a plasma factor deficient in von Willebrand's disease that is necessary for platelet aggregation. Relationship to factor VIII procoagulant activity and antigen content. J. Clin. Invest., *52*:2708, 1973.

Weiss, H. J.: Platelet physiology and abnormalities of platelet function. N. Engl. J. Med., *293*:531, 580, 1975.

White, J. C.: Platelet morphology. *In* Johnson, S. A. (ed.): The Circulating Platelet. New York, Academic Press, 1971, p. 45.

Williams, W. J., and Knight, R. H.: Platelet antigens and antibodies. *In* Williams, W. J., Beutler, E., Erslev, A. J., and Rundles, R. W. (eds.): Hematology. New York, McGraw-Hill Book Co., 1972, p. 1289.

Wilner, G. D., Nossel, H. L., and LeRoy, E. C.: Aggregation of platelets by collagen. J. Clin. Invest., *47*:2616, 1968.

Wintrobe, M. M., Lee, G. R., Boggs, D. R., Bithell, T. C., Athens, J. W., and Foerster, J.: Clinical Hematology, 7th ed. Philadelphia, Lea and Febiger, 1974.

Wright, H. P.: The adhesiveness of blood platelets in normal subjects with varying concentration of anticoagulants. J. Pathol., *53*:255, 1941.

Zucker, S., and Mielke, C. H.: Classification of thrombocytosis based on platelet function tests: Correlation with hemorrhagic and thrombotic complications. J. Lab. Clin. Med., *80*:385, 1972.

BLOOD COAGULATION AND ITS DISORDERS

Frederick R. Davey, M.D.

3

SYSTEMS OF COAGULATION AND FIBRINOLYSIS

The coagulation of blood is due to the enzymatic interaction of procoagulants (proteins of the coagulation system), phospholipids, and ions. The plasma proteins which are involved in coagulation circulate in the blood in an inert form. Vascular injury usually initiates the activation of these procoagulants, followed by the sequential proteolysis and further activation of other coagulation factors. This action culminates in the formation of an insoluble fibrin clot (Macfarlane, 1964; Davie, 1964).

PHYSICAL AND CHEMICAL PROPERTIES OF PROCOAGULANTS

NOMENCLATURE

Circulating procoagulants have been given descriptive names (fibrinogen, prothrombin, thrombin), functional names (labile and stable factors), and surnames of the kindreds in whom hereditary defects were first discovered (Hageman, Fletcher, and Stuart factors). In order to avoid confusion, an international committee established a nomenclature of blood clotting factors. Roman numerals were used to denote factors in order of their discovery without regard to their position in the sequence of the reactions. In addition, Factor VI was initially the activated form of Factor V. The term has since been dropped. Factor IV is not a circulating procoagulant but represents calcium ions. The non-activated factors have been assigned a Roman numeral (Table 33–1) and the activated forms are indicated by an appended "a". Factors V and VIII may not have activated forms.

CONTACT FACTORS

Factor XII, Factor XI, prekallikrein, and high molecular weight kininogen are plasma proteins involved in the earliest stages of blood coagulation. Because of their activation by glass and other foreign surfaces, they have been referred to as contact factors. Most of these factors are involved in the complex interaction among the coagulation, fibrinolytic, and kinin systems (Kaplan, 1976). The func-

Table 33-1. NOMENCLATURE FOR COAGULATION FACTORS

ROMAN NUMERAL	SYNONYMS
I	Fibrinogen
II	Prothrombin
III	Tissue factor, thromboplastin
IV	Calcium ions
V	Proaccelerin; labile factor
VII	Proconvertin; stable factor
VIII	Antihemophilic factor (AHF), antihemophilic globulin (AHG), antihemophilic factor A
IX	Plasma thromboplastin component (PTC), antihemophilic factor B, Christmas factor
X	Stuart factor, Prower factor
XI	Plasma thromboplastin antecedent (PTA)
XII	Hageman factor
XIII	Fibrin stabilizing factor
Prekallikrein	Fletcher factor
High molecular weight kininogen	Fitzgerald factor, Williams factor, Flaujeac factor

tion of contact factors is not dependent upon vitamin K.

Factor XII (Hageman factor) is a sialoglycoprotein with a molecular weight of 110,000 to 122,000 daltons (Table 33-2). It migrates as a β-globulin, is not consumed in a clot, is heat stable, and is not adsorbed by barium sulfate ($BaSO_4$) or aluminum hydroxide [$Al(OH)_3$].

Prekallikrein (Fletcher factor) is a plasma protein with a molecular weight of approximately 100,000 daltons. It is partially adsorbed by $BaSO_4$ and celite but not adsorbed by $Al(OH)_3$. Fletcher factor is resistant to heating at 56°C. for 30 minutes and is stable when stored in the cold or after lyophilization (Hathaway, 1965).

High molecular weight kininogen is a protein in normal plasma that shortens the prolonged partial thromboplastin time of plasma from patients with Fitzgerald trait, Flaujeac trait, and Williams trait (Donaldson, 1976; Saito, 1975b; Colman, 1975). It has a molecular weight of 200,000 daltons, migrates as an α-globulin, and accounts for 20 per cent of the total plasma kininogen (Mandle, 1976).

Factor XI has a molecular weight of 165,000 daltons and migrates as a β-globulin. Its activity is slightly decreased by adsorption with $Al(OH)_3$ or $BaSO_4$ and it is unstable at 56°C. Factor XI activity remains unchanged in the serum and is inhibited by diisopropylfluorophosphate (DFP), suggesting that Factor XI is a proteolytic enzyme with an active serine site (Bennett, 1977).

PROTHROMBIN FACTORS

Factors II, VII, IX, and X are considered part of the prothrombin complex. The function of all factors is dependent upon vitamin K. The prothrombin factors are adsorbed by $BaSO_4$ and $Al(OH)_3$ and, except for Factor II, are present in serum. The prothrombin complex factors have a molecular weight between 50,000 and 100,000 daltons. These factors are glycoproteins and migrate as α- or β-globulins. The activated forms are sensitive to DFP inhibition.

CONSUMABLE FACTORS

Factors I, V, VIII, and XIII are consumed during the coagulation process. Therefore, these factors are not present in serum. They are not dependent upon vitamin K for their activity and are not adsorbed from the plasma with $Al(OH)_3$ or $BaSO_4$. The consumable fac-

Table 33-2. PROPERTIES OF COAGULATION FACTORS

FACTORS	BIOCHEMISTRY	MOLECULAR WEIGHT (daltons)	CONCENTRATION IN PLASMA (mg/l)	BIOLOGIC HALF-LIFE (hours)	TURNOVER (mg/ml/day)	ADSORBED WITH $BaSO_4$ OR $Al(OH)_3$*	PRESENT IN AGED SERUM	VITAMIN K DEPENDENT
I	Glycoprotein	340,000	200–4000	72–120	500	No	No	No
II	Glycoprotein	70,000	100–150	48–96	40	Yes	No	Yes
V	Glycoprotein	300,000	10	15–24	10	No	No	No
VII	Glycoprotein	53,000	0.5–30	4–6	2	Yes	Yes	Yes
VIII	Glycoprotein	1,200,000	15	10–18	25	No	No	No
IX	Glycoprotein	60,000	3	18–30	2	Yes	Yes	Yes
X	Glycoprotein	55,000	15	40–60	6	Yes	Yes	Yes
XI	β or γ globulin	165,000	<5	45–54	<2	No	Yes	No
XII	Sialoglycoprotein	110,000	<5	48–96	<2	No	Yes	No
XIII	β or γ globulin	320,000	20	96	3	No	Reduced	No

* $BaSO_4$ = Barium sulfate
  $Al(OH)_3$ = Aluminum hydroxide

CASCADE MECHANISM OF BLOOD COAGULATION

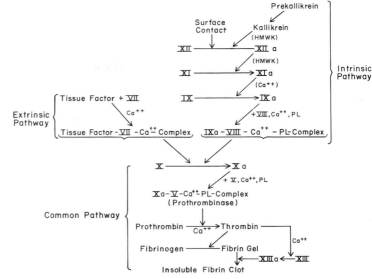

Figure 33–1. Diagram representing the interrelationship of the proteins active in the intrinsic, extrinsic, and common pathways of coagulation. HMWK = High Molecular Weight Kininogen; PL = Phospholipid. (Modified from Davie, 1964.)

tors are glycoproteins and migrate in an electrophoretic field as α- or β-globulins. Fibrinogen, Factor V, and Factor XIII have a molecular weight of approximately 320,000 daltons. Factor VIII is a larger molecule with a molecular weight of 1,200,000 daltons.

ACTIVATION OF COAGULATION FACTORS

The enzymatic activation of coagulation factors can be divided into two systems which are, in effect, alternative modes of activating Factor X (Fig. 33–1). In the *intrinsic pathway*, all of the procoagulants necessary for clot formation are within the circulating blood. In contrast, the *extrinsic pathway* requires the release of tissue factor from endothelial cells before activation can occur. Activation of either or both pathways results in the conversion of Factor X to Xa; the remaining reactions therefore form a common pathway and terminate in the formation of the insoluble fibrin clot (Fig. 33–1).

INTRINSIC PATHWAY

Activation of Factor XII can begin following damage of the vascular endothelium. Exposure of the blood to collagen, microfibrils, and basement membrane not only induces platelet adhesion but also brings about a con-

formational alteration in Factor XII that reveals a biologically active serine site. Thus, a surface is required for Factor XII activation. In addition, high molecular weight kininogen and prekallikrein are necessary to activate Factor XII at an optimal rate (Mandle, 1976).

A variety of substances act as surface agents and activate Factor XII (Table 33–3). The particulate activators of Factor XII carry high negative charges, which may be a critical characteristic (Nossel, 1976). Neutralization of these negative foci by positively charged substances prevents activation of Hageman factor. However, studies on the procoagulant action of collagen indicate that the free carboxyl groups (Wilner, 1968) as well as mainte-

Table 33–3. SURFACE CONTACT ACTIVATORS*

SURFACES PRESENT IN VIVO	OTHER ACTIVATORS
Collagen	Glass
Fatty acid	Celite
Skin	Kaolin
Uric acid	Ellagic acid
Homocystine	Barium carbonate
	Asbestos
	Carboxymethyl cellulose
	Cellulose sulphate
	Carrageenan
	Calcium pyrophosphate
	Spider webs

*Modified from Nossel, H. L.: The contact system. *In* Biggs, R. (ed.): Human Blood Coagulation, Haemostasis and Thrombosis. Oxford, Blackwell Scientific Publications, 1976.

ACTIVATION OF CONTACT FACTORS

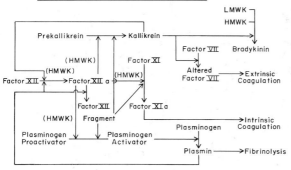

Figure 33–2. Diagram demonstrating the interrelationship among various contact factors and the kinin, coagulation, and fibrinolytic systems. HMWK = High Molecular Weight Kininogen; LMWK = Low Molecular Weight Kininogen. (Modified from Kaplan, 1976.)

nance of the triple helical structure are important properties in the activation of Factor XII (Nossel, 1976).

Factor XIIa hydrolyzes three different enzyme precursors (Fig. 33–2). It converts prekallikrein (Fletcher factor) to kallikrein, a serine protease which acts on kininogens, a group of plasma proteins. Both the high molecular weight kininogens (Fitzgerald, Williams, and Flaujeac factors) and the low molecular weight kininogens can serve as a substrate for kallikrein (Kaplan, 1976). However, high molecular weight kininogen is the preferred substrate. Kallikrein cleaves kininogen into small polypeptide fragments and releases a vasoactive decapeptide called bradykinin. This decapeptide causes vasodilation, lowers blood pressure, increases vascular permeability, produces local pain, and acts as a chemotactic factor (Saito, 1975b). Kallikrein also appears capable of altering Factor VII to increase its activity in the extrinsic pathway (Saito, 1975a). Thus, there is an interaction between Factors XIIa and VII mediated by kallikrein.

Factor XIIa also hydrolyzes plasminogen proactivator, converting the plasma protein into plasminogen activator. This enzyme in turn cleaves plasminogen to form plasmin, which is a potent fibrinolytic enzyme (Davidson, 1977).

Activated Hageman factor (XIIa) converts Factor XI into Factor XIa. This reaction requires the presence of high molecular weight kininogen. Factor XIa, a serine protease, activates Factor IX in the presence of Ca^{++} through the cleavage of a peptide bond (Fig. 33–1).

Kallikrein, plasmin, and Factor XIa with high molecular weight kininogen as a cofactor, cleave XII to produce more XIIa (Kaplan, 1976). In addition, plasmin can further digest

XIIa to form XII fragments (XIIf) which have the capacity to activate prekallikrein and promote coagulation (Davidson, 1977). Thus XIIa and XIIf can both activate prekallikrein, Factor XI, and plasminogen proactivator. This tends to amplify the effect of the initial activating agent.

In the next step Factor IXa [complexed with Factor VIII, phospholipid (PF$_3$), and calcium ions] converts Factor X to its activated form. It is postulated that factor VIII acts as a cofactor in this reaction. However, it has been demonstrated that the catalytic activity of Factor VIII can be accelerated after exposure to trace amounts of thrombin (Rapaport, 1963).

EXTRINSIC PATHWAY

Tissues contain a lipoprotein (tissue factor) that accelerates the coagulation of blood (Nemerson, 1972). Tissue factor binds with Factor VII to yield an enzymatically active complex which in the presence of calcium ions activates Factor X. It appears that Factor VII, a single-chain glycoprotein with a molecular weight of 53,000 daltons, provides the enzymatic activity and tissue factor serves as a catalyst (Radcliffe, 1975). Utilizing an immunoperoxidase method, tissue factor has been localized to the plasma membranes of endothelial cells in blood vessels (Zeldis, 1972). Thus, tissue factor probably plays a significant role in hemostasis and thrombosis.

COMMON PATHWAY

The common pathway begins with the activation of Factor X by either the intrinsic or extrinsic systems. In addition, Russell's viper venom and trypsin can activate Factor X di-

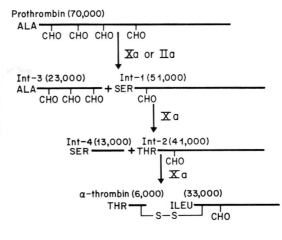

Figure 33-3. Schematic model for prothrombin activation. Prothrombin and the intermediate molecules (Int-1, Int-2, Int-3, Int-4) in the generation of thrombin are represented. The N-terminal amino acids and molecular weights are given for each. CHO indicates a carbohydrate side chain. (From Mann, K. G.: Prothrombin activation. Hum. Pathol., 5:377, 1974.)

rectly (Macfarlane, 1961). Factor X is a glycoprotein of 55,000 daltons and is composed of two chains connected by disulfide bonds. The activation of Factor X involves the cleavage of a glycopeptide of molecular weight 11,000 daltons from the amino terminal end of the heavy chain (Fujikawa, 1972). Activated Factor X (molecular weight 44,000 daltons) is a serine protease which interacts with Factor V, phospholipid (PF_3), and calcium ions to activate prothrombin.

Although Xa can convert prothrombin to thrombin directly, the reaction is very slow. In contrast, the reaction is accelerated a thousandfold if Factor Xa is in the presence of Factor V, calcium ions, and phospholipids.

The prothrombinase complex (Factor Xa, Factor V, calcium ions, and phospholipids) corresponds to a lipid micelle, with the activation occurring on an interface between a hydrophobic and a hydrophilic layer.

Prothrombin has a molecular weight of 70,000 daltons and has three to four carbohydrate side chains. The activation of prothrombin involves multiple cleavages of prothrombin by Xa or mixtures of Xa and thrombin (IIa) (Mann, 1974). Initially, prothrombin is cleaved to form intermediates 1 and 3. Intermediate 1 is subsequently cleaved to form intermediates 2 and 4. Finally, intermediate 2 is acted on by Xa to form a two-chain alpha-thrombin (Fig. 33-3).

The intermediate 3 segment serves in binding the prothrombin molecule to the pro-

thrombinase complex. This segment also acts as a potent inhibitor of the prothrombinase complex. Thus, intermediate 3 may act as a negative feedback regulator of thrombin generation.

The final series of reactions in the coagulation of blood involves the conversion of fibrinogen to fibrin and the insolubilization of the fibrin polymer. Fibrinogen is a glycoprotein with a molecular weight of 340,000 daltons. The molecule is composed of 3 pairs of polypeptide chains $\alpha(A)_2$, $\beta(B)_2$, and γ_2 (Blombäck, 1972). The three chains are cross-linked at the N-terminal portion of the molecule by disulfide bridges. Thus, the disulfide knot contains the N-terminal portion of each pair of chains and represents the site at which both halves of the fibrinogen molecule are joined.

Thrombin cleaves four arginyl-glycine bonds and splits off first a pair of fibrinopeptides A and then a pair of fibrinopeptides B from the amino terminal ends of α- and β-chains (Bailey, 1951, 1955). After the removal of fibrinopeptides, the fibrin monomers align themselves into a loose mesh and undergo hydrogen bonding. This fibrin polymer is soluble in 5M urea and 1 per cent monochloracetic acid. In addition, the venom of *Bothrops atrox* (Reptilase) and of the Malayan pit viper (Ancrod) can cleave fibrinopeptide A from fibrinogen with subsequent polymerization of the fibrin monomers (Blombäck, 1957; Pizzo, 1972).

This fibrin clot is made insoluble in 5M urea

and 1 per cent monochloracetic acid by the action of activated Factor XIII, a transamidase which catalyzes the reaction between ε-amino groups of lysine of one fibrin monomer and the γ-carboxamido groups of glutamine from another fibrin monomer (Pisano, 1972). Two chains line up in antiparallel fashion so that lysine is located opposite a glutamine residue. There are γ-γ and α-α cross-linkages (Chen, 1970). However, the γ-γ cross-links are primarily responsible for the stability of the fibrin clot in 5M urea and 1 per cent monochloracetic acid.

Factor XIII with a molecular weight of 320,000 daltons is composed of 2 α-chains (75,000 daltons) and two β-chains (85,000 daltons). Factor XIII is converted to Factor XIIIa through the proteolytic activity of thrombin, with release of a small molecular weight polypeptide (4,000 daltons) from the α-chain (Chung, 1972).

KINETICS OF COAGULATION FACTORS

The liver is the probable site of synthesis of all coagulation factors, with the possible exception of Factor VIII. Endothelial cells synthesize Factor VIII antigen and von Willebrand's factor. The exact site of synthesis of the procoagulant portion of Factor VIII remains unknown (Jaffe, 1973). In addition, there is evidence that the α-chain of Factor XIII, characteristically present in platelets, may be produced in megakaryocytes. However, plasma Factor XIII, containing both α- and β-chains, is probably synthesized in the liver (McDonagh, 1972).

Factors II, VII, IX, and X require vitamin K for their synthesis in the liver to a functional procoagulant (Suttie, 1973) (Fig. 33–4). Vitamin K has been shown to be necessary for the carboxylation of glutamic acid residues on precursor proteins to form γ-carboxyglutamyl residues (Suttie, 1977a). The evidence suggests that during the process of activation, Factors II, VII, IX, and X are bound to phospholipids, with Ca^{++} ion serving as a bridge between the

γ-carboxyglutamic acid residues on the procoagulants and negatively charged groups on the phospholipids. Without the carboxylation of glutamic acid residues or the presence of Ca^{++} ions, the precursor protein fails to bind to the phospholipid, and activation does not occur (Jackson, 1977). The precursor proteins are referred to as Proteins Induced by Vitamin K Absence (PIVKA proteins) (Hemker, 1968), and their presence in the plasma can be measured by immunologic techniques (Ganrot, 1968). Thus, the functional but not immunologic activity of Factors II, VII, IX, and X is reduced in patients deficient in vitamin K or in patients receiving coumarin drugs.

The plasma concentration of procoagulants is related to their rate of synthesis, rate of destruction, and distribution in the extravascular pool. The turnover of procoagulants can be measured by assaying the course of a transfused factor in a patient with a specific procoagulant deficiency or by assaying the loss of activity in the plasma of a purified factor labeled with a radioisotope. The biologic half-life of most factors has been measured in normal individuals, and this data is presented in Table 33–2.

NORMAL CONTROL MECHANISM OF COAGULATION

Normal physiologic and biochemical mechanisms are present to prevent continuous clot formation and to contain the size and spread of a thrombus once it has developed. The flow of blood removes inactivated procoagulants from a potential site of activation and dilutes activated procoagulants into a larger volume. The reticuloendothelial system and liver appear to remove activated procoagulants from the circulation. Procoagulants are also inhibited by the presence in the plasma of at least four inhibitors, including antithrombin III, $α_1$-antitrypsin, C_1 inactivators, and $α_2$-macroglobulin (Table 33–4).

Antithrombin III is a glycoprotein with a molecular weight of 65,000 daltons. It exists as a single polypeptide chain and migrates as an

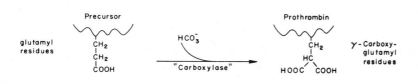

Figure 33–4. The vitamin K–dependent carboxylation reaction. (From Jackson, C. M., and Suttie, J. W.: Recent developments in understanding the mechanism of vitamin K and vitamin K-antagonistic drug action and the consequences of vitamin K action in blood coagulation. Prog. Hematol., *10*:333, 1977.)

Table 33–4. EFFECTS OF NATURALLY OCCURRING BIOCHEMICAL INHIBITORS*

	ANTITHROMBIN III	α_1-ANTITRYPSIN	C_1-INHIBITOR	α_2-MACROGLOBULIN
Factor XIIa	+	−	+	−
Factor XIa	+	+	+	−
Kallikrein	+	−	+	+
Plasminogen activator	?	−	−	+
Plasmin	+	+	+	+

*Modified from Kaplan, 1976. + indicates inhibitor is effective against the enzyme. − indicates inhibitor has no effect against active enzyme.

α_2-globulin. It neutralizes the action of Factors IXa, Xa, XIa, thrombin, and plasmin (Harpel, 1976). Arginine residues located on antithrombin III bind to a serine group on thrombin, thereby inhibiting the active site. Heparin binds to antithrombin III at ε-aminolysyl residues, causing a molecular alteration resulting in greater exposure of the arginine of antithrombin III (Fig. 33–5). Thus, the action of heparin accelerates the rate of thrombin inhibition by antithrombin III. Presumably, heparin also catalyzes the action of antithrombin III on Factors IXa, Xa, and XIa and plasmin.

Alpha$_1$-antitrypsin is a glycoprotein with a molecular weight of approximately 50,000 daltons which acts as a serine protease. Substrates for α_1-antitrypsin include Factor XIa, thrombin, plasmin, trypsin, chymotrypsin, and elastase (Bennett, 1977).

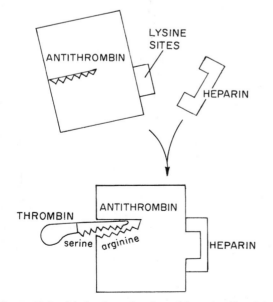

Figure 33–5. Mechanism of action of heparin. (Reprinted from Rosenberg, R. D.: Hemorrhagic disorders. I. Protein interactions of the clotting mechanism. *In* Beck, W. F. (ed.). Hematology, 2nd ed., 1977, by permission of the MIT Press, Cambridge, Massachusetts. Copyright 1977 by the Massachusetts Institute of Technology.)

C_1 inactivator is a glycoprotein with a molecular weight of 105,000 daltons. C_1 inactivator inhibits Factor XIIa and XIa and plasma kallikrein as well as C_1 esterase (Bennett, 1977).

Alpha$_2$-macroglobulin is a glycoprotein with a molecular weight of 725,000 daltons. It inhibits trypsin, thrombin, kallikrein, and chymotrypsin. In a manner similar to plasmin, α_2-macroglobulin can also digest fibrinogen. In addition, there is some evidence to suggest that plasmin may be a major substrate for α_2-macroglobulin (Harpel, 1976).

FIBRINOLYTIC SYSTEM

The fibrinolytic system has four components: plasminogen proactivator, plasminogen activators, plasminogen, and plasmin. Plasminogen proactivator is a plasma protein with a molecular weight of approximately 95,000 daltons. This inert protein is a substrate for the proteolytic activity of XIIa. Thus, plasminogen proactivator is converted to a plasminogen activator by the action of XIIa.

Plasminogen activators are a heterogeneous group of proteins which react with plasminogen to produce plasmin. Some of these activators are proteolytic enzymes found in lysosomes of most cells in the body. Other plasminogen activators are present in endothelial cells of blood vessels. A plasminogen activator known as urokinase can be found in the urine. Urokinase is a serine protease with a molecular weight of 54,000 daltons (Sherry, 1977). Following tissue destruction or vascular injury, plasminogen activators may be released into the blood.

Plasminogen is a single-chain protein with a molecular weight of 85,000 daltons. It circulates in the plasma at a concentration of 0.1 to 0.2 g/l and has a half-life of approximately 40 hours. Plasminogen is converted to plasmin by the action of plasminogen activators (Fig. 33–6). Proteolysis is accomplished by cleavage of arginine-valine and lysine-lysine bonds.

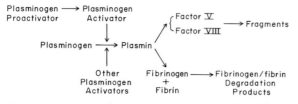

Figure 33–6. Interaction of the proteins of the plasminogen system.

Plasmin is a potent proteolytic enzyme which hydrolyzes the arginyl-lysyl bonds of fibrinogen and fibrin, resulting in the formation of fibrinogen/fibrin degradation products. In addition, plasmin also hydrolyzes Factors V and VIII and other serum proteins (Sherry, 1977).

Plasmin first cleaves a small polypeptide from the A chain of fibrinogen (Marder, 1971). This results in the formation of the X fragment with a molecular weight of approximately 270,000 daltons (Fig. 33–7). Plasmin further digests the X fragment with the production of a Y fragment (155,000 daltons) and a D fragment (83,000 daltons). Finally, the Y fragment is further split to form a second D fragment and an E fragment (50,000 daltons). The E fragment consists of the disulfide portion of the original fibrinogen molecule (Marder, 1974).

Fragments X, Y, D, and E are known as fibrinogen/fibrin degradation products. Fragment X can be acted upon by thrombin to form a fragile fibrin clot. The reaction occurs

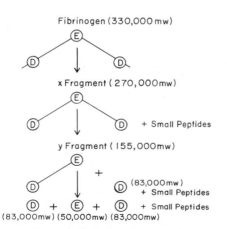

Figure 33–7. Diagram illustrating the proteolytic activity of plasmin on fibrinogen. See text. (Modified from Marder, 1968.)

slowly, delaying the formation of a clot. Fragments Y, D, and E do not form a clot (Fig. 33–7). However, fragments Y and D inhibit fibrin polymerization and E inhibits thrombin activity. In addition, fibrinogen/fibrin degradation products interfere with platelet function.

COAGULATION DISORDERS

INHERITED COAGULATION DISORDERS

Until the mid-1950's, it was the prevailing opinion that the inherited coagulopathies were due to an inability of the afflicted patients to synthesize normal amounts of a particular procoagulant. In 1956, Fantl demonstrated that one third of the patients with Christmas disease contained a plasma protein which cross-reacted with an antibody to Factor IX. Since that time similar findings have been verified in most of the inherited coagulopathies. It is now apparent that many of the inherited coagulopathies can be separated into at least two groups; patients unable to synthesize the deficient factor and patients unable to synthesize a biologically active procoagulant but able to produce a defective protein.

In the sections that follow, reference is made to the results of the general coagulation screening assays, the whole blood clotting time (p. 1155), the prothrombin time (p. 1156), the activated partial thromboplastin time (p. 1156), and the thrombin time (p. 1157). It may be useful to refer to the discussions of the principles and interpretations of these measurements and also to Figure 33–1 in order to visualize where they are involved in the coagulation mechanism.

AUTOSOMAL COAGULATION DISORDERS

Disorders of fibrinogen

Hereditary Afibrinogenemia. Hereditary afibrinogenemia is a disorder in which the plasma fibrinogen concentration is usually less than 0.05 g/l. It is a rare illness occurring in less than 0.5 per million individuals. Approximately 60 cases have been reported in the literature. The deficiency is inherited as an autosomal recessive trait, and more than 50 per cent of the patients are the offspring of consanguineous marriages. Heterozygotes are usually asymptomatic, and some have below-normal levels of fibrinogen (Ratnoff, 1972).

Hereditary afibrinogenemia is due to a diminished production of fibrinogen. In these patients the half-life of infused fibrinogen is usually normal, indicating no increased consumption of fibrinogen (Gitlin, 1953).

Patients with afibrinogenemia can have severe bleeding episodes. Hemorrhages tend to occur early in life, with bleeding from the umbilical cord or following circumcision. Hemorrhages tend to appear after minor trauma and eruption of deciduous teeth. Wound healing can be defective. Patients do not have hemarthrosis (Yamagata, 1968).

Laboratory studies usually show a lack of coagulation in most clotting assays. The bleeding time is prolonged in 50 per cent of cases. The thrombin time, prothrombin time, and partial thromboplastin time assays are prolonged and can be corrected by the addition of normal plasma. Fibrinogen cannot be demonstrated by clotting assays, immunologic methods, and heat-precipitable or salting-out techniques. Platelets from patients with afibrinogenemia show deficient platelet aggregation with ADP and epinephrine, decreased adhesiveness to glass beads, and occasionally a prolonged bleeding time (Weiss, 1971).

Hereditary Hypofibrinogenemia. Hereditary hypofibrinogenemia is also a very rare disorder. The fibrinogen levels usually range from 0.7 to 1.0 g/l. In some kinships the disorder is inherited as an autosomal recessive trait and in others as an autosomal dominant trait. Hereditary hypofibrinogenemia is a mild bleeding syndrome (Ratnoff, 1972). Since many individuals with hereditary hypofibrinogenemia have not been studied using a variety of immunologic and functional assays, some of the reported cases may represent heterozygotes of afibrinogenemia or even cases of dysfibrinogenemia.

Congenital Dysfibrinogenemia. As with other inherited coagulopathies, congenital dysfibrinogenemia is a rare disorder. Approximately 37 kinships have been recorded in the literature. The disorder is inherited as an autosomal trait.

Congenital dysfibrinogenemia is a heterogeneous disorder. Multiple alterations in fibrinogen structure exist. Ratnoff (1976) has divided the congenital dysfibrinogenemias into five groups (Table 33-5). There are cases of dysfibrinogenemia associated with (1) impaired release of fibrinopeptides by thrombin; (2) abnormal aggregation of fibrin monomers; (3) rapid thrombin time; (4) impaired fibrinogen cross-linkage; and (5) no known functional defect. In addition, some of the groups can be

Table 33-5. FUNCTIONAL CLASSIFICATION OF ABNORMAL FIBRINOGENS *

IMPAIRED PEPTIDE RELEASE	AGGREGATION DEFECTS	RAPID THROMBIN TIME	IMPAIRED CROSS-LINKAGE	FUNCTIONAL DEFECT UNKNOWN
Gissen	Manila	Oslo	Oklahoma	Vancouver
Cleveland II	Marburg		Tokyo	Iowa City
Baltimore	Paris II			Los Angeles
Detroit	Zurich I			Valencia
Bethesda I	St. Louis			Vienna
New York	Wiesbaden			Montreal II
Metz	Zurich II			
	Philadelphia			
	Montreal I			
	Leaven			
	Troyes			
	Alba/Geneva			
	Paris III			
	Paris I			
	Caracas			
	Nancy			
	Bethesda II			
	Buenos Aires			
	Cleveland I			
	Amsterdam			

* Modified from Ratnoff, 1976.

further subdivided based on the migration of the fibrinogens in an electromagnetic field. Some fibrinogens migrate normally, some anodally, and others cathodally.

In most patients the abnormality is discovered by chance. When symptoms exist, the hemorrhages are usually very mild. Individuals with disordered aggregation of fibrin monomers usually do not have a hemorrhagic tendency. In contrast, thrombotic episodes have been described in patients with fibrinogens Oslo, Baltimore, Paris II, Marburg, Paris III, and New York (Samama, 1977).

Laboratory studies usually reveal a prolonged prothrombin time, thrombin time, and reptilase clotting time. Plasma fibrinogen levels measured by a thrombin coagulation assay suggest low values. However, fibrinogen levels performed by immunologic methods are usually normal. In a few cases (fibrinogen Cleveland), both the coagulation and immunologic assays are reduced because of increased catabolism of the abnormal fibrinogen. In one kindred, an abnormal fibrinogen appeared to result in a rapid thrombin time and clinically excessive thrombosis (Egeberg, 1967). Two abnormal fibrinogens are characterized by defective fibrin polymer stabilization with solubility in 5M urea (Morton, 1970; Samori, 1975).

In the majority of cases the criterion for the diagnosis of dysfibrinogenemia is met when a prolonged thrombin clotting time is demonstrated on purified fibrinogen. The purification of fibrinogen, the measurement of fibrinopeptide release, and the analysis of fibrin monomer aggregation are usually performed in a coagulation research laboratory.

Congenital prothrombin deficiency

Congenital prothrombin deficiency is an extremely rare disorder inherited as an autosomal recessive trait. Two types of prothrombin deficiencies have been described. One type is characterized by diminished plasma concentration of procoagulant and antigenic material, indicating decreased synthesis of Factor II (Girolami, 1970b). The second group is recognized by diminished procoagulant activity but normal antigenic concentrations of prothrombin (Shapiro, 1969; Josso, 1971). These data suggest that in some cases there is synthesis of an abnormal prothrombin molecule.

Homozygous individuals usually have a functional prothrombin level of 10 per cent or less of normal. The bleeding manifestations of these patients include epistaxis, easy bruising, bleeding from gums, and bleeding after dental extractions. About one half of the patients have post-traumatic hemarthroses (Girolami, 1970b). The heterozygotes have a biologic activity of Factor II ranging from 40 to 60 per cent of normal and are asymptomatic.

Coagulation studies usually reveal normal bleeding time and thrombin time. The prothrombin and partial thromboplastin times are prolonged and can be corrected by incubation of an equal volume of patient's plasma with fresh plasma but not with serum or adsorbed plasma. The diagnosis of prothrombin deficiency can be documented by a specific factor assay.

Factor V deficiency (parahemophilia)

Congenital Factor V deficiency or parahemophilia was first described in 1947 by Owren. The disorder occurs in less than one per million individuals and is inherited either as an autosomal dominant with incomplete expressivity or as an autosomal recessive (Colman, 1976).

Parahemophilia may be due to deficient biosynthesis of Factor V protein, since antigenic material has not been found in the plasma of two affected individuals (Feinstein, 1970).

Patients with parahemophilia have a mild to moderately severe bleeding disorder. The most common symptoms include ecchymoses, epistaxes, oral hemorrhages, prolonged bleeding after minor lacerations, and menorrhagia (Freidman, 1961; Seeler, 1972).

Laboratory studies usually show a prolonged prothrombin time and partial thromboplastin time with a normal thrombin time. The prothrombin time can be corrected by mixing test plasma with an equal volume of adsorbed plasma or plasma from a patient on warfarin drugs, but not with aged serum. Factor V assays are performed using aged oxalated plasma or plasma from patients with parahemophilia as the substrate plasma.

Factor VII deficiency

Factor VII deficiency is a rare disorder (Alexander, 1951). Approximately 60 to 70 cases of hereditary Factor VII deficiency have been reported. The disorder is inherited as an autosomal recessive trait.

Studies employing immunodiffusion and antibody-neutralizing assays have disclosed that Factor VII deficiency is a heterogeneous disorder. Plasma from some patients contains material that cross-reacts with heterologous antiserum to Factor VII (Goodnight, 1971). Plasma from other patients has no Factor VII antigenic material (Prydz, 1965). These findings suggest that some patients make an abnormal Factor VII, whereas other patients fail to synthesize Factor VII.

Abnormal bleeding occurs in patients with a functional Factor VII procoagulant activity of 0 to 25 per cent of normal. Asymptomatic patients have Factor VII procoagulant levels between 25 and 75 per cent of normal. The most common hemorrhagic manifestations of this disorder include epistaxes, ecchymoses, menorrhagia, and post-partum and post-surgical hemorrhage (Marder, 1964).

The laboratory findings are characterized by a prolonged prothrombin time with a normal thrombin time and partial thromboplastin time. The prothrombin time can be corrected by mixing the patient's plasma with an equal volume of aged serum but not with adsorbed plasma. The Stypven time is normal (p. 1157). The diagnosis is confirmed by a specific Factor VII assay using plasma from a Factor VII-deficient patient as the substrate.

Factor X deficiency

Factor X deficiency was first described independently by Telfer (1956) and Hougie (1957). From the surnames of the two index families, the abnormalities have also been referred to as Prower-Stuart deficiency. The disorder is transmitted as an autosomal recessive trait (Lechler, 1965) and occurs in approximately one per million individuals. Immunologic and functional analysis of Factor X activity suggests that Factor X deficiency represents a heterogeneous group of abnormalities. As a result, some investigators have suggested that the term "Factor X defect" would be more appropriate. Immunodiffusion and antibody neutralization studies on plasma from patients with a functional Factor X deficiency have demonstrated that some plasma samples have normal antigenic concentrations of Factor X. Others have approximately one third normal levels, and still other plasmas have very low concentrations of Factor X antigen. In addition, there are at least two variants of abnormal Factor X present in the group of patients with the normal concentration of Factor X antigen. Plasma from the Prower kindred contains material which

cross-reacts with rabbit anti-human Factor X. This material fails to be activated by complete or partial thromboplastin or by Russell's viper venom (Stypven time) (Denson, 1970). The plasma from the Friuli kindred also contains cross-reacting material. In functional assays, however, Friuli Factor X can be activated by Russell's viper venom but not by thromboplastins (Girolami, 1970a). Plasma from the Stuart family exhibits no cross-reacting material and shows little activation with any reagent (Denson, 1970). Other variants of Factor X have been demonstrated by observing different patterns of reactivity between rabbit antibody against Factor X and plasma from Factor X-deficient patients in an Ouchterlony immunodiffusion chamber. Denson (1970) postulated at least five different variants of the Factor X.

Homozygous-deficient patients can have frequent epistaxes and increased bleeding following trauma and surgery. Prolonged hemorrhages after dental extraction have been described in several patients. Heterozygotes are usually asymptomatic.

The bleeding time and thrombin time are normal. The partial thromboplastin time and prothrombin time are prolonged and can be corrected by mixing with normal plasma and serum but not with adsorbed plasma. Equal mixtures of Factor VII-deficient plasma and test plasma produce a normal prothrombin time. Factor X assay using specific Factor X-deficient substrate plasma demonstrates the abnormality. The biologic activity of Factor X in homozygous-deficient patients is usually less than 10 per cent of normal, whereas in heterozygotes the level ranges from 40 to 68 per cent of normal.

Factor XI deficiency

The hereditary deficiency of Factor XI (plasma thromboplastin antecedent) is an uncommon hemorrhagic disorder (Rosenthal, 1955). Factor XI deficiency is inherited as an autosomal recessive trait. Homozygous individuals have a major defect with less than 20 per cent Factor XI and heterozygous individuals have a minor deficiency with levels ranging from 20 to 70 per cent (Leiba, 1965). This disorder has a relatively high frequency among persons of Jewish extraction.

Forbes (1972) found in a study of 10 patients with hereditary Factor XI deficiency that the plasma from all subjects contained diminished levels of Factor XI antigen. These data suggest that the abnormality is due to a decreased biosynthesis of Factor XI.

In general the bleeding diathesis observed in patients with Factor XI deficiency is milder than that in patients with Factor VIII or IX deficiencies. Spontaneous bleeding is rare; it tends to occur in homozygous rather than heterozygous subjects (Rapaport, 1961). Hemorrhages usually appear following dental extractions, trauma, or surgical procedures.

In the severe deficiencies, the whole blood clotting time and the activated partial thromboplastin time assays are prolonged (Rosenthal, 1955). In the mild disorders the whole blood clotting time and activated partial thromboplastin time are normal. The prothrombin time and thrombin time are normal. The bleeding time is rarely prolonged. The prolongation in the activated partial thromboplastin time is corrected by incubation of the patient's plasma with an equal volume of adsorbed plasma or serum. The diagnosis is dependent upon a Factor XI assay using Factor XI-deficient plasma as the substrate. Since contact with glass can activate Factor XI, it is preferable to collect blood samples in plastic tubes. In addition, the ability to discern deficiencies of Factor XI in plasma from heterozygous individuals may be lost following freezing of the plasma sample (Wintrobe, 1974).

Hageman trait

Hageman trait is a rare disorder occurring in approximately one individual per million. It is inherited as an autosomal recessive trait (Ratnoff, 1962). The disorder is probably due to a deficient biosynthesis of Factor XII, since immunologic studies show diminished Factor XII antigenic material in the plasma of patients with Hageman trait (Smink, 1967). With rare exceptions (Rizza, 1976), Factor XII deficiency is unassociated with hemorrhagic symptoms even after trauma, surgery, or childbirth (Ratnoff, 1966).

The prothrombin time and thrombin time assays are normal. The partial thromboplastin time is prolonged but is corrected by mixing patient's plasma in equal volumes with either serum or adsorbed plasma. The diagnosis is confirmed by performing a Factor XII assay. Normal levels of Factor XII vary from 36 to 152 per cent of normal (Ratnoff, 1972).

Fletcher factor deficiency

Fletcher factor deficiency is a rare disorder which is inherited as an autosomal recessive trait (Hathaway, 1965). The abnormality is due to a deficiency in prekallikrein (Wuepper, 1973). Plasma from subjects with this disorder shows diminished functional and antigenic activity of prekallikrein (Wuepper, 1973). As in Hageman trait, none of the subjects with Fletcher factor deficiency have excessive bleeding (Hathaway, 1965). The abnormality is characterized by a prolonged activated partial thromboplastin time which progressively normalizes as incubation times with surface-activating reagents are increased. The whole blood coagulation time is slightly prolonged in glass tubes and is moderately lengthened in plastic tubes. The prothrombin time and thrombin time assays are normal. *In vitro* studies of Fletcher factor-deficient plasma have indicated a diminished Hageman factor activation, fibrinolytic activity, kinin generation, and leukocyte chemotactic activity and decreased formation of permeability factor (Weiss, 1974).

Deficiency in high molecular weight kininogen

Plasma deficient in a coagulant factor has been reported in individuals with the surnames of Fitzgerald (Saito, 1975b), Flaujeac (Wuepper, 1975), and Williams (Colman, 1975). The disorder(s) is very rare and the mode of inheritance is not yet clear. However, it probably is transmitted as an autosomal recessive trait. Patients do not have a clinically significant bleeding disorder. Plasma from subjects with this abnormality have diminished activity of high molecular weight kininogen. In addition, plasma from some patients contains decreased amounts of low molecular weight kininogen as well as high molecular weight kininogen (Colman, 1975). Wuepper (1975) demonstrated that a small amount (9 per cent of normal) of material from Flaujeac plasma cross-reacted with sheep antiserum to human kininogen. When plasma from children of propositi were studied by electroimmunodiffusion, the average level of kininogen antigen was 51 per cent of normal, whereas the coagulation assay of kininogen revealed a mean value of 34 per cent. These data suggested that kininogen synthesis is diminished and that a small amount of an abnormal kininogen could be produced. The partial thromboplastin time is significantly prolonged and is not shortened by prolonged incubation with surface-activating reagents (Donaldson, 1976). Coagulation factor assay can be performed using plasma from deficient patients as a substrate. The prothrombin time and thrombin time are normal. In addition, plasma from affected subjects shows reduced kinin generation and fibrinolytic activity (Colman, 1976).

Passovoy factor deficiency

Hougie (1975) described a family five members of which had a mild hemorrhagic diathesis transmitted as an autosomal dominant disorder. The affected patients had prolonged partial thromboplastin times. The bleeding time, prothrombin time, thrombin time, and all known factor assays were within normal limits. The function of this defective or deficient coagulation factor is as yet unknown.

Factor XIII deficiency

Congenital Factor XIII deficiency is an uncommon disorder. In most families, the disorder is inherited as an autosomal recessive trait (Duckert, 1968). There is a high frequency of consanguinity in these families. Ratnoff (1972b) has postulated that the disorder is transmitted in a small subpopulation as a sex-linked disorder. Factor XIII is found in two forms, one in the plasma and the other in platelets. Plasma Factor XIII is a protein composed of two α-chains and two β-chains, whereas platelet Factor XIII is composed of only two α-chains. Factor XIII is activated by the enzymatic action of thrombin with the subsequent release of polypeptides from the α-chain. Israel (1973) has determined that patients with Factor XIII deficiency have no α-chain antigen but contain normal concentrations of β-chain antigen. These data suggest that the clot-stabilizing activity and thrombin-reactive sites are situated on the α-chain.

Duckert (1961) was the first to describe the hemorrhagic manifestations of Factor XIII deficiency. Patients with this disorder are often diagnosed during the neonatal period because of umbilical cord bleeding (Barry, 1965). There is a high frequency of hematomas, ecchymoses, and bleeding after minor trauma. Intracranial hemorrhages have occurred in 20 of 75 patients and have been responsible for the death of 4 of these individ-

uals (Duckert, 1972). In addition, wound healing is poor and sometimes leads to keloid formation.

In the laboratory, the plasma clot from a patient is soluble in 5M urea or 1 per cent monochloracetic acid. Specific quantitative assays for Factor XIII employ a technique measuring the covalent binding of monodansylcadaverine (a synthetic fluorescent amine) with casein by the action of activated Factor XIII; these assays are available in research laboratories. All other coagulation assays are normal. Utilizing a quantitative assay, heterozygous family members have Factor XIII levels intermediate between normal and homozygous values (McDonagh, 1974).

SEX-LINKED COAGULATION DISORDERS

Hemophilia A

Hemophilia A is inherited as a sex-linked recessive trait. It occurs in approximately one individual per 10,000. The disorder is the result of the synthesis of a dysfunctional Factor VIII molecule.

Factor VIII antigen is detected in about 10 per cent of hemophilic plasma when tested in a coagulation inhibitor neutralization assay utilizing a human antibody (Hoyer, 1968). However, normal levels of Factor VIII antigens are detected in virtually all cases of classic hemophilia when plasma is tested with an antibody raised in rabbits, using either the electroimmunoassay or a radioimmunoassay (Zimmerman, 1975; Hoyer, 1972). It now appears that the human antibody binds to a low molecular weight protein moiety responsible for the coagulant activity of Factor VIII. In contrast, the rabbit antibody reacts with a high molecular weight protein moiety which contains the von Willebrand's factor (Bloom, 1977b). The latter is necessary for the control of the bleeding time, platelet retention on glass beads, and ristocetin-induced platelet aggregation (Fig. 33-8). It is not yet certain if these two proteins are one molecule, two separate molecules, or a molecular complex (Bloom, 1977a).

Severe cases of hemophilia have less than 1 per cent functional Factor VIII (Table 33-6). These individuals have spontaneous hemorrhage early in childhood. They suffer from multiple hemarthroses which frequently result in ankylosis of large joints and destruction of

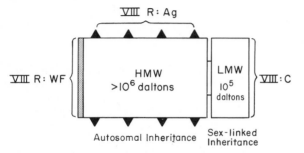

Figure 33–8. Diagram representing the Factor VIII complex. HMW represents the high molecular weight fragment and LMW the low molecular weight fragment. The Factor VIII procoagulant portion (VIII:C) can contain determinants that cross-react with homologous antibody. The Factor VIII-related antigen (VIII R:Ag) represents that portion of the HMW fragment which cross-reacts with heterologous antibodies. Von Willebrand's factor (VIII R:WF) corrects for prolonged bleeding time, abnormal platelet retention on glass beads, and abnormal ristocetin-induced platelet aggregation. (Redrawn from Meyer, 1977.)

small articulations. Spontaneous hemorrhages may occur into subcutaneous areas, intramuscular tissue, retroperitoneal compartments, gastrointestinal and genitourinary systems, and the brain. In moderately severe cases functional Factor VIII levels vary from 1 to 5 per cent of normal. In these individuals spontaneous bleeding, hemarthroses, and ankylosis are uncommon. However, patients may suffer serious hemorrhages following minor traumatic experiences. Mildly affected individuals (Factor VIII 5 to 25 per cent) rarely suffer bleeding episodes unless challenged by major surgery or trauma. Carrier females have an average Factor VIII level of 50 per cent of normal (Zimmerman, 1971). These women are usually free of the clinical manifestations of the bleeding disorder.

The bleeding time and the prothrombin time are normal. The whole blood clotting time is prolonged only in patients severely affected by the disorder. The partial thromboplastin time is prolonged in patients with hemophilia but usually normal in the carrier females. The prolonged partial thromboplastin time is corrected by incubating the patient's plasma with an equal mixture of adsorbed plasma but not with aged serum. The Factor VIII procoagulant assay shows reduced function, but Factor VIII antigen is present in normal amounts when tested with heterologous antiserum (Zimmerman, 1971). The marked discordance between the level of Factor VIII procoagulant and Factor VIII antigen (Factor VIII procoagulant/Factor VIII antigen ratio $\cong$ 0.01) serves to distinguish hemophilia A from severe von Willebrand's disease, in which both Factor VIII procoagulant and Factor VIII antigen levels are decreased (Factor VIII procoagulant/Factor VIII antigen ratio $\cong$ 1) (Meyer, 1977) (Fig. 33–9).

The measurement of Factor VIII procoagulant levels is not a reliable assay in the identification of carrier females, since many normal individuals have Factor VIII levels of 50 to 60 per cent. However, the availability of techniques which measure the level of Factor VIII antigen has greatly improved the ability to detect the carrier state. In normal individuals the ratio of Factor VIII procoagulant activity to Factor VIII antigen is approximately 1.0 but is only 0.5 in the carrier state. In von Willebrand's disease the Factor VIII procoagulant to Factor VIII antigen ratio may be significantly higher than that observed in normals (Chun-Yet Lian, 1976). Utilizing the ratio of Factor VIII procoagulant to Factor VIII antigen, it is possible to correctly classify from 72 to 94 per cent of female carriers (Klein, 1977).

In approximately 8 per cent of patients with hemophilia, an antibody will develop with

Table 33–6. LABORATORY FINDINGS IN HEMOPHILIA A

SEVERITY OF DISEASE	WHOLE BLOOD CLOTTING TIME	PARTIAL THROMBO-PLASTIN TIME (PTT)	PTT CORRECTED BY		FACTOR VIII ASSAY(%)*	FACTOR VIII ANTIGEN(%)*
			AGED SERUM	ADSORBED PLASMA		
Severe	prolonged	prolonged	no	yes	1	50–150
Moderate	normal	prolonged	no	yes	1–5	50–150
Mild	normal	prolonged	no	yes	5–25	50–150
Carriers	normal	normal	–	–	25–75	50–150

*Per cent of reference value (pooled normal plasma). Normal range 50 to 150 per cent.

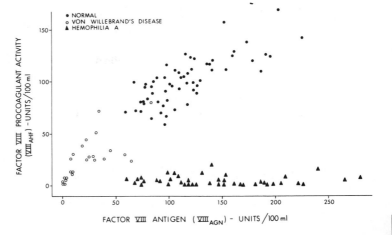

Figure 33-9. Comparison of Factor VIII procoagulant activity (VIII AHF) and Factor VIII antigen (VIII AGN). Data are given for 59 normal plasmas, 42 plasmas from patients with hemophilia A, and 24 plasmas from von Willebrand's disease. VIII AHF was measured by a one-stage assay; VIII AGN was measured by radioimmunoassay. (From Hoyer, L. W.: von Willebrand's disease. Prog. Hemostas. Thromb., 3:231–287, 1976.)

specificity against Factor VIII. The antibody is usually of the IgG class (Strauss, 1967), gamma G_3 and/or G_4 subclass (Andersen, 1968). The inhibitor is best demonstrated at 37°C. (p. 1162). In addition, test plasma should be incubated with pooled normal plasma for at least 60 minutes to demonstrate the presence of this inhibitor. The prolongation of partial thromboplastin time or the lack of response following adequate therapy may be the first sign of the presence of an inhibitor.

It is important to identify hemophilic patients with circulating antibodies against antihemophilic globulin because a high titer makes a patient refractory to therapy with cryoprecipitate and Factor VIII concentrates.

Christmas disease
(hemophilia B; Factor IX deficiency)

Christmas disease is inherited as a sex-linked recessive trait. It occurs in approximately one individual per 75,000 to 85,000. The clinical manifestations of Christmas disease are identical to those of hemophilia A (Aggeler, 1952; Biggs, 1952). Christmas disease is caused by any of several abnormal variants of the Factor IX molecule. Fantl (1956) was the first to describe a patient whose plasma contained greater Factor IX antigenic material (using an antibody neutralization assay) than Factor IX procoagulant activity. Hougie (1967) described a variant of Christmas disease called hemophilia B_m. These patients were distinguished from other patients with Christmas disease by a prolonged prothrombin time using thromboplastin prepared from bovine brain. He postulated that an abnormal Factor IX molecule was causing the

prolongation of bovine thromboplastin time. Kasper (1977) observed at least six groups of Christmas disease patients. Groups were determined on the basis of plasma level of Factor IX procoagulant activity, Factor IX antigen activity, and the bovine thromboplastin time (Table 33-7). The antibody neutralization assay using human antibody to Factor IX measured an equivalent concentration of Factor IX antigenic material as did the electroimmunoassay using rabbit anti-human Factor IX antibody. Kasper (1977) indicated that only one third of 92 hemophilia B patients had Factor IX antigen excess. In contrast, Meyer (1972) demonstrated antigenic Factor IX material in 21 of 22 hemophilia B patients using a rabbit antibody to Factor IX, whereas only 9 to 21 patients had antigenic material when measured against a human antibody.

Denson (1968) and Kasper (1977) demonstrated that incubation of hemophilia B_m plasma with a human or bovine Factor IX antibody abolishes the prolongation of bovine thromboplastin time. This supports Hougie's original hypothesis that the presence of an abnormal Factor IX produces the prolonged bovine thromboplastin time.

Veltkamp (1970) observed a form of Christmas disease (hemophilia B Leyden) with the presence of cross-reacting material to human antibody. A striking feature in this variant was the disappearance of bleeding symptoms paralleled by a rise in Factor IX activity with increasing age of the patients.

More recently a variant of Factor IX (Factor IX Chapel Hill) has been described (Roberts, 1975a) which, upon activation, does not undergo a reduction in molecular weight.

In the laboratory diagnosis of Christmas

Table 33-7. CLASSIFICATION OF PATIENTS WITH FUNCTIONAL FACTOR IX DEFICIENCY*

GROUP NO.	DEFICIENCY OF CLOTTING ACTIVITY	BOVINE THROMBOPLASTIN TIME	RANGE OF IMMUNOLOGIC ACTIVITY	RATIO OF CLOTTING ACTIVITY TO IMMUNOLOGIC ACTIVITY
I	Severe or moderate	Greatly prolonged	Normal	Severely decreased
II	Severe or moderate	Slightly prolonged	Slightly decreased to normal	Moderately to severely decreased
III	Severe or moderate	Normal	Slightly decreased to normal	Moderately to severely decreased
IV	Severe or moderate	Normal	Severely decreased	Normal
V	Mild	Normal	Slightly decreased to normal	Moderately decreased
VI	Mild	Normal	Moderately decreased	Normal

*Modified from Kasper, C. K., Østerud, B., Minyami, J. Y., Shonick, W., and Rapaport, S. I.: Hemophilia B: Characterization of genetic variants and detection of carriers. Blood, 50:351, 1977.

disease, the bleeding time, prothrombin time, and thrombin time are normal. The partial thromboplastin time is prolonged but is corrected by incubating the patient's plasma with an equal volume of serum. A specific Factor IX procoagulant assay, using plasma from a patient with known Christmas disease as the substrate, shows reduced Factor IX levels.

In approximately 7 per cent of patients with Christmas disease there develops an antibody to Factor IX (Weiss, 1975). These antibodies have been described as polyclonal (Reisner, 1977) and as monoclonal IgG_4 (Pike, 1972) in studies from the same laboratory. It is important to identify Christmas disease patients with Factor IX antibody because replacement therapy is generally reserved for severe hemorrhages.

Identification of the carrier state in Christmas disease is not as precise as in hemophilia A because approximately two thirds of carriers do not produce excessive Factor IX antigen. Although the carrier state is usually associated with reduced levels of functional Factor IX (Didisheim, 1962), normal levels of Christmas factor are not infrequent. A detailed analysis of the identification of the carrier state is provided by Kasper (1977).

ACQUIRED COAGULATION DISORDERS

VITAMIN K-DEFICIENT STATES

Vitamin K is necessary for the activity of a hepatic carboxylase, which is essential for the conversion of precursor proteins of Factors II, VII, IX, and X into biologically active procoagulants (Suttie, 1977a and b). When vitamin K is deficient, the liver synthesizes dysfunctional procoagulant proteins which can be detected by immunologic methods and can act as inhibitors of coagulation (Tullis, 1977).

Vitamin K is obtained from the diet and the synthetic action of intestinal bacteria. Vitamin K is fat-soluble and requires the presence of bile acid for absorption (Bowie, 1977).

Vitamin K deficient states are associated with a variety of disorders. *Hemorrhagic disease of the newborn* is a condition which occurs in 3- to 5-day-old infants. The disorder is characterized by bleeding from the gastrointestinal tract, umbilical stump, and skin. In untreated cases the fatality rate ranges from 5 to 30 per cent (Shapiro, 1977b). Between 0.1 and 1 mg of water-soluble vitamin K can prevent the disorder (Donaldson, 1974). Large doses of synthetic vitamin K, however, can result in hemolytic anemia.

Vitamin K deficiency has been described in sprue, cystic fibrosis, biliary obstruction, and cases of chronic diarrhea. Malnourished patients who receive antibiotics which sterilize the intestine may become vitamin K-deficient. In addition, warfarin and other coumarin drugs interfere with the function of vitamin K in the synthesis of prothrombin complex procoagulants (Bowie, 1977).

Coagulation assays include prolonged prothrombin and partial thromboplastin times but normal thrombin time. The prothrombin time and partial thromboplastin time are corrected by mixing an equal volume of normal or aged plasma to the test plasma. Adsorbed plasma will not correct the prolonged coagulation assays. Factor analyses reveal decreased levels of procoagulants II, VII, IX, and X. All coagulation assays return to normal following vitamin K therapy.

COAGULATION ABNORMALITIES ASSOCIATED WITH LIVER DISEASE

Bleeding frequently occurs in patients with severe liver disease. Clotting abnormalities associated with hepatic dysfunction are markedly diverse because the liver plays a variety of roles in the coagulation system. The liver is the site of synthesis of most if not all coagulation factors. Plasminogen, antithrombins, and antiplasmins are also synthesized in the liver. In addition, the liver has an important role in removing activated coagulation factors from the circulation (Roberts, 1972).

As hepatic dysfunction develops, there is a gradual decrease in Factors II, VII, IX, and X (vitamin K-dependent factors). In patients with acute hepatic failure, a good correlation exists between Factor VII level and recovery (Dymock, 1975). Patients with Factor VII activity exceeding 8 per cent survived, whereas others died. Factor VII is also shown to be diminished in other liver disorders (Green, 1976a).

In more severe hepatic disease, Factor V levels tend to decrease in the plasma. Factor V levels, however, are not a dependable measurement for assessing prognosis in acute liver failure. Factor V levels may be raised with acute inflammation, early hepatitis, and cholestasis. When hepatic dysfunction is associated with diffuse intravascular coagulation (DIC) and fibrinolysis, however, Factor V levels are reduced (Poller, 1977).

Factor VIII procoagulant and Factor VIII antigenic activities are elevated in patients with advanced cirrhosis (Green, 1974). In over 50 per cent of the cases, the elevation of Factor VIII antigen was significantly higher than that of procoagulant activity. The cause of the elevated Factor VIII in cirrhosis is not known. It may be due to (1) increased production related to a stress response, (2) increased release of Factor VIII from damaged hepatic cells, or (3) decreased catabolism of Factor VIII.

Green (1976b) described a high frequency of abnormal fibrin polymerization in patients with hepatic cirrhosis, acute liver failure, and chronic active liver disease. The disorder is suspected when there exists a prolongation of thrombin time with normal fibrinogen level. The diagnosis is confirmed by the demonstration of reduced clot opacity following the addition of reptilase to patients' plasma. Clinical improvement of the liver disease correlates with normalization of fibrin polymerization. The abnormalities are not observed in patients with surgical obstructive jaundice.

Primary fibrinolysis or fibrinolysis secondary to DIC is increased in some patients with hepatic disease (Poller, 1977). Primary fibrinolysis may arise from diminished synthesis of plasmin inhibitors by the liver; it is discussed on page 1149. In addition, DIC has been described in a variety of liver disorders (Horder, 1969).

Acquired dysfibrinogenemia has been described in the plasma of some patients with severe hepatic disease. Laboratory analysis usually reveals a prolonged thrombin time and reptilase clotting time (p. 1139). Reduced levels of D-galactose and increased amounts of sialic acid have been described in some of these abnormal fibrinogens. These results suggest a role for a carbohydrate moiety in conversion of fibrinogen to fibrin (Poller, 1977).

Thrombocytopenia is a common complication of liver disease. In most cases it is due to hypersplenism. Qualitative platelet abnormalities have also been described (Thomas, 1967).

DIFFUSE INTRAVASCULAR COAGULATION

Diffuse intravascular coagulation (DIC) is a hemorrhagic syndrome which occurs following the uncontrolled activation of procoagulants and fibrinolytic enzymes in the microvasculature. In this disorder fibrin is deposited in small vessels, causing tissue injury or necrosis (Rapaport, 1977). Platelets and procoagulants are consumed by the coagulation process, depleting their levels in the blood (Rodriguez-Erdmann, 1965). The disorder is further complicated by the presence of plasmin, a powerful proteolytic enzyme. Plasmin digests fibrinogen and fibrin clots, releasing fibrinogen/fibrin degradation products (FDP) which inhibit fibrin polymerization.

DIC can be localized or generalized. Renal allograft rejection is associated with intravascular coagulation localized to one organ. In contrast, intravascular coagulation occurring in malignancies usually involves multiple organs (Simpson, 1973).

DIC can be acute or chronic. In acute DIC the patient is profoundly ill and is usually bleeding. Multiple coagulation assays show marked abnormalities. In chronic DIC, the bleeding diathesis is less severe and the illness has a longer course. Although the procoagulant levels in the blood can be normal, some degree of thrombocytopenia is usually present (Kwaan, 1972).

Pathophysiology

Activation of Clotting. Diffuse intravascular coagulation (DIC) may be initiated by activation of the extrinsic or intrinsic coagulation system.

The extrinsic system is activated by the release of tissue thromboplastins from leukocytes, such as seen in sepsis and progranulocytic leukemia. Necrotic or injured tissues which result from a variety of disorders (Table 33-8) may release tissue thromboplastins into the blood.

Table 33-8. DISORDERS ASSOCIATED WITH DIFFUSE INTRAVASCULAR COAGULATION (DIC)

1. Infectious disease
   Bacterial (gram-negative and gram-positive septicemia)
   Mycotic (disseminated aspergillosis)
   Rickettsial (Rocky Mountain spotted fever)
   Viral (Korean hemorrhagic fever)
   Parasitic (*Plasmodium falciparum* malaria)
2. Malignant disorders
   Acute progranulocytic leukemia
   Metastatic carcinoma
3. Liver disease
   Severe hepatic necrosis
   Severe hepatic cirrhosis
4. Obstetrical disorders
   Amniotic fluid embolism
   Abruptio placentae
   Retained dead fetus
5. Neonatal disorders
   Intrauterine infections
   Idiopathic respiratory distress syndrome
   DIC in infant following abruptio placentae
6. Vascular Disorders
   Giant hemangioma
   Arterial aneurysms
   Pulmonary embolism
   Allergic vasculitis
   Cyanotic congenital heart disease
7. Miscellaneous disorders
   Shock
   Heatstroke
   Burns
   Snake venom

The intrinsic clotting system can be activated by damaged blood vessels and by the presence of endotoxins. In a variety of immunologic or infectious vasculitides, the damaged vascular surfaces can initiate clotting through activation of Hageman factor and aggregation of platelets by exposure to subendothelial collagen (Cash, 1977). Endotoxin directly activates Factor XII. In addition, endotoxins produce extensive endothelial vascular damage. Contact of the blood to exposed collagen then leads to the activation of Factor XII. Endotoxin may also cause a platelet injury, resulting in the release of platelet factor 3.

Deposition of Fibrin. The activation of procoagulants and platelets can result in the deposition of fibrin in the microvasculature. There is marked variation in the amount and localization of the fibrin deposits. The rate of blood flow, the extent of injury of the microvasculature, the blood levels of corticosteroids and catecholamines, the efficiency of local fibrinolysis, and the state of activity of reticuloendothelial system are factors which affect the degree of fibrin deposition in small vessels.

Fibrin deposition can produce varying degrees of tissue ischemia. In addition, erythrocytes can be fragmented by passage through fibrin strands, producing a hemolytic anemia.

Hemostatic Alterations. DIC alters the concentration of platelets, plasma procoagulants, and proteins associated with the fibrinolytic system. In acute DIC, there is usually a marked depletion in the consumable factors (I, V, VIII, and XIII) and platelets (Rodriguez-Erdmann, 1965; Harker, 1972). Sometimes the concentration of other circulating procoagulants is also reduced (Deykin, 1970).

In addition, the presence of fibrin in the microvasculature brings about the release of plasminogen activator from the endothelium. Plasminogen activator converts plasminogen to plasmin. The action of plasmin on fibrinogen and fibrin causes the release of fibrinogen/fibrin degradation products. These fragments form complexes with fibrin monomers and prevent fibrin polymerization. Thus, secondary fibrinolysis results in reduced levels of plasminogen and fibrinogen but elevated levels of fibrinogen/fibrin degradation products (Rapaport, 1977).

Clinical presentation

Two main forms of the disorder are observed. Acute DIC occurs in desperately ill patients and lasts from a few hours to days.

Subacute or chronic DIC occurs in chronically ill patients and ranges from days to weeks in duration (Mersky, 1967).

In acute DIC, bleeding and excessive bruising are common. The degree of bleeding is proportional to the degree of procoagulant deficiencies and thrombocytopenia. The presence of fibrin thrombi in small vessels also accounts for a portion of the clinical symptomatology. Fibrin thrombi in renal capillaries may result in renal cortical necrosis, and fibrin thrombi in the pulmonary vessels can result in pulmonary insufficiency. In addition, microangiopathic hemolytic anemia is a rare consequence of DIC.

In subacute or chronic DIC, the plasma levels of procoagulants may be normal or elevated. Thrombocytopenia is usually present but not as marked as in the acute form. Bleeding is less severe. Most patients with chronic DIC have an underlying malignant disorder.

Laboratory diagnosis

Routine laboratory assays help confirm the clinical impression of DIC (Table 33-9). The peripheral blood film usually indicates a thrombocytopenia, a finding which should be verified by a platelet count. The granulocyte count can be elevated, normal, or decreased. Toxic granulation of myeloid cells is sometimes present. In a small percentage of cases, fragmentation of erythrocytes, reticulocytosis, and leukoerythroblastosis may be present.

The whole blood clotting time, thrombin time, prothrombin time, and partial thromboplastin time are prolonged. When patient's plasma is mixed with an equal volume of pooled normal plasma, correction of thrombin time does not occur, owing to the presence of FDP. Fibrinogen and Factors V, VIII, and XIII are usually markedly reduced (Abildgaard, 1969).

Fibrinogen/fibrin degradation products in the serum (p. 1161) are elevated. The presence of fibrin monomers is demonstrated by a positive plasma paracoagulation assay (p. 1162). The whole blood clot lysis and euglobulin clot lysis assays (p. 1160) are usually normal.

The diagnosis of DIC can be difficult to verify at times. However, in an extremely ill patient, the diagnosis is most likely in the presence of thrombocytopenia, prolonged thrombin, prothrombin, and partial thromboplastin times, low fibrinogen, and elevated fibrinogen/fibrin degradation products. Sequential performance of these measurements will usually clarify an ambiguous set of results.

PRIMARY FIBRINOLYSIS

Primary fibrinolysis is a rare disorder. Plasminogen is present in human plasma in a concentration of 0.1 to 0.2 g/l (Davidson, 1977). It is converted to plasmin by the action of plasminogen activators when it is released from any of a number of tissues, especially blood vessel endothelium and prostate gland. Normally these plasminogen activators are inhibited by antiactivators synthesized in the liver. In certain disorders the balance between

Table 33-9. COMPARISON OF LABORATORY RESULTS IN DIFFUSE INTRAVASCULAR COAGULATION (DIC) AND IN PRIMARY FIBRINOLYSIS

ASSAY	ACUTE DIC	CHRONIC DIC	PRIMARY FIBRINOLYSIS
Platelet count	Low	Moderately low	Normal
Prothrombin time	Prolonged	Slightly prolonged	Prolonged
Partial thromboplastin time	Prolonged	Slightly prolonged	Prolonged
Thrombin time	Prolonged	Normal to slightly prolonged	Prolonged
Fibrinogen	Low	Slightly decreased to elevated	Low
Factor V	Low	Usually normal	Low
Factor VIII	Low	Usually normal	Low
Paracoagulation tests	Positive	Positive	Negative
Whole blood clot lysis	Normal or long	Normal	Rapid
Euglobulin clot lysis	Normal or long	Normal	Rapid
Fibrin plate lysis	Normal or slightly increased	Normal	Markedly increased
Fibrinogen/fibrin degradation products	Usually increased	Increased	Markedly increased

plasminogen activators and inhibitors is disturbed, as in some cases of carcinoma or hepatic insufficiency, and excessive fibrinolytic activity exists (Tagnon, 1953; Ratnoff, 1952).

The clinical hemorrhagic manifestations of primary fibrinolysis are similar to those of DIC. Laboratory differences are present, however (Table 33-9). In primary fibrinolysis, thrombocytopenia is unusual. The plasma protamine paracoagulation assay for fibrin monomers is negative. The whole blood clot lysis time, euglobulin lysis time, and fibrin plate assay indicate elevated levels of circulating plasmin. Since DIC and primary fibrinolysis may occur together, diagnostic difficulties arise under these circumstances.

PATHOLOGIC INHIBITION OF BLOOD COAGULATION

Natural inhibitors of coagulation include antithrombin III, α_2-macroglobulin, α_1-antitrypsin, and C_1 inactivator. These plasma proteins help regulate the normal concentration of activated procoagulants in blood. In contrast, acquired circulating inhibitors are present in some pathologic conditions and may result in a bleeding diathesis.

FACTOR VIII INHIBITORS

Factor VIII inhibitors are the most frequent of the pathologic anticoagulants. Approximately 8 per cent of hemophilic patients develop an inhibitor to Factor VIII. Inhibitors usually arise in severe hemophiliacs. The inhibitor is usually an IgG immunoglobulin. Most inhibitors in hemophilic individuals are of a single light chain type (Shapiro, 1968). Heavy chain typing shows a predominance of IgG_4 and IgG_3 subtypes (Shapiro, 1977a). The development of Factor VIII antibodies in hemophilic patients is related to frequency of transfusion with Factor VIII. After antibody has been detected, it tends to remain for prolonged periods of time. Infusion of Factor VIII is usually followed by rise in titer of Factor VIII antibody in 3 to 4 days.

Factor VIII inhibitors have been described in postpartum women, usually after the birth of their firstborn (Greenwood, 1967; Nilsson, 1958). The inhibitor may result in clinically significant bleeding, at times life-threatening. After a variable period of time, spontaneous disappearance of the inhibitor is characteristic of this disorder (Margolius, 1961).

Factor VIII inhibitors have been described in patients with collagen vascular disease and immunologic disorders (Robboy, 1970). In addition, Factor VIII inhibitors sometimes arise in elderly individuals without known underlying disease (Feinstein, 1972).

ACQUIRED VON WILLEBRAND'S DISEASE

At least 10 cases of acquired von Willebrand's disease have been reported. The diagnoses were based on the presence of prolonged bleeding time, low levels of procoagulant Factor VIII, and reduced platelet retention to glass beads in patients without a personal or family history of von Willebrand's disease (Mant, 1973; Handin, 1976; Simone, 1968; Ingram, 1973; Stableforth, 1976). Most patients had an underlying immunologic or collagen vascular disorder. In seven cases the anticoagulant did not inhibit the factor VIII procoagulant. One case (Handin, 1976) showed an inhibitor against von Willebrand's factor and in another case (Stableforth, 1976), antibodies were directed against Factor VIII procoagulant, Factor VIII antigen, and von Willebrand's factor. In one case the inhibitor was an IgG immunoglobulin (Handin, 1976) and in another the inhibitor was an IgG_3 λ paraprotein (Mant, 1973).

FACTOR IX INHIBITORS

Approximately 7 per cent of patients with Christmas disease develop inhibitors to Factor IX. The inhibitors have been described chemically as IgG immunoglobulins. One inhibitor was shown to be restricted to only IgG_4 λ immunoglobulin (Pike, 1972). However, in an additional case, the inhibitor was shown to be more heterogeneous (Reisner, 1977). The development of Factor IX antibody is correlated with intravenous exposure of Factor IX in patients with severe Christmas disease. The antibody titer may rise following transfusion of Factor IX.

In a few cases, Factor IX inhibitors have been described in patients with underlying disorders (Shapiro, 1975); in over 30 per cent of these, the patients had a collagen-vascular disease.

FACTOR V INHIBITORS

Acquired inhibitors to Factor V occur rarely in patients with no previous history of bleeding diathesis (Feinstein, 1970). Symptoms may vary from mild to severe. The clinical effects of the inhibitor are usually short-lived. Development of an inhibitor to Factor V is associated with exposure to streptomycin or major surgery. The inhibitor is usually an IgG immunoglobulin (Shapiro, 1975).

OTHER INHIBITORS

Acquired inhibitors have been described with specificity against fibrinogen and Factors X, XI, XII, and XIII (Bidwell, 1969; Roberts, 1975b). Underlying disorders include systemic lupus erythematosus, ill-defined collagen vascular diseases, infectious disorders, and malignancies. In some cases no primary disease is evident.

LUPUS INHIBITOR

Ten to fifty per cent of patients with systemic lupus erythematosus develop a coagulation inhibitor. In most cases the inhibitor is an IgG immunoglobulin, but in some cases an IgM immunoglobulin or both IgG and IgM immunoglobulins have been found. The specificity of the antibody is probably directed against phospholipid, thus inhibiting coagulation reactions in which phospholipid is required. Most patients with lupus inhibitor do not have abnormal bleeding (Feinstein, 1972).

Clinically significant hemorrhage in patients with lupus inhibitor is usually due to associated decrease of Factor II (prothrombin) and/or thrombocytopenia.

Laboratory measurements show a prolonged partial thromboplastin time and often a slightly prolonged prothrombin time. The thrombin time is usually normal. A mixture of equal volumes of normal plasma and test plasma does not correct the prolonged partial thromboplastin time. Prothrombin time assays performed with diluted thromboplastin show abnormally prolonged values. Specific procoagulant assays of Factors XII, XI, IX, and VIII may show erroneously low values if the one-stage assay is employed (Feinstein, 1972).

INHIBITORS ASSOCIATED WITH PARAPROTEINEMIAS

A variety of hemostatic abnormalities have been described in patients with multiple myeloma or Waldenström's macroglobulinemia (Perkins, 1970; Lackner, 1973). Prolonged bleeding time and abnormal platelet function assays have been described. Prolonged thrombin time, prothrombin time, and partial thromboplastin time assays are not uncommon (Perkins, 1970). There may be slight to moderate depression of most coagulation factors. The defect is probably due to a physiochemical interaction between the paraprotein and circulating procoagulants. The most frequently observed abnormality is the prolongation of the thrombin time, which appears to be due to the interference of fibrin polymerization by the paraprotein (Lackner, 1970). This results in formation of a structurally abnormal gelatinous clot (Coleman, 1972; Davey, 1976).

Clinically significant hemorrhage is unusual in these patients. Bleeding appears to correlate better with the elevated levels of blood viscosity, prolongation of bleeding time, and decreased platelet adhesiveness assays than with abnormal clotting assays (Perkins, 1970). Plasmapheresis is helpful in improving hemostasis.

THE LABORATORY MONITORING OF HEPARIN AND COUMARIN THERAPY

HEPARIN

Heparin is an acid mucopolysaccharide with a molecular weight of approximately 12,000 daltons. It is composed of uronic acid and glucosamine subunits (Lindahl, 1977). Heparin is normally present in mast cells located in the liver, lung, and intestine of man and in a variety of animals (Jaques, 1977).

Heparin is a powerful anticoagulant. Its action is to catalyze the neutralizing effects of antithrombin III on Xa, XIa, IXa, thrombin, and plasmin (Harpel, 1976). Heparin also inhibits platelet aggregation induced by thrombin.

Heparin is removed from the circulation through renal clearance and hepatic inactivation. The half-life of heparin in the blood is usually 90 minutes, with a range of 30 to 360 minutes (Genton, 1974). The half-life is dose-dependent. When 3,000 units of heparin is injected intravenously the half-life is 40 minutes, but when 10,000 units is given intravenously the half-life extends from 69 to 83 minutes.

Because heparin action neutralizes multiple factors, several clotting assays are prolonged.

It is typical to find prolongation of the whole blood clotting time, plasma recalcification time, partial thromboplastin time, prothrombin time, and thrombin time assays. However, there probably is no completely satisfactory assay for monitoring the *in vivo* effects of heparin. In fact, some investigators claim that it is not necessary to regulate heparin dosage based on any laboratory assay (Wessler, 1976). Traditionally, most physicians agree that sufficient heparin should be given to prolong the whole blood clotting time $1\frac{1}{2}$ to 3 times the control value (Wintrobe, 1974). Unfortunately, the whole blood clotting time lacks precision, and, at therapeutic levels of heparin, it requires 30 to 45 minutes for completion.

The activated partial thromboplastin time has gained popularity as an effective assay for following patients on heparin. The activated partial thromboplastin time is more reproducible and has a more rapid endpoint than the whole blood clotting time (Colman, 1970). Because the activated partial thromboplastin time is usually performed on blood anticoagulated with sodium citrate, the assay can be performed in a central laboratory and at a convenient time (Genton, 1974). As with whole blood clotting time, sufficient heparin should be administered to prolong the activated partial thromboplastin time $1\frac{1}{2}$ to $2\frac{1}{2}$ times the normal control. Difficulties with this assay exist, however. The commercially available partial thromboplastin reagents differ considerably in their sensitivity to heparin. The activated partial thromboplastin time can be infinite at high concentrations of heparin (Reno, 1974), so that monitoring peak levels of heparin is limited. During storage of some commercial evacuated blood collection tubes, the citrate anticoagulant consistently develops a substance with antiheparin activity which interferes with heparin monitoring (Hirsh, 1976).

An assay for the inactivation of Factor Xa (Yin, 1973) and quantitative heparin assays (Chen, 1975; Marder, 1970) have been advocated for following patients on heparin. However, they appear to be too cumbersome for most clinical laboratories.

Some investigators have used the thrombin time to monitor heparin. When commercial thrombin was diluted with calcium chloride to give a concentration of 7 NIH units/ml and to produce a normal thrombin time of 8 to 9 seconds, the sensitivity of the system was stabilized to produce a reliable assay of heparin between 0.1 to 6 units/ml (Penner, 1974).

The whole blood activated recalcification time (Reno, 1974) and the activated clotting time (Hattersley, 1966) assays have been shown to correlate well with the whole blood clotting time. The assays adequately reflect the degree of hypocoagulation in patients receiving therapeutic levels of intravenous heparin. In addition, they are more reproducible than the whole blood clotting time and have a shorter coagulation endpoint (Schriever, 1973; Hill, 1974).

At the present time, there is no general agreement on one clearly superior method for monitoring heparin therapy. If a coagulation assay is selected to monitor heparinized patients, special controls for the coagulation assay need to be established. The thromboplastin or activator of coagulation should be standardized for lot-to-lot variation. The sensitivity of the thromboplastin or activator to heparin should be determined before use (a 2- to $2\frac{1}{2}$-fold prolongation in whole blood clotting time corresponds to 0.2 to 0.3 units of heparin/ml). If an anticoagulant-containing evacuated tube is used to collect the blood samples, it is imperative that it contain no antiheparin activity.

COUMARIN

All oral agents that antagonize the normal synthesis of vitamin K-dependent procoagulants are derived from either 4-hydroxycoumarin or the 1,3-indanediones (Levine, 1975). These drugs are absorbed through the gastrointestinal system and then bound to protein (principally albumin) in the plasma. The drugs are transported to the liver, where they undergo hydroxylation and perhaps glucuronide conjugation (O'Reilly, 1976). They are then excreted into the bile, deconjugated in the intestinal tract, and reabsorbed in the blood. Finally, the drugs are re-excreted into the urine as unconjugated, hydroxylated metabolites. The rate of metabolism varies among individuals and among various oral preparations. The mean half-time of warfarin in plasma is 42 hours, with a range of 15 to 58 hours. Thus, the dosage and control of warfarin therapy must be individualized (O'Reilly, 1976).

The coumarin and indanedione drugs act in the hepatic cells to impair the function of vitamin K in the synthesis of Factors II, VII, IX, and X.

Vitamin K has been shown to be a cofactor for a carboxylase of the precursor proteins of

Figure 33-10. Action of vitamin K "epoxidase" and "epoxide reductase." Both of these enzymatic activities are present in the same microsomal preparations that will catalyze the vitamin K-dependent carboxylase. The reductase activity is inhibited by warfarin and other coumarin anticoagulants. (From Jackson, C. M., and Suttie, J. W.: Recent developments in understanding the mechanism of vitamin K and vitamin K–antagonistic drug action and the consequences of vitamin K action in blood coagulation. Prog. Hematol., 10:333, 1977.)

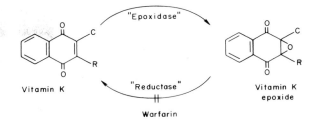

prothrombin and presumably of Factor VII, IX, and X. Without the carboxylase step, Factors II, VII, IX, and X circulate as non-functional proteins which may interfere with normal coagulation (Jackson, 1977).

The exact mechanism by which warfarin inhibits vitamin K function is unclear; many theories exist to explain its action. The most appealing hypothesis suggests that vitamin K is normally converted to vitamin K epoxide and then reduced to its active form by a reductase before it functions as a cofactor for the carboxylase (Fig. 33-10). Warfarin appears to inhibit the epoxide reduction, thus reducing the level of available active form of vitamin K (Suttie, 1977b).

Since the therapy with the indanediones is associated with a high incidence of adverse effects, the various coumarin drugs are most often used. Following the administration of coumarin drugs, the vitamin K factors decline in order of increasing half-life. Factor VII has the shortest half-life (6 hours), Factor IX (24 hours) and Factor X (40 hours) have intermediate half-lives, and prothrombin has the longest (60 hours). Some investigators believe that the antithrombogenic effects of coumarin drugs occur only after Factors IX and X are diminished. This may require three to four days. In addition, it has been shown that large loading doses have no greater effect in decreasing Factor IX and X than do small daily doses. O'Reilly (1976) suggests the administration of 10 to 15 mg of warfarin daily until the prothrombin time is within therapeutic range.

The regulation of therapy depends upon laboratory monitoring to determine the degree of hypocoagulation. Three different assays have been used in the past for laboratory control of coumarin therapy. They include the prothrombin time of Quick (1935), the prothrombin and proconvertin time (P and P test) of Owren (1951), and the thrombotest of Owren (1959).

The prothrombin time assay does not measure the effect of diminished levels of Factor IX and may be prolonged with decreased levels of Factor V and fibrinogen. Owren (1951) introduced the P and P test to overcome some of these difficulties, but it has not obtained widespread usage, owing in part to the difficulty in obtaining and standardizing the reagents, human brain thromboplastin, and ox adsorbed plasma.

The thrombotest reagent is composed of adsorbed bovine plasma, bovine thromboplastin, and cephalin. The thrombotest results depend on the levels of procoagulants II, VII, IX, and X and the effects of PIVKA (Proteins Induced by Vitamin K Absence). Excellent clinical results have been reported with this reagent by several investigators (Harker, 1974; O'Reilly, 1974).

The one-stage prothrombin assay, however, remains the most popular method of following patients on coumarin drugs in the United States and in Great Britain. It has been shown to be a reliable assay in the monitoring of patients on coumarin therapy (Biggs, 1967; Mersky, 1965). The popularity of the prothrombin time depends on its simplicity and availability of reagents. As a result, the assay has been readily adopted to automated methods (Davey, 1972; Miale, 1965). In a quest for a standardized prothrombin time assay, investigators in Great Britain have concentrated on the development of a standardized thromboplastin. The British Comparative Thromboplastin is made from a phenol-saline preparation of human brain and is used by each local laboratory to calibrate its own thromboplastin (Denson, 1971). The test procedure is performed in duplicate on four fresh normal samples and 20 different samples of fresh plasma from patients stabilized on coumarin therapy. Prothrombin time assays are performed on each sample using the British Comparative Thromboplastin and the local thromboplastin (usually commercial rabbit thromboplastin).

The prothrombin time ratios are calculated by dividing the prothrombin time of each test sample by the mean prothrombin time for the normal plasmas. The prothrombin time ratios of the British Comparative Thromboplastin are then plotted against clotting time ratios obtained with the test thromboplastin. From the best straight line drawn through the points, one can convert any observed prothrombin time ratio obtained with the local reagent to that obtained with the British Comparative Thromboplastin. Thus, a patient's coumarin therapy could be monitored safely by several different laboratories using different thromboplastins of varying sensitivity because the results are reported out in prothrombin time ratio using the British Comparative Thromboplastin (Dacie, 1975).

Miale doubted that it was possible to describe a significant mathematical relationship among the activities of the various thromboplastin reagents (Miale, 1969, 1972). He therefore recommended the use of standard reference plasmas. This proposal has been accepted by the Standards Committee of the College of American Pathologists. A therapeutic range for each thromboplastin can be determined by assaying prothrombin times on standardized plasmas with deficiencies in Factors II, VII, and X (ranging from 10 to 20 per cent of normal activities). Recently, Miale (1977) has indicated that the length of the prothrombin time of standard reference plasma using various commercial thromboplastins is related to the reciprocal of the level of Factor VII. He states that since Factor VII is the one factor most predictably depressed by oral anticoagulants, the therapeutic range of coumarin is equivalent to a Factor VII level of 10 to 20 per cent. The suggested therapeutic level for each thromboplastin is given in Table 33–10. As the various commercial companies change their thromboplastin preparations, so too will the given therapeutic range change.

The value of prothrombin time in monitoring patients on coumarin drugs is also related to the accuracy and precision of the prothrombin time assay. Each laboratory should define its own normal values and determine the precision of the assay. Using automated equipment, the precision of replicate values should yield a coefficient of variation of 4 per cent or less. In addition, the daily use of normal and abnormal plasma is also very helpful.

Coumarin anticoagulation is affected by a variety of disorders. Vitamin K deficiency,

Table 33–10. THERAPEUTIC LEVELS FOR VARIOUS COMMERCIAL THROMBOPLASTINS, REPRESENTING A REDUCTION OF THE FACTOR VII LEVEL TO 10 TO 20 PER CENT OF NORMAL

THROMBOPLASTIN	THERAPEUTIC RANGE (SEC.)
British Comparative	30–53
Hyland (dried) (1)	22–36
Simplastin (2)	22–36
Fibroplastin (3)	22–30
Simplastin A (2)	21–30
Ortho (4)	15–30
Dade (dried) (5)	17–26
Dade (activated) (5)	15–21

From Miale, J. B.: Laboratory Medicine: Hematology, 5th ed. St. Louis, The C. V. Mosby Co., 1977.
(1) Hyland, Division Travenol Laboratories, Costa Mesa, Cal.
(2) General Diagnostics, Division Warner-Lambert Co., Morris Plains, N.J.
(3) Baltimore Biological Laboratory (BBL), Baltimore, Md.
(4) Ortho Diagnostics, Raritan, N.J.
(5) Dade, Division, American Hospital Supply Corp., Miami, Fla.

hepatic insufficiency, and hypermetabolic states augment the response to coumarin drugs. In contrast, myxedematous patients have an increased dose requirement for oral anticoagulants (O'Reilly, 1974). In addition, a variety of drugs may either enhance or inhibit

Table 33–11. DRUGS INTERFERING WITH COUMARIN ANTICOAGULATION

DRUGS INCREASING COUMARIN SENSITIVITY	DRUGS DECREASING COUMARIN SENSITIVITY
Allopurinol	Antacids
Anabolic steroids	Ascorbic acid
Chloral hydrate	Barbiturates
Chloramphenicol	Carbamazepine
Clofibrate	Cholestyramine
Dextrothyroxine	Chlortetracycline
Disulfiram	Cortisone-prednisone
Glucagon	Estrogenic contraceptives
MAO-inhibitors	Ethchlorvynol
Mefenamic acid	Glutethimide
Methylphenidate	Griseofulvin
Neomycin	Haloperidol
Nortriptyline	Rifampin
Oxyphenbutazone	Xanthines
Phenylbutazone	
Phenyramidol	
Phenytoin	
Phytate	
Propylthiouracil	
Quinidine	
Salicylates	
Sulfonamides	

the hypoprothrombinemic effect of coumarin drugs; mechanisms are reviewed by Koch-Weser (1971). An incomplete listing of interfering drugs is presented in Table 33–11.

LABORATORY METHODS

ASSAYS OF COAGULATION

Whole blood clotting time

Principle. The whole blood clotting time is the time required for freshly collected blood to form a firm clot in standardized glass tubes at 37°C. Thus, the whole blood clotting time is a measure of the integrity of the intrinsic system.

Method (Lee, 1913, as modified by Tocantins, 1964). From a clean venipuncture withdraw 4 ml of blood. Start a timer the moment the blood enters the syringe. After the needle has been removed from the syringe, gently deliver 1 ml of blood into each of three glass 13 by 100 mm test tubes, labeled 1, 2, and 3, respectively. Place the tubes into a 37°C. waterbath. After 5 minutes have elapsed, tilt the third tube at a 45 degree angle every 30 seconds until blood is completely clotted. Record the time needed for blood to clot in the third tube. Repeat the procedure for the second, then for the first tube. The clotting time is reported as the time needed for the first tube to clot.

Interpretation. In normal individuals the whole blood clotting time ranges from 5 to 15 minutes. The whole blood clotting time is an insensitive screening test of factor deficiencies. Prolongation of whole blood clotting time is usually seen when deficient factors are less than 2 per cent of normal or an anticoagulant is present. The major use of the assay is in monitoring heparinized patients.

Activated coagulation time of whole blood

Principle. The activated coagulation time of whole blood is the time necessary for fresh blood to form a firm clot when incubated at 37°C. in the presence of surface contact activation. This assay, like the whole blood clotting time, measures overall activity of the intrinsic clotting system.

Method (Hattersley, 1966). Using a double syringe technique, draw 1 ml of blood from a fresh venipuncture, change syringes, then collect 2 ml blood in the second syringe. Place the 2 ml blood in a prewarmed 12 mm tube containing diatomaceous earth. At the moment blood appears in the tube, start a stopwatch. Invert the tube several times to mix the sample and then incubate at 37°C. At one minute and after each succeeding 5-second interval, remove the blood from the bath, tilt to 45 degrees, and examine for stability of clot. Time is recorded to the nearest 5 seconds, upon observation of a solid clot.

Interpretation. The normal range extends from 1 minute 21 seconds to 2 minutes 13 seconds. The precision of the assay has about a 4 per cent coefficient of variation. Although prolonged results have been described in a variety of inherited and acquired coagulopathies, its widest use appears to be in monitoring heparin therapy (Hattersley, 1976). The activated coagulation time of whole blood has been particularly helpful in following the degree of hypocoagulation of patients during extracorporeal circulation for open-heart surgery (Bull, 1975). A small portable machine with an automatic endpoint allows bedside determinations (Hill, 1974).

Plasma recalcification time

Principle. Plasma collected in sodium citrate forms a fibrin clot after the addition of calcium chloride. The plasma recalcification time assay, therefore, measures the intrinsic system, i.e., all circulating procoagulants except Factor VII and Factor XIII.

Method (Owen, 1955). Mix nine parts fresh venous blood with one part of a solution containing 1 volume 0.1 M citric acid and 3 volumes of 0.1 M trisodium citrate. Centrifuge at 2000 g for 20 minutes to obtain platelet-poor plasma. Mix 0.1 ml of plasma and 0.1 ml of 0.145 M sodium chloride in a 13 $\times$ 100 mm test tube; warm the mixture to 37°C. Add 0.1 ml of 0.025 M calcium chloride to the plasma mixture and start a stopwatch. Allow the reaction mixture to remain undisturbed at 37°C. for 90 seconds, then gently tilt the tube every 30 seconds and observe for clot.

Interpretation. Normal values usually range from 110 to 240 seconds. If platelet-rich plasma is used, the normal range is usually 90 to 120 seconds. However, it is difficult to obtain a consistent number of platelets. In addition, the plasma recalcification time will be shortened by prolonged exposure of plasma to glass surface.

Prolonged times are obtained in deficiencies of Factors I, II, V, VIII, IX, X, XI, and XII. In the presence of circulating inhibitors, prolonged clotting times are also observed. Since the assay measures the effect of platelets on coagulation, the plasma recalcification assays have been used to measure platelet thromboplastic activity (Weiss, 1967).

Activated partial thromboplastin time

Principle. The partial thromboplastin time assay is the time needed for plasma to form a fibrin clot following the addition of calcium and a phospholipid reagent (partial thromboplastin). The partial thromboplastin time is similar to the recalcification time except for the addition of the phospholipid reagent which substitutes for platelet phospholipid, i.e., platelet factor 3. In the activated partial thromboplastin time a contact activating agent such as ellagic acid, celite, or kaolin is added. As a result of optimal activation of the contact factors, the activated partial thromboplastin time is shorter and less variable than the partial thromboplastin time. Both assays measure the intrinsic system.

Method (Proctor, 1961). Platelet-poor plasma is obtained as described in the plasma recalcification time assay. Plasma should be kept at 5 to 10°C. until ready to use. Commercial thromboplastins are stable and provide satisfactory results. The stock kaolin suspension is made by suspending 2 g kaolin powder in 100 ml physiologic saline solution. Mix equal volume of thromboplastin reagent with kaolin solution and then deliver 0.2 ml of this mixture to a test tube containing 0.2 ml test or control plasma. Incubate the mixture of plasma and thromboplastin-kaolin at 37°C. After 3 minutes add 0.2 ml of 0.025 M calcium chloride and start the stopwatch. Gently swirl the tube for the first 30 seconds, then tilt the tube and examine for first signs of fibrin formation.

Interpretation. In normal individuals the activated partial thromboplastin time ranges from 32 to 51 seconds. Prolonged values can occur with any factor deficiency with the exception of Factor VII and Factor XIII. In general, the activated partial thromboplastin time can detect levels of 40 per cent or less of Factor VIII, 30 per cent or less of Factor IX, 15 per cent or less of Factor XI, and 10 per cent or less of Factor XII (Goulian, 1965). The sensitivity of the activated partial thromboplastin time to plasma levels of procoagulants varies markedly among different commercial thromboplastins (Sibley, 1973) and, in our experience, among lots of thromboplastin from the same manufacturer.

In the event that the activated partial thromboplastin time is prolonged, more specific information can be obtained by mixing equal volumes of test plasma with normal

Table 33–12. THE USE OF MIXING ASSAYS IN DEFINING FACTOR DEFICIENCIES

CAUSE OF PROLONGED ACTIVATED PARTIAL THROMBOPLASTIN TIME	CORRECTION OF TEST PLASMA WITH EQUAL VOLUME MIXTURE OF COMPONENT		
	Adsorbed Plasma	Aged Serum	Normal Plasma
Factor XII deficiency	+	+	+
Factor XI deficiency	+	+	+
Factor X deficiency	0	+	+
Factor IX deficiency	0	+	+
Factor VIII deficiency	+	0	+
Circulating anticoagulant	0	0	0

+ = Correction of prolonged activated partial thromboplastin time.

0 = No correction of prolonged activated partial thromboplastin time.

plasma, $Al(OH)_3$ or $BaSO_4$ adsorbed plasma, and aged serum (Table 33–12). The adsorbed plasma can be prepared (Owen, 1975) or obtained commercially.

Prothrombin time

Principle. The prothrombin time is the time needed for plasma to clot after adding calcium and tissue factor (brain or brain-lung extract). The complex formed between plasma Factor VII and tissue factor, in the presence of calcium, directly activates Factor X. The prothrombin time, therefore, measures the integrity of the extrinsic system. It is the most widely used measurement for monitoring patients on coumarin therapy.

Method (Quick, 1935). Platelet-poor plasma is obtained according to the method described in the plasma recalcification time assay. Keep the plasma on ice until ready to use. Commercially prepared thromboplastin can be purchased with or without calcium chloride. Both reagents are satisfactory for routine work. The thromboplastin reagent is usually maintained at 37°C. in a water bath or heating block. The patient's plasma or control plasma is incubated at 37°C. for two to three minutes prior to use. Mix 0.2 ml of thromboplastin calcium reagent with 0.1 ml of plasma. Gently tilt tube and examine for fibrin clot. If thromboplastin reagent and calcium chloride are obtained separately, mix 0.1 ml plasma with 0.1 ml thromboplastin reagent. One-tenth ml 0.025 M calcium chloride solution is added, the mixture is shaken, and the time for coagulation to occur is recorded.

Interpretation. Reference values may vary depending on the source of thromboplastin and type of sensing device used to measure clot formation. Manual methods usually give

Table 33–13. EFFECT OF PLASMA
COMPONENTS ON A PROLONGED
PROTHROMBIN TIME

CAUSE OF PROLONGED PROTHROMBIN TIME	CORRECTION OF TEST PLASMA WITH EQUAL VOLUME MIXTURE OF COMPONENT		
	Adsorbed Plasma	Aged Serum	Normal Plasma
Fibrinogen deficiency	+	0	+
Prothrombin deficiency	0	0	+
Factor V deficiency	+	0	+
Factor VII deficiency	0	+	+
Factor X deficiency	0	+	+
Circulating anticoagulant deficiency	0	0	0

+ = Correction of prolonged prothrombin time.
0 = No correction of prolonged prothrombin time.

longer reference values than automated techniques. In general the reference values for prothrombin time range from 12 to 15 seconds. Each laboratory should establish its own reference values. The prothrombin time is prolonged in deficiencies of fibrinogen, prothrombin, Factor V, Factor VII, or Factor X. The sensitivity of the prothrombin time to concentrations of Factor VII varies greatly among various commerical thromboplastin reagents (Singer, 1973).

When the prothrombin time is prolonged, incubating equal volumes of test plasma with normal plasma, $AL(OH)_3$ or $BaSO_4$ adsorbed plasma, and aged serum can yield more specific information (Table 33–13).

Standardization of the prothrombin time assay for following patients on anticoagulants is covered in the section on monitoring coumarin therapy.

A variation of the prothrombin time, the Stypven time, employs a mixture of Russell's viper venom and cephalin in place of tissue factor. This directly activates Factor X without the need for Factor VII. The Stypven time is therefore normal in Factor VII deficiency and abnormal in deficiency of Factor X, except in the Friuli variant (p. 1141).

Fibrinogen

Principle. Thrombin is added to plasma diluted with a buffer solution. Change in absorbance of the plasma solution is recorded by a spectrophotometer. The fibrinogen value is obtained comparing the absorbance results to a previously determined calibration curve.

Method **(Ellis and Stransky, 1961).** Five-tenths (0.5) ml citrated plasma is added to each of two 20 ml test tubes containing 10 ml of barbitol-saline buffer (0.1M/l at pH 7.2) and mixed. Six ml of the resulting solution is pipetted into cuvettes. To one cuvette two drops of calcium-thrombin solution (equal volumes of a stock thrombin solution prepared at a concentration of 33.8 NIH units/ml in physiologic saline (0.145 M NaCl) and 3.38 M calcium chloride solution) are added and mixed by gentle inversion for 15 seconds. The other sample without the calcium-thrombin solution is used as the blank. After 20 minutes incubation, the absorbance is read at 470 nm on a spectrophotometer.

A calibration curve is constructed by selecting six randomized plasma samples. From these samples the absorbance by the Ellis-Stransky method is plotted against fibrinogen concentration as determined by the Ratnoff-Menzie method (1951) on linear graph paper and a best fit line is constructed. Future fibrinogen concentrations can be determined by the Ellis-Stransky method alone by referring to this calibration curve. A new calibration curve must be constructed for each new batch of calcium-thrombin solution.

Reference Method **(Ratnoff and Menzie, 1951).** Dilute 0.5 ml citrated plasma with 10 ml 0.145 M saline and clot with thrombin. Harvest the clot and wash it three times with saline. Add 1 ml of 2.5 N sodium hydroxide with the tube in a bath of boiling water. Determine the tyrosine equivalent using the Folin-Ciocalteau phenol reagent. Correct the fibrinogen concentration for dilution with citrate buffer and express the results as g/l of plasma.

Interpretation. Normal values vary from 1.6 to 3.4 g/l. Low values are observed in congenital afibrinogenemia, hypofibrinogenemia, and dysfibrinogenemia. In addition, low values may be observed in diffuse intravascular coagulation (DIC) and primary fibrinolysis. Elevated levels of fibrinogen are observed in pregnancy, postoperative states, malignancies, and many inflammatory disorders.

Plasma thrombin time

Principle. The thrombin time is the time needed for a fibrin clot to form following the addition of a standard amount of bovine thrombin to a given volume of citrated plasma.

Method **(Rapaport, 1957).** A stock thrombin solution is prepared by diluting commercially obtained bovine thrombin with sufficient 0.145 M saline to provide a concentration of 100 NIH units/ml. This stock solution can be frozen in small volumes and is stable under these conditions for six months. A working thrombin solution is prepared by diluting stock thrombin with Owren's Veronal buffer to give a thrombin time of 18 to 25 seconds when pooled normal plasma is used as a substrate. The working thrombin solution is stable for only 20 minutes at 37°C. in a plastic tube. Two-tenths ml of a patient's platelet-poor citrated plasma is pre-warmed to 37°C. for 3 minutes. Add 0.2 ml of working thrombin solution to the patient's plasma, start the stopwatch, and record the time for a fibrin clot to form. The patient's thrombin time should be performed in duplicate, as should the normal control. Duplicate samples should not vary by more than two seconds.

Interpretation. A thrombin time greater than 1.3 times the normal control value is considered abnormal. Prolonged thrombin times are seen in patients receiving heparin; in hypofibrinogenemia less than 90 mg/dl (Didisheim, 1967); and in most cases of dysfibrinogenemia (Samama, 1977). Fibrinogen/fibrin degradation products interfere with the polymerization of fibrin. If these fragments are elevated, therefore, the thrombin time may be prolonged. The thrombin time is usually abnormal in cases of multiple myeloma and macroglobulinemia (Perkins, 1970). The paraprotein appears to interfere with normal polymerization of fibrin, resulting in a delayed thrombin time and abnormal clot formation. In addition, the thrombin time may be prolonged in some cases of liver disease in which fibrinogen levels are normal and fibrinogen/fibrin degradation products are not elevated. In these circumstances, it appears that a dysfunctional fibrinogen is synthesized and then fails to polymerize normally (Poller, 1977).

Reptilase coagulation time

Principle. Reptilase-R,* a snake venom of *Bothrops atrox*, cleaves the α-chain of fibrinogen, liberating fibrinopeptide A. This initiates the polymerization of fibrin independently of the action of thrombin. Because of this, the reptilase coagulation time may be useful in the presence of a circulating heparin.

Method (Funk, 1971). Mix 0.3 ml of platelet-poor citrated plasma with 0.1 ml reconstituted Reptilase-R and measure coagulation time at 37°C.

Interpretation. Reptilase coagulation time is normal in heparinized patients. In the presence of fibrinogen/fibrin degradation products, the reptilase time is less prolonged

---
*Reptilase-R, Abbott Scientific Products Division, 820 Mission St., South Pasadena, Cal., 91030.

than the thrombin time. However, in patients with congenital dysfibrinogenemia, the thrombin time is less prolonged than the reptilase coagulation time.

Factor XIII (fibrin stabilizing factor)

Principle. Factor XIII, activated by thrombin, acts in the presence of calcium ions to stabilize the fibrin clot by promoting the formation of covalent bonds between γ-γ and α-α fibrin chains through a process of transamidation. A stabilized fibrin clot is insoluble in 5M urea or 1 per cent monochloracetic acid.

Method (Duckert, 1961). Pipet 0.5 ml of citrated plasma into a 13 by 100 mm test tube. Add 0.5 ml of 0.025 M calcium chloride, mix, and incubate for 30 minutes at 37°C. Gently remove the resulting fibrin clot from the tube and place it into a second tube containing 5 ml of 5M urea or 3 ml of 1 per cent monochloracetic acid. Allow the clot to remain at room temperature. Observe for clot dissolution at 1, 2, 3, and 24 hours.

Interpretation. Dissolution of the clot in less than 24 hours is abnormal and indicates a severe deficiency, since clots from plasma with factor XIII levels over 1 per cent will not dissolve in 5M urea (Britten, 1967). Clot dissolution occurs therefore in homozygous Factor XIII deficiency but not in the heterozygous carrier. Abnormal solubility of the fibrin clot has also been described in some cases of dysfibrinogenemia. In these circumstances structural changes have been demonstrated on the fibrinogen molecule which correspond to sites of interaction with Factor XIII (Hampton, 1968).

One-stage assay for Factors II, V, VII, and X

Principle. The duration of the Quick one-stage prothrombin time (1935) is inversely proportional to the plasma concentrations of Factors II, V, VII, and X. Thus, the per cent activity of any one of these factors in a patient's plasma can be determined by measuring the degree of correction it provides when incubated with specific factor-deficient plasma in a prothrombin time.

Method (Modified from Quick, 1935). A calibration curve is made with serial dilutions of pooled normal plasma (collected from at least 20 normal individuals) in Owren's buffer ranging from 1:10 to 1:320. One-tenth (0.1) ml of each dilution is mixed with 0.1 ml of specific factor-deficient substrate plasma. A prothrombin time is performed in dupli-

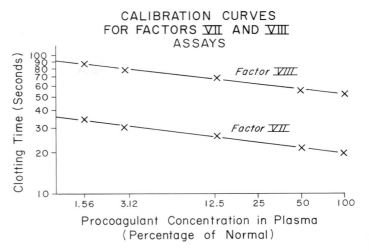

CALIBRATION CURVES
FOR FACTORS $\overline{VII}$ AND $\overline{VIII}$
ASSAYS

Figure 33–11. Representative calibration curves for assays of Factors VII and VIII.

cate on each dilution. The results of the duplicate pairs are averaged and the mean plotted on double-logarithmic paper with per cent of dilution on the abscissa and the time in seconds on the ordinate. A best fit straight line is drawn by connecting the points (Fig. 33–11). The ordinate points can be calculated using a linear regression analysis: $\hat{y}i = a + bxi$, where $\hat{y}i$ represents the calculated time in seconds, a is the y intercept, xi represents the factor concentration in the diluted plasma, and b is the slope. Calculations of slope and y-intercept are performed (Steel, 1960); a small calculator with this function is useful.*

Patients' blood should be collected in plastic using a two-syringe method. The specimen must be kept at 4 to 10°C. on melted ice and centrifuged at 20,000 g for 30 minutes. The sample must be used within two hours or should be stored at −85°C.

The patient's platelet-poor plasma is diluted 1:10 in Owren's buffer. One-tenth ml of this mixture is added to 0.1 ml of deficient substrate plasma, and a prothrombin time is performed. Triplicate values should be within 5 per cent and should be averaged. The concentration of factor in patient's plasma is determined by referring to the calibration curve or by calculating from the linear regression equation.

Interpretation. Reference values usually extend from 50 to 150 per cent, but should be established for each laboratory. In addition, a normal plasma and, if possible, known deficient plasma should be assayed as controls.

One-stage assay for Factors VIII, IX, XI, and XII

Principle. The activated partial thromboplastin time is sensitive to the plasma level of

Factors VIII, IX, XI, and XII. The plasma level of these procoagulants can be quantitated by measuring the ability of test plasma to correct the activated partial thromboplastin time of specific factor-deficient plasma. The activated partial thromboplastin time of this mixture is compared with a calibration curve made with various concentrations of pooled normal plasma.

Method. A calibration curve is constructed using serial dilutions of pooled normal plasma in Owren's buffer, starting at 1:5 and ending at 1:320. One-tenth (0.1) ml of each dilution is mixed with 0.1 ml of deficient substrate plasma and an activated partial thromboplastin time is done in duplicate on each dilution. The results of the duplicate pairs are averaged and then plotted on double-logarithmic paper. The per cent of dilution serves as the abscissa and the time in seconds represents the ordinate. A straight line is drawn connecting the points (Fig. 33–11). As in the case of assays based on the prothrombin time, the best fit ordinate points can be calculated using a linear regression analysis.

Patient's blood must be collected in plastic using a two-syringe technique. Keep the specimen at 4 to 10°C. prior to use and centrifuge at 20,000 g for 30 minutes. The sample should be used within two hours or stored at −85°C. until ready to perform assay.

The patient's platelet-poor plasma is diluted 1:5 in Owren's buffer. One tenth of this diluted plasma is mixed with 0.1 ml of deficient plasma. A partial thromboplastin time is performed in triplicate on the mixture, and the results are interpolated from the calibration curve or calculated using the linear regression equation.

Interpretation. Normal values usually extend from 50 to 150 per cent, but should be

---

*e.g., Texas Instruments SR-51 II, Texas Instruments Inc., Dallas, Texas 75222.

determined in each laboratory. The variability of these bioassays is great. Grant (1967) indicated that in the Factor VIII assay there is at least a 10 per cent error attributable to technical variation and an additional error of approximately 17 per cent due to day-to-day variation. Similar wide fluctuations in Factor VIII levels on a day-to-day basis using a semi-automated method have been described by Simone (1967). The source of this error is uncertain. For analysis of inherited deficiencies within families, therefore, it is best to collect the blood at one time and then to perform all of the assays on the same day.

Although there is an appreciable error, the assays are still clinically valuable. Marked differences or changes in Factor VIII levels are usually sought. In addition, the error is not as great at low plasma levels as it is for normal or elevated values (Grant, 1967).

Factor VIII antigen

Principle. Factor VIII antigen can be measured by the electroimmunodiffusion method of Laurell (1966). Test plasma is electrophoresed through an agarose gel containing Factor VIII antiserum. Rocket-shaped immunoprecipitation lines are formed where Factor VIII antigen combines with monospecific antisera. The maximal distance the immunoprecipitate has travelled from the origin (the height of the rocket) is proportional to the concentration of the antigen.

Method **(Zimmermann, 1975).** Factor VIII antiserum can be obtained commercially* or made in New Zealand white female rabbits. Add 0.175 ml of a 1:5 dilution of antisera to 10 ml of a 1 per cent solution of agarose in tris-barbital buffer pH 8.8. Pour agarose-antiserum mixture onto 8 by 8 cm glass slides. After gel has solidified, punch out a row of holes 2.5 mm in diameter, 6 mm apart, and 15 mm from the edge. The glass slide is put in the electrophoresis chamber filled with 1 liter of tris-barbital buffer. A calibration curve is established by applying 5 μl of undiluted, 1:2, 1:4, and 1:8 dilution of pooled normal plasma in tris-barbital buffer to the first four holes. Duplicate samples of a 1:2 dilution in tris-barbital buffer are placed in the remaining holes. The specimens are electrophoresed for 18 hours at 15°C. at 110 to 150 volts.

The immunoprecipitates are made visible by incubation of the plates in Coomassie blue stain (Fig.

---

*Anti-AHF can be obtained through Nordic Laboratories, Langestraet 57-61, P.O.B. 22, Tilburg, The Netherlands, or from Behring Diagnostics, American Hoechst Corporation, Somerville, N.J. 08876.

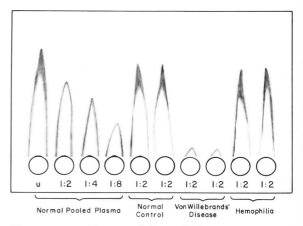

Figure 33–12. Diagram of Factor VIII immunoprecipitin reactions in agarose following electroimmunodiffusion. First four wells were filled with serial dilutions of pooled normal plasma. (U = undiluted plasma). The remaining wells contained 1:2 dilution in duplicate of plasma from normal control, von Willebrand's and hemophilic individuals.

33–12). After 30 minutes, clear with 7 per cent glacial acetic acid in distilled water. The rockets are then measured. A calibration curve is made on semilog paper by plotting the log of the length of rockets against the concentration of Factor VIII antigen. A best fit line connecting the points is made. The test results are obtained by reference to calibration curve and multiplying by dilution factor.

Control samples should include pooled normal plasma and von Willebrand's plasma. Different lots of Factor VIII antisera vary in titer. Thus, each lot of antisera should be tested against normal, hemophilic, and von Willebrand's plasma, to judge the appropriate concentration to mix with agarose solution.

Interpretation. Normal values range from 50 to 150 per cent. Hemophiliacs and carriers of hemophilia have normal values. Von Willebrand's patients have deficient to absent levels of Factor VIII antigen.

ASSAYS OF FIBRINOLYSIS

Whole blood clot lysis

Principle. A clot dissolves as a result of plasmin activity. Normally this does not occur in less than 72 hours because of the presence of plasma inhibitors which inactivate plasmin as it forms.

Method **(Owen, 1975).** Place 1 ml of whole blood from the patient into a 10 by 75 mm tube and allow blood to form a clot at 37°C. One of the tubes from the whole blood clotting time may be observed for clot retraction, then for lysis. Incubate the blood at 37°C. for at least 24 hours and examine periodically for lysis.

Interpretation. Lysis is complete when the clot is converted to the fluid state. This must be differentiated from clot retraction and the "fallout" of erythrocytes from the clot, which sometimes occurs in polycythemia. It may be helpful to pour the contents of the tube onto a paper towel and check for the presence of a clot. Lysis of a clot before 24 hours is abnormal and is usually associated with a fibrinolytic state. This is a gross estimate of fibrinolysis. More sensitive measurements shorten the normal lysis time by decreasing the influence of inhibitors, either by diluting the blood or by testing only the euglobulin fraction, as in the euglobulin clot lysis time.

Euglobulin clot lysis

Principle. The euglobulin fraction is precipitated from the plasma by the action of acetic acid. This plasma fraction contains fibrinogen, plasminogen activators, and plasminogen. Because inhibitors of the fibrinolytic system are not present in the euglobulin fraction, the time needed for dissolution of the euglobulin clot is a measure of the activity of plasminogen activators and plasmin on fibrinogen.

Method **(Buckell, 1958).** Collect 4.5 ml of blood with 0.5 ml citrate solution as anticoagulant (1 volume 0.1 M citric acid and 3 volumes 0.1 M trisodium citrate) and keep on ice. Obtain platelet-poor plasma by centrifugation at 2000 g for 6 minutes at 5°C. Mix 9.0 ml distilled water, 0.5 ml of plasma, and 0.1 ml of 1 per cent acetic acid. Refrigerate the mixture for 30 minutes at 4°C. to obtain the euglobulin fraction as a precipitate. Centrifuge the specimen for 5 minutes at 2000 g, decant, and invert the tube for 3 minutes to drain off the supernate containing inhibitors. Add 0.5 M of borate solution (9 g sodium chloride, 1 g sodium borate in 1 liter distilled water with pH 9.0), incubate at 37°C. and stir to dissolve clot. Next add 0.5 ml of 0.025 M calcium chloride and mix by inversion of tube. Record time of clot formation. Leave the tube at 37°C. and report time for clot lysis.

Interpretation. Normal clots usually lyse in two to four hours. Values of less than two hours usually indicate increased fibrinolysis, especially plasminogen activator activity.

Semiquantitative assay for fibrinogen/fibrin degradation products

Principle. Specific antiserum against human fibrinogen/fibrin fragments D and E (FDP) is adsorbed to latex beads. In the presence of a concentration of 2 μg/ml of FDP or greater, the latex beads clump together.

Method. Two ml of blood is collected into a tube containing 3600 NF units of soybean trypsin inhibitor and 20 NIH units of thrombin. The blood sample is mixed and then incubated at 37°C. for at least 30 minutes. If blood is collected from a heparinized patient, then add sufficient Reptilase-R to form a clot. Centrifuge the specimen, remove the serum, and prepare 1:5 and 1:20 dilutions of serum with a glycine saline buffer (7.5 g glycine, 8.5 g sodium chloride, 1.0 g sodium azide, and sufficient 0.2 N sodium hydroxide to obtain a pH of 8.2 in 1 liter distilled water).

Mix one drop of latex solution with one drop from each dilution of serum on a glass slide. Gently rock the slide for 2 minutes. Latex agglutination in the serum diluted at 1:5 will indicate the presence of at least 10 μg/ml of FDP, and agglutination at 1:20 dilution indicates at least 40 μg/ml of FDP.

Known negative and positive control sera should be analyzed with each series of tests.

All reagents are available in kit form (Wellcome Reagents Division, Burroughs Wellcome Co., Research Triangle Park, North Carolina 27709).

Interpretation. The concentration of FDP in the sera of normal individuals is less than 10 μg/ml. Elevated levels of FDP are present in many disorders, including diffuse intravascular coagulation, primary fibrinolysis, pulmonary embolism, myocardial infarction, post surgery, liver disease, and malignancies.

Quantitative assay for fibrinogen/fibrin degradation products

Principle. Dilutions of the patient's serum are incubated with rabbit serum containing a specific antibody against human fibrinogen. This antibody cross-reacts with fibrinogen antigen present on fibrinogen/fibrin degradation products (FDP). If fibrinogen antigen is not present in the serum, then the rabbit antibodies agglutinate tanned formalinized human erythrocytes previously coated with human fibrinogen. When fibrinogen antigen is in the patient's serum, it binds with rabbit anti-human fibrinogen antibody and prevents the agglutination of tanned erythrocytes. The assay is very specific for the fibrinogen antigen and is sensitive to 1.25 μg/ml of fibrinogen.

Method **(Merskey, 1966, as modified by Owen, 1975).** All reagents are commercially available (Wellcome Reagents, Burroughs Wellcome Co., Research Triangle Park, N.C. 27709).

Interpretation and Comment. Normal values are less than 10 μg/ml. Several other methods are available for measuring FDP. However, our experience indicates that the tanned red cell hemagglutination inhibition assay is the most reliable.

Plasma protamine paracoagulation test

Principle. When a dilute solution of protamine sulfate is added to citrated plasma incubated at 37°C., a precipitate forms in the presence of fibrin monomers or early fibrin degradation products.

Method **(Kidder, 1972).** Add 0.5 ml platelet-poor plasma to a 12 by 75 mm glass tube and incubate at 37°C. for 3 minutes. Inspect to be sure it is clear. Add 0.05 ml of a 1 per cent protamine sulfate* solution with a 50 μl disposable pipet (0.09 per cent final concentration). Gently mix the contents by tilting the tube several times. Then incubate for 15 minutes at 37°C. Tilt the tube gently at 3 minutes and 10 minutes after starting incubation. At the end of the incubation period observe for precipitation by placing the tube between a fluorescent light source and a concave mirror. By gently rocking the tube observe for the presence of fibrin web (strongly positive), a granular precipitate (positive), a fine precipitate which is difficult to see (weakly positive), or no precipitate (negative).

Interpretation. The assay must be performed with care. The sample must be obtained from a clean venipuncture and blood should be thoroughly mixed. The plasma must be incubated for at least 3 minutes at 37°C. before adding protamine to avoid precipitation of fibrinogen. When negative the test gives strong evidence against a diagnosis of disseminated intravascular coagulation. The assay is sensitive to 0.03 mg/ml of fibrin monomer. The presence of early fibrin degradation products but not fibrinogen degradation products is also detected. Since the presence of fibrin monomers and/or early fibrin degradation products implies the prior action of thrombin, this assay has been used to differentiate disseminated intravascular coagulation from primary fibrinolysis.

---

*Eli Lilly and Company, Indianapolis, Indiana.

ASSAYS OF INHIBITORS

Factor VIII inhibitor

Principle. The patient's plasma is mixed with a dilution of pooled normal plasma containing a known concentration of Factor VIII. After incubation for one hour at 37°C., a Factor VIII assay is performed on the mixture. A reduction in Factor VIII activity of 50 per cent is defined as 1 unit of inhibitor.

Method **(Strauss, 1967).** Construct a Factor VIII calibration curve as previously described (p. 1159). Perform a Factor VIII assay on patient's plasma and on pooled normal plasma. Dilute the pooled normal plasma with Owren's buffer to obtain approximately 50 per cent Factor VIII activity. Mix 0.2 ml of patient's plasma with 0.2 ml of diluted pooled normal plasma. Incubate for 60 minutes at 37°C. For a control, mix 0.2 ml of diluted normal plasma with 0.2 ml Owren's buffer and incubate for 60 minutes at 37°C. Since both the test and control plasmas contain $\frac{1}{4}$ volume of pooled normal plasma in their final dilutions, the Factor VIII level should be 25 per cent. This initial Factor VIII level is usually a little lower than expected, because of a loss of Factor VIII activity during the one-hour incubation period. Indeed, Strauss (1967) reported the initial Factor VIII level to be 21 ± 2 per cent.

Factor VIII levels of test plasma below 19 per cent usually indicate the presence of an inhibitor. An inhibitor unit is defined as the quantity contained in 1 ml of plasma that inactivates 50 per cent of the factor VIII activity during one hour of incubation at 37°C. Using semilog paper, the log of the per cent Factor VIII is plotted on the ordinate and the units of inhibitor on the abscissa. The line goes through the residual per cent Factor VIII of the control at zero units, and half of this value at one unit. The units of inhibitor in the patient's plasma are read from this graph for the residual per cent Factor VIII of the tube containing patient plasma. When residual Factor VIII activity is below 5 per cent, the unknown plasma sample is then sufficiently diluted with buffer to obtain a residual Factor VIII level of between 5 and 15 per cent. Units of inhibitor of the diluted sample are then multiplied by the dilution factor to express the total number of inhibitor units.

Interpretation. Clinically significant inhibitors exist at and above the 1 unit level.

Inhibitors of other factors

Inhibitor assays can be performed for Factors IX, XI, and XII utilizing the identical principle given for Factor VIII inhibitors. Of course substitution of appropriate factor assays is made in the method.

Assay for lupus anticoagulant (tissue inhibition test)

Principle. The lupus anticoagulant acts by inhibiting the activation of prothrombin by the complex composed of Factor Xa, Factor V, calcium, and phospholipid. The specific site of inhibition is probably with the phospholipid moiety. When a modified prothrombin time using diluted tissue thromboplastin (tissue thromboplastin inhibition test) is performed on plasma containing a lupus inhibitor, the clotting time is prolonged more than that of similarly treated pooled normal plasma. This may be due to an enhanced ratio of lupus antibody to phospholipid provided by the thromboplastin.

Method (Schleider, 1976). Tissue thromboplastin is diluted 1:50 and 1:500 with 0.145 M sodium chloride in distilled water and incubated at 37°C. for 5 minutes. One-tenth ml of patient's plasma and 0.1 ml of diluted tissue thromboplastin are mixed. After incubation for 5 minutes, 0.1 ml of 0.025 M calcium chloride is added and coagulation time is measured.

Interpretation. The results are considered abnormal when the patient's tissue thromboplastin inhibition test is at least 1.3-fold greater than the control. A lupus inhibitor is present when the activated partial thromplastin is prolonged, a mixture of pooled normal plasma with patient's plasma does not correct the activated partial thromboplastin time, and the tissue thromboplastin inhibition test is abnormal (Schleider, 1976).

Approximately 10 per cent of patients with systemic lupus erythematosus have a circulating inhibitor. Lupus-like anticoagulants are also present in a variety of malignant, immunologic, gynecologic, and miscellaneous disorders.

APPROACH TO THE DIAGNOSIS OF A BLEEDING PATIENT

A carefully obtained medical history and thoughtfully performed physical examination provide necessary information for the proper ordering of laboratory assays and subsequently for a reasonable interpretation of laboratory results.

Information regarding the type of bleeding gives valuable clues concerning the etiology of the disorder. Petechiae and purpura are usually signs associated with a platelet disorder. Non-traumatic hemarthroses and retroperitoneal hemorrhages are characteristics of procoagulant deficiencies. Hematomas are seen with both platelet and procoagulant disorders.

Questions concerning the time of onset of the bleeding problem are also important. Most inherited coagulopathies begin early in life, whereas acquired disorders may originate at any time.

Sometimes bleeding states are very mild and it is then difficult to differentiate an individual with a mild disorder from a normal individual. Thus, queries about hemostasis during and following previous surgery and tooth extractions may provide added evidence for the presence of an abnormality in a given patient. Sometimes it is helpful to ask patients specifically about the amount of blood lost or the necessity for transfusion during or following a common surgical procedure such as a tonsillectomy, circumcision, biopsy, and herniorrhaphy.

Patients should be questioned about the kinds of drugs they are taking. Numerous drugs interfere with platelet function. Some patients may be taking drugs that cause diminished platelet production. Patients sometimes take toxic levels of coumarins. In addition, some drugs may produce an allergic vasculitis associated with purpura.

It is also important to obtain a general medical history from the patient. Some systemic diseases are characteristically associated with a particular coagulation abnormality. In systemic lupus erythematosus, patients may have an acquired anticoagulant. Liver disease is often associated with diminished plasma concentration of prothrombin complex procoagulants.

A complete family history provides important data. Hemophilia A and Christmas disease are inherited as sex-linked disorders. Von Willebrand's syndrome is an autosomal dominant disease. Most of the other inherited procoagulant deficiencies are autosomal recessive traits; consanguineous marriages are more frequently observed than in the general population.

The physical examination helps to document the extent of the disease and often provides additional information. Petechiae suggest

3

platelet or vascular disorders. Palpable petechiae are often associated with allergic vasculitis, whereas non-palpable petechiae are usually due to thrombocytopenia. Mucosal and gastrointestinal hemorrhage are associated with thrombocytopenia and less often with vascular abnormalities. Bleeding into an elbow or knee joint is characteristic of hemophilia A and Christmas disease. The presence of splenomegaly may indicate a hepatic disorder or hematologic malignancy.

In assessing the cause of a bleeding disorder, it is important to choose coagulation assays that will screen most parameters of the coagulation system. The platelet count and bleeding time adequately detect abnormal platelet function. The activated partial thromboplastin time, prothrombin time, and thrombin time measure all aspects of the extrinsic and intrinsic coagulation systems. Observation of clot solubility in 5M urea will detect significant deficiency of Factor XIII. The 24-hour whole blood clot lysis test is a rough measurement of the fibrinolytic system. Results from these assays will allow selection of appropriate assays to specify the nature of a patient's problem.

In the assessment of platelet function, the bleeding time and platelet count together provide significant information. If the platelet count is low and bleeding time is markedly prolonged, then the thrombocytopenia is probably due to hypoproliferative thrombocytopenia or ineffective thrombopoiesis. If the platelet count is low and the bleeding time is only slightly prolonged, it is likely that the thrombocytopenia is due to a peripheral loss of platelets and that the bone marrow is responding normally with an adequate release of young platelets. When the platelet count is normal or elevated and the bleeding time is prolonged, von Willebrand's disease or some platelet functional disorder becomes a likely possibility. Assays for platelet adhesiveness, platelet aggregation, and Factor VIII procoagulant and antigen may now be required to define the patient's disorder.

Results from the thrombin time, prothrombin time, and partial thromboplastin time also aid in the differential diagnosis. When any of these tests is significantly prolonged, it should be repeated using a 1:1 mixture of patient's and control plasma. If the result returns to the normal range, the abnormality is likely to be a deficiency in clotting activity; if not, an inhibitor is more likely.

Normal thrombin time and partial thromboplastin time with prolonged prothrombin time are characteristic of a Factor VII deficiency. A normal thrombin time and prolonged partial thromboplastin and prothrombin times indicate diminished activity of the prothrombin complex factors or a deficiency in Factor V. A disproportionate prolongation of thrombin time with only slight prolongation of prothrombin time and partial thromboplastin time is sometimes seen in hypofibrinogenemia, dysfibrinogenemia, and paraproteinemias.

Prolongation of only the activated partial thromboplastin time is observed in deficiencies of Factors VIII, IX, XI, and XII. Factor XII deficiency is not associated with any clinically significant bleeding disorder. Mixture experiments of patient's plasma with adsorbed plasma and aged serum help to differentiate these disorders. Specific factor assays are used to confirm the diagnosis.

If the activated partial thromboplastin and (usually) the whole blood clotting time are prolonged, and all other routine coagulation tests and factor assays are normal, a deficiency in Fletcher factor, high molecular weight kininogen, or a new coagulation factor is possible. Sometimes inhibitors, such as the lupus inhibitor, masquerade as deficiencies of these factors.

Occasionally the thrombin time, prothrombin time, and partial thromboplastin time are markedly prolonged. In these circumstances, it is likely that there are multiple deficiencies of coagulation factors (diffuse intravascular coagulation, liver disease) or that the plasma contains an anticoagulant or inhibitor (heparin, paraprotein).

Excessive fibrinolytic activity can be measured by performing euglobulin clot lysis test and fibrinogen/fibrin degradation assay. In addition, kits for measurements of the immunologic activity of plasminogen* and the functional activity of plasmin† are commercially available.

---

*M-Partigen Plasminogen Kit, Behring Diagnostics, American Hoechst Corporation, Somerville, N.J. 08876.

†Enzo-diffusion(R) Fibrin Plate Test, Hyland Division, Travenol Laboratories, Costa Mesa, Cal. 92626.

REFERENCES

Abildgaard, C. F.: Recognition and treatment of intravascular coagulation. J. Pediatr., *74*:163, 1969.

Aggeler, P. M., White, S. G., Glendenning, M. B., Page, E. W., Leake, T. B., and Bates, G.: Plasma thromboplastin component (PTC) deficiency: A new disease resembling hemophilia. Proc. Soc. Exp. Biol. Med., *79*:692, 1952.

Alexander, B., Goldstein, R., Landwehr, G., and Cook, C. D.: Congenital SPCA deficiency: A hitherto unrecognized coagulation defect with hemorrhage rectified by serum and serum fractions. J. Clin. Invest., *30*:596, 1951.

Andersen, B. R., and Terry, W. D.: Gamma G$_4$-globulin antibody causing inhibition of clotting factor VIII. Nature, *217*:174, 1968.

Bailey, K., and Bettelheim, F. R.: The clotting of fibrinogen. I. The liberation of peptide material. Biochim. Biophys. Acta, *18*:495, 1955.

Bailey, K., Bettelheim, F. R., Lorand, L., and Middlebrook, W. R.: Action of thrombin in clotting of fibrinogen. Nature, *167*:233, 1951.

Barry, A., and Delâge, J. M.: Congenital deficiency of fibrin-stabilizing factor. Observation of a new case. N. Engl. J. Med., *272*:943, 1965.

Bennett, B.: Coagulation pathways: Interrelationships and control mechanisms. Semin. Hematol., *14*:301, 1977.

Bidwell, E.: Acquired inhibitors of coagulants. Ann. Rev. Med., *20*:63, 1969.

Biggs, R., and Denson, K. W. E.: Standardization of the one-stage prothrombin time for the control of anticoagulant therapy. Br. Med. J., *1*:84, 1967.

Biggs, R., Douglas, A. S., Macfarlane, R. G., Dacie, J. V., Pitney, W. R., Merskey, C., and O'Brien, J. R.: Christmas disease: A condition previously mistaken for hemophilia. Br. Med. J., *2*:1378, 1952.

Blombäck, B., and Blombäck, M.: The molecular structure of fibrinogen. Ann. N.Y. Acad. Sci., *202*:77, 1972.

Blombäck, B., Blombäck, M., and Nilsson, I. M.: Coagulation studies on reptilase, an extract of the venom from Bothrops Jararaca. Thromb. Diath. Haemorrh., *1*:76, 1957.

Bloom, A. L.: Physiology of factor VIII. In Poller, L. (ed.): Recent Advances in Coagulation, No. 2. Edinburgh, Churchill Livingstone, 1977a.

Bloom, A. L., and Peake, I. R.: Molecular genetics of factor VIII and its disorders. Semin. Hematol., *14*:319, 1977b.

Bowie, E. J. W., and Owen, C. A., Jr.: Hemostatic failure in clinical medicine. Semin. Hematol., *14*:341, 1977.

Britten, A. F. H.: Congenital deficiency of factor XIII (fibrin-stabilizing factor). Am. J. Med., *43*:751, 1967.

Buckwell, M.: The effect of citrate on euglobulin methods of estimating fibrinolytic activity. J. Clin. Pathol., *11*:403, 1958.

Bull, M. H., Huse, W. M., and Bull, B. S.: Evaluation of test used to monitor heparin therapy during extracorporeal circulation. Anesthesiology, *43*:346, 1975.

Cash, J. D.: Disseminated intravascular coagulation. In Poller, L. (ed.): Recent Advances in Blood Coagulation, No. 2. Edinburgh, Churchill Livingstone, 1977.

Chen, R., and Doolittle, R. F.: Isolation, characterization, and location of a donor-acceptor unit from cross-linked fibrin. Proc. Natl. Acad. Sci. U.S.A., *66*:472, 1970.

Chen, A. L., Hershgold, E. J., and Wilson, D. E.: One stage assay of heparin. J. Lab. Clin. Med., *85*:843, 1975.

Chung, S. I.: Comparative studies on tissue transglutaminase and factor XIII. Ann. N.Y. Acad. Sci., *202*:240, 1972.

Chun-Yet Lian, E., and Deykin, D.: *In vivo* dissociation of factor VIII (AHF) activity and factor VIII related antigen in von Willebrand's disease. Am. J. Hematol., *1*:71, 1976.

Coleman, M., Vigliano, E. M., Weksler, M. E., and Nachman, R. L.: Inhibition of fibrin monomer polymerization by lambda myeloma globulins. Blood, *39*:210, 1972.

Colman, R. W.: Factor V. Prog. Hemostasis Thromb., *3*:109, 1976.

Colman, R. W., Oxley, L., and Giannusa, R.: Statistical comparison of the automated activated partial thromboplastin time and the clotting time in the regulation of heparin therapy. Am. J. Clin. Pathol., *53*:904, 1970.

Colman, R. W., Bagdasarian, A., Talamo, R. C., Scott, G. F., Seavey, M., Guimaraes, J. A., Pierce, J. V., and Kaplan, A. P.: Williams trait. Human kininogen deficiency with diminished levels of plasminogen proactivator and prekallikrein associated with abnormalities of the Hageman-dependent pathways. J. Clin. Invest., *56*:1650, 1975.

Dacie, J. V., and Lewis, S. M.: Practical Hematology, 5th ed. Edinburgh, Churchill Livingstone, 1975.

Davey, F. R., Fiske, M. L., and Maltby, A.: Evaluation of a photoelectric automatic prothrombin analyzer. Am. J. Clin. Pathol., *58*:687, 1972.

Davey, F. R., Gordon, G. B., Boral, L. I., and Gottlieb, A. J.: Gamma globulin inhibition of fibrin clot formation. Ann. Clin. Lab. Sci., *6*:72, 1976.

Davidson, J. F.: Recent advances in fibrinolysis. In Poller, L. (ed.): Recent advances in blood coagulation, No. 2. Edinburgh, Churchill Livingstone, 1977.

Davie, E. W., and Ratnoff, O. D.: Waterfall sequence for intrinsic blood clotting. Science, *145*:1310, 1964.

Denson, K. W. E.: International and national standardization of control of anticoagulant therapy in patients receiving coumarin and indanedione drugs using calibrated thromboplastin preparations. J. Clin. Pathol., *24*:460, 1971.

Denson, K. W. E., Biggs, R., and Mannucci, P. M.: An investigation of three patients with Christmas disease due to an abnormal type of factor IX. J. Clin. Pathol., *21*:160, 1968.

Denson, K. W. E., Lurie, A., DeCataldo, F., and Mannucci, P. M.: The factor-X defect: Recognition of abnormal forms of factor X. Br. J. Haematol., *18*:317, 1970.

Deykin, D.: The clinical challenge of disseminated intravascular coagulation. N. Engl. J. Med., *282*:636, 1970.

Didisheim, P.: Screening tests for bleeding disorders. Am. J. Clin. Pathol., *47*:622, 1967.

Didisheim, P., and Vandervoort, R. L. E.: Detection of carriers for factor IX (PTC) deficiency. Blood, *20*:150, 1962.

Donaldson, V. H., and Kisker, C. T.: Blood coagulation in hemostasis. In Nathan, D. G., and Oski, F. A. (eds.): Hematology of Infancy and Childhood. Philadelphia, W. B. Saunders Company, 1974.

Donaldson, V. H., Glueck, H. I., Miller, M. A., Movat, H. Z., and Habal, F.: Kininogen deficiency in Fitzgerald trait: Role of high molecular weight kininogen in clotting and fibrinolysis. J. Lab. Clin. Med., *87*:327, 1976.

Duckert, F.: Documentation of the plasma factor XIII deficiency in man. Ann. N.Y. Acad. Sci., *202*:190, 1972.

Duckert, F., and Beck, E. A.: Clinical disorders due to the deficiency of factor XIII (fibrin stabilizing factor, fibrinase). Semin. Hematol., *5*:83, 1968.

Duckert, F., Jung, E., and Shmerling, D. H.: A hitherto undescribed congenital haemorrhagic diathesis probably due to fibrin stabilizing factor deficiency. Thromb. Diath. Haemorrh., *5*:179, 1961.

Dymock, I. W., Tucker, J. S., Woolf, I. L., Poller, L. and Thomson, J. M.: Coagulation studies as a prognostic index in acute liver failure. Br. J. Haematol., *29*:385, 1975.

Egeberg, O.: Inherited fibrinogen abnormality causing thrombophilia. Thromb. Diath. Haemorrh., *17*:176, 1967.

Ellis, B. C., and Stransky, A.: A quick and accurate method for the determination of fibrinogen in plasma. J. Lab. Clin. Med., *58*:477, 1961.

Fantl, P., Sawers, R. J., and Marr, A. G.: Investigation of a haemorrhagic disease due to beta-prothrombin deficiency complicated by a specific inhibitor of thromboplastin formation. Aust. Ann. Med., *5*:163, 1956.

Feinstein, D. I., and Rapaport, S. I.: Acquired inhibitors of blood coagulation. Prog. Hemostasis. Thromb., *1*:75, 1972.

Feinstein, D. I., Rapaport, S. I., McGehee, W. G., and Patch, M. J.: Factor V anticoagulants: Clinical, biochemical and immunological observations. J. Clin. Invest., *49*:1578, 1970.

Forbes, C. D., and Ratnoff, O. D.: Studies on plasma thromboplastin antecedent (factor XI), PTA deficiency and inhibition of PTA by plasma: Pharmacologic inhibitors and specific antiserum. J. Lab. Clin. Med., *79*:113, 1972.

Freidman, I. A., Quick, A. J., Higgins, F., Hussey, C. V., and Hickey, M. E.: Hereditary labile factor (factor V) deficiency. J.A.M.A., *175*:370, 1961.

Fujikawa, K., Legaz, M. E., and Davie, E. W.: Bovine factor X_1 and X_2 (Stuart factor) isolation and characterization. Biochemistry, *11*:4882, 1972.

Funk, C., Gmur, J., Herold, R., and Straub, P. W.: Reptilase-R—A new reagent in blood coagulation. Br. J. Haematol., *21*:43, 1971.

Ganrot, P. O., and Niléhn, J. E.: Plasma prothrombin during treatment with Dicumarol II. Demonstration of an abnormal prothrombin fraction. Scand. J. Clin. Invest., *22*:23, 1968.

Genton, E.: Guidelines for heparin therapy. Ann. Intern. Med., *80*:77, 1974.

Girolami, A., Molaro, G., Lazzarin, M., Scarpa, R., and Brunetti, A.: A 'new' congenital haemorrhagic condition due to the presence of an abnormal factor X (factor X Friuli): Study of a large kindred. Br. J. Haematol., *19*:179, 1970a.

Girolami, A., Sticchi, A., Lazzarin, M., and Scarpa, R.: Congenital hypothrombinemia. Acta. Haematol. (Basel), *44*:164, 1970b.

Gitlin, D., and Borges, W. H.: Studies on the metabolism of fibrinogen in two patients with congenital afibrinogenemia. Blood, *8*:679, 1953.

Goodnight, S. H., Feinstein, D. I., Østerud, B., and Rapaport, S. I.: Factor VII antibody-neutralizing material in hereditary and acquired factor VII deficiency. Blood, *38*:1, 1971.

Goulian, M., and Beck, W. S.: The partial thromboplastin time test. Modification of the procedure, and study of the sensitivity and optimal condition. Tech. Bull. Reg. Med. Technol., *35*:97, 1965.

Grant, J., and Biggs, R.: Experiments on the standardization of factor VII assay. Thromb. Diath. Haemorrh. (Suppl.), *26*:407, 1967.

Green, A. J., and Ratnoff, O. D.: Elevated antihemophilic factor (AHF, factor VIII) procoagulant activity and AHF-like antigen in alcoholic cirrhosis of the liver. J. Lab. Clin. Med., *83*:189, 1974.

Green, G., Poller, L., Thomson, J. M., and Dymock, I. W.: Factor VII as a marker of hepatocellular synthetic function in liver disease. J. Clin. Pathol., *29*:971, 1976a.

Green, G., Thomson, J. M., Dymock, I. W., and Poller, L.: Abnormal fibrin polymerization in liver disease. Br. J. Haematol., *34*:427, 1976b.

Greenwood, R. J., and Rabin, S. C.: Hemophilia-like postpartum bleeding. Obstet. Gynecol., *30*:362, 1967.

Hampton, J. W.: Qualitative fibrinogen defect associated with abnormal fibrin stabilization. J. Lab. Clin. Med., *72*:882, 1968.

Handin, R. I., Martin, V., and Moloney, W. C.: Antibody-induced von Willebrand's disease: A newly defined inhibitor syndrome. Blood, *48*:393, 1976.

Harker, L. A.: Hemostasis manual. Philadelphia, F. A. Davis Co., 1974.

Harker, L. A., and Slichter, S. J.: Platelet and fibrinogen consumption in man. N. Engl. J. Med., *287*:999, 1972.

Harpel, P. C., and Rosenberg, R. D.: α_2-macroglobulin and antithrombin-heparin cofactor: Modulators of hemostatic and inflammatory reactions. Prog. Hemostasis Thromb., *3*:145, 1976.

Hathaway, W. E., Belhasen, L. P., and Hathaway, H. S.: Evidence for a new plasma thromboplastin factor. I. Case report, coagulation studies and physiochemical properties. Blood, *26*:521, 1965.

Hattersley, P. G.: Activated coagulation time of whole blood. J.A.M.A., *196*:436, 1966.

Hattersley, P. G.: Progress report: The activated coagulation time of whole blood (ACT). Am. J. Clin. Pathol., *66*:899, 1976.

Hemker, H. C., Veltkamp, J. J., and Loeliger, E. A.: Kinetic aspects of the interaction of blood clotting enzymes. III. Demonstration of an inhibitor of prothrombin conversion in Vitamin K deficiency. Thromb. Diath. Haemorrh., *19*:346, 1968.

Hill, J. D., Dontigny, L., de Leval, M., and Mielke, C. H.: A simple method of heparin management during prolonged extracorporeal circulation. Ann. Thorac. Surg., *17*:129, 1974.

Hirsh, J., Bishop, J., Johnson, M., and Walker, C.: The development of antiheparin activity in stored vacutainer tubes. Blood, *48*:1004, 1976.

Hörder, M. H.: Consumptive coagulopathy in liver cirrhosis. Thromb. Diath. Haemorrh. (Suppl.), *36*:313, 1969.

Hougie, C., and Twomey, J.: Haemophilia B$_m$: A new type of Factor-IX deficiency. Lancet, *1*:698, 1967.

Hougie, C., Barrow, E. M., and Graham, J. B.: Stuart clotting defect. I. Segregation of an hereditary hemorrhagic state from the heterogeneous group heretofore called "stable factor" (SPCA, Proconvertin, factor VII) deficiency. J. Clin. Invest., *36*:485, 1957.

Hougie, C., McPherson, R. A., and Aronson, L.: Passovoy factor: A hitherto unrecognized factor necessary for haemostasis. Lancet, *2*:290, 1975.

Hoyer, L. W.: Immunologic studies of antihemophilic factor (AHF, factor VIII). IV. Radioimmunoassay of AHF antigen. J. Lab. Clin. Med., *80*:822, 1972.

Hoyer, L. W.: Von Willebrand's disease. Prog. Hemostas. Thromb., *3*:231, 1976.

Hoyer, L. W., and Breckenridge, R. T.: Immunologic studies of antihemophilic factor (AHF, factor VIII): Cross-reacting material in a genetic variant of hemophilia A. Blood, *32*:962, 1968.

Ingram, G. I. C., Prentice, C. R. M., Forbes, C. D., and Leslie, J.: Low factor VIII-like antigen in acquired von Willebrand's syndrome and response to treatment. Br. J. Haematol., *25*:137, 1973.

Israels, E. D., Parashevas, F., and Israels, L. G.: Immunological studies of coagulation factor XIII. J. Clin. Invest., *52*:2398, 1973.

Jackson, C. M., and Suttie, J. W.: Recent developments in understanding the mechanism of vitamin K and vitamin K-antagonistic drug action and the consequences of vitamin K action in blood coagulation. Prog. Hematol., *10*:333, 1977.

Jaffe, E. A., Hoyer, L. W., and Nachman, R. L.: Synthesis of antihemophilic factor antigen by cultured human endothelial cells. J. Clin. Invest., *52*:2757, 1973.

Jaques, L. B., Mahadoo, J., and Riley, J. F.: The mast cell/heparin paradox. Lancet, *1*:411, 1977.

Josso, F., Monasterio De Sanchez, J., Lavergne, J. M., Menache, D., and Soulier, J. P.: Congenital abnormality of the prothrombin molecule (Factor II) in four siblings: Prothrombin Barcelona. Blood, *38*:9, 1971.

Kaplan, A. P., Meier, H. L., and Mandle, R., Jr.: The Hageman factor dependent pathways of coagulation, fibrinolysis, and kinin-generation. Semin. Thromb. Hemostas., *3*:1, 1976.

Kasper, C. K., Østerud, B., Minami, J. Y., Shonick, W., and Rapaport, S. I.: Hemophilia B: Characterization of genetic variants and detection of carriers. Blood, *50*:351, 1977.

Kidder, W. R., Logan, L. J., Rapaport, S. I., and Patch, M. J.: The plasma protamine paracoagulation test: Clinical and laboratory evaluation. Am. J. Clin. Pathol., *58*:675, 1972.

Klein, H. G., Aledort, L. M., Bouma, B. N., Hoyer, L. W., Zimmerman, T. S., and DeMets, D. L.: A cooperative study for the detection of the carrier state of classic hemophilia. N. Engl. J. Med., *295*:959, 1977.

Koch-Weser, J., and Sellers, E. M.: Drug interactions with coumarin anticoagulants. N. Engl. J. Med., *285*:487, 547, 1971.

Kwaan, H. C.: Disseminated intravascular coagulation. Med. Clin. North Am., *56*:177, 1972.

Lackner, H.: Hemostatic abnormalities associated with dysproteinemias. Semin. Hematol., *10*:125, 1973.

Lackner, H., Hunt, V., Zucker, M. B., and Pearson, J.: Abnormal fibrin ultrastructure, polymerization, and clot retraction in multiple myeloma. Br. J. Haematol., *18*:625, 1970.

Laurell, C. B.: Quantitative estimation of proteins by electrophoresis in agarose gel containing antibodies. Anal. Biochem., *15*:45, 1966.

Lechler, E., Webster, W. P., Roberts, H. R., and Penick, G. D.: The inheritance of Stuart disease: Investigation of a family with factor X deficiency. Am. J. Med. Sci., *249*:291, 1965.

Lee, R. I., and White, P. D.: A clinical study of the coagulation times of blood. Am. J. Med. Sci., *145*:495, 1913.

Leiba, H., Ramot, B., and Many, A.: Heredity and coagulation studies in ten families with factor XI (plasma thromboplastin antecedent) deficiency. Br. J. Haematol., *11*:654, 1965.

Levine, W. G.: Anticoagulant, antithrombotic and thrombolytic drugs. *In* Goodman, L. S., and Gilman, A. (eds.): The Pharmacological Basis of Therapeutics. New York, MacMillan Publishing Co., Inc., 1975.

Lindahl, U. L., Höök, M., Bäckström, G., Jacobsson, I., Riesenfeld, J., Malmström, A., Rodén, L., and Feingold, D. S.: Structure and biosynthesis of heparin-like polysaccharides. Fed. Proc., *36*:19, 1977.

MacFarlane, R. G.: The coagulant action of Russell's viper venom; the use of antivenom in defining its reaction with a serum factor. Br. J. Haematol., *7*:496, 1961.

MacFarlane, R. G.: An enzyme cascade in the blood clotting mechanism, and its function as a biochemical amplifier. Nature, *202*:498, 1964.

Mandle, R. J., Colman, R. W., and Kaplan, A. P.: Identification of prekallikrein and high-molecular-weight kininogen as a complex in human plasma. Proc. Natl. Acad. Sci. U.S.A., *73*:4179, 1976.

Mann, K. G.: Prothrombin activation. Hum. Pathol., *5*:377, 1974.

Mant, M. J., Hirsh, J., Gauldie, J., Bienenstock, J., Pineo, G. F., and Luke, K. H.: Von Willebrand's syndrome presenting as an acquired bleeding disorder in association with a monoclonal gammopathy. Blood, *42*:429, 1973.

Marder, V. J.: A simple technique for the measurement of plasma heparin concentration during anticoagulant therapy. Thromb. Diath. Haemorrh., *24*:230, 1970.

Marder, V. J.: Identification and purification of fibrinogen degradation products produced by plasmin: Considerations on the structure of fibrinogen. Scand. J. Haematol. (Suppl.), *13*:21, 1971.

Marder, V. J., and Budzynski, A. Z.: The structure of fibrinogen degradation products. Prog. Hemostasis Thromb., *2*:141, 1974.

Marder, V. J., and Shulman, N. R.: Clinical aspects of congenital factor VII deficiency. Am. J. Med., *37*:182, 1964.

Margolius, A., Jackson, D. P., and Ratnoff, O. D.: Circulating anticoagulants: A study of 40 cases and a review of the literature. Medicine (Baltimore), *40*:145, 1961.

McDonagh, J., and Wagner, R. H.: Site of synthesis of plasma and platelet factor XIII. Ann. N.Y. Acad. Sci., *202*:31, 1972.

McDonagh, J., McDonagh, R. P., Myllylä, G., and Ikkala, E.: Factor XIII deficiency: A genetic study of two affected kindred in Finland. Blood, *43*:327, 1974.

Merskey, C., and Drapkin, A.: Anticoagulant therapy. Blood, *25*:567, 1965.

Merskey, C., Johnson, A. J., Kleiner, G. J., and Wohl, H.: The defibrination syndrome: Clinical features and laboratory diagnosis. Br. J. Haematol., *13*:528, 1967.

Mersky, C., Kleiner, G. J., and Johnson, A. J.: Quantitative estimation of split products of fibrinogen in human serum, relationship to diagnosis and treatment. Blood, *28*:1, 1966.

Meyer, D.: Von Willebrand's disease. *In* Poller, L. (ed.): Recent Advances in Blood Coagulation, No. 2. Edinburgh, Churchill Livingstone, 1977.

Meyer, D., Bidwell, E., and Larrieu, M. J.: Cross-reacting material in genetic variants of haemophilia B. J. Clin. Pathol., *25*:433, 1972.

Miale, J. B.: The fibrometer system for routine coagulation tests. Prothrombin time and partial thromboplastin time, macro and micro. Am. J. Clin. Pathol., *43*:475, 1965.

Miale, J. B.: Laboratory Medicine: Hematology. Saint Louis, The C. V. Mosby Co., 1977.

Miale, J. B., and Kent, J. W.: Standardization of the therapeutic range for control anticoagulants based on standard reference plasma. Am. J. Clin. Pathol., *57*:80, 1972.

Miale, J. B., and LaFond, D.: Prothrombin time standardization. Proposal of the Standards Committee, College of American Pathologists, Subcommittee on Coagulation Reagents. Am. J. Clin. Pathol., *52*:154, 1970.

Morton, R. O., and Hampton, J. W.: Fibrinogen Oklahoma—characterization of a familial bleeding diathesis. Clin. Res., *18*:533, 1970.

Nemerson, Y., and Pitlick, F. A.: The tissue factor pathway of blood coagulation. Prog. Hemostasis Thromb., *1*:1, 1972.

Nilsson, I. M., Skanse, B., Gydell, R.: Circulating anticoagulant after pregnancy and its response to ACTH. Acta Haematol. (Basel), *19*:40, 1958.

Nossel, H. L.: The contact system. *In* Biggs, R. (ed.): Human Blood Coagulation, Haemostasis and Thrombosis. Oxford, Blackwell Scientific Publications, 1976.

O'Reilly, R. A.: The pharmacodynamics of the oral anticoagulant drugs. Prog. Hemostasis Thromb., *2*:175, 1974.

Owen, C. A. Jr., Bowie, E. J. W., and Thompson, J. H.: The diagnosis of bleeding disorders. Boston, Little, Brown and Co., 1975.

Owen, C. A., Jr., Mann, F. D., Hurn, M. M., and Stickney, J. M.: Evaluation of disorders of blood coagulation in the clinical laboratory. Am. J. Clin. Pathol., *25*:1417, 1955.

Owren, P. A.: Parahemophilia. Hemorrhagic diathesis due to absence of a previously unknown clotting factor. Lancet, *1*:446, 1947.

Owren, P. A.: Thrombotest. A new method for controlling anticoagulant therapy. Lancet, *2*:754, 1959.

Owren, P. A., and Aas, K.: The control of dicumarol therapy and the quantitative determination of prothrombin and proconvertin. Scand. J. Clin. Lab. Invest., *3*:201, 1951.

Penner, J. A.: Experience with a thrombin clotting time assay for measuring heparin activity. Am. J. Clin. Pathol., *6*:645, 1974.

Perkins, H. A., MacKenzie, M. R., and Fudenberg, H. H.: Hemostatic defects in dysproteinemias. Blood, *35*:695, 1970.

Pike, I. M., Yount, W. J., Puritz, E. M., and Roberts, H. R.: Immunochemical characterization of a monoclonal γG_4, λ human antibody to factor IX. Blood, *40*:1, 1972.

Pisano, J. J., Bronzert, T. J., and Peyton, M. P.: ϵ-(γ-glutamyl) lysine cross-links: Determination in fibrin from normal and factor XIII–deficient individuals. Ann. N.Y. Acad. Sci., *202*:98, 1972.

Pizzo, S. V., Schwartz, M. L., Hill, R. L., and McKee, P. A.: Mechanism of ancrod anticoagulation: A direct proteolytic effect on fibrin. J. Clin. Invest., *51*:2841, 1972.

Poller, L.: Coagulation abnormalities in liver disease. *In* Poller, L. (ed.): Recent Advances in Blood Coagulation, No. 2. Edinburgh, Churchill Livingstone, 1977.

Proctor, R. R., and Rapaport, S. I.: The partial thromboplastin time with Kaolin. A simple screening test for first stage plasma clotting factor deficiencies. Am. J. Clin. Pathol., *36*:212, 1961.

Prydz, H.: Studies on proconvertin (Factor VII) VI. The production in rabbits of an antiserum against factor VII. Scand. J. Clin. Lab. Invest., *17*:66, 1965.

Quick, A. J., Stanley-Brown, M., and Bancroft, F. W.: A study of coagulation defect in hemophilia and in jaundice. Am. J. Med. Sci., *190*:501, 1935.

Radcliffe, R., and Nemerson, Y.: Activation of bovine factor VII by activated factor X and thrombin. Fed. Proc., *34*:259, 1975.

Rapaport, S. I.: Defibrination syndromes. *In* Williams, W. J., Beutler, E., Erslev, A. J., and Rundles, R. W. (eds.): Hematology, 2nd ed. New York, McGraw-Hill Book Co., 1977.

Rapaport, S. I., and Ames, S. B.: Clotting factor assays on plasma from patients receiving intramuscular or subcutaneous heparin. Am. J. Med. Sci., *234*:678, 1957.

Rapaport, S. I., Proctor, R. R., Patch, M. J., and Yettra, M.: The mode of inheritance of PTA deficiency: Evidence for the existence of major PTA deficiency and minor PTA deficiency. Blood, *18*:149, 1961.

Rapaport, S. I., Schiffman, S., Patch, M. J., and Ames, S. B.: The importance of activation of antihemophilic globulin and proaccelerin by traces of thrombin in the generation of intrinsic prothrombinase activity. Blood, *21*:221, 1963.

Ratnoff, O. D.: The biology and pathology of the initial stages of blood coagulation. Prog. Hematol., *5*:204, 1966.

Ratnoff, O. D.: The molecular basis of hereditary clotting disorders. Prog. Hemostasis Thromb. *1*:39, 1972a.

Ratnoff, O. D.: Studies on a proteolytic enzyme in human plasma. VII. A fatal hemorrhagic state associated with excessive plasma proteolytic activity in a patient undergoing surgery for carcinoma of head of pancreas. J. Clin. Invest., *31*:521, 1952.

Ratnoff, O. D., and Forman, W. B.: Criteria for the differentiation of dysfibrinogenemic states. Semin. Hematol., *13*:141, 1976.

Ratnoff, O. D., and Menzie, C.: A new method for the determination of fibrinogen in small samples of plasma. J. Lab. Clin. Med., *37*:316, 1951.

Ratnoff, O. D., and Steinberg, A. G.: Fibrin cross-linking and heredity. Ann. N.Y. Acad. Sci., *202*:186, 1972b.

Ratnoff, O. D., and Steinberg, A. G.: Further studies on the inheritance of Hageman trait. J. Lab. Clin. Med., *59*:980, 1962.

Reisner, H. M., Roberts, H. R., Krumholz, S., and Yount, W. J.: Immunochemical characterization of a polyclonal human antibody to factor IX. Blood, *50*:11, 1977.

Reno, W. J., Rotman, M., Grumbine, F. C., Dennis, L. H., and Mohler, E. R.: Evaluation of the Bart test (a modification of the whole-blood activated recalcification time test) as a means of monitoring heparin therapy. Am. J. Clin. Pathol., *61*:78, 1974.

Rizza, C. R.: The clinical features of clotting factor deficiencies. *In* Biggs, R. (ed.): Human Blood Coagulation, Haemostasis and Thrombosis. Oxford. Blackwell Scientific Publications, 1976.

Robboy, S. J., Lewis, E. J., Schur, P. H., and Colman, R. W.: Circulating anticoagulants to factor VIII. Am. J. Med., *49*:742, 1970.

Roberts, H. R., and Cederbaum, A. I.: The liver and blood coagulation: Physiology and pathology. Gastroenterology, *63*:297, 1972.

Roberts, H. R., and Cederbaum, A. I.: Molecular variants of factor IX. *In* Brinkhous, K. M., and Hemker, H. C. (eds.): Handbook of Hemophilia. New York, American Elsevier Publishing Co., Inc., 1975a.

Roberts, H. R., Cederbaum, A. I., and McMillian, C. W.: Immunology of acquired inhibitors to coagulation factors. *In* Brinkhous, K. M., and Hemker, H. C. (eds.): Handbook of Hemophilia. New York, American Elsevier Publishing Co., Inc., 1975b.

Rodriguez-Erdmann, F.: Bleeding due to increased intravascular blood coagulation. N. Engl. J. Med., *273*:1370, 1965.

Rosenberg, R. D.: Hemorrhagic disorders I. Protein interactions of the clotting mechanism. *In* Beck, W. S. (ed.): Hematology, 2nd ed. Cambridge, MIT Press, 1977.

Rosenthal, R. L., Dreskin, O. H., and Rosenthal, N.: Plasma thromboplastin antecedent (PTA) deficiency: Clinical coagulation, therapeutic and hereditary aspects of a new hemophilia-like disease. Blood, *10*:120, 1955.

Saito, H., and Ratnoff, O. D.: Alteration of factor VII activity by activated Fletcher factor (a plasma kallikrein): A potential link between the intrinsic and extrinsic blood-clotting systems. J. Lab. Clin. Med., *85*:405, 1975a.

Saito, H., Ratnoff, O. D., Waldmann, R., and Abraham, J. P.: Fitzgerald trait. Deficiency of a hitherto unrecognized agent. Fitzgerald factor, participating in surface-mediated reactions of clotting, fibrinolysis, generation of kinins, and the property of diluted plasma enhancing vascular permeability (PF/DIL). J. Clin. Invest., *55*:1082, 1975b.

Samama, M., Soria, J., and Soria, C.: Congenital and acquired dysfibrinogenaemia *In* Poller, L. (ed.): Recent Advance in Blood Coagulation, No. 2. Edinburgh, Churchill Livingstone, 1977.

Samori, T., Yatabe, M., Ukita, M., Fujimaki M., and Fukutake, K.: A new type of congenital dysfibrinogenemia (fibrinogen Tokyo) with defective stabilization of fibrin polymers. Thromb. Diath. Haemorrh., *34*:329, 1975.

Schleider, M. A., Nachman, R. L., Jaffe, E. A., and Coleman, M.: A clinical study of the lupus anticoagulant. Blood, *48*:499, 1976.

Schriever, H. G., Epstein, S. E., and Mintz, M. D.: Statistical correlation and heparin sensitivity of activated partial thromboplastin time, whole blood coagulation time, and automated coagulation time. Am. J. Clin. Pathol., *60*:233, 1973.

Seeler, R. A.: Parahemophilia. Factor V deficiency. Med. Clin. North Am., *56*:119, 1972.

Shapiro, S. S.: Acquired anticoagulants. *In* Williams, W. J., Beutler, E., Erslev, A. J., and Rundles, R. W. (eds.): Hematology, 2nd ed. New York, McGraw-Hill Book Co., 1977a.

Shapiro, S. S.: Disorders of the vitamin K-dependent coagulation factors. *In* Williams, W. J., Beutler, E., Erslev, A. J., Rundles, R. W. (eds.): Hematology, 2nd ed. New York, McGraw-Hill Book Co., 1977b.

Shapiro, S. S. and Carroll, K. S.: Acquired factor VIII antibodies. Further immunologic and electrophoretic studies. Science, *160*:786, 1968.

Shapiro, S. S., and Hultin, M.: Acquired inhibitors to the blood coagulation factors. Semin. Thromb. Hemostas., *1*:336, 1975.

Shapiro, S. S., Martinez, J., and Holburn, R. R.: Congenital dysprothrombinemia: An inherited structural disorder of human prothrombin. J. Clin. Invest., *48*:2251, 1969.

Sherry, S.: Fibrinolysis. *In* Williams, W. J., Beutler, E., Erslev, A. J., and Rundles, R. W. (eds.): Hematology, 2nd ed. New York, McGraw-Hill Book Co., 1977.

Sibley, C., Singer, J. W., and Wood, R. J.: Comparison of activated partial thromboplastin reagents. Am. J. Clin. Pathol., *59*:581, 1973.

Simone, J. V., Cornet, J. A., and Abildgaard, C. F.: Acquired von Willebrand's syndrome in systemic lupus erythematosus. Blood, *31*:806, 1968.

Simone, J. V., Vanderheiden, J., and Abildgaard, C. F.: A semiautomatic one-stage factor VIII assay with a commercially prepared standard. J. Lab. Clin. Med., *69*:706, 1967.

Simpson, J. G., and Stalker, A. L.: The concept of disseminated intravascular coagulation. Clin. Haematol., *2*:189, 1973.

Singer, J. W., and Sibley, C. A.: Sensitivity of commercial thromboplastins to factor VII. Am. J. Clin. Pathol., *59*:755, 1973.

Smink, M. McL., Daniel, T. M., Ratnoff, O. D., and Stavitsky, A. B.: Immunologic demonstration of a deficiency of Hageman factor-like material in Hageman trait. J. Lab. Clin. Med., *69*:819, 1967.

Stableforth, P., Tamagnini, G. L., and Dormandy, K. M.: Acquired von Willebrand syndrome with inhibitors both to factor VIII clotting activity and ristocetin-induced platelet aggregation. Br. J. Haematol., *33*:565, 1976.

Steel, R. G. D., and Torrie, J. H.: Principles and procedures of statistics, with special reference to biological sciences. New York, McGraw-Hill Book Co., 1960.

Stocker, K., and Straub, P. W.: Rapid detection of fibrinopeptides by bidimensional paper electrophoresis. Thromb. Diath. Haemorrh., *25*:248, 1970.

Strauss, H. S., and Merler, E.: Characterization and properties of an inhibitor of factor VIII in the plasma of patients with hemophilia A following repeated transfusions. Blood, *30*:137, 1967.

Suttie, J. W.: Mechanisms of action of vitamin K: Demonstration of a liver precursor of prothrombin. Science, *179*:192, 1973.

Suttie, J. W.: Oral anticoagulant therapy: The biosynthetic basis. Semin. Hematol., *14*:365, 1977a.

Suttie, J. W., Lehrman, S. R., Rich, D. H., and Whitlon, D. S.: Prothrombin biosynthesis: The vitamin-K dependent carboxylase. Thromb. Hemostas., *38*:51, 1977b.

Tagnon, H. J., Schulman, P., Whitmore, W. F., and Leone, L. A.: Prostatic fibrinolysin. Study of a case illustrating role in hemorrhagic diathesis of cancer of the prostate. Am. J. Med., *15*:875, 1953.

Telfer, T. P., Denson, K. W., and Wright, D. R.: A new coagulation defect. Br. J. Haematol., *2*:308, 1956.

Thomas, D. P., Ream, V. J., and Stuart, R. K.: Platelet aggregation in patients with Laennec's cirrhosis of the liver. N. Engl. J. Med., *276*:1344, 1967.

Tocantins, L. M. and Kazal, L. A.: Blood Coagulation, Hemorrhage and Thrombosis. New York, Grune & Stratton, Inc., 1964.

Tullis, J. L.: Clot. Springfield, Ill., Charles C Thomas, Publisher, 1976.

Veltkamp, J. J., Mielof, J., Remmelts, H. G., Van Der Vlerk, D., and Loeliger, E. A.: Another genetic variant of haemophilia B: Haemophilia B Leyden. Scand. J. Haematol., *7*:82, 1970.

Weiss, A. E.: Circulating inhibitors in Hemophilia A and B: Epidemiology and methods of dection. *In* Brinkhous, K. M., and Hemker, H. C. (eds): Handbook of Hemophilia. New York, American Elsevier Publishing Co., 1975.

Weiss, H. J.: Platelet aggregation, adhesion and adenosine diphosphate release in thrombopathia (platelet factor 3 deficiency). A comparison with Glanzmann's thrombasthenia and von Willebrand's disease. Am. J. Med., *43*:570, 1967.

Weiss, H. J., and Rogers, J.: Fibrinogen and platelets in the primary arrest of bleeding. Studies in two patients with congenital afibrinogenemia. N. Engl. J. Med., *285*:369, 1971.

Weiss, A. S., Gallin, J. I., and Kaplan, A. P.: Fletcher factor deficiency. A diminished rate of Hageman factor activation caused by absence of prekallikrein with abnormalities of coagulation, fibrinolysis, chemotactic activity and kinin generation. J. Clin. Invest., *53*:622, 1974.

Wessler, S., and Gitel, S.: Control of heparin therapy. Prog. Hemostasis Thromb., *3*:311, 1976.

Wilner, G. D., Nossel, H. L., and LeRoy, E. C.: Activation of Hageman factor by collagen. J. Clin. Invest., *47*:2608, 1968.

Wintrobe, M. M., Lee, R. G., Boggs, D. R., Bithell, T. C., Athens, J. W., and Foerster, J.: Clinical Hematology. Philadelphia, Lea and Febiger, 1974.

Wuepper, K. D.: Prekallikrein deficiency in man. J. Exp. Med., *138*:1345, 1973.

Wuepper, K. D., Miller, D. R., and Lacombe, M. J.: Flaujeac trait. Deficiency of human plasma kininogen. J. Clin. Invest., *56*:1663, 1975.

Yamagata, S., Mori, K., Kayaba, T., Hiratsuka, I., Kitamura, T., Ishimori, A., Takahashi, O., Tozawa, Y., Matsuyama, K., and Toyohara, M.: A case of congenital

3

afibrinogenemia and review of reported cases in Japan. Tohoku. J. Exp. Med., *96*:15, 1968.

Yin, E. T., Wessler, S., and Butler, J. V.: Plasma heparin: A unique, practical, submicrogram sensitive assay. J. Lab. Clin. Med., *81*:298, 1973.

Zeldis, S. M., Nemerson, Y., Pitlick, F. A., and Lentz, T. L.: Tissue factor (thromboplastin): Localization to plasma membranes by peroxidase-conjugated antibodies. Science, *175*:766, 1972.

Zimmerman, T. S., Hoyer, L. W., Dickson, L., and Edgington, T. S.: Determination of the von Willebrand's disease antigen (factor VIII-related antigen) in plasma by quantitative immunoelectrophoresis. J. Lab. Clin. Med., *86*:152, 1975.

Zimmerman, T. S., Ratnoff, O. D., and Littel, A. S.: Detection of carriers of classic hemophilia using an immunologic assay for antihemophilic factor (factor VIII). J. Clin. Invest., *50*:255, 1971.

INDEX

SUBJECT INDEX

i

GUIDELINES FOR ORDERING BLOOD FOR ELECTIVE SURGERY

These guidelines have been developed and are used at the State University of New York, Upstate Medical Center University Hospital (1978). Each institution is urged to generate its own guidelines, as described in the references. Variations to fit individual patient requirements are recognized and orders modified accordingly.

General Surgery

Amputation A/K, B/K	T&S*
Cholecystectomy and CD exploration	T&S
Gastrectomy with/without vagotomy:	
Subtotal	3
Total	3
Splenectomy	1
Sympathectomy	T&S
†Exploratory laparotomy	T&S
Esophageal resection	2–4
Breast biopsy	T&S
Mastectomy:	
Simple	T&S
Radical	1
Pancreatectomy:	
Partial	4
Radical (Whipple)	4
Thyroidectomy:	
Partial	T&S
Total	T&S
Parathyroidectomy	T&S
Parotidectomy	T&S
Colon Resection:	
Total large colon	2
Hemicolectomy	2
Sigmoidectomy	2
Anterior resection	2
Abdominal-perineal resection	3
Small bowel segment resection	1
Colostomy, Gastrostomy	T&S
Hemorrhoidectomy	T&S
Pilonidal cyst	T&S
Hernias:	
Inguinal	T&S
Incisional	T&S
Umbilical	T&S
Ventral	T&S
Hiatal	T&S
Vein stripping	T&S
Aneurysm resection	6
Femoropopliteal bypass	3
Portocaval shunt	4
Hepatectomy	6

Cardiopulmonary

Coronary vein graft:	
Single	4
Double	4
Triple	4
With other procedure	6
Valve replacement:	
Aortic	6
Mitral	5
Double valve	8(3)
Valve replacement plus single vein grafts	6
Atrial septal defect repair	3
Ventricular septal defect repair	4
Tetralogy of Fallot correction	6
Mitral commissurotomy	4
Pulmonary valvulotomy	3
Coarctation of the aorta correction	4
Aortic valvulotomy or annuloplasty	4
Pericardectomy	8
Thoracotomy:	
Pneumonectomy	2
Wedge resection, pulmonary	2
Esophagectomy	2
Bronchopleural fistula	2
Pectus excavatum	1
Tracheostomy	T&S
Embolectomy	2
Patent ductus arteriosus	4
Vascular tumors	4
Thoracic aneurysm	10(3)

Neurosurgery

Carpal tunnel procedures	T&S
Cranioplasty	1
†Craniotomy:	
Aneurysm	4–6
Subdural, epidural hematoma	2
Tumor	4–8
Cordotomy	T&S
†Laminectomy	T&S
Nerve repair	T&S
Hypophysectomy	T&S
Scalp and skull lesions (no intracranial communications)	T&S
Transphenoidal hypophysectomy	T&S
Ulnar nerve relocation	T&S
Ventricular peritoneal shunt	T&S

Otolaryngology

Branchial cleft cyst	T&S
Glossectomy	2
Laryngectomy	2
with radical neck dissection	4
Mandibulectomy	2
Ethmoidectomy	T&S
Caldwell-Luc operation	T&S
Orbital exploration	1
Mastoidectomy	2
Septoplasty	T&S
Tumor of palate	T&S
Maxillectomy	2
Jaw, neck, tongue dissection	4
Temporal bone resection	6